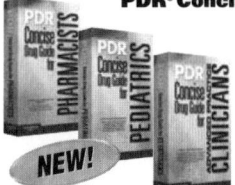

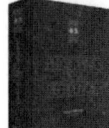

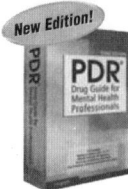

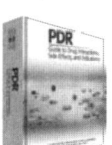

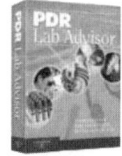

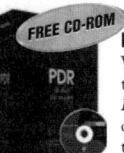

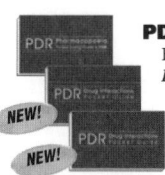

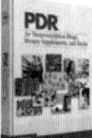

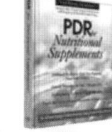

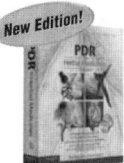

PDR®

FOR

Herbal Medicines

FOURTH EDITION

THOMSON™

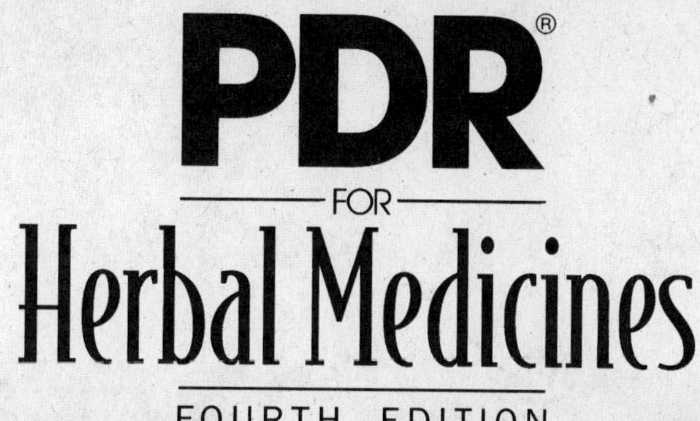

PDR® FOR Herbal Medicines

FOURTH EDITION

THOMSON™

Officers of Thomson Healthcare Inc.: *President and Chief Executive Officer:* Robert Cullen; *Chief Medical Officer:* Alan Ying, MD; *Senior Vice President and Chief Technology Officer:* Frank Licata; *Chief Strategy Officer:* Courtney Morris; *Executive Vice President, Payer Decision Support:* Jon Newpol; *Executive Vice President, Provider Markets:* Terry Cameron; *Executive Vice President, Marketing and Innovation:* Doug Schneider; *Senior Vice President, Finance:* Phil Buckingham; *Vice President, Human Resources:* Pamela M. Bilash; *General Counsel:* Darren Pocsik

ISBN: 1-56363-678-6

Contents

Foreword

Herbal medicines are preparations derived from naturally occurring plants with medicinal or preventive properties. The World Health Organization estimates that 4 billion people, amounting to 80% of the world's population, use herbal medicines for some aspect of primary health care. Herbal medicine is a major component in all indigenous peoples' traditional medicine and a common element in Ayurvedic, homeopathic, naturopathic, traditional oriental, and Native American medicine. The foods early humans ate contained a million different phytochemicals, and through modern science we are also recognizing some of these as functional foods (e.g., green tea catechins and pomegranate ellagitannins). Many spices such as cayenne and curcumin have medicinal properties in addition to their roles in flavoring foods. Today, we are rediscovering the utility of herbal medicines as botanical dietary supplements with potentially important preventive and medicinal effects. However, when patients talk about using herbal medicines, primary care physicians often lack the knowledge to provide informed advice on their use or misuse. This book is designed to fill that knowledge gap.

Herbs contain families of related compounds that interact, and the sum of these compounds' biological effects is often greater than the so-called "major active ingredient" in the herb or plant. For many herbal medicines, these families of compounds contribute to overall biological benefit by acting on several different targets simultaneously. For example, lycopene in a tomato plant is a potent antioxidant but also has effects in prostate cells on DNA and cellular communication. Recent research in animals demonstrated that isolated and purified lycopene did not have the same preventive activity against prostate cancer as tomato paste, which contains the plant's full complement of related phytochemicals including lycopene, phytoene, and phytofluene. Since toxicity is often related to the dose of the single most active constituent, the contributions of other analogs of the parent compound, or even unrelated compounds, to the biologically effective dose can lessen the risk of toxicity.

In human studies of Chinese Red Yeast Rice, our laboratory has found that eight monacolin analogs of monacolin K, or mevinolin, are metabolized differently than crystallized purified mevinolin, which is identical to the cholesterol-lowering drug lovastatin. Moreover, the red pigments in the yeast have biological activity when the monacolins are removed.

Today, the overall intake of natural foods and herbs has declined with the era of industrialization, which has filled our diets with what I call modern "white and beige" processed foods. For example, 25% of all vegetables eaten in America are French fries, and the traditional "spices" of Americans are ketchup and mustard. Without diversity in our diets, we have lost the benefits of herbals and plant foods. These benefits cannot always be addressed by pharmaceutical drugs, which have a single target or main mechanism of action, unlike herbal supplements, which typically have multiple targets.

Rather than concentrating on the isolation of chemicals from herbs and plants in order to develop drugs, the focus of modern research on herbal medicines and botanical dietary supplements should be the establishment of a sufficient science base to support definitive clinical trials using herbal supplements which are the complex matrices found in traditional herbals. Modern research techniques would include detailed phytochemical profiling using mass spectrometry, biological assays including gene expression analysis, and transgenic animal models of chronic disease. Also needed are toxicology and pharmacokinetic studies in animals and humans. In fact, the entire armamentarium of modern medical research can be brought to bear on these ancient herbal medicines to advance their use in modern times. Current problems with manufacturing, processing, contamination, and quality of botanical sources are all potentially soluble with adequate resources and talent over the next several decades.

In view of their preventive benefits and potential lack of toxicity when properly used, I view these botanicals as the medicines of the 21st century and predict they will ultimately be used for the prevention and treatment of many modern chronic diseases of aging. For anyone interested in current information on botanicals for preventive or medicinal purposes, this is an excellent reference book. It contains more than 700 monographs updated with newly recognized interactions. Another useful feature is the identification guide, which has clearly labeled, full-color photographs of medicinal plants. You'll also find a section on the most popular nutritional supplements, and information on the clinical management of interactions. Each monograph contains the common names of herbs followed by its official scientific name. A complete description of the herb is provided, including its medicinal parts (e.g., flower and fruit) and its unique characteristics. Additional common names and synonyms as well as a detailed summary of the active compounds are given. For each herb, indications and usage are given under any of six applicable categories: Commission E Approved; Chinese Medicine; Indian Medicine; Homeopathic; Unproven Uses; or Probable Efficacy. This reference is a great starting point for researchers interested in advancing the field or for practitioners who want a concise, accurate, and accessible reference on botanical medicines.

David Heber, MD, PhD, FACP, FACN
Professor of Medicine and Public Health
Director, UCLA Center for Human Nutrition
and UCLA Botanical Research Center
David Geffen School of Medicine at UCLA
Los Angeles, CA

How to Use This Book

In this completely updated fourth edition of *PDR® for Herbal Medicines*, we have significantly expanded both the range and depth of the first three volumes. Among the many improvements you'll find:

- **Expanded Coverage:** The book contains more than 700 botanicals, including extensive updates of the most commonly asked-about herbs such as Ginkgo, Green Tea, and St. John's Wort, plus new entries on herbs currently sparking interest, including Hoodia and Mangosteen.
- **Nutritional Supplements:** Because patients who try herbal remedies often use nutritional supplements, too, we've added the most recent studies and analyses on products such as Calcium, Folic Acid, and Probiotics.
- **More Research Data:** Entries have been augmented with additional information on safety, clinical trials (when available), and pharmacological effects, as well as accepted and unproven uses.
- **New Interactions Risk Categories:** The entries include updated information on herb-drug and herb-supplement interactions, which are now grouped according to risk level.
- **Better Organization:** Herbs appear under their more familiar common name, with each monograph cross-referenced by its botanical name.

One important aspect of the previous editions does, however, remain constant. Because it is still extremely hard to come by reliable information on unregulated herbal supplements, this new edition continues to provide you with the closest available analog to FDA-approved labeling—the findings of the German Regulatory Authority's herbal watchdog agency, commonly called "Commission E." This agency has conducted an intensive assessment of the peer-reviewed literature on more than 300 common botanicals, weighing the quality of the clinical evidence and identifying the uses for which the herb can reasonably be considered effective.

For the herbs not considered by Commission E, *PDR for Herbal Medicines* provides the results of a literature review conducted by the respected PhytoPharm U.S. Institute of Phytopharmaceuticals under the direction of noted botanist, Dr. Joerg Gruenwald. These additional monographs (more than 400 are included) provide a detailed introduction to an array of exotic botanicals that you'll be hard-pressed to find in any other source.

Additionally, we've added detailed information from the alternative medicine database maintained by our sister company, Thomson Micromedex. Their research covers recent clinical trials of herbs and nutritional supplements as well as literature reviews of warnings and drug interactions, including risk level.

To make the information in the monographs as useful and accessible as possible, *PDR®* has echoed the structure of standard U.S. product labeling. Each monograph contains up to 10 standard sections, covering considerations ranging from description to dosage. Here's a closer look at what you will find:

- **Title:** Each monograph begins with the herb's generally accepted common name, followed by its botanical name. In addition, all monographs are cross-referenced by their botanical designation.

- **Description:** This section provides a botanical overview of the herb, including information on its medicinal parts; flower and fruit; leaves, stem, and root; unique characteristics, habitat, production, related plants, and additional common names and synonyms.

- **Actions and Pharmacology:** Here you'll find data on the active compounds or heterogeneous mixtures found in the plant, followed by a summary of the herb's clinical effects. If various parts of the plant possess different pharmacological activity, the parts are discussed individually.

- **Clinical Trials:** Research findings that support—or contradict—popular use is summarized in this section.

- **Indications and Usage:** Information on the uses of the herb is listed under six categories, as applicable:
  — Approved by Commission E
  — Unproven Uses
  — Probable Efficacy
  — Chinese Medicine
  — Indian Medicine
  — Homeopathic

For nutritional supplements, we've included FDA-approved indications as well as unproven uses. Approved uses are presented in list fashion. Other uses are described with provisos as necessary regarding route and form of administration.

■ **Contraindications:** Although natural remedies can often be used under most circumstances, a few pharmacologically potent herbs must be avoided in the presence of certain medical conditions. Others must be avoided during pregnancy or breastfeeding. If any such contraindications exist, they are summarized here.

■ **Precautions and Adverse Reactions:** Found in this section are any cautions or special considerations regarding safe use of the herb, including any interactions with medications or food. Although information on known side effects is sometimes lacking, problems that have been reported in the available literature are noted here.

■ **Drug Interactions:** Some herbs and nutritional supplements may interact with prescription or over-the-counter medicines, resulting in unwanted effects such as bleeding or sedation. Awareness of these interactions helps minimize adverse events and facilitates appropriate clinical management. (For this reason, individuals are advised to inform their healthcare professionals about all medicines and supplements they use, especially before surgery.) This section provides herb-drug interactions and clinical management guidance from the Thomson Micromedex database. Further, drug interactions are evaluated as to their likelihood of occurrence and categorized by risk level—Major Risk, Moderate Risk, Minor Risk, and Potential Interactions.

■ **Overdosage:** As we all know, "natural" is not synonymous with "benign," and an overdose of certain herbs can have serious—even fatal—consequences. Whenever adverse effects of overdose have been found in the literature, they are reported here, along with suggested medical interventions to be undertaken when an overdose occurs.

■ **Dosage:** Listed here are common modes of administration, forms and strengths of available preparations, methods for preparing the natural herb, and representative dosage recommendations drawn from the literature. Note, however, that dosage recommendations can be used only as a general guide. Whenever applicable, we've included the common dosages used for treating specific medical conditions (e.g., diabetes, high blood pressure, etc.). The potency of individual preparations and extracts is subject to substantial variation, so the manufacturer's directions should be consulted whenever available.

■ **Literature:** This section provides you with a unique bibliography of the technical literature. Because German researchers have been particularly active in the herbal arena, you will find an unusual number of German-language citations. However, work in the English literature is included as well.

To assist you in quickly locating the information you require, the monographs have been indexed by name, therapeutic category, general indications, homeopathic indications, Asian indications, and side effects. To aid you in evaluating potential risk, a drug-herb interaction guide and a safety guide are also included. Here's an overview of what each index provides:

■ **Alphabetical Index:** This index includes both scientific and common names found in the herbal monographs, together with appropriate page numbers.

■ **Therapeutic Category Index:** This index lists the monographs and their page numbers, alphabetically by accepted common name, under appropriate therapeutic category headings. Herbs deemed effective by Commission E are flagged with a (•) symbol to their left. To facilitate comparison with prescription and nonprescription drugs, the *PDR* standard therapeutic categories are used throughout.

■ **Indications Index:** This index lists herbs and their page numbers, alphabetically by accepted common name, under their various indications. Herbs deemed effective for the indication by Commission E are flagged with a (•) symbol at their left. To help you quickly identify conventional alternatives, the indication headings match those found in the PDR Indications Index, which appears in the *PDR® Guide to Drug Interactions, Side Effects, and Indications* and the *PDR® Electronic Library* CD-ROM.

■ **Homeopathic Indications Index:** Included in this index are only the uses found in homeopathy. Herbs, which homeopaths typically prescribe by scientific name, are listed here in the same manner, followed by their accepted common name in parentheses. As in the main indications index, headings are chosen to match those in the *PDR Guide to Drug Interactions, Side Effects, and Indications.*

■ **Asian Indications Index:** Entries in this index are limited to uses found in Chinese and Indian medicine. (Chinese entries are signified with a "C," Indian entries with an "I.") Herbs are listed by accepted common name. Again, indication headings employ the nomenclature used in the *PDR Guide to Drug Interactions, Side Effects, and Indications.*

- **Side Effects Index:** In this index, you'll find a list of all herbs associated with a given adverse reaction. Herbs are listed alphabetically by accepted common name, with the scientific name and page number appended. Nomenclature employed in the side effect headings matches that used in the PDR Side Effects Index, another feature of the *PDR Guide to Drug Interactions, Side Effects, and Indications* and the *PDR Electronic Library* CD-ROM.

- **Drug/Herb Interactions Guide:** In this convenient reference, each potential interaction is listed under both the name of the drug and the name of the interacting herb. A brief description of the interaction's effect follows each item.

- **Safety Guide:** This section lists botanicals in three precautionary categories:
  — Not for use during pregnancy
  — Not for use while nursing
  — For use only under supervision

  Here, the scientific and common names of all herbs in each category are listed alphabetically, together with the appropriate page number for further information.

- **Herb Identification Guide:** Following the indices, just as in *PDR* itself, you'll find a full-color identification section. The guide includes photos of nearly 400 of the most widely used herbs and provides you with a truly unique reference unmatched in any other printed resource. We've also included a brief glossary of the unfamiliar terms found in the monographs.

PUBLISHER'S DISCLAIMER

PDR for Herbal Medicines is the product of one of the most thorough and inclusive examinations of the herbal literature ever undertaken. Nevertheless, it's important to remember that it merely summarizes and synthesizes key data from the underlying research reports, and of necessity includes neither every published report nor every recorded fact.

As in all scientific investigation, conclusions regarding the effectiveness of the herbs discussed in this compendium are based on the preponderance of current evidence and cannot be considered firm or final. The publisher does not warrant that any herb will unfailingly and uniformly exhibit the properties ascribed to it by Germany's Commission E or any other scientific authority.

In the United States, herbal products are marketed under the provisions of the Dietary Supplement Health and Education Act of 1994, which prohibits their sale for the diagnosis, treatment, cure, or prevention of disease. In 2007, the U.S. Food and Drug Administration (FDA) took further action toward protecting consumers' health when it issued a final rule establishing current good manufacturing practice requirements (CGMPs) for dietary supplements. Under the final rule, manufacturers are required to substantiate the identity, purity, quality, strength, and composition of dietary supplements, and, further, to report all serious dietary supplement adverse events to the FDA.

The compilation of monographs in this book should not be construed as a claim or warranty of their efficacy for any purpose. Furthermore, it should be understood that, just as omission of a product does not signify rejection, inclusion of a product does not imply endorsement, and that the publisher is not advocating the use of any product or substance described herein.

Please remember that dosing of herbal preparations is highly dependent on a variety of factors, such as cultivation and harvesting conditions, the specific parts of the plant to be processed, the extraction methods employed, and the dosage form chosen by the manufacturer. Appropriate dosing must also take into consideration an individual's age, weight, and general health status. Consequently, dosage ranges set forth in the book's monographs must be employed only as general guidelines.

In addition, the publisher does not guarantee that every possible hazard, adverse effect, contraindication, precaution, or consequence of overdose is included in the summaries presented here. The publisher has performed no independent verification of the data reported herein, and expressly disclaims responsibility for any error, whether inherent in the underlying literature or resulting from erroneous translation, transcription, or typography.

When patients approach you—as they surely will—for advice on the latest herbal "discovery" to hit the news, we hope that *PDR for Herbal Medicines* will provide you with all the facts you need to offer sound, rational guidance firmly grounded in fact. Certainly such counseling is the aim of every dedicated health care professional. And at *PDR*, we fully share that goal.

Alphabetical Index

Listed here are the scientific and common names found in the herbal monographs. Generally accepted common names that serve as monograph titles appear in bold type. Scientific names are shown in italic type. If an entry lists two page numbers, the first refers to a photograph of the plant or product in the Identification Guide, the second to the herbal monograph.

ALPHABETICAL INDEX

E

ALPHABETICAL INDEX

J

P

S

T

W

ALPHABETICAL INDEX

Therapeutic Category Index

Entries in this index are organized by prescribing category, enabling you to quickly identify botanicals with similar properties. Within each category, herbs are listed alphabetically by their accepted common name, with the scientific name shown in parentheses. Botanicals deemed effective by the German Regulatory Authority's "Commission E" are marked with a (•) symbol at their left. If an entry lists two page numbers, the first refers to a photograph of the plant in the Herb Identification Guide, the second to the herbal monograph. The index lists herbs by general category only. To locate botanicals considered appropriate for a specific indication, please consult the Indications Index.

• Denotes recommendation by Commission E.

• **Denotes recommendation by Commission E.**

Vervain (*Verbena officinalis*) G-25, 877
Watercress (*Nasturtium officinale*) 885
• White Fir (*Abies alba*) 889
• White Willow (*Salix species*) G-25, 894
Wild Indigo (*Baptisia tinctoria*) G-26, 897
Wild Mint (*Mentha aquatica*) G-26, 899
Wild Thyme (*Thymus serpyllum*) G-26, 900
Wild Yam (*Dioscorea villosa*) G-26, 902
Wintergreen (*Gaultheria procumbens*) 905
Winter's Bark (*Drimys winteri*) 904
Wood Anemone (*Anemone nemorosa*) 907
Wormwood (*Artemisia absinthium*) G-26, 912
Yellow Jessamine (*Gelsemium sempervirens*) 921

ANORECTAL PREPARATIONS

Bilberry (*Vaccinium myrtillus*) G-5, 78
• Butcher's Broom (*Ruscus aculeatus*) G-7, 140
• Poplar (*Populus species*) G-20, 664
• Psyllium (*Plantago ovata*) 669
• Sweet Clover (*Melilotus officinalis*) G-24, 829
• Tolu Balsam (*Myroxylon balsamum*) G-24, 848
• Witch Hazel (*Hamamelis virginiana*) G-26, 906

ANTACID PREPARATIONS

Barberry (*Berberis vulgaris*) G-4, 65
Congorosa (*Maytenus ilicifolia*) 225
European Five-Finger Grass (*Potentilla reptans*) G-11, 300
Lovage (*Levisticum officinale*) G-16, 536
Salep (*Orchis species*) 719
Wood Betony (*Betonica officinalis*) G-26, 908
Yellow Jessamine (*Gelsemium sempervirens*) 921

ANTHELMINTICS

Amargo (*Quassia amara*) G-3, 28
Balmony (*Chelone glabra*) G-4, 63
Behen (*Moringa oleifera*) 71
Black Hellebore (*Helleborus niger*) G-5, 102
Black Horehound (*Ballota nigra*) G-5, 103
Blue Cohosh (*Caulophyllum thalictroides*) 116
Burning Bush (*Dictamnus albus*) G-7, 139
Butternut (*Juglans cinerea*) 142
Calotropis (*Calotropis procera*) 149
Canadian Fleabane (*Erigeron canadensis*) G-7, 151
Castor Oil Plant (*Ricinus communis*) G-7, 166
Centaury (*Centaurium erythraea*) G-8, 183
Chives (*Allium schoenoprasum*) G-8, 196
Cinnamon (*Cinnamomum verum*) G-8, 197
Corn Cockle (*Agrostemma githago*) 229
Cowhage (*Mucuna pruriens*) 236
Eucalyptus (*Eucalyptus globulus*) G-11, 293
European Water Hemlock (*Cicuta virosa*) G-11, 310
Feverfew (*Tanacetum parthenium*) G-11, 321
Green Hellebore (*Helleborus viridis*) 413
Groundsel (*Senecio vulgaris*) 424
Indian Nettle (*Acalypha indica*) 467
Kamala (*Mallotus philippinensis*) 488
Kousso (*Hagenia abyssinica*) 500
Larkspur (*Delphinium consolida*) G-15, 511
Lavender Cotton (*Santolina chamaecyparissias*) G-16, 513
Male Fern (*Dryopteris filix-mas*) G-17, 553
Marigold (*Calendula officinalis*) G-17, 559
Morning Glory (*Ipomoea hederacea*) 585
Mugwort (*Artemisia vulgaris*) G-18, 591
Myrtle (*Myrtus communis*) G-18, 596
Neem (*Antelaea azadirachta*) G-18, 599
Papaya (*Carica papaya*) G-19, 627
Pineapple (*Ananas comosus*) 652
Pink Root (*Spigelia marilandica*) 653
Pomegranate (*Punica granatum*) G-20, 662
Pumpkin (*Cucurbita pepo*) G-20, 675
Quassia (*Picrasma excelsa*) 683
Rue (*Ruta graveolens*) G-21, 711
Sweet Gale (*Myrica gale*) G-24, 830
Tansy (*Tanacetum vulgare*) G-24, 837
Tree of Heaven (*Ailanthus altissima*) 859
Turmeric (*Curcuma domestica*) 864
Walnut (*Juglans regia*) G-25, 881
Water Germander (*Teucrium scordium*) 885
Wild Carrot (*Daucus carota*) G-25, 895
Wormseed (*Artemisia cina*) 910
Wormseed Oil (*Chenopodium ambrosioides*) G-26, 911
Wormwood (*Artemisia absinthium*) G-26, 912
Wormwood Grass (*Spigelia anthelmia*) 915
Yellow Lupin (*Lupinus luteus*) 922
Yew (*Taxus baccata*) G-26, 924

ANTIANXIETY AGENTS

Adonis (*Adonis vernalis*) G-3, 8
Aga (*Amanita muscaria*) G-3, 11

• Denotes recommendation by Commission E.

ANTIARRHYTHMICS

ANTICONVULSANTS

ANTIDEPRESSANTS

• Denotes recommendation by Commission E.

ANTIDIABETIC AGENTS

ANTIDIARRHEALS

THERAPEUTIC CATEGORY INDEX

• Denotes recommendation by Commission E.

Fever Bark (*Alstonia constricta*) 320
Fool's Parsley (*Aethusa cynapium*) G-12, 334
Gambir (*Uncaria species*) 343
Gotu Kola (*Centella asiatica*) G-13, 400
Great Burnet (*Sanguisorba officinalis*) G-13, 410
Green Tea (*Camellia sinensis*) G-13, 414
Ground Ivy (*Glechoma hederacea*) 422
Gum Arabic (*Acacia senegal*) 428
Herb Robert (*Geranium robertianum*) G-14, 441
Hogweed (*Heracleum sphondylium*) G-14, 444
Horehound (*Marrubium vulgare*) G-14, 452
Hound's Tongue (*Cynoglossum officinale*) 459
Houseleek (*Sempervivum tectorum*) G-14, 460
Jaborandi (*Pilocarpus microphyllus*) G-15, 472
• Jambol (*Syzygium cumini*) 475
Kudzu (*Pueraria lobata*) 501
• Lady's Mantle (*Alchemilla vulgaris*) G-15, 509
Levant Cotton (*Gossypium herbaceum*) G-16, 521
Logwood (*Haematoxylon campechianum*) 535
Loosestrife (*Lysimachia vulgaris*) G-16, 535
Lotus (*Nelumbo nucifera*) G-16, 536
Mangosteen (*Garcinia mangostana*) 556
Marshmallow (*Althaea officinalis*) 569
Matico (*Piper elongatum*) 573
Moneywort (*Lysimachia nummularia*) G-17, 583
Mountain Avens (*Dryas octopetala*) 587
Muira-Puama (*Ptychopetalum olacoides*) 592
Myrtle (*Myrtus communis*) G-18, 596
Nerve Root (*Cypripedium calceolus*) 600
• Oak (*Quercus robur*) G-18, 609
Oats (*Avena sativa*) G-18, 611
Pagoda Tree (*Sophora japonica*) 626
Pinus Bark (*Tsuga canadensis*) G-19, 653
Plantain (*Musa paradisiaca*) 656
Pomegranate (*Punica granatum*) G-20, 662
• Potentilla (*Potentilla anserina*) G-20, 667
• Psyllium (*Plantago ovata*) 669
• Psyllium Seed (*Plantago afra*) G-20, 673
Purple Loosestrife (*Lythrum salicaria*) G-20, 678
Quassia (*Picrasma excelsa*) 683
Quince (*Cydonia oblongata*) 685
Rhatany (*Krameria triandra*) 702
Rice (*Oryza sativa*) G-21, 705
Rue (*Ruta graveolens*) G-21, 711
Sage (*Salvia officinalis*) G-21, 717
Salep (*Orchis species*) 719
Sandarac (*Tetraclinis articulata*) 722
Self-Heal (*Prunella vulgaris*) G-22, 741
Simaruba (*Simaruba amara*) 753
Sloe (*Prunus spinosa*) G-22, 756
Smartweed (*Persicaria hydropiper*) 757
Sneezewort (*Achillea ptarmica*) 758
Southern Tsangshu (*Atractylodes lancea*) 763
Spanish-Chestnut (*Castanea sativa*) 778
Strawberry (*Fragaria vesca*) G-23, 821
Tree of Heaven (*Ailanthus altissima*) 859
Turmeric (*Curcuma domestica*) 864
• Uzara (*Xysmalobium undulatum*) 871
Water Avens (*Geum rivale*) G-25, 882
Water Germander (*Teucrium scordium*) 885
Wild Cherry (*Prunus serotina*) 896
Wild Daisy (*Bellis perennis*) G-26, 896
Wild Mint (*Mentha aquatica*) G-26, 899
Witch Hazel (*Hamamelis virginiana*) G-26, 906
Wood Betony (*Betonica officinalis*) G-26, 908
Yarrow (*Achillea millefolium*) G-26, 917

ANTIEMETICS

Adrue (*Cyperus articulatus*) G-3, 10
Almond (*Prunus dulcis*) 18
American Pawpaw (*Asimina triloba*) 32
Bilberry (*Vaccinium myrtillus*) G-5, 78
Black Hellebore (*Helleborus niger*) G-5, 102
Black Horehound (*Ballota nigra*) G-5, 103
British Elecampane (*Inula britannica*) 128
California Peppertree (*Schinus molle*) 147
Carob (*Ceratonia siliqua*) G-7, 158
Cascarilla (*Croton eluteria*) 164
Cayenne (*Capsicum annuum*) G-8, 173
Cola (*Cola acuminata*) 213
Common Kidney Vetch (*Anthyllis vulneraria*) G-9, 222
5-HTP (*Griffonia simplicifoclia*) 3
Gambir (*Uncaria species*) 343
Giant Milkweed (*Calotropis gigantea*) 364
• Ginger (*Zingiber officinale*) G-12, 365
Green Hellebore (*Helleborus viridis*) 413

• Denotes recommendation by Commission E.

ANTIFLATULENTS

ANTIFUNGALS

ANTIHISTAMINES

ANTIHYPERTENSIVE AGENTS

ANTI-INFECTIVES

• Denotes recommendation by Commission E.

ANTI-INFECTIVES & COMBINATIONS

ANTI-INFLAMMATORY AGENTS

ANTI-INFLAMMATORY AGENTS, SKIN AND MUCOUS MEMBRANE

ANTILIPIDEMIC AGENTS

ANTIMALARIAL AGENTS

ANTINEOPLASTICS

ANTIPANIC AGENTS

ANTIPARKINSONIAN AGENTS

ANTIPERSPIRANTS

ANTIPLATELET AGENTS

ANTIPRURITICS

ANTIPSORIATIC AGENTS

ANTIPSYCHOTIC AGENTS

ANTIRHEUMATIC AGENTS

• Denotes recommendation by Commission E.

THERAPEUTIC CATEGORY INDEX

ANTISEBORRHEIC AGENTS

ANTISPASMODICS

ANTITHYROID AGENTS

ANTITUBERCULOSIS AGENTS

ANTIVIRALS

APPETITE STIMULANTS

THERAPEUTIC CATEGORY INDEX

• Denotes recommendation by Commission E.

APPETITE SUPPRESSANTS

ASTRINGENTS

BENIGN PROSTATIC HYPERPLASIA (BPH) THERAPY

BLOOD MODIFIERS

BOWEL EVACUANTS

BURN PREPARATIONS

CALCIUM OXALATE STONE PREVENTION

• Denotes recommendation by Commission E.

CARDIOVASCULAR AGENTS

• Denotes recommendation by Commission E.

• Denotes recommendation by Commission E.

THERAPEUTIC CATEGORY INDEX

• Denotes recommendation by Commission E.

DIGESTIVE ENZYMES

DIURETIC AGENTS

• Denotes recommendation by Commission E.

EMOLLIENTS & MOISTURIZERS

ENEMAS

ENURESIS MANAGEMENT

ERECTILE DYSFUNCTION THERAPY

EXPECTORANTS & COMBINATIONS

FEVER REDUCERS

• Denotes recommendation by Commission E.

GASTRITIS AIDS

GASTROINTESTINAL AGENTS

• Denotes recommendation by Commission E.

• Denotes recommendation by Commission E.

GASTROINTESTINAL STIMULANTS

GOUT PREPARATIONS

THERAPEUTIC CATEGORY INDEX

• Denotes recommendation by Commission E.

• Denotes recommendation by Commission E.

LEPROSTATICS

LIVER PRODUCTS

THERAPEUTIC CATEGORY INDEX

LOCAL ANESTHETICS

MENOPAUSAL PREPARATIONS

MIGRAINE PREPARATIONS

• **Denotes recommendation by Commission E.**

MILK SUBSTITUTE

MOUTH & THROAT PRODUCTS

• Denotes recommendation by Commission E.

• **Denotes recommendation by Commission E.**

OPHTHALMIC PREPARATIONS

• Denotes recommendation by Commission E.

• Denotes recommendation by Commission E.

• Denotes recommendation by Commission E.

REVITALIZING AGENTS

SALIVA PRODUCTS

SCABICIDES & PEDICULICIDES

SEDATIVES & HYPNOTICS

• Denotes recommendation by Commission E.

SKELETAL MUSCLE RELAXANTS & COMBINATIONS

SKIN & MUCOUS MEMBRANE AGENTS

THERAPEUTIC CATEGORY INDEX

• Denotes recommendation by Commission E.

SMOKING CESSATION AIDS

SMOOTH MUSCLE RELAXANTS

STIMULANT LAXATIVES & COMBINATIONS

SUNBURN PREPARATIONS

TEETHING REMEDIES

TREMOR PREPARATIONS

URINARY ANTI-INFECTIVES & COMBINATIONS

• Denotes recommendation by Commission E.

URINARY TRACT AGENTS

• Denotes recommendation by Commission E.

VAGINAL PREPARATIONS

VASOPROTECTIVE AGENTS

VENOUS INSUFFICIENCY PRODUCTS

• Denotes recommendation by Commission E.

• Denotes recommendation by Commission E.

THERAPEUTIC CATEGORY INDEX

• Denotes recommendation by Commission E.

Indications Index

Entries in this index are organized by specific indication, enabling you to quickly review the botanical alternatives for a particular diagnosis. For ease of comparison with prescription and over-the-counter medications, the index employs the same nomenclature found in the Indications Index of the PDR Companion Guide™. *Under each heading, herbs are listed alphabetically by accepted common name, with the scientific name shown in parentheses. Botanicals deemed effective by the German Regulatory Authority's "Commission E" are marked with a (•) symbol at their left. If an entry lists two page numbers, the first refers to a photograph of the plant in the Herb Identification Guide, the second to the herbal monograph. For more information on both proven and traditional remedies, be sure to check the appropriate underlying monograph.*

• Denotes recommendation by Commission E.

• Denotes recommendation by Commission E.

BRONCHIAL ASTHMA

BRONCHIAL CONGESTION

BRONCHITIS

• Denotes recommendation by Commission E.

• Denotes recommendation by Commission E.

• Denotes recommendation by Commission E.

INDICATIONS INDEX

• Denotes recommendation by Commission E.

INDICATIONS INDEX

• Denotes recommendation by Commission E.

• Denotes recommendation by Commission E.

COUGH, WHOOPING

CRADLE CAP

CRAMPS, ABDOMINAL, SYMPTOMATIC RELIEF OF

CRAMPS, LEG

CRAMPS, TETANIC AND EPILEPTIC

CRAVINGS, AID IN CONTROL OF

CROUP

CUTS, MINOR, INFECTION FROM

CUTS, MINOR, PAIN ASSOCIATED WITH

CYSTITIS

• Denotes recommendation by Commission E.

• **Denotes recommendation by Commission E.**

Muira-Puama (*Ptychopetalum olacoides*) ... 592
Mullein (*Verbascum densiflorum*) ... G-18, 593
Rose (*Rosa centifolia*) ... 708
Southern Tsangshu (*Atractylodes lancea*) ... 763
Spanish-Chestnut (*Castanea sativa*) ... 778
Surinam Cherry (*Eugenia unifloria*) ... 827
Water Germander (*Teucrium scordium*) ... 885
White Willow (*Salix species*) ... G-25, 894
Wild Mint (*Mentha aquatica*) ... G-26, 899

DIARRHEA, BLOODY, SYMPTOMATIC RELIEF OF

Cumin (*Cuminum cyminum*) ... G-9, 244

DIARRHEA, CHRONIC

American White Pond Lily (*Nymphaea odorata*) ... G-3, 33
Dogwood (*Cornus florida*) ... G-10, 259

DIARRHEA, SYMPTOMATIC RELIEF OF

• Agrimony (*Agrimonia eupatoria*) ... G-3, 12
Alkanet (*Alkanna tinctoria*) ... G-3, 17
Amaranth (*Amaranthus hypochondriacus*) ... G-3, 28
Angostura (*Galipea officinalis*) ... 38
Apple Tree (*Malus domestica*) ... G-4, 40
Barberry (*Berberis vulgaris*) ... G-4, 65
Barley (*Hordeum distichon*) ... G-4, 67
Behen (*Moringa oleifera*) ... 71
Bennet's Root (*Geum urbanum*) ... G-4, 74
• Bilberry (*Vaccinium myrtillus*) ... G-5, 78
Bistort (*Persicaria bistorta*) ... G-5, 86
Black Catnip (*Phyllanthus amarus*) ... 94
Black Currant (*Ribes nigrum*) ... G-5, 100
• Blackberry (*Rubus fruticosus*) ... G-6, 109
Bog Bilberry (*Vaccinium uliginosum*) ... G-6, 119
Canadian Fleabane (*Erigeron canadensis*) ... G-7, 151
Carrageen (*Chondrus crispus*) ... 160
Cascarilla (*Croton eluteria*) ... 164
Cat's Claw (*Unicaria tomentosa*) ... 168
Cheken (*Eugenia chequen*) ... 188
• Cinquefoil (*Potentilla erecta*) ... G-8, 198
Cocoa (*Theobroma cacao*) ... G-8, 208
• Coffee (*Coffea arabica*) ... G-9, 210
Comfrey (*Symphytum officinale*) ... G-9, 219
Cranesbill (*Geranium maculatum*) ... 241
Dragon's Blood (*Daemonorops draco*) ... 263
Elephant-Ears (*Bergenia crassifolia*) ... 276
European Five-Finger Grass (*Potentilla reptans*) ... G-11, 300
European Mistletoe (*Viscum album*) ... G-11, 302
False Schisandra (*Kadsura japonica*) ... 316
Fool's Parsley (*Aethusa cynapium*) ... G-12, 334
Gambir (*Uncaria species*) ... 343
Goldenseal (*Hydrastis canadensis*) ... G-13, 395
Green Tea (*Camellia sinensis*) ... G-13, 414
Ground Ivy (*Glechoma hederacea*) ... 422
Herb Robert (*Geranium robertianum*) ... G-14, 441
Hogweed (*Heracleum sphondylium*) ... G-14, 444
Houseleek (*Sempervivum tectorum*) ... G-14, 460
Indian-Hemp (*Apocynum cannabinum*) ... 466
• Jambol (*Syzygium cumini*) ... 475
• Lady's Mantle (*Alchemilla vulgaris*) ... G-15, 509
Levant Cotton (*Gossypium herbaceum*) ... G-16, 521
Logwood (*Haematoxylon campechianum*) ... 535
Lotus (*Nelumbo nucifera*) ... G-16, 536
Marshmallow (*Althaea officinalis*) ... 569
Matico (*Piper elongatum*) ... 573
Moneywort (*Lysimachia nummularia*) ... G-17, 583
Myrtle (*Myrtus communis*) ... G-18, 596
Nutmeg (*Myristica fragrans*) ... G-18, 606
• Oak (*Quercus robur*) ... G-18, 609
Oats (*Avena sativa*) ... G-18, 611
Periwinkle (*Vinca minor*) ... 645
Pinus Bark (*Tsuga canadensis*) ... G-19, 653
Plantain (*Musa paradisiaca*) ... 656
Pomegranate (*Punica granatum*) ... G-20, 662
Poppyseed (*Papaver somniferum*) ... G-20, 666
• Potentilla (*Potentilla anserina*) ... G-20, 667
• Psyllium (*Plantago ovata*) ... 669
• Psyllium Seed (*Plantago afra*) ... G-20, 673
Purple Loosestrife (*Lythrum salicaria*) ... G-20, 678
Quassia (*Picrasma excelsa*) ... 683
Quince (*Cydonia oblongata*) ... 685
Rhatany (*Krameria triandra*) ... 702
Rue (*Ruta graveolens*) ... G-21, 711
Sage (*Salvia officinalis*) ... G-21, 717
Salep (*Orchis species*) ... 719
Sandarac (*Tetraclinis articulata*) ... 722
Self-Heal (*Prunella vulgaris*) ... G-22, 741
Simaruba (*Simaruba amara*) ... 753
Sloe (*Prunus spinosa*) ... G-22, 756
Sneezewort (*Achillea ptarmica*) ... 758

INDICATIONS INDEX

• Denotes recommendation by Commission E.

• Denotes recommendation by Commission E.

• Denotes recommendation by Commission E.

FEVER ASSOCIATED WITH COMMON COLD

FEVER, REDUCTION OF

• Denotes recommendation by Commission E.

INDICATIONS INDEX

FROSTBITE, POSSIBLY EFFECTIVE IN

FUNGAL INFECTIONS, SKIN

(*See under* Infections, mycotic, cutaneous)

FURUNCULOSIS

FURUNCULOSIS, SYMPTOMATIC RELIEF OF

GALLBLADDER DISORDERS, UNSPECIFIED

GALLSTONES

(*See under* Biliary calculi, chemical dissolution of)

GASTRIC HYPERACIDITY

(*See under* Hyperacidity, gastric)

GASTRITIS

• **Denotes recommendation by Commission E.**

• Denotes recommendation by Commission E.

• Denotes recommendation by Commission E.

• Denotes recommendation by Commission E.

HEMATEMESIS

HEMATURIA

HEMOPHILIA, UNSPECIFIED

HEMOPTYSIS

HEMORRHAGE, GASTROINTESTINAL, UNSPECIFIED

HEMORRHAGE, NASAL

HEMORRHAGE, POSTPARTUM

HEMORRHAGE, UNSPECIFIED

HEMORRHOIDS

HEMORRHOIDS, SYMPTOMATIC RELIEF OF

• Denotes recommendation by Commission E.

• Denotes recommendation by Commission E.

• Denotes recommendation by Commission E.

LIVER AND GALLBLADDER COMPLAINTS

LIVER DISORDERS

LUMPS IN THE BREAST

LYMPH NODES, INFLAMMATION OF

LYMPHEDEMA

INDICATIONS INDEX

• Denotes recommendation by Commission E.

• Denotes recommendation by Commission E.

MYALGIA, TOPICAL RELIEF OF
(*See under* Pain, topical relief of)

MYCOBACTERIUM LEPRAE INFECTIONS
(*See under* Leprosy)

MYOCARDITIS, UNSPECIFIED
Arnica (*Arnica montana*) 43

NARCOTIC ADDICTION, DETOXIFICATION TREATMENT OF
Oats (*Avena sativa*) G-18, 611

NASAL CONGESTION, SYMPTOMATIC RELIEF OF
Scotch Pine (*Pinus species*) G-22, 736

NAUSEA
(*See also under* Motion sickness)
Adrue (*Cyperus articulatus*) G-3, 10
Almond (*Prunus dulcis*) 18
Black Hellebore (*Helleborus niger*) G-5, 102
California Peppertree (*Schinus molle*) 147
Condurango (*Marsdenia condurango*) 224
Gambir (*Uncaria species*) 343
Green Hellebore (*Helleborus viridis*) 413
Jatamansi (*Nardostachys jatamansi*) 479
Levant Cotton (*Gossypium herbaceum*) G-16, 521
Marijuana (*Cannabis sativa*) G-17, 562
Peppermint (*Mentha piperita*) G-19, 640
Sneezewort (*Achillea ptarmica*) 758
Sweet Vernal Grass (*Anthoxanthum odoratum*) G-24, 833

NECK STIFFNESS
Hemlock (*Conium maculatum*) G-13, 436

NEPHRITIS, ACUTE
Black Hellebore (*Helleborus niger*) G-5, 102

NEPHROLITHIASIS, PREVENTION
Cranberry (*Vaccinium macrocarpon*) 238

NERVE INFLAMMATION
Lemon Balm (*Melissa officinalis*) G-16, 514
Levant Cotton (*Gossypium herbaceum*) G-16, 521
Rupturewort (*Herniaria glabra*) G-21, 713

NEURALGIA
(*See under* Pain, neurogenic)

NEURALGIA, TRIGEMINAL
Thuja (*Thuja occidentalis*) G-24, 844

NEURITIS, PERIPHERAL, ACUTE
(*See under* Pain, neurogenic)

NEUROLOGIC/PSYCHIATRIC DYSFUNCTION, DUE TO SEROTONIN DEFICIENCY
5-HTP (*Griffonia simplicifoclia*) 3

NEUROPATHY
California Poppy (*Eschscholtzia californica*) G-7, 148

NIGHT BLINDNESS
Southern Tsangshu (*Atractylodes lancea*) 763

NIGHT SWEATS
Asiatic Dogwood (*Cornus officinalis*) 54
False Schisandra (*Kadsura japonica*) 316

NIGHT VISION ENHANCER
Bilberry (*Vaccinium myrtillus*) G-5, 78

NUTRIENTS, DEFICIENCY OF
Arrowroot (*Maranta arundinacea*) 48
Jujube (*Zyzyphus jujube*) 484

NUTRIENTS, DEFICIENCY OF, STRESS-INDUCED
(*See under* Nutrients, deficiency of)

NUTRIENTS, DEFICIENCY OF, SURGERY-INDUCED
(*See under* Nutrients, deficiency of)

NUTRITION, INFANT
(*See under* Breast milk, replacement of or supplement to)

NYSTAGMUS
Fish Berry (*Anamirta cocculus*) 328

OBESITY, EXOGENOUS
Kava Kava (*Piper methysticum*) G-15, 489

OBESITY, UNSPECIFIED
Bladderwrack (*Fucus vesiculosus*) 110

OLIGURIA
Mate (*Ilex paraguariensis*) G-17, 572

OPHTHALMIA
Asarum (*Asarum europaeum*) 51
California Peppertree (*Schinus molle*) 147
Chickweed (*Stellaria media*) 189
Cornflower (*Centaurea cyanus*) G-9, 232
Eyebright (*Euphrasia officinalis*) 315

OPHTHALMIC DISORDERS
Congorosa (*Maytenus ilicifolia*) 225
Eyebright (*Euphrasia officinalis*) 315
Fennel (*Foeniculum vulgare*) G-11, 317
Nux Vomica (*Strychnos nux vomica*) G-18, 607
Oak (*Quercus robur*) G-18, 609
Oats (*Avena sativa*) G-18, 611
Pasque Flower (*Pulsatilla pratensis*) 633
Quince (*Cydonia oblongata*) 685
Red Maple (*Acer rubrum*) G-21, 697
Tomato (*Lycopersicon esculentum*) G-24, 849
Tropical Almond (*Terminalia chebula*) 861
Turmeric (*Curcuma domestica*) 864

• Denotes recommendation by Commission E.

• Denotes recommendation by Commission E.

• Denotes recommendation by Commission E.

INDICATIONS INDEX

RENAL IMPAIRMENT

RESPIRATORY SYMPTOMS, UPPER, RELIEF OF

(*See under* Influenza syndrome, symptomatic relief of)

RESPIRATORY TRACT DISORDERS

• Denotes recommendation by Commission E.

INDICATIONS INDEX

• Denotes recommendation by Commission E.

• Denotes recommendation by Commission E.

• Denotes recommendation by Commission E.

• Denotes recommendation by Commission E.

• Denotes recommendation by Commission E.

• Denotes recommendation by Commission E.

• Denotes recommendation by Commission E.

• **Denotes recommendation by Commission E.**

• Denotes recommendation by Commission E.

• **Denotes recommendation by Commission E.**

WOUNDS, SUPERFICIAL

• Denotes recommendation by Commission E.

Homeopathic Indications Index

Entries in this index are organized by specific indication, enabling you to quickly review the botanicals used by homeopaths for a particular diagnosis. For ease of comparison with prescription and over-the-counter medications, the index employs the same nomenclature found in the Indications Index of the PDR Companion Guide™. *Under each heading, herbs are listed alphabetically by scientific name, with the accepted common name shown in parentheses. If an entry lists two page numbers, the first refers to a photograph of the plant in the Herb Identification Guide, the second to the herbal monograph. For more information on any of these botanicals, be sure to check the appropriate underlying monograph.*

ABDOMINAL CRAMPS
(*See under* Cramps, abdominal, symptomatic relief of)

ABRASIONS, PAIN ASSOCIATED WITH
(*See under* Pain, topical relief of)

ACHES, MUSCULAR
(*See under* Pain, muscular, temporary relief of)

AIRWAY OBSTRUCTION DISORDERS
(*See under* Bronchial asthma)

AMENORRHEA, SECONDARY
(*See under* Menstrual disorders)

ANEMIA, UNSPECIFIED
Cinchona pubescens (Quinine) **G-20, 686**
Lycoperdon species (Puff Ball) **675**

ANGINA
(*See under* Angina pectoris)

ANGINA PECTORIS
Crataegus laevigata (English Hawthorn) **G-10, 279**
Nicotiana tabacum (Tobacco) **G-24, 847**
Spigelia anthelmia (Wormwood Grass) **915**

ANXIETY AND TENSION DUE TO MENOPAUSE
(*See under* Menopause, management of the manifestations of)

ANXIETY DISORDERS, MANAGEMENT OF
Aconitum napellus (Monkshood) **G-18, 584**
Amanita muscaria (Aga) **G-3, 11**
Anamirta cocculus (Fish Berry) **328**
Aquilegia vulgaris (Columbine) **G-9, 218**
Delphinium staphisagria (Stavesacre) **788**
Ferula sumbul (Sumbul) **G-23, 824**
Humulus lupulus (Hops) **G-14, 448**
Leonurus japonicus (Chinese Motherwort) **192**
Papaver rhoeas (Corn Poppy) **230**
Paris quadrifolia (Herb Paris) **G-14, 441**
Passiflora incarnata (Passion Flower) **G-19, 634**
Rhus toxicodendron (Poison Ivy) **658**
Spigelia marilandica (Pink Root) **653**
Strophanthus gratus (Strophanthus) **822**
Strophanthus hispidus (Kombé Seed) **499**
Strychnos ignatii (Ignatius Beans) **464**
Strychnos nux vomica (Nux Vomica) **G-18, 607**
Vitex agnus-castus (Chaste Tree) **G-8, 185**

ANXIETY, SHORT-TERM SYMPTOMATIC RELIEF OF
Camellia sinensis (Green Tea) **G-13, 414**
Myristica fragrans (Nutmeg) **G-18, 606**
Piper methysticum (Kava Kava) **G-15, 489**

APPETITE, SUPPRESSION OF
(*See under* Obesity, exogenous)

APPREHENSION
(*See under* Anxiety disorders, management of)

ARRHYTHMIAS
Crataegus laevigata (English Hawthorn) **G-10, 279**
Iberis amara (Bitter Candytuft) **87**
Viscum album (European Mistletoe) **G-11, 302**

Asian Indications Index

Entries in this index are organized by specific indication, enabling you to quickly review the botanicals used in Asian medicine for a particular diagnosis. For ease of comparison with prescription and over-the-counter medications, the index employs the same nomenclature found in the Indications Index of the PDR Companion Guide™. *Under each heading, herbs are listed alphabetically by accepted common name, with the scientific name shown in parentheses. An "I" in parentheses indicates Indian usage; a "C" denotes Chinese medical applications. If an entry lists two page numbers, the first refers to a photograph of the plant in the Herb Identification Guide, the second to the herbal monograph. For more information on any of these botanicals, be sure to check the appropriate underlying monograph.*

(I) denotes use in Indian medicine. (C) denotes use in Chinese medicine.

BITE WOUNDS
Bistort
(*Persicaria bistorta*) (C) ... G-5, 86
Great Burnet
(*Sanguisorba officinalis*) (C) G-13, 410
Scarlet Pimpernel
(*Anagallis arvensis*) (C) .. G-22, 729
Wormseed Oil
(*Chenopodium ambrosioides*) (C) G-26, 911

BITES, POISONOUS
Black Cohosh
(*Cimicifuga racemosa*) (C) . G-5, 95
Rauwolfia
(*Rauwolfia Serpentina*) (I) 691

BITTER TASTE
Chinese Thoroughwax
(*Bupleurum chinese*) (C) 194

BLEEDING ASSOCIATED WITH TOOTH EXTRACTION
(*See under* Bleeding, gingival)

BLEEDING, GINGIVAL
Henbane
(*Hyoscyamus niger*) (I) ... G-14, 438

BLEEDING, POSTPARTUM
Cane-Reed
(*Costus speciosa*) (I) 153

BLEEDING, VAGINAL, ASSOCIATED WITH PREGNANCY
European Mistletoe
(*Viscum album*) (C) G-11, 302

BLOODY STOOL
Pomegranate
(*Punica granatum*) (C) ... G-20, 662

BONE AND JOINT HEALTH
Lycium Berries
(*Lycium barbarum*) (C) 541

BREAST CANCER
(*See under* Carcinoma, breast)

BREAST CARCINOMA
(*See under* Carcinoma, breast)

BRONCHIAL ASTHMA
Arjun Tree
(*Terminalia arjuna*) (I) 42
Asa Foetida
(*Ferula foetida*) (I) 51
Bamboo
(*Arundinaria japonica*) (C) G-4, 63
Betel Nut (*Piper betle*) (I) .. G-4, 76
Black Nightshade
(*Solanum nigrum*) (I) G-6, 106
Black Pepper
(*Piper nigrum*) (I) G-6, 107
Cabbage
(*Brassica oleracea*) (I) ... G-7, 143
Calotropis
(*Calotropis procera*) (I) 149
Camphor Tree
(*Cinnamomum camphora*) (I) G-7, 150
Costus
(*Saussurea costus*) (I,C) 233
Garden Cress
(*Lepidium sativum*) (I) ... G-12, 345
Ginkgo
(*Ginkgo biloba*) (C) G-12, 371
Henbane
(*Hyoscyamus niger*) (I,C) . G-14, 438
Indian Squill
(*Urginea indica*) (I) 469
Jequirity
(*Abrus precatorius*) (I) 481
Jimson Weed
(*Datura stramonium*) (C) . G-15, 482
Ma-Huang
(*Ephedra sinica*) (C) G-16, 543
Northern Prickly Ash
(*Zanthoxylum americanum*) (I) 605
Nux Vomica
(*Strychnos nux vomica*) (I) G-18, 607
Rose (*Rosa centifolia*) (I) 708
Sumbul
(*Ferula sumbul*) (I) G-23, 824
Walnut (*Juglans regia*) (C) . G-25, 881
Zedoary
(*Curcuma zedoaria*) (I) .. G-26, 930

BRONCHIAL CONGESTION
Balloon-Flower
(*Platycodon grandiflorum*) (C) . 62

BRONCHITIS, ACUTE
Arjun Tree
(*Terminalia arjuna*) (I) 42
Arrowroot
(*Maranta arundinacea*) (I) 48
Betel Nut (*Piper betle*) (I) .. G-4, 76
Black Nightshade
(*Solanum nigrum*) (I) G-6, 106
Coconut Palm
(*Cocos nucifera*) (I) G-9, 209
Date Palm
(*Phoenix dactylifera*) (I) . G-10, 253
Fennel
(*Foeniculum vulgare*) (I) . G-11, 317
Fenugreek
(*Trigonella foenum-graecum*) (I) G-11, 319
Garlic (*Allium sativum*) (I) . G-12, 345
Henna
(*Lawsonia inermis*) (I) ... G-14, 440
Indian Nettle
(*Acalypha indica*) (I) 467
Japanese Mint
(*Mentha arvensis piperascens*) (I) 477
Jequirity
(*Abrus precatorius*) (C) 481
Lemongrass
(*Cymbopogon citratus*) (I) G-16, 515
Licorice
(*Glycyrrhiza glabra*) (I) . G-16, 522
Luffa (*Luffa aegyptica*) (I) . G-16, 538
Nux Vomica
(*Strychnos nux vomica*) (I) G-18, 607
Oak Gall
(*Quercus infectoria*) (I) 610
Papaya (*Carica papaya*) (I) . G-19, 627
Plantain
(*Musa paradisiaca*) (I) 656
Rose (*Rosa centifolia*) (I) 708
Saffron (*Crocus sativus*) (I) . G-21, 716
Zedoary
(*Curcuma zedoaria*) (I) .. G-26, 930

BRONCHITIS, CHRONIC
Black Nightshade
(*Solanum nigrum*) (C) G-6, 106
Indian Squill
(*Urginea indica*) (I) 469
Luffa (*Luffa aegyptica*) (C) . G-16, 538
Sumbul
(*Ferula sumbul*) (I) G-23, 824

BRONCHOSPASM, REVERSIBLE
(*See under* Bronchial asthma)

BRUISES
Black Nightshade (*Solanum nigrum*) (C) G-6, 106

BRUISES, TOPICAL RELIEF OF
(*See under* Pain, topical relief of)

BURNS, PAIN ASSOCIATED WITH
(*See under* Pain, topical relief of)

BURNS, WOUND HEALING OF
Hibiscus (*Hibiscus sabdariffa*) (C) . G-14, 442

CALCULOSIS
(*See under* Renal calculi)

CALLUSES
(*See under* Hyperkeratosis skin disorders)

CARCINOMA, BREAST
Reed Herb (*Phragmites communis*) (C) ... 700

CARCINOMA, LUNG, SMALL CELL
Astragalus (*Astragalus species*) (C) 56

CARCINOMA, STOMACH
Celandine (*Chelidonium majus*) (C) . G-8, 180

CARDIAC FAILURE
(*See under* Congestive heart failure, adjunct in)

CARDIOVASCULAR DISORDERS, UNSPECIFIED
Arjun Tree (*Terminalia arjuna*) (I) 42

CHEILITIS, ACTINIC
Areca Nut (*Areca catechu*) (I) G-4, 41

CHEST PAIN, SYMPTOMATIC RELIEF OF
Benzoin (*Styrax benzoin*) (C) 75
Chinese Thoroughwax (*Bupleurum chinese*) (C) 194
Croton Seeds (*Croton tiglium*) (C) 242
Green Tea (*Camellia sinensis*) (I) .. G-13, 414
Safflower (*Carthamus tinctorius*) (I) 715
Sandalwood (*Santalum album*) (C) 721
Siam Benzoin (*Styrax tonkinesis*) (C) 751
Sumatra Benzoin (*Styrax paralleloneurum*) (C) .. 823

CHICKENPOX
(*See under* Varicella, acute, treatment of)

CHOLERA
Cayenne (*Capsicum annuum*) (I) ... G-8, 173
Costus (*Saussurea costus*) (I,C) 233
Lotus (*Nelumbo nucifera*) (I) .. G-16, 536
Nutmeg (*Myristica fragrans*) (I) .. G-18, 606

CIRCULATORY DISORDERS
English Hawthorn (*Crataegus laevigata*) (C) G-10, 279

CIRRHOSIS, LIVER
Arjun Tree (*Terminalia arjuna*) (I) 42
Jasmine (*Jasminum officinale*) (C) . G-15, 478

COLD, COMMON, SYMPTOMATIC RELIEF OF
(*See also under* Influenza syndrome, symptomatic relief of)
Bitter Orange (*Citrus aurantium*) (C) G-5, 90
Ginger (*Zingiber officinale*) (C) .. G-12, 365
Oregano (*Origanum vulgare*) (C) .. G-19, 621
Perilla (*Perilla fructescens*) (C) 644

COLIC, SYMPTOMATIC RELIEF OF
Aloe (*Aloe barbadensis*) (I) .. G-3, 19
Aloe (*Aloe capensis*) (I) G-3, 19
Aloe (*Aloe vera*) (I) G-3, 19
Clove (*Syzygium aromaticum*) (I) G-8, 201
Dandelion (*Taraxacum officinale*) (I) G-9, 251
Northern Prickly Ash (*Zanthoxylum americanum*) (I) 605
Turmeric (*Curcuma domestica*) (I) 864
Walnut (*Juglans regia*) (I,C) G-25, 881

COLITIS
Fenugreek (*Trigonella foenum-graecum*) (I) G-11, 319

COLONOPATHY
Rice (*Oryza sativa*) (I) G-21, 705

CONGESTIVE HEART FAILURE, ADJUNCT IN
(*See also under* Edema, adjunctive therapy in)
Astragalus (*Astragalus species*) (C) 56

CONJUNCTIVITIS, UNSPECIFIED
Catechu (*Acacia catechu*) (I) ... 167
Hibiscus (*Hibiscus sabdariffa*) (C) . G-14, 442
Turmeric (*Curcuma domestica*) (I) 864

CONSTIPATION
Aloe (*Aloe barbadensis*) (I) .. G-3, 19
Aloe (*Aloe capensis*) (I) G-3, 19
Aloe (*Aloe vera*) (I) G-3, 19
Areca Nut (*Areca catechu*) (I) G-4, 41
Asa Foetida (*Ferula foetida*) (I) 51
Asparagus (*Asparagus officinalis*) (C) . G-4, 55
Cashew (*Anacardium occidentale*) (I) G-7, 164
Castor Oil Plant (*Ricinus communis*) (C) .. G-7, 166
Cotton (*Gossypium hirsutum*) (I) 234
Croton Seeds (*Croton tiglium*) (I,C) 242
Dong Quai (*Angelica sinensis*) (C) 260
Garlic (*Allium sativum*) (I) . G-12, 345
Golden Shower Tree (*Cassia fistula*) (I) G-13, 399
Guar Gum (*Cyamopsis tetragonoloba*) (I) . 428
Indian Nettle (*Acalypha indica*) (I) 467

(I) denotes use in Indian medicine. (C) denotes use in Chinese medicine.

Golden Shower Tree
(*Cassia fistula*) (I) G-13, 399
Green Tea
(*Camellia sinensis*) (I) ... G-13, 414
Henna
(*Lawsonia inermis*) (I) ... G-14, 440
Jambol (*Syzygium cumini*) (I) ... 475
Lemongrass
(*Cymbopogon citratus*) (I) G-16,515
Lotus
(*Nelumbo nucifera*) (I) ... G-16, 536
Lûffa (*Luffa aegyptica*) (I) G-16, 538
Lycium Bark
(*Lycium chinense*) (C) 540
Ma-Huang
(*Ephedra sinica*) (C) G-16, 543
Neem
(*Antelaea
azadirachta*) (I) G-18, 599
Northern Prickly Ash
(*Zanthoxylum americanum*)
(I) 605
Nutmeg
(*Myristica fragrans*) (I) .. G-18, 606
Nux Vomica
(*Strychnos nux
vomica*) (C) G-18, 607
Oak Gall
(*Quercus infectoria*) (I) 610
Oregano
(*Origanum vulgare*) (C) .. G-19, 621
Perilla
(*Perilla fructescens*) (C) 644
Picrorhiza
(*Picrorhiza kurroa*) (C) 649
Pineapple
(*Ananas comosus*) (I) 652
Quinine
(*Cinchona
pubescens*) (I,C) G-20, 686
Rauwolfia
(*Rauwolfia Serpentina*) (I) 691
Red Sandalwood
(*Pterocarpus santalinus*) (I) ... 698
Rehmannia
(*Rehmannia glutinosa*) (C) 701
Rose (*Rosa centifolia*) (I) 708
Saffron (*Crocus sativus*) (I) G-21, 716
Sandalwood
(*Santalum album*) (I) 721
Storax
(*Liquidambar
orientalis*) (I) G-23, 820
Tamarind
(*Tamarindus indica*) (I) 836
Zedoary
(*Curcuma zedoaria*) (I) ... G-26, 930

FEVER, UNSPECIFIED

Cashew
(*Anacardium
occidentale*) (I) G-7, 164

FLATULENCE, RELIEF OF

Asa Foetida
(*Ferula foetida*) (I) 51
Black Nightshade
(*Solanum nigrum*) (I) G-6, 106
Black Pepper
(*Piper nigrum*) (I) G-6, 107
Cardamom
(*Elettaria
cardamomum*) (C) G-7, 156
Chaulmoogra
(*Hydnocarpus species*) (I) 187
Clove
(*Syzygium
aromaticum*) (I) G-8, 201
Costus
(*Saussurea costus*) (I,C) 233
Dandelion
(*Taraxacum officinale*) (I) G-9,251
Golden Shower Tree
(*Cassia fistula*) (I) G-13, 399
Jatamansi
(*Nardostachys jatamansi*) (I) .. 479
Lemongrass
(*Cymbopogon
citratus*) (I) G-16, 515
Morning Glory
(*Ipomoea hederacea*) (I) 585
Northern Prickly Ash
(*Zanthoxylum americanum*)
(I) 605
Radish
(*Raphanus sativus*) (I) ... G-20, 688
Star Anise
(*Illicium verum*) (I) G-23, 787
Tomato
(*Lycopersicon
esculentum*) (I) G-24, 849
Tropical Almond
(*Terminalia chebula*) (I) 861
Turmeric
(*Curcuma domestica*) (I) 864
Wheat (*Triticum aestivum*) (I) ... 886
Wild Thyme
(*Thymus serpyllum*) (C) .. G-26, 900

FLU SYMPTOMS

(*See under* Influenza
syndrome, symptomatic
relief of)

FURUNCULOSIS

Bistort
(*Persicaria bistorta*) (C) ... G-5, 86
Black Nightshade
(*Solanum nigrum*) (C) G-6, 106
Bog Bean
(*Menyanthes trifoliata*) (C) G-6,118
Burdock
(*Arctium lappa*) (C) G-7, 136
Castor Oil Plant
(*Ricinus communis*) (C) .. G-7, 166
Chaulmoogra
(*Hydnocarpus species*) (C) 187
Croton Seeds
(*Croton tiglium*) (C) 242
Ground Ivy
(*Glechoma hederacea*) (C) 422
Hibiscus
(*Hibiscus sabdariffa*) (C) G-14, 442
Licorice
(*Glycyrrhiza glabra*) (C) G-16, 522
Myrrh
(*Commiphora molmol*) (C) G-18,595
Picrorhiza
(*Picrorhiza kurroa*) (C) 649
Plumbago
(*Plumbago zeylanica*) (C) 657
Red-Rooted Sage
(*Salvia miltiorrhiza*) (C) 698
Vervain
(*Verbena officinalis*) (C) G-25, 877
White Nettle
(*Lamium album*) (C) G-25, 893

GIST

(*See under* Tumors,
gastrointestinal stromal)

GALLBLADDER DISORDERS, UNSPECIFIED

Radish
(*Raphanus sativus*) (I) ... G-20, 688

GALLSTONES

(*See under* Biliary calculi,
chemical dissolution of)

GASTRITIS

Black Pepper (*Piper nigrum*) (C) G-6, 107
Psyllium (*Plantago ovata*) (I) ... 669
Tropical Almond (*Terminalia chebula*) (I) 861

GASTROINTESTINAL DISORDERS

Black Catnip (*Phyllanthus amarus*) (I) 94
Bog Bean (*Menyanthes trifoliata*) (C) G-6,118
Cabbage (*Brassica oleracea*) (I) ... G-7, 143
Clove (*Syzygium aromaticum*) (I) G-8, 201
Costus (*Saussurea costus*) (I,C) 233
Date Palm (*Phoenix dactylifera*) (I) . G-10, 253
Jatamansi (*Nardostachys jatamansi*) (I) .. 479
Lemongrass (*Cymbopogon citratus*) (I) G-16, 515
Oak Gall (*Quercus infectoria*) (I) 610
Pomegranate (*Punica granatum*) (I) ... G-20, 662
Poppyseed (*Papaver somniferum*) (C) G-20, 666
Schisandra (*Schisandra chinensis*) (C) 731
Southern Tsangshu (*Atractylodes lancea*) (C) 763
Tropical Almond (*Terminalia chebula*) (I,C) 861
Turmeric (*Curcuma domestica*) (C) 864

GASTROINTESTINAL STROMAL TUMORS

(*See under* Tumors, gastrointestinal stromal)

GASTROINTESTINAL TRACT, SMOOTH MUSCLE SPASM

(*See under* Spasm, smooth muscle)

GENITOURINARY TRACT, SMOOTH MUSCLE SPASM

(*See under* Spasm, smooth muscle)

GINGIVITIS

Basil (*Ocimum basilicum*) (C) ... G-4, 68
Tropical Almond (*Terminalia chebula*) (I) 861

GONORRHEA

Cotton (*Gossypium hirsutum*) (I) 234
Cowhage (*Mucuna pruriens*) (I) 236
Flax (*Linum usitatissimum*) (I) G-12, 329
Grape (*Vitis vinifera*) (I) .. G-13, 405
Knotweed (*Polygonum aviculare*) (C) G-15,498
Oak Gall (*Quercus infectoria*) (I) 610
Psyllium (*Plantago ovata*) (I) ... 669
Sandalwood (*Santalum album*) (I) 721

GOUT, MANAGEMENT OF SIGNS AND SYMPTOMS

Bog Bean (*Menyanthes trifoliata*) (C) G-6,118
Cabbage (*Brassica oleracea*) (I) ... G-7, 143
Cayenne (*Capsicum annuum*) (I) ... G-8, 173
Dandelion (*Taraxacum officinale*) (I) G-9, 251
Golden Shower Tree (*Cassia fistula*) (I) G-13, 399
Psyllium (*Plantago ovata*) (I) ... 669

HAIR LOSS

Cashew (*Anacardium occidentale*) (I) G-7, 164
Oriental Arborvitae (*Thuja orientalis*) (C) 623

HALITOSIS

Clove (*Syzygium aromaticum*) (I) G-8, 201

HALITOSIS, ADJUNCTIVE THERAPY IN

Dill (*Anethum graveolens*) (I) G-10, 256

HANSEN'S DISEASE

(*See under* Leprosy)

HEADACHE

Adrue (*Cyperus articulatus*) (C) .. G-3, 10
Bog Bean (*Menyanthes trifoliata*) (C) G-6,118
Chicory (*Cichorium intybus*) (I) ... G-8, 190
Cotton (*Gossypium hirsutum*) (I) 234
Date Palm (*Phoenix dactylifera*) (I) . G-10, 253
Grape (*Vitis vinifera*) (I) .. G-13, 405
Henna (*Lawsonia inermis*) (I) .. G-14, 440
Japanese Mint (*Mentha arvensis piperascens*) (I,C) 477
Jasmine (*Jasminum officinale*) (I) G-15, 478
Jatamansi (*Nardostachys jatamansi*) (I) .. 479
Licorice (*Glycyrrhiza glabra*) (I) . G-16, 522
Northern Prickly Ash (*Zanthoxylum americanum*) (I) 605
Nutmeg (*Myristica fragrans*) (I) . G-18, 606
Perilla (*Perilla fructescens*) (C) 644
Radish (*Raphanus sativus*) (I) ... G-20, 688
Red Sandalwood (*Pterocarpus santalinus*) (I) ... 698
Saffron (*Crocus sativus*) (I) G-21, 716

HEADACHE, MIGRAINE

Coffee (*Coffea arabica*) (I) G-9, 210
Green Tea (*Camellia sinensis*) (I,C) G-13, 414

HEADACHE, TENSION

(*See under* Pain, unspecified)

HEADACHE, VASCULAR

(*See under* Headache, migraine)

HEARING, IMPAIRMENT

Lycium Berries (*Lycium barbarum*) (C) 541
Rehmannia (*Rehmannia glutinosa*) (C) ... 701

HEART FAILURE
(*See under* Congestive heart failure, adjunct in)

HEART FAILURE, CONGESTIVE
(*See under* Congestive heart failure, adjunct in)

HEARTBURN
(*See under* Hyperacidity, gastric, symptomatic relief of)

HEAT STROKE
Sandalwood (*Santalum album*) (I) 721
Turmeric (*Curcuma domestica*) (C) 864

HELMINTHIASIS
Agrimony (*Agrimonia eupatoria*) (C) G-3, 12
Aloe (*Aloe barbadensis*) (I) .. G-3, 19
Aloe (*Aloe capensis*) (I) G-3, 19
Aloe (*Aloe vera*) (I) G-3, 19
Asa Foetida (*Ferula foetida*) (C) 51
Calamus (*Acorus calamus*) (I) G-7, 146
Croton Seeds (*Croton tiglium*) (I,C) 242
Dill (*Anethum graveolens*) (I) G-10, 256
Giant Milkweed (*Calotropis gigantea*) (I) 364
Henbane (*Hyoscyamus niger*) (I) .. G-14, 438
Indian Squill (*Urginea indica*) (I) 469
Kamala (*Mallotus philippinensis*) (I) .. 488
Knotweed (*Polygonum aviculare*) (C) G-15,498
Lemongrass (*Cymbopogon citratus*) (I) G-16,515
Lotus (*Nelumbo nucifera*) (I) .. G-16, 536
Morning Glory (*Ipomoea hederacea*) (I,C) 585
Neem (*Antelaea azadirachta*) (I) G-18,599
Northern Prickly Ash (*Zanthoxylum americanum*) (I) 605
Onion (*Allium cepa*) (C) ... G-19, 619
Papaya (*Carica papaya*) (I) G-19, 627
Plantain (*Musa paradisiaca*) (I) 656
Plumbago (*Plumbago zeylanica*) (C) 657
Pomegranate (*Punica granatum*) (C) ... G-20, 662
Tropical Almond (*Terminalia chebula*) (I) 861

HEMATEMESIS
Adrue (*Cyperus articulatus*) (C) .. G-3, 10
Henbane (*Hyoscyamus niger*) (I) ... G-14, 438
Lycium Bark (*Lycium chinense*) (C) 540
Pineapple (*Ananas comosus*) (I) 652
Red Sandalwood (*Pterocarpus santalinus*) (I) ... 698

HEMATURIA
Chocolate Vine (*Akebia quinata*) (C) 196
Cleavers (*Galium aparine*) (C) 200
Luffa (*Luffa aegyptica*) (I) G-16, 538
Oriental Arborvitae (*Thuja orientalis*) (C) 623

HEMOPTYSIS
Asparagus (*Asparagus officinalis*) (C) G-4, 55
Ginseng (*Panax ginseng*) (C) ... 384
Great Burnet (*Sanguisorba officinalis*) (C) G-13, 410
Oak Gall (*Quercus infectoria*) (I) 610
Oriental Arborvitae (*Thuja orientalis*) (C) 623
Pineapple (*Ananas comosus*) (I) 652
Turmeric (*Curcuma domestica*) (C) 864

HEMORRHAGE, NASAL
Coriander (*Coriandrum sativum*) (I) . G-9, 228
Great Burnet (*Sanguisorba officinalis*) (C) G-13, 410
Henbane (*Hyoscyamus niger*) (I) .. G-14, 438
Lycium Bark (*Lycium chinense*) (C) 540
Oriental Arborvitae (*Thuja orientalis*) (C) 623
Rehmannia (*Rehmannia glutinosa*) (C) 701
Turmeric (*Curcuma domestica*) (C) 864

HEMORRHAGE, UNSPECIFIED
Rehmannia (*Rehmannia glutinosa*) (C) 701

HEMORRHOIDS
Acacia (*Acacia arabica*) (I) 7
Black Pepper (*Piper nigrum*) (I) G-6, 107
Cabbage (*Brassica oleracea*) (I) ... G-7, 143
Carambola (*Averrhoa carambola*) (I) 154
Coriander (*Coriandrum sativum*) (I,C) G-9, 228
Garden Cress (*Lepidium sativum*) (I) .. G-12, 345
Grape (*Vitis vinifera*) (I) .. G-13, 405
Lycium Berries (*Lycium barbarum*) (I) 541
Oak Gall (*Quercus infectoria*) (I,C) 610
Oleander (*Nerium oleander*) (I) G-19, 616
Papaya (*Carica papaya*) (I) G-19, 627
Picrorhiza (*Picrorhiza kurroa*) (C) 649
Psyllium (*Plantago ovata*) (I) ... 669
Tamarind (*Tamarindus indica*) (I) 836
Tropical Almond (*Terminalia chebula*) (I) 861

HEMOSTASIS, AN AID IN
Agrimony (*Agrimonia eupatoria*) (C) G-3, 12
Basil (*Ocimum basilicum*) (C) ... G-4, 68

HEPATITIS, CHRONIC
Areca Nut (*Areca catechu*) (C) G-4, 41

HEPATITIS, UNSPECIFIED
Black Nightshade (*Solanum nigrum*) (C) G-6, 106

Jasmine
(*Jasminum officinale*) (C) . G-15, 478
Jequirity
(*Abrus precatorius*) (C) 481
Rehmannia
(*Rehmannia glutinosa*) (C) 701
Schisandra
(*Schisandra chinensis*) (C) 731

HERNIA, UNSPECIFIED
Fennel
(*Foeniculum vulgare*) (C) . G-11, 317
Fenugreek
(*Trigonella foenum-graecum*) (C) G-11, 319
Tobacco
(*Nicotiana tabacum*) (I) . . G-24, 847

HERPES ZOSTER INFECTIONS
Hibiscus
(*Hibiscus sabdariffa*) (C) . G-14, 442

HICCUP
Black Nightshade
(*Solanum nigrum*) (I) G-6, 106
Black Pepper
(*Piper nigrum*) (I) G-6, 107
Tropical Almond
(*Terminalia chebula*) (I) 861

HOARSENESS
Cayenne
(*Capsicum annuum*) (I) . . . G-8, 173

HYPERACIDITY, GASTRIC, SYMPTOMATIC RELIEF OF
Lemon (*Citrus limon*) (I) 513

HYPERCHOLESTEROLEMIA
Alisma
(*Alisma plantago-aquatica*) (C) G-3, 16

HYPERGLYCEMIA, CONTROL OF, ADJUNCT TO DIET
Alisma
(*Alisma plantago-aquatica*) (C) G-3, 16
Anemarrhena
(*Anemarrhena asphodeloides*) (C) 35
Arjun Tree
(*Terminalia arjuna*) (I) 42
Cashew
(*Anacardium occidentale*) (I) G-7, 164
Chaulmoogra
(*Hydnocarpus species*) (I) 187
Divi-Divi
(*Caesalpinia bonducella*) (I) . . 257
Fenugreek
(*Trigonella foenum-graecum*) (I) G-11, 319
Jambol (*Syzygium cumini*) (I) . . . 475
Lycium Bark
(*Lycium chinense*) (C) 540
Lycium Berries
(*Lycium barbarum*) (C) 541
Nux Vomica
(*Strychnos nux vomica*) (I) G-18, 607
Oak Gall
(*Quercus infectoria*) (I) 610
Red Sandalwood
(*Pterocarpus santalinus*) (I) . . . 698
Reed Herb
(*Phragmites communis*) (C) . . . 700
Rehmannia
(*Rehmannia glutinosa*) (C) 701
Rice (*Oryza sativa*) (C) G-21, 705
Salep (*Orchis species*) (I) 719

HYPERHIDROSIS
Arjun Tree
(*Terminalia arjuna*) (I) 42
Asiatic Dogwood
(*Cornus officinalis*) (C) 54
Lycium Bark
(*Lycium chinense*) (C) 540
Oak Gall
(*Quercus infectoria*) (I,C) 610
Rehmannia
(*Rehmannia glutinosa*) (C) 701
Rice (*Oryza sativa*) (C) G-21, 705
Rose (*Rosa centifolia*) (I) 708
Schisandra
(*Schisandra chinensis*) (C) 731
Soybean (*Glycine soja*) (C) . G-22, 765

HYPERKERATOSIS SKIN DISORDERS
Cashew
(*Anacardium occidentale*) (I) G-7, 164

HYPERTENSION
Alisma
(*Alisma plantago-aquatica*) (C) G-3, 16
Arjun Tree
(*Terminalia arjuna*) (I) 42
Dong Quai
(*Angelica sinensis*) (C) 260
Lycium Bark
(*Lycium chinense*) (C) 540
Rauwolfia
(*Rauwolfia Serpentina*) (I) 691
Sumbul
(*Ferula sumbul*) (I) G-23, 824

HYPERTENSION, ESSENTIAL
(*See under* Hypertension)

HYPERTENSIVE CRISES
(*See under* Hypertension)

HYPERTONIA
Ginkgo
(*Ginkgo biloba*) (C) G-12, 371

HYPNOTIC
(*See under* Sleep, induction of)

HYPOSALIVATION
Lemon-Wood
(*Schisandra sphenanthera*) (C) 519

IMMUNODEFICIENCY, UNSPECIFIED
(*See under* Infection, tendency to)

IMPETIGO CONTAGIOSA
Burning Bush
(*Dictamnus albus*) (C) . . . G-7, 139
Oak Gall
(*Quercus infectoria*) (I) 610

IMPOTENCE, MALE
(*See under* Erectile dysfunction)

INDIGESTION
(*See under* Digestive disorders, symptomatic relief of)

INFECTION, TENDENCY TO
Rehmannia
(*Rehmannia glutinosa*) (C) 701

INFECTIONS, EAR, NOSE AND THROAT
Kamala
(*Mallotus philippinensis*) (I) . . 488

INFECTIONS, FUNGAL, UNSPECIFIED
Aloe (*Aloe barbadensis*) (C) . G-3, 19
Aloe (*Aloe capensis*) (C) G-3, 19
Aloe (*Aloe vera*) (C) G-3, 19
Calamus
(*Acorus calamus*) (C) G-7, 146
Onion (*Allium cepa*) (C) . . G-19, 619

(I) denotes use in Indian medicine. (C) denotes use in Chinese medicine.

ASIAN INDICATIONS INDEX

(I) denotes use in Indian medicine. (C) denotes use in Chinese medicine.

(I) denotes use in Indian medicine. (C) denotes use in Chinese medicine.

Bitter Orange
(*Citrus aurantium*) (C) G-5, 90
Sandalwood
(*Santalum album*) (C) 721

PAIN, JOINT
Asiatic Dogwood
(*Cornus officinalis*) (C) 54
Birthwort
(*Aristolochia clematitis*) (C) G-5,84
Chinese Cinnamon
(*Cinnamomum aromaticum*)
(C) 191
Divi-Divi
(*Caesalpinia bonducella*) (I) .. 257
Duckweed
(*Lemna minor*) (C) G-10, 263
European Mistletoe
(*Viscum album*) (C) G-11, 302
Garlic (*Allium sativum*) (I) G-12, 345
Henbane
(*Hyoscyamus niger*) (C) .. G-14, 438
Japanese Mint
(*Mentha arvensis*
piperascens) (I) 477
Plumbago
(*Plumbago zeylanica*) (C) 657
Red-Rooted Sage
(*Salvia miltiorrhiza*) (C) 698
Scarlet Pimpernel
(*Anagallis arvensis*) (C) .. G-22, 729
Soybean (*Glycine soja*) (C) G-22, 765

PAIN, LUMBAR
Asiatic Dogwood
(*Cornus officinalis*) (C) 54
European Mistletoe
(*Viscum album*) (C) G-11, 302
Lycium Berries
(*Lycium barbarum*) (C) 541
Nux Vomica
(*Strychnos nux*
vomica) (I) G-18, 607
Walnut (*Juglans regia*) (C) G-25, 881
White Nettle
(*Lamium album*) (C) G-25, 893

PAIN, MENSTRUAL
False Schisandra
(*Kadsura japonica*) (C) 316
Red-Rooted Sage
(*Salvia miltiorrhiza*) (C) 698

PAIN, MUSCULAR, TEMPORARY RELIEF OF
Camphor Tree
(*Cinnamomum*
camphora) (I) G-7, 150

European Mistletoe
(*Viscum album*) (C) G-11, 302

PAIN, NEUROGENIC
Dong Quai
(*Angelica sinensis*) (C) 260
Jimson Weed
(*Datura stramonium*) (C) G-15, 482
Peanut
(*Arachis hypogaea*) (I) 636
Quinine
(*Cinchona pubescens*) (I) G-20, 686
Radish
(*Raphanus sativus*) (I) .. G-20, 688

PAIN, RENAL
Siberian Ginseng
(*Eleutherococcussenticosus*)
(C) 751

PAIN, STOMACH
Benzoin (*Styrax benzoin*) (C) 75
Birthwort
(*Aristolochia clematitis*) (C) G-5,84
Cardamom
(*Elettaria*
cardamomum) (C) G-7, 156
Croton Seeds
(*Croton tiglium*) (C) 242
False Schisandra
(*Kadsura japonica*) (C) 316
Henbane
(*Hyoscyamus niger*) (C) .. G-14, 438
Jambol (*Syzygium cumini*) (I) ... 475
Jasmine
(*Jasminum officinale*) (I) G-15, 478
Siam Benzoin
(*Styrax tonkinesis*) (C) 751
Sumatra Benzoin
(*Styrax paralleloneurum*) (C) .. 823

PAIN, TOOTH
Betel Nut (*Piper betle*) (I) .. G-4, 76
Calamus
(*Acorus calamus*) (I) G-7, 146
Catechu (*Acacia catechu*) (I) ... 167
Cinnamon
(*Cinnamomum verum*) (I) . G-8, 197
Clove
(*Syzygium*
aromaticum) (I) G-8, 201
Henbane
(*Hyoscyamus niger*) (I) .. G-14, 438

Japanese Mint
(*Mentha arvensis*
piperascens) (I,C) 477
Jasmine
(*Jasminum officinale*) (I) G-15, 478
Lycium Berries
(*Lycium barbarum*) (I) 541
Northern Prickly Ash
(*Zanthoxylum americanum*)
(I) 605
Pellitory
(*Anacyclus pyrethrum*) (I) 638
Red Sandalwood
(*Pterocarpus santalinus*) (I) ... 698
Tobacco
(*Nicotiana tabacum*) (I) .. G-24, 847
Wild Thyme
(*Thymus serpyllum*) (C) .. G-26, 900

PAIN, TOPICAL RELIEF OF
Indian Nettle
(*Acalypha indica*) (I) 467

PAIN, UNSPECIFIED
Henbane
(*Hyoscyamus niger*) (I) .. G-14, 438
Nux Vomica
(*Strychnos nux*
vomica) (C) G-18, 607
Onion (*Allium cepa*) (I) G-19, 619
Southern Tsangshu
(*Atractylodes lancea*) (C) 763
Wild Thyme
(*Thymus serpyllum*) (C) .. G-26, 900

PARALYSIS, UNSPECIFIED
Luffa (*Luffa aegyptica*) (C) G-16, 538
Northern Prickly Ash
(*Zanthoxylum americanum*)
(I) 605
Nux Vomica
(*Strychnos nux*
vomica) (I) G-18, 607
Salep (*Orchis species*) (I) 719

PEDICULOSIS, HUMAN
Fish Berry
(*Anamirta cocculus*) (I) 328

PERTUSSIS
Asa Foetida
(*Ferula foetida*) (I) 51

PHARYNGITIS, SYMPTOMATIC RELIEF OF
Balloon-Flower
(*Platycodon grandiflorum*) (C) . 62

(I) denotes use in Indian medicine. (C) denotes use in Chinese medicine.

(I) denotes use in Indian medicine. (C) denotes use in Chinese medicine.

(I) denotes use in Indian medicine. (C) denotes use in Chinese medicine.

WHOOPING COUGH

(*See under* Pertussis)

WOUND CARE, ADJUNCTIVE THERAPY IN

Black Catnip
(*Phyllanthus amarus*) (I) 94
Costus
(*Saussurea costus*) (I,C) 233
Henna
(*Lawsonia inermis*) (I) ... G-14, 440
Licorice
(*Glycyrrhiza glabra*) (I) .. G-16, 522
Myrrh
(*Commiphora molmol*) (I,C) G-18, 595
Oak Gall
(*Quercus infectoria*) (C) 610
Rauwolfia
(*Rauwolfia Serpentina*) (I) 691
Rose (*Rosa centifolia*) (I) 708
Safflower
(*Carthamus tinctorius*) (C) 715
Smartweed
(*Persicaria hydropiper*) (C) ... 757
Storax
(*Liquidambar orientalis*) (I) G-23, 820
Tropical Almond
(*Terminalia chebula*) (I) 861
Turmeric
(*Curcuma domestica*) (I) 864
White Nettle
(*Lamium album*) (C) G-25, 893
Zedoary
(*Curcuma zedoaria*) (I) .. G-26, 930

Side Effects Index

Presented here is an alphabetical list of every side effect cited in the herbal monographs. Under each heading, herbs associated with the reaction are listed alphabetically by accepted common name, with the scientific name shown in parentheses. For ease of comparison with prescription and over-the-counter medications, the index employs the same nomenclature found in the Side Effects Index of the PDR Companion Guide™. *If an entry lists two page numbers, the first refers to a photograph of the plant in the Herb Identification Guide, the second to the herbal monograph.*

Drug/Herb Interactions Guide

This section catalogs potentially adverse drug/herb combinations by both the generic name of the drug or drug category and the accepted common name of the herb. Under each bold-face drug entry you'll find a list of the herbs with which the agent may interact. Likewise, under a bold-face herb entry you'll find a list of potentially interactive drugs. A description of the interaction's effect follows each item in the list. Further information on each drug can be found in Physicians' Desk Reference®. *Information on each herb appears in the Herbal Monographs section of this book.*

ACARBOSE
Bitter Melon
(Concurrent use may result in an increased risk of hypoglycemia)
Kudzu
(P. lobata may lower blood glucose levels)

ACEBUTOLOL HYDROCHLORIDE
Kudzu
(P. lobata may interfere with antiarrhythmic agents)

ACHILLEA MILLEFOLIUM
(*See under* Yarrow)

ACITRETIN
St. John's Wort
(May result in unplanned pregnancy and birth defects)

ACRIVASTINE
Mangosteen
(G. mangostana may possibly be unsafe when used by patients taking antihistamines)

ADANSONIA DIGITATA
(*See under* Baobab)

ADENOSINE
Kudzu
(P. lobata may interfere with antiarrhythmic agents)

ADONIS
Calcium
(Increases action of Adonis)
Digoxin
(Increases action of Adonis)
Glucocorticoids
(Increases action of Adonis)
Laxatives
(Increases action of Adonis)
Quinidine
(Increases action of Adonis)
Saluretics
(Increases action of Adonis)

ADONIS VERNALIS
(*See under* Adonis)

AESCULUS HIPPOCASTANUM
(*See under* Horse Chestnut)

ALBENDAZOLE
Ginseng
(May alter the therapeutic efficacy of albendazole)

ALCOHOL
German Chamomile
(Additive effects of alcohol)
Kava Kava
(May increase sedative effect and risk of hepatotoxicity)
Marijuana
(Increased intoxication)
Rauwolfia
(Increases impairment of motor skills)
Valerian
(Additive depressive effects with Valerian)
White Willow
(Enhances toxicity of salicylates)

ALDESLEUKIN
Astragalus
(Increase in tumor killing activity)

ALFALFA
Anticoagulant drugs, unspecified
(May reduce effectiveness of anticoagulant and increase risk of bleeding)
Azathioprine
(May precipitate organ transplant rejection)
Cyclosporine
(May precipitate organ transplant rejection)
Prednisone
(May reduce effectiveness of prednisone)

ALKALINE DRUGS
Green Tea
(Decreased absorption of alkaline drugs due to tannin component in tea)

Oak
(Absorption of alkaline drugs may be reduced or inhibited)

ALKALOIDS

Oak
(Absorption of alkaloids may be reduced or inhibited)

ALLIUM SATIVUM

(*See under* Garlic)

ALOE

Antiarrhythmics
(Aloe-induced hypokalemia may affect cardiac rhythm)
Cardiac Glycosides
(Increases effect of cardiac glycosides)
Corticosteroids
(Increased potassium loss)
Licorice
(Increased potassium loss)
Thiazide Diuretics
(Increased potassium loss)
Antiarrhythmics
(Aloe-induced hypokalemia may affect cardiac rhythm)
Cardiac Glycosides
(Increases effect of cardiac glycosides)
Corticosteroids
(Increased potassium loss)
Licorice
(Increased potassium loss)
Thiazide Diuretics
(Increased potassium loss)
Antiarrhythmics
(Aloe-induced hypokalemia may affect cardiac rhythm)
Cardiac Glycosides
(Increases effect of cardiac glycosides)
Corticosteroids
(Increased potassium loss)
Licorice
(Increased potassium loss)
Thiazide Diuretics
(Increased potassium loss)

ALOE BARBADENSIS

(*See under* Aloe)

ALOE CAPENSIS

(*See under* Aloe)

ALOE VERA

(*See under* Aloe)

ALPHA ADRENERGIC BLOCKERS

Saw Palmetto
(Saw Palmetto has an additive alpha adrenergic blocking effect when given in combination with alpha blockers)

ALPINE CRANBERRY

Medication and Food that Increase Uric Acid Levels
(Decreases effect of Alpine Cranberry)

AMANTADINE HYDROCHLORIDE

Belladonna
(Increases anticholinergic effect of herb)
Chaste Tree
(Enhances dopaminergic adverse effects)
Henbane
(Increased anticholinergic action)
Scopolia
(Increased effect when given simultaneously with herb)

AMINOLEVULINIC ACID HYDROCHLORIDE

St. John's Wort
(May result in increased risk of phototoxic reaction)

AMIODARONE HYDROCHLORIDE

Kudzu
(P. lobata may interfere with antiarrhythmic agents)
St. John's Wort
(Extends risk for reducing amiodarone levels)

AMLODIPINE BESYLATE

Kudzu
(P. lobata may interfere with hypotensive agents)

AMPHETAMINE RESINS

Rhodiola
(May have additive effects with other stimulants)

ANANAS COMOSUS

(*See under* Pineapple)

ANDROGENS

Saw Palmetto
(Saw Palmetto antagonizes the effect of androgens)

ANGELICA SINENSIS

(*See under* Dong Quai)

ANISINDIONE

Mangosteen
(G. mangostana may possibly be unsafe when used by patients taking anticoagulants)

ANTACIDS, UNSPECIFIED

Ma-Huang
(Risk of ephedrine toxicity)

ANTIARRHYTHMICS

Aloe
(Aloe-induced hypokalemia may affect cardiac rhythm)
Buckthorn
(Increased effect due to potassium loss with chronic use of herb)
Cascara Sagrada
(Potentiates arrhythmias with prolonged use of Cascara)
English Hawthorn
(May increase activity)
Licorice
(Licorice-induced hypokalemia increases risk of arrhythmias)
Senna
(Senna-induced hypokalemia may increase risk of arrythmia)

ANTICHOLINERGICS

Jimson Weed
(Co-administration of Jimson Weed with other anticholinergic drugs may increase the frequency and/or severity of anticholinergic side effects such as dry mouth, constipation, drowsiness, and others)

ANTICOAGULANT DRUGS, UNSPECIFIED

Alfalfa
(May reduce effectiveness of anticoagulant and increase risk of bleeding)
Arnica
(Coumarin component in Arnica may increase anticoagulant effect)
Astragalus
(Astragalus may potentiate anticoagulant effects)
Bilberry
(Enhanced anti-aggretory mechanism)

Borage
(Increased risk of bleeding)
Dong Quai
(Increased risk of bleeding)
Garlic
(Increased risk of bleeding)
German Chamomile
(Increased risk of bleeding)
Ginger
(Increased risk of bleeding)
Ginkgo
(Increased risk of bleeding)
Ginseng
(May decrease INR)
Horse Chestnut
(Horse Chestnut has a coumarin componant and may interact with warfarin, salicylates and other drugs with anticoagulant properties)
Kava Kava
(May increase risk of bleeding)
Licorice
(May increase risk of bleeding)
Pineapple
(Increased nsL and bleeding)
Red Clover
(Increased risk of bleeding)
Siberian Ginseng
(May enchance effects)
St. John's Wort
(May result in reduced effectiveness of anticoagulants)
Valerian
(Increased risk of bleeding)

ANTICONVULSANTS

Evening Primrose
(Evening Primrose oil may lower seizure threshold and decrease effectiveness of anticonvulsant medications)
Ginkgo
(May precipitate seizures)

ANTIDIABETIC DRUGS, UNSPECIFIED

Licorice
(May reduce hypoglycemic effects)
Siberian Ginseng
(May potentiate effects)
St. John's Wort
(May result in hypoglycemia)

ANTIHISTAMINES

Henbane
(Increased anticholinergic action)

ANTIHYPERTENSIVE AGENTS, UNSPECIFIED

Licorice
(May reduce effectiveness)
Ma-Huang
(Decreased effectiveness)
Yohimbe Bark
(May need to adjust antihypertensive medications due to hypertensive effect of Yohimbe)

ANTIPLATELET DRUGS

Arnica
(Increased risk of bleeding)
Bilberry
(Enhanced anti-aggretory mechanism)
Borage
(Increased risk of bleeding)
English Hawthorn
(May increase risk of bleeding)
Garlic
(Increased risk of bleeding)
Ginger
(Increased risk of bleeding)
Ginkgo
(Increased risk of bleeding)
Kava Kava
(May increase risk of bleeding)
Licorice
(May increase risk of bleeding)
Siberian Ginseng
(May enchance effects)
Valerian
(Increased risk of bleeding)
White Willow
(Additive effect with salicylates)

ANTITHROMBOLYTIC DRUGS

Dong Quai
(Increased risk of bleeding)
Ginkgo
(Increases effect of antithrombolytic drugs)

ANTITHROMBOTIC AGENTS

Siberian Ginseng
(May enchance effects)

ARCTOSTAPHYLOS UVA-URSI

(*See under* Uva-Ursi)

ARDEPARIN SODIUM

Mangosteen
(G. mangostana may possibly be unsafe when used by patients taking anticoagulants)

ARNICA

Anticoagulant drugs, unspecified
(Coumarin component in Arnica may increase anticoagulant effect)
Antiplatelet Drugs
(Increased risk of bleeding)
Low Molecular Weight Heparins
(Increased risk of bleeding)
Thrombolytics
(Increased risk of bleeding)
Warfarin Sodium
(Additive anticoagulant effect)

ARNICA MONTANA

(*See under* Arnica)

ARTEMISIA ABSINTHIUM

(*See under* Wormwood)

ASPALATHUS LINEARIS

(*See under* Rooibos)

ASPIRIN

Cayenne
(Decreased bioavailability of aspirin)
Feverfew
(Increased antithrombotic effect)

ASTEMIZOLE

Mangosteen
(G. mangostana may possibly be unsafe when used by patients taking antihistamines)

ASTRAGALUS

Aldesleukin
(Increase in tumor killing activity)
Anticoagulant drugs, unspecified
(Astragalus may potentiate anticoagulant effects)
Cyclophosphamide
(Increase in tumor killing activity)
Immunosuppressants
(Decreased effectiveness of immunosuppressive effect due to immunostimulant effect of Astragalus)

ASTRAGALUS SPECIES

(*See under* Astragalus)

ATENOLOL

Kudzu
(P. lobata may interfere with hypotensive agents)

ATORVASTATIN CALCIUM

Bitter Melon
(Bitter melon may potentiate cholesterol-lowering drugs)

ATROPA BELLADONNA

(*See under* Belladonna)

AZATADINE MALEATE

Mangosteen
(G. mangostana may possibly be unsafe when used by patients taking antihistamines)

AZATHIOPRINE

Alfalfa
(May precipitate organ transplant rejection)

BAOBAB

(None cited in PDR database)

BARBITURATES

Hops
(May increase sedative action)
Kava Kava
(May increase CNS depression)
Marijuana
(Excessive CNS depression)
Rauwolfia
(Synergistic effect)
St. John's Wort
(May decrease the CNS depressant effect of barbiturates)
Valerian
(Increased CNS effects possible, especially sedation)
White Willow
(Enhances toxicity of salicylates)

BELLADONNA

Amantadine Hydrochloride
(Increases anticholinergic effect of herb)
Quinidine
(Increases anticholinergic effect of herb)
Tricyclic Antidepressants
(Increases anticholinergic effect of herb)

BENAZEPRIL HYDROCHLORIDE

Kudzu
(P. lobata may interfere with hypotensive agents)

BENDROFLUMETHIAZIDE

Kudzu
(P. lobata may interfere with hypotensive agents)

BENZODIAZEPINES

German Chamomile
(Additive effects of benzodiazepines)
Kava Kava
(May increase CNS depression)
St. John's Wort
(May result in reduced benzodiazepines effectiveness)
Valerian
(CNS effects may be increased)

BETA BLOCKERS

English Hawthorn
(May cause hypertension)
St. John's Wort
(May induce the metabolism of beta-blockers resulting in reduced drug concentrations and decreased effectiveness of beta-blockers)

BETAXOLOL HYDROCHLORIDE

Kudzu
(P. lobata may interfere with hypotensive agents)

BILBERRY

Anticoagulant drugs, unspecified
(Enhanced anti-aggretory mechanism)
Antiplatelet Drugs
(Enhanced anti-aggretory mechanism)
Salicylates
(Increases prothrombin time; caution should be observed when used concurrently)
Warfarin Sodium
(Increases prothrombin time; caution should be observed when used concurrently)

BISOPROLOL FUMARATE

Kudzu
(P. lobata may interfere with hypotensive agents)

BITTER MELON

Acarbose
(Concurrent use may result in an increased risk of hypoglycemia)
Atorvastatin Calcium
(Bitter melon may potentiate cholesterol-lowering drugs)
Cerivastatin Sodium
(Bitter melon may potentiate cholesterol-lowering drugs)
Chlorpropamide
(Concurrent use may result in an increased risk of hypoglycemia)
Cholestyramine
(Bitter melon may potentiate cholesterol-lowering drugs)
Clofibrate
(Bitter melon may potentiate cholesterol-lowering drugs)
Colestipol Hydrochloride
(Bitter melon may potentiate cholesterol-lowering drugs)
Fenofibrate
(Bitter melon may potentiate cholesterol-lowering drugs)
Fluvastatin Sodium
(Bitter melon may potentiate cholesterol-lowering drugs)
Gemfibrozil
(Bitter melon may potentiate cholesterol-lowering drugs)
Glimepiride
(Concurrent use may result in an increased risk of hypoglycemia)
Glipizide
(Concurrent use may result in an increased risk of hypoglycemia)
Glyburide
(Concurrent use may result in an increased risk of hypoglycemia)
Insulin
(Concurrent use may result in an increased risk of hypoglycemia)
Insulin Aspart
(Concurrent use may result in an increased risk of hypoglycemia)
Insulin Aspart Protamine, Human
(Concurrent use may result in an increased risk of hypoglycemia)
Insulin Aspart, Human
(Concurrent use may result in an increased risk of hypoglycemia)

Insulin Aspart, Human Regular
(Concurrent use may result in an increased risk of hypoglycemia)
Insulin Detemir (rDNA Origin)
(Concurrent use may result in an increased risk of hypoglycemia)
Insulin Glulisine
(Concurrent use may result in an increased risk of hypoglycemia)
Insulin Lispro Protamine, Human
(Concurrent use may result in an increased risk of hypoglycemia)
Insulin Lispro, Human
(Concurrent use may result in an increased risk of hypoglycemia)
Insulin glargine
(Concurrent use may result in an increased risk of hypoglycemia)
Insulin, Human (rDNA origin)
(Concurrent use may result in an increased risk of hypoglycemia)
Insulin, Human NPH
(Concurrent use may result in an increased risk of hypoglycemia)
Insulin, Human Regular
(Concurrent use may result in an increased risk of hypoglycemia)
Insulin, Human Regular and Human NPH Mixture
(Concurrent use may result in an increased risk of hypoglycemia)
Insulin, Human, Zinc Suspension
(Concurrent use may result in an increased risk of hypoglycemia)
Insulin, NPH
(Concurrent use may result in an increased risk of hypoglycemia)
Insulin, Regular
(Concurrent use may result in an increased risk of hypoglycemia)
Insulin, Regular and NPH mixture
(Concurrent use may result in an increased risk of hypoglycemia)
Insulin, Zinc Crystals
(Concurrent use may result in an increased risk of hypoglycemia)
Insulin, Zinc Suspension
(Concurrent use may result in an increased risk of hypoglycemia)
Lovastatin
(Bitter melon may potentiate cholesterol-lowering drugs)
Metformin Hydrochloride
(Concurrent use may result in an increased risk of hypoglycemia)
Miglitol
(Concurrent use may result in an increased risk of hypoglycemia)
Nateglinide
(Concurrent use may result in an increased risk of hypoglycemia)
Pioglitazone Hydrochloride
(Concurrent use may result in an increased risk of hypoglycemia)
Pravastatin Sodium
(Bitter melon may potentiate cholesterol-lowering drugs)
Probucol
(Bitter melon may potentiate cholesterol-lowering drugs)
Repaglinide
(Concurrent use may result in an increased risk of hypoglycemia)
Rosiglitazone Maleate
(Concurrent use may result in an increased risk of hypoglycemia)
Simvastatin
(Bitter melon may potentiate cholesterol-lowering drugs)
Sitagliptin Phosphate
(Concurrent use may result in an increased risk of hypoglycemia)
Tolazamide
(Concurrent use may result in an increased risk of hypoglycemia)
Tolbutamide
(Concurrent use may result in an increased risk of hypoglycemia)
Troglitazone
(Concurrent use may result in an increased risk of hypoglycemia)

BLADDERWRACK

Hypoglycemic Drugs
(Herb may have an additive hypoglycemic effect when taken with other hypoglycemic drugs)

BORAGE

Anticoagulant drugs, unspecified
(Increased risk of bleeding)
Antiplatelet Drugs
(Increased risk of bleeding)
Iron
(Increased risk of bleeding)

BORAGO OFFICINALIS

(*See under* Borage)

BRETYLIUM TOSYLATE

Kudzu
(P. lobata may interfere with antiarrhythmic agents)

BREWER'S YEAST

MAO Inhibitors
(Increase in blood pressure)

BROMODIPHENHYDRAMINE HYDROCHLORIDE

Mangosteen
(G. mangostana may possibly be unsafe when used by patients taking antihistamines)

BROMPHENIRAMINE MALEATE

Mangosteen
(G. mangostana may possibly be unsafe when used by patients taking antihistamines)

BUCKTHORN

Antiarrhythmics
(Increased effect due to potassium loss with chronic use of herb)
Cardiac Glycosides
(Increased effect due to potassium loss with chronic use of herb)
Corticosteroids
(Increases hypokalemic effects)
Digoxin
(Herb may cause hypokalemia, which may increase digoxin toxicity)
Licorice Root
(Increases hypokalemic effects)
Thiazide Diuretics
(Increases hypokalemic effects)

BUGLEWEED

Diagnostic Procedures Using Radioactive Isotopes
(Herb interferes with these isotopes)
Thyroid Preparations
(Effect not specified)

BUSPIRONE HYDROCHLORIDE

St. John's Wort
(May result in an increased risk of serotonin syndrome (hypertension, hyperthermia, myoclonus, mental status changes))

BUTTERNUT

Iron
(Adverse sequelae on blood components)

CAFFEINE

St. John's Wort
(May result in increased caffeine metabolism)

CALCIUM

Adonis
(Increases action of Adonis)

Lily-of-the-Valley
(Increases the effect of Lily-of-the-Valley)

Squill
(Increases effectiveness and side effects of herb)

CALCIUM CHANNEL BLOCKERS, UNSPECIFIED

St. John's Wort
(May result in decreased effectiveness of calcium channel blockers)

CALCIUM SALTS

Kombé Seed
(Increases effects and side effects of herb)

Oleander
(Increased efficacy and side effects when given simultaneously with herb)

Strophanthus
(Simultaneous administration with herb enhance both effects and side effects)

CAMELLIA SINENSIS

(*See under* Green Tea)

CANDESARTAN CILEXETIL

Kudzu
(P. lobata may interfere with hypotensive agents)

CANNABIS SATIVA

(*See under* Marijuana)

CAPSICUM ANNUUM

(*See under* Cayenne)

CAPTOPRIL

Kudzu
(P. lobata may interfere with hypotensive agents)

CARBAMAZEPINE

Psyllium
(Reduced bioavailability)

St. John's Wort
(May result in altered carbamazepine blood concentrations)

Yohimbe Bark
(Precipitates manic episodes in bipolar disorder)

CARBIDOPA

5-HTP
(Concurrent use may result in an increased risk of developing scleroderma-like illness in susceptible individuals; monitor for signs of skin changes, which may manifest as edema, tightness, and/or a burning sensation)

CARBONIC ANHYDRASE INHIBITORS

Ma-Huang
(Increased serum concentrations)

White Willow
(Potentiates action of salicylates)

CARDIAC GLYCOSIDES

Aloe
(Increases effect of cardiac glycosides)

Buckthorn
(Increased effect due to potassium loss with chronic use of herb)

Cascara Sagrada
(Increased effect due to potassium loss with chronic use of herb)

Chinese Rhubarb
(Increased effect due to potassium loss with chronic use of herb)

Frangula
(Increased effect due to potassium loss with chronic use of herb)

Guarana
(Increased effect due to potassium loss with chronic use of herb)

Ma-Huang
(Disturbance of heart rhythm)

CARDIOACTIVE STEROIDS

Castor Oil Plant
(Increased effect due to potassium loss with chronic use of herb)

CARICA PAPAYA

(*See under* Papaya)

CARTEOLOL HYDROCHLORIDE

Kudzu
(P. lobata may interfere with hypotensive agents)

CASCARA SAGRADA

Antiarrhythmics
(Potentiates arrhythmias with prolonged use of Cascara)

Cardiac Glycosides
(Increased effect due to potassium loss with chronic use of herb)

Corticosteroids
(Increases hypokalemic effect)

Digoxin
(Herb may cause hypokalemia, which may increase digoxin toxicity)

Indomethacin
(Decreases therapeutic effect of Cascara)

Thiazide Diuretics
(Increases hypokalemic effect)

CASSIA SENNA

(*See under* Senna)

CASTOR OIL PLANT

Cardioactive Steroids
(Increased effect due to potassium loss with chronic use of herb)

CAYENNE

Aspirin
(Decreased bioavailability of aspirin)

CENTRAL NERVOUS SYSTEM STIMULANTS

Ma-Huang
(Ma-Huang has an additive effect on the CNS when combined with CNS stimulants)

CERIVASTATIN SODIUM

Bitter Melon
(Bitter melon may potentiate cholesterol-lowering drugs)

CETIRIZINE HYDROCHLORIDE

Mangosteen
(G. mangostana may possibly be unsafe when used by patients taking antihistamines)

CHASTE TREE

Amantadine Hydrochloride
(Enhances dopaminergic adverse effects)

Dopamine Antagonists
(Enhances dopaminergic adverse effects)
Dopamine D2 Antagonists
(Decreased effectiveness of drug)
Levodopa
(Enhances dopaminergic adverse effects)
Pergolide Mesylate
(Enhances dopaminergic adverse effects)
Phenothiazines
(Enhances dopaminergic adverse effects)
Pramipexole Dihydrochloride
(Enhances dopaminergic adverse effects)
Ropinirole Hydrochloride
(Enhances dopaminergic adverse effects)

CHINESE RHUBARB
Cardiac Glycosides
(Increased effect due to potassium loss with chronic use of herb)
Digoxin
(Herb may cause hypokalemia, which may increase digoxin toxicity)

CHLOROTHIAZIDE
Kudzu
(P. lobata may interfere with hypotensive agents)

CHLOROTHIAZIDE SODIUM
Kudzu
(P. lobata may interfere with hypotensive agents)

CHLOROTRIANISENE
Kudzu
(P. lobata may inhibit the effects of estrogen therapy)
Pygeum
(Prunus may interact with estrogen or other hormones)

CHLORPHENIRAMINE MALEATE
Mangosteen
(G. mangostana may possibly be unsafe when used by patients taking antihistamines)

CHLORPHENIRAMINE POLISTIREX
Mangosteen
(G. mangostana may possibly be unsafe when used by patients taking antihistamines)

CHLORPHENIRAMINE TANNATE
Mangosteen
(G. mangostana may possibly be unsafe when used by patients taking antihistamines)

CHLORPROPAMIDE
Bitter Melon
(Concurrent use may result in an increased risk of hypoglycemia)
Kudzu
(P. lobata may lower blood glucose levels)

CHLORTHALIDONE
Kudzu
(P. lobata may interfere with hypotensive agents)

CHLORZOXAZONE
Garlic
(Increased metabolism of drug)
St. John's Wort
(May result in reduced chlorzoxazone effectiveness)

CHOLESTYRAMINE
Bitter Melon
(Bitter melon may potentiate cholesterol-lowering drugs)

CIMETIDINE
Cranberry
(Concurrent use may result in reduced effectiveness of the H2 blocker)

CIMETIDINE HYDROCHLORIDE
Cranberry
(Concurrent use may result in reduced effectiveness of the H2 blocker)

CINCHONA PUBESCENS
(*See under* Quinine)

CISAPRIDE
English Hawthorn
(May cause hyperkalemia)

CITALOPRAM HYDROBROMIDE
5-HTP
(Concurrent use may result in an increased risk of serotonin syndrome (hypertension, hyperthermia, myoclonus, mental status change); combining 5-HTP with SSRIs may increase the risk of serotonergic side effects)
Mangosteen
(G. mangostana may possibly be unsafe when used by patients taking selective serotonin reuptake inhibitors)

CLEMASTINE FUMARATE
Mangosteen
(G. mangostana may possibly be unsafe when used by patients taking antihistamines)

CLOFIBRATE
Bitter Melon
(Bitter melon may potentiate cholesterol-lowering drugs)

CLOMIPRAMINE HYDROCHLORIDE
Yohimbe Bark
(Increased risk of hypertension)

CLONIDINE
Kudzu
(P. lobata may interfere with hypotensive agents)
Ma-Huang
(Increased pressor response to ephedrine)
Yohimbe Bark
(Reduced effectiveness of clonidine)

CLONIDINE HYDROCHLORIDE
Kudzu
(P: lobata may interfere with hypotensive agents)

CLOZAPINE
St. John's Wort
(May decrease effectiveness of clozapine secondary to induction of drug-metabolizing enzymes in the liver)

CNS-ACTIVE DRUGS, UNSPECIFIED
Kava Kava
(May intensify effect)

COCAINE HYDROCHLORIDE
Marijuana
(Increased effects of cocaine)

COFFEA ARABICA
(*See under* Coffee)

COFFEE
Drugs, unspecified
(Hinders resorption of other drugs)

COLESTIPOL HYDROCHLORIDE

Bitter Melon
(Bitter melon may potentiate cholesterol-lowering drugs)

COLEUS FORSKOHLII

Garlic
(Platelet aggregation potentiated)

CONVALLARIA MAJALIS

(*See under* Lily-of-the-Valley)

CORTICOSTEROIDS

Aloe
(Increased potassium loss)
Buckthorn
(Increases hypokalemic effects)
Cascara Sagrada
(Increases hypokalemic effect)
Echinacea
(Echinacea may potentially interfere with the anti-cancer chemotherapeutic effect of corticosteroids)
Licorice
(Potentiates effects of corticosteroids)
Ma-Huang
(Increased metabolism of corticosteroids)

CRANBERRY

Cimetidine
(Concurrent use may result in reduced effectiveness of the H2 blocker)
Cimetidine Hydrochloride
(Concurrent use may result in reduced effectiveness of the H2 blocker)
Esomeprazole Magnesium
(Concurrent use may result in reduced effectiveness of proton pump inhibitors)
Famotidine
(Concurrent use may result in reduced effectiveness of the H2 blocker)
Lansoprazole
(Concurrent use may result in reduced effectiveness of proton pump inhibitors)
Nizatidine
(Concurrent use may result in reduced effectiveness of the H2 blocker)
Omeprazole
(Concurrent use may result in reduced effectiveness of proton pump inhibitors)
Pantoprazole Sodium
(Concurrent use may result in reduced effectiveness of proton pump inhibitors)
Rabeprazole Sodium
(Concurrent use may result in reduced effectiveness of proton pump inhibitors)
Ranitidine Bismuth Citrate
(Concurrent use may result in reduced effectiveness of the H2 blocker)
Ranitidine Hydrochloride
(Concurrent use may result in reduced effectiveness of the H2 blocker)
Warfarin Sodium
(Concurrent use may result in increased risk of bleeding)

CRATAEGUS LAEVIGATA

(*See under* English Hawthorn)

CREATINE PHOSPHATE

Ma-Huang
(Stroke risk)

CUCURBITA PEPO

(*See under* Pumpkin)

CYCLOPHOSPHAMIDE

Astragalus
(Increase in tumor killing activity)
St. John's Wort
(May result in reduced chyclophophamide effectiveness)

CYCLOSPORINE

Alfalfa
(May precipitate organ transplant rejection)
St. John's Wort
(May result in decreased cyclosporine levels and acute transplant rejection)

CYPROHEPTADINE HYDROCHLORIDE

Mangosteen
(G. mangostana may possibly be unsafe when used by patients taking antihistamines)

CYTISUS SCOPARIUS

(*See under* Scotch Broom)

DALTEPARIN SODIUM

Mangosteen
(G. mangostana may possibly be unsafe when used by patients taking anticoagulants)

DANAPAROID SODIUM

Mangosteen
(G. mangostana may possibly be unsafe when used by patients taking anticoagulants)

DATURA STRAMONIUM

(*See under* Jimson Weed)

DESERPIDINE

Kudzu
(P. lobata may interfere with hypotensive agents)

DEXCHLORPHENIRAMINE MALEATE

Mangosteen
(G. mangostana may possibly be unsafe when used by patients taking antihistamines)

DEXTROAMPHETAMINE SULFATE

Rhodiola
(May have additive effects with other stimulants)

DIAGNOSTIC PROCEDURES USING RADIOACTIVE ISOTOPES

Bugleweed
(Herb interferes with these isotopes)

DIAZOXIDE

Kudzu
(P. lobata may interfere with hypotensive agents)

DICHLORPHENAMIDE

Ma-Huang
(Decreased elimination of ephedrine)

DICUMAROL

Mangosteen
(G. mangostana may possibly be unsafe when used by patients taking anticoagulants)

DIENESTROL

Kudzu
(P. lobata may inhibit the effects of estrogen therapy)

Pygeum
(Prunus may interact with estrogen or other hormones)

DIETHYLSTILBESTROL

Kudzu
(P. lobata may inhibit the effects of estrogen therapy)
Pygeum
(Prunus may interact with estrogen or other hormones)

DIGITALIS

Methylxanthines
(Increases risk of cardiac arrhythmias)
Phosphodiesterase Inhibitors
(Increases risk of cardiac arrhythmias)
Quinidine
(Increases risk of cardiac arrhythmias)
Sympathomimetic Agents
(Increases risk of cardiac arrhythmias)

DIGITALIS GLYCOSIDE PREPARATIONS

Rauwolfia
(Severe bradycardia when used in combination with digitalis glycosides)
Senna
(Senna-induced hypokalemia may increase toxicity of digitalis preparations)

DIGITALIS PURPUREA

(*See under* Digitalis)

DIGOXIN

Adonis
(Increases action of Adonis)
Buckthorn
(Herb may cause hypokalemia, which may increase digoxin toxicity)
Cascara Sagrada
(Herb may cause hypokalemia, which may increase digoxin toxicity)
Chinese Rhubarb
(Herb may cause hypokalemia, which may increase digoxin toxicity)
English Hawthorn
(May increase effect of digoxin)
Guarana
(Herb may cause hypokalemia, which may increase digoxin toxicity)
Licorice
(Increased risk of hypokalemia)
Lily-of-the-Valley
(Increases the effect of Lily-of-the-Valley)
Ma-Huang
(Risk of arrhythmia)
Siberian Ginseng
(Elevated serum levels)
Squill
(Squill potentiates the positive inotropic and negative chronopic effects of digoxin)
St. John's Wort
(May result in significantly lower serum digoxin levels)
Uzara
(Herb contains cardiac glycosides and may have additive effect when taken with digoxin, possibly increasing digoxin toxicity)

DILTIAZEM HYDROCHLORIDE

Kudzu
(P. lobata may interfere with hypotensive agents)

DIOSCOREA VILLOSA

(*See under* Wild Yam)

DIPHENHYDRAMINE CITRATE

Mangosteen
(G. mangostana may possibly be unsafe when used by patients taking antihistamines)

DIPHENHYDRAMINE HYDROCHLORIDE

Mangosteen
(G. mangostana may possibly be unsafe when used by patients taking antihistamines)

DIPHENYLPYRALINE HYDROCHLORIDE

Mangosteen
(G. mangostana may possibly be unsafe when used by patients taking antihistamines)

DISOPYRAMIDE PHOSPHATE

Kudzu
(P. lobata may interfere with antiarrhythmic agents)

DISULFIRAM

Marijuana
(May induce hypomania reaction)

DIURETICS

Frangula
(Herb may cause hypokalemia, which may increase digoxin toxicity)
Kombé Seed
(Increases effects and side effects of herb)

DOFETILIDE

Kudzu
(P. lobata may interfere with antiarrhythmic agents)

DONG QUAI

Anticoagulant drugs, unspecified
(Increased risk of bleeding)
Antithrombolytic Drugs
(Increased risk of bleeding)
Low Molecular Weight Heparins
(Increased risk of bleeding)

DOPAMINE ANTAGONISTS

Chaste Tree
(Enhances dopaminergic adverse effects)
Kava Kava
(May decrease effectiveness of dopamine)

DOPAMINE D2 ANTAGONISTS

Chaste Tree
(Decreased effectiveness of drug)

DOXAZOSIN MESYLATE

Kudzu
(P. lobata may interfere with hypotensive agents)

DRUGS THAT CAUSE THROMBOCYTOPENIA

Quinine
(Herb increases risk of thrombocytopenia)

DRUGS, UNSPECIFIED

Coffee
(Hinders resorption of other drugs)
Flax
(Absorption of other drugs may be delayed when taken simultaneously)

Niauli
(Co-administration may result in decreased effect of drugs that undergo liver metabolism)
Psyllium
(Absorption of other drugs may be decreased if taken simultaneously with herb)
Psyllium Seed
(Absorption of other drugs may be decreased if taken simultaneously with herb)

ECHINACEA

Corticosteroids
(Echinacea may potentially interfere with the anti-cancer chemotherapeutic effect of corticosteroids)
Immunosuppressants
(The immune-stimulating effect of Echinacea may interfere with drugs that have immunosuppressant effects)

ECHINACEA ANGUSTIFOLIA

(*See under* Echinacea)

ELEUTHEROCOCCUS SENTICOSUS

(*See under* Siberian Ginseng)

ENALAPRIL MALEATE

Kudzu
(P. lobata may interfere with hypotensive agents)

ENALAPRILAT

Kudzu
(P. lobata may interfere with hypotensive agents)

ENGLISH HAWTHORN

Antiarrhythmics
(May increase activity)
Antiplatelet Drugs
(May increase risk of bleeding)
Beta Blockers
(May cause hypertension)
Cisapride
(May cause hyperkalemia)
Digoxin
(May increase effect of digoxin)

ENOXAPARIN SODIUM

Mangosteen
(G. mangostana may possibly be unsafe when used by patients taking anticoagulants)

ENOXIMONE

Mangosteen
(G. mangostana may possibly be unsafe when used by patients taking phosphodiesterase inhibitors)

EPHEDRA SINICA

(*See under* Ma-Huang)

EPROSARTAN MESYLATE

Kudzu
(P. lobata may interfere with hypotensive agents)

ESCITALOPRAM OXALATE

5-HTP
(Concurrent use may result in an increased risk of serotonin syndrome (hypertension, hyperthermia, myoclonus, mental status change); combining 5-HTP with SSRIs may increase the risk of serotonergic side effects)
Mangosteen
(G. mangostana may possibly be unsafe when used by patients taking selective serotonin reuptake inhibitors)

ESMOLOL HYDROCHLORIDE

Kudzu
(P. lobata may interfere with hypotensive agents)

ESOMEPRAZOLE MAGNESIUM

Cranberry
(Concurrent use may result in reduced effectiveness of proton pump inhibitors)

ESTRADIOL

Kudzu
(P. lobata may inhibit the effects of estrogen therapy)
Pygeum
(Prunus may interact with estrogen or other hormones)

ESTROGEN

Ginseng
(May enhance estrogen's effects)
Hops
(May increase estrogenic activity in patients with reduced ability to metabolize estrogen)
Red Clover
(Altered effectiveness or increased side effects)
Senna
(Senna decreases estrogen levels when taken with estrogen supplements)
Wild Yam
(Additive effect)

ESTROGENS, CONJUGATED

Kudzu
(P. lobata may inhibit the effects of estrogen therapy)
Pygeum
(Prunus may interact with estrogen or other hormones)

ESTROGENS, ESTERIFIED

Kudzu
(P. lobata may inhibit the effects of estrogen therapy)
Pygeum
(Prunus may interact with estrogen or other hormones)

ESTROPIPATE

Kudzu
(P. lobata may inhibit the effects of estrogen therapy)
Pygeum
(Prunus may interact with estrogen or other hormones)

ETHANOL

Yohimbe Bark
(Increased anxiogenic effects)

ETHINYL ESTRADIOL

Kudzu
(P. lobata may inhibit the effects of estrogen therapy)
Pygeum
(Prunus may interact with estrogen or other hormones)

ETOPOSIDE

St. John's Wort
(May result in reduced effectiveness of etoposide)

EVENING PRIMROSE

Anticonvulsants
(Evening Primrose oil may lower seizure threshold and decrease effectiveness of anticonvulsant medications)

FAMOTIDINE

Cranberry
(Concurrent use may result in reduced effectiveness of the H2 blocker)

FELODIPINE

Kudzu
(P. lobata may interfere with hypotensive agents)

FENOFIBRATE

Bitter Melon
(Bitter melon may potentiate cholesterol-lowering drugs)

FENUGREEK

Hypoglycemic Drugs
(Herb may have an additive hypoglycemic effect when taken with other hypoglycemic drugs)

FEVERFEW

Aspirin
(Increased antithrombotic effect)
Warfarin Sodium
(Increased antithrombotic effect)

FEXOFENADINE HYDROCHLORIDE

Mangosteen
(G. mangostana may possibly be unsafe when used by patients taking antihistamines)

5-HTP

Carbidopa
(Concurrent use may result in an increased risk of developing scleroderma-like illness in susceptible individuals; monitor for signs of skin changes, which may manifest as edema, tightness, and/or a burning sensation)
Citalopram Hydrobromide
(Concurrent use may result in an increased risk of serotonin syndrome (hypertension, hyperthermia, myoclonus, mental status change); combining 5-HTP with SSRIs may increase the risk of serotonergic side effects)
Escitalopram Oxalate
(Concurrent use may result in an increased risk of serotonin syndrome (hypertension, hyperthermia, myoclonus, mental status change); combining 5-HTP with SSRIs may increase the risk of serotonergic side effects)
Fluoxetine Hydrochloride
(Concurrent use may result in an increased risk of serotonin syndrome (hypertension, hyperthermia, myoclonus, mental status change); combining 5-HTP with SSRIs may increase the risk of serotonergic side effects)
Fluvoxamine Maleate
(Concurrent use may result in an increased risk of serotonin syndrome (hypertension, hyperthermia, myoclonus, mental status change); combining 5-HTP with SSRIs may increase the risk of serotonergic side effects)
Isocarboxazid
(Concurrent use may result in an increased risk of serotonin syndrome (hypertension, hyperthermia, myoclonus, mental status change))
Moclobemide
(Concurrent use may result in an increased risk of serotonin syndrome (hypertension, hyperthermia, myoclonus, mental status change))
Pargyline Hydrochloride
(Concurrent use may result in an increased risk of serotonin syndrome (hypertension, hyperthermia, myoclonus, mental status change))
Paroxetine Hydrochloride
(Concurrent use may result in an increased risk of serotonin syndrome (hypertension, hyperthermia, myoclonus, mental status change); combining 5-HTP with SSRIs may increase the risk of serotonergic side effects)
Phenelzine Sulfate
(Concurrent use may result in an increased risk of serotonin syndrome (hypertension, hyperthermia, myoclonus, mental status change))
Procarbazine Hydrochloride
(Concurrent use may result in an increased risk of serotonin syndrome (hypertension, hyperthermia, myoclonus, mental status change))
Rasagiline Mesylate
(Concurrent use may result in an increased risk of serotonin syndrome (hypertension, hyperthermia, myoclonus, mental status change))
Selegiline
(Concurrent use may result in an increased risk of serotonin syndrome (hypertension, hyperthermia, myoclonus, mental status change))
Selegiline Hydrochloride
(Concurrent use may result in an increased risk of serotonin syndrome (hypertension, hyperthermia, myoclonus, mental status change))
Sertraline Hydrochloride
(Concurrent use may result in an increased risk of serotonin syndrome (hypertension, hyperthermia, myoclonus, mental status change); combining 5-HTP with SSRIs may increase the risk of serotonergic side effects)
Tranylcypromine Sulfate
(Concurrent use may result in an increased risk of serotonin syndrome (hypertension, hyperthermia, myoclonus, mental status change))

FLAX

Drugs, unspecified
(Absorption of other drugs may be delayed when taken simultaneously)

FLECAINIDE ACETATE

Kudzu
(P. lobata may interfere with antiarrhythmic agents)

FLUOXETINE HYDROCHLORIDE

5-HTP
(Concurrent use may result in an increased risk of serotonin syndrome (hypertension, hyperthermia, myoclonus, mental status change); combining 5-HTP with SSRIs may increase the risk of serotonergic side effects)

Mangosteen
(G. mangostana may possibly be unsafe when used by patients taking selective serotonin reuptake inhibitors)

FLUVASTATIN SODIUM

Bitter Melon
(Bitter melon may potentiate cholesterol-lowering drugs)

FLUVOXAMINE MALEATE

5-HTP
(Concurrent use may result in an increased risk of serotonin syndrome (hypertension, hyperthermia, myoclonus, mental status change); combining 5-HTP with SSRIs may increase the risk of serotonergic side effects)

Mangosteen
(G. mangostana may possibly be unsafe when used by patients taking selective serotonin reuptake inhibitors)

FONDAPARINUX SODIUM

Mangosteen
(G. mangostana may possibly be unsafe when used by patients taking anticoagulants)

FOSINOPRIL SODIUM

Kudzu
(P. lobata may interfere with hypotensive agents)

FRANGULA

Cardiac Glycosides
(Increased effect due to potassium loss with chronic use of herb)

Diuretics
(Herb may cause hypokalemia, which may increase digoxin toxicity)

FUCUS VESICULOSUS

(*See under* Bladderwrack)

FUROSEMIDE

Kudzu
(P. lobata may interfere with hypotensive agents)

GALEGA OFFICINALIS

(*See under* Goat's Rue)

GARCINIA MANGOSTANA

(*See under* Mangosteen)

GARLIC

Anticoagulant drugs, unspecified
(Increased risk of bleeding)

Antiplatelet Drugs
(Increased risk of bleeding)

Chlorzoxazone
(Increased metabolism of drug)

Coleus Forskohlii
(Platelet aggregation potentiated)

Low Molecular Weight Heparins
(Increased risk of bleeding)

Nonsteroidal Anti-Inflammatory Drugs
(Increased bleeding time due to decreased platelet aggregation)

Protease Inhibitors
(Increased metabolism of drug)

Thrombolytics
(Increased risk of bleeding)

GEMFIBROZIL

Bitter Melon
(Bitter melon may potentiate cholesterol-lowering drugs)

GERMAN CHAMOMILE

Alcohol
(Additive effects of alcohol)

Anticoagulant drugs, unspecified
(Increased risk of bleeding)

Benzodiazepines
(Additive effects of benzodiazepines)

Warfarin Sodium
(Hydroxycoumarin component in Chamomile may elevate prothrombin times)

GINGER

Anticoagulant drugs, unspecified
(Increased risk of bleeding)

Antiplatelet Drugs
(Increased risk of bleeding)

Low Molecular Weight Heparins
(Increased risk of bleeding)

Thrombolytics
(Increased risk of bleeding)

GINKGO

Anticoagulant drugs, unspecified
(Increased risk of bleeding)

Anticonvulsants
(May precipitate seizures)

Antiplatelet Drugs
(Increased risk of bleeding)

Antithrombolytic Drugs
(Increases effect of antithrombolytic drugs)

Insulin
(May alter insulin requirements)

Low Molecular Weight Heparins
(Increased risk of bleeding)

MAO Inhibitors
(May potentiate MAOI effects)

Nicardipine
(May reduce the hypotensive effect of nicardipine)

Nifedipine
(May increase mean plasma concentrations of nifedipine)

Nonsteroidal Anti-Inflammatory Drugs
(Increased risk of bleeding)

Papaverine
(May increase the adverse effects of papaverine)

Selective Serotonin Reuptake Inhibitors
(May precipitate hypomania)

Thiazide Diuretics
(May increase blood pressure)

Thrombolytics
(Increased risk of bleeding)

GINKGO BILOBA

(*See under* Ginkgo)

GINKGO BILOBA

St. John's Wort
(May have precipitated a hypomanic episode in a case report)

GINSENG

Albendazole
(May alter the therapeutic efficacy of albendazole)

Anticoagulant drugs, unspecified
(May decrease INR)

Estrogen
(May enhance estrogen's effects)

Hypoglycemic Drugs
(Increases hypoglycemic effect)

Insulin
(May reduce hypoglycemic efforts)

Loop Diuretics
(Increases diuretic resistance)
MAO Inhibitors
(Combination increases chance for headache, tremors, mania)
Nifedipine
(May increase the plasma concentration of nifedipine)
Opioid Analgesics
(May suppress analgesic effects)

GLIMEPIRIDE
Bitter Melon
(Concurrent use may result in an increased risk of hypoglycemia)
Kudzu
(P. lobata may lower blood glucose levels)

GLIPIZIDE
Bitter Melon
(Concurrent use may result in an increased risk of hypoglycemia)
Kudzu
(P. lobata may lower blood glucose levels)

GLUCOCORTICOIDS
Adonis
(Increases action of Adonis)
Kombé Seed
(Increases effects and side effects of herb)
Licorice
(Licorice potentiates effect of glucocorticoids)
Lily-of-the-Valley
(Increases the effect of Lily-of-the-Valley)
Oleander
(Increased efficacy and side effects when given simultaneously with herb)
Squill
(Increases effectiveness and side effects of herb)
Strophanthus
(Simultaneous administration with herb enhance both effects and side effects)

GLYBURIDE
Bitter Melon
(Concurrent use may result in an increased risk of hypoglycemia)
Kudzu
(P. lobata may lower blood glucose levels)

GLYCINE SOJA
(*See under* Soybean)

GLYCYRRHIZA GLABRA
(*See under* Licorice)

GOAT'S RUE
Hypoglycemic Drugs
(Herb may have an additive hypoglycemic effect when taken with other hypoglycemic drugs)

GOLDENSEAL
Vitamin B Complex
(May decrease Vitamin B absorption)

GREEN TEA
Alkaline Drugs
(Decreased absorption of alkaline drugs due to tannin component in tea)

GRIFFONIA SIMPLICIFOCLIA
(*See under* 5-HTP)

GUANABENZ ACETATE
Kudzu
(P. lobata may interfere with hypotensive agents)
Yohimbe Bark
(May decrease hypotensive effect of Guanabenz)

GUANADREL SULFATE
Yohimbe Bark
(May decrease hypotensive effect of Guanadrel)

GUANETHIDINE
Ma-Huang
(Increased sympathomimetic effects)
Yohimbe Bark
(May decrease hypotensive effect of Guanethidine)

GUANETHIDINE MONOSULFATE
Kudzu
(P. lobata may interfere with hypotensive agents)

GUANFACINE HYDROCHLORIDE
Yohimbe Bark
(May decrease hypotensive effect of Guanfacine)

GUARANA
Ma-Huang
(Risk of hypertension, stroke, seizure, and cardiac arrhythmia)
Cardiac Glycosides
(Increased effect due to potassium loss with chronic use of herb)
Digoxin
(Herb may cause hypokalemia, which may increase digoxin toxicity)

HALOPERIDOL
Milk Thistle
(Silymarin in combination with haloperidol causes a decrease in lipid peroxidation)

HALOTHANE
Ma-Huang
(Disturbance of heart rhythm)

HENBANE
Amantadine Hydrochloride
(Increased anticholinergic action)
Antihistamines
(Increased anticholinergic action)
Phenothiazines
(Increased anticholinergic action)
Procainamide
(Increased anticholinergic action)
Quinidine
(Increased anticholinergic action)
Tricyclic Antidepressants
(Increased anticholinergic action)

HEPARIN CALCIUM
Mangosteen
(G. mangostana may possibly be unsafe when used by patients taking anticoagulants)

HEPARIN SODIUM
Mangosteen
(G. mangostana may possibly be unsafe when used by patients taking anticoagulants)

HEPATOTOXIC DRUGS, UNSPECIFIED
Kava Kava
(May increase toxicity)
Valerian
(May increase liver transaminases)

HERBAL MEDICINES, UNSPECIFIED
Pygeum
(Prunus may interact with herbs/ supplements containing chemicals with estrogen-like constituents)

HOODIA
(None cited in PDR database)

HOODIA GORDONII
(*See under* Hoodia)

HOPS
Barbiturates
(May increase sedative action)
Estrogen
(May increase estrogenic activity in patients with reduced ability to metabolize estrogen)

HORMONES, UNSPECIFIED
Pygeum
(Prunus may interact with estrogen or other hormones)

HORSE CHESTNUT
Anticoagulant drugs, unspecified
(Horse Chestnut has a coumarin componant and may interact with warfarin, salicylates and other drugs with anticoagulant properties)

HUMULUS LUPULUS
(*See under* Hops)

HYDRALAZINE HYDROCHLORIDE
Kudzu
(P. lobata may interfere with hypotensive agents)

HYDRASTIS CANADENSIS
(*See under* Goldenseal)

HYDROCHLOROTHIAZIDE
Kudzu
(P. lobata may interfere with hypotensive agents)

HYDROFLUMETHIAZIDE
Kudzu
(P. lobata may interfere with hypotensive agents)

HYOSCYAMUS NIGER
(*See under* Henbane)

HYPERICUM PERFORATUM
(*See under* St. John's Wort)

HYPNOTICS
Valerian
(Additive effect when taken with Valerian)

HYPOGLYCEMIC DRUGS
Bladderwrack
(Herb may have an additive hypoglycemic effect when taken with other hypoglycemic drugs)
Fenugreek
(Herb may have an additive hypoglycemic effect when taken with other hypoglycemic drugs)
Ginseng
(Increases hypoglycemic effect)
Goat's Rue
(Herb may have an additive hypoglycemic effect when taken with other hypoglycemic drugs)

IMATINIB MESYLATE
St. John's Wort
(May result in decreased imatinim effectiveness)

IMMUNOSUPPRESSANTS
Astragalus
(Decreased effectiveness of immunosuppressive effect due to immunostimulant effect of Astragalus)
Echinacea
(The immune-stimulating effect of Echinacea may interfere with drugs that have immunosuppressant effects)

INDAPAMIDE
Kudzu
(P. lobata may interfere with hypotensive agents)

INDIAN SQUILL
Methylxanthines
(Can increase the risk of cardic arrhythmias when given simultaneously with this herb)
Phosphodiesterase Inhibitors
(Can increase the risk of cardic arrhythmias when given simultaneously with this herb)
Quinidine
(Can increase the risk of cardic arrhythmias when given simultaneously with this herb)
Sympathomimetic Agents
(Can increase the risk of cardic arrhythmias when given simultaneously with this herb)

INDINAVIR SULFATE
St. John's Wort
(The herb induces the cytochrome P450 enzyme system and will lower indinavir serum levels)

INDOMETHACIN
Cascara Sagrada
(Decreases therapeutic effect of Cascara)
Senna
(Decreased therapeutic effect of Senna)
Wild Yam
(Wild Yam may decrease the anti-inflammatory effect of indomethacin)

INSULIN
Bitter Melon
(Concurrent use may result in an increased risk of hypoglycemia)
Ginkgo
(May alter insulin requirements)
Ginseng
(May reduce hypoglycemic efforts)
Kudzu
(P. lobata may lower blood glucose levels)
Licorice
(Increased risk of hypokalemia)
Psyllium
(Effect unspecified; insulin dose should be decreased)
Siberian Ginseng
(May potentiate effects)

INSULIN ASPART
Bitter Melon
(Concurrent use may result in an increased risk of hypoglycemia)
Kudzu
(P. lobata may lower blood glucose levels)

INSULIN ASPART PROTAMINE, HUMAN
Bitter Melon
(Concurrent use may result in an increased risk of hypoglycemia)
Kudzu
(P. lobata may lower blood glucose levels)

INSULIN ASPART, HUMAN

Bitter Melon
(Concurrent use may result in an increased risk of hypoglycemia)

Kudzu
(P. lobata may lower blood glucose levels)

INSULIN ASPART, HUMAN REGULAR

Bitter Melon
(Concurrent use may result in an increased risk of hypoglycemia)

Kudzu
(P. lobata may lower blood glucose levels)

INSULIN DETEMIR (RDNA ORIGIN)

Bitter Melon
(Concurrent use may result in an increased risk of hypoglycemia)

Kudzu
(P. lobata may lower blood glucose levels)

INSULIN GLULISINE

Bitter Melon
(Concurrent use may result in an increased risk of hypoglycemia)

Kudzu
(P. lobata may lower blood glucose levels)

INSULIN LISPRO PROTAMINE, HUMAN

Bitter Melon
(Concurrent use may result in an increased risk of hypoglycemia)

Kudzu
(P. lobata may lower blood glucose levels)

INSULIN LISPRO, HUMAN

Bitter Melon
(Concurrent use may result in an increased risk of hypoglycemia)

Kudzu
(P. lobata may lower blood glucose levels)

INSULIN GLARGINE

Bitter Melon
(Concurrent use may result in an increased risk of hypoglycemia)

Kudzu
(P. lobata may lower blood glucose levels)

INSULIN, HUMAN (RDNA ORIGIN)

Bitter Melon
(Concurrent use may result in an increased risk of hypoglycemia)

Kudzu
(P. lobata may lower blood glucose levels)

INSULIN, HUMAN NPH

Bitter Melon
(Concurrent use may result in an increased risk of hypoglycemia)

Kudzu
(P. lobata may lower blood glucose levels)

INSULIN, HUMAN REGULAR

Bitter Melon
(Concurrent use may result in an increased risk of hypoglycemia)

Kudzu
(P. lobata may lower blood glucose levels)

INSULIN, HUMAN REGULAR AND HUMAN NPH MIXTURE

Bitter Melon
(Concurrent use may result in an increased risk of hypoglycemia)

Kudzu
(P. lobata may lower blood glucose levels)

INSULIN, HUMAN, ZINC SUSPENSION

Bitter Melon
(Concurrent use may result in an increased risk of hypoglycemia)

Kudzu
(P. lobata may lower blood glucose levels)

INSULIN, NPH

Bitter Melon
(Concurrent use may result in an increased risk of hypoglycemia)

Kudzu
(P. lobata may lower blood glucose levels)

INSULIN, REGULAR

Bitter Melon
(Concurrent use may result in an increased risk of hypoglycemia)

Kudzu
(P. lobata may lower blood glucose levels)

INSULIN, REGULAR AND NPH MIXTURE

Bitter Melon
(Concurrent use may result in an increased risk of hypoglycemia)

Kudzu
(P. lobata may lower blood glucose levels)

INSULIN, ZINC CRYSTALS

Bitter Melon
(Concurrent use may result in an increased risk of hypoglycemia)

Kudzu
(P. lobata may lower blood glucose levels)

INSULIN, ZINC SUSPENSION

Bitter Melon
(Concurrent use may result in an increased risk of hypoglycemia)

Kudzu
(P. lobata may lower blood glucose levels)

IOBENGUANE SULFATE I-131

Ma-Huang
(Reduced uptake in neuroendocrine tumors)

IRBESARTAN

Kudzu
(P. lobata may interfere with hypotensive agents)

IRINOTECAN HYDROCHLORIDE

St. John's Wort
(May result in decreased imatinib effectiveness)

IRON

Borage
(Increased risk of bleeding)

Butternut
(Adverse sequelae on blood components)

Saw Palmetto
(May complex with saw palmetto, creating adverse sequelae on blood)

Slippery Elm
(Reduced absorption of iron)

Soybean
(May result in reduced absorption of iron)

St. John's Wort
(May result in non-absorbable insoluble complexes and may result in adverse sequelae on blood components)
Uva-Ursi
(May complex with iron and result in adverse sequelae on blood components)
Valerian
(May complex with iron and result in adverse sequelae on blood components)
Wormwood
(May complex with iron, resulting in adverse sequelae on blood components)
Yarrow
(May complex with iron, resulting in adverse sequelae on blood components)

ISOCARBOXAZID

5-HTP
(Concurrent use may result in an increased risk of serotonin syndrome (hypertension, hyperthermia, myoclonus, mental status change))

ISRADIPINE

Kudzu
(P. lobata may interfere with hypotensive agents)

JIMSON WEED

Anticholinergics
(Co-administration of Jimson Weed with other anticholinergic drugs may increase the frequency and/or severity of anticholinergic side effects such as dry mouth, constipation, drowsiness, and others)

JUGLANS CINEREA

(*See under* Butternut)

KAVA KAVA

Alcohol
(May increase sedative effect and risk of hepatotoxicity)
Anticoagulant drugs, unspecified
(May increase risk of bleeding)
Antiplatelet Drugs
(May increase risk of bleeding)
Barbiturates
(May increase CNS depression)
Benzodiazepines
(May increase CNS depression)
CNS-Active Drugs, unspecified
(May intensify effect)
Dopamine Antagonists
(May decrease effectiveness of dopamine)
Hepatotoxic Drugs, unspecified
(May increase toxicity)
Low Molecular Weight Heparins
(May increase risk of bleeding)
MAO Inhibitors
(May increase toxicity associated with excessive inhibition of MAOI)
Opium Preparations
(May increase sedative effects and CNS depression)
Phenothiazines
(May decrease effectiveness of dopamine)
Skeletal Muscle Relaxants
(May increase sedative effects and CNS depression)
Thrombolytics
(May increase risk of bleeding)

KOMBÉ SEED

Calcium Salts
(Increases effects and side effects of herb)
Diuretics
(Increases effects and side effects of herb)
Glucocorticoids
(Increases effects and side effects of herb)
Laxatives
(Increases effects and side effects of herb)
Quinidine
(Increases effects and side effects of herb)

KUDZU

Acarbose
(P. lobata may lower blood glucose levels)
Acebutolol Hydrochloride
(P. lobata may interfere with antiarrhythmic agents)
Adenosine
(P. lobata may interfere with antiarrhythmic agents)
Amiodarone Hydrochloride
(P. lobata may interfere with antiarrhythmic agents)
Amlodipine Besylate
(P. lobata may interfere with hypotensive agents)
Atenolol
(P. lobata may interfere with hypotensive agents)
Benazepril Hydrochloride
(P. lobata may interfere with hypotensive agents)
Bendroflumethiazide
(P. lobata may interfere with hypotensive agents)
Betaxolol Hydrochloride
(P. lobata may interfere with hypotensive agents)
Bisoprolol Fumarate
(P. lobata may interfere with hypotensive agents)
Bretylium Tosylate
(P. lobata may interfere with antiarrhythmic agents)
Candesartan Cilexetil
(P. lobata may interfere with hypotensive agents)
Captopril
(P. lobata may interfere with hypotensive agents)
Carteolol Hydrochloride
(P. lobata may interfere with hypotensive agents)
Chlorothiazide
(P. lobata may interfere with hypotensive agents)
Chlorothiazide Sodium
(P. lobata may interfere with hypotensive agents)
Chlorotrianisene
(P. lobata may inhibit the effects of estrogen therapy)
Chlorpropamide
(P. lobata may lower blood glucose levels)
Chlorthalidone
(P. lobata may interfere with hypotensive agents)

Clonidine
(P. lobata may interfere with hypotensive agents)
Clonidine Hydrochloride
(P. lobata may interfere with hypotensive agents)
Deserpidine
(P. lobata may interfere with hypotensive agents)
Diazoxide
(P. lobata may interfere with hypotensive agents)
Dienestrol
(P. lobata may inhibit the effects of estrogen therapy)
Diethylstilbestrol
(P. lobata may inhibit the effects of estrogen therapy)
Diltiazem Hydrochloride
(P. lobata may interfere with hypotensive agents)
Disopyramide Phosphate
(P. lobata may interfere with antiarrhythmic agents)
Dofetilide
(P. lobata may interfere with antiarrhythmic agents)
Doxazosin Mesylate
(P. lobata may interfere with hypotensive agents)
Enalapril Maleate
(P. lobata may interfere with hypotensive agents)
Enalaprilat
(P. lobata may interfere with hypotensive agents)
Eprosartan Mesylate
(P. lobata may interfere with hypotensive agents)
Esmolol Hydrochloride
(P. lobata may interfere with hypotensive agents)
Estradiol
(P. lobata may inhibit the effects of estrogen therapy)
Estrogens, Conjugated
(P. lobata may inhibit the effects of estrogen therapy)
Estrogens, Esterified
(P. lobata may inhibit the effects of estrogen therapy)
Estropipate
(P. lobata may inhibit the effects of estrogen therapy)
Ethinyl Estradiol
(P. lobata may inhibit the effects of estrogen therapy)
Felodipine
(P. lobata may interfere with hypotensive agents)
Flecainide Acetate
(P. lobata may interfere with antiarrhythmic agents)
Fosinopril Sodium
(P. lobata may interfere with hypotensive agents)
Furosemide
(P. lobata may interfere with hypotensive agents)
Glimepiride
(P. lobata may lower blood glucose levels)
Glipizide
(P. lobata may lower blood glucose levels)
Glyburide
(P. lobata may lower blood glucose levels)
Guanabenz Acetate
(P. lobata may interfere with hypotensive agents)
Guanethidine Monosulfate
(P. lobata may interfere with hypotensive agents)
Hydralazine Hydrochloride
(P. lobata may interfere with hypotensive agents)
Hydrochlorothiazide
(P. lobata may interfere with hypotensive agents)
Hydroflumethiazide
(P. lobata may interfere with hypotensive agents)
Indapamide
(P. lobata may interfere with hypotensive agents)
Insulin
(P. lobata may lower blood glucose levels)
Insulin Aspart
(P. lobata may lower blood glucose levels)
Insulin Aspart Protamine, Human
(P. lobata may lower blood glucose levels)
Insulin Aspart, Human
(P. lobata may lower blood glucose levels)
Insulin Aspart, Human Regular
(P. lobata may lower blood glucose levels)
Insulin Detemir (rDNA Origin)
(P. lobata may lower blood glucose levels)
Insulin Glulisine
(P. lobata may lower blood glucose levels)
Insulin Lispro Protamine, Human
(P. lobata may lower blood glucose levels)
Insulin Lispro, Human
(P. lobata may lower blood glucose levels)
Insulin glargine
(P. lobata may lower blood glucose levels)
Insulin, Human (rDNA origin)
(P. lobata may lower blood glucose levels)
Insulin, Human NPH
(P. lobata may lower blood glucose levels)
Insulin, Human Regular
(P. lobata may lower blood glucose levels)
Insulin, Human Regular and Human NPH Mixture
(P. lobata may lower blood glucose levels)
Insulin, Human, Zinc Suspension
(P. lobata may lower blood glucose levels)
Insulin, NPH
(P. lobata may lower blood glucose levels)
Insulin, Regular
(P. lobata may lower blood glucose levels)
Insulin, Regular and NPH mixture
(P. lobata may lower blood glucose levels)
Insulin, Zinc Crystals
(P. lobata may lower blood glucose levels)

Insulin, Zinc Suspension
(P. lobata may lower blood glucose levels)
Irbesartan
(P. lobata may interfere with hypotensive agents)
Isradipine
(P. lobata may interfere with hypotensive agents)
Labetalol Hydrochloride
(P. lobata may interfere with hypotensive agents)
Lidocaine Hydrochloride
(P. lobata may interfere with antiarrhythmic agents)
Lisinopril
(P. lobata may interfere with hypotensive agents)
Losartan Potassium
(P. lobata may interfere with hypotensive agents)
Mecamylamine Hydrochloride
(P. lobata may interfere with hypotensive agents)
Metformin Hydrochloride
(P. lobata may lower blood glucose levels)
Methyclothiazide
(P. lobata may interfere with hypotensive agents)
Methyldopa
(P. lobata may interfere with hypotensive agents)
Methyldopate Hydrochloride
(P. lobata may interfere with hypotensive agents)
Metolazone
(P. lobata may interfere with hypotensive agents)
Metoprolol Succinate
(P. lobata may interfere with hypotensive agents)
Metoprolol Tartrate
(P. lobata may interfere with hypotensive agents)
Metyrosine
(P. lobata may interfere with hypotensive agents)
Mexiletine Hydrochloride
(P. lobata may interfere with antiarrhythmic agents)
Mibefradil Dihydrochloride
(P. lobata may interfere with hypotensive agents)
Miglitol
(P. lobata may lower blood glucose levels)
Minoxidil
(P. lobata may interfere with hypotensive agents)
Moexipril Hydrochloride
(P. lobata may interfere with hypotensive agents)
Moricizine Hydrochloride
(P. lobata may interfere with antiarrhythmic agents)
Nadolol
(P. lobata may interfere with hypotensive agents)
Nateglinide
(P. lobata may lower blood glucose levels)
Nicardipine Hydrochloride
(P. lobata may interfere with hypotensive agents)
Nifedipine
(P. lobata may interfere with hypotensive agents)
Nisoldipine
(P. lobata may interfere with hypotensive agents)
Nitroglycerin
(P. lobata may interfere with hypotensive agents)
Penbutolol Sulfate
(P. lobata may interfere with hypotensive agents)
Perindopril Erbumine
(P. lobata may interfere with hypotensive agents)
Phenoxybenzamine Hydrochloride
(P. lobata may interfere with hypotensive agents)
Phentolamine Mesylate
(P. lobata may interfere with hypotensive agents)
Pindolol
(P. lobata may interfere with hypotensive agents)
Pioglitazone Hydrochloride
(P. lobata may lower blood glucose levels)
Polyestradiol Phosphate
(P. lobata may inhibit the effects of estrogen therapy)
Polythiazide
(P. lobata may interfere with hypotensive agents)
Prazosin Hydrochloride
(P. lobata may interfere with hypotensive agents)
Procainamide Hydrochloride
(P. lobata may interfere with antiarrhythmic agents)
Propafenone Hydrochloride
(P. lobata may interfere with antiarrhythmic agents)
Propranolol Hydrochloride
(P. lobata may interfere with antiarrhythmic agents)
Quinapril Hydrochloride
(P. lobata may interfere with hypotensive agents)
Quinestrol
(P. lobata may inhibit the effects of estrogen therapy)
Quinidine Gluconate
(P. lobata may interfere with antiarrhythmic agents)
Quinidine Polygalacturonate
(P. lobata may interfere with antiarrhythmic agents)
Quinidine Sulfate
(P. lobata may interfere with antiarrhythmic agents)
Ramipril
(P. lobata may interfere with hypotensive agents)
Rauwolfia Serpentina
(P. lobata may interfere with hypotensive agents)
Repaglinide
(P. lobata may lower blood glucose levels)
Rescinnamine
(P. lobata may interfere with hypotensive agents)
Reserpine
(P. lobata may interfere with hypotensive agents)
Rosiglitazone Maleate
(P. lobata may lower blood glucose levels)

Sitagliptin Phosphate
(P. lobata may lower blood glucose levels)
Sodium Nitroprusside
(P. lobata may interfere with hypotensive agents)
Sotalol Hydrochloride
(P. lobata may interfere with antiarrhythmic agents)
Spirapril Hydrochloride
(P. lobata may interfere with hypotensive agents)
Telmisartan
(P. lobata may interfere with hypotensive agents)
Terazosin Hydrochloride
(P. lobata may interfere with hypotensive agents)
Timolol Maleate
(P. lobata may interfere with hypotensive agents)
Tocainide Hydrochloride
(P. lobata may interfere with antiarrhythmic agents)
Tolazamide
(P. lobata may lower blood glucose levels)
Tolbutamide
(P. lobata may lower blood glucose levels)
Torsemide
(P. lobata may interfere with hypotensive agents)
Trandolapril
(P. lobata may interfere with hypotensive agents)
Trimethaphan Camsylate
(P. lobata may interfere with hypotensive agents)
Troglitazone
(P. lobata may lower blood glucose levels)
Valsartan
(P. lobata may interfere with hypotensive agents)
Verapamil Hydrochloride
(P. lobata may interfere with antiarrhythmic agents)

LABETALOL HYDROCHLORIDE

Kudzu
(P. lobata may interfere with hypotensive agents)

LANSOPRAZOLE

Cranberry
(Concurrent use may result in reduced effectiveness of proton pump inhibitors)

LAXATIVES

Adonis
(Increases action of Adonis)
Kombé Seed
(Increases effects and side effects of herb)
Licorice
(Increased risk of hypokalemia)
Lily-of-the-Valley
(Increases the effect of Lily-of-the-Valley)
Oleander
(Increased efficacy and side effects when given simultaneously with herb)
Squill
(Increases effectiveness and side effects of herb)
Strophanthus
(Simultaneous administration with herb enhance both effects and side effects)

LEVODOPA

Chaste Tree
(Enhances dopaminergic adverse effects)
Rauwolfia
(Decreased effect; increases in extra-pyramidal symptoms)

LEVOTHYROXINE SODIUM

Soybean
(May result in decreased effectiveness of Levothyroxine)

LICORICE

Aloe
(Increased potassium loss)
Antiarrhythmics
(Licorice-induced hypokalemia increases risk of arrhythmias)
Anticoagulant drugs, unspecified
(May increase risk of bleeding)
Antidiabetic Drugs, unspecified
(May reduce hypoglycemic effects)
Antihypertensive agents, unspecified
(May reduce effectiveness)
Antiplatelet Drugs
(May increase risk of bleeding)
Corticosteroids
(Potentiates effects of corticosteroids)
Digoxin
(Increased risk of hypokalemia)
Glucocorticoids
(Licorice potentiates effect of glucocorticoids)
Insulin
(Increased risk of hypokalemia)
Laxatives
(Increased risk of hypokalemia)
Loop Diuretics
(Additive effect of hypokalemia)
Low Molecular Weight Heparins
(May increase risk of bleeding)
MAO Inhibitors
(Increased risk of toxicity associated with inhibition of MAOIs)
Oral Contraceptives
(May precipitate rise in blood pressure or fluid retention)
Potassium Preparations
(Increased risk of hypokalemia)
Testosterone
(Reduced levels of testosterone)
Thiazide Diuretics
(Additive effect of hypokalemia)
Thrombolytics
(May increase risk of bleeding)

LICORICE ROOT

Buckthorn
(Increases hypokalemic effects)

LIDOCAINE HYDROCHLORIDE

Kudzu
(P. lobata may interfere with antiarrhythmic agents)

LILY-OF-THE-VALLEY

Calcium
(Increases the effect of Lily-of-the-Valley)
Digoxin
(Increases the effect of Lily-of-the-Valley)
Glucocorticoids
(Increases the effect of Lily-of-the-Valley)

Laxatives
(Increases the effect of Lily-of-the-Valley)
Quinidine
(Increases the effect of Lily-of-the-Valley)
Saluretics
(Increases the effect of Lily-of-the-Valley)

LINUM USITATISSIMUM
(*See under* Flax)

LISINOPRIL
Kudzu
(P. lobata may interfere with hypotensive agents)

LITHIUM
Psyllium
(Possible decreased levels of lithium)
Yohimbe Bark
(Precipitates manic episodes in bipolar disorder)

LOOP DIURETICS
Ginseng
(Increases diuretic resistance)
Licorice
(Additive effect of hypokalemia)
Uva-Ursi
(The sodium-sparing effect of Uva-Ursi may antagonize the diuretic effect of the loop diuretics)

LOPERAMIDE HYDROCHLORIDE
St. John's Wort
(May result in delirium with symptoms of confusion, agitation and disorientation)
Valerian
(May result in delirium, confusion, agitation or disorientation)

LORATADINE
Mangosteen
(G. mangostana may possibly be unsafe when used by patients taking antihistamines)

LOSARTAN POTASSIUM
Kudzu
(P. lobata may interfere with hypotensive agents)

LOVASTATIN
Bitter Melon
(Bitter melon may potentiate cholesterol-lowering drugs)

LOW MOLECULAR WEIGHT HEPARINS
Arnica
(Increased risk of bleeding)
Dong Quai
(Increased risk of bleeding)
Garlic
(Increased risk of bleeding)
Ginger
(Increased risk of bleeding)
Ginkgo
(Increased risk of bleeding)
Kava Kava
(May increase risk of bleeding)
Licorice
(May increase risk of bleeding)
Mangosteen
(G. mangostana may possibly be unsafe when used by patients taking anticoagulants)
Red Clover
(Increased risk of bleeding)

LYCOPUS VIRGINICUS
(*See under* Bugleweed)

MAO INHIBITORS
Brewer's Yeast
(Increase in blood pressure)
Ginkgo
(May potentiate MAOI effects)
Ginseng
(Combination increases chance for headache, tremors, mania)
Kava Kava
(May increase toxicity associated with excessive inhibition of MAOI)
Licorice
(Increased risk of toxicity associated with inhibition of MAOIs)
Ma-Huang
(Increases sympathomimetic effects of ephedrine)
Scotch Broom
(Increased risk of hypertensive crisis)
St. John's Wort
(Increased risk of serotonin syndrome (hypertension, hyperthermia, myoclonus, mental status changes) and/or an increased risk of hypertensive crisis)

MA-HUANG
Antacids, unspecified
(Risk of ephedrine toxicity)
Antihypertensive agents, unspecified
(Decreased effectiveness)
Carbonic Anhydrase Inhibitors
(Increased serum concentrations)
Cardiac Glycosides
(Disturbance of heart rhythm)
Central Nervous System Stimulants
(Ma-Huang has an additive effect on the CNS when combined with CNS stimulants)
Clonidine
(Increased pressor response to ephedrine)
Corticosteroids
(Increased metabolism of corticosteroids)
Creatine Phosphate
(Stroke risk)
Dichlorphenamide
(Decreased elimination of ephedrine)
Digoxin
(Risk of arrhythmia)
Guanethidine
(Increased sympathomimetic effects)
Guarana
(Risk of hypertension, stroke, seizure, and cardiac arrhythmia)
Halothane
(Disturbance of heart rhythm)
Iobenguane Sulfate I-131
(Reduced uptake in neuroendocrine tumors)
MAO Inhibitors
(Increases sympathomimetic effects of ephedrine)
Midodrine Hydrochloride
(Increased pressor effects)
Oxytocin
(Development of high blood pressure)

Phenylpropanolamine
(Risk of arrhythmia)
Pseudoephedrine Preparations
(Excessive andregenic stimulation)
Sympathomimetic Agents
(Increased effects of ephedrine)
Theophylline
(CNS and gastrointestinal adverse events)

MANGOSTEEN

Acrivastine
(G. mangostana may possibly be unsafe when used by patients taking antihistamines)
Anisindione
(G. mangostana may possibly be unsafe when used by patients taking anticoagulants)
Ardeparin Sodium
(G. mangostana may possibly be unsafe when used by patients taking anticoagulants)
Astemizole
(G. mangostana may possibly be unsafe when used by patients taking antihistamines)
Azatadine Maleate
(G. mangostana may possibly be unsafe when used by patients taking antihistamines)
Bromodiphenhydramine Hydrochloride
(G. mangostana may possibly be unsafe when used by patients taking antihistamines)
Brompheniramine Maleate
(G. mangostana may possibly be unsafe when used by patients taking antihistamines)
Cetirizine Hydrochloride
(G. mangostana may possibly be unsafe when used by patients taking antihistamines)
Chlorpheniramine Maleate
(G. mangostana may possibly be unsafe when used by patients taking antihistamines)
Chlorpheniramine Polistirex
(G. mangostana may possibly be unsafe when used by patients taking antihistamines)
Chlorpheniramine Tannate
(G. mangostana may possibly be unsafe when used by patients taking antihistamines)
Citalopram Hydrobromide
(G. mangostana may possibly be unsafe when used by patients taking selective serotonin reuptake inhibitors)
Clemastine Fumarate
(G. mangostana may possibly be unsafe when used by patients taking antihistamines)
Cyproheptadine Hydrochloride
(G. mangostana may possibly be unsafe when used by patients taking antihistamines)
Dalteparin Sodium
(G. mangostana may possibly be unsafe when used by patients taking anticoagulants)
Danaparoid Sodium
(G. mangostana may possibly be unsafe when used by patients taking anticoagulants)
Dexchlorpheniramine Maleate
(G. mangostana may possibly be unsafe when used by patients taking antihistamines)
Dicumarol
(G. mangostana may possibly be unsafe when used by patients taking anticoagulants)
Diphenhydramine Citrate
(G. mangostana may possibly be unsafe when used by patients taking antihistamines)
Diphenhydramine Hydrochloride
(G. mangostana may possibly be unsafe when used by patients taking antihistamines)
Diphenylpyraline Hydrochloride
(G. mangostana may possibly be unsafe when used by patients taking antihistamines)
Enoxaparin Sodium
(G. mangostana may possibly be unsafe when used by patients taking anticoagulants)
Enoximone
(G. mangostana may possibly be unsafe when used by patients taking phosphodiesterase inhibitors)
Escitalopram Oxalate
(G. mangostana may possibly be unsafe when used by patients taking selective serotonin reuptake inhibitors)
Fexofenadine Hydrochloride
(G. mangostana may possibly be unsafe when used by patients taking antihistamines)
Fluoxetine Hydrochloride
(G. mangostana may possibly be unsafe when used by patients taking selective serotonin reuptake inhibitors)
Fluvoxamine Maleate
(G. mangostana may possibly be unsafe when used by patients taking selective serotonin reuptake inhibitors)
Fondaparinux Sodium
(G. mangostana may possibly be unsafe when used by patients taking anticoagulants)
Heparin Calcium
(G. mangostana may possibly be unsafe when used by patients taking anticoagulants)
Heparin Sodium
(G. mangostana may possibly be unsafe when used by patients taking anticoagulants)
Loratadine
(G. mangostana may possibly be unsafe when used by patients taking antihistamines)
Low Molecular Weight Heparins
(G. mangostana may possibly be unsafe when used by patients taking anticoagulants)
Methdilazine Hydrochloride
(G. mangostana may possibly be unsafe when used by patients taking antihistamines)
Milrinone Lactate
(G. mangostana may possibly be unsafe when used by patients taking phosphodiesterase inhibitors)
Paroxetine Hydrochloride
(G. mangostana may possibly be unsafe when used by patients taking selective serotonin reuptake inhibitors)

Promethazine Hydrochloride
(G. mangostana may possibly be unsafe when used by patients taking antihistamines)
Pyrilamine Maleate
(G. mangostana may possibly be unsafe when used by patients taking antihistamines)
Pyrilamine Tannate
(G. mangostana may possibly be unsafe when used by patients taking antihistamines)
Sertraline Hydrochloride
(G. mangostana may possibly be unsafe when used by patients taking selective serotonin reuptake inhibitors)
Sildenafil Citrate
(G. mangostana may possibly be unsafe when used by patients taking phosphodiesterase inhibitors)
Tadalafil
(G. mangostana may possibly be unsafe when used by patients taking phosphodiesterase inhibitors)
Terfenadine
(G. mangostana may possibly be unsafe when used by patients taking antihistamines)
Tinzaparin Sodium
(G. mangostana may possibly be unsafe when used by patients taking anticoagulants)
Trimeprazine Tartrate
(G. mangostana may possibly be unsafe when used by patients taking antihistamines)
Tripelennamine Hydrochloride
(G. mangostana may possibly be unsafe when used by patients taking antihistamines)
Triprolidine Hydrochloride
(G. mangostana may possibly be unsafe when used by patients taking antihistamines)
Vardenafil Hydrochloride
(G. mangostana may possibly be unsafe when used by patients taking phosphodiesterase inhibitors)
Vinpocetine
(G. mangostana may possibly be unsafe when used by patients taking phosphodiesterase inhibitors)
Warfarin Sodium
(G. mangostana may possibly be unsafe when used by patients taking anticoagulants)

MARIJUANA

Alcohol
(Increased intoxication)
Barbiturates
(Excessive CNS depression)
Cocaine Hydrochloride
(Increased effects of cocaine)
Disulfiram
(May induce hypomania reaction)
Protease Inhibitors
(Reduced bioavailability of protease inhibitors)
Selective Serotonin Reuptake Inhibitors
(May induce manic symptoms)
Theophylline
(May require an increase in theophylline dosage)
Tricyclic Antidepressants
(Increased heart rate and delirium)

MATRICARIA RECUTITA

(*See under* German Chamomile)

MECAMYLAMINE HYDROCHLORIDE

Kudzu
(P. lobata may interfere with hypotensive agents)

MEDICAGO SATIVA

(*See under* Alfalfa)

MEDICATION AND FOOD THAT INCREASE URIC ACID LEVELS

Alpine Cranberry
(Decreases effect of Alpine Cranberry)
Uva-Ursi
(Decreases effect of herb)

MELALEUCEA VIRIDIFLORA

(*See under* Niauli)

METFORMIN HYDROCHLORIDE

Bitter Melon
(Concurrent use may result in an increased risk of hypoglycemia)
Kudzu
(P. lobata may lower blood glucose levels)

METHADONE HYDROCHLORIDE

St. John's Wort
(May result in reduced methadone levels and increased risk of withdrawal symptoms)

METHAMPHETAMINE HYDROCHLORIDE

Rhodiola
(May have additive effects with other stimulants)

METHDILAZINE HYDROCHLORIDE

Mangosteen
(G. mangostana may possibly be unsafe when used by patients taking antihistamines)

METHYCLOTHIAZIDE

Kudzu
(P. lobata may interfere with hypotensive agents)

METHYLDOPA

Kudzu
(P. lobata may interfere with hypotensive agents)

METHYLDOPATE HYDROCHLORIDE

Kudzu
(P. lobata may interfere with hypotensive agents)

METHYLPHENIDATE

Rhodiola
(May have additive effects with other stimulants)

METHYLPHENIDATE HYDROCHLORIDE

Rhodiola
(May have additive effects with other stimulants)

METHYLXANTHINES

Digitalis
(Increases risk of cardiac arrhythmias)
Indian Squill
(Can increase the risk of cardic arrhythmias when given simultaneously with this herb)
Squill
(Increases risk of cardiac arrhythmias)

METOLAZONE
Kudzu
(P. lobata may interfere with hypotensive agents)

METOPROLOL SUCCINATE
Kudzu
(P. lobata may interfere with hypotensive agents)

METOPROLOL TARTRATE
Kudzu
(P. lobata may interfere with hypotensive agents)

METYROSINE
Kudzu
(P. lobata may interfere with hypotensive agents)

MEXILETINE HYDROCHLORIDE
Kudzu
(P. lobata may interfere with antiarrhythmic agents)

MIBEFRADIL DIHYDROCHLORIDE
Kudzu
(P. lobata may interfere with hypotensive agents)

MIDODRINE HYDROCHLORIDE
Ma-Huang
(Increased pressor effects)

MIGLITOL
Bitter Melon
(Concurrent use may result in an increased risk of hypoglycemia)
Kudzu
(P. lobata may lower blood glucose levels)

MILK THISTLE
Haloperidol
(Silymarin in combination with haloperidol causes a decrease in lipid peroxidation)
Phenothiazines
(Silymarin in combination with phenothiazines causes a decrease in lipid peroxidation)
Phentolamine Mesylate
(Silymarin antagonizes the effect of phentolamine)
Yohimbine Hydrochloride
(Silymarin antagonizes the effect of yohimbine)

MILRINONE LACTATE
Mangosteen
(G. mangostana may possibly be unsafe when used by patients taking phosphodiesterase inhibitors)

MINOXIDIL
Kudzu
(P. lobata may interfere with hypotensive agents)
Yohimbe Bark
(May decrease hypotensive effect of Minoxidil)

MOCLOBEMIDE
5-HTP
(Concurrent use may result in an increased risk of serotonin syndrome (hypertension, hyperthermia, myoclonus, mental status change))

MOEXIPRIL HYDROCHLORIDE
Kudzu
(P. lobata may interfere with hypotensive agents)

MOMORDICA CHARANTIA
(*See under* Bitter Melon)

MORICIZINE HYDROCHLORIDE
Kudzu
(P. lobata may interfere with antiarrhythmic agents)

MORPHINE SULFATE
Yohimbe Bark
(Potentiates effects of morphine)

NADOLOL
Kudzu
(P. lobata may interfere with hypotensive agents)

NALOXONE HYDROCHLORIDE
Yohimbe Bark
(May increase symptoms of nervousness, anxiety, tremors, palpitations, nausea and hot flushes/cold flushes and increase plasma levels)

NALTREXONE HYDROCHLORIDE
Yohimbe Bark
(Potentiates Yohimbe side effects)

NATEGLINIDE
Bitter Melon
(Concurrent use may result in an increased risk of hypoglycemia)
Kudzu
(P. lobata may lower blood glucose levels)

NEFAZODONE HYDROCHLORIDE
St. John's Wort
(May result in serotonin syndrome manifested as anxiety, confusion, disorientation, diaphoresis, hyperreflexia, myoclonus, rigidity, seizures, tremor, hypertension, hyperthermia, and/or coma)

NERIUM OLEANDER
(*See under* Oleander)

NEUROLEPTICS
Rauwolfia
(Synergistic effect)

NIAULI
Drugs, unspecified
(Co-administration may result in decreased effect of drugs that undergo liver metabolism)

NICARDIPINE
Ginkgo
(May reduce the hypotensive effect of nicardipine)

NICARDIPINE HYDROCHLORIDE
Kudzu
(P. lobata may interfere with hypotensive agents)

NIFEDIPINE
Ginkgo
(May increase mean plasma concentrations of nifedipine)
Ginseng
(May increase the plasma concentration of nifedipine)
Kudzu
(P. lobata may interfere with hypotensive agents)
Senna
(Inhibits activity of Senna via calcium channel blockade)

NISOLDIPINE
Kudzu
(P. lobata may interfere with hypotensive agents)

NITROGLYCERIN

Kudzu
(P. lobata may interfere with hypotensive agents)

NIZATIDINE

Cranberry
(Concurrent use may result in reduced effectiveness of the H2 blocker)

NON-NUCLEOSIDE REVERSE TRANSCRIPTASE INHIBITORS

St. John's Wort
(May result in sub-therapeutic non-nucleoside reverse transcriptase inhibitor levels resulting in treatment failure and drug resistance)

NONSTEROIDAL ANTI-INFLAMMATORY DRUGS

Garlic
(Increased bleeding time due to decreased platelet aggregation)
Ginkgo
(Increased risk of bleeding)
White Willow
(Use with caution; effect not specified)

NORTRIPTYLINE HYDROCHLORIDE

St. John's Wort
(May result in decreased effectiveness of nortriptyline and possible increased risk of serotonin syndrome)

OTC STIMULANTS

Yohimbe Bark
(Potentiates hypertensive effect)

OAK

Alkaline Drugs
(Absorption of alkaline drugs may be reduced or inhibited)
Alkaloids
(Absorption of alkaloids may be reduced or inhibited)

OENOTHERA BIENNIS

(*See under* Evening Primrose)

OLEANDER

Calcium Salts
(Increased efficacy and side effects when given simultaneously with herb)
Glucocorticoids
(Increased efficacy and side effects when given simultaneously with herb)
Laxatives
(Increased efficacy and side effects when given simultaneously with herb)
Quinidine
(Increased efficacy and side effects when given simultaneously with herb)
Saluretics
(Increased efficacy and side effects when given simultaneously with herb)

OMEPRAZOLE

Cranberry
(Concurrent use may result in reduced effectiveness of proton pump inhibitors)

OPIOID ANALGESICS

Ginseng
(May suppress analgesic effects)
St. John's Wort
(May result in increased sedation)
Valerian
(May result in increased CNS depression)

OPIUM PREPARATIONS

Kava Kava
(May increase sedative effects and CNS depression)

ORAL CONTRACEPTIVES

Licorice
(May precipitate rise in blood pressure or fluid retention)
St. John's Wort
(Breakthrough bleeding has been reported with concomitant use of the herb with oral contraceptives)

OXYTOCIN

Ma-Huang
(Development of high blood pressure)

PACLITAXEL

St. John's Wort
(May result reduced paclitaxel effectiveness)

PANAX GINSENG

(*See under* Ginseng)

PANTOPRAZOLE SODIUM

Cranberry
(Concurrent use may result in reduced effectiveness of proton pump inhibitors)

PAPAVERINE

Ginkgo
(May increase the adverse effects of papaverine)

PAPAYA

Warfarin Sodium
(Increased risk of bleeding)

PARGYLINE HYDROCHLORIDE

5-HTP
(Concurrent use may result in an increased risk of serotonin syndrome (hypertension, hyperthermia, myoclonus, mental status change))

PAROXETINE HYDROCHLORIDE

5-HTP
(Concurrent use may result in an increased risk of serotonin syndrome (hypertension, hyperthermia, myoclonus, mental status change); combining 5-HTP with SSRIs may increase the risk of serotonergic side effects)
Mangosteen
(G. mangostana may possibly be unsafe when used by patients taking selective serotonin reuptake inhibitors)

PAULLINIA CUPANA

(*See under* Guarana)

PAUSINYSTALIA YOHIMBE

(*See under* Yohimbe Bark)

PEMOLINE

Rhodiola
(May have additive effects with other stimulants)

PENBUTOLOL SULFATE

Kudzu
(P. lobata may interfere with hypotensive agents)

PERGOLIDE MESYLATE
Chaste Tree
(Enhances dopaminergic adverse effects)

PERINDOPRIL ERBUMINE
Kudzu
(P. lobata may interfere with hypotensive agents)

PHENELZINE SULFATE
5-HTP
(Concurrent use may result in an increased risk of serotonin syndrome (hypertension, hyperthermia, myoclonus, mental status change))

PHENOTHIAZINES
Chaste Tree
(Enhances dopaminergic adverse effects)
Henbane
(Increased anticholinergic action)
Kava Kava
(May decrease effectiveness of dopamine)
Milk Thistle
(Silymarin in combination with phenothiazines causes a decrease in lipid peroxidation)
Wormwood
(Wormwood preparations should not be administered with drugs known to lower the seizure threshold)

PHENOXYBENZAMINE HYDROCHLORIDE
Kudzu
(P. lobata may interfere with hypotensive agents)

PHENTOLAMINE MESYLATE
Kudzu
(P. lobata may interfere with hypotensive agents)
Milk Thistle
(Silymarin antagonizes the effect of phentolamine)

PHENYLPROPANOLAMINE
Ma-Huang
(Risk of arrhythmia)

PHENYTOIN
St. John's Wort
(May result in reduced phenytoin effectiveness)

PHOSPHODIESTERASE INHIBITORS
Digitalis
(Increases risk of cardiac arrhythmias)
Indian Squill
(Can increase the risk of cardic arrhythmias when given simultaneously with this herb)
Squill
(Increases risk of cardiac arrhythmias)

PHOTOSENSITIZING AGENTS
St. John's Wort
(An additive photosensitizing effect is expected when the herb is used with photosensitizing drugs such as tetracyclines, sulfonamides, and thiazides)

PINDOLOL
Kudzu
(P. lobata may interfere with hypotensive agents)

PINEAPPLE
Anticoagulant drugs, unspecified
(Increased nsL and bleeding)
Tetracyclines, unspecified
(Elevated plasma and urine levels of drug)
Thrombolytics
(Increased nsL and bleeding)

PIOGLITAZONE HYDROCHLORIDE
Bitter Melon
(Concurrent use may result in an increased risk of hypoglycemia)
Kudzu
(P. lobata may lower blood glucose levels)

PIPER METHYSTICUM
(*See under* Kava Kava)

PLANTAGO AFRA
(*See under* Psyllium Seed)

PLANTAGO OVATA
(*See under* Psyllium)

POLYESTRADIOL PHOSPHATE
Kudzu
(P. lobata may inhibit the effects of estrogen therapy)
Pygeum
(Prunus may interact with estrogen or other hormones)

POLYTHIAZIDE
Kudzu
(P. lobata may interfere with hypotensive agents)

POTASSIUM PREPARATIONS
Licorice
(Increased risk of hypokalemia)

PRAMIPEXOLE DIHYDROCHLORIDE
Chaste Tree
(Enhances dopaminergic adverse effects)

PRAVASTATIN SODIUM
Bitter Melon
(Bitter melon may potentiate cholesterol-lowering drugs)

PRAZOSIN HYDROCHLORIDE
Kudzu
(P. lobata may interfere with hypotensive agents)

PREDNISONE
Alfalfa
(May reduce effectiveness of prednisone)

PROBUCOL
Bitter Melon
(Bitter melon may potentiate cholesterol-lowering drugs)

PROCAINAMIDE
Henbane
(Increased anticholinergic action)

PROCAINAMIDE HYDROCHLORIDE
Kudzu
(P. lobata may interfere with antiarrhythmic agents)

PROCARBAZINE HYDROCHLORIDE
5-HTP
(Concurrent use may result in an increased risk of serotonin syndrome (hypertension, hyperthermia, myoclonus, mental status change))

PROGESTERONE
Red Clover
(Decreased effectiveness of progesterone)

PROMETHAZINE HYDROCHLORIDE
Mangosteen
(G. mangostana may possibly be unsafe when used by patients taking antihistamines)

PROPAFENONE HYDROCHLORIDE
Kudzu
(P. lobata may interfere with antiarrhythmic agents)

PROPRANOLOL HYDROCHLORIDE
Kudzu
(P. lobata may interfere with antiarrhythmic agents)

PROTEASE INHIBITORS
Garlic
(Increased metabolism of drug)
Marijuana
(Reduced bioavailability of protease inhibitors)
St. John's Wort
(May result in sub-therapeutic protease inhibitor levels resulting in treatment failure and drug resistance)

PRUNUS AFRICANA
(*See under* Pygeum)

PSEUDOEPHEDRINE PREPARATIONS
Ma-Huang
(Excessive andregenic stimulation)

PSYLLIUM
Carbamazepine
(Reduced bioavailability)
Drugs, unspecified
(Absorption of other drugs may be decreased if taken simultaneously with herb)
Insulin
(Effect unspecified; insulin dose should be decreased)
Lithium
(Possible decreased levels of lithium)

PSYLLIUM SEED
Drugs, unspecified
(Absorption of other drugs may be decreased if taken simultaneously with herb)

PUERARIA LOBATA
(*See under* Kudzu)

PUMPKIN
Warfarin Sodium
(Increased risk of bleeding)

PYGEUM
Chlorotrianisene
(Prunus may interact with estrogen or other hormones)
Dienestrol
(Prunus may interact with estrogen or other hormones)
Diethylstilbestrol
(Prunus may interact with estrogen or other hormones)
Estradiol
(Prunus may interact with estrogen or other hormones)
Estrogens, Conjugated
(Prunus may interact with estrogen or other hormones)
Estrogens, Esterified
(Prunus may interact with estrogen or other hormones)
Estropipate
(Prunus may interact with estrogen or other hormones)
Ethinyl Estradiol
(Prunus may interact with estrogen or other hormones)
Herbal Medicines, unspecified
(Prunus may interact with herbs/ supplements containing chemicals with estrogen-like constituents)
Hormones, unspecified
(Prunus may interact with estrogen or other hormones)
Polyestradiol Phosphate
(Prunus may interact with estrogen or other hormones)
Quinestrol
(Prunus may interact with estrogen or other hormones)
Serenoa repens
(Caution in taking concomitantly with saw palmetto)

PYRILAMINE MALEATE
Mangosteen
(G. mangostana may possibly be unsafe when used by patients taking antihistamines)

PYRILAMINE TANNATE
Mangosteen
(G. mangostana may possibly be unsafe when used by patients taking antihistamines)

QUERCUS ROBUR
(*See under* Oak)

QUINAPRIL HYDROCHLORIDE
Kudzu
(P. lobata may interfere with hypotensive agents)

QUINESTROL
Kudzu
(P. lobata may inhibit the effects of estrogen therapy)
Pygeum
(Prunus may interact with estrogen or other hormones)

QUINIDINE
Adonis
(Increases action of Adonis)
Belladonna
(Increases anticholinergic effect of herb)
Digitalis
(Increases risk of cardiac arrhythmias)
Henbane
(Increased anticholinergic action)
Indian Squill
(Can increase the risk of cardic arrhythmias when given simultaneously with this herb)
Kombé Seed
(Increases effects and side effects of herb)
Lily-of-the-Valley
(Increases the effect of Lily-of-the-Valley)
Oleander
(Increased efficacy and side effects when given simultaneously with herb)
Scopolia
(Increased effect when given simultaneously with herb)
Squill
(Increases risk of cardiac arrhythmias; increases effectiveness and side effects of herb)
Strophanthus
(Simultaneous administration with herb enhance both effects and side effects)

QUINIDINE GLUCONATE
Kudzu
(P. lobata may interfere with antiarrhythmic agents)

QUINIDINE POLYGALACTURONATE
Kudzu
(P. lobata may interfere with antiarrhythmic agents)

QUINIDINE SULFATE
Kudzu
(P. lobata may interfere with antiarrhythmic agents)

QUININE
Drugs that Cause Thrombocytopenia
(Herb increases risk of thrombocytopenia)

RABEPRAZOLE SODIUM
Cranberry
(Concurrent use may result in reduced effectiveness of proton pump inhibitors)

RAMIPRIL
Kudzu
(P. lobata may interfere with hypotensive agents)

RANITIDINE BISMUTH CITRATE
Cranberry
(Concurrent use may result in reduced effectiveness of the H2 blocker)

RANITIDINE HYDROCHLORIDE
Cranberry
(Concurrent use may result in reduced effectiveness of the H2 blocker)

RASAGILINE MESYLATE
5-HTP
(Concurrent use may result in an increased risk of serotonin syndrome (hypertension, hyperthermia, myoclonus, mental status change))

RAUWOLFIA
Alcohol
(Increases impairment of motor skills)
Barbiturates
(Synergistic effect)
Digitalis Glycoside Preparations
(Severe bradycardia when used in combination with digitalis glycosides)
Levodopa
(Decreased effect; increases in extra-pyramidal symptoms)
Neuroleptics
(Synergistic effect)
Sympathomimetic Agents
(Increases blood pressure)

RAUWOLFIA SERPENTINA
Kudzu
(P. lobata may interfere with hypotensive agents)

RAUWOLFIA SERPENTINA
(*See under* Rauwolfia)

RED CLOVER
Anticoagulant drugs, unspecified
(Increased risk of bleeding)
Estrogen
(Altered effectiveness or increased side effects)
Low Molecular Weight Heparins
(Increased risk of bleeding)
Progesterone
(Decreased effectiveness of progesterone)
Tamoxifen Citrate
(Decreases effectiveness of tamoxifen citrate)
Thrombolytics
(Increased risk of bleeding)

REPAGLINIDE
Bitter Melon
(Concurrent use may result in an increased risk of hypoglycemia)
Kudzu
(P. lobata may lower blood glucose levels)

RESCINNAMINE
Kudzu
(P. lobata may interfere with hypotensive agents)

RESERPINE
Kudzu
(P. lobata may interfere with hypotensive agents)
St. John's Wort
(May result in reduced reserpine effectiveness)
Yohimbe Bark
(May reduce effectiveness of resperpine)

RHAMNUS CATHARTICUS
(*See under* Buckthorn)

RHAMNUS FRANGULA
(*See under* Frangula)

RHAMNUS PURSHIANA
(*See under* Cascara Sagrada)

RHEUM PALMATUM
(*See under* Chinese Rhubarb)

RHODIOLA
Amphetamine Resins
(May have additive effects with other stimulants)
Dextroamphetamine Sulfate
(May have additive effects with other stimulants)
Methamphetamine Hydrochloride
(May have additive effects with other stimulants)
Methylphenidate
(May have additive effects with other stimulants)
Methylphenidate Hydrochloride
(May have additive effects with other stimulants)
Pemoline
(May have additive effects with other stimulants)

RHODIOLA ROSEA
(*See under* Rhodiola)

RICINUS COMMUNIS
(*See under* Castor Oil Plant)

ROOIBOS
(None cited in PDR database)

ROPINIROLE HYDROCHLORIDE
Chaste Tree
(Enhances dopaminergic adverse effects)

ROSIGLITAZONE MALEATE
Bitter Melon
(Concurrent use may result in an increased risk of hypoglycemia)

Kudzu
(P. lobata may lower blood glucose levels)

SSRIS

St. John's Wort
(May result in an increased risk of serotonin syndrome)

SACCHAROMYCES CEREVISIAE

(*See under* Brewer's Yeast)

SALICYLATES

Bilberry
(Increases prothrombin time; caution should be observed when used concurrently)
White Willow
(Use with caution; effect not specified)

SALIX SPECIES

(*See under* White Willow)

SALURETICS

Adonis
(Increases action of Adonis)
Lily-of-the-Valley
(Increases the effect of Lily-of-the-Valley)
Oleander
(Increased efficacy and side effects when given simultaneously with herb)
Squill
(Increases effectiveness and side effects of herb)
Strophanthus
(Simultaneous administration with herb enhance both effects and side effects)

SAW PALMETTO

Alpha Adrenergic Blockers
(Saw Palmetto has an additive alpha adrenergic blocking effect when given in combination with alpha blockers)
Androgens
(Saw Palmetto antagonizes the effect of androgens)
Iron
(May complex with saw palmetto, creating adverse sequelae on blood)
Warfarin Sodium
(May increase risk of bleeding)

SCOPOLIA

Amantadine Hydrochloride
(Increased effect when given simultaneously with herb)
Quinidine
(Increased effect when given simultaneously with herb)
Tricyclic Antidepressants
(Increased effect when given simultaneously with herb)

SCOPOLIA CARNIOLICA

(*See under* Scopolia)

SCOTCH BROOM

MAO Inhibitors
(Increased risk of hypertensive crisis)

SELECTIVE SEROTONIN REUPTAKE INHIBITORS

Ginkgo
(May precipitate hypomania)
Marijuana
(May induce manic symptoms)
St. John's Wort
(Concomitant use with the herb will result in an additive serotonin effect and possible toxicity)

SELEGILINE

5-HTP
(Concurrent use may result in an increased risk of serotonin syndrome (hypertension, hyperthermia, myoclonus, mental status change))

SELEGILINE HYDROCHLORIDE

5-HTP
(Concurrent use may result in an increased risk of serotonin syndrome (hypertension, hyperthermia, myoclonus, mental status change))

SENNA

Antiarrhythmics
(Senna-induced hypokalemia may increase risk of arrythmia)
Digitalis Glycoside Preparations
(Senna-induced hypokalemia may increase toxicity of digitalis preparations)
Estrogen
(Senna decreases estrogen levels when taken with estrogen supplements)
Indomethacin
(Decreased therapeutic effect of Senna)
Nifedipine
(Inhibits activity of Senna via calcium channel blockade)

SERENOA REPENS

Pygeum
(Caution in taking concomitantly with saw palmetto)

SERENOA REPENS

(*See under* Saw Palmetto)

SERTRALINE HYDROCHLORIDE

5-HTP
(Concurrent use may result in an increased risk of serotonin syndrome (hypertension, hyperthermia, myoclonus, mental status change); combining 5-HTP with SSRIs may increase the risk of serotonergic side effects)
Mangosteen
(G. mangostana may possibly be unsafe when used by patients taking selective serotonin reuptake inhibitors)

SIBERIAN GINSENG

Anticoagulant drugs, unspecified
(May enchance effects)
Antidiabetic Drugs, unspecified
(May potentiate effects)
Antiplatelet Drugs
(May enchance effects)
Antithrombotic Agents
(May enchance effects)
Digoxin
(Elevated serum levels)
Insulin
(May potentiate effects)

SIBUTRAMINE HYDROCHLORIDE MONOHYDRATE

Yohimbe Bark
(May cause adverse cardiovascular effects)

SILDENAFIL CITRATE

Mangosteen
(G. mangostana may possibly be unsafe when used by patients taking phosphodiesterase inhibitors)

SILYBUM MARIANUM

(*See under* Milk Thistle)

SIMVASTATIN

Bitter Melon
(Bitter melon may potentiate cholesterol-lowering drugs)

SIROLIMUS

St. John's Wort
(May result in sub-therapeutic sirolimus levels resulting in possible transplant rejection)

SITAGLIPTIN PHOSPHATE

Bitter Melon
(Concurrent use may result in an increased risk of hypoglycemia)

Kudzu
(P. lobata may lower blood glucose levels)

SKELETAL MUSCLE RELAXANTS

Kava Kava
(May increase sedative effects and CNS depression)

SLIPPERY ELM

Iron
(Reduced absorption of iron)

SODIUM NITROPRUSSIDE

Kudzu
(P. lobata may interfere with hypotensive agents)

SOTALOL HYDROCHLORIDE

Kudzu
(P. lobata may interfere with antiarrhythmic agents)

SOYBEAN

Iron
(May result in reduced absorption of iron)

Levothyroxine Sodium
(May result in decreased effectiveness of Levothyroxine)

Tamoxifen Citrate
(May result in reduced effectiveness of Tamoxifen)

Warfarin Sodium
(May result in reduced effectiveness of Warfarin)

SPIRAPRIL HYDROCHLORIDE

Kudzu
(P. lobata may interfere with hypotensive agents)

SQUILL

Calcium
(Increases effectiveness and side effects of herb)

Digoxin
(Squill potentiates the positive inotropic and negative chronopic effects of digoxin)

Glucocorticoids
(Increases effectiveness and side effects of herb)

Laxatives
(Increases effectiveness and side effects of herb)

Methylxanthines
(Increases risk of cardiac arrhythmias)

Phosphodiesterase Inhibitors
(Increases risk of cardiac arrhythmias)

Quinidine
(Increases risk of cardiac arrhythmias; increases effectiveness and side effects of herb)

Saluretics
(Increases effectiveness and side effects of herb)

Sympathomimetic Agents
(Increases risk of cardiac arrhythmias)

ST. JOHN'S WORT

Acitretin
(May result in unplanned pregnancy and birth defects)

Aminolevulinic Acid Hydrochloride
(May result in increased risk of phototoxic reaction)

Amiodarone Hydrochloride
(Extends risk for reducing amiodarone levels)

Anticoagulant drugs, unspecified
(May result in reduced effectiveness of anticoagulants)

Antidiabetic Drugs, unspecified
(May result in hypoglycemia)

Barbiturates
(May decrease the CNS depressant effect of barbiturates)

Benzodiazepines
(May result in reduced benzodiazepines effectiveness)

Beta Blockers
(May induce the metabolism of beta-blockers resulting in reduced drug concentrations and decreased effectiveness of beta-blockers)

Buspirone Hydrochloride
(May result in an increased risk of serotonin syndrome (hypertension, hyperthermia, myoclonus, mental status changes))

Caffeine
(May result in increased caffeine metabolism)

Calcium Channel Blockers, Unspecified
(May result in decreased effectiveness of calcium channel blockers)

Carbamazepine
(May result in altered carbamazepine blood concentrations)

Chlorzoxazone
(May result in reduced chlorzoxazone effectiveness)

Clozapine
(May decrease effectiveness of clozapine secondary to induction of drug-metabolizing enzymes in the liver)

Cyclophosphamide
(May result in reduced chyclophophamide effectiveness)

Cyclosporine
(May result in decreased cyclosporine levels and acute transplant rejection)

Digoxin
(May result in significantly lower serum digoxin levels)

Etoposide
(May result in reduced effectiveness of etoposide)

Ginkgo biloba
(May have precipitated a hypomanic episode in a case report)
Imatinib Mesylate
(May result in decreased imatinim effectiveness)
Indinavir Sulfate
(The herb induces the cytochrome P450 enzyme system and will lower indinavir serum levels)
Irinotecan Hydrochloride
(May result in decreased imatinib effectiveness)
Iron
(May result in non-absorbable insoluble complexes and may result in adverse sequelae on blood components)
Loperamide Hydrochloride
(May result in delirium with symptoms of confusion, agitation and disorientation)
MAO Inhibitors
(Increased risk of serotonin syndrome (hypertension, hyperthermia, myoclonus, mental status changes) and/or an increased risk of hypertensive crisis)
Methadone Hydrochloride
(May result in reduced methadone levels and increased risk of withdrawal symptoms)
Nefazodone Hydrochloride
(May result in serotonin syndrome manifested as anxiety, confusion, disorientation, diaphoresis, hyperreflexia, myoclonus, rigidity, seizures, tremor, hypertension, hyperthermia, and/or coma)
Non-Nucleoside Reverse Transcriptase Inhibitors
(May result in sub-therapeutic non-nucleoside reverse transcriptase inhibitor levels resulting in treatment failure and drug resistance)
Nortriptyline Hydrochloride
(May result in decreased effectiveness of nortriptyline and possible increased risk of serotonin syndrome)
Opioid Analgesics
(May result in increased sedation)
Oral Contraceptives
(Breakthrough bleeding has been reported with concomitant use of the herb with oral contraceptives)
Paclitaxel
(May result reduced paclitaxel effectiveness)
Phenytoin
(May result in reduced phenytoin effectiveness)
Photosensitizing Agents
(An additive photosensitizing effect is expected when the herb is used with photosensitizing drugs such as tetracyclines, sulfonamides, and thiazides)
Protease Inhibitors
(May result in sub-therapeutic protease inhibitor levels resulting in treatment failure and drug resistance)
Reserpine
(May result in reduced reserpine effectiveness)
SSRIs
(May result in an increased risk of serotonin syndrome)
Selective Serotonin Reuptake Inhibitors
(Concomitant use with the herb will result in an additive serotonin effect and possible toxicity)
Sirolimus
(May result in sub-therapeutic sirolimus levels resulting in possible transplant rejection)
Statins
(May result in reduced effectiveness of statin drugs)
Sympathomimetic Agents
(St. John's Wort may have MAO inhibitor properties and caution should be used with sympathomimetic agents)
Tacrolimus
(May result in sub-therapeutic tacrolimus levels)
Tamoxifen Citrate
(May result in reduced tamoxifen effectiveness)
Theophylline
(May result in reduced theophylline efficacy)
Trazodone Hydrochloride
(May result in risk of serotonin syndrome (hypertension, hyperthermia, myoclonus, mental status changes) and/or coma)
Tricyclic Antidepressants
(May result in risk of serotonin syndrome (hypertension, hyperthermia, myoclonus, mental status changes) and/or coma)
Tyramine
(May result in increased risk of hypertensive crisis)
Venlafaxine Hydrochloride
(May result in risk of serotonin syndrome (hypertension, hyperthermia, myoclonus, mental status changes) and/or coma)

STATINS

St. John's Wort
(May result in reduced effectiveness of statin drugs)

STROPHANTHUS

Calcium Salts
(Simultaneous administration with herb enhance both effects and side effects)
Glucocorticoids
(Simultaneous administration with herb enhance both effects and side effects)
Laxatives
(Simultaneous administration with herb enhance both effects and side effects)
Quinidine
(Simultaneous administration with herb enhance both effects and side effects)
Saluretics
(Simultaneous administration with herb enhance both effects and side effects)
Calcium Salts
(Simultaneous administration with herb enhance both effects and side effects)

Glucocorticoids
(Simultaneous administration with herb enhance both effects and side effects)
Laxatives
(Simultaneous administration with herb enhance both effects and side effects)
Quinidine
(Simultaneous administration with herb enhance both effects and side effects)
Saluretics
(Simultaneous administration with herb enhance both effects and side effects)

STROPHANTHUS GRATUS
(*See under* Strophanthus)

STROPHANTHUS HISPIDUS
(*See under* Kombe Seed)

STROPHANTHUS KOMBE
(*See under* Strophanthus)

SYMPATHOMIMETIC AGENTS
Digitalis
(Increases risk of cardiac arrhythmias)
Indian Squill
(Can increase the risk of cardic arrhythmias when given simultaneously with this herb)
Ma-Huang
(Increased effects of ephedrine)
Rauwolfia
(Increases blood pressure)
Squill
(Increases risk of cardiac arrhythmias)
St. John's Wort
(St. John's Wort may have MAO inhibitor properties and caution should be used with sympathomimetic agents)

TACROLIMUS
St. John's Wort
(May result in sub-therapeutic tacrolimus levels)

TADALAFIL
Mangosteen
(G. mangostana may possibly be unsafe when used by patients taking phosphodiesterase inhibitors)

TAMOXIFEN CITRATE
Red Clover
(Decreases effectiveness of tamoxifen citrate)
Soybean
(May result in reduced effectiveness of Tamoxifen)
St. John's Wort
(May result in reduced tamoxifen effectiveness)

TANACETUM PARTHENIUM
(*See under* Feverfew)

TELMISARTAN
Kudzu
(P. lobata may interfere with hypotensive agents)

TERAZOSIN HYDROCHLORIDE
Kudzu
(P. lobata may interfere with hypotensive agents)

TERFENADINE
Mangosteen
(G. mangostana may possibly be unsafe when used by patients taking antihistamines)

TESTOSTERONE
Licorice
(Reduced levels of testosterone)

TETRACYCLINES, UNSPECIFIED
Pineapple
(Elevated plasma and urine levels of drug)

THEOPHYLLINE
Ma-Huang
(CNS and gastrointestinal adverse events)
Marijuana
(May require an increase in theophylline dosage)
St. John's Wort
(May result in reduced theophylline efficacy)

THIAZIDE DIURETICS
Aloe
(Increased potassium loss)
Buckthorn
(Increases hypokalemic effects)
Cascara Sagrada
(Increases hypokalemic effect)
Ginkgo
(May increase blood pressure)
Licorice
(Additive effect of hypokalemia)
Uva-Ursi
(The sodium-sparing effect of Uva-Ursi may antagonize the diuretic effect of thiazide diuretics)

THROMBOLYTICS
Arnica
(Increased risk of bleeding)
Garlic
(Increased risk of bleeding)
Ginger
(Increased risk of bleeding)
Ginkgo
(Increased risk of bleeding)
Kava Kava
(May increase risk of bleeding)
Licorice
(May increase risk of bleeding)
Pineapple
(Increased nsL and bleeding)
Red Clover
(Increased risk of bleeding)
Valerian
(Increased risk of bleeding)

THYROID PREPARATIONS
Bugleweed
(Effect not specified)

TIMOLOL MALEATE
Kudzu
(P. lobata may interfere with hypotensive agents)

TINZAPARIN SODIUM
Mangosteen
(G. mangostana may possibly be unsafe when used by patients taking anticoagulants)

TOCAINIDE HYDROCHLORIDE
Kudzu
(P. lobata may interfere with antiarrhythmic agents)

TOLAZAMIDE
Bitter Melon
(Concurrent use may result in an increased risk of hypoglycemia)

Kudzu
(P. lobata may lower blood glucose levels)

TOLBUTAMIDE
Bitter Melon
(Concurrent use may result in an increased risk of hypoglycemia)
Kudzu
(P. lobata may lower blood glucose levels)

TORSEMIDE
Kudzu
(P. lobata may interfere with hypotensive agents)

TRANDOLAPRIL
Kudzu
(P. lobata may interfere with hypotensive agents)

TRANYLCYPROMINE SULFATE
5-HTP
(Concurrent use may result in an increased risk of serotonin syndrome (hypertension, hyperthermia, myoclonus, mental status change))

TRAZODONE HYDROCHLORIDE
St. John's Wort
(May result in risk of serotonin syndrome (hypertension, hyperthermia, myoclonus, mental status changes) and/or coma)
Wormwood
(Wormwood preparations should not be administered with drugs known to lower the seizure threshold)

TRICYCLIC ANTIDEPRESSANTS
Belladonna
(Increases anticholinergic effect of herb)
Henbane
(Increased anticholinergic action)
Marijuana
(Increased heart rate and delirium)
Scopolia
(Increased effect when given simultaneously with herb)
St. John's Wort
(May result in risk of serotonin syndrome (hypertension, hyperthermia, myoclonus, mental status changes) and/or coma)
Wormwood
(Wormwood preparations should not be administered with drugs known to lower the seizure threshold)

TRIFOLIUM PRATENSE
(*See under* Red Clover)

TRIGONELLA FOENUM-GRAECUM
(*See under* Fenugreek)

TRIMEPRAZINE TARTRATE
Mangosteen
(G. mangostana may possibly be unsafe when used by patients taking antihistamines)

TRIMETHAPHAN CAMSYLATE
Kudzu
(P. lobata may interfere with hypotensive agents)

TRIPELENNAMINE HYDROCHLORIDE
Mangosteen
(G. mangostana may possibly be unsafe when used by patients taking antihistamines)

TRIPROLIDINE HYDROCHLORIDE
Mangosteen
(G. mangostana may possibly be unsafe when used by patients taking antihistamines)

TROGLITAZONE
Bitter Melon
(Concurrent use may result in an increased risk of hypoglycemia)
Kudzu
(P. lobata may lower blood glucose levels)

TYRAMINE
St. John's Wort
(May result in increased risk of hypertensive crisis)

ULMUS RUBRA
(*See under* Slippery Elm)

URGINEA INDICA
(*See under* Indian Squill)

URGINEA MARITIMA
(*See under* Squill)

URINARY TRACT ACIDIFIERS
Uva-Ursi
(Drugs or foods that acidify the urine will decrease the antibacterial effect of Uva-Ursi)

UVA-URSI
Iron
(May complex with iron and result in adverse sequelae on blood components)
Loop Diuretics
(The sodium-sparing effect of Uva-Ursi may antagonize the diuretic effect of the loop diuretics)
Medication and Food that Increase Uric Acid Levels
(Decreases effect of herb)
Thiazide Diuretics
(The sodium-sparing effect of Uva-Ursi may antagonize the diuretic effect of thiazide diuretics)
Urinary Tract Acidifiers
(Drugs or foods that acidify the urine will decrease the antibacterial effect of Uva-Ursi)

UZARA
Digoxin
(Herb contains cardiac glycosides and may have additive effect when taken with digoxin, possibly increasing digoxin toxicity)

VACCINIUM MACROCARPON
(*See under* Cranberry)

VACCINIUM MYRTILLUS
(*See under* Bilberry)

VACCINIUM VITIS-IDAEA
(*See under* Alpine Cranberry)

VALERIAN
Alcohol
(Additive depressive effects with Valerian)
Anticoagulant drugs, unspecified
(Increased risk of bleeding)
Antiplatelet Drugs
(Increased risk of bleeding)
Barbiturates
(Increased CNS effects possible, especially sedation)
Benzodiazepines
(CNS effects may be increased)
Hepatotoxic Drugs, unspecified
(May increase liver transaminases)

Hypnotics
(Additive effect when taken with Valerian)
Iron
(May complex with iron and result in adverse sequelae on blood components)
Loperamide Hydrochloride
(May result in delirium, confusion, agitation or disorientation)
Opioid Analgesics
(May result in increased CNS depression)
Thrombolytics
(Increased risk of bleeding)

VALERIANA OFFICINALIS
(*See under* Valerian)

VALPROIC ACID
Yohimbe Bark
(May predispose patients to manic episodes)

VALSARTAN
Kudzu
(P. lobata may interfere with hypotensive agents)

VARDENAFIL HYDROCHLORIDE
Mangosteen
(G. mangostana may possibly be unsafe when used by patients taking phosphodiesterase inhibitors)

VENLAFAXINE HYDROCHLORIDE
St. John's Wort
(May result in risk of serotonin syndrome (hypertension, hyperthermia, myoclonus, mental status changes) and/or coma)

VERAPAMIL HYDROCHLORIDE
Kudzu
(P. lobata may interfere with antiarrhythmic agents)

VINPOCETINE
Mangosteen
(G. mangostana may possibly be unsafe when used by patients taking phosphodiesterase inhibitors)

VITAMIN B COMPLEX
Goldenseal
(May decrease Vitamin B absorption)

VITEX AGNUS-CASTUS
(*See under* Chaste Tree)

WARFARIN SODIUM
Arnica
(Additive anticoagulant effect)
Bilberry
(Increases prothrombin time; caution should be observed when used concurrently)
Cranberry
(Concurrent use may result in increased risk of bleeding)
Feverfew
(Increased antithrombotic effect)
German Chamomile
(Hydroxycoumarin component in Chamomile may elevate prothrombin times)
Mangosteen
(G. mangostana may possibly be unsafe when used by patients taking anticoagulants)
Papaya
(Increased risk of bleeding)
Pumpkin
(Increased risk of bleeding)
Saw Palmetto
(May increase risk of bleeding)
Soybean
(May result in reduced effectiveness of Warfarin)

WHITE WILLOW
Alcohol
(Enhances toxicity of salicylates)
Antiplatelet Drugs
(Additive effect with salicylates)
Barbiturates
(Enhances toxicity of salicylates)
Carbonic Anhydrase Inhibitors
(Potentiates action of salicylates)
Nonsteroidal Anti-Inflammatory Drugs
(Use with caution; effect not specified)
Salicylates
(Use with caution; effect not specified)

WILD YAM
Estrogen
(Additive effect)
Indomethacin
(Wild Yam may decrease the anti-inflammatory effect of indomethacin)

WORMWOOD
Iron
(May complex with iron, resulting in adverse sequelae on blood components)
Phenothiazines
(Wormwood preparations should not be administered with drugs known to lower the seizure threshold)
Trazodone Hydrochloride
(Wormwood preparations should not be administered with drugs known to lower the seizure threshold)
Tricyclic Antidepressants
(Wormwood preparations should not be administered with drugs known to lower the seizure threshold)

XYSMALOBIUM UNDULATUM
(*See under* Uzara)

YARROW
Iron
(May complex with iron, resulting in adverse sequelae on blood components)

YOHIMBE BARK
Antihypertensive agents, unspecified
(May need to adjust antihypertensive medications due to hypertensive effect of Yohimbe)
Carbamazepine
(Precipitates manic episodes in bipolar disorder)
Clomipramine Hydrochloride
(Increased risk of hypertension)
Clonidine
(Reduced effectiveness of clonidine)
Ethanol
(Increased anxiogenic effects)

Guanabenz Acetate
(May decrease hypotensive effect of Guanabenz)
Guanadrel Sulfate
(May decrease hypotensive effect of Guanadrel)
Guanethidine
(May decrease hypotensive effect of Guanethidine)
Guanfacine Hydrochloride
(May decrease hypotensive effect of Guanfacine)
Lithium
(Precipitates manic episodes in bipolar disorder)
Minoxidil
(May decrease hypotensive effect of Minoxidil)
Morphine Sulfate
(Potentiates effects of morphine)
Naloxone Hydrochloride
(May increase symptoms of nervousness, anxiety, tremors, palpitations, nausea and hot flushes/cold flushes and increase plasma levels)
Naltrexone Hydrochloride
(Potentiates Yohimbe side effects)
OTC stimulants
(Potentiates hypertensive effect)
Reserpine
(May reduce effectiveness of resperpine)
Sibutramine Hydrochloride Monohydrate
(May cause adverse cardiovascular effects)
Valproic Acid
(May predispose patients to manic episodes)

YOHIMBINE HYDROCHLORIDE

Milk Thistle
(Silymarin antagonizes the effect of yohimbine)

ZINGIBER OFFICINALE

(*See under* Ginger)

Safety Guide

This guide lists botanicals in three precautionary categories:

- *Not for use during pregnancy*
- *Not for use while nursing*
- *For use only under supervision*

All common and scientific names of each potentially harmful botanical are listed alphabetically. Generally accepted common names that serve as monograph titles appear in bold type. Scientific names are shown in italic type. If an entry lists two page numbers, the first refers to a photograph of the plant or product in the Identification Guide, the second to the herbal monograph. For additional information on potential adverse effects, be sure to check the appropriate underlying monograph.

Not for use during pregnancy

Not for use while nursing

For use only under supervision

Common Herbal Terminology

Common Herbal Terminology

In this section, you'll find a brief glossary of the terms that frequently appear in discussions of herbs and herbal remedies. Some are familiar from the current medical literature. Others are now considered archaic, but can still be found in foreign herbal references.

abortifacient A drug or chemical that induces abortion.

achene A small 1-seeded fruit which has a pericarp attached to the seed at only one point.

acuminate Pointed, or tapering to a slender point.

adaptogen A preparation that acts to strengthen the body and increase resistance to disease.

alterative Any drug used to favorably alter the course of an ailment and to restore health. To improve the excretion of wastes from the circulatory system.

amarum Bitters.

androgynous In botany, flowers with stamen and pistil in the same bunch.

annual A plant that completes its growth cycle in one year.

anthelmintic An agent or drug that is destructive to worms.

anther The part of the stamen that contains pollen.

antiphlogistic An agent that prevents or counteracts inflammation and fever.

antisialagogue An agent that prevents or counteracts the formation or flow of saliva.

autumnalis In botany, referring to producing, gathering, or harvesting in the autumn.

bitter An alcoholic liquid prepared by maceration or distillation of a bitter herb or herb part that is often used to improve appetite or digestion.

blood purification Removal of undesirable agents from the blood.

bracteole A small leaf arising from the floral axis.

brightening agent A substance added to the active constituents.

calculosis The condition or formation of calculi.

calyx The outer set of floral leaves consisting of fused or separate sepals.

campanulate Shaped like a bell.

capitulum A rounded or flattened cluster of sessile flowers.

capsule A closed container that contains seeds or spores.

carminative An aid to relieve gas from the alimentary canal.An agent that acts to relieve colic.

carpel A small pistil or seed vessel comprising the innermost whorl of a flower.

cataplasm A poultice or soft external application.

catarrh An inflammation of the air passages usually involving the nose, throat, or lungs.

catkin A cattail-like inflorescence bearing scaly bracts.

cauline Growing on the upper portion of a stem.

cholagogue An agent that stimulates the flow of bile from the gallbladder to the duodenum.

choleretic An agent that stimulates the production of bile by the liver.

climacteric The syndrome of physical and psychic changes that occur during the transition to menopause.

comminuted Broken or crushed into small pieces.

cordate A heart-shaped leaf.

coriaceous Tough, strong, and leather-like.

corolla The inner set of floral leaves that consist of separate or fused leaves.

cortex In botany, the bark of a tree or the rind of a fruit.

cotyledon A seed leaf, or the first set of leaves from the embryo in seed plants.

crenate In reference to leaf structure, having a margin cut into rounded scallops.

cyme An inflorescence where the axes always end in a single flower.

deciduous A tree that sheds its leaves at the end of the growing season.

decoction A liquid substance prepared by boiling plant parts in water or some other liquid for a period of time.

decumbent A plant, stem, or shoot that lays on the ground but terminates with an ascending apex.

dentate Tooth-like projections on the margin of a leaf.

dessertspoon A unit of measure equal to about 2½ fluidrams.

diaphoretic An agent that causes sweating or excessive perspiration.

dioecious In botany, when a plant has either a stamen or a pistil on each flower.

downy Covered with soft hairs.

dromotropic An effect on nerve fiber conduction.

dropsy An abnormal accumulation of fluid in body tissues or cavities usually related to an underlying disease.

drupe A one-seeded fruit; as in an olive or a peach.

embrocation An external medication applied as a liniment or other liquid form.

emmenagogue A substance that renews or stimulates the menstrual flow.

endosperm The albumin of the seed.

epicalyx An external accessory calyx located outside the true calyx of the flower.

eructation The act of belching.

exocarp The outer wall of a fruit covering.

extraction The portion of a plant that is removed by solvents and used in drug preparations in solid or liquid form.

febrifuge An agent that counteracts fever; an antipyretic.

floret A little flower; one of the small individual flowers that form a cluster or head.

flos Flower.

fluidextract A hydroalcoholic preparation of a botanical drug where 1 ml of the preparation contains 1 gm of the standard botanical.

folium The leaf of a plant.

fructus Fruit.

furuncle A boil or sore caused by bacterial infection of the subcutaneous tissue.

galenic preparation Medications prepared from plants as opposed to refined chemicals.

glabrous Having a smooth surface; without hair or down.

globular Spherical.

hastate Plant leaves with a triangular shape with the base coming together on each side into an acute lobe.

hilum The scar on a seed which indicates its point of attachment.

homeopathic Substances that are administered in minute amounts with the theory that substances that may cause or mimic a disease in larger amounts can be used to treat or prevent disease if given in small amounts.

imbricate Overlapping flower petals; as in the bud.

indehiscent A fruit or grain that doesn't open spontaneously when ripe.

induration The process of hardening.

inflorescence The mode of disposition of flowers or the act of flowering. The spatial arrangement of flowers along the axis.

infusion The process of steeping or soaking plant matter in a liquid to extract its medicinal properties without boiling.

involucre A ring or rosette of leaves that surround the base of a flower cluster.

labiate A lip-like part of a plant; like a calyx or corolla.

lanceolate Lance-like or spear shaped; often referring to a long, tapering leaf.

lignum Woody tissue.

maceration The softening of a solid preparation by soakingit in a liquid.

meteorism The presence of gas in the intestine or stomach.

monoecious Having stamens and pistils in separate blossoms on the same plant.

mucilage 1. A viscid substance in a plant consisting of a gum dissolved in the juice of the plant. 2. A soothing application made from plant gums.

muscarinic An effect characterized by contraction of smooth muscle, excessive salivation and perspiration, abdominal colic and excessive bronchial secretion.

nutlet The stone in a drupe.

obstipation Persistent or intractable constipation.

panicle A loose, multiple flower cluster usually formed fromnumerous branches.

pedicel The stalk that supports a single flower in an inflores-cence of flowers arranged upon a common peduncle.

peduncle A stalk that bears a flower or flower cluster.

percolation A liquid containing the soluble portion of a drug that has been filtered or separated from the plant matter.

perennial A plant that grows for three or more years.

perianth The external envelope of a flower which does not include the calyx and corolla if they are distinguishable.

pericarp The wall of the ripened ovary of a flower containing the germ of the fruit.

petal One of the leaves of the corolla.

petiolate The footstalk of a leaf.

pinnate Compound leaves or leaflets that have a feather-like arrangement with leaves arranged on both sides of a common axis.

pinnatisect Cleft pinnately or almost to the midrib.

pistil The seed-bearing organ of flowering plants consisting of the ovary and the stigma; usually with a style.

plaster A viscous substance that is spread on linen or cloth and applied to a part of the body for healing purposes.

poultice A soft, moist mass of plant parts that are wrapped inmuslin or gauze and applied warm or hot to the skin.

pubescent In botany, having a fuzzy surface; covered with soft fine short hairs.

raceme An inflorescence where flowers are borne on stalks at an almost equal distance apart along an elongated axis that continues to grow with flowers opening in succession from below.

radix The root of a plant.

reniform When describing a leaf, kidney or bean shaped.

resin An amorphous, solid or semi-solid substance produced by plants usually as a result of terpene oxidation.

reticulate Veins, fibers, or lines crossing like a network across the surface of a leaf.

rhizome An underground stem.

roborant A tonic or substance that gives strength.

runners A plant that spreads or forms by means of runners.

scape A flower stalk or peduncle arising from the surface or from below the ground.

schizocarp A dry fruit that splits at maturity into several one-seeded carpels.

scrofulous Having an ulcerous or diseased appearance on the surface.

secretagogue An agent that promotes secretion.

secretolytic To inhibit or dry secretions.

semen A seed or seed-like fruit.

sepal One of the modified leaves comprising a calyx; usually positioned outside and surrounding the carpels.

serrate Having notched, teeth-like protrusions along the margin of a leaf that points toward the apex.

sessile Attached directly to the base of a main stem or branch without the aid of an intervening stalk.

stamen The organ of the flower that comprises the anther and filament and gives rise to the male gamete.

stipule A stalk.

stomachic An agent that promotes digestion and improves appetite.

subshrub A perennial plant which has woody stems with theexception of the terminal portion of new growth, which drops off annually.

sudorific Causing or inducing sweat.

tendril The portion of a stem, leaf, or stipule that modified into a slender, spiral-shaped, touch-sensitive specialized appendage, which acts as an anchor to aid in the plants ability to climb.

tepal Any of the modified leaves that combine to make up the perianth.

testa The hard outer coating of a seed; the exocarp.

tincture An alcoholic or hydroalcoholic mixture prepared from plant parts.

tomentose Covered with densely matted hairs.

tonic A medication used to fortify and provide increased vigor.

turiones A shoot or sprout which develops from a bud on a subterranean rootstock.

umbel Numerous flower stalks arising from the same point at the apex of the main stalk and terminating at an equal distance from the joining point.

undulate A wavy formation at the margin of a leaf, or bending in a gradual curve.

villous Having long, soft hairs.

vulnery A preparation applied externally.

wineglassful A measure equal to four fluid ounces.

Herb Identification Guide

In this full-color photo section, you'll find pictures of over 300 common medicinal plants. Each herb is labeled with its generally accepted common name immediately above the photo, and its scientific name immediately below. The pictures are arranged alphabetically by common name.

Please note that the plants are not reproduced in actual size, and that the scale of the photos varies. For the average dimensions of the plant and its component structures, please check the Description section of the corresponding herbal monograph.

ABSCESS ROOT

Polemonium reptans

AGRIMONY

Agrimonia eupatoria

ALOE

Aloe species

AMERICAN IVY

Parthenocissus quinquefolia

ADONIS

Adonis vernalis

ALFALFA

Medicago sativa

ALPINE CRANBERRY

Vaccinium vitis-idaea

AMERICAN WHITE POND LILY

Nymphaea odorata

ADRUE

Cyperus articulatus

ALISMA

Alisma plantago-aquatica

AMARANTH

Amaranthus species

ANGELICA

Angelica archangelica

AGA

Amanita muscaria

ALKANET

Alkanna tinctoria

AMARGO

Quassia amara

ANISE

Pimpinella anisum

APPLE TREE

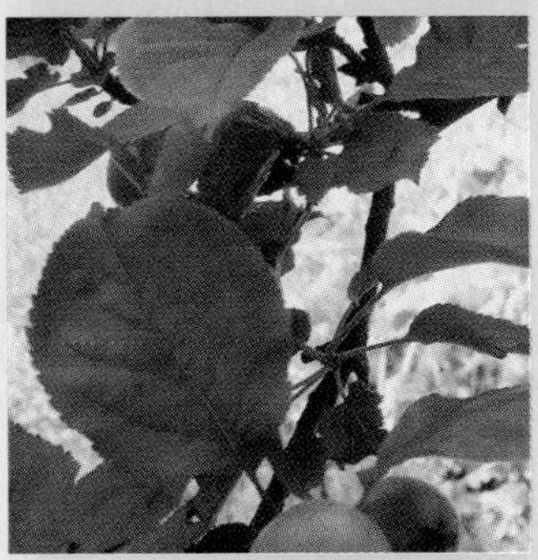

Malus domestica

ARECA NUT

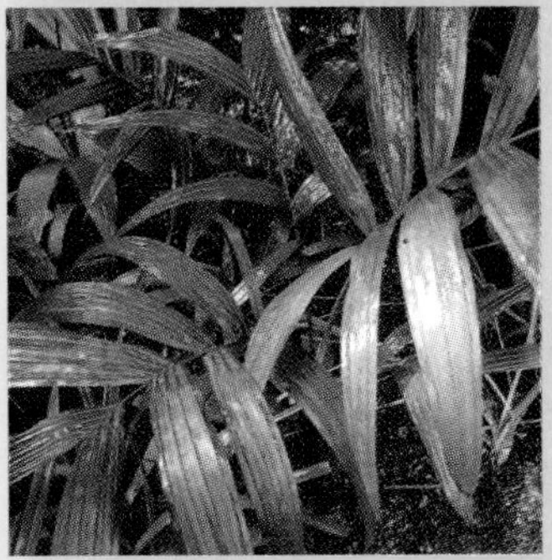

Areca catechu

ARTICHOKE

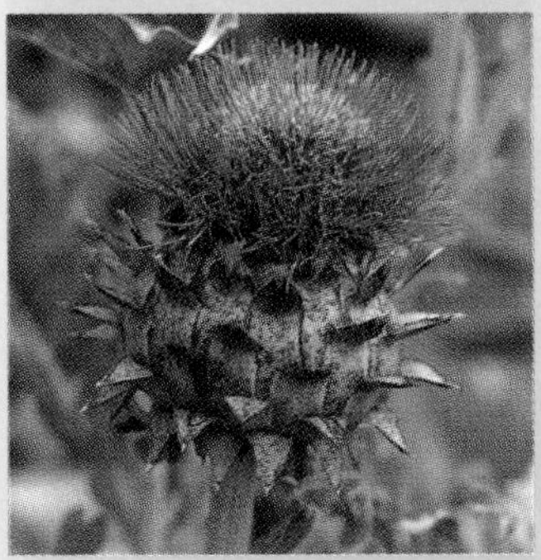

Cynara scolymus

ASH

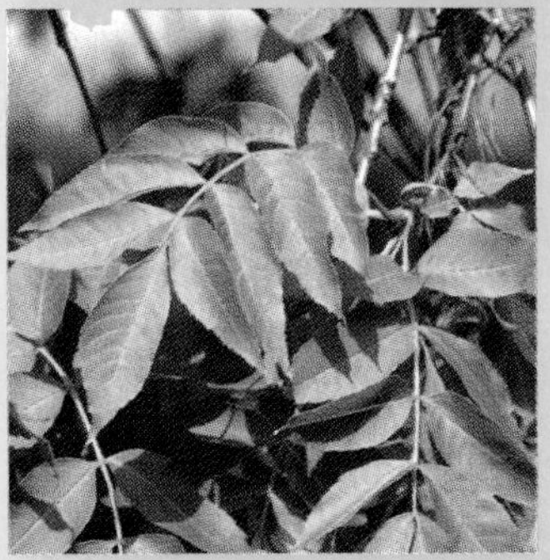

Fraxinus excelsior

ASPARAGUS

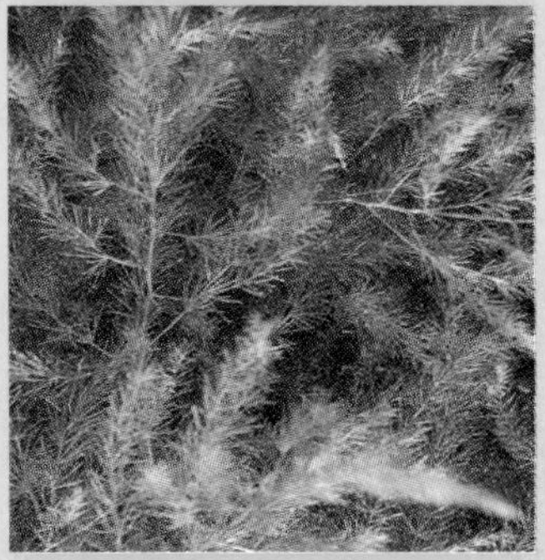

Asparagus officinalis

BALMONY

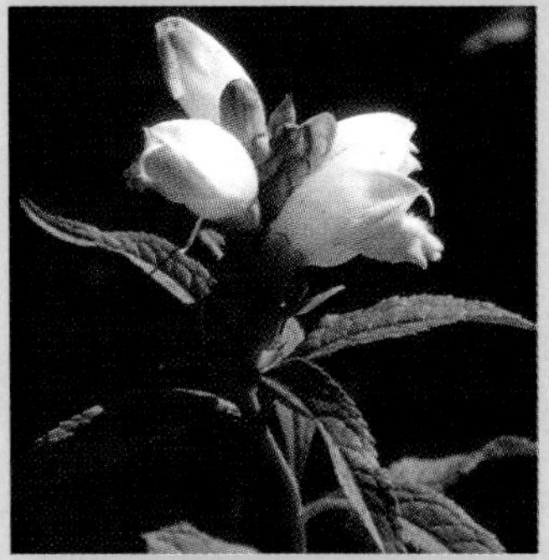

Chelone glabra

BAMBOO

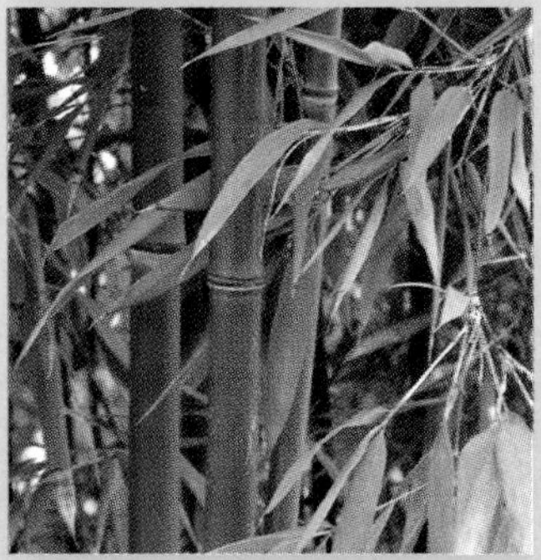

Arundinaria japonica

BARBERRY

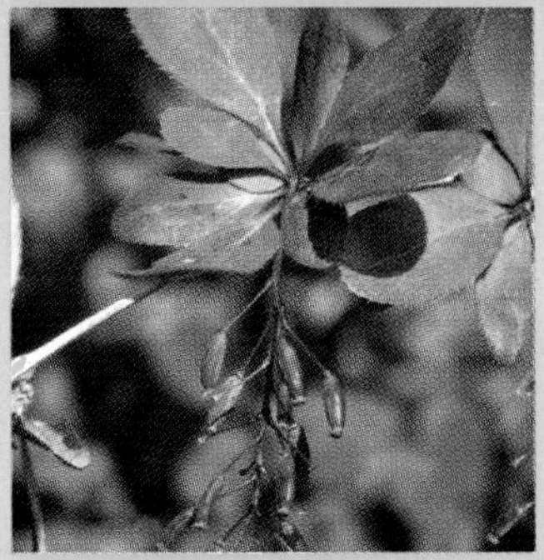

Berberis vulgaris

BARLEY

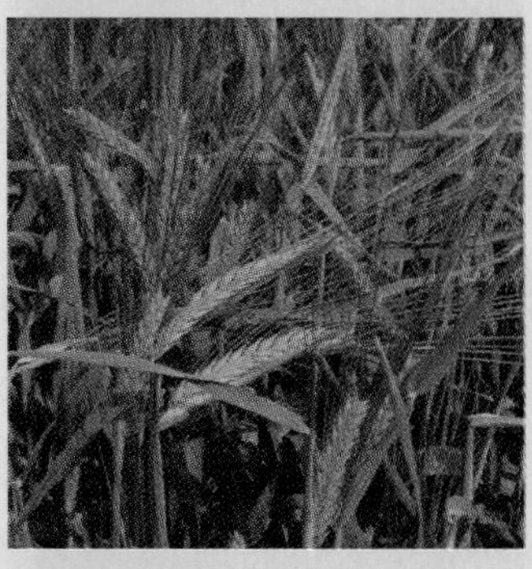

Hordeum species

BASIL

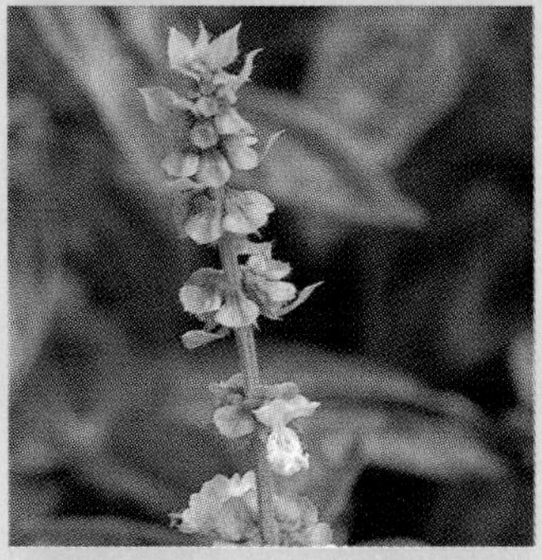

Ocimum basilicum

BEAN POD

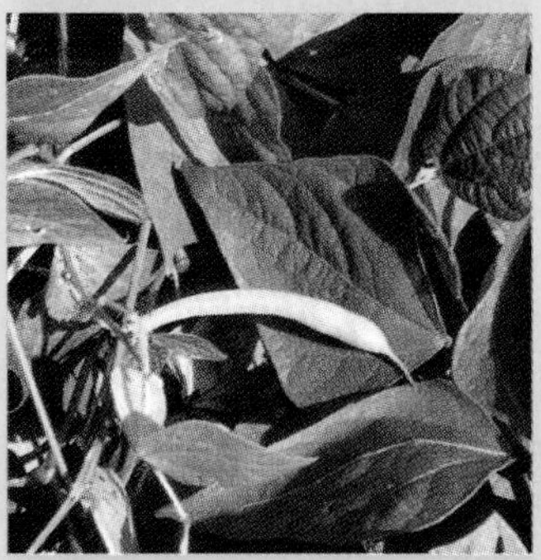

Phaseolus vulgaris

BEET

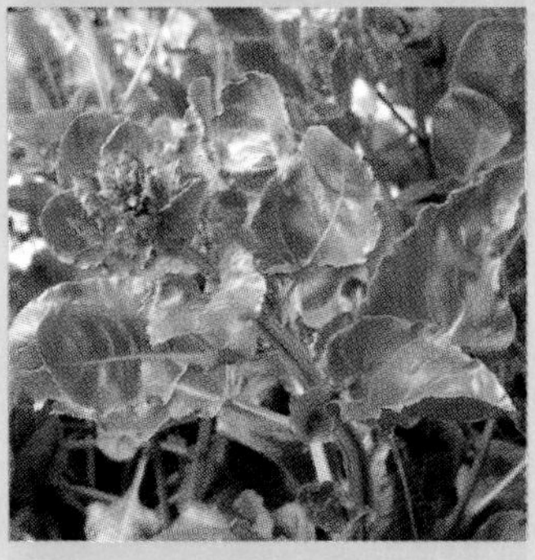

Beta vulgaris

BELLADONNA

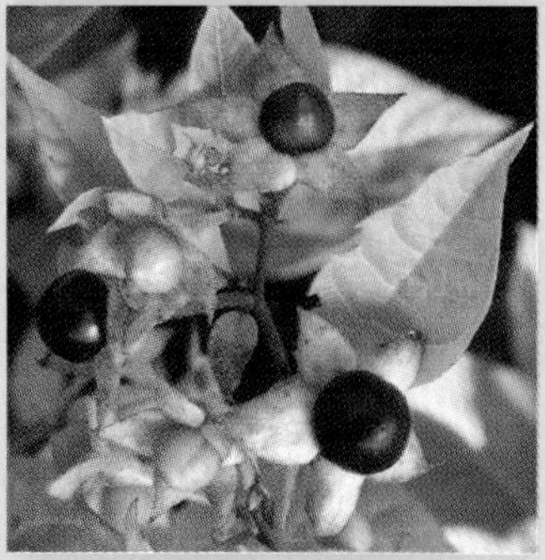

Atropa belladonna

BENNET'S ROOT

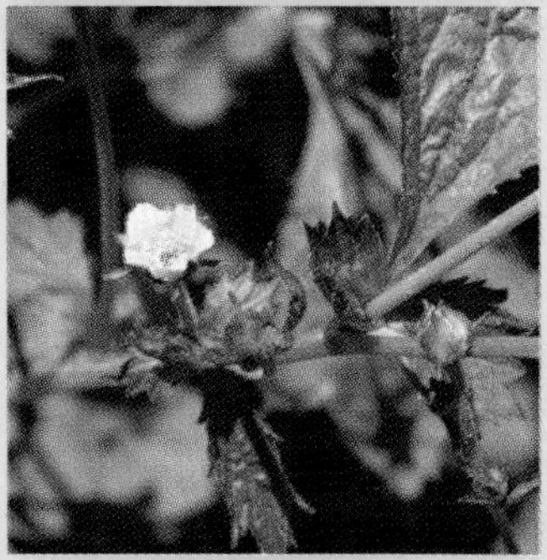

Geum urbanum

BETEL NUT

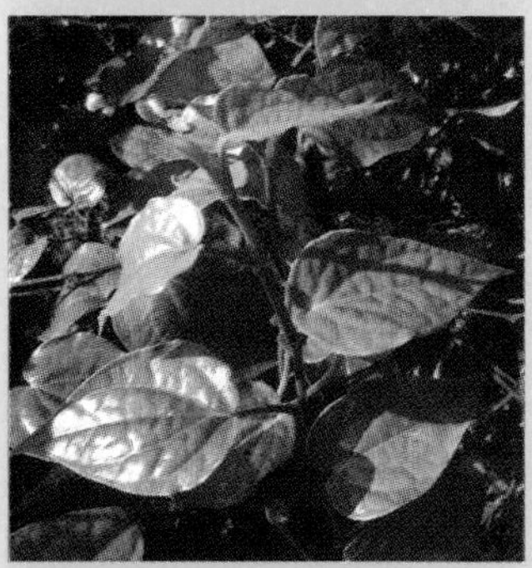

Piper betle

BETH ROOT

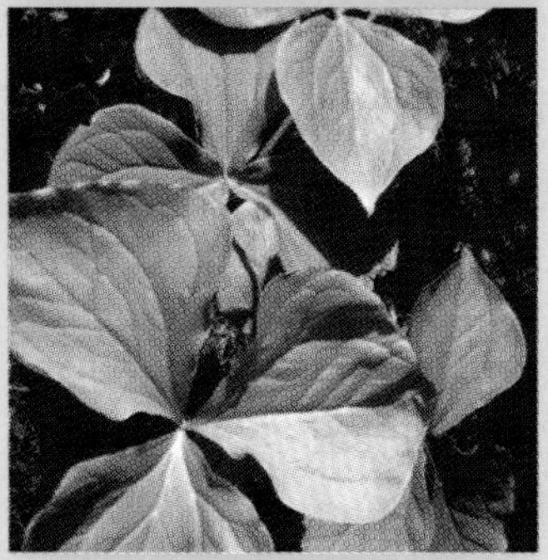

Trillium erectum

BILBERRY

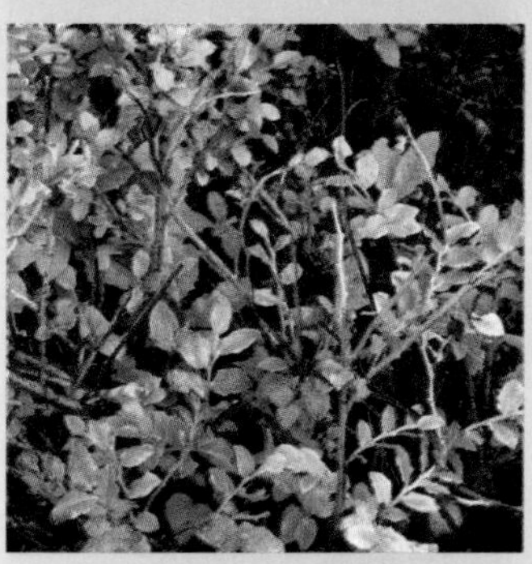

Vaccinium myrtillus

BIRCH

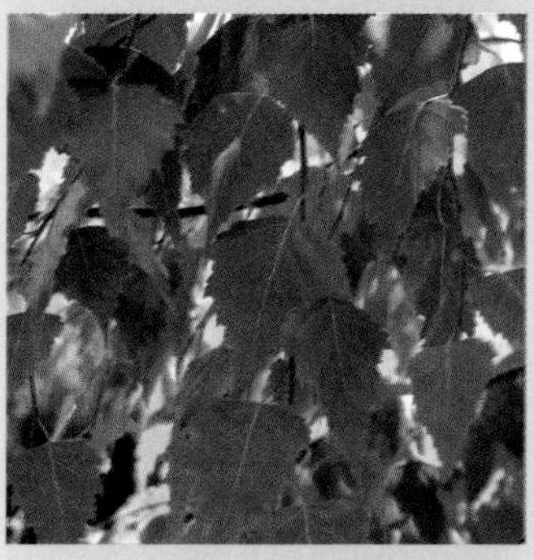

Betula species

BIRTHWORT

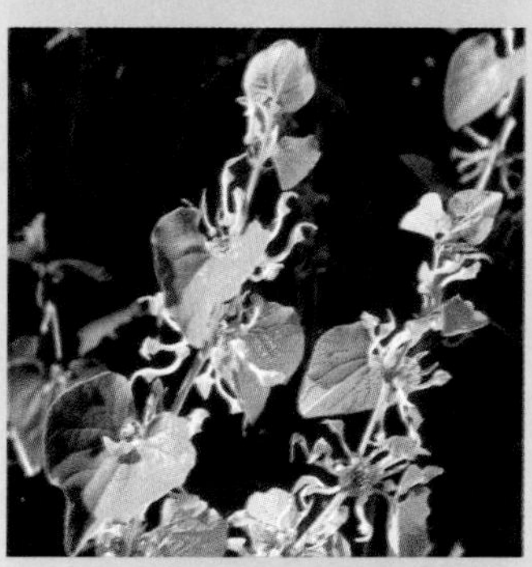

Aristolochia clematitis

BISHOP'S WEED

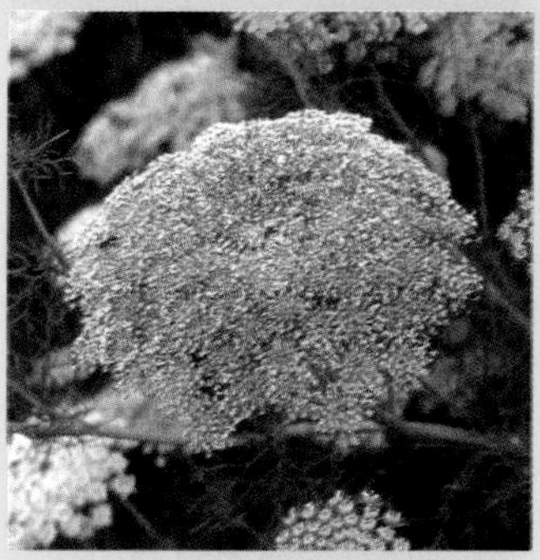

Ammi visnaga

BISTORT

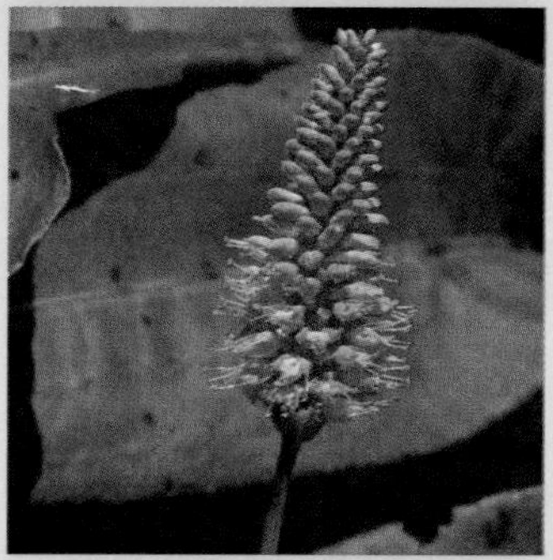

Persicaria bistorta

BITTER APPLE

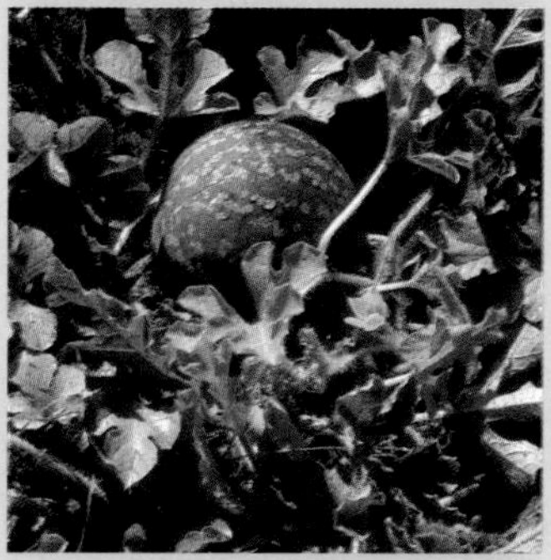

Citrullus colocynthis

BITTER ORANGE

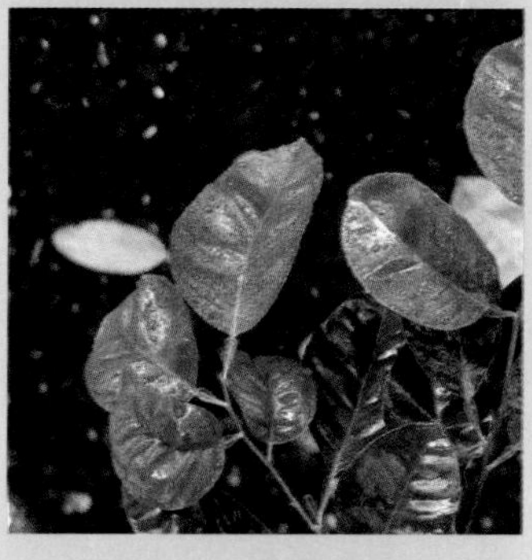

Citrus aurantium

BITTERSWEET NIGHTSHADE

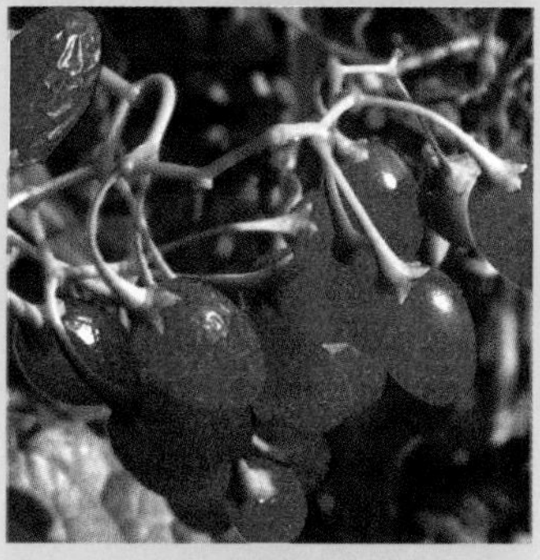

Solanum dulcamara

BLACK ALDER

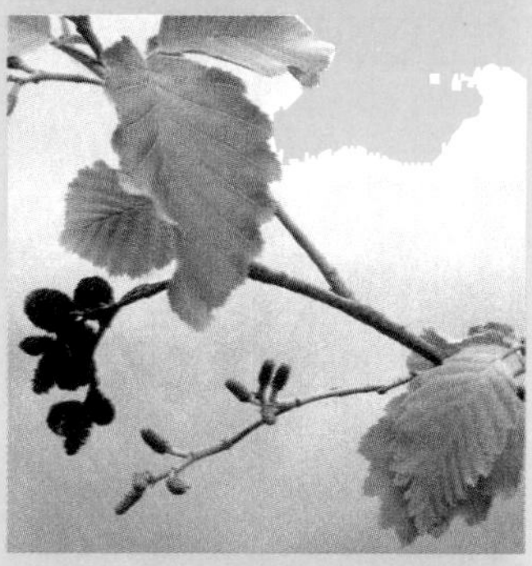

Alnus glutinosa

BLACK BRYONY

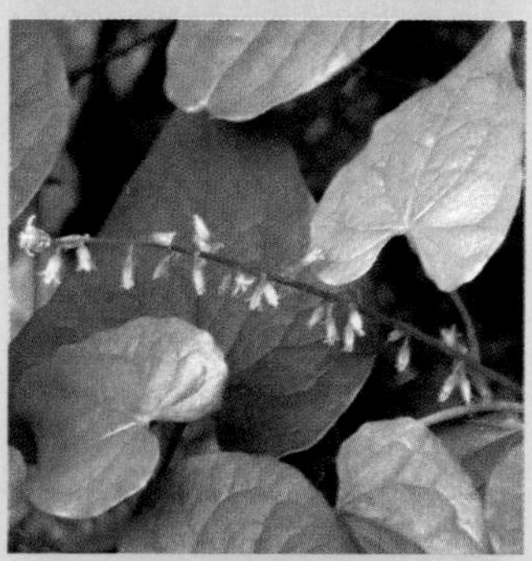

Tamus communis

BLACK COHOSH

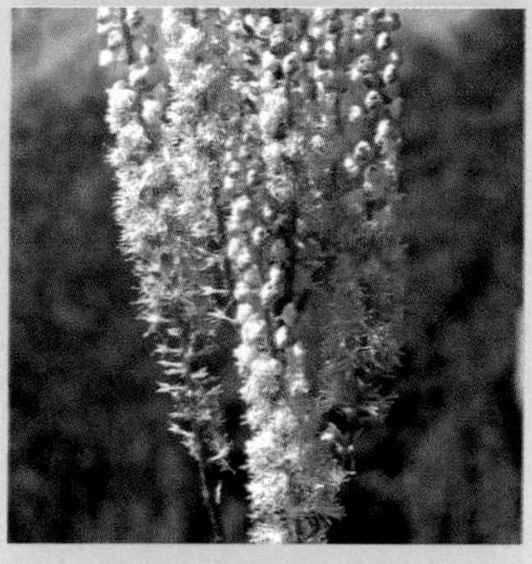

Cimicifuga racemosa

BLACK CURRANT

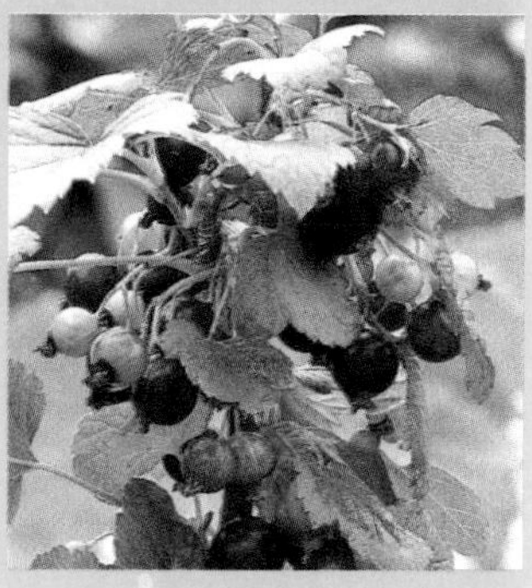

Ribes nigrum

BLACK HAW

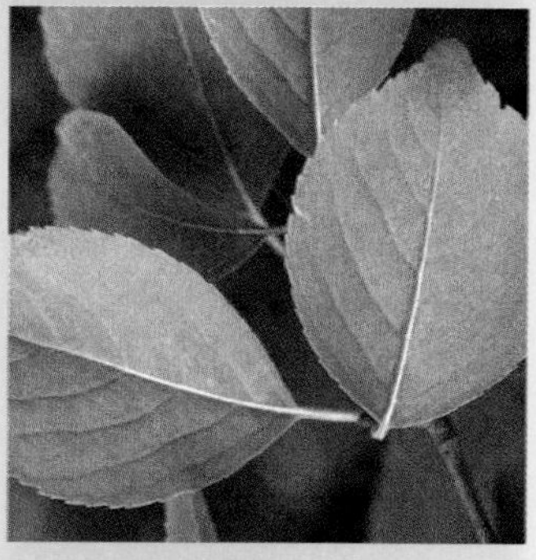

Viburnum prunifolium

BLACK HELLEBORE

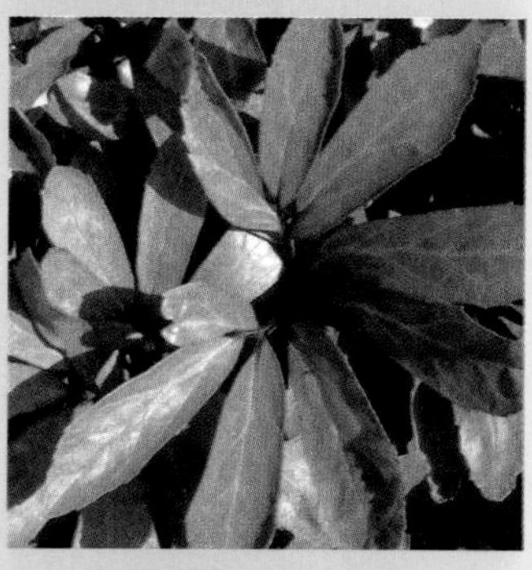

Helleborus niger

BLACK HOREHOUND

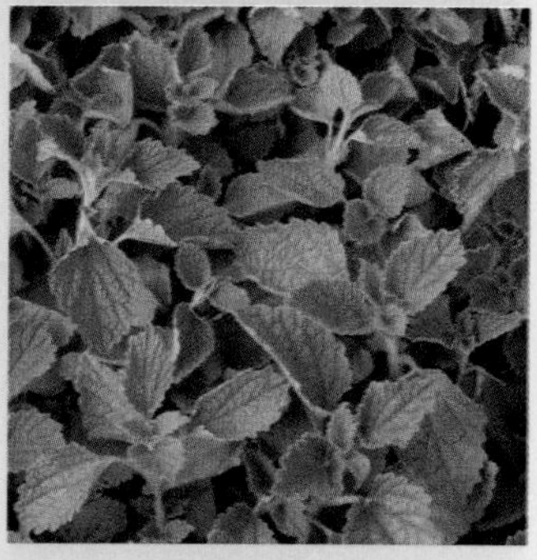

Ballota nigra

BLACK MUSTARD

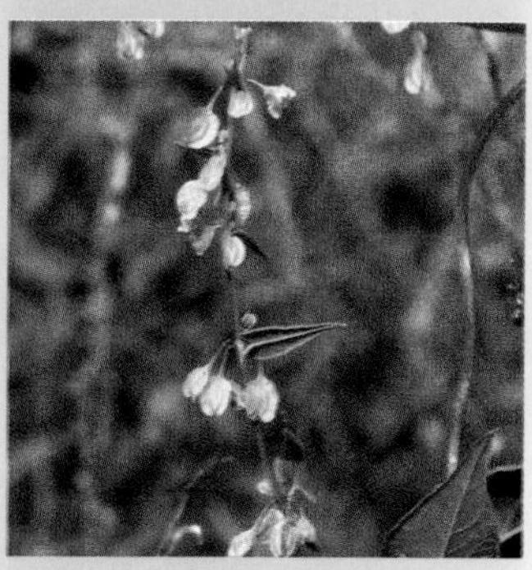

Brassica nigra

BLACK NIGHTSHADE

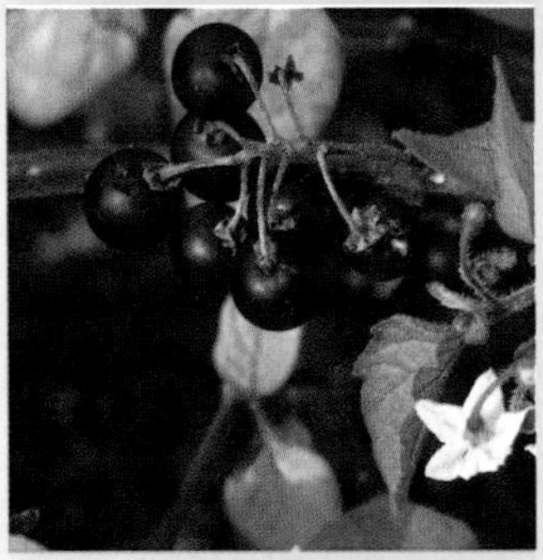

Solanum nigrum

BLACK PEPPER

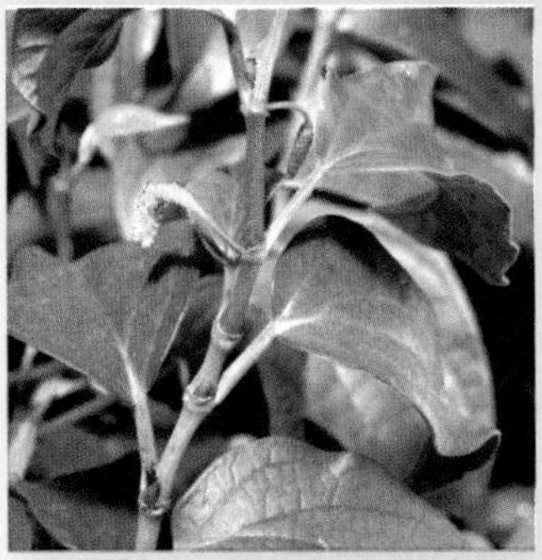

Piper nigrum

BLACKBERRY

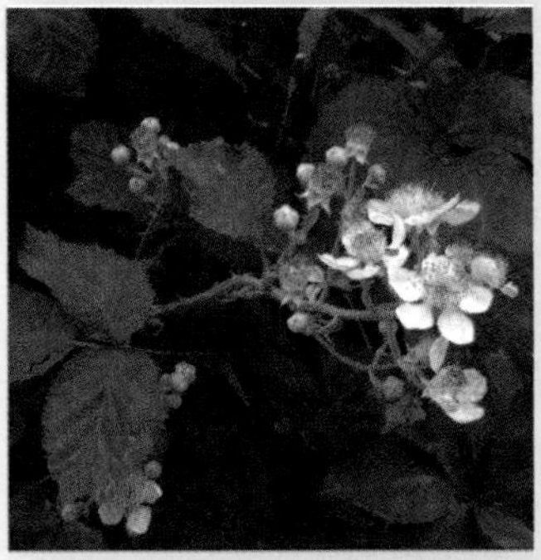

Rubus fruticosus

BLADDERWORT

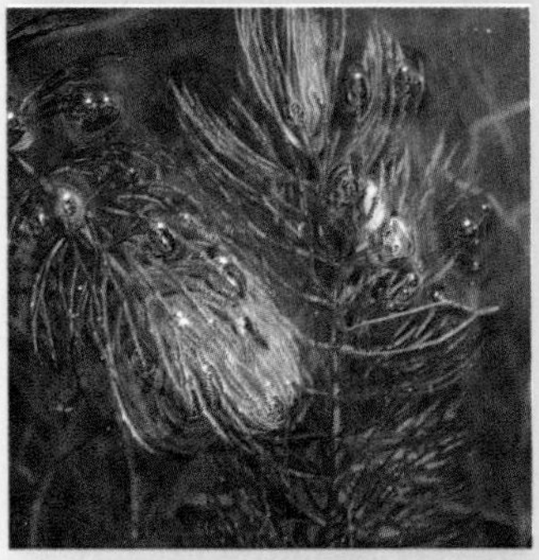

Utricularia vulgaris

BLESSED THISTLE

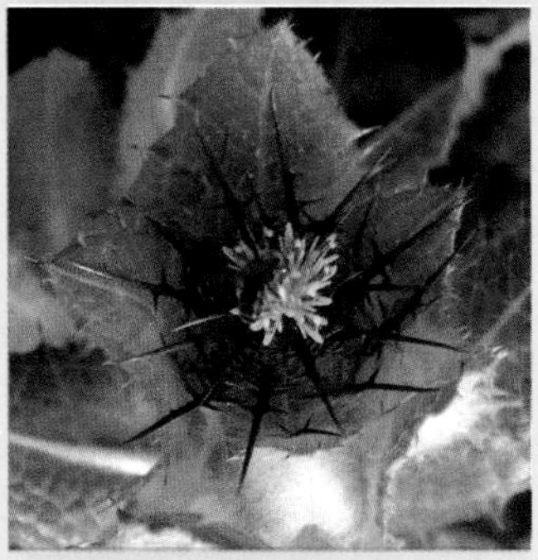

Cnicus benedictus

BOG BEAN

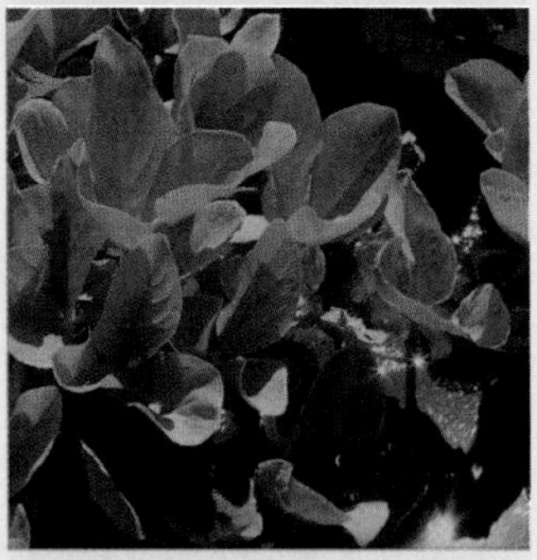

Menyanthes trifoliata

BOG BILBERRY

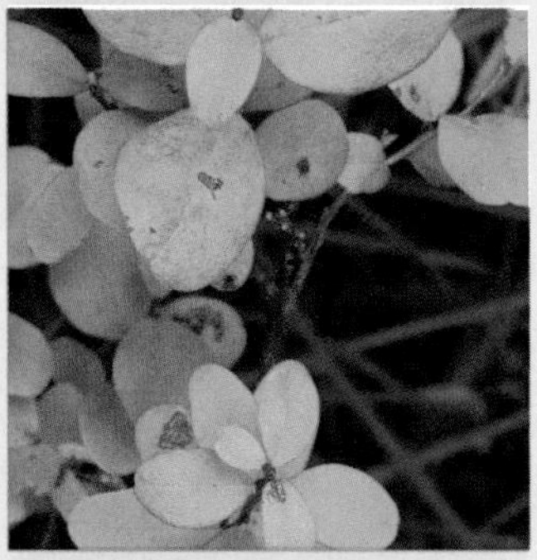

Vaccinium uliginosum

BOLDO

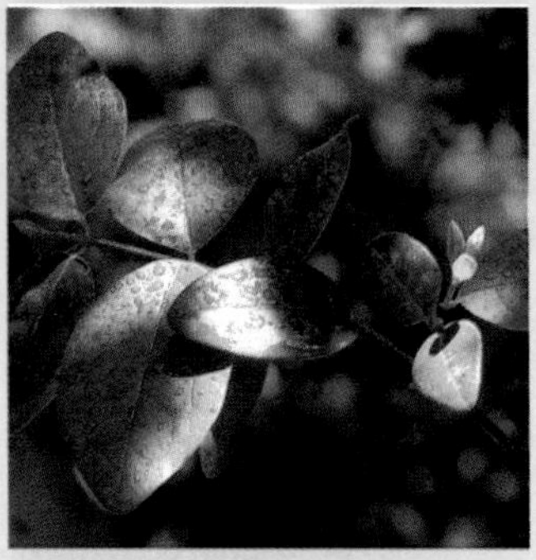

Peumus boldus

BONESET

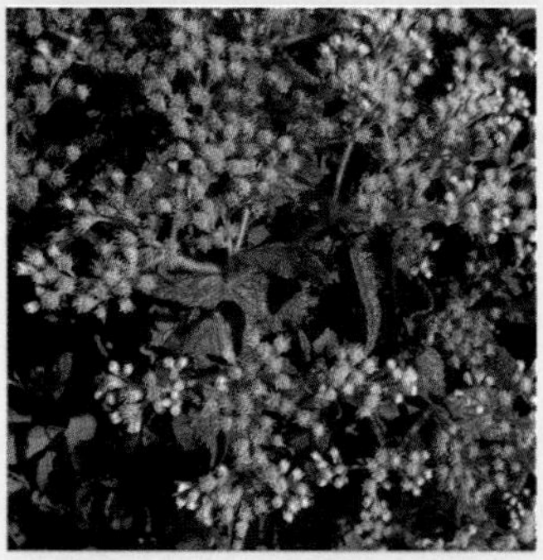

Eupatorium perfoliatum

BORAGE

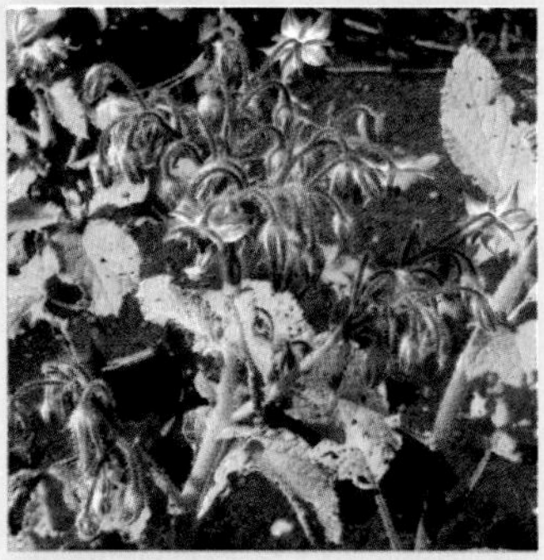

Borago officinalis

BOXWOOD

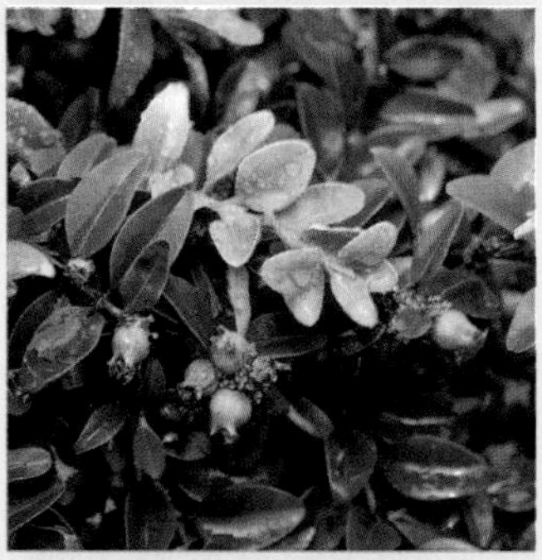

Buxus sempervirens

BROOKLIME

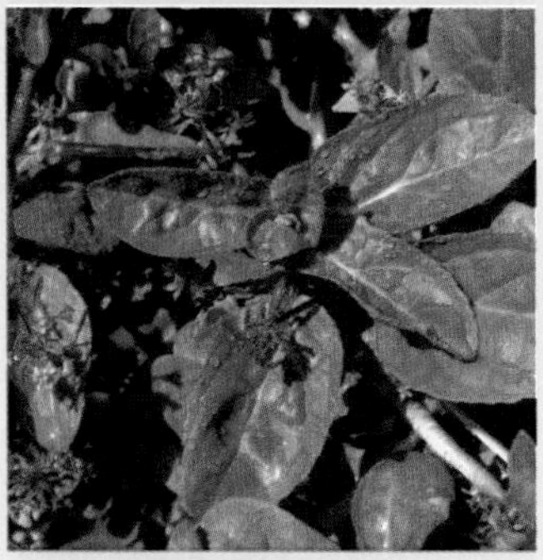

Veronica beccabunga

BUCKTHORN

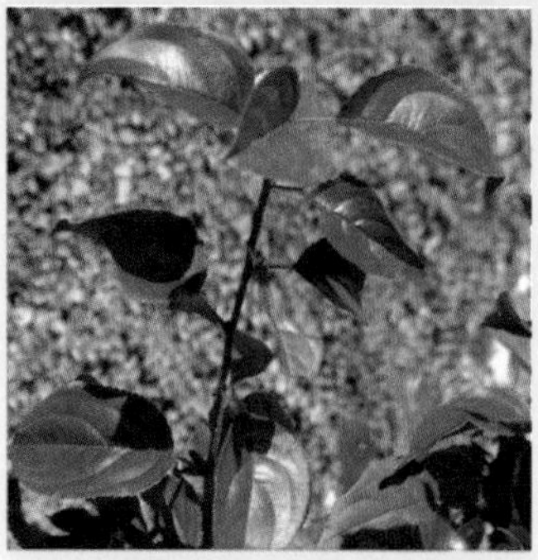

Rhamnus catharticus

BUCKWHEAT

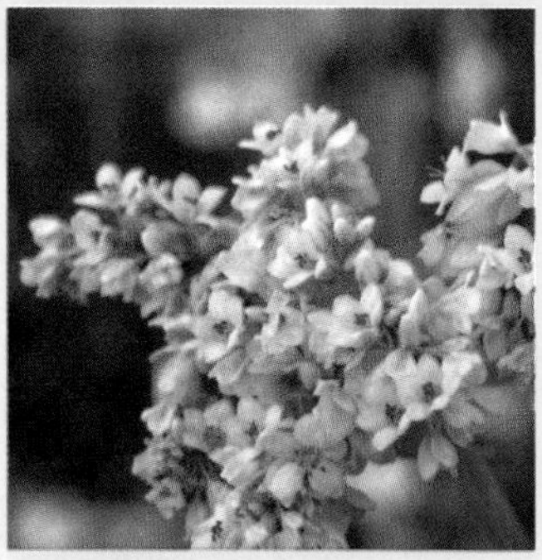

Fagopyrum esculentum

BUGLE

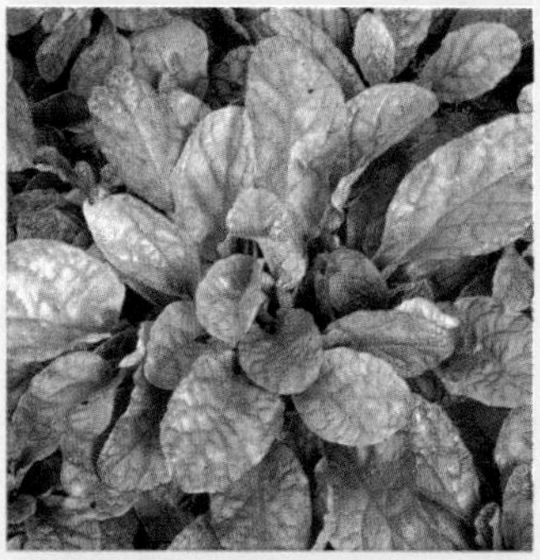

Ajuga reptans

BUGLEWEED

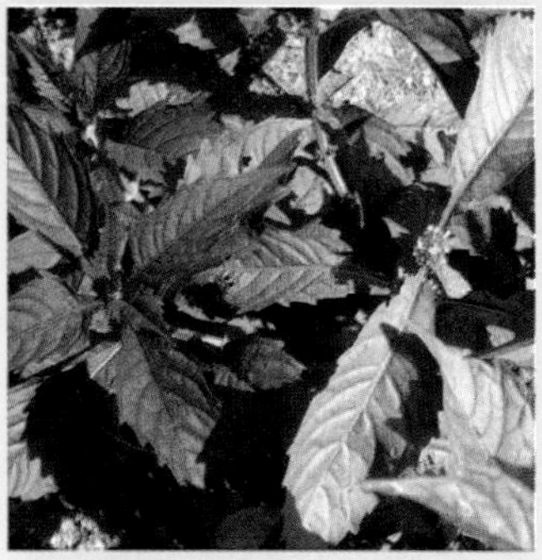

Lycopus virginicus

BURDOCK

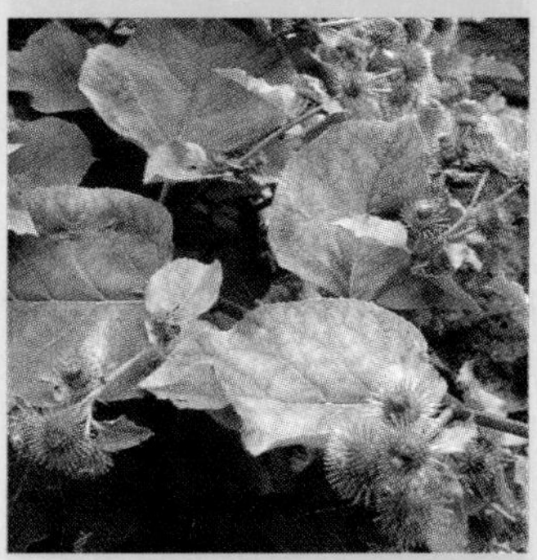

Arctium lappa

BURNING BUSH

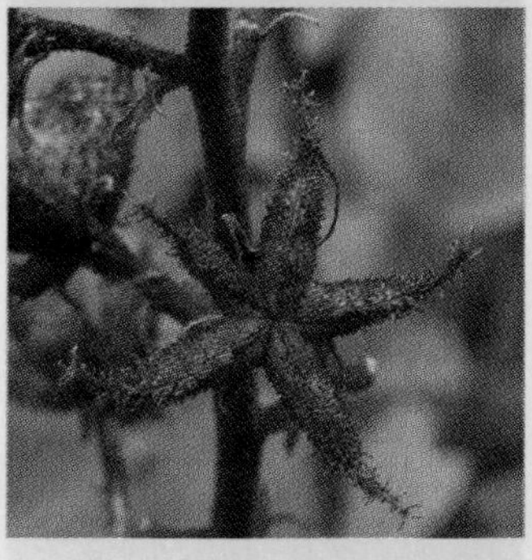

Dictamnus albus

BURR MARIGOLD

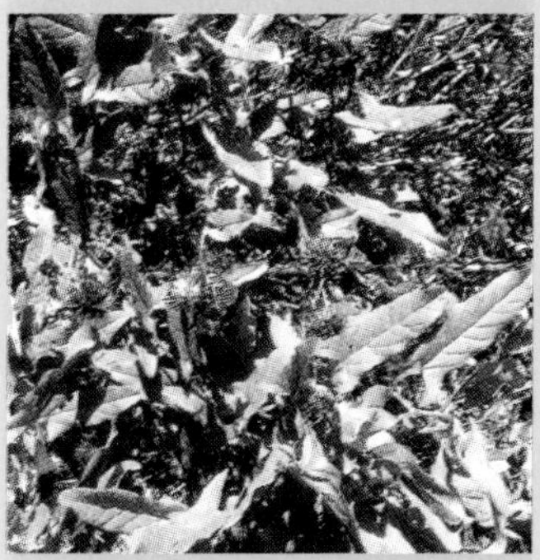

Bidens tripartita

BUTCHER'S BROOM

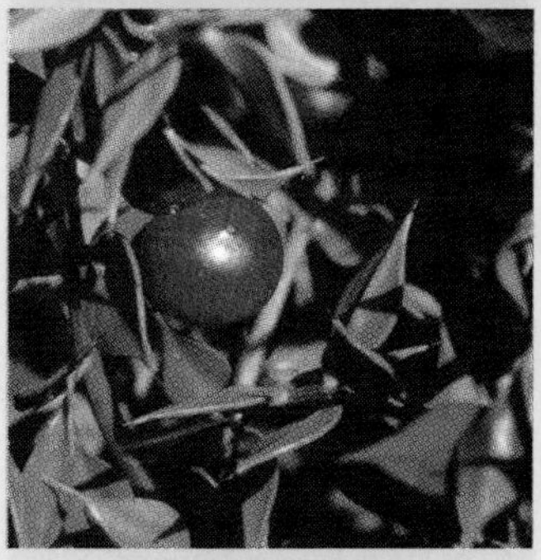

Ruscus aculeatus

CABBAGE

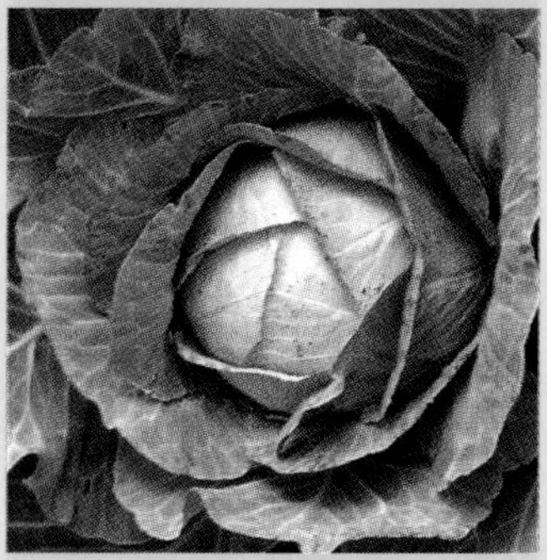

Brassica oleracea

CAJUPUT

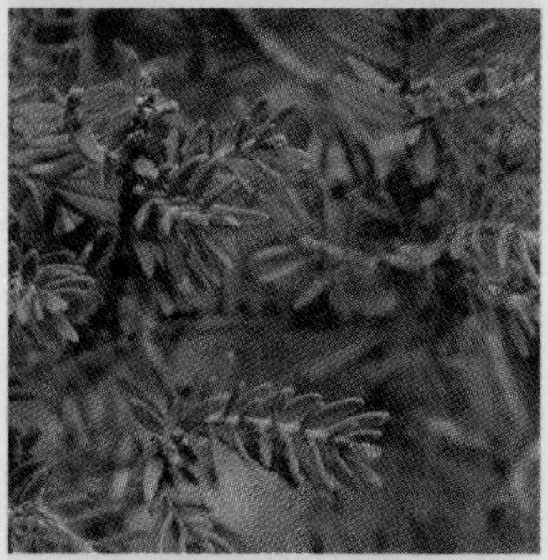

Melaleuca leucadendra

CALAMUS

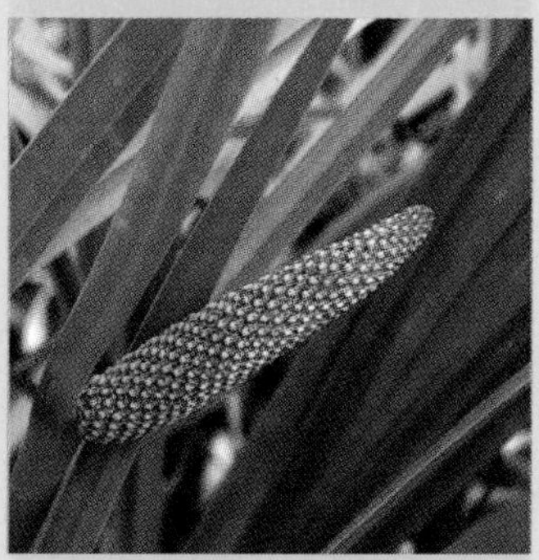

Acorus calamus

CALIFORNIA POPPY

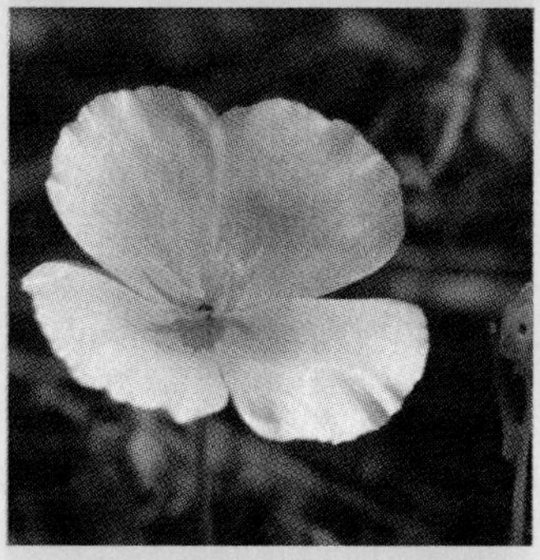

Eschscholtzia californica

CAMPHOR TREE

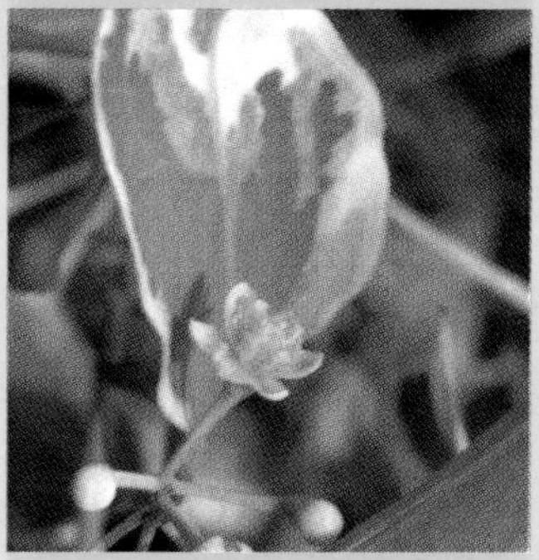

Cinnamomum camphora

CANADIAN FLEABANE

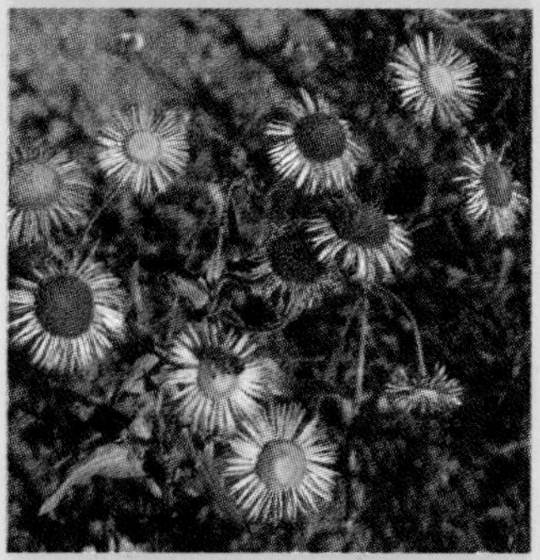

Erigeron canadensis

CARAWAY

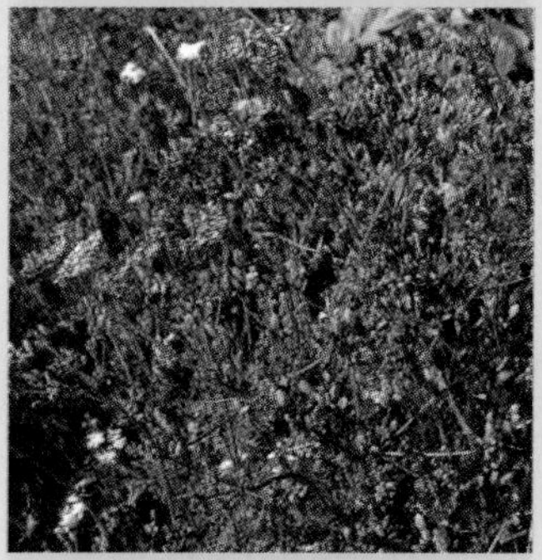

Carum carvi

CARDAMOM

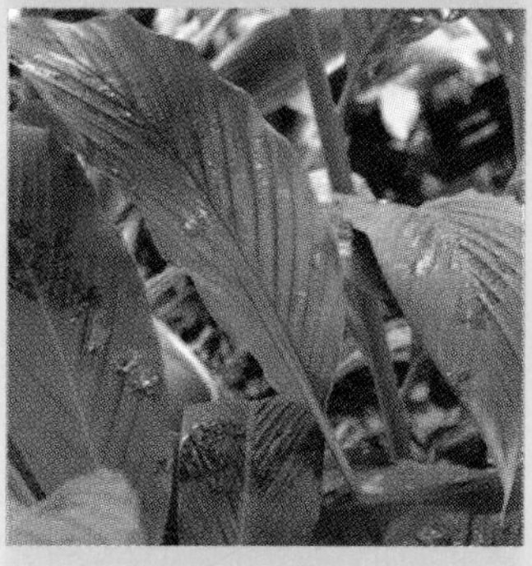

Elettaria cardamomum

CAROB

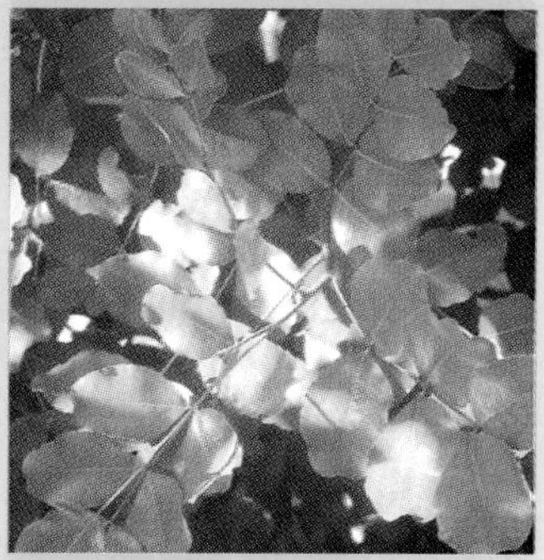

Ceratonia siliqua

CASCARA SAGRADA

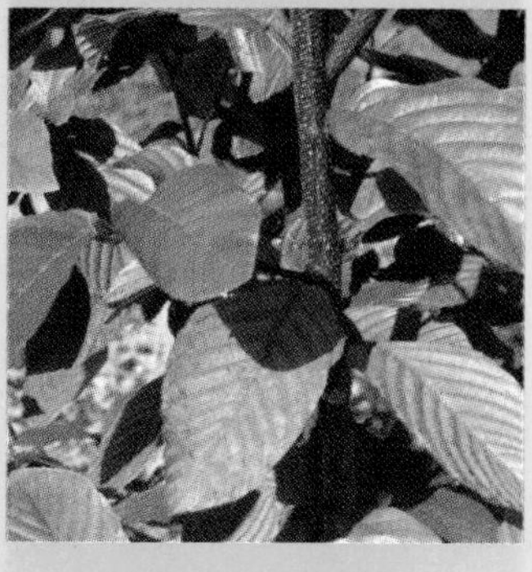

Rhamnus purshiana

CASHEW

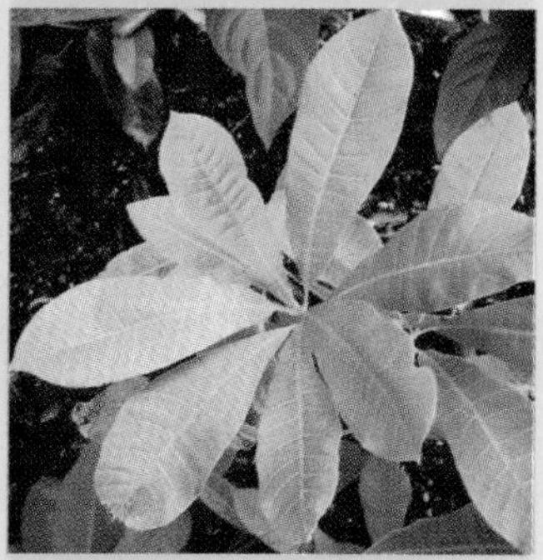

Anacardium occidentale

CASTOR OIL PLANT

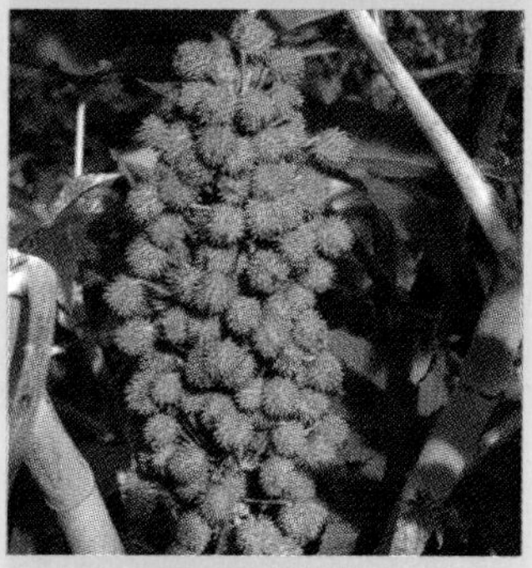

Ricinus communis

CATNIP

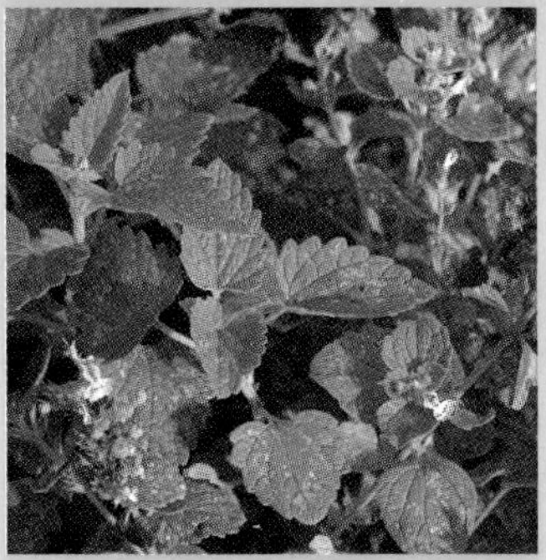

Nepeta cataria

CAT'S FOOT

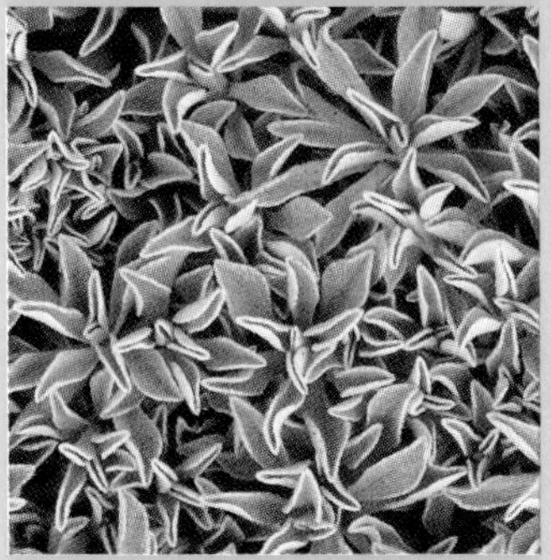

Antennaria dioica

CAYENNE

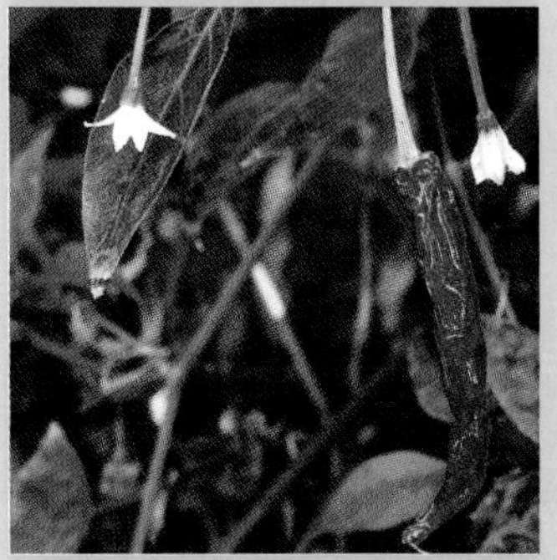

Capsicum annuum

CELANDINE

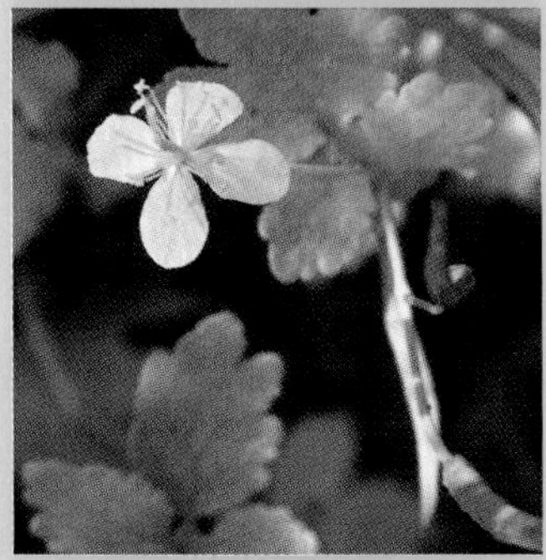

Chelidonium majus

CELERY

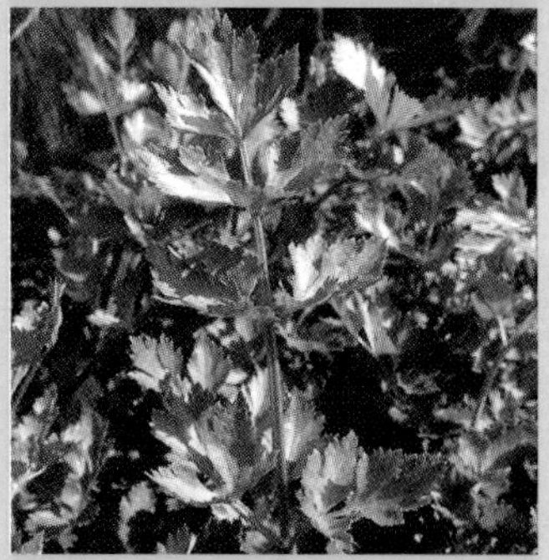

Apium graveolens

CENTAURY

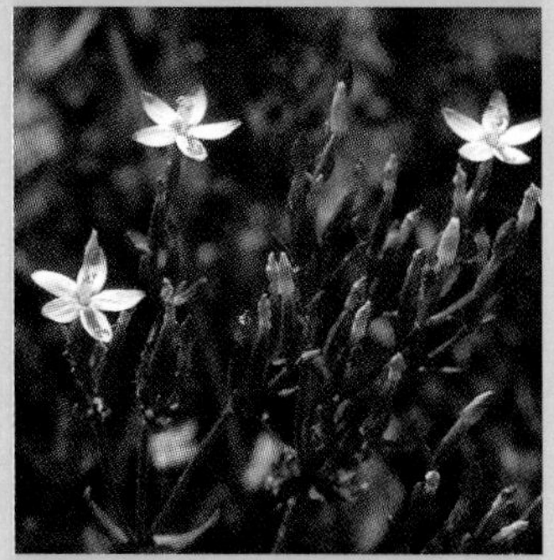

Centaurium erythraea

CHASTE TREE

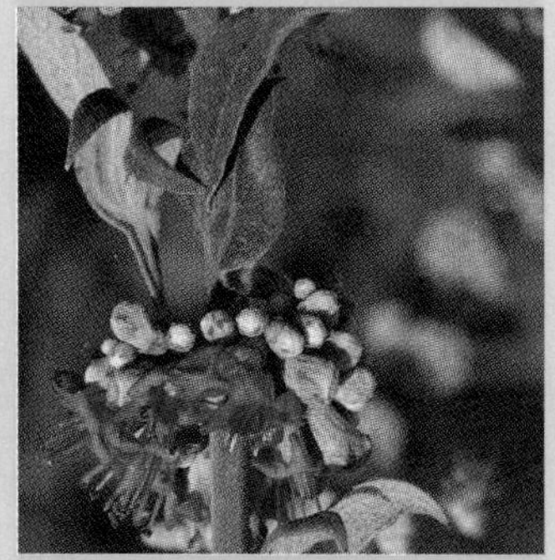

Vitex agnus-castus

CHERRY LAUREL

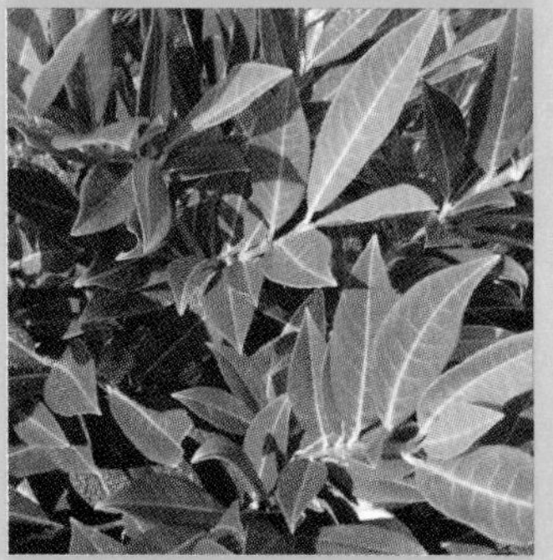

Prunus laurocerasus

CHICORY

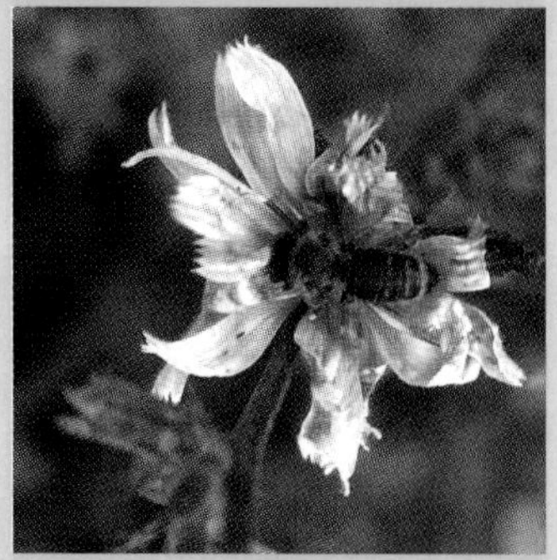

Cichorium intybus

CHINESE RHUBARB

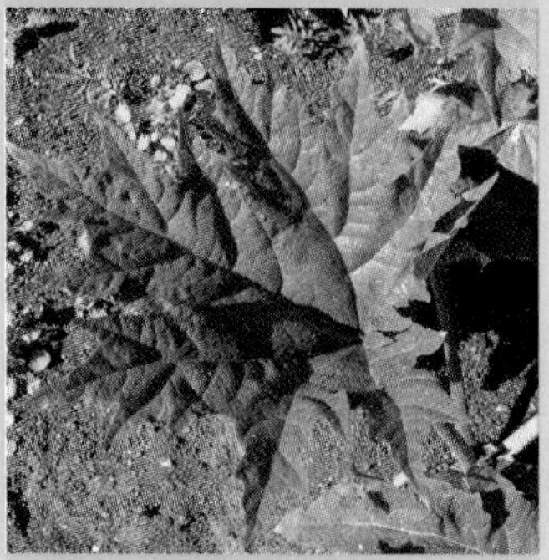

Rheum palmatum

CHIVE

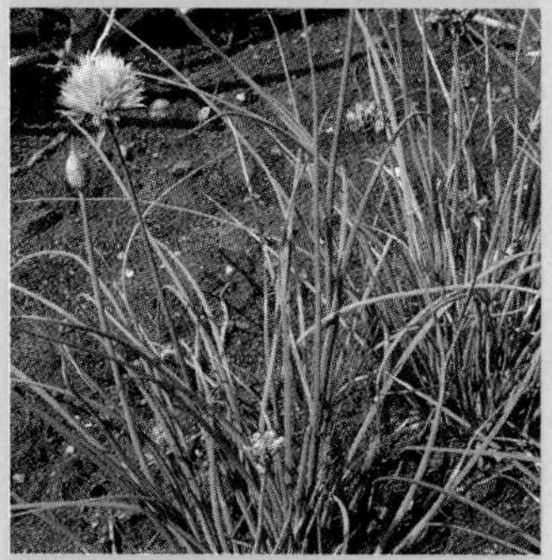

Allium schoenoprasum

CINNAMON

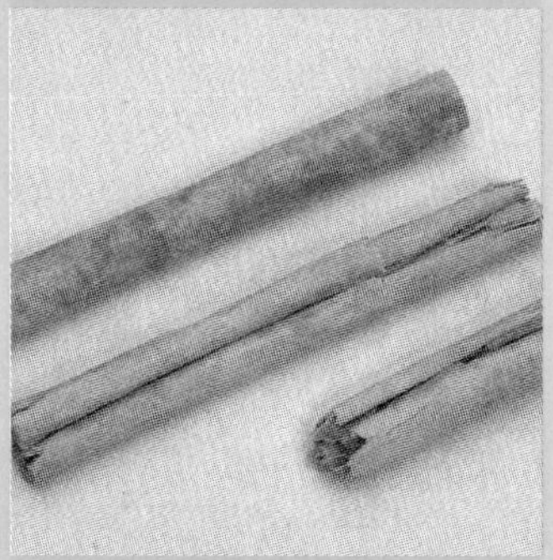

Cinnamomum verum

CINQUEFOIL

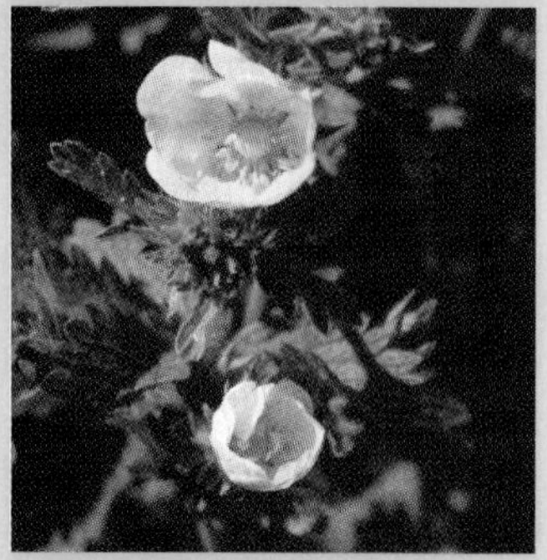

Potentilla erecta

CLEMATIS

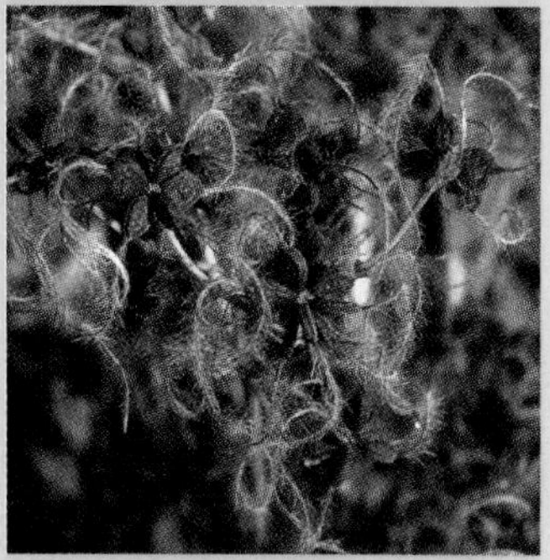

Clematis recta

CLOVE

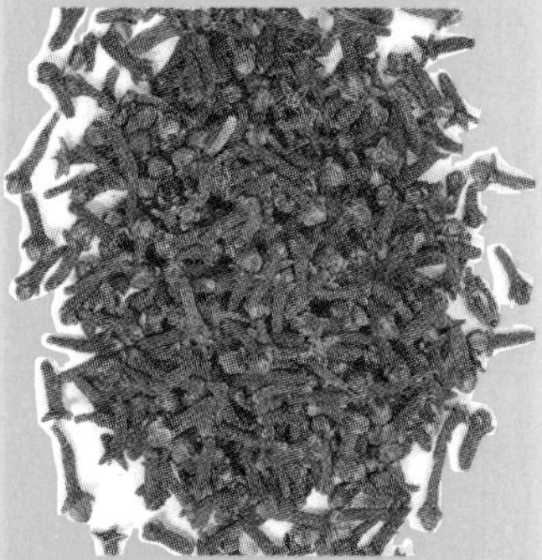

Syzygium aromaticum

COCOA

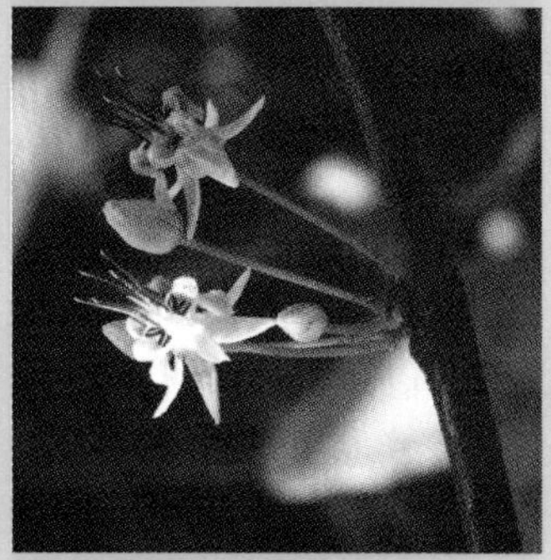

Theobroma cacao

COCONUT PALM

Cocos nucifera

COFFEE

Coffea arabica

COLCHICUM

Colchicum autumnale

COLT'S FOOT

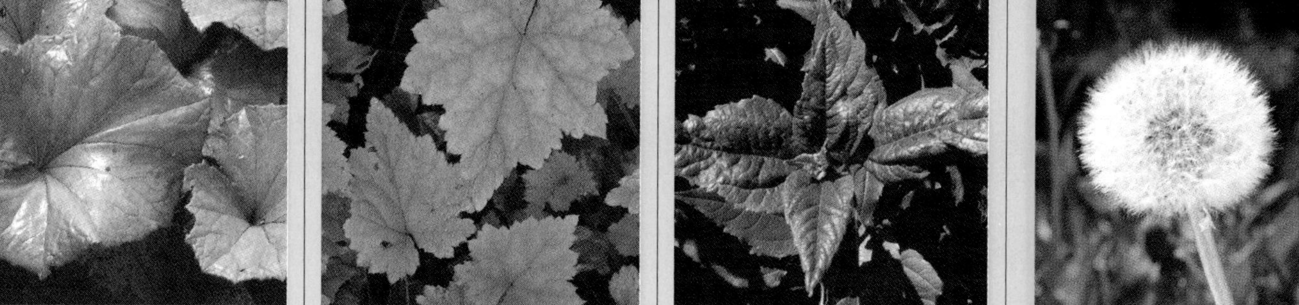

Tussilago farfara

COLUMBINE

Aquilegia vulgaris

COMFREY

Symphytum officinale

COMMON KIDNEY VETCH

Anthyllis vulneraria

COOLWORT

Tiarella cordifolia

CORIANDER

Coriandrum sativum

CORNFLOWER

Centaurea cyanus

CUMIN

Cuminum cyminum

CUP PLANT

Silphium perfoliatum

CURCUMA

Curcuma xanthorrhizia

CYPRESS

Cupressus sempervirens

CYPRESS SPURGE

Euphorbia cyparissias

DANDELION

Taraxacum officinale

DATE PALM

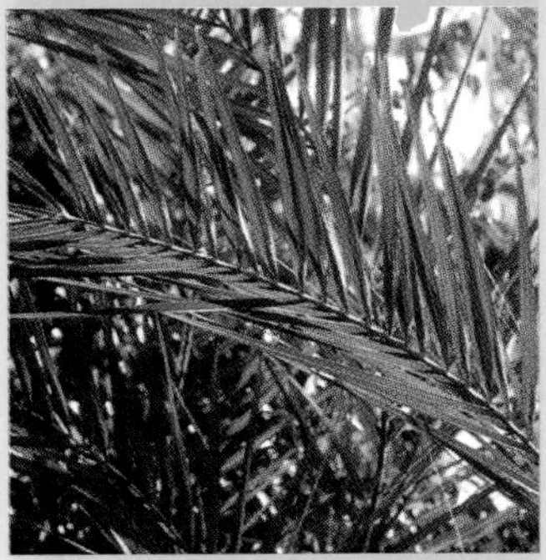

Phoenix dactylifera

DIGITALIS

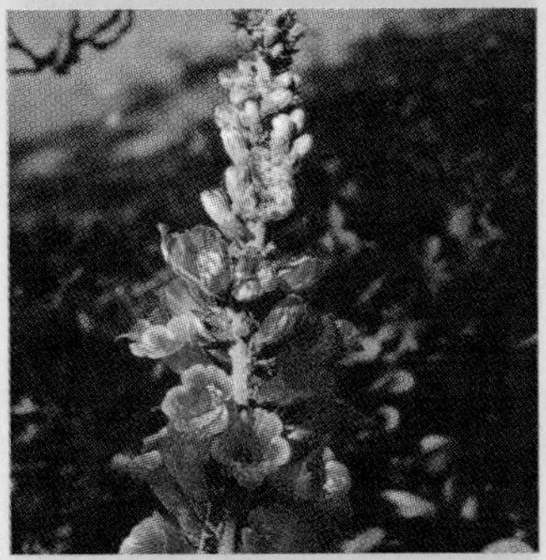

Digitalis purpurea

DILL

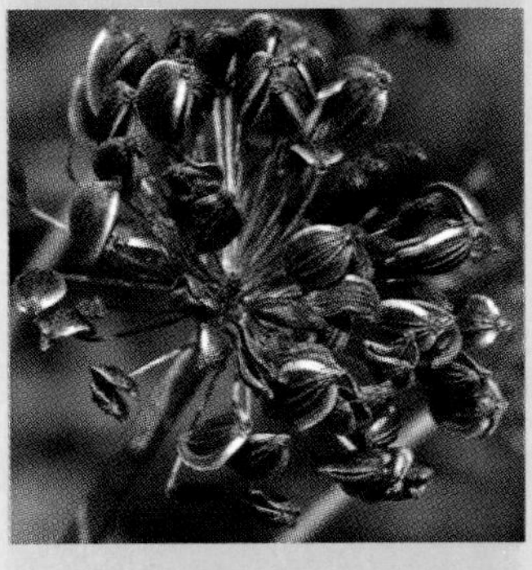

Anethum graveolens

DODDER

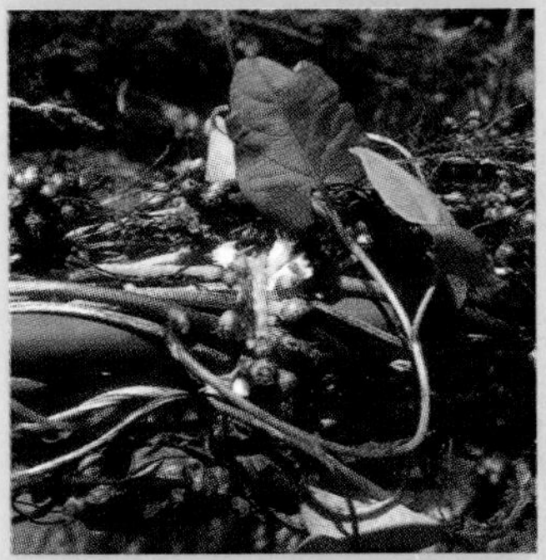

Cuscuta epithymum

DOG ROSE

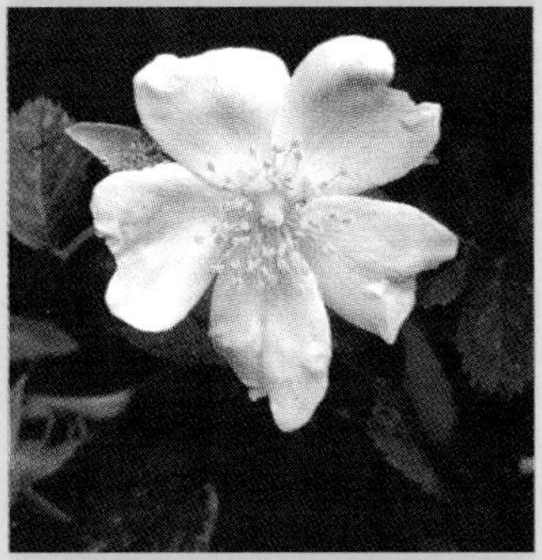

Rosa canina

DOGWOOD

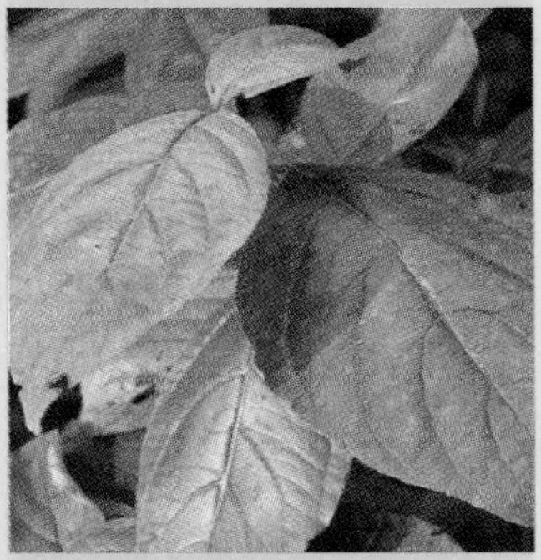

Cornus florida

DUCKWEED

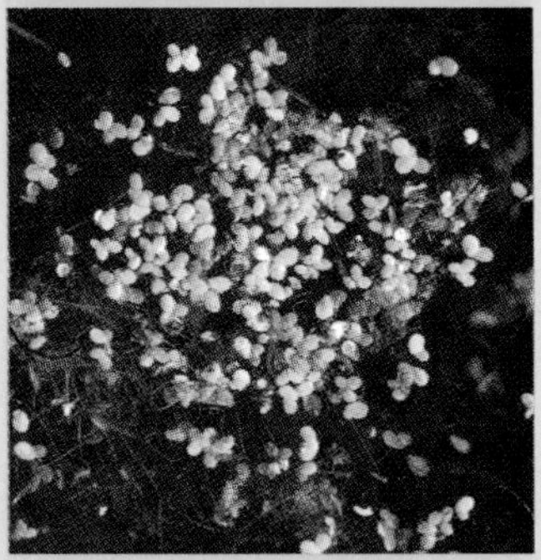

Lemna minor

DYER'S BROOM

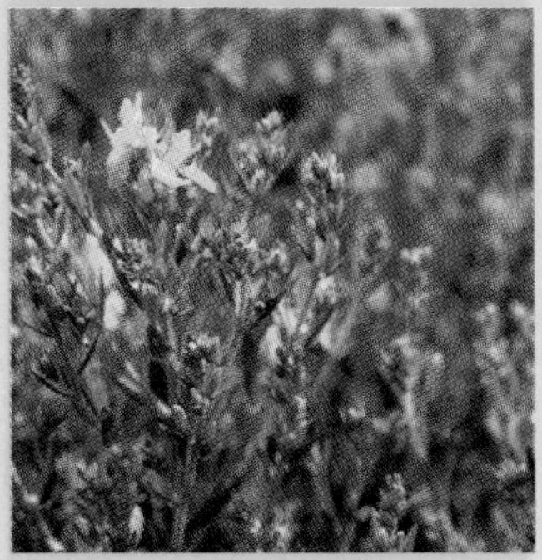

Genista tinctoria

ECHINACEA PURPUREA

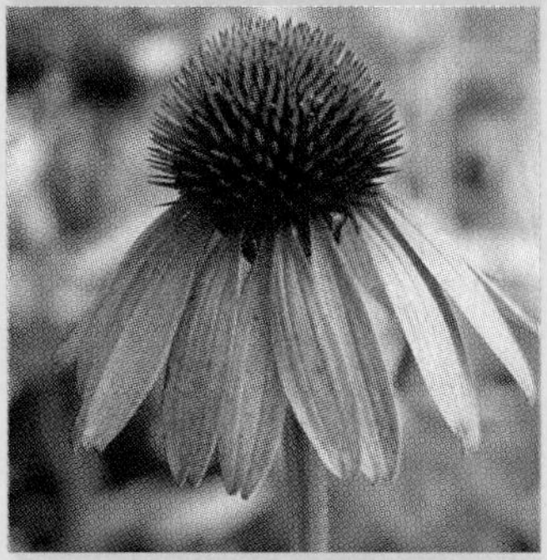

Echinacea purpurea

ELECAMPANE

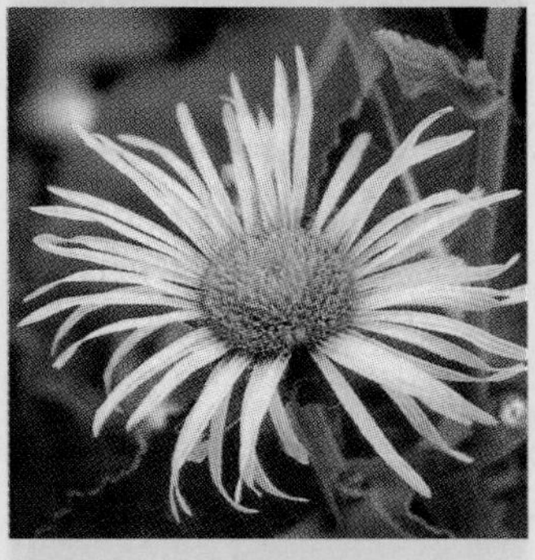

Inula helenium

ELM BARK

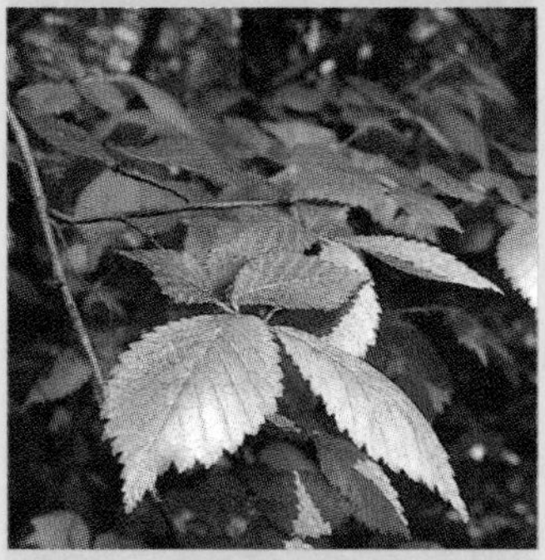

Ulmus minor

ENGLISH CHAMOMILE

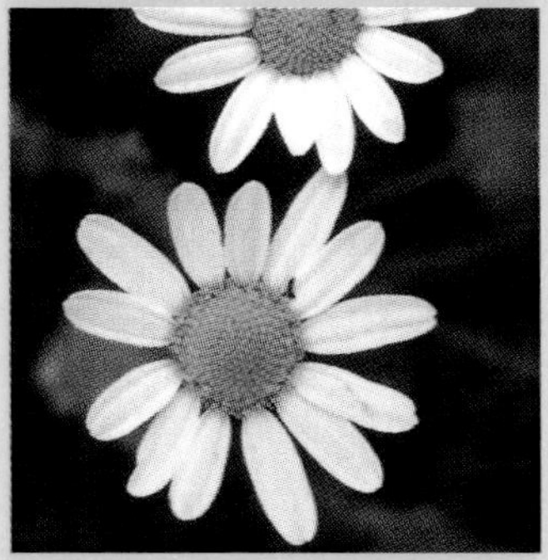

Chamaemelum nobile

ENGLISH HAWTHORN

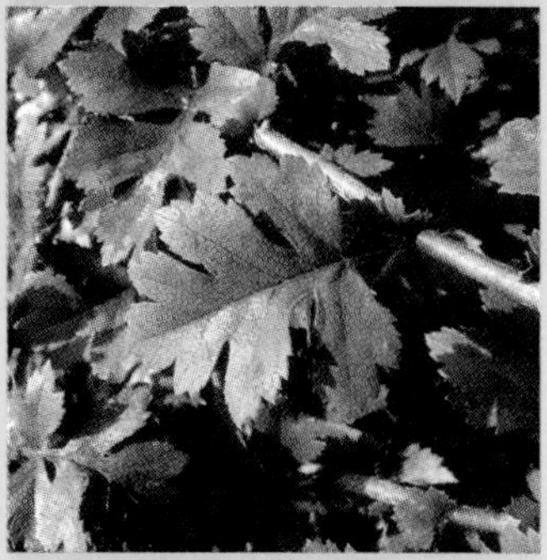

Crataegus laevigata

ENGLISH HORSEMINT

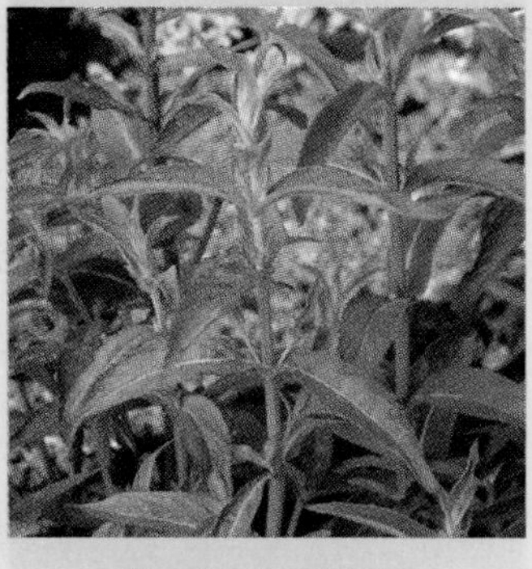

Mentha longifolia

ENGLISH IVY

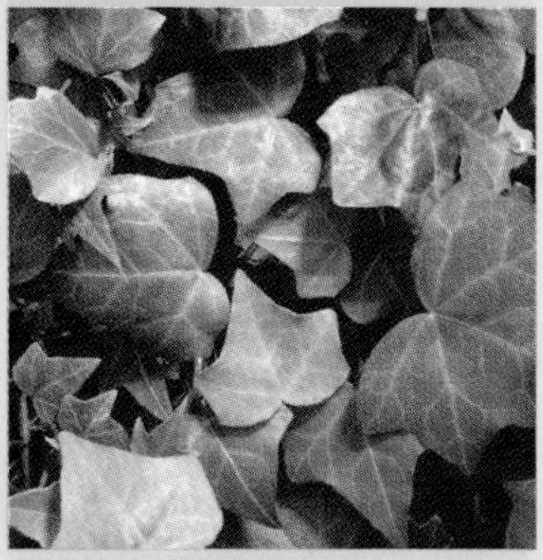

Hedera helix

ENGLISH LAVENDER

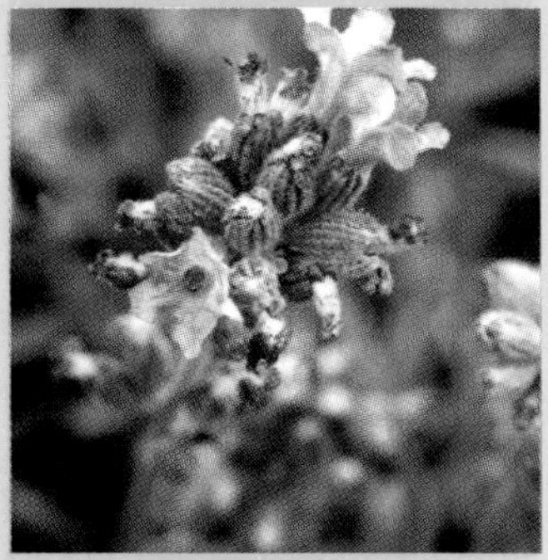

Lavandula angustifolia

ENGLISH PLANTAIN

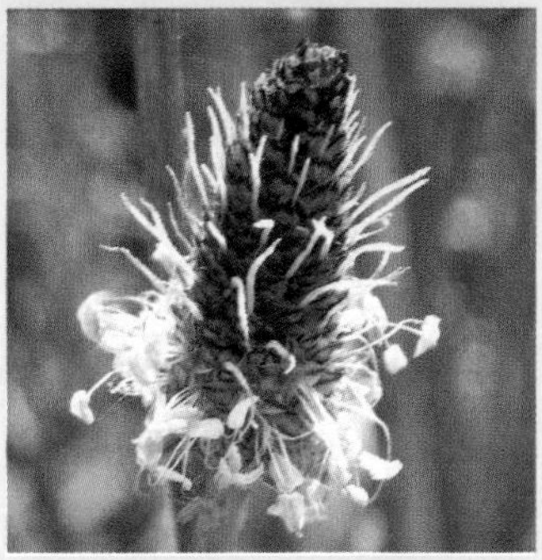

Plantago lanceolata

ERYNGO

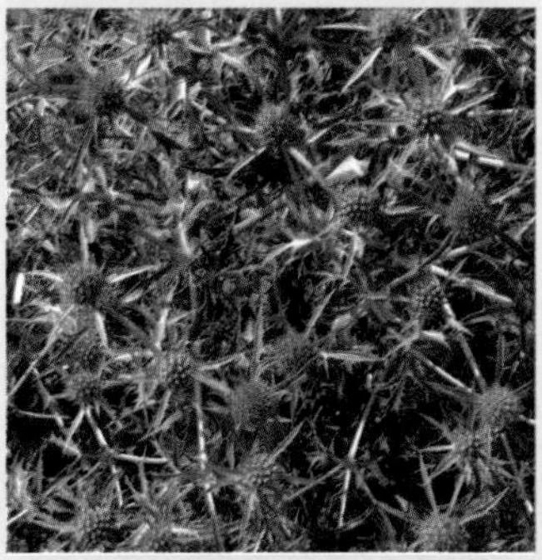

Eryngium campestre

EUCALYPTUS

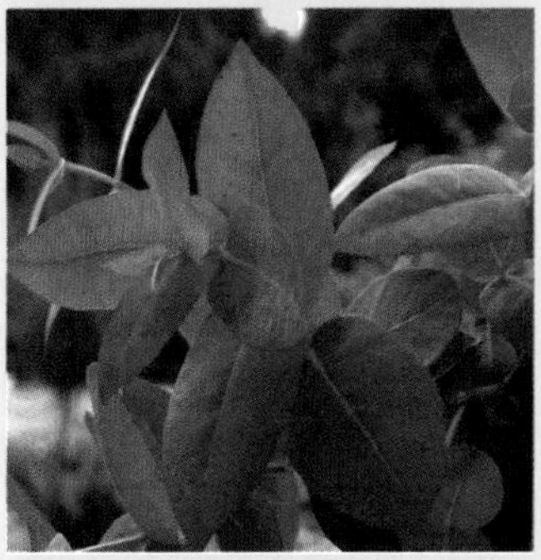

Eucalyptus globulus

EUROPEAN ELDER

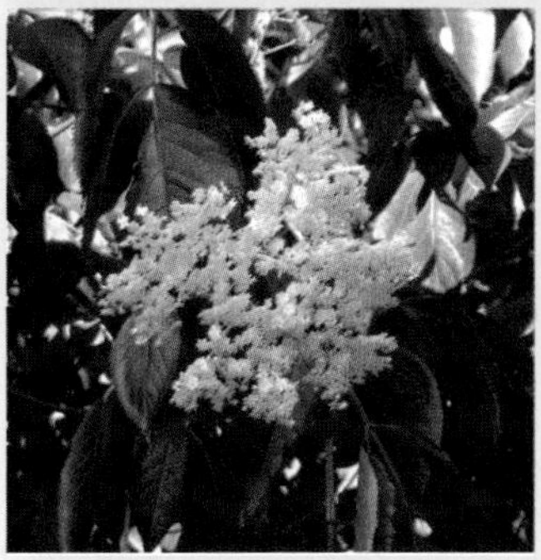

Sambucus nigra

EUROPEAN FIVE-FINGER GRASS

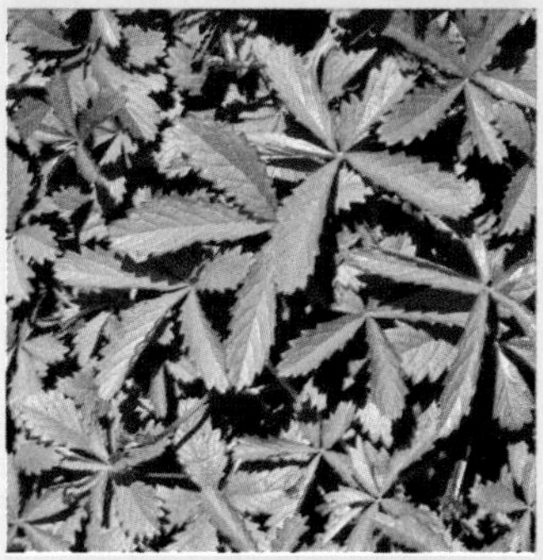

Potentilla reptans

EUROPEAN GOLDEN ROD

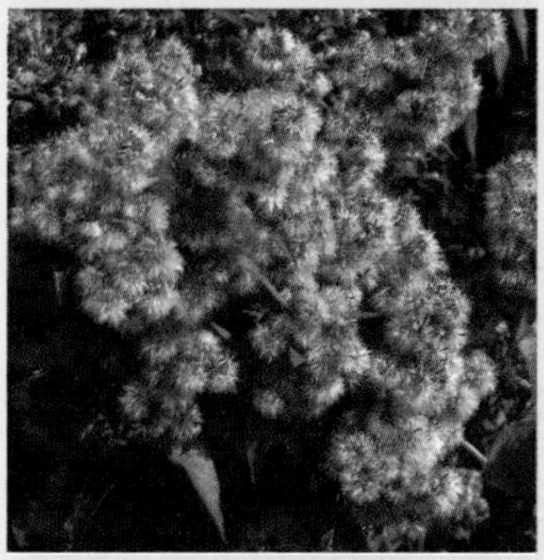

Solidago virgaurea

EUROPEAN MISTLETOE

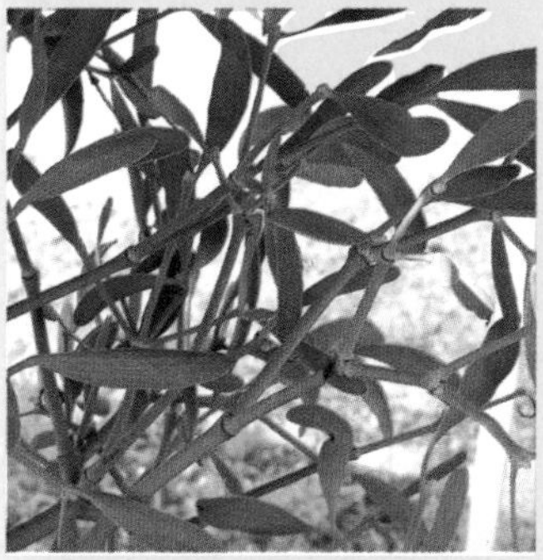

Viscum album

EUROPEAN PEONY

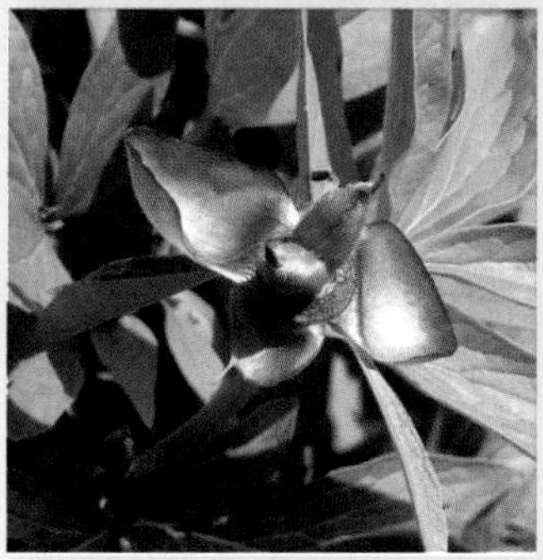

Paeonia officinalis

EUROPEAN WATER HEMLOCK

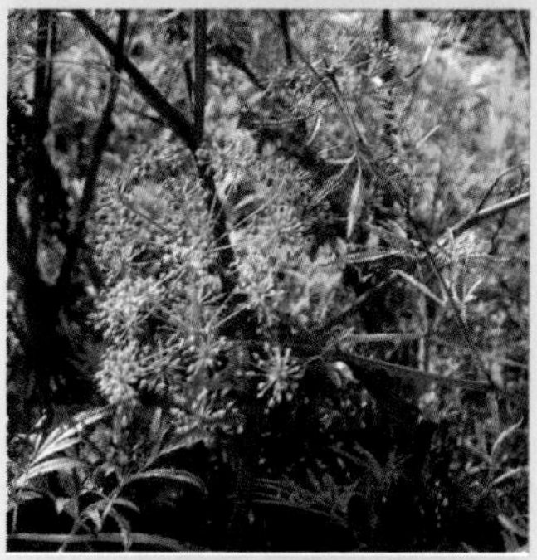

Cicuta virosa

EVENING PRIMROSE

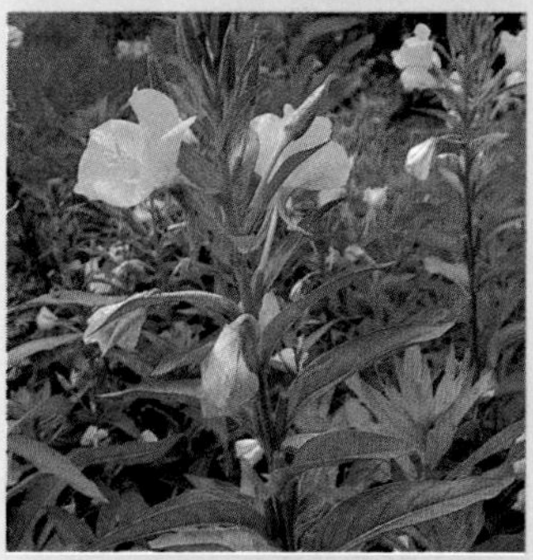

Oenothera biennis

FENNEL

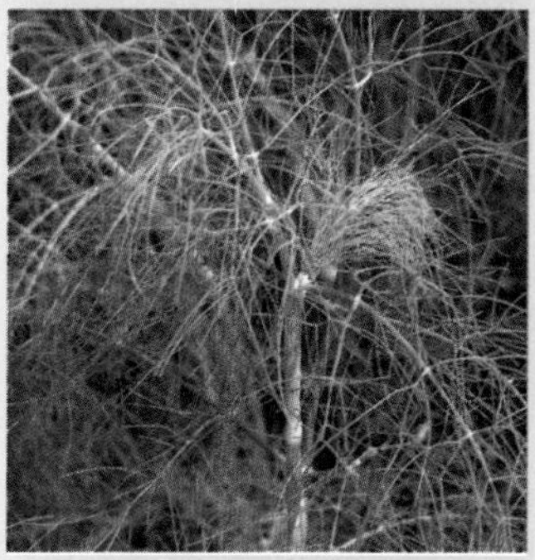

Foeniculum vulgare

FENUGREEK

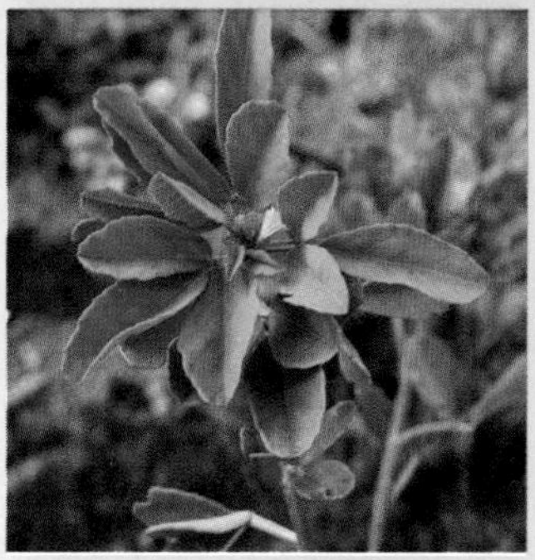

Trigonella foenum-graecum

FEVERFEW

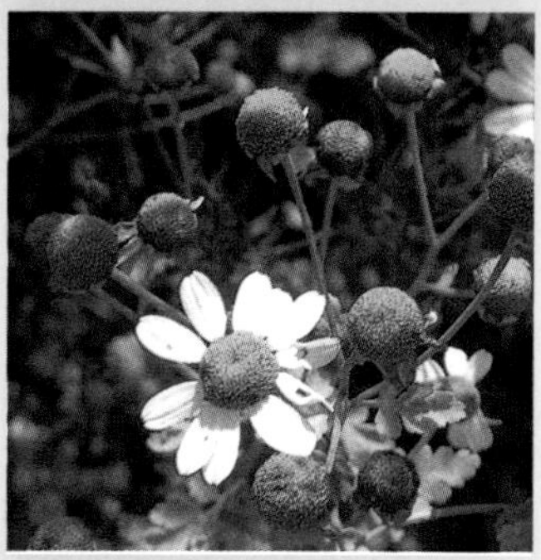

Tanacetum parthenium

FIELD SCABIOUS

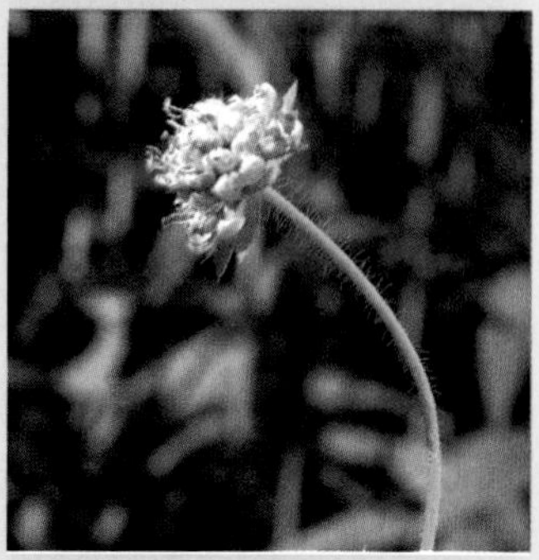

Knautia arvensis

FIGS

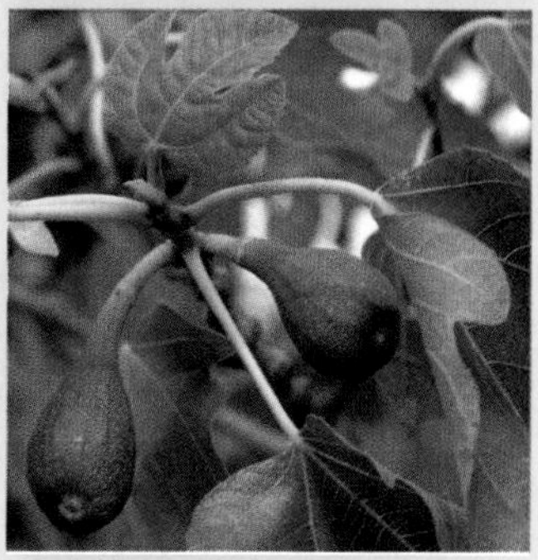

Ficus carica

FIGWORT

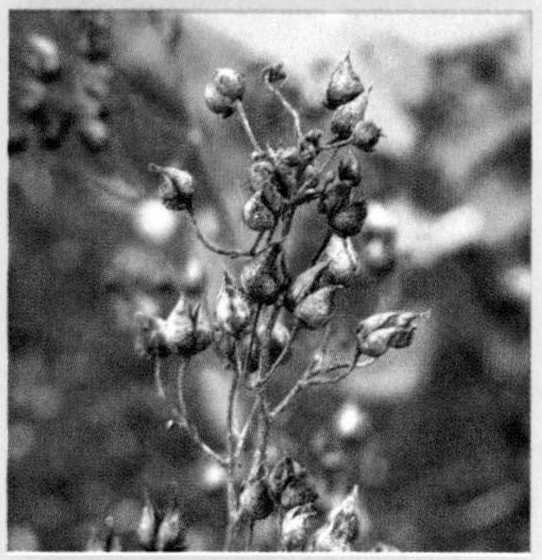

Scrophularia nodosa

FLAX

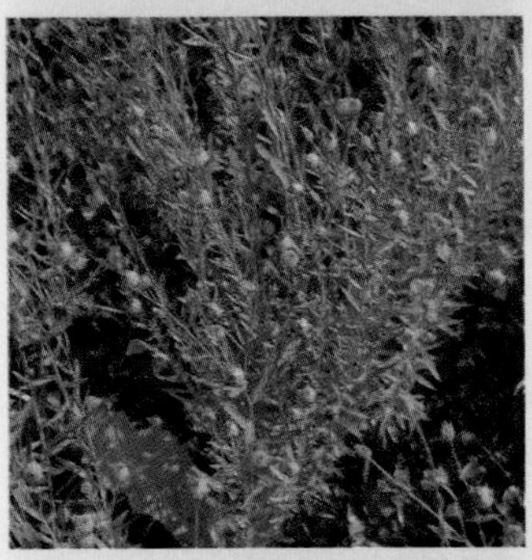

Linum usitatissimum

FOOL'S PARSLEY

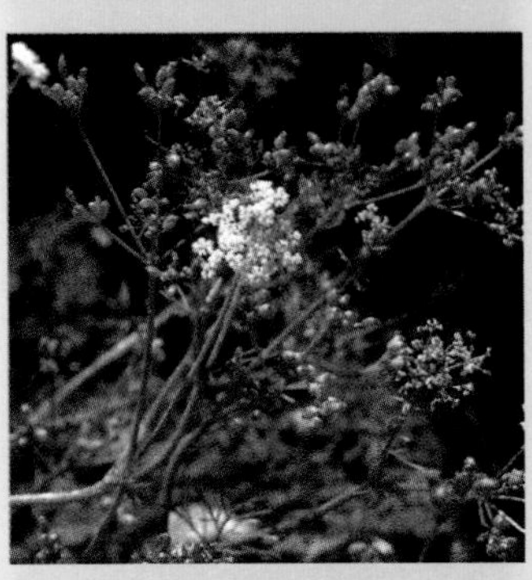

Aethusa cynapium

FORGET-ME-NOT

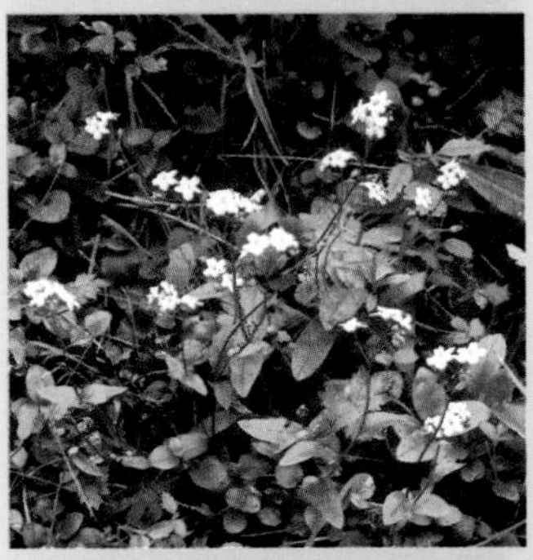

Myosotis arvensis

FRANGULA

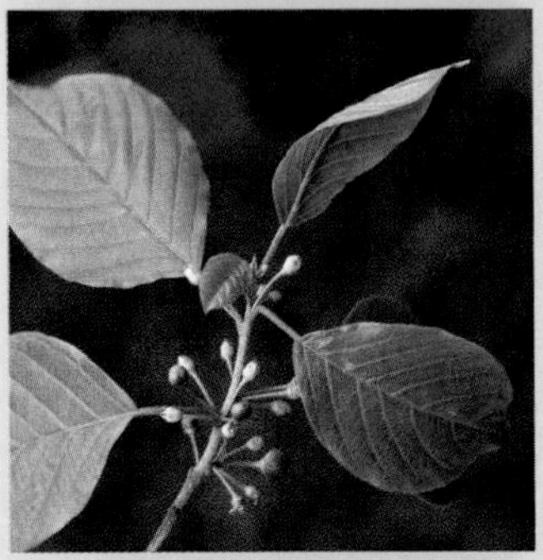

Rhamnus frangula

FRENCH TARRAGON

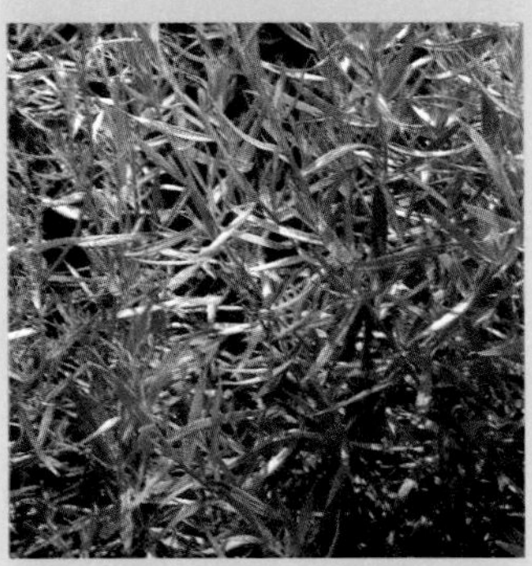

Artemisia dracunculus

FRINGETREE

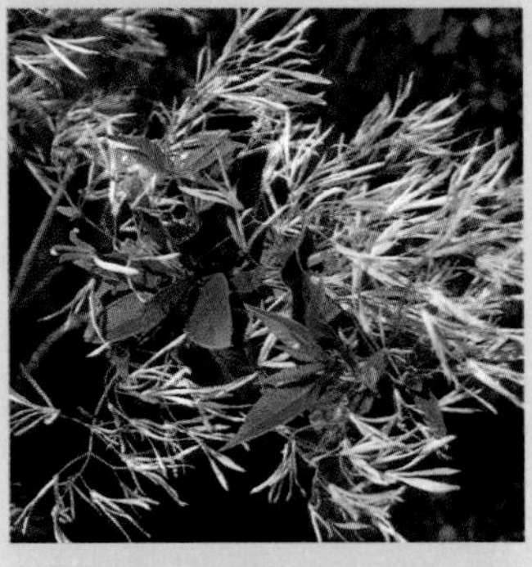

Chionanthus virginicus

FROSTWORT

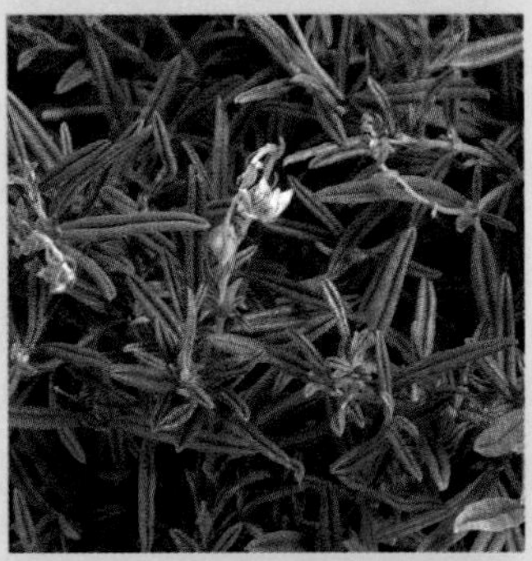

Helianthemum canadense

FUMITORY

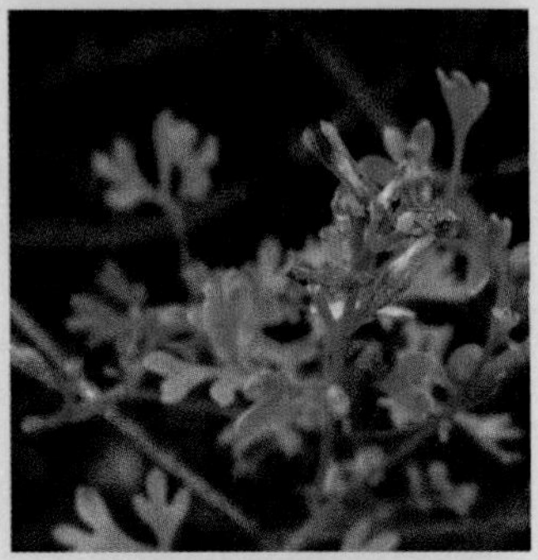

Fumaria officinalis

GAMBOGE

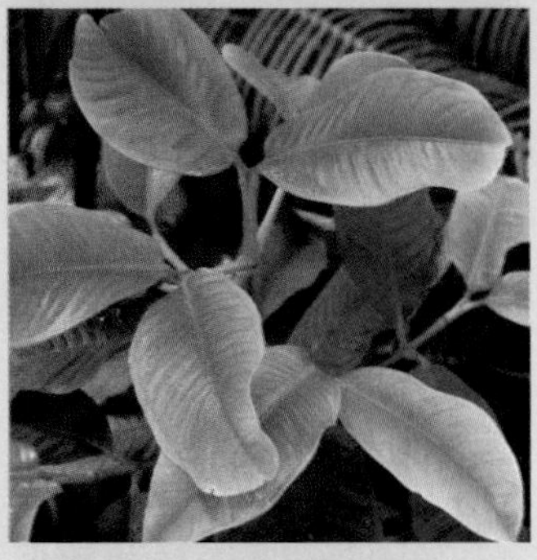

Garcinia hanburyi

GARDEN CRESS

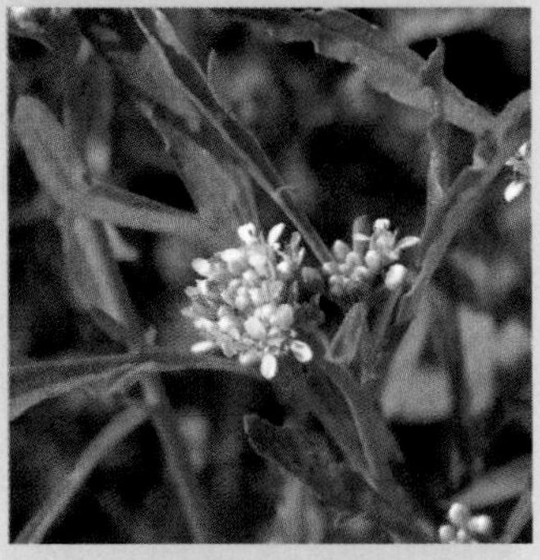

Lepidium sativum

GARLIC

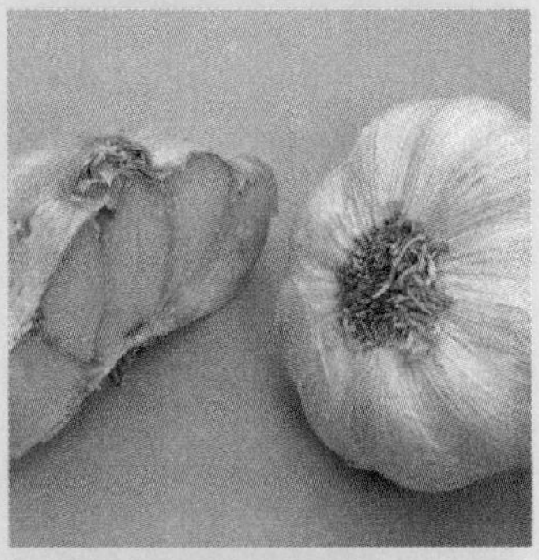

Allium sativum

GERMAN CHAMOMILE

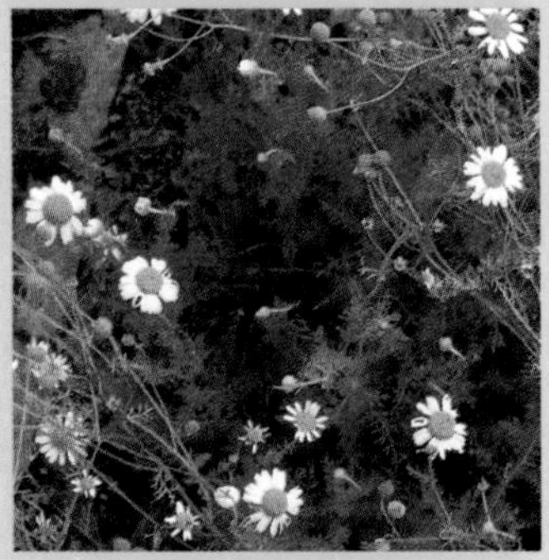

Matricaria recutita

GERMANDER

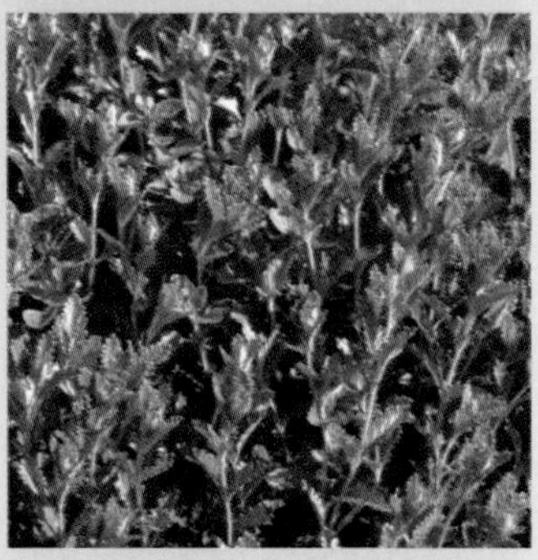

Teucrium chamaedrys

GINGER

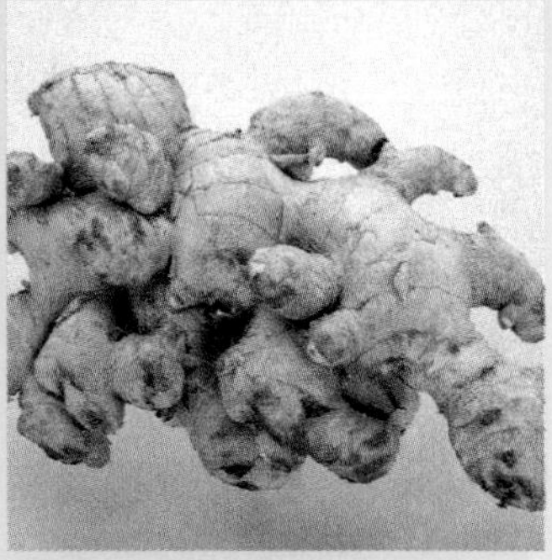

Zingiber officinale

GINKGO

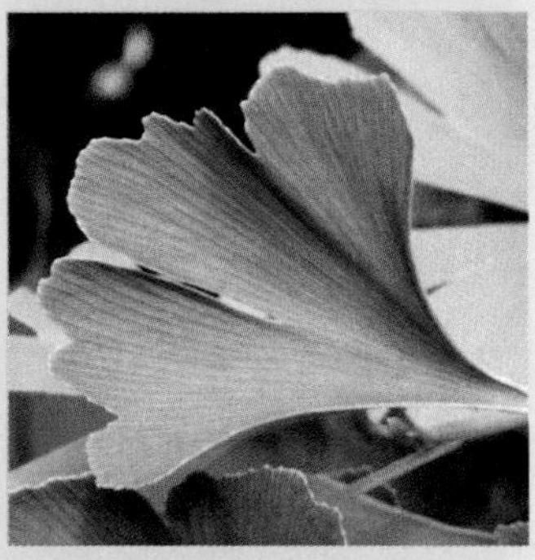

Ginkgo biloba

GLOBE FLOWER

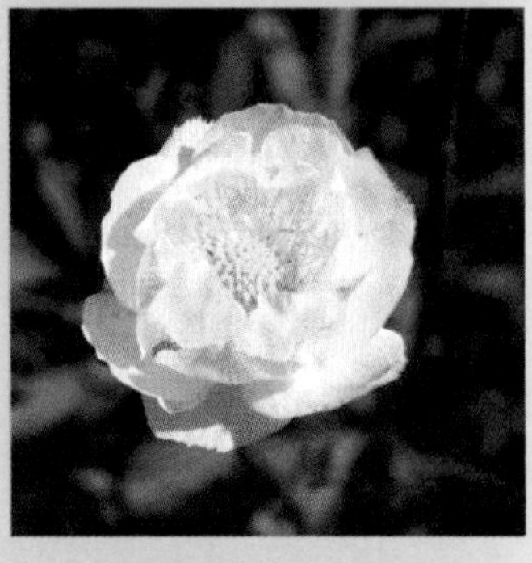

Trollius europaeus

GOAT'S RUE

Galega officinalis

GOLDEN SHOWER TREE

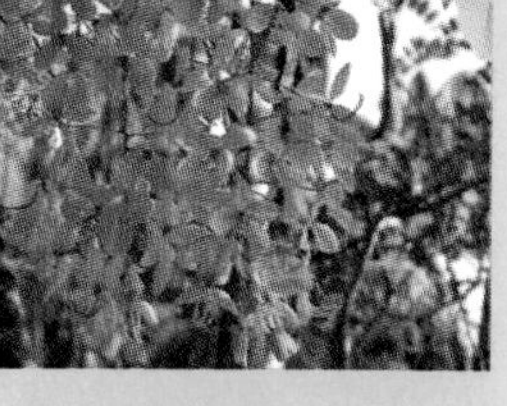

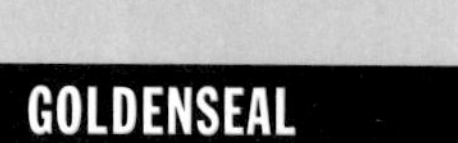

Cassia fistula

GOLDENSEAL

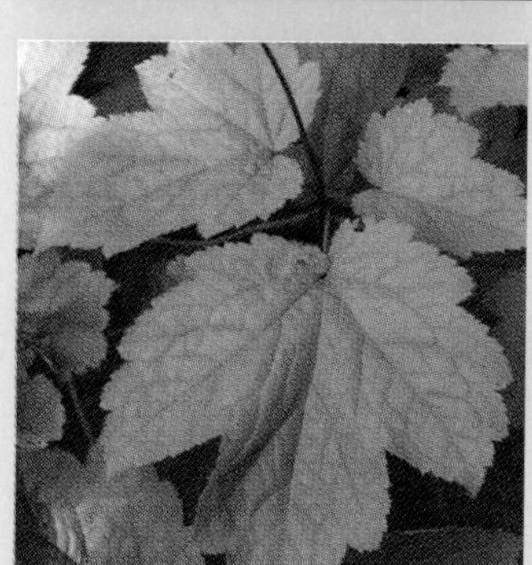

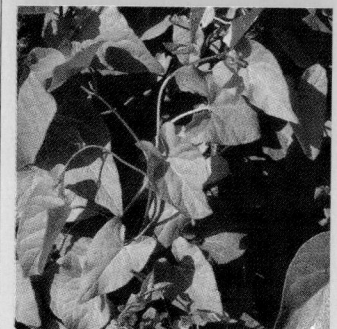

Hydrastis canadensis

GOTU KOLA

Centella asiatica

GOUTWEED

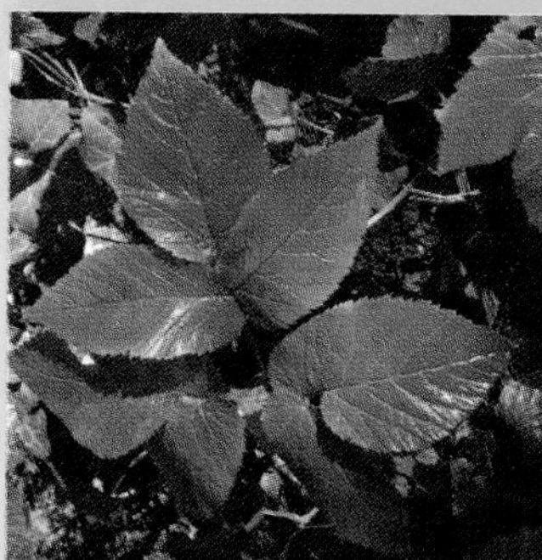

Aegopodium podagraria

GRAINS OF PARADISE

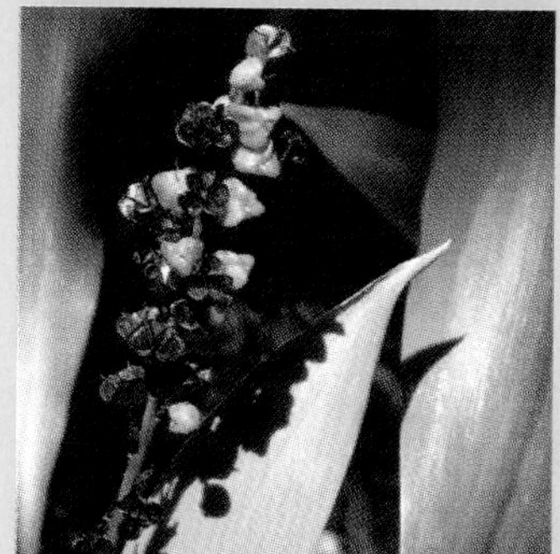

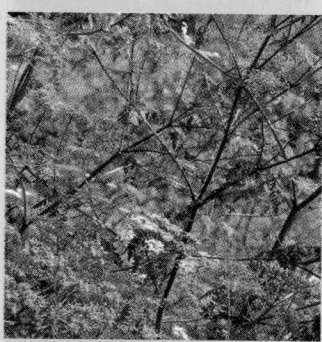

Aframomum melegueta

GRAPE

Vitis vinifera

GREAT BURNET

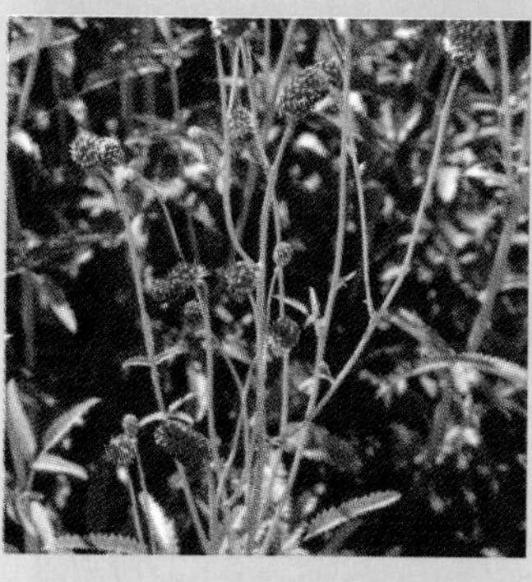

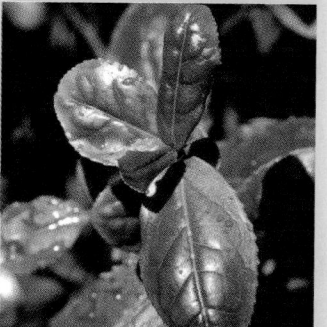

Sanguisorba officinalis

GREATER BINDWEED

Calystegia sepium

GREEN TEA

Camellia sinensis

GROUND PINE

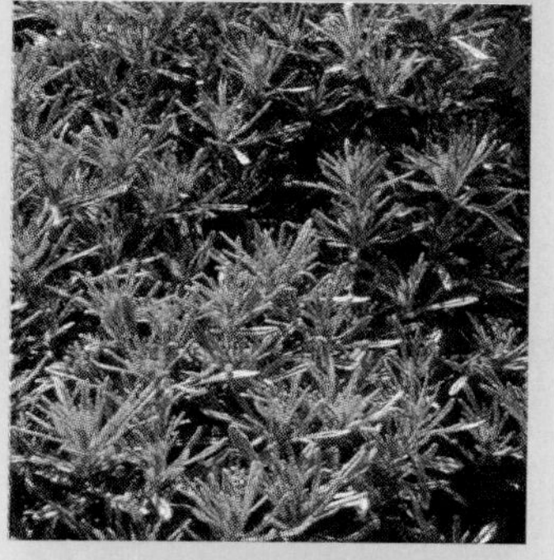

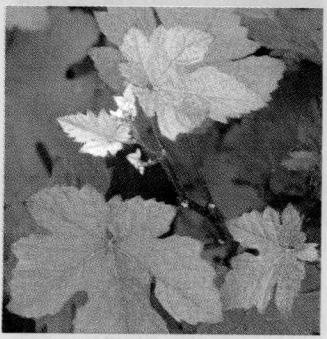

Ajuga chamaepitys

HEATHER

Calluna vulgaris

HEDGE-HYSSOP

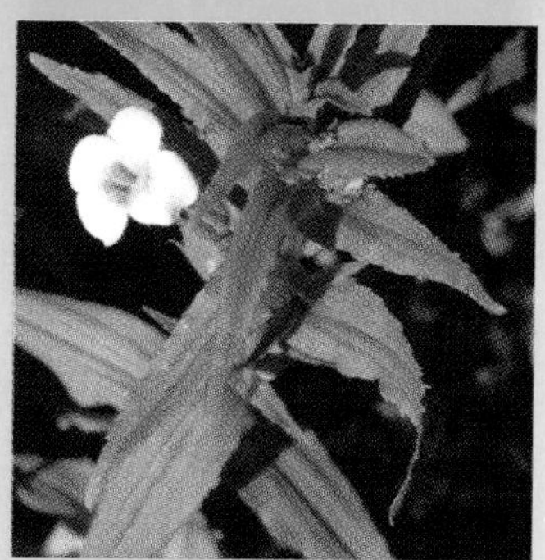

Gratiola officinalis

HEMLOCK

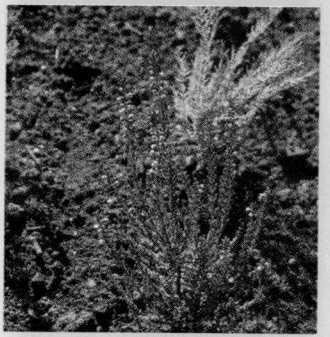

Conium maculatum

HEMP AGRIMONY

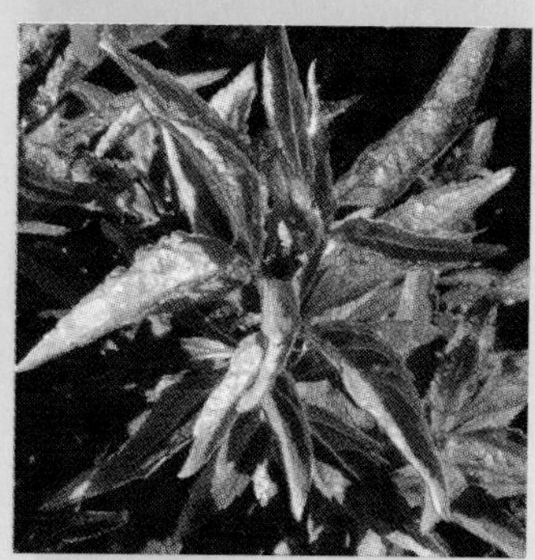

Eupatorium cannabinum

HEMPNETTLE

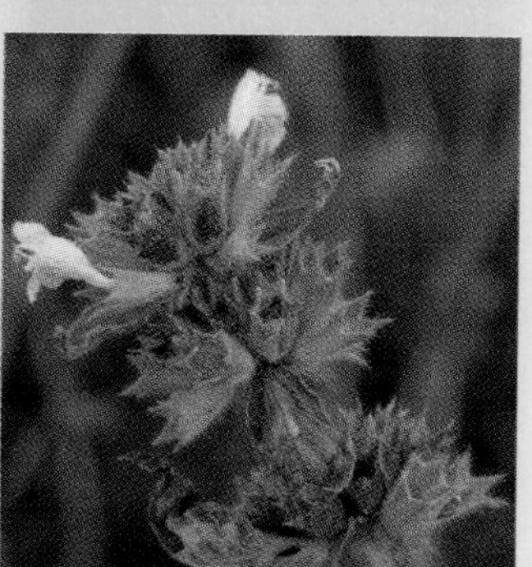

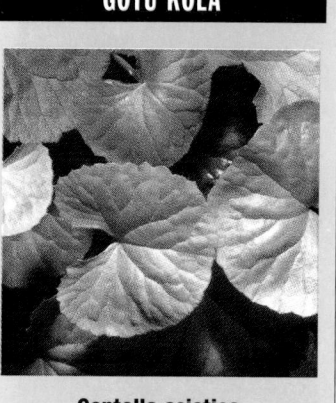

Galeopsis segetum

HENBANE

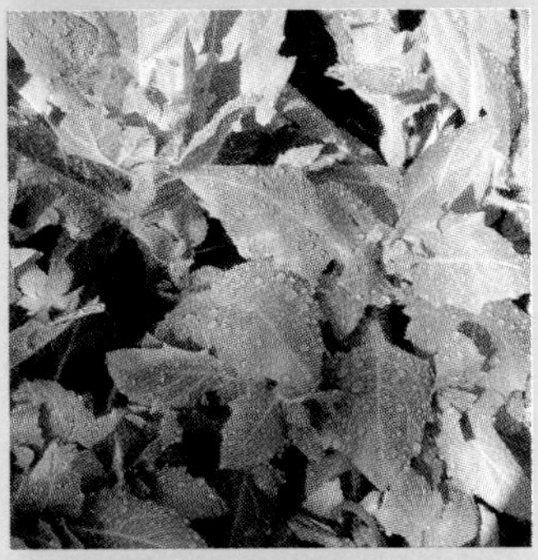

Hyoscyamus niger

HIBISCUS

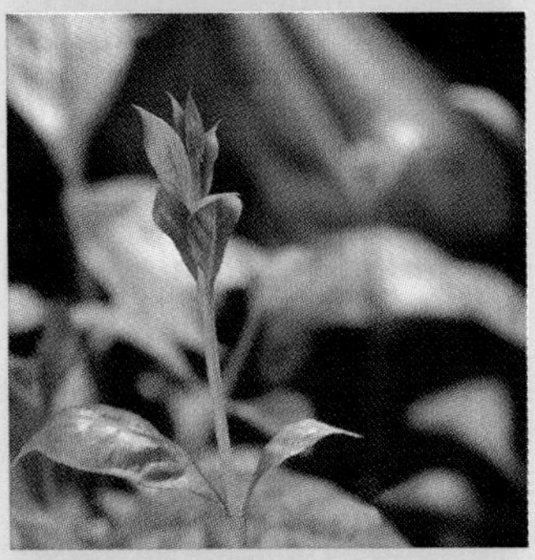

Hibiscus sabdariffa

HOLLYHOCK

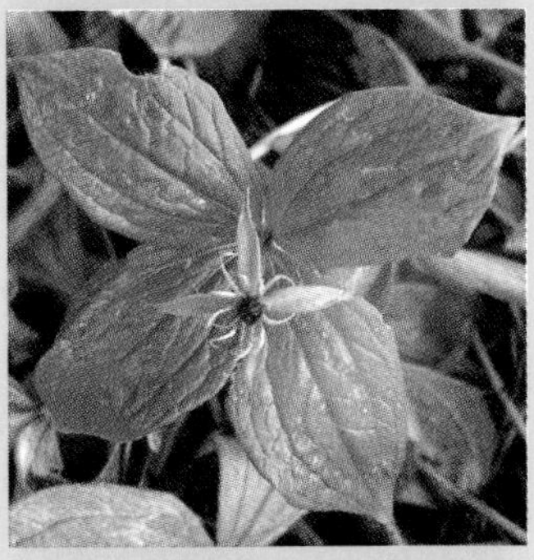

Alcea rosea

HORSERADISH

Armoracia rusticana

HENNA

Lawsonia inermis

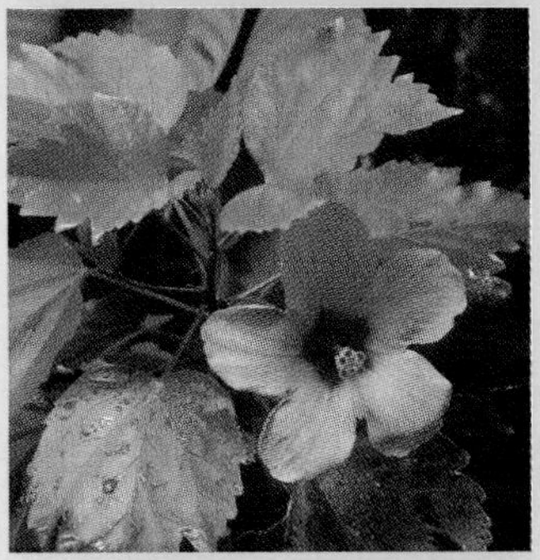

HIGH MALLOW

Malva sylvestris

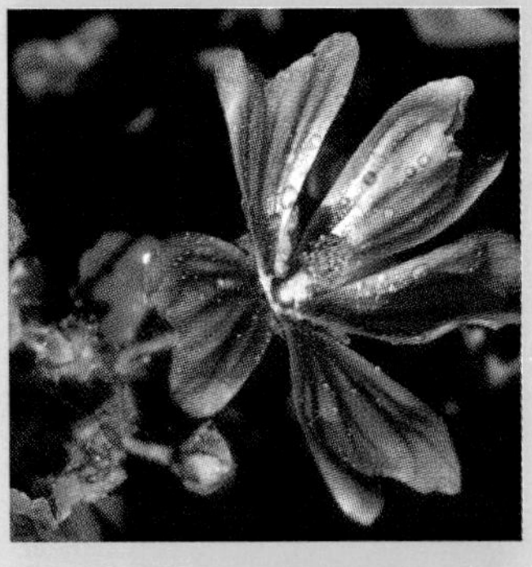

HOPS

Humulus lupulus

HORSETAIL

Equisetum arvense

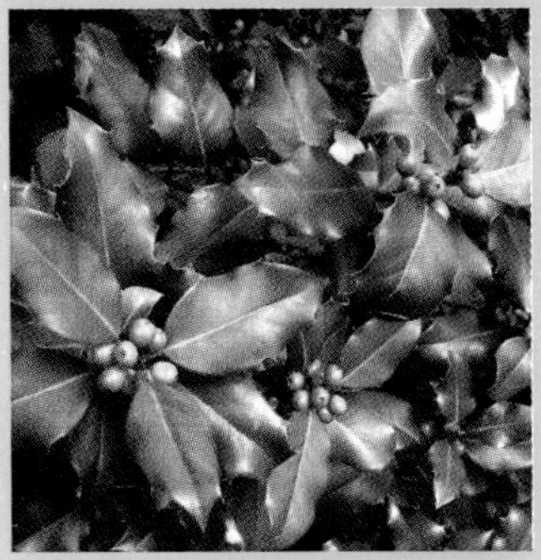

HERB PARIS

Paris quadrifolia

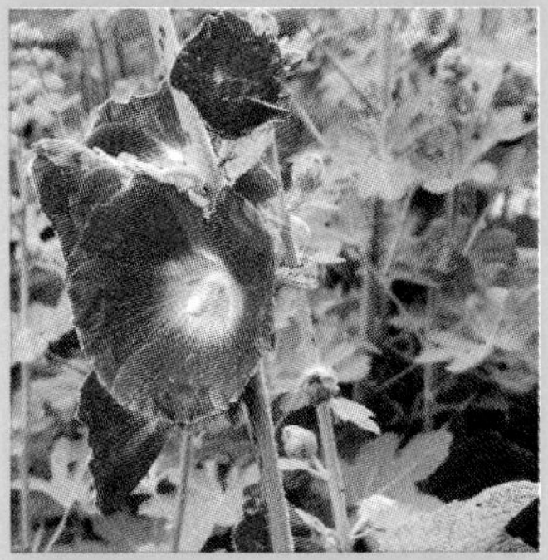

HOGWEED

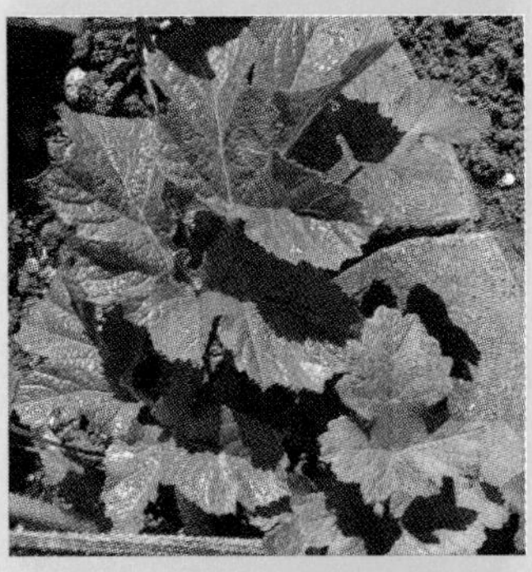

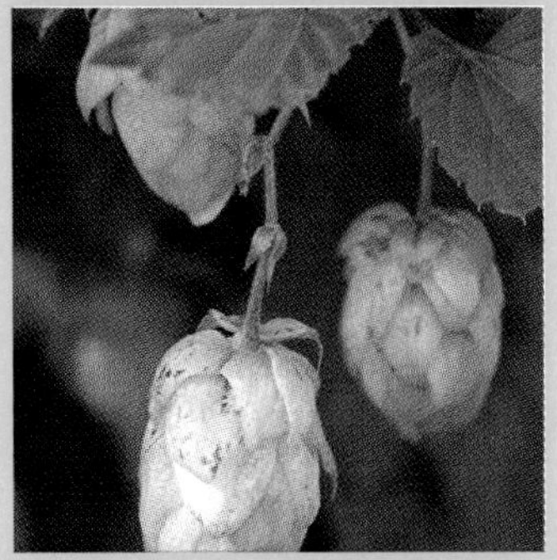

Heracleum sphondylium

HOREHOUND

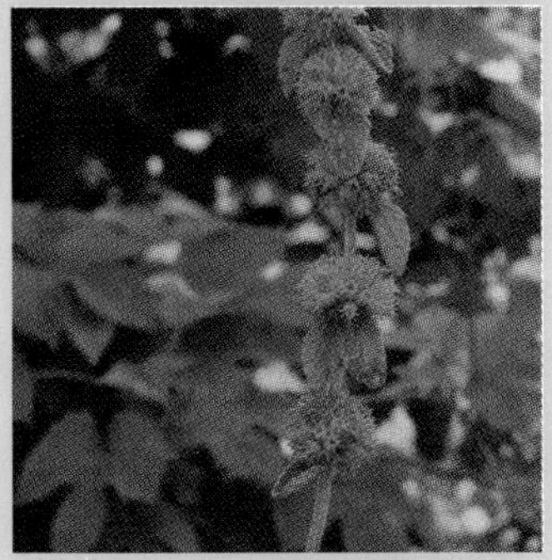

Marrubium vulgare

HOUSELEEK

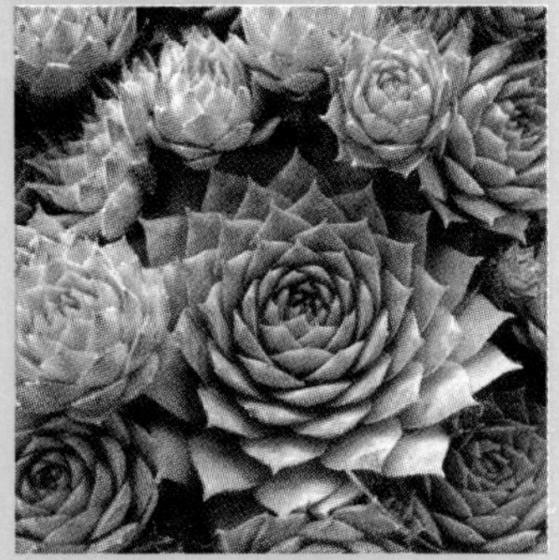

Sempervivum tectorum

HERB ROBERT

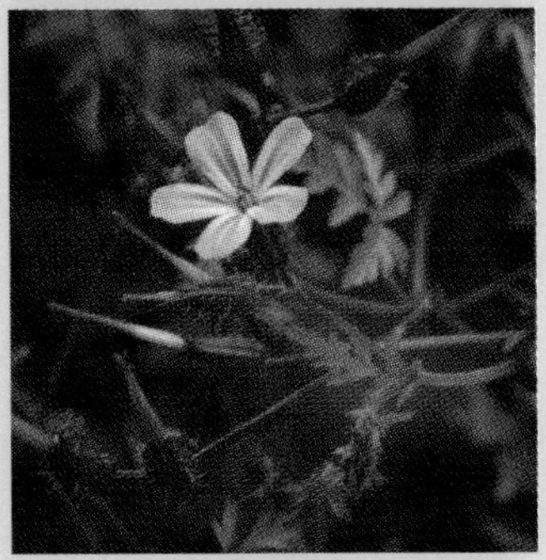

Geranium robertianum

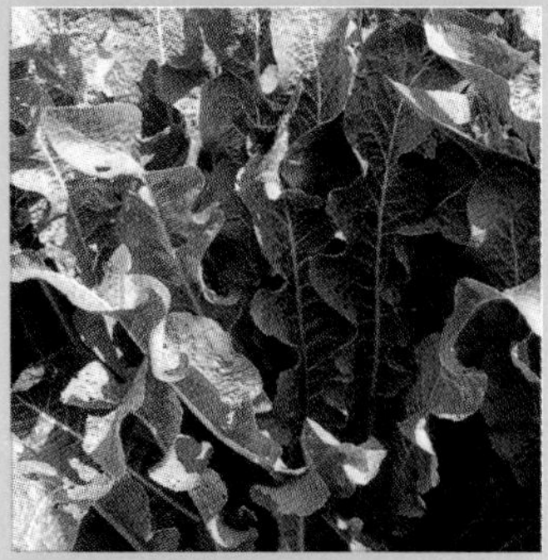

HOLLY

Ilex aquifolium

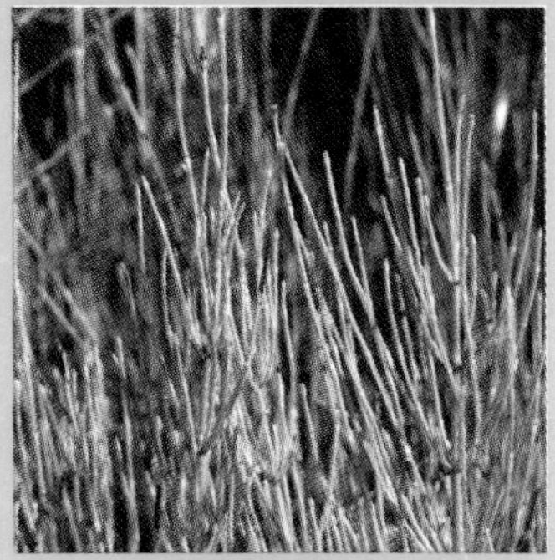

HORSE CHESTNUT

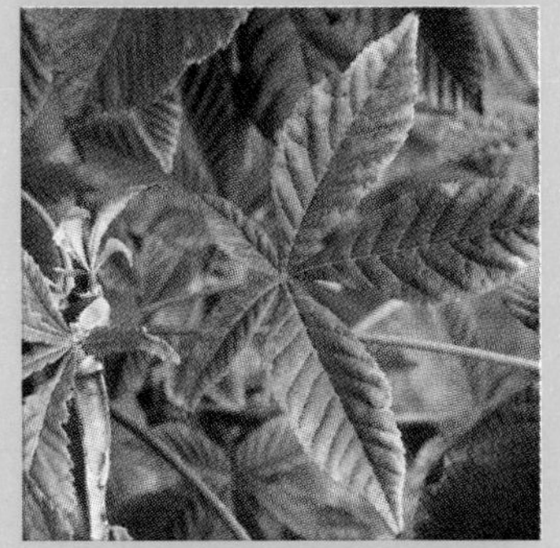

Aesculus hippocastanum

HYDRANGEA

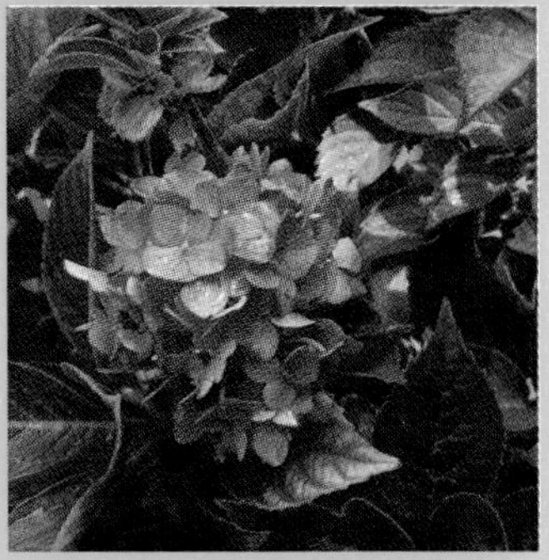

Hydrangea arborescens

HYSSOP

Hyssopus officinalis

JASMINE

Jasminum officinale

KAVA KAVA

Piper methysticum

LADY'S MANTLE

Alchemilla vulgaris

JABORANDI

Pilocarpus microphyllus

JIMSON WEED

Datura stramonium

KNOTWEED

Polygonum aviculare

LARCH

Larix decidua

JACOB'S LADDER

Polemonium caeruleum

JOJOBA

Simmondsia chinesis

LADY FERN

Athyrium filix-femina

LARKSPUR

Delphinium consolida

JALAP

Ipomoea purga

JUNIPER

Juniperus communis

LADY'S BEDSTRAW

Galium verum

LAUREL

Laurus nobilis

LAVENDER COTTON

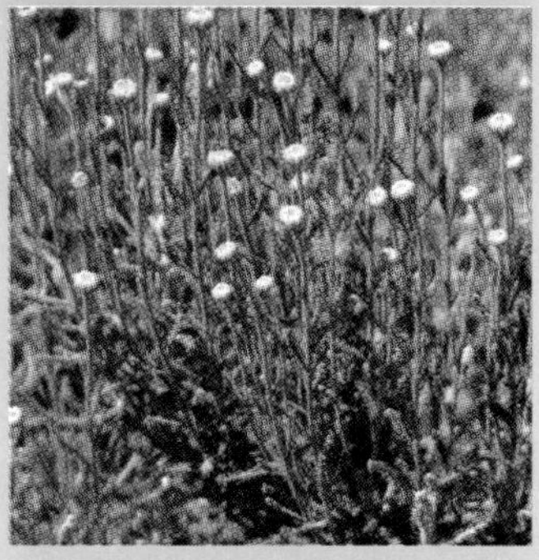

Santolina chamaecyparissias

LEMON BALM

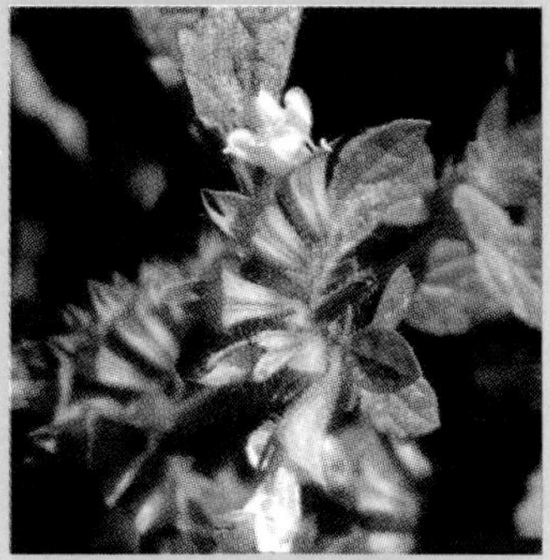

Melissa officinalis

LEMONGRASS

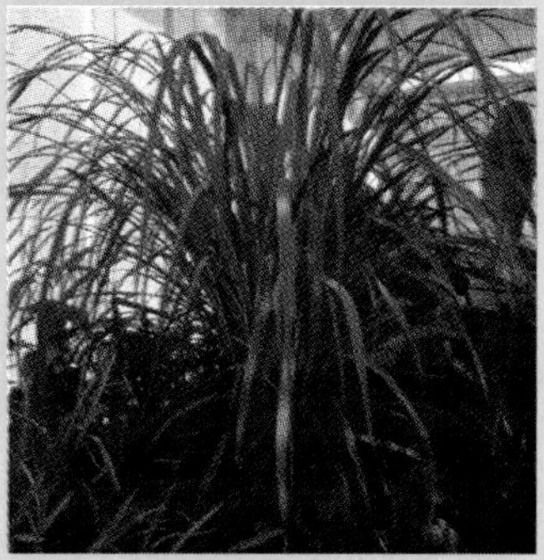

Cymbopogon citratus

LEVANT COTTON

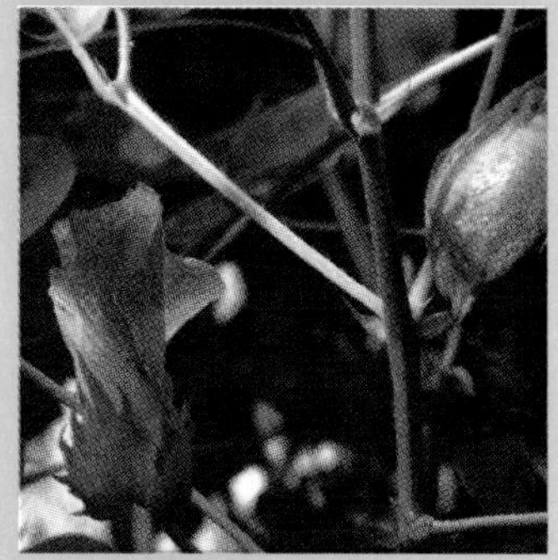

Gossypium herbaceum

LICORICE

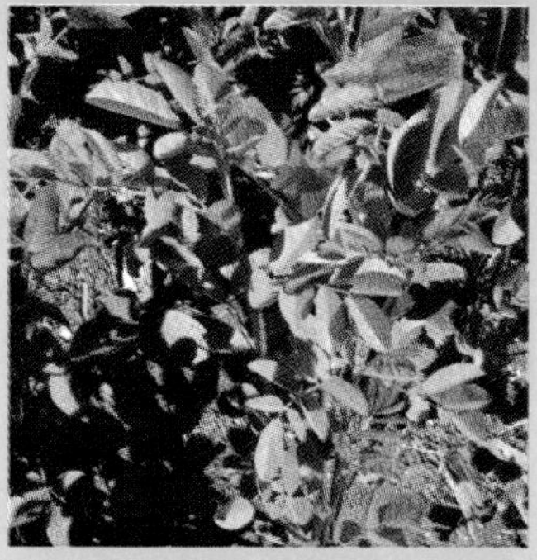

Glycyrrhiza glabra

LILY-OF-THE-VALLEY

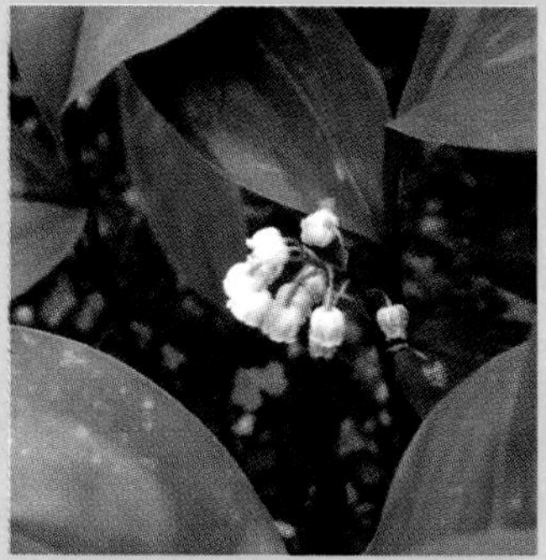

Convallaria majalis

LIME

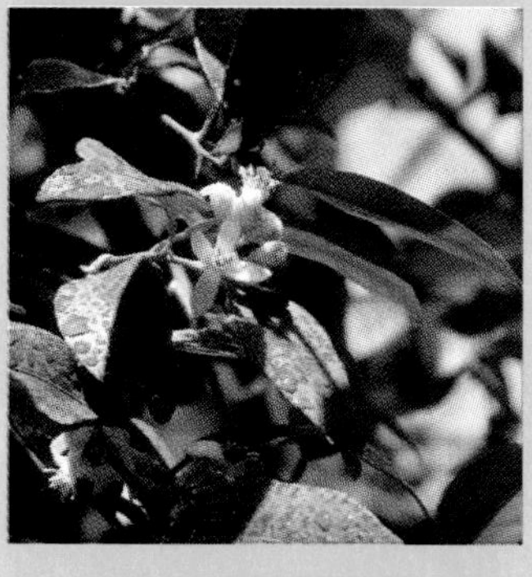

Citrus aurantifolia

LINDEN

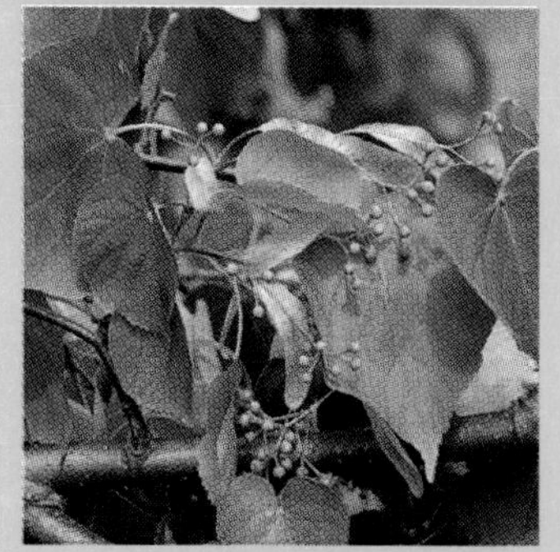

Tilia species

LOBELIA

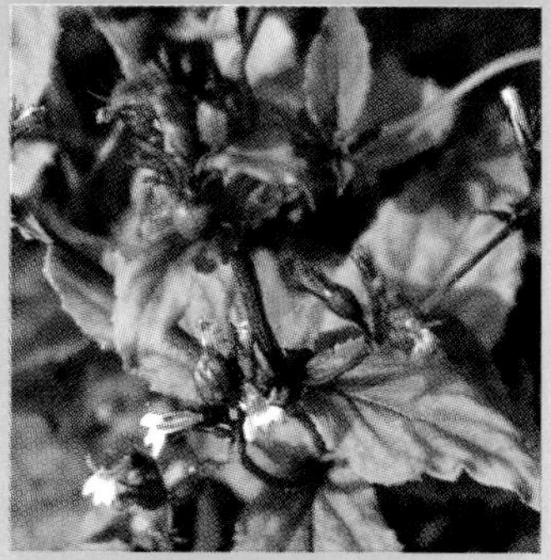

Lobelia inflata

LOOSESTRIFE

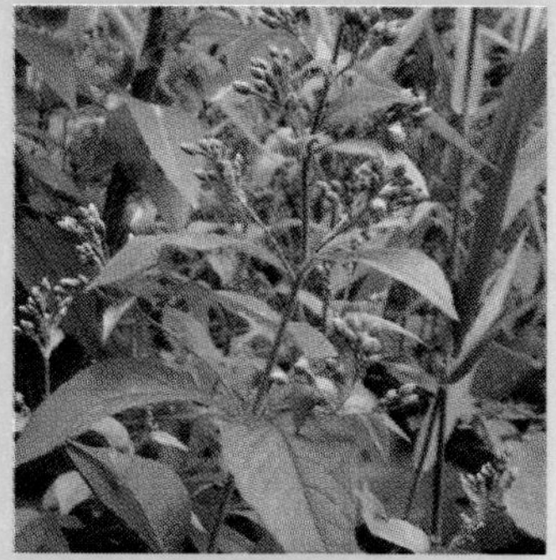

Lysimachia vulgaris

LOTUS

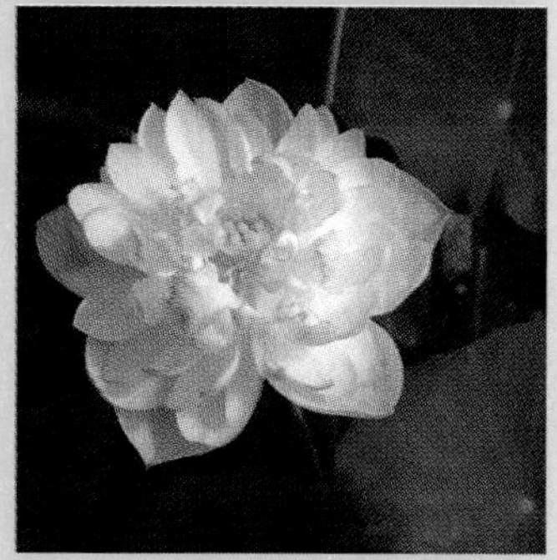

Nelumbo nucifera

LOVAGE

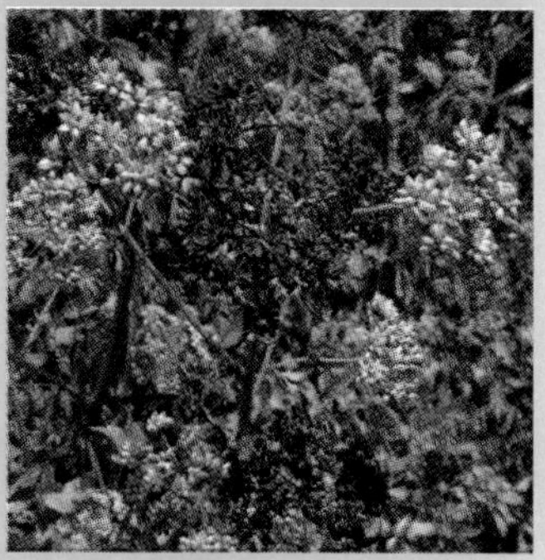

Levisticum officinale

LUFFA

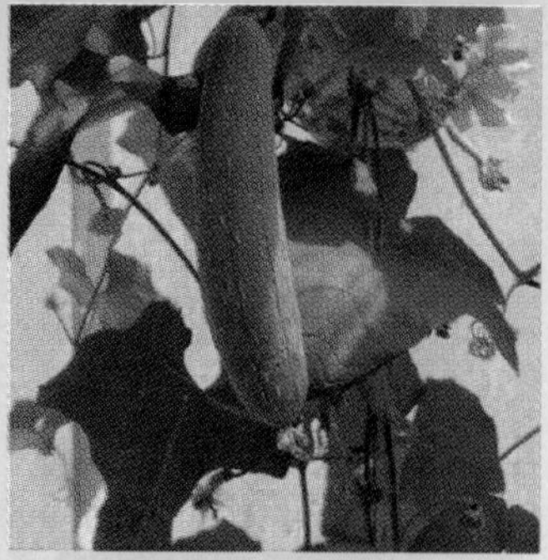

Luffa aegyptica

LUNGWORT

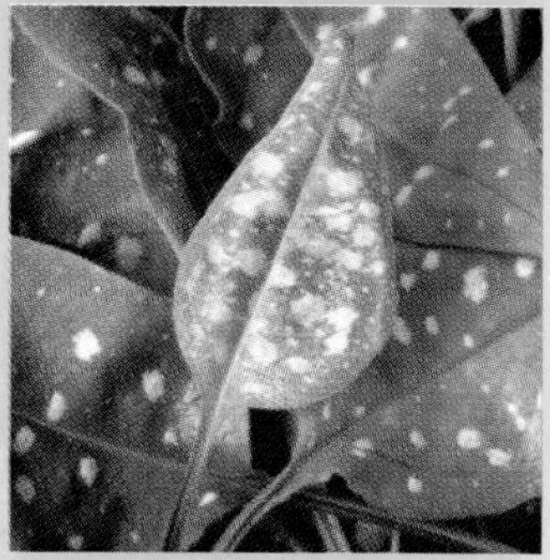

Pulmonaria officinalis

MADDER

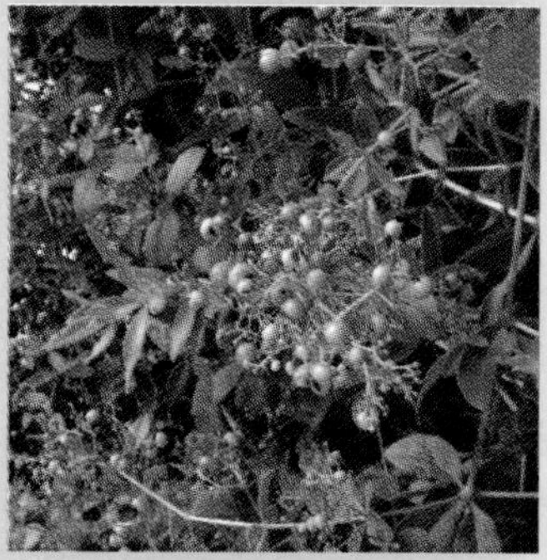

Rubia tinctorum

MA HUANG

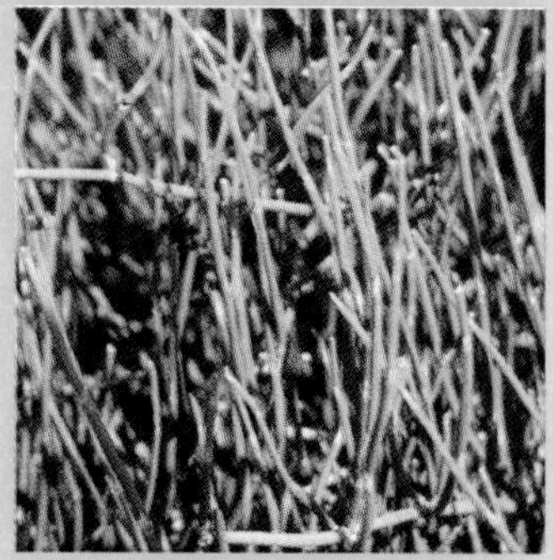

Ephedra sinica

MALABAR NUT

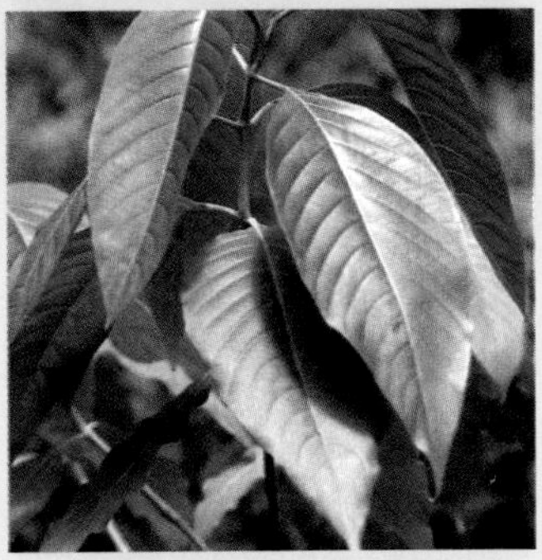

Justicia adhatoda

MALE FERN

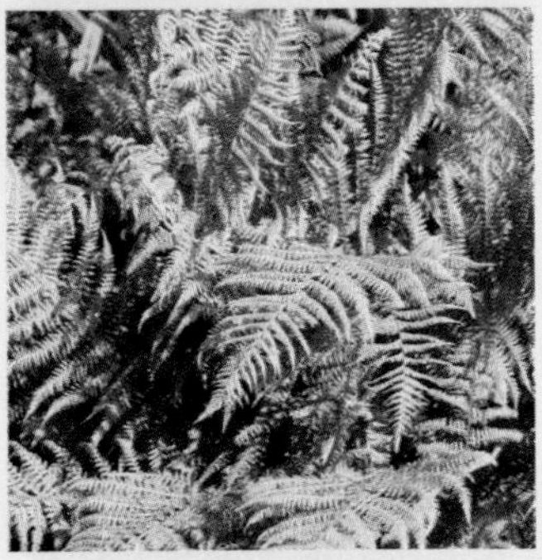

Dryopteris filix-mas

MANDRAKE

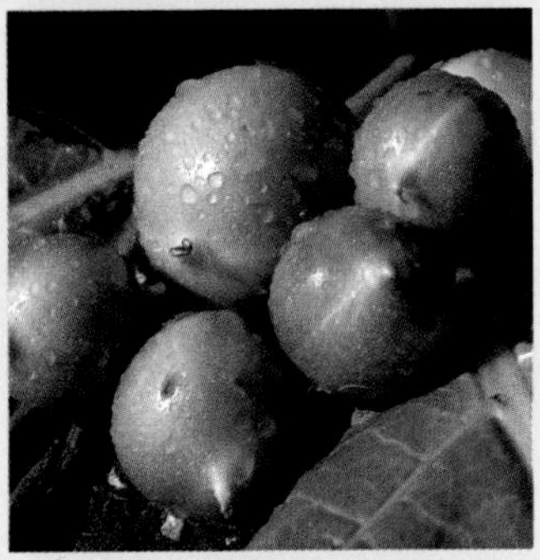

Mandragora officinarum

MANNA

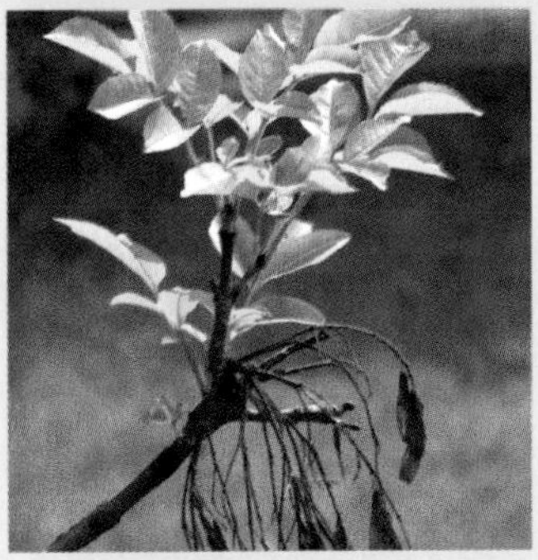

Fraxinus ornus

MARIGOLD

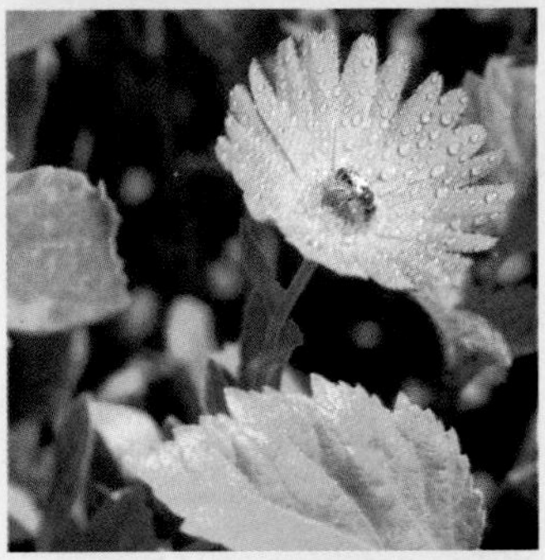

Calendula officinalis

MARIJUANA

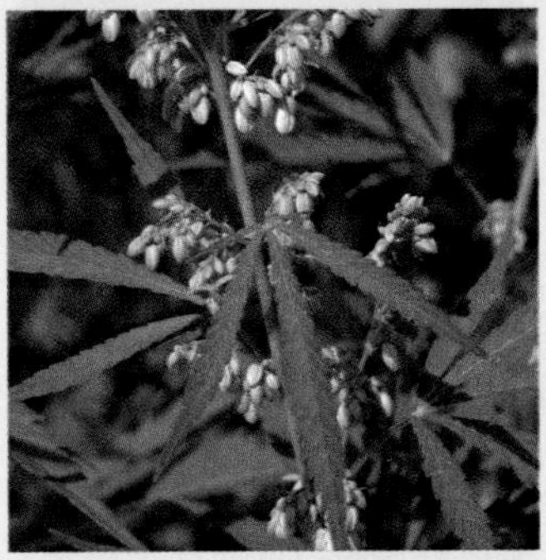

Cannabis sativa

MARSH BLAZING STAR

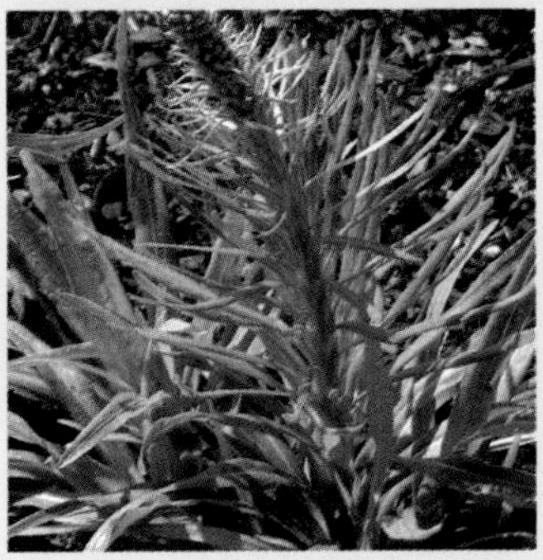

Liatris spicata

MARSH MARIGOLD

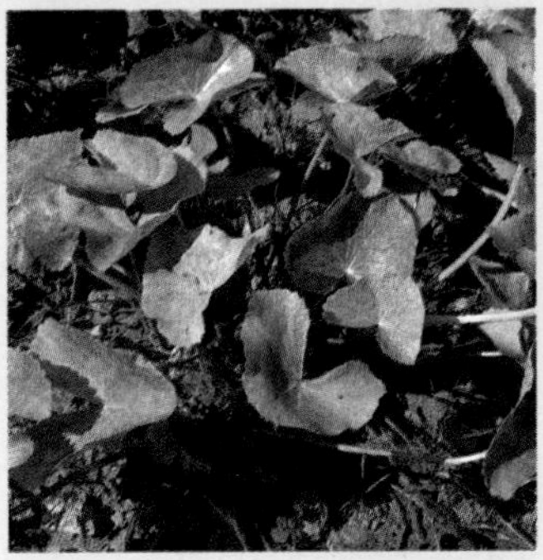

Caltha palustris

MASTIC TREE

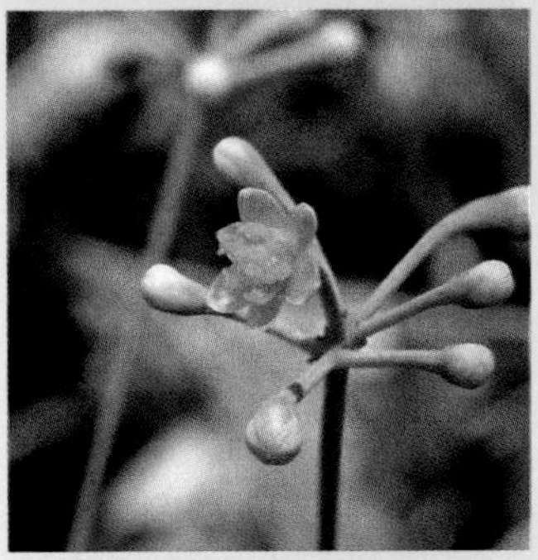

Pistacia lentiscus

MATÉ

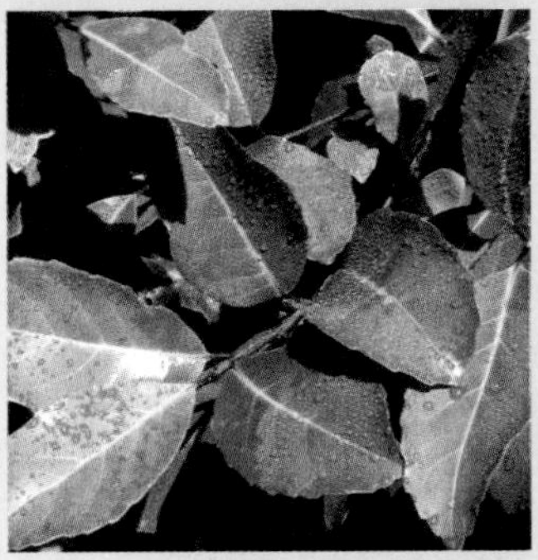

Ilex paraguariensis

MAYAPPLE

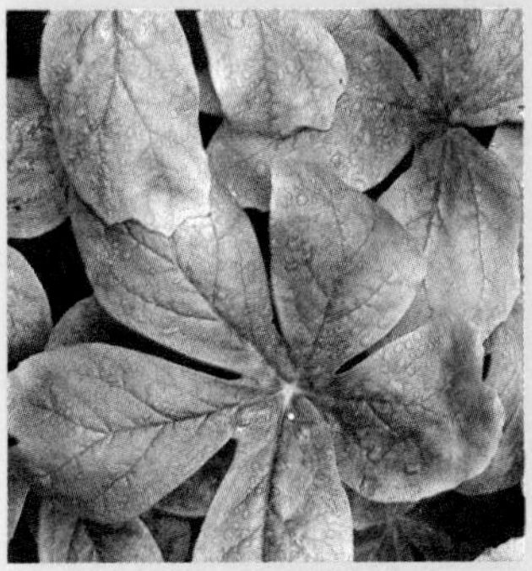

Podophylium peltatum

MEADOWSWEET

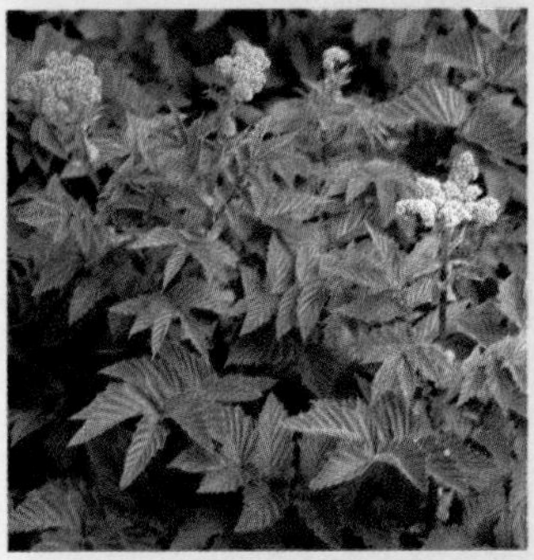

Filipendula ulmaria

MERCURY HERB

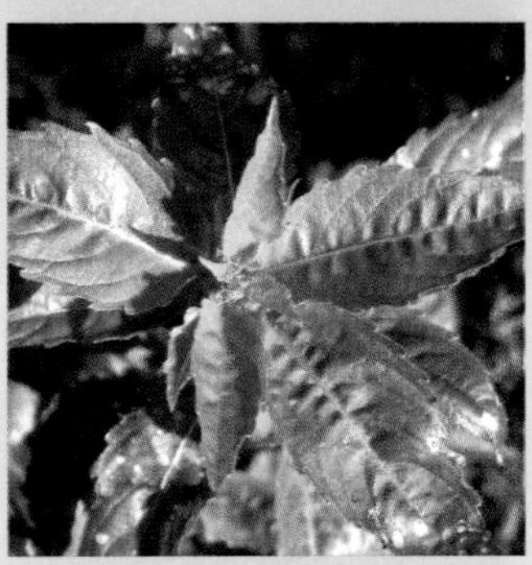

Mercurialis annua

MEZEREON

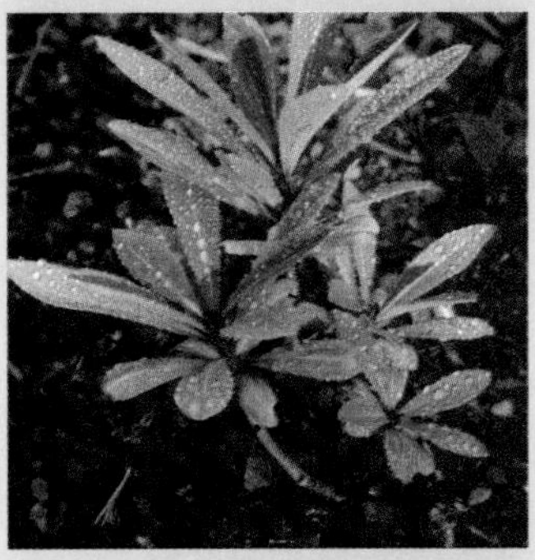

Daphne mezereum

MILK THISTLE

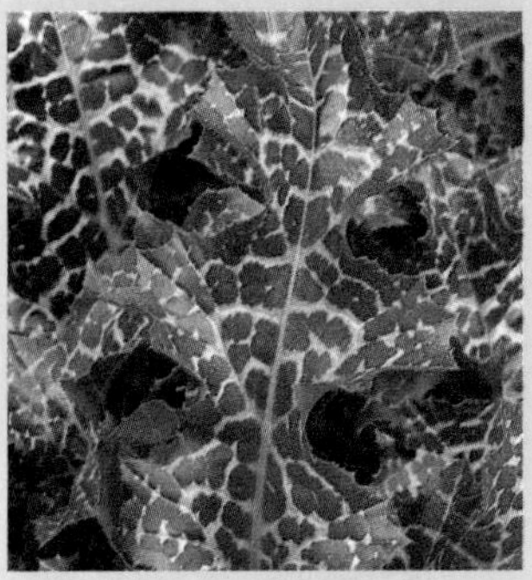

Silybum marianum

MONEYWORT

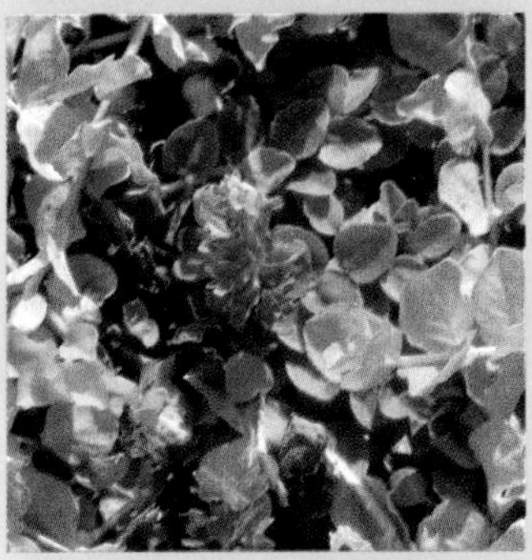

Lysimachia nummularia

MONKSHOOD

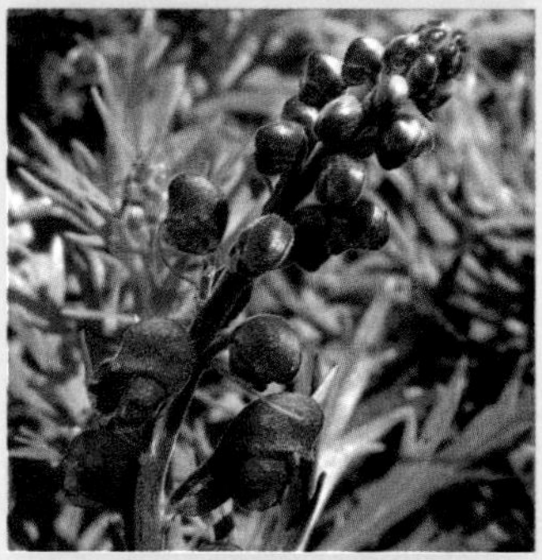

Aconitum napellus

MOTHERWORT

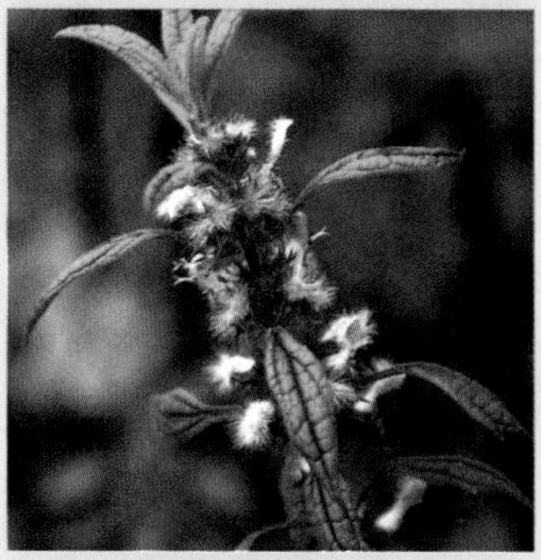

Leonurus cardiaca

MOUNTAIN ASH BERRY

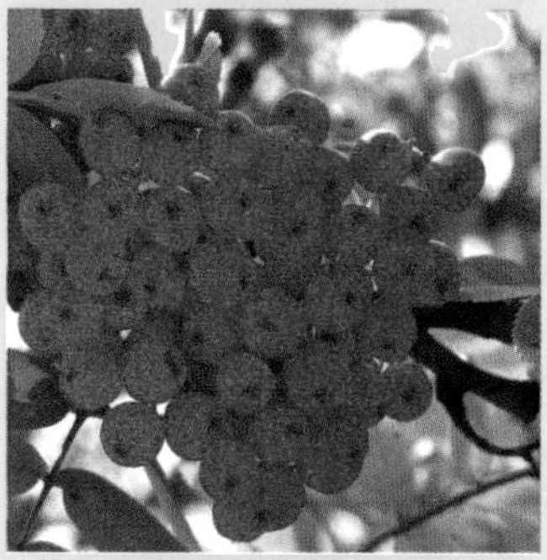

Sorbus aucuparia

MOUNTAIN GRAPE

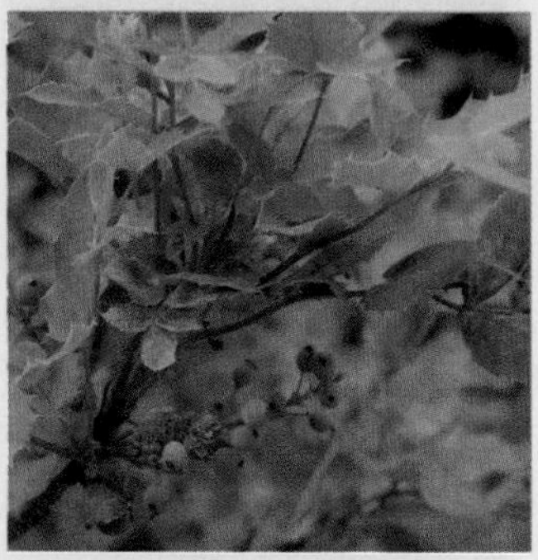

Mahonia aquifolium

MOUNTAIN LAUREL

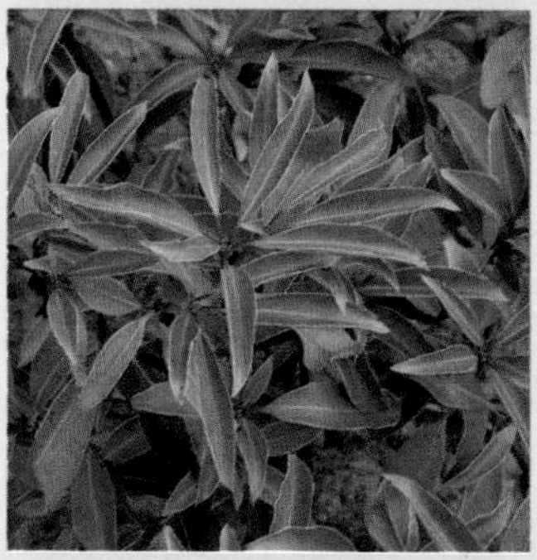

Kalmia latifolia

MUGWORT

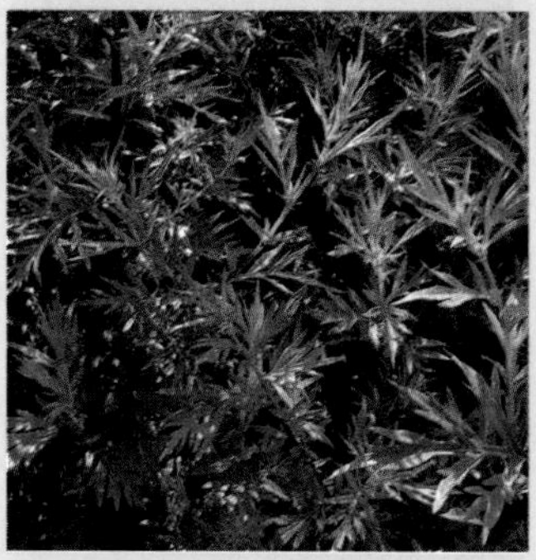

Artemisia vulgaris

MULLEIN

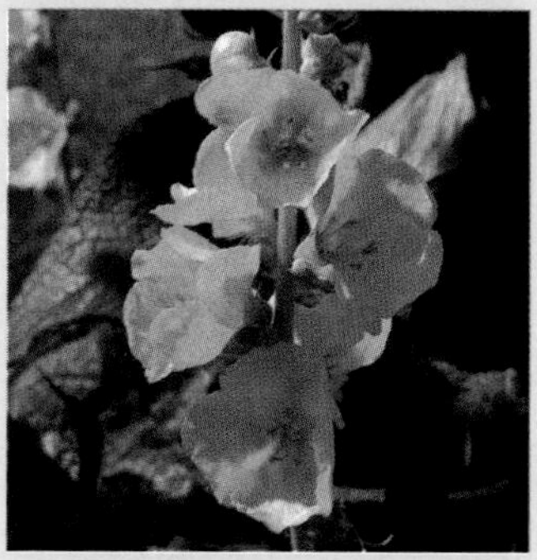

Verbascum densiflorum

MYRRH

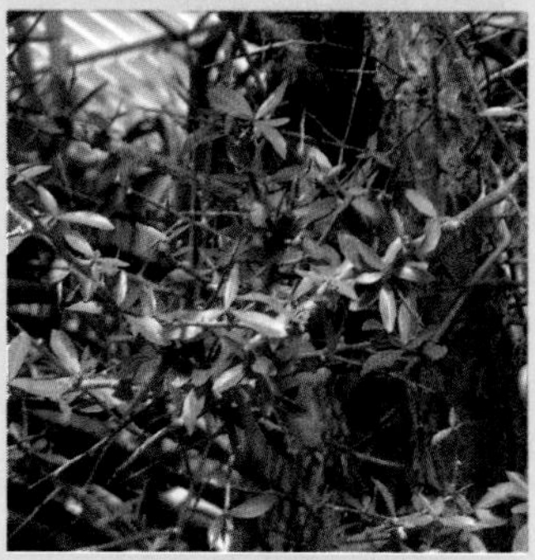

Commiphora molmol

MYRTLE

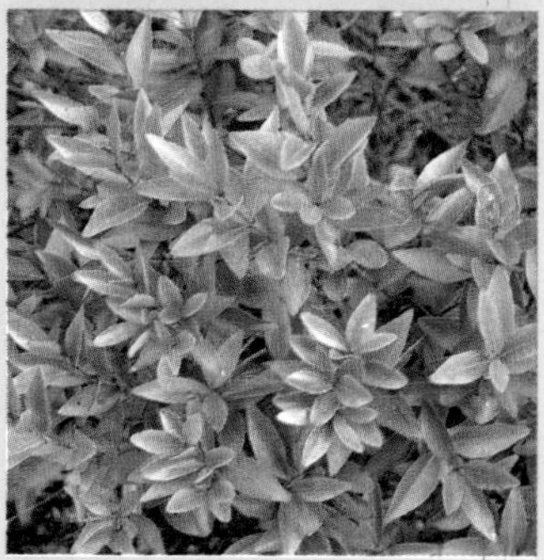

Myrtus communis

NASTURTIUM

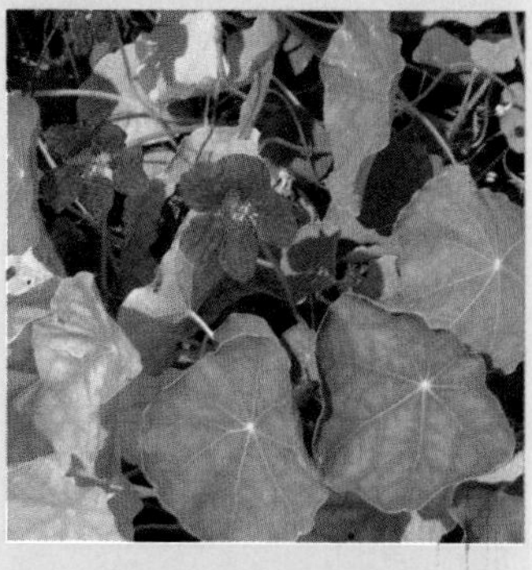

Tropaeolum majus

NEEM

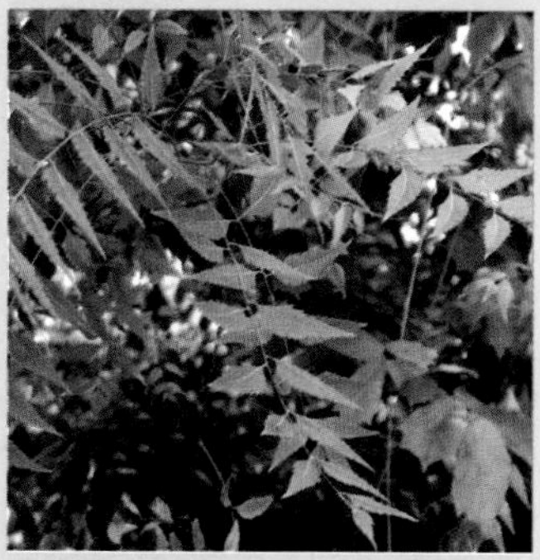

Antelaea azadirachta

NONI

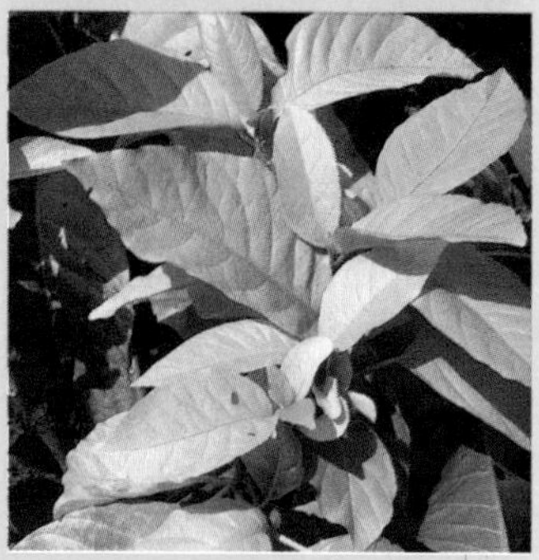

Morinda citrifolia

NUTMEG

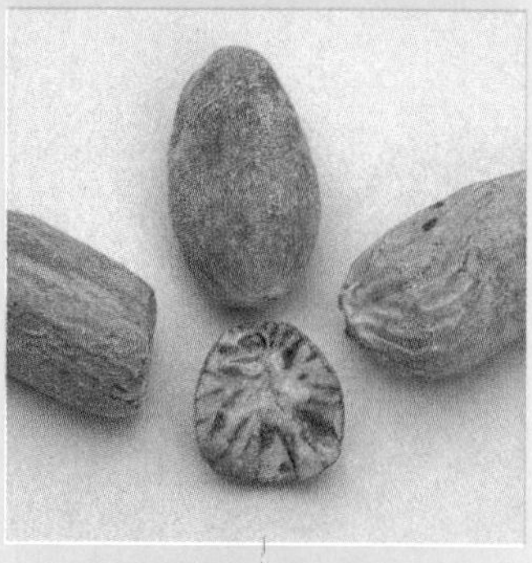

Myristica fragrans

NUX VOMICA

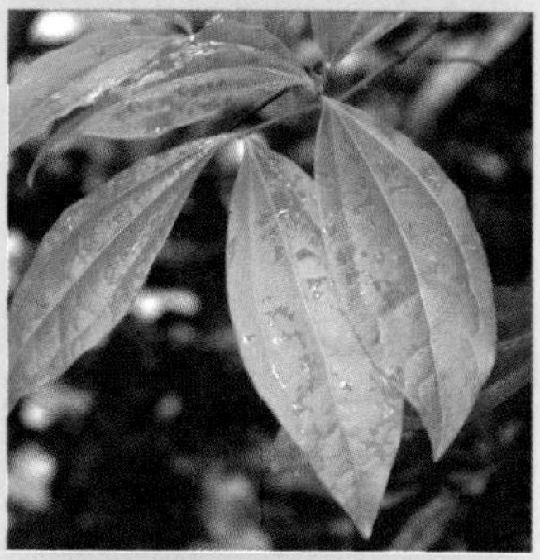

Strychnos nux vomica

OAK

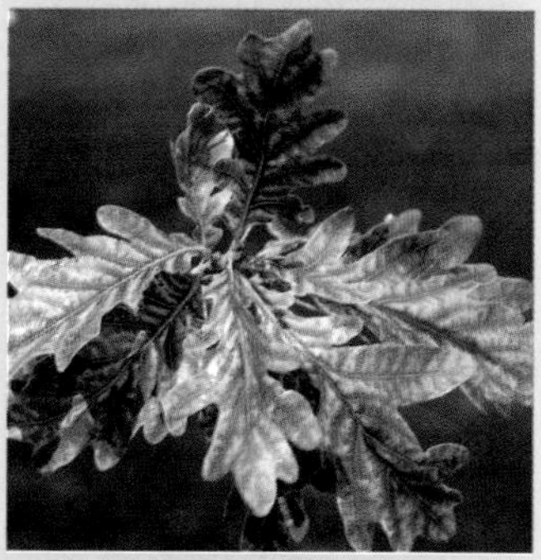

Quercus robur

OATS

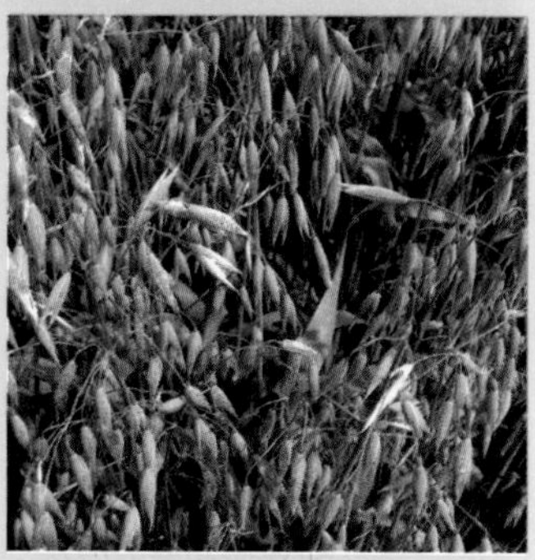

Avena sativa

OILSEED RAPE

Brassica napus

OREGANO

Origanum vulgare

PARSNIP

Pastinaca sativa

PETASITES

Petasites hybridus

OLEANDER LEAF

Nerium oleander

ORRIS

Iris species

PASSION FLOWER

Passiflora incarnata

PEYOTE

Lophophora williamsii

OLIVE

Olea europaea

PAPAYA

Carica papaya

PATCHOULI

Pogostemon cablin

PIMPINELLA

Pimpinella major

ONION

Allium cepa

PARSLEY

Petroselinum crispum

PEPPERMINT

Mentha piperita

PINUS BARK

Tsuga canadensis

PITCHER PLANT

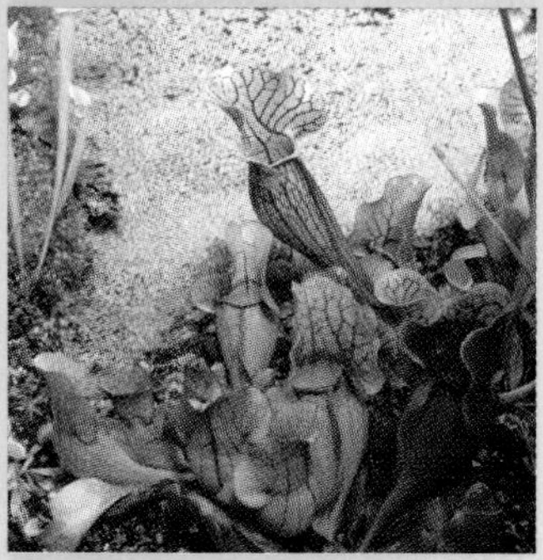

Sarracenia purpurea

PLEURISY ROOT

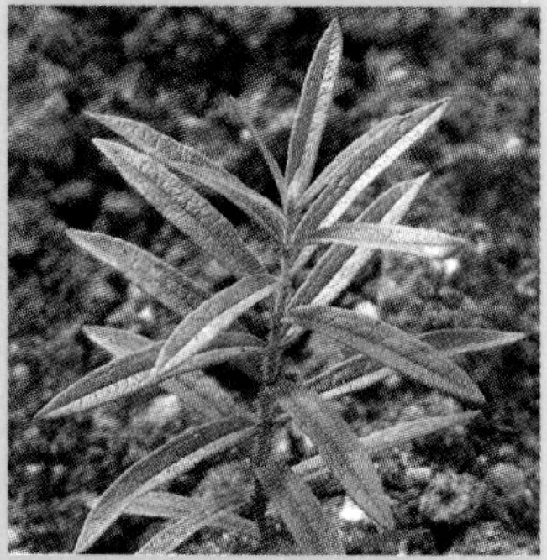

Asclepias tuberosa

POISONOUS BUTTERCUP

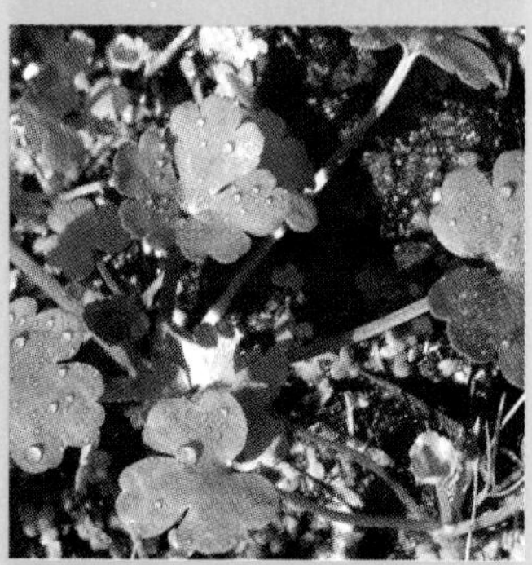

Ranunculus sceleratus

POKE

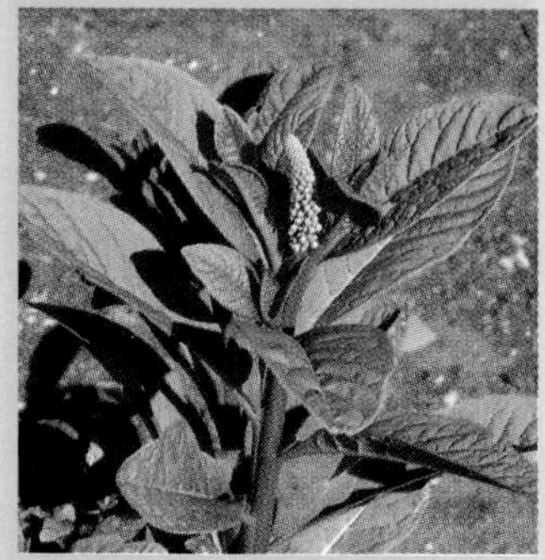

Phytolacca americana

POMEGRANATE

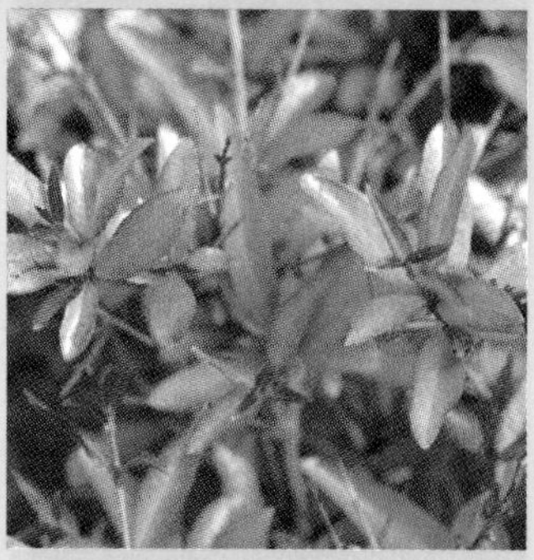

Punica granatum

POPLAR

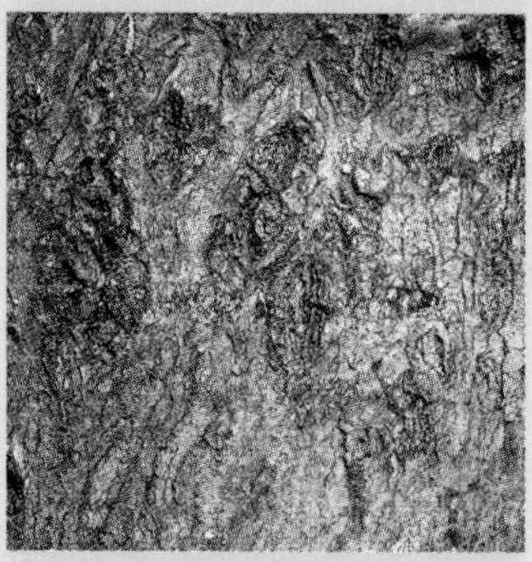

Populus species

POPPYSEED

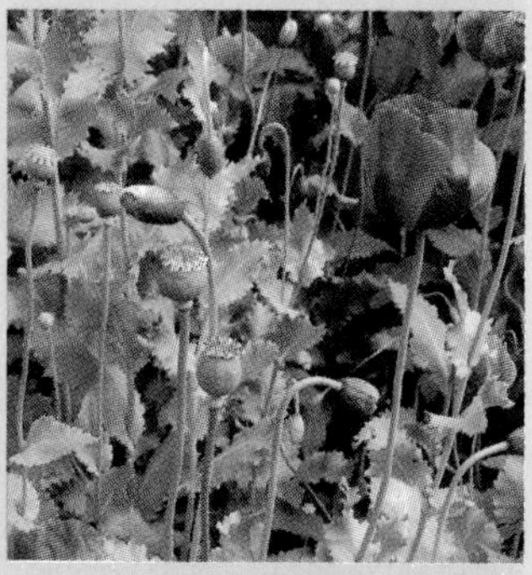

Papaver somniferum

POTENTILLA

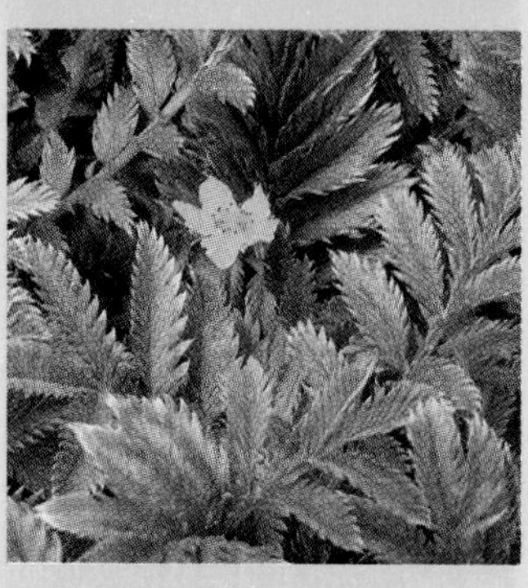

Potentilla anserina

PREMORSE

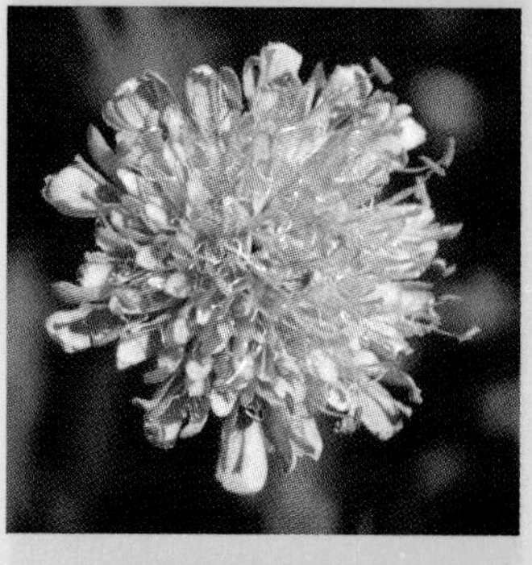

Scabiosa succisa

PSYLLIUM SEED

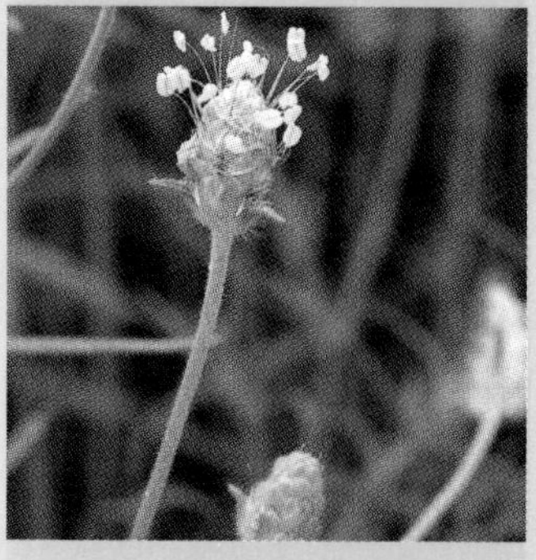

Plantago afra

PUMPKIN

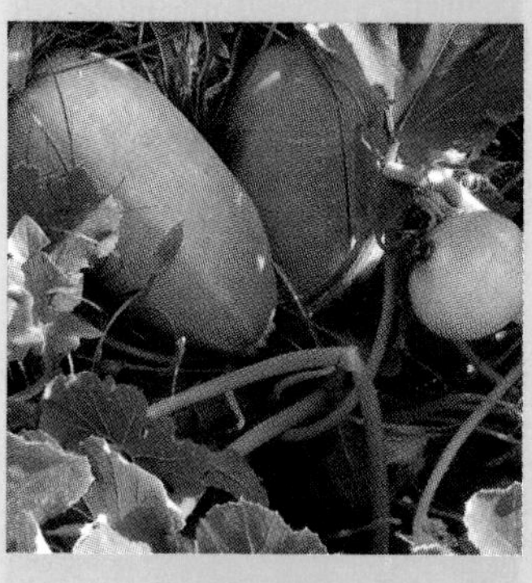

Cucurbita pepo

PURPLE LOOSESTRIFE

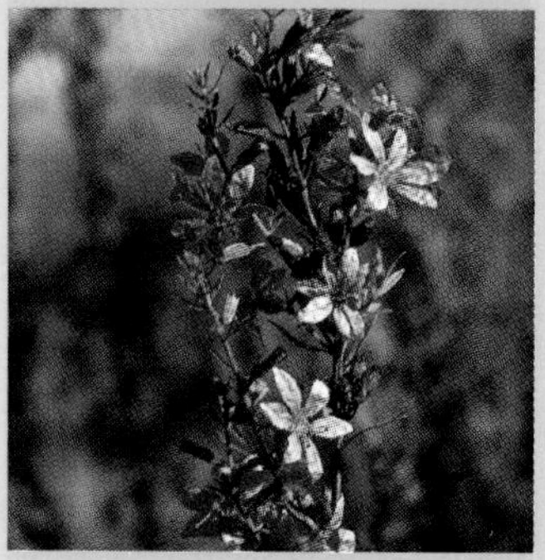

Lythrum salicaria

QUILLAJA

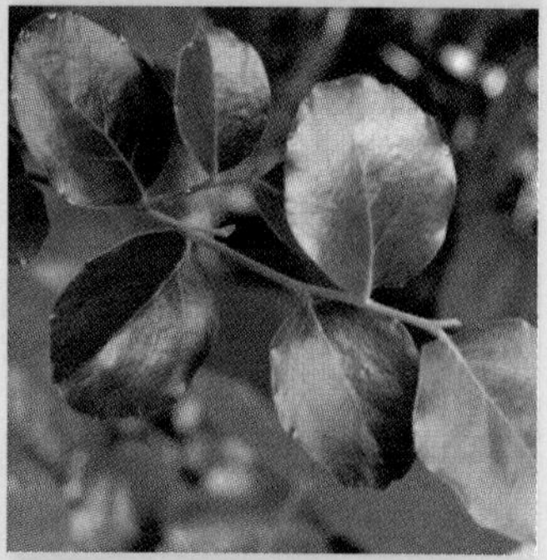

Quillaja saponaria

QUININE

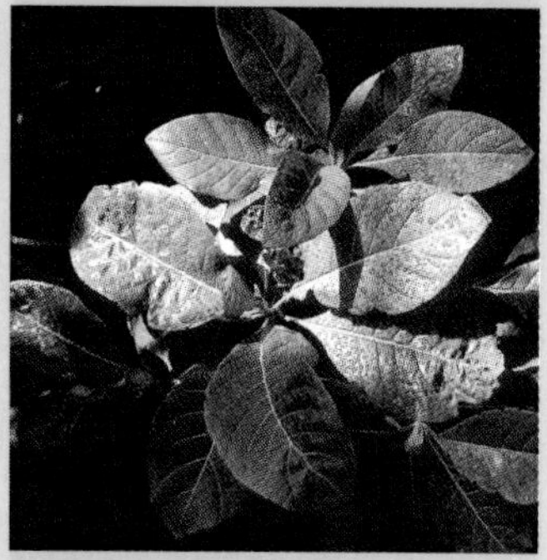

Cinchona pubescens

RADISH

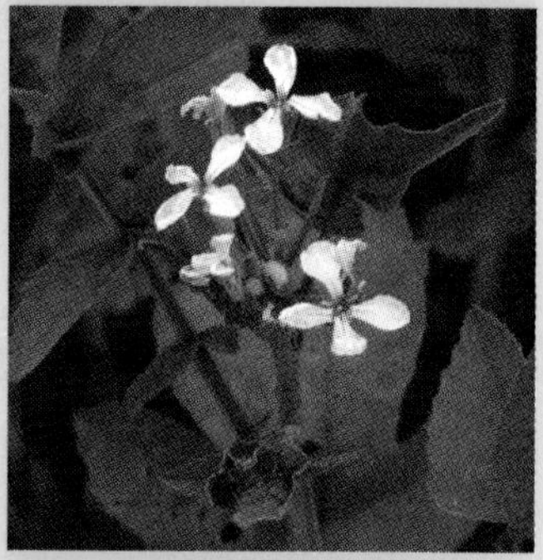

Raphanus sativus

RAGWORT

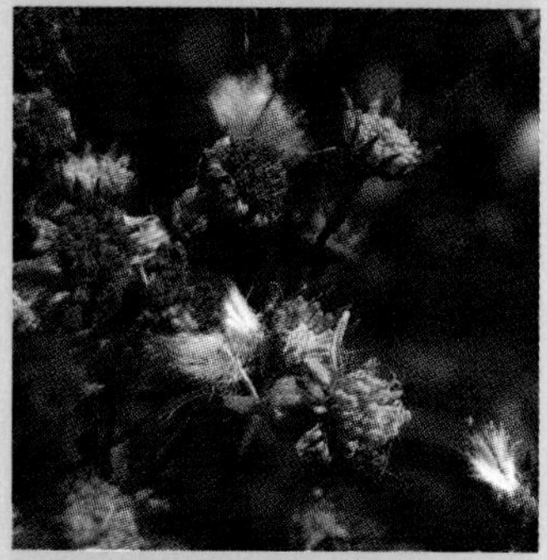

Senecio jacobaea

RASPBERRY

Rubus idaeus

RED CLOVER

Trifolium pratense

RED CURRANT

Ribes rubrum

RED MAPLE

Acer rubrum

RED-SPUR VALERIAN

Centranthus ruber

RICE

Oryza sativa

ROSEMARY

Rosmarinus officinalis

ROSINWEED

Silphium laciniatum

RUE

Ruta graveolens

RUPTUREWORT

Herniaria glabra

SAFFRON

Crocus sativus

SAGE

Salvia officinalis

SARSAPARILLA

Smilax species

SASSAFRAS

Sassafras albidum

SAVIN TOPS

Juniperus sabina

SAW PALMETTO

Serenoa repens

SCARLET PIMPERNEL

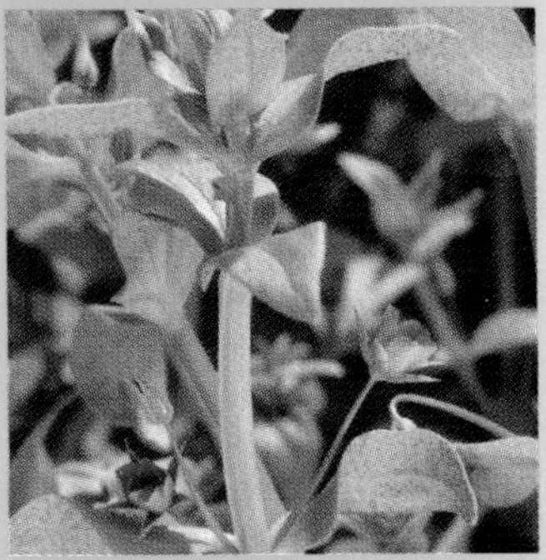

Anagallis arvensis

SCOTCH BROOM

Cytisus scoparius

SCOTCH PINE

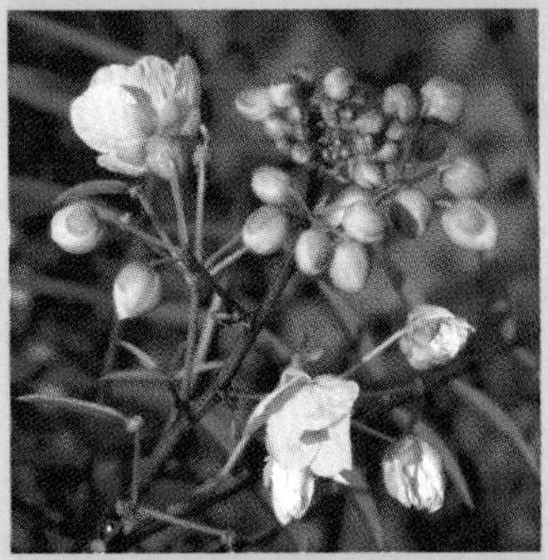

Pinus species

SCOTCH THISTLE

Onopordum acanthium

SCULLCAP

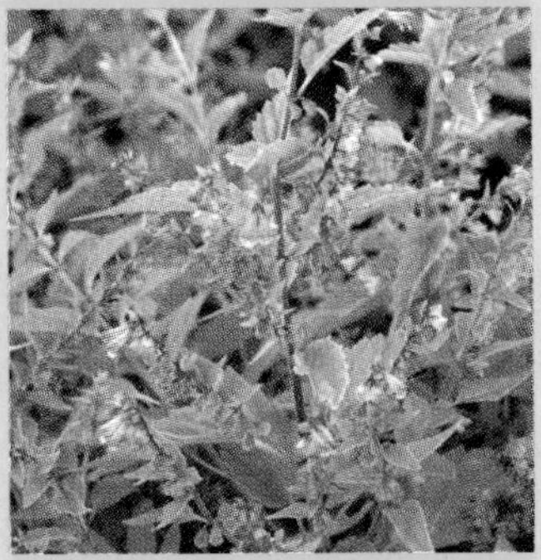

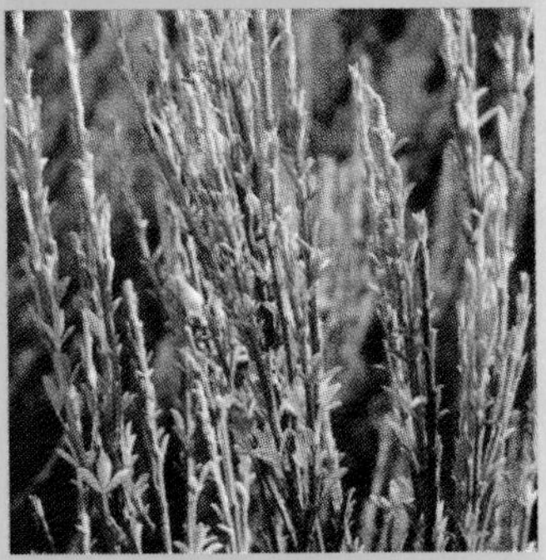

Scutellaria lateriflora

SCURVY GRASS

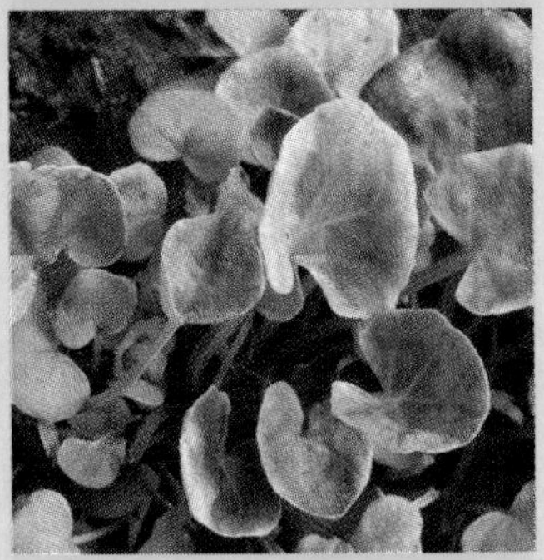

Cochlearia officinalis

SEA BUCKTHORN

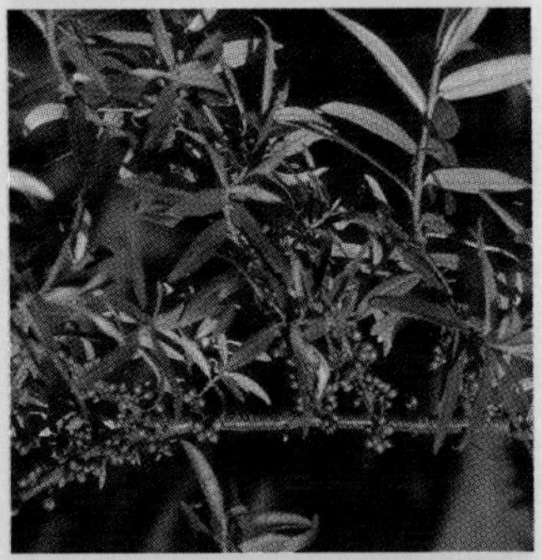

Hippophaë rhamnoides

SELF-HEAL

Prunella vulgaris

SENNA

Cassia senna

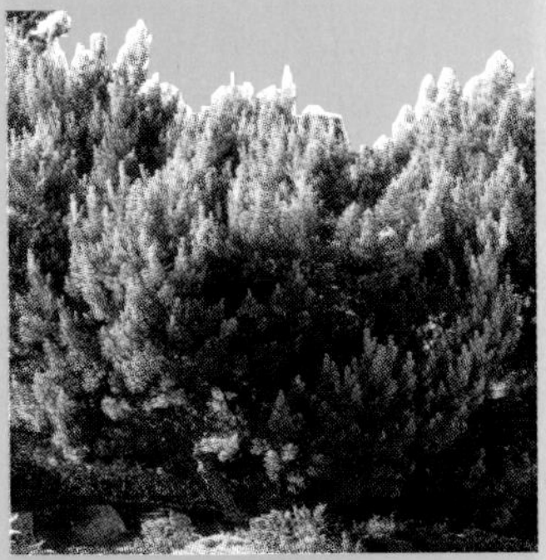

SHEPHERD'S PURSE

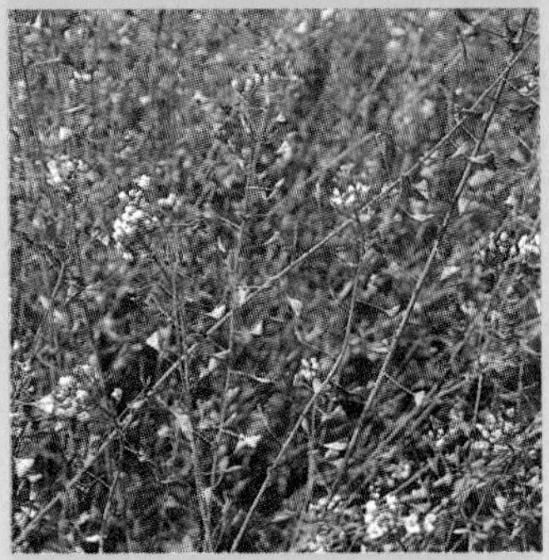

Capsella bursa-pastoris

SKIRRET

Sium sisarum

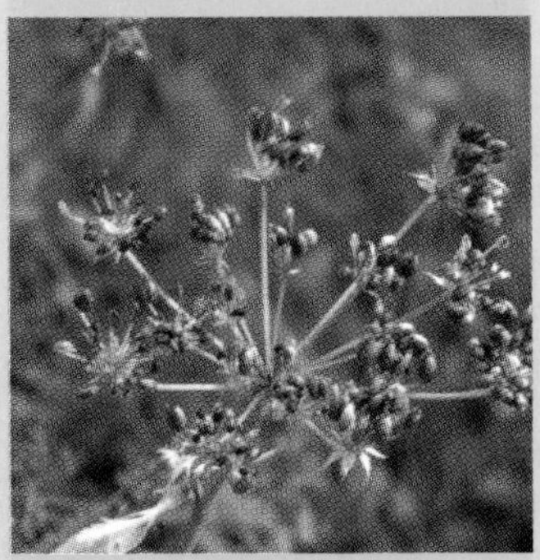

SLOE

Prunus spinosa

SOAPWORT

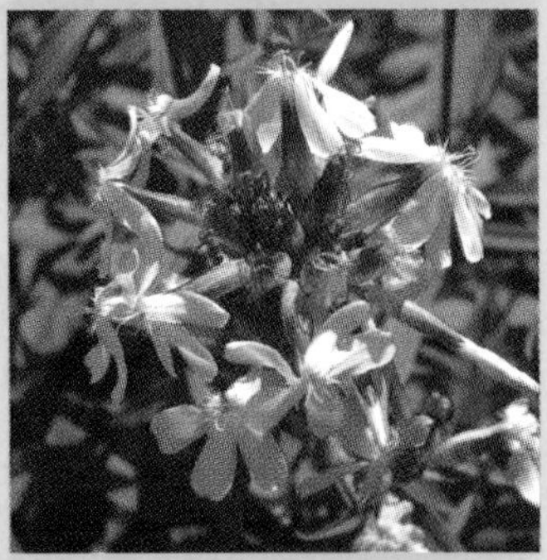

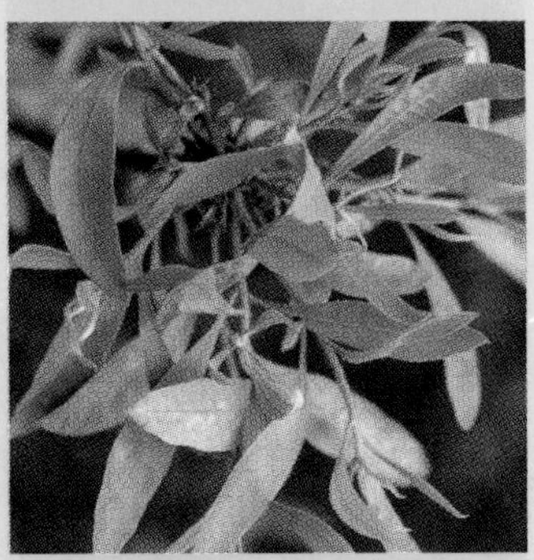

Saponaria officinalis

SOLOMON'S SEAL

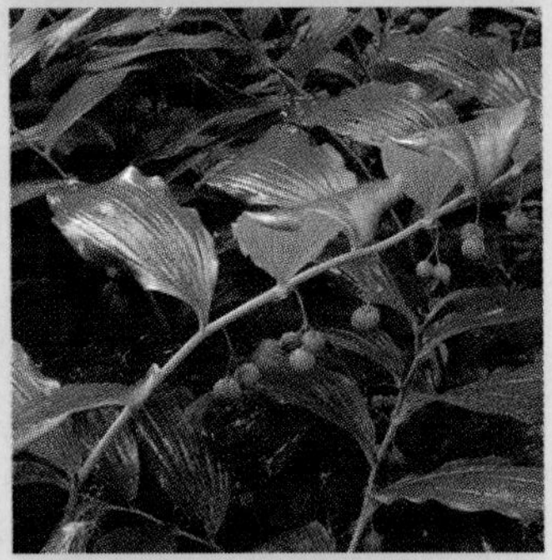

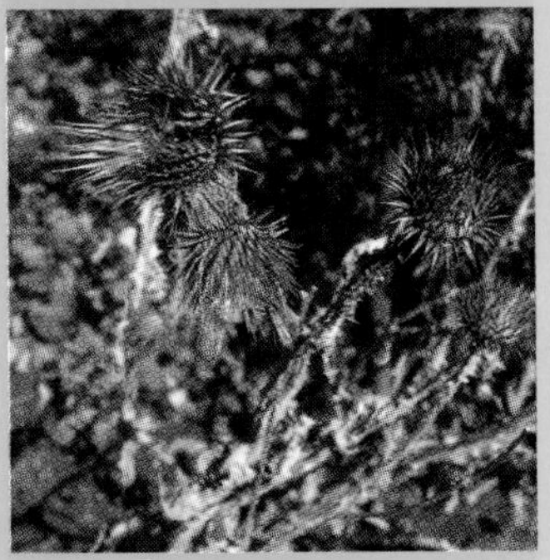

Polygonatum multiflorum

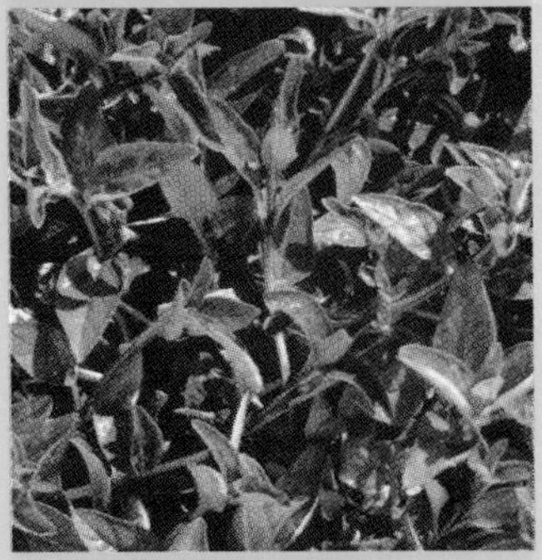

SOUTHERN BAYBERRY

Myrica cerifera

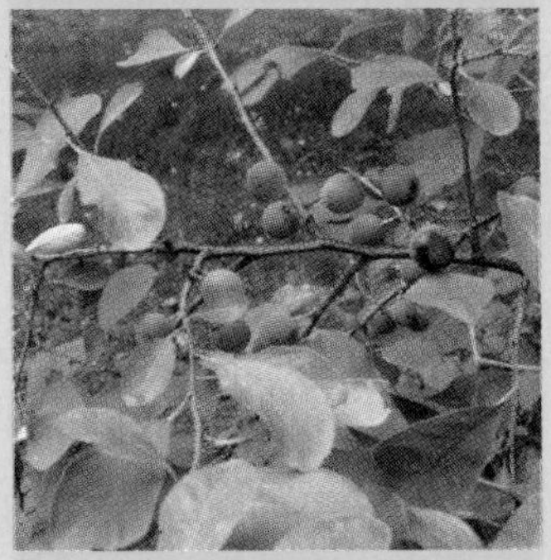

SOYBEAN

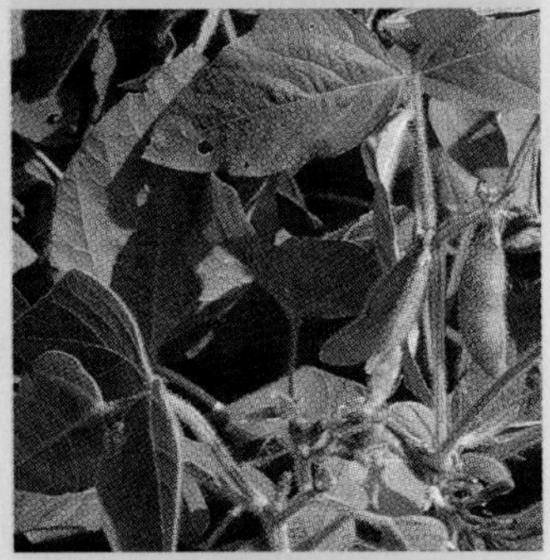

Glycine soja

SPEARMINT

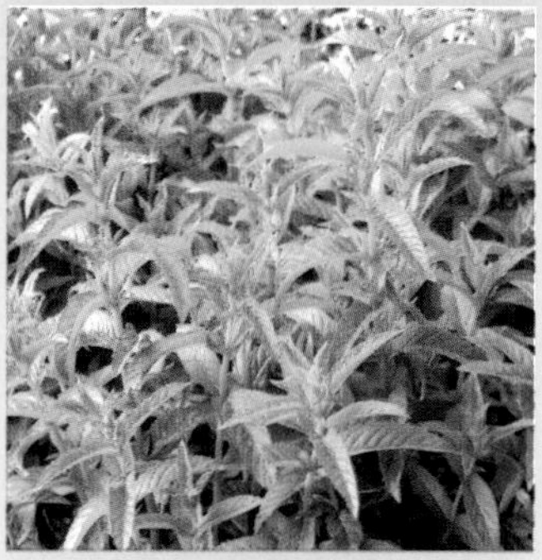

Mentha spicata

SPINY REST HARROW

Ononis spinosa

STINGING NETTLE

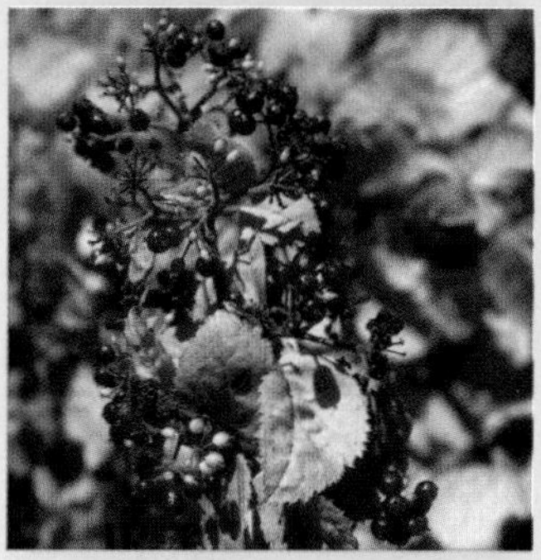

Urtica dioica

SUMBUL

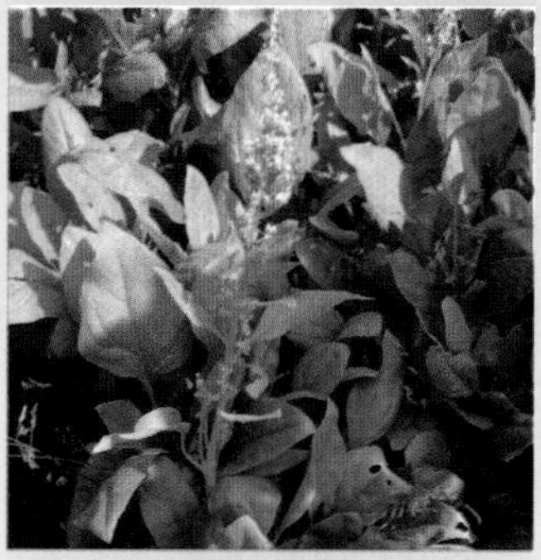

Ferula sumbul

SPEEDWELL

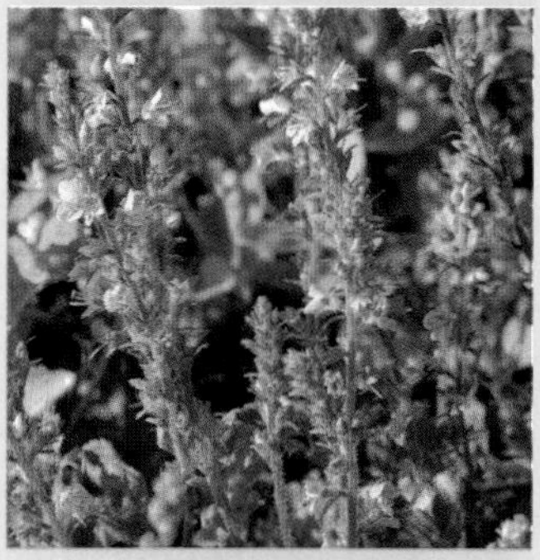

Veronica officinalis

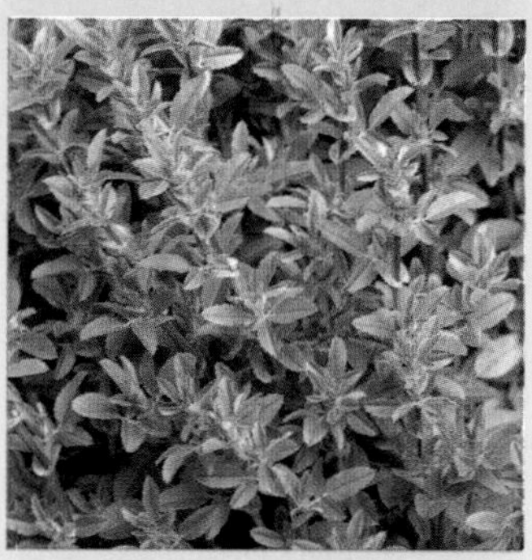

SQUILL

Urginea maritima

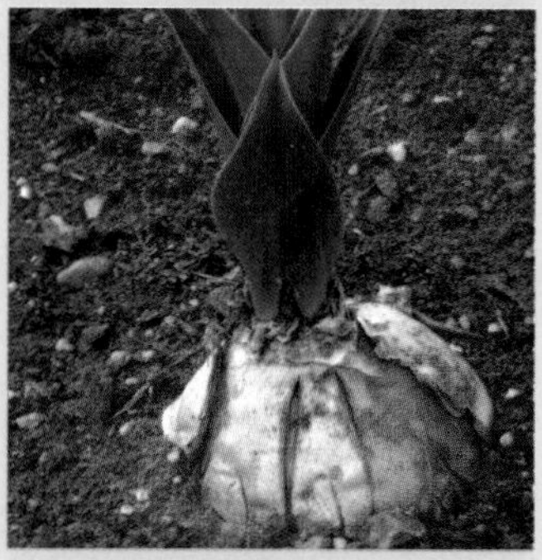

STONE ROOT

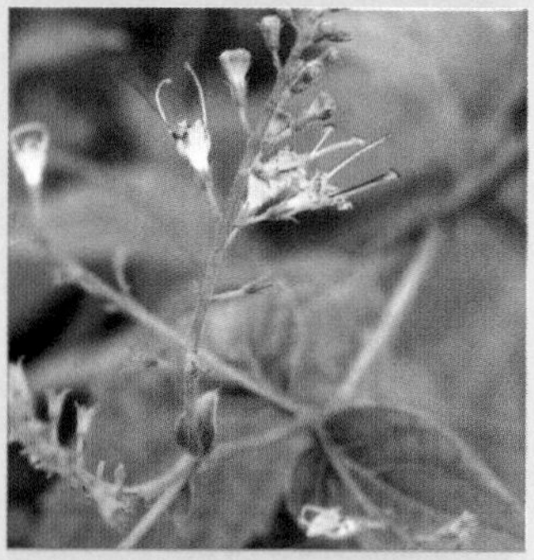

Collinsonia canadensis

SUMMER SAVORY

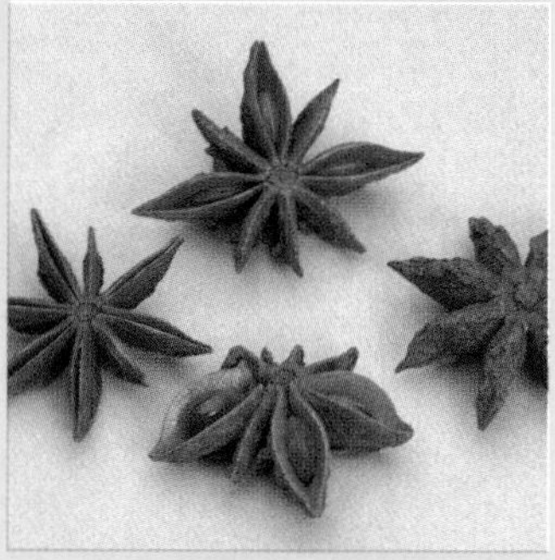

Satureja hortensis

SPIKENARD

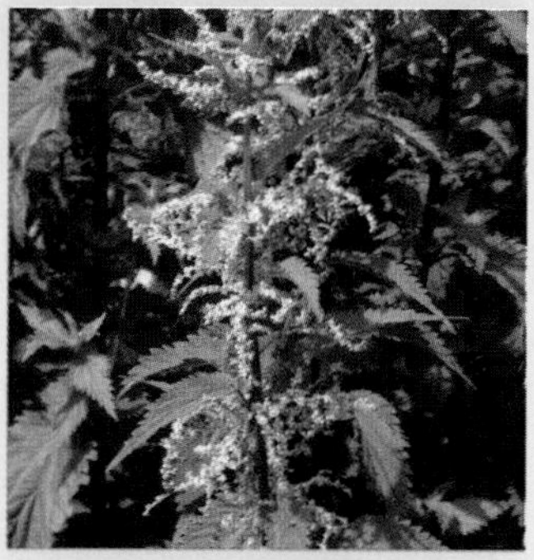

Aralia racemosa

ST. JOHN'S WORT

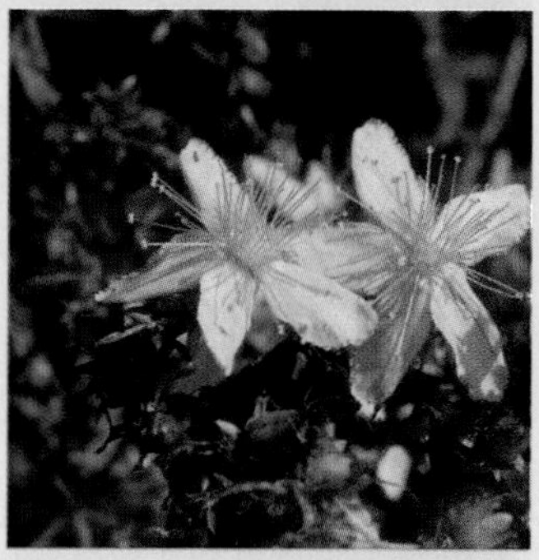

Hypericum perforatum

STORAX

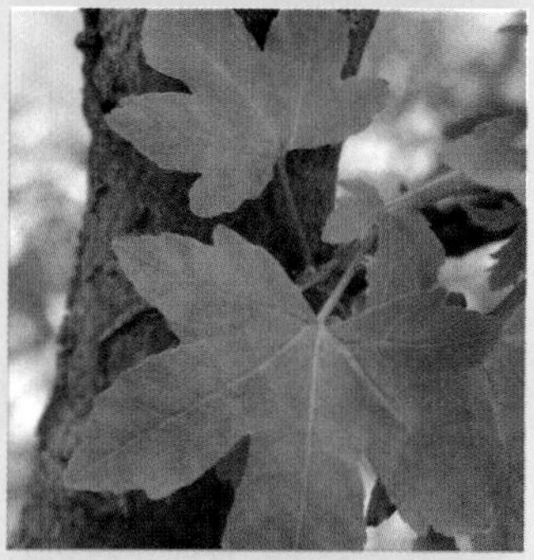

Liquidambar orientalis

SUNFLOWER

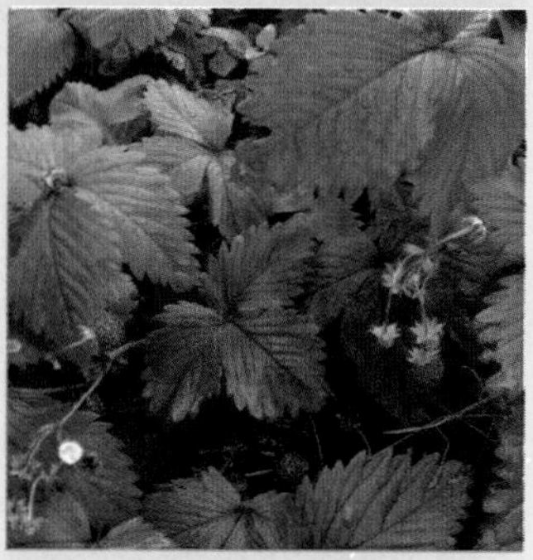

Helianthus annuus

SPINACH

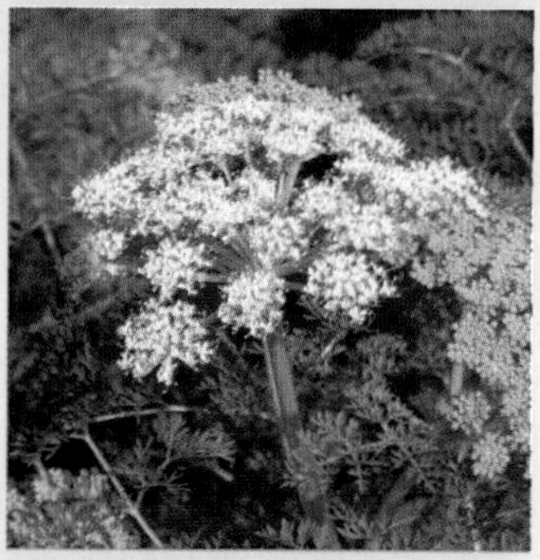

Spinacia oleracea

STAR ANISE

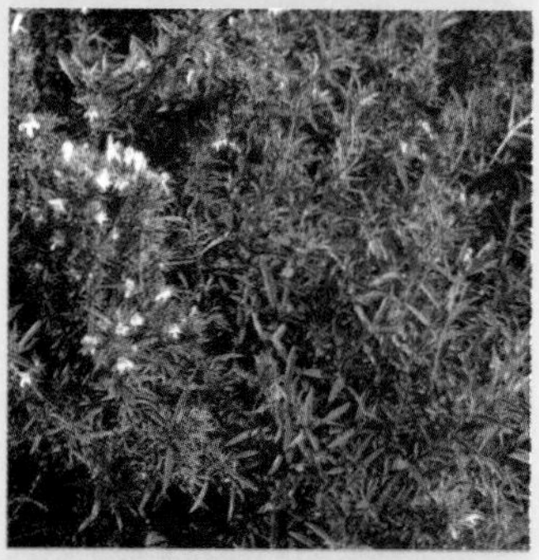

Illicium verum

STRAWBERRY

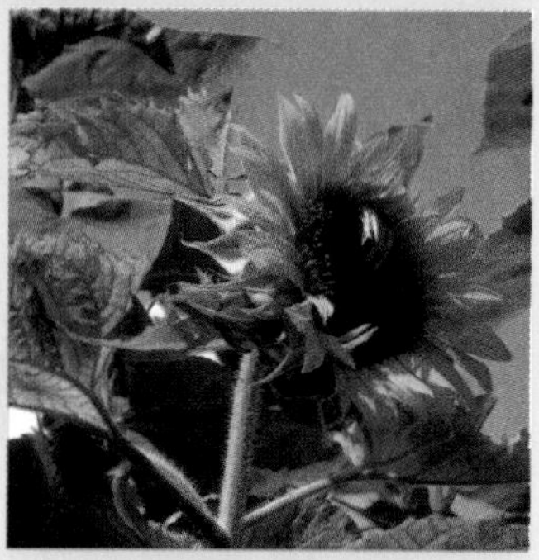

Fragaria vesca

SWAMP MILKWEED

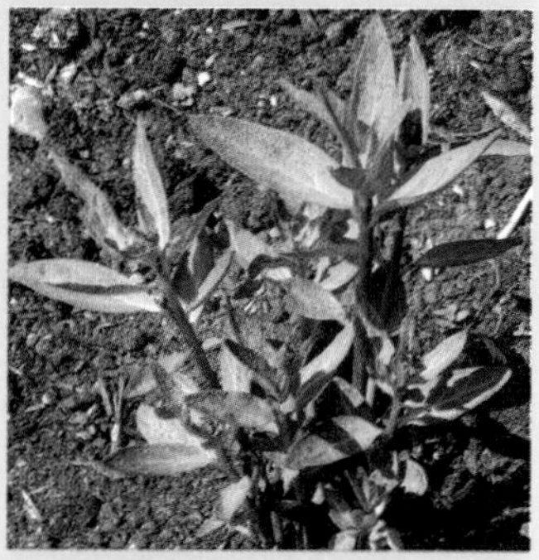

Asclepias incarnata

SWEET CICELY

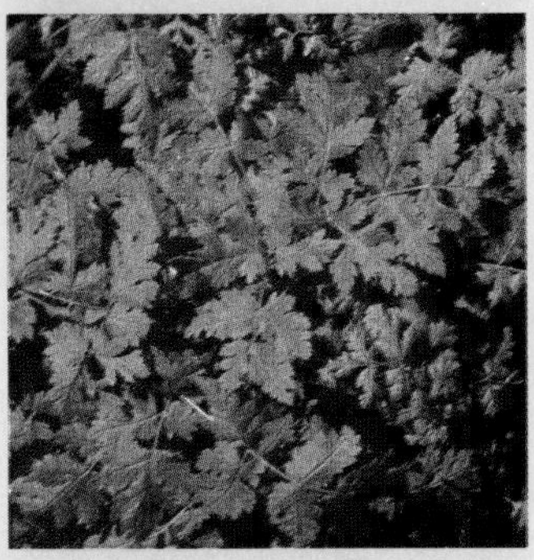

Myrrhis odorata

SWEET CLOVER

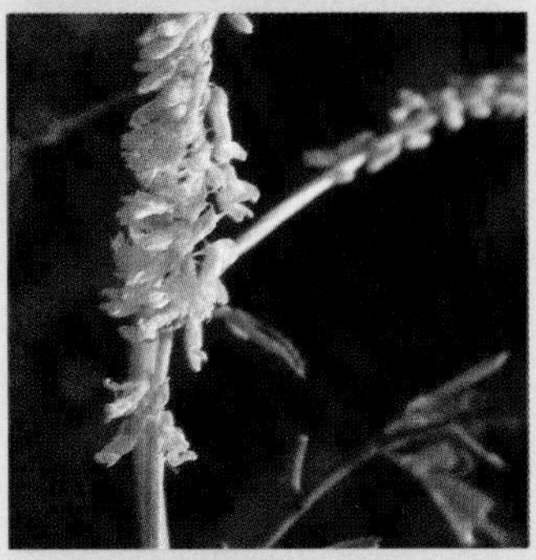

Melilotus officinalis

SWEET GALE

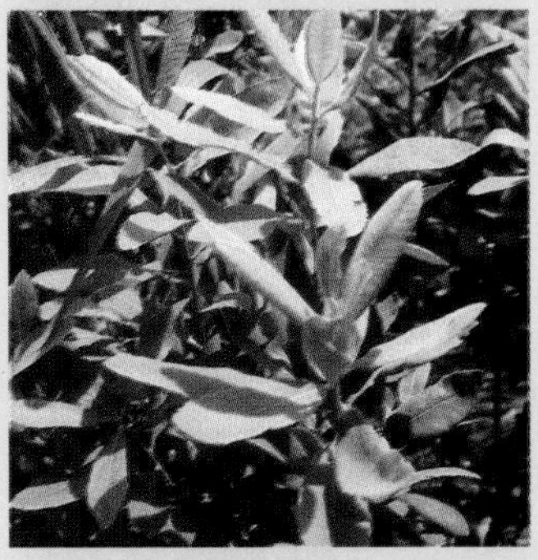

Myrica gale

SWEET MARJORAM

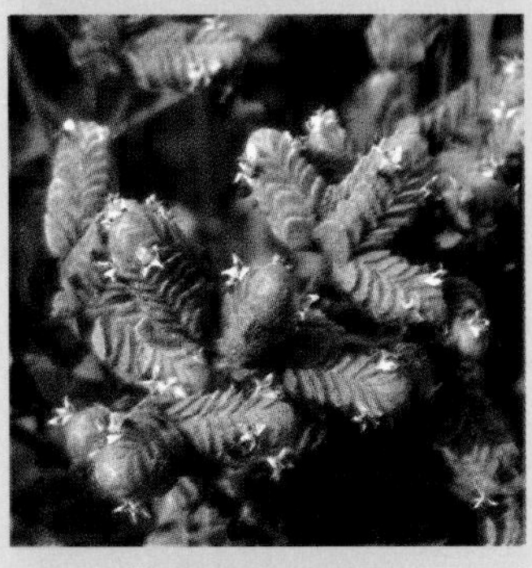

Origanum majorana

SWEET ORANGE

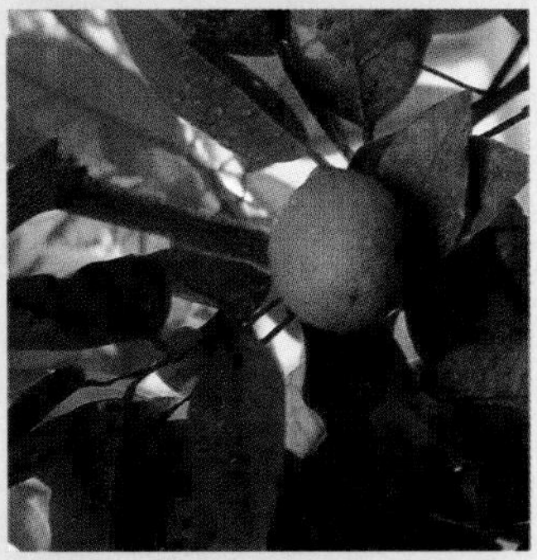

Citrus sinensis

SWEET VERNAL GRASS

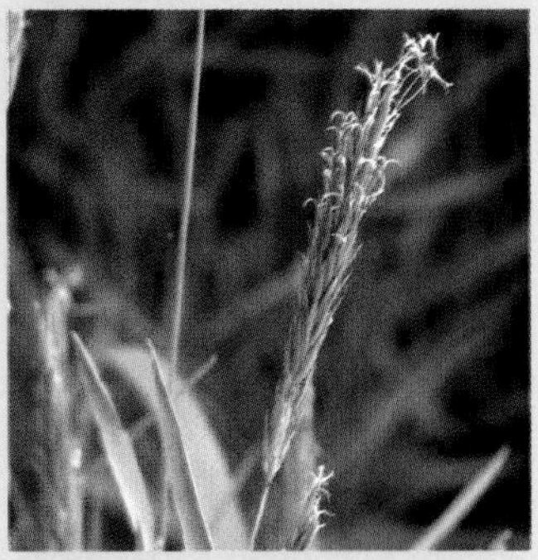

Anthoxanthum odoratum

SWEET VIOLET

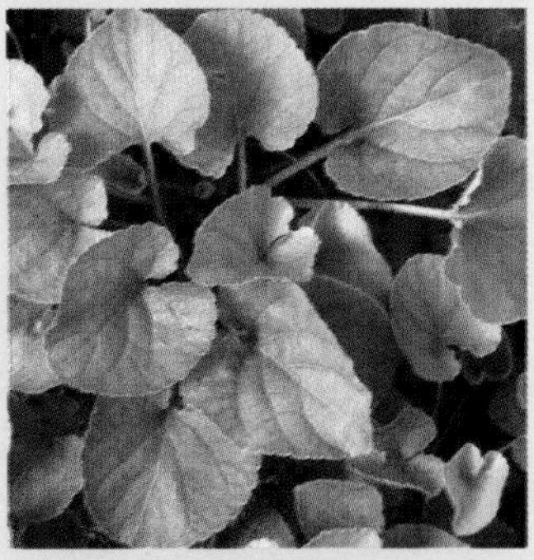

Viola odorata

SWEET WOODRUFF

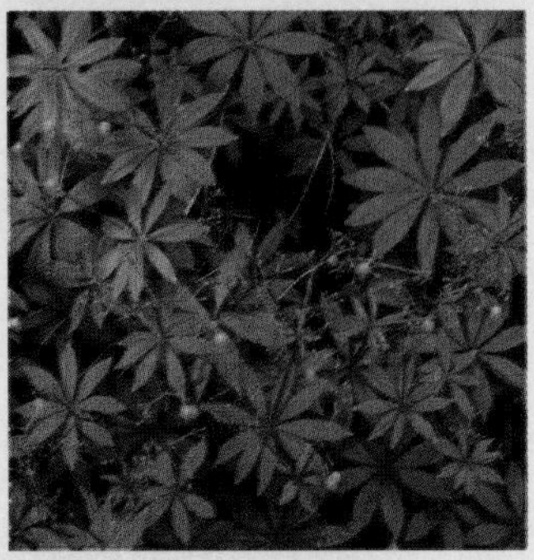

Galium odoratum

TANSY

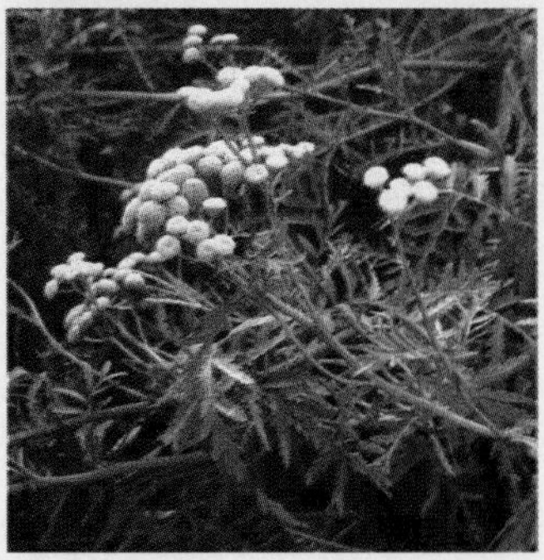

Tanacetum vulgare

TAUMELLOOLCH

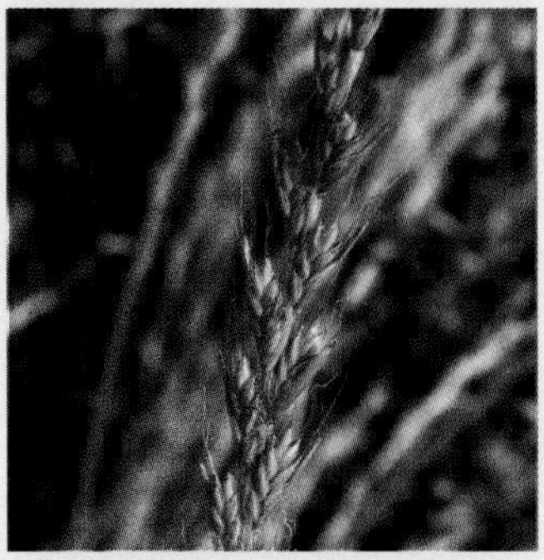

Lolium temulentum

TEAZLE

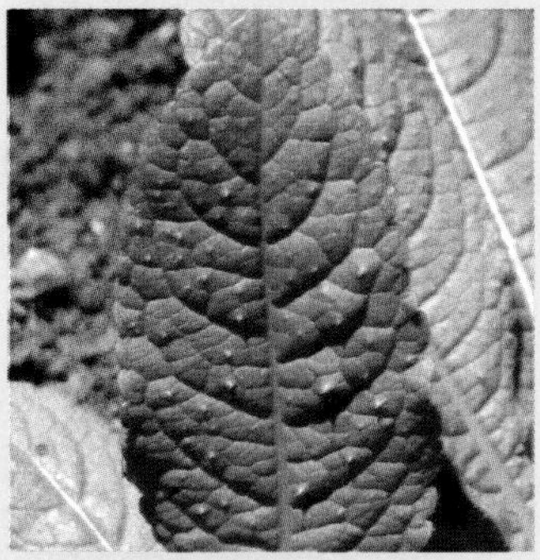

Dipsacus silvestris

THUJA

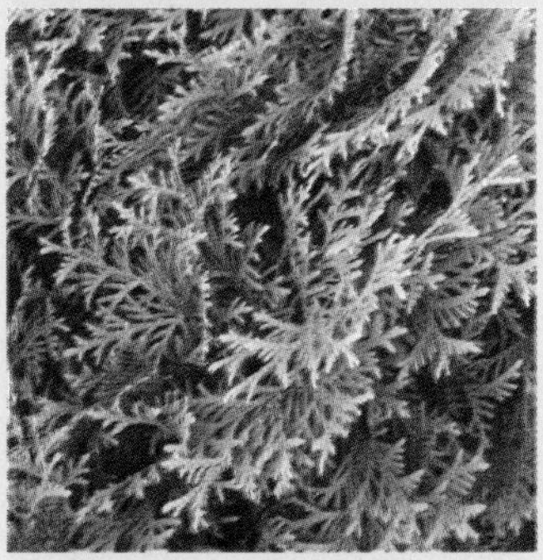

Thuja occidentalis

THYME

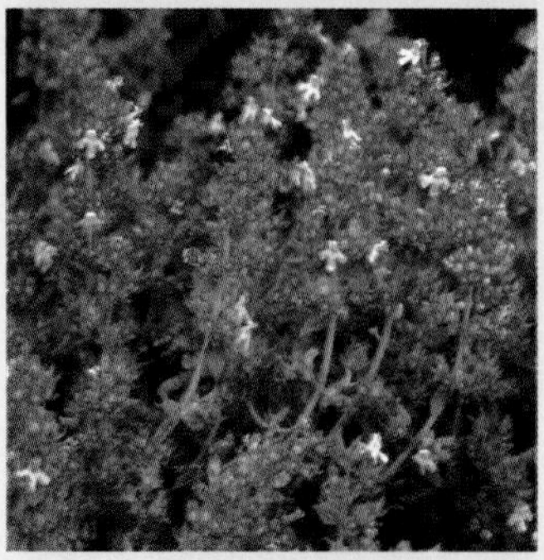

Thymus vulgaris

TOBACCO

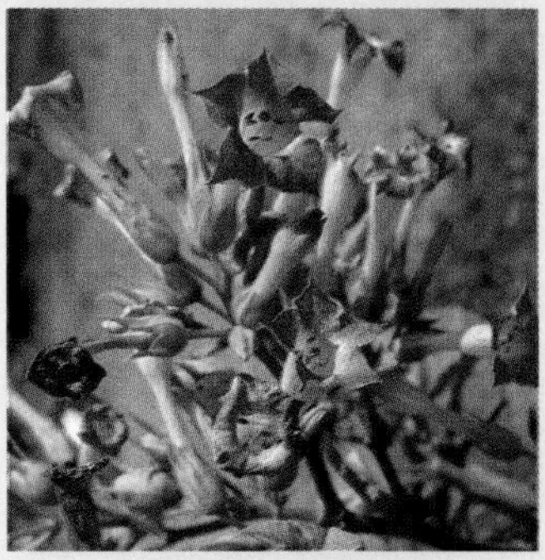

Nicotiana tabacum

TOLU BALSAM

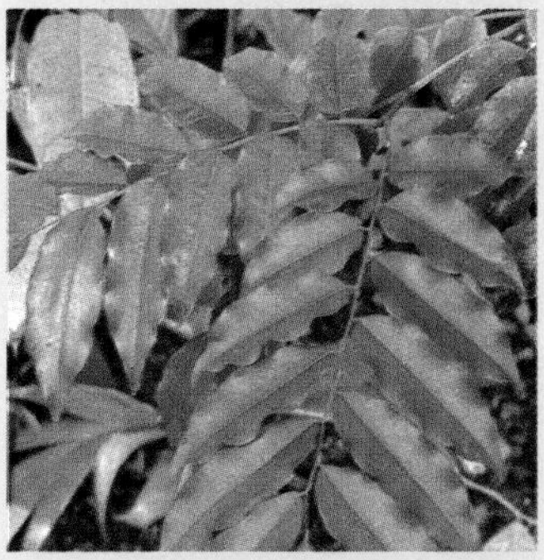

Myroxylon balsamum

TOMATO

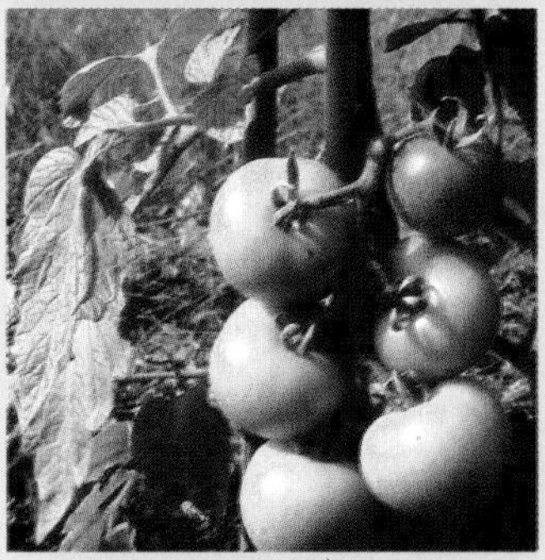

Lycopersicon esculentum

TRAVELLER'S JOY

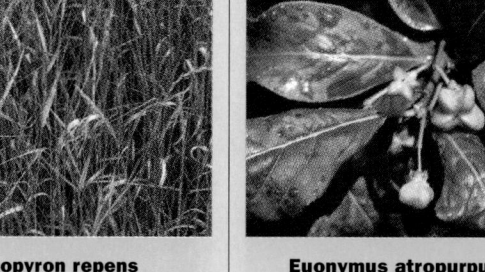

Clematis vitalba

TRITICUM

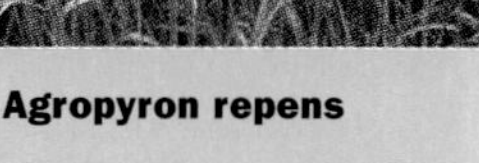

Agropyron repens

UVA-URSI

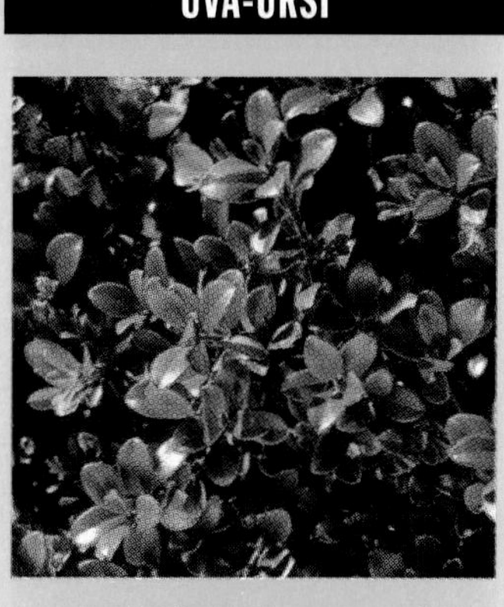

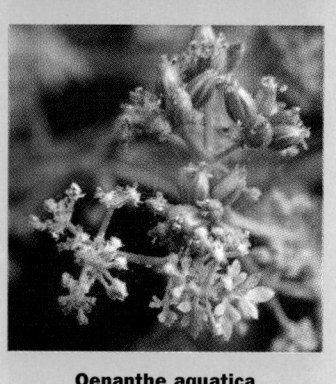

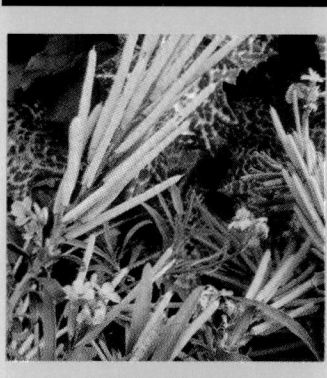

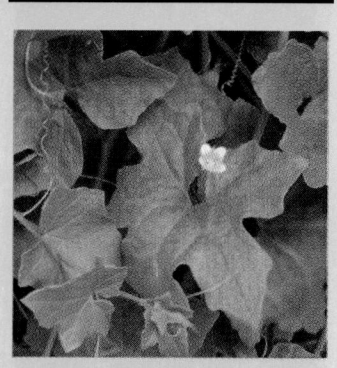

Arctostaphylos uva-ursi

VALERIAN

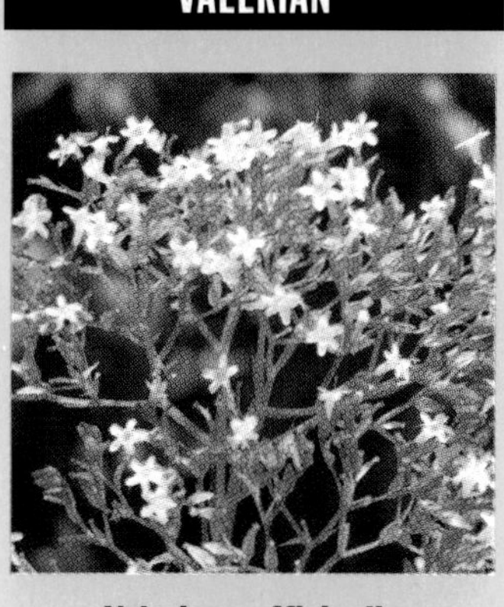

Valeriana officinalis

VERVAIN

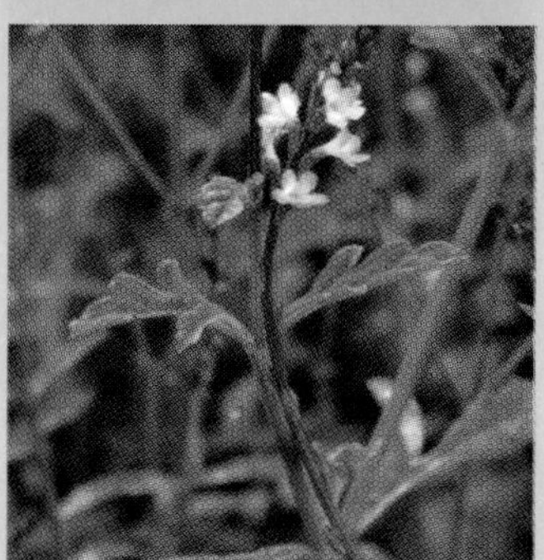

Verbena officinalis

WAHOO

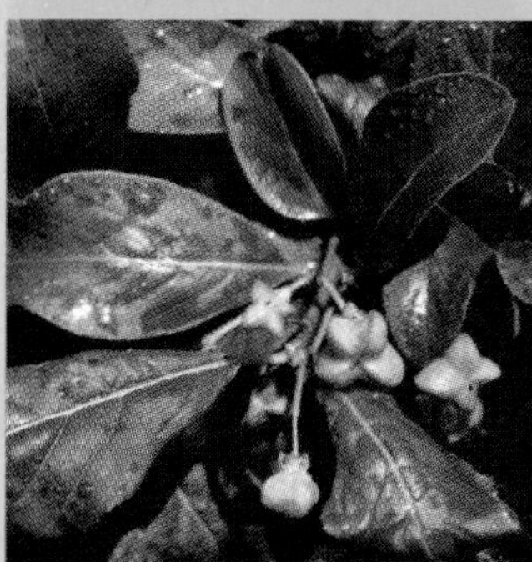

Euonymus atropurpurea

WALLFLOWER

Cheiranthus cheiri

WALNUT

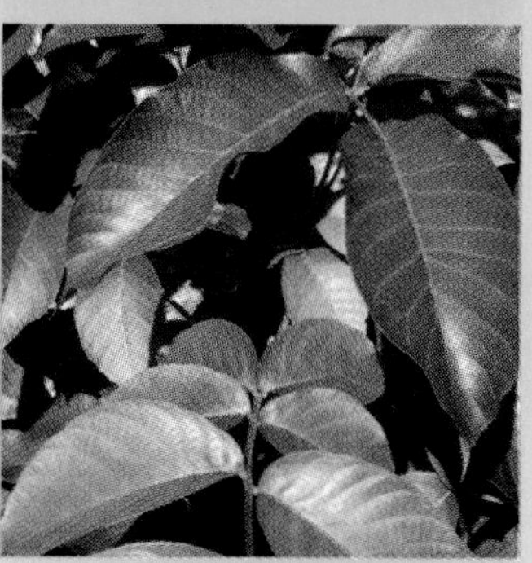

Juglans regia

WATER AVENS

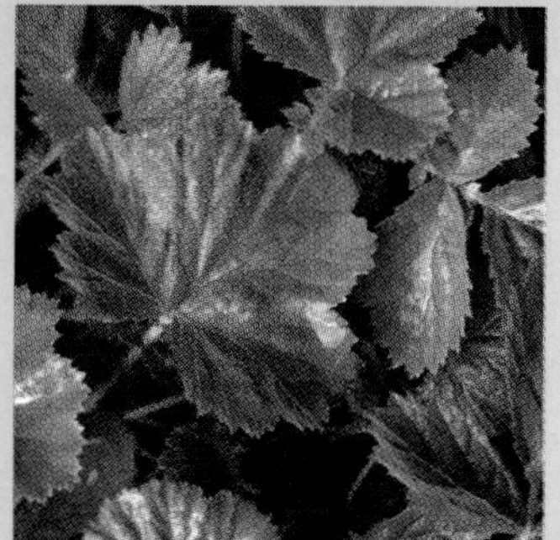

Geum rivale

WATER FENNEL

Oenanthe aquatica

WHITE BRYONY

Bryonia alba

WHITE HELLEBORE

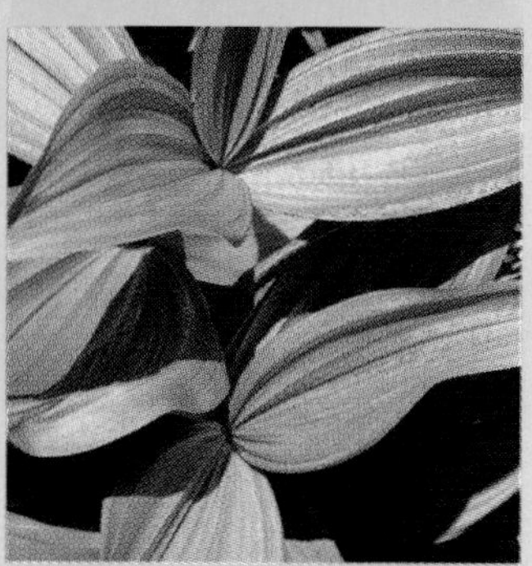

Veratrum album

WHITE MUSTARD

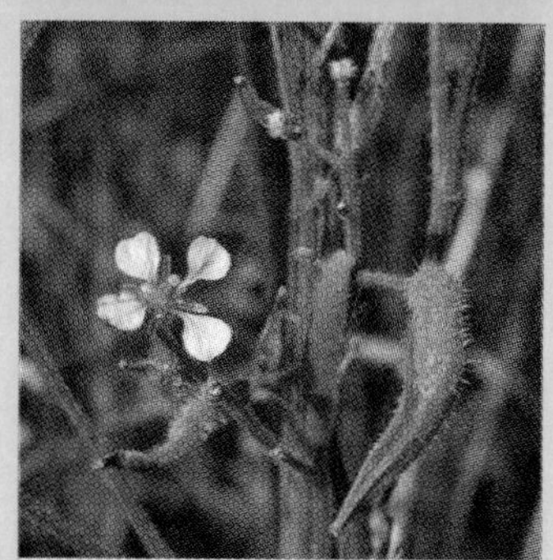

Sinapis alba

WHITE NETTLE

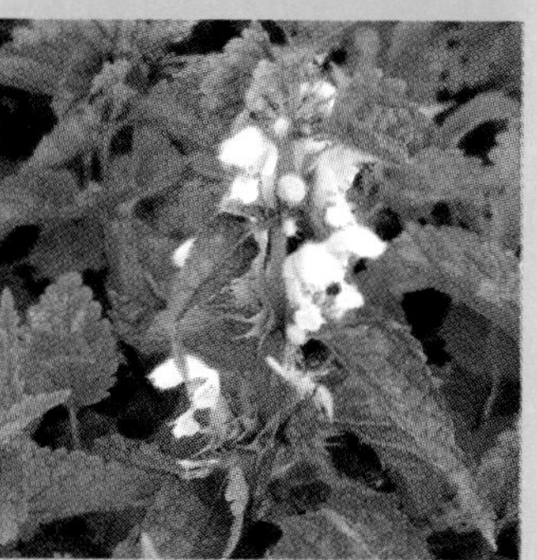

Lamium album

WHITE WILLOW

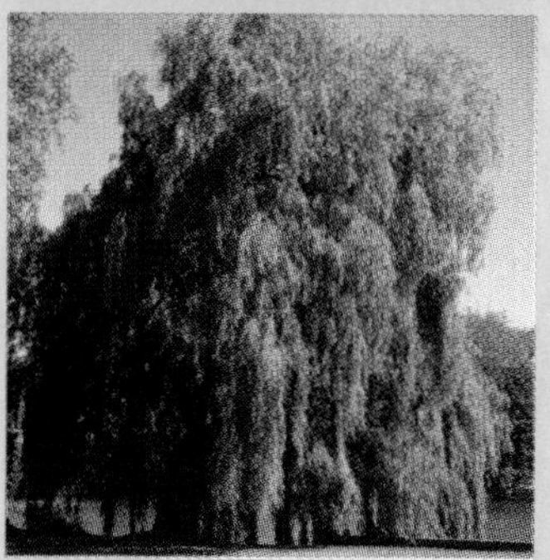

Salix species

WILD CARROT

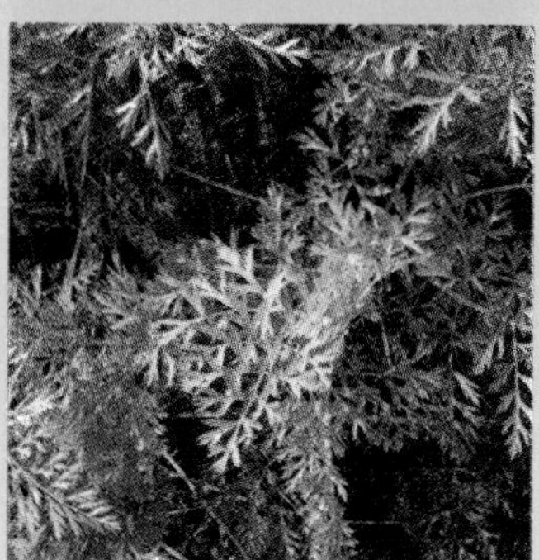

Daucus carota

WILD DAISY

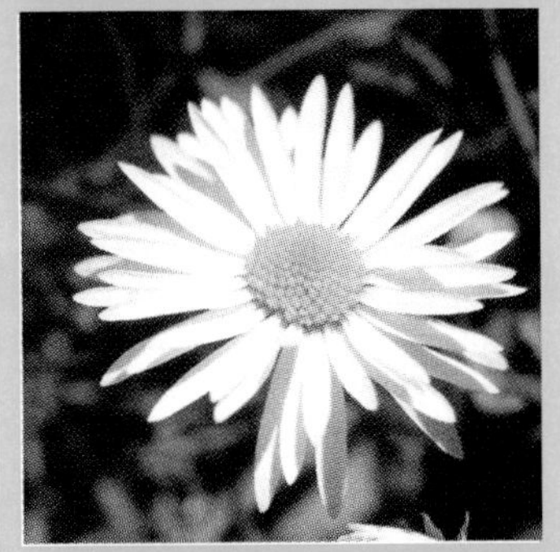

Bellis perennis

WILD INDIGO

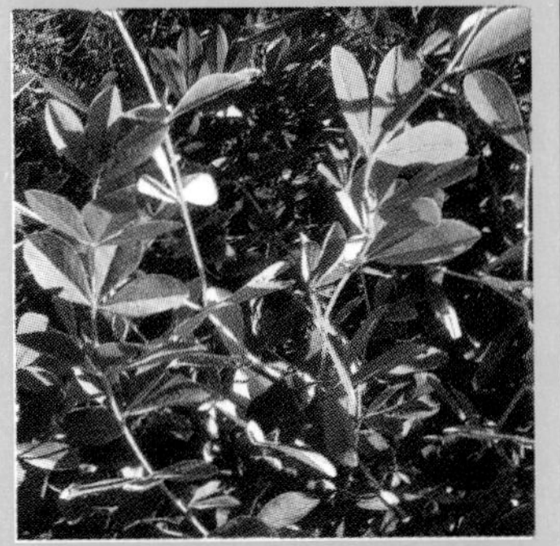

Baptisia tinctoria

WILD MINT

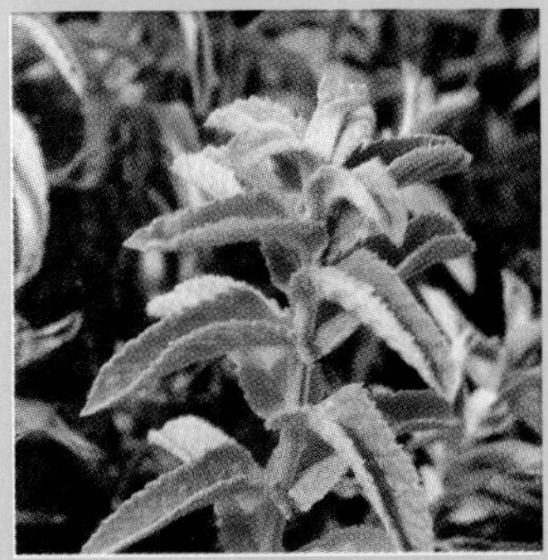

Mentha aquatica

WILD RADISH

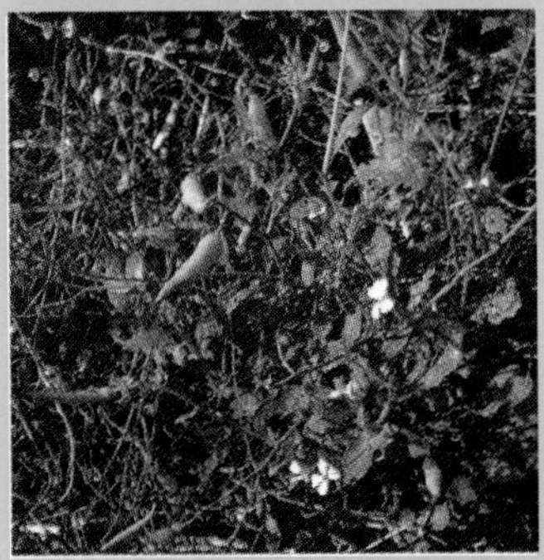

Raphanus raphanistrum

WILD THYME

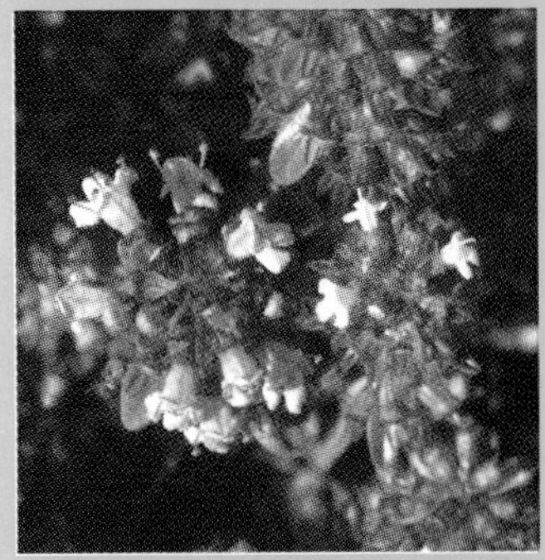

Thymus serpyllum

WILD YAM

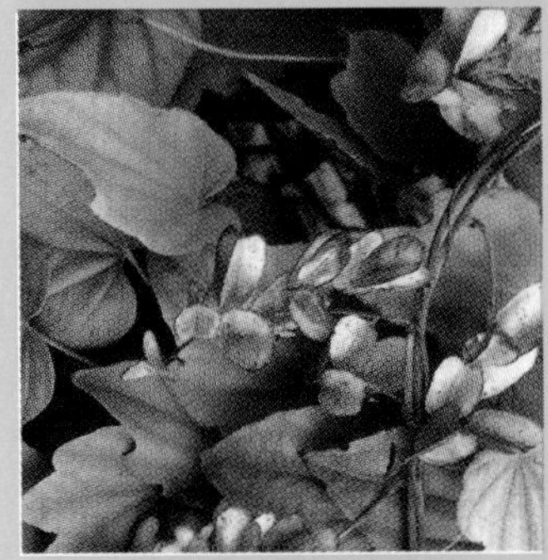

Dioscorea villosa

WILLOW HERB

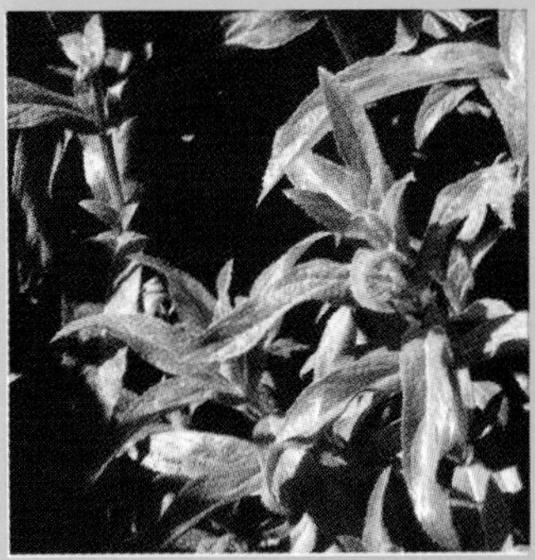

Epilobium angustifolium

WINTER CHERRY

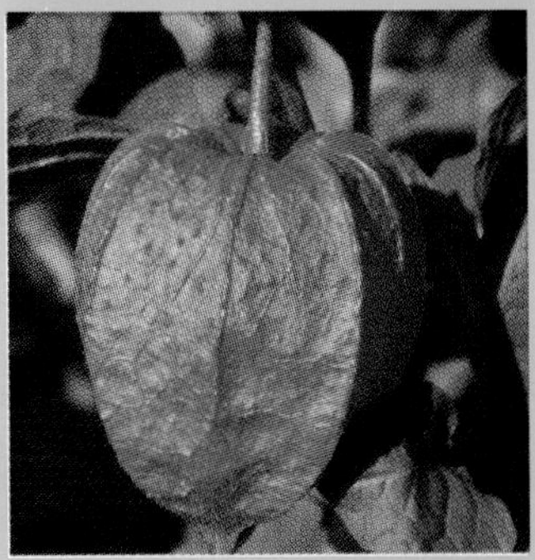

Physalis alkekengi

WITCH HAZEL

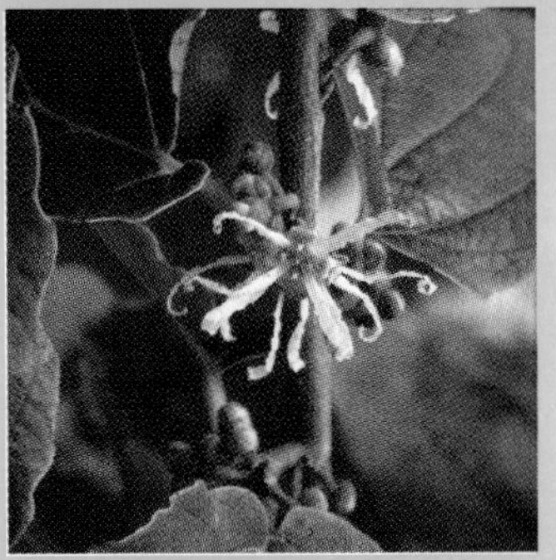

Hamamelis virginiana

WOOD BETONY

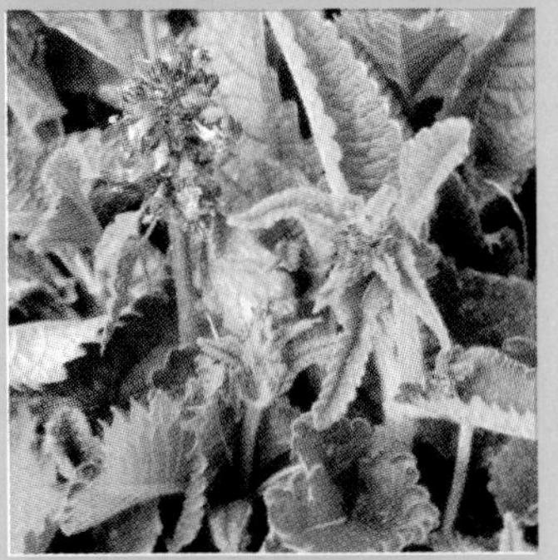

Betonica officinalis

WOOD SAGE

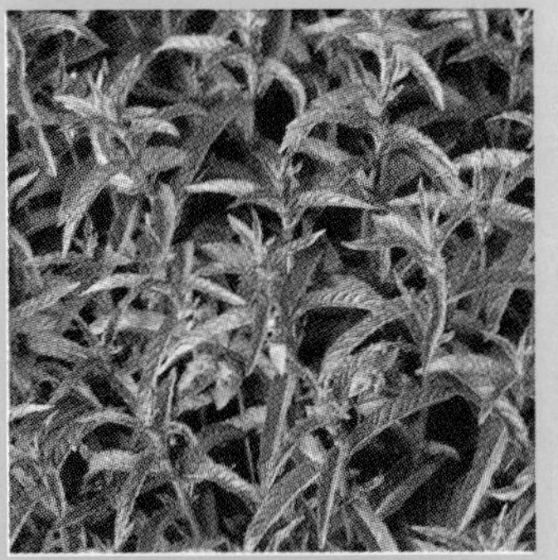

Teucrium scorodonia

WORMSEED OIL

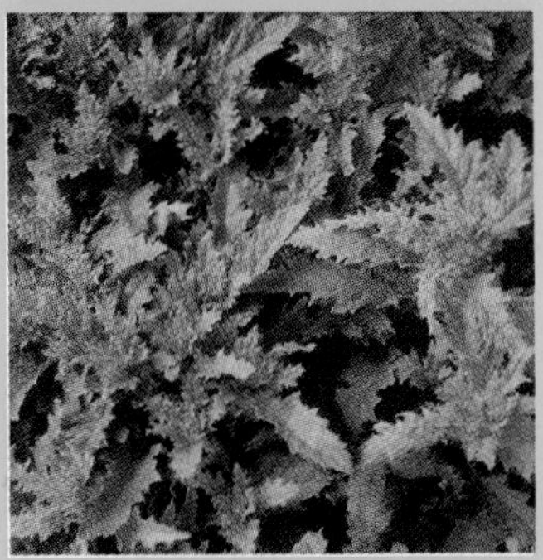

Chenopodium ambrosioides

WORMWOOD

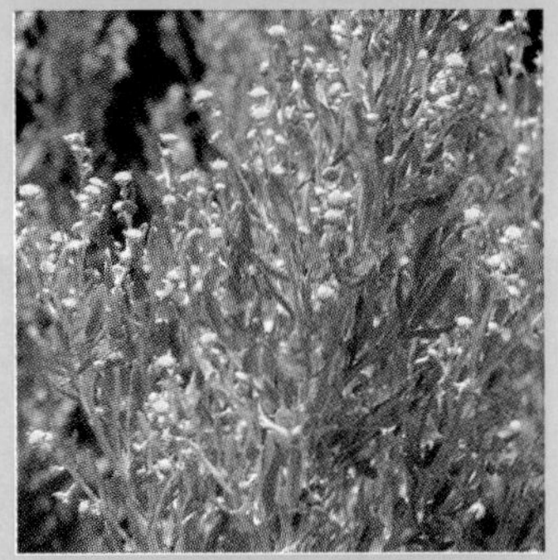

Artemisia absinthium

YARROW

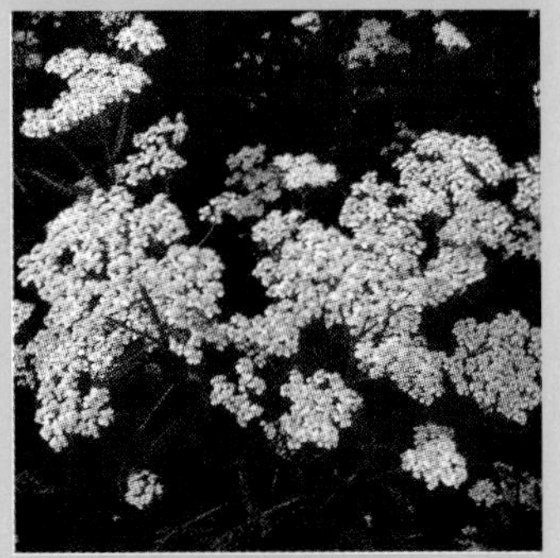

Achillea millefolium

YEW

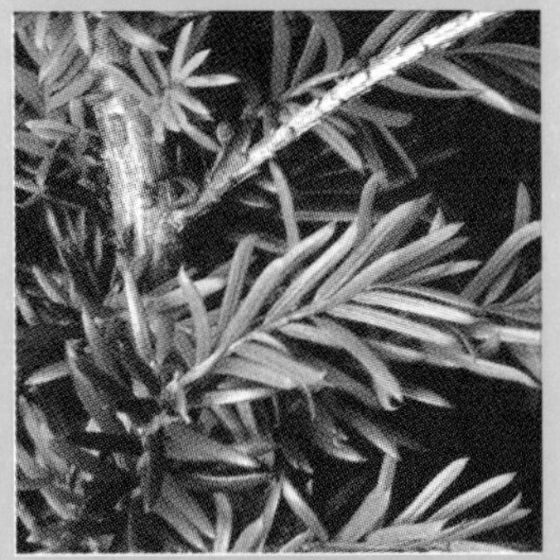

Taxus baccata

ZEDOARY

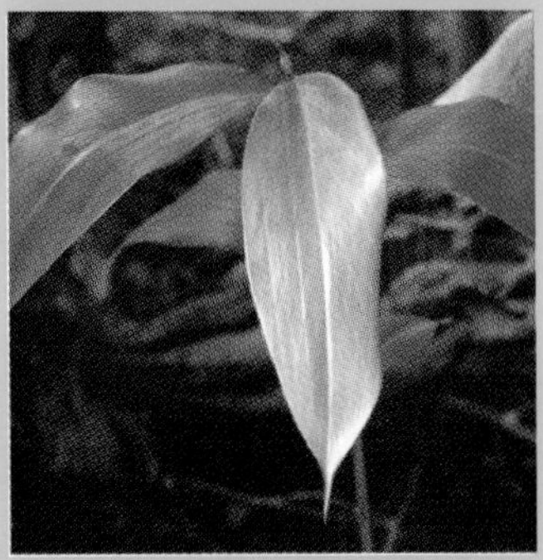

Curcuma zedoaria

Herbal Monographs

5-HTP

Griffonia simplicifolia

DESCRIPTION

Medicinal Parts: Brown-grey powdered seed with peppery odor.

Botanical Description: Stout, woody, climbing shrub growing to about 3 m with greenish flowers and inflated black pods.

Habitat: Occurs mainly in West-Central Africa in thickets, usually associated with mounds of the termite Macrotermes on plains, in forests, in secondary vegetation, and on old farms. It is evergreen, vigorous, and has wide adaptability.

Production: Wild crafted. 5-HTP is commercially produced by extraction from the seeds.

ACTIONS AND PHARMACOLOGY

COMPOUNDS

Griffonia contains several indole derivatives including 5-Hydroxy-L-tryptophan, indole-3-acetylaspartic acid and 5-hyrdroxy indole-3-acetic acid (5-HIAA).

EFFECTS

5-Hydroxytryptophan (5-HTP) is the intermediate metabolite of the amino acid L-tryptophan (LT) in the serotonin pathway. Therapeutic use of 5-HTP bypasses the conversion of LT into 5-HTP by the enzyme tryptophan hydrolase, which is the rate-limiting step in the synthesis of serotonin. Tryptophan hydrolase can be inhibited by numerous factors, including stress, insulin resistance, vitamin B6 deficiency, and insufficient magnesium. In addition, these same factors can increase the conversion of LT to kynurenine via tryptophan oxygenase, making LT unavailable for serotonin production. 5-HTP functions as an antioxidant; whereas LT can actually promote oxidative damage. 5-HTP is well absorbed from an oral dose, with about 70 percent ending up in the bloodstream. Absorption of 5-HTP is not affected by the presence of other amino acids; therefore it may be taken with meals without reducing its effectiveness. Unlike LT, 5-HTP cannot be shunted into niacin or protein production. Serotonin levels in the brain are highly dependent on levels of 5-HTP and LT in the central nervous system (CNS). 5-HTP easily crosses the blood-brain barrier, not requiring the presence of a transport molecule. LT, on the other hand, requires use of a transport molecule to gain access to the CNS. Since it shares this transport molecule with several other amino acids, the presence of these competing amino acids can inhibit LT transport into the brain. 5-HTP acts primarily by increasing levels of serotonin within the central nervous system. Other neurotransmitters and CNS chemicals, such as melatonin, dopamine, norepinephrine, and beta-endorphin, have also been shown to increase following oral administration of 5-HTP.

CLINICAL TRIALS

Depression

To date, some 40 studies have evaluated the clinical effects of 5-HTP on depression.

In an open trial design, a total of 107 patients with endogenous unipolar or bipolar depression were given daily oral dosages of 5-HTP from 50 to 300 mg. Significant improvement was observed in 74 of the patients (69%), and no significant side effects were reported. The response rate in most of these patients was quite rapid (less than two weeks). Speed of response was subsequently addressed in a study of 59 patients with eight different types of depression. 5-HTP was administered orally in dosages from 150 to 300 mg daily for a period of three weeks. Thirteen patients (22%) were markedly improved, and another 27 patients (45.8%) showed moderate improvement. Of these 40 patients who improved, 20 (50%) began to show improvement within three days, and 32 patients (80%) improved within two weeks of beginning treatment with 5-HTP (Sano, 1972).

Effectiveness of 5-hydroxy-L-trytophan as an antidepressant drug was studied in 59 patients with depressive symptoms in a double blind clinical study using a Rating Scale for Depression (Nakajima, 1978). A daily dose of 150–300 mg of 5-hydroxyl-L-tryptophan was administered for three weeks. Favorable responses were observed in 40 patients (67.8%), of whom 13 patients were markedly improved. These effects were noticed in 32 patients (80% of the improved patients) within a week of the treatment. Analysis indicated that endogenous depression and involutional or senile depression were the preferable indication of 5-hydroxy-L-tryptophan loading. The main side effects of 5-hydroxy-L-tryptophan were gastrointestinal disturbances which were minimized by the simultaneous administration of metoclopromide or trihexyphenidyl.

Employing positron-emission tomography, 8 healthy volunteers and 6 people diagnosed with major depression received infusions of radio labeled 5-HTP. Significantly less 5-HTP crossed the blood-brain barrier into the brains of the depressed subjects than into the brains of the normal controls. A significant reduction in anxiety was observed on three different scales designed to measure anxiety (Agren, 1991).

A double-blind clinical trial was carried out involving 26 hospitalized, depressed patients who were randomized into two groups and received chlorimipramine (50 mg/day), combined with L-5-HTP (300 mg/day) in Group A, and with placebo in Group B. For 28 days, patients were evaluated by HRSD each week, and by ZDSI and CGI at the beginning and end of treatment. The results for both types of pathology were quantitatively and qualitatively more positive for Group A than for Group B (Nardini, 1983).

5-HTP was administered to 24 patients hospitalized for depression. After two weeks of treatment, amelioration of depressive symptoms was observed in seven patients diagnosed with unipolar depression. A 30% increase in the levels of 5-hydroxyindolacetic acid, the primary metabolite of serotonin, was also noted in the patients' cerebrospinal fluid. This suggests that the exogenous 5-HTP was converted to serotonin within the CNS (Takahashi, 1975).

5-HTP was evaluated in comparison to an SSRI drug in a double-blind, multicenter study design (Poldinger, 1991). A total of 36 subjects, all of whom were diagnosed with some form of depression, received either 100 mg of 5-HTP three times per day, or 150 mg of fluvoxamine (an SSRI) three times daily. The subjects were evaluated at 0, 2, 4, and 6 weeks, using four evaluation tools: the Hamilton Rating Scale for Depression (HRSD), a standard depression rating scale; a patient-performed self-assessment; the investigator's assessment of severity; and a global clinical impression. Both treatment groups showed significant and nearly equal reductions in depression beginning at week two and continuing through week six. After four weeks, 15 of the 36 patients treated with 5-HTP, and 18 of the 33 patients treated with fluvoxamine had improved by at least 50 percent, according to the HRSD scores. By week six, the two groups had about equal numbers showing 50 percent improvement. When the numbers were totaled at the end of the study, the researchers found the mean percentage improvement from baseline to the final assessment was slightly greater for patients treated with 5-HTP. The number of treatment failures was higher in the fluvoxamine group (5/29, 17%) than in the 5-HTP group (2/34, 6%), although neither of these differences were statistically significant. All four evaluation tools yielded similar results. The study also looked at the incidence of adverse effects from both treatments, which were found to be rare and generally mild, usually occurring during the first few days of treatment and then disappearing. Overall, 5-HTP appeared to be slightly better tolerated than fluvoxamine, although the results did not reach the level of statistical significance. Tolerance was assessed as being ''good to very good'' in 34/36 patients receiving 5-HTP (94.5%), compared to 28/33 in the fluvoxamine group (84.8%). 5-HTP has also been compared in a few studies with conventional tricyclic antidepressants (chloripramine and imipramine)—the most effective drugs for treating depression until the development of the SSRIs.

Fibromyalgia

A double-blind, placebo-controlled study of the efficacy and tolerability of 5-hydroxytryptophan (5-HTP) was conducted in 50 patients with primary fibromyalgia syndrome. All the clinical parameters studied were significantly improved by treatment with 5-HTP and only mild and transient side-effects were reported (Caruso, 1990).

The efficacy and tolerability of 5-hydroxy-L-tryptophan (5-HTP) were studied in an open 90-day study in 50 patients affected by primary fibromyalgia syndrome. All clinical variables studied throughout the trial (number of tender points, anxiety, pain intensity, quality of sleep, fatigue) showed a significant improvement compared to baseline. The overall evaluation of the patient condition indicated a ''good'' or ''fair'' clinical improvement in nearly 50% of the patients during the treatment period. A total of 15 patients (30%) reported side-effects but only one patient was withdrawn from the treatment for this reason. No abnormality in the laboratory evaluation was observed (Puttini, 1992).

In a randomized, placebo-controlled study of 200 fibromyalgia patients who were also migraine sufferers, 5-HTP (400 mg/day) was compared to a tricyclic drug (amitriptyline) and a monoamine oxidase inhibitor (MAOI) drug (pargilyne or phenelzine). The combination of 5-HTP (200 mg/day) with an MAOI was also evaluated. Patients were treated for a total of 12 months and kept a daily pain diary by means of a visual analogic scale. At the end of the twelve-month trial period, all treatment regimens showed significant improvement over placebo ($p<0.0001$), although the combination of 5-HTP with the MAOI was the most effective. 5-HTP alone was as effective as the tricyclic or MAOI drugs. No patients withdrew from the study due to side effects; eight percent of the patients taking 5-HTP alone reported some degree of stomach upset (Nicolodi, 1996).

Obesity

In a placebo-controlled, double-blind trial the effects of 5-HTP (300 mg three times daily) on the eating habits and weight loss of 20 obese female patients were evaluated. All patients had a BMI between 30 and 40, and were determined to consume an excess of food daily, based on calculated energy needs. The 12-week study period was divided into two six-week sections. During the first six weeks, the patients took either 5-HTP or placebo, with no dietary restrictions. In the second six-week period, the patients were placed on a 1,200 calorie per day diet, while continuing to take either the 5-HTP or placebo. Subjects in the placebo group did not experience significant weight loss in either of the two periods (94.3 ± 5.6 kg vs. 93.2 ± 5.3 kg), while the subjects in the 5-HTP group showed significant weight loss in both the first period (99.7 ± 5.9 kg vs. 98.0 ± 5.0 kg, $p<0.03$) and the second period (98.0 ± 5.0 vs. 94.7 ± 5.1 kg, $p<0.02$). The placebo group also did not show significant change in their calorie intake, even in the second period when instructed to reduce food intake, while the 5-HTP group had a significant spontaneous dietary intake reduction during the first period, from 3,220 calories/day to 1879 calories/day ($p<0.001$), with carbohydrate intake falling by 50%. During the second period, the calorie intake of the 5-HTP group decreased further, to 1,268 calories/day ($p<0.01$), with further reductions in carbohydrates. The researchers interpreted these findings as supporting the theory that 5-HTP decreased carbohydrate cravings and binge eating, even in the absence of a structured diet. At this high dosage of 5-HTP (900 mg/day), about 80% of the subjects initially reported experiencing some nausea. However, this side effect was not severe enough to cause any of the subjects to drop out of the study, and was less frequent during the second six-week period, suggesting that this symptom may be a transitory effect of 5-HTP administration (Cangiano, 1992).

Insomnia

5-HTP has been shown to be beneficial in treating insomnia, especially in improving sleep quality by increasing REM sleep. Eight normal subjects were monitored to determine the effect of 5-HTP on rapid eye movement (REM) sleep. A total of 600 mg 5-HTP was administered to the subjects in the following manner: 200 mg at 9:15 pm, followed by 400 mg at 11:15 pm. A significant increase in the amount of REM sleep was observed while the subjects were taking 5-HTP (118 ± 14 min vs. 98 ± 11 min, p<0.005). A smaller dose of 200 mg also showed increases in REM sleep, but to a lesser degree (Wyatt, 1971).

Chronic Headache

In a large study of 124 subjects, the ability of 5-HTP to prevent migraines was compared to methysergide, one of the most commonly used migraine drugs. At a dosage of 600 mg daily for six months, 5-HTP totally prevented or substantially decreased the number of migraine attacks in 75 percent of the subjects. However, this difference was not determined to be statistically significant. In a study of 48 elementary and junior high school students, 5-HTP (4.5 mg/kg/day) produced a 70 percent decrease in headache frequency, compared to an 11 percent decrease in the placebo group (Giorgis, 1987).

INDICATIONS AND USAGE

Unproven Uses: Traditional African uses for the plant include the use of the stem and roots as chewing sticks, leaves to aid in the healing of wounds, while the leaf juice is used as an enema and for the treatment of kidney ailments. A decoction of the stems and leaves is also used to stop vomiting, to treat congestion of the pelvis, and as an aphrodisiac. The bark-pulp is applied as a plaster to soft chancres.

Probable Efficacy: L-5-Hydroxytryptophan is reported to be of greatest benefit in psychiatric and neurological disorders where there is a deficiency of neural serotonin. L-5-Hydroxytryptophan has also been indicated for its uses in alleviating the symptoms of a number of common syndromes such as anxiety and depression. It has been referred to as a natural relaxant, to help alleviate insomnia by inducing normal sleep, for the treatment of migraine and headaches, and to aid in the control of cravings such as in eating disorders. L-5-Hydroxytryptophan may stimulate the immune system and may help to reduce the risk of artery and heart spasms. L-5-Hydroxytryptophan has been used in the management of Parkinson's Disease and epilepsy.

CONTRAINDICATIONS

The use of 5-HTP in pregnancy or lactation has not been determined in controlled trials; therefore, it should not be used during pregnancy (Birdsall, 1998).

PRECAUTIONS AND ADVERSE REACTIONS

When administered orally, 5-HTP may cause the following adverse reactions: heartburn, stomach pain, flatulence, diarrhea and vomiting. 5-HTP may cause asymptomatic eosinophila.

DRUG INTERACTIONS

MODERATE RISK

Carbidopa: Concurrent use may result in an increased risk of developing scleroderma-like illness in susceptible individuals. *Clinical Management:* Patients taking 5-HTP and carbidopa concomitantly should be monitored for signs of skin changes, which may manifest as edema, tightness, and/or a burning sensation.

Monamine Oxidase Inhibitors (MAOIs): Concurrent use may result in an increased risk of serotonin syndrome (hypertension, hyperthermia, myoclonus, mental status changes). *Clinical Management:* Caution is advised if therapy with an MAOI is initiated with 5-HTP.

Selective Serotonin Repuptake Inhibitors (SSRIs): Concurrent use may result in an increased risk of serotonin syndrome (hypertension, hyperthermia, myoclonus, mental status changes). Combining 5-HTP with SSRIs may increase the risk of serotonergic side effects. *Clinical Management:* No cases have been reported of serotonin syndrome resulting from this combination. Caution is advised if 5-HTP and an SSRI are used concomitantly. Monitor the patient for early signs of serotonin syndrome, such as anxiety, confusion, and disorientation.

OVERDOSAGE

DOSAGE

Daily Dose: For depression, dosage may be 50 mg three times a day. For insomnia, the dosage is usually 100-300 mg before bedtime. In primary fibromyalgia syndrome (PFS), 100 mg three times daily has been used.

LITERATURE

Agren H, Reibring L, Hartvig P, et al. Low brain uptake of L-(11C)5-hydroxytryptophan in major depression: A positron emission tomography study on patients and healthy volunteers. Acta Psychiatr Scand. 1991;83:449-455.

Amer A, Breu J, McDermott J, Wurtman RJ, Maher TJ. 5-Hydroxy-L-tryptophan suppresses food intake in food-deprived and stressed rats. Pharmacol Biochem Behav 2004 Jan;77(1):137-43.

Anderson IM, Parry-Billings M, Newsholme EA, et al. Dieting reduces plasma tryptophan and alters brain 5-HT function in women. Psychol Med 1990;20:785-791

Angst J, Woggon B, Schoepf J. The treatment of depression with L-5-hydroxytryptophan versus imipramine. Results of two open and one double-blind study. Arch Psychiatr Nervenkr 1977;224:175-186.

Aviram M, Cogan U, Mokady S. Excessive dietary tryptophan enhances plasma lipid peroxidation in rats. Atherosclerosis 1991;88:29-34.

Benedittis de G, Massei R. Serotonin precursors in chronic primary headache. A double-blind cross-over study with L-5-hydroxytryptophan vs. placebo. J Neurosurg Sci 1985;29:239-248.

Boer den JA, Westenberg HG. Behavioral, neuroendocrine, and biochemical effects of 5-hydroxytryptophan administration in panic disorder. Psychiatry Res 1990;31:267-278.

Bono G, Criscuoli M, Martignoni E, et al. Serotonin precursors in migraine prophylaxis. Adv Neurol 1982;33:357-363.

Brodie HKH, Sack R, Siever L. Clinical studies of L-5-hydroxytryptophan in depression. In: Barchas J, Usdin E, eds. Serotonin and Behavior. New York: Academic Press; 1973:549-559

Bruni O, Ferri R, Miano S, Verrillo E. L -5-Hydroxytryptophan treatment of sleep terrors in children. Eur J Pediatr 2004 Jul;163(7):402-7. Epub 2004 May 14.

Cangiano C, Ceci F, Cairella M, et al. Effects of 5-hydroxytryptophan on eating behavior and adherence to dietary prescriptions in obese adult subjects. Adv Exp Med Biol 1991;294:591-593

Cangiano C, Ceci F, Cascino A, et al. Eating behavior and adherence to dietary prescriptions in obese adult subjects treated with 5-hydroxytryptophan. Am J Clin Nutr 1992;56:863-867.

Caruso I, Puttini PS, Cazzola M, Azzolini V. Double-blind study of 5-hydroxytryptophan versus placebo in the treatment of primary fibromyalgia syndrome. J Int Med Res 1990;18:201-209.

Ceci F, Cangiano C, Cairella M, et al. The effects of oral 5-hydroxytryptophan administration on feeding behavior in obese adult female subjects. J Neural Transm 1989;76:109-117.

Croonenberghs J, Verkerk R, Scharpe S, Deboutte D, Maes M. Serotonergic disturbances in autistic disorder: L-5-hydroxytryptophan administration to autistic youngsters increases the blood concentrations of serotonin in patients but not in controls. Life Sci 2005 Mar 25;76(19):2171-83.

Das YT, Bagchi M, Bagchi D, Preuss HG. Safety of 5-hydroxy-L-tryptophan. Toxicol Lett 2004 Apr 15;150(1):111-22.

Esteban S, Nicolaus C, Garmundi A, Rial RV, Rodriguez AB, Ortega E, Ibars CB. Effect of orally administered L-tryptophan on serotonin, melatonin, and the innate immune response in the rat. Mol Cell Biochem 2004 Dec;267(1-2):39-46.

Freeman MP, Helgason C, Hill RA. Selected integrative medicine treatments for depression: considerations for women. J Am Med Womens Assoc 2004 Summer;59(3):216-24.

Giorgis de G, Miletto R, Iannuccelli M, et al. Headache in association with sleep disorders in children: a psychodiagnostic evaluation and controlled clinical study L-5-HTP versus placebo. Drugs Exp Clin Res 1987;13:425-433

Guilleminault C, Cathala JP, Castaigne P. Effects of 5-hydroxytryptophan on sleep of a patient with a brain-stem lesion. Electroencephalogr Clin Neurophysiol 1973;34:177-184

Hiele van LJ. L-5-Hydroxytryptophan in depression: the first substitution therapy in psychiatry? The treatment of 99 out-patients with 'therapy-resistant' depressions. Neuropsychobiology 1980;6:230-240.

Isaac M. Serotonergic 5-HT2C receptors as a potential therapeutic target for the design antiepileptic drugs. Curr Top Med Chem 2005;5(1):59-67.

Katsuzaki H, Miyahara Y, Ota M, Imai K, Komiya T. Chemistry and antioxidative activity of hot water extract of Japanese radish (daikon). Biofactors 2004;21(1-4):211-4.

Keithahn C, Lerchl A. 5-hydroxytryptophan is a more potent in vitro hydroxyl radical scavenger than melatonin or vitamin C. J Pineal Res 2005 Jan;38(1):62-6.

Lance JW. 5-Hydroxytryptamine and its role in migraine. Eur Neurol 1991;31:279-281

Larmie ET, Poston L. The in vitro Effects of Griffonin and Ouabain on Erythrocyte Sodium Content Obtained from Normal Subjects and Sickle Cell Patients. Planta Med 1991, 57; 116-118

Longo G, Rudoi I, Iannuccelli M, et al. Treatment of essential headache in developmental age with L-5-HTP (cross over double-blind study versus placebo). Pediatr Med Chir 1984;6:241-245

Loo H, Zarifian E, Wirth IF, Deniker P. Open study of L-5-H.T.P. in melancholic depressed patients over 50 years of age. Encephale 1980;6:241-246.

Lopez-Ibor Alino JJ, Ayuso Guiterrez JL, Montejo Iglesias ML. 5-Hydroxytryptophan (5-HTP) and a MAOI (Nialamide) in the treat of depressions. Int Pharmacopsychiat 1976;11:8-15

Lynn-Bullock CP, Welshhans K, Pallas SL, Katz PS. The effect of oral 5-HTP administration on 5-HTP and 5-HT immunoreactivity in monoaminergic brain regions of rats. J Chem Neuroanat 2004 May;27(2):129-38.

Maron E, Toru I, Vasar V, Shlik J. The effect of 5-hydroxytryptophan on cholecystokinin-4-induced panic attacks in healthy volunteers. J Psychopharmacol 2004 Jun;18(2):194-9.

Martin TG. Serotonin Syndrome. Ann Emerg Med 1996;28:520-526.

Nakajima T, Kudo Y, Kaneko Z. Clinical evaluation of 5-hydroxy-L-tryptophan as an antidepressant drug. Folia Psychiatr Neurol Jpn 1978;32:223-230.

Nardini M, DeStefano R, Ianuccelli M, et al. Treatment of depression with l-5-hydroxytryptophan combined with chlomipramine: A double-blind study. J Clin Pharmacol Res 1983;3:239-250.

Poldinger W, Calanchini B, Schwarz W. A functional-dimensional approach to depression: serotonin deficiency as a target syndrome in a comparison of 5-hydroxytryptophan and fluvoxamine. Psychopathology 1991;24:53-81

Puttini PS, Caruso I. Primary fibromyalgia syndrome and 5-hydroxy-L-tryptophan: a 90-day open study. J Int Med Res 1992;20:182-189

Sano I. L-5-hydroxytryptophan-(L-5-HTP) therapy. Folia Psychiatr Neurol Jpn 1972;26:7-17.

Simic MG, al-Sheikhly M, Jovanovic SV. Inhibition of free radical processes by antioxidants-tryptophan and 5-hydroxytryptophan. Bibl Nutr Dieta 1989;43:288-296.

Soulairac A, Lambinet H. Effect of 5-hydroxytryptophan, a serotonin precursor, on sleep disorders. Ann Med Psychol 1977;1:792-798.

Takahashi S, Kondo H, Kato N. Effect of L-5-hydroxytryptophan on brain monoamine metabolism and evaluation of its clinical effect in depressed patients. J Psychiatr Res 1975;12:177-187.

Titus F, Davalos A, Alom J, Codina A. 5-Hydroxytryptophan versus methysergide in the prophylaxis of migraine. Randomized clinical trial. Eur Neurol 1986;25:327-329

Wyatt RJ, Zarcone V, Engelman K, et al. Effects of 5-hydroxytryptophan on the sleep of normal human subjects. Electroencephalogr Clin Neurophysiol 1971;30:505-509.

Yunus MB, Dailey JW, Aldag JC, et al. Plasma tryptophan and other amino acids in primary fibromyalgia: a controlled study. J Rheumatol 1992;19:90-94

Abelmoschus moschatus

See Muskmallow

Abies alba

See White Fir

Abrus precatorius

See Jequirity

Abscess Root

Polemonium reptans

DESCRIPTION

Medicinal Parts: The medicinal part is the dried root.

Flower and Fruit: The hanging blue flowers are in loose terminal, glandular-haired panicles.

Leaves, Stem and Root: The plant grows to about 25 cm. It has creeping roots and a thin rhizome, which produces numerous stems and numerous pale, thin, glabrous and brittle roots. The glabrous stems are heavily branched and bear alternate or opposite, pinnatifid leaves with 6 or 7 pairs of leaflets.

Habitat: The plant is found in the U.S.

Production: Abscess Root is the rhizome of Polemonium reptans.

Not to be Confused With: The plant is known as False Jacob's Ladder because it has an astringent action similar to true Jacob's Ladder.

Other Names: American Greek Valerian, Blue Bells, False Jacob's Ladder, Sweatroot

ACTIONS AND PHARMACOLOGY

COMPOUNDS

Triterpene saponins

EFFECTS

Abscess root has astringent, diaphoretic and expectorant effects.

INDICATIONS AND USAGE

Unproven Uses: The drug is used for febrile and inflammatory disorders.

PRECAUTIONS AND ADVERSE REACTIONS

No health hazards or side effects are known in conjunction with the proper administration of designated therapeutic dosages.

DOSAGE

Mode of Administration: It is ground as a drug for infusion.

LITERATURE

Hegnauer R, Chemotaxonomie der Pflanzen, Bde 1-11, Birkhäuser Verlag Basel, Boston, Berlin 1962-1997.

Acacia

Acacia arabica

DESCRIPTION

Medicinal Parts: The medicinal parts are the bark, the gum and the fruit of the plant.

Flower and Fruit: The flowers are yellow and sweetly scented. Two to 6 inflorescence peduncles with capitula-like inflorescences grow from the axils of the upper leaflets. The flowers have short calyces with numerous overlapping sepals. The completely fused petals are almost twice as large as the sepals. The fruit is a 12 to 16 cm long and 1.5 cm wide pod. The pod is straight or lightly curved, flat to convex, and pinched in to create segments. It is matte-black to dark-red. The seeds are 7 x 6 mm and the same color as the pod.

Leaves, Stem and Root: Acacia arabica is a 6 m high tree with a compact, round to flat crown. Older branches are bare, younger ones measuring 15 to 20 mm in diameter are covered in hairy down. The bark is black and fissured; the coloring in the fissure changes to red-brown. There are stipule thorns at the nodes. The leaflets of the double-pinnate leaves are in 3 to 12 pairs on the bare to downy petiole, which is covered with glands. The leaflets are oblong, blunt, and bare or thinly ciliate.

Habitat: The plant is indigenous to the Nile area, Ethiopia, East Africa, Angola, Mozambique, South Africa, Arabia, Iran, Afghanistan and India.

Production: The bark is collected from plants that are at least 7 years old and then left to mature for a year.

Not to be Confused With: The bark of the Australian species Acacia decurrens, which is commercially available under the same name.

Other Names: Acacia Bark, Babul Bark, Wattle Bark, Indian Gum, Black Wattle

ACTIONS AND PHARMACOLOGY

COMPOUNDS

Tannins

EFFECTS

The drug has an astringent effect.

INDICATIONS AND USAGE

Unproven Uses: The drug is used as a decoction for gum disease and inflammations of the mucous membrane of the mouth and throat (rarely used today).

Indian Medicine: Acacia is used as a decoction in the treatment of diarrhea and vaginal secretions, and as an enema for hemorrhoids.

PRECAUTIONS AND ADVERSE REACTIONS

Large doses taken internally can lead to indigestion and constipation.

LITERATURE

Berger F, Handbuch der Drogenkunde, W Maudrich Verlag Wien 1964.

Hänsel R, Keller K, Rimpler H, Schneider G (Hrsg.), Hagers Handbuch der Pharmazeutischen Praxis, 5. Aufl., Bde 4-6 (Drogen), Springer Verlag Berlin, Heidelberg, New York, 1992-1994.

Trease GE, Evans WC (Eds.), Pharmacognosy, 12th Ed., Bailliere Tindall 1983.

Acacia arabica

See Acacia

Acacia catechu

See Catechu

Acacia senegal

See Gum Arabic

Acalypha indica

See Indian Nettle

Acer rubrum

See Red Maple

Achillea millefolium

See Yarrow

Achillea ptarmica

See Sneezewort

Aconitum napellus

See Monkshood

Acorus calamus

See Calamus

Actaea spicata

See Baneberry

Adam's Needle

Yucca filamentosa

DESCRIPTION

Medicinal Parts: The medicinal parts are the leaves and the roots of nonflowering plants.

Flower and Fruit: The flowers are ivory-colored and located in nodding, many-blossomed terminal panicles. The perigone is simple, campanulate, tinged greenish on the outside, with 6 sepals. The flower has 6 stamens, and the stigma is trisectioned.

Leaves, Stem, and Root: The plant is 120 to 240 cm in height. The leaves are in a basal rosette. They are sword-shaped and erect with a recurved tip. They are short-thorned, broadly grooved, and covered on the margin with long, twisted, whitish or yellowish threads.

Habitat: The plant is indigenous to the southern United States and is cultivated mainly as an ornamental plant in Europe.

Production: Adam's Needle leaves are the leaves of *Yucca filamentosa.*

ACTIONS AND PHARMACOLOGY

COMPOUNDS

Steroid saponins (from the roots; the saponins from the leaves remain uninvestigated): protoyuccoside C, yuccoside B, yuccoside E, yuccoside C, aglycones including sarsapogenin, tigogenin

EFFECTS

No information is available.

INDICATIONS AND USAGE

Unproven Uses: The plant is used for liver and gallbladder disorders.

PRECAUTIONS AND ADVERSE REACTIONS

No health hazards or side effects are known in conjunction with the proper administration of designated therapeutic dosages. Intake can lead to stomach complaints because of the saponin content.

DOSAGE

Mode of Administration: Adam's Needle is available in ground form and in extracts.

LITERATURE

Kern W, List PH, Hörhammer L (Hrsg.), Hagers Handbuch der Pharmazeutischen Praxis, 4. Aufl., Bde. 1-8: Springer Verlag Berlin, Heidelberg, New York, 1969.

Madaus G, Lehrbuch der Biologischen Arzneimittel, Bde 1-3, Nachdruck, Georg Olms Verlag Hildesheim 1979.

Adansonia digitata

See Baobab

Adiantum capillus-veneris

See Maidenhair

Adonis

Adonis vernalis

DESCRIPTION

Medicinal Parts: The medicinal part is derived from the aerial parts of the herb, which are collected during the flowering season and dried.

Flower and Fruit: The erect, solitary, terminal flower is 4 to 7 cm in diameter and the 5 broad-ovate, downy sepals are half as long as the petals. The 10 to 20 petals are narrow, wedge-shaped, simple or finely serrated at the tip. They are 20 to 40 mm long and lemon-yellow, splayed, glossy, reddish on the outside or greenish-tinged. There are numerous stamens and carpels. The small fruit forms a globose capitulum. The fruit is tomentose, wrinkled, laterally veined and keeled with a sideways-facing, hook-shaped beak. The fruit are arranged on the spindle-shaped, oblong receptacle.

Leaves, Stem and Root: The plant is 10 to 40 cm high with a sturdy, black-brown rhizome. The stem is erect, undivided, covered with scales at the base, vertically grooved and succulent. There are few branches. The leaves have many slits and a curved, glabrous or sparsely haired tip. The middle leaves are half-clasping.

Characteristics: Adonis is a poisonous plant.

Habitat: This Siberian/east European plant is found in the north as far as the central Urals and southwest Sweden. In central Europe, it is limited to the basins of the Weichsel and the Oder as far as the Main and Rhine.

Production: The drug is gathered in forests and should be dried quickly.

Not to be Confused With: Other Adonis species may be added to Adonidis herba.

Other Names: False Hellebore, Yellow Pheasant's Eye, Ox-eye, Sweet Vernal, Pheasant's Eye, Red Morocco, Rose-a-Rubie

ACTIONS AND PHARMACOLOGY

COMPOUNDS

Cardioactive steroid gylcosides (cardenolids): including adonitoxin, k-strophanthoside, k-strophanthoside-β and cymarin

Flavonoids: including vitexin and luteolin

EFFECTS

Adonis has a positive inotropic effect. Animal tests demonstrated a tonic effect on the veins. The adonitoxin component is slightly more toxic than coumarin. The drug is insufficiently documented.

INDICATIONS AND USAGE

Approved by Commission E:

- Arrhythmia
- Nervous heart complaints

Unproven Uses: The drug is used for mild impairment of heart functions (NYHA I and II), especially when accompanied by nervous symptoms.

In Russian folk medicine, the drug is used for dehydration, cramps, fever and menstrual disorders, but efficacy is unproven.

Homeopathic Uses: Preparations of Adonis vernalis are used for cardiac insufficiency.

CONTRAINDICATIONS

Adonis is contraindicated in conjunction with digitalis glycoside therapy and also in potassium deficiency.

PRECAUTIONS AND ADVERSE REACTIONS

General: Despite the strong efficacy of the drug's cardioactive steroid gylcosides in parenteral application, serious poisoning in the course of per oral administration is hardly to be expected due to the low resorption rate.

DRUG INTERACTIONS

Digoxin: Concurrent use is contraindicated.

OVERDOSAGE

For possible symptoms of overdose and treatment of poisonings see *Digitalis folium.*

DOSAGE

Mode of Administration: Comminuted herb and preparations thereof for internal use.

Daily Dosage: The average daily dose is 0.6 gm of standardized Adonis powder. The maximum single dose is 1.0 gm; maximum daily dose is 3.0 gm.

Homeopathic Dosage: From D2: 5 to 10 drops, 1 tablet or 5 to 10 globules, 1 to 3 times daily; Injection solution: 1 ml once a week sc. From D4: Injection solution: 1 ml twice weekly sc.

Storage: Adonis herb and powder should be stored carefully. Adonis powder should be stored away from light in tightly sealed containers.

LITERATURE

Brevoort P, Der Heilpflanzenmarkt der USA - Ein Überblick. In: *ZPT 18*(3):155-162. 1997.

ESCOP-Monographs. In: ESCOP-Monographs Fascicule I and II. 1996.

Hiller KO, Rahlfs V, Therapeutische Äquivalenz eines hochdosierten Phytopharmakons mit Amytriptylin bei ängstlich-depressiven Versimmungen - Reanalyse einer randomisierten Studie unter besonderer Beachtung biometrischer und klinischer Aspekte. In: *Forsch.*

Lee MK, et al., Antihepatotoxic activity of Icariin, a major constituent of Epimedium koreanum. In: *PM* 61(6):523-526. 1995.

Loew, Buch. In: Loew D, Rietbrock N: Phytopharmaka II: Forschung und klinische Anwendung, Steinkopff Verlag, Darmstadt, 1996.

Loew DA, Loew AD, Pharmakokinetik von herzglykosidhaltigen Pflanzenextrakten. In: *ZPT* 15(4):197-202. 1994.

Loew D, Phytotherapie bei Herzinsuffizienz. In: *ZPT* 18(2):92-96. 1997.

Martinez-Vazquez M, Ramirez Apan TO, Hidemi Aguilar M, Bye R, Analgesic and antipyretic activities of an aqueous extract and of the flavone Linarin of Buddleia cordata. In: *PM* 62:137-140. 1996.

Reinhard KH, Uncaria tomentosa (WILLD.) DC. - Cat's claw, Una de gato oder Katzenkralle Protrait einer Arzneipflanze. In: *ZPT* 18(2):112-121. 1997.

Sandberg F, Thorsen R, (1962) *Lloydia* 25(3):201.

Schulz V, Hübner WD, Ploch M, Klinische Studien mit Psycho-Phytopharmaka. In: *ZPT* 18(3):141-154. 1997.

Winkler C and Wichtel M, (1985) *Pharm Acta Helv* 60(9/10): 234.

Adonis vernalis

See Adonis

Adrue

Cyperus articulatus

DESCRIPTION

Medicinal Parts: Adrue root is used in the West Indies for its anti-emetic properties.

Flower and Fruit: The tubers are blackish and top-shaped, with bristly remains of former leaves. The plant is sometimes connected in twos or threes by narrow underground stems. The transverse section is pale, showing a central column with darker vascular bundles.

Characteristics: Adrue has an aromatic odor and a bitter taste, reminiscent of Lavender.

Habitat: Turkey, region of the river Nile, Jamaica.

Production: Adrue root is the root of Cyperus articulatus. The roots are collected in the autumn, scalded or steamed, and then dried in the sun.

Other Names: Guinea Rush

ACTIONS AND PHARMACOLOGY

COMPOUNDS

Volatile oil: containing above all sesquiterpene hydrocarbons and sesqiterpene alcohols, including cyperenone

EFFECTS

Adrue has anti-emetic, carminative and sedative properties.

INDICATIONS AND USAGE

Unproven Uses: Preparations of the root are used for digestive disorders, nausea and flatulence.

Chinese Medicine: Used for pre- and post-natal headaches, epigastric pain, vomiting with bleeding, hematuria, leukorrhea, menstrual irregularities, tension and pain in the breasts and amenorrhea.

PRECAUTIONS AND ADVERSE REACTIONS

Health risks or side effects following the proper administration of designated therapeutic dosages are not recorded.

DOSAGE

Mode of Administration: Available as a liquid extract for internal use.

Daily Dosage: 6 to 9 gm of drug

Storage: Should be stored in a cool and dry place, protected from insects.

LITERATURE

Bum EN et al.; Extracts from rhizomes of Cyperus articulatus displace 3H CGP39653 and 3H glycine binding from cortical membranes and selectively inhibit NMDA receptor-mediated neurotransmission. *J Ethnopharmacol,* 54:103-11, 1996 Nov

Kern W, List PH, Hörhammer L (Hrsg.), Hagers Handbuch der Pharmazeutischen Praxis, 4. Aufl., Bde 1-8, Springer Verlag Berlin, Heidelberg, New York, 1969.

Mongelli E, Desmarchelier C, Coussio J, Ciccia G, Antimicrobial activity and interaction with DNA of medicinal plants from the Peruvian Amazon region. *Rev Argent Microbiol,* 27:199-203, 1995 Oct-Dec

Pinder AR, (1976) Tetrahedron 23:2172.

Aegle marmelos

See Bael

Aegopodium podagraria

See Goutweed

Aesculus hippocastanum

See Horse Chestnut

Aethusa cynapium

See Fool's Parsley

Aframomum melegueta

See Grains-of-Paradise

African Potato

Hypoxis rooperi

DESCRIPTION

Medicinal Parts: The medicinal part is the plant's rhizome tuber.

Flower and Fruit: Four to 10 flowers are arranged in racemes on a long peduncle; the pedicles are 1.2 to 2.5 cm long. The 6 tepals are approximately 18 mm long, elongate, free and yellow. There are 6 stamens, and the ovary is inferior, 3-chambered, top-shaped and thickly pubescent. The fruit is a densely pubescent capsule approximately 12 mm long and split in the middle. The seeds are black and warty.

Leaves, Stem and Root: The plant is a herbaceous perennial with 12 to 18 leaves that are 30 to 60 cm long, 2.4 to 4 cm wide, lanceolate, acuminate, firm with a ciliate margin and short hairs underneath. The leaves grow from a globose shoot, which has a diameter of 5 to 8 cm and is crowned with a ring of bristle-like hairs.

Habitat: Hypoxis rooperi is indigenous to South Africa.

Production: Bantu tulip is the fresh or dried rhizome tuber of Hypoxis rooperi. The plant is collected in the wild, cut and then dried in the sun.

Other Names: Bantu Tulip, Sterretjie

ACTIONS AND PHARMACOLOGY

COMPOUNDS

Lignans (3.5 to 4.5%): particularly hypoxoside (norlignan glucoside)

Steroids: sterols, including beta-sitosterol (ca. 0.2%), beta-sitosterol glucoside

Polysaccharides: starch

EFFECTS

The phytosterols, which have not as yet been more closely identified (beta-sitosterol is possibly the chief active ingredient), are said to have anti-exudative effects in animal experiments. The positive effect of the drug on benign prostate hyperplasia (reduction of the residual urine volume, increase of the uroflow, improvement of subjectively experienced complaints) is explained by the phytosterols' inhibition of local prostaglandin synthase.

INDICATIONS AND USAGE

Unproven Uses: Used internally for micturition complaints resulting from benign prostate hyperplasia, cystitis (South Africa/decoction) and lung disease (Botswana). It is used externally as a vulnerary (Africa). Efficacy for these indications has not yet been proved.

PRECAUTIONS AND ADVERSE REACTIONS

No health hazards are known in conjunction with the proper administration of designated therapeutic dosages.

DOSAGE

Mode of Administration: Whole and cut drug preparations for internal and external use.

How Supplied: Commercially produced capsules.

LITERATURE

Bräuer H, Schomann C, Tolerance of beta-sitosterin from Hypoxis rooperi in patients with limited liver function. Results of a controlled double-blind study, Fortschr *Med*, 96:833-4, 1978 Apr 20.

Hänsel R, Keller K, Rimpler H, Schneider G (Ed.), Hagers Handbuch der Pharmazeutischen Praxis, 5. Aufl., Bde 4 - 6 (Drogen), Springer Verlag Berlin, Heidelberg, New York, 1992-1994.

Aga

Amanita muscaria

DESCRIPTION

Medicinal Parts: The fungus is used to prepare homeopathic dilutions.

Flower and Fruit: Aga belongs to the group of lamella fungi, genus Amanita. The hymenium in the inside of the fruiting body is exposed by unfolding the cap on the underside.

Characteristics: The poisonous fungus has a basidia that is dirty white, as are the cuffs and underside of the cap. The mushroom's cap is orange at first, then strong red with a few dirty-white to yellow spots.

Habitat: Aga grows in the Northern Hemisphere as far north as the tundra and thrives in sandy, acid soils.

Production: Aga is the above-ground part of *Amanita muscaria.*

Other Names: Fly Agaric

ACTIONS AND PHARMACOLOGY

COMPOUNDS

Ibotenic acid (0.17% to 1%)

Muscimol

Muscarine (traces)

Muscazone

Betalains (skin pigment): muscaflavin, muscaaurins and muscapurpurins

Amavandin (compound containing vanadium)

EFFECTS

The drug, containing ibotenic acid, has a psychotropic and hallucinogenic effect and is toxic in higher doses. The decarboxylation product muscimol is similar in structure to the neurotransmitter GABA and attaches itself to the latter's receptor complex as a selective and direct antagonist. The drug is initially stimulating then paralyzing in its effect.

INDICATIONS AND USAGE

Homeopathic Uses: The fungus is used to treat neuralgias, fever, anxiety, alcohol poisoning, and joint pains.

PRECAUTIONS AND ADVERSE REACTIONS

The drug is highly toxic. Signs of poisoning include dizziness, vomiting, abdominal pain, movement disorders, muscle cramps and psychic stimulation, followed by deep sleep.

OVERDOSAGE

The intake of more than 10 g of the fresh mushroom can lead to coordination disorders, confusion, illusions and manic attacks. Higher dosages (over 100 g of fresh mushrooms) lead to unconsciousness, asphyxiation, coma, and death.

The treatment of poisoning includes emptying the gastrointestinal tract and the use of sedatives. In case of shock, a plasma volume expander should be used. Artificial respiration should be administered for respiratory arrest.

DOSAGE

Mode of Administration: In homeopathy, dilutions of the mother tincture are used.

LITERATURE

Hastings MH, et al., *Brain Res* 360:248. 1985.

Hatfield GM, Brady LR, *JNP* 38:36, 1975.

Marmo E, *Med Res Rev* 8:441, 1988.

Schwarz B, Ein Männlein steht im Walde. In: *PZ* 139(13):1040. 1994.

Agar

Gelidium amansii

DESCRIPTION

Medicinal Parts: The medicinal part of the plant is the seaweed's gelatinous extract known as Agar or Agar-Agar.

Flower and Fruit: This perennial seaweed grows up to 1 m long. The thallus sprouts from a permanent base every year and is heavily branched. It is cylindrical or flattened, pinnately subdivided and tough. The brownish-white, translucent thallus has prickly appendages on the branchings. The fruit is spherical.

Characteristics: Agar is colorless and tasteless. It is capable of absorbing up to 200 times its volume of water to form a jelly.

Habitat: The plant is indigenous to the Pacific coasts of Japan and China, Sri Lanka and also the South African coasts.

Production: Agar, or Agar-Agar, is the purified and bleached gel derived from algae mucilage of the *Rhodophyceae Gelidium amansii* (Lamour), which has been dried and cut into thread-like strips. An aqueous extract is obtained from the algae through autoclaving (pressure-cooking), using overheated steam. It is then chilled in ice cells and cooled into ice-blocks, which are crushed and thawed. Water separates from the gel during the thawing process. The gel mass is dried using warm air.

Other Names: Agar-Agar, Japanese Isinglass

ACTIONS AND PHARMACOLOGY

COMPOUNDS

Heteropolysaccharides: made up of D-galactose- and 3,6-anhydro-L-galactose- components, partially bearing sulfate or pyruvic acid residues, low-sulfate fraction designated agarose

EFFECTS

The drug has a laxative effect due to its ability, similar to that of cellulose, to absorb and retain large quantities of water and swell in the intestine. The mucilaginous substances cause an increase in the bulk of the content of the intestine that stimulates the intestinal muscles, thereby aiding peristalsis.

INDICATIONS AND USAGE

Unproven Uses: The drug is used as a mild laxative.

PRECAUTIONS AND ADVERSE REACTIONS

No health hazards or side effects are known in conjunction with the proper administration of designated therapeutic dosages.

DOSAGE

Mode of Administration: The drug is used internally.

Daily Dosage: Laxative: Take 1 to 2 teaspoons of the powder, always with some liquid, fruit, or jam before meals, 1 to 3 times daily. Never take dry!

Storage: Dried Agar can be kept tightly sealed for up to 5 years without being opened and tested.

LITERATURE

Ataki C, *Chem Soc Japan* 29:543. 1956.

Franz G (Hrsg.), Polysaccharide. Springer Verlag Berlin, Heidelberg, New York 1991.

Kern W, List PH, Hörhammer L (Hrsg.), Hagers Handbuch der Pharmazeutischen Praxis, 4. Aufl., Bde. 1-8, Springer Verlag Berlin, Heidelberg, New York, 1969.

Murano E et al., Pyruvate-rich agarose from the red alga Gracilaria dura. In: *PM* 58(Suppl. 7):A588. 1992.

Schmid OJ, Marina (Hamburg) 1:54. 1959.

$teinegger E, Hänsel R, Pharmakognosie, 5. Aufl., Springer Verlag Heidelberg 1992.

Teuscher E, Biogene Arzneimittel, 5. Aufl., Wiss. Verlagsges. Stuttgart 1997.

Vessal M, Mehrani HA, Omrani GH, Effects of an aqueous extract of Physalis alkekengi fruit on estrus cycle, reproduction and uterine craetive kinase BB-isoenzyme in rats. In: *ETH* 34(1):69-78. 1991.

Agrimonia eupatoria

See Agrimony

Agrimony

Agrimonia eupatoria

DESCRIPTION

Medicinal Parts: The drug consists of the flowering plant, which is cut a few fingers width above the ground and dried.

Flower and Fruit: The flowers are yellow, arranged along small, spike-like racemes. They have an epicalyx and 5 sepals, 5 ovate petals, 5 to 20 stamens and 2 ovaries. The calyx is rough-haired with deep furrows. The fruit is obconical and thorny (burdocks).

Leaves, Stem and Root: The plant is 50 to 100 cm high, with a villous, erect stem. The leaves are alternate and irregularly pinnate. The leaflets are deeply serrate and downy beneath.

Characteristics: Agrimony has a slight pleasant fragrance and a tangy, bitter taste.

Habitat: The plant is indigenous to middle and northern Europe, temperate Asia and North America.

Production: Agrimony herb consists of the dried, above-ground parts of *Agrimonia eupatoria* and/or *Agrimonia procera* gathered just before or during flowering, as well as its preparations in effective dosage.

Other Names: Stickwort, Cocklebur, Liverwort, Common Agrimony, Philanthropos, Church Steeples, Sticklewort

ACTIONS AND PHARMACOLOGY

COMPOUNDS

Catechin tannins

EFFECTS

Agrimony is an astringent.

INDICATIONS AND USAGE

Approved by Commission E:

- Diarrhea
- Inflammation of the skin
- Inflammation of the mouth and pharynx

Unproven Uses: Agrimony is used internally for mild, nonspecific, acute diarrhea, cholestasis, inflammation of oral and pharyngeal mucosa, inflammation of kidney and bladder, diabetes and childhood bedwetting; externally for poorly healing wounds, chronic pharyngitis, psoriasis, seborrhoeic eczema as well in hip-baths for lower abdominal conditions.

Chinese Medicine: Agrimony is used as a hemostyptic. It is also used for certain forms of cancer and as an anthelmintic.

PRECAUTIONS AND ADVERSE REACTIONS

No health hazards or side effects are known in conjunction with the proper administration of designated therapeutic dosages. Because of the constituent tannins, the intake of larger quantities could lead to digestive complaints and constipation.

DOSAGE

Daily Dosage: Internally, the average daily dose is 3 to 6 gm of herb or equivalent preparations. Externally, a poultice prepared from a decoction (10%) several times a day is applied.

LITERATURE

Bilai AR, et al., A flavonol glycoside from Agrimonia eupatoria. In: *PH* 32:1078. 1993.

Chon SC, et al., (1987) *Med Pharmacol Exp* 16(5):407-413.

Drozd GA, et al., (1983) *Khim Prir Soed* 1:106.

Patrascu V, et al., (1984) *Ser. Dermato-Venerol* 29(2):153-157.

Peter-Horvath M, et al., (1964) *Rev Med* 10(2):190-193.

Agropyron repens

See Triticum

Agrostemma githago

See Corn Cockle

Ailanthus altissima

See Tree of Heaven

Ajuga chamaepitys

See Ground Pine

Ajuga reptans

See Bugle

Akebia quinata

See Chocolate Vine (Mu-Tong)

Alcea rosea

See Hollyhock

Alchemilla vulgaris

See Lady's Mantle

Alchornea floribunda

See Iporuru

Aletris

Aletris farinosa

DESCRIPTION

Medicinal Parts: The medicinal part is the dried *Aletris farinosa* rhizome with roots. Fresh underground parts that are dug up after flowering are also used.

Flower and Fruit: The plant has numerous white, tubular-oblong, campanulate flowers. The flowers, with a few small bracts, are in terminal, spikelike racemes on stalks that reach up to 1 m. The perianth is tubular and covered in scales; it shrinks when ripe. Later, the perianth springs open in a beak shape. The fruit is an ovoid capsule containing many oblong ribbed seeds.

Leaves, Stem and Root: The leaves are erect-oblong, lanceolate and 2 to 20 cm long. The rhizome is brownish-gray, flattened and has a diameter of up to 1 cm, but usually measures less. The upper part is covered in leaf bases and stem scars. The fracture is floury and white.

Characteristics: The plant has a sweet taste, becoming bitter and soapy. The odor is mild.

Habitat: The plant is found in the northeast U.S., south to Gulf of Mexico, southern Canada.

Production: Aletris root is the rhizome of *Aletris farinosa*. It is gathered in the wild and air-dried in the shade.

Other Names: Star Grass, Colic-Root, Starwort, Blazing Star, Ague-Root, Aloe-Root, Ague Grass, Black-Root, Bitter Grass, Crow Corn, Bettie Grass, Devil's Bit, True Unicorn Star-Grass, True Unicorn Root

ACTIONS AND PHARMACOLOGY

COMPOUNDS

Saponins

Volatile oil

Resins

Bitter principles

Starch

EFFECTS

The active agents increase motility and act as a tonic. There may be an estrogenic principle but a possible estrogenic effect has not been sufficiently researched.

INDICATIONS AND USAGE

Unproven Uses: In the U.S., the plant is used for gynecological disorders or "female complaints," in particular dysmenorrhea, amenorrhea, and complaints associated with *prolapses vaginae.*

Preparations of Aletris are also used for loss of appetite, venous dyspepsia, flatulence, and nervous digestive complaints. In Argentina, it is used to treat chronic bronchitis.

Homeopathic Uses: Prolapsed uterus, gastrointestinal complaints.

PRECAUTIONS AND ADVERSE REACTIONS

No health hazards or side effects are known in conjunction with the proper administration of designated therapeutic dosages.

DOSAGE

Mode of Administration: Available in the forms of powdered root, liquid extract and infusions for internal use.

Preparation: To prepare an infusion, 1.5 gm of the drug is added to 100 mL of water. The fluid extract (1:1) is produced with ethanol water (45%).

Daily Dosage: Approximately 6 gm. The recommended single dose is 0.3 to 0.6 gm to be taken 3 times daily. Infusion: 1.5 gm of the drug to 100 mL water.

Homeopathic Dosage: 5 to 10 drops, 1 tablet, or 5 to 10 globules; injection solution: 1 mL once a week sc (HAB1).

LITERATURE

Costello CH, Lynn EV, (1950) *J Am Pharm Ass* 39:117.

Marker RE et al., (1940) *J Chem Soc* 60:2620.

Aletris farinosa

See Aletris

Alfalfa

Medicago sativa

DESCRIPTION

Medicinal Parts: The medicinal parts are the whole flowering plant or the germinating seeds.

Flower and Fruit: The cloverlike flowers can be yellow to violet-blue. They are 9 to 10 mm long and appear in oblong, many-blossomed racemes. The fruit is a spiraled pod with 2 or 3 twists; the center is hollow and not thorny.

Leaves, Stem, and Root: The annual, succulent plant grows from 45 to 100 cm high. The stems are erect, smooth, and sharply angled. The leaves are trifoliate, petiolate, and alternate. The leaflets are thorny-tipped, dentate toward the front, obovate, and villous beneath. The stipules are ovate, lanceolate, slightly dentate, and acuminate.

Characteristics: The taste is unpleasantly salty, bitter, and dry.

Habitat: The plant is indigenous to the Mediterranean region and has been widely cultivated elsewhere for centuries.

Other Names: Buffalo Herb, Lucerne, Purple Medic, Purple Medick, Purple Medicle

ACTIONS AND PHARMACOLOGY

COMPOUNDS: IN THE FOLIAGE

Carotinoids: including among others, lutein

Triterpene saponins: sojasapogenols A-E aglycones medicagenic acid, hederagenin

Isoflavonoids: including among others, formononetin glycosides, genistein, daidzein

Coumestans: coumestrol, 3′-methoxy coumestrol, lucernol, sativol, trifoliol

Triterpenes: including among others, stigmasterol, spinasterol

Cyanogenic glycosides: corresponding to less than 80 mg HCN/100 g

COMPOUNDS IN THE SEEDS

L-canavaine

Betaine: stachydrine, homostachydrine

Trigonelline

Fatty oil

EFFECTS

The saponin contents act on the cardiovascular, nervous, and digestive systems.

Antilipidemic Effects: Saponins and other components in alfalfa act synergistically to bind the bile acids required for cholesterol absorption from the gut. Saponins may also affect cholesterol metabolism indirectly, by interfering with the enterohepatic circulation of bile acids. Some saponins form large mixed micelles with bile acids. In humans, alfalfa has shown moderate ability to lower serum cholesterol concentrations, probably because of the saponins within it; if saponins are extracted, alfalfa loses its hypocholesterolemic effect (Molgaard et al, 1987).

Alfalfa exhibited hypoglycemic effects in mice rendered diabetic by administration of streptozotocin, which destroys pancreatic cells, while having no significant effect in nondiabetic mice (Gray & Flatt, 1997).

Antifungal Effects: Saponins have well-documented antifungal properties (Zehavi & Polacheck, 1996). When applied topically, a gluco derivative of medicagenic acid cured skin lesions of guinea pigs infected with the dermatophyte *Trichophyton mentagrophytes* and good skin tolerance was observed. Liposomes containing compound G2, the gluco derivative, were effective in a drug-delivery system to treat murine cryptococcosis and candidiasis (Zehavi & Polacheck, 1996).

Enzymatic Effects: In one investigation, alfalfa decreased trypsin and chymotrypsin activities (Dunaif & Schneeman, 1981), and lipase activities (Schneeman, 1978).

Prolactin-inhibiting Effects: A peptide with thyrotropin-releasing hormone (TRH) immunocharacteristics has been detected in alfalfa. Unlike TRH, which is a potent prolactin releaser, this peptide is a prolactin-inhibiting factor. Because TRH is highly resistant to degradation by gastrointestinal enzymes, this TRH-like peptide may be capable of producing systemic effects (Morley, 1982).

CLINICAL TRIALS

Hypercholesterolemia

In a short-term study involving three normolipidemic individuals given alfalfa seeds (80-60 g daily), serum cholesterol concentrations were reported to be reduced (Molgaard et al, 1987). In another small study in which heat-treated alfalfa seeds (40 g three times daily for eight weeks) were taken by eight type IIA hyperlipoproteinemic patients and three type IIB patients, a significant decrease was noted in total serum cholesterol concentrations, LDL cholesterol, and apolipoprotein B. The LDL cholesterol concentration fell by less than 5% in two of the 11 patients (Molgaard et al, 1987).

Alfalfa seeds added to the diet of 15 patients with type II hyperlipoproteinemia (HLP) decreased total plasma cholesterol, LDL cholesterol, and apolipoprotein B without changing the high-density lipoprotein (HDL) cholesterol concentrations. After treatment, patients with type II HLP manifested a maximal lowering of pretreatment median values of total plasma cholesterol from 9.58 to 8.00 mmol/L ($p<0.001$) and of LDL cholesterol from 7.69 to 6.33 mmol/L ($p<0.01$) which corresponds to 17% decreases of total plasma cholesterol and 18% decreases of LDL cholesterol. However, LDL cholesterol decreased less than 5% in 2 patients with hypercholesterolemia. In the same period apolipoprotein B decreased by 34% ($p<0.05$) in patients with type II HLP while apolipoprotein A-I did not change. After treatment ended, all lipoprotein concentrations returned to pretreatment levels (Molgaard et al, 1987).

INDICATIONS AND USAGE

Unproven Uses: In folk medicine, the drug is used in the treatment of diabetes and malfunctioning of the thyroid gland.

CONTRAINDICATIONS

Alfalfa is contraindicated in patients with gout and systemic lupus erythematosus.

Pregnancy: Not to be used during pregnancy.

PRECAUTIONS AND ADVERSE REACTIONS

In the United States and other countries, eating sprouts of alfalfa and other seeds has been associated with numerous culture-proven outbreaks of *Escherichia coli, Bacillus cereus,* and many serotypes of *Salmonella*. In addition, the sprouting process, which is characterized by high moisture and a temperature generally in the range of 21 to 25°C, provides an outstanding environment for microorganism propagation. Treating seeds or sprouts with chlorinated water or other disinfectants, diminishes but does not eradicate the pathogens. Gamma irradiation, on the other hand, controls *Salmonella* and *E coli* O157:H7 on alfalfa sprouts at doses approved for irradiating meat (which are higher than the 1.0 kiloGray dose used for fruits and vegetables) without affecting germination of seeds and constitutes the best preventive measure now available for decontaminating sprouts and other agricultural products (Taormina et al, 1999; Stephenson, 1997). One case of human listeriosis has been linked to consumption of alfalfa tablets (Farber et al, 1990).

Hypokalemia has been reported, and gastrointestinal disorders are possible, including *E. Coli, Salmonella*, and listerosis infections (see Precautions).

DRUG INTERACTIONS

MAJOR RISK

Azathioprine and Cyclosporine: Concurrent use may result in reduced immunosuppressive drug effectiveness and acute transplant rejection. *Clinical Management:* Advise patients taking azathioprine or cyclosporine for transplant maintenance to avoid alfalfa, including herbal teas and combination supplement products containing alfalfa. If the patients are taking alfalfa and either azathioprine or cyclosporine, discontinue alfalfa and evaluate for signs and symptoms of transplant rejection.

MODERATE RISK

Prednisone: Concurrent use may result in reduced prednisone effectiveness. *Clinical Management:* Patients with Systemic Lupus Erythematosus (SLE) should be advised to avoid use of alfalfa until the nature of this phenomenon (i.e., SLE activation) is known. Consumption of 8 to 15 tablets (dosage unspecified) daily has been associated with SLE activation overcoming the effect of established prednisone therapy.

MINOR RISK

Anticoagulants: Concurrent use may result in reduced anticoagulant effectiveness. *Clinical Management:* The amount of alfalfa taken in supplements and/or in the diet should be kept as constant as possible. Monitor the INR and adjust the dose of anticoagulant as necessary.

DOSAGE

How Supplied: Tablets, Ointment, Seeds, and Sprouted Seeds

Daily Dose: For hyperlipoproteinemia: 40 g of heat-prepared seeds 3 times a day at mealtimes.

LITERATURE

Boveris AD & Puntarulo S. Free-radical scavenging actions of natural antioxidants. *Nutr Res*; 18(9):1545-1557. 1998

Cheeke PR. Nutritional and physiological properties of saponins. *Nutr Rep Int*; 13(3):315-324. 1976

Dunaif G & Schneeman BO. The effect of dietary fiber on human pancreatic enzyme activity in vitro. *Am J Clin Nutr*; 34(6):1034-1035. 1981

Ehle FR, Robertson JB & Van Soest PJ. Influence of dietary fibers on fermentation in the human large intestine. *J Nutr*; 112(1):158-166. 1982

Farber JM, Carter AO, Varughese PV et al. Listeriosis traced to the consumption of alfalfa tablets and soft cheese. *N Engl J Med*; 332(5):338. 1990

Feingold RM. Should we fear ''health foods?'' *Arch Intern Med*; 159(13):1502. 1999

Gestetner B, *Phytochemistry* 10:2221. 1974

Gray AM & Flatt PR. Pancreatic and extra-pancreatic effects of the traditional anti-diabetic plant, *Medicago sativa* (lucerne). *Br J Nutr*; 78(2):325-334. 1997

Herbert V & Kasdan TS. Alfalfa, vitamin E, and autoimmune disorders. *Am J Clin Nutr*; 60:639-640. 1994

Jacobs LR. Relationship between dietary fiber and cancer: Metabolic, physiologic, and cellular mechanisms. *Proc Soc Exp Biol Med*; 183(3):299-310. 1986

Larher F et al., *Plant Sci Lett* 29(2/3):315. 1983

Light TD & Light JA. Acute renal transplant rejection possibly related to herbal medications. *Am J Transplant*; 3:1608-1609. 2003

Malinow MR et al. Prevention of elevated cholesterolemia in monkeys by alfalfa saponins. *Steroids*; 29: 105-11. 1977

Molgaard J, von Schenck H & Olsson AG. Alfalfa seeds lower low density lipoprotein cholesterol and apolipoprotein B concentrations in patients with type II hyperlipoproteinemia. *Atheroscler*; 65(1-2):173-179. 1987

Montanaro A & Bardana EJ Jr. Dietary amino acid-induced systemic lupus erythematosus. *Nutr Rheu Dis*; 17(2):323-332. 1991

Morley JE. Food peptides. A new class of hormones? *JAMA*; 247(17):2379-2380. 1982

Norred CL & Brinker F. Potential coagulation effects of preoperative complementary and alternative medicines. *Altern Ther Health Med*; 7(6): 58-67. 2001

Oakenfull D & Sidhu GS. Could saponins be a useful treatment for hypercholesterolaemia? *Eur J Clin Nutr*; 44(1):79-88. 1990

Sadovsky R. Foodborne disease and shiga toxin-producing *E coli. Am Fam Phys*; 61(7):2194. 2000

Schneeman BO. Effect of plant fiber on lipase, trypsin and chymotrypsin activity. *J Food Sci*; 43(2):634-635. 1978

Story JA. Dietary fiber and lipid metabolism. *Proc Soc Exp Biol Med*; 180(3):447-452. 1985

Swanston-Flatt SK et al. Traditional plant treatments for diabetes in normal and streptozotocin-diabetic mice. *Diabetologia*; 33: 462-464. 1990

Taormina PJ, Beuchat LR & Slutsker L. Infections associated with eating seed sprouts: An international concern. *Emerg Infect Dis*; 5(5):626-634. 1999

Van Beneden CA, Keene WE, Strang RA et al. Multinational outbreak of *Salmonella enterica* serotype Newport infections due to contaminated alfalfa sprouts. *JAMA*; 281(2):158-162. 1999

Wasan HS & Goodlad RA. Fibre-supplemented foods may damage your health. *Lancet*; 348(9023):319-320. 1996

Whittam J, Jensen C & Hudson T. Alfalfa, vitamin E, and autoimmune disorders. *Am J Clin Nutr*; 62(5):1025-1026. 1995

Zehavi U & Polacheck I. Saponins as antimycotic agents: Glycosides of medicagenic acid. *Adv Exp Med Biol*; 404:535-546. 1996

Zhao WS et al. Immunopotentiating effects of polysaccharides isolated from *Medicago sativa L. Acta Pharmacol Sinica*; 14: 273-276. 1993

Alisma (Ze-Xie)

Alisma plantago-aquatica

DESCRIPTION

Medicinal Parts: The medicinal part is the fresh rhizome.

Flower and Fruit: The peduncle is triangular. There are long-pedicled, white or reddish flowers in leafless, loose panicles. There are 3 sepals, 3 petals, and 3 stamens in the flower. The fruit is small and obtuse and is formed by 15 to 30 ovaries.

Leaves, Stem and Root: The water leaves are ribbonlike. There are long-stemmed, swimming leaves. The aerial leaves are basal, long-stemmed, and cordate, or oblong-ovate, and spoonlike.

Characteristics: The rootstock of Alisma has a bitter taste; it is poisonous when fresh.

Habitat: The plant is distributed widely throughout Europe, northern Asia and North America.

Other Names: Mad-Dog Weed, Water Plantain, Ze-Xie

ACTIONS AND PHARMACOLOGY

COMPOUNDS

Triterpenes: including alisol-A, alisol-B, alisol-C and their monoacetates

Sesquiterpenes (guaian type): alismol, alismol oxide

Flavone sulfate

Caffeic acid derivatives: chlorogenic acid sulfate

EFFECTS

No information is available.

INDICATIONS AND USAGE

Unproven Uses: Alisma is used for diseases of the bladder and urinary tract.

Chinese Medicine: The drug is used to lower blood sugar, blood pressure, and cholesterol levels; it is also used as a diuretic.

PRECAUTIONS AND ADVERSE REACTIONS

No health hazards or side effects are known in conjunction with the proper administration of designated therapeutic dosages.

DOSAGE

Mode of Administration: The drug is available as an extract for oral use. The root is also used in homeopathy.

LITERATURE

Kern W, List PH, Hörhammer L (Hrsg.), Hagers Handbuch der Pharmazeutischen Praxis, 4. Aufl., Bde 1-8, Springer Verlag Berlin, Heidelberg, New York, 1969.

Murata T et al., (1968) Tetrahedron Letteers 103:849.

Murata T et al., *Chem Pharm Bull* 18:1369. 1970.

Oshima Y et al., PH 22:183. 1983.

Alisma plantago-aquatica

See Alisma (Ze-Xie)

Alkanet

Alkanna tinctoria

DESCRIPTION

Medicinal Parts: The medicinal part is the root of the plant (the dried roots and rhizomes).

Flower and Fruit: The calyx is 4 to 5 mm in the flower, 5 to 6 mm in the fruit and eglandular. The corolla is blue and glabrous outside. The funnel is as long as or slightly longer than the calyx. The limb is 6 to 7 mm in diameter. There are 5 stamens, and the anthers are fused with the corolla tube. The nutlets are 2 mm in diameter, irregularly reticulate and tuberculate.

Leaves, Stem and Root: Alkanet is a short-bristled, perennial half-rosette shrub. The stems are 10 to 20 cm, procumbent or ascending and glandular. The basal leaves are 6 to 15 cm by 0.7 to 1.5 cm, linear-lanceolate; the lower ones are cauline, oblong-linear and cordate at base. The bracts are slightly longer than calyx and oblong-lanceolate. The neck of the root is covered with the remains of leaves and the stems. The root is spindle-shaped, curved, up to 25 cm long and 1.5 cm thick, with purplish root bark.

Habitat: The plant is indigenous to southeastern Europe and some parts of Turkey and Hungary. It is cultivated in other parts of Europe, Britain, and northern Africa.

Production: Alkanna rhizomes are the dried roots and rhizomes of Alkanna tinctoria Tausch.

Other Names: Anchusa, Dyer's Bugloss, Spanish Bugloss, Alkanet Root, Alkanna

ACTIONS AND PHARMACOLOGY

COMPOUNDS

Naphthazarine derivatives: including the ester of the (-)-alkannin (stained red)

Pyrrolizidine alkaloids

Tannins

EFFECTS

Antimicrobial action: In the agar diffusion test, Alkanet root extracts and Alkannin esters impaired the growth of *Staphylococcus aureus* and *Staphylococcus epidermidis*, however Alkannin worked only against *Candida albicans*.

Healing action for wounds: In a double-blind study, 72 patients suffering from ulcers of the leg (*Ulcus cruris*) caused by varicose veins, were treated with Histoplastin Red® over a period of 3 years. After 5 to 6 weeks of daily administration, 80% of the patients' ulcers had healed or were considerably reduced in size.

The results are difficult to assess, as details concerning the patients, the treatment pattern, and control groups are unavailable.

INDICATIONS AND USAGE

Unproven Uses: Used by the ancient Greeks to heal wounds; also for skin diseases and diarrhea.

PRECAUTIONS AND ADVERSE REACTIONS

Hepatotoxicity and carcinogenicity are expected due to the pyrrolizidine alkaloids with 1,2-unsaturated necic parent substances in its makeup. Alkanna should not be taken internally for this reason and is recommended for external use only. Not to be used during pregnancy or nursing.

DOSAGE

Mode of Administration: Seldom used as a drug. Internal administration is not recommended, due to the drugs toxic characteristics and its uncertain efficacy. Alkannin and extracts of the root are used externally in pharmacy.

Preparations: Extractum alcannae: almost black, green glistening mass (no extraction information).

Histoplastin Red® Ointment: The ointment, approved in Greece, contains 76.5 gm loosely defined ethereal oily Alkanet root extract with lipophil ointment base (beeswax, mastic rubber and olive oil q.s. ad 100 gm).

Daily Dosage: Maximum 0.1 mcg pyrrolizidine alkaloids with 1.2 unsaturated necin framework and their N-oxides.

LITERATURE

Majlathova L, (1971) Nahrung 15:505.

Papageorgiou VP, (1980) *Planta Med* 38(3):193-203.

Papageorgiou VP, PM 31:390-394. 1977.

Papageorgiou VP, Digenis GA, *PM* 39:81-84. 1980.

Röder E, Pyrrolizidinhaltige Arzneipflanzen. In: *DAZ* 132(45):2427-2435. 1992.

Röder E, et al., PH 23:2125-2126. 1984.

Wiedenfield H et al., (1985) *Arch Pharm* 318(4):294.

Alkanna tinctoria

See Alkanet

Allium cepa

See Onion

Allium sativum

See Garlic

Allium schoenoprasum

See Chives

Allium ursinum

See Bear's Garlic

Almond

Prunus species

DESCRIPTION

Medicinal Parts: The medicinal part is the ripe fruit.

Flower and Fruit: The short-petioled flowers appear in pairs before the leaves. The petals are 19 to 20 mm long, pale pink to whitish with dark veins. The fruit is oblong-ovoid, compressed, 3.5 to 4.6 cm long by 2.5 to 3 cm wide, gray-green, velvet-downy, and pubescent. The nutshell is yellow, hard, compressed, broad- and sharp-edged, punctated externally with irregular grooves; inside it's smooth and glossy, either thick- or thin-skinned. The seed is cinnamon brown, flattened, and 2 cm long by 1.2 to 1.5 cm wide.

Leaves, Stem and Root: The plant is of medium height, seldom reaching 12 m. It is a tree or shrub with mildly red-tinged branches, thorny in its wild form but not in the cultivated form. The leaves have a 1.2 to 1.5 cm long, glandular petiole, and glabrous, oblong-lanceolate-acuminate or serrate, tough, glossy, dark green blades.

Habitat: The tree is indigenous to Western Asia and is extensively cultivated in many regions.

Production: Bitter almonds are the fruits of *Prunus dulcis* var. amara (also of *Prunus armeniaca*).

Sweet almonds are the fruits of *Prunus amygdalus* var. dulcis.

Other Names: Greek Nuts, Jordan Almond, Bitter Almond, and Sweet Almond

ACTIONS AND PHARMACOLOGY

COMPOUNDS: BITTER ALMONDS

Cyanogenic glycosides, amygdalin, 0.2 to 8.5% (corresponding to 12 to 500 mg prussic acid per 100 gm)

Fatty oil (non-dehydrating, 38 to 60%): chief fatty acids oleic acid (77%) and linoleic acid (17 to 20%)

Mucilages (3%): arabinogalactans

Proteic substances (25 to 35%)

EFFECTS: BITTER ALMONDS

There is no reliable information available.

COMPOUNDS: SWEET ALMONDS

Fatty oil (non-dehydrating, 43 to 57%): chief fatty acids oleic acid (77%) and linoleic acid (17 to 20%)

Mucilages (3 to 4%): arabinogalactans

Proteic substances (20 to 25%)

EFFECTS: SWEET ALMONDS

Sweet Almonds have a demulcent effect.

INDICATIONS AND USAGE

BITTER ALMONDS

Unproven Uses: Bitter Almonds were used in the past as a remedy for coughs, vomiting and nausea in the form of bitter almond water.

SWEET ALMONDS

Unproven Uses: Sweet Almonds are used topically in skin care and liniments.

PRECAUTIONS AND ADVERSE REACTIONS

BITTER ALMONDS

To be used only under the supervision of an expert qualified in the appropriate use of this substance.

SWEET ALMONDS

No health hazards or side effects are known in conjunction with the proper administration of designated therapeutic topical dosages.

OVERDOSAGE

BITTER ALMONDS

10 bitter almonds are said to be fatal for a child, 60 for an adult (a fatal dosage would presumably be already reached at a lower level, given disadvantageous conditions, e.g., higher cyanide level in the almonds, intensive chewing). Recommended antidotes include injection of solutions of dicobalt-EDTA or thiosulfates or the application of methemoglobin-forming substances, such as amyl nitrite. At the same time, vomiting should be induced or the stomach emptied.

Circulation support measures and/or artificial respiration may be required.

DOSAGE

BITTER ALMONDS

Mode of Administration: The drug is obsolete and no longer used.

SWEET ALMONDS

Mode of Administration: Sweet Almonds fatty oil is used as an ointment base and in the production of natural cosmetics.

LITERATURE

BITTER ALMONDS

Fincke H, Z *Untersuch Lebensm* 52:423. 1926.

Le Quesne PW et al., *JNP* 48:496. 1985.

Opdyke DLJ, (1976) *Food Cosmet Toxicol*: 14.

Salvo F et al., Riv Ital Sostanze Grasse 57:24. 1980.

Saura-Calixto F et al., Fette, Seifen, Anstrichm 87:4. 1985.

SWEET ALMONDS

Fincke H, *Z Untersuch Lebensm* 52:423. 1926.

Le Quesne PW et al., *JNP* 48:496. 1985.

Opdyke DLJ, (1976) *Food Cosmet Toxicol*: 14.

Rosenthaler L, *Ber Pharm Ges* 30:13. 1920.

Salvo F et al., Riv Ital Sostanze Grasse 57:24. 1980.

Saura-Calixto F et al., Fette, Seifen, Anstrichm 87:4. 1985.

Sommer W, Dissertation Albrechts-Universität Kiel. 1984.

Alnus glutinosa

See Black Alder

Aloe

Aloe barbadensis/capensis/vera

DESCRIPTION

Medicinal Parts: The medicinal part of the plant is dried juice of the leaves.

Flower and Fruit: The inflorescence is forked once or twice and is 60 to 90 cm high. The raceme is dense, cylindrical and narrows toward the top. The terminal raceme is up to 40 cm high while the lower ones are somewhat shorter. The bracts are almost white, and the flowers are yellow, orange or red, and are 3 cm long.

Leaves, Stem, and Root: The lilylike succulent-leafed rosette shrub has a 25-cm stem or none at all. The stem has about 25 leaves in an upright dense rosette. The lanceolate leaf is thick and fleshy, 40 to 50 cm long and 6 to 7 cm wide at the base. The upper surface is concave, gray-green, often with a reddish tinge, which sometimes appears in patches in the young plants. The leaf margin has a pale pink edge and 2 mm long pale teeth.

Habitat: Aloe is thought to have originated in the Sudan and the Arabian Peninsula. Today the species is cultivated and found in the wild in northern Africa, the Near East, Asia, and in the southern Mediterranean region. The plant is cultivated in subtropical regions of the United States and Mexico, and on the Dutch Antilles, as well as coastal regions of Venezuela.

Production: Curacao Aloe consists of the dried latex of the leaves of *Aloe barbadensis* (syn. Aloe vera), as well as its preparations. Aloe is harvested from August until October. The juice is dried using various methods.

Not to be Confused With: Agave americana, known as American Aloe, which is not a true Aloe.

ACTIONS AND PHARMACOLOGY

COMPOUNDS: ALOE BARBADENSIS

Anthracene derivatives: particularly anthrone-10-C-glycosyls, including aloin A, aloin B, 7-hydroxyaloins A and B, and 1,8-dihydroxy ions, including Aloe-emodin, and 6′cinnamic acid esters of these compounds

2-alkylchromones: including Aloe resins B, C and D

Flavonoids

COMPOUNDS: ALOE CAPENSIS

Anthracene derivatives: particularly anthrone-10-C-glycosyls, including aloin A, aloin B, 5-hydroxyaloin, and 1,8-dihydroxy anthraquinones, including Aloe-emodin, and mixed anthrone-C- and O-glycosides, including aloinosides A and B

2-alkylchromones: including Aloe resins A, B, C and D

Flavonoids

EFFECTS

Antibacterial/Antiviral Effects: Aloe-emodin exerts dose-dependent growth inhibition of *Heliobacter pylori* through inhibition of arylamine N-acetyltransferase (NAT) activity (Wang, 1998). Aloe-emodin has shown antibacterial effects on four strains of methicillin-resistant *Staphylococcus aureus* (Hatano, 1999). Aloe emodin inactivates enveloped viruses and is directly viracidal to *herpes simplex virus type 1* and *type 2, varicella-zoster virus, pseudorabies virus*, and *influenza virus* (Sydiskis, 1991).

Anti-inflammatory effects: The anti-inflammatory effect of the Aloe gel may be due to the salicylates, inactivation of bradykinin (via carboxypeptidases), and inhibition of histamine formation (Briggs, 1995; Natow, 1986). It appears that various nonspecified components in the gel reduce the oxidation of arachidonic acid, thereby reducing prostaglandin synthesis and inflammation (Davis et al, 1987; Pennys, 1982).

Antineoplastic Effects: Emodin suppresses tyrosine kinase activity of HER-2/neu-encoded p185neu receptor tyrosine kinase resulting in antineoplastic effects. This is beneficial in controlling HER-2/neu overexpressing cancer cells (Zhang, 1998).

Laxative (Cathartic) Effects: Anthraquinones such as Aloe are colonic-specific stimulant laxatives that have a direct action on intestinal mucosa, increasing the rate of colonic motility, enhancing colonic transit time, and inhibiting water and electrolyte secretion (Klinik et al, 1993; Godding, 1988). In addition, the laxative effect is due to irritation and stimulation of the colon. Other ingredients include Aloe-emodin, Aloesin, Aloetic acid, anthracene, anthranol, barbaloin, beta-or isobarbaloin, chrysophanic acid, cinnamic acid ester, emodin, an ethereal oil, resins (resistannol), and saponins (Shelton, 1991; Holdsworth, 1971; McCarthy & Haynes, 1967). There is some evidence that endogenous nitric oxide modulates the diarrhea effect of Aloe. Studies demonstrate a laxative effect 9 hours after ingestion (Izzo, 1999).

Anthraquinones may also have stool softening properties and do not disrupt the usual pattern of defecation (Gilman et al, 1990; Godding, 1988). The onset of action may be in 6 to 12 hours, or delayed for up to 24 hours (Koch, 1993; Cohen, 1992). Aloe vera latex, the pericyclic cells of the leaf produce a bitter yellow latex which is dried to give a dark brown solid material called ''ALOEs'' in many older pharmacy texts. This material is a strong cathartic containing various anthraquinones usually designated as aloin, which is primarily 1,8-dihyroxy-3-(hydroymethyl)-p,10-anthracenedione (Briggs, 1995).

A partial purification (via ethanolic and aqueous extracts) of Aloe vera leaves was strongly antibacterial and inhibited the growth of *Bacillus subtilis*. The action of the antibiotic substance was thought to be inhibition of nucleic acid synthesis and subsequent protein synthesis (Levin et al, 1988).

The sugar and polysaccharide content of the Aloe gel may be antibiotic via osmotic inhibition of bacterial growth. An antibacterial action is still under investigation and studies may find there is no effect (Briggs, 1995).

Effects of Topical Aloe Plants: Aloe vera depresses potential generation and conduction at neuromuscular junction processes, which result in analgesic and anti-inflammatory effects (Friedman, 1999). Ultraviolet radiation (UV) suppresses delayed type hypersensitivity (DTH) by altering the function of immune cells in the skin and causing the release of immunoregulatory cytokines. Extracts of crude *Aloe barbadensis* gel inhibits this photosuppression by preventing suppression of DTH responses and reducing the amount of keratinocyte derived immunosuppressive cytokines (IL-2) (Byeon, 1998; Strickland, 1999). Aloe vera gel contains small molecular modulators that prevent UVB-induced immune suppression in the skin. The immunomodulators restore the UVB-induced damages on epidermal Langerham cells (Lee, 1999).

Aloe vera increases collagen content of the granulation tissue and its degree of crosslinking to contribute to wound healing (Chithra, 1998). Aloe vera acts as a modulatory system toward wounds with anti-inflammatory effects (Davis, 1991). The use of Aloe vera has been associated with a delay in wound healing compared to standard treatment (Schmidt, 1991). Aloe vera gel exerts anti-inflammatory activity through its inhibitory action on the arachidonic acid pathway via cyclooxygenase (Vazquez, 1996). Due to its anti-thromboxane effects, Aloe vera decreases the morbidity of progressive dermal ischemia in frostbite (Heggers, 1987). Aloe vera contains a carboxypeptidase that inactivates bradykinin, salicylates, and a substance that inhibits thromboxane formation (Fujita, 1976; Klein, 1988).

The exact mechanism for the wound healing abilities of Aloe is uncertain, but probably involves an anti-inflammatory effect involving consumption of complement 3, depletion of classical and alternative pathway complement activity, inhibition of free oxygen radicals by activating polymorphonuclear leucocytes, thromboxane inhibition, and bradykinin inhibition (Hart et al, 1989; Hart et al, 1988; Zachary et al, 1987)

CLINICAL TRIALS

Acne

A study involving Aloe vera preparations for acne was discussed in a larger review considering the empirical evidence for complementary and alternative treatments (topical and oral) for acne. While Aloe vera gel alone was only minimally effective in anti-acne activity, in one randomized controlled trial cited (n=84), its combination with Ocimum oil appeared to be synergistic—even more effective than the application of a standard acne prescription formula of 1% clindamycin. The study showed that the effectiveness of various concentrations of Aloe vera gel with and without *Ocimum gratissimum* oil (topical) were significantly better than placebo in reducing the number of acne lesions (Magin, 2006).

Constipation

A preparation containing celandin, Aloe vera, and psyllium produced more frequent bowel movements, softer stools, and less laxative dependence than controls in a double-blind, randomized, placebo-controlled study of 35 patients with chronic constipation. Symptoms during the last 2 weeks of this 28-day trial were compared with baseline figures obtained during the 2 weeks prior to the study initiation. Abdominal pain was not reduced in either group. A capsule of the preparation was given each day at the beginning of the study and, depending on response, was increased to 3 capsules during the study in some participants. Each capsule was 500 mg and consisted of celandin, Aloe vera, and psyllium in a 6:3:1 ratio. The part of the Aloe plant used was not mentioned. The preparations were not evaluated separately, only as the mixture. (Odes & Madar, 1991).

Herpes Simplex

Aloe vera whole leaf extract (0.5%) in hydrophilic cream (4.8 days) showed a statistically shorter mean duration of healing sores of genital herpes compared to Aloe vera gel (7 days) or placebo (14 days). The percentage of healed patients increased in the Aloe group as well (70%, 45%, and 7.5%, respectively). There were 120 male circumcised patients with their first episode of genital herpes and no previous history of herpes generalis. The subjects had a total of 1,496 lesions (mean of 12.5) that were present for less than 7 days (mean 4.3 days). Patients (n=120) were divided into three groups, one treated with the Aloe-containing cream, one with Aloe gel, the other a placebo cream. Application was 3 times a day with a protected finger, for 5 consecutive days per week for 2 weeks. Aloe vera extract and gel were both effective in reducing healing and duration of lesions, but Aloe vera in the cream form was statistically better in reducing mean lesion duration and healing compared to either the gel or the placebo. There were no significant side effects (Syed et al, 1996).

Aloe vera whole leaf extract (0.55) was found to be effective in treating first lesions of herpes simplex in 60 men with culture-confirmed herpes simplex genitalis who had lesions within 7 days of initial outbreak. The total number of lesions in the group was 738 (mean 12.3). Patients were randomly assigned to a placebo group and the same cream with aloe added. The cream was self-applied three times daily for 5 consecutive days for 3 weeks. Patients were examined twice weekly, and reepithelialized lesions with some residual erythema were considered "cured." The Aloe extract group had a significantly shorter mean time to healing than placebo (4.9 days as compared to 12 days) ($p<0.001$). There was also a 66.7% rate of healed patients in the aloe group, while only a 6.7% rate in the placebo group ($p<0.001$). There were 5 cases of mild itching that resolved in the first 24 hours; this did not result in patient withdrawal. "Cured" patients were followed for 20 months, and at the end of this time there was a 13% recurrence rate (Syed et al, 1997).

Irritable Bowel Syndrome

Fifty-eight patients with irritable bowel syndrome (IBS) were randomized to receive Aloe vera or a placebo during a 3-month period. Symptoms were assessed at baseline, 1 and 3 months. No evidence was found that Aloe vera benefits patients with IBS (Davis et al, 2006).

Psoriasis

Forty-one patients with stable plaque psoriasis took part in a randomized, double-blind, placebo-controlled right/left comparison study to test the effect of a commercial, preserved but otherwise untreated, Aloe vera gel. A 2-week wash-out period was followed by a 4-week treatment period with 2 daily applications and follow-up visits after 1 and 2 months. The score sum of erythema, infiltration, and desquamation decreased in 72.5% of Aloe vera-treated sites compared with 82% of placebo-treated areas from week 0 to week 4. The results indicate that the effect of the commercial Aloe vera gel on stable plaque psoriasis was modest and not better than placebo (Paulsen et al, 2005).

An earlier study shows, however, that Aloe vera (0.5%) whole leaf extract effectively ($p<0.001$) cured or reduced the signs of psoriasis in a double-blind, placebo-controlled study. Sixty patients with slight to moderate chronic plaque-type psoriasis were randomized into 2 groups, 1 using a placebo cream, the other using the cream with Aloe vera extract (with mineral oil and castor oil to solubilize the Aloe). The mean Psoriasis Area and Severity Index (PASI) score before treatment was 9.3 (range 4.8 to 16.7). Patients applied the creams topically, without occlusion or exposure to sunlight, to affected areas 3 times a day for 5 consecutive days per week for 4 weeks. Patients were examined weekly, for up to 16 weeks, for reduction of lesions, desquamation, decreased erythema, infiltration, and lowered PASI scores. Results showed that 83.3% of the patients had reduced or no psoriasis signs with Aloe, while only 6.6% of controls had a positive effect. Plaque was reduced by 82.8% for the Aloe group and only 7.7% for the control group ($p<0.001$). The PASI score in the treated group dropped to a mean of 2.2 (Syed et al, 1996).

Radiation-Induced Skin Toxicity

A phase III, double-blind, placebo-controlled study evaluated Aloe vera gel for use as a prophylactic agent for radiation-induced skin toxicity. A total of 194 women receiving breast or chest-wall irradiation were included in the study. Skin dermatitis was scored weekly during the trial by patients and by healthcare providers. Aloe vera gel did not protect against radiation therapy-induced dermatitis (Williams, 1996).

A double-blind, placebo-controlled study with 108 breast cancer patients that were treated with a minimum 50cGy radiation dose to the breast or chest wall were evaluated for dermatitis scores following the use of topical Aloe vera. Patients were stratified based on age, breast surgery, planned target radiation dose, and skin complexion, then randomized to a control group of no treatment or an Aloe vera treated (98% Aloe) group. The medications were applied to the treatment field twice daily starting within 3 days of radiation initiation. If radiation-induced dermatitis occurred, patients were instructed to apply a 1% hydrocortisone cream at least one hour either side of the Aloe or placebo application. The chest-wall skin was evaluated weekly by a physician or nurse, and the patients graded the skin reaction weekly via a questionnaire. Measures used to assess treatment efficacy included maximum reported severity of dermatitis, time to occurrence of severe (Grade 3 or greater) dermatitis, and duration of severe dermatitis. Treatment continued through the radiation therapy. The study reported no difference between the Aloe vera group and the group treated with placebo with respect to any of the assessments measured. (Williams et al, 1996).

In a literature review of novel approaches to radiotherapy-induced skin reactions, the authors cite research by the previous study author (Williams, 1996) and others, including data from a follow-up trial. In the study reviewed, the effects of Aloe vera gel plus mild soap versus mild soap alone as a means of preventing radiotherapy-induced dermatitis were assessed in a randomized controlled trial of 70 patients. The Aloe vera gel also included urea, vitamin E, preservatives, and a filler. Skin condition was evaluated weekly. There were no adverse effects from the use of Aloe vera gel, and its application was successful in preventing radio-dermatitis in some cases, particularly in patients who received relatively higher radiotherapy doses; the reaction was less severe and skin changes took longer to develop (Maddocks-Jennings, 2005).

In contrast, the authors of a systematic review and critical appraisal of evidence (including a previous systematic review, five randomized controlled trials, and two non-published randomized controlled trials) for the effectiveness of Aloe vera gel for radiation-induced skin reactions concluded that there is no evidence to indicate that topical Aloe vera preparations are effective in preventing or lessening these lesions (Richardson 2005).

No statistically significant difference was detected between treatment with Aloe vera and placebo for mild or moderate/severe mouth ulcers (mucositis) caused by radiation or chemotherapy for cancer in 58 subjects enrolled in a trial. The Aloe vera trial had been identified by authors of a larger review of interventions for preventing this common complication in people undergoing cancer treatment (Worthington 2007).

Radiotherapy Adjunct

A phase II, double-blind, prospective, randomized, placebo-controlled trial determined that Aloe vera gel was not a beneficial adjunct to head-and-neck radiotherapy. Patients (n=58) received biweekly examinations. At the end of treatment, it was shown that subjects taking Aloe vera had identical scores to those on placebo with regard to maximal grade of toxicity, duration of Grade 2 or worse mucositis, quality-of-life scores, percentage of weight loss, use of pain medications, hydration requirement, oral infections, and prolonged radiation breaks (Su et al, 2004).

Ulcerative Colitis

To investigate the efficacy and safety of Aloe vera gel for the treatment of mildly to moderately active ulcerative colitis, a double-blind, randomized, placebo-controlled trial was performed. Subjects (n=44) were given Aloe vera gel or placebo, 100 mL twice daily for 4 weeks, in a 2:1 ratio. Primary outcome measures were clinical remission, sigmoidoscopic remission, and histological remission. The results indicate that Aloe vera produced a clinical response more often than placebo, safely reducing the histological disease activity (Langmead et al, 2004).

Ulcers, Leg

Aloe vera gel was effective in healing long-term leg ulcers that other therapies had not been able to heal. Aloe vera gel was prepared from the fresh leaves and was applied locally (via an Aloe soaked gauze) to leg ulcers 3 to 5 times daily as a dressing after the wound had been cleansed with boric acid, hydrogen peroxide, and citrimide 1% solution (El Zawahry et al, 1973). There were no control ulcers, nor means of addressing the effect of Aloe separate from that of the wound cleansings.

Ulcers, Pressure

A review of wound cleansing options for care of pressure ulcers overall identified very little rigorous research (randomized and controlled trials). One study of reasonable quality included Aloe vera, however. The study of 126 subjects followed for 14 days showed statistically significant improvement in Pressure Sore Status tool scores (percentage reduction in pressure sore status) for wounds cleansed with a saline spray combination of Aloe vera, silver chloride, and decyl glucoside (Vulnopur), compared to wounds cleansed with isotonic saline (p=0.025) (Moore, 2007).

UV Light Damage

UVB light exposure was given to 12 volunteers for 1.5 minutes using an UVB light pen (250 to 450 nanometers light spectrum). Patients between 21 and 54 years of age had no peripheral vascular disease. Four sites (two on each arm) were irradiated, two sites on one arm and a nonirradiated control site were given topical aloe gel (directly from the plant leaf) application each hour. Measurement of blood flow were taken at these sites at 6 and 24 hours. Erythema was evaluated as either greater to, equal to, or less than that in the control area. There was no significant difference in blood flow between control sites and aloe gel treated sites exposed to ultraviolet light. This was true at 6 and 24 hours post-exposure. There was no qualitative difference in erythema. (Crowell et al, 1989).

Treatment of a dermabrasion with an Aloe gel resulted in accelerated healing by about 72 hours in one study (Fulton, 1990). Eighteen full-faced dermabrasions were performed and one-half of each face treated with the standard polyethylene oxide dressing (PEOD), the other side with the dressing saturated with Aloe vera gel. Within 24 to 48 hours the Aloe side showed considerable vasoconstriction and reduction in edema. By the third to fourth day the Aloe side had less crusting and exudate, and by the fifth and sixth day reepithelialization was almost complete (90%), while the PEOD site was only 40% to 50% complete. There was a slight stinging or burning sensation when the Aloe dressing was applied, but overall, there was less pain and throbbing.

Vitamin Absorption

Aloe vera preparations increased the absorption of vitamins C (water-soluble) and E (fat-soluble) in a randomized placebo-controlled double-blind crossover study involving 11 healthy individuals ranging in age from age 21 to 42. None were taking vitamin supplements. Both aloe preparations—a whole-leaf extract and an inner fillet gel—slowed the absorption and increased the duration of the vitamins in the subjects' plasma, with maximum concentrations 2 to 4 hours later than occurred in the control group. The Aloe gel extract was particularly effective in these regard to vitamin C (ascorbate) absorption after 8 and 24 hours (Vinson, 2005).

Wound Healing

Twenty-seven patients with a recent partial thickness burn injury and an individual confluent area of more than 2%, and no previous treatment, were treated with Aloe gel/gauze and found to have an improved healing rate versus controls that received petroleum jelly/gauze dressings. Cleaned wounds were divided into two parts, the first treated with either a transparent Aloe vera gel (85% Aloe gel with another unnamed ingredients), the second part with petroleum jelly. The materials were applied twice daily, topically, with a sterile glove. Wounds were inspected and photographed on day 1, 7, 14, 21, or until complete epithelialization. By the 14th day, most of the Aloe gel treated burn areas were completely healed. The mean healing time for the Aloe gel group was 11.89 days, the time for the petroleum jelly group was 18.18 days (p<0.002). Histology of the wounds via biopsy was done on days 1, 7, 14, and 21. On day 7 the ulcerated part of both treatment areas were covered with necrotic tissue debris and red blood cells, the petroleum jelly-treated sites also had an acute inflammatory exudate intermixed with necrotic tissue. Papillary and reticular dermis was infiltrated by acute and chronic inflammatory cells. Aloe-treated areas had full epithelialization developed by 14 days with newly formed squamous epithelium. On day 14, the petroleum jelly gauze areas had partially developed epithelialization at the wound edges (Visuthikosol et al, 1995).

Aloe vera gel produced a retardation in healing using a standard wound care protocol, with and without Aloe vera gel, in 21 women who had wound complications requiring additional healing after Cesarean delivery or laparotomy. Wounds treated with the standard protocol alone healed in 53 days (standard deviation of 24 days), while those treated with Aloe vera required 83 days (standard deviation of 28 days) (p=0.003). Patients were randomly assigned, and any with diabetes, cancer, or treatments requiring corticosteroids were excluded from the study. Incisions included in the study had opened spontaneously or had been drained to treat seroma, hematoma, or wound abscesses. The Aloe gel used was a commercial product (Carrington Dermal Wound Gel) and it was applied with a gloved finger, at each dressing change, to the granulation tissue in the wound bed at the level of the subcutaneous tissue and dermis (Schimidt & Greenspoon, 1991). The study was not performed on the original, non-complicated incisions, just on incisional cases with complications.

INDICATIONS AND USAGE

ALOE BARBADENSIS AND CAPENSIS

Approved by Commission E:

- Constipation

ALOE BARBADENSIS

Unproven Uses: The drug is used for evacuation relief in the presence of anal fissures after recto-anal operations. In European folk medicine the drug is employed for its ability to influence digestion.

Chinese Medicine: The most common use in Chinese medicine is for treatment of fungal diseases.

Indian Medicine: Uses in Indian medicine include stomach tumors, constipation, colic, skin diseases, amenorrhea, worm infestation, and infections.

ALOE CAPENSIS

Unproven Uses: Aloe capensis has been used as a stool softener in the presence of anal fissures, hemorrhoids, and after recto-anal operations. The fresh juice is used for eye inflammations and for syphillis in South Africa.

Homeopathic Uses: The herb is used for gastrointestinal disorders, hemorrhoids, and constipation.

CONTRAINDICATIONS

Aloe is contraindicated in cases of intestinal obstruction, acutely inflamed intestinal diseases (eg, Crohn's disease, ulcerative colitis), ileus of any kind (acute surgical abdomen, bowel obstruction, fecal impaction), appendicitis, and abdominal pain of unknown origin.

Pregnancy: Not to be used during pregnancy.

Breastfeeding: Not to be used while breastfeeding.

Pediatrics: Not to be given to children under 12 years of age.

PRECAUTIONS AND ADVERSE REACTIONS

Spasmodic gastrointestinal complaints are a side effect to the drug's purgative effect. Arrhythmias, nephropathies, edema, and accelerated bone deterioration may occur in rare cases. Prolonged use of Aloe may lead to pigmentation in the intestinal mucosa *(pseudomelanosis coli)*, a side effect that usually reverses upon discontinuation of the drug. Long-term use can also lead to albuminuria and hematuria. Hypersensitivity, manifested by generalized nummular eczematous and papular dermatitis, has been reported after long-term use of oral and topical Aloe preparations. Contact dermatitis to Aloe gel may be due to irritation of the skin by needlelike crystals. Use of the latex containing anthraquinones may result in absorption of these chemicals resulting in a brown discoloration of body fluids.

Effects on Plasma Electrolytes: Prolonged use of excessive laxative doses may lead to significant loss of electrolytes, in particular potassium, and electrolyte/fluid imbalance may occur. Potassium loss is partly due to direct loss in the feces and partly as secondary renal effect associated with sodium loss (Westendorff, 1993). Patients taking Aloe for more than 1-2 weeks may experience hypokalemia (signs and symptoms include lethargy, muscle cramps, headaches, paresthesias, tetany, peripheral edema, polyuria, breathlessness, and hypertension). The loss of potassium can result in hyperaldosteronism, inhibition of intestinal motility and enhancement of the effect of cardioactive medications. Prolonged use should be avoided (Bisset, 1994).

Gastrointestinal: Abdominal pain, excessive bowel activities, such as diarrhea, nausea, and perianal irritation are the primary adverse effects with anthraquinone laxatives such as Aloe (Bisset, 1994). Long-term laxative use may also include bloody diarrhea and, in toxic doses, possible kidney damage. Hemorrhoids may be exacerbated by taking the latex laxative orally (Briggs, 1995).

Malignancy: Prolonged use of anthracene drugs increases the relative risk of colon carcinoma (Siegers, 1993). Recent studies failed to demonstrate a connection between the administration of anthracene drugs and frequency of carcinomas in the colon (Schorkhuber, 1998). Low molecular weight compounds found in Aloe vera gel are cytotoxic (Avila, 1997). The component 1,8-dihydroxyanthraquinone inhibits the catalytic activity of topoisomerase II resulting in genotoxicity and mutagenicity (Mueller, 1999).

Tissue Damage: Chronic treatment with high doses of Aloe reduces vasoactive intestinal peptide and somatostatin levels, which may damage enteric nervous tissue (Tzavella, 1995).

Teratogenicity: Aloe latex contains anthraquinones that may stimulate uterine muscle activity, initiate premature labor, or possibly cause abortion when given orally. Mutagenic activity to lectins that are found in Aloe have been noted (Suzuki et al, 1979). A lectin found in whole Aloe arborescens leaves was shown to have mitogenic activity on lymphocytes (Suzuki et al, 1979).

DRUG INTERACTIONS

MODERATE RISK

Antidiabetic Agents: Increased risk of hypoglycemia. *Clinical Management:* Monitor blood glucose levels and signs and symptoms of hypoglycemia closely if Aloe and an antidiabetic agent are taken together.

Digoxin: Concurrent use may result in hypokalemia resulting in digoxin toxicity. *Clinical Management*: Patients who are taking digoxin should be advised to avoid concomitant use with Aloe. If digoxin toxicity occurs, potassium should be monitored and supplemented if necessary while discontinuing Aloe.

DOSAGE

Mode of Administration: Due to the side effects of the drug, it is rarely used internally and is not recommended. Aloe powder, aqueous- and aqueous-alcoholic extracts in powdered or liquid form are available for oral use.

How Supplied:

Capsules–250 mg, 470 mg

Cream

Gel–99%, 72%

Softgel–1000 mg

Preparation: A stabilized Aloe extract is prepared with hot water. The extract will have a content of 19% to 21% aloin.

Daily Dosage: The recommended daily dosage is 20 to 30 mg hydroxyanthracene derivatives/day, calculated as anhydrous aloin. The recommended single dosage is 0.05 g Aloe powder from Aloe barbadensis or 0.05 to 0.2 g Aloe powder of Aloe capensis in the evening. Aloe capensis can be given as a single dose of 0.1 g in the evening.

Homeopathic Dosage: For *Aloe capensis*, administer 5 drops, 1 tablet, 10 globules, or parenterally 1 to 2 mL three times daily (HAB1).

Note: The smallest dosage needed to maintain a soft stool should be used. Stimulating laxatives must not be used over an extended period of time (1 to 2 weeks) without medical advice.

Storage: Aloe should be protected from light and moisture.

LITERATURE

Anonym, Aloe und Aloine - Aktuelles über weltweit verwendete Arzneistoffe. In: *DAZ* 135(39):3644-3645. 1995

Avila H, Rivero J, Herrera F, Fraile G. Cytotoxicity of a low molecular weight fraction from Aloe vera *(Aloe barbadensis Miller)* gel. *Toxicon* Sep;35(9):1423-30. 1997

Blitz JJ, Smith JW & Gerard JR. Aloe vera gel in peptic ulcer therapy: preliminary report. *JAOAO*; 62:731-735. 1963

Briggs C. Herbal medicine: Aloe. *CPJ/RPC*; 128:48-50. 1995

Byeon SW, Pelley RP, Ullrich SE et al., *Aloe barbadensis* extracts reduce the production of interleukin-10 after exposure to ultraviolet radiation. *J Invest Dermatol* May;110(5):811-7. 1998

Cera LM, Heggers JP, Robson MC et al. The therapeutic efficacy of Aloe vera cream (Dermaide Aloe) in thermal injuries: two case reports. *J Am Anim Hosp Assoc*; 16:768-772. 1980

Che QM, Akao T, Hattori M, Kobashi K, Namba T, Metabolism of barbaloin by intestinal bacteria. 2. Isolation of human intestinal bacterium capable of tranforming barbaloin to Aloe-emodin anthrone. In: *PM* 57:15. 1991

Chithra P, Sajithlal GB, Chandrakasan G, Influence of Aloe vera on collagen turnover in healing of dermal wounds in rats. *Indian J Exp Biol* Sep;36(9):896-901. 1998

Cohen KB. Laxative update: concepts in patient care. *Am Druggist*; April:73-84. 1992

Crowell J, Hilsenbeck S & Penneys N. Aloe vera does not affect cutaneous erythema and blood flow following ultraviolet B exposure. *Photodermatology*; 6(5)237-239. 1989

Davis K, Philpott S, Kumar D, et al. Randomised double-blind placebo-controlled trial of aloe vera for irritable bowel syndrome. *Int J Clin Pract*; 60(9): 1080-1086. 2006.

Davis RH, Kabbani JM & Maro NP. Aloe vera and wound healing. *J Am Podiatr Med Assoc*; 77(4): 165-169. 1987

Davis RH, Parker WL, Samson RT, Murdoch DP, Isolation of a stimulatory system in an Aloe extract. *J Am Podiatr Med Assoc* 1991 Sep; 81(9): 473-8.

el-Zawahry M, Hegazy MR & Helal M. Use of Aloe in treating leg ulcers and dermatoses. *Int J Dermatol;* 12:69-73. 1973

Frumkin A. Aloe vera, salicyclic acid, and aspirin for burns (letter). *Plastic Reconstr Surg;* 83(1): 196. 1989

Fujita K, Ito S, Teradaira R, Beppu H, Properties of a carboxypeptidase from Aloe. *Biochem Pharmacol* Apr 1; 28(7). 1261. 1979

Fulton JE Jr. The stimulation of postdermabrasion wound healing with stabilized Aloe vera gel-polyethylene oxide dressing. J Dermatol Surg Oncol; 16(5): 460-467. 1990

Godding EW. Laxatives and the special role of senna. *Pharmacology*; 36(suppl 1):230-236. 1988

Gossel TA. Constipation? A treatment guide. *US Pharmacist*; June:30-34. 1991

Hatano T, Uebayashi H, Ito H et al., Phenolic constituents of Cassia seeds and antibacterial effect of some naphthalenes and anthraquinones on methicillin-resistant Staphylococcus aureus. *Chem Pharm Bull* (Tokyo) Aug;47(8):1121-7. 1999

Heggers JP, Robson MC, Manavalen K et al., Experimental and clinical observations on frostbite. *Ann Emerg Med* Sep;16(9):1056-62. 1987

Heggers JP, Elzaim H, Garfield R et al. Effect of the combination of Aloe vera, nitroglycerin, and L-NAME on wound healing in the rat excisional model. *J Altern Complement Med*; 3(2):149-153. 1997

Heggers JP, Kuchukcelebi A, Stabenau J et al. Wound healing effects of Aloe gel and other topical antibacterial agents on rat skin. *Phytother Res*; 9:455-457. 1995

Heggers JP, Kucukcelebi A, Listengarten D et al. Beneficial effects of aloe on wound healing in an excisional model. *J Altern Complement Med*; 2(2):271-277. 1996

Hirata T & Suga T. Biologically active constituents of leaves and roots of Aloe arborescens var natalensis. *Z Naturforsch* (C); 32(9-10):731-734. 1977

Holdsworth DK. Chromones in Aloe species, part 1: aloesin- C-glucosyl-7-hydroxychrome. Planta Med 1971; 19(4):322-325.

Hunter D & Frumkin A. Adverse reactions to vitamin E and Aloe vera preparations after dermabrasion and chemical peel. *Cutis*; 47(3):193-196. 1991

Hutter JA et al., Anti-inflammatory C-glucosyl chromone from *Aloe barbadensis*. In: *JNP* 59(5):541-543. 1996.

Izzo AA, Sautebin L, Borrelli F et al., The role of nitric oxide in aloe-induced diarrhoea in the rat. *Eur J Pharmacol* Feb 26;368(1):43-8. 1999

Klein AD, Penneys NS, Aloe vera. *J Am Acad Dermatol* Apr;18(4 Pt 1):714-20. 1988

Kloch A. Investigations on the laxative action of aloin in the human colon. *Planta Med*; 59(suppl):A689. 1993

Koch A, Investigations on the laxative action of aloin in the human colon. In: *PM* 59(7):A689. 1993

Koch A, Metabolisierung von Aloin. Korrelation zwischen In-vitro- und in-vivo-Versuchen. In: *DAZ* 135(13):1150-1152. 1995.

Langmead L. Feakins RM, Goldthorpe S, et al. Randomized, double-blind, placebo-controlled trial of the aloe vera gel for active ulcerative colitis. *Alimen Pharmacol Ther*; 19(7) 739-747. 2004.

Lee CK, Han SS, Shin YK et al., Prevention of ultraviolet radiation-induced suppression of contact hypersensitivity by Aloe vera gel components. *Int J Immunopharmacol* May;21(5):303-10. 1999

Lepik K. Safety of herbal medications in pregnancy. *Can Pharm J*; 130:29-33. 1997

Levin H, Hazenfratz R, Friedman J et al. Partial purification and some properties of an antibacterial compound from Aloe vera. Phytother Res; 2:67-69. 1988

Maddocks -Jennings W, Wilkinson JM, Shillington D. Novel approaches to radiotherapy-induced skin reactions: a literature review. *Comp Ther Clin Prac;* 11:224-231. 2005

Magin PJ, et al. Topical and oral CAM in acne: A review of the empirical evidence and a consideration of its context. *Comp Ther Med;* 14(1):62, 76. 2006

Magin PJ, et al. Complementary and alternative medicine therapies in acne, psoriasis, and atopic eczema: Results of a qualitative study of patients' experiences and perceptions. *J Alt Comp Med*; 12(5): 451, 457. 2006

McCauley RL, Heggers JP & Robson MC. Frostbite: methods to minimize tissue loss. *Postgrad Med;* 88(8):67-68,73-77. 1990

McCarthy TJ & Haynes LJ. The distribution of Aloesin in some South African Aloe species. *Planta Med*; 15(3):342-344. 1967

Moore ZEH, Cowman S. Wound cleansing for pressure ulcers. *Cochrane Database Syst Rev 4*: CD004983; 2005.

Morrow D, Rapaport M, Strick R. Hypersensitivity to aloe. *Arch Dermatol* Sep;116(9):1064-1065. 1980

Mueller S, Stopper H. Characterization of the genotoxicity of anthraquinones in mammalian cells. *Biochim Biophys Acta* Aug 5;1428(2-3):406-414. 1999

Muller-Lissner SA. Adverse effects of laxatives: facts and fiction. *Pathophysiology*; 47(suppl 1):138-145. 1993

Nath D, Sethi N, Singh RK et al. Commonly used Indian abortifacient plants with special reference to their teratological effects in rats. *J Ethnopharmacol*; 36(2):147-154. 1992

Natow AJ. Aloe vera, fiction or fact? *Cutis*; 37(2):106-108. 1986

Odes HS & Madar Z. A double-blind trial of a celandin, Aloe vera and psyllium laxative preparation in adult patients with constipation. *Digestion*; 49(2):65-71. 1991

Park MK et al., Neoaloesin A. A new C-glucofuranosyl chromone from *Aloe barbadensis*. In: *PM* 62(4):363-365. 1996.

Parry O & Wenyika J. The uterine relaxant effect of *Aloe chabaudii*. *Fitoterapia*; 65:253-259. 1994

Paulsen E, Korsholm L, Brandrup F. A double-blind, placebo-controlled study of a commercial Aloe vera gel in the treatment of slight to moderate psoriasis vulgaris. J Eur Dermatol Venereol; 19(3):326-331. 2005.

Penneys NS. Inhibition of arachidonic acid oxidation in vitro by vehicle components. *Acta Derm Vernereol* (Stockh); 62(1):59-61. 1982

Richardson J, et al. Aloe vera for preventing radiation-induced skin reactions: a systematic literature review. *Clin Oncol* 17(6):478-84. 2005.

Robson MC, DelBeccaro EJ & Heggers JP. Increasing dermal perfusion after burning by decreasing thromboxane production. *J Trauma*; 20(9):722-725. 1980

Schmidt JM, Greenspoon JS, Aloe vera dermal wound gel is associated with a delay in wound healing. *Obstet Gynecol* Jul;78(1):115-7. 1991

Shapiro W & Taubert K. Hypokalaemia and digoxin-induced arrhythmias. *Lancet*; 2:604-605. 1975

Shelton RM. Aloe vera: its chemical and therapeutic properties. *Int J Dermatol*; 30(10):679-683. 1991

Sigers C, von Hertzberg-Lottin E, Otte M, Schneider B. Anthranoid laxative abuse–a risk for colorectal cancer? *Gut* Aug;34(8):1099-101. 1993

Schorkhuber M, Richter M, Dutter A, et al. Effect of anthraquinone-laxatives on the proliferation and urokinase secretion of normal, premalignant and malignant colonic epithelial cells. *Eur J Cancer* Jun;34(7):1091-8. 1998

Strickland FM, Darvill A, Albersheim P et al., Inhibition of UV-induced immune suppression and interleukin-10 production by plant oligosaccharides and polysaccharides. *Photochem Photobiol* Feb;69(2):141-7. 1999

Su CK, Mehta V, Ravikumar L, et al. Phase II double-blind, randomized study comparing oral aloe vera versus placebo to prevent radiation-related mucositis in patients with head-and-neck neoplasms. *Int J Radiat Oncol Biol Phys*; 60 (1): 171-177. 2004.

Suzuki I, Saito H, Inoue S et al. Purification and characterization of two lectins from Aloe arborescens Mill. J Biochem (Tokyo) 1979; 85(1):163-171.

Sydiskis RJ, Owen DG, Lohr JL et al., Inactivation of enveloped viruses by anthraquinones extracted from plants. *Antimicrob Agents Chemother* 1991 Dec;35(12):2463-6.

Syed TA, Ahmad SA, Holt AH et al., Management of psoriasis with Aloe vera extract in a hydrophilic cream: a placebo-controlled, double-blind study. *Trop Med Int Health* 1996 Aug;1(4):505-9.

Syed TA, Afzal M, Ashfaq Ahmad S et al. Management of genital herpes in men with 0.5% Aloe vera extract in a hydrophilic cream:

a placebo-controlled double blind study. J Dermatol Treat; 8:99-102. 1997

't Hart LA, Nibbering PH, van den Barselaar MT et al. Effects of low molecular constituents from Aloe vera gel on oxidative metabolism and cytotoxic and bactericidal activities of human neutrophils. *Int J Immunopharmacol*; 12(4):427-434. 1990

't Hart LA, van den Berg AJJ, Kuis L et al. An anti-complementary polysaccharide with immunological adjuvant activity from the leaf parenchyma gel of Aloe vera. *Planta Med*; 55(6):509-512. 1989

't Hart LA, van Enckevort PH, van Dijk H et al. Two functionally and chemically distinct immunomodulatory compounds in the gel of Aloe vera. *J Ethnopharmacol*; 23(1):61-71. 1988

Tzavella K, Riepl RL, Klauser AG et al., Decreased substance P levels in rectal biopsies from patients with slow transit constipation. *Eur J Gastroenterol Hepatol* 1996 Dec;8(12):1207-1211.

Tzeng SH, Ko WC, Ko FN, Teng CM, Inhibition of platelet aggregation by some flavonoids. In: *Thromobosis Res* 64:91. 1991.

Vazquez B, Avila G, Segura D, Escalante B, Anti-inflammatory activity of extracts from Aloe vera gel. *J Ethnopharmacol* Dec;55(1):69-75. 1996

Vinson JA, Kharrat H, Andreoli L. Effect of Aloe vera preparations on the human bioavailability of vitamins C and E. *Phytomedicine* 12(10):760, 765. 2005.

Visuthikosol V, Chowchuen B, Sukwanarat Y et al. Effect of Aloe vera gel to healing of burn wound - a clinical and histologic study. *J Med Assoc Thai*; 78(8):403-408. 1995

Wang HH, Chung JG, Ho CC, Wu LT, Chang SH. Aloe-emodin effects on arylamine N-acetyltransferase activity in the bacterium *Helicobacter pylori. Planta Med* Mar;64(2):176-178. 1998

Williams MS, Burk M, Loprinzi CL et al., Phase III double-blind evaluation of an aloe vera gel as a prophylactic agent for radiation-induced skin toxicity. *J Radiat Oncol Biol Phys* Sep 1;36(2):345-9. 1996

Worthington HV, Clarkson JE, Eden OB. Interventions for preventing oral mucositis for patients with cancer receiving treatment. *Cochrane Database Syst Rev* 2:CD000978. 2006.

Yagi A, Shida T & Nishimura H. Effect of amino acids in Aloe extract on phagocytosis by peripheral neutrophil in adult bronchial asthma. *Arerugi*; 36(12):1094-1101. 1987

Yamaguchi I, Mega N & Sanada H. Components of the gel of Aloe vera (L.) burm-f. *Biosci Biotechnol Biochem;* 57(8):1350-1352. 1993

Yarnell, E, Abascal K. Herbs for treating herpes simplex infections. *Alt Comp Ther;* 11(2):83, 88. 2005.

Yoig A, Egusa T, Arase M, Tanabe M, Tsujitt, Isolation and characterization of the glycoprotein fraction with proliferation-promotory activity on human and hamster cells in vitro. In: *PM* 63:18-21. 1997.

Zachary LS, Smith DJ Jr, Heggers JP et al. The role of thromboxane in experimental inadvertent intra-arterial drug injections. *J Hand Surg* (Am); 12(2):240-245. 1987

Zhang L, Tizard IR, Activation of a mouse macrophage cell line by acemannan: the major carbohydrate fraction from Aloe vera gel. *Immunopharmacology* Nov;35(2):119-28. 1996

Aloysia triphylla

See Lemon Verbena

Alpine Cranberry

Vaccinium vitis-ideae

DESCRIPTION

Medicinal Parts: The medicinal parts are the dried leaves and the ripe dried fruit.

Flower and Fruit: The white to reddish-tinged flowers are in clusters of various sizes. The 10 stamens are pubescent at the base and the anthers are two-tipped and have no appendage. The white berries initially turn scarlet and contain numerous rust-brown seeds that are 1.5 to 2 mm.long.

Leaves, Stem and Root: The plant is a low shrub up to 30 cm high with scaly underground runners. The shoots sprout from the axillary buds of the runners. The sprouts are downy when young and later become glabrous. The leaves are alternate, short-petioled, obovate, and coriaceous. The upper surface is dark green and the under surface pale green and covered in glandular hairs.

Habitat: The plant is common in the Northern Hemisphere.

Production: Cranberry leaves are the foliage leaves of *Vaccinium vitis-ideae*. Collection takes place in uncultivated regions (Scandinavia, England). The leaves are dried in the open air.

Other Names: Cowberry, Lingonberry, Mountain Cranberry, Red Bilberry, Whortleberry

ACTIONS AND PHARMACOLOGY

COMPOUNDS

Hydroquinone glycosides: arbutin (3-5%), pyroside (6′-acetyl-arbutin), hydroquinone gentiobioside, 2-O-caffeoyl arbutin

Tannins (10-20%): chiefly condensed tannins, proanthocyanidine

Flavonoids: including among others, avicularin, hyperoside, quercitrin, isoquercitrin

Triterpenes: including among others, beta-amyrin, oleanolic acid, ursolic acid

EFFECTS

The drug is antiviral and a urine disinfectant due to the tannin fraction. It also raises cyclooxigenase activity through the flavonol glycosides.

INDICATIONS AND USAGE

Unproven Uses: Alpine Cranberry is used to treat urinary tract irritation, gout, rheumatism, and calculus (stone complaints). It is also considered a substitute for Bearberry leaves.

CONTRAINDICATIONS

The drug is contraindicated in pregnancy, nursing, and in children under 12 years of age.

PRECAUTIONS AND ADVERSE REACTIONS

No health hazards are known in conjunction with the proper administration of designated therapeutic dosages. Individuals with gastric sensitivity may experience queasiness and vomiting following intake of preparations made from the drug with high tannin content. Liver damage is conceivable with administration of the drug over extended periods, particularly with children, due to the possible hepatotoxicity of the hydroquinones released.

Because the urine-disinfecting effect of the hydroquinones released in the urinary tract only occurs in an alkaline environment, the simultaneous administration of medication and food that increases uric acid concentration in the bladder should be avoided.

DOSAGE

Mode of Administration: Available as whole, cut, and powdered drug.

Daily Dose: The internal dose is 2 gm as a single dose; as a decoction, the concentration is 2 gm per cup.

Storage: Store the drug in a tightly sealed container and protect it from light.

LITERATURE

Friedrich H, Naturwissenschaften 48:304. 1961.

Frohne D, Pfänder HJ, Giftpflanzen - Ein Handbuch für Apotheker, Toxikologen und Biologen, 4. Aufl., Wiss. Verlags-Ges. Stuttgart 1997.

Hänsel R, Keller K, Rimpler H, Schneider G (Hrsg.), Hagers Handbuch der Pharmazeutischen Praxis, 5. Aufl., Bde 4-6 (Drogen): Springer Verlag Berlin, Heidelberg, New York, 1992-1994.

Sticher O et al., *PM* 35:253. 1979.

Thieme H et al., *PA* 24:236. 1969.

Thieme H, Winkler HJ, *PA* 21:182. 1966.

Teuscher E, Biogene Arzneimittel, 5. Aufl., Wiss. Verlagsges. Stuttgart 1997.

Thompson RS et al., *J Chem Soc Perkin Tarns* I:1387. 1972.

Alpine Ragwort

Senecio nemorensis

DESCRIPTION

Medicinal Parts: The medicinal part is the herb.

Flower and Fruit: The composite flower heads are in a dense, usually heavily blossomed corymb. The involucre bracts are grass- or olive-green and often tinged greenish-black at the tips. The florets are yellow. The fruit is 4 mm long, long-stemmed and glabrous. During flowering, the pappus is only as long as the disc florets. By the time the fruit ripens, the pappus is 3 times as long as the fruit.

Leaves, Stem and Root: This geophytic perennial has runners that are fleshy, 20 cm long, and 5 cm thick. The stem is erect, 40 to 140 cm high with rounded ribs. The stem is green or, in particularly sunny locations, reddish-brown. The stem is glabrous to sparsely pubescent or short-downy. The foliage leaves are lanceolate-ovate, oblong-elliptic to oblong-lanceolate, acute or acuminate and serrate to double-serrate-dentate. The upper cauline leaves are usually petiolate, almost glabrous above to sparsely pubescent. The lower surface of the leaf is sparsely or moderately scattered and appressed pubescent.

Habitat: The plant grows in many regions of southern and western Europe and is cultivated in some eastern European countries.

Other Names: Squaw Weed, Life Root

ACTIONS AND PHARMACOLOGY

COMPOUNDS

Pyrrolizidine alkaloids (0.1-0.9%): including among others, senecionine, fuchsisencionine, 7-angeloylretronecin, bulgarsenine, nemorensin, platyphyllin, sarracin

Sesquiterpenes of the eremophilane-type: including among others, nemosenine A-D

Flavonoids: including among others, rutin, quercitrin

Hydroxycoumarins: including among others, esculetin

Volatile oil (0.1%)

EFFECTS

The drug is hemostyptic and hypoglycemic. The pyrrolizidine alkaloids are hepatotoxic and carcinogenic.

INDICATIONS AND USAGE

Unproven Uses: Folk medicine uses of the herb have included diabetes mellitus, hemorrhage, high blood pressure, spasms, and as a uterine stimulant. The drug is also used in bleeding as a result of tooth extraction.

PRECAUTIONS AND ADVERSE REACTIONS

Alpine Ragwort should not be taken internally. Hepatotoxicity and carcinogenicity are possible due to the presence of pyrrolizidine alkaloids with 1,2-unsaturated necic parent substances.

DOSAGE

Mode of Administration: Internal use is not recommended.

How Supplied: Forms of commercial pharmaceutical preparations include drops.

Preparation: To prepare a tea, pour boiling water over 1 teaspoonful (approximately 1 g) of finely cut drug, steep for 5 to 10 minutes, then strain.

Daily Dosage: A cup of the tea may be taken several times a day. (See precautions and adverse reactions).

LITERATURE

Gottlieb R et al., *DAZ* 130:285. 1990.

Röder E et al., *PH* 16:1462. 1977.

Röder E, Pyrrolizidinhaltige Arzneipflanzen. In: *DAZ* 132(45):2427-2435. 1992.

Wiedenfeld H et al., *Arch Pharm* 315:165. 1982.

Wiedenfeld H et al., *Arch Pharm* 318:294. 1985.

Wiedenfeld H et al., *PH* 18:1083. 1979.

Wiedenfeld H et al., *PM* 41:124. 1981.

Wiedenfeld H et al., *PM* 46:426. 1986.

Wiedenfeld H et al., *Sci Pharm* 57:97. 1989.

Alpinia officinarum

See Lesser Galangal

Alstonia constricta

See Fever Bark

Althaea officinalis

See Marshmallow

Amanita muscaria

See Aga

Amaranth

Amaranthus hypochondriacus

DESCRIPTION

Medicinal Parts: The entire plant is used medicinally

Flower and Fruit: The inflorescence is bifurcated, solitary, and oblong-spicate in dense spikelike terminal clusters with very short internodes, often composed of twigs. In some species they are all in the leaf axils. The plant is monoecious, dioecious, or mixed. Bracteoles are 4 to 6 mm, ovate, with a mucro that is about twice as long as the perianth. The perianth segments are narrowly ovate, usually acute and about as long as the fruit. The segments are dry-skinned, whitish- or reddish-green to red. The ovary is ovate. The fruit is one-seeded, ovate, dry-skinned, and forms a transversely dehiscing capsule. Seeds are lentil-shaped, erect, circular, smooth and usually black.

Leaves, Stem and Root: The plant is a tall, glabrous annual, occasionally perennial, and grows up to 2 m tall. It is erect, glabrous or sparsely pubescent above. The leaves are rhomboid-ovate and alternate, with occasionally undulating or ruffled margins.

Habitat: Amaranth is common in temperate and warm climates.

Production: Amaranth is the complete plant in flower of *Amaranthus hypochondriacus*.

Other Names: Lady Bleeding, Lovely Bleeding, Love-Lies-Bleeding, Red Cockscomb, Velvet Flower, Pilewort, Prince's Feather

ACTIONS AND PHARMACOLOGY

COMPOUNDS

Saponins

Betacyans

Protoalkaloids

EFFECTS

The drug is said to have an astringent effect (possibly due to the saponins, betacyans, and protoalkaloids). There are no studies available on efficacy.

INDICATIONS AND USAGE

Unproven Uses: Amaranth has been used for diarrhea, ulcers, and inflammation of the mouth and throat.

PRECAUTIONS AND ADVERSE REACTIONS

No health hazards or side effects are known in conjunction with the proper administration of designated therapeutic dosages.

DOSAGE

Mode of Administration: Amaranth is administered orally as a liquid extract.

LITERATURE

Martindale. The Extra Pharmacopoeia, 27th Ed. Pub. The Pharmaceutical Press (1977) UK.

Amaranthus hypochondriacus

See Amaranth

Amargo

Quassia amara

DESCRIPTION

Medicinal Parts: The medicinal part is the wood of the trunk and branches.

Flower and Fruit: The flowers are small and pale yellowish green. The sepals are round to ovate, fused at the base and imbricate. There are 5 petals, 10 stamens and 5 carpels. The style is fused from bottom to top. The fruit is a pea-sized drupe, which ripens from December to January. They are black, glossy, solitary, clavate, and have a thin skin.

Leaves, Stem and Root: The plant is a 15 to 30 m high tree with a diameter of 1 m. The bark is smooth and grayish. The alternate leaves are odd pinnate. The leaflets are opposite, oblong, acuminate and uneven at the base.

Habitat: The plant grows in Jamaica

Production: Quassia Wood is the wood of *Quassia amara* or *Picrasma excelsa*.

Not to be Confused With: The wood of Rhus metopium

Other Names: Bitter Wood, Jamaica Quassia, Surinam Quassia, Japanese Quassia, Bitter Ash

ACTIONS AND PHARMACOLOGY

COMPOUNDS

Triterpenes: decanor-triterpenes (picrasan derivatives, quassinoids, simaroubolides) chief components quassin (nigakilactone D, 0.1 to 0.2%), isoquassin (picrasmine), neoquassin and 18-hydroxyquassin

Indole alkaloids of: beta-carboline type, including n-methoxy-2-vinyl-beta-carboline; canthinone type, including 4-canthine-6-one-methoxy-5-hydroxycanthine-6-one

EFFECTS

The amaroid drug (quassinoids) stimulates secretion of gastric juices, increases appetite, and aids digestion. It may also have a choleretic effect.

INDICATIONS AND USAGE

Homeopathic Uses: Quassia amara is used for gallbladder complaints, as bitter tonic, purgative and as anthelmintic (for ascarid and threadworms).

CONTRAINDICATIONS

Contraindicated in pregnancy.

PRECAUTIONS AND ADVERSE REACTIONS

General: No health hazards or side effects are known in conjunction with the proper administration of designated therapeutic dosages. Internal administration can be followed occasionally by dizziness and headache, as well as by uterine pain.

Pregnancy: Not to be used during pregnancy.

OVERDOSAGE

Overdosage could lead to mucous membrane irritation, followed by vomiting. Use over prolonged periods of time may lead to weakened vision and total blindness.

DOSAGE

Mode of Administration: Quassia Wood is used in homeopathic dilutions and in commercial pharmaceutical preparations.

Daily Dosage: Tincture: 2-4 mL

Storage: Quassia should be protected from light and kept dry.

LITERATURE

Barbetti P et al., Quassinoids from Quassia amara. In: *PH* 32:1007. 1993.

Bray DH et al., (1987) *Phytother Res* 1 (1):22.

Geissmann T, (1964) *Ann Rev Pharmacol* 4:305.

Kupchan SM, Streelman DR, (1976) *J Org Chem* 41:3481.

Murae T et al., (1973) *Tetrahedron* 29:1515.

Murae T et al., (1975) *Chem Pharm* Bull 23 (9):2191.

Njar VCO et al., 2-Methoxycanthin-6-on: a new alkaloid from the stem wood of Quassia amara. In: PM 59(3):259. 1992.

Njar VCO et al., Antifertility activity of Quassia amara: Quassin inhibits the steroidgenesis in rat Leydig cells in vitro. In: PM 61(2):180-182. 1995.

Ohmoto T, Koike K. (1983) *Chem Pharm Bull* 31:3198.

Polonsky J, (1973) Fortschr. *Chem Org Naturst* 30. 101.

Wagner H et al., (1979) *Planta Med* 36:113.

Wagner H et al., (1980) *Planta Med* 38:204.

American Adder's Tongue

Erythronium americanum

DESCRIPTION

Medicinal Parts: The medicinal parts are the leaves and tubers.

Flower and Fruit: The flowers are terminal, large, hanging, and lilylike and are 2.5 cm in diameter. The bracts of the involucre are sharply revolute, bright yellow and often tinged purple and sprinkled at the base. There are 6 stamens. The fruit is a fusiform nodule about 2 cm long.

Leaves, Stem and Root: The plant grows from a small, ovate fern-colored corm to between 2 and 2.5 cm long. It is perennial with a bulbous light-brown root. The stem is thin and about 25 cm high. There are only 2 leaves, which are lanceolate and pale green. They have purplish or brownish spots, are about 6 cm long by 2 to 3 cm wide, minutely wrinkled, and with parallel veins. The petioles are 5 to 7.5 cm long.

Characteristics: The fresh leaves have emollient and antiscrofulous properties when applied as a poultice.

Habitat: The plant grows in the eastern U.S. as far south as Florida and as far north and west as Ontario and Arkansas.

Production: American Adder's Tongue leaves are the fresh leaves of *Erythronium americanum.*

Other Names: Dog's Tooth Violet, Erythronium, Lamb's Tongue, Rattlesnake Violet, Serpent's Tongue, Snake Leaf, Yellow Snakeleaf, Yellow Snowdrop

ACTIONS AND PHARMACOLOGY

COMPOUNDS

Alpha-methylene-gamma-butyrolactone-glucosides: tuliposides

EFFECTS

When used internally, the drug is emetic. Used externally, it is an emollient.

INDICATIONS AND USAGE

Unproven Uses: The plant is used externally for ulcers.

PRECAUTIONS AND ADVERSE REACTIONS

The plant has a strongly sensitizing effect. Reciprocal reactions occur with tulip, fritallaria, lily, alstroemeria and Bomarea species. Nothing is known regarding health hazards or side effects in connection with the administration of the drug.

DOSAGE

Mode of Administration: Fresh leaves are applied topically as a poultice or administered internally as an infusion.

LITERATURE

Cavallito CJ, Haskell TH, (1946) *J Am Chem Soc* 66:2332.

Hausen B, Allergiepflanzen, Pflanzenallergene, ecomed Verlagsgesellsch. mbH, Landsberg 1988.

Kern W, List PH, Hörhammer L (Hrsg.), Hagers Handbuch der Pharmazeutischen Praxis, 4. Aufl., Bde 1-8, Springer Verlag Berlin, Heidelberg, New York, 1969.

Teuscher E, Lindequist U, Biogene Gifte - Biologie, Chemie, Pharmakologie, 2. Aufl., Fischer Verlag Stuttgart 1994.

American Bittersweet

Celastrus scandens

DESCRIPTION

Medicinal Parts: The medicinal parts are the root and the bark of the plant.

Flower and Fruit: The twining shrub is up to 8 m tall. The leaves are 5 to 12.5 cm long, ovate to ovate-lanceolate and serrate. There are numerous very small greenish flowers on terminal racemes that are 10 cm long. The orange-yellow seed capsules are 1 cm in diameter.

Habitat: The plant is indigenous to North America.

Production: American Bittersweet root and bark are the root and bark of *Celastrus scandens*.

Other Names: Waxwork, False Bittersweet

ACTIONS AND PHARMACOLOGY

COMPOUNDS

Tannins

Celastrol (yellow quinoide nortriterpene)

EFFECTS

American Bittersweet has diuretic and diaphoretic effects.

INDICATIONS AND USAGE

Unproven Uses: The drug has been used for rheumatism, menstrual disorders, and liver disorders, but is rarely used today.

PRECAUTIONS AND ADVERSE REACTIONS

No health hazards or side effects are known in conjunction with the proper administration of designated therapeutic dosages.

DOSAGE

No information is available.

LITERATURE

Hegnauer R, Chemotaxonomie der Pflanzen, Bde 1-11, Birkhäuser Verlag Basel, Boston, Berlin 1962-1997.

Kern W, List PH, Hörhammer L (Hrsg.), Hagers Handbuch der Pharmazeutischen Praxis, 4. Aufl., Bde. 1-8, Springer Verlag Berlin, Heidelberg, New York, 1969.

American Hellebore

Veratrum viride

DESCRIPTION

Medicinal Parts: The medicinal parts are the dried rhizome and the roots.

Flower and Fruit: The terminal inflorescence is a panicle made up of spikelike racemes. The flowers are short-pedioled and often unisexual. The perigone has 6 tepals and is almost free. The anther is reniform. The fruit is capsulelike with numerous seeds and dividing membranes. The seeds are flattened, light-brown, and winged all around. The embryo is small and set in the tip of the fusiform endosperm.

Leaves, Stem and Root: The species are perennial herbs with strong leafy stems. The leaves are spiralled, broadly elliptical to linear-lanceolate, heavily ribbed and drawn together in a broad sheath. The leaves of *Veratrum viride* are oval to linear.

Characteristics: Characteristics of the species *Veratrum viride* is very similar to *Veratrum album*.

Habitat: The herb is indigenous to the swamps and moist ground from Canada to Georgia and westward to Minnesota.

Production: American Hellebore root is the rhizome of *Veratrum viride*.

Not to be Confused With: The rhizome from *Symplocarpus foetidus* is thicker than that of *Veratrum viride* and more porous.

Other Names: Bugbane, Devil's Bite, Earth Gall, Indian Poke, Itchweed, Tickleweed

ACTIONS AND PHARMACOLOGY

COMPOUNDS

Steroid alkaloids (1%): including among others, some of the solanidane-type, isorubijervine, rubijervine- C-nor-D-homo-sterane-type: including among others, protoverine, protoveratrine A and B. In contrast with *Veratrum album*, the less toxic alkaloids of the solanidane-type are the majority in this herb.

EFFECTS

The herb reduces blood pressure and slows down the pulse due to the alkaloid germitrin. When used externally, it is hyperemic, hyperalgic, and locally anaesthetic. The drug is extremely toxic.

INDICATIONS AND USAGE

Unproven Uses: The drug is obsolete due to the high risk of side effects. Historically, American Hellebore was used internally to treat pneumonia, peritonitis, epilepsy, pain, asthma, colds, cholera, croup, consumption, dyspepsia, fever, hypertension, herpes, gout, headache, inflammation, neuralgia, whooping cough, puerperal fever, scarlet fever, sciatica, rheumatism, shingles, toothache, scrofulous, tumors, and typhus. It was used externally for throat infections and tonsillitis (as a gargle solution), neuralgia, and skin irritations.

PRECAUTIONS AND ADVERSE REACTIONS

The drug is severely toxic and has numerous severe side effects, even in therapeutic dosages. It is no longer administered in allopathic medicine. The alkaloids are severely irritating to the mucous membranes, and because they inhibit inactivation of the sodium ion channels after resorption, the alkaloids have a paralyzing effect on numerous excitable cells, in particular those governing cardiac activity.

OVERDOSAGE

The first symptoms of poisoning are sneezing, lacrimation, salivation, vomiting, diarrhea, burning sensation in the mouth and pharyngeal space, and inability to swallow; then, following resorption: paresthesia, vertigo, possible blindness, paralysis of the limbs, also mild convulsions, lowering of cardiac frequency, cardiac arrhythmias and hypotension. Death occurs either through systolic cardiac arrest or through asphyxiation. The alkaloids can also be absorbed through uninjured skin.

Following gastrointestinal emptying (inducement of vomiting, gastric lavage with burgundy-colored potassium permanganate solution, sodium sulphate), installation of activated charcoal and shock prophylaxis (appropriate body position, quiet, warmth), the therapy for poisoning consists of treating spasms with diazepam or certain barbiturates (i.v.), bradycardia with atropine, and hypotension with peripherally active circulatory medications. Electrolyte substitution may be necessary and possible cases of acidosis should be treated with sodium bicarbonate infusions. Intubation and oxygen respiration may also be necessary.

DOSAGE

Mode of Administration: The herb can be found in whole and powdered forms.

Daily Dose: The daily dose is 100 mg.

Storage: The drug should be clearly labeled as ''poisonous'' and stored in a safe place.

LITERATURE

Brossi, B, In: Brossi A, Cordell GA (Eds), The Alkaloids. Vol. 41. Academic Press, 1250 Sixth Avenue, San Diego, CA 92101. 1992.

Frohne D, Pfänder HJ, Giftpflanzen - Ein Handbuch für Apotheker, Toxikologen und Biologen, 4. Aufl., Wiss. Verlags-Ges. Stuttgart 1997.

Kern W, List PH, Hörhammer L (Hrsg.), Hagers Handbuch der Pharmazeutischen Praxis, 4. Aufl., Bde 1-8: Springer Verlag Berlin, Heidelberg, New York, 1969.

Kupchan, S M et al., (1961) Lloydia 24(1):17.

Madaus G, Lehrbuch der Biologischen Arzneimittel, Bde 1-3, Nachdruck, Georg Olms Verlag Hildesheim 1979.

Roth L, Daunderer M, Kormann K, Giftpflanzen, Pflanzengifte, 4. Aufl., Ecomed Fachverlag Landsberg Lech 1993.

Teuscher E, Lindequist U, Biogene Gifte - Biologie, Chemie, Pharmakologie, 2. Aufl., Fischer Verlag Stuttgart 1994.

American Ivy

Parthenocissus quinquefolia

DESCRIPTION

Medicinal Parts: The medicinal parts are the bark, the branch tips, the fresh leaves, the berries, and the resin.

Flower and Fruit: The inflorescences are fairly small and appear in yellowish-green racemes. They produce dark purple, pea-sized berries; the seeds are cordate.

Leaves, Stem and Root: American Ivy is a high-climbing shrub with dark green branches, which sometimes develop adventitious roots. The flowering branches turn into regular, double-rowed creepers, which diminish toward the top. The leaves are long-petioled and divided into 5 elliptical, ovate or obovate, roughly serrate or dentate leaflets. The leaflets have broad, suddenly acuminate, and usually somewhat rounded-off teeth. The upper surface is dark green, and the undersurface is whitish-green and matte.

Habitat: Parthenocissus quinquefolia originated in North America and is cultivated worldwide.

Production: American Ivy bark is the bark of the trunk and branches of *Parthenocissus quinquefolia.*

Other Names: American Woodbine, Creeper, False Grapes, Five Leaves, Ivy, Virginia Creeper, Wild Woodbine, Wild Woodvine, Woody Climber

ACTIONS AND PHARMACOLOGY

COMPOUNDS

Up to 2% oxalic acid is contained in the berries, however there is no information available on the constituents of the rind.

EFFECTS

The plant is diaphoretic, astringent, and tonic.

INDICATIONS AND USAGE

Unproven Uses: American Ivy is used for digestive disorders.

PRECAUTIONS AND ADVERSE REACTIONS

The berries are considered poisonous, however no health hazards or side effects are known in conjunction with the proper administration of designated therapeutic dosages. Older scientific literature describes the death of a child following intake of the berries (Lewin, 1992).

DOSAGE

Mode of Administration: The drug is ground for use as an infusion.

How Supplied:

Capsules: 50 mg

Syrup

LITERATURE

Kern W, List PH, Hörhammer L (Hrsg.), Hagers Handbuch der Pharmazeutischen Praxis, 4. Aufl., Bde 1-8, Springer Verlag Berlin, Heidelberg, New York, 1969.

Lewin L, Gifte und Vergiftungen, 6. Aufl., Nachdruck, Haug Verlag, Heidelberg 1992.

Roth L, Daunderer M, Kormann K, Giftpflanzen, Pflanzengifte, 4. Aufl., Ecomed Fachverlag Landsberg Lech 1993.

American Liverwort

Hepatica nubilis

DESCRIPTION

Medicinal Parts: The drug is the herb, without roots, harvested at flowering season.

Flower and Fruit: The flowering stems are axillary, numerous, pubescent, and erect. They are usually reddish and have 3 entire-margined, ovate, unpetiolate, calyxlike bracts up to 1 cm long, directly under the upright flower. The 6 to 8 bracts are sky blue, paler on the outside, occasionally pink or white, narrow-ovate, entire-margined, and dropping. There are no nectaries. The stamens are almost white with red connective. The stigma is headlike. The fruit is oblong with a short beak fitted into the semiglobular receptacle.

Leaves, Stem and Root: The herb is a 7 to 15 cm high, a hardy perennial with a short, fibrous, dark-brown rhizome. The numerous leaves are basal, long-petioled, coriaceous, green above and usually violet beneath. They are cordate and three-lobed at the base, deeply indented, broadly ovate, with blunt to acute lobes. The young leaves, including the stems, are densely covered in silky white hairs. The leaves later become glabrous and appear after flowering. Liverwort is a protected species in Germany, Austria, Switzerland, Italy, the Czech Republic, Slovakia and Hungary.

Habitat: The plant is indigenous to almost all of Europe except the Atlantic regions, Denmark and northwest Germany. It is also indigenous to Korea, Japan, and temperate North America.

Production: American Liverwort consists of the fresh or dried above-ground parts of *Hepatica nobilis*. The herb is harvested when in bloom and air-dried in the shade. The roots must be left in the ground because they are a protected species.

Other Names: Herb Trinity, Kidneywort, Liverleaf, Liverweed, Round-Leaved Hepatica, Trefoil, Kidney Liverleaf

ACTIONS AND PHARMACOLOGY

COMPOUNDS

Protoanemonine-forming agents (0.07% in the freshly harvested plant, based on weight): presumably, the glycoside ranunculin changes enzymatically when the plant is cut into small pieces (and probably also during dehydration) into the pungent, volatile protoanemonine that quickly dimerizes to anemonine. Once dried, the plant is not capable of protoanemonine formation.

Flavonoids: including isoquercitrin, astragalin, quercimeritrin

Saponins

EFFECTS

The main active agents are lactone-forming glycosides, flavoglycosides and anthocyane. The fresh plant contains protoanemonine, which causes skin irritation.

INDICATIONS AND USAGE

Unproven Uses: Preparations of American Liverwort herb are used for liver ailments, liver diseases of all origins, jaundice, gallstones, and gravel.

PRECAUTIONS AND ADVERSE REACTIONS

Health risks or side effects following the proper administration of designated therapeutic dosages are not recorded.

Extended skin contact with the freshly harvested, bruised plant can lead to blister formation and cauterizations that are difficult to heal due to the resulting protoanemonine, which is severely irritating to the skin and mucous membranes. If taken internally, severe irritation to the gastrointestinal tract, combined with colic and diarrhea, as well as irritation of the urinary drainage passages, are possible.

Symptomatic treatment for external contact consists of mucilaginosa, following irrigation with diluted potassium permanganate solution. In case of internal contact, administration of activated charcoal should follow gastric lavage.

Pregnancy: Not to be used during pregnancy.

DOSAGE

Mode of Administration: The drug can be taken internally or used externally as a rinse. Also as a liniment made with added fats, oils, or alcohol.

Preparation: To make a rinse, a cataplasm can be made of the squeezed fresh plant; alcohol can be used if necessary.

Daily Dosage: When used internally, a single dose consists of 2 to 4 gm as an infusion, or 2 to 3 cups from a 3 to 6% infusion. The daily dosage is 4 teaspoonfuls, or 3.8 gm drug.

LITERATURE

Hänsel R, Keller K, Rimpler H, Schneider G (Hrsg.), Hagers Handbuch der Pharmazeutischen Praxis, 5. Aufl., Bde 4-6 (Drogen), Springer Verlag Berlin, Heidelberg, New York, 1992-1994.

Madaus G, Lehrbuch der Biologischen Arzneimittel, Bde 1-3, Nachdruck, Georg Olms Verlag Hildesheim 1979.

Roth L, Daunderer M, Kormann K: Giftpflanzen, Pflanzengifte, 4. Aufl., Ecomed Fachverlag Landsberg Lech 1993.

Ruijgrok HWL, PM 11:338-347. 1963.

Teuscher E, Lindequist U, Biogene Gifte - Biologie, Chemie, Pharmakologie, 2. Aufl., Fischer Verlag Stuttgart 1994.

American Pawpaw

Asimina triloba

DESCRIPTION

Medicinal Parts: The medicinal parts are the seeds, bark, and leaves.

Flower and Fruit: The axillary flowers are dull purple and solitary. They are about 3.5 cm wide. The petals are round, ovate, and marbled. The outer ones are almost circular and 3 to 4 times as long as the sepals. The fruit is yellowish and oblong-ovoid. The fleshy pods are about 7.5 by 2.5 cm and contain 3 flat, brown seeds. The seeds are slightly polished with darker brown lines on the surface. They are oblong-oval, with a grayish hilum at one end. The taste and smell are resinous.

Leaves, Stem and Root: The American Pawpaw grows up to 6 m in height. The young shoots and leaves are covered in rust-colored down and later become glabrous. The leaves are thin (20-25 cm long and 7 cm wide), smooth, entire, ovate and acuminate. The plant's leaves and flowers appear simultaneously.

Characteristics: The fruit has an unpleasant smell when unripe, but when it ripens after a frost, it smells, faintly of custard. This characteristic gives rise to one of its common names, Custard Apple.

Habitat: The plant is found in the west, south and central U.S., also India and parts of Asia and Africa.

Production: American Pawpaw seeds are the seeds of *Asimina triloba.*

Other Names: Custard Apple, Paw Paw Seeds

ACTIONS AND PHARMACOLOGY

COMPOUNDS

Benzyl isoquinoline alkaloids: including anolobine

Polyketides: including asimicine

Fatty oil

EFFECTS

No information is available.

INDICATIONS AND USAGE

Homeopathic Uses: In homeopathy, American Pawpaw is used in the treatment of scarlet fever, fevers, and vomiting as well as for mouth and throat inflammation.

PRECAUTIONS AND ADVERSE REACTIONS

The drug has a nauseant effect. Allergic individuals may be susceptible to severe urticaria.

DOSAGE

Mode of Administration: The mother tincture is used in homeopathic dilutions.

LITERATURE

He K, Shi G, Zhao GX, Zeng L, Ye Q, Schwedler JT, Wood KV, McLaughlin JL, Three new adjacent bis-tetrahydrofuran acetogenins with four hydroxyl groups from Asimina triloba. *J Nat Prod,* 59:1029-34, 1996.

He K, Zhao GX, Shi G, Zeng L, Chao JF, McLaughlin JL, Additional bioactive annonaceous acetogenins from *Asimina triloba* (Annonaceae). *Bioorg Med Chem,* 5:501-6, 1997.

Kern W, List PH, Hörhammer L (Hrsg.), Hagers Handbuch der Pharmazeutischen Praxis, 4. Aufl., Bde. 1-8, Springer Verlag Berlin, Heidelberg, New York, 1969.

Lewin L, Gifte und Vergiftungen, 6. Aufl., Nachdruck, Haug Verlag, Heidelberg 1992.

Oliver-Bever B (Ed.), Medicinal Plants of Tropical West Africa, Cambridge University Press Cambridge, London 1986.

Ratnayake S, Rupprecht JK, Potter WM, McLaughlin JL, Evaluation of various parts of the paw paw tree *Asimina triloba* (Annonaceae) as commercial sources of the pesticidal annonaceous acetogenins. *J Econ Entomol,* 55:2353-6, 1992.

Woo MH, Cho KY, Zhang Y, Zeng L, Gu ZM, McLaughlin JL, Asimilobin and cis- and trans-murisolinones novel bioactive Annonaceous acetogenins from the seeds of *Asimina triloba. J Nat Prod,* 4:1533-42, 1995.

Zhao G, Hui Y, Rupprecht JK, McLaughlin JL, Wood KV, Additional bioactive compounds and trilobacin a novel highly cytotoxic acetogenin from the bark of *Asimina triloba. J Nat Prod,* 55:347-56, 1992.

Zhao GX, Chao JF, Zeng L, McLaughlin JL, (24-cis)-asimicinone and (24-trans)-asimicinone: two novel bioactive ketolactone acetogenins from *Asimina triloba* (Annonaceae). *Nat Toxins,* 4:128-34, 1996.

Zhao GX, Chao JF, Zeng L, Rieser MJ, McLaughlin JL, The absolute configuration of adjacent bis-THF acetogenins and asiminocin a novel highly potent asimicin isomer from *Asimina triloba. Bioorg Med Chem,* 4:25-32, 1996.

American White Pond Lily

Nymphaea odorata

DESCRIPTION

Medicinal Parts: The medicinal parts are the cut and dried rhizome, the fresh rhizome and the rhizome with the roots.

Flower and Fruit: The androgynous flowers are solitary, 7 to 15 cm across and radial-symmetrical. They grow from the rhizome and extend above the water by means of a long stem. The 4 sepals are almost free, oblong-ovate, pale green on the outside and greenish-white on the inside. The pure white 23 to 32 petals are free, elliptical-lanceolate, narrower than the sepals and arranged on the axis like a screw. The numerous carpels are sunk into the beaker-shaped axis in a ring and are partially fused with it. The fruit is a berrylike capsule, which ripens under water. The seeds are small, ovate, approximately 2.5 mm long, smooth and have an aril. The flowers open as the sun rises, close a few hours later (before the intense midday heat) and remain closed until the next morning. The size of the plant varies according to depth of water.

Leaves, Stem and Root: The fragrant water lily is an aquatic plant with a strong horizontal rhizome, which grows under water. The leaves are swimming, alternate, long-petioled and have 4 air channels in the petiole. The lamina is oval-orbicular, large (15-30 cm long) and has a wedge-shaped deep indentation at the base. It is entire-margined, coriaceous, green above and purple-brown beneath. The petiole is greenish and is usually purple-tinged. The stipules are triangular to reniform.

Characteristics: The flowers have a sweet fragrance.

Habitat: The plant is indigenous to the eastern part of North America. It is found as far south as Mexico, El Salvador, and the West Indies and has been naturalized in parts of western Europe.

Production: American White Pond Lily root is the rhizome of *Nymphaea odorata* and other varieties. The drug is derived from the cut and dried rhizome and, in powdered form, is yellowish to gray-brown.

Other Names: Water Cabbage, Cow Cabbage, Water Lily, Water Nymph, Sweet-Scented Water Lily, White Pond Lily

ACTIONS AND PHARMACOLOGY

COMPOUNDS

Tannins (gallotannins, ellagitannins)

Only a very small amount of research work has been carried out on the drug, but American White Pond Lily root is known to contain large amounts of gallic and ellagic tannins.

EFFECTS

The astringent and antiseptic effects of the American White Pond Lily can be attributed to the high tannin content.

INDICATIONS AND USAGE

Unproven Uses: Chronic diarrhea is a common internal application. Externally, the plant has been used in the treatment of vaginal conditions and as a gargle in the treatment of diseases of the mouth and throat. Traditional folk medicine uses also included dysentery, gonorrhea, and leukorrhea, and the leaves and roots were applied as a mash poultice for boils, tumors, scrofulous sores and inflamed skin.

Homeopathic Uses: Morning diarrhea is one use in homeopathy.

PRECAUTIONS AND ADVERSE REACTIONS

No health hazards or side effects are known in conjunction with the proper administration of designated therapeutic dosages.

OVERDOSAGE

No poisonings have yet been observed among humans but animal experiments have been performed with fatal results. Even though very high dosages were used with the animals, these results should be taken as a warning to exercise care.

DOSAGE

Mode of Administration: As a decoction or liquid extract used for washes, poultices, and gargles or taken internally.

Preparation: The fluid extract is produced by percolation: 1:1 using ethanol 25%.

Daily Dosage: Internally: in a single dose of 1 to 2 g drug as an infusion; 1 to 4 mL of liquid extract.

Homeopathic Dosages: 5 drops, 1 tablet, or 10 globules every 30 to 60 minutes (acute) or 1 to 3 times daily (chronic); parenterally: 1 to 2 mL sc acute, 3 times daily; chronic: once a day (HAB1).

LITERATURE

Hänsel R, Keller K, Rimpler H, Schneider G (Hrsg.), Hagers Handbuch der Pharmazeutischen Praxis, 5. Aufl., Bde 4-6 (Drogen), Springer Verlag Berlin, Heidelberg, New York, 1992-1994.

Madaus G, Lehrbuch der Biologischen Arzneimittel, Bde 1-3, Nachdruck, Georg Olms Verlag Hildesheim 1979.

Odinstsova NV, (1960) *Farmakol i Toxicol* 23:132 (via CA 54:25303).

Roth L, Daunderer M, Kormann K, Giftpflanzen, Pflanzengifte, 4. Aufl., Ecomed Fachverlag Landsberg Lech 1993.

Su KL et al., (1983) *Lloydia* 36:72 and 80.

Ammi visnaga

See Bishop's Weed

Ammoniac Gum

Dorema ammoniacum

DESCRIPTION

Medicinal Parts: The medicinal part of the plant is a resin exuded from the flowers and stems.

Flower and Fruit: The inflorescence is an umbel that grows from the axils of the upper leaves. Because of the very short flower stems, the individual inflorescences appear very globular. The flower structures are in fives, the flowers radial and small, the calyx teeth indistinct, the petals white with revolute tips. There are 5 stamens. The ovary is inferior, two-chambered, densely haired, with a conical style cushion with two styles. The fruit is double achene.

Leaves, Stem and Root: This herbaceous perennial grows up to 2.5 m high. The leaves are arranged in spirals, with clearly developed sheaths, and the lamina is often only rudimentary. The stem is hollow, gnarled, blue-striped, and up to 5 cm thick. The taproot is tuberous.

Habitat: The plant is found growing in areas from Iran to southern Siberia.

Production: Ammoniac gum is the naturally exuding gum resin latex of *Dorema ammoniacum* hardened in the air and collected in the wild.

Not to be Confused With: Confusion may occur with North African and Cyrenian ammoniac.

ACTIONS AND PHARMACOLOGY

COMPOUNDS

Resin (60 to 70%): chief component ammoresinol

Water-soluble polysaccharides (10 to 20%)

Volatile oil (0.1 to 0.3%): chief components linalool, linalyl acetate, citronellyl acetate

EFFECTS

The drug is credited with being mildly diuretic, sudorific, spasmolytic, expectorate and menstruation-promoting in its effect, although research data regarding these effects is not available.

INDICATIONS AND USAGE

Unproven Uses: Uses dating back to ancient times include ingestion for its expectorant effect in chronic bronchitis, especially in the elderly. Because of the resin's purported diuretic, antispasmodic, and stimulant properties, it was often employed internally as a diaphoretic and emmenagogue as well as externally as a plaster for swellings of the joints and indolent tumors. In the late 19th century, it was used as an expectorant for chronic catarrh and externally in plasters to relieve hyperadenosis and in compresses for abscesses. More recently, internal folk medicine uses include chronic bronchitis, asthma, sciatica, and joint pain as well as conditions of the liver and spleen. Among external uses are treatment of wounds and abscesses and lymph node swelling.

Homeopathic Uses: Homeopathic uses include bronchitis.

CONTRAINDICATIONS

The drug is contraindicated during pregnancy due to the existence of indications of a menstruation-inducing effect.

PRECAUTIONS AND ADVERSE REACTIONS

According to older sources, repeated visual disorders and glaucomalike states appeared following ingestion of the drug, however no health hazards have been verified in conjunction with the proper administration of designated therapeutic dosages.

DOSAGE

Mode of Administration: Preparations for internal and external use

Preparation:

Ammoniacum depuratum: 1,000 parts coarse ammoniac powder are heated with 1,500 parts ethanol 60% in a steam bath while being constantly stirred until an emulsion is formed. It is then pressed through linen and evaporated until a few drops can be worked in the hand without becoming sticky.

Combination: Ammoniac emulsion: toluene: distilled water; 1:2:30

Daily Dosage: 0.3 to 1 g drug

Homeopathic Dosage: 5 drops, 1 tablet, or 10 globules every 30 to 60 minutes (acute) and 1 to 3 times daily (chronic); parenterally: 1 to mL sc acute: 3 times daily; chronic: once a day (HAB1); special doses for children

Storage: The drug should be stored over chalk in a container that protects it from light.

LITERATURE

Blaschek W, Hänsel R, Keller K, Reichling J, Rimpler G, Schneider G (Eds) Hagers Handbuch der Pharmazeutischen Praxis. Folgeb nde 1 und 2. Drogen A-Z. Springer. Berlin, Heidelberg 1998.

Amomum aromaticum

See Nepalese Cardamom

Anacardium occidentale

See Cashew

Anacyclus pyrethrum

See Pellitory

Anagallis arvensis

See Scarlet Pimpernel

Anamirta cocculus

See Fish Berry

Ananas comosus

See Pineapple

Andira araroba

See Goa Powder

Anemarrhena (Zhi-Mu)

Anemarrhena asphodeloides

DESCRIPTION

Medicinal Parts: The medicinal part of the plant is the rhizome.

Flower and Fruit: The inflorescence is spikelike, and the flowers are clustered and radial. The perianth structures are in sixes. The tepals are free and uniform. There are 3 stamens and a 3-carpeled, fused ovary, with 1 to 3 seeds in each chamber. The fruit is a globose capsule, which opens on 3 sides.

Leaves, Stem and Root: Anemarrhena asphodeloides is an herbaceous perennial, and extends up to 60 cm high. The leaves are grasslike and clustered at the base.

Habitat: The plant is native to northern China, Korea, and Japan.

Production: Zhi-Mu is the dried rhizome of *Anemarrhena asphodeloides*. It is best harvested in the third year of cultivation in spring or autumn. The rhizome is then air-dried.

ACTIONS AND PHARMACOLOGY

COMPOUNDS

Steroid saponins (6%): aglycones sarsapogenin, markogenin, neogitonin, particularly sarsapogenin-3-timobioside and markogenin-3-timobioside

Water-soluble polysaccharides: anemarans A to D

Lignans: hinoki resinol, among others

Xanthones: mangiferin (1.3%)

EFFECTS

A variety of experiments have been able to demonstrate antipyretic and cortisonelike effects for the drug with its steroid saponin content. In addition, inhibitions of platelet aggregation, of Na, K-ATP-ase and of DNA-polymerase were observed. The timosaponin A-III isolated from the drug reduced the serum levels of a 1-fetoprotein in animal experiments.

INDICATIONS AND USAGE

Chinese Medicine: In China, Zhi-Mu is used for febrile conditions and inflammation, diabetes, dry cough, ''bone fever'' and general dehydration, painful stool, and stranguria. It is also as a decoction for typhus, scarlet fever, and tuberculosis.

PRECAUTIONS AND ADVERSE REACTIONS

No health hazards are known in conjunction with the proper administration of designated therapeutic dosages.

OVERDOSAGE

The ingestion of large dosages of the drug may lead to gastroenteritis, intestinal colic, and diarrhea due to the saponin content. The drug is not to be administered in the presence of diarrhea.

DOSAGE

Mode of Administration: Whole and cut drug preparations for internal use.

Daily Dosage: 6 to 12 gm of drug often used with other herbs in teas.

Storage: Should be stored in a dry and well-aired place.

LITERATURE

Dong JX, Han GY, A new active steroidal saponin from Anemarrhena asphodeloides. *Planta Med*, 57:460-2, 1991 Oct.

Dong JX, Han GY, Studies on the active constituents of Anemarrhena asphodeloides bunge. *Yao Hsueh Hsueh Pao*, 27:26-32, 1992.

Hänsel R, Keller K, Rimpler H, Schneider G (Ed), Hagers Handbuch der Pharmazeutischen Praxis, 5. Aufl., Bde 4 - 6 (Drogen), Springer Verlag Berlin, Heidelberg, New York, 1992-1994.

Li PM, Zhong JL, Chen RQ, Zhang XK, Ho KL, Chiu JF, Huang DP, Zhi-mu saponin inhibits alpha-fetoprotein gene expression in developing rat liver. *Int J Biochem,* 21:15-22, 1989.

Liu JQ, Wu DW, 32 cases of postoperative osteogenic sarcoma treated by chemotherapy combined with Chinese medicinal herbs. *Planta Med,* 21: 1997.

Ma B, Wang B, Dong J, Yan X, Zhang H, Tu A, New spirostanol glycosides from Anemarrhena asphodeloides. Letter *Planta Med*, 63:376-9, 1997 Aug.

Miura T, Kako M, Ishihara E, Usami M, Yano H, Tanigawa K, Sudo K, Seino Y, Antidiabetic effect of seishin-kanro-to in KK-Ay mice. *Planta Med*, 21:320-2, 1997 Aug.

Nakashima N, Kimura I, Kimura M, Matsuura H, Isolation of pseudoprototimosaponin AIII from rhizomes of Anemarrhena asphodeloides and its hypoglycemic activity in streptozotocin-induced diabetic mice. *J Nat Prod*, 57:Kimura I, Matsuura H.

Takahashi M, Konno C, Hikino H, Isolation and hypoglycemic activity of anemarans A, B, C and D, glycans of Anemarrhena asphodeloides rhizomes. *Planta Med*, 57:100-2, 1985 Apr.

Anemarrhena asphodeloides

See Anemarrhena (Zhi-Mu)

Anemone nemorosa

See Wood Anemone

Anethum graveolens

See Dill

Angelica

Angelica archangelica

DESCRIPTION

Medicinal Parts: The medicinal parts are the seed, whole herb and root.

Flower and Fruit: The flowers are greenish-white to yellowish and are arranged in 20 to 40 rayed compact umbels without an involucre. The tiny epicalyx has numerous sepals with minute tips. The petals have an indented, indistinguishable tip. The elliptic fruit is 7 mm long by 4 mm wide and winged. The outer fruit membrane separates from the inner one.

Leaves, Stem and Root: The plant is 50 to 250 cm tall. The rhizome is short, strong, and fleshy and has long fibrous roots. The stem is erect, often as thick as an arm at the base. It is round, finely grooved, hollow, and tinged reddish below. The leaves are very large, 60 to 90 cm and tripinnate with a hollow petiole. Leaflets are ovate and unevenly serrate. The leaf sheaths are large and swollen.

Characteristics: The plant has a strong tangy odor. The taste is sweetish to burning tangy.

Habitat: Angelica is thought by some botanists to be indigenous to Syria, Holland, or Poland. Today it is found growing in the wild on the coasts of the North and Baltic Seas as far north as Lapland. It is a protected species in Iceland, and is cultivated in other regions. Other species are found in America (*A. atropurpurea*), in Europe (*A. sylvestris*) and in China/Asia (*A. sinensis*).

Production: Angelica seed consists of the fruit of Angelica archangelica, which is harvested from July onward. After drying in the air or in ovens, the umbels are threshed to separate the seeds. Angelica herb consists of the above-ground parts of Angelica archangelica. Angelica root is the dried root and rhizome of Angelica archangelica.

Other Names: European Angelica, Garden Angelica, Angel's Wort

ACTIONS AND PHARMACOLOGY

COMPOUNDS: ANGELICA FRUIT

Volatile oil: constituents include hexylmethyl phthalate, alpha-pinene, beta-phellandrene, borneol, camphene, beta-bisabolene, beta-caryophyllene, macrocyclic lactones (odor-determining) such as 15-oxypentadecenlactone

Furanocoumarins: including angelicin, bergaptene, imperatorin, oxypeucedanin, xantholtoxin

Fatty oil

Phytosterols: including beta-sitosterol, sigmasterol

EFFECTS: ANGELICA FRUIT

The furanocoumarins in the fruit are cytostatic and phototoxic. The spasmolytic, gastric juice-stimulating, and cholagogic effect of the herb could be explained by the aromatic-amaroid structure.

COMPOUNDS: ANGELICA LEAVES

Volatile Oil (0.015 to 0.1%): chief constituents myrcene (17 to 29%), p-cymene, limonene, cis-and trans-ocimene, alpha-phellandrene, beta-phellandrene, alpha-pinene

Furanocoumarins: including angelicin, bergaptene, imperatorin, isoimperatorin, oxypeucedanin, archangelicin

EFFECTS: ANGELICA LEAVES

The essential oils and furanocoumarins from the leaves have a strong irritant effect on the skin and mucous membranes (angelica dermatitis). The spasmolytic, gastric juice-stimulating and cholagogic effect of the herb could be explained by the aromatic-amaroid structure.

COMPOUNDS: ANGELICA ROOT

Volatile oil: chief components are alpha- and beta-phellandrenes, alpha-pinenes, macrocyclic lactones, including penta- and heptadecanolide

Furanocoumarins: including bergaptene, xanthotoxin, scopoletin, umbelliferone

Caffeic acid derivatives: including chlorogenic acid

Flavonoids

EFFECTS: ANGELICA ROOT

The root acts as an antispasmodic, cholagogue and stimulatory for secretion of gastric juices.

INDICATIONS AND USAGE

ANGELICA ROOT

Approved by Commission E:

- Dyspeptic complaints
- Loss of appetite

Unproven Uses: In folk medicine, preparations of the root are used as a mild rubefacient, for coughs, bronchitis, menstruation complaints, loss of appetite, dyspeptic complaints with mild gastrointestinal cramps, and liver and biliary duct conditions.

ANGELICA FRUIT

Unproven Uses: Preparations of angelica seed are used internally for conditions of the kidneys and efferent urinary tract, the intestinal tract and the respiratory tract, as well as for rheumatic and neuralgic complaints. Preparations are also used as a diaphoretic and have been used in the past for malaria. Externally, an ointment from the seeds is used for body lice.

ANGELICA LEAVES

Unproven Uses: Preparations from the leaves have been used as a diuretic and diaphoretic.

PRECAUTIONS AND ADVERSE REACTIONS

ANGELICA FRUIT AND HERB

General: No health hazards or side effects are known in conjunction with the proper administration of designated therapeutic dosages. Photodermatosis is possible following contact with the plant juice.

Pregnancy: Preparations are not to be used during pregnancy.

ANGELICA ROOT

No health hazards or side effects are known in conjunction with the proper administration of designated therapeutic dosages. The furocoumarins contained in angelica root sensitize the skin to light and can lead to inflammation of the skin in combination with UV rays. It is therefore advisable to avoid sunbathing and intensive UV radiation for the duration of treatment with Angelica or its preparations.

DRUG INTERACTIONS

MODERATE RISK

Anticoagulants and Thrombolytic Agents: Concurrent use may result in increased risk of bleeding. *Clinical Management:* Monitor for signs and symptoms of excessive bleeding.

MINOR RISK

Low Molecular Weight Heparins: Concurrent use may result in increased risk of bleeding. *Clinical Management:* Monitor for signs and symptoms of excessive bleeding.

DOSAGE

ANGELICA ROOT

Mode of Administration: Comminuted herb and other oral galenic preparations for internal use.

How Supplied:

Fluid Extract - 1:1

Oil

Tincture - 1:5

Preparation: There is no information on preparation in the literature.

Daily Dosage: 4.5 gm of drug, 1.5 to 3.0 gm of liquid extract (1:1); 1.5 gm of tincture (1:5); 10 to 20 drops of essential oil.

LITERATURE

ANGELICA FRUIT AND HERB

Heck, AM, DeWitt, BA, Lukes, AL. Potential interactions between alternative therapies and warfarin. *Am J Health Syst Pharm.* 2000;57(13):1221-1227.

Amling R, Phytotherapeutika in der Neurologie. In: *ZPT* 12(1):9. 1991.

Ashraf M et al., (1980) *Pak J Sci Ind Res* 23 (1-2):73.

Chang, EH et al., (Eds), Advances in Chinese Medicinal Materials Research, World Scientific Pub. Co. Singapore 1985.

Escher S, Keller U et al., (1979) *Helv Chim Acta* 62 (7):2061.

Glowniak K et al., Localisation and seasonal changes of psoralen in Angelica fruits. In: PM 62, Abstracts of the 44th Ann Congress of GA, 76. 1996.

Lemmich J et al., (1983) *Phytochemistry* 23 (2):553-555.

Leung AY, Encyclopedia of Common Natural Ingredients used in Food Drugs and Cosmetics, John Wiley & Sons Inc., New York, 1980.

Opdyke DLJ, (1975) *Food Cosmet Toxicol*: 13, Suppl 713.

Sethi OP, Shah AK, (1979) *Ind J Pharm Sci* 42 (6): C11.

Shimizu M, Matsuzawa T, Suzuki S, Yoshizaki M, Morita N, Evaluation of Angelicae radix (Touki) by inhibitory effect on platelet aggregation. In: *Chem Pharm Bull* 39:2046. 1991.

Taskinen J, (1975) *Acta Chem Scan* 29 (5):637 et (7) 757.

Tastrup O et al., (1983) *Phytochemistry* 22 (9):2035.

Zotikov YM et al., (1978) *Rastit Resur* 14 (4):579.

ANGELICA ROOT

Amling R, Phytotherapeutika in der Neurologie. In: ZPT 12(1):9. 1991.

Ashraf M et al., (1980) Pak J Sci Ind Res 23 (1-2):73.

Chang, EH et al., (Eds), Advances in Chinese Medicinal Materials Research, World Scientific Pub. Co., Singapore 1985.

Chalchat JC, Garry RPh, J Essent Oil Res 5:447. 1993.

Escher S, Keller U et al., (1979) Helv Chim Acta 62 (7):2061.

Glowniak K et al., Localisation and seasonal changes of psoralen in Angelica fruits. In: PM 62, Abstracts of the 44th Ann Congress of GA, 76. 1996.

Harkar S, Razdan TK, Waight ES, Steroids, chromoines and coumarins from Angelica officinalis. In: PH 23:419-426. 1983.

Härmälä P, Kaltia S, Vuorela H, PM 58:287. 1992.

Lemmich J et al., (1983) Phytochemistry 23 (2):553-555.

Leung AY, Encyclopedia of Common Natural Ingredients used in Food Drugs and Cosmetics, John Wiley & Sons Inc., New York, 1980.

Nykanen I et al., Essent Oil Res 3:229. 1991.

Opdyke DLJ, (1975) Food Cosmet Toxicol: 13, Suppl 713.

Sethi OP, Shah AK, (1979) Ind J Pharm Sci 42 (6):C11.

Shimizu M, Matsuzawa T, Suzuki S, Yoshizaki M, Morita N, Evaluation of Angelicae radix (Touki) by inhibitory effect on platelet aggregation. In: Chem Pharm Bull 39:2046. 1991.

Sun H, Jakupovic J, PA 41:888. 1986.

Taskinen J, (1975) Acta Chem Scan 29 (5):637 et (7) 757.

Tastrup O et al., (1983) Phytochemistry 22 (9):2035.

Zotikov YM et al., (1978) Rastit Resur 14 (4):579.

Angelica archangelica

See Angelica

Angelica sinensis

See Dong Quai

Angostura

Galipea officinalis

DESCRIPTION

Medicinal Parts: The medicinal part is the dried bark of the tree.

Flower and Fruit: The flowers are in terminal, peduncled and closed racemes. The fruit is a 5-valved capsule, of which 2 or 3 valves are often sterile. There are 2 round, black seeds in each capsule and usually only one seed is fertile.

Leaves, Stem and Root: Galipea officinalis is a small 4- to 5-m high tree, which is 7.5 to 12.5 cm in diameter and has a straight trunk and irregular branches. The bark is smooth and gray. It is slightly curved or quilled. The outer layer is sometimes soft and spongy; the inner surface is yellowish-gray. The transverse section is dark brown. The bright green leaves are smooth, glossy, alternate, and petiolate. They sometimes have white spots. The 3 leaflets are oblong, pointed and 4 cm long.

Characteristics: The flowers have a strong scent, which initially resembles that of tobacco. The taste is bitter.

Habitat: Angostura is indigenous to Venezuela and tropical regions of South America.

Production: Angostura is the whole or ground bark of *Galipea officinalis.*

Other Names: Cusparia Bark, True Angostura

ACTIONS AND PHARMACOLOGY

COMPOUNDS

Volatile oil: chief constitents galipol, (-)- cadinene, galipene

Quinolin alkaloids: including cusparine, galipine, galipoline, quinaldine, cuspareine, galipoidine, 1-methyl-2-quinolone

Angustorine (bitter iridoid glycoside)

EFFECTS

Angostura stimulates gastric juices and acts as a tonic. In larger doses, the drug also has an emetic and strong laxative effect.

INDICATIONS AND USAGE

Unproven Uses: Folk medicine indications include diarrhea; it is also used as a febrifuge.

PRECAUTIONS AND ADVERSE REACTIONS

No health hazards or side effects are known in conjunction with the proper administration of designated therapeutic dosages. The administration of larger doses can lead to nausea and vomiting.

LITERATURE

Brieskorn CH, Beck V, (1971) *Phytochemistry* 10:3205.

Hoppe HA, (1975-1987) Drogenkunde, 8. Aufl., Bde 1-3, W. de Gruyter Verlag, Berlin, New York.

Kern W, List PH, Hörhammer L (Hrsg.), Hagers Handbuch der Pharmazeutischen Praxis, 4. Aufl., Bde 1-8, Springer Verlag Berlin, Heidelberg, New York, 1969.

Leung AY, Encyclopedia of Common Natural Ingredients Used in Food Drugs and Cosmetics, John Wiley & Sons Inc. New York 1980.

Madaus G, Lehrbuch der Biologischen Arzneimittel, Bde 1-3, Nachdruck, Georg Olms Verlag Hildesheim 1979.

Roth L, Daunderer M, Kormann K, Giftpflanzen, Pflanzengifte, 4. Aufl., Ecomed Fachverlag Landsberg Lech 1993.

Anise

Pimpinella anisum

DESCRIPTION

Medicinal Parts: The medicinal parts are the essential oil from the ripe fruit and the dried fruit.

Flower and Fruit: The inflorescences are medium-sized umbels with about 7 to 15 scattered pubescent rays. There is usually no involucre, but sometimes there is a single bract. There are barely any sepals. The petals are white, about 15 mm long, and have a ciliate margin. They have small bristles on the outside and a long indented tip. The fruit is downy, ovate to oblong and flattened at the sides.

Leaves, Stem and Root: The plant is an annual herb about 0.5 m high; it is downy all over. The root is thin and fusiform, and the stem is erect, round, and grooved and branched above. The lower leaves are petiolate, orbicular-reniform, entire and coarsely dentate to lobed. The middle leaves are orbicular and 3-lobed, or 3-segmented with ovate or obovate segments. The upper leaves are short-petioled to sessile with narrow sheaths; they are pinnatisect with narrow tips.

Characteristics: The taste is sweet and the odor characteristic.

Habitat: The origin of the plant is unknown but it probably came from the Near East. Today, it is cultivated mainly in southern Europe, Turkey, central Asia, India, China, Japan, and Central and South America.

Production: Anise consists of the dried fruits of *Pimpinella anisum.*

ACTIONS AND PHARMACOLOGY

COMPOUNDS

Volatile oil (2 to 6%): chief constituent trans-anethole (94%), including as well chavicol methyl ether (estragole, 2%), anis aldehyde (1.4%)

Caffeic acid derivatives: including chlorogenic acid (0.1%), other caffeoyl quinic acids

Flavonoids: including apigenin-7-O-glucoside, isoorientin, isovitexin, luteolin-7-O-glucoside

Fatty oil (30%)

Proteic substances (20%)

EFFECTS

The drug is said to have an expectorant, mildly spasmolytic, and antibacterial effect based on the essential oil. The data is empirical and there are no recent studies available.

Aniseed oil (main constituent trans-anethol) has an antibacterial, antiviral, and insect repellent effect and in animal experiments it has been shown to be expectorant, spasmolytic, and estrogenic.

INDICATIONS AND USAGE

Approved by Commission E:

- Common cold
- Cough/bronchitis
- Fevers and colds
- Inflammation of the mouth and pharynx
- Dyspeptic complaints
- Loss of appetite

The drug is used internally for dyspeptic complaints. It is used both internally and externally for catarrhs of the respiratory tract.

Unproven Uses: In folk medicine, Anise is used internally for whooping cough, flatulence, coliclike pain, as a digestive, for menstruation disturbances, liver disease, and tuberculosis.

Homeopathic Uses: Pimpinella anisum is used for shoulder pain and lumbago.

CONTRAINDICATIONS

Anise is contraindicated in patients allergic to Anise and its chief constituent, anethole. Not to be used during pregnancy.

PRECAUTIONS AND ADVERSE REACTIONS

No health hazards or side effects are known in conjunction with the proper administration of designated therapeutic dosages. Sensitization has been observed very rarely. Allergic reactions of the skin, gastrointestinal tract, and breathing passages can occur occasionally.

DRUG INTERACTIONS

MODERATE RISK

Anticoagulants, Antiplatelet agents, Low molecular weight heparins, Thrombolytic agents: Concurrent use may result in increased risk of bleeding. *Clinical management:* Caution is advised. Monitor for signs and symptoms of increased bleeding.

DOSAGE

Mode of Administration: As a comminuted drug for infusions and other galenic preparations for internal use or for inhalation. The purpose of an external application of an Anise preparation is the inhalation of essential oil.

Daily Dosage: Internal average daily dose is 3 g drug (depending on the preparation).

Tea – Drink 1 cup mornings and/or evenings (expectorant); 1 dessertspoon per day (gastrointestinal complaints); infants 1 teaspoon (added to the bottle).

Infusion – single dose: 0.5 to 1 g before meals.

External application – inhalation of the essential oil.

Homeopathic Dosage: 5 drops, 1 tablet, or 10 globules every 30 to 60 minutes (acute) or 1 to 3 times daily (chronic); parenterally: 1 to 2 mL sc acute, 3 times daily; chronic: once a day (HAB1).

LITERATURE

Albert Puleo M, *J Ethnopharmacol*; 1980; 2(4):337.

Czygan FC, Anis (Anisi fructus DAB 10) - *Pimpinella anisum. ZPT*; 1992;13(3):101.

Drinkwater NR, Miller EC, Miller JA, Pitot HC, Hepatocarcinogenicity of estragole and 1′-hydroxyestragole in the mouse and mutagenicity of 1-acetoxystragole in bacteria. *J Natl Canc Inst*; 1976;57:1323-1331.

Garcia-Gonzales JJ, et al. Occupational rhinoconjunctivitis and food allergy because of aniseed sensitization. *Ann Allergy, Asthma & Immunol*; 2002;88:518-522.

Gershbein LL, *Food Cosmet Toxicol*; 1977;15(3):173.

Kartnig T et al., *Planta Med*; 1975;27:1.

Kubeczka KH, Formacek V, New Constituents from the Essential Oils of Pimpinella. In: Brunke EJ (Ed.) Progress in Essential Oil Research, Walter de Gruyter & Co, Berlin 1986.

Reichling J, Merkel B, Elicitor-Induced Formation of Coumarin Derivatives of Pimpinella anisum. *PM*; 1993;59(2):187.

Truhaut R, LeBourhis B, Attia M, Glomot R, Newman J, Caldwell J. Chronic toxicity/carcinogenicity study of trans-anethole in rats. *Food Chem Tox;* 1989;27:11-20.

Antelaea azadirachta

See Neem

Antennaria dioica

See Cat's Foot

Anthoxanthum odoratum

See Sweet Vernal Grass

Anthyllis vulneraria

See Common Kidney Vetch

Aphanes arvensis

See Parsley Piert

Apium graveolens

See Celery

Apocynum cannabinum

See Indian Hemp

Apple Tree

Malus domestica

DESCRIPTION

Medicinal Parts: The medicinal parts are the fresh false fruit, the dried fruit peels, and the inflorescences with their leaves and solid peduncles.

Flower and Fruit: The flowers are umbelled racemes with only a few blossoms. The petals are obovate, up to 2.5 cm long, stemmed, white, pink, or pink on the outside and white on the inside. The carpels are fused with the false fruit.

Leaves, Stem and Root: The plant is a 6- to 10-m high tree or shrub. Boughs and branches are initially villous-haired, later becoming glabrous. The leaves are alternate, ovate, usually shortly acuminate, and finely crenate-serrate.

Habitat: The plant is cultivated in the temperate regions of the Northern Hemisphere, and occasionally grows wild.

Production: Medicinal and pharmaceutical preparations of apples come in liquid and dried pectin forms. The source material is the apple residue with 10% to 20% pectin in the dried mass. The residue is extracted at pH 1.5 to 3 and 60° to 100° C.

ACTIONS AND PHARMACOLOGY

COMPOUNDS: IN THE FRUIT PULP

Fruit acids: the chief acid is malic acid (0.2 to 1.5%); in unripe apples quinic acid; including as well citric acid, succinic acid, lactic acid

Caffeic acid derivatives: including 5-caffeoyl quinic acid

Aromatic substances: in particular 2-trans-hexenal, 3-cis-hexenal, 2-trans-hexenol, 3-cis-hexenol, beta-damascenone, ethyl butyrate, methyl butyric acid hexylester; in some strains, 1-methoxy-4-(2-propenyl)benzole

Pectins

Tannins

Vitamins: in particular ascorbic acid (3 to 30 mg/100 gm)

COMPOUNDS: IN THE SEEDS

Cyanogenic glycoside: amygdalin (0.5 to 1.5%, corresponding to 30 to 90 mg HCN/100 gm)

Fatty oil

EFFECTS

Pectin is a swelling agent. Apple pectins have a mild binding effect.

INDICATIONS AND USAGE

Unproven Uses: Finely ground fruit or preparations that contain liquid or dry pectin are used for milder forms of dyspepsia, diarrhea, and digestive complaints, especially in children.

PRECAUTIONS AND ADVERSE REACTIONS

No health hazards or side effects are known in conjunction with the proper administration of designated therapeutic dosages.

DOSAGE

Mode of Administration: The fruit is available for oral use in the grated or chopped form. The peel can be used in teas. Medicinal and pharmaceutical preparations of apples come in liquid and dried pectin forms.

LITERATURE

Belitz HD, Grosch W, Lehrbuch der Lebensmittelchemie, 4. Aufl., Springer Verlag Berlin, Heidelberg, New York 1992.

Hänsel R, Keller K, Rimpler H, Schneider G (Hrsg.), Hagers Handbuch der Pharmazeutischen Praxis, 5. Aufl., Bde 4-6 (Drogen), Springer Verlag Berlin, Heidelberg, New York, 1992-1994.

Kern W, List PH, Hörhammer L (Hrsg.), Hagers Handbuch der Pharmazeutischen Praxis, 4. Aufl., Bde. 1-8, Springer Verlag Berlin, Heidelberg, New York, 1969.

Madaus G, Lehrbuch der Biologischen Arzneimittel, Bde 1-3, Nachdruck, Georg Olms Verlag Hildesheim 1979.

Roth L, Daunderer M, Kormann K, Giftpflanzen, Pflanzengifte, 4. Aufl., Ecomed Fachverlag Landsberg Lech 1993.

Teuscher E, Lindequist U, Biogene Gifte - Biologie, Chemie, Pharmakologie, 2. Aufl., Fischer Verlag Stuttgart 1994.

Aquilegia vulgaris

See Columbine

Arachis hypogaea

See Peanut

Aralia racemosa

See Spikenard

Arctium lappa

See Burdock

Arctostaphylos uva-ursi

See Uva-Ursi

Areca catechu

See Areca Nut

Areca Nut

Areca catechu

DESCRIPTION

Medicinal Parts: The medicinal part of the plant is the nut.

Flower and Fruit: The plant is an erect palm growing up to 30 m high. The trunk has a girth of about 50 cm. The numerous feathery leaflets are 30 to 60 cm long, confluent and glabrous. The flowers are on branching spadix. The male flowers are numerous and appear above, the female flowers are solitary and appear below. The ovoid drupe has a fibrous layer under the yellow shell and a one-seeded stone. The seeds are conical or nearly spherical and about 2.5 cm in diameter. They are very hard, and contain a deep brown testa with fawn marbling.

Characteristics: The taste is slightly acrid and astringent, and the odor faint.

Habitat: The plant is found in the East Indies, cultivated in parts of Asia and eastern Africa.

Production: Areca or Betel Nuts are the fresh seeds of *Areca catechu*.

Not to be Confused With: Piper Betel, also called Betel, the leaf of which is chewed.

Other Names: Betel Nut, Pinang

ACTIONS AND PHARMACOLOGY

COMPOUNDS

Pyridine alkaloids: arecoline, guvacoline (ester alkaloids), as well as arecaidine, guvacine

Tannins: catechin type

EFFECTS

The drug acts on the parasympathetic nervous system with an effect that is more muscarinic than nicotinic. It stimulates secretion in the salivary, bronchial, and intestinal glands and causes tremors and bradycardia. Chewing mouthfuls of betel leads to a saponification of the ester alkaloids and the resulting arecaidine produces euphoria. The drug also causes cramps in the muscles of intestinal parasites and stimulates the vagus nerve. Central nervous system stimulation has been observed in mice.

INDICATIONS AND USAGE

Unproven Uses: Betel Nut is no longer frequently prescribed in human medicine. Nevertheless, because of their intoxicating qualities, the nuts are chewed as a recreational drug by an estimated 450 million people. Fresh slices of the seed are part of the "betel titbit" used in eastern Asia. (Arecoline is converted in the central nervous system to the stimulant arecaidine through chewing.) That practice is being discouraged because of its link with some forms of oral cancer. In veterinary medicine, the drug is used as a vermifuge for tape worms in cattle and dogs, as well as for intestinal colic in horses.

Chinese Medicine: Uses in Chinese medicine include chronic hepatitis, edema, oliguria, diarrhea, and digestive problems.

Indian Medicine: The juice of young seeds is used as a laxative in Indian medicine. A decoction of the root is used for cracked lips.

PRECAUTIONS AND ADVERSE REACTIONS

Due to its arecoline content, the drug appears parasympathomimetic. It leads to increased salivation, in high doses to bradycardia, tremor, reflex excitability, spasms, and eventual paralysis. Long-term use of the drug as a stimulant can result in malignant tumors of the oral cavity through formation of nitrosamines. When the nuts are chewed, the mouth and lips are stained red, as are the feces.

OVERDOSAGE

The toxic dose for humans is 8 to 10 g of the drug. Atropine is given as the antidote. Chewing the ''nut'' leads to a saponification of the ester alkaloids. The resulting arecaidine produces euphoria.

DOSAGE

Mode of Administration: In the past, Areca Nut was used in chewing balm for gum disease and as a vermifuge. Today, it is used as a vermifuge only in veterinary medicine for house pets. Therapeutic use is insignificant.

Storage: Must be stored separately, protected from light and in well-sealed containers.

LITERATURE

Aue W, *Pharm Zentralhalle* 136:728. 1967.

Hirono I, *J Environ Sci Health* C3(2):145. 1985.

Huang JL, McLeish MJ, *J Chromatogr* 475:447. 1989.

Juptner H, (1968) Z Tropenmed Parasit 19:254.

Lewin L, Über Areca catechu, Chavica Betle und das Betelkauen. In: Monographie, Stuttgart, F. Enke, 1889.

Schneider E, *PUZ* 15:161. 1986.

Arenaria Rubra

Spergularia rubra

DESCRIPTION

Medicinal Parts: The medicinal part is the herb.

Flower and Fruit: The bracts of the inflorescence are almost as large as the leaves. The sepals and petals are 3 to 4 mm. The petals are usually pink, sometimes white. There are 5 to 10 stamens. The capsule is 4 to 5 mm and about equal in size to the sepals. The seeds are 0.45 to 0.55 mm, unwinged, dark brown, subtrigonal, and more or less flattened.

Leaves, Stem and Root: The plant is annual or perennial, with a slender to somewhat woody taproot, which is smooth and somewhat sticky. From beneath, it produces numerous 5- to 22-cm long, diffuse, decumbent or procumbent stems. The leaves are narrow, linear, and have very short, lanceolate, acute, silver, scarious stipules.

Habitat: The plant is common in Europe, Russia, Australia, North America and Asia.

Production: Arenaria Rubra is the aerial part of *Spergularia rubra.*

Other Names: Common Sandspurry, Sabline Rouge, Sandwort

ACTIONS AND PHARMACOLOGY

COMPOUNDS

Triterpene saponins

Resins

EFFECTS

The herb has diuretic effects.

INDICATIONS AND USAGE

Unproven Uses: Arenaria Rubra is used for conditions of the urinary tract, such as cystitis, dysuria, and urinary calculus.

PRECAUTIONS AND ADVERSE REACTIONS

No health hazards or side effects are known in conjunction with the proper administration of designated therapeutic dosages.

DOSAGE

Mode of Administration: The herb is used internally as a liquid extract.

LITERATURE

Kern W, List PH, Hörhammer L (Hrsg.), Hagers Handbuch der Pharmazeutischen Praxis, 4. Aufl., Bde 1-8: Springer Verlag Berlin, Heidelberg, New York, 1969.

Arisaema triphyllum

See Jack-in-the-Pulpit

Aristolochia clematitis

See Birthwort

Arjun Tree

Terminalia arjuna

DESCRIPTION

Medicinal Parts: The medicinal parts of the tree are the bark and fruit.

Flower and Fruit: The flowers are arranged in upright, apical panicles. The upper flowers of the panicles are usually only male. The flowers are small and fused; their structures are in fours or fives. The sepals are almost glabrous; the calyx tube has 4 to 5 short, triangular lobes. The petals are inconspicuous. There are 10 stamens and inferior, single-chambered, brownish or reddish pubescent ovary. The style is long and projects above the bud. The fruit is over 2-cm long, a glabrous, ovoid 4- to 5-sided drupe with 5 thick, narrow wings.

Leaves, Stem and Root: Arjun tree grows up to 30 m high. The leaves are opposite, 12 to 30 cm long and coriaceous with approximately 6-mm long petioles, which have 2 glands at the upper end. The lamina is elongate-elliptical, blunt or with a short tip. The base is narrow or cordate and has a finely crenate margin. The trunk is grooved with a thick bark.

Habitat: India

Production: Arjun Tree bark is the dried trunk bark of *Terminalia arjuna*. It is collected in wild areas.

Other Names: White Murda

ACTIONS AND PHARMACOLOGY

COMPOUNDS

Tannins: gallotannins, ellagitannins

Steroids: sterols, including beta-sitosterol

Triterpenes: arjunolic acid and its glucosides, oleanolic acid

Flavonoids: including arjunolon, baicalein

EFFECTS

Clinical experiments with the bark powder have demonstrated efficacy against congestive cardiac insufficiency and hypertonia. Various extracts caused lowered blood pressure, bradycardia, and positively inotropic effects in animal experiments. Spasmolytic and hemostyptic qualities have also been described. The substance is said to be sedative and potentiates the activity of barbiturates.

INDICATIONS AND USAGE

Indian Medicine: Arjun tree is used for fractures, ulcers, discharge of the urethra, leukorrhea, diabetes, anemia, cardiopathy, hyperhydrosis, asthma, bronchitis, states of exhaustion, tumors, dysentery, internal and external hemorrhaging, liver cirrhosis, and high blood pressure.

PRECAUTIONS AND ADVERSE REACTIONS

No health hazards are known in conjunction with the proper administration of designated therapeutic dosages.

DOSAGE

Mode of Administration: Powdered drug and liquid preparations for internal use.

Preparation: The following basic forms are used in Indian medicine in many compound preparations.

Arjunatvagadi – An aqueous decoction.

Pardhadyaristam – An aqueous decoction with grapes and final fermentation.

Arjunaghrtam – A paste of the powdered drug with purified butter, heated and filtered.

Arjunatvak – The powdered drug.

Daily Dosage: Since the Indian medicine is dosed according to the individual patient, there is no exact information available. There was, however, one study carried out with a daily dose of 3.88 gm powdered drug.

LITERATURE

Bharani A, Ganguly A, Bhargava KD, Salutary effect of Terminalia Arjuna in patients with severe refractory heart failure. *Int J Cardiol,* 49:191-9, 1995 May.

Chauhan S, Agarwal S, Mathur R, Vasal assault due to Terminalia arjuna W. & A. bark in albino rats. *Andrologia*, 53:491-4, 1990 Sep-Oct.

Dwivedi S, Jauhari R, Beneficial effects of Terminalia arjuna in coronary artery disease. *Indian Heart J*, 49:507-10, 1997 Sep-Oct.

Hänsel R, Keller K, Rimpler H, Schneider G (Ed), Hagers Handbuch der Pharmazeutischen Praxis, 5. Aufl., Bde 4 - 6 (Drogen), Springer Verlag Berlin, Heidelberg, New York, 1992-1994.

Kandil FE, Nassar MI, A tannin anti-cancer promoter from *Terminalia arjuna*. Phytochemistry, 53:1567-8, 1998 Apr.

Kaur S, Grover IS, Kumar S, Antimutagenic potential of ellagic acid isolated from *Terminalia arjuna. Indian J Exp Biol*, 53:478-82, 1997 May.

Pettit GR, Hoard MS, Doubek DL, Schmidt JM, Pettit RK, Tackett LP, Chapuis JC, Antineoplastic agents 338. The cancer cell growth inhibitory constituents of *Terminalia arjuna* (Combretaceae). *J Ethnopharmacol*, 53:57-63, 1996 Aug.

Pettit GR, Hoard MS, Doubek DL, Schmidt JM, Pettit RK, Tackett LP, Chapuis JC, Hypocholesterolaemic effects of Terminalia arjuna tree bark. *J Ethnopharmacol*, 53:165-9, 1997 Feb.

Pettit GR, Hoard MS, Doubek DL, Schmidt JM, Pettit RK, Tackett LP, Chapuis JC, On the ethnomedical significance of the Arjun tree, *Terminalia arjuna* (Roxb.) Wight & Arnot. *J Ethnopharmacol*, 53:173-90, 1987 Jul.

Seth SD, Maulik M, Katiyar CK, Maulik SK, Role of Lipistat in protection against isoproterenol induced myocardial necrosis in rats: a biochemical and histopathological study. *Indian J Physiol Pharmacol*, 42:101-6, 1998 Jan.

Singh N, Kapur KK, Singh SP, Shanker K, Sinha JN, Kohli RP, Mechanism of cardiovascular action of *Terminalia arjuna. Planta Med,* 53:102-4, 1982 Jun.

Srivastava N, Prakash D, Behl HM, Biochemical contents, their variation and changes in free amino acids during seed germination in *Terminalia arjuna. Int J Food Sci Nutr*, 53:215-9, 1997 May.

Armoracia rusticana

See Horseradish

Arnica

Arnica montana

DESCRIPTION

Medicinal Parts: The medicinal parts of Arnica are the ethereal oil of the flowers, the dried flowers, the leaves collected before flowering and dried, the roots, and the dried rhizome and roots.

Flower and Fruit: The terminal composite flower is found in the leaf axils of the upper pair of leaves. They have a diameter of 6 to 8 cm, are usually egg yolk-yellow to orange-yellow, but occasionally light yellow. The receptacle and epicalyx are hairy. The 10 to 20 female ray flowers are linguiform. In addition, there are about 100 disc flowers, which are tubular. The 5-ribbed fruit is black-brown and has a bristly tuft of hair.

Leaves, Stem, and Root: Arnica is an herbaceous plant growing 20 to 50 cm high. The brownish rhizome that is 0.5 cm thick by 10 cm long, usually unbranched, in 3 sections, and sympodial. The rhizome may also be 3-headed with many yellow-brown secondary roots. Leaves are in basal rosettes. They are in 2 to 3 crossed opposite pairs and are obovate and entire-margined with 5 protruding vertical ribs. The glandular-haired stem has 2 to 6 smaller leaves, which are ovate to lanceolate, entire-margined or somewhat dentate.

Characteristics: The flower heads are aromatic; the taste is bitter and irritating.

Habitat: Arnica is found in Europe from Scandinavia to southern Europe. It is also found in southern Russia and central Asia.

Production: Arnica flower consists of the fresh or dried inflorescence of *Arnica montana* or *Arnica chamissonis.* The flower should be dried quickly at 45° to 50°C.

Not to be Confused With: Other yellow-flowering Asteracea.

Other Names: Arnica Flowers, Arnica Root, Leopard's Bane, Mountain Tobacco, Wolfsbane

ACTIONS AND PHARMACOLOGY

COMPOUNDS

Sesquiterpene lactones of the pseudo-guaianolid-type: particularly esters of the helenalin- and 11,13-dihydrohelenalins with short-chained fatty acids such as acetic acid, isobutyric acid, 2- methyl-butyric acid, methylacrylic acid, isovaleric acid or tiglic acid

Volatile oil: with thymol, thymol esters, free fatty acids

Polyynes: including tri-dec-1-en-penta-3,5,7,9 11-in

Hydroxycumarines

Caffeic acid derivatives: including chlorogenic acid, 1,5-dicaffeoyl quinic acid

Flavonoids: numerous flavone and flavonol glycosides and their aglycones

EFFECTS

Arnica preparations have demonstrated wound-healing, antiseptic, and mild analgesic properties in animal and in vitro studies when applied topically. The flavonoid bonds, essential oils, and polyynes may also be involved. In cases of inflammation, Arnica preparations also show analgesic and antiseptic activity. The sesquiterpenes (helenalin) in the drug have an antimicrobial effect in vitro and an antiphlogistic effect in animal tests. A respiratory-analeptic, uterine tonic and cardiovascular effect (increase of contraction amplitude with simultaneous increase in frequency, i.e., positive inotropic effect) was demonstrated. Further in vitro and in vivo studies of Arnica preparations or isolated ingredients have shown antiaggregatory, immunostimulatory, cytotoxic, cardiotonic, and antioxidative effects. More controlled and comparative studies are necessary to define optimal therapies and to determine Arnica's place in therapy.

Analgesic Effects: The mild analgesic properties of Arnica flowers and its preparations are mainly attributed to the sesquiterpene lactones helenalin and dihydrohelenalin (Wichtl, 1997). Writhe reflex tests in mice demonstrated a marked analgesic action (Fachinformation Arthrosenex AR, 1998).

Anti-inflammatory Effects: The anti-inflammatory effect of the sesquiterpene lactone helenalin was found to be due to molecular mechanisms preventing the release of the transcription factor NF-kB (an immune regulator). Helenalin inhibited the release of IkB (an inhibitory subunit) by modification of the NF-kB/IkB complex, resulting in a suppression of the immune regulator NF-kB (Lyss et al, 1997; Schaffner, 1997). Helenalin inhibited the oxidative phosphorylation, chemotaxis, and mobility of human polymorphonuclear neutrophiles. It contributed to a reduction of the size of inflamed areas by stabilizing lysosomal membranes and was thought to possess therapeutic efficacy in the treatment of chronic arthritis. (Fachinformation Arthrosenex AR, 1998).

Antiseptic Effects: The wound-healing and antiseptic properties of Arnica flowers and its preparations are mainly attributed to the sesquiterpene lactones helenalin and dihydrohelenalin and related esters, which demonstrated bactericidal (e.g. salmonella) and fungicidal activity (Anon, 1998; Wichtl, 1997).

Immunostimulant Effects: Polysaccharides containing 65% to 100% galacturonic acid isolated from Arnica flowers caused a modification of the immune system response by inhibition of the complement system and a marked enhancement of phagocytic activity in vivo (Anon, 1998). Compounds of Arnica were found to stimulate macrophages to excrete tumor necrosis factor (Puhlmann et al, 1991).

CLINICAL TRIALS

Gonarthrosis

Gonarthrosis has been treated effectively by intra-articular injections of a combination preparation containing Arnica. Intra-articular injection of a homeopathic combination preparation containing extracts of *Arnica montana, Sanguinaria canadensis, Solanum dulcamara,* sulfur, and Toxicodendron quercifolium (Zeel comp®) had beneficial effects in the treatment of 446 patients with gonarthrosis. A mean dose of 2 injections per week was administered for a mean length of therapy of 4 to 5 weeks. Pain and joint stiffness improved in 90% of the patients. The combination preparation was tolerated well and had a favorable side effect profile compared to other commonly prescribed medications. No adverse effects have been recorded except for local reversible knee irritations (Anon, 1996).

Myalgia

Several double-blind, randomized, placebo-controlled studies failed to find beneficial effects of homeopathic Arnica preparations in the prevention and treatment of delayed-onset muscle soreness (Vickers et al, 1998; Vickers et al, 1997; Gulick et al, 1996).

Similar results were obtained with homeopathic Arnica 30X therapy of delayed onset muscle soreness in 519 runners in a double-blind, placebo-controlled randomized study. Five pills (either a placebo or Arnica) were taken two times daily starting the evening before the race for 5 days. The level of muscle soreness was determined by a 7-point Likert scale (a list of descriptives for level of muscle soreness). No differences between the Arnica group and the placebo group were found for Leikert scores or race time (Vickers et al, 1998).

Homeopathic therapy was ineffective in the treatment of delayed onset muscle soreness in a double-blind, placebo-controlled, randomized study of 68 volunteers who underwent a 10-minute period of bench stepping carrying a small weight. The patients were treated either with one tablet of a homeopathic complex of Arnica 30C, Rhus toxicodendron (Rhus tox) 30C, sarcolactic acid 30C three times daily, or placebo. Mean muscle soreness was assessed over a 5-day period following the exercise. No significant differences between homeopathic therapy and placebo were found (Vickers et al, 1997).

Neither topical *Arnica montana* ointment nor sublingual *Arnica montana* pellets have been effective in abating the signs and symptoms of delayed onset muscle soreness after forearm extensor muscle exercise on a Lido isokinetic dynamometer in a placebo-controlled, randomized study of 70 untrained volunteers. Patients were assigned to various treatment techniques. In the two Arnica groups, patients either received a thin layer (approximately 0.5 g) of 0.4% topical *Arnica montana* ointment on the posterior forearm every 8 hours or three sublingual *Arnica montana* pellets 6C every 8 hours for three days. Data on active and passive wrist flexion and extension, forearm girth, limb volume, visual analog pain scale, muscle soreness index, isometric strength, concentric and eccentric wrist total work, concentric and eccentric wrist average peak torque, and concentric and eccentric angle of peak torque were collected in the beginning and at the end of the exercise and 20 minutes, 24, 48 and 72 hours after treatment. No significant differences were found between the therapy regimens and the control group (Gulick et al, 1996).

Combination therapy consisting of Arnica and Rhus tox 30C produced beneficial effects in the treatment of delayed onset muscle soreness in a randomized, double-blind, placebo-controlled study of 50 volunteers undergoing vigorous bench stepping exercise. One tablet of the homeopathic preparation was administered 3 times daily, starting 24 hours before the exercise. The differences, however, between homeopathic therapy and placebo did not reach statistical significance (Jawara, 1997).

Pain Management

Three randomized, placebo-controlled, double-blind clinical trials were carried out sequentially at a single primary care unit specializing in knee surgery to determine the effectiveness of homeopathic Arnica on postoperative swelling and pain following knee surgery of one of the following three types: arthroscopy (ART; n=227), artificial knee joint implantation (AKJ; n=35), or cruciate ligament reconstruction (CLR; n=57). All participants received either placebo or homeopathic Arnica prior to the procedure (1 X 5 globules) of the homeopathic dilution 30x followed by 3 x 5 globules daily. Those randomized to receive the Arnica prior to the procedure showed a trend towards less postoperative swelling compared to patients receiving placebo—although this difference was only significant for the patients randomized to get homeopathic Arnica in the CLR group (Brinkhaus, 2006).

A small but statistically significant decrease in pain score compared to placebo was reported in a randomized trial of homeopathic Arnica for post-tonsillectomy analgesia at a tertiary referral center. The 190 tonsillectomy patients received either Arnica 30c or placebo (2 tablets 6 times in post-operative day followed by 2 tablets twice daily for subsequent 7 days). Questionnaires from 111 patients were available for analysis. A significantly ($p<0.05$) larger drop in pain score from postoperative day 1 to 14 (28.3) was recorded by the Arnica group compared to the placebo group (pain score 23.8). Variables such as quantity of analgesia and antibiotics used, number of days to return to work and or return to normal swallowing were not significantly different between the treatment to placebo group (Robertson, 2007).

No differences in pain or hand function improvement were detected after 21 days of treatment with either topical gel preparations of ibuprofen 5% or Arnica 50 g tincture/100g, DER 1:20 in a randomized, double-blind study in 204 individuals with confirmed and active osteoarthritis of interphalangeal joints of the hands. Adverse event rates were similar, with six patients using ibuprofen and five patients using Arnica reporting problems (Widrig, 2007).

A gel preparation of Arnica flowers applied externally to the limbs of 12 male volunteers was more effective than placebo in the treatment of muscle ache. In a randomized, double-blind, placebo-controlled study, 89 patients with venous insufficiency received Arnica gel (20% tincture) or placebo. It was reported that Arnica treatment produced improvements in venous tone, edema and in feeling of heaviness in the legs. (Barnes et al, 2002).

No significant differences in postoperative pain and infection management between homeopathic therapy with Arnica 30C and placebo were found in a randomized, placebo-controlled, double-blind study of 93 women undergoing total abdominal hysterectomy. Two doses of Arnica 30C or placebo were administered 24 hours before surgery followed by 3 daily doses for 5 days. With homeopathic treatment, 76% of the patients had to take additional antibiotics, compared to 71% in the placebo group; and mean pain scores were 32.6 for Arnica and 31.0 for placebo (Hart et al, 1997).

Homeopathic remedies including Arnica D30 have been ineffective in pain management of 24 patients undergoing oral surgical procedures in a randomized, double-blind, placebo-controlled study. Postoperative pain measured by visual analog scales and postoperative recovery assessed by swelling, bleeding, and the ability to open the mouth was not significantly affected by homeopathic therapy. The treatment regimen consisted of one dose of 3 tablets administered quarterly for the first 3 hours, thereafter 1 dose per hour until bedtime, and 2 doses on the following morning at an interval of 3 hours. Treatment continued with 4 daily doses (Loekken et al, 1995). Homeopathic Arnica preparations had no effect on surgically induced trauma after total abdominal hysterectomy or bilateral oral surgery.

Retinopathy, Diabetic

Two clinical studies demonstrated beneficial effects of homeopathic Arnica therapy in the treatment of diabetic retinopathy (Zicari et al, 1998; Zicari, 1997). Homeopathic Arnica 5CH therapy produced statistically significant improvement in retinal sensitivity and functional improvement in the peripheral retinal areas in a double-masked, randomized, placebo-controlled study of 29 insulin-dependent diabetes mellitus patients with diabetic retinopathy. Either 3 pearls of Arnica 5CH per day or placebo were administered three times daily for three months. No significant differences regarding intraocular pressure, ophthalmoscopic appearance, or metabolic condition between the placebo group and the Arnica group were recorded (Zicari et al, 1998; Zicari, 1997).

A statistically significant increase of red critical retinal flicker fusion was found in a study of 30 non-insulin-dependent diabetes mellitus patients after three months of therapy with Arnica 5CH. A daily dose of 3 pearls of Arnica 5CH or placebo was administered. Intraocular pressure and ophthalmoscopic appearance were not affected by Arnica therapy, but the metabolic condition improved during placebo therapy (Zicari, 1995).

Trauma

Homeopathic Arnica preparations had no effect on surgically induced trauma after total abdominal hysterectomy or bilateral oral surgery (Hart et al, 1997; Loekken et al, 1995).

INDICATIONS AND USAGE

Approved by Commission E:

- Fever and colds
- Inflammation of the skin
- Cough/bronchitis
- Inflammation of the mouth and pharynx
- Rheumatism
- Common cold
- Blunt injuries
- Tendency to infection

Unproven Uses: External folk medicine uses include consequences of injury such as traumatic edema, hematoma, contusions, as well as rheumatic muscle and joint problems. Other applications are inflammation of the oral and throat region, furunculosis, inflammation caused by insect bites and phlebitis. In Russian folk medicine, the drug is used to treat uterine hemorrhaging. Furthermore, the drug is used for myocarditis, arteriosclerosis, angina pectoris, exhaustion, cardiac insufficiency, sprains, and contusions and for hair loss due to psychological causes. While some uses are plausible, most have not been proved.

CONTRAINDICATIONS

Arnica is contraindicated in people with a known sensitivity to members of the daisy family, such as chamomile, marigold, or yarrow.

Pregnancy: Arnica preparations not to be used during pregnancy.

PRECAUTIONS AND ADVERSE REACTIONS

Arnica preparations should not be administered on mucous membranes, eyes, or damaged skin.

Frequent administration, in particular of the undiluted tincture, as well as with contacts with the plant, lead to sensitization. Prolonged topical administration on damaged skin, e.g., in injuries or ulcus cruris (indolent leg ulcers) may cause eczema and edematous dermatitis with the formation of pustules. Arnica preparations may cause cardiac arrhythmia, tremor, dizziness, and collapse when used internally at doses higher than those recommended. Oral administration is considered to be potentially unsafe, and ingestion of parts of the whole plant or of Arnica preparations has been reported to cause gastroenteritis, stomach pain, severe diarrhea, vomiting, cardiac arrest and death.

DRUG INTERACTIONS

MINOR RISK

Anticoagulants, Antiplatelets, Low Molecular Weight Heparins, and Thrombolytic Agents: Concomitant use of Arnica may result in increased risk of bleeding. *Clinical Management:* Arnica is generally used as a homeopathic or external preparation and may not be ingested in quantities large enough to cause an interaction. Due to limited data, monitor patients taking Arnica with antiplatelet agents for signs and symptoms of excessive bleeding.

OVERDOSAGE

Overdoses taken internally can lead to poisonings, characterized by severe mucous membrane irritation (vomiting, diarrhea, mucous membrane hemorrhage) and a brief stimulation of cardiac activity followed by cardiac muscle palsy. For that reason, internal administration of the drug is strongly discouraged. High dose Arnica therapy may cause arrhythmia and tachycardia.

DOSAGE

Mode of Administration: Arnica is used in the form of the whole herb, cut herb or herb powder for infusions, extracts, and tinctures; gel, oil, and poultice for external application.

How Supplied: Commercial pharmaceutical preparations include gels, ointments, tinctures, oils, and plasters.

Preparation: Arnica tincture (3x to 10x dilutions with water) is used to prepare a poultice. A tincture is prepared using 1 part Arnica flowers and 10 parts ethanol 70% v/v (according to DAB 10). Arnica oil is an extract of 1 part herb and 5 parts slightly warmed fatty oil. Ointments are made up with up to 15% Arnica oil or with 10 to 25% tinctures in a neutral ointment base. Mouthwashes are prepared as a tincture in 10x dilution.

Daily Dose: Tincture for cataplasm: tincture in 3x to 10x dilution. For mouth rinses: tincture in 10x dilution. Ointments should contain a maximum of 15% Arnica oil.

Storage: When stored, the drug should be tightly sealed and protected from light.

LITERATURE

Barnes J, Andersen LA, Phillipson Jd. Herbal Medicines. A Guide for Health Care Professionals, 2nd ed. London: Pharmaceutical Press. 2002

Beekman AC et al. Structure-cytotoxicity relationship of some helenanolide-type sesquiterpene lactones. In: *JNP* 60(3): 252-257. 1997

Brinkhaus B, Wilkens JM, Ludtke R, et al. Homeopathic arnica therapy in patients receiving knee surgery: Results of three randomized double-blind trials. *Complementary Therapies in Medicine;* 14, 237-247. 2006.

Ernst E. Possible interactions between synthetic and herbal medicinal products. Part I: a systematic review of the evidence. *Perfusion*; 13:4-15. 2000

Fachinformation: Arthrosenex(R) AR, ARNICA extract. Brenner-Efaka Pharma GmbH, Muenster, Germany, 1998

Gulick DT, Kimura IF, Sitler M et al. Various treatment techniques on signs and symptoms of delayed onset muscle soreness. *J Athletic Training*; 31:145-152. 1996

Haraguchi H, Ishikawa H, Sanchez Y et al. Antioxidative constituents in *Heterotheca inuloides. Bioorg Medicinal Chem*; 5(5):865-871. 1997

Hart O, Mullee MA, Lewith G et al. Double-blind, placebo-controlled randomized clinical trial of homeopathic Arnica C30 for pain and infection after total abdominal hysterectomy. *J R Soc Med*; 90(2): 73-78. 1997

Hausen BM. A 6-year experience with compositae mix. *Am J Contact Dermatitis*; 7(2):94-99. 1996

Hörmann HP, Kortin HC, Allergic acute contact dermatitis due to Arnica tincture self-medication. Phytomedicine 4:315-317. 1995

Jawara N, Lewith GT, Vickers AJ et al. Homeopathic Arnica and Rhus toxicodendron for delayed onset muscle soreness. *Br Hom J*; 86:10-15. 1997

Lokken P, Straumsheim PA, Tveiten D et al. Effect of homeopathy on pain and other events after acute trauma: placebo controlled trial with bilateral oral surgery. *BMJ*; 310(6992): 1439-1442. 1995

Lyss G, Schmidt TJ, Merfort I, Pahl HL. Helenalin an anti-inflammatory sesquiterpene lactone from Arnica selectively inhibits transcription factor NF-kappaB. *Biol Chem;* 378:951-61. 1997

Lyss G, Schmidt TJ, Merfort I, Pahl HL. Immunologic studies of plant combination preparations. In-vitro and in-vivo studies on the stimulation of phagocytosis. *Arzneimittelforschung;* 378:1072-6, 1991.

Lyss G, Schmidt TJ, Merfort I, Pahl HL, Postpartum homeopathic Arnica montana: a potency-finding pilot study. Br J Clin Pract; 378:951-61. 1997

Puhlmann J, Zenk MH & Wagner H. Immunologically active polysaccharides of Arnica montana cell cultures. *Phytochemistry*; 30(4): 1141-1145. 1991

Robertson A, Suryanarayanan R, Banerjee A. Homeopathic Arnica Montana for post-tonsillectomy analgesia: a randomized placebo control trial. *Homeopathy*; 96(1):17-21. 2007.

Robles M, Aregullin M, West J et al. Recent studies on the zoopharmacognosy, pharmacology and neurotoxicology of sesquiterpene lactones. *Planta Med*; 61:199-203. 1995

Schaffner W. Granny's remedy explained at the molecular level: helenalin inhibits NF-kappaB. *Biol Chem*; 378(9): 935. 1997

Schmidt Th J et al. Sesquiterpen lactones and inositol esters from *Arnica angustifolia*. In: *PM* 61(6): 544-550. 1995

Schroder H, Losche W, Strobach H et al. Helenalin and 11-alpha, 13-dihydrohelenalin, two constituents from *Arnica montana L.*, inhibit human platelet function via thiol-dependent pathways. *Thromb Res*; 57:839-845. 1990

Tveiten D, Bruseth S, Borchgrevink CF, L hne K. Effect of Arnica D 30 during hard physical exertion. A double-blind randomized trial during the Oslo Marathon 1990. *Tidsskr Nor Laegeforen;* 111:3630-1, Dec 10, 1991

Vickers AJ, Fisher P, Smith C et al. Homeopathic Arnica 30x is ineffective for muscle soreness after long-distance running: a randomized, double blind, placebo-controlled trial. *Clin J Pain*; 14(3): 227-231. 1998

Vickers AJ, Fisher P, Smith C et al. Homeopathy for delayed onset muscle soreness: a randomized double-blind placebo controlled trial. *Br J Sports Med*; 31(4):304-307. 1997

Weil D, Reuter HD, Einflu bβ von Arnika-Extrakt und Helenalin auf die Funktion menschlicher Blutplättchen. In: *ZPT* 9(1): 26. 1988

Weiss RF. Herbal Medicine. Gothenburg, Sweden: Ab Arcanum and Beaconsfield, UK: Beaconsfield Publishers Ltd,:169. 1988

Wichtl M. Arnicae flos. Herbal Drugs and Phytopharmaceuticals. CRC Press, Boca Raton, FL, USA, 1994:83-87. Willuhn G et al., *Planta Med* 50 (1): 35. 1984

Widrig R, et al. Choosing between NSAID and arnica for topical treatment of hand osteoarthritis in a randomised, double-blind study. *Rheumatol Int.* 27(6):585-91. 2007.

Willuhn G, Leven W, Luley C. Arnikablüten DAB 10. Untersuchung zur qualitativen und quantitativen Variabilität des Sesquiterepnelactongehaltes der offizinellen Arzneidroge. In: *DAZ* 134(42): 4077. 1994

Willuhn G, Leven W. Qualität von Arnikazubereitungen. In: *DAZ* 135(21): 1939-1942. 1995

Woerdenbag HJ et al. Cytotoxicity of flavonoids and sesquiterpene lactones from Arnica species. In: *PM* 59(7): A681. 1993

Woerdenbag H, Merfort I, Passreiter C et al. Cytotoxicity of flavonoids and sesquiterpene lactones from Arnica species against the GLC4 and the COLO 320 cell lines. *Planta Med*; 60(5):434-437. 1994

Zicari D, Comps P, Del Beato R et al. Arnica 5CH activity on retinal function. *Invest Ophthalmol Visual Science*; 38:767. 1997

Zicari D, Comps P, Del Beato R et al. Diabetic retinopathy treated with Arnica 5CH Microdoses. *Invest Ophthalmol Visual Science.* 1998

Arnica montana

See Arnica

Arrach

Chenopodium vulvaria

DESCRIPTION

Medicinal Parts: The whole fresh, flowering plant has medicinal properties.

Flower and Fruit: The flowers are small, yellow-green and inconspicuous. They grow in clusters in leafless, compact spikes at the tip of the stem. The fruit is enclosed by the involucre. The seeds are black and glossy.

Leaves, Stem and Root: The plant is 15 to 40 cm high. The stems are branched from low down. The leaves are broad, rhomboid, entire-margined and petiolate. The whole plant is floury-dusty.

Characteristics: Arrach has a distinctive unpleasant smell of musty herring brine.

Habitat: Europe, northern Africa and the Caucacus

Production: Arrach is the complete flowering plant of *Chenopodium vulvaria.*

Other Names: Stinking Arrach, Stinking Goosefoot, Dog's Arrach, Goat's Arrach, Goosefoot, Stinking Motherwort, Netchweed, Oraches

ACTIONS AND PHARMACOLOGY

COMPOUNDS

Mono-, di- and trimethylamine: only in the fresh plant due to their volatility

Betaine

Tannins

EFFECTS

No substantiated information is available.

INDICATIONS AND USAGE

Unproven Uses: Arrach is used internally and externally to relieve cramps and as an emmenagogue.

PRECAUTIONS AND ADVERSE REACTIONS

No health hazards or side effects are known in conjunction with the proper administration of designated therapeutic dosages. The offensive smell often precludes continued use.

DOSAGE

Mode of Administration: Arrach is used externally and as an extract.

LITERATURE

Roth L, Daunderer M, Kormann K, Giftpflanzen, Pflanzengifte, 4. Aufl., Ecomed Fachverlag Landsberg Lech 1993.

Arrowroot

Maranta arundinacea

DESCRIPTION

Medicinal Parts: The medicinal parts are the starch from the rhizome tubers and the dried rhizome.

Flower and Fruit: The flowers are in pairs, 3.5 cm long, and pedicled. They have 3 green, lanceolate sepals and a white, tubular-fused corolla with 1 hanging and 2 erect tips. The stamens are in 2 circles; the first consists of 2 petal-like staminoids, the second appears hoodlike. There is 1 thickened stamen partly developed like a petal. The ovary is inferior and 3-sectioned. Only 1 carpel is developed. The fruit is 1-valved and has 1 seed.

Leaves, Stem and Root: The plant is an herbaceous perennial, 1- to 2-m high with thin, reedlike, branched and canelike stems. The rhizome produces, along with the usual root, a sturdy, fusiform, swollen tuber up to 8 cm thick and 35 cm long. The tuber is thickly covered with whitish, scaly stipules. The leaves are obovate, light green, lightly pubescent, and short-petioled. They have long sheaths and ovate-lanceolate leaf blades up to 13 cm long.

Habitat: The plant is indigenous to Central America and is found today in all tropical regions around the world.

Production: Arrowroot is the rhizome of *Maranta arundinacea.* The drug itself is a white powder extracted from the rhizome. The rhizome is washed, peeled, and macerated, and the starch is then extracted, using water in a process of elutriation. The resulting starch mass is purified by repeated sieving and dried in the sun.

Not to be Confused With: Cheaper starches such as potato, maize, wheat, or rice starch. These are often used as substitutes.

Other Names: Maranta

ACTIONS AND PHARMACOLOGY

COMPOUNDS

Starch (25-27%, with respect to the fresh bulbs): as Marantae amylum, maranta starch, medicinal arrowroot

Other constituent elements are not known.

EFFECTS

Animal tests: In rats that received a Marantae-rich diet, a reduction in the increase of the cholesterol levels in the aorta and heart muscle was reported. The effect was put down to an increased elimination of bile acids.

In humans, the drug is a demulcent and soothing agent.

INDICATIONS AND USAGE

Unproven Uses: Arrowroot is used as a nutritive (nutritional foodstuff) for infants and convalescents, a dietary aid in gastrointestinal disorders, and also for diarrhea, especially in pediatrics. In folk medicine, it is used in acute diarrhea.

Indian Medicine: Arrowroot is used in dysentery, diarrhea, dyspepsia, bronchitis, coughs and as a particularly nourishing food for children, the chronically ill, and convalescents.

PRECAUTIONS AND ADVERSE REACTIONS

No health hazards or side effects are known in conjunction with the proper administration of designated therapeutic dosages.

DOSAGE

Mode of Administration: The powder is boiled with water.

Storage: Arrowroot should be stored in tightly sealed containers.

LITERATURE

Hänsel R, Keller K, Rimpler H, Schneider G (Hrsg.), Hagers Handbuch der Pharmazeutischen Praxis, 5. Aufl., Bde 4-6 (Drogen), Springer Verlag Berlin, Heidelberg, New York, 1992-1994.

Artemisia absinthium

See Wormwood

Artemisia cina

See Wormseed

Artemisia dracunculus

See French Tarragon

Artemisia vulgaris

See Mugwort

Artichoke

Cynara scolymus

DESCRIPTION

Medicinal Parts: The medicinal parts are the dried whole or cut basal leaves and the dried or fresh herb from the artichoke.

Flower and Fruit: Globose, thorny capituals of lingual florets grows at the end of the stem. The epicalyx is ovate to globose. The bracts are fleshy and taper into a flattened greenish or purple tip. The petals are blue, lilac, or white. The fruit is a pubescent achaene 4 to 5 mm in diameter and 7 to 8 mm long. It is flecked brown and glossy.

Leaves, Stem and Root: Cynara scolymus is a perennial plant with a short rhizome and a strong, erect, glabrous stalk. The stalk is up to 2 m high, thickly covered in lanceolate, prickly pinnate to double-pinnate leaves. The upper surface is bare and light green; the lower surface is gray and tomentose.

Habitat: The plant is found in the Mediterranean region, the Canary Islands, and South America. It is cultivated elsewhere.

Production: Artichoke root is the dried root of *Cynara scolymus*. Artichoke leaf consists of the fresh or dried basal leaves of *Cynara scolymus*. Artichoke is cultivated and dried with extreme care.

Other Names: Garden Artichoke, Globe Artichoke

ACTIONS AND PHARMACOLOGY

COMPOUNDS: ARTICHOKE LEAF

Caffeic acid derivatives: chlorogenic acid, neochlorogenic acid, cryptochlorogenic acid, cynarin

Flavonoids (0.5%): in particular rutin

Sesquiterpene lactones (0 to 4%): cynaropicrin, dehydrocynaropicrin, grossheimin, cynaratriol

COMPOUNDS: ARTICHOKE ROOT

Caffeic acid derivatives, including chlorogenic acid sesquiterpene lactones, are not contained in the rhizome.

EFFECTS: ARTICHOKE LEAF AND ROOT

The main active principles are sesquiterpenes (amaroids), hydroxy cinnamic acid, and flavonoids. The drug has a cholagogic, hepatotoxic, and lipid-reducing effect. A choleretic effect has been observed in rats (effect of the cinnamic acid). The cholesterol levels were reduced in the rats; a hepatostimulating and bitter effect on the gastrointestinal tract has also been documented.

INDICATIONS AND USAGE

ARTICHOKE LEAF

Approved by Commission E:

- Liver and gallbladder complaints
- Loss of appetite

ARTICHOKE LEAF AND ROOT

Unproven Uses: Artichoke is used for dyspeptic problems and also for prophylactic treatment against the return of gallstones.

In folk medicine, Artichoke is also used for digestion complaints and as a tonic in convalescence.

CONTRAINDICATIONS

ARTICHOKE LEAF AND ROOT

Because of the stimulating effect of the drug upon the biliary tract, it should not be administered if there is a bile duct blockage. Colic can occur where the patient suffers from gallstones.

PRECAUTIONS AND ADVERSE REACTIONS

ARTICHOKE LEAF AND ROOT

Health risks or side effects following the proper administration of designated therapeutic dosages are not recorded. The plant possesses a medium potential for sensitization through skin contact. Allergic reactions occur in particular when there is frequent on-the-job contact with artichokes. There are cross-reactions with other composites (including chrysanthemes, arnica pyrethrum).

DOSAGE

HOW SUPPLIED

Capsules: 170 mg, 320 mg

Liquid extract

ARTICHOKE LEAF

Mode of Administration: Dried, comminuted drug, pressed juice of fresh plant and other galenical preparations for internal use.

Daily Dosage: The average daily dose is 6 gm of drug; single dose is 500 mg of dry extract.

Storage: Artichoke should be protected from light and insects in well-sealed containers.

LITERATURE

Adzet T, Puigmacia M, *J Chromatogr* 348:447-453. 1985.

Brand N, Cynara scolymus L. - Die Artischocke. In: *ZPT* 11(5):169. 1990.

Fintelmann V, Antidyspetische und lipidsenkende Wirkung von Artischockenblätterextrakt. In: ZPT 17(5) Beilage ZFA. Zeitschrift für *Allgem Med.* 1996.

Fintelmann V, Menβen HG, Artischockenblätterextrakt Aktuelle Erkenntnis zur Wirkung als Lipidsenker und Antidyspeptikum. In: *DAZ* 136(17):1405-1414. 1996.

Hinou J, Harvala C, Philianos S, Polyphenolic substances of *Cynara scolymus* L. leaves. *Ann Pharm Fr*, 47:95-8, 1989

Khalkova Zh, Vangelova K, Zaikov Kh, An experimental study of the effect of an artichoke preparation on the activity of the sympathetic-adrenal system in carbon disulfide exposure. *Probl Khig*, 53:162-71, 1995

Kirchhoff R, Beckers CH, Kirchhoff GM, Trinczek-Gärtner H, Petrowicz O, Reimann HJ (1994) Increase in choleresis by means of artichoke extract. *Phytomedicine* 1:107-115.

Maros T, Seres-Sturm L, Racz G, Rettegi C, Kovacs VV, Hints M, Quantitative analysis of cynarin in the leaves of the artichoke (Cynara scolymus L.) *Farm Zh*, 18:56-9, 1965

Meding B, Allergic contact dermatitis from artichoke *Cynara scolymus*. Contact Dermatitis, 18:314, 1983 Jul

Reuter HD, Pflanzliche Gallentherapeutika (Teil I) und (Teil II). In: *ZPT* 16(1):13-20, 77-89. 1995.

Schilcher H, Pharmazeutische Aspekte pflanzlicher Gallentherapeutika. In: *ZPT* 16(4):211-222. 1995.

Schmidt M, Phytotherapie: Pflanzliche Gallenwegstherapeutika. In: *DAZ* 135(8):680-682. 1995.

Sokolova VE, Liubartseva LA, Vasilchenkoo EA, Effect of artichoke (*Synara scolymus*) on some aspects of nitrogen metabolism in animals. *Farmakol Toksikol*, 53:340-3, 1970 May-Jun

Wasielewski S, Artischockenblätterextrakt: Prävention der Arteriosklerose?. In: *DAZ* 137(24):2065-2067. 1997.

Arum

Arum maculatum

DESCRIPTION

Medicinal Parts: The medicinal part is the root of the plant.

Flower and Fruit: The flowers are pale yellowish-green. They are surrounded by a bulbous spath and therefore are not visible. A violet or brown-red spadix emerges from the bract with 2 circles of bristles underneath. Under the bristles are the male flowers; under these are the female flowers. The spath doubles the length of the spadix. The whole structure forms a typical insect trap. The fruit is a scarlet berry.

Leaves, Stem and Root: Arum maculatum is a 30 to 60 cm spit- to arrow-shaped plant. It is long-stemmed, glossy, often brown-speckled and basal. The petiole is spread to a sheath at the base. The root stock is tuberous, ovoid, and floury-fleshy, varying in size between that of a hazelnut and a pigeon's egg.

Characteristics: Arum maculatum bears attractive scarlet berries that yield an acrid juice that is poisonous and can be fatal if ingested by small children.

Habitat: The plant is indigenous to parts of Europe, Britain, and the U.S.

Production: Arum root is the fresh rhizome of *Arum maculatum* collected before removing the leaves.

Other Names: Adder's Root, Bobbins, Cocky Baby, Cuckoo Pint, Cypress Powder, Dragon Root, Friar's Cowl, Gaglee, Kings and Queens, Ladysmock, Lords and Ladies, Parson and Clerk, Portland Arrowroot, Quaker, Ramp, Wake Robin

ACTIONS AND PHARMACOLOGY

COMPOUNDS

Mucilages: glucomannane

Starch

Lectins

EFFECTS

The glucomannans, bassorin, and starch contained in the drug have a strong irritant and swelling effect on the mucous membranes. The diaphoretic and expectorant effect attributed to the drug may be due to the strong actions of these constituents.

INDICATIONS AND USAGE

Unproven Uses: Arum is used for colds and inflammation of the throat.

PRECAUTIONS AND ADVERSE REACTIONS

The intake of plant parts leads to severe mucous membrane irritations (swelling of the tongue, bloody vomiting, bloody diarrhea), presumably due to lesions of the membrane from the very sharp-edged oxalate needles and the introduction of impurities into the wounds. Decoctions of the roots in therapeutic dosages can be taken without risk. Caution is advised even though the level of cyanogenic glycosides is too low to be able to bring about signs of poisoning.

DOSAGE

No dosage information is available.

LITERATURE

Akhtardziev K et al., (1984) *Farmatsiya* 34(3):1.

Koch H, Steinegger E, Components of *Arum maculatum* L. (woven arrowroot). In: *Pharm Acta Helv* 54(2):33-36. 1979.

Mladenov IV, (1982) C R *Acad Bulg Sci* 35(8):116.

Mladenov I, Bulanov I, Stamenova M, Ribarova F, The composition and structure of isolectins from *Arum maculatum*. Eksp Med Morfol, 29:36-9, 1990.

Moore THS, *Vet Rec* 89:569. 1971.

Nahrstedt A, Triglochinin in *Arum maculatum*. In: *PH* 14(12):1870-1871. 1975.

Poisonous Plants in Britain and Their Effects on Animals and Man, Ministry of Agriculture, Fisheries and Food, Pub; HMSO (1984) UK.

Proliac A, Chaboud A, Raynaud J, Isolement et identification de trois C- glycosylflavonews dans les tiges feuilleés d'Arum dracunculus. In: *PA* :47:646-647. 1992.

Arum maculatum

See Arum

Arundinaria japonica

See Bamboo

Asa Foetida

Ferula foetida

DESCRIPTION

Medicinal Parts: The medicinal part is the oily gum-resin extracted from the plant.

Flower and Fruit: The flowers appear after 5 years in yellow umbels on a 10 cm thick naked stem. They are numerous, pale greenish-yellow to white. The fruit is ovate, flat, thin, flaky, and reddish-brown with distinct oil marks.

Leaves, Stem and Root: The plant is a herbaceous monoecious perennial, 1.5 to 2 m high with a large, fleshy rhizome, which is 14 cm thick at the crown. The leaves are large, bipinnate, and radical.

Characteristics: The fruit has milky juice and a strong smell.

Habitat: Afghanistan and eastern Iran.

Production: Asa foetida is the gum resin of Ferula foetida.

Other Names: Devil's Dung, Food of the Gods, Gum Asafoetida

ACTIONS AND PHARMACOLOGY

COMPOUNDS

Volatile oil: chief constituent is sec-propenyl-isobutyl disulphide

Gum resin: consisting mainly of ferulic acid esters, farnesiferol A, B, C and bassorinlike mucilage

Sesquiterpenoide coumarins: including asafoetida

EFFECTS

Asa foetida has a mild intestinal disinfectant effect; its sedative effect is uncertain. In animal experiments it has antitumoural and mild mutagenic effect on *Salmonella typhimurium.*

INDICATIONS AND USAGE

Unproven Uses: The drug is used for chronic gastritis, dyspepsia, and irritable colon.

Chinese Medicine: In China, the drug is used for infestation with intestinal parasites.

Indian Medicine: In India, Asa foetida is used to treat asthma, whooping cough, flatulence, constipation, diseases of the liver and spleen, and for epilepsy.

Homeopathic Uses: Ferula foetida is used for low acid levels in the stomach, stomach pressure, flatulence, and loose stools.

PRECAUTIONS AND ADVERSE REACTIONS

General: No health hazards or side effects are known in conjunction with the proper administration of designated therapeutic dosages. The intake of larger dosages can lead to swelling of the lips, digestive complaints (belching, flatulence, diarrhea), discomfort and headache. Convulsions are possible in susceptible individuals. Swelling of the genital organs has been observed following external administration on the abdomen.

Pregnancy: Not to be used during pregnancy.

DOSAGE

Mode of Administration: The drug is available as an extract.

Preparation: Gum-resin is obtained by incising the roots, which contain a fetid juice. This solidifies to a brown resin, sometimes with a pinkish tint, in sticky lumps. The final product has a pungent, acrid, persistent, alliaceous odor.

Daily Dosage: Tincture: 20 drops as a single dose.

Homeopathic Dosage: D3 and D4 dilutions.

LITERATURE

Buddrus J et al., (1985) *Phytochemistry* 24(4):869.

Kern W, List PH, Hörhammer L (Hrsg.), Hagers Handbuch der Pharmazeutischen Praxis, 4. Aufl., Bde 1-8, Springer Verlag Berlin, Heidelberg, New York, 1969.

Lewin L, Gifte und Vergiftungen, 6. Aufl., Nachdruck, Haug Verlag, Heidelberg 1992.

Madaus G, Lehrbuch der Biologischen Arzneimittel, Bde 1-3, Nachdruck, Georg Olms Verlag Hildesheim 1979.

Naimie H et al., (1972) *Collect Czec Chem Commun* 37:1166.

Rajanikanth B et al., (1984) *Phytochemistry* 23(4):899.

Roth L, Daunderer M, Kormann K, Giftpflanzen, Pflanzengifte, 4. Aufl., Ecomed Fachverlag Landsberg Lech 1993.

Asarum

Asarum europaeum

DESCRIPTION

Medicinal Parts: The primary medicinal part is the root of the plant. However, the leaves have been used to a lesser extent.

Flower and Fruit: The end of the stem forms a short-pedicled, slightly hanging flower. The perigone forms a campanulate tube with a 3- to 4-lobed margin. It is brownish on the outside, dark purple on the inside. There are 2 groups of 6 stamens on the ovaries, which are fused with the tube and are flattened above. The style is thick, short and solid; the stigma is 6-rayed. The fruit is a many-seeded, indehiscent capsule divided into many chambers by false membranes. Each capsule contains numerous boat-shaped seeds with a spongy appendage.

Leaves, Stem and Root: Asarum europaeum is a shaggy-haired perennial growing 4 to 10 cm high. It has a thin, creeping rhizome that is branched and usually has 3 to 4 scalelike, brownish-green stipules. It has an ascending short-scaled stem, with the terminal flower at the tip. There are 2 to 4 long-petioled, almost opposite, broad, reniform leaves. They are entire-margined, coriaceous, dark-green glossy above, pale and matte beneath, deeply reticulate and evergreen.

Characteristics: The rhizome has a pepperlike smell; the leaves and flowers have an unpleasant camphor smell. *Asarum europaeum* is a protected species.

Habitat: The plant is indigenous to the northern parts of southern Europe, central and east-central Europe as far as the Crimea and eastward into western Siberia as well as an enclave in the Atai. Asarum is cultivated in the U.S.

Production: Asarum root is the root of *Asarum europaeum*, which is gathered in August and air-dried in the shade. Asarum is primarily collected in the wild, but is cultivated in the U.S.

Not to be Confused With: Can be confused with other valerian types and with *Arnica montana, Genum urbanum, Valeriana officinalis* and *Viola ordorata*. Powder that is not made from *Asarum europaeum* can be identified by the presence of fibers, stone cells, oxalate filament agglomerations, and the absence of starch.

Other Names: Asarabacca, Coltsfoot, False Coltsfoot, Fole's Foot, Hazelwort, Public House Plant, Snakeroot, Wild Ginger, Wild Nard

ACTIONS AND PHARMACOLOGY

COMPOUNDS

Volatile oil: composition depends upon variety but possible constituents include asarone trans-isoasarone, trans-isoeugenol methyl ether, trans-isoelemicin or eudesmol, possibly in addition to sesquiterpene hydrocarbons, -alcohols, -furans,-carbonyl compounds

Caffeic acid derivatives: including chlorogenic acid, isochlorogenic acid

Flavonoids

EFFECTS

Asarum acts as an expectorant, bronchial spasmolytic, superficial relaxant, and local anesthetic. Studies of the plant's emetic action exist for Asari root and herb. However, self-experimentation with 100 gm trans-isoasaron taken orally caused severe vomiting.

The surface-tension-reducing effect of trans-isoasaron and trans-isomethyleugenol was studied in vitro, using stalagmometry. Both substances showed a concentration-dependent surface activity, which surpassed the effect of the control substance tyloxapol in a normal treatment concentration.

In studies of Asarum's spasmolytic effect, bronchial spasms induced in a guinea pig by histamine were inhibited in vivo by trans-isoasaron, depending on the dose. The survival rate was determined subsequent to the addition of a histamine-containing aerosol 30 minutes after trans-isoasarin had been administered. The control substance here was clemizole hydrochloride, which has a similarly inhibiting effect.

The action of trans-isoasaron and of isomethyleugenol as a local anesthetic was tested on 10 volunteer subjects, in order to compare it with benzocaine (anesthetic index AI = 1). The results showed a dose-related action for both drugs, with the following anesthetic indexes of AI = 0.72 for trans-isoasarin and AI = 0.47 for trans-isomethyleugenol.

The only available studies of Asarum's antibacterial effect are those carried out on Asari root and herb. A double-blind, placebo-controlled clinical trial was carried out on 30 patients with acute bronchitis, 30 with chronic bronchitis and an additional 30 with bronchial asthma. Eighty percent of the patients with acute bronchitis, 58% of the patients with chronic bronchitis, and 68% of the patients with bronchial asthma were cured or showed improvement in both their subjective and objective states. The contrast with the placebo groups was significant. The treatment consisted of a daily dose of 3 x 2 tablets, purified dry (GB) or powdered (US) extract (30 mg phenylpropanol derivatives) taken over an average of 7 days. However, to obtain conclusive results, further trials are needed over a longer period and with more patients. The drug's efficacy was also tested in a multicentric field trial, a clinically controlled study and an open bicentric study. However, the results are only useful to a small extent, as there is an absence of details about placebo groups, trial parameters, and statistical analysis.

INDICATIONS AND USAGE

Unproven Uses: The purified dry extract of *Asarum europaeum* rootstock is used for inflammatory conditions of the lower respiratory system (acute and chronic bronchitis), for various causes of bronchial spasms and for bronchial asthma. Asari root and Asari root with herb are used for similar indications in folk medicine. In the past, the drugs were used as emetics. Some other uses are as antitussives (cough remedies), sneezing-powder for chronic rhinitis, for inflammation of the eye, for pneumonia, angina pectoris, migraines, liver disease and jaundice, for dehydration, as an emmenagogue (menstrual stimulant) and for artificial abortion. The dried, powdered leaves have been used as an ingredient of some snuffs, helping to expel mucus from the respiratory passages.

Homeopathic Uses: Homeopathic uses include diarrhea and exhaustion.

PRECAUTIONS AND ADVERSE REACTIONS

Older scientific literature contains reports of signs of poisoning including burning of the tongue, gastroenteritis, diarrhea, erysipeloid skin rashes, and hemiparesis. An extremely susceptible mouse strain developed hepatoma after exposure to asarone. Administration of the drug is not advised.

CONTRAINDICATIONS

Asarum is not to be used during pregnancy.

DOSAGE

Mode of Administration: Asarum is taken as a sneezing-powder, or orally as a purified dry extract in the form of coated tablets and pills. It is obsolete as a drug.

How Supplied: Commercial pharmaceutical preparations include coated tablets and confectionery tea mixtures.

Preparation: The air-dried rootstock is extracted with an organic solvent, which can be mixed with water. The liquid extract is separated from the solvent by means of vacuum distillation. The watery portion remaining is diluted with an equal amount of distilled water, and further extraction takes place. Then the organic liquid extract is mixed with a suitable excipient according to the desired percentage of trans-isoasaron. Afterward, the extract is dried and rubbed. Trans-isoasaron can also be produced from asarylaldehyde by means of Perkin's cinnamic synthesis. As sneezing-powder, the average content of the drug is 20%.

Daily Dosage: The average daily oral dose of the dry extract for adults and children aged 13 and over is 30 mg, which corresponds to 30 mg phenylpropane derivatives and should be spread over 2 to 3 doses per day. Children aged 2 and over can take an extract corresponding to 5 mg phenylpropanol derivatives 3 times daily. The average single dose of the drug is 0.1 gm.

Homeopathic Dosage: 5 to 10 drops, 1 tablet, or 5 to 10 globules 1 to 3 times daily or 1 ml injection solution twice weekly sc; ointments 1 to 2 times daily; D1 and D2 should not be taken for longer than 1 month (HAB1).

Storage: Coated tablets and pills that contain the purified dry extract or the tincture from the rhizome can be stored for a period of 28 days in conditions of high temperature, humidity and light. Under preferred storage conditions (i.e. brown glass, away from light), they can be stored for up to 2 years, after which period stability should be checked.

LITERATURE

Doskotch RW, Vanevenhoven PW, (1967) *Lloydia* 30:141.

Gracza L, (1987) *Pharmazie* 42 (2):141.

Gracza L, In vitro studies on the expectorant effect of the phenylpropane derivatives from hazlewort. 12. The active agents in *Asarum europaeum*. In: *PM* 42(2):155. 1981.

Gracza L, Phytobiological (phytophamacological) studies on phenylpropane derivatives from *Asarum europaeum* L. 10. Actice principles of *Asarum europaeum* L. In: *Arzneim Forsch* 30(5):767-771. 1980.

Gracza L, Über die Wirkstoffe von *Asarum europaeum*. 16. Mitt., Die lokalanästhetische Wirkung der Phenylprpanderivate. In: *PM* 48(3):153-157. 1983.

Mose JR, Lukas G, (1961) Arzneim Forsch 11:33.

Rosch A, (1984) *Z Phytother* 5(6):964.

Trennheuser L, Dissertation Saarbrücken. 1961.

Asarum europaeum

See Asarum

Asclepias incarnata

See Swamp Milkweed

Asclepias tuberosa

See Pleurisy Root

Ash

Fraxinus excelsior

DESCRIPTION

Medicinal Parts: The medicinal parts are the dried leaves, the fresh bark, the branch bark, and the fresh leaves.

Flower and Fruit: The flowers are in richly blossomed panicles, the terminal ones appearing on the new flowering branches. They are usually androgynous, occasionally male, polygamous, or dioecious. They have no calyx or corolla. The anthers of the male flowers are dark purple and are on short filaments. The female flowers consist of 1 inferior ovary with a 2-lobed stigma and 2 split staminoids. The fruit is a narrow lanceolate to oblong-obovate nutlet hanging on a thin stem. The fruit is 25 to 50 mm long and 7 to 10 mm wide, glossy brown, 1-seeded with a veined winged border.

Leaves, Stem and Root: The ash is an impressive 15 to 30 m tall tree with a gray-brown, smooth, later fissured and wrinkled bark and large, black-brown, pubescent buds. The leaves are entire-margined, opposite, and odd pinnate. There are 9 to 15 leaflets. The leaflets are sessile, usually 5 to 11 cm long by 1 to 3 cm wide, oblong-ovate to lanceolate, long acuminate, finely and sharply serrate. They are glabrous above, rich green, loosely tomentose or almost glabrous, and greenish brown beneath.

Habitat: The plant is distributed in most parts of Europe except the northern, southern and eastern edges.

Production: Ash bark consists of the bark of young branches of *Fraxinus excelsior*. Ash leaf consists of the leaf of Fraxinus excelsior. The leaves are harvested in spring and air-dried.

Not to be Confused With: It may be confused with *Ailanthus glandulosa*.

Other Names: Bird's Tongue, European Ash, Common Ash, Weeping Ash

ACTIONS AND PHARMACOLOGY

COMPOUNDS: ASH LEAF

Flavonoids: including rutin (0.1-0.9%)

Tannins

Mucilages (10-20%)

Mannitol (16-28%)

Triterpenes, phytosterols

Iridoide monoterpenes: including syringoxide, deoxysyringoxidin

COMPOUNDS: ASH BARK

Hydroxycoumarins: aesculin, fraxin, aesculetin, fraxetin, fraxidin, isofraxidin, fraxinol, scopoletine

Tannins

Iridoide monoterpenes: including 10-hydroxyligstroside

EFFECTS: ASH BARK

The main active principle is coumarin. Preparations of fresh ash bark showed an analgesic, antioxidative, and antiphlogistic action. Cyclo AMP phosphodiesterase is inhibited and an antioxidative (radical trapping action) effect was proven for scopoletine, isofraxin, and fraxin.

INDICATIONS AND USAGE

ASH LEAF

Unproven Uses: Preparations of Ash leaf are used for arthritis, gout, bladder complaints, as well as a laxative and diuretic. In folk medicine Ash leaf is used internally for fever, rheumatism, gout, edema, stones, constipation, stomach symptoms, and worm infestation; and externally for lower leg ulcers and wounds.

ASH BARK

Unproven Uses: Preparations of Ash bark are used for fever and as a tonic.

PRECAUTIONS AND ADVERSE REACTIONS

Health risks or side effects following the proper administration of designated therapeutic dosages are not recorded.

DOSAGE

Mode of Administration: Since the efficacy for the claimed applications has not been documented, therapeutic application cannot be recommended. The efficacy of Ash in fixed combinations must be verified specifically for each preparation.

Preparation: Tea: Soak 3 teaspoons of the drug in 2 glasses of hot water.

Daily Dosage: Tea: Several time a day.

Storage: Should be protected from light.

LITERATURE

Carnat A, Lamaison JL, Dubnand F, *Plant Méd Phytothér* 24:145-151. 1990.

Genius OB, DAZ 120:1505-1506. 1980.

Jensen SR, Nielsen BJ, PH 15:221-223. 1976.

Marekov N et al., *Khim Ind* 58:132-135. 1986.

Tissut M, Ravane P, PH 19:2077-2081. 1980.

Yamagami I, Suzuki Y, Koichiro I, Pharmacological studies on the components of *Fraxinus japonica*. In: Nippon Yakurigaku Zasshi 64(6):714-729 (jap.). 1968.

Asiatic Dogwood

Cornus officinalis

DESCRIPTION

Medicinal Parts: The medicinal part of the tree is the fruit.

Flower and Fruit: The umbels contain 20 to 30 flowers surrounded by 4 yellow-green, 6 to 8 mm long, elliptical-acuminate bracts. The flower structures are in fours and the diameter of the flower is 4 to 5 mm, including the disc. The calyx is fused and has 4 tips. There are 4 free petals, 4 stamens and a 2-chambered ovary, with 1 ovule per chamber. The drupe is elongate-elliptical, approximately 15 mm long and red with an elongate, 2-chambered stone kernel.

Leaves and Branches: Cornus officinalis is shrub or tree that grows up to 4 m high. The leaves are opposite, simple, and 4 to 10 cm long. The petiole is 6 to 10 cm long. The lamina is ovate-elliptical or ovate, long acuminate, rounded at the base, yellow-brown and pubescent beneath. The branches are smooth, bluish-green, and the bark peels off.

Habitat: China, Japan

Production: Cornus fruit is the dried fruit pulp of *Cornus officinalis*. Fruits are harvested in the late autumn or the beginning of winter. They are scalded with boiling water or gently heated. Cleaning of the raw drug follows kernel extraction and drying.

ACTIONS AND PHARMACOLOGY

COMPOUNDS

Iridoids: iridoid glycosides, including loganin, cornuside, sweroside, morronoside

Tannins: gallotannins, including cornusiens-A to -G, tellimagrandin I and II, camptothins-A and -B

Triterpenes: including oleanolic acid, ursolic acid

Anthocyans

EFFECTS

The drug has an astringent effect due to its tannin content. It has exhibited diuretic, blood pressure-lowering and leukocytopoiesis-promoting effects in clinical tests.

INDICATIONS AND USAGE

Unproven Uses: In folk medicine, the drug has been used for impotency, loss of semen, lumbago-sciatica syndrome, night sweats, and vertigo.

Chinese Medicine: In China, Asiatic Dogwood is used for liver and renal disorders, tinnitus, hyperhidrosis, impotency, and lower back and knee pain.

PRECAUTIONS AND ADVERSE REACTIONS

No health hazards are known in conjunction with the proper administration of designated therapeutic dosages.

DOSAGE

Mode of Administration: Whole herb preparations and liquid preparations for internal use

Preparation: The fruit is boiled or steamed with wine until all the liquid has been drawn out.

Daily Dosage: 5 to 12 gm of drug.

Chinese Medicine Dosage: 3 to 9 gm of drug daily.

Storage: The herb should be protected from insects and stored in dry place.

LITERATURE

Hänsel R, Keller K, Rimpler H, Schneider G (Ed) Hagers Handbuch der Pharmazeutischen Praxis. 5. Aufl., Bde 4 - 6 (Drogen), Springer Verlag Berlin, Heidelberg, New York, 1992-1994.

Jeng H, Wu CM, Su SJ, Chang WC A substance isolated from *Cornus officinalis* enhances the motility of human sperm. *Am J Chin Med*, 25:301-6, 1997.

Jeng H, Wu CM, Su SJ, Chang WC Observations on the biological characteristics of *Cornus officinalis. Chung Yao Tung Pao*, 25:8-11, Jul, 1985.

Asimina triloba

See American Pawpaw

Aspalathus linearis

See Rooibos

Asparagus

Asparagus officinalis

DESCRIPTION

Medicinal Parts: The medicinal parts of the plant are the herb and the rhizome with roots.

Flower and Fruit: Thin pedicles measuring from 2 to 20 mm long produce 1 to 3 flowers from the nodes. The plants are usually dioecious. The perigone of the male flowers is about 5 mm long, funnel-shaped and whitish to greenish-yellow. The perigone is longer than the cauline leaves and has oblanceolate sections that are twice as long as the perigone tube. The stamens are oblong and almost as long the filaments. The perigone of the female flowers is much smaller. The fruit is a pea-sized, brick-red round berry that is up to 8 mm thick. The seeds are black with wrinkly stripes and are 3 to 4 mm wide.

Leaves, Stem and Root: Asparagus officinalis is a perennial with a short, woody root stock. In the wild, the plant typically reaches heights of 30 to 100 cm, but cultivated plants may grow to 150 cm. The stem is erect, glabrous, and smooth, later inclined with numerous erect to leaning branches. The scale sections at the base have short spurs. The round, needlelike phylloclades are in clusters of 4 to 15 that are 5 to 25 cm long and about 0.5 cm thick. The root stock produces a few ascending shoots that are as thick as a finger, fleshy, white, and red or blue-reddish tinged. (This is the edible asparagus.) The female plants are often slimmer than the male, which are shorter and stockier.

Characteristics: The fruit is considered to be poisonous, but that has not been substantiated.

Habitat: The plant grows in central and southern Europe, the Middle East, western Siberia, and northern Africa. It is cultivated in many places.

Production: Asparagus herb consists of the above-ground parts of *Asparagus officinalis*. Asparagus root consists of the rhizome with roots of *Asparagus officinalis,* which are dug up and air-dried in autumn, and also the fresh underground shoots.

Not to be Confused With: This variety is sometimes confused with other types of asparagus cultivated in the Mediterranean region.

Other Names: Sparrow Grass

ACTIONS AND PHARMACOLOGY

COMPOUNDS: ASPARAGUS HERB

Flavonoids: including rutin, hyperoside, isoquercitrin

Steroid saponins

EFFECTS: ASPARAGUS HERB

Animal experiments indicate the herb has a mild diuretic action.

COMPOUNDS: ASPARAGUS RHIZOME AND ROOT

Steroid saponins: including asparagosides A, B, D, F, G, H, I, the bitter steroid saponins, aspartic saponin I

Amino acids: among them sulphur-containing aspartic acid, the esters 3-mercapto- butyric acid, 3-methylthio-isobutyric acid, diisobutyric acid disulphide

Fructans: asparagose, asparagosine

EFFECTS: ASPARAGUS RHIZOME AND ROOT

Animal tests indicate that the root has a diuretic effect. The main active principles are flavonol glycoside and furostanol and spirostanol glycosides, mainly derivatives of sarsapogenin. The distinctive odor of the urine after an individual has eaten asparagus is believed to be caused by methylmercaptan.

INDICATIONS AND USAGE

ASPARAGUS HERB

Unproven Uses: Preparations of Asparagus are used as a diuretic, although the effectiveness for the claimed application has not been sufficiently documented.

ASPARAGUS RHIZOME AND ROOT

Approved by Commission E:

- Infections of the urinary tract
- Kidney and bladder stones

Unproven Uses: Traditional uses of the root include application for nonspecific inflammatory diseases of the urinary tract and for prevention of kidney and bladder stones (irrigation therapy). Among other folk medicine uses are dropsy, rheumatic conditions, liver disease, bronchial asthma, and gout. These applications have not been proved.

Chinese Medicine: The root is used to treat irritable cough, coughing with blood, dry mouth and throat, and constipation.

Homeopathic Uses: Uses in homeopathy include kidney stones and cardiac insufficiency.

CONTRAINDICATIONS

ASPARAGUS RHIZOME AND ROOT

Because of the irritating effect of saponin, the drug should not be administered in the presence of kidney diseases. In the case of reduced cardiac and/or kidney function, irrigation therapy should not be attempted.

PRECAUTIONS AND ADVERSE REACTIONS

ASPARAGUS HERB

No health hazards or side effects are known in conjunction with the proper administration of designated therapeutic dosages. The plant has a low sensitization potential through skin contact. The berries are considered poisonous, although there is no proof of this.

ASPARAGUS RHIZOME AND ROOT

No health hazards or side effects are known in conjunction with the proper administration of designated therapeutic dosages. When used in irrigation therapy, ensure ample fluid intake. There is a low sensitization potential, particularly among workers in canning factories who can become prone to asparagus scabies.

DOSAGE

ASPARAGUS RHIZOME AND ROOT

Mode of Administration: The cut rhizome is used for teas, as well as other galenic preparations for internal use. When used in flushing-out therapy, ensure ample fluid intake.

How Supplied:

Capsules: 170 mg, 320 mg

Liquid extract

Daily Dosage: 800 mg of the drug.

Homeopathic Dosage: 5 to 10 drops, 1 tablet, or 5 to 10 globules 1 to 3 times daily, or 1 mL injection solution twice weekly sc (HAB1).

LITERATURE

ASPARAGUS HERB

Goryanu GM et al., (1976) *Khim Prir Soed* 3: 400 et 6: 762.

Kawano K et al., (1975) *Agric Biol Chem* 39: 1999.

Shiomi N et al., (1976) *Agric Biol Chem* 40: 567.

Tagasuki M et al., (1975) *Chem Letters* 1: 43.

Woeldecke M, Hermann K, (1974) *Z Lebensm Forsch Unters* 25: 459.

ASPARAGUS RHIZOME AND ROOT

Goryanu GM et al., (1976) Khim Prir Soed 3: 400 et 6: 762.

Kawano K et al., Agric Biol Chem (Tokyo) 41:1. 1977.

Lazurevskii GV et al., Doklady Akademii Nauk SSSR 231:1479. 1976.

Pant G et al., PH 27:3324. 1988.

Shao Y et al., Steroidal saponins from Asparagus officinalis and their cytotoxic activity. In: PM 63(3):258-262. 1997.

Shiomi N et al., (1976) Agric Biol Chem 40: 567.

Tagasuki M et al., (1975) Chem Letters 1: 43.

Woeldecke M, Hermann K, (1974) Z Lebensm Untersuch Forsch 25: 459

Asparagus officinalis

See Asparagus

Aspidosperma quebracho-blanco

See Quebracho

Astragalus gummifer

See Tragacanth

Astragalus (Huang-Qi)

Astragalus species

DESCRIPTION

Medicinal Parts: The primary medicinal parts of the herb are the roots.

Flower and Fruit: The flower racemes are apical, and most are axillary. The inflorescenses have many small blue, purple, or blue-purple flowers. Two to three days following bloom, pods will develop in a square shape of a cross section with two chambers. There are 10 dark brown seeds in each chamber. The seeds are 6 to 13 mm long.

Leaves, Stem, and Root: The plant is a perennial and has several stems 1.5 to 2.0 m high. The stems are covered with pinnate leaves with T-shaped soft hairs. The primary root is thick, long, and contains many lateral roots. There is a secondary root beginning 20 to 30 feet below the soil surface.

Characteristics: The plant is cold tolerant and also able to grow in high temperatures.

Habitat: Astragalus australis is an endemic plant of the Olympic Mountains in Washington state. Other species are grown in northern and southern parts of China, Japan, and Korea.

Other Names: Astragali, Beg Kei, Bei Qi, Hwanggi, Membranous Milk Vetch, Tragacanth

ACTIONS AND PHARMACOLOGY

COMPOUNDS

Triterpene glycosides: brachyosides A, B, and C, and cyclocephaloside II, astrachrysoside A

Saponins: astragalosides I, II, and IV, isoastragaloside I, 3-0-beta-D-xylopyranosyl-cycloastragenol, cyclocanthoside E, soyasaponin I and cycloastragenol

Tragacanth (from the sap)

Sterols: daucosterol and beta-sitosterol

Fatty acids: including heptenoic acid, tetradecanoic acid, pentadecanoic acid, hexadecanoic acid, octadecenoic acid, octadecanoic acid, octadecadienoic acid, linolenic acid, eicosanoic acid, eicosenoic acid and docosanoic acid

Isoflavonoid compounds: astrasieversianin XV (II), 7,2′-dihydroxy-3′,4′-dimethoxy-isoflavane-7-O-beta-D-glucoside (III)

Amino acids: gamma-L-glutamyl-Se-methyl-seleno-L-cysteine, Se-methylseleno-L-cysteine

Polysaccharides

EFFECTS

Astragalus has immunostimulant, antioxidant, antiviral, hepatoprotective, and cardiotonic properties. Astragalus may also be useful for the prevention of thrombotic disorders (Zhang, 1997) and may have some protective effect against cochlear damage caused by gentamicin (Xuan, 1995). Other immunomodulating responses seen with the use of Astragalus include proliferation of B cells of the spleen, production of interleukin-6 and tumor necrosis factor from macrophages, polyclonal immunoglobulin production, and cytotoxic T lymphocyte activity (Yoshida, 1997).

Antioxidant Effects: Astragalus membranaceus inhibits lipid peroxidation in rat heart mitochondria (Hong, 1994).

Antiviral Effects: The broad array of immune stimulating characteristics of Astragalus has been widely used in treating patients with both acute and chronic infections, including viral myocarditis and viral hepatitis. *Astragalus membranaceus* inhibits the replication of coxsackie B-3 virus (CB3V)-RNA, a virus that causes myocarditis in animal models (Peng, 1995). The herb demonstrated significantly higher survival rates and lower abnormal action potential in animal models infected with CB3V, suggesting its possible use for prevention and treatment of acute myocarditis involving CB3V (Rui, 1994; Tianqing et al, 1995; Yang 1990). Astragalus has demonstrated immune-potentiating effects in human, animal, and in vitro studies and is often used as an adjunctive therapy in HIV-positive persons and those with AIDS (Bone, 1997).

Cardiovascular Effects: Astragalus membranaceus increases cardiac output in patients with angina pectoris (Lei, 1994). Astragaloside IV improves left ventricular end-diastolic volume and left ventricular end-systolic volume, and slows heart rate in heart failure. The compound also alleviates chest distress and dyspnea associated with heart failure (Luo, 1995). The herb has therapeutic effects on sodium and water retention in aortocaval fistula-induced heart failure, improving cardiac and renal functions in heart failure. The mechanism is partly through correction of abnormal mRNA expressions of hypothalmic arginine vasopresin system and aquaporin-2, and amelioration of blunted renal response to atrial natriuretic peptide (Ma, 1998). In human clinical trials, Astragalus was shown to have positive inotropic effects in patients with congestive heart failure (Luo, 1995), to significantly shorten ventricular late potentials (Shi, 1991), and to improve angina pectoris in EKG profiles along with the symptoms of ischemic heart disease (Li, 1995). Compounds in the root have demonstrated angiotensin-receptor down-regulating effects (Yarnell, 2007).

Chemoprotective Effects: A combination of *Astragalus membranaceus* and *Pyrola rotundifolia* protected against cochlear damage caused by gentamycin (Xuan et al, 1995).

Fertility Effects: A water extract of Astragalus membranaceus showed a significant stimulatory effect on human sperm motility (Hong, 1992).

Fibrinolytic Effects: The in vitro fibrinolytic/antithrombotic activity demonstrated by Astragalus is compatible with its use in patients with heart disease. Astragaloside IV increases the fibrinolytic potential of endothelial cells by up-regulating the expression of tissue-type plasminogen activator and by down-regulating the expression of plasminogen activator inhibitor type 1 (Zhang, 1997). In adition, Astragalus also appears to increase renal responsiveness to ANP-atrial natriuretic peptide (Ma & Peng, 1998) and reduce abnormal electrical activity of the myocardium (Shi et al, 1994).

Gastrointestinal Effects: The herb strengthens the movement and muscle tonus in the intestine, especially the jejunum, to increase movements in the digestive tract, as evidenced by positive effects on the cycle duration of interdigestive myoelectric complex (Lei, 1994).

Hepatoprotective Effects: Cytoprotective effects shown are prevention of liver fibrosis from carbon tetrachloride (Li CX et al. 1998) and decreased liver damage from stilbenemide (Zhang et al, 1990). An ethanol extract of the root of *Astragalus membranaceus* alleviated liver injury through a reduction of elevated SGPT levels and subacute toxicity. The herb also decreased loss of righting reflex and protected hepatic cells from pathological changes (Zhang, 1990).

Hypolipidemic Effects: A combination of *Astragalus mongholicus* and *Angelica sinensis* significantly lowered total serum cholesterol ($p<0.01$), triglycerides ($p<0.05$), low density lipoproteins (LDL) ($p<0.01$), and very low density (VLDL) lipoproteins ($p<0.05$) in rats with experimentally-induced nephrotic syndrome compared with untreated nephrotic rats (Jingzi et al, 2000).

Immunomodulating Effects: Multiple studies demonstrated that Astragalus potentiates the killing of tumor cells. The herb stimulates macrophages, promotes antibody formation, and increases T lymphocyte proliferation. F3, an immuno-regulatory component of the herb, reverses macrophage suppression induced by urological tumors (Rittenhouse, 1991). *Astragalus membranaceus* extracts enhance the antibody response to a T-dependent antigen associated with an increase of T-cell activity in normal and immunodepressed animal models (Zhao, 1990). A fractionated extract of *Astragalus membranaceus* potentiates lymphokine-activated killer (LAK) cell cytotoxicity generated by low-dose recombinant interleukin-2 (rIL-2). This immune response occurs through a 10-fold potentiation of rIL-2 activity manifested by tumor-cell killing activity resulting from LAK cell generation (Chu, 1990).

The immune stimulating effects of Astragalus are commonly used in cancer patients to both enhance the effectiveness and reduce the side effects of chemotherapy (Weng, 1995). It has also been used to stimulate interleukin-6 and tumor necrosis factor production by macrophages/monocytes (Yoshida et al, 1997; Zhao & Kong 1993); increase macrophage oxidative burst activity (Kajimura et al, 1996; Rittenhouse et al, 1991); improve mononuclear cell responsiveness (Chu et al, 1988); enhance lymphokine activated killer cells (LAK) cytotoxicity (Wang et al, 1992; Chu et al, 1994; Zhao, 1993; Chu et al, 1988b); stimulate the proliferation of B cells in the spleen (Yoshida et al, 1997); and increase antibody productions (Zhao et al, 1990).

A partially purified fraction from *Astragalus membranaceus* demonstrated immune potentiating effects in rats (Chu et al, 1988).

Memory-Enhancing Effects: Aqueous extracts of Astragalus demonstrated improvement of anisodine-induced impairment on memory acquisition as well as the alcohol-elicited deficit of memory retrieval (a reduction in errors and prolonged latent period) (Hong, 1994).

CLINICAL TRIALS

Cardiovascular Disease

The symptoms of ischemic heart disease in patients treated with Astragalus were significantly improved over controls in an open-label study ($p<0.05$) (Li et al, 1995). Astragaloside IV, a component of Astragalus, had positive inotropic effects in patients with congestive heart failure. Nineteen patients were treated by astragaloside IV injection for 2 weeks. Patients had decreased symptoms and radionucleide ventriculography showed improvements in left ventricular modeling and ejection (Luo et al, 1995). Injection of *Astragalus membranaceus* significantly shortened the duration of ventricular late potentials (VLPs) in a study of 313 patients. Body surface signal-averaged electrocardiogram (SAECG) was recorded on all patients studied, including 266 patients who were also monitored by 24-hour Holter EKG. VLPs were detected in 203 of those patients who had a history of angina pectoris, myocardial infarction, myocarditis, cardiomyopathy, or arrhythmia of unknown origin. Patients with VLPs were treated with either Mexilentine hydrochloride, lidocaine hydrochloride, or injection *of Astragalus membranaceus.* While none of the treatments resolved the VLPs, injection of *Astragalus membranaceus* significantly shortened the duration of the VLPs (39.8±3.3 ms versus 44.5±5.9 ms, $p<0.01$) (Shi, 1991).

The effect of *Astragalus membranaceus* on left ventricular function and oxygen free radicals was evaluated in 43 cardiac patients. All patients in the treatment group had experienced myocardial infarction within the past 36 hours. The herb demonstrated a strengthening of left ventricular function and an effect of anti-oxygen free radicals for a cardiotonic action. The herb decreased the ratio of pre-ejection period/left ventricular ejection time, increased the superoxide dismutase activity of red blood cells, and reduced lipid peroxidation content (Chen, 1995).

Chemotherapy Side Effects

A limited meta-analysis of 4 randomized clinical trials involving a total of 342 patients found some evidence of benefit from decoctions of traditional Chinese herbs containing Astragalus in counteracting the side effects of chemotherapy for colorectal cancer. These blends were prepared with the dried root of *Astragalus membranaceus* and *Astragalus mongolicus*, and with Huang-Qi compounds as the active ingredient. Four trials were included in the analysis. Subjects treated with chemotherapy and Huang-Qi decoctions as opposed to chemotherapy alone were less likely to develop nausea, vomiting, or low white blood cell counts. Huang-Qi compounds appeared to stimulate the immune system cells but did not alter antibody levels in the blood (Taixiang, 2007).

Immunomodulating Effects

Astragalus-based Chinese herbal medicine showed efficacy in increasing the effectiveness of platinum-based chemotherapy as compared to platinum-based chemotherapy alone in a meta-analysis of randomized trials for advanced non-small-cell lung cancer. The authors note that results of this meta-analysis of 34 randomized trials involving 2,815 patients require further confirmation with well-designed and rigorously controlled trials. Overall, inclusion of Astragalus was associated with reduced risk of death at 12 months (12 studies), improved tumor response data (30 studies), increased tumor response (3 studies) and reduced risk of death at 24 months (2 studies) (McCulloch, 2006).

The addition of Astragalus to a combined modality treatment for small-cell lung cancer improved survival rates compared with published survival rates. Fifty-four patients were treated with chemotherapy, radiotherapy, immunotherapy, and traditional Chinese medicine, which included Astragalus. Chemotherapy consisted of vincristine, cyclophosphamide, methotrexate, and carmustine. The overall response rate was 98.1% (Cha et al, 1994).

The effect of pure Astragalus preparation (PAP) in treating 115 patients with leukopenia was determined after 8 weeks of therapy. Group I was treated by a concentrated PAP (10 mL, equivalent to 15 g of Astragalus), and group II was treated with a different concentration of PAP (10 mL, equivalent to 5 g of Astragalus). Both treatment groups received a dose of 10 mL twice daily. The effectiveness was statistically different between the groups with 82.76% and 47.37% in Group I and II, respectively. The total effective rate was 65.22%. The average WBC counts of group I was significantly higher than that of group II with a significant rise of the WBC counts in both groups after treatment (Weng XS, 1995).

INDICATIONS AND USAGE

Unproven Uses: The herb has been used for respiratory infections, immune depression, cancer, heart failure, viral infections, liver disease, and kidney disease. Astragalus has also been used as a diuretic.

Chinese Medicine: The herb has been used alone and in combination for liver fibrosis, acute viral myocarditis, heart failure, small cell lung cancer, and amenorrhea, and as an antiviral agent.

CONTRAINDICATIONS:

Astragalus is contraindicated in patients with known autoimmune disease. Consider discontinuing Astragalus prior to elective surgery as Astragalus may increase the risk of bleeding.

PRECAUTIONS AND ADVERSE REACTIONS

Caution should be taken with patients receiving immunosuppressive therapy, such as transplant patients, due to the immunostimulating properties of Astragalgus. Extracts of *Astragalus lusitanicus* in animal models resulted in toxic excitatory cardiac effects and respiratory depression, involving skeletal muscle and neurological systems (Abdennebi, 1998; Yoshida et al, 1997).

DRUG INTERACTIONS

MODERATE RISK

Anticoagulants, Antiplatelet Agents, Thrombolytic Agents, Low Molecular Weight Heparins: Increased risk of bleeding with concomitant use. *Clinical Management:* Avoid concomitant use of Astragalus with these drugs. If Astragalus must be administered concomitantly with one of these agents, monitor closely for increased signs and symptoms of bleeding. Consider discontinuing Astragalus preoperatively to reduce the risk of surgical bleeding complications.

OVERDOSAGE

Due to the selenium content in Astragalus, toxic doses may result in neurological damage leading to paralysis.

DOSAGE

How Supplied:

Capsule-200 mg, 250 mg, 400 mg, 450 mg, 470 mg, 500 mg, 520 mg

Liquid

Tea Bags

Daily Dosage: The dried root is administered as 2-6 g daily, and the fluid extract as 4 to 12 mL daily. The powdered root capsule (250 mg-500 mg) has been administered as two capsules three times daily.

LITERATURE

Abdennebi EH, el Ouazzani N, Lamnaouer D. Clinical and analytical studies of sheep dosed with various preparations of *Astragalus lusitanicus. Vet Hum Toxicol* Dec;40(6):327-31. 1998

Bedir D. Calis I. Aquino R et al. Secondary metabolites from the roots of *Astragalus trojanus. J Nat Prod* Apr;62(4):563-8. 1999

Bedir E. Calis I. Aquino R et al. Cycloartane triterpene glycosides from the roots *of Astragalus brachypterus* and Astragalus microcephalus. *J Nat Prod* Dec;61(12):1469-72. 1998

Bone K. Clinical Applications of Ayurvedic and Chinese Herbs: Monographs for the Western Herbal Practitioner. Phytotherapy Press, Queensland, Australia 1997.

Cha RJ, Zeng DW & Chang QS. Non-surgical treatment of small cell lung cancer with chemo-radio-immunotherapy and traditional Chinese medicine. *Chung Hua Nei Ko Tsa Chih*; 33:462-466. 1994

Chen LX. Liao JZ. Guo WQ. Effects of *Astragalus membranaceus* on left ventricular function and oxygen free radical in acute myocardial infarction patients and mechanism of its cardiotonic action. *Chung Kuo Chung Hsi I Chieh Ho Tsa Chih* Mar;15(3):141-3. 1995

Chen M. Liu F. Chemical constituents of the seed oil of *Astragalus complanatus* R. Brown. *Chung Kuo Chung Yao Tsa Chih* Apr;15(4):225-6, 255. 1990

Chu D. Sun Y. Lin J et al. F3, a fractionated extract of *Astragalus membranaceus* potentiates lymphokine-activated killer cell cytotoxicity generated by low-dose recombinant interleukin-2. *Chung Hsi I Chieh Ho Tsa Chih* Jan;10(1):34-6, 5. 1990

Chu DT. Lin JR. Wong W. The in vitro potentiation of LAK cell cytotoxicity in cancer and aids patients induced by F3–a fractionated extract of *Astragalus membranaceus. Chung Hua Chung Liu Tsa Chih* May;16(3):167-71. 1994

Chu DT, Lepe-Zuniga J, Wong WL, et al. Fractionated extract of *Astragalus membranaceus*, a Chinese medicinal herb, potentiates LAK cell cytotoxicity generated by a low dose of recombinant interleukin-2. *J Clin Lab Immunol*:3-187. 1988

Chu D-T, Wong WL & Mavligit GM. Immunotherapy with Chinese medicinal herbs. I. Immune restoration of local xenogeneic graft-versus-host reaction in cancer patients by fractionated *Astragalus membranaceus* in vitro. *Clin Immunol*; 25:119-123. 1988

Chu D-T, Wong WL & Mavligit GM. Immunotherapy with Chinese medicinal herbs. II. Reversal of cyclophosphamide-induced immune suppression by administration of *fractionated Astragalus membranaceus* in vivo. *J Clin Lab Immunol*; 25:125-129. 1988

Foster S. Astragalus: A superior herb. *Herbs for Health*; Sept/Oct: 40-41. 1998

Guo XW. Zhang XX. Zhang ZM. Li FD. Characterization of *Astragalus sinicus* rhizobia by restriction fragment length polymorphism analysis of chromosomal and nodulation genes regions. *Curr Microbiol* Dec;39(6):358-0364. 1999

Hirotani M. Zhou Y. Rui H. Furuya T. Cycloartane triterpene glycosides from the hairy root cultures of *Astragalus membranaceus. Phytochemistry* Nov;37(5):1403-7. 1994

Hong CY. Lo YC. Tan FC et al. *Astragalus membranaceus* and *Polygonum multiflorum* protect rat heart mitochondria against lipid peroxidation. *Am J Chin Med* 1994;22(1):63-70.

Hong GX. Qin WC. Huang LS. Memory-improving effect of aqueous extract *of Astragalus membranaceus* (Fisch.) Bge. *Chung Kuo Chung Yao Tsa Chih* Nov;19(11):687-8, 704. 1994

Hong CY, Ku J & Wu P: *Astragalus membranaceus* stimulates human sperm motility in vitro. *Am J Chin Med*; 20(3-4):289-294. 1992

Jingzi LI, Lei YU, Ningjur LI et al. *Astragalus mongholicus* and *Angelica sinensis* compound alleviates nephrotic hyperlipidemia in rats. *Chin Med J*; 113(4):310-314. 2000

Kaye TN. From flowering to dispersal: reproductive ecology of an endemic plant, *Astragalus australis* var. olympicus (Fabaceae). *Am J Bot* Sep;86(9):1248. 1999

Khoo KS. Ang PT. Extract *of Astragalus membranaceus* and *ligustrum lucidum* does not prevent cyclophosphamide-induced myelosuppression. *Singapore Med J* Aug; 36(4):387-90. 1995

Lei ZY. Qin H. Liao JZ. Action of *Astragalus membranaceus* on left ventricular function of angina pectoris. *Chung Kuo Chung Hsi I Chieh Ho Tsa Chih* Apr;14(4):199-202, 195. 1994

Li SQ. Yuan RX. Gao H. Clinical observation on the treatment of ischemic heart disease with *Astragalus membranaceus. Chung Kuo Chung Hsi I Chieh Ho Tsa Chih* Feb;15(2):77-80. 1995

Luo HM. Dai RH. Li Y. Nuclear cardiology study on effective ingredients of *Astragalus membranaceus* in treating heart failure. *Chung Kuo Chung Hsi I Chieh Ho Tsa Chih* Dec; 15(12):707-9. 1995

Ma J. Peng A. Lin S. Mechanisms of the therapeutic effect of *Astragalus membranaceus* on sodium and water retention in experimental heart failure. *Chin Med J (Engl)* Jan;111(1):17-23. 1998

McCulloch M, See C, Shu XJ et al. Astragalus-based Chinese herbs and platinum-based chemotherapy for advanced non-small-cell lung cancer: meta-analysis of randomized trials. *J Clin Oncol;* 24:419-30. 2006.

Nigam SN. McConnell WB. Seleno amino compounds from *Astragalus bisulcatus*. Isolation and identification of gamma-L-glutamyl-Se-methyl-seleno-L-cysteine and Se-methylseleno-L-cysteine. *Biochim Biophys Acta* Nov 18;192(2):185-90. 1969

Norred CL & Finlayson CA. Hemorrhage after the preoperative use of complementary and alternative medicines. *AANA J*; 68(3):217-220. 2000

Panter KE, Hartley WJ, James LF, et al. Comparative toxicity of selenium from seleno-DL-methionine, sodium selenate, and *Astragalus bisulcatus* in pigs. *Fundam Appl Toxicol* Aug; 32(2):217-23. 1996

Peng T. Yang Y. Riesemann H; Kandolf R. The inhibitory effect of *Astragalus membranaceus* on coxsackie B-3 virus RNA replication. *Chin Med Sci J* Sep;10(3):146-50. 1995

Rittenhouse JR. Lui PD. Lau BH. Chinese medicinal herbs reverse macrophage suppression induced by urological tumors. *J Urol* Aug;146(2):486-90. 1991

Shi HM, Dai RH & Fan WH. Intervention of lidocaine and *Astragalus membranaceus* on ventricular late potentials. *Chung Kuo Chung Hsi I Chieh Ho Tsa Chih*; 14(10):598-600. 1994

Shi HM, Dai RH & Wang SY. Primary research on the clinical significance of ventricular late potentials (VLPs), and the impact of mexiletine, lidocaine, and Astragalus. *Chung His I Chieh Ho Tsa Chih,* May; 11(5): 259, 265-267. 1991

Rui T. Yang YZ. Zhou TS. Effect of *Astragalus membranaceus* on electrophysiological activities of acute experimental Coxsackie B3 viral myocarditis in mice. *Chung Kuo Chung Hsi I Chieh Ho Tsa Chih* May;14(5):292-4, 26. 1994

Taixiang, W., Munro, A. J., and Guanjian, L.: Chinese medical herbs for chemotherapy side effects in colorectal cancer patients. *Cochrane Database Syst Rev 1 (Online)*:CD004540. 2005.

Tianqing P, Yingzhen Y, Riesemann H et al. The inhibitory effect *of Astragalus membranaceus* on Coxsackie B-3 virus RNA replication. *Chin Med Sci J*; 10:146-150. 1995

Wang HK. He K. Xu HX, et al. The structure of astrachrysosid A and the study of 2D-NMR on astrasieversianin XV and 7,2′-dihydroxy-3’,4′-dimethoxy-isoflavane-7-O- beta-D-glycoside. *Yao Hsueh Hsueh Pao*;25(6):445-50. 1990

Weng XS. Treatment of leucopenia with pure Astragalus preparation–an analysis of 115 leucopenic cases. *Chung Kuo Chung Hsi I Chieh Ho Tsa Chih* Aug;15(8):462-4. 1995

Wong V, et al. A hospital clinic-based survey on traditional Chinese medicine usage among chronic hepatitis B patients. *Comp Ther Med*; 13:175-182. 2005.

Xuan W, Dong M & Dong M: Effects of compound injection of *Pyrola rotundifolia L and Astragalus membranaceus Bge* on experimental guinea pigs' gentamicin ototoxicity. *Ann Otol Rhinol Laryngol*; 104:374-380. 1995

Yang Y-z, Jin P-y, Guo Q et al. Treatment of experimental coxsackie B-3 viral myocarditis with *Astragalus membranaceus* in mice. *Chinese Med J*; 103:14-18. 1990

Yarnell, E. and Abascal, K: Herbs for relieving chronic renal failure. *Alt Comp Ther;* 13(1):18-23. 2007.

Yoshida Y, Wang MQ, Liu JN et al. Immunomodulating activity of Chinese medicinal herbs and *Oldenlandia diffusa* in particular. *Int J Immunopharm*; 19:359-370. 1997

Yuan W-l, Chen H-z, Yang, Y-z et al. Effect of *Astragalus membranaceus* on electric activities of cultured rat beating heart cells infected with Coxsackie B-2 virus. *Chinese Med J*; 103:177-182. 1990

Zhang WJ. Wojta J. Binder BR. Regulation of the fibrinolytic potential of cultured human umbilical vein endothelial cells: astragaloside IV downregulates plasminogen activator inhibitor-1 and upregulates tissue-type plasminogen activator expression. *J Vasc Res* Jul-Aug;34(4):273-80. 1997

Zhang ZL. Wen QZ. Liu CX. Hepatoprotective effects of Astragalus root. *J Ethnopharmacol* Sep;30(2):145-9. 1990

Zhang YD, Shen JP, Zhu SH et al. Effects of Astragalus (ASI, SK) on experimental liver injury. *Yao Hsueh Hsueh Pao*; 27(6):401-406. 1992

Zhao KS. Mancini C. Doria G. Enhancement of the immune response in mice *by Astragalus membranaceus* extracts. *Immunopharmacology* Nov-Dec;20(3):225-33. 1990

Zheng Z. Liu D. Song C et al. Studies on chemical constituents and immunological function activity of hairy root of *Astragalus membranaceus*. *Chin J Biotechnol*;14(2):93-7. 1998

Astragalus species

See Astragalus (Huang-Qi)

Athyrium filix-femina

See Lady Fern

Atractylodes japonica

See Japanese Atractylodes

Atractylodes lancea

See Southern Tsangshu (Cang-Zhu)

Atropa belladonna

See Belladonna

Avena sativa

See Oats

Averrhoa carambola

See Carambola

Avocado

Persea americana

DESCRIPTION

Medicinal Parts: The medicinal parts are the dried leaves, the fresh leaves, the whole fruit, including the seed and the oil extracted from the leaves.

Flower and Fruit: The flowers are in compact or loose racemes. They are 5 to 8.2 mm long and greenish. The inner and outer perianth circles are 4 to 6 mm long and elliptical to oval-elliptical. The anthers are 3.5 mm long, and the filaments are 2.3 mm. The ovary is oval or pear-shaped and downy. It develops into a drupe, which is green and fleshy and grows up to 18 cm long. The drupe is smooth with thick oily flesh and a very large seed.

Leaves, Stem and Root: The avocado is a tree up to 40 m in height and with a trunk 60 cm in diameter. The leaves are 6 to 30 cm long and 3.5 to 19 cm wide. They are narrow to broadly elliptical. The leaf surface is sticky, while the lower surface is downy.

Habitat: The plant originated in central and southern South America and is cultivated in all tropical and subtropical regions today.

Production: Avocado oil comes from the fruit of *Persea americana*. Avocado oil is recovered from the pericarp of *Persea americana* and refined if necessary.

ACTIONS AND PHARMACOLOGY

COMPOUNDS

Fatty oil: chief fatty acids oleic acid, palmitic acid, linoleic acid, palmitoleic acid (tocopherols, vitamin E)

EFFECTS

Avocado oil is an emollient, which improves rough ichtyotic skin.

INDICATIONS AND USAGE

Avocado is a main ingredient in lines of ''natural'' cosmetics.

PRECAUTIONS AND ADVERSE REACTIONS

No health hazards or side effects are known in conjunction with the proper administration of designated therapeutic dosages.

DOSAGE

Mode of Administration: As an active or inactive ingredient in various preparations (bath oils, ointments, etc.).

Storage: Oils from different batches should not be mixed. The drug should be stored in a sealed container away from light and moisture.

LITERATURE

Browse J. Antifugal compounds from idioblast cells isolated from avocado fruits. *Phytochem.* 54: 183-9. 2000

Kawagishi H, Fukumoto Y, Hatakeyama M, et al. Liver injury suppressing compounds from avocado (*Persea americana*): *J Agric Food Chem.*; 49: 2215-21. 2001

Kasai T. Acetyl-CoA carboxylase inhibitors from avocado (*Persea americana Mill*) fruits. *Biosci Biotechnol Biochem.* 65: 1656-8. 2001

Lequesne M, Maheu E, Cadet C, Dreisler RL. Structural effect of avocado/soybean usaponifiables on joint space loss in osteoarthritis of the hip. *Arthritis Rheum.* 47:50-58. 2002.

Kim OK, Murakami A, Nakamura Y, Takeda N, Yoshizumi H, Ohigashi H. Novel nitric oxide and superoxide generation inhibitors, persenone A and B, from avocado fruit. *J Agric Food Chem*; 48: 1557-63. 2000

Kut-Lassere C, Miller CC, Ejeil AL, et al. Effect of avocado and soybean unsaponifiables on gelatinase A (IMMP-2), stromelysin 1 (MMP-3), and tissue inhibitors of matrix metalloproteinase (TIMP-1 and TIMP-2) secretion by human fibroblasts in culture. *J Periodontol*; 72: 1685-94. 2001

Teuscher E, Biogene Arzneimittel, 5. Aufl., Wiss. Verlagsges. Stuttgart 1997.

Bael

Aegle marmelos

DESCRIPTION

Medicinal Parts: The medicinal parts are the unripe fruit, the root, leaves, and branches.

Flower and Fruit: The plant has greenish-white flowers. The yellow fruit is globular or ovoid, with a hard shell. The fruit is divided internally like an orange. The flesh is reddish, with numerous seeds covered in a layer of latex.

Characteristics: The taste is mucilaginous and slightly sour.

Habitat: This plant is native to India but has spread over wide areas of southeast Asia.

Other Names: Bel, Bengal Quince, Indian Bael

ACTIONS AND PHARMACOLOGY

COMPOUNDS

Tannins

Saccharides

Starch

Fatty oil

Furocoumarins

Furoquinolin alkaloids

EFFECTS

Bael has a digestive and an astringent effect.

INDICATIONS AND USAGE

Indian Medicine: Bael is used for digestive complaints and diarrhea.

PRECAUTIONS AND ADVERSE REACTIONS

No health hazards or side effects are known in conjunction with the proper administration of designated therapeutic dosages.

OVERDOSAGE

Digestive complaints and constipation are possible with the intake of large quantities, due to the constituent tannins.

DOSAGE

Mode of Administration: Available as a liquid extract for internal use.

LITERATURE

Oliver-Bever B (Ed., 1986), Medicinal Plants of Tropical West Africa, Cambridge University Press UK.

Sharma BR and Sharma P, (1981) *Planta Med* 43:102.

Schimmer O, Furochinolinalkaloide als biologisch aktive Naturstoffe. In: *ZPT* 12(5):151. 1991.

Balloon-Flower (Jie-Geng)

Platycodon grandiflorum

DESCRIPTION

Medicinal Parts: The medicinal parts of the plant are the main and secondary roots.

Flower and Fruit: The flowers are at the tip of the leading shoot. The flower structures are in fives and are fused. The calyx tube is appressed to the ovary; the corolla is 5-lobed, blue, occasionally white with a diameter of approximately 5 cm. The 5 stamens are free and the ovary inferior with numerous ovules. The fruit is an obovoid, multichambered, dehiscent capsule. The seeds are ovoid, light to dark brown, and smooth, 1.7 to 2.2 mm long, 1 to 1.2 mm wide and flattened.

Leaves, Stem, and Root: The plant is a herbaceous perennial growing to 90 cm high. The leaves are almost sessile with a simple lamina, bluish-green above and gray-green beneath, irregularly crenate-serrate and entire at the base. The plant has a hardy (approximately 3 cm thick) taproot and hardy secondary roots.

Habitat: Balloon-Flower is indigenous to China, Japan, Korea, and Siberia.

Production: The plant is collected in the wild and air-dried. Balloon-Flower root is the dried main and secondary root of *Platycodon grandiflorum.*

Other Names: Chinese Bell-Flower, Japanese Bell-Flower

ACTIONS AND PHARMACOLOGY

COMPOUNDS

Triterpene saponins (1.7%): including platycodin, platycodoside C, aglycone platycodigenin, including glycosides of polygalic acid, platycogenic acids A to C

Volatile oil (0.2 to 0.3%)

Steroids: sterols, including delta7-stigmasterol, alpha-spinasterol

EFFECTS

The saponin fraction contained in the drug has inhibiting effects upon gastric secretion and exhibits both ulcer-protective and ulcer-healing effects. In addition, a mild antibacterial effect has been demonstrated. The plant is said to have a sedative effective on the respiratory organs and encourages expectoration. The antitussive, anti-inflammator,y and sedative effects require further clinical testing for verification.

INDICATIONS AND USAGE

Chinese Medicine: Jie-Geng is mainly used as an expectorant for bronchitis, sore throat, tonsillitis, and other conditions of the respiratory tract. Efficacy as an expectorant is plausible due to the saponin content; efficacy for the other indications has not been proved.

PRECAUTIONS AND ADVERSE REACTIONS

No health hazards are known in conjunction with the proper administration of designated therapeutic dosages.

DOSAGE

Mode of Administration: Preparations of whole, cut and powdered drug are for internal use.

Preparation: Liquid extract: root powder 1:1 25% ethanol

Daily Dosage:

Powder – 6 g daily; 0.5 g as a single dose

Decoction – 1 g daily; 0.2 g as a single dose

Storage: Store tightly sealed and protected from light.

LITERATURE

Hänsel R, Keller K, Rimpler H, Schneider G (Ed), Hagers Handbuch der Pharmazeutischen Praxis, 5. Aufl., Bde 4 - 6 (Drogen), Springer Verlag Berlin, Heidelberg, New York, 1992-1994.

Kim KS, Ezaki O, Ikemoto S, Itakura H, Effects of *Platycodon grandiflorum* feeding on serum and liver lipid concentrations in rats with diet-induced hyperlipidemia. *J Nutr Sci Vitaminol* (Tokyo), 41:485-91, 1995 Aug.

Kim KS, Ezaki O, Ikemoto S, Itakura H, Effects of *Platycodon grandiflorum* feeding on serum and liver lipid concentrations in rats with diet-induced hyperlipidemia. *Yakugaku Zasshi,* 41:485-91, 1995 Aug.

Kim KS, Ezaki O, Ikemoto S, Itakura H Rat plasma corticosterone secretion-inducing activities of total saponin and prosapogenin methyl esters from the roots of *Platycodon grandiflorum* A.DC. *Yakugaku Zasshi*, 41:1191-4, 1995 Aug.

Ballota nigra

See Black Horehound

Balmony

Chelone glabra

DESCRIPTION

Medicinal Parts: The medicinal part is the fresh herb picked during the flowering season

Flower and Fruit: The inflorescence is a short terminal spike of bilabiate white, purple, cream, or pink flowers. The lower lip is awned in the tube and the cordate anthers are downy. The seeds are round and bitter.

Leaves, Stem, and Root: The plant is small and erect, and may reach up to 60 cm in height. It is a perennial herb with angular, smooth stems and a horizontally spreading root system. The leaves are opposite, oblong-lanceolate and grow on short petioles.

Characteristics: The leaves have a tea-like smell and an extremely bitter taste.

Habitat: Northeastern U.S. and Canada

Production: Balmony is the above-ground part of *Chelone glabra.*

Other Names: Turtlebloom, Turtle Head, Chelone, Shellflower, Salt-Rheum Weed, Bitter Herb, Hummingbird Tree, Snakehead

ACTIONS AND PHARMACOLOGY

COMPOUNDS

Iridoide monoterpenes: catalpol

Resin: (bitter-tasting)

EFFECTS

No information available.

INDICATIONS AND USAGE

Homeopathic Uses: Balmony is used in the treatment of liver disorders, digestive disorders, and worm infestation.

PRECAUTIONS AND ADVERSE REACTIONS

No health hazards or side effects are known in conjunction with the proper administration of designated therapeutic dosages.

DOSAGE

Mode of Administration: The herb is available in homeopathic dilutions.

LITERATURE

Belofsky G et al., *PH* 28:1601. 1989.

Kern W, List PH, Hörhammer L (Hrsg.), Hagers Handbuch der Pharmazeutischen Praxis, 4. Aufl., Bde. 1-8, Springer Verlag Berlin, Heidelberg, New York, 1969.

Bamboo

Arundinaria japonica

DESCRIPTION

Medicinal Parts: The medicinal parts are the young shoots of the plant.

Flower and Fruit: Greenish-yellow, round culms exceeding 3 m in height are surrounded at the culm nodes by dry leaf sheaths, which do not fall off. The upper surface of the leaves are shiny and dark green; the underside is matte and gray-green. The leaf margins are sharply serrated.

Habitat: The plant is indigenous to the tropics, southern subtropics and Asia.

Production: Bamboo sprouts are the young shoots of *Arundinaria japonica.*

ACTIONS AND PHARMACOLOGY

COMPOUNDS

Soluble mono-, oligo-, and polysaccharides

Silicic acid: to some extent water-soluble

EFFECTS

No information is available.

INDICATIONS AND USAGE

Bamboo is seldom used for medicinal purposes in Western medicine.

Indian Medicine: The drug is used for asthma, arthritis, and coughs.

PRECAUTIONS AND ADVERSE REACTIONS

No health hazards or side effects are known in conjunction with the proper administration of designated therapeutic dosages.

DOSAGE

Mode of Administration: The juice from the young shoots is hardened as bamboo sugar and used internally.

LITERATURE

No literature is available.

Baneberry

Actaea spicata

DESCRIPTION

Medicinal Parts: The medicinal part is the root.

Flower and Fruit: The white flowers are in ovate racemes. They have 4 to 6 bracts, white stamens and 1 ovary. The fruit is a black, many-seeded berry.

Leaves, Stem, and Root: The plant grows 30 to 60 cm tall. It is large, long-petioled, trifoliate, and pinnate. The leaflets are pinnatisect and serrate. The stem is erect and glabrous.

Characteristics: Baneberry is poisonous, as are several other plants with similar qualities.

Habitat: The plant grows in most of Europe and in moderate and arctic regions of Asia.

Production: Baneberry or Herb Christopher root is the root of *Actaea spicata.*

Not to be Confused With: Helleborus niger is occasionally used as a substitute by mistake.

Other Names: Bugbane, Herb Christopher, Toadroot

ACTIONS AND PHARMACOLOGY

COMPOUNDS

Isoquinoline alkaloids: magnoflorine, corytuberine

Triterpene glycosides: including actein

Trans-aconitic acid

EFFECTS

The drug, which contains alkaloids (magnoflorine) and saponins, was shown to inhibit growth of *Mycobacterium tuberculosis*. An antirheumatic effect is being investigated.

INDICATIONS AND USAGE

Unproven Uses: Baneberry is used as an emetic and purgative.

Homeopathic Uses: The drug is used in homeopathy for rheumatic conditions, especially those of the smaller joints.

PRECAUTIONS AND ADVERSE REACTIONS

No health hazards or side effects are known in conjunction with the proper administration of designated therapeutic dosages.

DOSAGE

Mode of Administration: In homeopathy, Baneberry is available as dilutions of the mother tincture.

LITERATURE

Fardella G, Corsano St, Preliminary study on actein biosynthesis. In: *Ann Chim* (Rom)63:333-337. 1973.

Frohne D, Pfänder HJ, Giftpflanzen - Ein Handbuch für Apotheker, Toxikologen und Biologen, 4. Aufl., Wiss. Verlags-Ges Stuttgart 1997.

Kern W, List PH, Hörhammer L (Hrsg.), Hagers Handbuch der Pharmazeutischen Praxis, 4. Aufl., Bde. 1-8, Springer Verlag Berlin, Heidelberg, New York, 1969.

Madaus G, Lehrbuch der Biologischen Arzneimittel, Bde 1-3, Nachdruck, Georg Olms Verlag Hildesheim 1979.

Nikonow GK, Syrkina SA, Chemische Untersuchungen der aktiven Prinzipien von Actaea spicata L. In: *Pharm Zentralhalle* 103(8):601. 1964.

Banisteriopsis caapi

See Yagé

Baobab

Adansonia digitata

DESCRIPTION

Medicinal Parts: Fruit pulp mixed with water, decoctions of bark and leaves.

Botanical Description: The African baobab tree is characterized by its massive size, reaching to a height of 18-25m and producing a rounded crown and showing a stiff branching habit. The trunk is swollen and stout, up to 10m in diameter, usually tapering or cylindrical and abruptly bottle-shaped; often buttressed. Branches are distributed irregularly and large. The bark is smooth, reddish brown to grey, soft and fibrous. The tree produces an extensive lateral root system and the roots end in tubers. Leaves are 2-3-foliate at the start of the season and they are early deciduous; more mature ones are 5-7(-9)-foliate. Leaves are alternate at the ends of branches or occur on short spurs on the trunk. Flowers are pendulous, solitary or paired in leaf axils, large and showy and produced during both wet and dry seasons. Fruits are very variable, usually globose to ovoid but sometimes oblong-cylindrical, often irregular in shape, 7.5-54cm long x 7.5-20cm wide, apex pointed or obtuse, covered by velvety yellowish hairs (sometimes greenish).

Habitat: African baobab occurs naturally in most countries south of the Sahara with notable absence in Liberia, Uganda, Djibouti and Burundi. Introduced in Gabon, Democratic Republic of the Congo, São Tomé, Madagascar and Comoros. Introduced by traders, it is also found in Réunion, Malaysia, Indonesia (Java), China-Taiwan, Philippines, Guyana, New Caledonia, Cuba, Haiti, Dominican Republic, Martinique, USA (Hawaii, Puerto Rico, Virgin Islands, and Florida), Jamaica, Montserrat, Netherlands Antilles, Dominica, St. Kitts and Nevis, St. Lucia, St. Vincent and the Grenadines, Trinidad and Tobago, and Barbados.

Other Names: Baobab, Monkey bread tree, Ethiopian sour gourd, Cream of tartar tree, Senegal calabash, Upside-down tree, pain de singe, arbre aux calebasses, arbre de mille ans, calebassier du Senégal, Cabaçevre, Buhibab, hamao-hamaraya, gangoleis, Habhab, Hamar, hamaraya, Teidoûm, humr, homeira, Dungwol, Trega, twega, toayga, Oro, Konian, ko, Sira, Babbe, boki, olohi, Sira, sito, Fromdo, Kouka, kuka, Goui, gouis, goui, lalo, boui, Bak, Boubakakou, Boki, bokki, Bamba, Hemmer, dumma, Mlonje, Mnambe, Mlambe, Mbuye.

ACTIONS AND PHARMACOLOGY

COMPOUNDS

Leaves: Young leaves contain (dry weight): 13-15% protein, 60-70% carbohydrate, 4-10% fat and around 11% fiber and 16% ash. Leaves are also known to be significant sources of minerals, especially magnesium and manganese. *Fruit:* Ripe fruit contain an average of 8.7% moisture with 2.7% protein, 0.2% fat, 73.7% carbohydrate, 8.9% fibres and 5.8% ash. High levels of Vitamin C. Sweetness is provided by fructose, saccharose and glucose contents. *A. digitata* is rich in tartaric acid and citric acid. Active principle is assumed to be one of the various flavonols such as quercetin-7-O-beta-D-xylopyranoside or triterpenoids such as 7-baueren-3-acetate. The plant contains also adansonin.

EFFECTS

Febrifuge (malaria), astringent, anti-inflammatory, refreshing, perspiration-reducing, weakly hypotensive, mildly irritating, rich in vitamin C, strophantus-like effects, expectorant, diaphoretic, antiasthmatic. The plant is reported to produce Strophantus-like activities. Aqueous and alcoholic extracts of the leaves produced a slight drop in blood pressure after IV administration to dogs. Adansonia-flavonoside is able to reduce capillary permeability in rabbits. A marked decrease of carotid pressure after IV application was also seen in dogs as was a countering of asthmatic crisis induced by histamine aerosol in guinea pigs.

INDICATIONS AND USAGE

Unproven Uses: In traditional South African medicine, the bark and leaves are considered anti-inflammatory and diaphoretic and are used for urinary disorders and mild diarrhea. The leaves are used against fever, to reduce excessive perspiration and as an astringent and expectorant. The bark has been sold commercially in Europe as a substitute for chinchona bark for the treatment of fever, especially that caused by malarial infection. The fruit pulp, an important source of ascorbic acid, is the basis for health beverages and is also used in the treatment of fever, diarrhea, and hemoptysis. The powdered seeds are recommended as a hiccup remedy for children.

CONTRAINDICATIONS

No information is available.

PRECAUTIONS AND ADVERSE REACTIONS

Alcoholic and aqueous extracts of the leaves showed a low order of toxicity in mice. The plant contains tartaric acid, which is mildly irritating in high concentrations.

DRUG INTERACTIONS

No human drug information is available.

DOSAGE

No information is available.

LITERATURE

Atawodi SE, Ameh DA, Ibrahim S, Andrew JN, Nzelibe HC, Onyike EO, Anigo KM, Abu EA, James DB, Njoku GC, Sallau AB. Indigenous knowledge system for treatment of trypanosomiasis in Kaduna state of Nigeria. J Ethnopharmacol. 2002 Feb;79(2):279-82.

Barminas JT, Charles M, Emmanuel D. Mineral composition of non-conventional leafy vegetables. Plant Foods Hum Nutr. 1998;53(1):29-36.

Chauhan JS, Kumar S, Chaturvedi R. A New Flavanonol Glycoside from Adansonia digitata Roots. Planta Med. 1984 Feb;50(1):113.

Eromosele IC, Eromosele CO, Kuzhkuzha DM. Evaluation of mineral elements and ascorbic acid contents in fruits of some wild plants. Plant Foods Hum Nutr. 1991 Apr;41(2):151-4.

Fabiyi JP, Kela SL, Tal KM, Istifanus WA. [Traditional therapy of dracunculiasis in the state of Bauchi - Nigeria] Dakar Med. 1993;38(2):193-5.

Le Grand A. [Anti-infective phytotherapies of the tree-savannah, Senegal (occidental Africa). III: A review of phytochemical substances and the antimicrobial activity of 43 species] J Ethnopharmacol. 1989 May;25(3):315-38.

Locher CP, Burch MT, Mower HF, Berestecky J, Davis H, Van Poel B, Lasure A, Vanden Berghe DA, Vlietinck AJ. Antimicrobial activity and anti-complement activity of extracts obtained from selected Hawaiian medicinal plants. J Ethnopharmacol. 1995 Nov 17;49(1):23-32.

Obizoba IC, Anyika JU. Nutritive value of baobab milk (gubdi) and mixtures of baobab (Adansonia digitata L.) and hungry rice, acha (Digitaria exilis) flours. Plant Foods Hum Nutr. 1994 Sep;46(2):157-65.

Osman MA. Chemical and nutrient analysis of baobab (Adansonia digitata) fruit and seed protein solubility. Plant Foods Hum Nutr. 2004 Winter;59(1):29-33.

Sidibe, M. and Williams, J. T. (2002) Baobab. Adansonia digitata. International Centre for Underutilised Crops, Southampton, UK.

Tal-Dia A, Toure K, Sarr O, Sarr M, Cisse MF, Garnier P, Wone I. [A baobab solution for the prevention and treatment of acute dehydration in infantile diarrhea] Dakar Med. 1997;42(1):68-73.

Baptisia tinctoria

See Wild Indigo

barbadensis/capensis/vera

See Aloe

Barberry

Berberis vulgaris

DESCRIPTION

Medicinal Parts: The medicinal part is the fruit and the root bark.

Flower and Fruit: The flowers are 5 to 7 cm long in yellow, dense, hanging clusters. The 6 sepals are yellow and the 6 petals have orange-colored honey glands at the base. The 6 stamens burst open at the side. The ovary is superior with a flat stigma. The edible fruit is a bright scarlet, oblong-cylindrical berry, 10 to 12 mm long and 6 mm thick. The exocarp is membranous-coriaceous. There are usually 2 seeds.

Leaves, Stem, and Root: Barberry is a deciduous, heavily branched, thorny bush up to 2 m high. The thorny branches are angular, deeply grooved, initially brownish yellow, then more whitish gray. The thorns are 1 to 2 cm long and stick out horizontally. The leaves are in bunches and are obovate to elliptoid, 2 to 4 cm long and narrow. They are dark green and reticulate; the margin is dentate.

Characteristics: The flowers have a repulsive smell; the stamens lie on the carpels at the slightest touch. The flesh of the fruit is juicy and sour.

Habitat: Europe, northern Africa, and parts of America and central Asia.

Production: Barberries are the ripe fruit of *Berberis vulgaris.* Barberry root bark or berberis bark is the dried root bark of *Berberis vulgaris. Berberis aquifolium* is a closely related American variety that is often used in commercially available Oregon Grape products.

Not to be Confused With: There is a possibility of confusion with the fruits of other berberidis types. The commercial drug often consists of admixtures; between 15% and 50% of branch and trunk bark.

Other Names: Berberry, Pipperidge, Jaundice Berry, Sow Berry, Mountain Grape, Oregon Grape

ACTIONS AND PHARMACOLOGY

COMPOUNDS: BARBERRY FRUIT

Isoquinoline alkaloids (at the most, traces)

Anthocyans

Chlorogenic acid

Malic acid, acetic acid

EFFECTS: BARBERRY ROOT BARK

Source of vitamin C. In various metabolic processes, vitamin C increases immune system activity, stimulates iron absorption, and prevents scurvy. There is a mild diuretic effect due to the acid content.

COMPOUNDS: BARBERRY ROOT BARK

Isoquinoline alkaloids: in particular berberine, berbamine, oxyacanthin, further to include columbamine, palmatine, jatrorrhizine, magnoflorine.

EFFECTS: BARBERRY ROOT BARK

Cardiovascular effect: Fractions from the root extracts, which contain 80% berberine and other alkaloids, have been shown to reduce the blood pressure of cats for several hours. With varying doses, both positive and negative inotropic effects on the cats' hearts were recorded.

Cholagogue effect: A homeopathic mother tincture increased the bile flow in guinea pigs by an average of 20%. An extract with 80% berberine and additional alkaloids stimulated the bile excretion of rats by 72%.

Antipyretic effect: Aqueous tinctures have an anti-febrile effect on a feverish rabbit.

Antibiotic effect

Stimulation of intestinal peristalsis

INDICATIONS AND USAGE

BARBERRY FRUIT

Unproven uses: Decoction or alcoholic extract for lung, spleen, and liver diseases. Jam or wine made from the fresh berries can relieve constipation and stimulate the appetite. Alcoholic extracts have been used for heartburn and stomach cramps. Extracts have also been used for susceptibility to infection, feverish colds, and diseases of the urinary tract. Used in the pharmaceutical industry as a syrup for masking flavor.

BARBERRY ROOT BARK

Unproven uses: Barberry has been used for opium or morphine withdrawal. In folk medicine, the bark is used for liver malfunctions, gallbladder disease, jaundice, splenopathy, indigestion, diarrhea, tuberculosis, piles, renal disease, urinary tract disorders, gout, rheumatism, arthritis, lumbago, malaria, and leishmaniasis.

Homeopathic: The drug is used for kidney stones, gout, rheumatism, liver and gallbladder disorders, and dry skin diseases

PRECAUTIONS AND ADVERSE REACTIONS

BARBERRY FRUIT AND ROOT BARK

No health hazards or side effects are known in conjunction with the proper administration of designated therapeutic dosages.

OVERDOSAGE

BARBERRY ROOT BARK

Dosages over 4 mg will bring about light stupor, nosebleeds, vomiting, diarrhea, and kidney irritation. The treatment for poisonings is to be carried out symptomatically.

DOSAGE

BARBERRY FRUIT

Mode of Administration: Barberry is used internally in tea mixtures and combination preparations.

Preparation: To prepare a tea infusion, pour approximately 150 ml of hot water into 1 to 2 teaspoons of whole or squashed Barberries and strain after 10 to 15 minutes.

BARBERRY ROOT BARK

How Supplied:

Liquid extract–1:1, 1:5

Tea

Preparation: A tincture 1:10 is prepared according to the German Pharmacopeia 10th ed.

To extract the pure alkaloids from berberis roots, use 0.3% sulphuric acid mixed with 10% sodium chloride. The precipitated berberine hydrochloride is washed with mildly hydrochloric water and dried. It is then dissolved in water (pH 8) and filtered. The filtrate is heated to 70° C and set to pH 2.0 using hydrochloric acid. The precipitate of pure berberine hydrochloride is then washed and dried.

Daily Dosage: The dosage of the infusion is 2 g in 250 ml water, to be sipped. The tincture dosage is 20 to 40 drops daily.

Homeopathic Dosage: 5 drops, 1 tablet, or 10 globules every 30 to 60 minutes (acute) or 1 to 3 times daily (chronic);

parenterally: 1 to mL 3 times a day; suppositories: 2 to 3 times daily; ointment: 1 to 2 times daily (HAB).

LITERATURE

Andronescu E et al., (1973) *Clujul. Med* 46: 627.

Chen MQ et al., (1965) *Acta Pharm Sinica* 12 (3): 185.

Cordell GA, Farnsworth NR, (1977) *Lloydia* 40: 1.

Ikram M, (1975) *Planta Med* 28: 253.

Lahiri SC et al., (1958) *Ann Biochem Exp Med India* 18: 95.

Liu CX et al., (1979) Chinese Traditional and Herbal Drugs Communications 9: 36.

Naidovich LP et al., (1976) *Farmatsiya* 24: 33.

Subbaiah TV, Amin AH, (1967) *Nature* 215: 527.

Ubebaba K et al., (1984) *Jpn J Pharmacol* 36 (Suppl): 352.

Willaman JJ, Hui-Li L, (1970) *Lloydia* 33 (3A): 1.

Barley

Hordeum distichon

DESCRIPTION

Medicinal Parts: The medicinal part is the polished grain without the husk.

Flower and Fruit: The spike is 7 to 15 cm long. The long form is nodding and the shorter one erect and compressed on the side that does not bear spikelets. The spike spindle is tough and loosens the spikelets when ripe. The lateral spikelets are unbearded, male, or sexless. The middle spikelet is seed-bearing, with a beard up to 15 cm long.

Leaves, Stem, and Root: The plant is an annual that grows 60 to 130 cm high. It has a long hollow stalk and lanceolate leaves. The leaflets are very wide, long, and glabrous.

Habitat: Barley is cultivated worldwide.

Production: Barley seeds are the seeds of *Hordeum distichon.*

Other Names: Pearl Barley, Pot Barley, Scotch Barley

ACTIONS AND PHARMACOLOGY

COMPOUNDS

Polysaccharides: starch (50%), fructans

Mono- and oligosaccharides: saccharose, raffinose, glucodifructose, glucose, fructose

Proteins (10%): including, among others, prolamines: hordein- glutelins: hordenine (not to be confused with the amine of the same name, see below)- albumins and globulins

Prolamines: hordein

Glutelins: hordenine (not to be confused with the amine of the same name, see below)

Albumins and globulins

Fatty oil (2%): chief fatty acids linoleic and oleic acid

Vitamins: Vitamin E, nicotinic acid, pantothenic acid, vitamins B6, B2, folic acid

Hydroxycoumarins (only in the stalks): including, among others, umbelliferone, scopoletin, herniarin, aesculetin (in the sprouts)

Amines: tyramine, hordenine (dimethyltyramine), gramine also with certain strains (dimethy- laminomethylindol)

EFFECTS

Barley is soothing on the alimentary tract.

INDICATIONS AND USAGE

Unproven Uses: Barley has been used for convalescents and in the treatment of diarrhea, gastritis, and inflammatory bowel conditions.

PRECAUTIONS AND ADVERSE REACTIONS

General: No health hazards or side effects are known in conjunction with the proper administration of designated therapeutic dosages.

Pregnancy: Not to be used during pregnancy.

DOSAGE

Mode of Administration: Barley is used as a malt extract, in preparations and in combinations.

How Supplied:

Capsules - 450 mg

LITERATURE

Bergantino E, Sandon'a D, Cugini D, Bassi R, The photosystem II subunit CP29 can be phosphorylated in both C3 and C4 plants as suggested by sequence analysis. *Plant Mol Biol*, 36:11-22, 1998 Jan

Davies TG, Theodoulou FL, Hallahan DL, Forde BG, Cloning and characterisation of a novel P-glycoprotein homologue from barley. *Gene*, 199:195-202, 1997 Oct 15

Dhar ML et al., (1968) Indian J Exp Biol 6:232.

Kern W, List PH, Hörhammer L (Hrsg.), Hagers Handbuch der Pharmazeutischen Praxis, 4. Aufl., Bde. 1-8, Springer Verlag Berlin, Heidelberg, New York, 1969.

Labbe M, (1936) *J Canad Med Assoc* 34:141.

Oliver-Bever B (Ed), Medicinal Plants of Tropical West Africa. Cambridge University Press, Cambridge, London 1986

Pajuelo P, Pajuelo E, Forde BG, Marquez AJ, Regulation of the expression of ferredoxin-glutamate synthase in barley. *Planta*, 203:517-25, 1997 Dec

Rudi H et al., A (His)6-tagged recombinant barley endosperm ADP-glucose pyrophosphorylase expressed in the baculovirus-insect cell system is insensitive to allosteric regulation by 3-phosphoglycerate and inorganic phosphate. *FEBS Lett*, 419, 1997

Schuurink RC, Shartzer SF, Fath A, Jones RL, Characterization of a calmodulin-binding transporter from the plasma membrane of barley aleurone. *Proc Natl Acad Sci* U S A, 95:1944-9, 1998 Feb 17

Barosma species

See Short Buchu

Basil

Ocimum basilicum

DESCRIPTION

Medicinal Parts: The medicinal parts of the plant are the fresh or dried herb as well as the oil extracted from the dried aerial parts.

Flower and Fruit: The white, labiate flowers are in 6-blossomed, pedicled, almost sessile axillary false whorls. The calyx is bilabiate, and the corolla is 4-lobed. The 4 stamens lie on the simple lower lip.

Leaves, Stem, and Root: The plant grows from 20 to 40 cm high. The stem is erect, branched from the base up, and downy. The leaves are ovate or oblong. They are long-petioled, acuminate, irregularly dentate, or entire-margined.

Characteristics: Basil has a characteristic odor and sharp taste.

Habitat: The plant probably originated in India, Afghanistan, Pakistan, and northern India, and now is cultivated worldwide.

Production: Basil herb consists of the dried, above-ground parts of *Ocimum basilicum.* Oil of basil is the essential oil extracted from the dried aerial parts of *Ocimum basilicum* by steam distillation.

Other Names: St. Josephwort

ACTIONS AND PHARMACOLOGY

COMPOUNDS: BASIL HERB

Volatile oil: chief constituents are chavicol methyl ether (estragole), linalool and eugenol

Caffeic acid derivatives

Flavonoids

EFFECTS: BASIL HERB

In vitro, Basil is antimicrobial.

COMPOUNDS: BASIL OIL

Chief constituents: estragole (chavicol methyl ether), linalool, eugenol

EFFECTS: BASILOIL

In vitro, the oil demonstrates an antimicrobial effect.

INDICATIONS AND USAGE

BASIL HERB

Unproven Uses: Preparations of basil are used for supportive therapy for feelings of fullness and flatulence, for the stimulation of appetite and digestion, and as a diuretic.

Chinese Medicine: Basil herb is used for disturbances of renal function, gum ulcers, stomach cramps, and as a hemostyptic both before and after birth.

Indian Medicine: Among uses in Indian medicine are ear-aches, rheumatoid arthritis, anorexia, itching, and skin diseases, amenorrhea and dysmenorrhea, malaria, and other febrile illnesses.

BASIL OIL

Unproven Uses: Among traditional uses for the oil are wounds, rheumatic complaints, colds and chills, contusions, joint pains, and depression.

PRECAUTIONS AND ADVERSE REACTIONS

BASIL HERB

General: No health hazards or side effects are known in conjunction with the proper administration of designated therapeutic dosages.

Pregnancy: The herb contains about 0.5% essential oil with up to 85% estragole. Because of the high estragole content in the essential oil, the herb should not be taken during pregnancy.

BASIL OIL

General: No health hazards or side effects are known in conjunction with the proper administration of designated therapeutic dosages. However, pending final determination of basil oil's carcinogenic potential, one should completely forgo administration of the drug.

Pregnancy: Because a mutagenic effect in vitro and a carcinogenic effect in animal experiments have been demonstrated for estragole, oil of basil should not be administered during pregnancy or while nursing.

Pediatric Use: Basil oil should not be given to infants or small children.

DOSAGE

Basil Herb:

Tea: 3 g of drug with 150 mL hot water.

Basil Oil: Until the final determination of the drug's carcinogenic potential, one should completely forgo its administration.

LITERATURE

Balambal R et al., (1985) *J Assoc Phys* (India) 33(8):507.

Czygan FCh, Balsilikum - *Ocimum basilicum* L. Portrait einer Arzneipflanze. In: *ZPT* 18(1):58-66. 1997.

Hussein, Ayoub SM. Antibacterial and antifungal activities of some Libyan aromatic plants. *Planta Med.* 56:644-645. 1990.

Jain ML, Jain SR, (1972) *Planta Med* 22:66.

Lemberkovics É et al., Formation of essential oil and phenolic compounds during the vegetation period in *Ocimum basilicum.* In: *PM* 59(7):A700. 1993.

Miller EC et al., (1983) *Cancer Res* 43:1124.

Morton, JF. Mucilaginous plants and their uses in medicine. *J Ethnopharmacol.* 29:245-266. 1990.

Opdyke DLJ, (1973) *Food Cosmet Toxicol* 11:867.

Wagner H, Nörr H, Winterhoff H, Drogen mit ''Adaptogenwirkung'' zur Stärkung der Widerstandskräfte. In: *ZPT* 13(2):42. 1992.

Bean Pod

Phaseolus vulgaris

DESCRIPTION

Medicinal Parts: The medicinal parts are the ripe, dried pods and the beans.

Flower and Fruit: The white, pink and lilac flowers are in lightly blossomed, peduncled racemes, which are shorter than their leaves. The calyx is bilabiate. The carina, stamens, and style are twisted in a spiral. The fruit is a straight, smooth, hanging pod with a number of reniform seeds.

Leaves, Stem, and Root: The annual plant grows from 30 to 60 cm high. It is heavily branched but not twining. The leaves are trifoliate, the leaflets are broad ovate and acuminate. The terminal leaflet is rhomboid.

Habitat: The plant is indigenous to America and is cultivated worldwide today.

Production: The seed-free pods of *Phaseolus vulgaris* are collected during the harvest season.

Other Names: Common Bean, Green Bean, Kidney Bean, Navy Bean, Pinto Bean, Snap Bean, String Bean, Wax Bean

ACTIONS AND PHARMACOLOGY

COMPOUNDS

Lectins: complex termed phytomitogen (tetrameric glycoproteins)

Saponins

L-pipecolic acid

Flavonoids

EFFECTS

A weak diuretic action has been demonstrated in animal and human experiments. Chromium salts present in the Bean Pod may produce an antidiabetic effect. The starch from garden beans reduced overall cholesterol levels in rats. The polyphenols it contains exhibited antimutagenic effect in vitro.

INDICATIONS AND USAGE

Approved by Commission E:

- Infections of the urinary tract
- Kidney and bladder stones

Unproven Uses: Bean Pod is used as a supportive treatment for inability to urinate. In folk medicine, it is used as a diuretic and antidiabetic.

PRECAUTIONS AND ADVERSE REACTIONS

No health hazards or side effects are known in conjunction with the proper administration of designated therapeutic dosages, in the form of heated infusions.

OVERDOSAGE

Poisonings following the intake of large quantities of fresh green bean husks (or of raw green beans) are not to be entirely ruled out, due to the lectins content, which varies greatly among the individual species. Symptoms include vomiting, diarrhea, and gastroenteritis. The lectins are destroyed in the process of cooking.

DOSAGE

Mode of Administration: As a comminuted herb for decoctions and other galenic preparations for internal use. The drug is a component of various kidney and bladder teas and of standardized preparations of natural diuretics and antidiabetics.

Preparation: To make an infusion, pour boiling water over 2.5 g drug and strain after 10 to 15 minutes while still covered (1 teaspoonful = 1.5 g drug).

Daily Dosage: The recommended daily dosage is 5 to 15 g of herb.

LITERATURE

Atta-ur-Rahman Zaman K. Medicinal plants with hypoglycemic activity. *J Ethnopharmacol*. 26:1-55. 1989.

Cardador-Martinez A, Castano-Tostado E, Lorca-Pina G. Antimutagenic activity of natural phenolic compounds present in the common bean (*Phaseolus vulgaris*) against alfatoxin B1. *Food Add Contam*. 19:62-69. 2002.

Fukushima M, Ohashi T, Kojima M, et al. Low density lipoprotein receptor mRNA in rat liver is affected by resistant starch in beans. *Lipids*. 36:129-134. 2001.

Madaus G, Lehrbuch der Biologischen Arzneimittel, Bde 1-3, Nachdruck, Georg Olms Verlag Hildesheim 1979.

Pusztai A et al., Recent advances in the study of the nutrtional toxicity of kidney bean (*Phaseolus vulgaris*) lectins in rat. In: Toxicon 20(1): R195. 1982.

Bear's Garlic

Allium ursinum

DESCRIPTION

Medicinal Parts: The fresh herb and fresh bulb are the medicinal parts of the plant.

Flower and Fruit: The sheath of the terminal inflorescence is made up of 3 ovate-lanceolate, acute, early-falling leaves, which are almost as long as the peduncle. The inflorescence is a loose, flat, 2.5 to 6 cm wide cyme with 6 to 20 florets. The florets are erect, outward-inclined, pointed or blunt. They are pure white and have 6 star-shaped, splayed petals. Six stamens are wedge-shaped, only fused at the base and only half as long as the involucre. One superior ovary is formed out of 3 carpels and 3 deep grooves. The 3-valved capsule contains black, angular seeds.

Leaves, Stem, and Root: The plant's compact stem is upright, 10 to 50 cm high, double-edged, half-cylindrical or triangular-to-round in shape. The leaf blade is flat, narrow-elliptical-lanceolate to narrow-ovate and acute. It is 6 to 20 cm long and thin, with a base that is rounded to cordate and narrows suddenly to a 5 to 20 cm long petiole. The leaf's dark-green underside is covered with irregular horizontal veins that face upward, leaving the paler upper surface facing toward the ground. The bulb is almost cylindrical, 2 to 6 cm long, about 1 cm wide and surrounded by transparent or white skins.

Characteristics: Bear's garlic forms many bulbs and has a distinctive leek odor.

Habitat: Bear's Garlic is indigenous to almost all of Europe and Turkey, but not in the Hungarian plain and the evergreen Mediterranean region. It is also found in the Caucasus and Siberia as far as Kamtschatka.

Production: Bear's garlic is fresh or dried herb of *Allium ursinum.*

Not to be Confused With: One case was reported of confusion with colchicum leaves.

Other Names: Ramsons, Broad-Leaved Garlic

ACTIONS AND PHARMACOLOGY

COMPOUNDS

Alliins (alkylcysteine sulphoxides): in particular methyl alliin (methyl-L-(+)-cysteine sulphoxide) and allylalliin (allyl-L-(+)-cysteine sulphoxide) and presumably their gamma-glutamyl conjugates, that readily transform into the so-called alliaceous oils, for example into dimethyl-disulphide-mono-S-oxide, allicin (diallyl-disulphide-mono-S-oxide) and allyl-methyl-disulphide mono-S-oxide and the corresponding dialkyldi- or oligosulphides

EFFECTS

In both in vitro and and animal experiments, similar to Allium sativum, the drug has exhibited lipid-reducing and hypotensive effects, aggregation-inhibiting effects, and cardioprotective effects.

INDICATIONS AND USAGE

Unproven Uses: The drug is used internally for gastrointestinal complaints, fermentative dyspepsia, flatulence, high blood pressure and arteriosclerosis; externally for chronic rashes.

Homeopathic Uses: Uses in homeopathy include digestive disorders.

PRECAUTIONS AND ADVERSE REACTIONS

No health hazards or side effects are known in conjunction with the proper administration of designated therapeutic dosages.

DOSAGE

Mode of Administration: The drug is used internally as well as externally.

Preparation: Extract of bear's garlic.

Daily Dosage: Due to low concentration of the active substance, the drug must be administered in higher doses than Allium sativum.

Homeopathic Dosage: 5 drops, 1 tablet, 10 globules every 30 to 60 minutes for acute conditions, and 1 to 3 times daily for chronic; parenterally: 1 to 2 ml daily sc (HAB1).

LITERATURE

Landshuter J et al., Comparative biochemical studies on a purified C-S-lyase preparation from wild garlic. In: *PM* 58(7):A666. 1992.

Pruess HG, Clouatre M, Mohamadi A, and Jarrell ST. Wild garlic has a greater effect than regular garlic on blood pressure and blood chemistries of rats. *Int Uro Nephrol.* 32:525-530. 2001

Rietz B, Insensee H, Strobach H, Makdessi S, and Jacob R. Cardioprotective actions of wild garlic (*allium ursinium*) in ischemia and reperfusion. *Mol Cell Biochem.* 119:143-150. 1993

Sendl A, Bärlauch: Alternative zu Knoblauch. In: *Naturw. Rdsch* 7/94. 1994.

Sendl A, Phytotherapie: Bärlauch und Knoblauch im Vergleich. In: *DAZ* 133(5):392. 1993.

Veit M, Bärlauch (*Allium ursinum*) als Ersatz für Knoblauch (*Allium sativum*). In: *ZPT* 13(6):201. 1993.

Wagner H, Ebl G, Lotter H, Guinea M, Evaluation of natural products as inhibitors of angiotensin I-converting enzyme (ACE). In: *Pharm Pharmacol Letters* 1(1):15-18. 1991.

Wagner H, Sendl A, Bärlauch und Knoblauch. In: *DAZ* 130(33):1809. 1990.

Beet

Beta vulgaris

DESCRIPTION

Medicinal Parts: The root is the medicinal part.

Flower and Fruit: The flowers bloom in clusters of 2 to 4 in paniclelike leafy inflorescences.

Leaves, Stem, and Root: The beet is a 0.5 to 1.5 m perennial with a swollen, edible tuber that is red or white. The large, upright leaves have long stalks and grow in rosettes that arise basally from the top of the tuber. They are deep green and tinged with red.

Habitat: The Beet is indigenous to the coastal regions of Europe, North Africa, and Asia from Turkey to India. Red Beets, Sugar Beets and the white variety are all widely cultivated.

Other Names: Chard

ACTIONS AND PHARMACOLOGY

COMPOUNDS

Saccharose (up to 27% in the pressed sugar beet)

Other oligosaccharides: refined sugar, ketose

Polysaccharides: including galactans, arabans, pectin

Fruit acids: including L(-)-malic acid, D(+)-tartaric acid, oxaluric acid, adipic acid, citric acid, glycolic acid, glutaric acid

Amino acids: including asparagine, glutamine

Betaine (trimethylglycine)

Triterpene saponins

EFFECTS

Beet is said to have antihepatotoxic effects; in animal tests, the drug effectively keeps fat from depositing in the liver. This is probably due to the herb's concentration of betaine, which is a methyl group donor in the liver's transmethylation process.

INDICATIONS AND USAGE

Unproven Uses: Beet is used as supportive therapy in diseases of the liver and fatty liver.

Indian Medicine: The drug is used for coughs and infections.

PRECAUTIONS AND ADVERSE REACTIONS

No health hazards or side effects are known in conjunction with the proper administration of designated therapeutic dosages.

OVERDOSAGE

Taking very large quantities could lead to hypocalcemia and kidney damage because of the drug's oxaluric acid content.

DOSAGE

Mode of Administration: Beet is available as a granular powder in standardized form.

Daily Dosage: For the first 14 days, take 10 gm of drug after meals throughout the course of the day. For long-term treatment, the dose is 5 gm per day for at least 3 months.

LITERATURE

Atta-ur-Rahman Zaman K. Medicinal plants with hypoglycemic activity. *J Ethnopharmacol.* 26:1-55. 1989.

Kern W, List PH, Hörhammer L (Hrsg.), Hagers Handbuch der Pharmazeutischen Praxis, 4. Aufl., Bde 1-8, Springer Verlag Berlin, Heidelberg, New York, 1969.

Behen

Moringa oleifera

DESCRIPTION

Medicinal Parts: The medicinal parts of the plant are the leaves, bark, nuts and root, which have had numerous uses in traditional medicine.

Flower and Fruit: The inflorescence is a leaf-axillary panicle. The flowers are zygomorphic with their structures in fives and a bowel-shaped receptacle. The sepals are linear-lanceolate, irregular, and revolute. The petals are spatulate, veined, irregular and white or yellow. There are 5 stamens, and a superior ovary developing from 3 fused carpals. The fruit is a hanging capsule opening on 3 sides, up to 1.2 m long and triangular with 9 ribs. The seeds are triangular, light brown to black, with 3 thin, whitish wings, approximately the size of a hazelnut.

Leaves, Stem and Root: The leaves of the tree are alternate, 30 to 60 cm long, and incompletely triple-pinnate. The leaflets are 12 to 20 mm long and elliptical. The branches are slim.

Characteristics: The flowers are extremely fragrant, and the leaves, root, and fruit taste like horseradish.

Habitat: The tree is indigenous to India.

Production: Behen root is the fresh or dried root of *Moringa oleifera*. Behen nuts are the ripe unpeeled seeds of *Moringa oleifera*.

Other Names: Ben Nut Tree, Drumstick Tree, Indian Horseradish

ACTIONS AND PHARMACOLOGY

COMPOUNDS: BEHEN ROOT

Glucosinolates: 4-(alpha-L-rhamnosyloxy)benzyl glucosinolate (ca. 1%), yielding 4-(alpha-L-rhamnosyloxy)benzyl isothiocyanate following enzymatic segregation with myrosinase, glucotropaeolin (ca. 0.05%), yielding benzyl isothiocyanate

EFFECTS: BEHEN ROOT

The root is antimicrobial in effect, due to the mustard oils it contains. Applied as a cataplasm, it triggers local hyperemias due to the irritating effect of the isothiocyanates. Dried extracts of the root are abortive and contraceptive in their effect.

COMPOUNDS: BEHEN SEEDS

Glucosinolates (up to 9% in the defatted seeds): 4-(alpha-L-rhamnosyloxy)benzyl glucosinolate, yielding 4-(alpha-L-rhamnosyloxy)benzyl isothiocyanate following enzymatic segregation with myrosinase

Phenol carboxylic acids: 1-beta-D-glucosyl-2,6-dimethyl benzoate

Fatty oil (20 to 50%): chief fatty acids oleic acid (60 to 70%), palmitic acid (3 to 12%), stearic acid (3 to 12%), including as well behenic acid, eicosanoic acid, lignoceric acid

EFFECTS: BEHEN SEEDS

The seeds are antimicrobial in effect, due to the mustard oils they contain.

INDICATIONS AND USAGE

BEHEN ROOT

Unproven Uses: The root has been used internally in folk medicine for gastrointestinal complaints, epilepsy, paralyses, cardiac and blood pressure disturbances, fever (particularly intermittent), scurvy, dizziness, and colds. External indications include gingivitis, worm diseases, snake bites, abscesses, inflammation, rheumatism, and poorly healing wounds. Root paste has been used to treat worms, rheumatism, and headaches.

Indian Medicine: Indications have included smallpox and rheumatism. Efficacy for rheumatism seems plausible because of the stimulating effect of the isothiocyanates. Efficacy for the other indications has not yet been proved.

BEHEN SEEDS

Unproven Uses: Folk medicine indications for internal use are constipation, warts, and worms (Central America); for diarrhea (Chad); for splenomegaly, colic, dyspepsia, fever, inflammation of the skin, edema, diabetes, abdominal tumors, paralyses, and lumbago (Saudi Arabia). The seeds are used externally for dandruff in Nigeria.

Indian Medicine: Behen seeds are used for fever and as an aphrodisiac. Efficacy for these indications has not yet been proved.

PRECAUTIONS AND ADVERSE REACTIONS

BEHEN ROOT

No health hazards are known in conjunction with the proper administration of designated therapeutic dosages. The ingestion of larger quantities can lead to nausea, dizziness and vomiting.

BEHEN SEEDS

No health hazards are known in conjunction with the proper administration of designated therapeutic dosages.

The single peroral administration of a dosage of 5 g of the drug/kg body weight to a mouse led to hyperkeratosis in the stomach and to liver cell steatosis. Administration of 22 to 50 mg/kg body weight, parenterally, of the glucosinolate mentioned above proved to be fatal for mice.

CONTRAINDICATIONS

BEHEN ROOT

Behen preparations are contraindicated during pregnancy because of their possible abortive effect.

DOSAGE

BEHEN ROOT

Mode of Administration: Preparations of the whole and powdered root are administered internally and externally.

BEHEN SEEDS

Mode of Administration: Preparations of the seed are used internally and externally.

LITERATURE

Gilani AH, Aftab K, Suria A, Siddiqi S, SalemR, Siddiqi BS, Faizi S. Pharmacologic studies on hypertensive and spasmolytic activities of pure compounds of *Moringa oleifera.* 8(2):87-91. 1994.

Hänsel R, Keller K, Rimpler H, *Phytother Res* Schneider G (Ed), Hagers Handbuch der Pharmazeutischen Praxis, 5. Aufl., Bde 4 - 6 (Drogen), Springer Verlag Berlin, Heidelberg, New York, 1992-1994.

Belladonna

Atropa belladonna

DESCRIPTION

Medicinal Parts: The medicinal parts are the leaves and roots.

Flower and Fruit: The flowers are solitary and hanging. The calyx is fused at the base, has 5 divisions and is spread like a star when the fruit ripens. The violet corolla is a campanulate tube, 2.5 to 3.5 cm long, dirty yellow on the inside with crimson veins. There are 5 stamens and 1 style with a 2-lobed stigma. The ovary is superior. The fruit is a cherry-sized globose berry. The fruit is initially green, then becomes black and glossy with numerous black, ovoid seeds.

Leaves, Stem, and Root: Atropa belladonna is a perennial, herbacious plant 1 to 2 m high with a many-headed cylindrical rhizome. The woody stem is erect, branched, bluntly angular and hairy. The leaves are ovately pointed, entire-margined, downy and up to 15 cm long. The lower leaves are alternate. Near the inflorescence the leaves are in pairs of one large and one small.

Characteristics: Belladonna has a strong narcotic smell, a sharp and bitter taste, and is poisonous.

Habitat: The plant is found throughout western, central and southern Europe, in the Balkans, southeast Asia, Iran, northern Africa, Denmark, Sweden, and Ireland. It is cultivated in other countries, particularly England, France, and the U.S.

Production: Belladonna leaf consists of the dried leaves, or the dried leaves together with the flowering branch tips, of *Atropa belladonna.* The leaves are collected in the wild from May to July. They are dried at a temperature not exceeding 60°C. Belladonna root consists of the dried roots and rhizomes of *Atropa belladonna.* The roots of 2- to 4-year-old plants are dug up in mid-October to mid-November or shortly before the start of the flowering season. They are cleaned and dried at a maximum temperature of 50° C.

Not to be Confused With: Belladonna leaf should not be confused with *Ailanthus altissimus, Phytolacca americana* or *Scopolia carniolica.* Belladonna root should not be confused with *Atropa acuminata.* It is sometimes adulterated with *Phytolacca americana* and *Scopolia cariolica.*

Other Names: Deadly Nightshade, Devil's Cherries, Devil's Herb, Divale, Dwale, Dwayberry, Great Morel, Naughty Man's Cherries, Poison Black Cherry

ACTIONS AND PHARMACOLOGY

COMPOUNDS: BELLADONNA LEAF

Tropan alkaloids: chief alkaloid (-)-hyoscyamine, which during drying transforms to some extent into atropine, as well as apoatropine, scopolamine and tropine

Flavonoids

Hydroxycoumarins: including scopoline, scopoletine

Tannins

COMPOUNDS: BELLADONNA ROOT

Tropan alkaloids: chief alkaloid (-)-hyoscyamine, in drying transformed to some extent during dehydration into atropine as well as apoatropine, 3alpha-phenylacetoxytropane, tropine, cuskhygrine, scopolamine, pseudotropine

EFFECTS: BELLADONNA LEAF AND ROOT

The tropane alkaloids in the drug (atropine, scopolamine, tropine etc.) are responsible for the anti-cholinergic-parasympatholytic, spasmolytic, positive, dromotropic and chronotropic effect. Atropa belladonna preparations act as a parasympatholytic or anticholinergic via a competitive antagonism of the neuromuscular transmitter acetylcholine. This antagonism concerns mainly the muscarine-like effect of acetylcholine and less the nicotine-like effects on the ganglions and the neuromuscular end plate. *Atropa belladonna* preparations release peripheral effects targeted on the vegetative nervous system and the smooth muscle system, as well as the central nervous system. Because of the parasympatholytic properties, the drug can cause relaxation of organs with smooth muscles and relieve spastic conditions, especially in the gastrointestinal tract and bile ducts. Additionally, Belladonna use may result in muscular tremor or rigidity due to effects on the central nervous system. *Atropa belladonna* preparations have a positive dromotropic as well as a positive chronotropic effect on the heart. The drug has always been important in folk medicine for its hallucinogenic effect.

INDICATIONS AND USAGE

BELLADONNA LEAF

Approved by Commission E:

- Liver and gall bladder complaints

Unproven Uses: Belladonna leaf is used for spasms and coliclike pain in the gastrointestinal tract and bile ducts. External uses include gout and ulcers. In folk medicine, the drug is contained in medicinal plasters and is applied for neurovegetative disorders, hyperkinesis, hyperhydrosis, and bronchial asthma.

Homeopathic Uses: Homeopathic uses include meningitis as well as inflammations (accompanied by fever) of the tonsils, respiratory organs, the urogenital tract, the skin, the joints and the gastrointestinal tract.

BELLADONNA ROOT

Approved by Commission E:

- Liver and gall bladder complaints

Unproven Uses: The drug is used for arrhythmia, cardiac insufficiency NYHA I and II, nervous heart complaints, and coliclike pains in the gastrointestinal tract and bile ducts. In folk medicine, a drug from the leaves is preferred for pain in the gastrointestinal area, for asthma, bronchitis, and muscular pain. (Also see Belladonna leaf.)

PRECAUTIONS AND ADVERSE REACTIONS

BELLADONNA LEAF AND ROOT

General: No health hazards are known in conjunction with the proper administration of designated therapeutic dosages. The following could occur as side effects, particularly with overdoses: erubescence, dryness of the mouth, mydriasis, and tachycardiac arrhythmias. These are early signs of atropine poisoning. Other side effects may include hypocycloses, heat accumulation through reduction of perspiration, micturation difficulties and obstipation. Because of potential ramifications, Belladonna should be used only under the supervision of an expert familiar with the appropriate use of this substance.

Pediatric Use: The fatal dose in children is considerably less than that of adults.

DRUG INTERACTIONS

MODERATE RISK

Phenothiazines: Concurrent use may result in additive anticholinergic effects. *Clinical Management:* Do not administer concomitantly; alternatives include barbiturates, chloral hydrates, or benzodiazepines.

MINOR RISK

Amantadine, Atropine, Benztropine, Biperiden, Brompheniramine, Chlorpheniramine, Cisapride, Clemastine, Clidinium, Clozapine, Cyclopentolate, Cyproheptadine, Dicyclomine, Diphenhydramine, Haloperidol, Homatropine, Hyoscyamine, Ipratropium, Loxapine, Molindone, Olanzapine, Oxybutynin, Pimozide, Procyclidine, Quinidine, Scopolamine, Thiothixene, Tricyclic Antidepressants, Trihexyphenidyl, Trimeprazine, Triprolidine: Concurrent use may result in increased anticholinergic activity (severe dry mouth, constipation, decreased urination, excessive sedation, blurred vision). *Clinical Management:* Excessive anticholinergic activity may be manifested by dry mouth, constipation, urinary retention, tachycardia, decreased sweating, mydriasis, blurred vision, elevated temperature, muscular weakness, and sedation. If such effects are noted, belladonna should be discontinued immediately. In severe cases, paralytic ileus, confusion, psychoses, agitation, delusions, delirium, and paranoia may be encountered as well as tachycardia, dysrhythmia, and hypertension. In severe cases, immediate medical attention should be obtained.

Bethanechol: Concurrent use may result in reduced effectiveness of bethanechol. *Clinical Management:* If a patient does take both agents together, monitor closely for reduced effectiveness of both agents.

Procainamide: Concurrent use may result in antivagal effect on A-V nodal conduction. *Clinical Management:* Monitor heart rate and EDG in patients given procainamide concomitantly with an anticholinergic medication.

OVERDOSAGE

BELLADONNA LEAF AND ROOT

High dosages lead to central excitation that may produce restlessness, talkativeness, hallucinations, delirium, and manic attacks, followed by exhaustion and sleep. The fatal dose depends on the atropine content; asphyxiation can occur with 100 mg atropine, which corresponds to 5 to 50 g of Belladonna. Treatment of poisonings consists of gastric lavage, application of wet cloths to reduce body temperature (avoid antipyretics), oxygen respiration for breathing distress, intubation, parenteral physostigmine salts as an antidote, diazepam for spasm, and chlorpromazine for serious excitation. (Also see side effects listed under PRECAUTIONS AND ADVERSE REACTIONS, which may be early signs of poisoning.)

DOSAGE

BELLADONNA LEAF

Mode of Administration: The comminuted drug is used for decoctions and dried extracts, and the powdered drug is used internally for galenic preparations. Due to the toxicity, the drug must be handled with care.

How Supplied: Forms of commercial pharmaceutical preparations include coated and uncoated tablets, drops, tea, juice, syrup, ampules, capsules, suppositories, plaster, and ophthalmic drops.

Daily Dosage: When using Belladonna powder (belladonnae pulvis normatus-total alkaloid content 0.28% to 0.32% German pharmacopoeia 10), the average single dose is 0.05 to 0.10 g. The maximum single dose is 0.20 g, which is equivalent to 0.60 mg total alkaloids, calculated as hyoscyamine. The maximum daily dosage is 0.60 g, which is equivalent to 1.8 mg total alkaloids, calculated as hyoscyamine.

For Belladonna extract, the maximum daily dosage is 0.15 g, which is equivalent to 2.2 mg total alkaloids, calculated as hyoscyamine.

Storage: Belladonna leaves and various leaf preparations have specific storage requirements. Store leaves and powders tightly sealed and protected from light. Extracts require protection from moisture and light as well as a temperature of approximately 30°C. Store tinctures tightly sealed without exposure to direct sunlight or extreme heat to attain a shelf life of approximately 3.5 years.

BELLADONNA ROOT

Mode of Administration: As a comminuted drug for infusions and dried extracts and as a powdered drug for other galenic preparations for internal use.

Daily Dosage: The average daily dosage is 0.3 g, which is equivalent to 1.5 mg total alkaloids, calculated as hyoscyamine. Single doses range from 0.05 g to a maximum of 0.1 g.

For Belladonna extract, the total alkaloids range from 1.3% to 1.45% (German pharmacopoeia 10). Single doses of the extract range from 0.01 g to 0.05 g. The maximum daily dosage is 0.15 g, which is equivalent to 2.2 mg total alkaloids, calculated as hyoscyamine.

For Belladonna tincture, a single dose of 0.5 to 2 ml is given 3 times daily.

Homeopathic Dosage: 5 to 10 drops, 1 tablet, 5 to 10 globules, 1 to 3 times daily or 1 ml injection solution twice weekly sc. From D3: one suppository 2 to 3 times daily; ointments 1 to 2 times daily (HAB1).

Storage: Belladonna root should be stored for a maximum of 3 years in well-sealed containers protected from light and insects.

LITERATURE

BELLADONNA LEAF AND ROOT

Fintelmann V, Phytopharmaka in der Gastroenterologie. In: *ZPT* 15(3):137. 1994.

Hartmann Th et al., Reinvestigation of the alkaloid composition of Atropa belladonna plants, roots cultures, and cell suspension. In: PM 53:390-395. 1986.

Phillipson JD et al., (1975) *Phytochemistry* 14: 999-1003.

BELLADONNA ROOT

Fintelmann V, Phytopharmaka in der Gastroenterologie. In: ZPT 15(3):137. 1994.

Hartmann Th et al., Reinvestigation of the alkaloid composition of Atropa belladonna plants, roots cultures, and cell suspension. In: PM 53:390-395. 1986.

Phillipson JD et al., (1975) Phytochemistry 14: 999.

Bellis perennis

See Wild Daisy

Bennet's Root

Geum urbanum

DESCRIPTION

Medicinal Parts: The medicinal parts of the plant are the dried flowering herb, the dried or fresh underground parts, and the roots.

Flower and Fruit: The inflorescence is a loose panicled, umbelled cyme with a few terminal and erect flowers. The pedicles are short-haired. The sepals are 3 to 8 cm long with long tips, pubescent on the outside and glabrous on the inside, except for a tomentose border. The epicalyx bracts are half as long as the sepals, pubescent on both sides and narrowly lanceolate. The yellow petals are 3 to 7 mm long, slightly stemmed, and drop easily. The style is jointed and the stigma flat. The small fruits have no stems and are pubescent.

Leaves, Stem and Root: The plant is a semi-rosette shrub with a primary root that dies off early and is replaced by adventitious roots. The rhizome is simple, thick, cylindrical, and crooked. The stem is erect, soft-haired, 15 to 70 cm high; it sprouts from the basal rosette. The basal leaves are rosettelike and pinnate. The cauline leaves are trifoliate to tripinnate and the stipules are small, fused with the stem in the lower part, and ovate-lanceolate roughly dentate to pinnatesect.

Characteristics: The plant's root has a clovelike scent.

Habitat: Bennet's Root is found in central and southern Europe, central Asia and North America.

Production: Bennet's Root herb is the aerial part of *Geum urbanum*. Bennet's Root (root) is the root of *Geum urbanum*, which is usually harvested in May and then air-dried or dried artificially at a maximum of 35° C.

Other Names: Avens Root, Colewort, Herb Bennet, City Avens, Wild Rye, Way Bennet, Goldy Star, Geum, European Avens, Blessed Herb, Star of the Earth, Yellow Avens

ACTIONS AND PHARMACOLOGY

COMPOUNDS: BENNET'S ROOT HERB

Tannins: gallo tannins, ellagitannins, including sanguiin H-6, casuarictin, pendunculagin, potentillin, tellimagrandin I

EFFECTS: BENNET'S ROOT HERB

The drug has an astringent effect.

COMPOUNDS: BENNET'S ROOT (ROOT)

In the freshly harvested rhizome:

Tannins

Gein (eugenol-vicianose): transformed through drying or size reduction into eugenol

In the dried rhizome and the roots:

Volatile oil (traces): chief components - eugenol, additionally cis- and trans-myrtanal, cis- and trans-myrtanol

EFFECTS: BENNET'S ROOT (ROOT)

The drug has an astringent effect.

INDICATIONS AND USAGE

BENNET'S ROOT HERB

Unproven Uses: Although rarely used today, folk medicine indications have included use of the drug for digestive complaints and diarrhea, febrile illnesses, and for muscle and nerve pain. Use as a bath additive for hemorrhoids seems plausible due the astringent content.

BENNET'S ROOT (ROOT)

Unproven Uses: Internal folk medicine applications include use for digestive problems such as loss of appetite and diarrhea. The root of Bennet's Root has been used externally as a gargle for gum and mucous membrane inflammations and as a bath additive or poultice for frostbite, hemorrhoids, and skin diseases. Efficacy appears plausible due to the astringent properties of the tannins.

Homeopathic Uses: Homeopathic applications include use for inflammations of the bladder and urinary tract.

PRECAUTIONS AND ADVERSE REACTIONS

Health risks or side effects following the proper administration of designated therapeutic dosages are not recorded.

DOSAGE

BENNET'S ROOT HERB

The herb is rarely used medicinally today. It is found in some pharmaceutical preparations.

BENNET'S ROOT (ROOT)

Mode of Administration: Infusions are drunk or applied as an external wash or poultice.

Preparation: To prepare an internal infusion, boil 1/2 to 1 teaspoon coarsely powdered drug in water for 10 minutes and filter. Prepare an external infusion by adding 1 teaspoon coarsely powdered drug to cold water, bringing it briefly to the boil, leaving it to steep for 10 minutes and then straining.

Daily Dosage: Infusion (internal): 1 cup lukewarm several times a day. Infusion (external): Use several times a day for washes or poultices.

Homeopathic Dosage: 5 drops, 1 tablet or 10 globules every 30 to 60 minutes (acute) or 1 to 3 times a day (chronic); parenterally: 1 to 2 ml sc acute, 3 times daily; chronic: once a day (HAB1).

LITERATURE

BENNET'S ROOT HERB

Hänsel R, Keller K, Rimpler H, Schneider G (Hrsg.), Hagers Handbuch der Pharmazeutischen Praxis, 5. Aufl., Bde 4-6 (Drogen), Springer Verlag Berlin, Heidelberg, New York, 1992-1994.

Madaus G, Lehrbuch der Biologischen Arzneimittel, Bde 1-3, Nachdruck, Georg Olms Verlag Hildesheim 1979.

Psenăk M et al., (1970) *Planta Med* 19(2):154.

Vollmann C, Schultze W, Nelkenwurz. In: *DAZ* 135(14):1238-1248. 1995.

Vollmann C, Untersuchung der Nelkenwurz. In: *DAZ* 131(40):2081. 1991.

BENNET'S ROOT (ROOT)

Hänsel R, Keller K, Rimpler H, Schneider G (Hrsg.), Hagers Handbuch der Pharmazeutischen Praxis, 5. Aufl., Bde 4-6 (Drogen), Springer Verlag Berlin, Heidelberg, New York, 1992-1994.

Madaus G, Lehrbuch der Biologischen Arzneimittel, Bde 1-3, Nachdruck, Georg Olms Verlag Hildesheim 1979.

Psenăk M et al., (1970) *Planta Med* 19(2):154.

Wichtl M (Hrsg.), Teedrogen, 4. Aufl., Wiss. Verlagsges. Stuttgart 1997.

Vollmann C, Schultze W, Nelkenwurz. In: *DAZ* 135(14):1238-1248. 1995.

Vollmann C, Untersuchung der Nelkenwurz. In: *DAZ* 131(40):2081. 1991.

Benzoin

Styrax benzoin

DESCRIPTION

Medicinal Parts: The medicinal part of the plant is the balsamic resin obtained from the mechanically damaged trunk.

Flower and Fruit: The flowers are in terminal or axillary panicled racemes. The flowers are fused and their structures are in fives. The calyx is campanulate, weakly 5 toothed, densely silky tomentose and red-brown on the inside. The corolla is 6 to 11 mm long with 5 tips, brown-red, silky tomentose on the outside and at the margin. There are 8 to 10 stamens fused below to a tube and a 1-chambered ovary above and 2- to 3-chambered ovary below. The fruit is nutlike, appressed pubescent with a diameter of up to 3 cm. The seeds are light brown with 6 longitudinal stripes and are up to 2 cm long.

Leaves, Stem, and Root: Styrax benzoin is an evergreen tree, which grows up to 30 m high. The leaves are alternate and the petioles are rust brown-downy pubescent. They are approximately 1 cm long. The lamina is 8 to 13 cm long, 2.5 to 5 cm wide, ovate or elongate with a rounded base and irregularly curved-dentate margin. The lamina is covered with white and brown star hairs beneath. The bark is wine-red and the wood is white.

Characteristics: The flowers have a strong fragrance.

Habitat: The plant is native to western Java and Sumatra.

Production: Sumatra benzoin (Gum benzoin) is the balsamic resin from the damaged trunk of *Styrax benzoin* and *Styrax paralleloneurum*. The optimal age of trees to be harvested is 7 years. The tree is cut, causing it to exude resin to heal the cuts. The resin is then collected in a vessel and left to melt to a homogenous mass in the sun.

Other Names: Benjamin Tree

ACTIONS AND PHARMACOLOGY

COMPOUNDS

Ester mixture (70 to 80%): composed of coniferyl benzoate and cinnamyl benzoate, as well as cinnamyl cinnamoate (styracin), propyl cinnamoate

Phenylacrylic acids: cinnamic acid (10%)

Benzoic acid (to 30%)

Resins

EFFECTS

The expectorant effect with which the drug is credited could not be proved experimentally (it possibly originated in connection with an ''aroma therapy,'' due to its vanilla content).

INDICATIONS AND USAGE

Unproven Uses: Benzoin is used for respiratory catarrh.

Chinese Medicine: In China, benzoin is used for stroke, syncopes, post partal syncope due to heavy loss of blood, and for chest and stomach pain.

PRECAUTIONS AND ADVERSE REACTIONS

No health hazards are known in conjunction with the proper administration of designated therapeutic dosages.

DOSAGE

Mode of Administration: Whole herb preparations are for internal use.

Storage: Benzoin should be tightly sealed and stored below 25°C.

LITERATURE

Bacchi EM, Sertié JA, Villa N, Katz H, delta7-stigmasteryl-3 betaD-glucoside from Styrax officinalis. Part II. *Planta Med*, 61:221-2, 1976 Nov

Bacchi EM, Sertié JA, Villa N, Katz H, Preliminary investigations on the herba of Styrax officinalis. I. *Planta Med*, 61:290-3, 1973 Nov

Hänsel R, Keller K, Rimpler H, Schneider G (Ed), Hagers Handbuch der Pharmazeutischen Praxis, 5. Aufl., Bde 4 - 6 (Drogen), Springer Verlag Berlin, Heidelberg, New York, 1992-1994

James WD, White SW, Yanklowitz B, Allergic contact dermatitis to compound tincture of benzoin. *J Am Acad Dermatol*, 11:847-50, 1984 Nov

Berberis vulgaris

See Barberry

Bergenia crassifolia

See Elephant-Ears

Beta vulgaris

See Beet

Betel Nut

Piper betle

DESCRIPTION

Medicinal Parts: The main medicinal parts are the dried leaves; the roots and the fruit are also used.

Flower and Fruit: The inflorescences are compact, hanging, cylindrical and 3.5 to 5 cm long spikes of yellow-green flowers. There are 2 stamens in the male flowers. The female stamens have an ovary, which is pubescent at the top and has 3 to 5 stigmas. The fruit is globular, fleshy and about 6 mm in diameter. The fruit is yellow and becomes red when ripe. The seeds are also globular.

Leaves, Stem and Root: The plant is a dioecious or monoecious woody climber that can grow to 15 m. It has numerous small and short adventitious roots. The stem is thickened at the nodes, and the younger parts are glabrous. The leaves have a 2.5 to 5 cm long petiole, are broadly cordate, 5 to 18 cm long and half as wide. The leaves are glabrous, light green and glossy on both surfaces with 5 to 7 radiating ribs.

Habitat: Piper betle is found in tropical southern Asia and has been introduced to east Africa, Madagascar and the West Indies.

Production: Betel Nut leaves are the leaves of Piper betle. When the leaves are green, they are gathered, pressed and dried.

Other Names: Betel

ACTIONS AND PHARMACOLOGY

COMPOUNDS

Volatile oil (0.8-1.8%): chief components- chavibetol (betel phenol), eugenol, additionally allylpyrocatechol (hydroxychavicol), allylpyrocatechol-mono and -diacetate, anethole, chavibetolacetate, chavicol, methyl eugenol, safrol

Neolignans: including crotepoxide, piperbetol, piperol, among others

EFFECTS

The essential oils are antimicrobial and immune-modulating. The Betel leaf is centrally sedating.

INDICATIONS AND USAGE

Unproven Uses: In folk medicine, Betel Nut is used for coughs, as an expectorant for stomach ailments, diphtheria and inflammation of the middle ear.

Indian Medicine: In India, Betel Nut is used to treat asthma, bronchitis, coughs, dyspepsia, rheumatism, leprosy, severe thirst, alcoholism, syncopes, toothache and impotency.

PRECAUTIONS AND ADVERSE REACTIONS

No health hazards or side effects are known in conjunction with the proper administration of designated therapeutic dosages.

DOSAGE

Mode of Administration: Today, the drug is obsolete.

LITERATURE

Das PC, Sarkar AK, (1979) *Acta Physiol Pol.* 30(3):389.

Rawat AKS et al., Ind Perf 31:146-149. 1987.

Sen S, Talukder G, Sharma A. Betel cytotoxicity. *J Ethnopharmacol.* 26:217-247. 1989.

Sharma ML et al., *Ind Perf* 26:134-137. 1982.

Beth Root Stock

Trillium erectum

DESCRIPTION

Medicinal Parts: The medicinal parts are the rhizome, the dried root, and the leaves.

Flower and Fruit: The plant has solitary, terminal, hanging flowers. The 3 green, persistent sepals and the 3 large, white to red or yellow, wilting sepals are characteristic.

Leaves, Stem, and Root: The plant is a perennial, smooth herb with an erect stem, which grows from 25 to 40 cm high. It bears 3 whorled, terminal leaves under the flower, which are broad, rhomboid and lightly curled. The rhizome is matte brown, subconical, more or less compressed, 3 to 5 cm long and 2 to 3 cm in diameter. It is often ringed with oblique lines and with numerous wrinkled root fibers on the upper surface.

Characteristics: The taste is sweetish then acrid and the odor is characteristic.

Habitat: The plant is indigenous to the central and western U.S.

Production: Beth Root Stock is the rhizome of *Trillium erectum, Trillium pendulum* and other varieties.

Other Names: Birthroot, Indian Shamrock, Lamb's Quarters, Wake-Robin, Indian Balm, Ground Lily, Coughroot, Jew's-Harp Plant, Milk Ipecac, Pariswort, Rattlesnake Root, Snake-bite, Three-Leaved, Nightshade

ACTIONS AND PHARMACOLOGY

COMPOUNDS

Steroid saponins: including among others, trillin (disogenin monoglucoside), trillarin (disogenin diglucoside), aglycones including cryptogenin, chlorogenin, nologenin

Tannins

EFFECTS

The drug has astringent and expectorant properties. It can severely irritate the area to which it has been applied; the irritation can cause vomiting.

INDICATIONS AND USAGE

Unproven Uses: Internally, Beth Root is used internally for long and heavy menstruation. Externally, it is used for varicose veins, ulcers, hematoma, and hemorrhoidal bleeding.

CONTRAINDICATIONS

The drug should not be used during pregnancy.

PRECAUTIONS AND ADVERSE REACTIONS

No health hazards or side effects are known in conjunction with the proper administration of designated therapeutic dosages. In higher dosages, the drug is said to be nauseant, and to have the effect of promoting labor and menstruation.

Pregnancy: In high dosages, the drug promotes labor; therefore, it should not be used during pregnancy.

DOSAGE

Mode of Administration: The ground drug and liquid extract are used for infusions and poultices.

Daily Dosage: The usual dose is 2 to 4 gm dissolved in liquid as an infusion.

LITERATURE

Fukuda N et al., (1981) *Chem Pharm Bull* 29 (2):325.

Hegnauer R, Chemotaxonomie der Pflanzen, Bde 1-11: Birkhäuser Verlag Basel, Boston, Berlin 1962-1997.

Kern W, List PH, Hörhammer L (Hrsg.), Hagers Handbuch der Pharmazeutischen Praxis, 4. Aufl., Bde. 1-8: Springer Verlag Berlin, Heidelberg, New York, 1969.

Madaus G, Lehrbuch der Biologischen Arzneimittel, Bde 1-3, Nachdruck, Georg Olms Verlag Hildesheim 1979.

Nakano K et al., (1982) *J Chem Soc Chem Commun.* 789.

Nakano K et al., (1982) Yakugaku Zasshi 102(11):1031.

Nakano K et al., (1983) *Phytochemistry* 22 (5):1249.

Roth L, Daunderer M, Kormann K, Giftpflanzen, Pflanzengifte, 4. Aufl., Ecomed Fachverlag Landsberg Lech 1993.

Wolters B, Zierpflanzen aus Nordamerika. In: *DAZ* 137(26):2253-2261. 1997.

Betonica officinalis

See Wood Betony

Betula species

See Birch

Bidens tripartita

See Burr Marigold

Bilberry

Vaccinium myrtillus

DESCRIPTION

Medicinal Parts: The medicinal parts are the dried leaves, the ripe, dried fruit, and the ripe fresh fruit.

Flower and Fruit: The flowers are axillary and solitary. They are 4 to 7 mm long, short-pedicled, greenish tinged with pale pink. The calyx is fused to the ovary, persistent, and indistinctly 5-lobed. The corolla is globular-jug-shaped and has 5 tips. There are 8 to 10 stamens, which are enclosed and shorter than the styles. They have glabrous filaments that widen toward the base and 2 hornlike yellow-brown anthers with an erect spurred appendage. The fruit is a globular, blue-black, frosted, many-seeded berry with purple pulp.

Leaves, Stem, and Root: The plant is a deciduous, dwarf shrub with sharp-edged, green branches 15 to 50 cm high. The leaves are alternate, ovate or oblong-ovate, acuminate and finely serrate.

Habitat: The plant is common to central and northern Europe, Asia and North America.

Production: The leaves and fruit of Bilberry are collected in the wild from July to August and dried in the shade.

Not to be Confused With: Myrtilli folium should not be confused with the fruits of *Vaccinium uliginosum.*

Other Names: Airelle, Black Whortles, Bleaberry, Blueberry, Burren myrtle, Dyeberry, Huckleberry, Hurtleberry, Wineberry Hurts, Trackleberry, Whortleberry

ACTIONS AND PHARMACOLOGY

COMPOUNDS: BILBERRY LEAF

Catechin tannins (1 to 7%): including oligomeric proanthocyandins

Flavonoids: including among others, avicularin, hyperoside, isoquercitrin, quercitrin, meratine, astragaline

Iridoide monoterpenes: asperuloside, monotropein

Caffeic acid derivatives: chlorogenic acid

Phenolic acids: including among others, salicylic acid, gentisic acid

Quinolizidine alkaloids: myrtine, epimyrtine (hybrids of Vaccinium myrtillus x V. vitis-idaea contain arbutin [hydroquine glucosides]).

EFFECTS: BILBERRY LEAF

The drug is astringent and useful for treating diarrhea due to the catechin tannin content. The drug is antiviral and, in animal experiments, lipid-lowering.

COMPOUNDS: BILBERRY FRUIT

Fruit acids: including among others, quinic acid (3-5%), malic acid, citric acid

Tannins (5-12%): chiefly catechin tannins, including oligomeric procyanidins

Anthocyanoides (0.1% -0.5%): chief components delphinidine-3-O-arabinoside, delphinidine-3-O-galactoside, delphinidine-3-O-glucoside, cyanidin, petunidin, peonidin, malvidin

Flavonoids: including among others, hyperoside, isoquercitrin, quercitrin, astragaline

Iridoids: including asperuloside, onotropein (only in the unripe fruits)

Caffeic acid derivatives: chlorogenic acid

Pectins

EFFECTS: BILBERRY FRUIT

Bilberry is stated to possess astringent, tonic, antioxidant, and antiseptic properties. Several pharmacological activities, such as ophthalmic, wound healing, anti-ulcer, anti-atherosclerotic, and vasoprotective activities have been documented for Bilberry. Anthocyanins have also been reported to inhibit platelet aggregation. The hypolipidemic and hypoglycemic activity of oral administration of dried hydroalcoholic extract of the leaf of *Vaccinium myrtillus* has been demonstrated in animal studies. Extracts of *Vaccinium myrtillus* leaves have demonstrated antibacterial activity against several species, including *Staphylococcus aureus* and *Escherichia coli.*

Antineoplastic Effects: Components of Bilberry have been reported to exhibit potential anticarcinogenic activity in vitro as demonstrated by inhibition of the induction of ornithine decarboxylase (ODC) by the tumor promoter phorbol 12 myristate 13-acetate (TPA) (Bomser J et al, 1996).

Antioxidant Effects: Bilberry *(Vaccinium myrtillus)* extract exhibited potent antioxidant activity and protected plasma low-density lipoproteins (LDL) from copper- or photo-induced oxidative modifications and vitamin E consumption in vitro. Oxidation of these cellular components has been implicated in vascular pathology and chronic diseases, such as atherosclerosis, carcinogenesis, and other cardiovascular diseases (Laplaud, 1997, Rasetti, 1996/97, Viana, 1996).

Antiulcer Effects: Inhibition of histamine-induced capillary hyperpermeability and protection from capillary fragility were demonstrated potential mechanisms for the observed wound healing of Bilberry (Cristoni & Magistretti, 1987). The influence of Bilberry extract on mucopolysaccharides may be responsible for its antiulcer effects (Cristoni & Magistretti, 1987).

Microvascular Integrity Effects: Anthocyanosides induce relaxation of splenic arteries in vitro. The effect is present after pretreatment with beta-blockers and diminishes after pretreatment with indomethacin or lysine acetylsalicylate (Bettini et al, 1985).

Platelet Aggregation Effects: Bilberry anthocyanosides increased in intracellular concentrations of cyclic AMP or decreased the concentration of thromboxane A2 in platelets, or both (Pulliero et al, 1989, Bottecchia et al, 1987). The anthocyanoside component of Bilberry extract is responsible for the antiplatelet activity and stimulates the production of a prostacyclin (PGI 2)-like substance (Morazzoni & Magistretti, 1990, Morazzoni & Magistretti, 1986).

Wound-Healing Effects: Inhibition of histamine-induced capillary hyperpermeability and protection from capillary fragility were demonstrated as a potential mechanisms for the observed wound healing of Bilberry. The influence of Bilberry extract on mucopolysaccharides may be responsible for its wound healing effects (Cristoni & Magistretti, 1987).

CLINICAL TRIALS

Antiplatelet Aggregation

A study involving 30 healthy subjects with normal platelet aggregation investigated the effects of administration of *Vaccinium myrtillus* anthocyanins (Myrtocyan 480 mg) daily, ascorbic acid 3 g daily and *Vaccinium myrtillus* anthocyanins plus ascorbic acid on collagen- and ADP-induced platelet aggregation (Pulliero G et al, 1989). Platelet aggregation in blood samples taken from participants after 30 and 60 days' treatment was clearly reduced in all subjects compared with baseline values. The reduction in platelet aggregation was greater in subjects who received *Vaccinium myrtillus* anthocyanins alone than in those who received ascorbic acid alone and was most marked in subjects who received both preparations. Platelet aggregation returned to baseline values when tested 120 days after discontinuation of treatment (Pulliero G et al, 1989).

Diabetic Retinopathy

Forty patients with diabetic and/or hypertensive retinopathy received 160 mg Myrtocyan twice daily or placebo for 1 month. It was reported that 77% to 90% of treated patients experienced improvement compared with the pretreatment period, as determined by ophthalmoscopy and fluorescein fundus angiography. However, there does not appear to have been a statistical comparison between the treatment and placebo groups studied (Repossi P et al., 1987).

A Bilberry anthocyanoside preparation (Tegens 160 mg/capsule) given twice a day for 12 months significantly improved retinal condition in a placebo-controlled trial of 40 patients with retinopathy in its initial stages. Improvement was seen in 50% of the treatment group as compared with 20% of controls; 30% remained unchanged in the treatment group and 20% of the group got worse as compared to the control group, in which 45% were unchanged and 35% got worse (Repossi et al, 1987).

Twelve diabetic patients were treated with 600 mg anthocyanosides/day for 2 months. The use of radio-labeled amino acids demonstrated a significant decrease in biosynthesis, especially polymeric collagen. Anthocyanosides may help to prevent diabetic patients from injuries caused by malfunction of synthesis activities during normal diabetic treatment (Boniface, 1996).

Retinal improvement was demonstrated in a small trial of 40 patients. Ophthalmoscopic examination and descriptions of the fluoroangiographic investigation of patients with diabetic or hypertensive vascular retinopathy was performed in a double-blind, randomized, controlled study with specific exclusion criteria. Patients were given one capsule of Tegens®, containing 160 mg of Bilberry anthocyanosides, 2 times daily for approximately 1 month. Seventy-nine percent demonstrated retinal improvement. Of the 28 patients with ophthalmoscopic abnormalities and of 13 patients in the treatment group given anthocyanosides, 1 patient was much improved (8%), 9 patients were improved (69%), and 3 were unchanged (23%). None of the 15 patients in the placebo group exhibited retinal changes until they were treated with Tegens, at which time 12 patients (80%) were improved and 3 (20%) showed no improvement. Similar results were obtained in the fluoroangiographic investigation (Perossini et al, 1987).

Significant retinal improvement with a decrease or disappearance of hemorrhage was noted in a small study of 10 patients with varying levels of diabetic retinopathy related to type 2 diabetes. Tegens, containing 80 mg of Bilberry anthocyanosides/capsule, was given in an oral dose of 6 capsules/day in 3 divided doses for 6 months (Orsucci et al, 1983).

Diabetic retinopathy has been linked to abnormally increased synthesis of connective tissue. One study in diabetic patients using radio labeled amino acids demonstrated a significant decrease in biosynthesis activity, especially polymeric collagen after 2 months of 600 milligrams of anthocyanosides/day. Low luminance visual acuity was evaluated in diabetic patients with retinal pathologies. Retinal function was improved after administration of anthocyanoside-purified extract (Forte, 1996).

Cataracts

Bilberry prevented the development of further lens opacity in 97% of the eyes of 50 patients with mild senile cortical cataracts in a randomized, double blind, placebo-controlled trial. A Bilberry extract of 180 mg of Bilberry and 100 milligrams vitamin E was given orally twice a day for 8 months (Bravetti et al, 1989).

In a randomized, double-blind trial involving 51 patients with mild senile cortical cataracts who received *Vaccinium myrtillus* anthocyanins plus vitamin E twice daily for 4 months, treated patients showed significant improvements in lens opacity compared with placebo recipients (Bravetti et al, 1989).

Dysmenorrhea

A randomized, double-blind, placebo-controlled trial of *Vaccinium myrtillus* anthocyanins 320 mg/day taken for 3 days before menstruation was conducted involving 30 patients with chronic primary dysmenorrhea. Significant differences between the active treatment and placebo groups were reported for several symptoms investigated, including nausea and vomiting and breast tenderness. There was no effect on headache (Colombo & Vescovini, 1985).

Gastric Ulcers

Gastric mucosal prostaglandin E2 (PGE2) concentrations and release increased significantly without affecting stomach acid or fluid secretion in a controlled trial. Eight males, 20 to 36 years of age with no history of ulcers, were given 600 mg anthocyanin pigment occurring in Bilberry twice daily for ten days. One subject reported increased salivation and prolonged sleep pattern (Mertz-Nielsen et al, 1990).

Myopia

Improvement in retinal sensitivity, as measured by computerized central perimetry, was found in 32 of 42 adult eyes with myopia (-4 D to -25 D). Twenty-four patients received 3 tablets, each containing 50 milligrams of dry hydroalcoholic Bilberry extract, for 15 days. Subjective analyses showed that 58% of those tested experienced a decrease in dazzling, 79.1% showed an improvement in clarity of visual images, and 54.1% had an improvement in twilight vision (Virno et al, 1986).

Night-Vision Enhancement

A systematic review of placebo-controlled trials in subjects with normal or above average eyesight demonstrated no positive effects of anthocyanosides of *Vaccinium myrtillus* in night vision. Twelve trials met the inclusion criteria for this review. Four randomized/controlled studies demonstrated no significant effects of Bilberry on reduced-light vision. Seven placebo-controlled but nonrandomized trials and one randomized, controlled trial reported positive effects on at least one outcome measure relevant to reduced-light vision. The authors concluded that results should be cautiously interpreted due to methodological rigor, dose, geographical variations in extract composition, and other factors (Canter & Ernst, 2004).

Pupillary dynamics improved in some patients who received Bilberry in a double-blind, placebo-controlled trial. Forty adults received either 240 mg Bilberry anthocyanosides or placebo. Fifteen of the 20 subjects who received the drug demonstrated improvement in pupillary dynamics. The greatest improvements were observed 2 hours after administration ($p<0.05$). The response of the pupil to light was demonstrated as greater contraction, faster movement, and greater acceleration in less time. Those taking placebos exhibited similar responses but did not exhibit greater contraction (Vannini et al, 1986).

Night visual acuity (NVA) and contrast sensitivity (CS) were not improved in males in a double-blind, placebo-controlled, crossover trial. Participants (25 to 47 years) were treated with 160 mg Bilberry extract (containing 25% anthocyanosides) (n=8) or placebo (n=7) 3 times daily for 3 weeks. After a 1-month washout period, the groups were crossed. No improvements were noted for NVA or CS during the 3-month treatment period (Muth et al, 2000).

Macular recovery time and night vision were significantly improved in eight subjects after oral administration of two 30 mg tablets of Bilberry anthocyanosides for 1 week. Significant improvement ($p<0.05$) was noted in the reading of optotypes with medium-high angle between 0.85 and 0.22 degrees (Paronzini & Indemini, 1988).

Venous Insufficiency

In a controlled study of 54 pregnant women between 24 and 37 years, significant improvements ($p<0.01$) were observed for complaints related to venous insufficiency due to capillary fragility (pain, paresthesias, burning, heaviness, and leg cramps). The women received 320 milligrams Bilberry anthocyanosides (Tegens) daily for 60 to 80 days beginning in their sixth month of pregnancy (Grismondi, 1980).

Bilberry supplementation improved symptoms in patients with varicose veins of the legs. Forty-seven patients participated in the study. Half of the patients were treated with Bilberry anthocyanosides, 6 capsules of Tegens 80 mg each for 30 days. The other half of the group was treated with the same dose of Bilberry after saphenectomy. Significant improvements were found in symptoms, such as edema, feeling of heaviness, burning, pain, leg cramps, pruritis, paresthesias, cutaneous dystrophy, and dyschromia, and potential for hemorrhagic suffusion (especially in the second group). No study patient took diuretics or other medications (Ghiringhelli et al, 1977).

INDICATIONS AND USAGE

BILBERRY LEAF

Unproven Uses: Bilberry has been used in diabetes mellitus (for prevention and treatment); complaints of the gastrointestinal tract, kidneys, and urinary tract, and for arthritis, gout, and dermatitis. External uses include inflammation of the oral mucosa, eye inflammation, burns and skin diseases.

BILBERRY FRUIT

Approved by Commission E:

- Diarrhea
- Inflammation of the mouth and pharynx

Internally, Bilberry is used for nonspecific, acute diarrhea (particularly in light cases of enteritis). Externally the berry is used for mild inflammation of the mucous membranes of mouth and throat.

Unproven Uses: Folk medicine uses include internal use for vision impairment, vomiting, bleeding, and hemorrhoids, and external use for poorly healing skin ulcers and wound healing.

CONTRAINDICATIONS

Pregnancy: Not to be used during pregnancy.

Breastfeeding: Not to be used while breastfeeding.

PRECAUTIONS AND ADVERSE REACTIONS

Side effects may include those relating to the skin, gastrointestinal, and nervous systems. High doses and prolonged use of Bilberry may lead to chronic intoxication. Digestive complaints, including nausea due to the high tannin content were reported. Chronic administration of high doses (1.5 g/kg per day or more) to animals has been reported to be fatal.

DRUG INTERACTIONS

MODERATE RISK

Anticoagulants, and Antiplatelet and Thrombolytic Agents, Low Molecular Weight Heparins: Increased risk of bleeding with concomitant use. *Clinical Management*: Monitor the patient closely for signs and symptoms of bleeding. Adjust the anticoagulant dose only if the patient is consistently taking Bilberry with a consistent and standardized product.

DOSAGE

BILBERRY LEAF

No reliable dosing data.

BILBERRY FRUIT

Mode of Administration: Tablets, capsules, macerated drug for infusions for internal use and local application.

How Supplied: Most commercially available capsules and tablets are standardized at 25 to 36% anthocyanoside content.

Capsule—40 mg, 60 mg, 80 mg, 125 mg, 160 mg, 310 mg, 320 mg, 375 mg, 400 mg, 500 mg, 1000 mg

Tablet—40 mg

Preparation: To prepare an infusion, use 5 to 10 g mashed drug in cold water; bring to a simmer for 10 minutes, then strain (1 teaspoonful = 4 g drug). A 10% decoction is prepared for external use.

Daily Dose: 20 to 60 g of unprocessed fruit for internal use. Externally use a 10% infusion. For commercially available tablets and capsules that are standardized to 36% anthocyanosides, the recommended dose is 60 to 160 mg three times daily.

LITERATURE

Alexeeff T. Circulatory insufficiency: A historical and modern review of three classic herbs. *Aust J Med Herbalism*; 10(4):135-140. 1998

Bettini V, Aragno R, Bettini MB et al. Facilitating influence of *Vaccinium myrtillus* anthocyanosides on the acetylcholine-induced relaxation of isolated coronary arteries: role of the endothelium-derived relaxing factor. *Fitoterapia*; LXIV (1):45-57. 1993

Bettini V, Aragno R, Bettini MB et al. Vasodilator and inhibitory effects of *Vaccinium myrtillus* anthocyanosides on the contractile responses of coronary artery segments to acetylcholine: Role of the prostacyclins and of the endothelium-derived relaxing factor. *Fitoterapia*; LXII (1):15-28. 1991

Bettini V, Fiori A, Martino R et al. Study of the mechanism whereby anthocyanosides potentiate the effect of catecholamines on coronary vessels. *Fitoterapia;* LVI (2):67-72. 1985a

Bettini V, Guerra B, Martino R et al. Contractile responses of isolated rat stomach to stimulation of post-ganglionic cholinergic fibers in the presence of *Vaccinium myrtillus* anthocyanosides. *Fitoterapia;* LVII (4):211-216. 1986

Bettini V, Mayellaro F, Pilla I et al. Mechanical responses of isolated coronary arteries to barium in the presence of *Vaccinium myrtillus* anthocyanosides. *Fitoterapia*; LVI (1):3-10. 1985

Bettini V, Mayellaro F, Ton P et al. Effects of *Vaccinium myrtillus* anthocyanosides on vascular smooth muscle. *Fitoterapia*; 15:265-272. 1984

Bomser J et al. In vitro anticancer activity of fruit extracts from *Vaccinium* species. In: *PM* 62(3):212-216. 1996

Bottecchia D et al. Preliminary report on the inhibitory effect of *Vaccinium myrtillus* anthocyanosides on platelet aggregation and clot retraction. *Fitoterapia*; 58: 3-8. 1987

Bomser J et al. In vitro anticancer activity of fruit extracts from *Vaccinium* species. *Planta Med*; 62: 212-216. 1996

Bone K & Morgan M. Bilberry - The vision herb. MediHerb Professional Review; 59:1-4. 1997

Boniface R, Miskulin M, Robert L et al. Pharmacological properties of myrtillus anthocyanosides: correlation with results of treatment of diabetic microangiopathy. *Flavonoids Bioflavonoids*; 293-301. 1985

Boniface R & Robert AM. Influence of anthocyanosides on human connective tissue metabolism (German). *Klin Monatsbl Augenheilkd*; 209(6):368-372. 1996

Bosio E et al. *Ginkgo biloba L.* and *Vaccinium myrtillus L.* extracts prevent photo-induced oxidation of low density lipoproteins. In: *PM* 62, Abstracts of the 44th Ann Congress of GA, 24. 1996

Brantner A, Grein E. Antibacterial activity of plant extracts used externally in traditional medicine. *J Ethnopharmacol*; 44: 35-40. 1994

Bravetti GO et al. Preventive medical treatment of senile cataract with vitamin E and Vaccinium myrtillus anthocianosides: clinical evaluation. *Ann Ottal Clin Ocul*; 115: 109-116. 1989

Canter P & Ernst E: Anthocyanosides of *Vaccinium myrtillus* (Bilberry) for night vision-a systematic review of placebo-controlled trials. *Surv Ophthalmol*; 49(1):38-50. 2004

Cignarella A, Bertozzi D, Pinna C, Puglisi L, Hypolipidemic activity of *Vaccinium myrtillus* leaves on an model of genetically hyperlipidemic rat. In: *PM* 58(Suppl. 7):A581. 1992

Colombo D, Vescovini R. Studio clinico controllato sull'efficacia degli antocianosidi del mirtillo cel trattamento della dismenorrea essenziale. *Giorn It Ost Gin*; 7: 1033-1038. 1985

Colantuoni A, Bertuglia S, Magistretti MJ, Donato L. Effects of *Vaccinium Myrtillus* anthocyanosides on arterial vasomotion. *Arzneimittelforschung*; 84:905-9, Sep, 1991

Corsi C, Pollastri M, Tesi C et al. Contribution to the study of the activity of anthocyanosides on the microcirculation: Flowmeter evaluations in chronic venous insufficiency. S. Chiara Nursing Home:23-31. 1981

Cristoni A & Magistretti M. Antiulcer and healing activity of Vaccinium myrtillus anthocyanosides. *Farmaco*; 42(2):29-43. 1987

Detre Z, Jellinek H, Miskulin M et al. Studies on vascular permeability in hypertension: action of anthocyanosides. *Clin Physiol Biochem*; 4(2):143-149. 1986

Dombrowicz E, Zadernowski R, Swiatek L. Phenolic acids in leaves of *Arctostaphylos uva ursi L., Vaccinium vitis idaea L.* and *Vaccinium myrtillus L. Pharmazie*, 84:680-1, Sep, 1991

Forte R et al. Fitotherapy and ophthalmology: considerations on dynamized myrtillus retinal effects with low luminance visual acuity. *Ann Ottal Clin Ocul*; 122: 325-333. 1996

Ghiringhelli C, Gregoratti L & Marastoni F. Capillarotropic activity of anthocyanosides in high doses in phlebopathic stasis. *Estratto Minerva Cardioangiologica*: 1-31. 1977

Gomez Trillo JT. Varices of the lower legs: Symptomatic treatment with the new vascular drug. *Prensa Med Mex*; 38:293-296. 1973

Grismondi G. Treatment of pregnancy-induced phlebopathies. *Estratto Minerva Ginecologic;* 1-14. 1980

Laplaud PM et al. Antioxidant action of *Vaccinium myrtillus* extract on human low-density lipoproteins in vitro: initial observations. *Fund Clin Pharmacol*; 11: 35-40. 1997

Lietti A, Cristoni A & Picci M. Studies on *Vaccinium myrtillus* anthocyanosides, 1: vasoprotective and antiinflammatory activity. *Arzneimittelforschung*; 26(5):829-832. 1976

Lietti A & Forni G. Studies on *Vaccinum myrtilus* anthocyanosides, II: aspects of anthocyanin pharmacokinetics in the rat. *Arzneimittelforschung*; 26(5):832-835. 1976

Magistretti MJ et al. Antiulcer activity of an anthocyanidin from *Vaccinium myrtillus. Arzneimittelforschung*; 38: 686-690. 1988

Mertz-Nielsen A, Munck LK, Bukhave K et al. A natural flavonoid, IdB 1027, increases gastric luminal release of prostaglandin E2 in healthy subjects. *Ital J Gastroenterol*; 22:288-290. 1990

Morazzoni P & Bombardelli E. Vaccinium myrtillus. *Fitoterapia*; 48(1):3-29. 1995

Morazzoni P & Magistretti MJ. Activity of Myrtocyan®, an anthocyanoside complex from *Vaccinium myrtillus* (VMA), on platelet aggregation and adhesiveness. *Fitoterapia*; LXI (1):13-21. 1990

Morazzoni P & Magistretti MJ. Effects of *Vaccinium myrtillus* anthocyanosides on the prostacyclin-like activity in rat arterial tissue. *Fitoterapia*; LVII (1): 11-14. 1986

Paronzini S & Indemini P. Modifications of the macular recovery tests in normal subjects after administration of anthocyanosides. *Bollettino Oculistica*; 67(suppl 4):185-188. 1988

Pezzangora V, Barina R, De Stefani R et al. Medical therapy with Bilberry anthocyanosides in patients submitted to hemorrhoidectomy. *Gaz Med It - Arch Sc Med*; 143:405-409. 1984

Pulliero G, Montin S, Bettini V et al. Ex vivo study of the inhibitory effects *of Vaccinium myrtillus* anthocyanosides on human platelet aggregation. *Fitoterapia*; LX(1):69-75. 1989

Rasetti M, Caruso D, Galli G et al. Extracts of *Ginkgo bilboba L.* leaves and *Vaccinium myrtillus L.* fruits prevent photo induced oxidation of low density lipoprotein cholesterol. *Phytomedicine*; 3(4):335-338. 1996/1997

Repossi P et al. The role of anthocyanosides on vascular permeability in diabetic retinopathy. *Ann Ottal Clin Ocul*; 113: 357-361. 1987

Teglio L, Mazzanti C, Tronconi R et al: *Vaccinium myrtillus* anthocyanosides (Tegens®) in the treatment of venous insufficiency of lower limbs and acute piles in pregnancy. *Quaderni Clinica Ostetrica Ginecologica*; 42(May-June):221-231. 1987

Tori A & D'Errico F. *Vaccinium myrtillus* anthocyanosides in the treatment of stasis venous diseases of the lower limbs. *Gazzetta Medica Italiana*; 139:217-224. 1980

Viana M, Barbas C, Bonet B et al. In vitro effects of a flavonoid-rich extract on LDL oxidation. *Atherosclerosis*; 123(1-2):83-91. 1996

Virno M, Motolese E, Garofalo G et al. Effect of Bilberry anthocyanosides on retinal sensitivity of myopic patients assessed by computerized perimetry. *Bollettino Oculistica*; 65(7-8):789-795. 1986

Birch

Betula species

DESCRIPTION

Medicinal Parts: The medicinal parts are the bark, leaves and buds.

Flower and Fruit: The male flowers of *Betula pendula* are sessile and oblong-cylindrical 6 to 10 cm long. The female catkins are petioled, cylindrical and 2 to 4 cm long by 8 to 10 mm thick when fully grown. They are densely flowered, first yellow-green, later light green. The fruit scales are brownish and pubescent or glabrous. The middle lobes are small, short-triangular and shorter than the broad, always revolute side lobes. The fruit wings are half-oval and 2 to 3 times as broad as the fruit.

The male catkins of *Betula pubescens* are sessile and oblong-cylindrical. They are initially upright, later hanging, 2.5 to 4 cm long and 6 to 10 mm thick, greenish to light brown. The middle lobes of the fruit scales protrude clearly, are usually linguiform-elogated and generally longer than the usually sharp-cornered, clearly evolute side lobes. The fruit scales are about as broad as the fruit.

Leaves, Stem, and Root: Betula pendula is a tree that grows up to 30 cm high, with a snow white bark that usually peels off in horizontal strips or changes into a black, stony, hard bark. Young branches are glabrous and thickly covered in warty resin glands. The petioled leaves are dark green above, a lighter gray-green below. They have serrate margins and particularly tightly packed veins. The lamina are about 3 to 7 cm long by 2 to 5 cm wide, rhomboid-triangular, acuminate, glabrous, densely covered in glands, and have a doubly serrate margin. They are dark green and glabrous above and a lighter green below; they are initially downy and later pubescent in the vein axils.

Habitat: Betula pendula and *Betula pubescens* are indigenous to Europe from the northern Mediterranean regions to Siberia and to temperate regions of Asia.

Production: Birch leaf consists of the fresh or dried leaf of *Betula pendula* (syn. *Betula verrucosa*), *Betula pubescens*, or of both species. The leaves are collected in the wild during the spring and dried at room temperature in the shade. Birch tar (*Betulae oleum empyreumaticum retificatum*) is a clear, dark brown oil obtained from *Betula pendula* or *Betula pubescens* through a distillation process.

Other names: Common Birch, Silver Birch, White Birch

ACTIONS AND PHARMACOLOGY

COMPOUNDS: BIRCH LEAF

Triterpene alcohol ester with saponinlike effect: betula-triterpene saponins

Flavonoids: including hyperoside, quercetin, myricetin digalactosides

Proanthocyanidins

Volatile oil: including sesquiterpene oxide

Monoterpene glucosides: including betula alboside A and B, roseoside

Caffeic acid derivatives: including chlorogenic acid

Ascorbic acid

3,4'-dihydroxy propiophenone-3-beta-D-glucoside

EFFECTS: BIRCH LEAF

Birch leaves have a mild saluretic effect and are antipyretic. In animal tests, they have been shown to increase the amount of urine.

COMPOUNDS: BIRCH TAR

Phenols (6%): including among others guaiacol, cresole, catechol, pyrogallol, 5-propyl-pyrogallol dimethyl ether and 5-methyl-pyrogallol dimethyl ether

EFFECTS: BIRCH TAR

The aliphatic and aromatic hydrocarbons in birch tar are irritating to the skin and have an antiparasitic effect. Its use for diverse skin conditions and for parasitic infestation such as scabies seems plausible.

INDICATIONS AND USAGE

BIRCH LEAVES

Unproven Uses: The leaves are used in flushing-out therapy for bacterial and inflammatory diseases of the urinary tract and for kidney gravel. They are also used in adjunct therapy for rheumatic ailments, for increasing amount of urine. In folk medicine, the leaves are used as a blood purifier, and for gout and rheumatism. Externally, the leaves are used for hair loss and dandruff.

BIRCH TAR

Unproven Uses: External birch tar uses include parasitic infestation of the skin with subsequent hair loss, rheumatism and gout (ointment); dry eczema and dermatoses (liquid preparations), psoriasis and other chronic skin diseases. Birch tar is a constituent of ''Unguentum contra scabiem'' that is used for the treatment of scabies.

CONTRAINDICATIONS

BIRCH LEAF

The drug should not be used for edema when there is reduced cardiac or kidney function.

PRECAUTIONS AND ADVERSE REACTIONS

BIRCH LEAF

No health hazards or side effects are known in conjunction with the proper administration of designated therapeutic dosages.

BIRCH TAR

No health hazards are known in conjunction with the proper administration of designated therapeutic dosages. Birch tar can cause irritations on sensitive skin. Administration of the drug is not advisable, due to the possible presence of carcinogenic hydrocarbons.

DOSAGE

BIRCH LEAF

Mode of Administration: Comminuted herb or dry extracts are used for teas; other galenic preparations and freshly pressed plant juices can also be used internally.

Preparation: Tea is prepared by pouring 150 mL hot water over 1 to 2 dessertspoons of drug and then straining the leaves out after 15 minutes.

Daily Dosage: The average daily dose is 2 to 3 g drug several times a day with a caution to ensure ample intake of fluid (minimum 2 liters per day). A fresh cup of tea is taken between meals 3 to 4 times a day.

Storage: Birch leaf should be stored in sealed containers protected from light and moisture.

BIRCH TAR

Mode of Administration: Birch Tar is used in combination preparations as external ointments and liniments.

Storage: Birch tar should be stored in tightly sealed containers.

LITERATURE

BIRCH LEAF

Anonym, Phytotherapie: Pflanzliche Antirheumatika - was bringen sie. In: DAZ 136(45):4012-4015. 1996.

Bufe A, Spangfort MD, Kahlert H, Schlaak M, Becker WM, The major birch pollen allergen Bet v 1 shows ribonuclease activity. *Planta*, 175:413-5, 1996.

Cadot P, LeJoly M, Van Hoeyveld EM, Stevens EA, Influence of the pH of the extraction medium on the composition of birch (*Betula verrucosa*) pollen extracts. *Allergy*, 108:431-7, 1995 May.

Carnat A, Lacouture I, Fraisse D, Lamaison JL, Standardization of the birch leaf. *Ann Pharm Fr*, 175:231-5, 1996.

Cirla AM, Sforza N, Roffi GP, Alessandrini A, Stanizzi R, Dorigo N, Sala E, Della Torre F, Preseasonal intranasal immunotherapy in birch-alder allergic rhinitis. A double-blind study. *Allergy*, 175:299-305, 1996 May.

Czygan FC, Betula pendula - Die Birke. Z Phytother 10(1989): 135-139.

Davidov MI, Goriunov VG, Kubarikov PG, Phytoperfusion of the bladder after adenomectomy. *Urol Nefrol* (Mosk), 175:19-20, 1995 Sep-Oct.

Fountain DW, Berggren B, Nilsson S, Einarsson R, Expression of birch pollen-specific IgE-binding activity in seeds and other plant parts of birch trees (Betula verrucosa Ehrh.). *Int Arch Allergy Immunol*, 98:370-6, 1992.

Hasler A et al., High-performance liquid chromatographic determination of five widespread flavonoid aglycones. *J Chromatogr*. 508, 1(1990): 236-40.

Hiller K, Pharmazeutische Bewertung ausgewählter Teedrogen. In: *DAZ* 135(16):1425-1440. 1995.

Hörhammer L, Wagner H, Luck R, *Arch Pharm* 290:338-341. 1957.

Karatodorof K, Kalarova R, (1977) Izn Durzh Inst Kontrol Lek Sredstva 10:103-9.

Keinanen M, Comparison of methods for extraction of flavonoids from birch leaves carried out using high-performance liquid chromatography. *J Agric Food Chem*. 41, 11(1993): 1986-90.

Kiiskinen M, Korhonen M, Kangasjaervi J, Immunological study of the HLA class II antigen associated with birch pollen allergy. Nippon Jibiinkoka Gakkai Kaiho, 35:541-50, 1992 Apr.

Lee MW et al., Phenolic compounds of the leaves of Betula. *Arch Pharmaceutical Res*. 15, 3(1992): 211-14.

Olsen OT et al., A double-blind randomized study investigating the efficacy and specificity of immunotherapy with Artemisia vulgaris or Phleum pratense/betula verrucosa. Allergol Immunopathol (Madr), 23:73-8, 1995 Mar-Apr.

Ossipov V et al., HPLC isolation and identification of flavonoids from white birch. *Biochem Syst Ecol*. 23, 3(1995): 213-22.

Pietta PG et al., HPLC determination of the flavonoid glycosides from *Betulae folium*. *Chromatographia*, 28, 5-6(1989): 311-12.

Pisha E et al., Discovery of betulinic acid as a selective inhibitor of human melanoma that functions by induction of apoptosis. In: *Nature Medicine* 1:1046-1051. 1995.

Ramirez J, Carpizo JA, Ipsen H, Carreira J, Lombardero M, Quantification in mass units of Bet v 1 the main allergen of *Betula verrucosa* pollen by a monoclonal antibody based-ELISA. *Clin Exp Allergy*, 27:926-31, 1997 Aug.

Rickling B, Glombitza KW, Saponins in the leaves of birch? Hemolytic dammarane triterpenoids esters of Betula pendula. *Planta Med* 59 (1993), 77.

Schilcher H, Boesel R, Effenberger ST Segebrecht S, Neuere Untersuchungsergebnisse mit aquaretisch, antibakteriell und prostatotrop wirksamen Arzneipflanzen. In: *ZPT* 10(3):77. 1989.

Schilcher H, Rau H, Nachweis der aquaretischen Wirkung von Birkenblätter- und Goldrutenauszügen im Tierversuch. *Urologe B* 28(1988): 274-280.

Sökeland J, Phytotherapie in der Urologie. In: *ZPT* 10(1):8. 1989.

Spangfort MD, Ipsen H, Sparholt SH, Aasmul-Olsen S, Osmark P, Poulsen FM, Larsen M, M rtz E, Roepstorff P, Larsen JN, Characterisation of recombinant isoforms of birch pollen allergen Bet v 1. *Adv Exp Med Biol*, 175:251-4, 1996.

Tschesche R, Ciper F, Breitmeier E, *Chem Ber* 110:3111-3117. 1977.

Valenta R, Duchene M, Ebner C, Valent P, Sillaber C, Deviller P, Ferreira F, TeJkl M, Edelmann H, Kraft D, et al., Profilins constitute a novel family of functional plant pan-allergens. *J Exp Med*, 175:377-85, 1992 Feb 1.

BIRCH TAR

Kreitmair H, PA 8:534-536. 1953.

Nowak GA, Am Perf Cosmet 81:37-39. 1966.

Birthwort

Aristolochia clematitis

DESCRIPTION

Medicinal Parts: The medicinal parts are the aerial portion (when in blossom) and the root.

Flower and Fruit: The plant has dirty yellow flowers, usually in axillary groups of 7. The perigone forms a straight tube, which is bulbous beneath and has a linguiform, oblong-ovate, obtuse border. There are 6 stamens, the style is upward growing, and the stigma is 6-lobed. The flower briefly traps the insects that pollinate it. The fruit is a globose, pear-shaped capsule.

Leaves, Stem, and Root: The plant grows to a height of 30 to 100 cm. The stem is erect, simple, grooved, and glabrous. The leaves are alternate, long-petioled, cordate-reniform, yellow-green with prominent ribs.

Characteristics: The plant has a fruitlike fragrance and is poisonous.

Habitat: Indigenous to Mediterranean regions, Asia Minor and the Caucasus, but is also found in numerous other regions.

Production: Birthwort is the aerial part of *Aristolochia clematitis*.

ACTIONS AND PHARMACOLOGY

COMPOUNDS

Aristolochic acids (10-nitro-phenanthrene-1-acids): in particular aristolochic acids I and II

Isoquinoline alkaloids: including magnoflorin, corytuberin

Volatile oil (0.03 to 0.2%): chief constituents alpha-pinene, alpha-terpineol

EFFECTS

The aristolochic acids have a phagocytosis- and metabolism-activating effect. They are also thought to improve the production of lymphokinins. Activation of phagocytes has been demonstrated in animal tests in rabbits and guinea pigs, along with an increase in serum bactericides and stimulation of β-lysine. In addition, in animal tests, immune resistance to Herpes simplex viruses of the eye was proved. In the ring test, stimulation and formation of granulation tissue was demonstrated in rats. In mice, there was a clear increase in the survival rate in cases of general infection. No significant results were recorded in cases where infections had no or only a low leucocytic immune reaction. The drug's pure aristolochic acid acts similarly to colchicine; it is nephrotoxic, carcinogenic and mutagenic.

INDICATIONS AND USAGE

Unproven Uses: Birthwort is used to stimulate the immune system and in the treatment of allergically caused gastrointestinal and gallbladder colic. The plant is used in a wide variety of ways in the folk medicine of nearly all European countries.

Chinese Medicine: Uses in Chinese medicine include joint pain, stomachache, malaria and abscesses.

Homeopathic Uses: Homeopathic indications include gynecological disorders and climacteric symptoms, as well as the treatment of wounds and ulcers. It is also used as a treatment after major surgery and in ear-nose-throat treatments.

CONTRAINDICATIONS

Birthwort is contraindicated during pregnancy.

PRECAUTIONS AND ADVERSE REACTIONS

General: Birthwort is highly toxic. The intake of acutely toxic doses leads to vomiting, gastroenteritis, spasms, severe kidney damage, and eventually to death by kidney failure. The chronic intake of low dosages among both humans and laboratory animals led to the development of tumors. Because of the genotoxic and carcinogenic effects of the aristolochic acids, the drug is not to be administered even in small dosages. Only to be used under the supervision of an expert qualified in its appropriate use.

Pregnancy: Birthwort is not to be used during pregnancy.

DOSAGE

Mode of Administration: Birthwort is used as a tincture in an ethanol solution. No further information is available.

How Supplied: Birthwort is available in homeopathic dilutions of D11.

LITERATURE

Che CT et al., (1984) J Nat Prod 47(2):331.

Fanselow G, Der Einfluβ von Pflanzenextrakten (Echinacea purpurea, Aristolochia clematitis) und homöopathischen Medikamenten auf die Phagocytoseleistung humaner Granulocyten in vitro. In: Dissertation Berlin. 1981.

Henrickson CU, (1970) *Z Immunitäts Forsch* 5:425.

Mengs U, Klein M, Genotoxic Effects of Aristolochic Acid in the Mouse Micronucleus Test. In: *PM* 52(6):502. 1988.

Mix DB et al., (1982) *J Nat Prod* 45(6):657.

Siess M, Seybold G, Untersuchungen über die Wirkung von Pulsatilla pratensis, Cimicifuga racemosa und Aristolochia clematis auf den Östrus infantiler und kastrierter weiβer Mäuse. In: Arzneim Forsch 10:514. 1960.

Strauch R, Hiller K, (1974) *Pharmazie* 29(10/11):656.

Tympner KD, (1981) *Z Angew Phytother* 5:181.

Bishop's Weed

Ammi visnaga

DESCRIPTION

Medicinal Parts: The medicinal part is the fruit.

Flower and Fruit: The rays are slender and patent in the flower, becoming erect, thickened and indurate in the fruit. The bracts are 1 to 2-pinnatisect, equaling or exceeding the rays, and the bracteoles are subulate. The pedicles are erect, stout and rigid in the fruit. The fruit is 2 to 2.5 mm long.

Leaves, Stem and Root: Bishop's Weed is a robust annual or biennial that grows up to 100 cm tall. The lower leaves are pinnate, the others are 2 to 3 pinnate. All of the leaves have narrow linear or filform lobes.

Habitat: The plant grows in the Mediterranean region, and is cultivated in the U.S., Mexico, Chile and Argentina.

Production: Bishop's Weed fruit consists of the dried, ripe fruits of Ammi visnaga.

Other Names: Khella, Khella Fruits, Greater Ammi

ACTIONS AND PHARMACOLOGY

COMPOUNDS

Furochromones: particularly khellin, visnagin, khellol and khellol glucoside

Pyranocoumarins: particularly visnadin and samidin

Flavonoids: including quercetin and isohamnetin and their 3-sulfates

Volatile oil

Fatty oil

EFFECTS

The drug intensifies coronary and myocardial circulation, acting as a mild positive ionotrope. It has an antispasmodic effect on smooth muscles.

INDICATIONS AND USAGE

Unproven Uses: Bishop's Weed has been used for angina pectoris, cardiac insufficiency, paroxysmal tachycardia, extra systoles, hypertonia, asthma, whooping cough and cramp-like complaints of the abdomen.

PRECAUTIONS AND ADVERSE REACTIONS

Infrequently, a cholestatic jaundice (reversible) is observed following administration of the drug. The drug also possesses a phototoxic effect.

DOSAGE

Median dose corresponding to 20 mg g-pyrone derivatives, calculated as khellin.

Liquid extract: (1:1) 0.5 mL

Tincture: (1:10) 4 mL

Tea: 0.5 gm in one cup of water, taken several times a day.

OVERDOSAGE

Long-term use or overdose of the drug can lead to queasiness, dizziness, loss of appetite, headache or sleep disorders. Very high dosages, corresponding to over 100 mg khellin, may cause elevated levels (reversible) of liver enzymes in blood plasma.

DOSAGE

No information is available.

LITERATURE

Duarte J et al., Effects of visnadine on rat vascular smooth muscle. In: PM 63(3):233-236. 1997.

El-Domiaty MM. Improved high-performance liquid chromatographic determination of khellin and visnagin in *Ammi visnaga* fruits and pharmaceutical formulations. *J Pharm Sci.* 81:475-478. 1981.

Greinwald R, Stobernack HP, Ammi visnaga - Das Bischhofskraut. In: ZPT 11(2):65. 1990.

Le Quesne PW et al., JNP 48:496. 1985.

Martelli P et al., J Chromatogr 301:297. 1984.

Trunzler G, Phytotherapeutische Möglichkeiten bei Herz- und arteriellen Gefäßerkrankungen. In: ZPT 10(5):147. 1989.

Bistort

Persicaria bistorta

DESCRIPTION

Medicinal Parts: The medicinal parts are the leaves and the rhizome.

Flower and Fruit: The flowering stem terminates in a compact, cylindrical, false spike of flesh-colored flowers without a terminal bud. The pedicle is winged. The flowers consist of 5 sepals, 8 stamens and an ovary with 2 to 3 styles. The flowers are in pairs, one of which is complete, the other only having a rudimentary ovary. Only the latter ripens. The complete flowers can be cross-pollinated by insects. The fruit is a three-seeded achene. The ripe seeds are small, brown, and glossy.

Leaves, Stem, and Root: The plant is a perennial, 30 cm to 1 m high herb on a thick, somewhat flattened and twisted S-shaped rhizome. The radical, oval leaves grow out of the rhizome to form basal rosette leaves with cordate bases, which are blue-green above and somewhat undulate.

Habitat: The plant is indigenous to Europe, North America and Asia.

Production: Bistort root and rhizome is the subterranean part of *Persicaria bistorta.* The root stocks of the older plants are harvested, cleaned, and freed from green parts and rootlets. The stronger parts are then cut up, and this material is dried in the sun.

Other Names: Adderwort, Dragonwort, Easter Giant, Easter Mangiant, Oderwort, Osterick, Patience Dock, Red Legs, Snakeweed, Sweet Dock

ACTIONS AND PHARMACOLOGY

COMPOUNDS

Tannins (15-36%): chiefly catechin tannins, small quantity of gallo tannins

Starch (in the root 30%)

EFFECTS

The active agents are the galenic tannin substance, starch, catechin and silicic acid. Higher concentrations of the root cause an increase in the formation of mucous. It is also an astringent.

INDICATIONS AND USAGE

Unproven Uses: The herb is used in the treatment of digestive disorders, particularly diarrhea and for internal bleeding. Externally, it is used as a gargle for mouth and throat infections and as an ointment for wounds.

Chinese Medicine: Preparations from the rhizome are used for epilepsy, fever, tetanus, carbuncles, snake and mosquito bites, scrofulous and cramps in the hands and feet.

PRECAUTIONS AND ADVERSE REACTIONS

No health hazards or side effects are known in conjunction with the proper administration of designated therapeutic dosages.

DOSAGE

Mode of Administration: Internally as a powdered drug for infusion, or externally as an extract or ointment.

Preparation:

Infusion (internal) – Macerate 50 g drug in 1 l water for 6 hours, percolate and sweeten as required (Penso, 1987).

Infusion (external) – Boil 60 g drug with 1 l water for 15 minutes, percolate and cool (Penso, 1987).

Liquid extract – drug 1:1 in 25% ethanol (BHP83).

Tincture – drug 1:5 in 25% ethanol (BHP83).

Daily Dosage:

Internal Dosage

Powder – in the form of 0.25 g gelatine capsules, 2 to 4 capsules every 3 hours.

Decoction – 1 to 2 g for each decoction, 3 times a day.

Infusion – 200 ml every 3 hours.

Liquid extract – 1 to 2 ml 3 times daily.

Tincture – 1 to 3 ml 3 times daily.

External Dosage

Decoction – poultice applied every 2 hours.

LITERATURE

Gonnet JF, (1981) *Biochem Syst Ecol* 9(4):299.

Kern W, List PH, Hörhammer L (Hrsg.), Hagers Handbuch der Pharmazeutischen Praxis, 4. Aufl., Bde. 1-8, Springer Verlag Berlin, Heidelberg, New York, 1969.

Penso G, Medico Farmaceutica, Milano, 1987.

Rao PRSP, Rao EV, (1977) *Curr Sci* 48(18):640.

Bitter Apple

Citrullus colocynthis

DESCRIPTION

Medicinal Parts: The medicinal part of the plant is the dried pulp.

Flower and Fruit: The flowers are yellow and appear singly in the leaf axils. The fruit is about the size of an apple. It is yellow, smooth, dry, and very bitter. When ripe, the fruit contains white spongy flesh within the coriaceous peel, with numerous ovate, white or brownish seeds. The seeds are 0.75 cm long and 0.5 cm wide, ovate, compressed, without an edge, oily and somewhat shiny.

Leaves, Stem, and Root: Bitter Apple is an annual similar to a watermelon plant. The stems are leafy and rough-haired. The leaves are alternate on long petioles. They are triangular, divided, variously indented, obtuse and pubescent. The upper surface is delicate green, the lower surface rough and pale.

Characteristics: Bitter Apple (the drug) is highly poisonous.

Habitat: Bitter Apple is indigenous to Turkey and southern Mediterranean countries. It is also found in Sri Lanka, Egypt, Syria, and the Arabian Gulf.

Production: Bitter Apples are the ripe fruits of *Citrullus colocynthis* that have been removed from the harder outer layer.

Other Names: Colocynth Pulp, Bitter Cucumber

ACTIONS AND PHARMACOLOGY

COMPOUNDS

Cucurbitacins: including cucurbitacin E-, J-, L-glucosides

Caffeic acid derivatives: chlorogenic acid

Fatty oil (in the seeds)

EFFECTS

Bitter Apple irritates the intestinal mucous membrane, increasing liquid production.

INDICATIONS AND USAGE

Unproven Uses: Preparations of Bitter Apple are used as a drastic (painful) purgative in fixed combinations in the treatment of acute and chronic constipation with various causes.

Indian Medicine: Acitis and elephantiasis are among the conditions treated with Bitter Apple in Indian medicine.

PRECAUTIONS AND ADVERSE REACTIONS

The drug is severely poisonous. It has a strongly irritating (and painful) effect on mucous membranes due to its cucurbitacin glycoside content, out of which cucurbitacins are released in watery environments.

OVERDOSAGE

Vomiting, bloody diarrhea, colic, and kidney irritation follow the intake of toxic dosages (0.6 to 1 g), and then increased diuresis that progresses to anuria. Lethal dosages (starting at 2 g) lead to convulsions, paralysis and, if untreated, to death through circulatory collapse. The treatment for poisonings should proceed symptomatically following gastric lavage. Administration in allopathic dosages is no longer defensible.

LITERATURE

Habs M et al., (1984) *J Cancer Res Clin Oncol* 108(1):154.

Konopa J et al., In: Advances in Antimicrobial and Antineoplastic Chemotherapy, Vol. 2, Ed. M. Semonsky, Avicenna Press Prague 1972.

Lavie D et al., (1964) *Phytochemistry* 3:52.

Rawson MD, (1966) *Lancet* 1:1121.

Bitter Candytuft

Iberis amara

DESCRIPTION

Medicinal Parts: The medicinal parts are the ripe seeds and the whole flowering plant.

Flower and Fruit: The stemmed flowers are arranged in racemes; there are 4 orbicular, diagonally splayed sepals approximately 2 mm long with white or reddish membranous margins and 4 obovate-elongate white petals, the outer ones approximately 6 mm, the inner ones 3 mm long. The plant has 2 short and 4 long stamens and a superior 4-carpeled ovary; the carpels are fused. The fruit is a small pod, 4 to 5 mm long, almost circular with wide-winged fruit sides and a tough margin. Each of the 2 chambers has only 1 seed. The seeds are semi-ovoid, 2.5 to 3 mm long, flat and approximately 1 mm thick. They are usually narrow-winged at the margin, brown and smooth.

Leaves, Stem, and Root: The plant is an herb, occasionally biennial, up to 40 cm high. The leaves are elongate-cuneiform and obtuse. The lower leaves are often spatulate and narrow toward the petiole. The upper leaves are sessile, usually with 2 to 4 blunt teeth at wide intervals and a ciliate margin. The stem is upright with splayed branches and downy-haired at the edges.

Habitat: The plant is found in most parts of western, central and southern Europe, in the Caucasus, and also in Algeria.

Production: Bitter Candytuft seeds are the ripe seeds of *Iberis amara*, which are collected in the wild and cultivated. Bitter Candytuft herb is the fresh, whole flowering plant of cultivated *Iberis amara*.

Other Names: Clown's Mustard, White Candytuft

ACTIONS AND PHARMACOLOGY

COMPOUNDS: BITTER CANDYTUFT SEEDS

Cucurbitacins (0.2 to 0.4%): particularly cucurbitacin E and cucurbitacin I

Glucosinolates (1%): glucoiberin, glucocheiroline, glucoiberviridine

Fatty oil (12%): chief fatty acids are behenic acid (45%), oleic acid (20%), palmitic acid (10%) and linolenic acid (10%)

EFFECTS: BITTER CANDYTUFT SEEDS

The cucurbitacins contained in the seeds are toxic, cytotoxic and generally irritating to the small and large intestines. Furthermore, the seeds exhibit a mildly antimicrobial and fungistatic effect,

COMPOUNDS: BITTER CANDYTUFT HERB

Cucurbitacins: particularly cucurbitacins E and I

Flavonoids: including kempferol-3-O-arabinosido-7-O-rhamnoside, kempferol-7-O-rhamnoside, quercetin-3-O-glucosido-7-O-rhamnoside (high concentration in the flowers)

EFFECTS: BITTER CANDYTUFT HERB

The chief active ingredients of the fresh plant are cucurbitacins. A significant anti-edematous effect was exhibited in animal experiments. Its nature as a bitter substance makes its administration both as a choleretic and for stimulating the secretion of gastric juices appear plausible.

INDICATIONS AND USAGE

BITTER CANDYTUFT SEEDS

Unproven Uses: In folk medicine, the drug is used for digestive problems

Homeopathic Uses: Homeopathic uses include cardiac arrhythmia and insufficiency.

BITTER CANDYTUFT HERB

Unproven Uses: Folk medicine usage includes digestion problems.

PRECAUTIONS AND ADVERSE REACTIONS

BITTER CANDYTUFT SEEDS

The drug is toxic, due to its cucurbitacin content. Symptoms of poisoning could include vomiting, diarrhea, colic and kidney irritation. Cases of poisonings, however, have not been documented.

BITTER CANDYTUFT HERB

No risks are known in connection with the administration of homeopathic dosages of the drug. The drug is mildly toxic due to its (low) level of cucurbitacins. Symptoms of poisoning could include vomiting, diarrhea, colic and kidney irritation. Cases of poisonings have, however, never been documented.

OVERDOSAGE

BITTER CANDYTUFT SEEDS

In case vomiting has not already occurred, gastric lavage should be induced using burgundy-colored potassium permanganate solution and sodium sulfate.

Following gastrointestinal emptying and installation of activated charcoal, begin therapy for poisoning. Diazepam (i.v.) for muscle spasm may be necessary, along with electrolyte substitution and treatment for possible cases of acidosis with sodium bicarbonate infusions. In the event of shock, plasma volume expanders should be infused. Monitoring of kidney function is imperative. Intubation and oxygen respiration also may be necessary.

DOSAGE

BITTER CANDYTUFT SEEDS

How Supplied: Commercially prepared pharmaceutical compounds only.

Homeopathic Dosage: 5 drops, 1 tablet, 10 globules, every 30 to 60 minutes (acute) and 1 to 3 times daily (chronic); parenterally: 1 ml sc: 3 times daily (acute); 1 ml sc once a day (chronic) (HAB1).

BITTER CANDYTUFT HERB

How Supplied: Only available in commercial pharmaceutical compound preparations.

LITERATURE

Hänsel R, Keller K, Rimpler H, Schneider G (Ed), Hagers Handbuch der Pharmazeutischen Praxis, 5. Aufl., Bde 4 - 6 (Drogen), Springer Verlag Berlin, Heidelberg, New York, 1992-1994.

Kowalewski Z, Wierzbicka K, Flavonoid compounds in the blossoms *of Iberis amara, L. Planta Med*, 20:328-39, 1971 Dec.

Uhlenbruck G, Dahr W, Studies on lectins with a broad agglutination spectrum. XII. N-acetyl-D-galactosamine specific lectins from the seeds of *Soja hispida, Bauhinia purpurea, Iberis amara, Moluccella laevis* and *Vicia graminea. Vox Sang,* 21:338-51, 1971 Oct.

Bitter Melon

Momordica charantia

DESCRIPTION

Botanical Description: It is a slender, climbing annual vine with long-stalked leaves and yellow, solitary male and female flowers borne on the leaf axils. The fruit, usually oblong, resembles a a warty gourd or a small cucumber. The young fruit is emerald green, turning to orange-yellow when ripe. At maturity, the fruit splits into three irregular valves that curl backwards and release numerous reddish-brown or white seeds encased in scarlet arils.

Habitat: Bitter melon grows in tropical areas, including parts of the Amazon, East Africa, India, Asia, and the Caribbean.

Other Names: bitter gourd, bitter apple, bitter cucumber, balsam pear, carella fruit (USA), karela (India), fu kwa (China), ampalaya (Phillipines).

ACTIONS AND PHARMACOLOGY

COMPOUNDS

Bitter melon contains an array of biologically active plant chemicals including triterpenes, proteins, and steroids.

EFFECTS

In numerous studies, at least three different groups of constituents found in all parts of bitter melon have clinically demonstrated hypoglycemic (blood sugar lowering) properties or other actions of potential benefit against diabetes mellitus. The chemicals that lower blood sugar include a mixture of steroidal saponins known as charantins, insulin-like peptides, and alkaloids. The hypoglycemic effect is more pronounced in the fruit of bitter melon where these chemicals are found in greater abundance.

CLINICAL TRIALS

Diabetes mellitus

The effect of *Momordica charantia* extracts on fasting and postprandial serum glucose levels were investigated in 100 cases of moderate non-insulin dependent diabetic subjects. Drinking of the aqueous homogenized suspension of the vegetable pulp led to significant reduction ($p<0.001$) of both fasting and postprandial serum glucose levels. This hypoglycemic action was observed in 86 cases. Five cases showed reduced fasting serum glucose only (Ahmad et al, 1999).

A controlled randomized trial was conducted to evaluate the efficacy of *Momordica charantia* as a hypoglycemic agent. Fifty patients with moderate type 2 diabetes mellitus were enrolled and randomly assigned to receive either bitter gourd tablets (n=26) or placebo (n=24) over a period of 4 weeks. No significant changes in blood sugar or fructosamine levels could be found in both treatment groups (John et al, 2003).

Supplemental cancer treatment

Cancer patients have compromised defective immune systems. There is a decrease of total white blood cell count including lymphocytes and natural killer (NK) cells. NK cells, one type of lymphocyte, play a role in eliminating cancer cells by an antibody-dependent, cell-mediated cytotoxicity (ADCC) mechanism. Previous studies have shown that P-glycoprotein (170 kDa, transmembrane protein) may be a transporter for cytokine-releasing in ADCC mechanism. One study explored the role of bitter melon intake in cervical cancer patients undergoing radiotherapy. Control and treatment groups were cervical cancer patients (stage II or III) treated with radiotherapy (without or with bitter melon ingestion). Blood samples of patient control and patient treatment groups were analyzed for NK cells percentage and P-glycoprotein level. Bitter melon ingestion did not affect NK cell level but it did affect the decrease of P-gp level on NK cell membrane (Pongnikorn et al, 2003).

INDICATIONS AND USAGE

Unproven Uses: viruses, colds and flu, cancer and tumors, high cholesterol, and psoriasis.

Probable Efficacy: diabetes.

CONTRAINDICATIONS

Pregnancy: Bitter melon traditionally has been used as an abortive and has been documented with weak uterine stimulant activity; therefore, it is contraindicated during pregnancy. This plant has been documented to reduce fertility in both males and females and should therefore not be used by those undergoing fertility treatment or seeking pregnancy.

Hypoglycemia: All parts of bitter melon (especially the fruit and seed) have demonstrated in numerous in vivo studies that they lower blood sugar levels. As such, it is contraindicated in persons with hypoglycemia.

Lactation: The active chemicals in bitter melon can be transferred through breast milk; therefore, it is contraindicated in women who are breast feeding.

PRECAUTIONS AND ADVERSE REACTIONS

Diabetics should check with their physicians before using this plant and use with caution while monitoring their blood sugar levels regularly as the dosage of insulin medications may need adjusting.

Many in vivo clinical studies have demonstrated the relatively low toxicity of all parts of the bitter melon plant when ingested orally. Other studies have shown extracts of the fruit and leaf (ingested orally) to be safe during pregnancy.

DRUG INTERACTIONS

MODERATE RISK

Antidiabetic Agents: Concurrent use may result in an increased risk of hypoglycemia. *Clinical Management:* If bitter melon and an antidiabetic agent are used together, blood glucose levels should be monitored regularly.

POTENTIAL INTERACTIONS

Cholesterol-lowering drugs: Bitter melon may potentiate cholesterol-lowering drugs. *Clinical Management:* Caution is advised.

DOSAGE

How Supplied: Fruit juice or concentrate. Concentrated fruit and seed extracts can be found in capsules and tablets, as well as whole herb/vine powders and extracts in capsules and tinctures.

Daily Dose: 1g/day

LITERATURE

Ahmad N, Hassan, MR, Halder H, Bennoor KS. Effect of Momordica charantia (Karolla) extracts on fasting and postprandial serum glucose levels in NIDDM patients. Bangladesh Med Res Counc Bull; 25(1): 11-13. 1999.

Basch E, Gabardi S, Ulbricht C. Bitter melon (Momordica charantia): a review of efficacy and safety. Am J Health Syst Pharm 2003;60(4):356-359.

Chen Q, Chan LL, Li ET. Bitter melon (Momordica charantia) reduces adiposity, lowers serum insulin and normalizes glucose tolerance in rats fed a high fat diet. J Nutr 2003;133(4):1088-1093.

John AJ, Cherian R, Subhash HS, Cherian AM. Evaluation of the efficacy of bitter gourd (Momordica charantia) as an oral hypoglemic agent — a randomized controlled clinical trial. Indian J Physiol Pharmacol; 47(3): 363-365. 2003.

Lee-Huang S, Huang PL, Chen HC, et al. Anti-HIV and anti-tumor activities of recombinant MAP30 from bitter melon. Gene 1995;161(2):151-156.

Lee-Huang S, Huang PL, Huang PL, et al. Inhibition of the integrase of human immunodeficiency virus (HIV) type 1 by anti-

HIV plant proteins MAP30 and GAP31. Proc Natl Acad Sci U S A 1995;92(19):8818-8822.

Lee-Huang S, Huang PL, Sun Y, et al. Inhibition of MDA-MB-231 human breast tumor xenografts and HER2 expression by anti-tumor agents GAP31 and MAP30. Anticancer Res 2000;20(2A):653-659.

Miura T, Itoh C, Iwamoto N, et al. Hypoglycemic activity of the fruit of the Momordica charantia in type 2 diabetic mice. J Nutr Sci Vitaminol (Tokyo) 2001;47(5):340-344.

Pongnikorn S, Fongmoon D, Kasinrerk W, Limtrakul PN. Effect of bitter melon (Momordica charantia Linn) on level and function of natural killer cells in cervical cancer patients with radiotherapy. J Med Assoc Thai. 2003 Jan;86(1):61-8.

Raman A, Lau C. Anti-diabetic properties and phytochemistry of Momordica charantia L. (Cucurbitaceae). Phytomedicine 1996;2(4):349-362.

Rathi SS, Grover JK, Vats V. The effect of Momordica charantia and Mucuna pruriens in experimental diabetes and their effect on key metabolic enzymes involved in carbohydrate metabolism. Phytother Res 2002;16(3):236-243.

Schreiber CA, Wan L, Sun Y, et al. The antiviral agents, MAP30 and GAP31, are not toxic to human spermatozoa and may be useful in preventing the sexual transmission of human immunodeficiency virus type 1. Fertil Steril 1999;72(4):686-690.

Tennekoon KH, Jeevathayaparan S, Angunawala P, et al. Effect of Momordica charantia on key hepatic enzymes. J Ethnopharmacol 1994;44(2):93-97.

Virdi J, Sivakami S, Shahani S, et al. Antihyperglycemic effects of three extracts from Momordica charantia. J Ethnopharmacol 2003;88(1):107-111.

Wang YX, Jacob J, Wingfield PT, et al. Anti-HIV and anti-tumor protein MAP30, a 30 kDa single-strand type-I RIP, shares similar secondary structure and beta-sheet topology with the A chain of ricin, a type-II RIP. Protein Sci 2000;9(1):138-144.

Wang YX, Neamati N, Jacob J, et al. Solution structure of anti-HIV-1 and anti-tumor protein MAP30: structural insights into its multiple functions. Cell 1999;99(4):433-442.

Bitter Milkwort

Polygala amara

DESCRIPTION

Medicinal Parts: The medicinal part is the flowering plant with root.

Flower and Fruit: The blue or occasionally white or pink flowers are in many-blossomed racemes. Of the 5 sepals, the 2 lateral ones are large, petal-like, patent and 3-veined. The other 3 are smaller; the middle vein is green. The 3 petals are fused together with the stamens. These form 2 clusters in 2 green pockets on the larger, lower petal. The 2 upper petals form a kind of upper lip. The ovary is superior and bilocular with a spoonlike style. The fruit is an obcordate capsule, compressed at the sides and enclosed in the sepals.

Leaves, Stem and Root: The plant grows from 5 to 15 cm high. The stems are branched at the base, decumbent, or ascending. The basal leaves form a rosette, while the cauline leaves are alternate, oblong-cuneate or obovate-lanceolate.

Habitat: The plant is indigenous to Europe.

Production: Bitter Milkwort herb, including its roots, is the complete plant of *Polygala amara*.

Other Names: European Bitter Polygala, European Senega Snakeroot, Evergreen Snakeroot, Flowering Wintergreen, Little Pollom

ACTIONS AND PHARMACOLOGY

COMPOUNDS

Saponins (1-2%)

Bitter principles: polygalin (polygamarin)

Phenol glycosides: monotropitoside (methyl salicylic acid-primveroside)

Polygalite (acerite, 1,5-anhydrosorbite)

EFFECTS

The drug is mildly expectorant.

INDICATIONS AND USAGE

Unproven Uses: Bitter Milkwort is used for conditions of the respiratory tract, cough, and bronchitis.

PRECAUTIONS AND ADVERSE REACTIONS

No health hazards or side effects are known in conjunction with the proper administration of designated therapeutic dosages.

DOSAGE

Preparation: The drug is contained in tea for the treatment of bronchitis.

LITERATURE

Hegnauer R, Chemotaxonomie der Pflanzen, Bde 1-11, Birkhäuser Verlag Basel, Boston, Berlin 1962-1997.

Kern W, List PH, Hörhammer L (Hrsg.), Hagers Handbuch der Pharmazeutischen Praxis, 4. Aufl., Bde. 1-8, Springer Verlag Berlin, Heidelberg, New York, 1969.

Madaus G, Lehrbuch der Biologischen Arzneimittel, Bde 1-3, Nachdruck, Georg Olms Verlag Hildesheim 1979.

Bitter Orange

Citrus aurantium

DESCRIPTION

Medicinal Parts: The medicinal parts are the fresh and dried fruit peel, the flowers, the seed,s and the extracted essential oil.

Flower and Fruit: The flowers are arranged singly or in clusters in the axils, and are very fragrant. The calyx is cup-shaped, and the 5 thick fleshy petals are an intense white and revolute. The fruit is about 7.5 cm in diameter (similar in size to a cherry), subglobose, slightly flattened at both ends, and 10- to 12-locular. The peel is thick, rough, and orange when ripe. The fruit pulp is acidic. The core is hollow when ripe.

Leaves, Stem, and Root: Bitter Orange is an evergreen tree with a rounded crown and smooth grayish-brown bark. The branches are angular when young, then become terete and glabrous, with a few stout but flexible axillary spines. The alternate leaves are 7.5 to 10 cm, broadly elliptoid, subacute at the apex, cuneate or rounded below. The upper surface is a shiny dark green and the underside paler. Petioles are broadly winged, tapering to a wingless base.

Habitat: The plant is indigenous to tropical Asia but is widely cultivated in other regions today, such as the Mediterranean.

Production: Bitter Orange flower consists of the dried flowers of *Citrus aurantium*. The oil is obtained by steam distillation of the fresh, fully opened flowers. Bitter Orange peel consists of the dried outer peel of ripe fruits of *Citrus aurantium* separated from the white pulp layer.

Other Names: Orange, Neroli, Bigarade Orange

ACTIONS AND PHARMACOLOGY

COMPOUNDS: BITTER ORANGE FLOWER AND FLOWER OIL

Volatile oil: chief constituents linalool, linalyl acetate, alpha-pinenes, limonene, nerol

Methyl anthranilate

Limonoids: (triterpenoide bitter principles)

Flavonoids

EFFECTS: BITTER ORANGE FLOWER AND FLOWER OIL

No substantiated information available. Efficacy of the use of an extraction of the blossoms as a neurostimulant is not confirmed.

COMPOUNDS: BITTER ORANGE PEEL

Volatile oil: chief constituents (+) -limonene, nerol, geraniol, linalool, linalyl-, neryl-, geranyl- and citronellyl acetate, typical constituent methyl anthranilate

Flavonoids: among them the bitter compounds neohesperidin dyhydrochalcone and naringin as well as the lipophilic compounds sinensetin, nobiletin, tangeretin

Furocoumarins

EFFECTS: BITTER ORANGE PEEL

Bitter Orange has a mild spasmolytic effect on the gastrointestinal tract and increases gastric juice secretion.

INDICATIONS AND USAGE

BITTER ORANGE FLOWER AND FLOWER OIL

Unproven Uses: Preparations of Bitter Orange flower and flower oil are used as a preventive measure for gastric and nervous complaints, gout, sore throat, as a sedative for nervous tension and sleeplessness. Folk medicine uses include chronic bronchitis.

Chinese Medicine: Uses in Chinese medicine include pain in the epigastrum, vomiting, and anorexia.

BITTER ORANGE PEEL

Approved by Commission E:

■ Loss of appetite

■ Dyspeptic complaints

Unproven Uses: Folk medicine uses include loss of appetite and dyspeptic symptoms.

Chinese Medicine: Bitter Orange peel is used for coughs, colds, anorexia, to reduce apathy, and for uterine and anal prolapse.

PRECAUTIONS AND ADVERSE REACTIONS

BITTER ORANGE FLOWER AND FLOWER OIL

No health hazards or side effects are known in conjunction with the proper administration of designated therapeutic dosages.

BITTER ORANGE PEEL

No health hazards or side effects are known in conjunction with the proper administration of designated therapeutic dosages. An elevation of UV-sensitivity is possible with light-skinned individuals due to the phototoxic effect of the furocoumarins. Frequent contact with the drug or with the volatile oil (such as the exposure experienced by workers in the liquor industry) can cause a sensitization that results in erythema, swelling, blisters, pustules, dermatoses leading to scab formation and pigment spots.

DOSAGE

BITTER ORANGE FLOWER AND FLOWER OIL

No reliable dosing information available.

BITTER ORANGE PEEL

Mode of Administration: Cut and coarsely powdered drug for teas, other bitter-tasting galenic preparations for oral application.

How Supplied: Commercial pharmaceutical preparations include drops, tonics and tea mixtures.

Preparation: To prepare a tea, add 1 tsp of drug to 150 ml of hot water, let stand for 10 minutes, then strain.

Daily Dosage:

Drug: 4 to 6 g

Extract: 1 to 2 g

Tea: 1 cup half-hour before meals

Tincture: (1:5) 2 to 3 g

LITERATURE

BITTER ORANGE FLOWER AND OIL

Slater CA, (1961) *J Sci Agric Food* 12:732.

Stanley WL, Jurd L, (1971) *J Agric Food Chem* 19:1106.

Tatum JH, Berry RE, (1977) *Phytochemistry* 16:109.

BITTER ORANGE PEEL

Clavarano I, *Essenze Deriv. Agrum* 36:5. 1966.

Horowitz RM, Gentili B, *Tetrahedron* 19:773. 1963.

Morimoto I, Watanabe F, Osawa T, Okitsu T, Kada T. Mutagenicity screening of crude drugs with *Bacillus subtilus* rec-assay and Salmonella/microsome reversion assay. *Mutation Res.* 97:81-102. 1982

Slater CA, (1961) *J Sci Agric Food* 12:732.

Stanley WL, Jurd L, (1971) *J Agric Food Chem* 19:1106.

Tatum JH, Berry RE, (1977) *Phytochemistry* 16, 109.

Bittersweet Nightshade

Solanum dulcamara

DESCRIPTION

Medicinal Parts: The medicinal part is the stem of the plant.

Flower and Fruit: The violet flowers are arranged in 10 to 20 blossomed, hanging, long-peduncled, paniclelike forms. The calyx is fused, 5-tipped and does not drop. The corolla has a very short tube and 5 long tips, which become revolute when mature. At the base of each tip, there are 2 green spots surrounded by white. There are 5 stamens with golden yellow anthers, which lean toward each other, and 1 superior ovary. The fruit is an oblong, scarlet, and many-seeded berry.

Leaves, Stem, and Root: The plant is a subshrub from 30 to 150 cm in height with a creeping, branched rhizome. The stem is twining or creeping, woody below, angular and usually glabrous. The leaves are petiolate, the upper and lower ones are usually cordate and acute. The middle leaves are usually pinnatesect with one pair of lateral segments and a large terminal segment.

Habitat: The plant is common in Europe, northern Africa, eastern and western Asia, and North America.

Production: Bittersweet Nightshade consists of the dried, 2- to 3-year-old stems of *Solanum dulcamara* harvested in spring prior to leafing, or late autumn after the leaves have dropped.

Other Names: Bittersweet, Dulcamara, Felonwort, Felonwood, Felonwort, Scarlet Berry, Violet Bloom, Blue Nightshade, Fever Twig, Nightshade, Woody, Staff Vine, Climbing Nightshade

ACTIONS AND PHARMACOLOGY

COMPOUNDS

Steroid alkaloid glycosides: (0.07 to 0.4%) the alkaloid spectrum varies widely with the variety

Tomatidenol variety–alpha-solamarine, beta-solamarine

Soladulcidine variety–soladulcidinetetraoside

Solasodine variety–solasonine, solamargine

Steroid saponins

Mixed varieties also occur.

EFFECTS

The main active principles are the steroid alkaloid glycosides whose resorption is probably promoted by the saponins. They stimulate phagocytosis, are hemolytic, cytotoxic, antiviral, anticholinergic and have local anaesthetic properties.

Solasodin has a cortisonelike effect. A desensitizing and cardiotonic effect has been observed in clinical trials with patients suffering from rheumatic polyarthritis.

Its use as an expectorant may be due to the saponin content.

INDICATIONS AND USAGE

Approved by Commission E:

- Eczema
- Furuncles
- Acne
- Warts

Unproven Uses: In folk medicine, Bittersweet Nightshade is used internally for nose bleeds, rheumatic conditions, asthma, and bronchitis, and to stimulate the immune system; externally for herpes, eczema, abscesses, and contusions.

Homeopathic Uses: Solanum dulcamara is used for inflammation of the respiratory and gastrointestinal tracts, the joints and skin, and for febrile infections. Efficacy has not been proved.

CONTRAINDICATIONS

Bittersweet Nightshade is contraindicated in pregnancy and nursing mothers.

PRECAUTIONS AND ADVERSE REACTIONS

Health risks or side effects following the proper administration of designated therapeutic dosages are not recorded. Toxic effects should not be seen in dosages under approximately 25 gm due to the low alkaloid content of the stem.

OVERDOSAGE

The unripe berries have caused poisonings among children. More than 10 berries cause nausea, vomiting, dilated pupils, and diarrhea. Lethal dosage is estimated to be 200 berries.

DOSAGE

Mode of Administration: Comminuted herb is used in teas and other galenic preparations for internal use. The drug is also used externally in compresses and rinses.

Preparation: A decoction is prepared by adding 1 to 2 g of drug to 250 mL water.

Daily Dosage: The average daily internal dose is 1 to 3 gm of the drug. Externally, the herb is used as infusions or decoctions that have strengths equivalent to 1 to 2 gm of the drug per 250 mL of water.

Homeopathic Dosage: 5 drops, 1 tablet, or 10 globules every 30 to 60 minutes (acute) or 1 to 3 times a day (chronic); parenterally: 1 to 2 mL, sc, acute: 3 times daily; chronic: once a day (HAB1)

LITERATURE

Frohne D, (1992) *Solanum dulcamara L.* - Der Bittersüße Nachtschatten. Portrait einer Arzneipflanze. Z Phytother 14: 337-342.

Hölzer I, (1992) Dulcamara-Extrakt bei Neurodermitis und chronischem Ekzem. Ergebnisse einer klinischen Prüfung. *Jatros Dermatologie* 6: 32-36.

JNP 56(3):430-431. 1993.

Kumar P, Dixit VP, Khanna P. Antifertility studies of kaempferol: Isolation and identification from tissue culture of some medicinally important plant species. *Plant Med et Phyt.* 23:193-201. 1989

Kupchan SM et al., (1965) Science 150:1827.

Lee YY, Hashimoto F, Yahara S, Nohara T, Yoshida N. Steroidal glycosides from *Solanum dulcamara. Chem Pharm Bull.* 42:707-709. 1994.

Rönsch H, Schreiber K, Stubbe H, Naturwissenschaften 55:182. 1968.

Schopke T, Bartlakowski J, Hiller K. Critical micellar concentrations of a number of triterpenoid saponins of different structure types. *Pharmazie* 50(11): 771. 1995.

Willaman JJ, Hui-Li L, (1970) *Lloydia* 33 (3A):1.

Willuhn G, Kothe U, (1983) *Arch Pharm* 316(8):678-687.

Willuhn G, Phytopharmaka in der Dermatologie. In: *ZPT* 16(6):325-342. 1995.

Wolters B, Antibiotische Wirkung von *Solanum dulcamara.* In: Naturwissenschaften 51:111. 1964.

Wolters B, Der Anteil der Steroidsaponine an der antibiotischen Wirkung von Solanum dulcamara. In: PM 13:2. 1965.

Wolters B, (1965) *Planta Med* 13:189.

Black Alder

Alnus glutinosa

DESCRIPTION

Medicinal Parts: The medicinal parts of the plant are the bark and leaves.

Flower and Fruit: Black Alder is monoecious. Male flowers are arranged in stemmed catkins. Female flowers form ovoid fruit, which turns woody and remains on the tree the whole year.

Leaves, Stem, and Root: The plants grow as a shrub or tree extending up to 25 m high. Black Alder has gray branches and orange-colored wood. The obovate leaves have double-serrate margins; the young leaves are very sticky.

Habitat: Black Alder originated in the damp regions of Europe, Asia, and North America. The plant now grows in much of the Northern Hemisphere.

Production: Black (English) Alder bark is the bark and branch rind of *Alnus glutinosa*. It is gathered from the shrubs or trees growing wild.

Other Names: Common Alder, Owler, Tag Alder

ACTIONS AND PHARMACOLOGY

COMPOUNDS

Tannins

Flavonoids: in particular hypericin

Steroids: beta-sitosterol

Triterpenes: especially alpha-amyrenone, lupenone, taraxerol, glutenone

EFFECTS

The decoction is a tonic and has astringent and hemostatic properties, which may be due to the tannins (20%), flavone glycosides, and triterpenes.

INDICATIONS AND USAGE

Unproven Uses: Black Alder is used as a decoction for gargles in the treatment of streptococcal sore throat and pharyngitis, and for intestinal bleeding. The bark is considered to be effective for intermittent fever.

PRECAUTIONS AND ADVERSE REACTIONS

No health hazards or side effects are known in conjunction with the proper administration of designated therapeutic dosages.

DOSAGE

Mode of Administration: Leaves and bark are prepared as infusions and decoctions for internal and local use. Mention is made of an ophthalmic powder.

Preparations: The bark is prepared as a decoction.

LITERATURE

Freudenberg K, Weinges K. *Tetrahedron Letters* 17: 19. 1967

Hänsel R, Keller K, Rimpler H, Schneider G (Hrsg.), Hagers Handbuch der Pharmazeutischen Praxis, 5. Aufl., Bde 4-6 (Drogen), Springer Verlag Berlin, Heidelberg, New York, 1992-1994.

Hoppe, HA. Drogenkunde, 8. Aufl., Bde 1-3, W. de Gruyter Verlag, Berlin, New York. 1975-1987

Black Bryony

Tamus communis

DESCRIPTION

Medicinal Parts: The medicinal part is the root.

Flower and Fruit: The flowers are small greenish-white and in loose clusters. They consist of 6 petals and are found on various plants in fertile and infertile form. The fertile flowers develop into crimson berries.

Leaves, Stem, and Root: Tamus communis is a glabrous climber. The stem dies back in winter but the root is perennial. The leaves are cordate, smooth, acute, and glossy. The root is almost cylindrical with a diameter of 2 to 3 cm. The root is 6 to 8 cm long and has scattered, thin root fibers. Externally, the root is blackish-brown. Internally, it is whitish and produces a slimy paste when it is peeled.

Characteristics: The taste of the root is acrid and the odor is slightly earthy.

Habitat: The plant is indigenous to parts of Europe.

Production: Black Bryony root is the root of *Tamus communis*. The roots are gathered at the end of the vegetation period. They are dug up and the bark is peeled off and cut into slices or pieces. During this procedure, gloves should be worn to protect the hands, as the fresh roots cause serious reddening of the skin.

Other Names: Blackeye Root

ACTIONS AND PHARMACOLOGY

COMPOUNDS

Histamine-oxalate: in the form of skin- and mucous membrane-irritating needles

Mucilages (2.5-5%)

Volatile oil (1%)

Phenanthrene derivatives

Steroid saponins, aglycone diosgenin

EFFECTS

Black Bryony stimulates the external nerve ends. A substance similar to histamine increases blood circulation in areas of the skin to which it is applied.

INDICATIONS AND USAGE

Unproven Uses: The herb stimulates and reddens the skin. It is used for bruises, strains, torn muscles, gout and other rheumatic disorders. Black Bryony is also used for irritation of the intestine mucous membrane and as an emetic. It is also used as a tonic for hair loss, as it improves blood circulation to the scalp.

PRECAUTIONS AND ADVERSE REACTIONS

Skin contact with the fresh plant leads to the formation of rashes, swelling, pustules, and wheals, due to the skin- and mucous membrane-irritating oxalate needles and histamine. Internal administration triggers signs of severe irritation in the mouth, pharyngeal space, and gastrointestinal tract, combined with vomiting and intense diarrhea. Extracts from the plant are toxicologically harmless. Skin lesions are treated with cortisone foam and sterile coverings; tetanus prophylaxis might be required. If taken by mouth, following gastric lavage with burgundy-colored potassium permanganate solution and administration of activated charcoal, treat spasms with diazepam (IV) and colic with atropine. Monitoring of kidney function is essential. Intubation and oxygen respiration may also be necessary.

DOSAGE

Mode of Administration: The ground root is applied externally as a lotion.

LITERATURE

Aquino R, Conti C, DiSimone F, Orsi N, Pizza C, Stein ML. Antiviral activity of constituents of *Tammis communis. J Chemother*. 3:305-309. 1991

Aquino R et al., (1985) *J Nat Prod* 48(5):811.

Barbakadze V, Usov AI, Isolation and characterisation of glucans from roots of *Tamus communis L.* In: *PM* 62, Abstracts of the 44th Ann Congress of GA, 127. 1996.

Frohne D, Pfänder HJ, Giftpflanzen - Ein Handbuch für Apotheker, Toxikologen und Biologen, 4. Aufl., Wiss. Verlags-Ges. Stuttgart 1997.

Ireland CR et al., (1981) *Phytochemistry* 20:1569.

Kern W, List PH, Hörhammer L (Hrsg.), Hagers Handbuch der Pharmazeutischen Praxis, 4. Aufl., Bde. 1-8: Springer Verlag Berlin, Heidelberg, New York, 1969.

Lewin L, Gifte und Vergiftungen, 6. Aufl., Nachdruck, Haug Verlag, Heidelberg 1992.

Roth L, Daunderer M, Kormann K, Giftpflanzen, Pflanzengifte, 4. Aufl., Ecomed Fachverlag Landsberg Lech 1993.

Teuscher E, Lindequist U, Biogene Gifte - Biologie, Chemie, Pharmakologie, 2. Aufl., Fischer Verlag Stuttgart 1994.

Black Catnip

Phyllanthus amarus

DESCRIPTION

Medicinal Parts: The whole, dried herb is the medicinal part.

Flower and Fruit: The flowers are axillary. The male flower has 5, 0.5 mm long, acute, pale-green sepals with a white margin. There are 3 stamens with the filaments forming a 0.2 mm high column. The female flowers have an apically thickened pedicle and 5 ovate-elongate, up to 1 mm long, yellowish-green sepals. The ovary is 0.3 mm in diameter and 3-chambered. The fruit is ochre to olive with 3 pressed lobes, 2 mm in diameter and 1 mm long.

Leaves and Stem: Black catnip is a monoecious, occasionally dioecious, upright or ascending herb, which grows up to 60 cm high, or occasionally higher. The bracts and stipules are linear-lanceolate, 1 mm long, cream with a brownish middle rib. The stem is round, greenish or reddish, glabrous and woody at the base.

Habitat: Africa, Asia and America.

Production: Black catnip herb is the aerial part of *Phyllanthus amarus*. The harvested herb is dried.

Not to be Confused With: May be confused with *Phyllanthus urinaria, P niruri, P debilis* and *P fraternus*.

ACTIONS AND PHARMACOLOGY

COMPOUNDS

Tannins: gallotannins, including amarine, phyllanthusin D, geraniine, corilagin, elaecarpusin

Flavonoids: including rutin, quercetin-3-O-glucoside

Lignans: phyllantin (0.8%, extremely bitter), hypophyllanthin

EFFECTS

The drug, which contains tannins and lignans, is antiviral and antimicrobial in effect.

INDICATIONS AND USAGE

Unproven Uses: The herb is used for fever (Cuba, Nigeria), for malaria (Cuba, Bahamas), diarrhea, tachycardia and female sterility (Congo), constipation with spasms and colic, as a diuretic (Nigeria) and for diabetes (Dominican Republic).

Indian Medicine: Black catnip is used for stomach conditions, ascites, jaundice, diarrhea, dysentery, intermittent fever, conditions of the urogenital tract, eye disease, scabies, ulcers, and wounds.

PRECAUTIONS AND ADVERSE REACTIONS

No health hazards are known in conjunction with the proper administration of designated therapeutic dosages.

DOSAGE

Mode of Administration: Whole herb preparations for internal and external use.

Preparation: Decoction: 10 plants to 1 liter of water

Daily Dosage: No exact doses are known.

LITERATURE

Blaschek W, Hänsel R, Keller K, Reichling J, Rimpler G, Schneider G (Eds), Hagers Handbuch der Pharmazeutischen Praxis. Folgebände 1 und 2. Drogen A-Z. Springer. Berlin, Heidelberg 1998.

Blumberg BS, Millman I, Venkateswaran PS, Thyagarajan SP, Hepatitis B virus and hepatocellular carcinoma - treatment of HBV carriers with Phyllanthus amarus. Cancer Detect Prev, 14:195-201, 1989.

Blumberg BS, Millman I, Venkateswaran PS, Thyagarajan SP, Hepatitis B virus and primary hepatocellular carcinoma: treatment of HBV carriers with Phyllanthus amarus. Vaccine, 8 Suppl: 86-92, 1990 Mar.

Bratati Datta PC. Pharmacognostic evaluation of *Phyllanthus amarus. Int J Crude Drug Res.* 29(2):81-88. 1991

Lee CD, Ott M, Thyagarajan SP, Shafritz DA, Burk RD, Gupta S, Phyllanthus amarus down-regulates hepatitis B virus mRNA transcription and replication. Eur J Clin Invest, 26:1069-76, 1996 Dec.

Leelarasamee A, Trakulsomboon S, Maunwongyathi P, Somanabandhu A, Pidetcha P, Matrakool B, Lebnak T, Ridthimat W, Chandanayingyong D, Failure of Phyllanthus amarus to eradicate hepatitis B surface antigen from symptomless carriers. Lancet, 2:1600-1, 1990 Jun 30.

Niu JZ, Wang YY, Qiao M, Gowans E, Edwards P, Thyagarajan SP, Gust I, Locarnini S, Effect of Phyllanthus amarus on duck hepatitis B virus replication in vivo. J Med Virol, 32:212-8, 1990 Dec.

Ott M, Thyagarajan SP, Gupta S, Phyllanthus amarus suppresses hepatitis B virus by interrupting interactions between HBV enhancer I and cellular transcription factors. Eur J Clin Invest, 27:908-15, 1997 Nov.

Srividya N, Periwal S, Diuretic, hypotensive and hypoglycaemic effect of Phyllanthus amarus. Indian J Exp Biol, 74:861-4, 1995 Nov.

Thamlikitkul V, Wasuwat S, Kanchanapee P, Efficacy of Phyllanthus amarus for eradication of hepatitis B virus in chronic carriers. J Med Assoc Thai, 74:381-5, 1991 Sep.

Thyagarajan SP, Jayaram S, Valliammai T, Madanagopalan N, Pal VG, Jayaraman K, Phyllanthus amarus and hepatitis B. Lancet, 2:949-50, 1990 Oct 13.

Thyagarajan SP, Subramanian S, Thirunalasundari T, Venkateswaran PS, Blumberg BS, Beneficial effects of Phyllanthus amarus for chronic hepatitis B. J Hepatol, 2:405-6, 1991 May.

Thyagarajan SP, Subramanian S, Thirunalasundari T, Venkateswaran PS, Blumberg BS, Effect of Phyllanthus amarus on chronic carriers of hepatitis B virus. Lancet, 2:764-6, 1988 Oct 1.

Thyagarajan SP, Subramanian S, Thirunalasundari T, Venkateswaran PS, Blumberg BS, In vitro effect of Phyllanthus amarus on hepatitis B virus. Indian J Med Res, 2:71-3, 1991 Mar.

Black Cohosh

Cimicifuga racemosa

DESCRIPTION

Medicinal Parts: The medicinal part is the fresh and dried root.

Flower and Fruit: The inflorescence is a long-peduncled, drooping raceme, 30 to 90 cm long with white flowers. There are 3 to 8 petals without nectaries, and the sepals enclose the flower bud.

Leaves, Stem, and Root: The plant grows 1 to 1.5 m high. It is leafy, with a sturdy, blackish rhizome, which is cylindrical, tough, and knotty. The straight, grooved, dark-brown roots sprout from the underground rhizome and are roughly quadrangular. The transverse root section shows wedge-shaped bundles of white wood. The rhizome section shows a large black medulla surrounded by a ring of paler, woodier wedges. The leaves are double-pinnate, smooth, and crenate-serrate.

Habitat: Black Cohosh is native to Canada and the U.S.; it is cultivated in Europe.

Production: The medicinally used part of the plant consists of the dried rhizome of *Cimicifuga racemosa* with attached roots.

Other Names: Black Snake Root, Bugbane, Bugwort, Cimicifuga, Rattleroot, Rattleweed, Richweed, Squaw Root

ACTIONS AND PHARMACOLOGY

COMPOUNDS

Triterpenes: triterpene glycoside, including actein, 27-deoxyactein, cimifugoside

Quinolizidine alkaloids: cytisine, methyl cytisine

Phenylpropane derivatives: including isoferulic acid

EFFECTS

The active ingredients in the root are the triterpine glycosides such as cimifugaside, 27-deoxyactein, and actein. The increase in luteinizing hormone (LH) that occurs as estrogen levels decrease is implicated as the cause of menopausal symptoms. Compounds of the rootstock of *Cimicifuga racemosa* bind to the estrogen receptor where it selectively suppresses LH secretion with no effect on FSH. The result is an estrogenic effect, which will decrease climacteric symptoms such as hot flashes, diaphoresis and psychological disturbances (Duker, 1991, Lehmann-Wilenbrock, 1988). The improvement in premenstrual symptoms, dysmenorrheal, and menopause may be due to the relaxing of uterine tissue (Tyler, 1997).

There have been some conflicting reports stating *Cimicifuga racemosa* has no estrogenlike action (Einer-Jensen, 1996; Liske, 1998). The herb did not appear to have an effect on levels of LH, FSH, sex hormone-binding globulin (SHBG), prolactin, and estradiol in a study that concluded the therapeutic effects seen are not attributable to estrogenic or other endocrine-system effects (Liske, 1998).

Other reported effects in animal trials include analgesic, antidepressant, and anti-inflammatory activities.

Analgesic Effects: Methanol extract of Cimicifuga rhizome demonstrated significant anti-nociceptive activity in rats (Kim & Kim, 2000).

Antidepressant Effects: An extract of Black Cohosh exhibited antidepressant activity when administered to female mice. Tail suspension test (TST) was used as a screening test for antidepressant activity in this study. Black cohosh extract significantly reduced the period of immobility, a result comparable to that of imipramine, another antidepressant drug (Winterhoff et al, 2003).

Anti-Inflammatory Effects: Methanol extract of *Cimicifuga* rhizome demonstrated significant anti-inflammatory activity in rats (Kim & Kim, 2000). Virus-infected mice were found to have lowered interleukin-8 levels and reduced numbers of exuded neutrophils (obtained by bronchoalveolar lavage) after treatment with ferulic acid, isoferulic acid, or a *Cimicifuga* extract, as compared to the control group (Hirabayashi et al, 1995).

Hormonal Effects: In vitro data suggest that black cohosh has antagonistic effects on estrogen receptor-positive human breast cancer cells and it may act as a selective estrogen receptor modulator (SERM) (Bodinet & Freudenstein, 2002). An in vitro assay demonstrated antiestrogenic activity from the rhizome of *Cimicifuga racemosa*. It antagonized estradiol-induced activities in an experimental model (Zierau et al, 2002). At high concentrations, *Cimicifuga racemosa* inhibited the proliferation of human breast adenocarcinoma cells (MCF-7). In addition, estrogen-induced proliferation of MCF-7 was reduced in the presence of *Cimicifuga racemosa* extract, an effect that was reversible with increased concentrations of estradiol. Another in vitro study failed to demonstrate any significant binding to estrogen or progesterone receptors as well as estrogenic effect of Black Cohosh (Zava et al, 1998).

Extract of *Cimicifuga racemosa* in doses up to 100-fold the human therapeutic dose did not exert estrogenic activity in rats with experimentally induced, hormone-responsive mammary tumors. The *Cimicifuga racemosa* extract did not have a direct effect on uterine tissue proliferation or an indirect effect on pituitary-secreted, estrogen-regulated hormones (Freudenstein et al, 2002). Black Cohosh extract did not promote the growth of an estrogen-dependent breast cancer cell line (MCF-7) in animal cells. Black cohosh did not significantly transactivate through human estrogen receptor (hER)-alpha or hER-beta (Amato et al, 2002).

An extract of *Cimicifuga racemosa* (CR) exhibited an estrogen-antagonistic effect on estrogen receptor-positive breast cancer cells. At high concentrations, CR inhibited the proliferation of human breast adenocarcinoma cells (MCF-7). In addition, estrogen-induced proliferation of MCF-7 was reduced in the presence of CR-extract, an effect that was reversible with increased concentrations of estradiol. Results from additional studies suggested that CR-extract may act as a selective estrogen receptor modulator (SERM) (Bodinet & Freudenstein, 2002).

CLINICAL TRIALS

Cancer

In a pharmaco-epidemiologic, observational, retrospective cohort study, it was shown that women treated with an isopropanolic black cohosh extract were no more likely than women not treated with the herb to experience an increased risk of breast cancer recurrence. The study showed that treatment with black cohosh was associated with prolonged disease-free survival (Zepelin et al, 2007).

The effects of the isopropanolic extract of black cohosh on mammographic breast density and breast epithelial proliferation was evaluated in a prospective, open, uncontrolled drug safety study of healthy postmenopausal women with climacteric symptoms. During the 6- month treatment, no adverse effects on breast tissue were caused by black cohosh extracts and no endometrial or general safety concerns were detected (Hirschberg et al, 2007).

Four hundred postmenopausal women with symptoms related to estrogen deficiency were enrolled in a prospective, open-label, multinational, multicenter study. For one year, participants received a daily special black cohosh extract corresponding to 40 mg of herbal drug. Endometrial safety was determined by assessment of endometrial biopsy samples. After one year, no endometrial proliferation could be found. An improvement of climacteric complaints as well as only few gynecologic organ-related adverse events were reported (Raus et al, 2006).

Menopausal Symptoms

A rigorous, systematic review of placebo-controlled randomized clinical trials of Black Cohosh and other nonhormonal therapies for menopausal symptoms indicated that, while the herb has been studied in numerous trials, the quality of the trials vary widely and results are mixed (Tice, 2007).

Most randomized, placebo-controlled trials of Black Cohosh for relief of menopausal symptoms have been relatively short in duration (12 weeks or less) and somewhat small in terms of participants. In contrast, the Herbal Alternatives for Menopause Trial (HALT), the results of which were published in the *Annals of Internal Medicine* in 2006, was a comparatively large and lengthy trial. It found that Black Cohosh has little potential as a therapy for relieving menopausal hot flushes or night sweats, neither reducing their frequency or severity—whether used alone or as part of a blend. The 12-month, randomized, and double-blind, placebo-controlled trial involved 351 women who reported two or more hot flashes daily. The participants were randomly assigned to one of three herbal regimens: Black Cohosh 160 mg daily, a multi-botanical preparation containing 200 mg of Black Cohosh plus 9 other ingredients, or multi-botanicals plus increased intake of foods containing soy. Other women were randomized to hormone therapy (estrogen with or without progesterone), or placebo. Neither Black Cohosh nor the other herbal regimens provided any clinically meaningful relief of hot flushes. At 3, 6, and 12 months, participants taking the botanical treatments experienced the same change in hot flushes as those taking the placebo. Those taking estrogen, however, had substantially decreased vasomotor symptoms. The study involved too few people to catch possible small changes in the frequency of hot flashes (fewer than 1.5 per day) (Nelson, 2006).

Similar results for the efficacy of black cohosh for the treatment of hot flashes were obtained in a double-blind, randomized, crossover trial of 132 women. The mean decrease in hot flash score and hot flash frequency was not significantly different between the black cohosh group and placebo. The study failed to provide evidence that black cohosh reduced hot flashes more than placebo (Pockaj et al, 2006).

A review of treatments for menopausal symptoms published in *The Lancet* in 2005 cites evidence that overall, results of randomized controlled trials do not suggest that Black Cohosh is useful for hot flashes, although there are exceptions. A high-dose of Black Cohosh in women with breast cancer and taking tamoxifen did reduce the number of hot flashes significantly more than those not taking Black Cohosh, for example (Hickey 2005).

Similarly, a discussion on managing menopausal symptoms published in the *New England Journal of Medicine* in 2006 identified mixed but primarily negative evidence for the effectiveness of Black Cohosh in regard to its ability to improve the frequency or severity of menopausal hot flashes. The author points out that Black Cohosh could possibly bind estrogen receptors and pose the same risk for adverse outcomes that estrogen poses; studies have not been of size or duration to fully document the safety of Black Cohosh (Grady, 2006).

A 2006 update in *Alternative & Complementary Therapies* notes that while several studies in 2005 and 2006 provide new information on Black Cohosh, two indicated positive effects on menopausal symptoms, while one had mixed results and one indicated no effect at all (Hudson, 2006).

A positive finding for Black Cohosh was reported in a 2006 trial in which the herb was combined with St. John's wort (*Hypericum perforatum*) in 301 women with menopausal complaints that included a psychological component. The 16-week, double-blind and randomized trial found the combination to be superior to placebo in alleviating the symptoms and the related depression as well, with the Menopause Rating Scale score decreasing 50% in those randomized to the combination treatment as compared to 19.6% of those taking placebo, and the Hamilton Depression Rating Scale decreasing 41.8% versus12.7%, respectively. Each treatment combination tablet contained Black Cohosh extract standardized to 1 mg trierpene glycosides and St. John's Wort extract standardized to 0.25 mg total hypericine; the participants randomized to this group started with a double dose (2x2 tablets per day) for the first 8 weeks of treatment followed by 2x1 tablets per day for the second study phase (Uebelhack, 2006).

Positive results were also demonstrated in a multicenter, randomized, placebo-controlled, double-blind, parallel-group study which investigated the efficacy and safety of the black cohosh root extract Cr 99 in 122 menopausal women with climacteric complaints. The 12-week study demonstrated a superiority of the *Cimicifuga racemosa* extract compared to placebo in the subgroup of patients with menopausal disorders of at least moderate intensity according to a Kupperman Index of 20 or greater, but not in the intention-to-treat population (Frei-Kleiner et al, 2005).

In a post-marketing surveillance study, 2,016 women (40-65 y) with a Kupperman Index of 20 were treated with an isopropanol extract of *Cimicifuga racemosa*. Changes of subjective symptoms of menopause were evaluated at the start and at the end of 4, 8, and 12 weeks of treatment. Based on weighted symptom scores, hot flashes, sweating, insomnia, and anxiety decreased significantly. Kupperman Index decreased, on average, 17.64 points (P(.001). Thus, the extract was found to be effective in the alleviation of menopausal symptoms (Vermes et al, 2005).

To investigate the efficacy of an isopropanolic aqueous extract of *Cimicifuga racemosa* on climacteric complaints in comparison with low-dose transdermal estradiol, 64 postmenopausal women were chosen to take part in a 3-month, randomized clinical trial. It was found that Cimicifuga racemosa may be a valid alternative to low-dose estradiol in the management of climacteric complaints, especially in those women who refuse or who cannot be treated with conventional medication (Nappi et al, 2005).

A placebo-controlled, open study was conducted to determine the effects of commercially available *Cimicifuga racemosa* extract (Remifemin) on LH and FSH secretion in 110 menopausal women. After 2 months of therapy with 8 mg daily of the drug, FSH levels in the Remifemin treatment group and placebo group were similar. LH secretion was significantly reduced in the Remifemin treatment group, which points to the estrogenic effect of *Cimicifuga racemosa* preparations (Duker, 1991).

There was no difference in the reduction of menopausal symptoms between a standard dose of 39 mg/day Remifemin and a high dose of 127.3 mg/day of Black Cohosh extract administered to perimenopausal and postmenopausal women in a 12-week randomized, double-blind, parallel group study. Neither dose exerted estrogenlike effects to the uterus. At 12-weeks the percentage of patients with a favorable therapeutic response (Kupperman Menopause Index score of less than 15) was 70% and 72% for the standard-dose and high dose groups, respectively (Liske et al, 2002).

Neither conjugated estrogens nor Black Cohosh were different from placebo in reducing menopausal symptoms in a 12-week this double-blind, randomized, placebo-controlled multicenter study; however, Black Cohosh lacked the undesired effects to the uterus seen with conjugated estrogens (Wuttke et al, 2003).

In an open-label study, 60 hysterectomized patients under 40 years of age with at least one intact ovary were involved in a study to determine the effect of *Cimicifuga racemosa* extract (Remifemen 8 mg), estriol (1 mg), conjugated estrogens (1.25 mg), and an estrogen-gestagen product on menopausal symptoms. *Cimicifuga racemosa* was as effective as the estrogen products in decreasing menopausal symptoms in young patients who have undergone a hysterectomy (Lehmann-Willenbrock, 1988).

Eighty percent of women experiencing menopausal symptoms improved or resolved in a multicenter study of 629 patients (mean age 51 years) who were treated with Black Cohosh. Patients tolerated the black cohosh well with mild gastrointestinal complaints recorded in 7% of the patients studied. (Stolze, 1982).

Menopausal Symptoms: Breast Cancer Survivors

A significant reduction in frequency and severity of hot flushes in premenopausal breast cancer survivors was observed following a 12-month treatment with Black Cohosh. Severe hot flushes included 5 or more daily episodes of heat, accompanied by sweating, sleep disturbances, irritation, and anxiety. At the end of the 12-month study, 46.7% of participants in the Black Cohosh group were free of hot flushes compared with none in the control group; 24.4% still suffered from severe symptoms compared with the control group (73.9%), and 28.9% experienced moderate symptoms compared to 26.1% in the control group (Munoz & Pluchino, 2003).

Black Cohosh was assessed in a randomized, double-blind, placebo-controlled trial involving 85 women with a history of breast cancer. Both treatment and placebo groups reported decreases in the number and intensity of hot flushes, compared with baseline values. There were no statistically significant differences between the two groups, and a subgroup analysis of tamoxifen users and nonusers did not reveal any statistically significant differences (Jacobson, 2001).

Osteoporosis

Positive effects on bone metabolism were observed in postmenopausal women following a 12-week treatment with Black Cohosh extract. Black Cohosh increased the levels of bone-specific alkaline phosphatase at week 12 (p=0.0358), which is a metabolic marker for bone formation, while the same marker remained unchanged in those received either conjugated estrogen and placebo. Black Cohosh and placebo appeared to increase osteoblast activity. Both Black Cohosh and conjugated estrogen increased serum triglycerides. No other serious adverse reactions were reported (Wuttke et al, 2003).

INDICATIONS AND USAGE

Approved by Commission E:

- Climacteric complaints
- Premenstrual syndrome (PMS)

Unproven Uses: In folk medicine, the plant is used for rheumatism, sore throats, and bronchitis. The tincture is also used as a sedative, for choreic states (involuntary, rapid motions), fever, lumbago, and snakebite. The herb is also available commercially in combination with St. John's Wort for depressive moods associated with premenstrual and menopausal symptoms.

Chinese Medicine: The Chinese have used Black Cohosh for the above indications as well as for measles in the pre-exanthem stage.

CONTRAINDICATIONS

Pregnancy: The use of Black Cohosh is contraindicated during pregnancy due to an increased risk of spontaneous abortion.

Breastfeeding: Not to be used during breastfeeding.

PRECAUTIONS AND ADVERSE REACTIONS

Cimicifuga racemosa should not be substituted for hormone replacement therapy with estrogen. There is no information to date that the herb contains cardioprotective effects or protective effects against osteoporosis.

Safety beyond use for 6 months is not yet determined (Hickey, 2005). Although no serious health hazards were reported in conjunction with the proper administration of designated therapeutic dosages, there are adverse events associated with the use of Black Cohosh, including gastroenteritis, nausea, and vomiting. A case of muscle damage was linked to the use of Black Cohosh in one individual (Minciullo, 2006).

DRUG INTERACTIONS

MAJOR RISK

Azathioprine: Concurrent use may result in reduced immunosuppressive drug effectiveness and acute transplant rejection. *Clinical management*: Black cohosh should not be used concurrently with azathioprine. Advise patients taking azathioprine for transplant maintenance to avoid black cohosh, including herbal teas and combination supplement products containing black cohosh. If patients are found to be taking black cohosh and azathioprine, discontinue black cohosh and evaluate the patient for signs and symptoms of transplant rejection.

Cyclosporine: Concurrent use may result in reduced immunosuppressive drug effectiveness and acute transplant rejection. *Clinical management:* Black cohosh should not be used concurrently with cyclosporine. Advise patients taking cyclosporine for transplant maintenance to avoid black cohosh, including herbal teas and combination supplement products containing black cohosh. If patients are found to be taking black cohosh and cyclosporine, discontinue black cohosh and evaluate the patient for signs and symptoms of transplant rejection.

POTENTIAL INTERACTIONS

Antihypertensives: Black Cohosh can potentiate the effect of antihypertensive medications. *Clinical Management:* Avoid concomitant use.

Tamoxifen: Cimicifuga racemosa extract may enhance effects of tamoxifen. Under estrogen-deprived conditions, dilutions of CR-extract significantly inhibited human breast adenocarcinoma (MCF-7) cells in vitro. This had an additive effect when combined with tamoxifen (Bodinet & Freudenstein, 2002).

Iron-Containing Products: The tannin content of black cohosh may complex with concomitantly administered iron, resulting in nonabsorbable insoluble complexes.*Clinical Management:* Patients who need iron supplementation should be advised to separate administration times of these two compounds by a minimum of 2 hours.

OVERDOSAGE

An intake of very high dosages of the drug (5 g) or an extract (12 g) leads to vomiting, headache, dizziness, limb pain, and hypotension.

DOSAGE

Mode of Administration: Galenic preparations for internal use.

How Supplied:

Capsules - 60 mg, 80 mg, 450 mg, 540 mg, 545 mg

Drops

Solutions

Tablets - 60 mg, 120 mg

Daily Dosage: Alcoholic-aqueous extracts (ethanolic-aqueous 40-60% (V/V) or isopropanolic-aqueous 40% (V/V)) corresponding to 40 mg drug. The herb is not recommended for treatment longer than 6 months unless advised by a physician.

Menopause symptoms: 40 to 200 mg daily (powdered rhizome); 0.4 to 2 mL daily (tincture, 1:10 in 60% alcohol).

Hot flushes due to tamoxifen therapy: 20 mg-tablet twice daily.

LITERATURE

Amato P, Christophe S & Mellon PL. Estrogenic activity of herbs commonly used as remedies for menopausal symptoms. *Menopause*; 9(2):145-150. 2002

Bodinet C & Freudenstein J. Influence of *Cimicifuga racemosa* on the proliferation of estrogen receptor-positive human breast cancer cells. *Breast Cancer Res Treat*; 76(1):1-10. 2002

Düker EM, Kopanski L, Jarry H, Wuttke W. Effects of extracts from *cimicifuga racemosa* on gonadotropin release in menopausal women and ovariectomized rats. *Planta Med*; 57:420-424. 1991

Einer-Jensen N, Zhao J, Andersen KP, Kristoffersen K. Cimicifuga and Melbrosia lack oestrogenic effects in mice and rats. In: *Maturitas;* 25:149-153. 1996. 1995

Frei-Kleiner S, Schaffner W, Rahlfs VW, et al. *Cimicifuga* racemosa dried ethanolic extract in menopausal disorders. *Maturitas*; 51(4): 397-404. 2005.

Freudenstein J, Dasenbrock C & Niblein T. Lack of promotion of estrogen-dependent mammary gland tumors in vivo by an isopropanolic *Cimicifuga racemosa* extract. *Cancer Res*; 62(12):3448-3452. 2002

Grady D. Management of menopausal symptoms. *N Eng J Med*; 355:2338-2347. 2006.

Hickey M, Davis SR, Sturdee D. Treatment of menopausal symptoms: what shall we do now? *Lancet*; 366(9483):409-21. 2005.

Hirabayashi T, Ochiai H, Sakai S et al. Inhibitory effect of ferulic acid and isoferulic acid on murine interleukin-8 production in response to influenza virus infections in vitro and in vivo. *Planta Med*; 61(3):221-226. 1995

Hirschberg AL, Edlund M, Svane G, et al. An isopropanolic extract of black cohosh does not increase mammographic breast density of breast cell proliferation in postmenopausal women. *Menopause*; 14(1): 89-96. 2007.

Hudson T. Black Cohosh Update. Does it work? Is it hepatotoxic? *Alt Comp Ther*; 132-135. 2006.

Jacobson JS, Troxel AB, Evans J et al. Randomized trial of black cohosh for the treatment of hot flashes among women with a history of breast cancer. *J Clin Oncol*; 19(10):2739-2745. 2001

Kim SJ & Kim MS. Inhibitory effects of Cimicifugae rhizome extracts on histamine, bradykinin and COX-2 mediated inflammatory actions. *Phytother Res*; 14 (8):596-600. 2000

Lehmann-Willenbrock E, Riedel HH. Clinical and endocrinologic studies of the treatment of ovarian insufficiency manifestations following hysterectomy with intact adnexa. *Zentralbl Gynakol;* 110 10):611-8. 1988

Liske E. Therapeutic efficacy and safety of *Cimicifuga racemosa* for gynecologic disorders. *Adv Ther* Jan-Feb;15(1):45-53. 1998

Liske E & Wustenberg P. Efficacy and safety of phytomedicines with particular references *to Cimicifuga racemosa. J Med Assoc Thai*; Jan:S108. 1998

Liske E, Hanggi W, Henneicke-Von Zepelin HH et al. Physiological investigation of a unique extract of black cohosh (Cimicifuga racemosae rhizome): A 6-month clinical study demonstrates no systemic estrogenic effect. *J Womens Health Gen Based Med*; 11(2):163-174. 2002

Minciullo PI, Saija A, Patafi M, et al. Muscle damage induced by black cohosh (Cimicifuga racemosa*). Phytomedicine*; 13(1-2):115-8.2006.

Munoz GH & Pluchino S. *Cimicifuga racemosa* for the treatment of hot flushes in women surviving breast cancer. *Maturitas*; 44(Suppl 1):S59-S65. 2003

Nappi RE, Malavasi B, Brundu B, et al. Efficacy of Cimicifuga racemosa on climacteric complaints: a randomized study versus low-dose transdermal estradiol. *Gynecol Endocrinol*; 20(1): 30-35. 2005.

Nelson, HD, Vesco KK, Haney E, et al. Nonhormonal therapies for menopausal hot flashes: systemic review and meta-analysis, JAMA;295(10):2057-2071. 2006

Pockaj BA, Gallagher JG, Loprinzi CL, et al. Phase III double-blind, randomized, placebo-controlled crossover trial of black cohosh in the management of hot flashes: NCCTG Trial N01CC1. J Clin Oncol; 24(18): 2836-2841. 2006.

Raus K, Brucker C, Gorkow C, et al. First-time proof of endometrial safety of the special black cohosh extract (Actacea or Cimicifuga racemosa extract) CR BNO 1055. *Menopause*; 13(4): 678-691. 2006.

Stolze H. Der andere Weg klimakterische Beschwerden zu behandeln. In: *Gyne;* 3:14-16. 1982

Tice J, Grady D. Alternatives to estrogen for treatment of hot flashes. Are they effective and safe*? JAMA*; 295(17): 2076-2078. 2006.

Tyler VE. The bright side of black cohosh. *Prevention Magazine;* April 1997

Tyler VE, Brady LR & Robbers JE. Pharmacognosy, 8th ed. Lea and Febiger, Philadelphia, PA; 1981. Vorberg G, Treatment of menopausal symptoms. *ZFA*;60:626-629. 1984

Uebelhack R, Blohmer JU, Graubaum HJ, et al. Black Cohosh and St. John's Wort for climacteric complaints: A randomized trial. *Obstet Gynecol; 107:247*-55. 2006.

Vermes G, Banhidy F, Acs N. The effects of remifemin on subjective symptoms of menopause. Adv Ther; 22(2): 148-154. 2005.

Winterhoff H. Arzneipflanzen mit endokriner Wirksamkeit. Z *Phytother;* 14:83-94. 1993

Winterhoff H, Spengler B, Christoffel V et al. Cimicifuga extract BNO 1055: reduction of hot flushes and hints on antidepressant activity. *Maturitas*; 44(suppl 1):S51-S58. 2003

Wuttke W, Seidlova-Wuttke D & Gorkow C. The Cimicifuga preparation BNO 1055 vs conjugated estrogens in a double-blind placebo-controlled study: effects on menopause symptoms and bone markers. *Maturitas*; 44(suppl 1):S67-S77. 2003

Zava D, Dollbaum CM & Blen M. Estrogen and progestin bioactivity of foods, herbs, and spices. *Proc Soc Exp Biol Med*; 217(3):369-378. 1998

Zepelin HH, Meden H, Kostev, et al. Isopropanolic black cohosh extract and recurrence-free survival after breast cancer. *Int J Clin Pharmacol Ther*; 45(3): 143-154. 2007.

Zierau O, Bodinet C, Kolba S et al. Antiestrogenic activities of *Cimicifuga racemosa* extracts. *J Steroid Biochem Mol Biol*; 80(1):125-130. 2002

Black Currant

Ribes nigrum

DESCRIPTION

Medicinal Parts: The medicinal parts are the leaves collected after the flowering season and dried, the fresh ripe fruit with the tops and stems and the fresh leaves collected in summer.

Flower and Fruit: The flowers form richly blossomed racemes. Each is in the axil of a pubescent bract, which is shorter than the petiole. The petiole is pinnate has 2 small bracteoles. The sepals are situated together with the 5 small stamens on the campanulate flower axis within which sits the single-valved ovary and the divided style. The hanging flowers are self-pollinating. The multiseeded, black, glandular punctuate berries develop from the ovary.

Leaves, Stem, and Root: The plant is a sturdy perennial bush up to 2 m high. The branches are pale, hard, and initially pubescent. The leaves are alternate, petiolate, becoming quickly glabrous on the upper surface and have numerous yellow resin glands on the undersurface. The 3- to 5-lobed leaf blade has a cordate base and doubly dentate margin.

Habitat: The plant is indigenous to Eurasian forests as far as the Himalayas, Canada and Australia and is cultivated in many regions.

Production: Black currant leaves are the leaves of *Ribes nigrum* collected during or shortly after the flowering season. Leaves are harvested from cultivated crops during or shortly after flowering. They are air-dried in the shade or carefully at a maximum temperature of 60° C.

Black currant fruits are the ripe fruits, with stalks attached, of *Ribes nigrum.* Fruits are harvested when fully ripe, and utilized immediately or deep frozen.

Other Names: Quinsy Berries, Squinancy Berries

ACTIONS AND PHARMACOLOGY

COMPOUNDS: BLACK CURRANT LEAVES

Flavonoids: including astragalin, isoquercitrin, rutin

Oligomeric proanthocyanidins

Ascorbic acid (vitamin C, 0.1 to 0.27% of fresh weight)

Volatile oil (traces)

EFFECTS: BLACK CURRANT LEAVES

A salidiuretic effect is attributed to the drug through a "diuretic factor" that is not closely defined. In animal experiments, a hypotensive, anti-exudative and prostaglandin-release inhibiting effect has been proved.

COMPOUNDS: BLACK CURRANT FRUITS

Ascorbic acid (vitamin C, 0.1 to 0.3%)

Anthocyans: chiefly cyanidin-3-O-rutinoside and delphinidin-3-O-rutinoside

Phenol caroboxylic acid derivatives: caffeoyl-, p-cumaroyl- and feruloyl-quinic acids; p-cumaroyl and feruloyl glucoses

Flavonoids: chief components isoquercitrin, myricetin glucoside, rutin

Fruit acids (3.5%): malic acid, citric acid, isocitric acid

Invert sugar

Pectins

COMPOUNDS: BLACK CURRANT SEEDS
Fatty oil (30%) with high gamma linolenic acid content

Monosaccharides: invert sugar

EFFECTS: BLACK CURRANT FRUIT AND SEEDS
The extract of the drug that contains anthocyane has a hypotensive and spasmolytic effect in animal experiments. In addition, an antimicrobial and xanthine-oxidase and lipoperoxidase inhibiting effect has been proved.

INDICATIONS AND USAGE

BLACK CURRANT LEAVES
Unproven Uses: Black Currant leaves are used internally to increase micturition. In folk medicine they are used internally for arthritis, gout and rheumatism, diarrhea, colic, jaundice and liver ailments, painful micturition, urinary stones, convulsive coughs, and whooping cough. Black Currant is used externally for treatment of wounds and insect bites.

BLACK CURRANT FRUITS
Unproven Uses: In folk medicine Black Currant fruit is used internally to relieve colds, hoarseness and coughs, diarrhea and stomachache. It is also used as a source of vitamin C. Preparations are used on mucous membranes as a gargle for hoarseness, strep throat and other inflammations of the oral cavity.

Black currant dried berries are used for bladder complaints, venous insufficiency, hemorrhoids, bruising and petechiae

CONTRAINDICATIONS

BLACK CURRANT LEAVES
Contraindicated in edema resulting from reduced cardiac and renal activity.

PRECAUTIONS AND ADVERSE REACTIONS

BLACK CURRANT LEAVES AND FRUITS
No health hazards or side effects are known in conjunction with the proper administration of designated therapeutic dosages.

DOSAGE

BLACK CURRANT LEAVES
Mode of Administration: Black currant leaves are available as whole, crude and powder drug for internal use.

Preparation: To prepare a tea, add 1 to 2 heaped teaspoons (2 to 4 gm) Black currant leaves to boiling water (150 ml), and strain after 10 minutes.

Daily Dosage:

Tea – 1 cup to be drunk several times a day.

Poultice – freshly rubbed Black Currant leaves or leaves soaked in warm water are dried and used as a compress. Place dried drug on wounds and fresh rubbed leaves on insect bites.

Storage: Should be protected from light and moisture

BLACK CURRANT FRUITS
Mode of Administration: Black Currant fruit is available as whole drug for internal use.

Daily Dosage:

Syrup – 5 to 10 ml, by the tablespoon, taken several times daily, or eaten as jelly or sweets.

Gargle – with the juice and equal parts of warm water.

LITERATURE

BLACK CURRANT LEAVES
Constantino L, Albasini A, Rastelli G, Benvenuti S. Activity of polyphenolic crude extracts as scavengers of superoxide radicals and inhibitors of xanthine oxidase. *Planta Med.* 58:342-344. 1992.

Declume C. Anti-inflammatory evaluation of a hydroalcoholic extract of black currant leaves (*ribes nigrum*). *J Ethnopharmacol.* 27:91-98. 1989.

Kyerematen G, Sandberg F, (1986) *Acta Pharm Suecica* 23:101.

Lietti A et al., (1976) Arzneim Forsch 26(5):829.

Senchute GV, Boruch IF, (1976) Rastit Resur 12(1):113.

BLACK CURRANT FRUITS
Declume C. Anti-inflammatory evaluation of a hydroalcoholic extract of black currant leaves (*ribes nigrum*). *J Ethnopharmacol.* 27:91-98. 1989.

Fernandes JB, Griffiths DW, Bain H. The evaluation of capillary zone and micellar electrokinetic capillary chromatographic techniques for the simultaneous determination of flavonoids, cinnamic, and phenolic acids in black currant (*ribes nigrum*) bud extracts. *Phytochem Anal.* 7:97-103. 1996.

Kyerematen G, Sandberg F, (1986) Acta Pharm Suecica 23:101.

Lietti A et al., (1976) Arzneim Forsch 26(5):829.

Senchute GV, Boruch IF, (1976) Rastit Resur 12(1):113.

Black Haw

Viburnum prunifolium

DESCRIPTION

Medicinal Parts: The medicinal part is the bark and the root.

Flower and Fruit: The flowers of the Viburnum species are white and in richly blossomed, flat, apical cymes. The central florets are campanulate and fertile; the lateral ones are much larger, rotate, and infertile. The calyx margin is small and 5-tipped. The corolla of the fertile florets is campanulate and 5-petalled. There are 5 stamens, a semi-inferior ovary, and 3 sessile stigmas. The fruit of the Black Haw is a shiny, black, juicy berry. The fruit of *Viburnum opulus* is red.

Leaves, Stem and Root: Black Haw is a deciduous tree 5 m tall. It has gray-brown bark and green, grooved branches. The leaves are opposite, petiolate, 3 to 5 lobed, roughly dentate, green on both surfaces and softly pubescent beneath.

Habitat: The plant is indigenous to the eastern and central U.S.

Production: Black Haw bark is the bark of the trunk and branches of *Viburnum prunifolium.*

Other Names: Stagbush, American Sloe, European Cranberry, Cramp Bark, Guelder Rose, Snowball Tree, King's Crown, High Cranberry, Red Elder, Rose Elder, Water Elder, May Rose, Whitsun Rose, Dog Rowan Tree, Whitsun Bosses, Silver Bells, Wild Guelder Rose

ACTIONS AND PHARMACOLOGY

COMPOUNDS

Flavonoids: amentoflavon (a biflavone)

Triterpenes: including among others oleanolic acid, ursolic acid as well as their acetates

Hydroxycoumarins: scopoletin, aesculetin, scoplin

Caffeic acid derivatives: chlorogenic acid, isochlorogenic acid

Phenol carboxylic acids: salicylic acid, salicin

Tannins (2%)

Arbutin (traces)

EFFECTS

The drug has a spasmolytic and, to date, an undefined effect on the uterus.

INDICATIONS AND USAGE

Unproven Uses: Black Haw is used for complaints of dysmenorrhea.

PRECAUTIONS AND ADVERSE REACTIONS

No health hazards or side effects are known in conjunction with the proper administration of designated therapeutic dosages.

DOSAGE

Mode of Administration: An extract is used as a constituent of a tea mixture made from Black Haw bark, Camomile flowers, and Peppermint leaves.

How Supplied

Liquid Extract

Tincture

Daily Dose: 2.5 to 5 gm of the drug as an infusion or decoction; 4 to 8 mL of fluid extract; 5 to 10 mL of tincture.

LITERATURE

Handjieva N et al., PH 27:3175. 1988.

Hörhammer L, Wagner H, Reinhardt H, Chemistry, pharmacology, and pharmaceutics of the components of Viburnum prunifolium and V. opulus. In: *Botan Mag* (Tokyo) 79(Oct./Nov.): 510-525. 1966.

Jarboe CH et al., (1967) *J Med Chem* 10: 448.

Jarboe CH et al., (1969) *J Org Chem* 34: 4202.

Jensen SR et al., *PH* 24:487. 1985.

Black Hellebore

Helleborus niger

DESCRIPTION

Medicinal Parts: The medicinal parts of the plant are the dried rhizome with or without roots and the fresh underground parts.

Flower and Fruit: The flower is white with a greenish margin, reddish on the outside. It is hanging and splayed. There are 5 broadly ovate, campanualate bracts with red-brown borders, which tend toward each other. The petals are altered to nectaries. There are numerous yellow stamens. The fruit is a podlike, many-seeded follicle with a curved beak and horizontal stripes. The seeds are matte black, ovate, and have a long swelling on them.

Leaves, Stem, and Root: The plant is a perennial subshrub up to 50 cm high. The stem is erect, glabrous, branched, woody at the base, and almost leafless. The basal leaves are long-petioled, thickish, coriaceous, glabrous, and dark green above with a lighter underside.

Characteristics: The plant is poisonous; rhizome is black-brown.

Habitat: The plant is indigenous to the forests of southern and central Europe.

Production: Black Hellebore root is the root of *Helleborus niger.*

Not to be Confused With: Helleborus foetidus, Helleborus niger and *Helleborus viridis* are different plants with different active compounds. They may be confused with the subterranean parts of *Trollius eurpaeus, Aconitum napellus, Astrantia major, Actaea spicata* and *Adonis vernalis.*

Other Names: Christe Herbe, Christmas Rose, Melampode

ACTIONS AND PHARMACOLOGY

COMPOUNDS: HELLEBORUS FOETIDUS

Steroid saponins: mixture known as helleborin

COMPOUNDS: HELLEBORUS NIGER

Steroid saponins: mixture known as helleborin

Cardioactive steroid glycosides (bufadienolide): including hellebrin, deglucohellebrin (only traces)

Alkaloids: celliamine, sprintillamine

COMPOUNDS: HELLEBORUS VIRIDIS

Steroid saponins: mixture known as helleborin

Cardioactive steroid glycosides (bufadienolide): including hellebrin, deglucohellebrin

Alkaloids: celliamine, sprintillamine, sprintillin

EFFECTS: ALL SPECIES

The plant is said to have a typical saponin effect (irritates mucous membranes) and is in general extremely toxic.

Note that other varieties of *Helleborus* also contain hellebrin with a digitalislike effect.

INDICATIONS AND USAGE

Unproven Uses: In folk medicine, Black Hellebore is used as a laxative, for nausea, worm infestation, to regulate menstruation, and as an abortifacient, as well as for acute nephritis. Also used in the treatment of head colds.

Homeopathic Uses: Used to treat acute diarrhea, encephalitis, cephalitis, kidney inflammation, and states of confusion.

PRECAUTIONS AND ADVERSE REACTIONS

General: The mucous membrane-irritating saponin effect of the drug is the chief focus in cases of poisoning. Symptoms include scratchy feeling in mouth and throat, salivation, nausea, vomiting, diarrhea, dizziness, shortness of breath, possible spasm, and asphyxiation. Cardiac arrhythmias are to be expected with large intakes of the rhizome of *Helleborus viridis*. Poisonings are recorded among the animals that feed on the plant. Following stomach and intestinal emptying (gastric lavage, sodium sulfate) and the administration of activated charcoal, therapy for poisonings consists of diazepam for spasm and electrolyte replenishment and sodium bicarbonate infusions for any acidosis that may arise. Intubation and oxygen respiration may also be necessary.

Pregnancy: In folk medicine, Black Hellebore is used as an abortifacient.

DOSAGE

Mode of Administration: Black Hellebore is obsolete and dangerous as a drug in allopathic doses.

Daily Dosage: The average dose is 0.05 gm; the maximum single dose is 0.2 gm; the largest daily dose is 1.0 gm. A powder with a medium content of 10% is used for head colds.

Homeopathic Dosage: 5 drops, 1 tablet or 10 globules every 30 to 60 minutes (acute) or 1 to 3 times daily (chronic); parenterally: 1 to 2 ml sc acute, 3 times daily; chronic: once a day (HAB34).

LITERATURE

Frohne D, Pfänder HJ, Giftpflanzen - Ein Handbuch für Apotheker, Toxikologen und Biologen, 4. Aufl., Wiss. Verlagsges. mbH Stuttgart 1997.

Glombitza KW et al., Do roots of *Helleborus niger* contain cardioactive substances. In: *PM* 55:107. 1989.

Hänsel R, Keller K, Rimpler H, Schneider G (Hrsg.), Hagers Handbuch der Pharmazeutischen Praxis, 5. Aufl., Bde 4-6 (Drogen), Springer Verlag Berlin, Heidelberg, New York, 1992-1994.

Kaij-a-Kamb M, Amoros M, Girre L. Search for new antiviral agents of plant origin. *Pharm Acta Helv*. 67:130-147. 1992.

Lewin L, Gifte und Vergiftungen, 6. Aufl., Nachdruck, Haug Verlag, Heidelberg 1992.

Madaus G, Lehrbuch der Biologischen Arzneimittel, Bde 1-3, Nachdruck, Georg Olms Verlag Hildesheim 1979.

Petricic J et al., *Acta Pharm Jugosl* 27:127. 1977.

Petricic J, *Acta Pharm Jugosl* 24:179. 1974.

Poisonous Plants in Britain and their effects on Animals and Man, Ministry of Agriculture Fisheries and Food, Pub; HMSO, UK 1984.

Roth L, Daunderer M, Kormann K, Giftpflanzen, Pflanzengifte, 4. Aufl., Ecomed Fachverlag Landsberg Lech 1993.

Teuscher E, Lindequist U, Biogene Gifte - Biologie, Chemie, Pharmakologie, 2. Aufl., Fischer Verlag Stuttgart 1994.

Wiβner W, Kating H, Botanische und phytochemische Untersuchung an europäischen und kleinasiatischen Arten der Gattung Helleborus. In: PM 26:128-143, 228-249, 364-374. 1974.

Black Horehound

Ballota nigra

DESCRIPTION

Medicinal Parts: The aerial parts of the plant are used medicinally.

Flower and Fruit: The clearly stemmed flowers are 1 to 1.5 cm long. They are arranged in 4 to 10 fairly loose and often short-stemmed cymes in the axils of the cauline leaves. The bracteoles are arrow-shaped and soft. They are half as long as the funnel-shaped calyx, which is downy to silky-shaggy haired. The calyx has 5 awned tips. The corolla is usually reddish-lilac, occasionally white. It contains a straight tube that grows out of the calyx tube and has a ring of hairs at the base. It has an elliptoid, slightly domed upper lip, which is slightly compressed from the outside. There is an equally long, downward hanging, white-marked lower lip, and an obovate, often edged or weakly dentate middle lip. The stamens are slightly hairy at the base and have small, distinctly spreading pollen sacks. The plant produces a hard fruit. The 12 mm long nuts are ovoid and quite smooth.

Leaves, Stem, and Root: Horehound is a perennial 0.30 to 1 m high shrub with a short creeping rhizome and upright, sturdy, angular, branched stems. The whole plant is pubescent and fresh green. In the autumn, the plant is often tinged brown-violet. The opposite leaves have a 0.5 to 1 cm long petiole. The lower leaves are larger and have an ovate to almost round, 2 cm long by 1.5 to 3.5 cm wide leaf blade. They are weakly cordate, blunt or wedge-shaped at the base, and finely crenate to roughly and unevenly serrate. Both sides are pubescent, the upper surface often becoming glabrous and somewhat glossy.

Characteristics: The whole plant has an unpleasant smell of essential oil.

Habitat: The plant is considered to be a weed in western, central and northern Europe, but was intentionally introduced to the U.S.

Production: Black Horehound is the aerial part of *Ballota nigra*, gathered when in bloom. It is collected in the wild or from cultivated plants propagated by sowing seeds or planting cuttings at the end of winter. The harvest is in July and August. There are no special conditions for drying.

Not to be Confused With: The drug can be confused with *Folia melissae*. Adulterations with hybrids of *Marubium vulgare* have been found on the market.

Other Names: Black (Stinking) Horehound, Black Hemp Nettle

ACTIONS AND PHARMACOLOGY

COMPOUNDS

Diterpenes, marrubiin: 7-acetoxymarrubiin, ballotinon, ballotenol, ballonigrin (to some extent bitter principles)

Volatile oil (traces, unpleasant smell)

Caffeic and ferulic acid derivatives: including chlorogenic acid

Tannins

EFFECTS

Horehound acts as a stimulant, antiemetic, and antispasmodic; however, the mode of action has not been satisfactorily explained. According to older literature, a drop in arterial blood pressure and bradycardia occurred in a dog when it was injected intravenously with an infusion (2.5 g infusion per kg body weight). When a decoction of the fresh plant was administered intravenously, the volume of gall secretions tripled within 30 minutes.

INDICATIONS AND USAGE

Unproven Uses: In folk medicine, the drug is used as a sedative, for stomach cramps and complaints, menopause symptoms, whooping cough, and to increase bile flow. Also used as an enema and as suppositories for worm infestation.

PRECAUTIONS AND ADVERSE REACTIONS

No health hazards or side effects are known in conjunction with the proper administration of designated therapeutic dosages.

DOSAGE

Mode of Administration: The drug is used internally in the form of liquid extracts and tinctures. It is also used externally.

Preparation: Liquid extract: 1:1 in 25% ethanol. Tincture: 1:10 with 45% ethanol. Alcohol tincture from the fresh plant with 90% alcohol.

Daily Dose: Single dose of the drug is 2 to 4 g (as an infusion); Liquid extract: 1 to 3 mL; Tincture: 1 to 2 mL.

LITERATURE

Balansard J, Compt Rend Soc Biol 115:1295-1297. 1933.

Kooiman P, (1972) *Acta Bot Nederl* 21 (4): 417.

Savona G et al., (1976) *J Chem Soc* (P) 1: 1607-1609.

Savona G et al., (1977) *J Chem Soc* (P) 1: 322-324 et 497-499.

Savona G et al., La chimica e líndustria 58:378. 1976.

Seidel V et al., Phenylpropanoid glycosides from Ballota nigra. In: *PM* 62(2):186-187. 1997.

Black Mulberry

Morus nigra

DESCRIPTION

Medicinal Parts: The medicinal parts are the ripe berries and the root bark.

Flower and Fruit: The plant is monoecious or dioecious. The greenish flowers are in catkinlike inflorescences. The male flowers are ovate to cylindrical; the female flowers ovate or globular. The flowers have a 4-bract involucre, which enlarges and becomes fleshy in the female flowers. The female flowers have 2 stigmas, the male flowers have 4 stamens. All of the fruit from the catkins develops into blackberrylike false berries, which are really a series of fleshy drupes that are edible and pleasant-tasting.

Leaves, Stem, and Root: The tree grows from 6 to 12 m high. The bark is gray-brown. The leaves are alternate with flat-grooved, somewhat hairy petioles. They are cordate or ovate, sessile, unevenly lobed, and serrate with short rough hairs on the upper surface.

Habitat: The plant is cultivated worldwide in temperate regions.

Other Names: Purple Mulberry, White Mulberry

ACTIONS AND PHARMACOLOGY

COMPOUNDS: IN THE FRUIT

Fruit acids (1.9%): including malic acid, citric acid

Saccharose (10%)

Pectins

Ascorbic acid (0.17%)

Flavonoids: including, among others rutin

COMPOUNDS: IN THE LEAVES

Flavonoids: including among others rutin (2-6%)

The constituents of the rhizome rind are not known.

EFFECTS

The active agents are sugar, acids, pectin and rutin, but there is no information available regarding their effects.

INDICATIONS AND USAGE

Unproven Uses: The drug is used as a mild laxative and in the treatment of inflammations of the mucous membranes of the respiratory system.

PRECAUTIONS AND ADVERSE REACTIONS

No health hazards or side effects are known in conjunction with the proper administration of designated therapeutic dosages.

DOSAGE

Mode of Administration: The drug is used internally as a comminuted drug, juice or syrup.

Daily Dosage: The average daily dose is 2 to 4 ml of syrup.

LITERATURE

Atta-ur-Rahman Zaman K. Medicinal plants with hypoglycemic activity. *J Ethnopharmacol*. 26:1-55. 1989.

Deshpande VH, (1968) Tetrahedron Lett 1715.

Kern W, List PH, Hörhammer L (Hrsg.), Hagers Handbuch der Pharmazeutischen Praxis, 4. Aufl., Bde 1-8, Springer Verlag Berlin, Heidelberg, New York, 1969.

Kimura Y et al., (1986) *J Nat Prod* 94(4):639.

Madaus G, Lehrbuch der Biologischen Arzneimittel, Bde 1-3, Nachdruck, Georg Olms Verlag Hildesheim 1979.

Marles RJ and Farnsworth NR. Antidiabetic plants and their active constituents. *Phytomedicine* 2(2):137-189. 1995.

Nomura T et al., (1983) *Planta Med* 47:151.

Oliver-Bever B (Ed.), Medicinal Plants of Tropical West Africa, Cambridge University Press, Cambridge 1986.

Black Mustard

Brassica nigra

DESCRIPTION

Medicinal Parts: The medicinal parts are the seeds from which oil is extracted.

Flower and Fruit: The inflorescences are terminal or axillary and compressed into a semisphere. The flowers have 4 free sepals, 4 free petals, 6 stamens, and 1 ovary. The sepals are 3.5 to 4.5 mm long and appear linear because of slits on the edge. They are yellowish-green, usually glabrous, upright, and slightly splayed. The yellow petals are twice as long as the calyx, obovate, rounded at the tip and narrowed to a stem at the base. The ovary is on the receptacle. The style is thin and has a semiglobose, cushionlike stigma. The fruit is an erect pod, which is linear and rounded or angular with a thin dividing wall. It is 10 to 25 mm long and pressed onto the stem. The seed is globose, brown, matte, and punctate.

Leaves, Stem, and Root: Black Mustard is an annual that grows up to 1 m tall and is slim-branched with thin fusiform roots. The stem grows up to 1 m. It is almost round and bristly haired at the base, with a bluish bloom toward the top. The stem is glabrous with upright branches almost in bushels. The leaves are petiolate, up to 12 cm long and 5 cm wide. The lower leaves are grass-green and covered in 1 mm long bristles. They are pinnatifid and densely dentate, with 2 to 4 obtuse lobes on each side and a large end section. The upper stem and branch leaves are smaller, usually glabrous and blue-green, ovate or lanceolate and slightly dentate.

Habitat: Black Mustard grows in temperate regions worldwide.

Production: Mustard seeds are the seeds of *Brassica nigra*.

Other names: Brown mustard, Red Mustard, Mustard Seed

ACTIONS AND PHARMACOLOGY

COMPOUNDS

Glucosinolates: chiefly sinigrin (allylglucosinolates, 1-5%); grinding the seeds into powder and then rubbing with warm water (not with hot water because enzymes would be destroyed), as well as chewing, releases the volatile mustard oil allylisothiocyanate

Fatty oil (30-35%)

Proteins (40%)

Phenyl propane derivatives: including sinapine (choline ester of sinapic acid, 1%)

EFFECTS

The hyperemic effect is the main effect and is employed for various indications where increased blood flow is desired. The drug contains glucosinolates whose main constituent, sinigrin, is converted through enzymatic hydrolysis to allyl mustard oil. This causes a stabbing pain and an intense reddening of the skin. Upon contact with the skin, Allylsen oil causes the severity of the inflammation to increase, potentially to the extent were blisters and necrosis may occur.

INDICATIONS AND USAGE

Unproven Uses: External uses include bronchial pneumonia, sinusitis, pleurisy, lumbago, and sciatica for which a mustard poultice is applied, sometimes to achieve an antirheumatic effect (mustard spirit 2%). Foot baths and full baths are used to prompt increased circulation (headaches and mild glaucoma) or to stimulate the cardiopulmonary system (frost bite and vascular disease).

Homeopathic Uses: Uses in homeopathy include irritation of the upper respiratory tract and the gastrointestinal tract.

CONTRAINDICATIONS

Use of Black Mustard is contraindicated in individuals with gastrointestinal ulcers or inflammatory kidney diseases.

PRECAUTIONS AND ADVERSE REACTIONS

General: No health hazards or side effects are known in conjunction with the proper administration of designated therapeutic dosages. Gastrointestinal complaints (and, rarely, kidney irritation) could occur following internal administration, due to the mucous membrane-irritating effect of the mustard oil. The drug possesses minimal potential for sensitization; contact allergies have been observed. The draining effect associated with the drug's administration makes it inadvisable in the presence of varicosis and venous disorder.

Sneezing, coughing, and possible asthmatic attacks can result from breathing the allylisothiocyanate that arises with the preparation and application of mustard poultices. Eyes should be protected when preparing or using the poultices because the vapors can cause eye irritation. Long-term external application or too-intensive reactions upon the skin can lead to injury such as blister formation, suppurating ulcerations, and necroses. Mustard poultices are to be removed after no more than 30 minutes.

Pediatric Use: Black Mustard should not be administered to children under 6 years of age.

DRUG INTERACTIONS

POTENTIAL INTERACTIONS

Avoid concomitant use of preparations containing ammonia, because ammonia with mustard oil forms inactive thiosinamine.

OVERDOSAGE

Internal overdosage can lead to vomiting, stomach pain, and diarrhea. In severe cases, these can be accompanied by somnolence, cardiac weakness, breathing difficulties, and even to death. Following installation of activated charcoal and shock prophylaxis (suitable body position, quiet, warmth), the therapy for poisonings consists of administering mucilaginosa for the protection of mucous membranes and generous amounts of fluids. Possible cases of acidosis should be treated with sodium bicarbonate infusions. In case of shock, plasma volume expanders should be infused. Cardiac massage, intubation, and oxygen respiration may also be necessary.

DOSAGE

Mode of Administration: Used externally as a mustard plaster, foot bath or full bath. On rare occasions, Black Mustard is used as a constituent in antirheumatic preparations and cardiac ointments.

How Supplied: Allyl mustard oil: 1 to 3% solution, ointments, emulsions and other rubs (including a rheumatism liniment) are available from commercial sources.

Preparation: To prepare a mustard poultice, mix approximately 100 g mustard flour with lukewarm water and pack in linen. Use on the chest should not exceed 10 minutes (with a maximum of 3 to 5 minutes for children over 6 years of age). Limit use on the face to 3 to 4 minutes and take care to avoid the eye area. When mustard paper is used, it is immersed in warm water and then placed on the painful area of skin.

To prepare a full mustard bath, mix 100 to 200 g mustard flour with cold water and press through a cloth into the warm bath. A mustard footbath should be prepared in a bucket or other container that allows the warm water to extend up the leg to the desired position. Add 1 to 3 dessertspoons of mustard flour and stir.

Daily Dosage: The poultice is placed on the chest for about 10 minutes (with a maximum of 3 to 5 minutes for children). Foot bath use should be limited to 10 minutes.

Homeopathic Dosage: 5 drops, 1 tablet, 10 globules every 30 to 60 minutes (acute) or 1 to 3 times daily (chronic); parenterally: 1 to 2 mL sc; acute: 3 times daily; chronic once a day (HAB34).

Storage: The stored drug should be protected from light.

LITERATURE

Alwan AH, Jawad AM, Al-Bana AS, Ali KF. Antiviral activity of some Iraqi indigenous plants. *Int J Crude Drug Res.* 26:107-111. 1988.

Cao G, Sofic E, Prior RL. Antioxidant capacity of common tea and vegetables. *J Agric Food Chem.* 44(11):3426-3431. 1996

Constabel F. Medicinal Plant Biotechnology. *Plant Med.* 56:421-425. 1990.

Halva S et al., *Agric Sci Finl* 58:157. 1986.

Hänsel R, Keller K, Rimpler H, Schneider G (Hrsg.), Hagers Handbuch der Pharmazeutischen Praxis, 5. Aufl., Bde 4-6 (Drogen): Springer Verlag Berlin, Heidelberg, New York, 1992-1994.

Hill CB et al., J Am Soc Hort Sci 112(2):309. 1987.

Leung AY, Encyclopedia of Common Natural Ingredients Used in Food Drugs, Cosmetics, John Wiley & Sons Inc., New York 1980.

Madaus G, Lehrbuch der Biologischen Arzneimittel, Bde 1-3, Nachdruck, Georg Olms Verlag Hildesheim 1979.

Roth L, Daunderer M, Kormann K, Giftpflanzen, Pflanzengifte, 4. Aufl., Ecomed Fachverlag Landsberg Lech 1993.

Steinegger E, Hänsel R, Pharmakognosie, 5. Aufl., Springer Verlag Heidelberg 1992.

Teuscher E, Lindequist U, Biogene Gifte - Biologie, Chemie, Pharmakologie, 2. Aufl., Fischer Verlag Stuttgart 1994.

Teuscher E, Biogene Arzneimittel, 5. Aufl., Wiss. Verlagsges. Stuttgart 1997.

Wichtl M (Hrsg.), Teedrogen, 4. Aufl., Wiss. Verlagsges. Stuttgart 1997.

Black Nightshade

Solanum nigrum

DESCRIPTION

Medicinal Parts: The medicinal parts are the dried herb collected during the flowering season

Flower and Fruit: The small white flowers are in 6- to 10-blossomed, umbel-like, nodding, axillary inflorescences. The calyx is 5-tipped and does not drop. The corolla is 5-tipped with a short tube. There are 5 stamens with clavate anthers inclining toward each other. The corolla is rotate and has 1 superior ovary. The fruit is a pea-sized black, occasionally green or yellow, berry.

Leaves, Stem and Root: Solanum nigrum is an annual plant 10 to 50 cm in height. The stem is erect, leafy and angular with outward-inclined branches. The leaves are fleshy, petiolate, rhomboid or ovate. They narrow to a cuneate base, which is crenate-dentate and glabrous or sparsely pubescent.

Characteristics: The plant has a musklike odor when wilting and is poisonous.

Habitat: The plant is found worldwide.

Production: Black Nightshade is the herb of *Solanum nigrum* picked in uncultivated regions (the wild) and dried in the open air.

Not to be Confused With: Black Nightshade was often called Petty (a corruption of ''petit'') Morel, to distinguish it from the Deadly Nightshade, or Great Morel, as it is also poisonous but apparently less so.

Other Names: Garden Nightshade, Petty Morel, Poisonberry

ACTIONS AND PHARMACOLOGY

COMPOUNDS

Steroid alkaloid glycosides: in the foliage and in unripe fruits (0-2.0%). Ripe fruits are, as a rule, free of alkaloids.

Chief alkaloids: solasonine, solamargine, β-solamargine

Steroid saponins: with tigogenin as an aglycone

EFFECTS

According to folk medicine, the herb should work as an antispasmodic, pain reliever, sedative and narcotic; however, there are no studies available. In animal experiments, the steroid alkaloid glycosides have a local anesthetic effect, increase sleep duration and significantly inhibit the occurrence of acetlysalicylic acid-induced stomach ulcers. The effect is attributed to the inhibition of pepsin and hydrochloric acid secretion.

INDICATIONS AND USAGE

Unproven Uses: Internally, Black Nightshade is used for gastric irritation, cramps, and whooping cough. Externally, the herb is used for psoriasis, hemorrhoids, abscesses, eczema, and bruising.

Chinese Medicine: Black Nightshade is used for furuncles, carbuncles, abscesses, erysipelas, sprains, strains, contusions, chronic bronchitis, and acute hepatitis.

Indian Medicine: Black Nightshade is used for rheumatic pain, coughs, asthma, bronchitis, wounds, swellings, ulcers, flatulence, dyspeptic complaints, vomiting, dysuria, earache, hiccups, eye disease, leprosy, and skin diseases.

Homeopathic Uses: Black Nightshade is used for cerebral and meningeal irritation.

PRECAUTIONS AND ADVERSE REACTIONS

No health hazards or side effects are known in conjunction with the proper administration of designated therapeutic dosages.

OVERDOSAGE

Overdoses resulting from the intake of large quantities of fresh foliage with high alkaloid content could lead to gastrointestinal signs of irritation, characterized by queasiness, vomiting, headache and, in rare cases, mydriasis.

DOSAGE

Mode of Administration: The herb is available as a ground drug, tincture and liquid extract for internal and external use.

Preparation: To prepare a rinse or moist compress, add a handful of drug to 1 liter of water and boil for 10 minutes. A tincture is prepared in a ratio of 1:1 with 95% ethanol.

Daily Dosage: Externally, use as a compress or rinse. Internally, the dose is 10 drops of liquid extract 2 to 3 times daily, or 5 to 10 gm of tincture daily.

Homeopathic Dosage: 5 drops, 1 tablet, or 10 globules every 30 to 60 minutes (acute) or 1 to 3 times daily (chronic); parenterally: 1 to 2 mL sc; acute, 3 times daily; chronic: once a day (HAB34)

LITERATURE

Akhtar MS and Munir M. Evaluation of gastric antiulcerogenic effects of Brassica oleracea and Ocimum basilicum in rats. *J Ethnopharmacol.* 27:1630176. 1989.

El Mekkawy S, Meselhy MR, Kusumoto IT, Kadota S, Hattori M, Namba T. Inhibitory effect of Egyptian folk medicines on human immunodeficiency virus (HIV) reverse transcriptase. *Chem Pharm Bull.* 43(4):641-648. 1995.

Frohne D, Pfänder HJ, Giftpflanzen - Ein Handbuch für Apotheker, Toxikologen und Biologen, 4. Aufl., Wiss. Verlags-Ges. Stuttgart 1997.

Hänsel R, Keller K, Rimpler H, Schneider G (Hrsg.), Hagers Handbuch der Pharmazeutischen Praxis, 5. Aufl., Bde 4-6 (Drogen): Springer Verlag Berlin, Heidelberg, New York, 1992-1994.

Johnson R, Lee JS, Ryan CA, Regulation of expression of a wound-inducible tomato inhibitor I gene in transgenic nightshade plants. *Plant Mol Biol*, 45:349-56, 1990 Mar.

Lewin L, Gifte und Vergiftungen, 6. Aufl., Nachdruck, Haug Verlag, Heidelberg 1992.

Madaus G, Lehrbuch der Biologischen Arzneimittel, Bde 1-3, Nachdruck, Georg Olms Verlag Hildesheim 1979.

Moundipa PF, Domngang FM, Effect of the leafy vegetable Solanum nigrum on the activities of some liver drug-metabolizing enzymes after aflatoxin B1 treatment in female rats. *Br J Nutr*, 45:81-91, 1991 Jan.

Ridout CL et al., *PA* 44:732. 1989.

Roth L, Daunderer M, Kormann K, Giftpflanzen, Pflanzengifte, 4. Aufl., Ecomed Fachverlag Landsberg Lech 1993.

Schreiber K, Kulturpflanze 11:451-501. 1963.

Sultana S, Perwaiz S, Iqbal M, Athar M, Crude extracts of hepatoprotective plants Solanum nigrum and Cichorium intybus inhibit free radical-mediated DNA damage. *J Ethnopharmacol*, 45:189-92, 1995 Mar.

Teuscher E, Biogene Arzneimittel, 5. Aufl., Wiss. Verlagsges. Stuttgart 1997.

Black Pepper

Piper nigrum

DESCRIPTION

Medicinal Parts: The medicinal parts are the berries, which have been freed from the pericarp, and the dried berrylike fruit, which has been collected before ripening.

Flower and Fruit: The inflorescences are pendulous, axillary spikes 5 to 15 cm long containing over 100 inconspicuous white florets. The florets have 1 large ovary with 3 stigmas, 2 stamens and a reduced perianth. Red berrylike drupes form the 30 to 50 flowers, which are fertilized.

Leaves, Stem, and Root: The plant is actually a liane, which in cultivation is trained on posts or wire. It can grow to over 6 m. The stem is strong and woody, and the leaves are cordate, glossy and pale green. The leaves are 5 to 10 cm wide, 8 to 18 cm long and are on 5 cm long petioles.

Habitat: The plant grows wild in southern India and is cultivated in tropical Asia and the Caribbean.

Production: Black Peppers are the dried fruits of *Piper nigrum*, harvested before ripening. The whole ears are plucked and separated from spindles that have been dried, or the fruit is first brushed from the spindles and then dried. Once the shell has been removed, the green stonefruit is sun-dried or roasted, after which it blackens.

Not to be Confused With: Foreign fruits of the *Piperacae* family. It is most frequently confused with peppershells, pepper spindles or stiles, i.e., byproducts of the extraction of white pepper from black pepper.

Other Names: Piper, Pepper Bark

ACTIONS AND PHARMACOLOGY

COMPOUNDS

Volatile oil (1.2-2.6%): chief components- sabinene (15-25%), limonene (15-20%), caryophyllene (10-15%), beta-pinene (10-12%), alpha-pinene (8-12%), delta3-carene (5%)

Acid amides (pungent substances): chief components- piperine, additionally including among others piperylin, piperolein A and B, cumaperine

3,4-dihydroxy phenyl ethanol glycosides (substratum for the enzymatic black colouring of the fresh fruits)

Polysaccharides (45%)

Fatty oil (10%)

EFFECTS

The drug stimulates the thermal receptors and increases secretion of saliva and gastric mucus. It has an antimicrobial effect. It influences liver and metabolic functions, and has an insecticidal effect.

INDICATIONS AND USAGE

Unproven Uses: Folk medicine uses include stomach disorders and digestion problems, neuralgia, and scabies.

Chinese Medicine: Black Pepper is used for vomiting, diarrhea, and gastric symptoms.

Indian Medicine: Indian uses include arthritis, asthma, fever, coughs, catarrh, dysentery, dyspepsia, flatulence, hemorrhoids, hiccoughs, urethral discharge, and skin damage.

Homeopathic Uses: Black Pepper is used for irritation of the mucous membranes and galactorrhea.

PRECAUTIONS AND ADVERSE REACTIONS

No health hazards or side effects are known in conjunction with the proper administration of designated therapeutic dosages.

DOSAGE

Mode of Administration: Black Pepper is used internally for stomach disorders and externally as an irritant ointment for neuralgia and scabies.

Daily Dosage: Single doses range from 0.3 to 0.6 gm. The daily dosage is 1.5 gm.

Homeopathic Dosage: 5 to 10 drops, 1 tablet, or 5 to 10 globules 1 to 3 times a day or from D4: 1 mL injection solution sc twice weekly (HAB1).

LITERATURE

Atal CK et al., (1975) *Lloydia* 38:256.

Aye-Than Kulkarni HJ, Wut-Hmone Tha SJ. Anti-diarrhoeal efficacy of some Burmese indigenous drug formulations in experimental diarrhoeal test models. *Int J Crude Drug Res.* 27:195-200. 1989.

Bano G, Amla V, Raino RK, Zutshi U, Chopra CL. The effect of piperine on pharmacokinetics of phenytoin on healthy volunteers. *Plant Med.* 53:568-569. 1987.

Bock Rde Gyssens I, Peetermans M, Noldard N. Aspergillus in pepper. *Lancet II.* 331-332. 1989.

Freist W, Der scharfe Geschmack des Pfeffers - Ein altes Rätsel, nur teilweise gelöst. In: *Chemie i.u. Zeit* 23(3):135-142. 1991.

Kapil A, Piperine. A Potent Inhibitor of Leishmania donovani Promastigotes in vitro. In: *PM* 59(5):474. 1993.

Koul IB, Kapil A, Evaluation of the Liver Protective Potential of Piperine, an Active Principle of Black and Long Peppers. In: *PM* 59(5):413. 1993.

Raina ML et al., (1976) *Planta Med* 30:198.

Richard ML et al., (1976) *J Food Sci* 36:584.

Schröder, Buch. In: Schröder R: Kaffee, Tee und Kardamom, Ulmer-Verlag, Stuttgart. 1991.

Traxter JT, (1971) *J Agric Food Chem* 19:1135.

Black Root

Leptandra virginica

DESCRIPTION

Medicinal Parts: The medicinal part is the dried rhizome with the roots. The roots have a very different action according to whether they are used fresh or dry. The dried root is milder.

Flower and Fruit: The stems end in terminal, 15 to 25 cm long spikes of white flowers.

Leaves, Stem, and Root: The plant is a perennial herb, which grows to about 120 cm high. The rhizome is horizontal, cylindrical, branched and dark red to dark purple-brown on the outside. The simple, erect stems grow in intervals of 1.2 to 3.2 cm from the rhizome. They are smooth and finely downy. The leaves are whorled (4 to 7 in one whorl), lançeolate, on short petioles, pointed, and finely serrate.

Habitat: Indigenous to the eastern U.S. but grows elsewhere.

Production: Black Root and its rhizome are the complete underground parts of *Leptandra virginica*.

Other Names: Bowman's Root, Physic Root, Hini, Oxadoddy, Tall Speedwell, Tall Veronica, Whorlywort, Culveris Root

ACTIONS AND PHARMACOLOGY

COMPOUNDS

Volatile oil: composition unknown

Cinnamic acid derivatives: including among others 4-methoxycinnamic acid, 3,4-dimethoxycinnamic acid and their esters

Tannins

The constituents of the drug have not been fully investigated.

EFFECTS

The drug has diaphoretic, carminative, and cathartic effects. It is also a cholagogue and a laxative.

INDICATIONS AND USAGE

Unproven Uses: Black Root is used for chronic constipation and liver and gallbladder disorders. It is also used as an emetic.

Homeopathic Uses: The drug is used for diarrhea and inflammation of the liver and gallbladder.

PRECAUTIONS AND ADVERSE REACTIONS

No health hazards are known in conjunction with the proper administration of designated therapeutic dosages. The emetic and laxative effects of the drug are used therapeutically.

DOSAGE

Homeopathic Dosage: 5 drops, 1 tablet, or 10 globules every 30 to 60 minutes (acute) or 1 to 3 times daily (chronic); parenterally: 1 to 2 mL sc, acute: 3 times daily; chronic: once a day (HAB1).

LITERATURE

Hänsel R, Keller K, Rimpler H, Schneider G (Hrsg.), Hagers Handbuch der Pharmazeutischen Praxis, 5. Aufl., Bde 4-6 (Drogen), Springer Verlag Berlin, Heidelberg, New York, 1992-1994 (unter *Veronica virginica*).

Lewin L, Gifte und Vergiftungen, 6. Aufl., Nachdruck, Haug Verlag, Heidelberg 1992.

Madaus G, Lehrbuch der Biologischen Arzneimittel, Bde 1-3, Nachdruck, Georg Olms Verlag Hildesheim 1979.

Wagner H, Wiesenauer M, Phytotherapie. Phytopharmaka und pflanzliche Homöopathika, Fischer-Verlag, Stuttgart, Jena, New York 1995.

Blackberry

Rubus fruticosus

DESCRIPTION

Medicinal Parts: The medicinal parts are the leaves, roots and berries.

Flower and Fruit: The white or sometimes pale pink flowers are in cymes. The calyx is 5-sepaled, the corolla is 5-petalled. There are numerous stamens and ovaries. The small fruit forms a black or reddish-black aggregate fruit.

Leaves, Stem, and Root: The plant is a fast-growing, thorny bush up to 2 m high. The generally blunt stems are densely covered in tough thorns that creep or curve backward. The leaves are usually 5-paired pinnate, glabrous above, and gray-to-white tomentose beneath.

Habitat: The plant is indigenous to Europe and has naturalized in America and Australia.

Production: Blackberry root consists of the underground parts of *Rubus fruticosus* as well as its preparations. Blackberry leaf consists of the dried, fermented, or unfermented leaf gathered during the flowering period of *Rubus fruticosus* as well as its preparations.

Other Names: American Blackberry, Dewberry, Bramble, Goutberry, High Blackberry, Thimbleberry

ACTIONS AND PHARMACOLOGY

COMPOUNDS: BLACKBERRY ROOT

Saponins

Tannins

EFFECTS: BLACKBERRY ROOT

There is no reliable information available.

COMPOUNDS: BLACKBERRY LEAF

Fruit acids: including citric acid, isocitric acid

Flavonoids

Tannins (8 to 14%): gallo tannins, dimeric ellagitannins

EFFECTS: BLACKBERRY LEAF

Blackberry leaf has astringent and antidiarrheal effects due to the high tannin content.

INDICATIONS AND USAGE

BLACKBERRY ROOT

Unproven Uses: Blackberry root is used in folk medicine as a prophylaxis for dropsy. It is also used in gastrointestinal conditions.

BLACKBERRY LEAF

Approved by Commission E:

- Diarrhea
- Inflammation of the mouth and pharynx

Blackberry leaf is used for nonspecific, acute diarrhea and mild inflammation of the mucosa of the oral cavity and throat.

PRECAUTIONS AND ADVERSE REACTIONS

BLACKBERRY ROOT AND LEAF

No health hazards or side effects are known in conjunction with the proper administration of designated therapeutic dosages.

DOSAGE

BLACKBERRY ROOT

No information is available

BLACKBERRY LEAF

Mode of Administration: Blackberry leaf is available as crude drug for infusions and other preparations for internal use, as well as for mouthwashes. The drug is a component of various tea mixtures.

Daily Dosage: 2 to 5 gm drug. To prepare a tea, scald 1.5 gm drug, steep for 10 to 15 minutes, strain (1 teaspoon equivalent to approximately 0.6 gm drug).

LITERATURE

BLACKBERRY LEAF

Brantner A and Grein E. Antibacterial activity of plant extracts used externally in traditional medicine. *J Ethnopharmacol.* 44:35-40. 1994.

Brown JP. A review of the genetic effects of naturally occurring flavonoids, anthraquinones, and related compounds. *Mutation Res.* 75:243-277. 1980.

Henning W, (1981) Lebensm Unters Forsch 173:180.

Gupta RK et al., *J Chem Soc Perkin* I:2525. 1982.

Mukherjee M et al., *PH* 23:2881. 1984.

Wollmann Ch et al., *PA* 19:456. 1964.

BLACKBERRY ROOT

Brantner A and Grein E. Antibacterial activity of plant extracts used externally in traditional medicine. *J Ethnopharmacol.* 44:35-40. 1994.

Brown JP. A review of the genetic effects of naturally occurring flavonoids, anthraquinones, and related compounds. *Mutation Res.* 75:243-277. 1980.

Henning W, (1981) *Lebensm Unters Forsch* 173:180.

Bladderwort

Utricularia vulgaris

DESCRIPTION

Medicinal Parts: The medicinal part is the whole plant.

Flower and Fruit: The vertical peduncle is 10 to 35 cm high and bears 4 to 15 flowers in a loose raceme. The petioles are short and campanulate, 13 to 20 mm long with a bilabiate margin.

Leaves, Stem and Root: Utricularia vulgaris is a water plant. The water shoot is 60 cm long with double-rowed leaves facing all directions. The water leaves are 1 to 8 cm long and have 2 to 3 large lobes. Each lobe is pinnatifid and ends in numerous tips. There are 8 to 209 tubes per leaf.

Habitat: Europe

Production: Bladderwort is the whole plant of *Utricularia vulgaris*.

ACTIONS AND PHARMACOLOGY

COMPOUNDS

Iridoids: including globularin, scutellarioside II

Phenylpropane derivatives: 1-p-cumaroyl-glucoside

EFFECTS

The plant has diuretic, antispasmodic, and anti-inflammatory effects.

INDICATIONS AND USAGE

The drug was formerly used internally in the treatment of urinary tract disorders and externally for burns. The active substances in Bladderwort increase gallbladder secretions; consequently, the drug is used to treat skin and mucous membrane inflammation.

PRECAUTIONS AND ADVERSE REACTIONS

No health hazards or side effects are known in conjunction with the proper administration of designated therapeutic dosages.

DOSAGE

Mode of Administration: The drug is obsolete in many parts of Germany. Bladderwort is used internally and externally in other parts of the world.

Preparation: To prepare a diuretic infusion for internal use, add 2 gm of drug per 100 mL of water. To prepare an anti-inflammatory infusion for external use, add 6 gm of drug per 100 mL of water.

Daily Dosage: Internally, as a diuretic infusion, drink two small cups daily. Externally, the anti-inflammatory infusion is used in mouthwashes, cleansers, cosmetics, and face packs.

LITERATURE

Baumgartner DL, Laboratory evaluation of the bladderwort plant, Utricularia vulgaris (Lentibulariaceae), as a predator of late instar Culex pipiens and assessment of its biocontrol potential. J Am Mosq Control Assoc, 23:504-7, 1987 Sep.

Hegnauer R, Chemotaxonomie der Pflanzen, Bde 1-11: Birkhäuser Verlag Basel, Boston, Berlin 1962-1997.

Bladderwrack

Fucus vesiculosus

DESCRIPTION

Medicinal Parts: The medicinal parts are the dried thallus and the fresh thallus of Bladderwrack.

Flower and Fruit: The reproductive organs are found at the end of the grainy-looking thalli. The fructifications consisting of 3-cm long ovoid receptacles are found in the tips of these thalli. They are either cordate or ovately flattened with grainy bladders.

Leaves, Stem, and Root: The plant is often over 1 m long, olive green when fresh, and black-brown when dry. The stem of the thallus is flat, repeatedly bifurcated and has a midrib along the whole length. Beside this midrib there are often scattered pores and numerous air-filled bladders.

Habitat: The plant is found on the North Sea coast, the western Baltic coast, and on the Atlantic and Pacific coasts.

Production: Bladderwrack consists of the dried thalli of *Fucus vesiculosus, Ascophyllum nodosum*, or of both species, as well as their preparations. The algae are harvested when the tide is out, then washed in fresh water and dried at 60° C.

Other Names: Black-Tang, Bladder Fucus, Cutweed, Fucus, Kelpware, Kelp-Ware, Quercus marina, Rockwrack, Seawrack

ACTIONS AND PHARMACOLOGY

COMPOUNDS

Inorganic iodine salts

Organically-bound iodine: in particular in proteins and lipids, also present as diiodothyrosine

Polysaccharides: including alginic acid, fucane, fucoidine (strongly sulfated)

Polyphenold: Phlorotannins

EFFECTS

The efficacy of Bladderwrack in any therapeutic area is unknown as there are no human studies reported to substantiate or refute its potential applications. In vitro and animal studies suggest Bladderwrack may possess antiviral, anti-inflammatory, antilipidemic, and hypoglycemic activity. It is rarely used alone for any condition because of its mild effects. Bladderwrack has been used in a variety of herbal formulations in Traditional Chinese Medicine (Lee et al, 1998; Liu XY, 1995).

Antibacterial Effects: An unnamed mucopolysaccharide/lectin isolated from Bladderwrack was shown to have bactericidal effects on Escherichia coli and Neisseria meningitidis but not other Enterobacteriaceae in vitro. The minimum bactericidal concentration was 10 mcg/mL. Bacteriostatic effects were observed at 5 mcg/mL. Rates of growth inhibition were 55% to 95% compared to controls at various concentrations; a dose-dependent effect was clearly demonstrated (Criado & Ferreiros, 1984).

Anticoagulant Effects: Fucoidan exhibits anticoagulant activity in vitro mediated by heparin cofactor II. Heparin cofactor II is a potent thrombin inhibitor. Modification of lysyl residues on the fucoidan interfered with its antithrombin activity similarly to such modifications of heparin (Church et al, 1989). Higher fibrinolytic activity was also measured in the more anticoagulant fractions (Durig et al, 1997).

Anti-Inflammatory Effects: Fucoidan reduced pulmonary neutrophil accumulation in rabbit models of acute respiratory distress syndrome and peritonitis, indicating it possesses anti-inflammatory effect (Shimaoka et al, 1996). In three murine models of inflammation, fucoidan inhibited leukocyte migration (Bartlett et al, 1994). Fucoidan largely prevented development of symptomatic demyelinating disease in a rat model (Willenborg & Parish, 1988).

Antilipidemic Effects: Bladderwrack polysaccharides were shown to interfere with hepatic synthesis of low-density lipoprotein (LDL) cholesterol and triglycerides and increase high-density lipoprotein (HDL) cholesterol levels in hyperlipidemic rats. Normolipidemic rats fed 5 mg/kg Bladderwrack extract had no changes in their serum lipid levels compared to untreated controls while those fed 2.5 mg/kg and 10 mg/kg showed reductions in their serum LDL cholesterol levels compared to controls ($p<0.01$ to 0.05). This argued against a dose-dependent effect in healthy rats (Vazquez-Freire et al, 1996b).

Hyperlipidemia was reduced in rats by each of three different polysaccharide fractions of Bladderwrack (Lamela et al, 1996). Orally administered, polysaccharide-rich extracts of Bladderwrack showed minimal hypocholesterolemic and no effect on lowering triglycerides in normal rabbits compared to untreated controls (Lamela et al, 1989).

Antiviral Effects: Fucoidan demonstrated human immunodeficiency virus (HIV) reverse transcriptase (RT) inhibitory activity in vitro. Cells infected with HIV and then exposed to fucoidan or dextran sulfate showed significant decreases in RT activity compared to untreated HIV-infected cells. Incubation of fucoidan with HIV directly also led to a reduction in RT activity. A synergistic depressive effect on RT activity was found when fucoidan and zidovudine (AZT) were added to HIV-infected human cells in vitro. The concentrations used were believed to be attainable in human subjects if fucoidan was administered intramuscularly (Sugawara et al, 1989). Several fractions and constituents in Bladderwrack were shown to inhibit human immunodeficiency virus (HIV), reverse transcriptase (RT), and/or syncytium formation in vitro (Beress et al, 1993).

Hypoglycemic Effects: Polysaccharides from Bladderwrack extracted in a calcium chloride solution lowered plasma glucose levels in normal rabbits compared to untreated subjects. Eight hours after injection, 5 mg/kg and 10 mg/kg of this solution lowered glucose levels 10% to 14%. A polysaccharide extract extracted with hydrochloric acid solution showed hyperglycemic activity. Both solutions were administered intravenously. The calcium chloride solution extract showed a dose-dependent effect. The mechanism of action in this study was not determined (Vazquez-Freire et al, 1996a).

CLINICAL TRIALS

There are no human studies conducted and/or reported using Bladderwrack in any therapeutic applications.

INDICATIONS AND USAGE

Unproven Uses: Preparations of Bladderwrack are used internally for diseases of the thyroid, obesity, overweight, arteriosclerosis, and digestive disorders and externally for sprains. With the availability of prescription thyroid medications that can be dosed precisely and predictably, the use of Bladderwrack in thyroid disease is no longer justifiable.

Homeopathic Uses: In Homeopathy Fucus vesiculosus is used for obesity and goitre.

CONTRAINDICATIONS

Bladderwrack may exacerbate or induce hyperthyroidism, therefore it is contraindicated in patients with known hyperthyroidism.

Pregnancy: Not to be used during pregnancy.

Breastfeeding: Not to be used while breastfeeding.

PRECAUTIONS AND ADVERSE REACTIONS

The long-term use of Bladderwrack is not recommended. Iodine supplements should not be used while taking Bladderwrack.

Exacerbation or induction of hyperthyroidism may occur with Bladderwrack ingestion. Some Bladderwrack products may be contaminated with heavy metals that could cause severe problems such as renal failure. Acne has also been reported with the use of Bladderwrack. Allergic reactions have also been known to occur.

DRUG INTERACTIONS

MODERATE RISK

Anticoagulants, Antiplatelet and Thrombolytic agents, and Low Molecular Weight Heparins: Concurrent use may result in increased risk of bleeding. *Clinical Management:* Avoid simultaneous use.

POTENTIAL INTERACTIONS

Hypoglycemic Medications: Bladderwrack has a hypoglycemic effect. Theoretically, there may be an interaction with other antihyperglycemic medications. *Clinical Management*: Monitor patients carefully if they are concurrently using glucose-lowering agents and Bladderwrack.

DOSAGE

Mode of Administration: Bladderwrack is available as drops and fluid extract for internal use.

How Supplied: Fluid Extract: 1:1

Daily Dosage:

Infusion - single dose: 5 to 10 g 3 times daily.

Extract - single dose: 4 to 8 mL 3 times daily.

Homeopathic Dosage: 5 drops, 1 tablet, or 10 globules every 30 to 60 minutes (acute) and 1 to 3 times daily (chronic); parenterally: 1 to 2 ml sc acute: 3 times daily; chronic: once a day (HAB34).

Maximum daily intake of iodine is limited to 120 mcg.

Storage: Should be protected from light.

LITERATURE

Bartlett MRE, Warren HS, Cowden WB et al. Effects of the anti-inflammatory compounds castanospermine, mannose-6-phosphate and fucoidan on allograft rejection and elicited peritoneal exudates. *Immunol Cell Biol*; 72:367-374. 1994

Béress A, Wassermann O, Bruhn T, Béress L. A new procedure for the isolation of anti-HIV compounds (polysaccharides and polyphenols) from the marine alga *Fucus vesiculosus*. In: *JNP* 56(4):478-488. 1993

Church FC, Meade JB, Treanor RE et al. Antithrombin activity of fucoidan. The interaction of fucoidan with heparin cofactor II, antithrombin III, and thrombin. *J Biol Chem*; 264:3618-3623. 1989

Conz PA, La Greca G, Benedetti P et al. *Fucus vesiculosus:* a nephrotoxic alga. *Nephrol Dial Transplant*; 13:526-527. 1998

Criado MT & Ferreiros CM. Toxicity of an algal mucopolysaccharide for *Escherichia coli* and *Neisseria meningitidis* strains. *Rev Esp Fisiol*; 40:227-230. 1984

Durig J, Bruhn T, Zurborn KH et al. Anticoagulant fucoidan fractions from *Fucus vesiculosus* induce platelet activation in vitro. *Thromb Res*; 85(6):479-91. 1997

Harrell BL & Rudolph AH. Kelp diet: a cause of acneiform eruption. *Arch Dermatol*; 112:560. 1976

Lamela M, Vazquez-Freire MJ & Calleja JM. Isolation and effects on serum lipids of polysaccharide fractions from *Fucus vesiculosus*. *Phytother Res*; 10:S175-176. 1996

Lee EH, Kim NK, Hwang CY et al. Activation of inducible nitric oxide synthase by Yongdam-Sagan-Tang in mouse peritoneal macrophages. *J Ethnopharmacol*; 60(1):61-69. 1998

Liewendahl K & Turula M. Iodide-induced goitre and hypothyroidism in a patient with chronic lymmphocytic tyroiditis. *Acta Endocrinologica*; 71:289-296. 1972

Liu XY. Therapeutic effect of chai-ling-tang (sairei-to) on the steroid-dependent nephrotic syndrome in children. *Am J Chin Med*; 23(3-4):255-60. 1995

Norred CL & Brinker F. Potential coagulation effects of preoperative complementary and alternative medicines. *Alt Ther*; 7(6):58-67. 2001

Okamura K, Inoue K & Omae T. A case of Hashimoto's thyroiditis with thyroid immunological abnormality manifested after habitual ingestion of seaweed. *Acta Endocrinologia*; 88:703-712. 1978

Sharp GJ, Samant HS & Vaidya OC. Selected metal levels of commercially valuable seaweeds adjacent to and distant from point sources of contamination in Nova Scotia and New Brunswick. *Bull Environ Contam Toxicol*; 40:724-730. 1988

Shimaoka M, Ikeda M, Iida T et al. Fucoidan: A potent inhibitor of leukocyte rolling, prevents neutrophil influx into phorbol-ester-induced inflammatory sites in rabbits lungs. *Am J Respir Crit Care Med*; 153:307-311. 1996

Sugawara I & Ishiazaka S. Polysaccharides with sulfate groups are human T-cell mitogens and murine polyclonal B-cell activators (PBAs). I. Fucoidan and heparin. *Cell Immunol*; 74:162-171. 1982

Sugawara I, Itoh W, Mori S et al. Further characterization of sulfated homopolysaccharides as anti-HIV agents. *Experientia*; 45:996-998. 1989

Usui T, Asari K & Mizuno T. Isolation of highly purified ''fucoidan'' from *Eisenia bicyclis* and its anticoagulant and antitumor activities. *Agric Biol Chem*; 44:1965-1966. 1980

Vazquez-Freire MJ, Lamela M & Calleja JM. A preliminary study of hypoglycaemic activity of several polysaccharide extracts from brown algae: *Fucus vesiculosus, Saccorhiza polyschides* and *Laminaria ochroleuca*. *Phytother Res*; 10:S184-185. 1996aVazquez-Freire MJ, Lamela M & Calleja JM. Hypolipidaemic activity of a polysaccharide extract from *Fucus vesiculosus L. Phytother Res*; 10:647-650. 1996b

Willenborg DO & Parish CR. Inhibition of allergic encephalomyelitis in rats by treatment with sulfated polysaccharides. *J Immunol*; 140:3401-3405. 1988

Blessed Thistle

Cnicus benedictus

DESCRIPTION

Medicinal Parts: The dried leaves and upper stems, including the inflorescence, and the flowering parts of the plant.

Flower and Fruit: The blossom is a pale yellow composite, its solitary flower sessile on the tips of the twigs. The florets are tubular. The few lateral florets are sterile, have 3-part borders and are smaller than the numerous androgynous florets. The epicalyx is ovate. The inner bracts end in a long, rigid and pinnatifid thorn. The outer bracts terminate in a simple thorn. They are broad, leafy, and connected with the cordate-oblong leaflets of the epicalyx by numerous weblike hairs. The fruit has a tuft of hair.

Leaves, Stem, and Root: The thistle grows to 30 to 50 cm high. The stems are heavily branched, thistlelike, villous, and glutinous pubescent. The leaves are oblong, emarginate to pinnatifid, thorny-dentate, and roughly reticulate.

Characteristics: The plant has a strong and bitter taste.

Habitat: The thistle comes from southern Europe but is cultivated in other regions of the continent.

Production: Blessed Thistle herb consists of the dried leaves and upper stems, including inflorescence, of *Cnicus benedictus*.

Other Names: St. Benedicts Thistle, Cardin, Holy Thistle, Spotted Thistle

ACTIONS AND PHARMACOLOGY

COMPOUNDS

Sesquiterpene lactone-bitter principles: chief components cnicin, additionally, salonitenolide, artemisiifolin

Lignans (also bitter): trachelogenin, arctigenin, nortracheloside

Volatile oil: components including n-nonane, n-undecane, n-tridecane, dodeca-1,11-dien-3,5,7,9-tetrain (polyyne), p-cymene, fenchon, citral, cinnamaldehyde

Triterpenes: alpha-amyrin, multiflorenol

Flavonoides: including apigenin-7-O-glucoside, luteolin, astragalin

EFFECTS

The main constituent is the amaroid cnicin, which is antimicrobial, cytotoxic and antitumoural. The amaroids stimulate the secretion of saliva and gastric juices. In animal tests an anti-edemic effect was demonstrated.

INDICATIONS AND USAGE

Approved by Commission E:

- Dyspeptic complaints
- Loss of appetite

Unproven Uses: The drug is used as a cholagogue. Internal folk medicine applications include loss of appetite, anorexia, fever and colds, and as a diuretic. External application for wounds and ulcers is noted.

CONTRAINDICATIONS

Not to be used during pregnancy.

PRECAUTIONS AND ADVERSE REACTIONS

Health risks or side effects following the proper administration of designated therapeutic dosages are not recorded. The drug exhibits a strong potential for sensitization (cross-reactions with mugwort and cornflower, among others); however, allergic reactions have been seen only rarely.

DOSAGE

Mode of Administration: Comminuted drug and dried extracts for infusions or other bitter-tasting galenic preparations for internal use.

How Supplied:

Capsules – 340 mg, 360 mg

Extract – 1:1

Tablets

Preparation: The tea is prepared by pouring 150 mL boiling water over 1.5 to 2 gm of drug, allowing to set 5 to 10 minutes.

Daily Dosage: Four to 6 gm of drug. The dosage for the aromatic bitter is 1 cup 1/2 hour before meals. One cup of tea is taken 3 times a day.

LITERATURE

Banhaelen M, Vanhaelen-Fastre R, (1975) *Phytochemistry* 14: 2709.

Farnsworth NR et al., (1975) *J Pharm Sci* 64(4):535.

Harnischfeger G, Stolze H, notabene medici 11:652. 1981.

Urzúa A, Acuna P, (1983) *Fitoterapia* 4:175

Vanhaelen-Fastre R, *PM* 24:165. 1973.

Vanhaelen-Fastre R, Vanhaelen M, (1976) *Planta Med* 29:179.

Bloodroot

Sanguinaria canadensis

DESCRIPTION

Medicinal Parts: The medicinal parts are roots and the whole plant.

Flower and Fruit: The plant bears a white flower with 8 to 12 petals on a 15-cm long scape. It is waxlike and has golden stamens. The seed is an oblong, narrow capsule approximately 2.5 cm long.

Leaves, Stem, and Root: The perennial plant grows to about 15 cm high. The rhizome is thick, round, fleshy and slightly curved at the end. It is 2.5 to 10 cm long and has orange-red rootlets. The 1 basal palmately lobed leaf appears when the flower dies. The down-covered, grayish green leaf is clasping,

15 to 25 cm long, and has 5 to 9 lobes. Protruding ribs are recognizable on the underside.

Habitat: The plant is indigenous to the northeastern U.S.

Production: Canadian Bloodroot is the root stock (rhizome) of *Sanguinaria canadensis.*

Other Names: Indian Paint, Tetterwort, Red Root, Paucon, Coon Root, Snakebite, Sweet Slumber, Indian Plant, Pauson, Sanguinaria

ACTIONS AND PHARMACOLOGY

COMPOUNDS

Isoquinoline alkaloids of the benzophenanthridine type (4-7%): chief alkaloid sanguinarine, further including among others, chelerythrine, oxysanguinarine; protoberberine-type. berberine, coptisine; protopine-type. protopine, alpha- and beta-allocryptopine

Resins

Starch

EFFECTS

Activities documented for Bloodroot are principally attributable to the isoquinoline alkaloid constituents, in particular sanguinarine The basis of sanguinarine activity results from reactions with nucleophiles such as sulfhydryl enzymes. These reactions may produce inhibition of oxidative decarboxylation of pyruvate (Becci et al, 1987). Sanguinarin has been shown to have antimicrobial, anti-inflammatory, and antiplaque properties. Its use as an antiplaque agent and for gingivitis is plausible and has been documented in diverse studies. The alkaloids initially act as a narcotic, causing severe cramping that is followed by a local paralysis of sensitive nerve endings.

Antibiotic Effects: The benzo-(c)phenthridine alkaloids in Bloodroot have antimicrobial action in vitro, but the in vivo effect appears to be weaker (Caolo & Stermitz, 1979; Karjalainen et al, 1988). Electron microscope examination of bacteria exposed to a 1:1 mixture of sanguinarine and chelerythrine showed bacteria aggregation and irregular morphology (Godowski, 1989). Antimicrobial activity of the alkaloid sanguinarine has been documented against both gram-positive and gram-negative bacteria, Candida, and dermatophytes, and Trichomonas (Godowski KC, 1989).

The antibacterial effects of sanguinaria extract are enhanced by zinc and by pH. The optimum pH (in vitro) was 6.5, and the minimum inhibitory concentration (MIC) values were 4 to 8 mcg/mL. When a combination product containing 300 mcg sanguinaria/mL and zinc chloride 0.2% was used, all strains were inhibited (Eisenberg et al, 1991).

Anti-inflammatory Effects: Sanguinarine appears to have greater anti-inflammatory action than does chelerythrine (another benzophenthridine alkaloid) when tested in a carrageenan edema test model (Lenfeld et al, 1981). In another animal study, the number of leukocytes was significantly reduced by a Sanguinaria extract concentration of 0.03%.

Antiplaque Effects: The alkaloid sanguinarine converts to an iminium ion that is negatively charged and is then able to bind to plaques (Fetrow & Avila, 1999) A preparation containing 0.03% sanguinaria extract has been reported to reduce plaque by 20% to 40% by some (Southard et al, 1985; Wennstrom & Lindhe, 1985), and found to have no effect by others.

Sanguinaria has been shown to inhibit several oral microbial isolates that may play a part in plaque formation (Dzink et al, 1985). Glycolysis in saliva is also inhibited. Salivary glycolysis inhibition by sanguinaria was greater than that of chlorhexidine, cetylpyridinium chloride (Cepacol®), etylpyridinium chloride, domiphene bromide (Scope®, and thymol-menthol (Listerine®) (Yankell, 1984; Boulware et al, 1984). Sanguinarine is retained in plaque above the minimum inhibitory concentration (MIC) for up to 2 hours after administration, and levels in plaque may be up to 100 times its level in saliva. In theory, this may kill plaque micro-organism without changing the rest of the oral flora (Swanbom & Davison, 1987; Southard et al, 1984).

Sanguinaria was assayed against 52 reference strains for oral bacteria. Additionally, 129 subgingival plaque isolates were taken from periodontal pockets and tested to determine the minimum inhibitory concentrations (MIC). Sanguinarine was found to have a minimum inhibitory concentration (MIC) of 1 to 16 micrograms/milliliters (mcg/mL) in 98% of the organisms tested. Ninety-eight percent of isolates were killed at 32 mcg/mL (Dzink & Socransky, 1985). Examples of various MICs include Actinobacillus species (8 to 16 micrograms/milliliter) (mcg/mL).

Bone Resorption Effects: Collagenase formation and subsequent bone resorption stimulated by parathyroid hormone was inhibited in cultures of mouse calvaria bone treated with 20 mmol/liter of sanguinarine (Sakamoto, 1986). In vitro inhibition of bone resorption and collagenase has been documented (Godowski KC, 1989).

Effects on Enzymes: Sanguinarine inhibits a variety of enzymes such as collagenase, aminotransferase, and butyryl- and acetylcholinesterases (Keller & Meyer, 1989; Ulrichova et al, 1983; Ulrichova et al, 1983a). Sanguinarine is an inhibitor of the transcription nuclear factor kappa B (NF-kB). Activation of NF-kB may result in inflammation, viral replication, and growth changes (Chaturvedi et al, 1997). Sanguinarine was an inhibitor of liver alanine (ALT) and aspartate (AST) aminotransferase in rat liver postmitochondrial supernatant (Walterova et al, 1981).

CLINICAL TRIALS

Many studies have investigated the efficacy of Bloodroot extracts in oral hygiene. Preparations containing Bloodroot extracts, such as oral rinses and toothpastes, have been reported to significantly lower plaque, gingival, and bleeding indices. Alteration of the oral microbial flora, or development of resistant microbial strains, has not been observed with the use of Bloodroot extracts.

Dental Plaque

Benzophenanthridine alkaloids were found to be better retained in plaque if the period of rinsing with a Bloodroot-containing rinse was increased (Harkrader et al, 1990). In another study by the same investigator the percent of total benzophenanthridine alkaloids retained did not change significantly when the concentration of sanguinarine in a dental rinse was increased, but the total amount of alkaloid retained and total plaque retention of the alkaloids did increase (Harkrader et al, 1990).

In a 6-month, double-blind, 4-cell, placebo-controlled, parallel study of 120 subjects, products containing sanguinaria extract and zinc chloride were statistically ($p<0.0001$) superior as antiplaque agents when compared with controls (Kopczyk et al, 1991).

In a double-blind, placebo-controlled study, the differences between rinses and either the baseline levels or controls was significant at the $p<0.05$ level. Rinses were given to subjects and compared to controls. The level of sanguinarine in both plague and saliva varied from person to person, and day to day, but in general sanguinarine levels were greater in plague than in saliva (Southard et al, 1984).

In a double-blind, randomized, multicenter, crossover study involving 60 subjects who used a sanguinaria-containing toothpaste followed by a sanguinaria-containing rinse, 80% had measurable improvement in plaque. This compares to a 17% improvement, using the same procedures, with commercial toothpaste and tap water rinse (Greenfield & Cuchel, 1984).

A sanguinarine-containing dentifrice was not more effective antiplaque agent than regular toothpaste in one placebo-controlled study (Schonfeld et al, 1986). Sanguinarine-containing mouthwash was not found to reduce gingivitis in a 21-day study of subjects with clean teeth and healthy gums who refrained from oral hygiene for the 21 days of the study (Siegrist et al, 1986).

INDICATIONS AND USAGE

Unproven Uses: The drug was formerly used as an expectorant, but due to its potential toxicity it is no longer considered for this purpose. Bloodroot is an active antiplaque agent, and an effective mouthwash. Taken internally Bloodroot is used to treat bacterial overgrowth in the small bowel. Its high alkaloid and tannin content account for most of Sanguinaria's strong antibacterial properties. Bloodroot is also used in bronchitis, asthma, croup, in certain neoplastic diseases, and topically as anti-inflammatory agent.

CONTRAINDICATIONS

Pregnancy: Not to be used during pregnancy.

PRECAUTIONS AND ADVERSE REACTIONS

Note: The FDA has ruled Bloodroot to be unsafe for use in foods, drugs, herbals, and beverages (Fetrow & Avila, 1999). Dizziness, vertigo, nausea, and vomiting are all possible side effects of Bloodroot.

OVERDOSE

The drug has an emetic effect in dosages above 0.03 g. Vomiting after an overdose may limit more serious signs of toxicity. Shock, hypotension, and coma have been reported in overdoses given to animals. In addition, high dosages of the drug severely irritate the mucous membranes and may cause diarrhea, intestinal colic, and possible collapse. In vitro toxicity studies using cultured cells lines derived from human oral tissues showed that a 3-hour exposure to sanguinarine ($\geq$0.1274 mmol) caused damage to the plasma membranes of the cells and caused leakage of lactic acid dehydrogenase. The toxicity was increased as the pH was increased from 6 to 7.8 (Babich et al, 1996).

DOSAGE

Mode of Administration: The drug is obsolete in most countries. Bloodroot is still used in homeopathic preparations, as an ingredient in some pharmaceutical preparations, and as a component of toothpaste and mouthwashes.

How Supplied: Liquid extract

LITERATURE

Arnason JT, Guerin B, Kraml MM et al. Phototoxic and photochemical properties of sanguinarine. *Photochem Photobiol*; 55(1):35-38. 1992

Babich H, Zuckerbraun HI, Barber IB et al. Cytotoxicity of sanguinarine chloride to cultured human cells form oral tissue. *Pharmacol Toxicol*; 78(6):397-403. 1996

Becci PJ, Schwartz H, Barnes HH et al. Short-term toxicity studies of sanguinarine and of two alkaloid extracts of *Sanguinaria canadensis L. J Toxicol Environ Health*; 20(1-2):199-208. 1987

Bodalski T, Pelczarska H & Vjec M. Action of some alkaloids of *C. majus* on *Trichomonas vaginalis* in vitro. *Arch Immunol Ter Dosw*; 6:705-711. 1958

Boulware RT, Southard GL, Walborn D et al. Salivary glycolysis testing of sanguinarine chloride, chlorhexidine and other antimicrobials (abstract 1274, IADR/AADR). *J Dent*; 63(special issue):312. 1984

Caolo MR & Stermitz FR. Benzophenanthridinium salt equilibria. *Heterocycles*; 12(1):11-15. 1979

Chaturvedi MM, Kumar A, Darnay BG et al. Sanguinarine (pseudochelerythrine) is a potent inhibitor of NF-kB activation, IkBa phosphorylation, and degradation. *J Biol Chem*; 272(48):30129-30134. 1997

Dzink JL, Socransky SS, Boulware RT et al. Comparative in vitro activity of sanguinarine against oral microbial isolates. *J Dent Res*; 64(special issue):212. 1985

Eisenberg AD, Young DA, Fan-Hsu J et al. Interactions of sanguinarine and zinc on oral streptococci and *Actinomyces* species. *Caries Res*; 25(3):185-190. 1991

Fetro CW and Avila JR (eds). Professional's Handbook of Complementary and Alternative Medicine. Springhouse Corp., Springhouse, PA. 1999

Frankos VH, Brusick DJ, Johnson EM et al. Safety of Sanguinaria extract as used in commercial toothpaste and oral rinse products. *J Can Dent Assoc*; 56(7 suppl):41-47. 1990

Godowski KC. Antimicrobial actions of sanguinarine. *J Clin Dent*; 1(4):96-101. 1989

Greenfield W & Cuchel SJ. The use of an oral rinse and dentifrice as a system for reducing dental plaque. *Compend Contin Educ Dent*; Suppl 5:82-86. 1984

Harkrader RJ, Reinhart PC, Rogers JA et al. The history, chemistry and pharmacokinetics of sanguinaria extract. *J Can Dent Assoc*; 56(suppl 7):7-12. 1990

Karjalainen K, Kaivosoja S, Seppa S et al. Effects of sanguinaria extract on leucocytes and fibroblasts. Proc Finn Dent Soc; 84(3):161-165. 1988

Karlowsky JA. Bloodroot. *Sanguinaria canadensis L. CPJ/RPC*; May:260-267. 1991

Keller KA & Meyer DL. Reproductive and developmental toxicology evaluation of sanguinaria extract. *J Clin Dent*; 1(3):59-66. 1989

Kopczyk RA, Abrams H, Brown AT et al. Clinical and microbiological effects of a sanguinarine-containing mouthrinse and dentifrice with and without fluoride during 6 months of use. *J Periodontol*; 62(10):617-622. 1991

Lenfeld J, Kroutil M, Marsalek E et al. Antiinflammatory activity of quaternary benzophenanthridine alkaloids from *Chelidonium majus. Planta Med*; 43(2):161-165. 1981

Nandi R, Maiti M, Chaudhuri K et al. Sensitivity of vibrios to sanguinarine. *Experientia*; 39(5):524. 1983

Palcanis KG, Sarbin AG, Koertge TE et al. Longitudinal evaluation of the effect of sanguinarine on plaque and gingivitis. *Gen Dent*; 38(1):17-19. 1990

Sakamoto S. Studies of sanguinarine in bone resorption models. *Compend Contin Educ Dent*; Suppl 7:S221-S223,S226. 1986

Schonfeld SE, Farnoush A & Wilson SG. In vivo antiplaque activity of a sanguinarine-containing dentifrice comparison with conventional toothpastes. *J Periodont Res*; 21(3):298-303. 1986

Schwartz HG. Safety profile of sanguinarine and Sanguinaria extract. *Compend Cont Educ Dent Suppl*; 7. S212-S217. 1986

Siegrist BE, Gusberti FA, Brecx M et al. Efficacy of supervised rinsing with chlorhexidine digluconate in comparison to phenolic and plant alkaloid compounds. *J Periodont Res*; 21(suppl):60-73. 1986

Southard GL, Boulware RT, Walborn DR et al. Sanguinarine, a new antiplaque agent, retention and plaque specificity. *J Am Dent Assoc*; 108(3):338-341. 1984Southard GL, Parsons LG & Thomas LG. The antiplaque efficacy of a sanguinarine oral rinse. (IAD/AADR abstract 549*). J Dent Res*; 64:236. 1985

Straub KD & Carver P. Sanguinarine, inhibitor of Na-K-dependent ATP'ase. *Biochem Biophys Res Commun*; 62(4):913-922. 1975

Swanbom DD & Davison CO. Crevicular delivery of sanguinaria to control gingivitis. *J Am Dent Assoc*; 114(5):591-594. 1987

Tin-Wa M, Farnsworth NR, Fong HHS et al. Biological and phytochemical evaluation of plants. VIII (8). isolation of a new alkaloid from Sanguinaria canadensis. *Lloydia*; 33(2):267-269. 1970

Ulrichova J, Walterova D, Preininger V et al. Inhibition of acteylcholinesterase activity by some isoquinolone alkaloids. *Planta Med*; 48(2):111-115. 1983a

Ulrichova J, Walterova D, Preininger V et al. Inhibition of butyrylcholinesterase activity by some isoquinioline alkaloids. *Planta Med*; 48(3):174-177. 1983

Walterova D, Ulrichova J, Preininger V et al. Inhibition of liver alanine aminotransferase activity by some benzophenanthridine alkaloids. *J Med Chem*; 24(9):1100-1103. 1981

Wennstrom J & Lindhe J. Some effects of a Sanguinarine-containing mouthrinse on developing plaque and gingivitis. *J Clin Periodontol*; 12(10):867-872. 1985

Yankell SL. Saliva glycolysis and plaque. *Compend Contin Educ Dent*; Suppl 5:57-60. 1984

Blue Cohosh

Caulophyllum thalictroides

DESCRIPTION

Medicinal Parts: Medicinal parts are the dried rhizome and roots and preparations of the fresh roots.

Flower and Fruit: The inflorescence on the terminal leaf is panicled, 3 to 6 cm long and surrounded by a leaflike bract. The flowers are yellowish-green to purple and are 1 cm in diameter. The 6 sepals are arranged in 2 rows. The 6 petals are markedly reduced, inconspicuous, and glandlike. The 6 stamens are as long as the petals. The ovary opens before it is ripe and contains 2 dark blue, 5- to 8-mm long, roundish seeds on solid stems. These resemble drupes because of the fleshy seed-shell.

Leaves, Stem, and Root: The plant is a leafy, 30- to 70-cm high erect perennial with a brownish-gray, branched rhizome. The leaves are inserted in the middle of the shoot with a large, almost sessile leaf, which is tripinnate. The leaflets are stemmed, obovate, and finely divided into 3 lobes; they are wedge-shaped at the base.

Characteristics: Taste is sweetish, then bitter; almost odorless.

Habitat: The plant is found in the damp woods of the eastern part of North America.

Production: Blue Cohosh is the dried root and rootstock of *Caulophyllum thalictroides*. It is collected in the wild.

Other Names: Beechdrops, Blue Ginseng, Blueberry Root, Papoose Root, Squawroot, Yellow Ginseng

ACTIONS AND PHARMACOLOGY

COMPOUNDS

Quinolizidine alkaloids: main alkaloids (-)-anagyrines, (-)-N-methyl-cytisines, and (-)-baptifoline

Isoquinoline alkaloids: magnoflorine

Triterpene saponins: caulophyllosaponin

Caulosapogenin

EFFECTS

A number of different alkaloids have been identified in the roots and rhizomes, namely the lupin alkaloids methylcytisine, baptifoline, and anagyrine, and the aporphine alkaloid magnoflorine. Animal or in vitro studies have shown some contraceptive, oxytocic, nicotinic, and partus preparatory properties. When evaluating this herb differentiate between the herb itself and studies of its alkaloids and glycosides constituents.

Nicotinic Effects: Methylcytisine, an alkaloid found in Blue Cohosh, was found to have pharmacologic actions similar to, but weaker than (1/25), those of nicotine, causing an elevation in blood pressure and stimulating both respiration and intestinal motility (Betz et al, 1998). Anagyrine and other such alkaloids have shown affinity for both the nicotinic and muscurinic receptor. Anagyrine displaced 50% of the ligands from the binding site at a concentration of about 2096 mmol for the nicotinic site and 132 mmol at the muscarinic receptor. Thus it is a stronger muscarinic than nicotinic agent (Schmeller et al, 1994). Methylcytisine is stated to have a nicotinic-like action, causing an elevation in blood pressure and stimulating both respiration and intestinal motility (Tyler et al 1993).

Uterine Stimulant Effects: Blue Cohosh infusions in concentrations of 500:1 or 1000:1, and fluid Caulosaponin and caulophyllosaponin, two glycosides found in Blue Cohosh, are uterine stimulants via smooth muscle contraction and appear to produce pharmacological effects similar to oxytocin (McFarlin et al, 1999; Jones & Lawson, 1998).

Antifertility actions documented in rats were reported to be caused by inhibition of ovulation and by interruption of implantation. (Chaudrasekhar et al. 1974). Smooth muscle stimulation has been documented for a crystalline glycoside constituent the coronary blood vessels (in vivo) of various small mammals (Ferguson, et al 1954) Caulosaponin is reported to possess oxytocic properties. (Tyler VE, 1993)

CLINICAL TRIALS

No human clinical trials of Blue Cohosh are recorded.

INDICATIONS AND USAGE

Unproven Uses: Native Americans used the herb for amenorrhea, dysmenorrhea, threatened miscarriage, contraction-like spasms, rheumatic symptoms, and conditions resulting from uterus atonia. None of these uses have been proved.

Homeopathic Uses: Uses include problems of menstruation and labor, as well as rheumatism of the fingers and toes.

CONTRAINDICATIONS

Blue Cohosh is contraindicated in the presence of heart disease.

Pregnancy: Not to be used during pregnancy.

PRECAUTIONS AND ADVERSE REACTIONS

Blue Cohosh may cause cardiac toxicity (Jones & Lawson, 1998). Tachycardia and myocardial infarction was reported with the association of Blue Cohosh. The most common adverse reactions reported with the use of Blue Cohosh are nausea, vomiting, abdominal pain, intestinal spasm, diarrhea, weakness, ketonuria, dermatitis, and diaphoresis.

DRUG INTERACTIONS

No drug interaction data is available.

OVERDOSAGE

Toxic effects of the Blue Cohosh constituent methylcytisine include tachycardia, hypotension, increased gastrointestinal motility, coronary vasoconstriction, and respiratory depression due to a curare-like muscle paralysis (Jones & Lawson, 1998).

DOSAGE

Mode of Administration: The drug is used internally as a decoction or a liquid extract.

How Supplied:

Liquid – 1:1

Preparation: Infusion (no specifications); liquid extract 1:1 in ethanol 70% (V/V)

Daily Dosage: The average single dose is 0.3 to 1 g of drug; 0.5 to 1 mL of liquid extract.

Homeopathic Dosage: 5 drops, 1 tablet, 10 globules 30 to 60 minutes (acute) or 1 to 3 times a day (chronic); parenterally: 1 to 2 mL 3 times a day sc (HAB34).

LITERATURE

Baillie N & Rasmussen P. Black and blue cohosh in labour. *N Z Med J*; 110(1036):20-21. 1997

Benoit PS et al, *Lloydia;* 39:160. 1976

Betz JM, Andrzejewski D, Troy A et al. Gas chromatographic determination of toxic quinolizidine alkaloids in blue cohosh *Caulophyllum thalictroides* (L.) Michx. *Phytochem Anal*; 9:232-236. 1998

Chaudrasekhar K, Raa Vishwanath C. Studies on the effect of Caulophyllum on implantation in rats. *J Reprod Fertil*; 38:245-246. 1974

Chaudrasekhar K, Sarma GHR. Observations on the effect of low and high doses of Caulophyllum on the ovaries and the consequential changes in the uterus and thyroid in rats. *J Reprod Fertil*; 38:236-237. 1974

Di Carlo FI et al., *J Reticuloendothelial Soc*; 1:224.1964

Farnsworth NR. Potential value of plants as sources of new antifertility agents I. *J Pharm Sci*; 64:535-598. 1975

Ferguson HC, Edwards LD. A pharmacological study of a crystalline glycoside *of Caulophyllum thalictroides. J Am Pharm Assoc*; 43:16-21. 1954

Flom MS, Doskotch RW & Beal JL. Isolation and characterization of alkaloids *from Caulophyllum thalictroides. J Pharm Sci*; 56(11):1515-1517. 1967

Flynn TJ, Kennelly EJ, Mazzola EP et al. Screening of the dietary supplement blue cohosh for potentially teratogenic alkaloids using rat embryo culture. *Teratology*; 57:219. 1998

Gunn TR & Wright MR. The use of black and blue cohosh in labour. *N Z Med J*; 109(1032): 410-411. 1996

Jones TK & Lawson BM. Profound neonatal congestive heart failure caused by maternal consumption of blue cohosh herbal medication. *J Pediatr*; 132(3 pt 1):550-552. 1998

Lepik K. Safety of herbal medications in pregnancy. *CPJ-RPC*; April: 29-33. 1997

McFarlin BL, Gibson MH, O'Rear J et al. A national survey of herbal preparation use by nurse-midwives for labor stimulation: review of the literature and recommendations for practice. *J Nurse Midwifery*; 44(3):205-216. 1999

McShefferty J & Stenlake JB. Caulosapogenin and its identity with hederagenin. *J Chem Soc*; 62(pt 2):2314-2316. 1956

Ortega JA & Lazerson J. Anagyrine-induced red cell aplasia, vascular anomaly, and skeletal dysplasia. *J Pediatr*; 111(1):87-89. 1987

Rao RB, Hoffman RS, Desiderio R et al: Nicotinic toxicity from tincture of blue cohosh (Caulophyllum thalictroides) used as an abortifaciant. *J Toxicol Clin Toxicol*; 36(5):455. 1998

Schmeller T, Sauerwein M, Sporer F et al. Binding of quinozolidine alkaloids to nicotinic and muscarinic acetylcholine receptors. *J Nat Prod*; 57(9):1316-1319. 1994

Scott CC & Chen KK. The pharmacological action of N-methylcytisine. *J Pharmacol Exp Ther*; 79(4):334-339. 1943

Bog Bean

Menyanthes trifoliata

DESCRIPTION

Medicinal Parts: The medicinal part of the plant is the dried herb.

Flower and Fruit: The flowers are white or reddish-white, medium-sized, and have many blossomed racemes on long, leafless peduncles. There are 5 sepals. The corolla is fused with 5 tips and is pubescent inside. There are 5 reddish stamens and 1 superior ovary. The fruit is an ovate capsule.

Leaves, Stem, and Root: Menyanthes trifoliata is a perennial green, glabrous aquatic plant that grows from 15 to 30 cm high. The herb has a small, finger-thick creeping rhizome. The decumbent stem varies in length according to conditions. Leaf sheaths surround the stem. The leaves are on long, fleshy, grooved petioles. They are trifoliate, 5 cm long and 2.5 cm wide, and have obovate leaflets.

Characteristics: The herb has a strong bitter taste.

Habitat: The plant is indigenous to Europe, Asia and America.

Production: Bog Bean leaf consists of the leaf of *Menyanthes trifoliata.*

Other Names: Buck Bean, Bog Myrtle, Brook Bean, Marsh Clover, Moonflower, Trefoil, Water Shamrock

ACTIONS AND PHARMACOLOGY

COMPOUNDS

Iridoide monoterpenes (bitter principles): chief components 7′, 8′-dihydrofoliamenthin, additionally including among others sweroside, loganin, menthiafolin, foliomenthin

Monoterpene alkaloids: including gentianin E

Flavonoids: including among others rutin, hyperoside, trifolin

Hydroxycoumarins: scopoletin

Caffeic acid derivatives

Pyrridine alkaloids: including gentianine, gentianidine

Triterpene glycosides: lupeol, beta-amyrenol, betulin, betulinic acid, alpha-spinasterol, stigmast-7-enol

EFFECTS

The drug stimulates saliva and gastric juice secretion. An antimicrobial effect has been demonstrated in vitro.

INDICATIONS AND USAGE

Approved by Commission E:

- Dyspeptic complaints
- Loss of appetite

Because it is a bitter and promotes gastric secretion, the drug is used for loss of appetite and peptic discomfort.

Unproven Uses: Folk medicine uses, particularly in European countries, include diseases of the digestive system and fevers.

Chinese Medicine: Insomnia, weak stomach and intestines, spleen disorders, intermittent fever, headache, breathing difficulties, amenorrhea, ear ache, jaundice, edema, gout, scabies, and furuncles are among the applications in Chinese medicine.

CONTRAINDICATIONS

Use of the drug is contraindicated for patients with diarrhea, dysentery, or colitis.

PRECAUTIONS AND ADVERSE REACTIONS

No health hazards or side effects are known in conjunction with the proper administration of designated therapeutic dosages.

OVERDOSAGE

Symptoms of overdose include vomiting and diarrhea.

DOSAGE

Mode of Administration: Comminuted herb for teas and other bitter-tasting preparations for internal use.

Preparation: Pour boiling water over 0.5 to 1 g of the finely cut drug (1 teaspoonful = 0.9 g) or place the drug in cold water and bring rapidly to a boil. Allow either preparation to steep for 5 to 10 minutes, then strain.

How Supplied: The drug is a component of standardized preparations of various tonics.

Daily Dosage: The average daily dose is 1.5 to 3 g of the drug. The dosage for the infusion is 1/2 cup, unsweetened, before each meal.

LITERATURE

Adamczyk U, Brown SA, Lewars EG, Swiatek L. Lactones of *Menyanthes trifoliate. Plant Med et Phyte*. 24:73-78. 1990.

Brantner A and Grein E. Antibacterial activity of plant extracts used externally in traditional medicine. *J Ethnopharmacol*. 44:35-40. 1994.

Battersby AR et al., (1967) *J Chem Soc Chem Commun*. 1277.

Ciaceri G, (1972) *Fitoterapia* 43:134.

Janeczko Z et al., A triterpenoid glycoside from Menyanthes trifoliata. In: *PH* 29(12):3885-3887. 1990.

Junior P, Weitere Untersuchungen zur Verteilung und Straktur der Bitterstoffe von *Menyanthes trifoliata*. In: *PM* 32(12):112. 1989.

Phillipson JD, Anderson LA, (1984) *Pharm J* 233:80 et 111.

Swaitek L et al., (1986) *Planta Med* 6:60P.

Tumón H et al., The effect of *Menyanthes trifolita L.* on acute renal failure might due to PAF-inhibition. In: *Phytomedicine* 1:39-45. 1994.

Bog Bilberry

Vaccinium uliginosum

DESCRIPTION

Medicinal Parts: The medicinal part is the dried ripe fruit.

Flower and Fruit: The flowers are arranged in axils of small leaves at the end of short lateral branches. They are hanging and white or reddish in color. The pedicle is encircled at the base with a light brown bud husk. The calyx is fused with the ovary. The fruit is a round or pear-shaped, blue-frosted, 7 to 10 cm long, multiseeded berry. The light brown seeds are sickle-shaped, with sharp ends and punctate-reticulate skin.

Leaves, Stem, and Root: The plant is an angular shrub up to 80 cm high with round, gray-brown, glabrous branches and a creeping rhizome. The leaves are deciduous, obovate or oblong, entire, tough and short-petioled. The undersurface has a protruding, reticulate vein system and is blue-green. The upper surface of the leaves is light matte-green to almost white.

Habitat: The plant is common throughout the Northern Hemisphere.

Production: Bog Bilberries and leaves are the ripe fruit and leaves of *Vaccinium uliginosum*. The collection or picking occurs in uncultivated regions. The drug is either air-dried in the shade or dried artificially.

Not to be Confused With: The Bog Bilberry has smaller flowers and berries than the common Bilberry (*Vaccinium myrtillus*; see separate entry).

ACTIONS AND PHARMACOLOGY

COMPOUNDS: IN THE LEAVES

Tannins: catechin tannins

Triterpenes: alpha-amyrin, friedelin, ursolic acid

Sterols: beta-sitosterol, beta-sitosterol-3-O-beta-glucoside

Flavonoids: including hyperoside

COMPOUNDS: IN THE FRUITS

Anthocyans: including chief components: malvidin-3-O-glucoside, delphinidine-3-O-glucoside, delphinidine-3-O-arabinoside

Organic acids: including benzoic acid

Flavonoids: including hyperoside, myricetin, myricetin-5′-methyl ether

EFFECTS

No information is available.

INDICATIONS AND USAGE

Unproven Uses: Bog Bilberry is used for gastric and intestinal catarrh, diarrhea, and bladder complaints.

PRECAUTIONS AND ADVERSE REACTIONS

No health hazards or side effects are known in conjunction with the proper administration of designated therapeutic dosages.

OVERDOSAGE

Signs of poisoning following consumption of large quantities of the fruits have occurred very rarely. Signs include nausea, vomiting, states of intoxication, feelings of weakness, and visual disorders. Presumably, these poisonings can be traced back to the plant being infested with the lower fungus *Sclerotinia megalospora*.

DOSAGE

Mode of Administration: The drug is used internally as a liquid extract (tea).

Preparation: To prepare a tea, pour 250 mL of cold water over 2 heaping teaspoons of drug; steep for 10 to 12 hours and strain.

Daily Dosage: Drink 1 cup of the prepared tea, unsweetened, once or twice a day.

LITERATURE

Frohne D, Pfänder HJ, Giftpflanzen - Ein Handbuch für Apotheker, Toxikologen und Biologen, 4. Aufl., Wiss. Verlags-Ges. Stuttgart 1997.

Hänsel R, Keller K, Rimpler H, Schneider G (Hrsg.), Hagers Handbuch der Pharmazeutischen Praxis, 5. Aufl., Bde 4-6 (Drogen): Springer Verlag Berlin, Heidelberg, New York, 1992-1994.

Lewin L, Gifte und Vergiftungen, 6. Aufl., Nachdruck, Haug Verlag, Heidelberg 1992.

Roth L, Daunderer M, Kormann K, Giftpflanzen, Pflanzengifte, 4. Aufl., Ecomed Fachverlag Landsberg Lech 1993.

Teuscher E, Lindequist U, Giftstoffe mikrobieller Endo- und Epiphyten. Gefahren für Mensch und Tier. In: *DAZ* 132(42):2231. 1992.

Boldo

Peumus boldo

DESCRIPTION

Medicinal Parts: The medicinal parts are the leaves.

Flower and Fruit: The inflorescences are racemes of whitish or pinkish campanulate flowers. The berries are small, yellowish-green and edible.

Leaves, Stem, and Root: The plant is a strongly aromatic, heavily branched evergreen shrub 5 to 6 m tall. The leaves are sessile, opposite, oval, about 5 cm long with an entire and slightly revolute margin. They are rather thick and coriaceous with a protruding midrib and a row of small glands on the upper surface. Both surfaces are slightly pubescent.

Characteristics: Boldo has a bitter, aromatic odor and a camphoraceous, lemony taste.

Habitat: The plant is indigenous to Chile and Peru. It is naturalized in mountainous Mediterranean regions and on the western coast of the U.S.

Production: Boldo leaf consists of the dried leaves of *Peumus boldus*.

Other Names: Boldu, Boldus

ACTIONS AND PHARMACOLOGY

COMPOUNDS

Isoquinoline alkaloids of the aporphine type (0.25-0.5%): main alkaloid boldine (0.1%)

Volatile oil (2-3%): chief components are p-cymene, cineol, ascaridiole

Flavonoids: including rhamnetin-3-O-arabinoside-3′-O-rhamnoside (peumoside), isorhamnetin-3-O-glucoside-7-O-rhamnoside (boldoside), isorhamnetin dirhamnoside (fragroside)

EFFECTS

Boldo has been shown to be antispasmodic, choleretic, and to increase gastric secretions.

INDICATIONS AND USAGE

Approved by Commission E:

- Dyspeptic complaints

CONTRAINDICATIONS

Boldo is contraindicated in patients with bile duct obstruction and those with severe liver diseases. Patients who have gallstones should consult a physician before using the drug.

PRECAUTIONS AND ADVERSE REACTIONS

No health hazards or side effects are known in conjunction with the proper administration of designated therapeutic dosages. The volatile oil should not be used, because it contains up to 40% of the toxin ascaridole.

OVERDOSAGE

Signs of paralysis are reported to appear following intake of very high dosages. A case is described in the older scientific literature in which depression, color hallucinations, sound hallucinations and partial motor aphasia occurred following the consumption of boldine over a period of months.

DOSAGE

Mode of Administration: Comminuted herb for infusions and other, virtually ascaridol-free preparations for internal application. Because of the ascaridol content, essential oil and distillates of Boldo leaf should not be used.

Preparation: Pour 150 mL of hot water over 1 to 2 gm of the drug, steep for 10 to 15 minutes.

Daily Dosage: The average daily dosage is 4.5 gm. Tea: 1 cup 2 to 3 times daily.

LITERATURE

Betts TJ, *J Chromatogr* 511:373. 1990.

Bombardelli E et al., (1976) *Fitoterapia* 47:3.

Gotteland A, Jimenez I, Brunser O, Guzman L, Romero S, Cassels BK, Speisky H. Protective effect of boldine in experimental colitis. *Planta Med* 63(4): 311-315. 1997.

Hue B, Corronc Hle Kuballa B, Anton R. Effects of the natural alkaloid boldine on cholinergic receptors of the insect central nervous system. *Pharm Pharmacol Lett* 3: 169-172. 1994

Kern W, List PH, Hörhammer L (Eds.), Hagers Handbuch der Pharmazeutischen Praxis, 4. Aufl., Bde. 1-8, Springer Verlag Berlin, Heidelberg, New York, 1969.

Kreitmar H, (1952) *Pharmazie* 7:507.

Leung AY, Encyclopedia of Common Natural Ingredients Used in Food Drugs and Cosmetics, John Wiley & Sons Inc., New York 1980.

Madaus G, Lehrbuch der Biologischen Arzneimittel, Bde 1-3, Nachdruck, Georg Olms Verlag Hildesheim 1979.

Reuter HD, Pflanzliche Gallentherapeutika (Teil I) und (Teil II). In: *ZPT* 16(1):13-20 u. 77-89. 1995.

Roth L, Daunderer M, Kormann K, Giftpflanzen, Pflanzengifte, 4. Aufl., Ecomed Fachverlag Landsberg Lech 1993.

Schulz R, Hänsel R, Rationale Phytotherapie, Springer Verlag Heidelberg 1996.

Steinegger E, Hänsel R, Pharmakognosie, 5. Aufl., Springer Verlag Heidelberg 1992.

Teuscher E, Biogene Arzneimittel, 5. Aufl., Wiss. Verlagsges. Stuttgart 1997.

Urzúa A, Acuna P, (1983) Fitoterapia 4:175.

Wichtl M (Eds.), Teedrogen, 4. Aufl., Wiss. Verlagsges. Stuttgart 1997.

Wolters B, Arzneipflanzen und Volksmedizin Chiles. In: *DAZ* 134(39):3693. 1994.

Boneset

Eupatorium perfoliatum

DESCRIPTION

Medicinal Parts: The medicinal part is the herb after flowering.

Flower and Fruit: There are numerous flower heads in terminal, large, and slightly convex cymose-paniculate inflorescences. They consist of 10 to 12 white, inconspicuous florets with bristly pappus whose hairs are arranged in a single row. The fruit is a tufted achene.

Leaves, Stem, and Root: Eupatorium perfoliatum is a perennial herb with a horizontal hairy rootstock. The stems are rough-haired and grow to about 1.5 m. The leaves are opposite, 10 to 15 cm long, lanceolate, crenate, tapering to narrow point and fused at the base. They have shiny yellow points due to the resin glands, which are visible on the undersurface.

Characteristics: The taste is astringent and persistently bitter.

Habitat: The herb is indigenous to the eastern U.S.

Production: Boneset is the complete aerial part of *Eupatorium perfoliatum.*

Other Names: Agueweed, Crosswort, Feverwort, Indian Sage, Sweating Plant, Teasel, Thoroughwort, Vegetable Antimony

ACTIONS AND PHARMACOLOGY

COMPOUNDS

Flavonoids: including eupatorin, astragalin, rutin, hyperoside

Sesquiterpene lactones: including eupafolin, euperfolitin, eufoliatin, eufoliatorin, euperfolide

Immunostimulating polysaccharides (heteroxylans)

EFFECTS

The herb acts as an antiphlogistic, a diaphoretic, and a bitter, in addition to stimulating the body's immune system. In a comparative study of the homeopathic preparation Eupatorium D2 with aspirin in the treatment of feverish catarrh, a similar positive tendency was observed. In vitro, the phagocytic action of granulocytes was increased.

INDICATIONS AND USAGE

Unproven Uses: On rare occasions, Boneset is used in folk medicine.

Homeopathic Uses: Boneset is used as a treatment for flu and febrile diseases.

PRECAUTIONS AND ADVERSE REACTIONS

Health risks or side effects following the proper administration of designated therapeutic dosages are not recorded. Sensitization after skin contact with the plant is possible. Older scientific literature (Lewin) calls attention to the fact that the drug can lead to enhanced outbreaks of sweat and diarrhea in therapeutic use.

DOSAGE

How Supplied:

Liquid Extract

Mode of Administration: Boneset is used in homeopathic preparations and dilutions.

LITERATURE

Antibiotika und Immunabwehr. In: *Symbiose* 4(2):20. 1992.

Benoit PS et al., (1976) *Lloydia* 39:160.

Bohlmann F et al., (1977) *Phytochemistry* 16:1973.

Elsässer-Beile U, Willenbacher W, Bartsch HH, Gallati H, Schulte Mönting J, Kleist von S et al., Cytokine production in leukocyte cultures during therapy with echinacea extract. In: *J Clin Lab Analysis* 10(6):441-445. 1996.

Franz G. Polysaccharides in pharmacy: Current applications and future concepts. *Planta Med* 55:493-497. 1989.

Herz W et al., (1977) *J Org Chem* 42(13):2264.

Vollmar A et al., (1986) *Phytochemistry* 25:377.

Wagner H (1972) *Phytochemistry* 11:1504.

Röder E, Pyrrolizidinhaltige Arzneipflanzen. In: *DAZ* 132(45):2427-2435. 1992.

Woerdenbag HJ, Eupatorium perfoliatum L.- der ''durchwachsene'' Wasserhanf. In: *ZPT* 13(4):134-139. 1992.

Borage

Borago officinalis

DESCRIPTION

Medicinal Parts: The medicinal parts are the dried Borage flowers and the dried or fresh foliage, stems, and leaves.

Flower and Fruit: The flowers are in separate, terminal, erect, leafy racemes. The calyx is divided almost to the base into 5 rough-haired tips. The corolla is 1.5 to 2.5 cm wide, usually sky blue (occasionally white), and has a short tube. The scales of the tube are white. The 5 stamens have a broadened filament and a violet, spurlike appendage. The anthers are black-violet. The style is thread-like with a headlike stigma. The ovary is divided into 4 valves. The small nut is elongate-ovate, about 7 to 10 mm long, light brown, keeled, ribbed, warty, and rough.

Leaves, Stem, and Root: Borage is an annual, succulent, bristly-haired herb that is 15 to 60 cm high. The erect, vertically grooved stems are covered in rough, whitish hairs. The leaves are alternate, clasping, solitary, entire-margined, and hairy. They are also folded, curved in at the margins, green on top and whitish on the underside. The leaves are 3 to 10 cm long and elliptoid to ovate.

Characteristics: Borage has a taste similar to cucumber.

Habitat: Borage originated in the Mediterranean region, but is now found all over Europe and the U.S.

Production: Borage oil is the fatty oil of the seeds of *Borago officinalis.* Borage leaves are the dried leaves and inflorescence of *Borago officinalis.* The herb most often grows wild, but is cultivated on a small scale in Yugoslavia, Rumania, Bulgaria, and Turkey. Borage is harvested during the flowering period. Due to the plant's very high water content, it should be artificially dried at 40°C.

Not to be Confused With: Echium vulgare.

Other Names: Bugloss, Burage, Burrage

ACTIONS AND PHARMACOLOGY

COMPOUNDS: BORAGE OIL

Fatty oil: Chief fatty acid is gamma-linolenic acid (17-25%), linoleic acid

COMPOUNDS: BORAGE LEAF

Pyrrolizidine alkaloids: supinin, lycopsamin, 7-acetyl-lycopsamin, intermedin, 7-acetyl- intermedine, amabiline, thesinine

Silicic acid (to some extent water-soluble)

Mucilages

Tannins

EFFECTS

BORAGE LEAF AND OIL

Borage seed oil appears to have anti-inflammatory properties. Animal trials suggest beneficial effects for some cardiovascular effects. Borage oil (starflower oil) is used as an alternative source to evening primrose oil for gamma-linolenic acid (GLA). The tannins in Borage leaves have an astringent effect and the mucins a sequestering effect.

Antihypertensive Effects: Studies on rats (Engler et al, 1992, 1993, 1998) indicate an antihypertensive effect in dietary Borage oil, presumably related to Borage's GLA content.

Anti-inflammatory Effects: Animal studies show that Borage oil and other oils containing polyunsaturated fatty acids may be beneficial in inflammatory skin disorders due to increases in epidermal 15-lipoxygenase products, which suppress the generation of proinflammatory leukotrienes (Miller et al, 1991). Elevated levels of dihomogamma-linoleic acid (DGLA) resulting from a diet containing Borage oil leads to an increase in series 1 prostaglandins. PGE-1 has been shown to cause signs of acute inflammation, yet also has a negative feedback role in the case of chronic inflammation. PGE-1 also inhibits the inflammatory process through the increase in cyclic AMP it produces, which in turn decreases leukocyte chemotaxis, margination, and adherence (Belch & Hill, 2000).

Effects in Cystic Fibrosis: Borage oil administered orally produced small but statistically insignificant increases in vital capacity and forced expiratory volume in patients with cystic fibrosis (Christophe et al, 1994).

Effects in Dermatitis: Topical application of an emulsion containing Borage oil and sunflower seed oil for 4 weeks improved ceramide 1 linoleate levels (Conti et al, 1996). The beneficial effects of topical Borage oil in the treatment of dermatitis may be due to the uptake of GLA by the stratum corneum with an increased water binding capacity of the stratum corneum and fluidization of the lipids resulting in a smooth surface (Nissen et al, 1995).

Immunomodulatory Effects: Orally administered Borage oil demonstrated a dose-dependent inhibition of calcium ionophore-induced polymorphonuclear neutrophil generation of proinflammatory leukotriene B4 in vitro (Ziboh & Fletcher, 1992). Gamma-linolenic acid (GLA) supplementation through oral administration of Borage oil caused a marked accumulation of dihomogamma-linolenic acid (DGLA) in human neutrophils (Chilton-Lopez et al, 1996).

Platelet Aggregation Effects: Oral administration of Borage oil to 6 healthy male subjects in a dose of 71.6 mg/kg daily for 42 days significantly ($p<0.05$) increased platelet aggregation, which was not associated with a significant rise in thromboxane A2, PGE-1, or PGE-2 despite a significantly increased DGLA/AA ratio in platelet phospholipids (Barre et al, 1993).

CLINICAL TRIALS

Alcohol Hangover

A systematic review of randomized, controlled trials on interventions for preventing or treating alcohol hangover identified a trial involving treatment with GLA from *Borago officinalis*. Forty healthy subjects ingested 140 to 160 ml alcohol as part of the parallel, double-blind trial. As compared to placebo, the subjects assigned to take the 1000 mg GLA directly before the alcohol challenge reported a significant reduction in the overall severity of hangover and symptoms of headache, lethargy, and fatigue. However, the review overall found no compelling evidence to indicate that any complementary or conventional intervention effectively treats or prevents alcohol hangover (Pittler, 2005).

Atopic Dermatitis/Eczema

Multiple randomized, placebo-controlled studies of orally administered or topically applied Borage oil failed to show improvement in symptoms of atopic dermatitis and atopic eczema (Takwale et al, 2003; Henz et al, 1999; Bahmer & Schaefer, 1992; Kiehl et al, 1994; Borelli et al, 1994). Treatment with Borage oil capsules was effective in relieving symptoms of mild-to-moderate atopic dermatitis in a 12-week, randomized, placebo-controlled, double-blind study of 32 patients.

Treatment with 1000 mg Borage oil twice daily resulted in a significantly reduced Atopic Dermatitis Area Severity Index (ADASI) score in 14 of 18 patients (78%; $p<0.05$ as compared to placebo, 43%) (Buslau & Thaci, 1996).

A cream containing 3% Borage oil reduced skin roughness and transepidermal water loss (TEWL) when applied to dermatitis induced by treatment with 5% sodium lauryl sulfate in 20 humans. The cream containing Borage oil significantly ($p<0.05$) decreased skin roughness and TEWL at 7 and 14 days compared with the other preparations. The cream with

Borage oil also had similar effects on normal skin (Nissen et al, 1995).

Diabetic Neuropathy

Twenty-two patients with distal diabetic neuropathy were studied in a double-blind, placebo-controlled trial where the active treatment consisted of 360 mg of GLA for 6 months. Compared to the placebo group, the active treatment group showed statistically significant improvement in neuropathy symptoms scores ($p<0.01$) (Jamal & Carmichael, 1990).

Infantile Seborrheic Dermatitis

Topical administration of Borage oil successfully treated 48 children with infantile seborrheic dermatitis. Borage oil, 0.5 milliliters, was applied to the scalp region twice daily. Skin lesions cleared within 10 to 12 days, even in areas where oil was not applied, suggesting percutaneous absorption. Discontinuation of treatment resulted in recurrence of lesions within 1 week (Tollesson & Frithz, 1993; Tollesson et al, 1997).

Rheumatoid Arthritis

Patients with rheumatoid arthritis had significant and clinically relevant improvement in signs and symptoms with 6 to 12 months of orally administered GLA obtained from Borage seed oil. Evaluation of patients at 15 months after study entry, however, showed that most patients had experienced an exacerbation of their disease (Zurier et al, 1996).

GLA in the form of Borage seed oil capsules administered orally to 37 patients with rheumatoid arthritis and active synovitis for 24 weeks resulted in clinically important reductions in signs and symptoms in a double-blind trial. The GLA-treated group showed significant ($p<0.05$) improvement from baseline in the joint tenderness score, joint swelling score, and platelet count. No GLA treated patients showed deterioration (Leventhal et al, 1993).

In patients with active synovitis, oral administration of Borage oil in a single dose of 2.4 g GLA or a dose of 1.2 g twice daily for a period of 11 to 24 weeks resulted in suppression of T lymphocyte proliferation in vitro. Lymphocyte proliferation returns to pre-treatment levels by 3 months after discontinuation (Rossetti et al, 1997).

Orally administered Borage seed oil can have an immunomodulatory function through effects on cytokine production. Subjects consumed 15 milliliters of refined Borage seed oil orally daily for 12 weeks and had peripheral blood collected and peripheral blood mononuclear cells separated prior to the oil and at 4, 8, and 12 weeks. An increased production of phytohemagglutinin (PHA)-induced transforming growth factor beta and decreased PHA-induced interleukin-4 production and anti-CD3-induced interleukin-10 production was observed. No significant change in proliferation of lymphocytes was noted in this study (Fisher & Harbige, 1997).

INDICATIONS AND USAGE

BORAGE OIL

Unproven Uses: The oil is used for neurodermatitis and as a food supplement.

BORAGE LEAF

Unproven Uses: In folk medicine, Borage is used as a sequestering and mucilaginous agent for coughs and throat illnesses and as a bronchial treatment. It is also used as an anti-inflammatory agent for kidney and bladder disorders, as an astringent and to treat rheumatism, and for atopic disease such as diabetic neuropathy, eczema, infantile seborrheic dermatosis, and for hypertension. Preparations using Borage are also used for blood purification and dehydration; the prevention of chest and peritoneal inflammation and rheumatism of the joints; as a pain-relieving, cardiotonic, sedative, sudorific; as a performance-enhancing agent; and for phlebitis and menopausal complaints.

CONTRAINDICATIONS

Borage oil is contraindicated in schizophrenic and/or epileptic patients and in those receiving epileptogenic drugs, because Borage oil may cause temporal lobe epilepsy (Newall et al, 1996).

Pregnancy: Not to be used during pregnancy.

Breastfeeding: Not to be used while breastfeeding.

PRECAUTIONS AND ADVERSE REACTIONS

Side effects of Borage use may include gastrointestinal discomfort. Excessive or prolonged ingestion of Borage should also be avoided due to its toxic pyrrolizidine alkaloid constituents.

DRUG INTERACTIONS

MODERATE RISK

Anticoagulants, Antiplatelet Agents, Thrombolytic Agents, Low Molecular Weight Heparins. Borage oil may increase the risk of bleeding if taken with anticoagulants, antiplatelet agents, thrombolytic agents or low molecular weight heparins. *Clinical Management:* Caution is advised if Borage oil is taken concomitantly with these medications. Monitor the patient closely for signs and symptoms of bleeding.

POTENTIAL INTERACTIONS

Iron: The tannin content of borage may complex with concomitantly administered iron, resulting in nonabsorbable insoluble complexes, which may result in adverse sequelae on blood components. *Clinical Management:* Patients who need iron supplementation should be advised to separate administration times of these two compounds by one to two hours.

DOSAGE

BORAGE OIL

Mode of Administration: In capsules, sometimes in combination with vitamins.

How Supplied.

Capsules – 500 mg, 1000 mg

Atopic Dermatitis/Eczema: 2 to 3 g Borage oil daily in divided doses (Buslau & Thaci, 1996; Bahmer & Schaefer, 1992).

Rheumatoid Arthritis: 6 to 7 g of Borage oil (equivalent to 1.4 g of GLA content) daily in 3 divided doses after meals (Leventhal et al, 1993).

Topical: Atopic Dermatitis/Eczema: Cream containing 3% to 10% Borage oil content: apply twice daily (Nissen et al, 1995; Borelli et al, 1994).

BORAGE LEAF

Storage: The drug should be protected from light and moisture.

LITERATURE

Bahmer FA & Schaefer J. Die Behandlung der atopischen Dermatitis mit Borretschsamen-Oel (Glandol(R)) - eine zeitreihenanalytische Studie. *Kinderaerztl Praxis*; 1992;60(7):199-202.

Bard JM, Luc G, Jude B et al. A therapeutic dosage (3 g/day) of Borage oil supplementation has no effect on platelet aggregation in healthy volunteers. *Fundam Clin Pharmacol*; 1997;11(2):143-144.

Barre DE & Holub BJ. The effect of Borage oil consumption on the composition of individual phospholipids in human platelets. *Lipids*; 1992;27(5):315-320.

Barre DE, Holub BJ & Chapkin RS. The effect of Borage oil supplementation on human platelet aggregation, thromboxane B2, prostaglandin E1 and E2 formation. *Nutr Res*; 1993;13:739-751.

Belch JJF & Hill A. Evening primrose oil and Borage oil in rheumatologic conditions. *Am J Clin Nutr*; 2000;71(suppl):352S-356S.

Borelli S, Bresser H & Belsan I. Externe Therpie mit Gamma-Linolensaeure - Ergebnis einer Doppelblindstudie. *H G Z Hautkr*; 1994;69(8):523-524.

Buslau M & Thaci D. Atopische Dermatitis. Borretschoel zur systemischen Therapie. *Z Dermatol*; 1996;182(3):131-132, 134-136.

Chilton-Lopez T, Surette ME, Swan DD et al. Metabolism of gamma-linolenic acid in human neutrophils. *J Immunol*; 1996;156(8):2941-2947.

Cotter MA, Dines KC & Cameron NE. Omega-6 essential fatty acid dysmetabolism and gamma-linolenic acid in experimental diabetic neuropathy. In. Hotta N, Greene DA, Ward AAF et al (eds). Diabetic Neuropathy. New Concepts and Insights. Elsevier Science, New York, NY, 1995: 257-262.

Christophe A, Robberecht E, Franckx H et al. Effect of administration of gamma-linolenic acid on the fatty acid composition of serum phospholipids and cholesteryl esters in patients with cystic fibrosis. *Ann Nutr Metab*; 1994;38(1):40-47.

Engler MM. Comparative study of diets enriched with evening primrose, black currant, Borage or fungal oils on blood pressure and pressor responses in spontaneously hypertensive rats. *Prostaglandins Leukot Essent Fatty Acids*; 1993;49(4):804-809.

Engler MM. Effects of dietary gamma-linolenic acid on blood pressure and adrenal angiotensin receptors in hypertensive rats. *Proc Soc Exp Biol Med*; 1998;218(3):234-237.

Engler MM, Engler MB, Erickson SK et al. Dietary gamma-linolenic acid lowers blood pressure and alters aortic reactivity and cholesterol metabolism in hypertension. *J Hypertens*; 1992;10(10):1197-1204.

Fan YY, Chapkin RS & Ramos KS. Dietary lipid source alters murine macrophage/vascular smooth muscle cell interactions in vitro. *J Nutr*; 1996;126(9):2083-2088.

Fisher BAC & Harbige LS. Effect of omega-6 lipid-rich Borage oil feeding on immune function in healthy volunteers. *Biochem Soc Trans*; 1997;25(2):343S.

Guivernau M, Meza M, Barja P et al. Clinicial and experimental study on the long-term effect of dietary gamma-linolenic acid on plasma lipids, platelet aggregation, thromboxane formation, and prostacyclin production. *Prostaglandin Leukot Essent Fatty Acids*; 1994;51:311-316.

Henz BM, Jablonska S, Van De Kerkhof PCM et al. Double-blind, multicentre analysis of the efficacy of Borage oil in patients with atopic eczema. *Br J Dermatol*; 1994;140(4):685-688.

Hoffman D. The Herb Users Guide, the Basic Skills of Medical Herbalism. Wellingborough. Thorsons, 1987. Ippen H, Gamma-Linolensäure besser aus Nachtkerzen- oder aus Borretschöl? *ZPT;* 1995;16(3):167-170.

Jamal GA & Carmichael H. The effect of gamma-linolenic acid on human diabetic peripheral neuropathy, a double-blind placebo-controlled trial. *Diabet Med*; 1990;7(4):319-323.

Kiehl R, Ionescu G, Manuel Ph et al. Klinische, immune- und lipidmodulatorische Effekte einer Behandlung mitungesaettigten Fettsaeuren bei atopischer. *Dermatitis. Z Hautkr*; 1994;69(1):42-48.

Leventhal LJ, Boyce EG & Zurier RB. Treatment of rheumatoid arthritis with gammalinolenic acid. *Ann Intern Med*; 1993;119(9):867-873.

Luthy J et al. *Pharm Acta Helv*; 1984;59: (9/10). 242.

Mills DE. Dietary fatty acid supplementation alters stress reactivity and performance in man. *J Hum Hypertens*; 1989;3:111-116.

Miller CC, Tang W, Ziboh VA et al. Dietary supplementation with ethyl ester concentrates of fish oil (n-3) and Borage oil (n-6) polyunsaturated fatty acids induces epidermal generation of local putative anti-inflammatory metabolites. *J Invest Dermatol*; 1991;96(1):98-103.

Mills DE, Mah M, Ward RP et al. Alteration of baroreflex control of forearm vascular resistance by dietary fatty acids. *Am J Physiol*; 1990;259(6 pt 2):R1164-R1171.

Mills DE, Prkachin KM, Harvey KA et al. Dietary fatty acid supplementation alters stress reactivity and performance in man. *J Hum Hypertens*; 1989;3(2):111-116.

Nissen HP, Biltz H & Muggli R. Borage Oil. gamma-linolenic acid in the oil decreases skin roughness and TEWL and increases skin moisture in normal and irritated human skin. *Cosmetics Toiletries Mag*; 1995;110:71-73,76.

Norred CL & Brinker F. Potential coagulation effects of preoperative complementary and alternative medicines. *Alt Ther*; 2001;7(6):58-67.

Pittler M, Verster JC, Ernst E. Interventions for preventing or treating alcohol hangover: systematic review of randomized controlled trials. *BMJ;* 331:1515-1518. 2005.

Rossetti RG, Seiler CM, DeLuca P et al. Oral administration of unsaturated fatty acids. effects on human peripheral blood T lymphocyte proliferation. *J Leukoc Biol*; 1997;62(4):438-443.

Takwale A, Tan E, Agarwal S et al. Efficacy and tolerability of Borage oil in adults and children with atopic eczema. Randomised, double blind, placebo controlled, parallel group trial. *BMJ*; 2003;327(7428):1385-1388.

Takwale A, Tan E, Agarwal S et al. Efficacy and tolerability of Borage oil in adults and children with atopic eczema. randomised, double blind, placebo-controlled, parallel group trial. *BMJ*; 2003;327(7428):1-4.

Tollesson A, Frithz A & Stenlund K. Malassezia furfur in infantile seborrheic dermatitis. *Pediatr Dermatol*; 1997;14(6):423-425.

Zurier RB, Rossetti RG, Jacobson EW et al. Gamma-linolenic acid treatment of rheumatoid arthritis, a randomized, placebo-controlled trial. *Arthritis Rheum*; 1996;39(11):1808-1817.

Borago officinalis

See Borage

Boswellia carteri

See Frankincense

Boxwood

Buxus sempervirens

DESCRIPTION

Medicinal Parts: The medicinal parts are the dried Boxwood tree leaves and the woody aerial parts of the plant.

Flower and Fruit: Clusters of axillary yellow flowers open in early spring. The male flowers are evenly shaped and have 4 tepals, 4 stamens, and a small rudimentary ovary. The female flowers have 4 to 8 tepals, 3 fused carpels with 3 free, short, thick styles. The fruit is a capsule with oblong, 5 to 6 mm long seeds.

Leaves, Stem, and Root: Boxwood is an evergreen monoecious shrub or tree growing to a height of 6 m with variable forms and leaf shapes. The green branches are initially pubescent, later glabrous, olive green, angular, and densely covered with ovate leaves, which are usually opposite. The upper surface of the leaves is smooth, coriaceous, dark green, and very glossy. The lower surface is lighter in shade, and the lamina margin is smooth.

Characteristics: The leaves have a nauseous taste.

Habitat: The plant is found mainly in southern and central Europe with a clear division into east and west regions, i.e., northwest Spain and southern France in the west and the Balkans to northern Greece and Asia Minor in the east. It is otherwise extensively cultivated.

Production: Boxwood leaves are the leaves of *Buxus sempervirens*. They are collected from the wild.

Other Names: Dudgeon, Bush Tree

ACTIONS AND PHARMACOLOGY

COMPOUNDS

Steroid alkaloids: including cyclobuxine-D, cyclobuxine-B, cycloprotobuxine-A, cycloprotobu

EFFECTS

The cycloprotobuxine in the drug was shown to have a cytotoxic effect in vitro as well as an inhibitory effect on the growth of *mycobacterium tuberculosis*.

In animal tests, an inhibition of motility, including tetanus, spinal paralysis and respiratory paralysis, was demonstrated.

A hypotensive effect has been described.

INDICATIONS AND USAGE

Unproven Uses: In folk medicine preparations were used internally for rheumatism and constipation (decoction), as a diaphoretic (aqueous extract), for malaria (tincture) and pneumonia (ethanol extract), and externally for rashes, hair loss, gout, and rheumatic complaints (ointment)

Homeopathic Uses: Buxus sempervirens is used for greasy scalp with dandruff and for hair loss.

PRECAUTIONS AND ADVERSE REACTIONS

No health hazards or side effects are known in conjunction with the proper administration of designated therapeutic dosages. Contact dermatitis, in particular through contact with the freshly harvested plant, is possible.

OVERDOSAGE

The intake of toxic dosages of the drug leads to vomiting, diarrhea, severe colonic spasms, eventually to signs of paralysis and ultimately to fatal asphyxiation. The fatal dosage in dogs is 0.1 gm of the alkaloid mixture/kg body weight (approximately 5 to 10 gm of the drug/kg body weight). The treatment for poisonings proceeds through suppression of the spasms with diazepam or barbiturates (no more than absolutely necessary) followed by gastric lavage and possible oxygen respiration. Phenothiazines and analeptics are not to be administered.

DOSAGE

Mode of Administration: Boxwood is obsolete as a drug.

Homeopathic Dosage: 5 to 10 drops, 1 tablet, 5 to 10 globules, 1 rubbed knife-tip 1 to 3 times daily or 1 mL injection solution sc twice weekly. (HAB34)

LITERATURE

Atta-ur-Rahman et al., Alkaloids from Buxus species. In: *PH* 31(8):2933-2935. 1992.

Atta-ur-Rahman et al., New alkaloids from Buxus sempervirens. In: *JNP* 52:1319-1322. 1989.

Atta-ur-Rahman et al., Steroidal alkaloids from leaves of *Buxus sempervirens*. In: *PH* 30(4):1295-1298. 1991.

Durant, Chantre, Gonzalez, Vandermander, et al. Efficacy and safety of *Buxus sempervirens* L preparations (SVP30) in HIV-infected asymptomatic patients: a multicentre, randomized, double-blind, placebo-controlled trial. *Phytomedicine* 5(1):1-10. 1998.

Frohne D, Pfänder HJ, Giftpflanzen - Ein Handbuch für Apotheker, Toxikologen und Biologen, 4. Aufl., Wiss. Verlags-Ges Stuttgart 1997.

Hänsel R, Keller K, Rimpler H, Schneider G (Hrsg.), Hagers Handbuch der Pharmazeutischen Praxis, 5. Aufl., Bde 4-6 (Drogen), Springer Verlag Berlin, Heidelberg, New York, 1992-1994.

Khodshaev BU et al., (1984) *Khim Prir Soedin* 6:802.

Lewin L, Gifte und Vergiftungen, 6. Aufl., Nachdruck, Haug Verlag, Heidelberg 1992.

Roth L, Daunderer M, Kormann K, Giftpflanzen, Pflanzengifte, 4. Aufl., Ecomed Fachverlag Landsberg Lech 1993.

Teuscher E, Lindequist U, Biogene Gifte - Biologie, Chemie, Pharmakologie, 2. Aufl., Fischer Verlag Stuttgart 1994.

Willaman JJ, Hui-Li L, (1970) *Lloydia* 33(3A):1.

Brassica napus

See Oilseed Rape

Brassica nigra

See Black Mustard

Brassica oleracea

See Cabbage

Brassica rapa

See Wild Turnip

Brazilian Pepper Tree

Schinus terebinthifolius

DESCRIPTION

Medicinal Parts: Medicinal properties have been attributed to the bark, leaves, fruit, and seeds.

Flower and Fruit: The flowers are in panicles up to 15 cm long. The flowers are small, ivory white to greenish, and the structures are in five. The calyx is 5-tipped. There are 5 petals, 10 stamens, a superior ovary developing from a single carpel, and a style in 3 sections. The fruit is a bright pink to red, glossy, single-drupe with a diameter of approximately 5 mm, a thin pergamentlike exocarp, an oleo-resin-rich mesocarp and a hard endocarp.

Leaves, Stem, and Root: The leaves are alternate, up to 40 cm long, odd pinnate, with 7 to 13 leaflets up to 8 cm long, 1 to 2 cm wide, sessile, elongate, glossy, finely serrate, or jagged-edged. The branches do not hang down.

Characteristics: The fruit is aromatic and sweetish.

Habitat: Indigenous to Central America and South America.

Production: Brazilian peppers (Pink peppers) are the ripe unpeeled seeds of *Schinus terebinthifolius Raddi*, which are harvested in winter (May to August) and then air- or freeze-dried.

Other Names: Christmas-Berry Tree, Florida Holly

ACTIONS AND PHARMACOLOGY

COMPOUNDS

Volatile oil (2.0 to 10.0%): chief components including limonene, alpha-phellandrene, beta-phellandrene, alpha-pinene, beta-pinene, including as well p-cymol, sabinene, terpinolene, in some chemical varieties up to 50% delta3-carene

Alkyl phenols (0.1%): cardanols, cardols, 2-methyl cardolenes

Fatty oil (in the seeds 20 to 60%)

Flavonoids: including biflavonoids, for example amentoflavone

Triterpenes: masticadienonic acid, 3-epimasticadienonic acid

EFFECTS

The ''antibiotic activity'' with which the drug is credited has not yet been proved. Its use on wounds and inflammatory alterations of the skin appears plausible, due to the antimicrobial, astringent, and anti-inflammatory characteristics of the gallic acid it contains.

INDICATIONS AND USAGE

Unproven Uses: Internal folk medicine uses have included treatment of tumors and as a diuretic. In Brazil, a liquid extract and tincture are prepared from the bark and used internally as a stimulant, tonic, and astringent, and externally for rheumatism, gout, and syphilis. The leaf and fruit have been added to baths for wounds and ulcers. (Hager, 1949.) The effect seems plausible due to the gallic acid content but has not yet been sufficiently clinically proved.

PRECAUTIONS AND ADVERSE REACTIONS

No health hazards are known in conjunction with the proper administration of designated therapeutic dosages, although there is some danger of sensitization (alkyl phenols). Sensitizations occur particularly frequently in North America. Stomach upset and vomiting have been observed following the ingestion of a number of the fruits.

CONTRAINDICATIONS

Should not be administered to individuals with a pre-existing sensitivity to alkyl phenols.

DOSAGE

Mode of Administration: Whole drug, tincture, and extract for internal and external use.

Daily Dosage: There is no information in the literature.

Storage: Store tightly sealed and protected from light in a cool, dry place.

LITERATURE

Hänsel R, Keller K, Rimpler H, Schneider G (Ed), Hagers Handbuch der Pharmazeutischen Praxis, 5. Aufl., Bde 4 - 6 (Drogen), Springer Verlag Berlin, Heidelberg, New York, 1992-1994.

Hayashi T, Nagayama K, Arisawa M, Shimizu M, Suzuki S, Yoshizaki M, Morita N, Ferro E, Basualdo I, Berganza LH,

Pentagalloylglucose, a xanthine oxidase inhibitor from a Paraguayan crude drug, Molle-i (*Schinus terebinthifolius*). *J Nat Prod*, 39:210-1, 1989 Jan-Feb.

Jain MK, Yu BZ, Rogers JM, Smith AE, Boger ET, Ostrander RL, Rheingold AL, Specific competitive inhibitor of secreted phospholipase A2 from berries of Schinus terebinthifolius. *Phytochemistry*, 39:537-47, 1995 Jun.

Ramos Ruiz A, De la Torre RA, Alonso N, Villaescusa A, Betancourt J, Vizoso A, Screening of medicinal plants for induction of somatic segregation activity in Aspergillus nidulans. *J Ethnopharmacol*, 39:123-7, 1996 Jul 5.

Wagner H. Search for new plant constituents with potential antiphlogistic and antiallergic activity. *Planta Med* 55: 235-241. 1989.

Brewer's Yeast

Saccharomyces cerevisiae

DESCRIPTION

Medicinal Parts: The medicinal part is the mature, debittered, bottom-fermented Brewer's Yeast.

Flower and Fruit: The cells may be single, in pairs, in chains or aggregate. On a suitable solid fertile base the individual cell colonies have smooth margins, are slightly convex to flat and are whitish to cream-yellow. Older individual colonies are slightly raised, smooth, or slightly lobed (sometimes in sections), or folded, and are yellowish to light brown. The vegetative reproduction is via multilateral budding. Ascospores are produced from the vegetative cells. There are normally 1 to 4, occasionally more, round, smooth-walled ascospores per ascus.

Characteristics: Brewer's Yeast is found extensively in the wild, and it lives as a saprophytic parasite or symbiotically.

Habitat: Brewer's Yeast is grown worldwide.

Production: Medicinal yeast consists of fresh or dried cells of *Saccharomyces cerevisiae* and/or of *Candida utilis.*

ACTIONS AND PHARMACOLOGY

COMPOUNDS

Vitamins of the B group (per 100 gm): thiamin 8-15 mg, riboflavin 4-8 mg, nicotinic acid amide 45-90 mg, pantothenic acid 7-25 mg, pyridoxine 4-10 mg, biotin 20 βg, folic acid 1-5 mg, vitamin B-12 20 βg

Polysaccharides: mannans, glucans

Proteins

Amines

Sterols: ergosterol, zymosterol

EFFECTS

The yeast is antibacterial and stimulates phagocytosis.

INDICATIONS AND USAGE

Approved by Commission E:

- Dyspeptic complaints
- Eczema, furuncles, acne
- Loss of appetite

Unproven Uses: Brewer's Yeast is used for constipation, itching skin diseases, and eczema.

PRECAUTIONS AND ADVERSE REACTIONS

General: Health risks or side effects following the proper administration of designated therapeutic dosages are not recorded. The intake of large quantities can cause gas. Allergic intolerance reactions are possible (itching, urticaria, exanthema, Quinck's disease). Migraine headaches can be triggered in susceptible patients.

DRUG INTERACTIONS

POTENTIAL INTERACTIONS

Monoamine Oxidase Inhibitors: Concurrent use may cause an increase in blood pressure.

DOSAGE

Mode of Administration: Medicinal yeast and galenic preparations are available for internal use. Pharmaceutical forms include tablets and compound preparations.

How Supplied:

Powder

Tablets

Daily Dosage: The average daily dosage is 6 gm.

Storage: Store in airtight containers protected from light.

LITERATURE

Aflmann C, Mikroorganismen:Biotherapeutika bei Infektionskrankheiten. In: *DAZ* 136(46):4136-4137. 1996.

Anonym, Hefepräparate haben sich bewährt. In: *PTA* 5(9):433. 1991.

Böckeler W, Thomas G, (1989): In-vitro-Studien zur destabilisierenden Wirkung lyophilisierter Saccharomyces cerevisiae Hansen CBS 5926-Zellen auf Enterobakterien. Läßt sich diese Eigenschaft biochemisch erklären? In, Müller J, Ottenjann R, Seifert J (Hrsg), Ökosystem Darm, Springer Verlag, S 142-153.

Czerucka D, Roux l, Rampal P, (1994) Saccharomyces boulardii inhibits sectretagogue-mediated adenosin-cyclic monophosphate induction in intestinal cells. Gastroenterology 106:65-72.

Ewe K, (1983) Obstipation - Pathophysiologie, Klinik, *Therapie. Int Welt* 6:286-292.

Gedek B, Hagenhoff G, (1989) Orale Verabreichung von lebensfähigen Zellen des Hefestammes *Saccharomyces cerevisiae* Hansen CBS 5926 und deren Schicksal während der Magen-Darm-Passage. Therapiewoche 38 (Sonderheft): 33-40.

Höchter W, Chase D, Hagenhoff G, (1990) *Saccharomyces boulardii* bei akuter Erwachsenediarrhoe. *Münch Med Wschr* 132: 188-192.

Hojgaard L, Arffmann S, Jorgeasen M, Krag E, (1981) Tea consumption, a cause of constipation. *BMJ* 282: 864.

Jahn HU, Zeitz M, (1991) Immunmodulàtorische Wirkung von *Saccharomyces boulardii* beim Menschen. In: Seifert J, Ottenjann

R, Zeitz M, Bockemühl J (Hrsg) Ökosystem Darm III. Springer-Verlag, S 159-164.

Kollaritsch HH, Tobüren D, Scheiner O, Wiedermann G, (1988) Prophylaxe der Reisediarrhoe. *Münch Med Wschr* 130: 671-673.

Massot J, Desconclois M, Astoin J, (1982) Protection par Saccharomyces boulardii de la diarrhée à *Escherichia coli* du souriceau. *Ann Pharm Fr* 40: 445-449.

Plein K, Hotz J, (1993) Therapeutic effect of *Saccaromyces boulardii* on mild residual symptoms in a stable phase of Crohn's disease with special respect to chronic diarrhea - a pilot study. *Z Gastroenterol* 31: 129-134.

Schmidt CH, (1977) Unspezifische Steigerung der Phagozytoseaktivitäten von Peritoneal-makrophagen nach oraler Gabe verschiedener Hefepräparationen. Dissertation Freie Universität Berlin.

Sinai Y, Kaplan A, Hai Y et al., (1974) Enhancement of resistance to infectious disease by oral administration of Brewer's Yeast. *Infection Immunol* 9: 781-787

Surawicz Ch, Elmer GW, Speelman P, McFarland LV, Chinn J, van Belle G, (1989) Die Prophylaxe Antibiotika-assoziierter Diarrhöen mit Saccharomyces boulardii. Eine prospektive Studie. *Gastroenterol* 96: 981-988.

Tempé JD, Steidel AL, Blehaut H, Hasselmann M, Lutun PH, Maurier F, (1983) Prévention par *Saccharomyces boulardii* des diarrhées de l'alimentation entérale à débit continu. La Semaine des Hopitaux de Paris 59: 1409-1412.

Weber R, Regio Seminar Pharma: Reisemedizinische Beratung. In: *DAZ* 135(25):2352-2354. 1995.

British Elecampane (Xuan-Fu-Hua)

Inula britannica

DESCRIPTION

Medicinal Parts: The medicinal part is the flower.

Flower and Fruit: The semi-globose composite flowers are surrounded by bracts; they have a diameter of 2.5 to 5 cm, are single or in umbelliferous racemes with bracts arranged in a number of rows. The lingual florets are yellow and up to 1 mm wide, the tubular florets are 5-tipped, androgenous, and numerous. The anther has an appendage tail. The fruit is a cylindrical, long-ribbed, 1.3 mm long achene. The pappus is single-rowed, approximately 5 mm long and consists of fine, rough bristles.

Leaves, Stem, and Root: This herbaceous perennial grows up to 60 cm high. The leaves are alternate and simple. The lower leaves narrow into the short petiole, entire or dentate. The upper leaves are sessile and rounded at the base, lanceolate, sparsely pubescent above, and are covered below in dense silky hairs or almost glabrous. The stem is upright, round, weakly ribbed, silky-haired to almost glabrous. The root is creeping.

Habitat: The plant is indigenous to Asia and Europe.

Production: Elecampane flowers are the inflorescences of *Inula britannica* and *Inula japonica*, dried in the sun or shade after harvesting.

Not to be Confused With: Arnicae flos

Other Names: Alant-Okleuveasis

ACTIONS AND PHARMACOLOGY

COMPOUNDS

Sesquiterpenes: sesquiterpene lactones, particularly gaillardin but also including britanin

Flavonoids: including isoquercitrin

Caffeic acid derivatives: including chlorogenic acid

EFFECTS

It has been reported that a watery extract of the sesquiterpene-containing drug inhibits in vitro cAMP-phosphodiesterase up to 60%, and prevents the infection of human embryo muscle cells with the herpes simplex virus II. The drug is also assumed to possess potential for sensitization, due to the sesquiterpene lactones with exocyclic methylene groups it contains. The secretolytic and emetic effect with which the drug is credited has not been documented. The flower of the East Asian species is used as a depurative.

INDICATIONS AND USAGE

Unproven Uses: Indications in folk medicine include feelings of fullness in the chest and diaphragm area, vomiting, coughs, and symptoms of the efferent urinary tract.

PRECAUTIONS AND ADVERSE REACTIONS

No health hazards are known in conjunction with the proper administration of designated therapeutic dosages. The drug is presumed to possess potential for sensibilization, due to the sesquiterpene lactones with exocyclic methyene groups it contains.

DOSAGE

Mode of Administration: Whole and powdered drug.

Preparation: The drug is roasted with a honey solution until it is no longer sticky. A decoction is prepared by boiling 3 to 9 g drug in a sealed sachet.

Storage: Store in a dry place.

LITERATURE

Hänsel R, Keller K, Rimpler H, Schneider G (Ed), Hagers Handbuch der Pharmazeutischen Praxis, 5. Aufl., Bde 4 - 6 (Drogen), Springer Verlag Berlin, Heidelberg, New York, 1992-1994.

Iijima K, Kiyohara H, Tanaka M, Matsumoto T, Cyong JC, Yamada H Preventive effect of taraxasteryl acetate from Inula britannica subsp. japonica on experimental hepatitis in vivo. *Planta Med*, 61:50-3, 1995 Feb.

Nikaido et al. Inhibitors of cyclic AMP phosphodiesterase in medicinal plants. *Planta Med* 43:18-23. 1981

Broad Bean

Vicia faba

DESCRIPTION

Medicinal Parts: The medicinal part is the fresh flower.

Flower and Fruit: The white or bluish short-pedicled flowers have black spots on the standard. They are arranged in groups of 2 to 4 in the upper leaf axils. The calyx tips are uneven, with the upper ones shorter than the lower. The pod is leathery and velvety on the flat surface. The brown seeds are large, flat, ovate or oblong.

Leaves, Stem and Root: The plant is 60 to 125 cm high. The stem is erect and has no climbers. The leaves are pinnate and the leaflets elliptical, fleshy, blue-green, and terminate acutely. The stipules are ovate and semi-saggitate.

Habitat: The plant is indigenous to the temperate regions of the world.

Production: Broad Beans are the seeds of *Vicia faba.*

ACTIONS AND PHARMACOLOGY

COMPOUNDS

Pyrimidine derivatives: vicine (vicioside, 0.4-0.8%), convicine (0.1-0.6%)

Lectins: The isolectins mixture is referred to as favine

L-3,4-dihydroxyphenylalanine (L-DOPA, up to 8%)

Starch

Proteins (26%)

Tannins (2%)

EFFECTS

No information is available.

INDICATIONS AND USAGE

Unproven Uses: Formerly, Broad Bean flowers were used in the treatment of coughs and kidney and genital complaints. Externally, they are used as a poultice for skin inflammation, warts, and burns.

Homeopathic Uses: An essence of the fresh plant after flowering is used in homeopathy.

PRECAUTIONS AND ADVERSE REACTIONS

No health hazards or side effects are known in conjunction with the proper administration of designated therapeutic dosages. Following division of the glycosides in the intestine resorption and oxidation through dehydration of SH-groups in the erythrocyte membrane, the pyrimidine derivatives can, in high dosages, lead to hemolysis.

OVERDOSAGE

The intake of large quantities of raw or only briefly cooked seeds can lead to queasiness, vomiting, diarrhea, and feelings of vertigo. In severe cases, overdosage may lead to acute hemolytic anemia with fever, icterus, hemoglobinuria, oliguria, and anuria, particularly among individuals with genetically caused glucose-6-phosphate-dehydrogenase deficiency (inadequate protection of the erythrocytes by glutathione), which is also known as favism. Favism is treated by transfusion of washed erythrocytes and administration of prednisone. Elevations in blood pressure are also possible due to the L-DOPA content of the seeds.

DOSAGE

Mode of Administration: Broad Bean preparations are now obsolete.

LITERATURE

Caceres A, Cano O, Samayoa B, Aguilar L. Plants used in Guatemala for the treatment of gastrointestinal disorders. 1. Screening of 84 plants against Enterobacteria. *J Ethnopharmacol* 30: 55-73, 1990.

Capitanio M, Cappelletti EM, Filippi R. Traditional antileukodermic herbal remedies in the Mediterranean area. *J Ethnopharmacol* 27:193-211. 1989.

Chevion M, Maer J, Glaser G, Naturally occurring food toxicant: favism-producing agents. In: CRC Handbook of Naturally Occurring Food Toxicants, CRC Press, Boca Raton, Florida. 1983.

Kern W, List PH, Hörhammer L (Hrsg.), Hagers Handbuch der Pharmazeutischen Praxis, 4. Aufl., Bde. 1-8: Springer Verlag Berlin, Heidelberg, New York, 1969.

Teuscher E, Lindequist U, Biogene Gifte - Biologie, Chemie, Pharmakologie, 2. Aufl., Fischer Verlag Stuttgart 1994.

Vered Y et al., The influence of Vicia faba (Broad bean) seedlings on urinary sodium excretion. In: *PM* 63(3):237-240. 1997.

Brooklime

Veronica beccabunga

DESCRIPTION

Medicinal Parts: The medicinal parts are the fresh flowering plant freed from the root, the fresh aerial parts collected during the flowering season and the whole plant.

Flower and Fruit: The flowers are in loose, axillary, diagonal clusters. The accompanying leaves are linear, as long as or shorter than the flowers. The peduncles and pedicles are glabrous. The calyx is dorsiventral and divided into four. The sepals are lanceolate to spatulate and acuminate; the front ones are larger than those in the back. The corolla is rotate with a very short tube, 4 to 9 mm wide and azure blue. The ovary is green and the stigma capitual-like. The fruit is a cordate, almost globular, narrow-winged capsule. The seeds are 0.6 mm long and 0.45 mm wide. They are yellow, oval and flatly convex with a fairly smooth back.

Leaves, Stem, and Root: The plant is a perennial with a creeping rhizome. The stem is ascending, up to 50 cm high, round and filled with latex. The leaves are petiolate, ovate, or broad elliptical, obtuse, narrowly serrate, glabrous and glossy.

Habitat: The plant is indigenous to almost all of Europe, western and northern Asia and northern Africa, and is naturalized in eastern North America.

Production: Brooklime is the aerial part of *Veronica beccabunga.* The collection or picking occurs in uncultivated regions in Europe, west and north Asia, North Africa and North America.

Other Names: Beccabunga, Mouth-Smart, Neckweed, Speedwell, Water Purslane, Water Pimpernel

ACTIONS AND PHARMACOLOGY

COMPOUNDS

Iridoide monoterpenes: aucubin (0.8%)

Flavonoids: including among others scutellarin glycosides

The drug has not been extensively investigated.

EFFECTS

Brooklime has a diuretic effect.

INDICATIONS AND USAGE

Unproven Uses: Brooklime is used to lessen the elimination of urine. It is also used for constipation, liver complaints, dysentery, and lung conditions. The drug has also been reported to be effective against bleeding of the gums.

PRECAUTIONS AND ADVERSE REACTIONS

No health hazards or side effects are known in conjunction with the proper administration of designated therapeutic dosages.

LITERATURE

Hänsel R, Keller K, Rimpler H, Schneider G (Hrsg.), Hagers Handbuch der Pharmazeutischen Praxis, 5. Aufl., Bde 4-6 (Drogen): Springer Verlag Berlin, Heidelberg, New York, 1992-1994.

Inouye H et al., (1974) *Planta Med* 25:285.

Kato Y, (1946) *Folia Pharmacol Jap* 42:37 (via CA 47: 1843).

Swiatek L et al., *Acta Pol Pharm* 25:597. 1968.

Broomcorn

Sorghum vulgare

DESCRIPTION

Medicinal Parts: The medicinal parts are the seeds.

Flower and Fruit: The flowers and inflorescences are large spadixlike and solitary. They may also be in pairs and terminal on long, stiff, indistinct panicles. The panicles may be bushy-branched or occasionally tangled-branched. The individual spikelets are usually ovate to round, and the spelts are usually broad-lanceolate. The spelts become hard, shiny, and dentated at the tip. The seeds are small, round, and white.

Leaves, Stem, and Root: The plant is reedlike and similar to maize but is not as tall.

Habitat: The plant is common in Spain, Italy and southern Europe. It is widely cultivated in the U.S.

Production: Broomcorn seeds are the seeds of *Sorghum vulgare.*

Other Names: Darri, Durri, Guinea Corn, Sorghum

ACTIONS AND PHARMACOLOGY

COMPOUNDS

Cyanogenic glycosides: dhurrin (in the fruits, in contrast with the foliage [250-700 mg/100 gm] only in very low concentrations: 0.005-5 mg/100 gm)

Starch (70%)

Proteins (10%)

Fatty oil (3%)

Vitamins of the B group: thiamin (B1), riboflavine (B2)

EFFECTS

Broomcorn is a demulcent that is soothing to the alimentary tract.

INDICATIONS AND USAGE

Unproven Uses: Preparations of the seeds are used for digestive disorders, but it is mainly used as a cereal grain.

PRECAUTIONS AND ADVERSE REACTIONS

No health hazards or side effects are known in conjunction with the proper administration of designated therapeutic dosages.

DOSAGE

Mode of Administration: Broomcorn can be administered as an infusion, but is mostly used as a cereal grain.

LITERATURE

Erb N et al. *PM* 41:84. 1981.

Kern W, List PH, Hörhammer L (Hrsg.), Hagers Handbuch der Pharmazeutischen Praxis, 4. Aufl., Bde. 1-8: Springer Verlag Berlin, Heidelberg, New York, 1969.

Seigler D, Cyanogene Glykoside (Vortragsref.). In: *DAZ* 132(25):1365. 1992.

Teuscher E, Lindequist U, Biogene Gifte - Biologie, Chemie, Pharmakologie, 2. Aufl., Fischer Verlag Stuttgart 1994.

Brown Kelp

Macrocystis pyrifera

DESCRIPTION

Medicinal Parts: The medicinal part is the thallus.

Flower and Fruit: This brown algae grows up to 100 m long. Generations switch between sporophyte and gametophyte. The haploid male or female gametophytes are tiny plantlets. The 50 to 100 m long sporophyte is made up of rootlike rhizoids, a ropelike cauloid, and phylloids that are leaflike, coriaceous-thick sections with a large elongate to pear-shaped air-bladder at the base. The rhizoids form a conical adhesive disc of up to 1 m in diameter. The phylloids grow up to 1 m long, are attached to the cauloidlike leaflets and are covered with sporangia.

Habitat: Found along the west coast of United States (primarily California) and along the coast of Chile.

Production: Brown algae thallus is the dried thallus, usually only the phylloid, of *Macrocystis pyrifera.* (*Macrocystis integrifolia* may be added.) The algae are harvested using vessels called mowing ships.

Other Names: Giant Kelp, Long-Bladder Kelp, Sea Kelp

ACTIONS AND PHARMACOLOGY

COMPOUNDS

Alginic acid (15 to 20%)

Polysaccharides: fucoidan, laminaran

Iodine (0.1 to 0.5%): to some extent organically bound

Proteins

Cyclitols: laminitol (4-C-methyl-meso-inositol)

Sugar alcohols: mannitol

EFFECTS

Brown algae thallus serves chiefly as a source of iodine. The drug has also been demonstrated to have an influence on the immune system, as well as antiviral qualities. In a study with 400 women, the daily intake of 5.5 g of macrocystis powder over a period of 6 to 8 weeks led to an elevation of hemoglobin levels of 86% over normal values. Although licensed as a substance to aid weight loss, no adequate experimental data are available to support that effect.

INDICATIONS AND USAGE

Unproven Uses: Folk medicine uses include weight reduction. The drug is used as a commercial pharmaceutical preparation in the U.S. for anemia in pregnancy. In Japan the drug is used for hypertension.

PRECAUTIONS AND ADVERSE REACTIONS

No health hazards are known in conjunction with the proper administration of designated therapeutic dosages.

CONTRAINDICATIONS

Brown Kelp should not be used by individuals with a familial disposition to thyroid illness or hyperthyroidism.

OVERDOSAGE

Long-term administration of daily dosages that exceed 150 mcg iodine carry with them the danger of worsening an existing hyperthyroidism. Quantities over 300 mcg iodine per day can precipitate hyperthyroidism.

DOSAGE

Mode of Administration: Brown Kelp preparations are available for internal use.

Storage: Store in tightly sealed container.

LITERATURE

Hänsel R, Keller K, Rimpler H, Schneider G (Ed), Hagers Handbuch der Pharmazeutischen Praxis, 5. Aufl., Bde 4 - 6 (Drogen), Springer Verlag Berlin, Heidelberg, New York, 1992-1994.

Zeller SG, Gray GR, Analysis of Macrocystis pyrifera and Pseudomonas aeruginosa alginic acids by the reductive-cleavage method. Carbohydr Res, 226:313-26, 1992 Mar 30.

Brunfelsia hopeana

See Manaca

Bryonia alba

See White Bryony

Bryonia cretica

See Red Bryony

Buckthorn

Rhamnus catharticus

DESCRIPTION

Medicinal Parts: The medicinal parts are the whole, ripe, dried fruit and the fresh ripe fruit.

Flower and Fruit: The small, dioecious, greenish-yellow flowers are in axillary cymes. The calyx is fused, has 4 segments and droops. The petals are small and are on the edge of the calyx tube, which has short stamens. The ovary is 4-valved with a style that is divided in 4. The fruit is a pea-sized, blackberrylike drupe. The seeds are 5 mm long and triangular with a narrow split, which separates slightly at the end and is surrounded by a cartilaginous margin.

Leaves, Stem, and Root: The plant occurs in a variety of forms, usually as a bush that is up to 3 m in height, but occasionally as a tree with a bent trunk that grows up to 8 m. The boughs are usually stiffly spread; the branches are more or less clearly opposite, glossy, glabrous or occasionally pubescent and end in a thorn. The leaves are clustered on the older branches, opposite on the younger ones. They are ovate or elliptical, finely serrate with 2 to 3 lateral ribs curved toward the midrib.

Characteristics: The flowers are fragrant. The heartwood is orange-red.

Habitat: The plant is common all over Europe, Western Asia, and North Africa.

Production: Buckthorn, consists of the dried ripe berries of *Rhamni catharticus* and its preparations. Buckthorn is harvested in uncultivated regions in autumn and dried.

Not to be Confused With: May be confused with the fruit of *Frangula alnus.*

Other Names: Hartsthorn, Common Buckthorn, Purging Buckthorn, Waythorn, Highwaythorn, Ramsthorn

ACTIONS AND PHARMACOLOGY

COMPOUNDS

Anthracene derivatives (2 to 7%): anthranoids, chief components glucofrangulin A, diacetylglucofrangulin, frangulin A

Flavonoids (1 to 2%): including catharticin (rhamnocitrin-3-O-rhamnoside), xanthorhamnine (rhamnetin-3-O-rhamnoside)

Tannins (3 to 4%): oligomeric proanthocyanidins

EFFECTS

The drug has a laxative effect because of the anthranoid content. Anthranoids have an anti-absorptive hydrogogic effect resulting in a more liquid stool and an increase in volume of the content of the intestine.

INDICATIONS AND USAGE

Approved by Commission E:

- Constipation

Buckthorn is used internally for constipation and for bowel movement relief in cases of anal fissures and hemorrhoids. It is used after recto-anal surgery and in preparation for diagnostic intervention in the gastrointestinal tract and to achieve softer stool.

Unproven Uses: In folk medicine it is used as a diuretic (in ''blood-purifying'' remedies).

Homeopathic Uses: Rhamnus catharticus is used for poor digestion.

CONTRAINDICATIONS

Contraindicated in intestinal obstruction, acute inflammatory intestinal diseases, appendicitis, and abdominal pain of unknown origin. Use during pregnancy or while nursing only after consulting a physician. The drug is not to be administered to children under 12 years of age.

PRECAUTIONS AND ADVERSE REACTIONS

General: Spasmodic gastrointestinal complaints could occur as a side effect to the drug's purgative effect. Long-term use leads to loss of electrolytes, especially potassium ions. This may lead to hyperaldosteronism, inhibition of intestinal motility and enhancement of the effect of cardioactive steroids, which in rare cases may result in cardiac arrhythmias. Nephropathies, edema, and accelerated bone deterioration may be the result of long-term use.

Drug-Interactions: Resorption of other medications could be reduced due to the laxative effect. In the case of chronic use/overuse, a potassium deficiency leads to an increase in the effect of cardiac glycosides as well as effecting heartbeat-regulating drugs. Potassium deficiency can be increased by the simultaneous use of thiazide diuretics, corticosteroids, and licorice root.

Pregnancy: Not to be used during pregnancy or while nursing.

OVERDOSAGE

The intake of large quantities of the fresh berries could lead to European cholera or kidney irritation. The question of the increase in probability of developing colonic carcinomas following long-term administration of anthracene drugs has not yet been fully clarified. Recent studies show no connection between the administration of anthracene drugs and the frequency of carcinoma of the colon.

DOSAGE

Mode of Administration: Buckthorn is available in solid pharmaceutical forms and in commercial compounded preparations for oral intake. It is also available parenterally for homeopathic use.

Preparation: To prepare a tea, pour boiling water over 2 gm cut drug and strain after 10 to 15 minutes or put the drug in cold water, bring to boil, boil for 2 to 3 minutes and strain while still warm.

Daily Dosage: 2 to 5 gm drug corresponding to 20 to 30 mg hydroxyanthracene derivative per day calculated as glucofrangulin A

Tea – 1 cup mornings and evenings.

The individual dose is the minimum dose required to produce a soft stool. Administration should be limited to a few days.

Homeopathic Dosage: from D3: 5 drops, 1 tablet, or 10 globules every 30 to 60 minutes (acute) or 1 to 3 times daily (chronic); parenterally: 1 to 2 ml sc acute: 3 times daily; chronic: once a day (HAB1)

Storage: Buckthorn should be protected from light.

LITERATURE

Anonym, Abwehr von Arzneimittelrisiken, Stufe II. In: *DAZ* 136(38):3253-2354. 1996.

Anonym, Anwendungseinschränkungen für Anthranoid-haltige Abführmittel angeordnet. In: *PUZ* 25(6):341-342. 1996.

BGA, Arzneimittelrisiken: Anthranoide. In: *DAZ* 132(21):1164. 1992.

Belkin M et al., (1952) *J Nat Cancer Inst* 13:742.

Coskun M. *Int J Pharmacogn* 30:151. 1992.

Demirezer LÖ, Glucofrangulinanthrone A/B, deren Oxidationsformen und davon abgeleitete Zuckerester aus Rhamnus-Arten. In: Dissertation Universität Frankfurt/Main. 1991.

Klimpel BE et al., Anthranoidhaltige Laxantien - ein Risiko für die Entwicklung von Tumoren der ableitenden Harnwege. In: *PUZ* 26(1):33, Jahrestagung der DPhG, Berlin, 1996. 1997.

Rauwald HW Just, J-D, (1981) *Planta Med* 42:244.

Thesen R, Phytotherapeutika - nicht immer harmlos. In: *ZPT* 9(49):105. 1988.

Buckwheat

Fagopyrum esculentum

DESCRIPTION

Medicinal Parts: The medicinal parts are the fresh aerial parts, and the leaves and flowers collected during the flowering season and later dried.

Flower and Fruit: Short, compact, long-peduncled thryses form in the leaf axils and at the end of the branches. The involucre is 3 to 4 mm long. It has 5 bracts, is pink or white and usually green at the base. The floret has 8 stamens with golden yellow nectaries at the base. The fruit is a sharply triangular achaene.

Leaves, Stem, and Root: Buckwheat is a 15 to 60 cm annual with an erect, usually red stem covered in alternating sagittate and sessile leaves. The lobes are obtuse or rounded with sweeping borders. The lower leaves are petioled, the upper ones less so. The root is fusiform. Tatar Buckwheat (*Fagopyrum tataricum*), which is used in the pharmaceutical industry, is easily distinguishable from *Fagopyrum esculentum* by its green flowers, usually green stems, and curved, dentated and squat achaenes.

Habitat: The plant is indigenous to central Asia and is cultivated in Europe.

Production: Buckwheat herb consists of the flower and leaves of *Fagopyrum esculentum,* which are harvested during flowering season and dried. The harvest takes place 50 to 60 days after sowing and before the fruit forms. There is a slight loss of rutin if it is quickly dried (20 to 40 minutes) at high temperatures (105° to 135° C).

ACTIONS AND PHARMACOLOGY

COMPOUNDS

Flavonoids: rutin (up to 8% in the leaves), quercitrin, hyperoside

Anthracene derivatives (naphthadianthrones, chiefly in the blossoms): fagopyrine (0.01%), protofagopyrine

EFFECTS

Buckwheat increases the venous tone (antiedemic, capillary sealing), which can be attributed to the rutin in the herb.

INDICATIONS AND USAGE

Unproven Uses: In folk medicine, the drug is used as a venous and capillary tonic and as a prophylaxis to prevent general hardening of the arteries. The drug alleviates venous stasis and varicose veins.

Homeopathic Uses: Buckwheat is used to treat skin and liver diseases with itching and headache.

PRECAUTIONS AND ADVERSE REACTIONS

Health risks or side effects following the proper administration of designated therapeutic dosages are not recorded.

OVERDOSAGE

The intake of large quantities of the Buckwheat plant leads to phototoxicoses in animals due to the photosensitizing effect of the naphthadianthrones. There are no dangers for humans in the application of therapeutic dosages.

DOSAGE

Mode of Administration: Buckwheat is taken orally as tablets and in teas.

Preparation: Follow package instructions for making Buckwheat tea.

Homeopathic Dosage: 5 drops, 1 tablet or 10 globules every 30 to 60 minutes (acute) or 1 to 3 times daily (chronic); from D6: parenterally: 1 to 2 mL sc, acute, 3 times daily; chronic: once a day (HAB1).

LITERATURE

Adamek B, Drozdzik M, Samochowiec L, Wojcicki J, Clinical effect of buckwheat herb, Ruscus extract and troxerutin on retinopathy and lipids in diabetic patients. In: *Phytotherapy Res* 10(8):659-662. 1996.

Anonym, Nicht-Brotgetreidearten: Alternative Körner unter der Lupe. In: *DAZ* 136(38):3229-2330. 1996.

Bässler R, PA 12:758-772 et 834-841. 1985.

Couch JF, Naghski J, Krewson CF, *Science* 103:197-198. 1974.

Gaidies I, Buchweizen, eine Venenhilfe. In: PTA 6(7):439. 1992.

Hagels H et al., Two anthraquinones and a bianthraquinone from *Fagopyrum tataricum.* In: PM 62, Abstracts of the 44th Ann Congress of GA, 125. 1996.

Ihme N et al., Leg oedema protection from a buckwheat herb tea in patients with chronic venous insufficiency: A single centre, randomised, double blind, placebo controlled clinical trial. In: *European J Clin Pharmacol* 50(6)443-447. 1996.

Koscielny J, Radtke H, Hoffmann KH, Jung F, Müller A, Grützner KI, Kiesewetter H, Fagorutin-Tee bei chronisch venöser Insuffizienz (CVI). In: *ZPT* 17(3):145-159. 1996.

Oomah BD and Mazza G. Flavonoids and antioxidant activities of buckwheat. *J Agric Food Chem.* 44(7):1746-1750. 1996.

Samel D, DonlaDeana A, Witte Pde. The effect of purified extract of *Fagopyrum esculentum* (buckwheat) on protein kinases involved in signal transduction pathways. *Planta Med* 62(2):106-110. 1996.

Samel D, de Witte P, Fagopyrins from Fagopyrum esculentum and their PTK inhibitory activity. In: *PM* 61(Abstracts of 43rd Ann Congr):67. 1995.

Theurer C, Gruetzner K, Freeman S, Koetter U. In vitro phototoxicity of hypericin, fagopyrin rich and fagopyrin free buckwheat herb extracts. *Pharm Pharmacol Lett* 7(2/3):113-155. 1997

Bugle

Ajuga reptans

DESCRIPTION

Medicinal Parts: The medicinal parts are the aerial parts collected during the flowering season and dried.

Flower and Fruit: The flowers are 1 to 1.5 cm long. The flowers are in spikes. They are located in the axils of undivided bracts at the end of the stem. The 5-tipped, hairy calyx is short-stemmed, erect, labiate, and campanulate. The tips are triangular and about as long as the tube. The corolla is bright violet-blue, pink, or white. It is downy-haired on the outside with a long straight tube, which has a circle of hairs under the stamen. There are 4 stamens with yellow anthers. The 4 mericarps are 2 mm long and finely reticulate.

Leaves, Stem and Root: Ajuga reptans is a shrub, up to 30 cm high with overground rooting runners sprouting from the rosettelike basal leaves. The flower stem is quadrangular, villous above and glabrous below. The rest of the plant is glabrous. The basal leaves are large, long-petioled, spatulate, and dentate. The cauline leaves are crossed opposite, short-petioled, small, and oval. The lowest or at least the third-lowest stem is flower-bearing. There are some upper false whorls, which are compressed into a false spike.

Habitat: The plant is found in Europe, Britain, and parts of Asia and northern Africa.

Production: The aerial parts of *Ajuga reptans* are picked when in bloom and dried. Gathered in uncultivated areas (the wild).

Other Names: Bugula, Middle Comfrey, Middle Confound, Sicklewort, Carpenter's Herb

ACTIONS AND PHARMACOLOGY

COMPOUNDS

Iridoid glycosides and ajugols

Phytoecdysone: ajugalactone

Diterpene bitter principles

Caffeic acid derivatives: including rosemary acid

EFFECTS

There is no information available.

INDICATIONS AND USAGE

Unproven Uses: Internally, Bugle is used as an astringent for inflammation of the mouth and larynx. It is also used for gallbladder and stomach disorders. Externally, the plant is used for the treatment of wounds.

PRECAUTIONS AND ADVERSE REACTIONS

No health hazards or side effects are known in conjunction with the proper administration of designated therapeutic dosages.

DOSAGE

Mode of Administration: Bugle is used topically, in alcoholic extracts, as a water infusion and in teas.

LITERATURE

Breschi M, Martinotti E, Catalano S, Flamini G, Morelli I, Pagni A, Vasoconstrictor activity of 8-O-Acetylharpagide from Ajuga reptans. In: *JNP* 55: 1145-1148. 1992.

Calcagno MP, Camps F, Coll J, Mele E, Sanchez-Baeza F. New phytoecdysteroids from roots of *Ajuga reptans* varieties. *Tetrehedon* 52:10137-10146. 1996

Camps F, et al., (1985) *An Quim* 81C(1):74-75.

Camps F, et al., (1981) *Rev Latinoamj Quim* 12:81-88. 1981.

Camps F, Coll J, (1993) Insect allochemicals from Ajuga plants. In: PH 32:1361.

Hänsel R, Keller K, Rimpler H, Schneider G (Hrsg.), Hagers Handbuch der Pharmazeutischen Praxis, 5. Aufl., Bde 4-6 (Drogen), Springer Verlag Berlin, Heidelberg, New York, 1992-1994.

Komissarenko NF, et al., (1976) *Khim Prir Soedin* 11:109-110. 1976.

Kooiman P, (1972) *Acta Bot Nederl*. 21(4):417.

Ruhdorfer J, Rimpler H, (1981) *Z Naturforsch* 36c:697-707. 1981.

Terahara N et al. Triacylated anthocyanins from *Ajuga reptans* flowers and cell cultures. *Phytochemistry* 55:199-203. 1996, May.

Bugleweed

Lycopus virginicus

DESCRIPTION

Medicinal Parts: The medicinal part is the fresh or dried herb collected during the flowering season.

Flower and Fruit: The flowers are small, almost radial in dense axillary whorls. The calyx is campanulate with a glabrous tube and 4 or 5 regular, usually erect, tips. The corolla is whitish with the tube only partly showing and a few uneven lobes. The epicalyx and calyx sepals are shorter than in the European variety. There are only 2 fertile stamens with initially parallel, then spreading, pollen sacs. The upper stamens are reduced to staminoids or completely disappear. The fruit is a flattened, rectangular, stunted, and smooth nutlet.

Leaves, Stem, and Root: The plant is a herbaceous perennial with runners. The quadrangular, 60 cm high smooth stems grow from the perennial creeping root. The stems bear pairs of opposite, short-petioled leaves. The upper ones are dentate and pointed; the lower ones wedge-shaped to entire-margined. They are glabrous and glandular-punctate on the lower surface.

Habitat: The plant grows in North America. *Lycopus europaeus*, Gypsywort, is a close European relative.

Production: Bugleweed consists of the fresh or dried, above-ground parts of *Lycopus europaeus* and/or *Lycopus virginicus*, as well as preparations collected in the wild and air-dried.

Other Names: Sweet Bugle, Water Bugle, Virginia Water Horehound, Gypsywort

ACTIONS AND PHARMACOLOGY

COMPOUNDS

Caffeic acid derivatives: rosmaric acid, lithospermic acid and their oligomerics created through oxidation.

Flavonoids: including acacetine-, apigenein-, luteolin glycosides, among them cosmosiin, genkwanin, pilloin, apigenin-, acacetine- and luteolin-7-O-glucuronides.

Diterpenes: tetrahydroxy-delta8(9)-pimaric acid methyl ester

Volatile oil (0.1%)

EFFECTS

Bugleweed has antigonadotropic and antithyrotropic effects. It inhibits the peripheral de-iodination of T4. The phenolic constituents of the drug have an antigonadotropic effect. They cause a lowering of the prolactin level and have a depressant effect on the thyroid as a result of an inhibition of iodine transport and the release of preformed thyroid hormone.

INDICATIONS AND USAGE

Approved by Commission E:

- Nervousness and insomnia
- Premenstrual syndrome (PMS)

Unproven Uses: Bugleweed is used for mild thyroid hyperfunction associated with disturbances of the autonomic nervous system. It is also used for tension and pain in the breast (mastodynia). In folk medicine, it is used for functional and organic cardiac conditions, and liver and kidney disease.

Homeopathic Uses: Lycopus virginicus is used to treat hyperthyroidism in homeopathic preparations.

CONTRAINDICATIONS

The drug is contraindicated in hypofunction of the thyroid and thyroid gland enlargement without function disturbance. There should not be any simultaneous administration of thyroid hormone preparations.

PRECAUTIONS AND ADVERSE REACTIONS

General: No health hazards or side effects are known in conjunction with the proper administration of designated therapeutic dosages.

DRUG INTERACTIONS

POTENTIAL INTERACTIONS

Thyroid Medications: Concurrent use may decrease thyroid activity and counteract the effects of medication used to treat hypothyroidism.

OVERDOSAGE

Enlargement of the thyroid gland is possible only through administration of the drug in very high dosage. Sudden discontinuation of *Lycopus* preparation can lead to a rebound phenomenon with increased TSH secretion and prolactin secretion, as well as an increase of the hyperthyroid symptom complex and mastodynia.

DOSAGE

Mode of Administration: Comminuted herb, freshly pressed juice and other galenic preparations for internal use.

How supplied:

Liquid Extract

Daily Dosage: The average daily dose is 1 to 2 gm of the drug for teas, and water-ethanol extracts containing the equivalent of 20 mg of the drug.

Each patient has his own individual optimal level of thyroid hormone. Only rough estimations of dosage are possible for thyroid disorders, in which age and weight must be considered.

Homeopathic Dosage: 5 drops, 1 tablet, or 10 globules every 30 to 60 minutes (acute) or 1 to 3 times daily (chronic); parenterally: 1 to 2 ml sc acute, 3 times daily; chronic: once a day (HAB1)

LITERATURE

Auf'mkolk M, (1985) *Endocrinology* 116(5):1687.

Bucar R et al., Flavonoid glycosides from *Lycopus europaeus.* In: *PM* 61(5):489. 1995.

Frömbling-Borges A, (1987) Intrathyreoidale Wirkung von *Lycopus europaeus*, Pflanzensäuren, Tyrosinen, Thyroninen und Lithiumchlorid. Darstellung einer Schilddrüsensekretions-blockade. Inauguraldissertation. Westfälische Wilhelms-Universtität Münster.

Frömbling-Borges A, Intrathyreoidale Wirkung von Lycopus europaeus, Pflanzensäuren, Kaliumjodid und Lithiumchlorid. In: *ZPT* 10(1):1. 1990.

Gumbinger HG et al., (1981) *Contraception* 23(6):661.

Hegnauer R, Kooiman P, (1978) *Planta Med* 33(1):13.

Jeremic D et al., (1985) *Tetrahedron* 41(2):357.

John M, Gumbinger HG, Winterhoff H, The oxidation of caffeic acid derivatives as model reaction for the formation of potent gonadotropin inhibitors in plant extracts. In: *PM* 59(3):195. 1993.

Jung F, Kiesewetter H, Mrowietz C, Pindur G, Heiden M, Miyashita C, Wenzel E, Akutwirkungen eines zusammengesetzten Knoblauchpräparates auf die Fließfähigkeit des Blutes. In: *ZPT* 10(3):87. 1989.

Kartnig T, Bucar F, Neuhold S. Flavonoids from the above-ground parts of *Lycopus virginicus. Planta Med* 59:563-564. 1993

Kern W, List PH, Hörhammer L (Hrsg.), Hagers Handbuch der Pharmazeutischen Praxis, 4. Aufl., Bde. 1-8, Springer Verlag Berlin, Heidelberg, New York, 1969.

Schulz R, Hänsel R, Rationale Phytotherapie, Springer Verlag Heidelberg 1996.

Kooiman P, (1972) *Acta Bot Neerl* 21(4)417.

Sourgens H et al., (1982) *Planta Med* 45:78.

Wagner H, Wiesenauer M, Phytotherapie. Phytopharmaka und pflanzliche Homöopathika, Fischer-Verlag, Stuttgart, Jena, New York 1995.

Winterhoff H, Gumbinger H, Sourgens H. On the antigonadotropic activity of *Lithospermum* and *Lycopus* species and some of their phenolic constituents. *Planta Med* 54:101-106. 1988.

Bulbous Buttercup

Ranunculus bulbosus

DESCRIPTION

Medicinal Parts: The medicinal parts are the latex and the fresh flowering herb with root.

Flower and Fruit: The large golden yellow flowers consist of 5 sepals hanging down, 5 petals on grooved stems and numerous stamens and ovaries. The small fruit has a short, curved beak.

Leaves, Stem, and Root: The plant grows from 10 to 30 cm high and has a tuber on the underground part of the stem. The basal leaves are long-petioled, trifoliate with orbicular and pinnasect leaflets. The middle one has a longer petiole and is sheathlike at the base. The stems are branched and tuberously thickened at the base. The plant is appressed pubescent above and patently pubescent below.

Habitat: The plant grows in the northern parts of Europe and in the northeastern U.S.

Production: Bulbous Buttercup is the whole plant in flower of *Ranunculus bulbosus* with root.

Other Names: Crowfoot, Cuckoo Buds, Frogwort, King's Cup, Meadowbloom, Pilewort, St. Anthony's Turnip, Frogsfoot, Goldcup

ACTIONS AND PHARMACOLOGY

COMPOUNDS

The glycoside ranunculin: changes enzymatically when the plant is cut into small pieces, and probably also when it is dried, into the pungent, volatile protoanemonine that quickly dimerizes to non-mucous-membrane irritating anemonine. When dried, the plant is not capable of protoanemonine formation.

EFFECTS

The active agents cause signs of toxic irritation; the drug is also said to cause symptoms of drowsiness and tiredness.

INDICATIONS AND USAGE

Homeopathic Uses: The herb is used for skin diseases, rheumatism, gout, neuralgia, influenza, and meningitis.

CONTRAINDICATIONS

The administration of the drug during pregnancy is absolutely contraindicated.

PRECAUTIONS AND ADVERSE REACTIONS

General: No health hazards or side effects are known in conjunction with the proper administration of designated therapeutic dosages of the dehydrated drug.

Extended skin contact with the freshly harvested, bruised plant can lead to blister formation and cauterizations that are difficult to heal due to the resulting protoanemonine, which is severely irritating to skin and mucous membranes. If taken internally may cause severe irritation to the gastrointestinal tract, combined with colic and diarrhea, as well as irritation of the urinary drainage passages. Symptomatic treatment for external contact should consist of mucilage, after irrigation with diluted potassium permanganate solution; in case of internal contact, activated charcoal should follow gastric lavage.

Pregnancy: The administration of the drug during pregnancy is absolutely contraindicated.

OVERDOSAGE

Death by asphyxiation following the intake of large quantities of protoanemonine-forming plants has been observed in animal experiments.

DOSAGE

Mode of Administration: The herb is used as an extract in homeopathic dilutions.

LITERATURE

Bonora A et al., *PH* 26:2277. 1987.

Didry N, Dubreiil L, Pinkas M. Microbiological properties of protoanemonin isolated from *Ranunculus bulbosus. Phytother Res.* 7(1):21-24. 1993.

Didry N, Dubreiil L, Pinkas M. New procedure for direct bioautographic TLC assay as applied to a tincture of *Ranunculus bulbosus. J Ethnopharmacol.* 29:283-290. 1990.

Frohne D, Pfänder HJ, Giftpflanzen - Ein Handbuch für Apotheker, Toxikologen und Biologen, 4. Aufl., Wiss. Verlags-Ges. Stuttgart 1997.

Kern W, List PH, Hörhammer L (Hrsg.), Hagers Handbuch der Pharmazeutischen Praxis, 4. Aufl., Bde. 1-8: Springer Verlag Berlin, Heidelberg, New York, 1969.

Madaus G, Lehrbuch der Biologischen Arzneimittel, Bde 1-3, Nachdruck, Georg Olms Verlag Hildesheim 1979.

Roth L, Daunderer M, Kormann K, Giftpflanzen, Pflanzengifte, 4. Aufl., Ecomed Fachverlag Landsberg Lech 1993.

Ruijgrok HWL, *PM* 11:338-347. 1963.

Teuscher E, Lindequist U, Biogene Gifte - Biologie, Chemie, Pharmakologie, 2. Aufl., Fischer Verlag Stuttgart 1994.

Bupleurum chinense

See Chinese Thoroughwax (Chai-Hu)

Burdock

Arctium lappa

DESCRIPTION

Medicinal Parts: The medicinal parts of the plant are the ripe seed and the fresh or dried roots.

Flower and Fruit: The crimson flowers grow in long-peduncled, loose cymes. The heads are fairly large, globose, and almost glabrous. All flowers are funnel-shaped and androgynous. The bracts are green and coriaceous with a barb-shaped, inward-curving tip. The fruit is compressed and has a bristly tuft, which falls off easily. The fruits separate from their stems on ripening.

Leaves, Stem, and Root: The plant grows to a height of 80 to 150 cm. The stem is erect, rigid, grooved, branched, and downy to wooly. The leaves are alternate, petiolate, broad to ovate-cordate. They are blunt and slightly wooly to hairy on the underside. The lowest leaves are very large and have a latex-filled stem.

Habitat: Burdock grows in Europe, northern Asia, and North America.

Production: Burdock root consists of the fresh or dried underground parts of *Arctium lappa, Arctium minus,* and/or *Arctium tomentosum.* Roots are gathered in the autumn of the plant's first year or the early part of the second year.

Other Names: Bardana, Beggar's Buttons, Burr Seed, Clot-Bur, Cockle Buttons, Cocklebur, Fox's Clote, Great Burr, Happy Major, Hardock, Hareburr, Lappa, Love Leaves, Personata, Philanthropium, Thorny Burr

ACTIONS AND PHARMACOLOGY

COMPOUNDS

Volatile oil (small amounts) of very complex make-up: including, among others, phenylacetaldehyde, benzaldehyde, 2-alkyl-3-methoxy-pyrazines

Lignans: neoarchtiin A

Sesquiterpene lactones

Polyynes: chief components are trideca-1, 11-dien-3, 5,7,9-tetrain, as well as sulfur derivatives

Caffeic acid derivatives: including chlorogenic acid, isochlorogenic acid

Polysaccharides: insulin (fructose), mucilage's (xyloglucans, acidic xylans)

Triterpenes: including alpha-amyrin, omega-taraxasterol, present to some extent as acetic acid ester

Phytosterols: beta-sitosterol, stigmasterol, campesterol and their esters

Tannins

EFFECTS

There are no human clinical trials validating the use of burdock root for any indication. Animal and in vitro data report that burdock may have antibacterial, antineoplastic, antioxidant, antiretroviral, and anti-inflammatory and hepatoprotective properties. The most extensive in vitro and animal research has been on the antineoplastic activity of burdock (Ryu et al, 1995; Umehara et al, 1993; Morita et al, 1984; Dombradi, 1970). Burdock exhibited antibacterial activity in vitro (Izzo et al, 1995) and inhibits human immunodeficiency virus (HIV-1) in vitro (Collins et al, 1997).

Antibacterial Effects: Eighty-percent ethanol extracts of aerial portions of burdock showed activity against *Bacillus subtilis* and *Salmonella typhi H* but not *Staphylococcus*, *Streptococcus*, *Escherichia coli*, *Klebsiella*, *Pseudomonas*, or *Proteus* (Izzo et al, 1995). The antimicrobial activity documented for burdock has been attributed to the polyacetylene constituents, (Schulte et al, 1967) although only traces of these compounds are found in the dried commercial herb (Wagner et al, 1983). No antibacterial activity was noted for the butyrolactone lignan glycoside arctiin and its aglycone, arctigenin, isolated from burdock achenes, against a variety of gram-positive and -negative organisms in vitro (Ryu et al, 1995).

Anti-Inflammatory Effects: A hot aqueous extract of achenes of burdock exhibited significant activity at inhibiting platelet-activating factor (PAF) binding to platelets in vitro (Iwakami et al, 1992). Methanol extracts from burdock achenes showed anticomplementary activity at a concentration of 0.05 g crude material/mL (6.3 mg/mL of the extract) in vitro. The active constituents were shown to be lignans such as lappaols B and H, arctigenin, matairesinol, and arctiin found in the ethyl acetate eluate of the methanol extract (Oshima et al, 1988).

Antineoplastic Effects: The burdock achene-derived butyrolactone lignan glycoside arctiin and its aglycone, arctigenin, exhibited antiproliferative activity against five human cancer cell lines in vitro. The activity of these constituents was significantly less than that of podophyllotoxin but similar to that of cisplatin and doxorubicin. These lignans bear structural similarity to podophyllotoxin (Ryu et al, 1995).

Lignans, such as arctigenin from the achenes of burdock, induced normalizing differentiation of a murine myeloid leukemia cell line into non-neoplastic phagocytic cells in vitro at concentrations of 5 micromolar. Sesquilignans and dilignans from burdock showed much weaker activity. Similar activity was not seen in a human leukemia cell line (Umehara et al, 1993).

An unidentified constituent of a fresh juice extract of burdock root showed antimutagenic activity against a wide range of mutagens in vitro. The compound was active against mutagens requiring metabolic activation as well as those that did not. Heating and exposure to proteolytic enzymes did not eliminate the antimutagenic activity. Manganese chloride eliminated the antimutagenicity of the extract. The active constituent was a polyanionic substance of high molecular weight (Morita et al, 1984).

Antioxidant Effects: Hot aqueous burdock root extracts showed superoxide dismutase-like activity and quenched hydroxyl radicals in vitro (Lin et al, 1996). Five caffeoylquinic acid compounds from the root of burdock showed more potent antioxidant activity than alpha-tocopherol, caffeic acid, or chlorogenic acid in vitro (Maruta et al, 1995).

Antiretroviral Effects: Aqueous extracts of achenes of burdock showed 90% inhibition of human immunodeficiency virus (HIV)-1 gp120 protein binding to the CD4 receptor in vitro (Collins et al, 1997).

Hepatoprotective Effects: Compared to untreated carbon tetrachloride-exposed controls, serum glutamic oxaloacetic transaminase (GOT) and glutamic pyruvic transaminase (GPT) levels were significantly lower in animals treated with any level of burdock extract ($p<0.01$ to 0.05). There was a clear dose-response effect. Liver histology was also markedly less abnormal in the animals given burdock extract. The burdock extracts, at a concentration of 300 and 1000 mg/kg, showed a superior ability to maintain normal serum GOT and GPT levels compared to 25 mg/kg silymarin (no statistical analysis provided). The authors suggest the activity was due to burdock's antioxidant properties (Lin et al, 1996).

CLINICAL TRIALS

There are no controlled and/or open-label clinical trials validating the use of burdock root for any indication.

INDICATION AND USAGE

Unproven Uses: Preparations of Burdock Root are used for ailments and complaints of the gastrointestinal tract, as a diaphoretic and diuretic, and for blood purifying. Externally, it is used for ichthyosis, psoriasis, and seborrhea of the scalp. The claimed efficacies have not been documented.

Chinese Medicine: Burdock is used to treat carbuncles, ulcers and erythema of the skin as well as sore throats. Efficacy has not been proved.

CONTRAINDICATIONS

Pregnancy: The achene or fruit of Burdock should not be used during the first trimester of pregnancy.

PRECAUTIONS AND ADVERSE REACTIONS

No health hazards or side effects are known in conjunction with the proper administration of designated therapeutic dosages. There is a slight potential for sensitization via skin contact with the drug. Anti-cholinergic symptoms have been reported in multiple cases related to consumption of burdock products (Bryson et al, 1978; Rhoads et al, 1984-1985). These were due to adulteration of the products with atropine-containing herbs and not due to any constituents or properties inherent to burdock (De Smet, 1993a).

Burdock can be safely combined with pharmaceutical drugs other than the combination of any Burdock tincture or alcohol extract with disulfiram or metronidazole due to the alcohol content.

DRUG INTERACTIONS

No interaction data is available.

DOSAGE

Mode of Administration: Administered as a drug and, for external use, in the form of burdock oil (extract with fat oil).

Preparation: Tea: steep 2.5 g (1 teaspoon) of the drug with 150 mL boiling water.

How Supplied:

Capsules – 460 mg and 475 mg

Fluid Extract – 1:1

Daily Dose: Tea. 1 cup 1 to 2 times a day.

LITERATURE

Bever BO, Zahnd GR. Plants with oral hypoglycaemic action. *Q J Crude Drug Res*; 17:139-196. 1979

Bryson PD, Watanabe AS, Rumack BH et al. Burdock root tea poisoning. case report involving a commercial preparation. *JAMA*; 239(20):2157. 1978

Cappelletti EM et al. External antirheumatic and antineuralgic herbal remedies in the traditional medicine of North-eastern Italy. *J Ethnopharmacol*; 6:161-190. 1982

Collins RA, Ng TB, Fong WP et al. A comparison of human immunodeficiency virus type 1 inhibition by partially purified aqueous extracts of Chinese medicinal herbs. *Life Sci*; 60:345-351. 1997

DeSmet PAGM, Keller K, Hansel R et al (eds). Legislatory outlook on the safety of herbal remedies. In. Adverse Effects of Herbal Drugs, vol 2. Springer-Verlag, Berlin, Germany:1-90. 1993b

Dombradi GA. Tumour-growth inhibiting substances of plant origin. II. The experimental animal tumour-pharmacology of arctigenin-mustard. *Chemotherapy*; 15:250-265. 1970

Izzo AA, Di Carlo G, Biscari D et al. Biological screening of Italian medicinal plants for antibacterial activity. *Phytother Res*; 9:281-286. 1995

Iwakami S, Wu JB, Ebizuka Y et al. Platelet activating factor (PAF) antagonist contained in medicinal plants. Lignans and sesquiterpenes. *Chem Pharm Bull* (Tokyo); 40:1196-1198. 1992

Lin CC, Lin JM, Yan JJ et al. Anti-inflammatory and radical scavenge effects of *Arctium lappa*. *Am J Chin Med*; 24:127-137. 1996

Morita K, Kada T & Namiki M. A desmutagenic factor isolated from burdock (*Arctium lappa Linne*). *Mutat Res*; 129:25-31. 1984

Maruta Y, Kawabata J, Niki R. Antioxidant caffeolyquinic acid derivatives in the roots of burdock (*Arcticum lappa L*). *J Agric Food Chem;* 43:2592-2592. 1995

Oshima Y, Suzuki K & Hikino H. Anticomplementary activity of lignan-analogs of *Arctium lappa* achenes. *Shoyakugaku Zasshi*; 42:337-338. 1988

Rhoads PM, Tong TG, Banner W Jr et al. Anticholinergic poisonings associated with commercial burdock root tea. *J Toxicol Clin Toxicol*; 22(6):581-584. 1984-1985

Rodriguez P et al. Allergic contact dermatitis due to burdock (*Arcticum lappa*). *Contact Dermatitis;* 343:134-135. 1995

Ryu SY, Ahn JW, Kang YH et al. Antiproliferative effect of actigenin and arctiin. *Arch Pharm Res*; 18:462-263. 1995

Schulte KE et al. Polyacetylenes in burdock root. *Arzneimittelforschung*; 17. 829-833. 1967

Umehara K, Sugawa A, Kuroyanagi M et al. Studies on differentiation-inducers from *Arctium fructus*. *Chem Pharm Bull* (Tokyo); 41:1774-1779. 1993

Yamada Y et al., *Phytochemistry;* 14:582. 1975

Yamanouchi S et al., *Yakugaku Zasshi;* 96(12):1992. 1976

Further information in.

Hausen B, Allergiepflanzen, Pflanzenallergene, ecomed Verlagsgesellsch. mbH, Landsberg, 1988.

Kern W, List PH, Hörhammer L (Hrsg.), Hagers Handbuch der Pharmazeutischen Praxis, 4. Aufl., Bde. 1-8, Springer Verlag Berlin, Heidelberg, New York, 1969.

Leung AY, Encyclopedia of Common Natural Ingredients Used in Food, Drugs and Cosmetics, John Wiley & Sons Inc., New York, 1980.

Madaus G, Lehrbuch der Biologischen Arzneimittel, Bde 1-3, Nachdruck, Georg Olms Verlag Hildesheim, 1979.

Moore M. Medicinal Plants of the Mountain West. Museum of New Mexico Press, Santa Fe, NM, 1979.

Wagner H et al. Plant Drug Analysis. Berlin. Springer-Verlag, 1983.

Wichtl M (Hrsg.), Teedrogen, 4. Aufl., Wiss. Verlagsges. Stuttgart, 1997.

Burning Bush

Dictamnus albus

DESCRIPTION

Medicinal Parts: The medicinal parts are the dried and occasionally the fresh leaves, the fresh or dried root, and the fresh or dried root rind.

Flower and Fruit: The flowers are terminal racemes and pink with dark veins. They are large and irregular, with 5 sepals and 5 petals. There are 2 bracteoles that are slightly zygomorphous. The 10 stamens are long, threadlike, and bent forward. The ovaries have 5 carpels fused at the base on a short gynophore. The fruit is a capsule that bursts open into mericarps ejecting the seeds.

Leaves, Stem, and Root: The plant is a 0.5 to 1.5 m high perennial. Numerous erect, unbranched and sticky-glandular-haired shoots grow from the root. The leaves are alternate, odd, 7 to 11 pinnate, and transparently punctuated with oil glands.

Characteristics: The plant has a strong lemon or cinnamon fragrance. The oil is easily inflammable.

Habitat: The plant is indigenous to central Europe and parts of Asia, and is cultivated in the northern U.S.

Not to be Confused With: Burning Bush herb can be confused with that of the herb *Dictamni cretici*. Previous sources cite confusion between Burning Bush root and Carophyllaceen root.

Other Names: Fraxinella, Dittany, Gas Plant, Diptam

ACTIONS AND PHARMACOLOGY

COMPOUNDS: BURNING BUSH ROOT

Volatile oil: chief components are the fraxinellone derivatives, thymol methylether, beta-pinene, pregeijerene, geijerene

Furoquinoline alkaloids: including skimmianine, gamma-fagarine, dictamnine

Limonoids: including limonin, obacunone, dictamdiol, limonin diosphenol

EFFECTS: BURNING BUSH ROOT

In vitro, a mutagenic effect on *Salmonella typhimurum* and a phototoxic effect on bacteria and yeasts have been observed.

In animal tests, a contraceptive effect was observed through the inhibition of implantation, as well as a slight increase in hair growth of shaved mice after the application of an alcoholic extract.

COMPOUNDS: BURNING BUSH HERB

Volatile oil: chief components (according to breed) anethole (+) estragole, anethole (+) myrcene, limonene, 1,8-cineol, p-cymene (+) estragole

Furoquinoline alkaloids: including skimmianine, gamma-fagarine, dictamnine

Furocoumarins: including psoralen, xanthotoxin, auraptene, bergaptenE

Limonoids: including limonin, obacunone, obacunone acid

Flavonoids: including rutin, diosmin, isoquercitrin

EFFECTS: BURNING BUSH HERB

See Burning Bush root.

A 40% reduction in egg-laying by *Clonorchis sinensis* (Chinese liver fluke) was observed when infected rabbits were given an evaporated extract of the drug.

INDICATIONS AND USAGE

BURNING BUSH ROOT

Unproven Uses: Infusion of the root is used to treat stomach disorders, cramps and worm infestation, and to promote menstruation.

In Greece, it is used as a tonic and a stimulant.

Chinese Medicine: Burning Bush root is used for jaundice, inflammation of the skin, rheumatic ailments, fever, hemorrhage of the womb, thread fungus, as a sedative, tonic, and for nervous crying in children. It is also found in decoctions for the external treatment of eczema, impetigo, and scabies.

Indian Medicine: Burning Bush root is used for amenorrhea and the regulation of labor.

BURNING BUSH HERB

Unproven Uses: In the Middle Ages, the drug was used as a cure or remedy for wounds, to promote menstruation and to aid the expulsion of afterbirth. It served as a urinary aid and was used in the treatment of epilepsy, in combination with mistletoe and peony.

At the end of the 19th century, the drug was applied as an ointment for rheumatism. The infusion is used as a remedy for worm infestation, to treat stomach disorders and cramps and to promote menstruation. In Greece, it is used as a tonic and stimulant.

PRECAUTIONS AND ADVERSE REACTIONS

BURNING BUSH ROOT AND HERB

Health risks or side effects following the proper administration of designated therapeutic dosages are not recorded. The plant can trigger phototoxicoses through skin contact. The furoquinoline derivatives have a mutagenic effect in the Ames test.

DOSAGE

BURNING BUSH ROOT

Mode of Administration: Mostly obsolete as a drug. It is occasionally used in tea mixtures.

Preparation: To prepare a tea infusion, add 1 teaspoon of drug to 2 glasses of hot water.

Daily Dosage: Drink the tea preparation throughout the day.

BURNING BUSH HERB

Mode of Administration: Mostly obsolete as a drug. The herb is sometimes used internally as an infusion.

Preparation: An infusion is prepared by adding 20 gm of dried herb to 1 liter of water; or 1 gm fresh or 2 gm dried herb to 1 cup of water.

Daily Dosage: Drink one cup of the infusion 2 to 3 times daily after meals.

LITERATURE

Can Baser KH, Cosar M, Malyer H, Ozek T. The essential oil composition of *Dictamnus ablus* from Turkey. *Planta Med.* 481-482. 1994.

Inaoka Y et al. Studies on active substances in herbs used for hair treatment. I. Effects of herb extracts on hair growth and isolation of an active substance from *Polyporus umbellatus F. Chem Pharm Bull* 42:530-533. 1994.

Kanamori H, Sakamoto I, Mizuta M, *Chem Pharm Bull* 34:1826. 1986.

Reisch J, *PM* 15:320. 1967.

Szenedrei K, Novak I, Varga E, Buzas G, *PA* 23:76-77. 1968.

Burr Marigold

Bidens tripartita

DESCRIPTION

Medicinal Parts: The whole Burr Marigold plant is used medicinally.

Flower and Fruit: The flower heads are solitary, erect or inclined, 15 to 25 mm long and wide, generally with no lingual blossoms. There are two rows of bracts. The inner row is ovate and brownish-yellow; the outer is oblong and green. The petals are brownish-yellow. The fruit is glabrous, distinctly compressed, brownish-green, with thorny edges and 2 to 4 awns.

Leaves, Stem, and Root: Bidens tripartita is an erect annual growing 15 to 100 cm high with a fibrous fusiform root. The stem is erect, heavily branched, glabrous or somewhat downy, and often brownish-red. The leaves are dark green, opposite and narrow to a short, winged petiole. The leaves are usually 3 to 5 lobed, ovate-rhomboid to lanceolate with pointed, roughly dentate tips and straight or narrowly curved teeth.

Habitat: The plant is found in damp regions throughout Europe.

Production: Burr Marigold is the aerial part of *Bidens tripartita*.

Other Names: Water Agrimony

ACTIONS AND PHARMACOLOGY

COMPOUNDS

Flavonoids: including isookanin-7-O-glucoside and tridecane derivatives such as trideca-1,12-dien-3,5,7,9-tetrain

Hydroxycoumarins: including umbelliferone, scopoletin

Polyynes (tridecane derivatives): including trideca-1,12-dien-3,5,7,9-tetrain

Water-soluble polysaccharides

Bitter principles

Tannins

Volatile oil: including eugenol, ocimene, cosmene

EFFECTS

Astringent, diaphoretic, and diuretic effects are attributed to the plant, but remain unproved. In a study that has not been described in detail, a choleretic effect caused by the flavones and flavonoids was proved.

INDICATIONS AND USAGE

Unproven Uses: Folk medicine uses include gout, hematuria, colitis, and loss of hair.

PRECAUTIONS AND ADVERSE REACTIONS

No health hazards or side effects are known in conjunction with the proper administration of designated therapeutic dosages.

DOSAGE

No information is available.

LITERATURE

Bauer R, Neues von ''immunmodulierenden Drogen'' und ''Drogen mit antiallergischer und antiinflammatorischer Wirkung''. In: *ZPT* 14(1):23-24. 1993.

Ben'ko GN, (1983) *Rastit Resur* 19 (4),516.

Morozova SS et al., (1981) *Rastit Resur* 17 (1),101.

Butcher's Broom

Ruscus aculeatus

DESCRIPTION

Medicinal Parts: The medicinal parts are the herb and the rhizome.

Flower and Fruit: The small greenish white flowers are solitary or in a few clusters and grow from the middle of the leaves. They are dioecious. The corolla is deeply divided into 6 segments. In one variety the stamens are fused at the base. In fertile varieties the style is surrounded by a honey gland. The fertile flowers develop into cherry-sized, scarlet berries, which ripen in September and remain on the tree all winter.

Leaves, Stem, and Root: The plant is a perennial evergreen subshrub that grows 20 to 80 cm high. The stems are erect, woody, and heavily branched. The leaves are small, brown-membranous, triangular to lanceolate, and scalelike. The phylloclades (short shoots spread like leaves) are oblong, stiff, double-rowed, up to 2.5 cm long and terminate in a sharp tip.

Habitat: The plant is indigenous to almost all of Europe, western Asia and North Africa.

Production: Butcher's Broom consists of the dried rhizome and root of *Ruscus aculeatus*.

Other Names: Kneeholm, Pettigree, Sweet Broom, Knee Holly, Jew's Myrtle

ACTIONS AND PHARMACOLOGY

COMPOUNDS

Steroid saponins (4-6%): chief components, ruscine, ruscoside, aglycones neoruscogenin, ruscogenin

Benzofuranes: euparone, ruscodibenzofurane

EFFECTS

In animal tests, there was an increase in venous tone and an electrolytelike reaction on the cell wall of capillaries. Butcher's Broom is antiphlogistic and diuretic.

INDICATIONS AND USAGE

Approved by Commission E:

- Hemorrhoids
- Venous conditions

The herb is used as supportive therapy for discomfort of chronic venous insufficiency, such as pain and heaviness, as well as cramps in the legs, itching, and swelling. Butcher's Broom also is used as therapy for hemorrhoid complaints, such as itching and burning.

PRECAUTIONS AND ADVERSE REACTIONS

No health hazards or side effects are known in conjunction with the proper administration of designated therapeutic dosages. Stomach complaints and queasiness can occur in rare cases.

DOSAGE

Mode of Administration: Extracts and their preparations for internal use.

How Supplied:

Capsules – 75 mg, 370 mg, 470 mg, 475 mg

Liquid extract

Daily Dosage: Raw extract, equivalent to 7 to 11 mg total ruscogenin (determined as the sum of neoruscogenin and ruscogenin obtained after fermentation or acid hydrolysis).

LITERATURE

Adamek B, Drozdzik M, Samochowiec L, Wojcicki J, Clinical effect of buckwheat herb, Ruscus extract and troxerutin on retinopathy and lipids in diabetic patients. In: *Phytotherapy Res* 10(8):659-662. 1996.

Dunaouau CH et al., Triterpenes and sterols from Ruscus aculeatus. In: *PM* 62(2):189-190. 1997.

Landa N, Aguirre A, Goday J, Raton JA, Diaz-Perez JL. Allergic contact dermatitis from a vasoconstrictor cream. *Contact Dermatitis* 22:290-291. 1990.

Maffei Facino R, Carini M, Stefani R, Aldini G, Saibene L. Anti-elastase and anti-hyaluronidase activities of saponins and sapogenins from *Hedera helix, Aesculus hippocastanum*, and *Ruscus aculeatus*: Factors contributing to their efficacy in treatment of venous insufficiency. *Arch Pharm* (Weinheim) 328:720-722.

Mimaki Y et al. Steroidal saponins from the underground parts of *Ruscus aculeatus* and their cytostatic activity on HL-60 cells. *Phytochemistry* 48(3):485-493. 1998.

Nikolov S and Gussev C. Sulphated steroidal derivatives from *Ruscus aculeatus. Phytochemistry* 42(3) 895-897. 1998

Rauwald HW, Janβen B, Desglucoruscin and Desglucoruscosid als Leitstoffe des Ruscus-aculeatus-Wurzelstock. Analytische Kennzeichnung mittel HPLC und DC. In: *PZW* 133(1):61-68. 1988.

Schiebel-Schlosser G, Stechender Mäusedorn, eine Venenhilfe. In: *PTA* 8(7):586. 1994.

Vanhoutte PM (1986) in: Advances in Medicinal Phytochemistry, Ed. D Barton, WD Ollis, Pub. John Wiley 1986.

Buttercup

Ranunculus acris

DESCRIPTION

Medicinal Parts: The medicinal part is the herb.

Flower and Fruit: The golden-yellow, medium-sized flowers are on long, round pedicles. The 5 sepals and 5 petals are close. There are numerous stamens and ovaries. The broad obovate petals are very glossy and have a broad scale on the surface. The small fruit is in an almost globular capitulum.

Leaves, Stem and Root: The leafy plant grows from 30 to 80 cm. The erect stem has few branches. The petioles and pedicles are appressed and downy. The basal leaves are long-petioled and palmate with rhomboid tips, which are divided into 2 or 3 sections. The similar cauline leaves have shorter-petioles.

Characteristics: The fresh herb is spicy and poisonous; once dried, it is no longer poisonous.

Habitat: The plant is indigenous to northern Europe.

Production: Buttercup is the fresh herb *Ranunculus acris.*

Other Names: Acrid Crowfoot, Batchelor's Buttons, Blister-weed, Burrwort, Globe Amaranth, Gold Cup, Meadowbloom, Yellows, Yellowweed

ACTIONS AND PHARMACOLOGY

COMPOUNDS

Glycoside ranunculin: as protoanemonine-forming agent in the freshly harvested plant (0.36-2.66% of the fresh weight) that changes enzymatically when the plant is cut into small pieces (and probably also while it is drying) into the pungent, volatile protoanemonine, which quickly dimerizes to non-mucous-membrane-irritating anemonine. Once dried, the plant may not be capable of protoanemonine formation.

Saponins

EFFECTS

The active agents are ranunculin, protoanemonin, and anemonin. On contact with the skin, the juice of the plant causes redness, swelling, and blisters. If taken internally, it can lead to burning in the mouth, vomiting, stomachache, and pains in the liver.

INDICATIONS AND USAGE

Unproven Uses: Buttercup is used for bronchitis, chronic skin complaints, neuralgia, and rheumatism.

PRECAUTIONS AND ADVERSE REACTIONS

No health hazards or side effects are known in conjunction with the proper administration of designated therapeutic dosages of the dehydrated drug. Extended skin contact with the freshly harvested, bruised plant can lead to blister formation and cauterizations that are difficult to heal due to the resulting protoanemonine, which is severely irritating to skin and mucous membranes. If taken internally, severe irritation to the gastrointestinal tract, combined with colic and diarrhea, as well as irritation of the urinary drainage passages, may occur.

Symptomatic treatment for external contact should consist of mucilaginosa, after irrigation with diluted potassium permanganate solution. In case of internal contact, administration of activated charcoal should follow gastric lavage.

OVERDOSAGE

Death by asphyxiation following the intake of large quantities of protoanemonine-forming plants has been observed in animal experiments.

DOSAGE

Mode of Administration: Buttercup is available as a ground dried herb and as an extract.

LITERATURE

Bonora A et al., *PH* 26:2277. 1987.

Frohne D, Pfänder HJ: Giftpflanzen - Ein Handbuch für Apotheker, Toxikologen und Biologen, 4. Aufl., Wiss. Verlags-Ges. Stuttgart 1997

Hegnauer R, Chemotaxonomie der Pflanzen, Bde 1-11: Birkhäuser Verlag Basel, Boston, Berlin 1962-1997.

Kern W, List PH, Hörhammer L (Hrsg.), Hagers Handbuch der Pharmazeutischen Praxis, 4. Aufl., Bde. 1-8: Springer Verlag Berlin, Heidelberg, New York, 1969.

Roth L, Daunderer M, Kormann K, Giftpflanzen, Pflanzengifte, 4. Aufl., Ecomed Fachverlag Landsberg Lech 1993.

Ruijgrok HWL, *PM* 11:338-347. 1963.

Teuscher E, Lindequist U: Biogene Gifte - Biologie, Chemie, Pharmakologie, 2. Aufl., Fischer Verlag Stuttgart 1994.

Butternut

Juglans cinerea

DESCRIPTION

Medicinal Parts: The medicinal parts are the bark of the tree and root.

Flower and Fruit: The tree has male catkins and female flowers. The male catkins are 5 to 8 cm long. The fruit is 4 to 6.5 cm and ovoid-oblong. The fruit is pubescent, viscid and strong smelling. The hard nut is ovoid-oblong with 4 prominent and 4 less prominent sharp ridges and many broken grooves between them.

Leaves, Stem, and Root: Butternut tree grows up to 30 m tall. The bark is gray and deeply fissured. The leaf scars have a prominent pubescent band on their upper edge. The 6- to 12-cm long leaflets are oblong-lanceolate, acuminate, and appressed-serrate. They are finely pubescent above, glandular, and pubescent beneath.

Habitat: Butternut is indigenous to the forests of the U.S.

Production: Butternut bark is the inner rind of *Juglans cinerea.*

Other Names: Black Walnut, Lemon Walnut, Oil Nut, White Walnut

ACTIONS AND PHARMACOLOGY

COMPOUNDS

Fatty oil

Tannins

Juglone

Juglandis folium

EFFECTS

Butternut is said to be a vermifuge, laxative, and tonic. Sedative and antitumor effects have been shown in animal and in vitro studies (Girzu et al, 1998, Sugie et al, 1998; Yu & Reed, 1995; Frew et al, 1995).

Antifungal Effects: Juglone was observed to have antifungal activity against the yeasts *Candida albicans, Saccharomyces cerevisiae,* and *Cryptococcus neoformans* in a quantitative and qualitative assay study of various microorganisms. Relatively effective activity was observed against *Aspergillus flavus* and *Aspergillus fumigatus* (Clark et al, 1990).

Antitumor Effects: Naphthoquinones juglone and plumbagin were found to be promising agents for the treatment of intestinal cancer in a study evaluating intestinal carcinogenesis in 160 rats (Sugie et al, 1998). Juglone isolated from black walnut and methyljuglone was found to inhibit protein kinase C (PKC) in an in vivo study conducted to investigate antitumor activity of naphthoquinones and quinoline quinones (Frew et al, 1995). Juglans and solanum in concentrations up to 1 mcg/mL inhibited the growth curve of human ovarian cancer cells in an in vitro study. A liquid preparation of juglan and solanum did not demonstrate any cytotoxic effects on the cancer cells (Yu & Reed, 1995).

Sedative Effects: Juglone was shown to have sedative activity in mice in a controlled and blinded study (Girzu et al, 1998).

CLINICAL TRIALS

There are no clinical studies reported using black walnut herb (*Juglans cinerea*).

INDICATIONS AND USAGE

Approved by Commission E

■ Inflammation of the skin

■ Excessive perspiration of the hands and feet

Unproven Uses: Preparations of the bark are used for disorders of the gallbladder, for hemorrhoids and in the treatment of skin diseases. Juglone has antimicrobial, antineoplastic, and antiparasitic properties as well as being a gentle laxative.

CONTRAINDICATIONS

Black walnut should be avoided in patients with liver disease due to the risk of hepatotoxicity.

Pregnancy: Not to be used during pregnancy.

Breastfeeding: Not to be used while breastfeeding.

PRECAUTIONS AND ADVERSE REACTIONS

No health hazards or side effects are known in conjunction with the proper administration of designated therapeutic dosages. Contact dermatitis has been documented following exposure to the juice. Long-term use is not advised as it has shown carcinogenic effects in humans.

DRUG INTERACTIONS

POTENTIAL INTERACTIONS

Iron: The tannin content of Butternut leaf may complex with concomitantly administered iron, resulting in nonabsorbable insoluble complexes that may result in adverse sequelae on blood components. *Clinical Management:* Patients who need iron supplementation should be advised to separate administration times of these two compounds by one to two hours.

DOSAGE

Mode of Administration: Available preparations include liquid and dry extracts that are used internally and externally.

How Supplied:

Capsules – 95 mg, 500 mg, 3.5 g

Fluid Extract - 1:1

LITERATURE

Chung KT, Wong TY, Wei CI et al. Tannins and human health: a review. *Crit Rev Food Sci Nutrition*; 38:421-464. 1998

Clark A, Jurgens T, and Hufford C. Antimicrobial activity of juglone. *Phytotherapy Research*; 4(1):11-14. 1990

Craton D and Williams R. Juglone dermatitis: allergy or irritant? Indiana Academy of Science 1980; 90: 98-102.

Frew T, Powis G, Berggren M et al. Novel quinone antiproliferative inhibitors of phosphatidylinositol-3-kinase. *Anti-Cancer Drug Design*; 10(4):347-359. 1995

Galey FD, Whitely HE, Goetz TE. Black Walnut (*Juglans nigra*) toxicosis: a model for equine laminitis. *J Comp Path*; 104(3):313-326. 1991

Girzu M, Carnat A, Privat AM. Sedative effect of walnut leaf extract and juglone, an isolated constituent. *Pharmaceutical Biology*; 36 (4):280-286. 1998

Koren G, Boichis H & Keren G. Effects of tea on the absorption of pharmacological doses of an oral iron preparation. Sci Meet Israel 1982; 18:547. Madaus G, Lehrbuch der Biologischen Arzneimittel, Bde 1-3, Nachdruck, Georg Olms Verlag Hildesheim 1979.

Pizarro F, Olivares M, Hertrampf E et al. Factors which modify the nutritional state of iron: tannin content of herbal teas. *Arch Latinoam Nutr*; 44:277-280. 1944

Siegel J. Dermatitis due to black walnut juice. AMA Archives of Dermatology and Syphilology 1954; 70(4):511-513.

Sugie S, Okamoto K, Rahman W. Inhibitory effects of plumbagin and juglone on azoxymethane-induced intestinal carcinogenesis in rats. *Cancer Letters*; 127(1-2):177-183. 1998

Yu J & Reed E. Preliminary study of the effect of selected Chinese natural drugs on human ovarian cancer cells. *Oncology Reports*; 2:571-575. 1995

Buxus sempervirens

See Boxwood

Cabbage

Brassica oleracea

DESCRIPTION

Medicinal Parts: The medicinal parts of the plant are the fresh cabbage head and juice derived from the fresh leaves.

Flower and Fruit: The inflorescences have long-pedicled flowers. The flowers are large and have 4 erect, narrowly elliptoid sepals 6 to 12 mm long. The 4 petals are about twice as long as the calyx and are sulphur yellow. The margin broadens at the tip and narrows at the base to an equally long wedge-shaped funicle stem. The stamens are erect and close to the ovary. The central honey gland is almost erect. The fruit is oblong, podlike, almost cylindrical, and has a domed lid. The dividing wall of the fruit is thin as well as pitted and folded between the dark brown seeds, which have a diameter of 1.5 to 4 mm.

Leaves, Stem, and Root: The plant can be annual, biennial, or perennial. It is about 2 m high and has thin roots. The stem is woody from the first year and is covered in leaf nodes. It has a bluish bloom and is branched toward the top. The leaves are fleshy, blue-green, and glabrous. The lower leaves are petiolate, lyre-shaped, pinnatifid or simple. The upper leaves are oblong to linear-oblong, usually entire-margined and narrowed to rounded at the base and sessile.

Habitat: Wild Cabbage was originally found in the Mediterranean region. Today it grows wild as far north as southern England and Helgoland, and cultivated varieties are found in temperate and damp climates worldwide.

Production: White cabbage juice is the juice of *Brassica oleracea.*

Other Names: Colewort

ACTIONS AND PHARMACOLOGY

COMPOUNDS

Mustard oils (breakdown products of the glucosinolates accompanying cell destruction): allyl mustard oil, methyl sulfinyl alkyl isothiocyanates, methyl sulfonyl alkyl isothiocyanates

3-hydroxy-methyl-indole

5-vinyl-oxazolidine-2-thion (goitrin)

Rhodanides

Alkyl nitriles

Amino acids: including S-methyl cysteine sulphoxide, S-methyl methionine sulphoxide and, when extracted from red cabbage, also anthocyans, including cyanidine-5-0-glucoside-3-0-sophoroside

EFFECTS

Cabbage protects the mucous membrane of the stomach from gastric hydrochloric acid. The gastroprotective effect of the juice is attributed to the regenerative ability of the mucous membrane that is caused by an anti-ulcer factor (vitamin U).

INDICATIONS AND USAGE

Unproven Uses: Folk medicine uses include drinking the juice for gastritis, gastric and duodenal ulcers.

Homeopathic Uses: Preparations of the flowering herb are used for hypothyroidism.

Indian Medicine: Cabbage leaves are used for disorders of the thyroid, gastrointestinal tract, itching and cough, as well as for asthma, gout, and hemorrhoids.

PRECAUTIONS AND ADVERSE REACTIONS

No health hazards or side effects are known in conjunction with the proper administration of designated therapeutic dosages.

DOSAGE

Mode of Administration: The drug is available as a standard preparation or prepared from chopped and pressed Cabbage for internal use. Also available in homeopathic preparations.

How Supplied:

Tablet – 500 mg

Preparation: White cabbage (*Brassica Oleracea Var. Capitata*) extract is prepared by processing leaves by mashing or using a centrifuge. The resulting mass is pressed through a linen cloth.

Daily Dosage: To augment a bland diet take 1 liter of juice daily for at least 3 weeks but not more than 6 weeks as a dietary additive.

Homeopathic Dosage: 5 drops, 1 tablet, 10 globules every 30 to 60 minutes (acute) or 1 to 3 times daily (chronic); parenterally: 1 to 2 mL sc; acute: 3 times daily; chronic: once a day (HAB34).

Storage: The fresh juice will keep for approximately 24 hours if kept cool.

LITERATURE

Akhtar MS, Munir M. Evaluation of the gastric antiulcerogenic effect of 482 1989 *Brassica oleracea* and *Ocimum basilicum* in rats. *J Ethnopharmacol*. 27:163-176. 1989.

Brown JP. A review of the genetic effects of naturally occurring flavonoids, anthraquinones, and related compounds. *Mutation Res.* 75:243-277. 1980.

Fischer J. Sulphur- and nitrogen-containing volatile components of kohlrabi (*Brassica oleracea var. gongylodes L.*) *Z Lebensm Unters Forsch*. 194:259-262. 1992.

Kaoulla N et al., *PH* 19:1053-1056. 1980.

Larson KM, Stermitz FR, *JNP* 47(4):747-748. 1984.

Petroski RJ, Tookey HL, *PH* 21:1903-1905. 1982.

Slominski BA, Campbell LD, *J Agric Food Chem* 37:1297-1302. 1989.

Caesalpinia bonducella

See Divi-Divi

Cajuput

Melaleuca leucadendra

DESCRIPTION

Medicinal Parts: The medicinal part is the oil distilled from the fresh leaves and twigs.

Flower and Fruit: The tree has racemes of small, sessile, creamy white flowers on long terminal spikes up to 15 cm long, which themselves terminate in a tuft of leaves. The flowers have numerous stamens extending to 15 mm.

Leaves, Stem and Root: Melaleuca leucadendra is a large tree up to 40 m tall with a flexible trunk and irregular pendulous branches. The tree is covered in a pale, lamellate bark, which is soft and spongy and occasionally peels off its layers. The leaves are alternate, entire-margined, oblong-lanceolate, tapering, ash-colored and on short petioles.

Characteristic: It has an odor reminiscent of camphor and eucalyptus.

Habitat: The plant is indigenous to Southeast Asia and the tropical regions of Australia. It is cultivated elsewhere.

Production: Cajuput oil consists of the essential oil of *Melaleuca leucadendra*. It is extracted from the fresh leaves and twig tips of a number of varieties collected from the wild or from cultivation, followed by air-drying and aqueous steam distillation.

Other Names: White Tea Tree, Swamp Tea Tree, Paperbark Tree, White Wood

ACTIONS AND PHARMACOLOGY

COMPOUNDS

Chief constituents: cineol, (+)-alpha-terpineol, (-)-alpha-terpineol, (+)-alpha-terpineol valerate, (-)- alpha-terpineol valerate, furthermore alpha-pinenes and bicyclic sesquiterpenes, non-rectified oils also contain 3,5-dimethyl-4, 6-di-O-methyl-phloroacetophenone

EFFECTS

In vitro, the drug has an antimicrobial and a rubefacient effect.

INDICATIONS AND USAGE

Approved by Commission E:

- Rheumatism
- Neurogenic pain
- Temporary relief of muscular pain
- Tendency to infection
- Wounds and burns

Unproven Uses: The drug is used for painful muscles and joints in rheumatic disorders, sciatica, lumbago, slipped disk, and low back pain. Cajuput is also used for muscular tension and pain following sports injuries such as sprains, bruising, and pulled muscles or ligaments.

CONTRAINDICATIONS

No internal administration of the drug should take place in the presence of inflammatory illnesses of the gastrointestinal area or of the biliary ducts, nor in the presence of severe liver diseases. Preparations containing the oil should not be applied to the faces of infants or small children (glottal spasm or bronchial spasm or even asthmalike attacks or respiratory failure might occur).

PRECAUTIONS AND ADVERSE REACTIONS

General: No health hazards or side effects are known in conjunction with the proper administration of designated therapeutic dosages; however, contact dermatitis is possible.

Pediatric Use: The drug should not be applied to the facial area, in particular not around the nose, of infants and small children (glottal spasms could occur).

OVERDOSAGE

Overdoses of cajuput oil (more than 10 gm) could lead to life-threatening poisonings due to the high cineole content. Symptoms include including loss of blood pressure, circulatory disorders, collapse, and respiratory failure. Vomiting is not to be induced in the case of poisoning, because of the danger of aspiration. Following administration of activated charcoal, the therapy for poisonings consists of treating spasms with diazepam (i.v.), treating colic with atropine, electrolyte substitution and treating possible cases of acidosis with sodium bicarbonate infusions. Intubation and oxygen respiration may also be necessary.

DOSAGE

Mode of Administration: Cajuput oil is used only for external purposes. It is often found in combination with a number of other essential oils, including pine, rosemary, peppermint, camphor, menthol, clove, sage, and eucalyptus.

LITERATURE

Fenaroli's Handbook of Flavor Ingredients, Vol. 1. 2nd Ed., CRC Press 1975.

Kern W, List PH, Hörhammer L (Hrsg.), Hagers Handbuch der Pharmazeutischen Praxis, 4. Aufl., Bde 1-8, Springer Verlag Berlin, Heidelberg, New York, 1969.

Leung AY, Encyclopedia of Common Natural Ingredients Used in Food Drugs and Cosmetics, John Wiley & Sons Inc., New York 1980.

Lowry JB, (1973) *Nature* 241:61.

Opdyke DLJ, (1976) *Food Cosmet Toxicol*:14.

Steinegger E, Hänsel R, Pharmakognosie, 5. Aufl., Springer Verlag Heidelberg 1992.

Teuscher E, Biogene Arzneimittel, 5. Aufl., Wiss. Verlagsges. Stuttgart 1997.

Calabar Bean

Physostigma venenosum

DESCRIPTION

Medicinal Parts: The medicinal parts are the seeds.

Flower and Fruit: The inflorescences are pendulous racemes of beanlike flowers. The fruit is a dark brown pod up to 15 cm long containing 2 or 3 dark brown or blackish kidney-shaped seeds that are about 2.5 cm long. They are rounded at the ends, uneven, and somewhat polished with the hilum extending along the whole convex side. The cotyledons are whitish.

Leaves, Stem and Root: The plant is a large, perennial, twining, woody climber with large, pinnate, trifoliate leaves.

Habitat: The plant is indigenous to western Africa and is cultivated in India and parts of South America.

Production: The Calabar Bean is the seed of *Physostigma venenosum.*

Other Names: Chop Nut, Ordeal Bean

ACTIONS AND PHARMACOLOGY

COMPOUNDS

Indole alkaloide (0.3 - 0.5%): main alkaloid physostigmine, secondary alkaloids include physovenine, geneserine, eseramine

Starch (up to 50%)

Proteic substances

Fatty oil

EFFECTS

The main alkaloid, physostigmine, is miotic, spasmogenic, negatively chronotropic and curare-antagonistic. It causes an increase in tone in the parasympathetic system and the striated muscles. In particular, it causes the pupils to contract, thus reducing intraocular pressure. It is a glandular stimulant and increases peristalsis of the gastrointestinal tract. It reduces heart rate and is a curare antidote.

INDICATIONS AND USAGE

Unproven Uses: The drug is frequently used in the treatment of glaucoma. It is also a poison antidote. Studies of its use in the treatment of Alzheimer's disease to reduce memory loss and confusion have not shown it to be of any more significance than placebo.

PRECAUTIONS AND ADVERSE REACTIONS

Calabar Bean is extremely poisonous. The drug is only used in the extraction of physostigmine. Symptoms of poisoning include: diarrhea, dizziness, nausea, salivation, stupor, signs of exhaustion, sweats, chills in the extremities, muscle paralysis, and vomiting. Poisonings are possible through inappropriate administration of physostigmine eye drops due to drainage into the mouth or nose.

OVERDOSAGE

Lethal doses can cause muscle twitching, spasms, tachycardia, and cyanosis through asphyxiation. Following gastric lavage, poisonings are treated with atropine; in the case of spasms, diazepam is also used. Forced diuresis can be useful. The lethal dose for an adult is 6 to 10 mg of physostigmine (corresponding to approximately 2 to 3 Calabar Beans).

DOSAGE

Mode of Administration: As an eye medication, in drops and ointments. It is used as an antidote in the form of an injection solution. For gastrointestinal use, it has been replaced by synthetic prostigmine.

Daily Dosage: Apply 1 to 2 eye drops 3 times daily to the conjunctival sac.

LITERATURE

Coelho Filho JM and Birks J. Physostigmine for Alzheimer's disease. The Cochrane Library. Oxford 2; 2002.

Die G, 125 Jahre Physostigmin. In: *ZPT* 11(2):7. 1990.

Morbus A, Was gibt es Neues aus der Forschung? In: *DAZ* 133(23):2090. 1993.

Kern W, List PH, Hörhammer L (Eds.), Hagers Handbuch der Pharmazeutischen Praxis, 4. Aufl., Bde. 1-8, Springer Verlag Berlin, Heidelberg, New York, 1969.

Madaus G, Lehrbuch der Biologischen Arzneimittel, Bde 1-3, Nachdruck, Georg Olms Verlag Hildesheim 1979.

Roth L, Daunderer M, Kormann K, Giftpflanzen, Pflanzengifte, 4. Aufl., Ecomed Fachverlag Landsberg Lech 1993.

Steinegger E, Hänsel R, Pharmakognosie, 5. Aufl., Springer Verlag Heidelberg 1992.

Teuscher E, Lindequist U, Biogene Gifte - Biologie, Chemie, Pharmakologie, 2. Aufl., Fischer Verlag Stuttgart 1994.

Teuscher E, Biogene Arzneimittel, 5. Aufl., Wiss. Verlagsges. Stuttgart 1997.

Calamint

Calamintha nepeta

DESCRIPTION

Medicinal Parts: The medicinal parts are the dried foliage, stems, leaves, and flowers.

Flower and Fruit: The medium-sized to large flowers are 5 to 20 blossomed cymes. The pedicle is 0 to 22 mm long and the tubular calyx is 3 to 7 mm by 1 to 1.5 mm in size and slightly downy to very downy on the inside. The upper tips are 0.5 to 1.5 mm and the lower ones are 1 to 2 mm, downy. They occasionally have long, ciliate hairs. The corolla is white to lilac and purple.

Leaves, Stem, and Root: Calamint is a perennial, 30 to 80 cm high, slightly to densely downy shrub. The leaves are oval, obtuse, almost entire-margined or lightly to deeply crenate-serrate, with 9 teeth on each side.

Habitat: Britain, Europe, northern Africa

Production: Calamint is the above-ground part of *Calamintha nepeta*. It is collected in the wild.

Other Names: Basil Thyme, Mountain Mint, Mountain Balm, Mill Mountain

ACTIONS AND PHARMACOLOGY

COMPOUNDS

Volatile oil (0.35%): including pulegone, menthone, menthol and its ester, β-bisobolen, cineol, thymol

Triterpenes: including calaminthadiol, ursolic acid

EFFECTS

The drug is a diaphoretic and expectorant.

INDICATIONS AND USAGE

Unproven Uses: Calamint has been used for febrile colds and respiratory diseases. The drug is also used in folk medicine for hiccups, tinnitus, as a diuretic and for stomach complaints.

PRECAUTIONS AND ADVERSE REACTIONS

No health hazards or side effects are known in conjunction with the proper administration of designated therapeutic dosages.

DOSAGE

No information is available.

LITERATURE

de Pooter HL, Goetghebeur P. Schamp P, *PH* 26(12):3355-3356. 1987.

Hänsel R, Keller K, Rimpler H, Schneider G (Hrsg.), Hagers Handbuch der Pharmazeutischen Praxis, 5. Aufl., Bde 4-6 (Drogen), Springer Verlag Berlin, Heidelberg, New York, 1992-1994.

Kokkalo E, Stefanaou E. The volatile oil of Calamintha nepeta (L) savi (Labies). *Plant Med et Phyte*. 24:203-213. 1990

Perrucci S et al. In vitro antifungal activity of essential oils against some isolates of *Microsporum canis* and *Microsporum gypseum*. *Planta Med* 60:184-187. 1994.

Calamintha nepeta

See Calamint

Calamus

Acorus calamus

DESCRIPTION

Medicinal Parts: The medicinal part is the rhizome after the removal of all other material.

Flower and Fruit: Green flowers, like small dice, form a tightly packed, slim, conical spadix. The plant doesn't bear fruit and propagates from the rhizome.

Leaves, Stem, and Root: The plant grows from 60 to 100 cm tall. The stem is triangular and sprouts from a horizontal, round rootstock, which has the thickness of a thumb. The upper shoot forms a grooved flower sheath. The leaves are oblong, sword-shaped, and arranged in two rows. The leaves have no stems.

Characteristics: The rhizome has an intensely aromatic fragrance and a tangy, pungent and bitter taste. The leaves often undulate on the margins.

Habitat: Today Calamus is found all over the world. It probably originated in India and North America.

Production: Calamus rootstock is the dried, coarsely ground and mostly peeled, rootstock of *Acorus calamus*. Calamus oil is extracted from the same plant.

Other Names: Sweet Flag, Sweet Sedge, Grass Myrtle, Myrtle Flag, Sweet Grass, Sweet Myrtle, Sweet Rush, Sweet Root, Sweet Cane, Gladdon, Myrtle Sedge, Cinnamon Sedge

ACTIONS AND PHARMACOLOGY

COMPOUNDS

Volatile oil: chief constituents are heavily dependent upon the chemical strain (di-, tri-, tetraploid); beta-asarone (cis-isoasarone), alpha- and gamma-asarone, beta- gurjuns, acorone (bitter), ZZ-Deca-4,7-dienal (odor-determining)

EFFECTS

In vitro, the essential oil (main constituent—cis-isoaron) blocks the aggregation of human blood platelets, influences glucose transport, and has a vermicidal and insecticidal effect. In animal experiments it had a spasmolytic effect, a possible CNS effect (sedative, anti-aggressive, reduction of spontaneous activity), and caused a reduction in the ulcer index. Its use as a stomachic seems plausible because of the amaroid content and the spasmolytic effect of the essential oil. Externally, it has a hyperemic effect.

INDICATIONS AND USAGE

Unproven Uses: The drug is used in the form of teas, for dyspeptic disorders, gastritis and ulcers. It is used externally for rheumatism, gum disease and tonsillitis.

Indian Medicine: Calamus is used for dyspeptic complaints, worms, pain syndrome and toothache.

Chinese Medicine: Acorus calamus stimulates peptic juices for disorders of the gastrointestinal tract. It is used externally for fungal infections.

PRECAUTIONS AND ADVERSE REACTIONS

No health hazards or side effects are known in conjunction with the proper administration of designated therapeutic dosages. Long-term use of this drug should be avoided. Malignant tumors appeared in rats that received Indian Calmus oils over an extended period (tetraploid strain, over 80% β-asarone in volatile oil).

DOSAGE

Mode of Administration: Calamus preparations are for internal and external use. Preparations are used as a bitter, stomachic, carminative, digestant, sedative, rubefacient, balneotherapeutic, and corrigent. Calamus is available in tea mixtures, as an oil or extract and as a bath oil.

Preparation: Steep with hot water to make a tea. For use in a bath, add 250 to 500 g of the drug to the bath water.

Storage: Store for a maximum of 18 months. If in powder form, however, do not keep for more than 24 hours.

LITERATURE

Azad Chowdhury AK, Ara T, Faisal Hasim M, Ahmed M. A new phenyl derivative from *Acorus calamus*. *Pharmazie* 48:786-787. 1993.

Keller K et al., *Planta Med* 51(1):6. 1985

Keller K, Stahl E, Composition of the essential oil from beta-asarone free calamus. In: *PM* 47(2):71. 1983.

Mazza G, Gas chromatographic and mass spectrometric studies of the constituents of the rhizome of calamus. In: *J Chromatogr* 328:179-206. 1985.

Rohr M, Naegeli P, *Phytochemistry* 18(2):279 and 328. 1979

Saxena DB, Phenyl indane from *Acorus calamus*. In: *PH* 25(2):553. 1986.

Shukla PK, et al. Protective effect of *Acorus calamus* against acrylamide induced neurotoxicity. *Phyther Res.* 16:256-260. 2002

Stahl E, Keller K, Classification of typical commercial Calamus drugs. In: PM 43(2):128-140. 1981.

Taylor JM et al., Toxicity of oil of calamus (Jammu variety). In: *Toxicol Appl Pharmacol* 10:405 (Abstract). 1967.

Calendula officinalis

See Marigold

California Peppertree

Schinus molle

DESCRIPTION

Medicinal Parts: Medicinal properties have been attributed to the plant's leaves, bark, fruit, and gum resin.

Flower and Fruit: The flowers are in apical, heavily branched, hanging, 5 to 30 cm long panicles. The flowers are small, yellowish-white, and their structures are in fives. The calyx has 5 tips. The flower has 5 petals, 10 stamens, and a superior ovary that develops from a carpel. The style is divided into three. The fruit is a coral red, single-seeded drupe with a diameter of approximately 7 mm, a thin pergamentlike exocarp, an oleo-resin-rich mesocarp, and a hard endocarp.

Leaves, Stem and Root: The tree is an evergreen, up to 15 m high. The leaves are alternate, up to 25 cm long and odd pinnate. There are 17 to 35 leaflets, 1.6 to 6 cm long, 2 to 8 mm wide, sessile, linear-lanceolate, punctate with oil glands and dentate. The branches hang down.

Characteristics: The leaves give off a pepper-like smell when rubbed; the fruit is aromatic and somewhat sweet.

Habitat: The tree is indigenous to Central America and South America.

Production: California Peppertree (or Peruvian Peppertree) leaves are the leaflets of *Schinus molle*. California Peppertree fruits are ripe unpeeled drupes of Schinus mollek, which are air- or freeze-dried.

Not to be Confused With: Other *Schinus* species.

Other Names: Australian Pepper Tree, Brazilian Pepper Tree, False Pepper, Peruvian Mastix Tree, Peruvian Peppertree, Weeping Pepper Tree

ACTIONS AND PHARMACOLOGY

COMPOUNDS: CALIFORNIA PEPPERTREE LEAVES

Volatile oil (0.2 to 1.0%): chief components including alpha-phellandrene, beta-phellandrene, limonene, including as well T-cadinol, elemol, germacrene D, gamma-eudesmol

Flavonoids: including kaempferol, myricetin, quercetin

Resins

Mucilages

EFFECTS: CALIFORNIA PEPPERTREE LEAVES

The leaves contain unknown bitter substances and tannins, which make administration for inflammatory alterations of the skin and oral mucous membranes plausible.

COMPOUNDS: CALIFORNIA PEPPERTREE FRUIT

Volatile oil (2.0 to 5.0%): chief components including alpha-phellandrene, beta-phellandrene, limonene, alpha-pinene, beta-pinene, including as well camphene, carvacrol, p-cymol, 4-ethyl phenol

Triterpenes: including 3-epiisomasticadienolalic acid, 3-epi-masticadienolic acid, isomasticadienonic acid, masticadienonic acid

Fatty oil (in the seeds 6 to 14%)

Resins (with long-chained fatty acids, C22 to C28)

EFFECTS: CALIFORNIA PEPPERTREE FRUIT

The fruit resin is purgative in effect. The essential oil is fungicidal and is said to be excreted primarily through the lungs and the kidneys. No experimental data are available for the traditional areas of administration.

INDICATIONS AND USAGE

CALIFORNIA PEPPERTREE LEAVES

Unproven Uses: Internal uses in folk medicine include infections of the pharynx, respiratory tract conditions, rheumatism (decoction), for leukorrhea, suppuration of the mucous membranes and hypertension (infusion), for swellings, loss of teeth, conjunctivitis (leaf juice), and as a diuretic. External indications are considered to include uterus prolapse, eye inflammations, joint pains, colds (used as healing baths), as a vulnerary and for rheumatism.

CALIFORNIA PEPPERTREE FRUIT

Unproven Uses: Used internally as a stomachic, tonic, for nausea, vomiting, anuria, gastric complaints, loss of appetite, conditions of the respiratory tract, blennorrhagia, for muscular pain and as a diuretic. Preparations from the fruit are used externally for rheumatism.

PRECAUTIONS AND ADVERSE REACTIONS

CALIFORNIA PEPPERTREE LEAVES AND FRUIT

No health hazards are known in conjunction with the proper administration of designated therapeutic dosages.

DOSAGE

CALIFORNIA PEPPERTREE LEAVES

Preparation: To prepare an infusion, use 30 g drug to 500 mL water.

Daily Dosage: For inflammation of the mucous membranes, gargle with infusion 3 times daily. For wound cleansing, wash wounds with infusion.

CALIFORNIA PEPPERTREE FRUIT

Mode of Administration: Whole and cut drug are used in preparations for internal and external use.

Daily Dosage: No information is given in the literature.

Storage: Tightly sealed, cool, dry and protected from light.

LITERATURE

Maffei M, Chialva F. Essential Oils from Schinus molle L. Berries and Leaves. *Flav Fragr J.* 5; 49-52 (1990)

Dikshit A, Naqvi AA, Husain A, Schinus molle: a new source of natural fungitoxicant. *Appl Environ Microbiol*, 38:1085-8, 1986 May.

Hänsel R, Keller K, Rimpler H, Schneider G (Ed), Hagers Handbuch der Pharmazeutischen Praxis, 5. Aufl., Bde 4 - 6 (Drogen), Springer Verlag Berlin, Heidelberg, New York, 1992-1994.

Olafsson K, Jaroszewski JW, Wagner-Smitt U, Nyman U. Isolation of Angiotensin Converting Enzyme (ACE) Inhibiting Triterpenes from *Schinus molle. Planta Med.* 63 (4); 352-355 (1997).

Vargas Correa JB, Sβnchez Sol s L, Farfβn Ale JA, Noguchi H, Moguel Banos MT, Vargas de la Peña MI, Allergological study of pollen of mango (Magnifera indica) and cross reactivity with pollen of piru (Schinus molle). *Rev Alerg*, 38:134-8, 1991 Sep-Oct.

California Poppy

Eschscholtzia californica

DESCRIPTION

Medicinal Parts: The medicinal parts of *Eschscholtzia californica* are the aerial parts collected during the flowering season and dried.

Flower and Fruit: The bright yellow-to-orange flowers are solitary, axillary, and long-pedicled. They are 2.5 to 4 cm in diameter with a cup-shaped receptacle. The sepals are fused. Four crenate petals, orange-red at the base, form an open dish. The stigma is threadlike. There are numerous yellow stamens. The fruit is an oblong, 4 to 6 cm podlike exploding capsule, which spreads small globular seeds.

Leaves, Stem and Root: Eschscholtzia californica is a bluish-green annual or perennial that grows 30 to 60 cm high. The leaves are sparse. The strongly pinnatifid leaves have linear sections and taper to a thin tip.

Habitat: The plant grows in California and is cultivated in central Europe and southern France.

Production: The Californian Poppy herb consists of the aerial parts of *Eschscholtzia californica*. It is collected in uncultivated regions.

ACTIONS AND PHARMACOLOGY

COMPOUNDS

Isoquinoline alkaloids: The main alkaloid is californidine. Included are others, such as eschscholzine (escholzine), protopine, alpha-allocryptopine, beta-allocryptopine.

Cyanogenic glycosides (in the freshly-harvested plant)

EFFECTS

The main active principle californidine has sleep-inducing, sedative, anxiolytic, and spasmolytic effects. In mice, a hot water extract had a significant sleep-inducing effect. In other animal experiments an anxiolytic and spasmolytic effect was proven.

INDICATIONS AND USAGE

Unproven Uses: Preparations of the drug are used for insomnia, aches, nervous agitation, enuresis nocturna in children, diseases of the bladder and liver, reactive agitative and masked depressions, melancholia, neurasthenia, neuropathy, organic neuroses, vegetative-dystonic disorders, mood swings, weather sensitivity, vasomotor dysfunctions, vegetative-endocrine syndrome, constitutional weakness of the nervous system, and vasomotor cephalgia. The tea is used as a sedative.

Homeopathic Uses: Eschscholtzia californica is used to treat insomnia.

PRECAUTIONS AND ADVERSE REACTIONS

General: Health risks or side effects following the proper administration of designated therapeutic dosages are not recorded.

Pregnancy: Not to be used during pregnancy.

DOSAGE

Mode of Administration: The drug is rarely prescribed, yet is a component of some standardized preparations in combination with plant sedatives. Medical or clinical documentation and other experimental material about phytotherapeutic application of the Californian Poppy herb are unavailable. As the efficacy of the claimed uses has not been documented, a therapeutic application cannot be justified.

Preparation: The tea is prepared using 2 gm herb per 150 ml water. The liquid extract (Extractum *Eschscholziae*) should be prepared according to the German Pharmacopoeia (DAB)10.

Daily Dosage: The tea is taken as a drink. The average single dose for the liquid extract is 1 to 2 ml.

Homeopathic Dosage: from D2: 5 drops, 1 tablet, or 10 globules every 30 to 60 minutes (acute) or 1 to 3 times daily (chronic); from D4: parenterally: 1 to 2 mL sc acute: 3 times daily; chronic: once a day (PF X).

LITERATURE

Hänsel R, Keller K, Rimpler H, Schneider G (Hrsg.), Hagers Handbuch der Pharmazeutischen Praxis, 5. Aufl., Bde 4-6 (Drogen), Springer Verlag Berlin, Heidelberg, New York, 1992-1994.

Jain L et al., Alkaloids of *Eschscholtzia californica*. In: *PM* 62(2):188. 1997.

Lewin L, Gifte und Vergiftungen, 6. Aufl., Nachdruck, Haug Verlag, Heidelberg 1992.

Roth L, Daunderer M, Kormann K, Giftpflanzen, Pflanzengifte, 4. Aufl., Ecomed Fachverlag Landsberg Lech 1993.

Sturm S, Stuppner H, Mulinacci N, Vincieri F, Capillary zone electrophoretic analysis of the main alkaloids from *Eschscholtzia californica*. In: *PM* 59(7):A625. 1993.

Teuscher E, Lindequist U, Biogene Gifte - Biologie, Chemie, Pharmakologie, 2. Aufl., Fischer Verlag Stuttgart 1994.

Weischer ML, Okpanyi SN, Pharmakologie eines pflanzlichen Schlafmittels. In: *ZPT* 15(5):257-262. 1994.

Calluna vulgaris

See Heather

Calotropis

Calotropis procera

DESCRIPTION

Medicinal Parts: The medicinal parts are the dried root and root bark. The bark with its outer cork layer removed is known as Mudar, and is used medicinally.

Flower and Fruit: The fragrant flowers are 2.5 cm in diameter and form umbel-like flower clusters. The erect petals are whitish and have purple spots on the upper half. The bracts of the corolla are smooth or downy with a divided tip. The ovate follicles are 7.5 to 10 cm long by 5 to 7.5 cm wide. The seeds have a tuft of silky hair.

Leaves, Stem, and Root: This upright herbacious perennial normally grows to a height of 1.8 to 2.4 m. The leaves are short-petioled, 6 to 15 cm long by 4.5 to 8 cm wide, oblong-elliptoid to broadly ovate. The bark appears in irregular short pieces, slightly quilled or curved and about 0.3 to 0.5 cm thick. The external portion is grayish-yellow, soft and spongy. The internal portion is yellowish-white. The fracture is short.

Characteristics: The taste is acrid and bitter.

Habitat: Indigenous to parts of Asia, India, Africa, Pakistan and on the Sunda Islands

Production: Calotropis bark is the dried root bark of *Calotropis procera*.

Other Names: Mudar Bark, Mudar Yercum

ACTIONS AND PHARMACOLOGY

COMPOUNDS

Cardioactive steroids (cardenolids): including calotropin, calactin, uscharidin

EFFECTS

The cardenolid glycocides calotropine shows an anti-tumor effect in vitro on human epidermoid carcinoma cells of the rhinopharynx. It is also works as an expectorant and a diuretic.

INDICATIONS AND USAGE

Unproven Uses: The powdered root bark is used to treat dysentery. It has a similar effect to that of the ipecacuanha root. In Indian and African folk medicine, the bark is used to treat epilepsy, hysteria, cramps, cancer, warts, leprosy, elephantitis, worms, fever, gout and snake bites. In particular, the milky juice is used against boils, ulcers, swellings and rheumatism. In Africa, it is used to treat toothache, syphilis, digestive disorders and diarrhea.

Indian Medicine: The smoke (fumes) from the bark is used for coughs and asthma and as a sudorific.

Homeopathic Uses: Calotropis procera is used for obesity.

PRECAUTIONS AND ADVERSE REACTIONS

No health hazards or side effects are known in conjunction with the proper administration of designated therapeutic dosages.

OVERDOSAGE

The drug is highly toxic. Higher dosages cause vomiting, diarrhea, bradycardia, and convulsions. Very high dosages may cause death. Following gastric lavage, treatment for poisonings should proceed symptomatically (for further measures, see Digitalis).

DOSAGE

Mode of Administration: Calotropis is used in a ground form, as a powder, as smoke (fume) and also topically.

Daily Dosage: As an expectorant and diaphoretic 200 mg to 600 mg; as an emetic 2 gm to 4 gm.

Homeopathic Dosage: from D4: 5 to 10 drops, 1 tablet, 5 to 10 globules 1 to 3 times daily; from D6: 1 ml injection solution sc twice weekly (HAB1).

LITERATURE

Abraham KI, Joshi PN. Isolation of Calotropain FI. *J Chromatogr.* 168; 284-289 (1979)

Ali M, Gupta J, Neguerulea MV, Perez-Alonso MJ. New ursan-type triterpenic esters from the roots of *Calotropis gigantea. Pharmazie* 53 (10); 718-721 (1998).

Banu MJ, Nellaiappan K, Dhandayuthapani S. Mitochondrial Malate Dehydrogenase and Malic Enzyme of a Fialrial Worm *Setaria digitata*: Some Properties and Effects of Drugs and Herbal Extracts. *Jap J Med Sci Biol.* 45; 137-150 (1992).

Dewan S, Sangraula H, Kumar VL. Preliminary studies on the analgesic activity of latex of *Calotropis procera. J Ethnopharmacol.* 73(1,2); 307-311.2000.

Hänsel R, Keller K, Rimpler H, Schneider G (Hrsg.), Hagers Handbuch der Pharmazeutischen Praxis, 5. Aufl., Bde 4-6 (Drogen), Springer Verlag Berlin, Heidelberg, New York, 1992-1994.

Sasidharan VK. Search for antibacterial and antifungal Activity of some Plants Kerala. *Acta Pharm.* 47; 47-51 (1997).

Willaman JJ, Hui-Li L, (1970) *Lloydia* 33(3A):1.

Calotropis gigantea

See Giant Milkweed

Calotropis procera

See Calotropis

Caltha palustris

See Marsh Marigold

Calystegia sepium

See Greater Bindweed

Camellia sinensis

See Green Tea

Camphor Tree

Cinnamomum camphora

DESCRIPTION

Medicinal Parts: The medicinal part is camphor oil extracted from the tree.

Flower and Fruit: The flowers are small, white, and sessile on 1 to 1.5 mm long pedicles. The petals are pubescent on the inside. The flowers are caespitose, on long axillary petioles. The 1.5 mm stamens form 3 circles and are pubescent with broad, sessile-cordate glands. The fruit is a purple-black, 1-seeded, 10 to 12 mm oval drupe.

Leaves, Stem, and Root: The plant is an evergreen tree growing up to 50 m tall and 5 m in diameter. The trunk is erect at the lower part and knottily branched above. The leaves are alternate on long petioles, oval-lanceolate, acuminate, grooved, and glossy. They are light yellowish-green above and paler beneath; they grow to 5 to 11 cm long by 5 cm across.

Habitat: Camphor trees are indigenous to Vietnam and an area extending from southern China to southern Japan.

Production: Purified camphor is obtained from the chipped wood of the *Cinnamomum camphora* tree using steam distillation followed by sublimation to yield the oil.

Other Names: Gum Camphor, Laurel Camphor, Cemphire

ACTIONS AND PHARMACOLOGY

COMPOUNDS

Camphora is a single substance: D(+) -camphor ((1R,4R)-1,7,7-trimethyl-bicyclo[2.2.1]heptan-2-on), extracted from the volatile oil of the trunk of the camphor tree, Cinnamomum camphora. L(-)-camphor also occurs in nature. Synthetic camphor is DL-camphor.

EFFECTS

Used externally, camphor acts as a bronchial secretolytic and hyperemic. Internally, the effect is that of a respiratory analeptic and bronchospasmolytic. It should be noted that the effect only sets in at dosages considered toxic. An antibacterial effect has been noted in vitro, with cineol the main active principle.

INDICATIONS AND USAGE

Approved by Commission E:

- Arrhythmia
- Cough/bronchitis
- Hypotension
- Nervous heart complaints
- Rheumatism

Unproven Uses: External uses in folk medicine include muscular rheumatism and cardiac symptoms. Among internal uses are hypotonic circulatory regulation disorders, and digestive complaints. Inflammation of respiratory-tract mucous membranes is treated with both internal and external applications.

Indian Medicine: Uses include muscle pain, cardiac insufficiency, and asthma.

CONTRAINDICATIONS

Camphor should not be used during pregnancy.

PRECAUTIONS AND ADVERSE REACTIONS

General: Local administration can lead to skin irritation, as well as to resorbent and/or airborne poisonings. Contact eczema occasionally appears following the application of oily salves containing camphor.

Pediatric Use: Camphor salves should not be administered to infants.

OVERDOSAGE

Symptoms of poisonings that have been seen, particularly in children, include intoxicated states, delirium, spasms and respiratory control disturbances. Treatment proceeds symptomatically. Less than 1 g can be a lethal dosage for young children. For adults, the lethal dosage is considered to be approximately 20 g. However, toxicity in adults has been noted after use of as little as 2 g.

DOSAGE

Mode of Administration: As a liquid (camphor spirit) for topical application or inhalation, and also semi-solid ointments, and liniments.

How Supplied: Commercial pharmaceutical preparations include creams, ointments, balms, and gels.

Daily Dosage: For external use, camphor spirit (DAB10) 9.5 to 10.5% camphor to be rubbed in several times a day. Depending on prescribed application, concentrations generally are not higher than 25% for adults and no higher than 5% for small children. Ointments and liniments should contain 10% to 20% camphor, but no more than 25%.

Storage: Camphor should be stored in containers filled so there is no empty air space left and also should be protected from light.

LITERATURE

Bean NE, Camphora -curriculum vitae of a perverse terpene. In: *Chem in Brain* 8(9):386. 1972.

Burrow A, Eccles R, Jones AS, (1983) The effects of camphor, eucalyptus and menthol vapor on nasal resistance to airflow and nasal sensation. *Acta Otolaryng* (Stockholm) 96:157-161.

Leow YH, Ng SK, Wong WK, Goh CL. Contact Allergic Potential of Topical Traditional Chinese Medicaments in Singapore. *Am J Contact Dermatitis* 6 (1); 4-8 (1995).

Medici D de, Pieretti S, Salvatore G, Nicoletti M, Rasoanaivo P. Chemical Analysis of Essential Oils of Madagasy Medicinal Plants by Gas Chromatography and NMR Spectroscopy. *Flav Fragr J.* 7; 275-281 (1992).

Stone JE, Blundell MJ, (1951) *Anal Chem* 23:771.

Canadian Fleabane

Erigeron canadensis

DESCRIPTION

Medicinal Parts: The medicinal parts are the dried aerial parts of the plant and the fresh aerial parts of the flowering plant.

Flower and Fruit: Canadian Fleabane has very small yellowish-white composite flowers in long, terminal, branched paniclelike inflorescences. The involucre is in a number of rows. The composite head has numerous florets. The ray florets are linguiform, female, white or reddish. The disc florets are tubular and androgynous. The stamens are fused. The fruit is an achaene, 1.2 to 1.5 mm long, brownish and has short appressed hair.

Leaves, Stem, and Root: Erigeron canadensis is an annual or biennial 30 to 100 cm high. The root is thin and fusiform, the stem erect, roundish, slightly ribbed, greenish with paler ribs and is covered in scattered patent hairs. It is branched from the peduncle. The leaves are alternate, pointed, ciliate, narrowly lanceolate and up to 10 cm wide and tapering to the petiole.

Habitat: The plant is indigenous to America but is found globally today.

Production: Canadian Fleabane is the flowering plant and seeds (without the root) of *Erigeron canadensis*. The plant is collected in the wild in high summer, then hung in bundles to dry.

Other Names: Coltstail, Flea Wort, Horseweed, Prideweed

ACTIONS AND PHARMACOLOGY

COMPOUNDS

Volatile oil: including (+)-limonene, alpha-cis-bergamots, beta-trans-farnesene, beta-pinenes, myrcene, cis, cis-matricariamethyl ester (polyyne)

Tannins

EFFECTS

The drug is reported to have antiedemic and antiphlogistic effects.

INDICATIONS AND USAGE

Unproven Uses: The drug is used for diarrhea, dysentery, as an antithelmintic, a mild hemostyptic, for uterine bleeding, gout, rheumatic symptoms, dropsy, tumors, and bronchitis. In African folk medicine, it is used in the treatment of granuloma annulare, sore throats, urinary tract infections, and is used for medicinal baths.

Homeopathic Uses: Erigeron canadensis is used for bleeding of the bladder, hemorrhoids, menorrhagia and metrorrhagia, gastritis, hepatitis, and cholecystitis

PRECAUTIONS AND ADVERSE REACTIONS

Health risks or side effects following the proper administration of designated therapeutic dosages are not recorded.

DOSAGE

Mode of Administration: The drug is used topically and in alcoholic extracts.

Daily Dosage: Tea: 3 cups daily after meals; Liquid extract: approximately 2 teaspoons.

Homeopathic Dosage: 5 drops, 1 tablet or 10 globules every 30 to 60 minutes (acute) or 1 to 3 times daily (chronic); parenterally: 1 to 2 mL 3 times daily sc (HAB1).

LITERATURE

Grancia D et al., (1985) *Ceskoslov Farm* 34(6):209.

Hänsel R, Keller K, Rimpler H, Schneider G (Hrsg.), Hagers Handbuch der Pharmazeutischen Praxis, 5. Aufl., Bde 4-6 (Drogen), Springer Verlag Berlin, Heidelberg, New York, 1992-1994 (unter Conyza).

Lasser B et al., (1983) *Naturwissenschaften* 70:95.

Madaus G, Lehrbuch der Biologischen Arzneimittel, Bde 1-3, Nachdruck, Georg Olms Verlag Hildesheim 1979.

Wagner H, Wiesenauer M, Phytotherapie. Phytopharmaka und pflanzliche Homöopathika, Fischer-Verlag, Stuttgart, Jena, New York 1995.

Canadian Golden Rod

Solidago canadensis

DESCRIPTION

Medicinal Parts: The medicinal parts are the dried aerial parts collected during the flowering season, the fresh inflorescences, and the flowering twigs.

Flower and Fruit: The yellow composite flowers are in erect racemes facing all directions and are simple or compound. They are medium-sized. The involucral bracts are imbricate and arranged in numerous rows. The ray florets are narrow, lingual, and female. The disc florets are funnel-shaped, 5-tipped, and androgynous. The fruit is an achene, which is cylindrical with numerous ribs. It is brown, sparsely pubescent, and 3.5 to 4.5 mm long with a tuft of hair.

Leaves, Stem, and Root: The plant is a perennial that ranges in size from a few centimeters to over 1 m. The rhizome is cylindrical, noded, diagonally ascending and short. The stem is erect, canelike, angularly grooved above, usually red-tinged beneath, and glabrous to loosely appressed pubescent higher up. The basal leaves are long-petioled, elliptical, acuminate, and narrowing to the winged stem. The lower ones are serrate and the upper ones entire-margined.

Habitat: The plant is indigenous to Europe, Asia and North America.

Production: Golden Rod is the aerial part of *Solidago virgaurea*. It occurs in the wild in Hungary, former Yugoslavia, Bulgaria, and Poland. Golden Rod herb consists of the above-ground parts of *Solidago serotina* (synonym *S. gigantea*). *Solidago canadensis* and its hybrids are gathered during the flowering season and carefully dried.

Not to be Confused With: Despite qualitative and quantitative differences in their effects, drugs containing *Solidago gigantea* or *Solidago canadensis* are exchanged with *Solidago virgaurea* on the market; confusions with *Senecio* species are also conceivable.

Other Names: Aaron's Rod, Woundwort

ACTIONS AND PHARMACOLOGY

COMPOUNDS: CANADIAN GOLDEN ROD

Triterpene saponins: bisdemosides of the bayogenin, bearing acylglycosidically-bound arabino residue

Polysaccharides (water-soluble): beta-1,2-fructans, acidic polysaccharides

Volatile oil (0.6%): chief components curlone, germacrene D, alpha-pinene, beta-sesquiphellandrene, limonene

Diterpenes of the trans-clerodane and ladanum types

Carotenoids (as blossom pigments)

Flavonoids (2.4%): rutin (1.4%), including as well hyperoside, quercitrin, astragalin

Caffeic acid derivatives: including chlorogenic acid

COMPOUNDS: CANADIAN GOLDEN ROD (GIGANTEA VARIETY)

Triterpene saponins (9%): bisdesmoside of the bayogenins: GS1-GS4

Volatile oil (0.5%): chief components gamma-cadinene-diterpenes of the cis-clerodane-type, including among others 6-deoxysolidagolactone IV-18,19-olide

Carotenoids (as blossom pigments)

Flavonoids (3.8%): quercitrin (1.3%), further including among others hyperoside, rutin, isoquercitrin

Caffeic acid derivatives: including among others chlorogenic acid

EFFECTS: CANADIAN GOLDEN ROD

Canadian Golden Rod is diuretic, weakly spasmolytic and, because of the saponin componant, antiphlogistic.

INDICATIONS AND USAGE

Approved by Commission E:

- Infections of the urinary tract
- Kidney and bladder stones

Unproven Uses: The herb is used as a flushing-out therapy for inflammatory diseases of the lower urinary tract.

CONTRAINDICATIONS

Irrigation therapy is contraindicated in cases of edema resulting from reduced cardiac and/or kidney function.

PRECAUTIONS AND ADVERSE REACTIONS

No health hazards or side effects are known in conjunction with the proper administration of designated therapeutic dosages. The drug possesses a weak potential for sensitization. Care must be taken in patients with chronic renal diseases, and the drug should be used in this patient population only under the supervision of a doctor.

DOSAGE

Mode of Administration: As chopped drug by itself or in combination preparations.

Daily Dosage: The daily dosage is 6 to 12 gm of comminuted drug prepared as an infusion. Fluid intake of at least 2 liters daily is recommended.

Storage: The drug must be protected from light and moisture.

LITERATURE

Budzianowski J, Skrzypczak L, Wesolowska M. Flavonoids and Leiocarposide in Four Solidago Taxa. *Sci Pharm.* 58; 15-23 (1990).

Cantrell CL, Fischer NH, Urbatsch L, McGuire MS, Franzblau SG. Antimycobacterial crude plant extracts from South, Central, and North America. *Phytomedicine* 5 (2); 137-145 (1998).

Lu T, Menelaou MA, Vargas D, Fronczek FR, Fischer NH. Polyacetylenes and Diterpenes from *Solidago canadensis. Phytochemistry* 32; 1483-1488 (1993).

Reznicek G et al., *Tetrahedron Lett* 30:4097. 1989.

Reznicek G, Freiler M, Schader M, Schmidt U, Determination of the content and the composition of the main saponins from Solidago gigantea AIT. Using high-perfomance liquid chromatography. In: *J Chromatogr A* 755(1):133-37. 1996.

Tiansheng L et al., Polyacetylenes and diterpenes from *Solidå canadensis*. In: *PH* 32:1483. 1993.

Weyerstahl P, Marshall H, Christiansen C, Kalemba D, Góra J, Constituents of the essential oil of *Solidago canadensis* (''Goldenrod'') from Poland. In: *PM* 59(3):281. 1993.

Canarium species

See Chinese Olive

Cane-Reed

Costus specious

DESCRIPTION

Medicinal Parts: The medicinal part of the plant is the rhizome.

Flower and Fruit: The inflorescence is ovoid, apical, and 4 to 7 cm long. The zygomorphic flowers are each supported by one narrow, ovate, acuminate, coriaceous, thickly haired, red to red-brown bract. There is a bracteole, which is approximately 2 cm long, violet to brown-red and sparsely pubescent. The calyx is approximately 2.5 cm long, green to red-brown and tubular. The 3 petals are approximately 6 cm long, white to pale pink and silky haired. The corolla tube is approximately 1.5 cm long. The lobes are elliptical to ovate and 6 to 7 cm long. The lobes are white to pale pink, with a yellow lip in the center made up of 5 stamens. When spread out, the lobe is broad obviate and crenate. There is 1 fertile stamen, which is white to yellowish and up to 5 cm long. The style is threadlike and the ovary 3-chambered and inferior. The fruit is a light red, loculicidal capsule. The seeds are black, 2 to 4 mm wide, with a narrow, fleshy aril.

Leaves, Stem, and Root: Costus specious is a herbaceous perennial, upright, up to 3 m high. The leaves have tubular sheaths, which are 0.7 to 1.2 cm in diameter and a pubescent to glabrous. The ligula is 1 to 2 mm long; the leaves are 12 to 25 cm long, 3 to 6 cm wide, narrow elliptical, thorny-tipped, glabrous above and downy-haired beneath. The stem is upright. The rhizome is up to 50-cm long, 3 cm thick and rich in starch.

Habitat: India

Production: Kust or costus root is the dried rhizome of *Costus speciosus.*

Not to be Confused With: Confusion may occur with *Saussurea lappa* and *Canella winterana.* The drug itself is used to adulterate *Gloroisa superba.*

ACTIONS AND PHARMACOLOGY

COMPOUNDS

Steroid saponins (1 to 4%): chief components dioscin and gracillin, aglycones diosgenin, tigogenin

Steroids: sterols, including beta-sitosterol, beta-sitosterol glucoside

Curcuminoids (3 %): including curcumin

EFFECTS

The saponin fraction of the drug exhibits estrogenic, antiexudative, spasmolytic, choleretic, and anesthesia-prolonging effects.

INDICATIONS AND USAGE

Indian Medicine: for febrile conditions, coughs, skin conditions, retention of the placenta, postpartum bleeding, threatening abortion, insufficient uterine contractility, and snake bites.

PRECAUTIONS AND ADVERSE REACTIONS

No health hazards are known in conjunction with the proper administration of designated therapeutic dosages. It is conceivable that gastric complaints and nausea might be experienced, as well as kidney irritation, due to the high level of saponin content.

OVERDOSAGE

Overdose could lead to European cholera, increased diuresis, and shock.

DOSAGE

Mode of Administration: Whole herb preparations, cut and powdered drug for internal use.

LITERATURE

Hänsel R, Keller K, Rimpler H, Schneider G (Ed) Hagers Handbuch der Pharmazeutischen Praxis. 5. Aufl., Bde 4 - 6 (Drogen), Springer Verlag Berlin, Heidelberg, New York, 1992-1994

Canella

Canella winterana

DESCRIPTION

Medicinal Parts: The medicinal part is the bark of the tree.

Flower and Fruit: The flowers are small and seldom open. They are violet and fused in clusters to the tips of the branches. The involucre is sometimes fused at the base. The stamens are fused to form a pollen tube. The fruit is an elongate berry with 4 reniform seeds. The fruit changes color from green to blue and then to a shiny black.

Leaves, Stem, and Root: Canella winterana is a tree that grows up to 15 m and is only branched at the top. The bark is whitish-yellowish on the outside and chalklike on the inside. The leaves are alternate, oblong, thick, and are a dark, intense laurel-green shade.

Habitat: The tree is indigenous to the Caribbean and Florida.

Not to be Confused With: It is often sold as the rarer *Cortex winteranus*.

Other Names: Canella alba, White Cinnamon, White Wood, Wild Cinnamon

ACTIONS AND PHARMACOLOGY

COMPOUNDS

Volatile oil (1%): chief components eugenol, cineol, pinene, caryophyllene, myristicin

Resins (8%)

Sesquiterpenes: including muzigadial, warburganal (pungent-tasting dialdehydes)

Mannitol (6-8%)

Starch (12%)

EFFECTS

Canella has a stimulant and tonic effect. The sesquiterpenes contained in the bark have antimycotic and molluscacidal effects.

INDICATIONS AND USAGE

Unproven Uses: In Central and South America, Canella is used internally to treat upset stomach, fever, and conditions of the mouth and throat; it is used externally for rheumatism. In the West Indies, it is used to treat scurvy and as a spice.

PRECAUTIONS AND ADVERSE REACTIONS

No health hazards or side effects are known in conjunction with the proper administration of designated therapeutic dosages.

DOSAGE

Mode of Administration: Canella is available in whole, cut and powdered forms.

LITERATURE

El Feraly M et al., (1980) *J Nat Prod.* 43:407.

Kern W, List PH, Hörhammer L (Hrsg.), Hagers Handbuch der Pharmazeutischen Praxis, 4. Aufl., Bde 1-8, Springer Verlag Berlin, Heidelberg, New York, 1969.

Morton JF, An Atlas of Medicinal Plants of Middle America, Charles C. Thomas USA 1981.

Canella winterana

See Canella

Cannabis sativa

See Marijuana

Capsella bursa-pastoris

See Shepherd's Purse

Capsicum species

See Cayenne

Carambola

Averrhoa carambola

DESCRIPTION

Medicinal Parts: The medicinal part is the fruit.

Flower and Fruit: Cymose inflorescences grow from the trunk. The flowers are radial, and their structures are arranged in fives. The petals are free; there are 10 stamens and a 5-chambered ovary. The fruit is a berry, approximately 10 cm long. The berry is acuminate, 5-sided and star-shaped in cross-section. It is translucently amber-yellow.

Leaves, Stem and Root: Averrhoa carambola is a tree that grows up to 5 m high. The leaves are alternate, odd pinnate, and 10 to 12 cm long.

Habitat: India

Production: The fruit of the Carambola tree is the ripe fruit of *Averrhoa carambola.*

ACTIONS AND PHARMACOLOGY

COMPOUNDS

Oxalic acid (0.3% of fresh weight)

Vitamin C (0.05% of fresh weight)

Monosaccharides/polysaccharides

Carotinoids

EFFECTS

No definitive data available.

INDICATIONS AND USAGE

Indian Medicine: Carambola is used for diarrhea, vomiting, severe thirst, hemorrhoids, intermittent fever, scabies, and liver pain.

PRECAUTIONS AND ADVERSE REACTIONS

There is no evidence of any health risks connected with limited consumption of the fruit or the preserves made from them. Nevertheless, due to the high oxalate content, which corresponds approximately to that of rhubarb stalks, the ingestion of large amounts over extended periods should be avoided.

DOSAGE

No information is available.

LITERATURE

Frôhlich O, Schreier P. Additional Volatile Constituents of Carambola (*Averrhoa carambola L.*) Fruit. *Flav Fragr J.* 4; 177-184 (1989).

Neto MM, Robl F, Netto JC, Depressant action of *Averrhoa carambola. Med J Malaysia.* 13:279-80, 1980 Mar.

Neto MM, Robl F, Netto JC, Intoxication by star fruit (*Averrhoa carambola*) in six dialysis patients? (Preliminary report) news. *Nephrol Dial Transplant.* 13:570-2, 1998 Mar.

Caraway

Carum carvi

DESCRIPTION

Medicinal Parts: The medicinal part is the fruit and the oil obtained from the squashed fruit when ripe.

Flower and Fruit: The main trunk and the side branches each terminate in a compound flowering umbel of 8 to 16 umbel rays. The epicalyx and calyx are almost nonexistent. The florets are white or reddish and very small. The fruit is a schizocarp that is glabrous, oblong, and elliptoid. It consists of 2 mericarps that are 3 to 6 mm long, sickle-shaped, brownish with 5 lighter, angular main ribs (caraway seeds).

Leaves, Stem and Root: Carum carvi is usually a biennial, 30 to 100 cm high plant with a fleshy, fusiform tap root. The stem is erect, angular, grooved, filled with latex, glabrous and branched from the ground up. The rosette leaves and the cauline leaves are glabrous and in part tripinnate. The lower pinnae are typically crossed.

Characteristics: The plant has a caraway taste and an aromatic smell.

Habitat: Caraway is found in Europe, Siberia, the Caucasus, the Near East, the Himalayas, Mongolia and Morocco. Found wild in North America after being introduced.

Production: Caraway oil consists of the essential oil extracted from the ripe fruits of *Carum carvi*. Caraway is harvested when completely ripe and threshed 3 weeks later. The oil is recovered from the crushed seeds by a process of aqueous steam distillation.

Not to be Confused With: Carvon is occasionally added in synthetic form.

ACTIONS AND PHARMACOLOGY

COMPOUNDS

In the berries: volatile oil, fatty oil, polysaccharides, proteins, furocoumarins (traces)

In volatile oil: in particular D-(+)-carvone and D-(+)-limonene

EFFECTS

In animal tests the drug had a spasmolytic effect. The antimicrobial effect has been demonstrated against *bacillus, pseudomonas*, *aspergillus* and *candida* species; *dermatomyces* are also inhibited.

INDICATIONS AND USAGE

Approved by Commission E:

■ Dyspeptic complaints

Unproven Uses: Caraway is used for gastrointestinal cramps, flatulence and feelings of fullness, as well as nervous cardiac-gastric complaints.

In folk medicine, Caraway is used to improve lactation in nursing mothers, as an emmenagogue, and to settle the stomach. The essential oil is used as constituent in mouthwashes and bath additives.

PRECAUTIONS AND ADVERSE REACTIONS

No health hazards or side effects are known in conjunction with the proper administration of designated therapeutic dosages.

OVERDOSAGE

An intake of larger dosages of the volatile oil (see for example in caraway liquor) for extended periods can lead to kidney and liver damage.

DOSAGE

Mode of Administration: Preparations from the essential oil are for internal use. The comminuted fresh drug is used for infusions and other galenic preparations.

How Supplied: Powder, capsules, film tablets, coated tablets, drops, and tea.

Preparation: An infusion is prepared by pressing 1 to 2 teaspoonfuls of seeds before using and pouring 150 mL of hot water over it, draining after 10 to 15 minutes.

Daily Dosage: The average single dose of oil is 2 to 3 drops on sugar; caraway, 1 to 5 gm. The average daily dose of oil is 3 to 6 drops; caraway, 1.5 to 6 gm.

Storage: Protect from light and moisture in glass or metal containers.

LITERATURE

Bouwmeester HJ, Davies JAR, Toxopeus H. Enantiomeric Composition of Carvone, Limonene, and Carveols in Seeds of Dill and Annual and Biennial Caraway Varieties. *J Agric Food Chem.* 43 (12); 3057-3064. 1995.

Brown JP. A Review of the Genetic Effects of Naturally Occuring Flavonoids, Anthraquinones and Related Compounds. *Mutation Res.* 75; 243-277.1980.

Salveson A et al., *Sci Pharm.* 46(2):93-100. 1978.

Zheng G, Kenney PM, Lam LK. Anethofuran, Carvone, and Limonene: Potential Cancer Chemopreventive Agents from Dill Weed Oil and Caraway Oil. *Planta Med.* 58; 338-341. 1992.

Cardamom

Elettaria cardamomum

DESCRIPTION

Medicinal Parts: The medicinal parts are the oil extracted from the seeds and fruit plus seeds harvested shortly after ripening.

Flower and Fruit: The flowering shoots grow on the stem very close to the ground. The panicle branches can grow up to 8 cm. The flowers are alternate and covered by sheathlike bracts before opening. The calyx is slightly wider above, finely striped, obtusely triple-tipped, and does not droop. The corolla is greenish white. The lobes are rounded, somewhat curly, white with a yellowish border with blue veins and lines in the center. The only fertile stamen is set into the edge of the petals. The sterile stamens are arranged beside the styles on the receptacle. The pollen is globular and prickly. The ovary is inferior, oblong, obovate with 3 valves, each with 12 horizontal ovules. The fruit is 6 to 18 mm long, 6 to 10 mm thick, short-stemmed, ovate, or elliptical to oblong. The seeds are light brown, gray, or dark red brownish. They are very roughly wrinkled, 4 to 5 mm long, irregular edged and the whole seed is surrounded by an almost colorless seed coat. Mysore and Malabar cardamoms are usually blanched pale and have a smooth surface. They are sold commercially less often than the Green Aleppy or Ceylon varieties.

Leaves, Stem, and Root: Elettaria cardamomum is a perennial with a thick, tuberous rhizome and numerous long roots. There are up to 30 erect, glabrous, green stems that are 2 to 3 m high. The leaves are in 2 rows with a leaf membrane at the end of a soft-haired sheath. The leaf surface is lanceolate, clearly acuminate, and up to 60 cm long. The leaves are entire-margined, downy above, silky-haired beneath and punctuated by numerous small oil cells. The seeds are about 4 mm diameter and dark-reddish-brown.

Characteristics: Cardamom has an aromatic and pleasant odor. The taste is aromatic and pungent.

Habitat: The plant is indigenous in southern India and Sri Lanka and is cultivated in tropical regions in southeast Asia and Guatamala.

Production: Cardamom consists of the dried, almost ripe, greenish to yellow-gray fruit of *Elettaria cardamomum.* Medicinal use is limited to the seed, which is removed from its fruit capsule. The main harvest is in October and November of the third year after planting. The fruit is then dried either in the sun or in so-called "curing houses" and then sorted according to size, form, color, etc.

ACTIONS AND PHARMACOLOGY

COMPOUNDS

Volatile oil: composition varies according to the specific strain, chief components 1,8-cineol, alpha-terpinyl acetate, linaloyl acetate

Starch (20% to 40%)

EFFECTS

The drug is a cholagogue and has virustatic properties. The essential oil (monoterpene) of the drug is antibacterial and antimycotic. In animal experiments the essential oil caused an increase in the secretion of bile and a reduction of gastric juice production.

INDICATIONS AND USAGE

Approved by Commission E:

- Dyspepsia

Unproven Uses: Cardamom is also used for in folk medicine for digestive complaints, vomiting and diarrhea, morning sickness, and loss of appetite as well as Roemheld syndrome.

Chinese Medicine: Cardamom is used for stomachache, nausea, vomiting, and flatulence.

Indian Medicine: In Indian medicine, Cardamom is used for disorders of the efferent urinary tract.

PRECAUTIONS AND ADVERSE REACTIONS

No health hazards or side effects are known in conjunction with the proper administration of designated therapeutic dosages. The drug can trigger gallstone colic, due to its motility-enhancing effect.

DOSAGE

Mode of Administration: Ground seeds, as well as galenic preparations for internal use.

How Supplied:

Liquid Extract

Powder

Daily Dosage: The average daily dosage is 1.5 gm of drug. When using a tincture, the dosage range is 1 to 2 gm.

Storage: Cardamom should be stored in a cool, dry place protected from light in tightly sealed containers. The powder can be stored for a maximum of 24 hours. Loose seeds without the testa cannot be stored.

LITERATURE

Aye-Than Kulkarni HJ, Wut-Hmone Tha SJ. Anti-diarrhoeal Efficacy of Some Burmese Indigenous Drug Formulations in Experimental Diarrhoeal Test Models. *Int J Crude Drug Res.* 27; 195-200. 1989.

Fenaroli's Handbook of Flavor Ingredients, Vol. 1, 2nd Ed., CRC Press 1975.

Hänsel R, Keller K, Rimpler H, Schneider G (Hrsg.), Hagers Handbuch der Pharmazeutischen Praxis, 5. Aufl., Bde 4-6 (Drogen), Springer Verlag Berlin, Heidelberg, New York, 1992-1994.

Leung AY, Encyclopedia of Common Natural Ingredients Used in Food, Drugs and Cosmetics, John Wiley & Sons Inc., New York 1980.

Lewis YS, Nambuduri ES, Philip T. *Perfum Essent Oli Res.* 57:623-628. 1966.

Paranjpe P, Patki P, Patwardhan B. Ayurvedic Treatment of Obesity: a Randomised double-blind, placebo-controlled clinical trial. *J Ethnopharmacol.* 29; 1-11. 1990.

Teuscher E, Biogene Arzneimittel, 5. Aufl., Wiss. Verlagsges. mbH Stuttgart 1997.

Wagner H, Wiesenauer M, Phytotherapie. Phytopharmaka und pflanzliche Homöopathika, Fischer-Verlag, Stuttgart, Jena, New York 1995.

Carex arenaria

See German Sarsaparilla

Carica papaya

See Papaya

Carlina acaulis

See Carline Thistle

Carline Thistle

Carlina acaulis

DESCRIPTION

Medicinal Parts: The medicinal part is the root.

Flower and Fruit: The flowers are made up of individual heads that are 7 to 13 cm in diameter. The disc florets are androgynous, pink to violet, and have a 5-tipped radial corolla. The outer bracts are thorny. The middle bracts consist of glossy white, acuminate, 3 to 4 cm long leaves. The stamens have bristly-tipped appendages. The styles are cylindrical with short stigma lobes. The fruit is 5 mm long, obclavate to cylindrical, and bluntly angular with bifurcated hairs at the tip.

Leaves, Stem, and Root: Carlina acaulis is a 30 cm high thistlelike, leafy plant with milky latex. The stem is compressed and under 5 cm long. The whorled to alternate leaves are flat or slightly frilled and a little tough, 10 to 20 cm long, pinnatifid to pinnatisect with broad, thorny tips. The rhizome is finger thick and has 1 or more heads.

Habitat: The plant extends from Spain, Italy and the Balkans across central Europe to central Russia.

Production: Carline Thistle (Dwarf Thistle) is the root of *Carlina acaulis* collected in autumn and dried. It is collected in the wild.

Not to be Confused With: Sometimes Carline Thistle is adulterated by addition of other Carlina species.

Other Names: Stemless Carlina Root, Dwarf Carline, Ground Thistle, Southernwood Root

ACTIONS AND PHARMACOLOGY

COMPOUNDS

Volatile oil: chief components carlina oxide

Inulin (18 to 20%) (fructosan)

Tannins

EFFECTS

There is no valid data on the mode of action. The essential oil hinders the growth of *Staphylococcus aureus* up to a dilution of 1:2 X 105. Carline Thistle has mild diuretic, spasmolytic, and diaphoretic effects.

INDICATIONS AND USAGE

Unproven Uses: The drug is used internally for atonic gastritis, dyspepsia, diseases of the biliary tract, and colds and fevers.

Externally, it is used as a wash for dermatosis, and to rinse wounds and ulcers; as a mouthwash to alleviate symptoms associated with cancer of the tongue.

PRECAUTIONS AND ADVERSE REACTIONS

No health hazards or side effects are known in conjunction with the proper administration of designated therapeutic dosages.

DOSAGE

Mode of Administration: Carline Thistle is used both internally and externally.

Daily Dosage: Common preparations and doses are:

Decoction: Boil 3 gm of drug in 150 mL of water for 5 minutes. Drink 3 cups daily.

Infusion: 2 teaspoons of the drug to be boiled in 1 cup of water for 10 minutes, leave to draw for half an hour, take 3 to 4 cups daily between mealtimes.

Tincture: 20 gm of chopped drug, left to draw for 10 days in 80 gm of ethanol 60%, use 40 to 50 drops, 4 to 5 times daily.

Externally it is used as a decoction; 30 gm of the drug added to 1 L of water.

Storage: Should be stored in tightly sealed containers.

LITERATURE

Capitanio M, Cappelletti EM, Filippini R. Traditional antileukodermic herbal Remedies in the Mediterranean Area. *J Ethnopharmacol.* 27; 193-211. 1989.

Hänsel R, Keller K, Rimpler H, Schneider G (Hrsg.), Hagers Handbuch der Pharmazeutischen Praxis, 5. Aufl., Bde 4-6 (Drogen), Springer Verlag Berlin, Heidelberg, New York, 1992-1994.

Schimmer O, Kröger A, Paulini H, Haefele F. An evaluation of 55 commercial plant extracts in the Ames mutagenicity test. *Pharmazie.* 49; 448-451. 1994.

Wichtl M (Hrsg.), Teedrogen, 4. Aufl., Wiss. Verlagsges. Stuttgart 1997.

Carob

Ceratonia siliqua

DESCRIPTION

Medicinal Parts: The medicinal parts are the fruit and the bark.

Flower and Fruit: The inflorescence is erect and lateral in old wood. It is often bushy, clustered,or catkinlike, and unisexual with erect receptacles. There is no corolla. The male flowers have 5 long filaments with long slits and opening pollen tubes. The female flowers have short-stemmed ovaries. The pods are 10 to 20 cm by 2 cm, tough leathery, brown-violet, flat and often rounded to a horn shape. There are numerous, lumpy, and glossy brown seeds.

Leaves, Stem, and Root: This walnutlike tree is usually under 6 m high, broad-crowned, sparsely branched, and with cracked gray-brown bark. There are 2 to 4 paired pinnate leaves. The leaflets are obovate, 4 to 5 cm long, curved, glabrous, glossy dark green above and red-brown beneath.

Habitat: Indigenous to southeastern Europe and west Asia, otherwise cultivated.

Production: Carob seed flour is the ground endosperm of the seeds of *Ceratonia siliqua*.

Not to be Confused With: Carob Tree, *Jacaranda procera* or *Jacaranda caroba*.

Other Names: St. John's Bread, Locust Bean, Locust Pods, Sugar Pods

ACTIONS AND PHARMACOLOGY

COMPOUNDS

Mucilages: chiefly made up of galactomannanes

Proteic substances

Flavonoids: including isoschaftoside, neoschaftoside, schaftoside

EFFECTS

In various test series and studies, the effect of carob gum on the serum glucose level, the secretion and activity of digestive enzymes, the secretion of gastrointestinal hormones as well as on the serum lipid level was proved. The hypoglycaemic and hypolipidaemic effect is attributed to an increase in viscosity of the gastrointestinal content.

Effects on nitrogen balance, efficacy in infantile diarrhea, as well as an antiexudative, anticoagulant, and antiviral effects have been demonstrated.

CLINICAL TRIALS

Hypercholesterolemia/Diabetes/Obesity

Using an ultrasound method, researchers investigated if the gastric emptying in healthy subjects could be influenced by adding locust bean gum or water directly into a nutrient semisolid test meal. The viscosity of a basic test meal (300 g rice pudding, 330 kcal) was increased by adding Nestargel (6 g, 2.4 kcal), containing viscous dietary fibers (96.5%) provided as seed flour of locust bean gum, and decreased by adding 100 ml of water. Gastric emptying of these three test meals was evaluated in 15 healthy, non-smoking volunteers, using ultrasound measurements of the gastric antral area to estimate the gastric emptying rate (GER). The median value of GER with the basic test meal (rice pudding) was estimated at 63%. Increasing the viscosity of the rice pudding by adding Nestargel resulted in significantly lower gastric emptying rates ($p < 0.01$), median GER 54%. When the viscosity of the rice pudding was decreased (basic test meal added with water), the difference in median GER 65% was not significantly different ($p = 0.28$) compared to the GER of the basic test meal. The addition of locust bean gum (carob) to a nutrient semisolid meal has a major impact on gastric emptying by delaying the emptying rate in healthy subjects (Darwiche, 2003).

Dose-dependent effects of the consumption of carob fiber were investigated in a randomized, single-blind, crossover study in 20 healthy subjects, age 22-62 years. Plasma total and acylated ghrelin, triglycerides, serum insulin, and nonesterified fatty acids (NEFA) levels were repeatedly assessed before and after ingestion of an isocaloric standardized liquid meal with 0, 5, 10, or 20 g of carob fiber over a 300-min period. The respiratory quotient (RQ) was determined after consumption of 0 or 20 g of carob fiber. Carob fiber intake lowered acylated ghrelin to 49.1%, triglycerides to 97.2%, and NEFA to 67.2% compared with the control meal ($P < 0.001$). Total ghrelin and insulin concentrations were not affected by consumption of a carob fiber-enriched liquid meal. Postprandial energy expenditure was increased by 42.3% and RQ was reduced by 99.9% after a liquid meal with carob fiber compared with a control meal ($P < 0.001$). It was shown that the consumption of a carob pulp preparation decreased postprandial responses of acylated ghrelin, triglycerides, and NEFA, and alters RQ, suggesting a change toward increased fatty acid oxidation. These results indicate that carob fiber might exert beneficial effects in energy intake and body weight (Gruendel, 2006).

Over 8 weeks, 47 volunteers suffering from mild to moderate hypercholesterolemia (total cholesterol: 232–302 mg/dl) consumed three portions per day of 5 g carob fiber each administered in three different products (breakfast cereal, fruit muesli bar, drink powder) as supplements to the habitual diet. After 4 weeks of treatment, the mean total cholesterol and LDL-cholesterol levels of initially 261.4 mg/dl and 171.2 mg/dl were reduced by 7.1 % and 10.6 %, respectively, and after 6 weeks by 7.8 % and 12.1 % ($p < 0,001$ in all cases). HDL-cholesterol and triglyceride levels remained unchanged. Three drop-outs were reported (Zunft et al., 2001).

A total of 58 volunteers with hypercholesterolemia were recruited to participate in a randomized, double-blind, placebo-controlled and parallel-arm clinical study with a 6- week intervention phase. Each day, subjects consumed both bread (two servings) and a fruit-bar (one serving), either with or without a total amount of 15 g/d of a carob pulp preparation. Serum concentrations of total, LDL and HDL cholesterol, and triglycerides were assessed at baseline and after week 4 and week 6. The consumption of carob fiber reduced LDL cholesterol ($p = 0.010$). The LDL:HDL cholesterol ratio was marginally decreased in the carob fiber group compared to the placebo group ($p = 0.058$). Carob fiber consumption also lowered triglycerides in females ($p = 0.030$). Lipid lowering effects were more pronounced in females than in males (Zunft et al., 2003).

Gastroesophageal Reflux in Children

The efficacy of anti-regurgitant milk (AR milk) with reduced concentration of locust bean gum (LBG) compared with a commercially available concentration of this thickener was evaluated in thirty infants with daily regurgitation but no other medical problems who were randomly assigned to one of two groups. Infants in group A (n = 16) were fed either HL-450, an AR milk thickened with a commonly used concentration of LBG (0.45 g/100 mL), or control milk (HL-00; no LBG) in a crossover manner for periods of 1 week. Infants in group B (n=14) were fed HL-350, an AR milk with a reduced LBG concentration (0.35 g/100 mL), or HL-00 in the same crossover fashion. The number of episodes of regurgitation, feeding time, and body weight gain were recorded. Three infants in group B did not complete the protocol and were excluded. Both AR formulas decreased the number of regurgitation episodes by approximately 50% compared with control. Five mothers who gave their infants HL-450 and no mothers who fed their children HL-350 reported that the infants had difficulty sucking the formula through the nipple. Thirteen (81.3%) mothers who used HL-450 and 9 (81.8%) mothers who used HL-350 preferred the AR milk to the control milk (Miyazawa, 2004).

To study the effect of carob bean gum on gastric emptying and the symptoms of regurgitation, 20 infants (mean age=13.4+/-7 week; mean body weight=4943+/-1272gm) without pathological gastroesophageal reflux were recruited. Initially, half-time gastric emptying (T 1/2 GET) was determined by Tc99m radioscintigraphy method (mean T 1/2 GET=116.1+/-72 min) in infants consuming standard infant cow's milk formula for 2 weeks. Afterwards, carob bean infant formula was given for 2-4 weeks. Weight gain, vomiting symptoms, night cough, colic, flatus, defecation character, and T 1/2 GET were assessed. There were statistically significant improvements in symptoms of vomiting (quantity $P<0.001$ and frequency $P<0.0001$) and improvements in weight gain per week ($P=0.005$) when infants consumed the carob bean formula. However, there was no significance difference in gastric emptying half-time ($P=0.154$) (Vivatvakin, 2003).

The aim of a randomized, placebo-controlled crossover study was to examine the influence of formula thickened with carob bean gum on acid and nonacid gastroesophageal reflux. Infants with recurrent regurgitation and without other symptoms were fed alternately (A-B-A-B-A-B) with thickened (A) and nonthickened (B) but otherwise identical formula. Documentation of reflux episodes during the study was performed by simultaneous intraesophageal impedance measurement (intraluminal electrical impedance, or IMP) and pH monitoring. Fourteen infants (42 +/- 32 days old) were examined during 6 feeding intervals each for a total measuring time of 342 hours. A total of 1,183 reflux episodes and 83 episodes of regurgitation were registered. Regurgitation frequency (15 vs 68 episodes) and amount (severity score 0.6 vs. 1.8) were significantly lower after feedings with thickened formula. The difference regarding the occurrence of reflux documented by IMP was also pronounced (536 vs 647 episodes). Although not statistically significant, maximal height reached by the refluxate in the esophagus was decreased after thickened feedings. Mean reflux duration and the frequency of acid (pH <4) reflux were not altered. Thickened feeding has a significant effect on the reduction of regurgitation frequency and amount in otherwise healthy infants. This effect is caused by a reduction in the number of nonacid (pH >4) GER episodes, but also because of a decrease of mean reflux height reached in the esophagus. However, the occurrence of acid reflux is not reduced (Wenzl, 2003)

INDICATIONS AND USAGE

Unproven Uses: Carob is used in dietary agents for acute nutritional disorders, diarrhea, dyspepsia, entero-colitis, celiac disease, and sprue. It is also used for habitual vomiting in babies, acetonemic vomiting, rumination, retching cough, and vomiting.

Carob seed flour is used in the production of gluten-free starch bread, which is used for vomiting during pregnancy, celiac disease and obesity. In cases of elevated cholesterol, it is used as part of a low-cholesterol, low-fat diet.

PRECAUTIONS AND ADVERSE REACTIONS

No health hazards or side effects are known in conjunction with the proper administration of designated therapeutic dosages.

Caution is advised for patients taking Vitamin A who ingest large amounts of carob foods.

DRUG INTERACTIONS

MODERATE RISK

Digoxin: Concurrent use may result in increased digoxin toxicity. *Clinical Management:* Monitor closely for symptoms of digoxin toxicity and consider measuring serum digoxin.

DOSAGE

Mode of Administration: It is obsolete as a drug but is included in thickening powders and as a baking aid for gluten-free starch bread.

Preparation: As a baking aid or thickening agent, dissolve in cold liquid, boil for 1 to 2 minutes, cool and mix into the prepared baby food.

Daily Dosage: For a 3 to 10% arabon preparation, add 20 to 30 mg of drug to water, tea or milk, to be drunk during the course of the day. As a baking agent in gluten-free bread for babies, add 1/4 to 1/2 gm of drug (max. 2 gm) to 100 mL liquid; adults 1% to 3% additive to low-calorie starters and desserts.

LITERATURE

Darwiche G, Bjorgell O, Almer LO. The addition of locust bean gum but not water delayed the gastric emptying rate of a nutrient semisolid meal in healthy subjects. *BMC Gastroenterol* 2003 Jun 6;3(1):12.

Gruendel S, Garcia AL, Otto B, Mueller C, Steiniger J, Weickert MO, Speth M, Katz N, Koebnick C. Carob pulp preparation rich in insoluble dietary fiber and polyphenols enhances lipid oxidation and lowers postprandial acylated ghrelin in humans. *J Nutr.* 2006 Jun;136(6):1533-8.

Kern W, List PH, Hörhammer L (Hrsg.), Hagers Handbuch der Pharmazeutischen Praxis, 4. Aufl., Bde 1-8, Springer Verlag Berlin, Heidelberg, New York, 1969.

Leung AY, Encyclopedia of Common Natural Ingredients Used in Food Drugs and Cosmetics, John Wiley & Sons Inc., New York 1980.

Miyazawa R, Tomomasa T, Kaneko H, Morikawa A. Effect of locust bean gum in anti-regurgitant milk on the regurgitation in uncomplicated gastroesophageal reflux. *J Pediatr Gastroenterol Nutr* 2004 May;38(5):479-83.

Tang W, Eisenbrand G, Chinese Drugs of Plant Origin, Springer Verlag Heidelberg 1992.

Teuscher E, Biogene Arzneimittel, 5. Aufl., Wiss. Verlagsges. mbH Stuttgart 1997.

Vivatvakin B, Buachum V. Effect of carob bean on gastric emptying time in Thai infants. *Asia Pac J Clin Nutr* 2003;12(2):193-7.

Wenzl TG, Schneider S, Scheele F, Silny J, Heimann G, Skopnik H. Effects of thickened feeding on gastroesophageal reflux in infants: a placebo-controlled crossover study using intraluminal impedance. *Pediatrics* 2003 Apr;111(4 Pt 1):e355-9.

Zunft HJ, Luder W, Harde A, Haber B, Graubaum HJ, Gruenwald J. Carob pulp preparation for treatment of hypercholesterolemia. *Adv Ther* 2001 Sep-Oct;18(5):230-6.

Zunft HJ, Luder W, Harde A, Haber B, Graubaum HJ, Koebnick C, Grunwald J. Carob pulp preparation rich in insoluble fibre lowers total and LDL cholesterol in hypercholesterolemic patients. *Eur J Nutr* 2003 Oct;42(5):235-42.

Carrageen

Chondrus crispus

DESCRIPTION

Medicinal Parts: The medicinal part of carrageen, the Irish seaweed, is the thallus that has been freed from the adhesive disc then dried and bleached in the sun.

Flower and Fruit: Gamatangia: The spematangia are colorless and are at the end of the younger thallus lobes. The spermatia are 7.5 to 10 +l mm long and 4 to 5 + l mm wide; the carposporangia are 20 to 20 + l mm long and 14 to 25 + l mm wide and have no outer threads. The tetrasporangia, along with the cruciform arranged tatra spores, are in the medulla of the short side branches.

Thallus: *Chondrus crispus* is a perennial red algae that grows in waters up to 25 m deep. The thallus is usually yellow-green to purplish-brown when fresh, white to yellow and translucent after drying. Thallus fronds are 10 to 30 cm long on an adhesive disc, arising from a subcylindrical stem. They then become flattened, curled, and sometimes bifid. The segments are linear and usually 3 to 8 mm wide. The margin is linguiform, later repeatedly dividing into bifid thallus lobes. The thallus is cartilaginous and double-layered. The internal tissue is made up of reticulately linked cells. The bark layer is at right angles to the thallus. The bifurcated cell strings are like strings of pearls that are spread radially.

Habitat: Carrageen is found from the coast of Iceland to the Baltic, from northern Russia to the south of Spain, Morocco and the Cape Verde Islands, and also in parts of North America and some Japanese coastal regions.

Production: Carrageen is the dried and bleached thalli of *Chondrus crispus* as well as other varieties of Gigartina species. After being cleaned, the algae are left to bleach in the sun, then dried.

Not to be Confused With: Confusion can arise with related species of *Gigartina stellata* and *Gigartina pistillata.*

Other Names: Irish Moss, Chondrus, Carrahan, Carrageennan

ACTIONS AND PHARMACOLOGY

COMPOUNDS

Carrageenans: (carrageenine): in particular kappa-, iota- and lambda-carrageenan (muciform galactane sulphates)

Proteins

Mineral salts: including iodides and bromides

EFFECTS

The drug contains hydrocolloids of the carrageenan type. Carrageen is considered mucilaginous because it hinders the effect of peptides in digestive enzymes. It also acts as an expectorant and secretory agent. In animal experiments the drug was not absorbed. There are no studies available on absorption in humans. The drug's purported demulcent and antitussive effects have not been confirmed.

INDICATIONS AND USAGE

Unproven Uses: Folk medicine internal uses of Carrageen include as roughage for constipation and as a mucilage for diarrhea, as well as for peptic ulcers. Sometimes a decoction is used for coughs, bronchitis, and tuberculosis.

PRECAUTIONS AND ADVERSE REACTIONS

No health hazards or side effects are known in conjunction with the proper administration of designated therapeutic dosages. Intracutaneous injections of solutions, however, can trigger local inflammations.

DOSAGE

Mode of Administration: Seldom used as a drug, but is included in compound preparations as syrup and granules.

Preparation: Irish moss extract is prepared using a diluted, almost boiling alkali solution. Filtration and vacuum inspissation follow prior to extensive dehydration. A decoction is prepared by combining 1.5 g drug with 1 cup water.

Storage: The drug should be stored in tightly sealed containers.

LITERATURE

Chapman B, Chapman VJ, Chapman DJ, Seaweeds and their uses. Chapmann and Hall, London, New York 1980.

Marcus R, Watt J. Potential Hazard of Carrageenan. *Lancet.* 8168; 602. 1980.

Sarett HP. Safety of Carrageenan used in Foods. *Lancet* I. 151-152. 1981.

Thomson AW, Horne CHW. *Brit J Exp Pathol.* 57:455. 1976.

Carthamus tinctorius

See Safflower

Carum carvi

See Caraway

Cascara Sagrada

Rhamnus purshiana

DESCRIPTION

Medicinal Parts: The medicinal part is the dried bark.

Flower and Fruit: The flowers are in richly blossomed axillary racemes. The receptacles are green and the sepals are larger than the petals. Both receptacles and sepals are white. The ovary is longer than the style and is trilocular. The fruit is dark purple and top-shaped. The seeds are ovate, black, glossy, domed on the outside, and have a distinct line on the inside.

Leaves, Stem, and Root: The plant is either a bush or a 6 to 18 m tall tree with branches which are gray tomentose when young. The leaves are oblong-ovate, rounded at the base or sometimes narrowing at the petiole. On the longer shoots they are up to 17 cm long and 7.5 cm wide with an 8 to 18 mm long petiole. The margins are finely dentate and the young leaves are tomentose, later becoming dark-green but not coriaceous even in autumn.

Habitat: The plant is indigenous to the western part of North America and is cultivated on the Pacific coast of the U.S., Canada, and in eastern Africa.

Production: Cascara Sagrada bark consists of the dried bark of *Rhamnus purshiana.*

Not to be Confused With: The bark of other Rhamnus species.

Other Names: Bitter Bark, California Buckthorn, Cascara Buckthorn, Chittem Bark, Dogwood Bark, Purshiana Bark, Sacred Bark, Sagrada Bark, Yellow Bark

ACTIONS AND PHARMACOLOGY

COMPOUNDS

Anthracene derivatives (8-10%): anthranoids, chief components cascarosides A and B (stereoisomeric aloin-8-glucosides), C and D (stereoisomeric 11-deoxy-aloin-8-glucosides), E and F (C-glucosyl-emodin-anthron-8-glucosides), further including aloin, 11-deoxyaloin

EFFECTS

Cascara has laxative effects, which appears to be caused by inducing the synthesis of nitric oxide (Izzo, 1997).

Laxative Effects

Water and electrolyte absorption and secretion are influenced by the anthraquinones (de Witte & Lemli, 1990). The anthranoids are anti-absorptive, hydrogogic and inhibit the absorption of electrolytes and water from the colon. The proposed mechanisms include inhibition of epithelial sodium- and potassium-ATPase increased mucosal permeability of the colonic mucosa, possibly caused by an uncoupling activity of anthraquinones on mitochondria, an influence on Meissner's plexus, and a prostaglandin-mediated mechanism. The laxative effect is caused by an increase in the volume of the intestinal contents with the resulting increase in pressure and stimulation of intestinal peristalsis. In addition, stimulation of the active chloride secretion into the intestine by nitric-oxide-donating compounds or nitric oxide itself increases water and electrolyte content (Izzo, 1998). Aloin and other anthranoid derivatives stimulate prostaglandin production in isolated segments of intestinal tissue, thus contributing to the cathartic action (Cohen, 1982; Capasso, 1983).

CLINICAL TRIALS

Bowel Preparation

In a prospective, randomized clinical trial was conducted to determine the side effects, patient acceptance, residual liquid and stool during colonoscopy and also quality of examination of three colon cleansing methods. Three hundred ambulatory patients were randomly assigned to one of the following three groups for colon preparation: Group 1, (4 liters of GoLytely), group 2, (2 liters of GoLytely combined with Cascara-Salax), and group 3, (X-Prep (a Senna preparation) combined with an enema). X-Prep caused significantly more abdominal cramps than Group 1 or Group 2. Vomiting was most frequent with Group 1, and the patients preferred X-Prep to 4 liters of GoLytely. The cleanest colon was obtained with 4 liters of GoLytely; 2 liters of GoLytely with Cascara-Salax was least effective. The quality of the examination was equal in groups 1 and 3, which were both significantly better than group 2 (Hangartner, 1989). Other studies have shown similar results (Borkje et al, 1991; Hangartner et al, 1989; Phillip et al, 1990).

In patients undergoing gallium scans, daily oral administration of cascara 5 mL plus milk of magnesia 30 mL did not speed removal of gallium from the intestine, improved scan quality, or reduced the number of days needed to obtain a diagnostic scan (Silberstein et al, 1981).

Constipation

Studies involving elderly patients suggest that cascara treatment, compared with placebo, leads to relief of constipation and increased bowel movements. Many authors recommend cascara for the relief of narcotic-related constipation (Hammack & Loprinzi, 1994; Cameron, 1992; Levy, 1991; Maguire et al, 1981).

INDICATIONS AND USAGE

Approved by Commission E:

- Constipation

Cascara Segrada is used for constipation, relief of defecation with anal fissures, hemorrhoids, and as a recto-anal post-operative treatment. The herb is also used in preparation of diagnostic procedures of the gastrointestinal tract and to obtain a soft stool.

Unproven Uses: In folk medicine, Cascara is used as a tonic and for cleaning wounds.

Homeopathic Uses: The herb is used for rheumatism and as a digestive aid.

CONTRAINDICATIONS

The drug is contraindicated in intestinal and bowel obstruction, acute inflammatory intestinal disease (colitis, Crohn's disease, irritable bowel), fecal impaction, nausea, vomiting, appendicitis, and abdominal pain of unknown origin.

Pregnancy: Not to be used during pregnancy.

Breastfeeding: Not to be used while breastfeeding.

Pediatrics: Cascara drug is not to be administered to children under 12 years of age.

PRECAUTIONS AND ADVERSE REACTIONS

Spasmodic gastrointestinal complaints can occur as a side effect to the drug's purgative effect. In rare cases, prolonged use may lead to heart arrhythmias, nephropathies, edema, and accelerated bone deterioration. Intake of the fresh rind could lead to European cholera, intestinal colic, bloody diarrhea, and kidney irritation. A benign melanotic pigmentation of the colonic mucosa (pseudomelanosis coli) may occur with prolonged use of the anthraquinones. Cascara sagrada may produce discoloration of acid urine to yellow-brown or discoloration of alkaline urine to pink-red, red-violet, or red-brown.

Excessive laxative use or inadequate fluid intake may lead to significant fluid and electrolyte imbalance. Prolonged use should also be avoided. Longer than 1 week is not recommended. Hyperaldosteronism, albuminuria, hematuria, inhibition of intestinal motility, and muscle weakness may occur with long-term use.

Metabolic Effects: Electrolyte abnormalities and fluid imbalance resulting from excessive catharsis may occur with anthraquinone laxatives (Olin, 1991). Hypokalemia is the most common finding (Muller-Lissner, 1993). This is caused by fecal loss, which is aggravated by hyperaldosteronism due to losses of water and sodium. Enhancement of cardioactive steroids and antiarhhythmics may also occur as a consequense of hypokalemia.

Carcinogenesis: The probability of carcinomas in the colon following long-term administration of anthracene drugs has not yet been fully clarified. Cascara glycoside may act as weak promoters in colon carcinogenesis in animal models (Mereto, 1996). Anthraquinone glycosides from cascara were shown to be weak promoters of colon cancer in rats (Mereto et al, 1996). Based on data from 2 studies, it was determined that anthraquinone laxative users may be at risk for colorectal cancer (Siegers et al, 1993). Authors calculated a risk for colorectal cancer in anthraquinone laxative abusers of 3.04 (95% confidence interval of 1.18 to 4.9). One study determined aloin-enriched diets did not promote incidence and growth of adenomas, carcinomas or significant hepatotoxicity after 20 weeks (Siegers, 1993a). Anthranoid laxative abuse is a risk factor for colorectal cancer (Siegerss, 1993b).

DRUG INTERACTIONS

MODERATE RISK

Digoxin: With prolonged use or abuse of Cascara Sagrada bark, potassium loss may potentiate digoxin toxicity. *Clinical Management:* Patients who are taking digoxin should be advised to avoid concomitant use with Cascara Sagrada bark. If digoxin toxicity occurs, potassium should be monitored and supplemented if necessary while discontinuing Cascara Sagrada bark.

OVERDOSAGE

Patients taking Cascara Sagrada bark for more than 1 to 2 weeks may experience hypokalemia (signs and symptoms include lethargy, muscle cramps, headaches, paresthesias, tetany, peripheral edema, polyuria, breathlessness, and hypertension).

Large doses of anthraquinones may cause nephritis.

DOSAGE

Mode of Administration: Liquid or solid forms of medication are exclusively for oral use. The drug is used as comminuted drug, powder or dry extracts for infusions, decoction, and as a cold maceration or elixir.

How Supplied:

Capsule – 425 mg, 440 mg, 450 mg, 850 mg

Preparation: To prepare an infusion, add 2 g finely cut drug to boiling water and strain after 10 minutes. (1 teaspoonful = 2.5 g drug)

Daily Dosage: Administer 20 to 30 mg hydroxyanthracene derivatives daily, calculated as cascaroside A.

Tea: Take 1 fresh cup mornings and evenings.

Homeopathic Dosage: from D3: 5 drops, 1 tablet, or 10 globules every 30 to 60 minutes (acute) or 1 to 3 times daily (chronic); parenterally: 1 to 2 mL sc acute: 3 times daily; chronic: once a day (HAB34)

Note: The individually correct dosage is the smallest dosage necessary to maintain a soft stool. Stimulating laxatives must not be used over a period of more than 1 to 2 weeks without medical advice.

LITERATURE

Bernardi M, D'Intino PE, Trevisani F et al. Effects of prolonged ingestion of graded doses of licorice by healthy volunteers. *Life Sci*; 55(11):863-872. 1994

Blachley JD & Knochel JP. Tobacco chewer's hypokalemia: licorice revisited. *N Engl J Med*; 302(14):784-785. 1980

Borkje B; Pedersen R; Lund GM et al. Effectiveness and acceptability of three bowel cleansing regimens. *Scand J Gastroenterol* Feb;26(2):162-6. 1991

Brouwers JRBJ, van Ouwerkerk WPL, de Boer SM et al. A controlled trial of senna preparations and other laxatives used for bowel cleansing prior to radiological examination. Pharmacology; 20(suppl 1):58-64. 1980

Cameron JC. Constipation related to narcotic therapy: a protocol for nurses and patients. *Cancer Nurs*; 15(5):372-377. 1992

Capasso F; Mascolo N; Autore G; Duraccio MR. Effect of indomethacin on aloin and 1,8 dioxianthraquinone-induced production of prostaglandins in rat isolated colon. *Prostaglandins* Oct;26(4):557-62. 1983

Cohen MM. The effect of cathartics on prostaglandin synthesis by rat gastrointestinal tract. *Prostaglandins Leukot Med* Apr;8(4):389-97. 1982

Connolly P, Hughes IW & Ryan G. Comparison of "Duphalac" and "irritant" laxatives during and after treatment of chronic constipation a preliminary study. *Curr Med Res Opin*; 2(10):620-625. 1975

Corsi FM, Galgani S, Gasparini C et al. Acute hypokalemic myopathy due to chronic licorice ingestion: report of a case. *Ital J Neurol Sci*; 4(4):493-497. 1983

Dellow EL, Unwin RJ & Honour JW. Pontefract cakes can be bad for you: refractory hypertension and liquorice excess. *Nephrol Dial Transplant*; 14:218-220. 1999

de Witte P, Cuveele J, Lemli J. Bicascarosides in fluid extracts of Cascara. In: *PM* 57:440. 1991.

de Witte P; Lemli L. The metabolism of anthranoid laxatives. *Hepatogastroenterology* Dec;37(6):601-5. 1990

Griffini A et al. Isolation and characterization of pure Cascarosides A, B, C, and D. In. *PM;* 58(Suppl.7):A593. 1992

Hagemann TM. Gastrointestinal medications and breastfeeding. *J Hum Lact* Sep;14(3):259-62. 1998

Hammack JE & Loprinzi CL. Use of orally administered opioid for cancer related pain. *Mayo Clin Proc*; 69(4):384-390. 1994

Hangartner PJ; Munch R; Meier J et al. Comparison of three colon-cleansing methods: evaluation of a randomized clinical trial with 300 ambulatory patients. *Endoscopy* Nov; 21(6): 272-5. 1989

Helmholz H, Ruge A, Piasecki A, Schröder S, Westendorf J, Genotoxizität der Faulbaumrinde. In: *PZ;* 138(43):3478. 1993

Hussain RM. The sweet cake that reaches parts other cakes can't! *Postgrad Med J*; 79:115-116. 2003

Izzo AA; Mascolo N; Capasso F. Nitric oxide as a modulator of intestinal water and electrolyte transport. *Dig Dis Sci* Aug; 43(8):1605-20. 1998

Izzo AA, Sautebin L, Rombola L et al. The role of constitutive and inducible nitric oxide synthase in senna- and cascara-induced diarrhea in the rat. *Eur J Pharmacol*; 323(1):93-97. 1997

Kato H, Kanaoka M, Yano S et al. 3-Monoglucuronyl-glycyrrhetinic acids is a major metabolite that causes licorice-induced pseudoaldosteronism. *J Clin Endocrinol Metab*; 80(6):1929-1933. 1995

Kageyama K, Watanobe H, Nishie M et al. A case of pseudoaldosteronism induced by a mouth refresher containing licorice. *Endocr J*; 44(4): 631-632.1997

Klimpel BE et al. Anthranoidhaltige Laxantien - ein Risiko für die Entwicklung von Tumoren der ableitenden Harnwege. In: *PUZ* 26(1): 33, Jahrestagung der DPhG, Berlin, 1996. 1997

Koren G, Boichis H & Keren G. Effects of tea on the absorption of pharmacological doses of an oral iron preparation. *Sci Meet Israel*; 18:547. 1982

Levy MH. Constipation and diarrhea in cancer patients. *Cancer Bull*; 43:412-422. 1991

Lin SH, Yang SS, Chau T et al. An unusual cause of hypokalemic paralysis: chronic licorice ingestion. *Am J Med Sci*; 325(3):153-156. 2003

Maguire LC, Yon JL & Muller E: Prevention of narcotic-induced constipation (letter). *N Engl J Med*; 305(27):1651. 1981

Manitto P et al. Studies on cascara, part 2. Structure of cascarosides E and F. In: *JNP;* 58(3): 419-423. 1995

Mereto E, Ghia M, Brambilla G. Evaluation of the potential carcinogenic activity of Senna and Cascara glycosides for the rat colon. *Cancer Lett* Mar, 19;101(1):79-83. 1996

Merhav H, Amitai Y & Palti H. Tea drinking and microcytic anemia in infants. *Am J Clin Nutrition*; 41:1210-1213. 1985

Muller-Lissner SA: Adverse effects of laxatives: fact and fiction. *Pharmacology*; 47(suppl 1):138-145. 1993

Perkin JM. Constipation in childhood: a controlled comparison between lactulose and standardized senna. *Curr Med Res Opin*; 4(8):540-543. 1977

Shapiro W & Taubert K. Letter: Hypokalaemia and digoxin-induced arrhythmias. *Lancet*; 2(7935):604-5. 1975

Shintani S, Murase H, Tsukagoshi H et al. Glycyrrhizin (Licorice)-induced hypokalemic myopathy. Eur Neurol; 32(1):44-51. 1992

Siegers CP; Siemers J; Baretton G. Sennosides and aloin do not promote dimethylhydrazine-induced colorectal tumors in mice. *Pharmacology* Oct; 47 Suppl 1:205-8. 1993a

Siegers CP, von Hertzberg-Lottin E, Otte M, Schneider B. Anthranoid laxative abuse–a risk for colorectal cancer? *Gut* Aug; 34(8):1099-101. 1993b

Silberstein EB, Fernandez-Ulloa M & Hall J. Are oral cathartics of value in optimizing the gallium scan? Concise communication. *J Nucl Med*; 22(5):424-427. 1981

Slanger A. Comparative study of a standardized senna liquid and castor oil in preparing patients for radiographic examination of the colon. *Dis Colon Rectum*; 22(5):356-359. 1979

Steiness E & Olesen KH. Cardiac arrhythmias induced by hypokalemia and potassium loss during maintenance digoxin therapy. *Br Heart J*; 38:167-172. 1976

Walker BR & Edwards CRW. Licorice-induced hypertension and syndromes of apparent mineralocorticoid excess. *Endocrinol Metab Clinic N America*; 23:359-377. 1994

Wash LK & Bernard JD. Licorice-induced pseudoaldosteronism. *Am J Hosp Pharm*; 32(1):73-74. 1975

Cascarilla

Croton eluteria

DESCRIPTION

Medicinal Parts: The medicinal part is the dried bark.

Flower and Fruit: The flowers are small, with white petals and a pleasant fragrance.

Leaves, Stem, and Root: The plant is a small tree that rarely grows to more than 6 m. It has small, opposite, ovate-lanceolate leaves about 5 cm long. Scales beneath densely cover the leaves, giving them a silver-bronze appearance. Above, the scales are scattered and white. The bark occurs in short quilled pieces, usually with a chalky, more or less cracked, white surface, with black dots due to the fruit of lichens. The transverse fracture is reddish-brown.

Characteristics: The taste is aromatic and bitter.

Habitat: Indigenous to the West Indies, also grown in tropical areas of America.

Production: Cascarilla bark is the bark of *Croton eluteria.*

Other Names: Sweet Wood Bark, Sweet Bark, Bahama Cascarilla

ACTIONS AND PHARMACOLOGY

COMPOUNDS

Volatile oil (1.5 to 3%): chief components are p-cymene, limonene, alpha-thujone, pinenes, linalool, myrcene, terpeni-nol-4

Diterpene bitter principles: including Cascarillin A (15%)

Resins (25%)

EFFECTS

Cascarilla is a stimulant and a tonic.

INDICATIONS AND USAGE

Unproven Uses: Cascarilla is used for digestive disorders, diarrhea, and vomiting.

PRECAUTIONS AND ADVERSE REACTIONS

Health risks or side effects following the proper administration of designated therapeutic dosages are not recorded.

DOSAGE

Mode of Administration: Available as a powder, liquid extract, or tincture.

LITERATURE

Fenaroli's Handbook of Flavor Ingredients, Vol. 1, 2nd Ed., CRC Press 1975.

Hegnauer R, Chemotaxonomie der Pflanzen, Bde 1-11, Birkhäuser Verlag Basel, Boston, Berlin 1962-1997.

Kern W, List PH, Hörhammer L (Hrsg.), Hagers Handbuch der Pharmazeutischen Praxis, 4. Aufl., Bde 1-8, Springer Verlag Berlin, Heidelberg, New York, 1969.

Leung AY, Encyclopedia of Common Natural Ingredients Used in Food Drugs and Cosmetics, John Wiley & Sons Inc., New York 1980.

Mc Echean CE et al., *J Chem Soc.* 166B:633. 1966.

Steinegger E, Hänsel R, Pharmakognosie, 5. Aufl., Springer Verlag Heidelberg 1992.

Cashew

Anacardium occidentale

DESCRIPTION

Medicinal Parts: The medicinal parts are the finely chopped bark, the cashew nut, the fresh leaves, and extracted cashew oil.

Flower and Fruit: Flowers are in terminal, cymelike, 10 to 20 cm long panicles and are polygamous. The pedicles are 2 to 3 mm long. The calyx is deeply divided into five sepals, which are lanceolate, erect, imbricate, glabrous inside and covered on the outside with short, thick, gray hairs. The corolla is 5-petaled. The petals are lineal-lanceolate, 7 to 8 mm long by 1 mm wide, acute, soft and gray-haired on the outside. The petals are glabrous and yellow with a red stripe on the inside that curls outward in the later stages. Seven to 10 stamens are fused at the base, but only one 8 to 9 mm long stamen is fertile; the sterile ones are shorter. Anthers are yellowish-white, oblong-ovate and burst open along a vertical slit. The gynoecium is obovate, 2 mm long, one-valved and elongates to a 4 mm long wedge-shaped style with a spotlike stigma. The flowers are followed by a fleshy, edible receptacle, which partly encloses the fruit. The fruit is reniform, with a smooth, pale grayish-brown drupe, about 2 to 3 cm long and 1 cm thick.

Leaves, Stem, and Root: The Cashew is a broad evergreen tree from 6 to 10 m high with smooth glabrous branches, densely leafed toward the tops. It has short-petioled leaves that are alternate, coriaceous and entire-margined. The leaf blade is obovate, 12 to 14 cm by 6 to 8 cm with a prominent midrib and 10 to 14 veins that are almost parallel.

Habitat: The plant grows in the Caribbean and Central and South America; it is cultivated everywhere in the tropics, especially in Africa and India.

Production: Fruit of the Cashew tree is harvested with the stem removed.

Other Names: East Indian Almond

ACTIONS AND PHARMACOLOGY

COMPOUNDS: IN THE SEED CASE

Alkyl phenoles

Anacardic acid

Cardol

Methyl cardol

COMPOUNDS: IN THE SEEDS

Fatty oil

Chief fatty acids: oleic acid and linolenic acid

Proteins

Starch

EFFECTS

It has been demonstrated in vitro that the dried extract prepared with ethanol is effective against the gram-positive bacteria *Bacillus subtilis* and *Staphylococcus aureus.* It also acts as an astringent and cauterizing agent due to the phenolic skin stimulant (anacardic acid) found mostly in the skin of the fruit. The fruit itself exhibits antimicrobial, molluscacidal, vermicidal, and antitumoral effects.

INDICATIONS AND USAGE

Unproven Uses: Cashew is used for gastrointestinal ailments in Brazil and Nigeria. Cashew shell oil and cashew fruit are used as skin stimulants and cauterizing agents for ulcers, warts and corns. In Brazil and Nigeria, the bark is used to make an astringent decoction to treat toothache and inflammation of the gums. Young leaves are used in the Philippines in the treatment of diarrhea, dysentery and hemorrhoids; older leaves are used as hot poultices for burns and skin disorders. Efficacy for these indications has not been documented.

Indian Medicine: Cashew bark is used for fevers, as a laxative and anthelmintic, and to treat diabetes insipidus. One particular form is used to treat snake bites. Cashew shell oil is used as a rubefacient and skin stimulant in the treatment of leprosy, elephantitis, psoriasis, and ringworm, in addition to warts and corns.

Homeopathic Uses: Cashew is used to treat severely itching rashes with blistering and also facial erysipelas.

PRECAUTIONS AND ADVERSE REACTIONS

The alkyl phenoles contained in the seed case of the nut are strong skin irritants. Contact between the seed case and skin can lead to erythemas with nodule and blister formation. Frequent contact can lead to rimose exanthemas. The roasted seeds eaten as cashew nuts are free of alkyl phenoles, as is the plant stalk.

DOSAGE

Mode of Administration: Available preparations include acajou oil, cashew oil, oleum anacardiae and fatty oil extracted from the seeds.

Preparation: Preparations are often compounds, particularly in homeopathy.

Homeopathic Dosage: Daily dosage is 5 drops, 1 tablet, 10 globules, every 30 to 60 minutes for acute conditions; or one of those options 1 to 3 times daily for chronic conditions. Parenterally: 1 to 2 mL 3 times daily; Ointments, rinses and poultices: 1 dessertspoon: 1/4L water 1 to 2 times daily (HAB34).

LITERATURE

Bedello PG, Goitre M, Cane D, Roncarolo G, Alovisi V. Allergic contact dermatitis to cashew nut. *Contact Dermatitis.* 12; 235. 1985.

Banerjee S, Rao AR, Promoting action of cashew nut shell oil in DMBA-initiated mouse skin tumour model system. *Cancer Lett.* 47:149-52, 1992 Feb 29.

Caceres A, Cano O, Samayoa B, Aguilar L. Plants used in Guatemala for the Treatment of Gastrointestinal Disorders. 1.Screening of 84 Plants against *Enterobacteria. J Ethnopharmacol.* 30; 55-73. 1990.

de Souza CP, Mendes NM, Jannotti-Passos LK, Pereira JP. The use of the shell of the cashew nut *Anacardium occidentale* as an alternative molluscacide. *Rev Inst Med Trop Sao Paulo.* 34:459-66, Sep-Oct. 1992.

Diogenes MJN, Morais SMde Carvalho FF. Contact dermatitis among cashew nut workers. *Contact Dermatitis.* 35; 114-115. 1996.

George J, Kuttan R. Mutagenic carcinogenic and cocarcinogenic activity of cashew nut shell liquid. *Cancer Lett.* 47:11-6, Jan 15. 1997.

Kubo I, et al., Tyrosinase inhibitors from *Anacardium occidentale.* In: *JNP.* 57(4):545. 1994.

Nagaraja KV. *Plant Foods Hum Nutr.* 37:307-311. 1987.

Neuwinger HD, Arzneipflanzen Schwarzafrikas. In: DAZ 134(6):453. 1994.

Knight TE, Boll P, Epstein WL, Prasad AK. Resorcinols and Catechols: A Clinical Study of Cross-sensitivity. *Am J Contact Dermatitis*. 7 (3); 138-145. 1996.

Smit HF, Woerdenbag HJ, Singh RH, Meulenbeld GJ, Labadie RP, Zwaving JH, Ayurvedic herbal drugs with possible cytostatic activity. *J Ethnopharmacol*. 47:75-84, 1995 Jul 7.

Cassia fistula

See Golden Shower Tree

Cassia species

See Senna

Castanea sativa

See Spanish Chestnut

Castor Oil Plant

Ricinus communis

DESCRIPTION

Medicinal Parts: The medicinal parts are the oil extracted from the seeds, the fat extracted from the oil, and the ripe and dried seeds.

Flower and Fruit: The inflorescences are terminal and almost panicled and 15 to 50 cm long. The pedicled female flowers are in the upper section and the male flowers are clustered in the lower section of the inflorescence. The male ones have a 3 to 5 part perianth with numerous, heavily branched stamens, which bear up to 1,000 separate bursting anthers. The female perianth is divided in 5. The ovary is trilocular. The style has 3 red, doubly split stigma branches.

The fruit capsule is soft prickly or smooth and grooved, 1 to 2.5 cm in diameter. The capsule bursts open when ripe flinging out the large brightly speckled seeds.

Leaves, Stem and Root: Ricinus communis is an annual plant in Central Europe, a biennial or triennial shrub in Southern Europe and a perennial tree in the tropics. There is a taproot and lateral roots near the surface. The stem is erect and hollow. As it grows older, the stem becomes green or brownish-red. The leaves are petioled, greenish or reddish, often frosted blue, and arranged in a spiral. The leaf blade is peltate, 10 to 60 cm long, and wide. The blade is usually divided into palmate, ovate-oblong or lanceolate lobes. The ribs are palmate and the margins are irregularly serrate.

Habitat: The plant is cultivated widely today in the tropics and subtropics and in temperate latitudes where maize thrives.

Production: Castor Oil is fatty oil obtained from the seeds of *Ricinus communis*. It is obtained by mechanical harvesting followed by sorting. Fruits that open by bursting when ripen, must be harvested before ripening and then threshed.

Not to be Confused With: May be confused with the poisonous seeds of other *Euphorbiaceae*.

Other Names: Castor Bean, Mexico Seed, Castor Oil Bush, Palma Christi

ACTIONS AND PHARMACOLOGY

COMPOUNDS

CASTOR OIL SEEDS

Fatty oil (42 to 55%, see below for constituents)

Proteic substances (20 to 25%)

Lectins (0.1 to 0.7%): including ricin D (RCA-60, severely toxic), RCA-120 (less toxic)

Pyrridine alkaloids: ricinine (up to 0.3%)

Triglycerides: chief fatty acids ricinoleic acid (12-hydroxy-oleic acid, 85 to 90%)

Tocopherols (vitamin E)

EFFECTS

The laxative principle of Castor Oil is the ricinolic acid. Ricinolic acid is anti-absorptive and secretogogic. In animal experiments, stimulation of PgE2 synthesis in the small intestine was proven. The possible reason for effectiveness of ricini semen is the antimicrobial activity of the seeds (ricin is highly toxic).

INDICATIONS AND USAGE

Unproven Uses: Castor Oil is used internally in folk medicine for acute constipation, intestinal inflammation, for removal of worms, and as a form of birth control. The oil is used externally for inflammatory skin disorders, furuncles, carbuncles, abscesses, inflammation of the middle ear and headaches (poultice.)

Chinese Medicine: In China, Castor Oil is used to treat sore throat, facial paralysis, dry stool, furuncles, ulcers, and festering inflammation of the skin.

Indian Medicine: In India, the drug is used for dyspeptic complaints and joint pains.

Homeopathic Uses: Ricinus communis is used to treat diarrhea.

CONTRAINDICATIONS

Castor Oil is contraindicated in intestinal obstruction, acute inflammatory intestinal diseases, appendicitis, abdominal pain of unknown origin, during pregnancy and while nursing. The drug is not to be administered to children under 12 years of age.

PRECAUTIONS AND ADVERSE REACTIONS

General: No health hazards or side effects are known in conjunction with the proper administration of designated therapeutic dosages of Castor Oil. Allergic skin rashes have been observed in rare cases.

Pregnancy: Not to be used during pregnancy.

OVERDOSAGE

Overdosage can lead to gastric irritation with nausea, vomiting, colic, and severe diarrhea. Long-term use leads to loss of electrolytes, especially potassium ions. This effect may lead to hyperaldosteronism, inhibition of intestinal motility, and enhancement of the effect of cardioactive steroids.

Castor beans are severely poisonous due to the toxic lectin content. The ricinus lectins disturb the function of ribosomes and thereby prevent protein synthesis. Twelve castor beans are believed to be fatal for an adult. Symptoms include severe gastroenteritis with bloody vomiting and bloody diarrhea, kidney inflammation, loss of fluid and electrolytes and ultimately circulatory collapse. Death is usually the result of hypovolemic shock.

Following gastrointestinal emptying (inducement of vomiting, gastric lavage with burgundy-colored potassium permanganate solution, sodium sulfate) and installation of medicinal charcoal, the therapy for castor bean poisoning includes treating spasms with diazepam (IV) generous supplies of fluids, electrolyte substitution and treating possible cases of acidosis with sodium bicarbonate infusions. In case of shock, plasma volume expanders should be infused. Monitoring of kidney function and blood coagulation is essential. Papain activated with H2-S has been attempted as an antidote.

DOSAGE

Mode of Administration: Castor Oil is available as whole drug, in solid, semisolid and in compounded pharmaceutical preparations for internal and external use.

Preparation: Industrial production using specific procedures.

Daily Dosage:

Internally — for acute constipation or as a laxative against worms, at least 5 (x2 g) or 10 (x1 g) capsules must be taken; Caster Oil is also available in compound preparations.

Externally — a paste made of ground seeds is applied to the affected skin areas twice daily. A course of treatment takes up to 15 days.

Homeopathic Dosage: 5 drops, 1 tablet or 10 globules every 30 to 60 minutes (acute) or 1 to 3 times daily (chronic); parenterally: 1 to 2 ml sc acute: 3 times daily; chronic: once a day (HAB34)

LITERATURE

Gelfand D, Chen Y, Ott D. Colonic cleansing for radiographic detection of neoplasia: Efficacy of the magnesium citrate/castor oil cleansing enema regimen. *Am. J. Roentgenol.* 151: 705-708. 1988.

Gould S, Williams C. Castor oil or senna preparation bevor colonoscopy for inactive chronic ulcerate colitis. *Gastrointest Endosc.* 28: 6-8. 1982.

Kolts B, Lyles W, Achem S, et al., A comparison of the effectivenes and patient tolerance of oral sodium phosphate, castor oil, and standard electrolyte lavage for colonoscopy or sigmoidoscopy preparation. *Am. J. Gastroenterol.* 88: 1218-1223. 1993.

Mascolo N, Autore G, Borrelli F et al. Diarrhoea and mucosal injury evoked by castor oil are dependent events. *Nt J Parmacognosy.* 34: 91-95. 1996

Scarpa A, Guerci A, Various uses of the castor oil plant (*Ricinus communis L.*), a review. In: *ETH* 5(2):117. 1982.

Catechu

Acacia catechu

DESCRIPTION

Medicinal Parts: Black catechu is extracted from the heartwood in a process of distillation and is used in a variety of preparations.

Flower and Fruit: The flowers grow in closely sitting spikes from the leaf axils. The calyx is about 1 to 2 mm and covered in gray hairs. The corolla is yellow. The pod is about 10 to 15 cm long, dark brown and veined with 6 to 8 seeds.

Leaves, Stem, and Root: Acacia catechu is a medium-sized tree with brown bark and downy-haired branches. The leaf stems of the double-pinnate leaves are about 15 cm long and have glands at the base and between the upper 5 to 7 cm long fronds. The leaflets are sessile, close, pale green, and smaller than 1 cm. There are a few short thorns in pairs.

Habitat: The plant is indigenous to India and Burma.

Production: The heartwood is ground and boiled in water for 12 hours. The wood residue is removed and the extract steamed to the consistency of syrup. The syrup is stirred and cooled in molds. The dried mass is broken up into irregular pieces.

Not to be Confused With: Haematoxylon campechium and the seeds of Areca catechu, tar products and admixtures of earth, alumen, iron carbonate, and sand.

Other Names: Cutch

ACTIONS AND PHARMACOLOGY

COMPOUNDS

Catechins (2-12%): (+)- and (-)-catechin, (+)- and (-)-epicatechin

Catechin tannins (20-60%)

EFFECTS

Catechu is an astringent and antiseptic.

INDICATIONS AND USAGE

Unproven Uses: Internally, Catechu is used for chronic catarrh of the mucous membranes, dysentery, and bleeding. Externally, Catechu is a constituent of tooth tinctures, mouthwashes, and gargles. It is used externally in hemostatic powders, dressing solutions, and injection solutions. It is also used for colitis mucosa, gingivitis, stomatitis, and pharyngitis.

Indian Medicine: Catechu is a constituent of preparations for mouth ulcers, throat infections, toothache, and conjunctivitis.

Chinese Medicine: The drug is used for poorly healing ulcers, weeping skin diseases, oral ulcers with bleeding and traumatic injuries.

PRECAUTIONS AND ADVERSE REACTIONS

No health hazards or side effects are known in conjunction with the proper administration of designated therapeutic dosages. Large internal doses could lead to indigestion or constipation.

DOSAGE

Mode of Administration: Catechu tincture can be painted on mucous membranes or used for mouthwashes.

Preparation: Catechu tincture.

Daily Dosage: The average daily dose of the drug is 0.3 to 2 gm to be taken orally, 3 times daily; single dose is 0.5 gm.

Twenty drops of Catechu tincture is added to a glass of lukewarm water for use as a mouthwash, or the tincture may be applied with a brush in undiluted form to affected mucous membranes.

LITERATURE

Kuchandy E, Rao MN. Generation of superoxide anion and hydrogen peroxide by (+)-cyanidanol-3. *Int J Pharmaceut.* 65; 261-263. 1990.

Moushumi L, Sumati B. Studies on Possible Protective Effect of Plant Derived Phenols and the Vitamin Precursors- Beta-Carotene and Alpha-Tocopherol on 7,12 dimethylbenz (a) Anthracene Induced Tumour Initiation Events. *Phytother Res.* 8 (4); 237-240. 1994.

Cat's Claw

Uncaria tomentosa

DESCRIPTION

Medicinal Parts: The medicinal part is the root bark.

Flower and Fruit: The flowers are bisexual and sessil. The calyx is tubular 1 to 2 mm in length and 1 mm in diameter. The corolla is 7 to 12 mm long, 4 mm in diameter, and contains 5 roundish lobes. The stamens are in fives and fused. The anthers are 1 mm in length; the stigma elliptical. The ovary is inferior. The fruits are elliptical, 6-8 mm in length and 4 to 6 mm wide.

Leaves, Stem, and Root: Uncaria tomentosa is a large woody vine that sometimes reaches heights of 100 feet. The bark has longitudinal fissures that range from yellow to yellow-green in color. The leaves are simple, opposite, elliptic, or ovate. They range in size from 7 to 18 cm in length and from 4 to 13 cm wide. The margins of the leaf are entire, with a roundish base. The spines are woody and occur in pairs. They are curved like a cat's and thorn-like.

Characteristics: The sap of *Uncaria tomentosa* is watery and has an astringent taste.

Habitat: Cat's Claw is indigenous to the rainforest areas of Central and South America.

Production: Cat's Claw is harvested in the wild.

Not to be Confused With: There are several plants with the common name of Una de Gato. Confusion can occur with *Anadenanthera flava, Bauhinia aculeata, Berberis goudotii, Celtis uguanae, Doxantha ungis catti, Mimosa albida, Pisonia aculeata, Rubus urticaefolius,* the various *Smilax* species, and *Zanthoxylum panamensis* (Obregon, 1995).

Other Names: Garbato, Paraguaya, Tambor hausca, Toron, Una de Gato

ACTIONS AND PHARMACOLOGY

Alkaloids: including 5-alpha-carboxystrictosidine, isopteropodine, mitraphylline, isomitraphyllin, isorynchophylline, rynchophylline.

Triterpenes

Organic acids: oleanolic acid, ursolic acid

Glycosides: quinovic acid glycosides

Procyanidins: (-)-epicatechin, cinchonain 1 a, cinchonain 1b

Sterols: beta-sitosterol (60%), stigmasterol, capesterol

EFFECTS

Various components (alkaloids, triterpenes, glycosides, and procyanidins) of Cat's Claw are stated to possess antiviral, anti-inflammatory, antioxidant, contraceptive, anticancer, and immunostimulatory activities.

Anti-Inflammatory Effects: Cat's Claw appears to inhibit Tumor Necrosis Factor alpha, as well as function as an antioxidant, which may explain its mechanism of action in treating inflammatory disorders such as osteoarthritis, arthritis, and gastritis in traditional settings in South America (Hardin, 2007). In addition, the sterol components of Cat's Claw (beta-sitosterol, stigmasterol, and campesterol) have been found to have anti-inflammatory activity (Senatore et al, 1989). Anti-inflammatory activity has also been noted with some procyanins, but the exact compound responsible for the anti-inflammatory effect is not known (Wirth & Wagner, 1997).

In vitro use of oxindol alkaloids has shown increased phagocytosis. Pentacyclic oxindole alkaloids derived from *Uncaria tomentosa* induced production of lymphocyte-proliferation factors from human endothelial cells. Tetracyclic oxindole alkaloids antagonized the effect of the pentacyclic oxindole alkaloids (Wurm et al, 1998). The oxindol alkaloids of *Uncaria tomentosa* have been shown to increase phagocytosis in both in vitro tests and in vivo-carbon clearance tests (Wagner et al, 1985).

Cat's Claw root bark extract was shown to protect cells against oxidative stress (Sandoval et al, 1997a). Peroxynitrite-induced oxidative stress was reduced when measured in colonic (T84) and macrophage (RAW 264.7) cell lines with cell viability measured using trypan blue dye exclusion (Sandoval et al, 1997a). In vitro antioxidant activity was noted when testing several extracts of Cat's Claw root and bark. (Desmarchelier et al, 1997).

Cat's Claw extract, administered in drinking water, prevented indomethacin induced disruption of jejunal mucosal architecture in rats. The liver metallothionein levels in rats receiving Cat's Claw extract in addition to indomethacin were significantly lower than in rats receiving only indomethacin ($p<0.05$) (Sandoval-Chacon et al, 1998).

Cat's Claw root bark extract administered to rats was shown to have a beneficial effect on nonsteroidal anti-inflammatory enteropathy. Rats given Cat's Claw root bark extract and the indomethacin injections had reduced MT levels ($p<0.05$) than those receiving indomethacin alone (Sandoval et al, 1997). Extracts corresponding to 2 g of dried root bark were found to have an anti-inflammatory effect when tested in the carrageenan-induced edema rat paw model (Aquino et al, 1991).

Antineoplastic Effects: Uncaria tomentosa extract has been shown to induce apoptosis and inhibit proliferation of human tumor cells. Aqueous extracts of *Uncaria tomentosa* suppressed cell growth through induction of apoptosis in two different human leukemic cell lines (Sheng et al, 1998). Extracts from Cat's Claw have shown cytostatic activity, but dosages are unknown (Rizzi et al, 1993).

In vitro antitumor activity of water extracts of *Uncaria tomentosa* has been shown in a human leukemic cell line (HL-60) and a human Epstein-Barr virus (EBV)-transformed B lymphoma cell line (Sheng et al, 1998). *In vitro*, aqueous extracts of *Uncaria tomentosa* bark appear to interact with estrogen receptor-binding sites (Salazar & Jayme, 1998).

Antioxidant Effects: In vitro antioxidant activity of stem bark and root extracts of *Uncaria tomentosa* has been demonstrated in an assay using tert-butylhydroperoxide-initiated chemoluminescence in rat liver homogenates (Desmarchelier et al, 1997). Extracts also prevented free radical-mediated DNA sugar damage (Desmarchelier et al, 1997). Extracts and fractions of *Uncaria tomentosa* bark have shown no mutagenic effect but demonstrated a protective antimutagenic effect in vitro against 8 methoxypsoralen- and UVA-induced photomutagenesis in *Salmonella typhimurium* TA102 (Rizzi et al, 1993).

Antiviral Effects: Antiviral activity from the chloroform extract of Cat's Claw and from the quinovic acid glycosides in the plant has been demonstrated. Quinovic acid glycosides have been shown to have antiviral activity against vesicular stomatitis virus (VSV) but not against rhinovirus type 1B HRV 1B (RV) in HeLa cell cultures (Aquino et al, 1989). Quinovic acid glycosides have demonstrated antiviral activity in in vitro tests against the RNA virus vesicular stomatitis virus (Aquino et al, 1989). Two quinovic acid glycosides also demonstrated in vitro activity against rhinovirus type 1B (Aquino et al, 1989).

Cardiovascular Effects: Hirsutine has antihypertensive effects. This effect can partly be explained by the ability of hirsutine to reduce intracellular calcium levels by inhibiting calcium release from the calcium store and increasing calcium uptake into the calcium store. Hirsutine was also found to exhibit calcium-channel blocking activity by inhibiting the calcium influx through voltage dependent calcium channels in the rat aorta (Horie et al., 1992).

Contraceptive Effects: There is only limited evidence of the use of Cat's Claw in the prevention of pregnancy. In Peru, it has been used for this purpose for years in some rainforest tribes, but the amount of drug used would be considered very high. A decoction prepared from 11 to 13 pounds of the root is reduced to about 1 cup and taken at the time of menstruation. It is claimed that sterility can be maintained for 3 to 4 years after one dose (Cabieses, 1994). Contraceptive activity has been shown for Cat's Claw extract, dose and species unknown (Rizzi et al, 1993).

Effects on Serotonin and Dopamine: In one study, rhynchophylline increased the serotonin levels in the hypothalamus and cortex of rat brain and reduced the dopamine levels in the cortex, amygdala, and spinal cord (Shi et al, 1993). Receptor-binding assays using dihydrocorynantheine isolated from the branchlet and hook of *Uncaria sinensis* (and also found in *Uncaria tomentosa*) have shown that this alkaloid is a partial agonist for serotonin receptors (Kanatani et al, 1985). Hirsutine, an alkaloid present in *Uncaria tomentosa* has a potent ganglion-blocking effect. Hirsutine was found to block nicotine induced dopamine release in rat pheochromocytoma cells. Hirsutine was found to be equipotent to hexamethonium in blocking the inward current activated by nicotine (Nakazawa, et al, 1991).

Immunomodulating Effects: Uncaria tomentosa extract stimulates interleukin-1 (IL-1) and interleukin-6 (IL-6) production by alveolar macrophages. IL-1 and IL-6 are both known to be initiators of a cascade of immunologic defense mechanisms (Lemaire et al, 1999). Certain oxindole alkaloids isolated in *Uncaria tomentosa* (isopteropodine, pteropodine, isomitraphylline, isorhynchophylline) have been shown to enhance phagocytosis markedly in vitro (Wagner et al, 1985). Pentacyclic oxindole alkaloids from *Uncaria tomentosa* have been reported to induce the release of a lymphocyte proliferation-regulating factor from human endothelial cells; tetracyclic oxindole alkaloids were found to reduce the activity of pentacyclic oxindole alkaloids on these cells in a dose-dependent manner (Keplinger et al, 1999; Wurm et al, 1985). Stem bark extracts of *Uncaria tomentosa* have also been shown to stimulate IL-1 and IL-6 production in vitro in rat alveolar macrophages in a dose-dependent manner (range 0.025 to 0.1 mg/mL) and to potentiate the production of IL-1 and IL-6 in lipopolysaccharide-stimulated macrophages (LemaireI et al, 1999).

CLINICAL TRIALS

Analgesia

A 2005 review of the toxicological aspects of Cat's Claw and other South American herbs cited controlled clinical trials that show reduction in pain associated with intake of the herb in individuals with myriad chronic inflammatory disorders. However, the authors conclude that overall, data are insufficient to make firm conclusions regarding Cats Claws' anti-inflammatory actions—which have been attributed to the oxindole alkaloids from the root bark. Conflicting trial results regarding anti-inflammatory properties may be due to the activity of additional or unknown substances in Cats Claw, they noted (Gonzales, 2005).

Anti-Cancer

While *in vitro* data suggest effectiveness of Cat's Claw for treatment of various types of cancer, and some animal *in vivo* studies support this finding as well, further preclinical research clearly needs to be carried out to fully describe the plant's anti-cancer potential (Gonzales, 2006).

One *in vivo* antimutagenic test showed a decrease of mutagenic potential at the end of the treatment with Cat's Claw. Two individuals were given a decoction of *Uncaria tomentosa* each day for 15 days (as would be prescribed by a traditional Peruvian healer). One of the subject's was a nonsmoker while the other subject was a pack-a-day smoker who had smoked for 15 years. Both volunteers were 35 years of age and in good health. A bacterium was added to the urine samples to test for mutagenicity. This test determines whether there is evidence that genetic mutagenic activity is occurring which could possibly lead to certain types of cancers. The nonsmoker's urine did not show any mutagenic activity before, during, or after Cat's Claw treatment. By comparison, the smoker's urine had mutagenic activity before treatment and a decrease of mutagenic potential at the end of the treatment, persisting until 8 days after the end of the treatment (Rizzi, 1993).

Immune support

In an uncontrolled study, 13 HIV-positive individuals who refused to receive other therapies ingested 20 mg daily of an extract of *Uncaria tomentosa* root (containing 12 mg total pentacyclic oxindole alkaloids per gram) for 2.2 to 5 months. The total leukocyte number in the group was unchanged, compared with pretreatment values, whereas the relative and absolute lymphocyte count increased significantly. No significant changes in T4/T8 cell ratios were observed (Keplinger et al, 1999).

INDICATIONS AND USAGE

Unproven Uses: The effects that have some scientific evidence of efficacy include antiviral, immunostimulating, and anti-inflammatory properties. Cat's Claw has been used in folk medicine for rheumatic complaints, diarrhea, gastritis, treatment of wounds, as an adjunct to cancer treatment, asthma, menstrual irregularity, and as a contraceptive.

CONTRAINDICATIONS

Due to the immune stimulating properties of Cat's Claw, it should be avoided or used with great caution in patients with autoimmune disease or who are on immunosuppressants to prevent rejection of implanted organs, including bone marrow transplants (Reinhard, 1999).

Pregnancy: Not to be used during pregnancy.

Breastfeeding: Not to be used while breastfeeding.

PRECAUTIONS AND ADVERSE REACTIONS

Serum estradiol and progesterone levels may be reduced after long-term Cat's Claw use. In one study, long-term use (8 weeks) of *Uncaria tomentosa* resulted in a precipitous drop in both estradiol and progesterone serum levels (Rodriguez et al, 1998).

Cat's Claw inhibited cytochrome P450 3A4 in vitro (Budzinski et al, 2000); caution is advised if Cat's Claw is administered with drugs metabolized by this enzyme.

Renal failure following ingestion of Cat's Claw has been reported.

DRUG INTERACTIONS

MODERATE RISK

Anticoagulants, antiplatelet and thrombolytic agents, and low molecular weight heparins: Cat's Claw may increase the risk of bleeding if taken with these medications. Cat's Claw contains rhynochophylline, which may inhibit platelet aggregation. *Clinical Management:* Avoid concomitant use. Monitor the patient closely for signs and symptoms of bleeding.

DOSAGE

Mode of Administration: Cat's Claw is available in a powder form, capsules, and liquid for internal administration.

Preparation: To prepare a decoction, add 30 g of powder to 800 mL water; allow to simmer on the stove for 45 minutes or until there is about 500 mL liquid remaining. Allow to cool, then strain and refrigerate (Schauss, 1998).

How Supplied:

Capsule – 250 mg, 350 mg, 400 mg, 440 mg, 500 mg, 505 mg, 540 mg

Liquid – 4:1

Daily Dosage: The daily dosage is 250 to 1000 mg daily. The total alkaloid equivalent should be 10 to 30 mg. Decoction dosage is 60 ml once daily in the morning on an empty stomach (Schauss, 1998).

Storage: Cat's Claw should be stored at room temperature away from heat, moisture, and direct light.

LITERATURE

Aquino R, De Feo V, De Simone F et al. Plant metabolites: new compounds and anti-inflammatory activity of *Uncaria tomentosa. J Nat Prod* 54(2):453-459. 1991

Aquino R et al. Plant metabolites. Structure and in vitro antiviral activity of quinovic acid glycosides from *Uncaria tomentosa* and *Guettarda platypoda. J Nat Prod*; 52:679-685. 1989

Chen C, et al. Inhibitory effect of rhynchophylline on platelet aggregation and thrombosis. In: *Chung Kuo Yao Li Hsueh Pao;* 13(2);126-30, Mar, 1992

Cabieses, Fernando, The saga of the Cat's Claw, In: Via Lactera Editores: Lima, Peru, 1994

Desmarchelier C et al. Evaluation of the in vitro antioxidant activity in extracts of *Uncaria tomentosa* (Willd.) DC. *Phytother Res*; 11:254-256. 1997

Gonzales GF, Valerio LG. Toxicological aspects of the South American herbs cat's claw (Uncaria tomentosa) and Maca (Lepidium meyenii): a critical synopsis. *Toxicol Rev. 24(*1):11-35. 2005.

Gonzales GF, Valerio LG. Medicinal plants from Peru: a review of plants as potential agents against cancer. *Anti-Cancer Agents in Medicinal Chemistry;* 6(5): 429-444. 2006.

Hardin SR. Cat's Claw: An Amazonian vine decreases inflammation in osteoarthritis. *Comp Ther Clin Pract* 13;25-28. 2007.

Hilepo JN, Bellucci AG & Mossey RT. Acute renal failure caused by "cat's claw" herbal remedy in a patient with systemic lupus erythematosus (letter). *Nephron;* 77(3):361-369. 1997

Horie S, et al. Effects of hirsutine, an antihypertensive indole alkaloid from *Uncaria rhynchophylla*, on intracellular calcium in rat thoracic aorta. In: *Life Sci*; 50(7):491-8. 1992

Jin RM et al. Effect of rhynchophylline on platelet aggregation and experimental thrombosis. *Acta Pharm Sin*; 26:246-249. 1991

Kanatani H et al. The active principles of the branchlet and hook of *Uncaria sinensis Oliv*. examined with a 5-hydroxytryptamine receptor binding assay. *J Pharm Pharmacol*; 37:401-404. 1985

Keplinger K et al. *Uncaria tomentosa* (Willd.) DC. - ethnomedicinal use and new pharmacological, toxicological and botanical results. *J Ethnopharmacol*; 64:23-34. 1999

Kowalak JF & Mills EJ (Eds): Professional Guide to Complementary & Alternative Therapies. Springhouse Corp., Bethlehem Pike, PA; 2001

Lee KK et al. Bioactive indole alkaloids from the bark of *Uncaria guianensis. Planta Med*; 65: 759-760. 1999

Lemaire I, Assinewe V, Cano P et al. Stimulation of interleukin-1 and -6 production in alveolar macrophages by the neotropical liana, *Uncaria tomentosa* (una de gato). *J Ethnopharmacol;* 64(2):109-115. 1999

Nakazawa K, et al. Inhibition of ion channels by hirsutine in rat pheochromocytoma cells. In: *Jpn J Pharmacol;* 57(4):507-15, Dec. 1991

Obregon LE. Identificacion correcta de "una de gato" (genero Uncaria). *Natura Medicatrix;* 40(summer):28-30. 1995

Paulsen SM. Use of herbal products and dietary supplements by oncology patients - informed decisions? *Highlights Oncol Pract*; 15(4):94-106. 1998

Reinhard KH: Uncaria tomentosa (Willd.) DC: Cat's Claw, Una de Gato, or Saventaro. *J Altern Complement Med*; 5(2):143-151. 1999

Rizzi R et al. Mutagenic and antimutagenic activities of Uncaria tomentosa and its extracts. *J Ethnopharmacol*; 38:63-77. 1993

Rodriguez H, Massey PJ, Rodriguez K et al. Inhibition of steroid hormone production by a nutrition supplement "una de gato" or "cat's claw." *Biol Reprod;* 58(1):208. 1998

Salazar EL & Jayme V. Depletion of specific binding sites for estrogen receptor by *Uncaria tomentosa. Proc Western Pharmacol Soc;* 41:123-124. 1998

Sandoval-Chacon M et al. Antiinflammatory actions of cat's claw: the role of NF-kB. *Aliment Pharmacol Ther*; 12:1279-1289. 1998

Sandoval M, Mannick EE, Mishra J et al. Cat's Claw (*Uncaria tomentosa*) protects against oxidative stress and indomethacin-induced intestinal inflammation. *Gastroenterology*; 112(suppl):A1081. 1997

Sandoval M, Ronzio RA, Muanza DN et al. Protection from peroxynitrite-induced apoptosis by plant-derived antioxidants. *FASEB J*; 11(3):A648. 1997a

Santa Maria A, Lopez A, Diaz MM et al. Evaluation of the toxicity of *Unicaria tomentosa* by bioassay in vitro. *J Ethnopharmacol;* 57(3):183-187. 1997

Schauss AG. Cat's Claw (*Uncaria tomentosa*). *Nat Med J*; 1(2):16-19. 1998

Senatore A, Cataldo A, Iaccarino FP et al. Ricerche fitochimiche e biologiche sull? *Uncaria tomentosa* (Italian). *Boll Soc Ital Biol Sper;* 65:517-520. 1989

Sheng Y, Pero RW, Amiri A et al. Induction of apoptosis and inhibition of proliferation in human tumor cells treated with extracts of *Uncaria tomentosa. Anticancer Res;* 18(5A):3363-3368. 1998

Shi J, et al. Effects of rhynchophylline on motor activity of mice and serotonin and dopamine in rat brain. In: *Chung Kuo Yao Li Hsueh Pao*, 14(2):114-117, Mar, 1993

Shi JS et al. Hypotensive and hemodynamic effects of isorhynchophylline in conscious rats and anesthetised dogs. *Chin J Pharmacol Toxicol*; 3:205 210. 1989

Wagner H et al. Die alkaloide von *Uncaria tomentosa* und ihre Phagozytose steigernde Wirkung. *Planta Med*; 51:419-423. 1985

Wirth C & Wagner H. Pharmacologically active procyanidines from the bark of *Uncaria tomentosa. Phytomedicine*; 4(3):265-266. 1997

Wurm M, Kacani L, Laus G et al: Pentacyclic oxindole alkaloids from *Uncaria tomentosa* induce human endothelial cells to release a lymphocyte-proliferation-regulating factor. *Planta Med*; 64(8):701-704. 1998

Zhang W, Liu G-X. Effects of rhynchophylline on myocardial contractility in anesthetized dogs and cats. *Acta Pharmacol Sin*; 7:426-428. 1986

Zhu Y et al. Negatively chronotropic and inotropic effects of rhynchophylline and isorhynchophylline on isolated guinea pig atria. *Chin J Pharmacol Toxicol*; 7:117-121. 1993

Cat's Foot

Antennaria dioica

DESCRIPTION

Medicinal Parts: The medicinal part is the flower.

Flower and Fruit: The plant has bright red and white, dioecious composite flowers. They are very small and are in terminal cymes. The female flowers are bright red with threadlike, cylindrical corolla. The male flowers are white with a funnel-shaped corolla. The bracts of the male are white, the female, pink. The fruit has a tuft of hair.

Leaves, Stem, and Root: The plant is 7 to 20 cm tall, with leafy rooting runners. The stem is erect with basal leaves that are spatulate, green above, gray beneath, cauline, linear and erect.

Habitat: Cat's Foot is found in Europe, Asia and America as far north as the Arctic.

Production: Cat's Foot flower consists of the fresh or dried flowers of *Antennaria dioica*.

Not to be Confused With: Occasional confusion occurs with the flower heads of *Helichrysum stoechas* or *Helichrysum angustifolium*.

Other Names: Mountain Everlasting, Life Everlasting, Cudweed

ACTIONS AND PHARMACOLOGY

COMPOUNDS

Anthracene derivatives

Flavonoids: including luteolin and its glucosides

Bitter substances

Mucilages

Saponins

Tannins

EFFECTS

In animal tests, a mild spasmolytic and choleric effect has been reported.

INDICATIONS AND USAGE

Unproven Uses: In folk medicine, preparations of Cat's Foot flower are used intestinal diseases, gallbladder complaints, and as a diuretic.

PRECAUTIONS AND ADVERSE REACTIONS

No health hazards or side effects are known in conjunction with the proper administration of designated therapeutic dosages.

DOSAGE

Mode of Administration: Since the efficacy for the claimed uses is not documented, a therapeutic application cannot be recommended.

Preparation: To prepare an infusion, pour 150 mL boiling water over 1 gm finely cut drug, then strain after 5 to 10 minutes. Take 1 cup 3 to 4 times daily.

LITERATURE

Delaveau P, et al., *Planta Med* 40:49. 1980.

Didry N, et al., *Ann Pharm Fr* 40 (1):75. 1982

Swiatek L, et al., *Planta Med* 30:153, 12P. 1982.

Catha edulis

See Khat

Catnip

Nepeta cataria

DESCRIPTION

Medicinal Parts: The medicinal parts are the aerial parts of the plant.

Flower and Fruit: The inflorescence is spikelike and the lower verticillasters distant from each other. The small individual flowers are on short pedicles. The bracts are 1.5 to 3 mm and linear-awl-shaped. The sepals are 5 to 6.5 mm long and ovate. The tips are 1.5 to 2.5 mm long, linear-lanceolate and patent. The corolla is 7 to 10 mm long, slightly longer than the calyx and white with small purple spots.

Leaves, Stem, and Root: The root of the plant is perennial. The stems are up to 1 m high, angular, erect, and branched. They are leafy and gray-pubescent to tomentose, which gives the entire plant a whitish-gray appearance. The leaves are 2 to 8 cm, ovate, cordate at the base, crenate or serrate and gray-tomentose beneath. The petiole is 0.5 to 4 cm in length.

Characteristics: The plant has a characteristic aromatic scent, reminiscent of Mint and Pennyroyal.

Habitat: Catnip is indigenous to Europe and naturalized in the U.S.

Production: Catnip is the aerial part of *Nepeta cataria*. The harvesting of uncultivated plants takes place during the flowering season. The drug is manually cut during dry and sunny weather. The woodless parts of the plant are sorted out and the usable material is then left to dry in the shade.

Other Names: Catnep, Catrup, Catmint, Catswort, Field Balm

ACTIONS AND PHARMACOLOGY

COMPOUNDS

Volatile oil (0.2-0.7%): chief components are nepetalactone (share 80-95%), additionally including among others epinepetalactone, caryophyllene, camphor, thymol, carvacrol, pulegone

EFFECTS

Active agents are bitter and tannin substances, as well as essential oil. Catnip is considered to have antipyretic, refrigerant, antispasmodic, sedative, and diaphoretic effects. The tea has a diuretic effect and increases gallbladder activity.

INDICATIONS AND USAGE

Unproven Uses: Folk medicine uses include treatment of colds, colic and fevers. It is also used for nervous disorders and migraine, since preparations from the mint have a calming effect. It is also used in the treatment of gynecological disorders. Catnip has a long tradition in England and France as a kitchen and medicinal herb and was used occasionally as a stimulating drink until the introduction of black tea.

CONTRAINDICATIONS

Catnip is not to be taken during pregnancy.

PRECAUTIONS AND ADVERSE REACTIONS

No health hazards or side effects are known in conjunction with the proper administration of designated therapeutic dosages.

DOSAGE

Mode of Administration: Orally in ground and dried forms. Flowers are usually ingested in tea form, because the important constituent elements are to some extent volatile.

How Supplied:

Capsules – 380 mg

Fluid extract – 1:1

Liquid – 1:01

Preparation: To prepare an infusion (tea), add 10 dessert-spoonfuls per liter of water, leave this to steep for 20 minutes, then strain.

Daily Dosage: 3 cups of the tea daily.

LITERATURE

Clark IM, Forde BG, Hallahan DL. Spatially distinct expression of two new cytochrome P450s in leaves of Nepeta racemosa: identification of a trichome-specific isoform. *Plant Mol Biol,* 33:875-85, Mar. 1997.

Hallahan DL. Purification and characterization of an acyclic monoterpene primary alcohol:NADP+ oxidoreductase from catmint (*Nepeta racemosa). Arch Biochem Biophys*, 33:105-12, Apr 1. 1995

Margolis JS, In: Complete Book of Recreational Drugs, Cliff House Books USA 1978.

Massoco CO, Silva MR, Gorniak SL, Spinosa MS, Bernardi MM. Behavioral effects of acute and long-term administration of catnip (*Nepeta cataria*) in mice. *Vet Hum Toxicol*, 33:530-3, Dec. 1995

Roitman JN, (1981) *Lancet* I:944.

Tagawa M, Murai F, (1983) *Planta Med* 47:109.

Young LA et al., In: Recreational Drugs, Berkeley Publishing Co. USA 1977.

Caulophyllum thalictroides

See Blue Cohosh

Cayenne

Capsicum species

DESCRIPTION

Medicinal Parts: The fresh or dried fruits of different Capsicum species are used medicinally.

Flower and Fruit: The flowers are usually solitary, but may occasionally be in pairs or in threes. They are hanging and long-pedicled. The calyx is semiglobose to campanulate and has 5 to 7 tips. The corolla is wheel-shaped with a short tube, varying in color from white to yellow, occasionally from purple to violet with whitish-green or violet markings. There are 5 to 6 stamens with violet anthers and 5 small papillous staminoids. The ovary is superior. The dividing walls are partially underdeveloped. The seed carriers at the top are attached to the walls and fused to a column below. The berry is 1.5 to 5 cm long and up to 9 cm thick; it varies in form. The wall of the fruit is tough and leathery and may be red, yellow-green, or brownish. The seeds are numerous, light, yellowish-white, flat, circular or kidney-shaped and thickened at the margins. The surface is pitted.

Leaves, Stem, and Root: Capsicum annum is an annual (perennial in the tropics) 20 to 100 cm high plant with an erect stem, which is somewhat woody and angular. It is sparsely branched higher up. The leaves are usually solitary, long-petioled, oval, lanceolate to ovate, obtusely accuminate, wedge-shaped at the base, entire-margined or slightly curved and glabrous.

Habitat: The herb is indigenous to Mexico and Central America and is cultivated today in warmer regions of the globe.

Production: Paprika consists of the dried ripe fruit of *Capsicum anuum* or *Capsicum fructescens*. The fruit is harvested when completely ripe and dried at a maximum temperature of 35° C.

Not to be Confused With: Other varieties of Capsicum anuum.

Other Names: African Pepper, Bird Pepper, Capsicum Chili Pepper, Chilies, Chili, Goat's Pod, Grains of Paradise, Hungarian Pepper, Red Pepper, Paprika, Sweet Pepper, Tabasco Pepper, Zanzibar Pepper

ACTIONS AND PHARMACOLOGY

COMPOUNDS

Capsaicinoids (amides of the vanillyl amine with C8 - C13-fatty acids): chief components capsaicin (32-38%), dihydrocapsaicin (18-52%)

Carotinoids (0.3-0.8%): in particular capsanthin (dark red), alpha-carotin, violaxanthine, free or as fatty acid esters

Flavonoids: including apiin, luteolin-7-O-glucoside

Steroid saponins: mixture referred to as capsicidine, in the seeds

Volatile oil (0.1%): 2-methoxy-3-isobutyl pyrazine and N-(13-methyl tetradecyl)acetamide (capsiamide)

EFFECTS

Capsaicin relieves pain by depleting neuropeptides which initiate pain perception (Appendino & Szallasi, 1997; Fusco & Giacovazzo, 1997). Conflicting evidence exists concerning the role of capsaicin as a chemopreventive agent or a cancer-inducing agent (Surh & Lee, 1996; Surh & Lee, 1995). Similarly confusing are reports of gastroprotective (Kang et al, 1996) versus gastric-damaging effects (Myers et al, 1987). Capsaicin also demonstrates antimicrobial activity in vitro (Jones et al, 1997).

Efficacy of the drug has to date not been demonstrated for the claimed indications, especially internal applications, using the valid criteria for the clinical testing of drug substances. The significant tendency toward hyperemia caused by the content of irritant constituents in the drug does, however, provide antinoceptive and antiphlogistic effects with external administration, which could be used in the treatment of rheumatic illnesses, neuralgia, and myalgia.

Analgesic Effects: The most important active ingredient in the herb is the capsaicin, which exerts hyperemic effects. Cutaneous nociceptors are also known as peripheral sensory neurons of primary sensory neurons activated by noxious stimuli (Biro, 1997; Nakamura, 1999). Peripheral fibers produce a local response consisting of edema, redness, and vasodilation while afferent fibers relay nociceptive information to the central nervous system resulting in the perception of pain and burning. Long-term desensitization of the fibers occurs after repeated exposure to capsaicin, and results in a subsequent loss of pain sensation (Appendino, 1997; Fusco & Giacovazzo, 1997).

Capsaicin binds to the C-type vanilloid receptor (VR1) and opens a cationic channel allowing the influx of calcium. The calcium influx is an excitatory response, which initiates release of neuropeptides (substance P). The neuropeptides are responsible for chemogenic pain, thermoregulation and neurogenic inflammation. By blocking the calcium channel, there will be a depletion of substance P in the sensory nerves and loss of pain (Appendino, 1997; Biro, 1997; Fusco & Giacovazzo, 1997; Jung, 1999).

The pain relief observed with topical capsaicin is unlike anesthetics in that pain is blocked without effects on other sensations, such as touch and vibration (Bernstein et al, 1989; Fitzgerald, 1983).

The degeneration of epidermal nerve fibers contributes to the analgesia accredited to capsaicin. Discontinuation of capsaicin has resulted in reinnervation of the epidermis over a 6-week period in one trial (Nolano et al, 1999).

Antimicrobial: Various extracts of Cayenne as well as isolated capsaicin have shown inhibitory potential in vitro against Bacillus cereus, Bacillus subtilis, Clostridium sporogenes, Clostridium tetani, and *Streptococcus pyogenes* (Cichewicz, 1996). Capsaicin has shown bactericidal activity against *Helicobacter pylori* and therefore could have a protective effect against *H pylori*-associated gastroduodenal disease (Jones, 1997). It did not inhibit growth or kill nonpathogenic *Escherichia coli.*

A study using capsaicin from jalapeno peppers did not support the role for jalapenos in the treatment of *H pylori* infection (Graham, 1999).

Antineoplastic: Capsaicin, once thought to be carcinogenic, has been shown not to cause any significant increase in papilloma formation, abnormal hyperplasia, or inflammatory lesions. The drug does not induce the epidermal ornithine decarboxylase activity, suggesting that it lacks tumor-promotional activity (Park, 1997; Park, 1998). Chemoprotective effects of capsaicin and dihydrocapsaicin include the inhibition of microsomal monooxygenases involved in carcinogen activation (Surh, 1995).

Inhibition of the enzyme CYP2E1 may prevent activation of small molecular weight chemical carcinogens such as dimethylnitrosamine. Additionally, capsaicin may have a protective effect on metabolism, DNA binding, and mutagenicity of selected chemical carcinogens, including aflatoxin and tobacco-specific nitrosamine. These data suggest a chemoprotective effect of capsaicin (Surh & Lee, 1996; Surh & Lee, 1995).

In a case-control study conducted in Mexico City, a significant correlation was found between consumption of hot pepper and gastric cancer (Lopez-Carrillo et al, 1994).

Detoxification/Gastroprotective/Thrombolytic Effects: Capsaicin and dihydrocapsaicin have detoxification activity with pharmacologically active substances by interacting irreversibly with hepatic drug-metabolizing enzymes (Surh, 1995). Capsaicin has a gastroprotective effect against gastric mucosal injury caused by aspirin (Yeoh, 1995). Capsicum has been found to induce increased fibrinolytic activity and simultaneously cause hypocoagulability of blood (Visudhiphan, 1982).

CLINICAL TRIALS

Analgesic

A Chochrane Collaboration Review of herbal medicines for nonspecific low back pain cited a study involving Cayenne in plaster form, which in the study was found to reduce pain more than placebo did—and approximately the same amount as a homeopathic gel called Spiroflor SLR. The adverse effects reported were primarily mild and transient, and gastrointestinal in nature. However, the review failed to provide convincing data to substantiate the safety and effectiveness of Cayenne and other herbal medicines for long-term use as analgesics (Gagnier, 2007).

In an earlier double-blind, placebo-controlled study, capsaicin cream reduced neuropathic pain in patients with diabetes mellitus. All patients (n=277) had moderate-to-severe pain due to peripheral neuropathy or radiculopathy. Throughout the study, the placebo response was high, up to 58.1% on the physician global evaluation scale and 45.4% on the VAS pain relief scale used by patients. Based on this study, capsaicin cream is effective in some patients with diabetic neuropathy but burning is a frequent side effect which may lead to treatment discontinuation (Anon, 1991).

The efficacy of topical capsaicin was determined in 22 patients with chronic, severe painful diabetic neuropathy over an 8-week study period in a randomized, placebo-controlled study. Significant improvement was seen with capsaicin 0.75% applied 4 times daily for the overall clinical improvement of pain status, as measured by physician's global evaluation and by a categorical pain severity scale. The capsaicin treatment group had a 44.6% decrease in mean pain relief on VAS versus 23.2% decrease with the placebo group. Approximately 50% of subjects reported improved pain control or were cured in a follow-up, open-label study, and 25% were unchanged or worse (Tandan, 1992).

Arthritis

In a small study (n=21), capsaicin cream improved tenderness and pain in joints with osteoarthritis (OA) but had no beneficial effect in patients with rheumatoid arthritis (RA). All patients had arthritic pain in the small joints of the hands.

Treatment was randomly allocated and blinded; it consisted of application of vehicle or capsaicin cream 0.075% 4 times daily for 4 weeks. Tenderness and pain scores were reduced significantly at 4 weeks in patients with OA (n=14); however, other parameters including swelling, grip strength, duration of morning stiffness, subjective pain, and function were not improved. Patients with RA (n=5, completed study) had no response to capsaicin cream. This study suffered from several deficiencies including a small sample size and potential loss of blinding due to burning after capsaicin application (McCarthy & McCarty, 1992).

Patients with osteoarthritis (OA) (n=70) and rheumatoid arthritis (RA) (n=31) had a reduction in knee pain during treatment with capsaicin cream. Capsaicin appears useful as an adjunct to standard therapy to increase pain relief at a limited number of joints with intense pain (Deal et al, 1991).

Chilblains

Ten adult patients with chilblains, also known as perniosis, had complete healing of all lesions after 10 days of treatment with capsaicin. All patients were in the edematous, erythematous phase of chilblains. Few therapies have been effective for treating chilblains; therefore, capsaicin, if effective in larger, controlled studies, would be a useful new therapy for this condition. The mechanism by which capsaicin has beneficial effects is unknown but may be due to effects of a vasoactive neuropeptide in regulating blood flow and fibrinolytic activity in the skin (Cappugi et al, 1995).

Cough Sensitivity Test

Children with recurrent cough showed a heightened response to the capsaicin cough sensitivity test compared with children with asthma, cystic fibrosis, or normal airways. After controlling for age, sex, and spirometry, the dose at which capsaicin induced cough was significantly lower than in the other groups (Chang et al, 1997a).

Energy metabolism

In a randomized, crossover, intervention study, the metabolic effects of a chili meal containing cayenne after the consumption of a bland diet and a diet supplemented with a chili-blend (30 g/day; 55% cayenne chili) was investigated. Thirty-six subjects participated in the trial with 2 dietary periods (chili and bland) of 4 weeks. The postprandial effects of a bland meal after a bland diet, a chili meal after a bland diet, and a chili meal after a chili-containing diet were evaluated. Serum insulin, C-peptide, and glucose concentrations and energy expenditure were measured at fasting and up to 120 min postprandially. Results showed that regular consumption of chili containing cayenne may attenuate postprandial hyperinsulinemia (Ahuja et al, 2006). The same authors also studied the effect of 4-week chili supplementation on metabolic and arterial function, but did not find obvious beneficial or harmful effects on metabolic parameters. However, their findings suggest that cayenne may reduce resting heart rate and increase effective myocardial perfusion pressure time in men (Ahuja et al, 2007).

Gastroprotective Effects

The efficacy of capsaicin as a gastroprotective agent was determined in 18 healthy volunteers with normal index endoscopies. The volunteers underwent two studies 4 weeks apart to evaluate the effect of capsaicin against aspirin-induced gastric mucosal injury. The median gastric injury score in the chili group was significantly less than that of the aspirin group, demonstrating a gastroprotective effect of chili in human subjects (Yeoh, 1995). In a crossover study of 18 healthy subjects, treatment with capsaicin prior to aspirin administration significantly decreased gastric mucosal damage as compared with aspirin alone (Yeoh et al, 1995).

Nausea and Vomiting, Postoperative

In a double-blind, placebo-controlled study, postoperative nausea and vomiting occurred with lower frequency in women undergoing abdominal hysterectomy who were treated with a capsaicin-containing plaster than in those treated with an unmedicated plaster (Kim et al, 2002).

Neurogenic Bladder

Excellent or satisfactory improvement in urinary incontinence occurred in about 80% of patients treated with intravesical capsaicin. Patients with spinal cord disease primarily due to multiple sclerosis and those who had a failure to adequately respond to other therapy received capsaicin after a filling cystometrogram. Results of this and other studies indicate that patients with residual lower-limb function and strong motivation to overcome incontinence receive the greatest benefit from intravesical capsaicin (de Ridder et al, 1997).

Postherpetic Neuralgia

In a double-blind study, Capsaicin cream 0.075% applied 4 times per day gave pain relief to elderly patients suffering from chronic postherpetic neuralgia. Clinical improvement was reported in 77% receiving capsaicin and in 31% receiving placebo. More patients (54%) in the capsaicin group experienced 40% or greater pain relief than in the placebo group (6%). Burning, stinging, and erythema were reported in 5 patients treated with capsaicin and in 2 receiving placebo. These local effects usually subsided with continued application (Bernstein et al, 1989).

Pruritis

In a study, 19 of 22 patients with hemodialysis-related pruritus had relief of pruritus following treatment with capsaicin for 4 weeks (Cho et al, 1997).

Surgical Neuropathy

Topical capsaicin reduced the pain of post-surgery neuropathy in a majority of subjects in a double-blind, placebo-controlled crossover trial. There was a tendency for pain relief to be greater with post-mastectomy pain than with pain from other sources (amputation, thoracotomy). Patients who received capsaicin in the first 8 weeks maintained their level of pain relief during the placebo period (Ellison et al, 1997).

INDICATIONS AND USAGE

Approved by Commission E:

- Muscular tensions
- Rheumatism

Unproven Uses: Cayenne is used for painful muscle spasms in areas of shoulder, arm, and spine. In folk medicine the herb is used for frostbite, chronic lumbago, and as a gargle for hoarseness, sore throats, and infected throats. The drug is also used internally for gastrointestinal disorders, seasickness, and as prophylactic therapy for arteriosclerosis, stroke, and heart disease.

The herb is used in cream form for circulation and as a female orgasm stimulant. Use should be limited to 2 days, and should only be used again after 2 weeks. Longer usage can cause festering dermatitis, blistering, and ulceration (See PRECAUTIONS).

Indian Medicine: Cayenne is used for gout, arthritis, sciatica, coughs, and hoarseness. It has been used for lowering the temperature in malaria, yellow fever, scarlet fever, and typhus. It is used for cholera, edema, and anorexia nervosa. It is used in compound preparations for loss of appetite, dyspepsia, and diarrhea (tablets 1:1:1; Cayenne pepper, rhubarb and ginger root) and for alcoholism as an infusion (Cayenne pepper with sugar and cinnamon) to reduce the desire for alcohol.

Homeopathic Uses: The herb is used for inflammation of the efferent urinary tract, the alimentary canal, the mouth and throat, and middle ear infection.

CONTRAINDICATIONS

Capsaicin cream should not be applied to open wounds or to the eyes. Other contraindications include stomach ulcers or stomach inflammation, chronic irritable bowel, and inhalation. Avoid use in patients with gastrointestinal and renal disease (Palevitch & Craker, 1993).

PRECAUTIONS AND ADVERSE REACTIONS

Burning, stinging, and redness of skin are all possible side effects of Cayenne use. This is a normal action of capsaicin and these effects almost always lessen and disappear over a few days time with repeated application. Accidental transfer of the cream to the eyes or mucous membranes can cause temporary burning. If worsening occurs or no improvement occurs after 7 days, stop using the product. Wash hands immediately after use unless treating the hands.

There has not yet been a final determination of possible health hazards or side effects in conjunction with the proper administration of designated therapeutic dosages. Internal administration may increase gastrointestinal peristalsis resulting in diarrhea, intestinal, and gallstone colics. Besides the intended stimulating effect, external applications can lead to blister and ulcer formation. Investigations into mutagenicity, teratogenicity, and carcinogenicity yielded contradictory results.

Warning: Use should be limited to 2 days and should only be used again after 2 weeks. Keep away from the eyes!

Carcinogenicity: High intake of cayenne peppers as food has been correlated to an increased risk of gastric carcinoma in one case-control study of 972 persons in Mexico (Lopez-Carrillo et al, 1994). Any consumption of chilies was correlated with an odds ratio of 5.49 for risk of stomach cancer and 17.11 for those who self-rated in the highest tertile of intake. The dose-response curve was inexplicably flat in this study. A related review of the literature summarizes available data by stating that low doses of cayenne may be anticarcinogenic while higher doses may be carcinogenic (Surh & Lee, 1996).

Central Nervous System Effects: Topical capsaicin in concentrations of 1% or greater has been associated with neurotoxicity and thermal hyperalgesia (Reynolds, 1991; Robertson & George, 1990).

Dermatologic Effects: Local discomfort characterized by burning, stinging, and redness of the skin occurs frequently after application of topical capsaicin; local discomfort is increased when capsaicin cream is applied fewer than 3 to 4 times daily. Local reactions usually subside within 72 hours of beginning regularly scheduled use of topical capsaicin (Bernstein et al, 1989; Bernstein et al, 1987).

Hematologic Effects: Capsicum has been found to induce increased fibrinolytic activity and simultaneously cause hypocoagulability of blood (Visudhiphan, 1982).

Hypersensitivity: Anaphylaxis and rhinoconjunctivitis symptoms have been associated with the herb due to its antigenic components (Jensen-Jarolim, 1998; Vega de la Osada, 1998). Contact dermatitis has been reported from the direct handling of chili peppers containing capsaicin (Williams, 1995). A hypersensitivity reaction known as plasma cell gingivitis may occur with the herb, and may cause severe gingival inflammation, discomfort, and bleeding (Serio, 1991). One study suggests the allergy is rarely an autonomous sensitization, but rather a consequence of pollen allergy on the basis of immunologic cross-reactivity (Ebner, 1998).

Iron Absorption

Three experiments were conducted in healthy young women (n=10 per study) to evaluate the effect of chili pepper and turmeric on iron absorption, and to identify a possible effect of chili on gastric function. Freeze-dried, ground chili pepper within the range of habitual chili intake by Thai adults (14.2 g fresh wt; 25 mg polyphenols as gallic acid equivalents) reduced iron absorption from a basic meal of vegetables and rice by 38%, but the authors note that the findings don't necessarily show that chili intake is a risk factor for iron depletion. (Turmeric, in contrast, did not inhibit iron absorption.) The authors conclude that both the quality and quantity of the phenol compounds in plants determine their iron-absorptive inhibitory powers (Tuntipopipat, 2006).

Respiratory Effects: Chronic exposure to chili peppers has been associated with an increase in cough (Blanc, 1991). Capsaicin inhalation has been associated with cough and a transient increase in airway resistance. These effects are likely related to stimulation of sensory airway nerves (Fuller, 1991). Cough induced by inhaled capsaicin has been exacerbated by pretreatment with angiotensin converting enzyme (ACE) inhibitors (O'Hollaren & Porter, 1990).

DRUG INTERACTIONS

MODERATE RISK

Angiotensin converting enzyme (ACE) inhibitors: May result in increased risk of cough when used concurrently with topical capsaicin. *Clinical management*: Patients should be advised to discontinue capsaicin use if they experience cough while taking capsaicin and an ACE inhibitor. Since the incidence of this effect is not yet known and it is presently not possible to predict which patients will experience this adverse effect, complete avoidance of the combination is not recommended at this time.

Anticoagulants, antiplatelet agents, thrombolytic agents, and low molecular weight heparins: Concurrent use of capsaicin with these medications may increase the risk of bleeding. The clinical significance of capsaicin's effect on platelet aggregation and fibrinolytic activity is unknown. *Clinical Management*: Signs and symptoms of excessive bleeding should be monitored closely if capsaicin and any of these agents are taken concomitantly. It is advisable to discontinue appreciable intake of capsaicin (or large amounts of red pepper) prior to administration of anticoagulants, antiplatelet agents, low molecular weight heparins, or thrombolytic agents.

Barbiturates: Concurrent use may result in increased or decreased effect of the barbiturate, depending on the length of time capsaicin is administered. *Clinical Management:* Until the clinical significance of this interaction is better studied in humans, patients prescribed barbiturates are advised to avoid concomitant use of capsaicin.

Theophylline: Concomitant use of capsaicin and theophylline may result in an increased risk of theophylline toxicity and should be undertaken with caution. *Clinical Management:* Theophylline levels and signs and symptoms of theophylline toxicity should be monitored closely if these agents are administered concomitantly.

POTENTIAL INTERACTIONS

Aspirin and salicylic acid compounds: The bioavailability of aspirin (acetylsalicylic acid) and of salicylic acid was reduced when given concomitantly with *Capsicum annuum* extract containing 100 mg of capsaicin per gram as a result of the gastrointestinal effects of capsaicin (Cruz, 1999).

OVERDOSAGE

Toxic dosages lead to life-threatening hypothermia by affecting the thermoreceptors. High doses of the drug (or the herb) administered over extended periods can cause chronic gastritis, kidney damage, liver damage, and neurotoxic effects. The treatment for poisonings proceeds symptomatically.

DOSAGE

Mode of Administration: Preparations of Cayenne are exclusively for external indications in antirheumatic ointments and plasters.

How Supplied:

Capsules–400 mg, 445 mg, 450 mg, 455 mg, 500 mg

Cream–0.25% capsaicin, 0.75% capsaicin

Liquid Extract

Preparation: A liquid extract is prepared by percolating 100 g drug with 60 g ethanol. Other formulations include: Capsicum-oleoresin with 90% ethanol and a tincture with 90% ethanol.

Daily Dosage: External daily dose: 10 g drug; Tincture: (1:10); Semisolid preparations: maximum 50 mg capsaicin in 100 g neutral base. The cream is applied to the affected area not more than 3 or 4 times daily (Zostrix Package Insert, 1998).

Internal application: Decoction: 1/2 liter water with 5 g powdered drug, 3 g powdered cascarilla bark and 5 g powdered rhubarb root; 2 cups per day.

Homeopathic Dosage: 5 drops, 1 tablet, or 10 globules every 30 to 60 minutes (acute) or 1 to 3 times a day (chronic); ointment: once or twice daily (HAB1)

Storage: Should be well sealed and protected from light.

LITERATURE

Ahuja KD, Robertson IK, Geraghety DP, Ball MJ. Effects of chili consumption on postprandial glucose, insulin, and energy metabolism. *Am J Clin Nutr*; 84(1): 63-69. 2006.

Ahuja KD, Robertson IK, Geraghety DP, Ball MJ. The effect of 4-week chili supplementation on metabolic and arterial function in humans. *Eur J Clin Nutr*; 61(3): 326-333. 2007.

Anonym. Behandlung chronischer Schmerzen. Capsaicin - Lichtblick für Schmerzpatienten. In: *DAZ* 137(13):1027-1028. 1997

Anonym. Phytotherapie. Pflanzliche Antirheumatika - was bringen sie? In: *DAZ* 136(45):4012-4015. 1996

Anonym. Treatment of painful diabetic neuropathy with topical capsaicin: a multicenter, double-blind, vehicle-controlled study: The Capsaicin Study Group. *Arch Intern Med*; 151(11):2225-2229. 1991

Appendino G & Szallasi A. Euphorbium. modern research on its active principle, resiniferatoxin, revives an ancient medicine. *Life Sci*; 60(10):681-696. 1997

Bascom R, Kageysobotka A, Prous D. Effect of intranasal capsaicin on symptoms and mediator release. In: *J Pharmacol Exp Ther;* 259(3):1323. 1991

Bernstein JE, Bickers DR, Dahl MV et al. Treatment of chronic postherpetic neuralgia with topical capsaicin: a preliminary study. *J Am Acad Dermatol*; 17(1):93-96. 1987

Bernstein JE, Korman NJ, Bickers DR et al. Topical capsaicin treatment of chronic postherpetic neuralgia. *J Am Acad Dermatol*; 21(2 pt 1):265-270. 1989

Bernstein JE, Parish LC, Rapaport M et al. Effects of topically applied capsaicin on moderate and severe psoriasis vulgaris. *J Am Acad Dermatol*; 15(3):504-507.1986

Biro T, Acs G, Acs P et al. Receptor advances in understanding of vanilloid receptors: a therapeutic target for treatment of pain and inflammation in skin. *J Invest Dermatol*; 2:56-60. 1997

Blanc P, Liu D, Juarez C, Boushey HA. Cough in hot pepper workers. *Chest* Jan; 99(1):27-32. 1991

Brinker F. Herb Contraindications and Drug Interactions, 2nd ed. Eclectic Medical Publications, Sandy, OR, USA. 1998

Camara B, Moneger R. *Phytochemistry;* 17:91. 1978

Cappugi P, Zippi P, Isolani D et al. Topical capsaicin as useful therapy in the treatment of chilblains. *Pain Clinic*; 8(4):347-351. 1995

Chang AB, Phelan PD, Sawyer SM et al. Cough sensitivity in children with asthma, recurrent cough, and cystic fibrosis. *Arch Dis Child*; 77(4):331-334. 1997a

Cho YL, Liu HN, Huang TP et al. Uremic pruritus: roles of parathyroid hormone and substance P. *J Am Acad Dermatol*; 36(4):538-543. 1997

Cichewicz RH, Thorpe PA. The antimicrobial properties of chili peppers (*Capsicum* species) and their uses in Mayan medicine. *J Ethnopharmacol*; 52:61-70. 1996

Cruz L, Castaneda-Hernandez G, Navarrete A et al. Ingestion of chili pepper (*Capsicum annuum*) reduces salicylate bioavailability after oral aspirin administration in the rat. *Can J Physiol Pharmacol* Jun;77(6):441-6. 1999

Deal CL, Schnitzer TJ, Lipstein E et al. Treatment of arthritis with topical capsaicin: a double-blind trial. *Clin Ther*; 13(3):383-395. 1991

De Ridder D, Chandiramani V, Dasgupta P et al. Intravesical capsaicin as a treatment for refractory detrusor hyperreflexia: a dual-center study with long-term followup. *J Urol*; 158(6):2087-2092. 1997

Ebner C, Jensen-Jarolim E, Leitner A, Breiteneder H. Characterization of allergens in plant-derived spices: *Apiaceae* spices, pepper (*Piperaceae*), and paprika (bell peppers, *Solanaceae*). *Allergy*; 53(46 Suppl):52-4. 1998

Ellison N, Loprinzi CL, Kugler J et al. Phase III placebo-controlled trial of capsaicin cream in the management of surgical neuropathic pain in cancer patients. *J Clin Oncol*; 15(8):2974-2980. 1997

Fitzgerald M. Capsaicin and sensory neurons - a review. *Pain*; 15(2):109-130. 1983

Fuller RW. Pharmacology of inhaled capsaicin. *Respir Med*; 85(suppl A):31-34. 1991

Fusco BM, Fiore G, Gallo F et al. "Capsaicin-sensitive" sensory neurons in cluster headache: pathophysiological aspects and therapeutic indication. *Headache* Mar; 34(3):132-7. 1994

Fusco BM & Giacovazzo M. Peppers and pain: the promise of capsaicin. Drugs; 53(6):909-914. 1997

Gagnier JJ, van Tulder M, Berman B, et al. Herbal medicine for low back pain (Review). Cochrane Database of Syst Rev 2: CD004504, Apr 19, 2006.

Graham DY, Anderson SY, Lang T et al. Garlic or jalapeno peppers for treatment of *Helicobacter pylori* infection. *Am J Gastroenterol* May; 94(5):1200-1202. 1999

Hakas JF Jr. Topical capsaicin induces cough in patient receiving ACE inhibitor (letter). *Ann Allergy*; 65(4):322-323. 1990

Heck AM, DeWitt BA & Lukes AL. Potential interactions between alternative therapies and warfarin. *Am J Health Syst Pharm*; 57(13):1221-1227. 2000

Jensen-Jarolim E, Santner B, Leitner A et al. Bell peppers (*Capsicum annuum*) express allergens (profilin, pathogenesis-related protein P23 and Bet v 1) depending on the horticultural strain. *Int Arch Allergy Immunol* Jun; 116(2):103-9. 1998

Jones NL, Shabib S & Sherman PM. Capsaicin as an inhibitor of the growth of the gastric pathogen Helicobacter pylori. FEMS *Microbiol Lett*; 146(2):223-227. 1997

Jung J, Hwang S, Kwak J et al. Capsaicin binds to the intracellular domain of the capsaicin-activated ion channel. *J Neurosci* Jan 15; 19(2):529-38. 1999

Kang JY, Teng CH & Chen FC. Effect of capsaicin and cimetidine on the healing of acetic acid induced gastric ulceration in the rat. *Gut*; 38(6):832-836. 1996

Kim KS, Koo MS, Jeon JW et al. Capsicum plaster at the Korean hand acupuncture point reduces postoperative nausea and vomiting after abdominal hysterectomy. *Anesth Analg*; 95:1103-1107. 2002

Kohane D, Kuang Y, Lu N et al. Vanilloid receptor agonists potentiate the in vivo local anesthetic activity of percutaneously injected site 1 sodium channel blockers. *Anesthesiology* Feb; 90(2):524-34. 1999

Kreymeier J, Rheumatherapie mit Phytopharmaka. In: *DAZ* 137(8):611-613. 1997

Lopez-Carrillo L, Hernandez Avila M & Dubrow R. Chili pepper consumption and gastric cancer in Mexico: a case-control study. *Am J Epidemiol*; 139(3):263-271. 1994

Marques S, Olliveira NG, Chaveca T, Rueff J. Micronuclei and sister chromatid exchanges induced by capsaicin in human lymphocyted. *Mut Res*; 517:39-46. 2002

McCarthy GM & McCarty DJ. Effect of topical capsaicin in the therapy of painful osteoarthritis of the hands. *J Rheumatol*; 19(4):604-607. 1992

Monsereenusorn Y et al. *Crit Rev Toxicol*; 10:321. 1982

Myers BM, Smith JL & Graham DY. Effect of red pepper and black pepper on the stomach. Am J Gastroenterol; 82(3):211-214. 1987

Nakamura A, Shiomi H, Recent advances in neuropharmacology of cutaneous nociceptors. *Jpn J Pharmacol* Apr; 79(4):427-31. 1999

Nolano M, Simone DA, Wendelschafer-Crabb G et al. Topical capsaicin in humans: parallel loss of epidermal nerve fibers and pain sensation. *Pain*; 81(1-2):135-145. 1999

Norred CL & Brinker F. Potential coagulation effects of preoperative complementary and alternative medicines. *Alt Ther*; 7(6):58-67. 2001

O'Hollaren MT & Porter GA. Angiotensin converting enzyme inhibitors and the allergist. *Ann Allergy*; 64(6):503-506. 1990

Palevitch D & Craker LE. Nutritional and medical importance of red peppers. *Herb Spice Medicinal Plant Dig*; 11(3):1-4. 1993

Park KK, Surh YJ, Effects of capsaicin on chemically induced two-stage mouse skin carcinogenesis. *Cancer Lett Mar* 19; 114(1-2):183-4. 1997

Park K, Chun K, Yook, Surh Y, Lack of tumor promoting activity of capsaicin, a principal pungent ingredient of red pepper, in mouse skin carcinogenesis. *Anticancer Res* Nov-Dec; 18(6A):4201-4205. 1998

Product Information. Zostrix(R)/Zostrix-HP(R), capsaicin. GenDerm Corporation, Lincolnshire, IL, USA. 1998

Robertson DRC & George CF. Treatment of post-herpetic neuralgia in the elderly. *Br Med Bull*; 46(1):113-123. 1990

Ross DR & Varipapa RJ. Treatment of painful diabetic neuropathy with topical capsaicin (letter). *N Engl J Med*; 321(7):474-475. 1989

Surh YJ & Lee SS, Capsaicin, a double-edged sword: toxicity, metabolism and chemopreventive potential. *Life Sci*; 56:1845-1855. 1995

Surh YJ, Lee RC, Park KK, Mayne ST et al. Chemoprotective effects of capsaicin and diallyl sulfide against mutagenesis or tumorigenesis by vinyl carbamate and N-nitrosodimethylamine. *Carcinogenesis* Oct;16(10): 2467-71. 1995

Surh YJ, Ahn SH, Kim KC et al. Metabolism of capsaicinoids: evidence for aliphatic hydroxylation and its pharmacological implications. *Life Sci Mar* 10; 56(16):PL305-11. 1995

Surh YJ & Lee SS, Capsaicin in hot chili pepper: carcinogen, co-carcinogen or anticarcinogen? Fd Chem Toxic; 34:313-316. 1996

Tuntipopipat S, Judprasong K, Zeder C, et al. Chili, but not turmeric, inhibits iron absorption in young women from an iron-fortified composite meal. *J Nutr;* 136: 2970-2974. 2006.

Vega de la Osada F, Esteve Drauel P, Alonso Lebrero E et al. Sensitization to paprika: anaphylaxis after intake and rhinoconjunctivitis after contact through airways. *Med Clin* (Barc) Sep 12; 111(7):263-6. 1998

Visudhiphan S, Poolsuppasit S, Piboonnukarintr O et al. The relationship between high fibrinolytic activity and daily capsicum ingestion in Thais. *Am J Clin Nutrition*; 35:1452-1458. 1982

Wasantapruek S, Poolsuppasit S & Piolnukarintr O. Enhanced fibrinolytic activity after capsicum ingestion. *N Engl J Med*; 290:1259-1260. 1974

Watson CPN, Evans RJ & Watt VR. Post-herpetic neuralgia and topical capsaicin. *Pain*; 33(3):333-340. 1988

Watson WA, Stremel KR & Westdorp EJ. Oleoresin capsicum (Cap-Stun®) toxicity from aerosol exposure. *Ann Pharmacother*; 30(7-8):733-735. 1996

Williams S, Clark R, Dunford J, Contact dermatitis associated with capsaicin. Hunan hand syndrome. *Ann Emerg Med* May; 25(5):713-5. 1995

Yeoh KG, Kang JY, Yap I et al. Chili protects against aspirin-induced gastroduodenal mucosal injury in humans. *Dig Dis Sci* Mar; 40(3):580-3. 1995

Ceanothus americanus

See New Jersey Tea

Cedar

Cedrus libani

DESCRIPTION

Medicinal Parts: The medicinal parts are the leaves, wood, and oil.

Flower and Fruit: The male cones are 3 to 5 cm; the female cones are 7 to 12 cm and almost cylindrical-truncate or umbilicate at the apex.

Leaves, Stem, and Root: The cedar is a majestic tree that grows up to 40 m in height with a rigid leading shoot and a flat crown. The young branches are glabrous. The needlelike leaves are dark green and 20 to 30 mm long.

Habitat: The Lebanon Cedar is indigenous to the Lebanese mountains and the southwest of Turkey, Cyprus, the Atlas Mountains and the Himalayas. The tree is also found in Asia and Africa.

Production: Cedar oil is the essential oil extracted from the leaves and wood of *Cedrus libani*.

ACTIONS AND PHARMACOLOGY

COMPOUNDS

When extracted from Cedrus libani (true cedarwood oil): borneol

When extracted from Cedrus atlantica (atlas cedarwood oil): cadinene, alpha- and gamma-atlantone

When extracted from Cedrus deodora (Himalayan cedarwood oil): alpha- and gamma-atlantone, p-methyl-delta-3-tetrahydroacetophenone, (+)-longiborneol, himachalol, allohimachalol

EFFECTS

Cedar has an expectorant effect.

INDICATIONS AND USAGE

Unproven Uses: Cedar wood oil is used for catarrhal conditions of the respiratory tract.

PRECAUTIONS AND ADVERSE REACTIONS

No health hazards or side effects are known in conjunction with the proper administration of designated therapeutic dosages.

DOSAGE

Mode of Administration: Externally, the drug is used as a rub (Bormelin balm). It is also used internally as an inhalation.

LITERATURE

Kern W, List PH, Hörhammer L (Hrsg.), Hagers Handbuch der Pharmazeutischen Praxis, 4. Aufl., Bde. 1-8, Springer Verlag Berlin, Heidelberg, New York, 1969.

Cedrus libani

See Cedar

Celandine

Chelidonium majus

DESCRIPTION

Medicinal Parts: The medicinal parts are the aerial parts that have been collected during the flowering season and dried. The root, which has been collected in late autumn and dried, and the fresh rhizome are also used medicinally.

Flower and Fruit: The plant has yellow flowers arranged in umbels. There are 2 sepals, 4 petals, numerous yellow stamens and 1 ovary. The fruit is pod-like and many-seeded. The seeds are black-brown and glossy.

Leaves, Stem and Root: Celandine is a 30 to 120 cm high plant with an erect stem. The stem has irregularly bifurcated, thickened nodes. The leaves are alternate and indent-pinnatifid. The upper leaves are pinnatisect, dull green above, sea-green beneath. The plant contains a dark-yellow latex.

Characteristics: Celandine has a hot and bitter taste. The latex has a narcotic fragrance.

Habitat: Celandine is found throughout Europe and the temperate and subarctic regions of Asia.

Production: Celandine herb consists of the dried, above ground parts of Chelidonium majus gathered during flowering season. The herb is collected in the wild during the flowering season and dried at high temperatures.

Greater Celandine root is the root, harvested between August and October, of Chelidonium majus. The herb is gathered in uncultivated regions and harvested commercially.

Other Names: Tetterwort

ACTIONS AND PHARMACOLOGY

COMPOUNDS: CELANDINE HERB

Isoquinoline alkaloids of the protoberberine type: including coptisine (main alkaloid), berberine

Isoquinoline alkaloids of the benzophenanthridine type: including chelidonine, sanguinarine, chelerythrine

Isoquinoline alkaloids of the protopine type: including protopin, cryptopine

Caffeic acid derivatives: including 2-(-)-coffeoyl-D-glyceric acid, coffeoyl-L-malic acid

EFFECTS: CELANDINE HERB

Celandine has mild analgesic, cholagogic, antimicrobial, oncostatic and central-sedative effects. It also acts as a spasmolytic on smooth muscles. In animal tests, Celandine is a cytostatic. It also has a nonspecific immune-stimulating effect.

Note: The blood pressure-lowering effects and the therapeutic efficacy for mild forms of hypertonia (borderline hypertonia) need further investigation.

COMPOUNDS: CELANDINE ROOT

Isoquinoline alkaloids of the protoberberine type: including coptisine (main alkaloid), berberine

Isoquinoline alkaloids of the benzophenanthridine type: including chelidonine, sanguinarine, chelerythrin

Isoquinoline alkaloids of the protopine-type: including protopin, cryptopine

Caffeic acid derivatives: including 2-(-)-coffeoyl-D-glyceric acid, coffeoyl-L-malic acid

EFFECTS: CELANDINE ROOT

Only clinical studies and experiments on the fresh plants are available. However, previous studies have shown that the extract, with an alkaloid content of 80%, should have similar effects to those of the fresh leaves. These effects include immobilization in mice, when it was applied subcutaneously and orally. On rabbit intestines it caused limpness; and in higher doses, tone reduction. When applied to the rabbit uterus, it caused contraction of the smooth muscle. Positive inotropic effects were observed in isolated cat and frog hearts; in a canine heart-lung preparation it stimulated the heart, raised blood pressure and widened the arteries.

Experimental data are unavailable, therefore the results must be considered unofficial.

An oncostatic effect was observed through the cytotoxic results of Eagle's 9 KB carcinoma of the naso-pharynx in cell cultures.

INDICATIONS AND USAGE

CELANDINE HERB

Approved by Commission E:

- Liver and gallbladder complaints

Unproven Uses: Celandine is used for spasmodic pain of the bile ducts and the gastrointestinal tract. In folk medicine, it was used for skin conditions such as blister rashes, scabies and warts. It is said to be effective in the treatment of cholecystitis, chloelithiasis, catarrhal jaundice, gastroenteritis, and diffuse latent liver and gall bladder complaints. It has also been used for intestinal polyps and breast lumps. Other uses include angina pectoris, cramps, asthma, arteriosclerosis, high blood pressure, stomach cancer, gout, edema and hepatitis.

Chinese Medicine: Celandine is used for inflammation of the rim of the eyelid, febrile and ulcerating dermatitis, warts, edema, ascites, jaundice and stomach carcinomas

CELANDINE ROOT

Unproven Uses: In folk medicine, the fresh roots are chewed to alleviate toothache, and a powder derived from the roots is applied to ease tooth extraction.

Chinese Medicine: Preparations are used for irregular menstruation.

Homeopathic Uses: Chelidonium majus is used for inflammation, stones and chronic disorders of the hepatobiliary system, rheumatism and inflammation of the lungs and pleura.

PRECAUTIONS AND ADVERSE REACTIONS

CELANDINE HERB

General: No health hazards or side effects are known in conjunction with the proper administration of designated therapeutic dosages. Older scientific literature credits the plant with toxicity (burning in the mouth, nausea, vomiting, bloody diarrhea, hematuria, stupor), but recent studies offer no clear proof of this; animal experiments yielded no results.

No symptoms of inflammation were observed in the eyes of rabbits following introduction of the chyle. Nevertheless, contact between it and the eyes should be avoided.

Pregnancy: Not to be used during pregnancy.

CELANDINE ROOT

No health hazards or side effects are known in conjunction with the proper administration of designated therapeutic dosages. Older scientific literature credits the plant with toxicity (burning in the mouth, nausea, vomiting, bloody diarrhea, hematuria, stupor), but recent studies offer no clear proof of this. Animal experiments yielded no examples of toxicity.

DOSAGE

CELANDINE HERB

Mode of Administration: Comminuted and powdered drug for infusions and decoctions; dried extracts for liquid and solid medicinal forms for internal use.

Preparations:

Fluid extract: 1:1 in 25% ethanol.

Tincture: 1:10 in 45% ethanol (BHP83).

Tea: allow 1$^1/_2$ dessertspoonfuls to draw in boiling water for 10 minutes.

Infusion: 15 gm dried herb to 1 liter of water, leave to draw for 15 minutes.

Daily Dosage: The average daily dose is 2 to 4 gm of drug in liquid or solid extracts, equivalent to 12 to 30 mg total alkaloids calculated as chelidonine; fluid extract, 1 to 2 ml three times daily; decoction, 3 cups daily; infusion, 3 cups between meals.

Storage: Celandine herb should be protected carefully from light.

CELANDINE ROOT

Mode of Administration: Most standardized and compound preparations contain the extract of Celandine herb; various homeopathic preparations also contain dilutions of the fresh herb Greater Celandine.

Daily Dosage: The standard dose is 0.5 gm of drug.

Homeopathic Dosage: 5 drops, 1 tablet, 10 globules every 30 to 60 minutes (acute) or 1 to 3 times daily (chronic); parenterally: 1 to 2 ml sc acute: 3 times daily; chronic: once daily (HAB1).

Storage: Preparations must be stored carefully.

LITERATURE

CELANDINE HERB

Äberlein H et al., Chelidonium majus L, Components with in vitro affinity for GABA A receptor: Positive cooperation of alkaloids. In: PM 62(3):227-231. 1996.

Anonym, Brennpunkt ZNS. In: DAZ 137(25):2166-2167. 1997.

Arnason JT, Gurein B, Kraml MM, Mehta B, Rehmond JC, Scaiano JC, Phototoxic and photochemical properties of sanguinarin. In: Photochemistry and Photobiology 55(1):35. 1992.

Baumann J, (1975) Über die Wirkung von Chelidonium, Curcuma, Absinth und Carduus marianus auf die Galle- und Pankreassekretion bei Hepatopathien. Med Mschr 29:173.

Boegge SC et al., Reduction of ACh-induced contraction of rat isolated ileum by Coptisin, Caffeoylmalic acid, Chelidonium majus, and Corydalis lutea extracts. In: PM 62(2):173-174. 1997.

Diener H, Schöllkraut. In: PTA 8(2):145. 1994.

Dostãl J et al., Structure of chelerythrine base. In: JNP 58(5):723-729. 1995.

Fulde G, Wichtl M, Analytik von Schöllkraut, Hauptalkaloid Coptisin. In: DAZ 134(12):1031. 1994.

Hahn R, Nahrstedt A, Hydroxycinnamic acid derivatives, caffeoylmalic and new caffeoylaldonic acid esters, from Chelidonium majus. In: PM 59(1):71. 1993.

Hamacher H, Haben Phytopharmaka eine Zukunft? In: DAZ 131(42):2155. 1991.

Kim DJ, Ahn B, Han BS, Tsuda H, Potential preventive effects of Chelidonium majus L (Papaveraceae) herb extract on glandular stomach tumor development in rats treated with N-methyl-N'-nitro-N nitrosoguanidine (MNNG) and hypertonic sodium chloride. In: Can.

Mitra S et al., Effect of Chelidonium majus L. on experimetal hepatic tissue injury. In: Phytother Res 10(4):354-356. 1996.

Reuter HD, Pflanzliche Gallentherapeutika (Teil I) und (Teil II). In: ZPT 16(1):13-20 u. 77-89. 1995.

Schilcher H, Pharmazeutische Aspekte pflanzlicher Gallentherapeutika. In: ZPT 16(4):211-222. 1995.

Schmidt M, Phytotherapie: Pflanzliche Gallenwegstherapeutika. In: DAZ 135(8):680-682. 1995.

Tãborskã E et al., The alkaloids of Chelidonium majus L. and their variability. In: PM 62, Abstracts of the 44th Ann Congress of GA, 145. 1996.

Vahlensiek U et al., The effect of Chelidonium majus herb extract on the choleresis in the isolated perfused rat liver. In: PH 61(3):267-270. 1995.

Vavreckova C, Gawlik I, Müller K, Benzophenanthridine alkaloids of Chelidonium majus: I. Inhibition of 5- and 12-lipoxygenase by a non-redox mechanism. In: PM 62(5):397-401. 1996.

Willaman JJ and Hui-Li L, (1970) Lloydia 33 (3A):1.

Celastrus scandens

See American Bittersweet

Celery

Apium graveolens

DESCRIPTION

Medicinal Parts: The medicinal parts are the root, above-ground foliage and stems, the fruit (seeds) of the plant, and the oil extracted from the seeds.

Flower and Fruit: The umbels are greenish-white, small, 6 to 12 rayed, star-shaped and splayed. Some umbels are top-heavy, short petioled or sessile, and some are terminal and more or less long-petioled with no involucre. Petals are usually 0.5 mm, white or greenish to yellowish, cordate at the base and have indented tips. The fruit is almost spherical and somewhat compressed at the side. The 5 mm mericarps are rounded in section. They are 5-cornered with 5 equal, weakly protruding, bow-shaped main ribs. The edge of the ribs form the edge of the mericarps. The fruit axis is bristly and slightly crenate at the tip.

Leaves, Stem, and Root: The glabrous plant is a biennial and reaches a height of 30 to 100 cm. The root of the wild variety is fusiform, about 5 to 7 mm thick, branched and becomes woody in the second year. The root of the cultivated variety is fleshy, roundly tuberous and reaches a diameter of over 15 cm. The stem is erect, with edged grooves, often hollow and branched. The leaves are glossy and rich green. The basal and lower cauline leaves are more or less long-petioled and pinnatifid. The upper cauline leaves are sometimes opposite. They are on short white-membrane-edged sheaths and are almost sessile and tri-pinnate. The lower leaves are roundish, almost blunt at the base with broad, lozenge-shaped, indented-serrate, blunt and short-thorned tips. The upper cauline leaves are wedge-shaped and acuminate, also 3-lobed or pinnate or lanceolate and entire-margined.

Characteristics: The plant has a strong odor.

Habitat: Celery is found in Europe from England and Lapland to southern Russia. The plant also grows in western Asia as far as eastern India; in northern and southern Africa and South America; and is cultivated and grows wild in North America, Mexico and Argentina.

Production: Celery seed consists of the fruit of *Apium graveolons*; celery herb consists of the fresh or dried above-ground parts of the plant; and celery root is the plant's fresh or dried underground parts.

Other Names: Smallage

ACTIONS AND PHARMACOLOGY

COMPOUNDS: CELERY SEED (FRUIT)

Volatile oil: chief constituents ((+) - limonene, beta-selinene, phthalides among them 3-butyliden phthalide, 3-butyl phthalide, 3-isovaleryliden-3a, 4-dihydrophthalid, 3-isobutyliden phthalide, sedanoid, neocnidilid)

Flavonoids: graveobioside A and B, apiin, isoquercitrin

Furocoumarins: including bergapten, isoimperatorin, isopimpinellin

Fatty oil

EFFECTS: CELERY FRUIT

In animal tests, a sedative and anticonvulsive effect was demonstrated; a diuretic effect could not be proved. The essential oil contained in the drug had a mildly inhibiting effect on bacteria and fungi.

COMPOUNDS: CELERY HERB

Volatile oil: including (+)-limonene, myrcene, beta-selinene, alpha-terpineol, carveol, dihydrocarvone, geranyl acetate, phthalides (including 3-butyliden phthalid, 3-butyl phthalid, 3-isobutyliden dihydrophthalid)

Flavonoids: including apiin, luteolin-7-O-apiosyl glucoside, chrysoeriol glucoside

Furocoumarins: including bergaptene, xanthotoxin, isopimpinellin

Caffeic acid derivatives: including chlorogenic acid

EFFECTS: CELERY HERB

See Celery herb

COMPOUNDS: CELERY ROOT

Volatile oil: chief constituents (+)-limonene, beta-pinene, p-cymene, cis-, 3-methyl-4-ethyl-hexane), phthalides (including 3-butyliden phthalid, 3-butyl phthalid, ligustilid, neocnidilid)

Flavonoids: including apiin, luteolin-7-O-apiosyl glucoside

Furocoumarins: including bergaptene

Polyyne: including falcarinol, falcarindiol

EFFECTS: CELERY ROOT

See Celery herb.

INDICATIONS AND USAGE

CELERY FRUIT, HERB, AND ROOT

Unproven Uses: Folk medicine use of celery and preparations of celery are used as a diuretic, for regulating the bowels, for glandular stimulation, rheumatic complaints, gout, gallstones, and kidney stones. Other traditional uses include as a prophylactic for nervous agitation, for loss of appetite and exhaustion. Celery is also used as a cough treatment and as a helminthic.

Homeopathic Uses: Celery preparations are used in homeopathy for ailments of the ovaries and rheumatism.

CONTRAINDICATIONS

CELERY SEED (FRUIT)

The drug should not be used during pregnancy. Also, because of the kidney-irritating effect of the volatile oil, the drug should not be administered to individuals with kidney infections.

PRECAUTIONS AND ADVERSE REACTIONS

CELERY FRUIT, HERB AND ROOT:

No health hazards or side effects are known in conjunction with the proper administration of designated therapeutic dosages. Nevertheless, because of the kidney-irritating effect of the volatile oil, the drug should not be administered in the presence of kidney infections. Latent yeast infections of the plant could cause the furanocoumarin content of the fresh root to rise to 200 times its original level under storage conditions. For this reason, the relatively large amounts of furanocoumarins frequently to be found in stored celeriac bulbs, or in incorrectly dehydrated drug samples, could lead to phototoxicoses.

DOSAGE

CELERY SEED (FRUIT)

Mode of Administration: Whole and powdered drug, liquid extract, and as a component in a variety of tea mixtures.

How Supplied:

Capsules: 450 and 505 mg

Fluid Extract: 1:1

Preparation: To prepare a liquid extract, percolate 1 kg of seed in a specula process to 1 liter of fluid extract. The essential oil is removed after filtration with paper soaked in alcohol. For an infusion, pour boiling water on 1 g of the squeezed drug and strain after 5 to 10 minutes. Decoctions are prepared in a 1:5 ratio.

Daily Dosage: The daily dosage of the seeds is 1.2 to 4 g and as an infusion, 1 g drug.

Homeopathic Dosage: 5 to 10 drops, 1 tablet, or 5 to 10 globules 1 to 3 times daily or 1 mL injection solution twice weekly sc (HAB34).

Storage: Celery seed should be kept tightly sealed, away from light and moisture.

CELERY HERB

Mode of Administration: Whole and cut drug as well as a variety of tea mixtures.

Preparation: Celery is contained in a variety of tea mixtures (kidney and bladder teas).

Daily Dosage: Pressed juice of the fresh plant: 23 g (15 ml) 3 times daily.

Homeopathic Dosage: 5 to 10 drops, 1 tablet, or 5 to 10 globules 1 to 3 times daily or 1 ml injection solution twice weekly sc (HAB34).

Storage: The herb should be kept sealed, away from light and moisture.

CELERY ROOT

Mode of Administration: The drug is available in a few combination preparations for internal use.

Preparation: A cough mixture is prepared by boiling the root juice with sugar.

Dosage: Pressed juice of the fresh plant: 23 g (15 mL) 3 times daily.

Homeopathic Dosage: 5 to 10 drops, 1 tablet, or 5 to 10 globules 1 to 3 times daily or 1 mL injection solution twice weekly sc (HAB1).

Storage: Celery root should be kept sealed, away from light and moisture.

LITERATURE

Beier RS, Oertli EH, Psoralen and other phytoalexins in celery. In: *PH* 22(11):2595. 1983.

Broda B, Grzybek J. Preparation of herbal mixtures / Studies on herbs with designed sedative activity. Z *Phytother*. 14; 307-314. 1993.

Cao G, Sofic E, Prior RL. Antioxidant Capacity of Tea and Common Vegetables. *J Agric Food Chem*. 44 (11); 3426-3431. 1996.

Dyas L, Threlfall DR, Goad LJ. The Sterol Composition of five Plant Species grown as Cell Suspension Cultures. *Phytochemistry* 35; 655-660. 1994.

Garg SK et al., (1980) *Planta Med* 38:363.

Jankiewicz A, Aulepp H, Altmann F, Fötisch K, Vieths S. Serological investigation of 30 Celery-allergic patients with particular consideration of the thermal stability of IgE-bindung celery allergens. *Allergo-J*. 7 (2); 87-95. 1998.

Lewis DA et al., (1985) *Int J Crude Drug Res* 28 (1):27.

Mac Leod G, Ames JM, Volatile components of celery and celeriac. In: *PH* 28(7):1817-1824. 1989.

Nigg HN, Strandberg JO, Beier RC, Petersen HD, Harrison JM, Furanocoumarins in Florida celery varieties increased by fungicide treatment. In: *J Agricult Food Chem* 45(4):1430-1436. 1997.

Tsi D et al., Effects of aqueous celery (*Apium graveolens*) extract on lipid parameters of rats fed a high fat diet. In: *PM* 61(1):18-21. 1995.

Uhlig, JW, Chang A, Jen JJ, Effect of phthalides on celery flavor. In: *J Food Sci* 52(3):658-660. 1987.

Centaurea cyanus

See Cornflower

Centaurium erythraea

See Centaury

Centaury

Centaurium erythraea

DESCRIPTION

Medicinal Parts: The medicinal parts are the dried, aerial parts of the flowering plant.

Flower and Fruit: The different-sized flowers form a dense or loose cyme. They are purple to pink-red, seldom white. The calyx tube is pentangular with awl-shaped tips. There are 5 petals fused into a tube, 5 stamens mostly fused to the corolla and 1 superior, narrowly linear ovary. The stigma is 2-lobed. The fruit is a large, yellow, many-seeded capsule.

Leaves, Stem, and Root: The plant is an annual that grows to between 5 and 30 cm high. The stem is erect, quadrangular, and unbranched. The cauline leaves are crossed opposite, fleshy, oblong-ovate to lanceolate, and sessile. The basal leaves are rosettelike, obovate and narrowed to a petiole.

Characteristics: Centaury has a very bitter taste.

Habitat: The plant is found in the Mediterranean region and as far as Britain and Scandinavia. It is cultivated in the U.S.

Production: Centaury consists of the dried aerial parts, in flower, of *Centaurium erythraea*. The plant is harvested during the flowering season and dried quickly to retain the flower color.

Not to be Confused With: Other *Centaurium* varieties.

Other Names: Feverwort, Centaury Gentian, Filwort, Centory, Christ's Ladder, Bitter Herb, Bitterbloom, Bitter Clover, Eyebright, Rose Pink, Wild Succory, Canchalagua

ACTIONS AND PHARMACOLOGY

COMPOUNDS

Iridoide bitter principles (monoterpenes): in particular swertiamarin, including among others gentiopicrin, sweroside

Pyrridine alkaloids: gentianine, gentianidine

Xanthones: including methyl bellidifoline

EFFECTS

Centaury increases gastric secretion and salivation because of the typical bitter reaction, also antiphlogistic and antipyretic effects have been studied in various animal experiments. The effect for loss of appetite, stomach complaints, and dyspepsia can also be attributed to the amaroids.

INDICATIONS AND USAGE

Approved by Commission E:

- Dyspeptic complaints
- Loss of appetite

Unproven Uses: The drug is used for loss of appetite, dyspepsia, and poor gastric secretion. In folk medicine, it is used for fever, worm infestation, and as a hypotensive. It is also used for diabetes in Mallorca, and for expelling kidney stones in Egypt. Externally, it is used in the treatment of wounds.

CONTRAINDICATIONS

Because of its secretion-activating effect, the drug should not be administered in the presence of stomach or intestinal ulcers.

PRECAUTIONS AND ADVERSE REACTIONS

No health hazards or side effects are known in conjunction with the proper administration of designated therapeutic dosages.

DOSAGE

Mode of Administration: Comminuted herb for infusions and other bitter-tasting preparations for internal use.

Preparation: Tea: Brew 2 to 3 gm drug with 150 ml boiling water and strain after 15 minutes; Centaurium Extract: extract of 1 part drug to 10 parts water and 1 part 98% ethanol steamed till thickened (EB6).

How Supplied

Liquid extract: 1:1 25% ethanol (V/V) (BHP83).

Daily Dosage: The average daily dose is 6 gm of drug or 1 to 2 gm of extract; single dose is 1 gm. The powdered drug is taken 3 times daily on a wafer with honey; the infusion is taken 1/2 hour before meals. The daily dose of extractum *Centaurii fluidum* is 2 to 5 mL.

Storage: Keep protected from light and moisture in sealed containers.

LITERATURE

Delitheos A, Tiligada E, Yannitsaros A, Bazos I. Antiphage activity in extracts of plants growing in Greece. *Phytomedicine* 4 (2); 117-124. 1997.

Schimmer O, Mauthner H, Polymethoxylated xanthones from the herb of Centaurium erythraea with strong antimutagenic properties in Salmonella typhimurium. In: *PM* 62(6):561-564. 1996.

Schimmer O, Mauthner H. Centaurium erythraea RAFN. Tausendgüldenkraut / Portrait einer Arzneipflanze. Z Phytother. 15; 297-304. 1994.

Schimmer O, Mauthner H, Centaurium erythraea RAFN. Tausendgüldenkraut. In: ZPT 15(5):299-304. 1994.

Centella asiatica

See Gotu Kola

Centranthus ruber

See Red-Spur Valerian

Cephaelis ipecacuanha

See Ipecac

Ceratonia siliqua

See Carob

Cetraria islandica

See Iceland Moss

Chamaemelum nobile

See English Chamomile

Chaste Tree

Vitex agnus-castus

DESCRIPTION

Medicinal Parts: The medicinal parts are the ripe dried fruit and the dried leaves.

Flower and Fruit: The 8 to 10 cm, blue, occasionally pink flowers form terminal, branched, spikelike inflorescences. The calyx and epicalyx of the bilabiate corolla are pubescent. The fruit is a globular to oblong, 3 to 4 mm, reddish black, 4-seeded drupe. It is surrounded up to two-thirds in cuplike fashion by the calyx. The exocarp has short-stemmed, glandular hairs.

Leaves, Stem, and Root: The plant is a 1 to 6 m high bush or tree with quadrangular, gray, tomentose, young branches. The leaves are deciduous, crossed-opposite, long-petioled, and palmate. They have 5 to 7 entire-margined, lanceolate leaflets up to 10 cm long. The under surface of the leaf is white and tomentose.

Habitat: The plant is indigenous to the Mediterranean region as far as western Asia.

Production: Chaste Tree fruits consist of the ripe, dried fruits of *Vitex agnus-castus*.

ACTIONS AND PHARMACOLOGY

COMPOUNDS

Iridoid glycosides: agnoside, aucubin

Flavonoids: including casticin, 3,6,7,4′-tetramethylether, 6 - hydroxy - kempferol - 3, 6, 7, 4′ - tetramethylether, 6-hydroxy-kempferol-3,6,7-trimethylether (penduletin), quercetagenin-3,6,7-trimethylether (chrysosplenol D)

Volatile oil (0.8-1.6%): including among others, 1,8-cineole, lime, alpha-pinene, beta-pinene, as well as bornyl acetate, camphor, p-cymol, sabinene

Fatty oils

EFFECTS

Chaste Tree may be effective for menstrual cycle disorders secondary to hyperprolactinemia and premenstrual syndrome. Data are inconclusive for its use for acne. A study failed to demonstrate a homeopathic preparation of Vitex was effective for female infertility. Homeopathic preparations have been somewhat effective in the treatment of mastalgia, but further trials are warranted.

A mechanism of action and pharmacologically active constituents have not been conclusively identified for *Vitex agnus castus*. It may act upon the pituitary-hypothalamic axis. Some study results indicated that it inhibited prolactin release while not affecting follicle stimulating hormone (FSH) or luteinizing hormone (LH) levels (Milewicz et al, 1993), while others claimed that it inhibited prolactin secretion while increasing LH release, resulting in increased progesterone levels (Lauritzen et al, 1997). One study suggested the effect on prolactin is dose dependent, increasing secretion with lower doses and decreasing prolactin with higher doses (Loew et al, 1996; Merz et al, 1996). Prolactin inhibition may be due to a dopaminergic effect since *Vitex agnus castus* binds at D2 receptor sites (Jarry et al, 1994).

Hormonal Effects: Chaste Tree extract and a homeopathic preparation (containing Vitex agnus castus D1, Caulophyllum thalictroides D4, Cyclamen D4, Ignatia D6, Iris D2, Lilium tigrinum D3 in an ethanolic solution) significantly inhibited basal and TRH-stimulated prolactin secretion by rat pituitary cells in vitro (Sliutz et al, 1993).

Effects on Female Infertility: A partially homeopathic preparation (containing Vitex agnus castus D1, Caulophyllum thalictroides D4, Cyclamen D4, Ignatia D6, Iris D2, and Lilium tigrinum D3 in 53% ethanol) achieved some positive, but not statistically significant, results in the treatment of female infertility in a prospective, double-blind, placebo-controlled trial (Gerhard et al, 1998).

Effects on Mastalgia: A partially homeopathic preparation (containing Vitex agnus castus D1, Caulophyllum thalictroides D4, Cyclamen D4, Ignatia D6, Iris D2, and Lilium tigrinum D3 in 53% ethanol) was effective in treating cyclical mastalgia in a multicenter, randomized, placebo-controlled, double-blind study. Since a combination product was used, it cannot definitely be concluded that the Vitex agnus castus ingredient was the effective constituent (Wuttke et al, 1997).

Premenstrual Syndrome: Chaste Tree extract was effective in women with premenstrual syndrome (PMS) diagnosed according to the DSM III criteria in a randomized, placebo-controlled trial (Schellenberg, 2001).

CLINICAL TRIALS

Premenstrual Syndrome (PMS)

An extract of chasteberry (*Vitex agnus castus* extract BNO 1095, equivalent to 40 mg herbal drug) was found to be effective and well tolerated in treating moderate to severe PMS in this prospective, open, non-comparative study of women (n=118), mean age 29.7. Severity of symptoms consistently lessened during treatment, according to the PMS diaries and self-assessments maintained by the participants over the course of three menstrual cycles. Response to treatment was positively recorded in 67.8% of participants during the third menstrual cycle treatment. Seven participants discontinued Chasteberry in this trial due to side effects, but no serious adverse events were reported. Of the side effects recorded, itching and erythema were the most frequent complaints. Whereas previous controlled trials focused on women with mild to moderate PMS, this trial involved women with moderate to severe PMS. The authors conclude that a placebo-controlled trial is merited (Prilepskaya, 2006).

Similarly, Chaste Tree extract was effective in women with PMS diagnosed according to the DSM III criteria in a randomized, placebo-controlled trial. One hundred and seventy women (mean age 36 years) with PMS symptoms were supplemented with either one 20 mg tablet *Vitex agnus castus* (fruit extract Ze 440: 60% ethanol m/m, extract ratio 6 to 12:1; standardized for casticin) (n=86) or placebo (n=84) orally daily for 3 menstrual cycles. Active group subjects reported improvement in irritability, mood alteration, breast fullness, anger, and other menstrual symptoms compared to placebo ($p<0.001$). Responder rate was 52% for the active group and 24% for the placebo group, as determined by self-assessment (Schellenberg, 2001).

Mastalgia

A partially homeopathic preparation (containing *Vitex agnus castus* D1, Caulophyllum thalictroides D4, Cyclamen D4, Ignatia D6, Iris D2, and Lilium tigrinum D3 in 53% ethanol) was effective in treating cyclical mastalgia in a multicenter, randomized, placebo-controlled, double-blind study. Significant improvements were noted in the treatment groups during the first and second treatment cycles. The number of pain-free days, as recorded by patients, increased by 15% in the treatment groups and by 8% in the placebo groups. There were no clinically significant effects on progesterone, FSH, or LH levels (Wuttke et al, 1997).

INDICATIONS AND USAGE

Approved by Commission E:

- Menstrual cycle irregularities
- Premenstrual syndrome (PMS)
- Mastalgia/mastodynia

Chaste Tree preparations are used to treat irregularities of the menstrual cycle, premenstrual complaints, and mastalgia/ mastodynia.

Unproven Uses: Insufficient milk production and menstrual disturbances caused by corpus luteum insufficiency. It is also used to control libido, increase milk flow, reduce flatulence, suppress appetite, and induce sleep. Additional uses include the treatment of impotency, spermatorrhea, prostatitis, swelling of the testes, sexual neurasthenia, sterility, amenorrhea, uterine pain, and swelling of the ovaries. Chaste Tree is also used to induce menstruation.

Homeopathic Uses: Chaste Tree is used for male sexual disturbances, disturbances of milk flow, and nervous depression.

CONTRAINDICATIONS

Pregnancy: Not to be used during pregnancy

Breastfeeding: Not to be used while breastfeeding.

PRECAUTIONS AND ADVERSE REACTIONS

General: Occasionally, the administration of the drug leads to the formation of rashes. Itching, nausea, vomiting, dry mouth, headache, dizziness, drowsiness, confusion, and agitation have been reported.

DRUG INTERACTIONS

MINOR RISK

Dopamine Agonists (e.g., levodopa, phenothiazines, pergolide, bromocriptine, amantadine, pramipexole, ropinirole): Concurrent use may result in increased dopaminergic side effects. *Clinical Management:* Avoid concomitant use of Vitex with a dopamine agonist. If the patient chooses to take Vitex, monitor closely for symptoms of additive dopamine agonism such as nausea, headache, dizziness, fatigue, vomiting, and postural hypotension.

Dopamine-2 Antagonists: Concurrent use may result in decreased effectiveness of dopamine antagonists. Theoretically, the dopamine agonist activity of chasteberry may oppose that of dopamine antagonists, decreasing their effectiveness. *Clinical Management:* If therapy is initiated with Vitex and a dopamine antagonist, monitor closely for return of symptoms previously controlled by the dopamine antagonist.

DOSAGE

Mode of Administration: Whole and powdered drug available as capsules, drops, film tablets, and compound preparations.

How Supplied:

Capsules – 40 mg, 100 mg

Liquid Extract – 1:1

Preparation: For the dried extract, preparations of 100 g contain 0.2 g dried extract in a ratio of 1:5, in either ethanol or water.

Daily Dosage: The daily dosage of aqueous-alcoholic extracts is 30 to 40 mg of the drug.

PMS: 20 mg daily (Schellenberg 2001; Berger 2000)

Menstrual cycle disorders: 20 mg to 1 g 3 times daily (Blumenthal et al, 1998; Newall et al, 1996).

Homeopathic Dosage: 5 to 10 drops, 1 tablet, or 5 to 10 globules, 1 to 3 times a day; parenterally: 1 mL injection solution sc twice weekly (HAB1).

LITERATURE

Antolic A & Males Z. Quantitative analysis of the polyphenols and tannins of *Vitex agnus-castus L.* In: *Acta Pharm*; 47(3):207-211, 1997

BAnz (Federal German Gazette) No. 50; published May 15, 1985; replaced Dec 2, 1992.

Becker H. Hemmung der Prolaktinsekretion. In: T W *Gynäkologie* 6:2-10. 1991

Berger D, Schaffner W, Schrader E et al. Efficacy of Vitex agnus castus L. extract Ze 440 in patients with pre-menstrual syndrome (PMS). *Arch Gynecol Obstet* 264 (3):150-153. 2000

Böhnert KJ, Hahn G. *Erfahrungsheilkunde* 39:494-502c. 1990

Dittmann FW, Böhnert KJ, Peeters M, Albrecht M, Lamertz M, Schmidt U. Prämenstruelles Syndrom. Behandlung mit einem Phytopharmakon. In: TW *Gynäkologie* 5:60-68. 1992

Feldmann HU, Albrecht M, Lamertz M, Böhnert KJ. Therapie bei Gelbkörperschwäche bzw. prämenstruellem Syndrom mit *Vitex-agnus-castus*-Tinktur. In: *Gyne* 11:421-425. 1990

Gerhard I, Patek A, Monga B et al. Mastodynon® bei weiblicher Sterilitaet. *Forsch Komplementaermed*; 5:272-278, 1998

Jarry H, Leonhardt S, Wuttke W, Behr B, Gorkow C. Agnus castus als dopaminerges Wirkprinzip in Mastodynon N. *Z Phytother;* 12:77-82, 1991

Kustrac D et al. The composition of the essential oil of *Vitex agnus-castus*. In: *PM;* 58(7):A681. 1992

Lal R, Sankaranarayanan A, Mathur VS et al. Antifertility and oxytocic activity of Vitex agnus-castus (seeds) in female albino rats. In: *Bull PGI*; 19(2):44-47. 1985

Lauritzen CH, Reuter HD, Repges R et al. Treatment of premenstrual tension syndrome with Vitex agnus castus. Controlled, double-blind study versus pyridoxine. In: *Phytomedicine*; 4(3):183-189, 1997

Pepeljnjak S, Antolic A & Kustrak D. Antibacterial and antifungal activities of the *Vitex agnus-castus L.* extracts. In: *Acta Pharm*; 46(3):201-206. 1996

Prilepskaya V, Ledina AV, Tagiyeva AV, et al. Vitex agnus castus: Successful treatment of moderate to severe premenstrual syndrome. In: *Maturitas*. 55S: S55-S63. 2006.

Reuter HD, Böhnert KJ, Schmidt U, Die Therapie des prämenstruellen Syndroms mit Vitex agnus castus. Kontrollierte Doppelblindstudie gegen Pyridoxin. *Z Phytother Abstractband*, S.7. 1995

Schellenberg R. Treatment for the premenstrual syndrome with agnus castus fruit extract: prospective, randomized, placebo controlled study. In: *BMJ*; 322(7279):134-137. 2001

Sliutz G, Speiser P, Schultz AM et al. *Agnus castus* extracts inhibit prolactin secretion of rat pituitary cells. In: *Horm Metab Res*; 25(5):253-255, 1993

Wuttke W, Gorkow Ch, Jarry J. Dopaminergic Compounds in Vitex Agnus Castus. In, Loew D, Rietbrock N (Hrsg) Phytopharmaka in Forschung und klinischer Anwendung. Steinkopff Verlag, Darmstadt, S. 81-91. 1995

Wuttke W, Splitt G, Gorkow C et al. Behandlung zyklusabhaengiger Brustschmerzen mit einem Agnus castus-haltigen Arzneimittel. Ergebnisse einer randomisierten, plazebo-kontrollierten Doppelblindstudie. *Geburtsh u Frauenheilk*; 57(10):569-574. 1997

Chaulmoogra

Hydnocarpus species

DESCRIPTION

Medicinal Parts: Chaulmoogra is found in all of the named species. The expressed oil is known as Gynocardia oil in Britain and Oleum Chaulmoograe in the U.S.

Flower and Fruit: The grayish seeds are about 2 to 3 cm long and 1.5 cm in diameter. They are irregularly angular with rounded ends. The kernel is oily and encloses two thin, heart-shaped, 3-veined cotyledons and a straight radical.

Characteristics: The taste is acrid and the odor disagreeable.

Habitat: Malaysia, Indian subcontinent.

Production: Chaulmoogra seeds are the seeds of various *Hydnocarpus* varieties. Chaulmoogra oil is the fatty oil extracted from the seeds.

Other Names: Hydnocarpus

ACTIONS AND PHARMACOLOGY

COMPOUNDS: CHAULMOOGRA SEEDS

Fatty oil (30%-40%, bitter-type consistency)

Proteins (25%)

Cyanogenic glycosides

Flavolignans

EFFECTS: CHAULMOOGRA SEEDS

The chaulmoogric acid in the drug is antimicrobial. The drug has sedative, febrifuge, and dermatic effects. The flavonol lignans hydnocarpin, hydnowightin, and neohydnocarpin isolated from the seeds are lipid lowering, anti-inflammatory, and antitumoral in animal experiments.

COMPOUNDS: CHAULMOOGRA OIL

Triglycerides: chief fatty acids D-hydnocarpic acid, D-chaulmoogric acid, D-gorli acid (cyclopentene fatty acids)

EFFECTS: CHAULMOOGRA OIL

The chaulmoogric acid in the drug is antimicrobial.

INDICATIONS AND USAGE

Unproven Uses: Externally, preparations of Hydnocarpus are used in the treatment of various skin conditions such as psoriasis and eczema. It is also used as an injection in the treatment of leprosy.

Chinese Medicine: In China, Chaulmoogra is used for leprosy, scabies and furuncles.

Indian Medicine: Uses include leprosy, skin diseases, itching, leucoderma, eczema, flatulence, and diabetes.

PRECAUTIONS AND ADVERSE REACTIONS

Coughing, dyspnea, laryngospasms, kidney damage, visual disorders, head and muscle pain, and central paralyses are side effects following intake of the oil. It is severely irritating in local application.

OVERDOSAGE

Following stomach and intestinal emptying (inducement of vomiting, gastric lavage with burgundy-colored potassium permanganate solution, sodium sulfate), the treatment for poisonings consists of the instillation of activated charcoal and shock prophylaxis (quiet, warmth), and of electrolyte substitution and the countering of any acidosis imbalance that may appear through sodium bicarbonate infusions. In the event of shock, plasma volume expanders should be infused. Monitoring of kidney function is necessary. Intubation and oxygen respiration may also be required.

The seeds are severely poisonous due to their cynagenic glycoside content. Antidotes include injections of solutions of Dicobalt-EDTA or of thiosulfates, or administration of methemoglobin-forming agents, such as amyl nitrite. Induce vomiting and begin gastric lavage in a parallel fashion. Circulatory support measures and artificial respiration may be required.

DOSAGE

Mode of Administration: The seeds and oil in various preparations, as powder, oil, emulsion, and ointments.

LITERATURE

Kern W, List PH, Hörhammer L (Hrsg.), Hagers Handbuch der Pharmazeutischen Praxis, 4. Aufl., Bde 1-8, Springer Verlag Berlin, Heidelberg, New York, 1969.

Lefort D et al., (1969) *Planta Med* 17:261.

Madaus G, Lehrbuch der Biologischen Arzneimittel, Bde 1-3, Nachdruck, Georg Olms Verlag Hildesheim 1979.

Roth L, Daunderer M, Kormann K, Giftpflanzen, Pflanzengifte, 4. Aufl., Ecomed Fachverlag Landsberg Lech 1993.

Sleumer, (1947) *Pharm Ztg* 83:165.

Teuscher E, Biogene Arzneimittel, 5. Aufl., Wiss. Verlagsges. Stuttgart 1997.

Cheiranthus cheiri

See Wallflower

Cheken

Eugenia chequen

DESCRIPTION

Medicinal Parts: The medicinal parts are the dried leaves.

Flower and Fruit: The flowers are usually solitary, occasionally in threes. The receptacle is top-shaped and pubescent. There are 4 pubescent or ciliate sepals. The petals are white, oval and 5 to 8 mm long. The stamens are numerous but small. The ovary is glabrous. The fruit is a red or black-violet, glabrous, globular berry, 6 to 8 mm in diameter. It has 2 to 3 seeds, which are dark, lentil-shaped, and are about 4 mm in diameter.

Leaves, Stem, and Root: The plant is an evergreen tree, which grows up to 15 m high and sometimes looks like a shrub. The leaves are coriaceous, ovate, about 1 to 1.5 cm long, 0.5 to 1 cm wide, entire-margined, and with very short petioles with numerous minute, round, translucent oil-cells.

Characteristics: The leaves have a bitter taste that is astringent and aromatic, reminiscent of bay leaves. The odor is slight and they contain an essential oil.

Habitat: Eugenia chequen grows in Chile.

Production: Cheken leaves are the leaves of *Eugenia chequen*.

Other Names: Arryan, Myrtus Chekan

ACTIONS AND PHARMACOLOGY

COMPOUNDS

Bitter substances

Volatile oil: including alpha-pinene, 1,8-cineol

EFFECTS

The ethanol extract inhibits xanthinoxydasis. The essential oil has a similar effect on germinating salad seeds such as auxin. An antibacterial and antimycotic effect has also been demonstrated. In the agar diffusion test, the leaf oil was effective against *Pseudomonas acruginsosa*, *Trichophyton mentagrophytes* and *Asperigillus niger*. It also affects fat metabolism: the oil is used against hyperlipoprotinemia. It is used as a tonic, a diuretic and an expectorant.

INDICATIONS AND USAGE

Unproven Uses: In South American folk medicine, a decoction of the leaves is used in the treatment of diarrhea, fever, gout, as a tonic, diuretic, an antihypertensive, and as a digestive aid.

PRECAUTIONS AND ADVERSE REACTIONS

Health risks or side effects following the proper administration of designated therapeutic dosages are not recorded.

DOSAGE

Mode of Administration: As a decoction and as a liquid extract.

LITERATURE

No literature is available.

Chelidonium majus

See Celandine

Chelone glabra

See Balmony

Chenopodium ambrosioides

See Wormseed Oil

Chenopodium vulvaria

See Arrach

Cherry Laurel

Prunus laurocerasus

DESCRIPTION

Medicinal Parts: The medicinal parts are the dried leaves.

Flower and Fruit: The flowers are erect and in slender racemes 10 to 12 cm long with 3-mm pedicles. The petals are white, obovate, and 3 mm long. The fruit is black and globular-ovoid. The smooth kernel within the fruit is ovoid and acute, with a long black weal.

Leaves, Stem, and Root: The plant is an evergreen shrub or tree, completely glabrous, and grows up to 6 m high. The bud scales drop early. The petioles are 1 cm long and glandless. The leaf blades are obovate-lanceolate and 8 to 15 cm long. They are curved, entire or with a finely serrated margin, coriaceous, and bright green. The upper surface of the leaves is glossy. The lower surface has 1 to 4 protruding nectaries in the axils of the ribs.

Characteristics: Poisonous. The fruit is similar to black cherries, and smells of hydrocyanic acid.

Habitat: The plant is indigenous to parts of Asia and is cultivated in many temperate areas.

Production: Cherry Laurel leaves are the leaves of *Prunus laurocerasus.*

Not to be Confused With: Other forms of *Prunus* species.

Other Names: Cherry-Bay

ACTIONS AND PHARMACOLOGY

COMPOUNDS

Cyanogenic glycosides: prunasin (corresponding to 0.5-2.5%, 50-210 mg HCN/100 gm)

EFFECTS

The drug acts as a tonic for the stomach, an anti-irritant, and a sedative.

INDICATIONS AND USAGE

Unproven Uses: Cherry Laurel is used to treat coughs and the common cold.

Homeopathic Uses: Cherry Laurel is used for dry coughs, whooping cough, cyanosis, and spasms.

PRECAUTIONS AND ADVERSE REACTIONS

No health hazards or side effects are known in conjunction with the proper administration of designated therapeutic dosages.

OVERDOSAGE

Overdoses of Cherry Laurel water prepared from the drug can lead to fatal poisonings. Ingestion of the leathery leaves and the seeds is improbable; the fruit pulp is low in cyanogenic glycosides (yielding 5-20 mg HCN/100 gm). The recommended antidotes include the injection of solutions of Dicobalt-EDTA or thiosulfates, or the administration of methemoglobin-forming agents, e.g., amyl nitrite, 4-dimethyl aminophenol. The inducement of vomiting or gastric lavage should be done in parallel fashion. Circulatory support and artificial respiration may also be required.

DOSAGE

Mode of Administration: The drug is available as a watery extract, an aromatic, a breathing stimulant, and an antispasmodic.

LITERATURE

Frohne D, Pfänder HJ, Giftpflanzen - Ein Handbuch für Apotheker, Toxikologen und Biologen, 4. Aufl., Wiss. Verlags-Ges. Stuttgart 1997.

Kern W, List PH, Hörhammer L (Hrsg.), Hagers Handbuch der Pharmazeutischen Praxis, 4. Aufl., Bde. 1-8, Springer Verlag Berlin, Heidelberg, New York, 1969.

Leung AY, Encyclopedia of Common Natural Ingredients Used in Food Drugs and Cosmetics, John Wiley & Sons Inc., New York. 1980.

Madaus G, Lehrbuch der Biologischen Arzneimittel, Bde 1-3, Nachdruck, Georg Olms Verlag Hildesheim. 1979.

Roth L, Daunderer M, Kormann K, Giftpflanzen, Pflanzengifte, 4. Aufl., Ecomed Fachverlag Landsberg Lech. 1993.

Sommer W, Dissertation Universität Kiel. 1984.

Steinegger E, Hänsel R, Pharmakognosie, 5. Aufl., Springer Verlag Heidelberg 1992.

Teuscher E, Lindequist U, Biogene Gifte - Biologie, Chemie, Pharmakologie, 2. Aufl., Fischer Verlag Stuttgart 1994.

Teuscher E, Biogene Arzneimittel, 5. Aufl., Wiss. Verlagsges. Stuttgart 1997.

Wagner H, Wiesenauer M, Phytotherapie. Phytopharmaka und pflanzliche Homöopathika, Fischer-Verlag, Stuttgart, Jena, New York 1995.

Chickweed

Stellaria media

DESCRIPTION

Medicinal Parts: The medicinal part is the fresh flowering or dried herb.

Flower and Fruit: The solitary white flowers are located in the leaf or branch axils. They open at 9 a.m. and, in good weather, remain open for 12 hours. The 5 double petals are shorter than the oblong-lanceolate sepals. There are 2 to 5 stamens and 3 stigma. The fruit is globular or ovate and covered in teeth. It opens when ripe and the seeds are shaken out through the movement of the plant.

Leaves, Stem, and Root: The plant is 5 to 30 cm high. The stem is decumbent and weak, heavily branched and often grows to an impressive length. It creeps along the ground, is fleshy, pale green, and slightly thickened at the nodes. The leaves are opposite and orbicular-ovate. The lower ones have long petioles and the upper ones are sessile. They are 1.25 cm long and 0.70 cm wide and sit in pairs on the stem.

Characteristics: The stem is pubescent on one side.

Habitat: The plant is found worldwide as a weed.

Production: Chickweed is the fresh herb in flower of *Stellaria media.*

Other Names: Adder's Mouth, Passerina, Satin Flower, Starweed, Starwort, Stitchwort, Tongue-Grass, Winterweed

ACTIONS AND PHARMACOLOGY

COMPOUNDS

Flavonoids: including, among others, rutin

Ascorbic acid (vitamin C, 0.1-0.15%)

Alkaloids

INDICATIONS AND USAGE

Unproven Uses: Internally, Chickweed is used for rheumatism, gout, stiffness of the joints, tuberculosis, and diseases of the blood. Externally, it is used for poorly healing wounds, hemorrhoids, inflammation of the eyes, eczema, and other diverse skin diseases.

PRECAUTIONS AND ADVERSE REACTIONS

No health hazards or side effects are known in conjunction with the proper administration of designated therapeutic dosages.

DOSAGE

Mode of Administration: The herb is used as a tea or in the form of juice for poultices, and in baths for medicinal purposes.

How Supplied

Capsules: 450 mg

Liquid Extract

LITERATURE

Budzianowski J, Pakulski G, Robak J. Studies on antioxidative activity of some C-glycosylflavones. *Pol J Pharmacol Pharm,* 1991; 43:395-401, Sep-Oct.

Guil JL, Torija ME, Gimenez JJ, Rodriguez-Garcia I, Gimenez A. Oxalic Acid and Calcium Determination in Wild Edible Plants. *J Agric Food Chem.* 1996; 44 (7); 1821-1823.

Watt JM, Breyer-Brandwijk MG, The Medicinal, Poisonous Plants of Southern, Eastern Africa, 2nd Ed, Livingstone 1962.

Chicory

Cichorium intybus

DESCRIPTION

Medicinal Parts: The medicinal parts of the plant are the dried leaves and roots, which are collected in autumn; the whole plant collected and dried in the flowering season; and the fresh plant and root.

Flower and Fruit: Size: The numerous flower heads are 3 to 4 cm in diameter and are terminal or axillary, solitary or in groups, sessile or short-pedioled. The epicalyx bracts are bristly ciliate, often glandular-haired. The inner bracts are oblong-lanceolate and erect, the outer ones ovate, splayed and half as long as the inner ones. The androgynous lingual florets are usually light blue, but occasionally white or pink. The fruit is an achaene 2 to 3 mm in length. It has no hair tuft and is ovate and straw yellow to blackish.

Leaves, Stem, and Root: The plant can grow to a height of 2 m and has a hardy, 10 to 30 cm long, thick root. The stem is rigidly erect, sparsely branched above and often bristly. The leaves are 10 to 30 cm long and 1 to 5 cm wide. They are obovate, oblong, shaped like a crosscut saw or slit, with numerous stiff hairs beneath. The lowest leaves in a basal rosette are petiolate. The upper ones as well as those near the inflorescences are alternate, oblong to lanceolate, crenate-dentate and sessile.

Characteristics: Chicory has a bitter taste.

Habitat: The plant is found in Europe, the Middle East as far as Iran, north and South Africa, all of America, Australia, and New Zealand.

Production: Chicory consists of the dried leaves and underground parts of *Cichorium intybus,* which are collected in autumn in the wild and air-dried.

Other Names: Succory, Hendibeh

ACTIONS AND PHARMACOLOGY

COMPOUNDS

Sesquiterpenes: sesquiterpene lactones, especially lactucin, lactucopicrin, 8-desoxy lactucin, guaianolid glycosides, including chicoroisides B and C, sonchuside C

Caffeic acid derivatives: chiroric acid, chlorogenic acid, isochlorogenic acid, dicaffeoyl tartaric acid

Hydroxycoumarins: including umbelliferone

Flavonoids: including hyperoside

Polyynes

EFFECTS

An antiexudative, choleretic, negatively chronotropic, and negatively inotropic effect has been described due to the plant's sesquiterpene lactones, cinnamic acid derivatives, and flavonoids. Animal studies have noted a distinct reduction of pulse rate and contractility; a mildly cholagogic effect; and lowered cholesteral levels in rats' livers and plasma. Application for dyspeptic complaints seems plausible because of the amaroid (guaianolide) content.

INDICATIONS AND USAGE

Approved by Commission E:

- Loss of appetite
- Dyspeptic complaints

Unproven Uses: In Folk medicine, the herb as a laxative for children, for loss of appetite, and dyspepsia.

Indian Medicine: Medicinal uses include headaches, dyspeptic symptoms, skin allergies, vomiting, and diarrhea.

PRECAUTIONS AND ADVERSE REACTIONS

No health hazards or side effects are known in conjunction with the proper administration of designated therapeutic dosages. There is a slight potential for sensitization via skin contact with the drug.

DOSAGE

Mode of Administration: Comminuted drug for infusions as well as other bitter-tasting preparations for internal use.

How Supplied: Commercial pharmaceutical preparations include drops and compound preparations.

Preparation: Prepare an infusion by scalding 2 g to 4 g drug with boiling water, allowing it to stand for 10 minutes, then straining. A tea is prepared by brewing 2 to 4 g of the whole herb with 150 to 250 ml boiling water and then straining it after 10 minutes.

Daily Dosage: 3 g comminuted drug. Single dose: 2 to 4 g whole herb for an infusion.

LITERATURE

Barlianto H, Maier HG. Acids in cichory roots and malt / II. Determination of acids derived from carbohydrates. Z Lebensm Unters Forsch. 1995; 200: 273-277.

Gilani AH, Janbaz KH. Evaluation of the liver protective potential of Cichorium intybus seed extract on Acetaminophen and CCL4-induced damage. Phytomedicine 1994; 1:193-197.

Piet DP, Schrijvers R, Franssen MCR, Groot Ade. Biotransformation of germacrane epoxides by Cichorium intybus. Tetrahedron 51 1995; (22):6303-6314.

Proliac A, Blanc M, (1976) Helv Chem Acta 58:2503.

Wagner, H, In "The Biology and Chemistry of the Compositae," Eds V. N. Heywood et al. Academic Press, London 1977.

Chimaphila umbellata

See Pipsissewa

Chinese Cinnamon

Cinnamomum aromaticum

DESCRIPTION

Medicinal Parts: The medicinal parts are the flowers collected and dried after they have finished blossoming, and the whole or partly peeled, dried bark of thin and young branches, as well the oil extracted from them.

Flower and Fruit: The flowers are small on short, slender, silky pedicles. They are arranged in threes in panicles in the leaf axils and in larger panicles at the end of the branches. The perianth is slightly silky, about 3 mm long, with oblong-lanceolate petals. The fruit is a juicy, pea-sized, elliptoid, smooth drupe.

Leaves, Stem, and Root: This evergreen tree grows up to 7 m tall with aromatic bark and angular branches. The bark is brown, in quilled pieces, sometimes with the remains of the outer layer present. The 7.5 to 10 cm long leaves are oblanceolate and pubescent on 6 to 8 cm long petioles, more or less tapered toward the base. They are coriaceous, alternate, and brown underneath.

Habitat: Indigenous and cultivated in southern China, Vietnam, Laos, and Burma.

Production: Chinese Cinnamon consists of the completely or partly peeled, dried stem bark from the aboveground or thin-branched axis of *Cinnamomum aromaticum*. The drug, from branches 2 to 3 cm thick, is peeled with horn knives, freed from cork and outer rind, and dried in the sun for 24 hours.

Not to be Confused With: Chinese Cinnamon should not be confused with waste products from the production process or other barks and materials, nor with the skins of horse chestnut seeds.

Other Names: Cassia, False Cinnamon, Bastard Cinnamon, *Cassia Lignea*, Cassia Bark, *Cassia aromaticum*, Canton Cassia

ACTIONS AND PHARMACOLOGY

COMPOUNDS

Volatile oil: chief components are cinnamaldehyde, weiterhin cinnamylacetate, cinnamyl alcohol, o-methoxycinnamaldehyde, cinnamic acid, coumarin

Diterpenes: cinnzeylanoles, cinncassioles A to E

Tannins: catechin tannins

Oligomere proanthocyanidins

Mucilages

EFFECTS

The essential oil and its main constituent cinnamaldehyde are antibacterial, fungistatic, improve immune resistance in animal tests (inhibiting allergic reactions Type I and II), promote motility, inhibit ulcers, and act on the digestive tract (tannin content).

INDICATIONS AND USAGE

Approved by Commission E:

- Loss of appetite
- Dyspeptic complaints

Unproven Uses: Folk medicine uses include symptomatic treatment of gastrointestinal disorders (mild, colicky upsets of the gastrointestinal tract, bloating, flatulence and diarrhea), as well as for loss of appetite. Efficacy has been sufficiently proved for gastric complaints and it is plausible for diarrhea, but the evidence is not sufficient for the other indications.

Chinese Medicine: Among uses in Chinese medicine are diarrhea, rheumatic conditions, amenorrhea, stomach ache, exhaustion, and to stabilize immunity.

Indian Medicine: Digestive complaints, vomiting, and diarrhea are the most common uses in Indian medicine.

CONTRAINDICATIONS

Use of medicinal preparations of Chinese Cinnamon is contraindicated during pregnancy.

PRECAUTIONS AND ADVERSE REACTIONS

General: No health hazards or side effects are known in conjunction with the proper administration of designated therapeutic dosages. The drug possesses a medium potential for sensitization, primarily due to the cinnamaldehyde.

Pregnancy: The drug is not to be administered in time of pregnancy.

DOSAGE

Mode of Administration: Comminuted bark for infusions, essential oil, as well as other galenic preparations for internal use.

Preparation: To prepare a tincture of Chinese Cinnamon, moisten 200 parts cinnamon bark evenly with ethanol and percolate to produce 1,000 parts tincture.

Daily Dosage: 2 to 4 g drug; 0.05 to 0.2 g essential oil. The average single dose is 1 g.

Storage: Chinese Cinnamon should be stored in a cool, dry environment in tightly sealed containers.

LITERATURE

Anon. Structure of potent antiulcerogenic compounds from *Cinnamomum cassia*. Tetrahedron 44 (1988), 4703.

Hikino H, Economic and Medicinal Plant Research, Vol I., Academic Press UK 1985.

Nagai H et al., (1982) Jpn J Pharmacol 32(5):813.

Nohara T et al., *Cinncassiol E,* a diterpene from the bark of *Cinnamomum cassia.* In: PH 24:1849. 1985.

Nohara T et al., PH 21:2130-2132. 1982.

Otsuka H et al., (1982) Yakugaku Zasshi 102:162.

Sagara K et al., J Chromatogr 409:365-370. 1987.

Senayake UM et al., (1978) *J Agric Food Chem* 20:822.

Structure of potent antiulcerogenic compounds from Cinnamomum cassia, Tetrahedron 44:4703. 1988.

Chinese Motherwort

Leonurus japonicus

DESCRIPTION

Medicinal Parts: The fruit is said to have medicinal properties.

Flower and Fruit: The inflorescence is long with whorls of a few widely spaced flowers. The bracts are short and usually have a thornlike awn. The flowers are sessile and dorsiventral. The calyx is narrow clavate, approximately 8 mm long and short-haired. The calyx teeth are upright, the lower 2 are longer than the 3 upper ones. The corolla is bilabiate, made up of 5 fused petals, approximately 10 mm long, lilac to pink. The upper lip has a purple middle lobe and the lower lip is divided into 3. There are 2 long and 2 short stamens. The ovary is superior, 2-carpled and 4-chambered. The fruit breaks up into 4 black, 3-edged, approximately 2 mm long, 1-seeded mericarps.

Leaves, Stem, and Root: This herbaceous perennial grows to a height of up to 1 m. The leaves are petiolate, 5 to 10 cm long, ovate to cordate, narrowing cuneiformly at the base. The lower leaves are palmately divided to the middle; the sections are pinnatifid with linear-acuminate lobes. The upper leaves are decussate opposite, simple, lanceolate, entire and pubescent on both surfaces. The stem is gray-green, upright, branched and square; the surface is grooved, and the ribs are pubescent.

Habitat: Leonurus japonicus is found in China, North and South Korea, and Japan.

Production: Chinese Motherwort fruit is the dried fruit of *Leonurus japonicus.*

ACTIONS AND PHARMACOLOGY

COMPOUNDS

Diterpenes: including leonurine

Fatty oil: chief fatty acids oleic acid and linolenic acid

EFFECTS

When taken internally, the alkaloid-containing drug (chief active ingredient leonurine) is said to have a contracting effect upon the uterus and to have generally anti-inflammatory effects upon various organ systems.

Topical application is said to reduce edema connected with injuries.

Watery drug extracts reduce blood pressure in animal experiments.

INDICATIONS AND USAGE

Chinese Medicine: Chinese Motherwort is used internally for inflammation of the kidney, the throat and the retina, for disturbances of menstruation, and in obstetrics for lochia. Externaily, the fruit is used for swelling of the tissue after trauma.

PRECAUTIONS AND ADVERSE REACTIONS

No health hazards are known in conjunction with the proper administration of designated therapeutic dosages.

OVERDOSAGE

Feelings of weakness, outbreaks of sweating, enhanced sensitivity to pain and feelings of closeness in the chest can all follow intake of higher dosages of the drug (starting at 30 g).

CONTRAINDICATIONS

Not to be used during pregnancy.

DOSAGE

Mode of Administration: Whole and powdered drug. Preparations are administered internally and externally

Preparation: Infusion: 4 to 10 g drug

Daily Dosage: Not specified in the literature

LITERATURE

Hänsel R, Keller K, Rimpler H, Schneider G (Ed), Hagers Handbuch der Pharmazeutischen Praxis, 5. Aufl., Bde 4 - 6 (Drogen), Springer Verlag Berlin, Heidelberg, New York, 1992-1994.

Chinese Olive

Canarium species

DESCRIPTION

Medicinal Parts: The medicinal part of the plant is the resin.

Flower and Fruit: The flowers are arranged in helicoid or scorpiod cymes; the structures are in threes. The 3 petals are thick and often coriaceous; the 3 sepals are usually fused into a cup- or jug-shaped calyx. There are 6 stamens, and the ovary is 3-chambered with an ovule in each chamber; the stigma is 3-lobed. The fruit is an ovoid drupe with a thin, resin-rich mesocarp.

Leaves, Stem, and Root: The tree is monoclinous or diclinous, reaching heights up to 15 m. The leaves are odd-pinnate. The leaflets are short-petiolate and very irregular. The stipules are round or slit.

Habitat: The tree is indigenous to the Spice Islands, Philippines, China, Melanesia, and Moluccas.

Production: Elemi is the oleoresin (soft) exuding from fresh cuts made in *Canarium luzonicum* and the residual resin (hard) left to dry on the tree. The soft elemi is obtained by cutting split secretion channels and, after knocking off the hard elemi, collecting the resin, which dries on the tree.

Other Names: Elemi

ACTIONS AND PHARMACOLOGY

COMPOUNDS

Triterpenes (70 to 80%): particularly alpha- and beta-amyrin, including alpha-, beta-, gamma-, delta-elemic acid, brein, maniladiol

Volatile oil (20 to 30%): chief component limonene (25%), also including alpha-phellandrene, elemol, eudesmol, carvacrol, methyl eugenol

EFFECTS

The resin is credited with promoting the healing of wounds. An immunostimulating effect was demonstrated in animal experiments. Topical administration causes skin irritation.

INDICATIONS AND USAGE

Unproven Uses: The resin is used in folk medicine as an expectorant for coughs as well as for gastric complaints, ulcers, and rheumatism (plaster).

PRECAUTIONS AND ADVERSE REACTIONS

No health hazards are known in conjunction with the proper administration of designated therapeutic dosages. According to older sources, stomach complaints, kidney irritation, and hemorrhagic erosions have been observed following administration of the essential oil. Topical application causes skin irritation.

DOSAGE

Mode of Administration: Preparations of the resin are used topically.

Preparation: Elemi resin is prepared by melting the resin at low heat and then putting it through a filter. This cleaning process results in a somewhat darker elemi. Plasters are prepared using 25% drug in ointment.

Storage: Store in well-sealed tins protected from light.

LITERATURE

Blaschek W, Hänsel R, Keller K, Reichling J, Rimpler G, Schneider G (Eds), Hagers Handbuch der Pharmazeutischen Praxis. Folgebände 1 und 2. Drogen A-Z. Springer. Berlin, Heidelberg 1998.

Chinese Rhubarb (Da-Huang)

Rheum palmatum

DESCRIPTION

Medicinal Parts: The medicinal parts are the dried underground parts, and most of the root bark in the dried form.

Flower and Fruit: The inflorescence is an erect panicle foliated to the tip. The flowers have narrow, red, pink or whitish yellow tepals. The tepals are curved and located far back in the mature flowers to facilitate wind pollination. The fruit is red-brown to brown, and oval. The fruit is angular, about to 7.8 mm to 10.2 mm wide and usually has scarious wings. The nutlet is 6 to 10 mm long and 7 mm in diameter.

Leaves, Stem, and Root: The plant is a large, sturdy herbaceous perennial. The stem grows to over 1.5 m high. The leaves are orbicular-cordate, palmate lobed, somewhat rough on the upper surface and 3 to 5 ribbed. The lobes are oblong-ovate to lanceolate, dentate, or pinnatisect. The root system consists of a tuber, which after a number of years measures 10 to 15 cm in diameter and has arm-thick lateral roots.

Habitat: The plant is indigenous to the western and north-western provinces of China and is cultivated in many regions around the world. The main producers are China and Russia.

Production: Chinese Rhubarb consists of the dried underground parts of *Rheum palmatum, Rheum officinale* or of both species. Stem parts, roots and most of the bark are removed from the rhizomes.

Not to be Confused With: Other Rheum species such as *Rheum rhaponticum* or *Rheum rhabarbarum.* Garden Rhubarb is *Rheum ponticum.*

Other Names: Rhubarb, Russian Rhubarb, East Indian Rhubarb, Indian Rhubarb

ACTIONS AND PHARMACOLOGY

COMPOUNDS

Anthracene derivatives (3-12%): chief components 1- or 8-O-β-glucosides of the aglycones rheumemodin, aloe-emodin, rhein, chrysophanol, physcion (together 60-80%), 8,8′-diglucosides of dianthrones (10-25%), including among others, sennosides A and B

Tannins: gallo tannins, including among others galloyl glucose, galloyl saccharose, lindleyine, isolindleyine

Flavonoids (2-3%)

Naphthohydroquinone glycosides

EFFECTS

Main active principles: hydroxyanthracene derivatives, tannins, and a small proportion of flavonoids

The laxative effect is due to the hydrogogic and anti-absorptive properties of the anthranoids. This effect causes an increase in the volume of the intestinal contents resulting in pressure and stimulation of intestinal peristalsis.

INDICATIONS AND USAGE

Approved by Commission E:

- Constipation

Unproven Uses: Rhubarb is used as an appetite stimulant and for digestion problems, gastrointestinal catarrh, and painful teething (children). External uses include burn treatment and skin conditions.

Chinese Medicine: In China, Rhubarb is used for delirium, tenesmus, edema, amenorrhea, and abdominal pain. Efficacy for digestion problems is plausible because of the tannin content but not without risk because of the toxicity of the anthranoids; efficacy for the other indications has not been proved.

Homeopathic Uses: Homeopathic uses include diarrhea and teething.

CONTRAINDICATIONS

Chinese Rhubarb is contraindicated in cases of intestinal obstruction, acute inflammatory intestinal disease, appendicitis, and abdominal pain of unknown origin.

PRECAUTIONS AND ADVERSE REACTIONS

General: Spasmodic gastrointestinal complaints can occur as a side effect to the drug's purgative effect. Long-term use leads to losses of electrolytes, in particular potassium ions. The loss of electrolytes may lead to hyperaldosteronism, inhibition of intestinal motility and enhancement of the effect of cardioactive steroids. Long-term use may lead to heart arrhythmias, nephropathies, edema, and accelerated bone deterioration.

The increased incidence of carcinoma of the colon following long-term administration of anthracene drugs has not yet been fully clarified. Recent studies show no association between the administration of anthracene drugs and the frequency of carcinoma of the colon.

Stimulating laxatives must not be used over an extended period (1 to 2 weeks) without medical advice.

Pregnancy: Use during pregnancy or while nursing only after consulting a physician.

Pediatric Use: The drug is not to be administered to children under 12 years of age.

DRUG INTERACTIONS

POTENTIAL INTERACTIONS

Long-term use of Chinese Rhubarb may lead to a potassium deficiency, which may cause an increase in the effect of cardiac glycosides.

DOSAGE

Mode of Administration: Liquid or solid forms of medication are exclusively for oral use. The drug is available as comminuted drug, powder or dry extracts for teas, decoctions, cold macerations or elixirs. Extracts of the drug are often constituents of laxatives, cholagogics, and gastrointestinal remedies, and are found in ''slimming cures,'' ''springtime tonics'' and ''blood purifying'' teas.

Preparation: To prepare an infusion to be used as a laxative, use 1.0 to 2.0 gm coarse powdered drug; for a stomachic, 0.1 to 0.2 gm powdered drug stirred with sufficient liquid (may be flavored with cinnamon, ginger, or peppermint oil) or scald and strain after 5 minutes. (1 teaspoonful = approximately 2.5 gm drug)

Daily Dosage: As a laxative, the dose is 1.0 to 2.0 gm of drug prepared according to instructions above. As an astringent and stomachic, the dose is 0.1-0.2 gm.

Tea – 1 cup mornings and/or evenings

Extract – Single dose: 0.3 to 1 gm

Laxatives should be used for the shortest possible time (maximum 1 to 2 weeks)

Homeopathic Dosage: 5 drops, 1 tablet, or 10 globules every 30 to 60 minutes (acute) or 1 to 3 times daily (chronic); parenterally: 1 to 2 mL sc acute: 3 times daily; chronic: once a day (HAB1).

LITERATURE

Amagaya S, Umeda M, Ogihara Y. Inhibitory Action of Shosaikoto and Daisaikoto (Traditional Chinese Medicine) on Collagen-Induced Platelet Aggregation and Prostaglandin Biosynthesis. *Planta Med.* 1986;52; 345-349.

BGA, Arzneimittelrisiken: Anthranoide. In: *DAZ* 132(21):1164. 1992.

Foust B, In: Foust MC. Rhubarb: The Wondrous Drug. Princeton University Press, Princeton, NJ 1992.

Heisig W, Wichtl M. The Identification of Anthraquinone and Flavonoid Drugs with Two Dimensional Thin-Layer-Chromatrography Using the TLC-Reaction-Box-Process. *Planta Med.* 1989; 55:614-615.

Iida K et al., Potent inhibitors of tyrosinase activity and melanin biosynthesis from *Rheum officinale*. In: *PM* 61(5):425-428. 1995.

Kashiwada Y et al., (1984) *Chem Pharm Bull* 32(9):3461.

Sanches EF, Feritas TV, Ferreiraalves DL, Velarde DT, Diniz MR, Cordeiro MN, Agostinicotta G, Biological activities of venoms from South American snakes. In: *Toxicon* 30(1):95. 1992.

Chinese Thoroughwax (Chai-Hu)

Bupleurum chinense

DESCRIPTION

Medicinal Parts: The medicinal part of the plant is the root.

Flower and Fruit: The inflorescence is a compound umbel. The flower structures are arranged in fives. The flowers are radial and small; the petals are yellowish, almost orbicular; the calyx teeth are insignificant. The ovary is inferior and 2-chambered. The fruit is a double achaene.

Leaves, Stem, and Root: Thoroughwax is an upright herbaceous perennial, which grows about 30 to 70 cm high. The leaves are alternate, arranged in spirals, simple, and entire. The stem is hollow, gnarled, and branched.

Habitat: China, Japan and central Europe

Production: Bupleuri roots are the dried roots of *Bupleurum chinense*. They are collected in the wild.

Not to be Confused With: May be confused with *Bupleurum longiradiatum*.

Other Names: Chai Hu

ACTIONS AND PHARMACOLOGY

COMPOUNDS

Triterpene saponins (saikosides, 1.2 to 4.9%, content declining with the diameter of the root): saikosaponins a, b1, b2, c and d, aglycones are the so-called saikogenins

Steroids: sterols, including alpha-spinasterol, stigmasterol

Polyynes: saikodiine A, B and C

EFFECTS

The drug is not usually used alone, but rather used in various drug mixtures.

The saiko saponins or saikogenins that the drug contains have exhibited antipyretic, edema-protective and anti-inflammatory effects in animal experiments. At the same time, an inducement of the depletion of corticosterone and a liver-protective effect could be demonstrated, as could a sedative and an analgesic effect. The drug is also credited with antitussive, anti-ulcerogenic and blood-pressure lowering characteristics.

INDICATIONS AND USAGE

Unproven Uses: Chinese Thoroughwax is used for inflammatory conditions (oriental regions).

Chinese Medicine: Preparations are used for shivering and fever, jaundice, chest pain, bitter taste in the mouth, nausea, vomiting, malaria, and deafness.

PRECAUTIONS AND ADVERSE REACTIONS

General: No health hazards are known in conjunction with the proper administration of designated therapeutic dosages.

Pregnancy: The drug is not to be administered during pregnancy.

OVERDOSAGE

The ingestion of larger dosages of the drug may lead to gastroenteritis, intestinal colic, and diarrhea, due to the saponin content.

DOSAGE

Mode of Administration: Whole drug and cut drug preparations for internal and external use.

Preparation: The drug is usually only used in Chinese and Japanese medicine in compounded preparations.

Storage: Should be well sealed (to protect against insects) and air dried.

LITERATURE

Hänsel R, Keller K, Rimpler H, Schneider G (Ed), Hagers Handbuch der Pharmazeutischen Praxis, 5. Aufl., Bde 4 - 6 (Drogen), Springer Verlag Berlin, Heidelberg, New York, 1992-1994.

Iwama H, Amagaya S, Ogihara Y. Effects of Kamphozai (Chinese Traditional Medicines) on the Immune Responses; I. In vivo Studies of Hochuekkito, Juzendaihoto and Tokisakuyakusan Using Sheep Red Blood Cell as Antigen in Mice. *Planta Med.* 1986; 52:247-250.

Izumi S, Ohno N, KawakitamT, Nomoto K, Yadomae T. Participation of free amino acids and reducing sugars in the interactions of constituents during preparation of a traditional Chinese herbal medicine, Xiao-Chai-Hu-Tang (Japanese name: Sho-saiko-To). *Pharm Pharmacol Lett.* 1996:6(1);37-41.

Jin RL, Shi L, Kuang Y, Comparative studies on the roots of wild and cultured *Bupleurum chinense. DC Chung Yao Tung Pao*, 20:11-3, 61, 1988 Apr.

Ohtsu S, Izumi S, Iwanaga S, Ohno N, Yadomae T, Analysis of mitogenic substances in *Bupleurum chinense* by ESR spectroscopy. *Biol Pharm Bull*, 20:97-100, 1997 Jan.

Zhang J, Comparison on saikosaponin levels in the root of *Bupleurum chinense* of various sizes. *Chung Yao Tung Pao*, 20:13-4, 1985 Apr.

Chionanthus virginicus

See Fringetree

Chiretta

Swertia chirata

DESCRIPTION

Medicinal Parts: The medicinal part is the herb, which is cut and dried when the seed is ripe.

Flower and Fruit: The numerous flowers are small and form a yellow panicle. The fruit is a single-valved capsule, which tastes very bitter and is odorless.

Leaves, Stem, and Root: The plant is an annual and grows up to 90 cm high. The branching stem is brown or purplish, 2 to 4 mm thick, cylindrical below and becoming quadrangular toward the top. The leaves are smooth, opposite, lanceolate or ovate, and entire-margined with 3 to 7 longitudinal ribs.

Habitat: The plant is indigenous to northern India and Nepal.

Production: Chiretta is the aerial part of *Swertia chirata*.

Other Names: Chirata, Chirayta, Indian Balmony, Indian Gentian

ACTIONS AND PHARMACOLOGY

COMPOUNDS

Iridoide monoterpenes as bitter substances (1.3%): chief components swertiamarin (0.4%), sweroside (0.2%), including as well gentiopicrin, amarogentin, amaroswerin

Xanthone derivatives: including mangiferin (0.12%), swerchirin (methyl bellidifoline), swertianin, 7-O-methyl swertianin, chiratol, swertiapunicoside, chiratanin

EFFECTS

Chiretta stimulates the secretion of gastric juices. In animal experiments, an anticholinergic (due to swertiamarin), antiphlogistic, hypoglycemic (due to xanthone derivatives), and centrally suppressing effect has been described.

INDICATIONS AND USAGE

Unproven Uses: Chiretta is used for dyspeptic disorders, loss of appetite, problems with the production of gastric juices, and disorders of the digestive system.

CONTRAINDICATIONS

The drug should not be used in patients who have gastric or duodenal ulcers due to the drug's stimulation of gastric juice secretion.

PRECAUTIONS AND ADVERSE REACTIONS

No health hazards or side effects are known in conjunction with the proper administration of designated therapeutic dosages.

DOSAGE

Mode of Administration: The drug is a constituent part of various preparations, especially drops.

Daily Dosage: The daily dosage is 15 to 20 drops, 3 times daily before meals. For nervous disorders, 10 to 15 drops are taken daily between meals.

LITERATURE

Atta-Ur-Rahman Zaman K. Medicinal Plants with Hypoglycemic Activity. *J Ethnopharmacol.* 1989; 26:1-55.

Ivorra MD, Paya M, Villar A. A Review of Natural Products and Plants as Potential Antidiabetic Drugs. *J Ethnopharmacol.* 1989; 27:243-275.

Ray S et al. Amarogentin, a naturally occuring secoiridoid glycoside and a newly recognized inhibitor of topoisomerase I from *Leishmania donovani.* In: *JNP* 59(1):27-29. 1996.

Chives

Allium schoenoprasum

DESCRIPTION

Medicinal Parts: The medicinal parts are the fresh or dried aerial parts of the plant.

Flower and Fruit: The cyme has numerous florets. The sheath of the inflorescence has 2 or 3 flaps. The flap is broad-ovate and shorter than the inflorescence; it is white or reddish. The florets are dense and globose with no bulbils. The petals of the perianth are lanceolate-ovate and acute or pointed. They are 7 to 11 mm long, bluish or white to yellowish, and have a dark middle stripe. The stamens are shorter than the perianth. They are awl-shaped and fused with each other and the perianth petals at the base. The perianth surrounds the capsule like a balloon.

Leaves, Stem, and Root: Allium schoenoprasum is a perennial, 15 to 30 cm high plant. The base is branched with numerous erect, closely packed leaves. Thin sheaths form incomplete, oblong bulbs. The bulb skin is thin, white, and splits when mature. The stem is round, usually smooth and leafy from the lower third. The compact leaves are completely hollow, round, somewhat elastic, and gray or gray-green.

Habitat: Chives grow wild in the temperate regions of Europe and North America and are cultivated in Europe, Turkistan, North America, and from Siberia to Japan.

Production: Chives are the complete aerial parts of *Allium schoenoprasum,* which are harvested before flowering.

Other Names: Cive Garlic, Civet, Chive

ACTIONS AND PHARMACOLOGY

COMPOUNDS

Alliins (alkyl cysteine sulfoxides): in particular, methyl alliin (S-methyl-L-(+)-cysteine sulfoxide) and pentyl alliin (S-pentyl-L-(+)-cysteine sulfoxide), as well as their gamma-glutamyl conjugates; in the course of cutting up the fresh foliage, the allins undergo a transformation (triggered by fermentation) into the so-called alliaceous oils, e.g., dimethyl-disulfide-mono-S-oxide

EFFECTS

The volatile and nonvolatile sulphur bonds are said to be anthelmintic. However, efficacy has not been documented in scientific studies.

INDICATIONS AND USAGE

Unproven Uses: The drug is used to expel worms and intestinal parasites.

PRECAUTIONS AND ADVERSE REACTIONS

No health hazards or side effects are known in conjunction with the proper administration of designated therapeutic dosages. The intake of large quantities can lead to stomach irritation.

DOSAGE

Mode of Administration: Chives are used fresh or dried, as a cut drug.

LITERATURE

Kameoka H, Hashimoto S, Two sulfur containing constituents from *Allium schoenoprasum.* In: *PH* 22:294-295. 1983.

Hänsel R, Keller K, Rimpler H, Schneider G (Hrsg.), Hagers Handbuch der Pharmazeutischen Praxis, 5. Aufl., Bde 4-6 (Drogen): Springer Verlag Berlin, Heidelberg, New York, 1992-1994.

Hashimoto S et al., *Food Sci* 48:1858. 1983.

Chocolate Vine (Mu-Tong)

Akebia quinata

DESCRIPTION

Medicinal Parts: The dried stems and fruits of the *Akebia quinata* are frequently used in medicine.

Flower and Fruit: The inflorescence is racemose, hanging, 5 to 9 cm long, with 1 to 3 female flowers. The pedicle is 3 to 5 cm long. There are 3 to 4 violet to pink-violet sepals up to 1.5 cm long and 5 to 7 apocarpic, blue-violet carpels. There are 4 to 15 male flowers with 3 violet to lilac sepals and 6 to 7 violet to black stamens. The fruit is an elongate pome, 6 to 9 cm long, dark violet when ripe with white spots and a coriaceous cupule. The seeds are numerous, red-brown to black, ovoid, approximately 6 mm long and embedded in jellylike tissue.

Leaves, Stem, and Root: Akebia quinata is a climbing shrub that grows up to 10 m high. The shrub is deciduous, diclinous and monoecious. The leaves are alternate and arranged in fives. The petiole and the stems of the leaflets are approximately 2 cm long. The leaflets are up to 2.5 cm long, rounded at the base and entire. The trunk is silvery or gray, with cork warts.

Characteristics: The fruit is edible.

Habitat: Japan, China, Korea

Production: Chocolate vine is the dried stem of *Akebia quinata.*

Other Names: Five-Leaflet Akebia, Mu Tong

ACTIONS AND PHARMACOLOGY

COMPOUNDS

Triterpene saponins: akebosides, aglycones oleanolic acid and hederagenin

Steroids: sterols, including beta-sitosterol, beta-sitosterol glucoside, betulin

Monosaccharides/oligosaccharides: saccharose

Cyclitols: meso-inositol

EFFECTS

Animal experiments have demonstrated an antiedemic effect attributed to the saponin mixture contained in the drug. In addition, diuretic, uricosuric, centrally depressant, antipyretic, mild analgesic and motility-inhibiting (intestinal) effects have been reported, although no results of controlled clinical studies have as yet been published.

INDICATIONS AND USAGE

Unproven Uses: Preparations of the plant have been used for acute urinary tract infections and ascites.

Chinese Medicine: Mu Tong is used for laryngitis and dry coughs, urinary stones, disturbances of bladder function, galacturia, convulsions, anemia, and hematuria.

PRECAUTIONS AND ADVERSE REACTIONS

No health hazards are known in conjunction with the proper administration of designated therapeutic dosages. The ingestion of larger dosages of the drug may lead to gastroenteritis, intestinal colic and diarrhea, due to the saponin content. The drug is not to be administered during pregnancy.

DOSAGE

Mode of Administration: Liquid preparations for internal use.

Daily Dosage: 3 to 9 gm in the form of a decoction.

LITERATURE

Hänsel R, Keller K, Rimpler H, Schneider G (Ed), Hagers Handbuch der Pharmazeutischen Praxis, 5. Aufl., Bde 4 - 6 (Drogen), Springer Verlag Berlin, Heidelberg, New York, 1992-1994.

Yang DJ, The study of the constituents of Clematis and Akebia spp. II. On the saponins isolated from the stem of *Akebia quinata Decne.* (1) (author's transl) Yakugaku Zasshi, 9:194-8, 1974 Feb.

Yang DJ, Tinnitus treated with combined traditional Chinese medicine and Western medicine. *Chung Hsi I Chieh Ho Tsa Chih,* 9:270-1, 259-60, 1989 May.

Chondrodendron tomentosum

See Pareira

Chondrus crispus

See Carrageen

Chrysanthemum cinerariifolium

See Pyrethrum

Chrysanthemum leucanthemum

See Ox-Eye Daisy

Cichorium intybus

See Chicory

Cicuta virosa

See European Water Hemlock

Cimicifuga racemosa

See Black Cohosh

Cinchona pubescens

See Quinine

Cinnamomum aromaticum

See Chinese Cinnamon

Cinnamomum camphora

See Camphor Tree

Cinnamomum verum

See Cinnamon

Cinnamon

Cinnamomum verum

DESCRIPTION

Medicinal Parts: The medicinal parts are the cinnamon oil extracted from the bark, the cinnamon bark of younger branches, and the cinnamon leaf oil.

Flower and Fruit: The flowers are whitish-green, inconspicuous and have an unpleasant smell. They are about 0.5 cm long; arranged in loose, axillary or terminal panicles; and covered in silky hairs. The fruit is berrylike, ovoid-oblong, short-thorned, and half-enclosed by the attached epicalyx.

Leaves, Stem, and Root: The plant is a heavily foliated evergreen tree 6.5 to 12 m tall with a pale brown bark in thin quills, several rolled inside one another. The branches are cylindrical with a gray-brown bark. The tough leaves, which are opposite and splayed horizontally to leaning, are initially red then turn green. They are about 12 cm by 5 cm, roundish-ovate or ovate-lanceolate to oblong, more or less acuminate and entire-margined. The leaves smell like cloves.

Habitat: Cinnamon is indigenous to Sri Lanka and southwest India.

Production: Cinnamon consists of the dried tree bark, separated from the cork and outer rind, of young shoots growing on the branches of *Cinnamomum verum*. The tree is widely cultivated, and the harvested bark is dried in the shade.

Not to be Confused With: Confusion can arise with other powdered cinnamon varieties.

Other Names: Ceylon Cinnamon

ACTIONS AND PHARMACOLOGY

COMPOUNDS

Volatile oil: chief components - cinnamaldehyde, weiterhin eugenol, cinnamylacetate, cinnamyl alcohol, o-methoxycinnamaldehyde, cinnamic acid

Diterpenes: cinnzeylanol, cinnzeylanin

Oligomeric proanthocyanidins

Mucilages

EFFECTS

The cinnmaldehyde in the cinnamon bark's essential oil is antibacterial, fungistatic, and promotes motility. It has a mildly positive estrogen effect on the genital system of animals in tests, although the constituent responsible is unidentified. Cinnamon increases gastric secretions slightly and is an insecticide due to the diterpenes cinnzeylanin and cinnceylanol.

INDICATIONS AND USAGE

Approved by Commission E:

- Loss of appetite
- Dyspeptic complaints

Unproven Uses: In addition, folk medicine internal uses include flatulence and exhaustion.

Indian Medicine: Uses in Indian medicine include toothache, nausea and vomiting, and dyspepsia.

CONTRAINDICATIONS

Use of the drug is contraindicated during pregnancy.

PRECAUTIONS AND ADVERSE REACTIONS

General: No health hazards or side effects are known in conjunction with the proper administration of designated therapeutic dosages. The drug possesses a medium potential for sensitization because of the cinnamaldehyde content.

Pregnancy: The drug is not to be administered to pregnant women.

DOSAGE

Mode of Administration: Comminuted drug for infusions; essential oil, as well as other galenic preparations for internal use. Bath additives, drops and compound preparations for external use.

How Supplied:

Extract – 1:1

Preparation: To prepare a tea, pour hot water over 0.5 to 1 g cinnamon bark and strain after 10 minutes. A tincture is made from a maceration of 200 parts cinnamon bark + 100 parts 70% ethanol V/V (ÖAB90).

Daily Dosage: 2 to 4 g drug; 0.05 to 0.2 g essential oil. One cup of tea/infusion is taken 2 to3 times daily at mealtimes

Storage: Protect from light and moisture in non-synthetic containers.

LITERATURE

Buchalter L, (1971) J Pharm Sci 60: 144.

Isogai A et al., (1977) Agric Biol Chem 41: 1779.

Kato Y, (1975) Koryo 113: 17, et 24.

Kaul R, Pflanzliche Procyanidine. Vorkommen, Klassifikation und pharmakologische Wirkungen. In: PUZ 25(4):175-185. 1996.

Schneider E, Cinnamomum verum - Der Zimt. In: ZPT 9(6):193. 1988.

Schröder, Buch. In: Schröder R: Kaffee, Tee und Kardamom, Ulmer-Verlag, Stuttgart. 1991.

Cinqefoil

Potentilla erecta

DESCRIPTION

Medicinal Parts: The medicinal parts are the rhizome freed from the roots, the fresh underground parts collected in the spring, the dried rhizome and the rhizome gathered in the spring.

Flower and Fruit: The small, yellow, long-pedicled flowers grow opposite the leaves or at branching points on the stem. The 4 sepals have a 4-bract epicalyx. There are 4 free petals, which are obcordate and somewhat darker at the base. There are usually 16 stamens and numerous ovaries with threadlike styles. The receptacle is domed. The fruit is nutlike, hard, 1 seeded, ovate, grooved and occasionally smooth.

Leaves, Stem, and Root: The rhizomatus herbacious perennial plant is about 30 cm high. The rhizome is 1 to 3 cm thick, irregular, gnarled to cylindrical, woody, dark-brown outside and blood red inside. The stem is erect or decumbent, never rooting, branching. The trifoliate rosettelike basal leaves wilt early and are gone before flowering. The cauline leaves are sessile, trifoliate, and appear to be in fives because of 2 stipules

Characteristics: The plant is odorless and has an astringent taste.

Habitat: The plant is found as far north as Northern Scandinavia and as far south as Northwest Africa, Italy, Central Spain, and the Balkans.

Production: Cinquefoil rhizome consists of the dried rhizome, freed from the roots, of *Potentilla erecta* (syn: *Potentilla tormentilla N.*) and its preparations. After harvesting the rhizome is air-dried.

Not to be Confused With: May be confused with *Radix bistortae* and the rhizomes of *Geum* species.

Other Names: Septfoil, Thormantle, Biscuits, Bloodroot, Earthbank, Ewe Daisy, Flesh and Blood, Shepherd's Knapperty, Shepherd's Knot, English Sarsaparilla

ACTIONS AND PHARMACOLOGY

COMPOUNDS

Catechins: including (-)-gallocatechin gallate, (-)-epigallocatechin gallate, dimerics and trimerics of the catechin derivatives

Catechin tannins (15 to 20%), transformed under storage conditions into non-water soluble tanner's reds (phlobaphenes)

Flavonoids: including kaempferol

Gallo tannins (3.5%), including agrimonine, pedunculagin, levigatines B and F proanthocyanidins

Tannins (5 to 10%)

Triterpenes: including tormentoside, ursolic acid, e-epi-pomolic acid

EFFECTS

The drug is astringent, antimicrobial, and molluscidal because of the tannin complex (gallic tannins and ellagic tannins). In animal experiments an antihypertensive, anti-allergic, immune-stimulating, antiviral, and interferon-inducing effect has been demonstrated.

INDICATIONS AND USAGE

Approved by Commission E:

- Diarrhea
- Inflammation of the mouth and pharynx
- Premenstrual syndrome

Unproven Uses: In folk medicine, the drug is used internally for diarrhea and inflammation of the oral and pharyngeal mucosa; externally for poorly healing wounds.

PRECAUTIONS

No health hazards are known in conjunction with the proper administration of designated therapeutic dosages. There are reports in the literature of gastric complaints or vomiting following intake of the drug or its extracts.

DOSAGE

Mode of Administration: Cinquefoil is available in solid, liquid, and compounded preparations for internal and external use.

Preparation: To prepare a tea, 2 to 3 gm finely cut or coarsely powdered drug is added to cold water, and rapidly brought to a boil, steep for some time and then strain. A cold-water decoction may be used to avoid loss of tannin strength that occurs during the boiling process (1 teaspoon is equivalent to approximately 4 gm drug).

To prepare a tincture, 1 part cut rhizome is percolated with 5 parts 70% ethanol (V/V) (DAB10)

Daily Dosage: 4 to 6 gm drug

Tincture (1:10): 10 to 20 drops to one glass of water as a rinse several times a day

Tea: 1 cup to be taken several times a day between meals.

Storage: The herb should be protected from light.

LITERATURE

Bilia AR, Ctalano S, Fontana C, Morelli I, Palme E, A new saponin from *Potentilla tormentilla*. In: *PM* 58(7):A723. 1992.

Geiger C et al., Ellagitannins from Alchemilla xanthochlora and *Potentilla erecta*. In: *PM* 60(4):384. 1994.

Schimmer O, Lindenbaum M. Tannins with antimutagenic properties in the herb of *Alchemilla* species and *Potentilla anserina*. *Planta Med* 61 (1995), 141-145.

Vennat B et al., J Pharm Belg 47:485. 1992.

Citrullus colocynthis

See Bitter Apple

Citrus aurantifolia

See Lime

Citrus aurantium

See Bitter Orange

Citrus limon

See Lemon

Citrus sinensis

See Sweet Orange

Cladonia pyxidata

See Cupmoss

Claviceps purpurea

See Ergot

Cleavers

Galium aparine

DESCRIPTION

Medicinal Parts: The medicinal parts are the aerial parts collected during the flowering season and dried, as well as the fresh, flowering herb and the fresh or dried whole plant.

Flower and Fruit: There are a few small white or greenish flowers in axillary, peduncled cymes. The corolla is about 1.5 to 1.7 mm long and has a pointed tip. The pedicles do not turn back before the fruit ripens. The 4 to 7 mm long mericarps are covered in barbed bristles.

Leaves, Stem, and Root: The plant is 60 to 150 cm high. The stem is decumbent or climbing, sharply quadrangular even to the point of being winged and branched. There are long, cauline leaves. The margins and midrib of the leaves are thorny. The foliage leaves are arranged in false whorls of 6 or 8. They are lanceolate from a wedge-shaped base, 30 to 60 mm long and 3 to 8 mm wide, obtuse, and thorny tipped.

Habitat: A common wild plant throughout Europe, in Asia from Siberia to the Himalayas, and in North and South America.

Production: Cleavers is the flowering herb of the aerial part of *Galium aparine*, which is gathered and then dried.

Other Names: Clivers, Goosegrass, Barweed, Hedgeheriff, Hayriffe, Eriffe, Grip Grass, Hayruff, Catchweed, Scratweed, Mutton Chops, Robin-Run-in-the-Grass, Love-Man, Goosebill, Everlasting Friendship, Bedstraw, Coachweed, Cleaverwort, Goose Grass, Gosling Weed, Hedge-Burs, Stick-a-Back, Sweethearts

ACTIONS AND PHARMACOLOGY

COMPOUNDS

Iridoide monoterpenes: asperuloside

Benzyl isoquinoline alkaloids: including protopine

Beta-carbolin alkaloids: harmine

Quinazoline alkaloids: 1-hydroxydesoxypeganin, 8-hydroxy-2,3-dehydrodesoxypeganin

Flavonoids

EFFECTS

No information is available.

INDICATIONS AND USAGE

The drug is used internally as well as externally for ulcers, festering glands, lumps in the breast and skin rashes. It is also used for lithuresis and calculosis and as a diuretic for dropsy, bladder catarrh, and retention of urine (ischuria). Efficacy has not been proved.

Chinese Medicine: Used for internal and external injuries, disorders of the efferent urinary tract, and hematuria.

Homeopathic: Used for kidney stones and ulcers (particularly of the tongue).

PRECAUTIONS AND ADVERSE REACTIONS

Health risks or side effects following the proper administration of designated therapeutic dosages are not recorded.

DOSAGE

Mode of Administration: Used topically in alcoholic extracts. Internally as a tea and juice.

How Supplied

Liquid Extract

Tea

Daily Dosage: As a tea, add 4 teaspoonfuls (3.3 to 4.4 gm) of the drug to 2 glasses of hot water. Drink in sips during the course of the day.

Homeopathic: 5 drops, 1 tablet, or 10 globules every 30 to 60 minutes and 1 to 3 times daily (chronic); parenterally, 1 to 2 mL sc 3 times daily (acute); chronic: once a day (HAB1).

LITERATURE

Berkowitz, WF et al., (1982) *J Org Chem* 47:824.

Bhan MK et al., (1976) *Ind J Chem* 14:475.

Buckova et al., (1970) *Acta Fac Pharm Univ Comeniana* 19:7.

Burnett AR, Thomsom RH, (1968) *J Clin Soc* (6):854.

Corrigan D et al., (1978) *Phytochemistry* 17:1131.

Hänsel R, Keller K, Rimpler H, Schneider G (Hrsg.), Hagers Handbuch der Pharmazeutischen Praxis, 5. Aufl., Bde 4-6 (Drogen), Springer Verlag Berlin, Heidelberg, New York, 1992-1994.

Hegnauer R, Chemotaxonomie der Pflanzen, Bde 1-11, Birkhäuser Verlag Basel, Boston, Berlin 1962-1997.

Inouye H et al., (1974) *Planta Med* 25:285.

Madaus G, Lehrbuch der Biologischen Arzneimittel, Bde 1-3, Nachdruck, Georg Olms Verlag Hildesheim 1979.

Clematis

Clematis recta

DESCRIPTION

Medicinal Parts: The medicinal part is the fresh, flowering plant.

Flower and Fruit: The flowers are in many blossomed terminal cymes. The individual blossoms are white and similar to *Clematis vitalba*, except that the bracts are only downy on the edges. The nutlet is glabrous, with a thickened edge and a long tail.

Leaves, Stem, and Root: The plant grows to about 50 to 125 cm high. The stem is nonclimbing, erect, leafy, and glabrous. The leaves are pinnatifid. The leaflets are smaller than those of *Clematis vitalba*.

Characteristics: The plant is poisonous.

Habitat: The plant grows in Europe.

Production: Clematis herb is the whole fresh flowering plant of *Clematis recta*. The herb is gathered when the plant is in full flower. It is turned regularly while being dried in the shade.

Other Names: Upright Virgin's Bower

ACTIONS AND PHARMACOLOGY

COMPOUNDS

Protoanemonine-forming agents in the freshly harvested plant: presumably, the glycoside ranunculin changes enzymatically when the plant is cut into small pieces (and probably also when it is dried) into the pungent, volatile protoanemonine, which quickly dimerises to anemonine. Once dried, the plant may not be capable of protoanemonine formation.

Saponins

EFFECTS

The fresh plant induces blistering on the skin and mucous membranes and is a fungicide. Sun plants are more effective than shade plants.

INDICATIONS AND USAGE

Unproven Uses: Clematis was formerly used as a remedy for venereal diseases (syphilis), chronic skin conditions, gout, rheumatism, and bone disorders, as well as a diuretic. In the pharmaceutical industry, it is used for rheumatic pains, headaches, and varicose veins. In folk medicine, it is used for blisters and as a poultice for festering wounds and ulcers.

Homeopathic Uses: Clematis is used in homeopathic dilutions for ulcers and poor wound healing.

PRECAUTIONS AND ADVERSE REACTIONS

No health hazards or side effects are known in conjunction with the proper administration of designated therapeutic dosages of the dehydrated drug. Extended skin contact with the freshly harvested, bruised plant can lead to blister formation and cauterizations that heal poorly, due to the released protoanemonine, which is severely irritating to the skin and mucous membranes. If taken internally, severe irritation to the gastrointestinal tract, combined with colic and diarrhea, as well as irritation of the urinary drainage passages, are possible.

Symptomatic treatment for external contact consists of mucilaginosa, after irrigation with diluted potassium permanganate solution. In case of internal contact, administration of activated charcoal should follow gastric lavage.

OVERDOSAGE

Death by asphyxiation following the intake of large quantities of protoanemonine-forming plants has been observed in animal experiments. The risk associated with use of this plant is less than that of many other Ranunculaceae (e.g., Anemones nemorosae) due to the relatively low levels of protoanemonine-forming agents.

DOSAGE

Mode of Administration: The drug is seldom used today. It is available in the form of decoctions, which are used for poultices, as well as extracts and drops.

Storage: The herb should be stored in tightly sealed containers.

LITERATURE

But PP, Cheng L, Kwok IM. Instant methods to spot-check poisonous podophyllum root in herb samples of clematis root. *Vet Hum Toxicol*, 200:366, 1997 Dec.

Kizu H, Shimana H, Tomimori T, Studies on the constituents of Clematis species. VI. The constituents of Clematis stans Sieb. et Zucc. *Chem Pharm Bull* (Tokyo), 43:2187-94, 1995 Dec.

Ruijgrok HWL, *PM* 11:338-347. 1963.

Shropshire CM, Stauber E, Arai M, Evaluation of selected plants for acute toxicosis in budgerigars. *J Am Vet Med Assoc*, 200:936-9, 1992 Apr 1.

Southwell IA et al., Protoanemonin in Australian Clematis. In: *PH* 33:1099. 1993.

Clematis recta

See Clematis

Clematis vitalba

See Traveller's Joy

Clove

Syzygium aromaticum

DESCRIPTION

Medicinal Parts: The medicinal parts are the oil extracted from the whole or macerated flower buds, the pedicles and leaves, the dried flower buds, and the not-quite-ripe fruit.

Flower and Fruit: The flowers are in triple-branched cymes. They are short-pedicled, whitish-pink, approximately 6 mm wide, and have 2 scalelike bracteoles. The calyx tube is 1 to 1.5 cm long and cylindrical. The 4 sepals are fleshy and there are 4 petals. The fruit is 2 to 2.5 cm long, 1.3 to 1.5 cm wide, and is crowned by 4 curved sepals. The fruit has a single seed.

Leaves, Stem, and Root: The plant is a 20 m high, pyramid-shaped evergreen tree. The diameter of the trunk is 40 cm. The branches are almost round. The leaves are 9 to 12 cm long and 3.5 cm wide. They are coriaceous, elliptical to lanceolate, short, obtusely tipped, and narrowing in a cuneate form to the petiole, which is 2.5 cm long. There is 1 main rib and more than 20 lateral ones.

Characteristics: The taste and odor are characteristic.

Habitat: The plant is indigenous to the Molucca Islands and is cultivated there and in Tanzania, Madagascar, Brazil, and other tropical regions.

Production: Cloves consist of the hand-picked and dried flower buds of *Syzygium aromaticum* (syn. *Jambosa caryophyllus, Eugenia caryophyllata*).

ACTIONS AND PHARMACOLOGY

COMPOUNDS

Volatile oil (15-21%): chief components eugenol (70-90%), eugenyl acetate (aceteugenol, up to 17%), beta-caryophyllene (5-12%)

Flavonoids: including astragalin, isoquercitrin, hyperoside, quercetin-3,4′-di-O-glycoside

Tannins (10%): ellagitannins, including eugenin

Triterpenes: oleanolic acid (1%), crataegolic acid (maslic acid, 0.15%)

Steroids: sterols, including beta-sitosterol

EFFECTS

Very few clinical trials have been done using clove; however, the preclinical data looks promising for the use of clove extracts as an antimicrobial/antiviral agent, antithrombotic, and hepatoprotective agent. Extract from clove has been historically used to prevent dental pain. One clinical trial showed that a topical cream containing clove was effective in relieving headache when rubbed on the temples (Schattner & Randerson, 1996).

Clove oil has been found to be an inhibitor of cyclooxygenase thus altering arachidonic acid metabolism. This activity is also seen in drugs used to treat arthritis, thrombosis and atherosclerosis, dysmenorrhea, and cancer (Mustafa & Srivastava, 1990). It also has an effect on drug metabolizing enzymes; however, it is not yet established whether this is a positive or negative effect.

The main constituent of clove is eugenol. Clove and/or eugenol are also found in the chewing product, betel quid, as well as clove cigarettes also known as kretek. Eugenol is also high in cinnamon, nutmeg, and basil.

Analgesic Effects: Patch-clamp experiments showed that eugenol reversibly activates calcium ion channels and chloride ion channels in dorsal root ganglion cells from rats. The response was partially blocked by a capsaicin receptor antagonist. Eugenol action may have two mechanisms, one through interaction with capsaicin receptors and one independent of capsaicin-receptors. Eugenol concentrations used were from 0.125 to 1 mmol/liter (Ohkubo & Kitamura, 1997).

Anti-inflammatory Effects: Eugenol from clove oil inhibited neutrophil migration to the chemo-attractant, N-formyl methionyl-leucyl-phenylalanine (FMLP). Inhibition was concentration-dependent, reversible and did not disrupt membrane integrity. Of the phenolic compounds tested, thymol, menthol, eugenol, safrole, guaiacol, and veratrole; eugenol was the most potent (Azuma et al, 1986).

Antimicrobial: Both an aqueous and an ethanol extract of clove had antimicrobial activity against penicillin-resistant *Staphylococcus aureus.* (Perez & Anesini, 1994). Several compounds isolated from clove exhibited growth-inhibitory activity towards oral pathogens associated with dental caries and periodontal disease (Cai & Wu, 1996). Oil of clove showed a wide spectrum of antibacterial activity towards enteropathogenic and spoilage bacterial strains. Clove oil was most effective against *Branhamella catarrhalis* with a minimum inhibitory concentration of 0.025 mg/mL. Activity was also demonstrated against *Staphylococcus aureus, Sarcina lutea, Bacillus subtillis, Klebsiella pneumoniae, Escherichia coli, Bordetella bronchiseptica*, and *Moraxella glucidolytica* (Ramanoelina et al, 1987).

Both oil of clove and purified eugenol demonstrated antimicrobial activity *towards Candida albicans, Staphlococcus aureus, Klebsiella pneumoniae, Escherichia coli, Pseudomonas aeruginosa*, and *Clostridium perfringens* (Briozzo et al, 1989).

Antiviral Effects: The active ingredient from both cloves (*Syzygium aromaticum*) and *Geum japonica* was found to be the phenolic compound eugeniin. Its mode of action was shown to be inhibition of viral DNA polymerase. Purified eugeniin exhibited antiviral activity by reducing the viral yield of four different strains of HSV-1, with a 50% effective dose of 5 mg/mL. The cytotoxic dose was much higher at 66 to 77 mg/mL. Eugeniin inhibited both DNA and protein synthesis in these viral strains. Furthermore, eugeniin was found to inhibit partially purified HSV-1 DNA polymerase and to a lesser extent, cellular DNA polymerases alpha and beta. These studies suggest that the mode of action of eugeniin may be different from the herpes drugs acyclovir or phosphonoacetic acid and thus may be useful in combination (Kurokawa et al, 1998).

Aqueous extract of clove exhibited an effect against HSV-1 activity in mice by decreasing skin lesions and delaying death (Kurokawa et al, 1995). In a separate study, aqueous extracts from clove inhibited recurrent HSV-1 infection in mice (Kurokawa et al, 1997).

Chemopreventive Effects: Eugenol, a component of clove oil, was found to be antimutagenic in the Ames Salmonella assay system against tobacco extract (Sukumaran & Kuttan, 1995). In a separate study, methanol extracts from clove inhibited cell growth and induced differentiation of myeloid leukemia cell lines into macrophages. The active ingredients were found to be oleanolic acid and crategolic acid. Both displayed optimum activity at a concentration of 20 micromolar. Induction of differentiation to a normal cell type can define an anticancer agent (Umehara et al, 1992).

Hepatoprotective Effects: Eugenol may protect the liver from damage by certain chemicals, including carbon tetrachloride and iron overload. The mechanism may involve eugenol acting both as an antioxidant to prevent lipid peroxidation and by scavenging free radicals by conjugating with glutathione. In an animal study, eugenol reduced the hepatic injury caused by iron overload. Eugenol lowered liver lipid peroxidation by 38% and serum lipid peroxidation by 30% in iron-treated rats (Reddy & Lokesh, 1996).

Neuroprotective Effects: In vitro studies indicate that clove oil may be neuroprotective. Eugenol provided neuroprotection against N-methyl-D-aspartate (NMDA)-induced and xanthine/xanthine oxidase-induced neurotoxicity in mice cortical cell cultures (Wie et al, 1997).

Platelet Aggregation Inhibition: Animal and in vitro data indicate that clove oil may be useful as an antithrombotic agent. Rabbits pretreated with clove oil were protected from sudden death caused by injection of arachidonic acid or platelet activating factor (PAF). This indicates a potential use of clove oil as an antithrombotic agent (Saeed & Gilani, 1994).

CLINICAL TRIALS

Dry Socket Pain

A clinical trial found that a collagen paste (Formula K) was more effective than the traditional zinc oxide mixed with oil of clove, or eugenol, for the treatment of dry socket. Following removal of a tooth, 151 patients who presented with dry socket were treated; 100 had their gum cavity filled with Formula K and 51 had their gum cavity filled with zinc oxide/eugenol pack. Fewer percentage of the patients in the Formula K group had pain or returned for repacking their socket, while a greater percentage of the zinc oxide/eugenol group had a tissue reaction. The authors note that although the Formula K probably provides a good biological matrix for tissue growth, it has no antibacterial qualities (Mitchell, 1986).

Headache Pain

A randomized, double-blind clinical trial showed that a clove oil-containing ointment was effective in treating tension headache. Fifty-seven patients were randomized to receive either the topical clove oil-containing ointment known as Tiger Balm, placebo topical treatment containing mint essence, or the drug paracetamol given orally. Patients rubbed the ointment onto the temple at 0, 30, and 60 minutes. The paracetamol treatment group took a single dose of 1000 mg. Patients recorded their results in a questionnaire at 5, 15, and 30 minutes and 1, 2, and 3 hours after treatment began. The Tiger Balm treatment group showed significant ($p<0.05$) improvement in headache compared to placebo from 5 minutes to 2 hours. Although both the Tiger Balm group and the paracetamol group received relief from symptoms, the Tiger Balm group had a more rapid decrease in headache symptoms. No adverse effects were found in any treatment group (Schattner & Randerson, 1996).

INDICATIONS AND USAGE

Approved by Commission E:

- Dental analgesic
- Inflammation of the mouth and pharynx

Unproven Uses: Clove oil is used internally for stomach ulcers and externally for colds and headaches. It is also used externally as a local analgesic and dental antiseptic.

Indian Medicine: The drug is used for halitosis, toothache, eye disease, flatulence, colic, gastropathy, and anorexia.

PRECAUTIONS AND ADVERSE REACTIONS

No health hazards or side effects are known in conjunction with the proper administration of designated therapeutic dosages. Allergic reactions to eugenol occur rarely. In concentrated form, oil of clove may be irritating to mucosal tissues (Blumenthal et al, 1998). Contact dermatitis is also possible.

Most of the adverse effects reported are due to the ingestion or inhalation of clove oil (Guidotti et al, 1987; Hartnoll et al, 1993; Brown et al, 1992). Mild hypertension has resulted in dogs after receiving 0.05 mL of eugenol.

Cytotoxic Effects: Cytotoxicity of eugenol was reduced by the use of antioxidants. Eugenol at 2 millimolar was lethal to human salivary gland tumor cell line and human oral squamous carcinoma cell line (Satoh et al, 1998). Eugenol can form an adduct with the amino acids lysine and arginine as well as with glutathione. This explains a possible mechanism of conjugation for eugenol to proteins and thus a toxicological reaction involving eugenol or its oxidation products (Medeiros et al, 1996).

Eugenol inhibited in vitro growth of dental pulp cells by 50% at a concentration of 0.6 millimolar (Kasugai et al, 1990). Higher levels of eugenol were cytotoxic to oral mucosal fibroblasts, whereas lower concentrations provided anti-oxidant activity (Jeng et al, 1994).

Hypersensitivity: Cloves can initiate both immediate and delayed-type hypersensitivity. Twelve percent of patients ($n=103$) suspected of contact allergy reacted positively for cloves (van den Akker et al, 1990). Out of 21 industrial workers exposed to clove, 16 (76%) had symptoms. These included smarting of the nostrils and eyes and a cough. These symptoms were transient and went away when the workers were home. The workers were mostly involved in grinding spices (Uragoda, 1992).

Respiratory Effects: A 17-year-old male high-school student died of rapidly progressive inflammatory lung disease that developed hours after smoking a clove cigarette. The student was recovering from a lower respiratory infection at the time. The California Department of Health Service and Centers for Disease Control collected 110 cases of clove cigarette toxicity by 1984, two of which were fatal. Clove cigarettes have been reported to cause acute respiratory problems in humans that rapidly progress to hemorrhagic pulmonary edema or pneumonia (Guidotti et al, 1987). During 1984 and 1985, the Centers for Disease Control received 11 case reports of clove cigarette smoking-associated acute respiratory system injury in adolescents and young adults; two deaths were also reported. The reported respiratory adverse effects included hemoptysis, bronchospasm, hemorrhagic and nonhemorrhagic pulmonary edema, pleural effusion, respiratory insufficiency, respiratory infection, and aspiration of foreign material (Pruitt et al, 1991; CDC, 1985). Clove affects cellular respiration as well. Eugenol inhibits cytochrome oxidase, thus poisoning the mitochondria (Guidotti et al, 1987).

DRUG INTERACTIONS

MODERATE RISK

Anticoagulants, Antiplatelet Agents, Thrombolytic Agents, and Low Molecular Weight Heparins: Concurrent use may result in increased risk of bleeding. *Clinical Management:* Avoid concomitant use. If both are taken together monitor the patient closely for signs and symptoms of bleeding.

Phenytoin Assay: May result in a false increase in phenytoin levels. *Clinical Management:* A different assay method may be necessary.

OVERDOSAGE

The 50% lethal dose (LD50) of eugenol for mice was found to be 1110 mg/kg of body weight for intraperitoneal injection. No lethality was found when eugenol was administered orally to mice (Woolverton et al, 1986).

DOSAGE

Mode of Administration: As a powdered, ground, or whole herb for the recovery of the essential oil, and other galenic preparations for topical use.

Daily Dosage: Aqueous solutions corresponding to 1 to 5% essential oil are used externally for mouthwashes. In dentistry, the undiluted essential oil is used. Toothache or gum inflammation: apply oil of clove directly to the site (Curtis, 1990). For headache pain, apply Tiger Balm ointment directly to temples (Schattner & Randerson, 1996).

Storage: Do not store the drug in plastic containers, and protect it from light.

LITERATURE

Anon. Council on Scientific Affairs: Evaluation of the health hazard of clove cigarettes. *JAMA* 260(24):3641-3644. 1988

Azuma Y, Ozasa N, Ueda Y et al. Pharmacological studies on the anti-inflammatory action of phenolic compounds. *J Dent Res* 1986; 65(1):53-56. 1986

Babich H, Stern A, Borenfreund E, Eugenol cytotoxicity evaluated with continuous cell lines. Toxic In Vitro; 7:105-109. 1993

Bodell WJ, Ye Q, Pathak DN et al. Oxidation of eugenol to form DNA adducts and 8-hydroxy-2′-deoxyguanosine: role of quinone methide derivative in DNA adduct formation. *Carcinogenesis;* 19(3):437-443. 1998

Briozzo J, Nunez L, Chirife J, et al. Antimicrobial activity of clove oil dispersed in a concentrated sugar solution. *J Appl Bacteriol;* 66(1):69-75. 1989

Brown SA, Biggerstaff J, Savidge GF. Disseminated intravascular coagulation and hepatocellular necrosis due to clove oil. *Blood Coagul Fibrinolysis;* 3(5):665-668. 1992

Cai L, Wu C. Compounds from *Syzygium aromaticum* possessing growth inhibitory activity against oral pathogens. *J Nat Prod;* 59:987-990. 1996

Centers for Disease Control (CDC). Clove cigarettes associated illness. *MMWR;* 34:297-299. 1985

Curtis EK. In pursuit of palliation: oil of cloves in the art of dentistry. *Bull Hist Dent;* 38(2):9-14. 1990

Debelmas AM, Rochat J. *Plant Med Phytother;* 1:23. 1967

Deiniger R. Gewürznelken (*Syzygium aromaticum*) und Nelkenöl - aktuelle Phytopharmaka. ZPT; 12(6):205. 1992

Fischer IU, von Unruh GE, Dengler HJ. The metabolism of eugenol in man. *Xenobiotica;* 20(2):209-222. 1990

Guidotti TL, Binder S, Stratton JW et al. Clove cigarettes: development of the fad and evidence for health effects. In: Hollinger MA (ed): Current Topics in Pulmonary Pharmacology and Toxicology, Vol 2. Elsevier Science Publishing Co, Inc, New York, NY, USA. 1-19. 1987

Hartnoll G, Moore D, Douek D. Near-fatal ingestion of oil of cloves. *Arch Dis Child;* 69(3):392-393. 1993

Jeng JH, Hahn LJ, Lu FJ et al. Eugenol triggers different pathobiological effects on human oral mucosal fibroblasts. *J Dent Res;* 73(5):1050-1055. 1994

Jones MD Jr., Helfer RE. A teething lotion resulting in the misdiagnosis of diphenylhydantoin administration. *Am J Dis Child;* 122(3):259-60. 1971

Kasugai S, Hasegawa N, Ogura H. A simple in vitro cytotoxicity test using the MTT (3-(4,5)-dimethylthiazol-2-yl)-2,5-diphenyl tetrazolium bromide) colorimetric assay: analysis of eugenol toxicity on dental pulp cells (RPC-C2A). *Jpn J Pharmacol;* 52(1):95-100. 1990

Kumaravelu P, Dakshinamoorthy DP, Subramaniam S, et al. Effect of eugenol on drug-metabolizing enzymes of carbon tetrachloride-intoxicated rat liver. *Biochem Pharmacol;* 49(11):1703-1707. 1995

Kumari MVR. Modulatory influences of clove (*Caryophyllus aromaticus, L*) on hepatic detoxification systems and bone marrow genotoxicity in male Swiss albino mice. *Cancer Lett;* 60(1):67-73. 1991

Kurokawa M, Nagasaka K, Hirabayashi T, et al. Efficacy of traditional herbal medicines in combination with acyclovir against herpes simplex virus type 1 infection in vitro and in vivo. *Antiviral Res;* 27(1-2):19-37. 1995

Kurokawa M, Nakano M, Ohyama H, et al. Prophylactic efficacy of traditional herbal medicines against recurrent herpes simplex virus type 1 infection from latently infected ganglia in mice. *J Dermatol Sci;* 14(1):76-84. 1997

Kurokawa M, Hozumi T, Basnet P et al. Purification and characterization of eugeniin as an anti-herpes virus compound from *Geum japonicum* and *Syzygium aromaticum. J Pharmacol Exp Ther;* 284(2):728-735. 1998

Lane BW, Ellenhorn MJ, Hulbert TV, et al. Clove oil ingestion in an infant. *Hum Exp Toxicol;* 10(4):291-294. 1991

Ludvigson HW, Rottman TR. Effects of ambient odors of lavender and cloves on cognition, memory, affect and mood. *Chem Senses;* 14:525-536. 1989

Medeiros MHG, Di Mascio P, Pinto AP et al. Horseradish peroxidase-catalyzed conjugation of eugenol with basic amino acids. *Free Radic Res;* 25(1):5-12. 1996

Mitchell R. Treatment of fibrinolytic alveolitis by a collagen paste (Formula K): a preliminary study. *Int J Oral Maxillofac Surg;* 15(2):127-133. 1986

Mizutani T, Satoh K, Nomura H et al. Hepatotoxicity of eugenol in mice depleted of glutathione by treatment with DL-buthionine sulfoximine. *Res Commun Chem Pathol Pharmacol;* 71(2):219-230. 1991

Mustafa T, Srivastava KC. Possible leads for arachidonic acid metabolism altering drugs from natural products. *J Drug Dev;* 3:47-60. 1990

Nagababu E, Sesikeran B, Lakshmaiah N. The protective effects of eugenol on carbon tetrachloride induced hepatotoxicity in rats. *Free Radic Res;* 23(6):617-627. 1995

Naidu KA. Eugenol - an inhibitor of lipoxygenase-dependent lipid peroxidation. *Prostaglandins Leukot Essent Fatty Acids;* 53(3):381-383. 1995

Narayanan CS, Matthew AG. *Ind Perf;* 29(1/2):15. 1985

Norred CL, Brinker F. Potential coagulation effects of preoperative complementary and alternative medicines. *Alt Ther;* 7(6):58-67. 2001

Ohkubo T, Kitamura K. Eugenol activates Ca(2+)-permeable currents in rat dorsal root ganglion cells. *J Dent Res;* 76(11):1737-1744. 1997

Perez C, Anesini C. Antibacterial activity of alimentary plants against Staphylococcus aureus growth. *Am J Chin Med;* 22(2):169-174. 1994

Phillips DH. Further evidence that eugenol does not bind to DNA in vivo. *Mutat Res;* 245(1):23-26. 1990

Pruitt AW, Jacobs EA, Schydlower M et al. Hazards of clove cigarettes. *Pediatrics;* 88:395-396. 1991

Ramanoelina AP, Terrom GP, Bianchini JP, et al. Contribution a l'etude de l'action antibacterienne de quelques huiles essentielles extraites de plantes malgaches. *Arch Inst Pasteur Madagascar;* 53(1):217-226. 1987

Reddy AP, Lokesh BR. Effect of curcumin and eugenol on iron-induced hepatic toxicity in rats. *Toxicology;* 107(1):39-45. 1996

Reddy AP, Lokesh BR. Studies on anti-inflammatory activity of spice principles and dietary n-3 polyunsaturated fatty acids on carrageenan-induced inflammation in rats. *Ann Nutr Metab;* 38(6):349-358. 1994

Reddy AP, Lokesh BR. Studies on spice principles as antioxidants in the inhibition of lipid peroxidation of rat liver microsomes. *Mol Cell Biochem;* 111(1-2):117-124. 1992

Reynolds JEF (ed). Martindale. The Extra Pharmacopoeia (electronic version). MICROMEDEX, Inc., Englewood, Colorado, USA. 1999

Rompelberg CM, Evertz SJ, Bruijntjes-Rozier GM et al. Effect of eugenol on the genotoxicity of established mutagens in the liver. *Food Chem Toxicol;* 34(1):33-42. 1996

Rompelberg CM, Ploemen JM, Jespersen S et al. Inhibition of rat, mouse, and human glutathione S-transferase by eugenol and its oxidation products. *Chem Biol Interact;* 99(1-3):85-97. 1996

Rompelberg CM, Vogels JE, de Vogel N et al. Effect of short-term dietary administration of eugenol in humans. *Hum Exp Toxicol;* 15(2):129-135. 1996

Saeed SA, Gilani AH. Antithrombotic activity of clove oil. *J Pak Med Assoc;* 44(5):112-115. 1994

Satoh K, Sakagami H, Yokoe I et al. Interaction between eugenol-related compounds and radicals. *Anticancer Res;* 18(1A):425-428. 1998

Schattner P, Randerson D. Tiger Balm(R) as a treatment of tension headache: a clinical trial in general practice. *Aust Fam Physician;* 25(2):216-222. 1996

Sharma JN, Srivastava KC, Gan EK. Suppressive effects of eugenol and ginger oil on arthritic rats. *Pharmacology;* 49(5):314-318. 1994

Srivastava KC. Antiplatelet components from common food spice clove (*Eugenia caryophyllata*) and their effects on prostanoid metabolism. *Planta Med;* 56:501-502. 1990

Srivastava KC. Antiplatelet principles from a food spice clove (*Syzgium-aromaticum L*). *Prostaglandins Leukot Essent Fatty Acids;* 48(5):363-372. 1993

Srivastava KC, Justesen U. Inhibition of platelet aggregation and reduced formation of thromboxane and lipoxygenase products in platelets by oil of cloves. *Prostaglandins Leukot Essent Fatty Acids;* 29(1):11-18. 1987

Srivastava KC, Malhotra N. Acetyl eugenol, a component of oil of cloves (*Syzygium aromaticum L*) inhibits aggregation and alters arachidonic acid metabolism in human blood platelets. *Prostaglandins Leukot Essent Fatty Acids;* 42(1): 73-81.1991

Sukumaran K, Kuttan R. Inhibition of tobacco-induced mutagenesis by eugenol and plant extracts. *Mutat Res;* 343(1):25-30. 1995

Tanaka T, Orii Y, Nonaka GI et al. Syziginins A and B, two ellegitannins from *Syzygium aromaticum;* PH 43(6)1345-1348. 1996

Umehara K, Takagi R Kuroyanagi M et al. Studies on differentiation-inducing activities of triterpenes. *Chem Pharm Bull;* (Tokyo) 40(2):401-405. 1992

Uragoda CG. Symptoms in spice workers. *J Trop Med Hyg;* 95(2):136-139. 1992

Van den Akker TW, Roesyanto-Mahadi ID, van Toorenenbergen AW, et al. Contact allergy to spices. *Contact Dermatitis;* 22(5):267-272. 1990

Warin RP, Smith RJ. Chronic urticaria investigations with patch and challenge tests. *Contact Dermatitis;* 8(2):117-121. 1982

Wie M-B, Won M-H, Lee K-H et al. Eugenol protects neuronal cells from excitoxic and oxidative injury in primary cortical cultures. *Neurosci Lett;* 225(2):93-96. 1997

Woolverton C, Fotos P, Mokas MJ et al. Evaluation of eugenol for mutagenicity by the mouse micronucleus test. *J Oral Pathol;* 15(8):450-453. 1986

Wright SE, Baron DA, Heffner JE. Intravenous eugenol causes hemorrhagic lung edema in rats: proposed oxidant mechanisms. *J Lab Clin Med;* 125(2):257-264. 1995

Yukawa TA, Kurokawa M, Sato H et al. Prophylactic treatment of cytomegalovirus infection with traditional herbs. *Antiviral Res;* 32(2):63-70.1996

Club Moss

Lycopodium clavatum

DESCRIPTION

Medicinal Parts: The medicinal parts are the spores and the fresh plant.

Flower and Fruit: Sulfur yellow, minute spores, carried in large numbers in 2 to 3 cylindrical yellow-green cones, develop in August at the ends of leafy, 15-cm high stalks extending from aerial branches.

Leaves, Stem and Root: The plant has a 1 m long, procumbent stem with only a few roots. It is covered with yellowish-green leaves, densely arranged in spirals, which are entire-margined, linear, smooth, and end in a long, white, upwardly bent hair tip. There are numerous erect, circular, 5 cm high branches on the main stem.

Habitat: The plant is found worldwide, but it originated in China and Eastern Europe.

Production: Club Moss is the aerial part *Lycopodium clavatum.* It is collected in the uncultivated regions and air-dried or dried artificially at a maximum of 40° C.

Other Names: Stags Horn, Witch Meal, Wolfs Claw, Vegetable Sulfur

ACTIONS AND PHARMACOLOGY

COMPOUNDS

Alkaloids (0.2%): including among others those of the lycopodine- and lycodan-types (derived from piperidine alkaloids), chief alkaloids lycopodine and dihydrolycopodine, in traces also nicotine.

Triterpenes: including alpha-onocerin, lycoclavatol, lycoclavanol, serratendiol (demonstrated in plants of Japanese origin)

Steroids: including beta-sitosterol, campesterol and stigmasterol

Flavonoids: including among others chrysoeriol, luteolin

EFFECTS

Club Moss has a diuretic effect.

INDICATIONS AND USAGE

Unproven Uses: In folk medicine, it is used internally for bladder and kidney complaints, also for pharyngeal catarrh and tonsillitis, menstruation complaints, rheumatism, and impotence; externally for wounds, itching and suppurating eczema of the skin.

Homeopathic Uses: Herb and spores are used in liver and gallbladder complaints, general blood poisoning, inflammation of the respiratory tract, disorders of the intestinal tract, varicose veins, metabolic diseases, chronic and acute skin conditions, inflammation of the female genital organs and menstruation complaints, as well as behavioral and mood disturbances.

PRECAUTIONS AND ADVERSE REACTIONS

No health hazards or side effects are known in conjunction with the proper administration of designated therapeutic dosages. Irritations should be expected with extended used of the drug.

OVERDOSAGE

Despite the toxicity of the alkaloids, no poisonings have been recorded.

DOSAGE

Mode of Administration: In folk medicine, chopped drug is used in teas.

How Supplied:

Tablets: 50 mg

Liquid Extract

Daily Dosage: Single dose: 1.5 gm drug. Tea: 1 cup to be taken 2 to 3 times daily.

Homeopathic Dosage: 5 drops, 1 tablet, or 10 globules every 30 to 60 minutes (acute) or 1 to 3 times daily (chronic); parenterally; 1 to 2 mL sc acute, 3 times daily; chronic: once a day (HAB1)

LITERATURE

Ansari FR, Ansari WH, Rahman W, Seligmann O, Chari VM, Wagner H, Österdahl BG. A New Acylated Apigenin 4'-O-?-D-glucoside from the Leaves of Lycopocium clavatum L., *Planta Med.* 1979; 36:196-199.

Blumenkopf TA, Heathcock CH, The Alkaloids, Vol. 5, Ed. SW Pelletier, John Wiley 1985.

Kern W, List PH, Hörhammer L (Hrsg.), Hagers Handbuch der Pharmazeutischen Praxis, 4. Aufl., Bde. 1-8, Springer Verlag Berlin, Heidelberg, New York, 1969.

Leete E, The Alkaloids, Vol. 1, Ed. SW Pelletier, John Wiley 1983.

Madaus G, Lehrbuch der Biologischen Arzneimittel, Bde 1-3, Nachdruck, Georg Olms Verlag Hildesheim 1979.

Wichtl M (Hrsg.), Teedrogen, 4. Aufl., Wiss. Verlagsges. Stuttgart 1997.

Cnicus benedictus

See Blessed Thistle

Coca

Erythroxylum coca

DESCRIPTION

Medicinal Parts: The medicinal parts are the leaves of the coca bush.

Flower and Fruit: The flowers are small and greenish white. They are in axillary clusters. The fruit is a red almost 1 cm long drupe with 1 seed.

Leaves, Stem, and Root: Erythroxylum coca is a small shrublike tree up to 5 m tall. The leaves are brownish-green, oval, thin but tough, up to 5 cm long and 2.5 cm wide with two lines on the surface parallel to the midrib. The margins are entire; the apex rounded. There are 2 faint projecting lines on the upper surface parallel to the midrib, which stiffen the leaf. There are small stipules in the leaf axils, which later become brown and hard.

Habitat: The plant is indigenous to the Andes region of South America; it is cultivated in Indonesia, India and Sri Lanka.

Production: Coca leaves are the dried leaves of *Erythroxylum coca.*

Other Names: Bolivian Coca, Cocaine, Cuca, Peruvian Coca

ACTIONS AND PHARMACOLOGY

COMPOUNDS

Tropane alkaloids: main alkaloid (-)-cocaine, including, among others, cis-cinnamoyl cocaine, trans-cinnamoyl cocaine, also including alpha-truxillin, beta-truxillin, benzoylecgonin

EFFECTS

The leaves act as a local anesthetic and stimulate the central nervous system. In high doses, the drug causes paralysis of motor neuron fibers.

INDICATIONS AND USAGE

Unproven Uses: The plant is used in the manufacture of the local anesthetic cocaine hydrochloride. It is a model for synthetic local anesthetics. Cocaine is still occasionally used in ophthalmology and for toothache and oral and pharyngeal mucosa irritation (as a gargle).

PRECAUTIONS AND ADVERSE REACTIONS

General: Chewing an excessively large quantity of the leaves can cause psychic disturbances and hallucinations. Chronic use can lead to poor nutritional states and disinterest in work, due to the suppression of feelings of hunger and the resulting reduction in food intake. The enhanced vulnerability to illness and the reduced life expectancy are also conditioned by the immunosuppressive effect of the drug. Beyond that, the drug is probably carcinogenic in effect, embryotoxic and sensitizing. The observed dependence on the drug (cocoaism) is mainly psychically conditioned, although withdrawal symptoms are also known (need for sleep, bulimia, anxiety, irritability, tremor). For the toxicology of cocaine, consult publications (Lewin, Teuscher).

Pregnancy: Cocaine passes into the embryo or fetus and is embryotoxic.

Nursing Mothers: Cocaine passes into the mother's milk.

DOSAGE

Mode of Administration: Use of Erythroxylum coca is obsolete except for use in 2% eyedrops.

LITERATURE

Aynilian G et al., (1974) *J Pharm Sci* 63:1938.

Brustschmerzen und Atherosklerose durch Cocain. In: *DAZ* 130(49):2723. 1990.

Chen GJ, Pillai R, Erickson JR, Martinez F, Estrada ALÖ, Watso RR, Cocaine immunotoxicity - abnormal cytokine production in hispanic drug users. In: *Toxicol Lett* 59(1-3):81. 1991.

Evans WC, *ETH* 3:265. 1981.

Grieb G, Mißbildungen: Schädigt Cocain menschliche Spermien? In: *DAZ* 132(12):578. 1992.

Homstedt B et al., (1977) *Phytochemistry* 16:1753.

Moore JM et al., 1-Hydroxytropacocaine: an abundant alkaloid of *Erythroxylum novogranatense* var. *novogranatense* and var. *truxillense*. In: *PH* 36(2):357. 1994.

Novak M, Salemink C, (1987) *Planta Med* 53(1):113.

Novak M, Salemink CA, Khan I, *ETH* 10:261. 1984.

Sukrasno N, Yeoman MM, Phenylpropanoid metabolism during growth and development of *Capsicum frutescens* fruits. In: *PH* 32:839. 1993.

Tuerner CE, Ma C, Elsohly *MA*, ETH 3:293. 1981.

Wiggins RC, Pharmacokinetics of Cocaine in pregnancy and effects on fetal maturation. In: *Clinical Pharmacokinetics* 22(2):85. 1992.

Cochlearia officinalis

See Scurvy Grass

Cochlospermum gossypium

See Cotton Tree

Cocillana Tree

Guraea rusbyi

DESCRIPTION

Medicinal Parts: The medicinal part of the plant is the bark.

Flower and Fruit: The flowers are radial, and their structures are in fives. They are white to yellowish and inconspicuous. The ovary is superior.

Leaves, Stem and Root: The plant grows as a tree, rising up to 5 m high. The leaves are large and pinnatifid.

Habitat: Guraea rusbyi is indigenous to Cuba, Brazil and Bolivia.

Production: Cocillana bark is the bark of the trunk of *Guarea rusbyi*, which is collected in the wild.

ACTIONS AND PHARMACOLOGY

COMPOUNDS

Volatile oil

Steroids: sterols, including beta-sitosterol

Tannin

Alkaloids

EFFECTS

The drug is said to be expectorate, emetic, and laxative in effect. In higher dosages, it is said to induce menstruation. The emetic effect is credited to the alkaloid fraction, which has not been more precisely defined. Experimental data have not been made available. The bark of the tree induces vomiting and can frequently bring on a feeling of weakness and nausea. But it can also provide a stimulatory expectorant and has been used successfully in the treatment of bronchitis and respiratory illnesses.

INDICATIONS AND USAGE

Unproven Uses: Uses in folk medicine have included treatment of chronic bronchitis and coughs and also as an emetic.

PRECAUTIONS AND ADVERSE REACTIONS

No health hazards are known in conjunction with the proper administration of designated therapeutic dosages. The drug is said to induce vomiting and diarrhea in high dosages.

CONTRAINDICATION

Because it is said to induce menstruation, it should not be administered to anyone who is pregnant.

DOSAGE

Mode of Administration: Whole, cut and powdered drug preparations for internal use.

Preparation: Tinctures are prepared using drug 1:10 60% ethanol (V/V) (BHP83). Liquid extracts contain drug 1:1 60% ethanol (V/V) (BHP83).

Daily Dosage:

Decoction: from 0.5 to 1 g drug, 3 times daily
Liquid extract: 0.5 to 1 mL, 3 times daily
Tincture: 5 to 10 mL, 3 times daily
Syrup: 2 to 4 mL, 3 times daily
Dose for children: 1/4 to 1/3 of the above doses.

LITERATURE

Blaschek W, Hänsel R, Keller K, Reichling J, Rimpler G, Schneider G (Eds), Hagers Handbuch der Pharmazeutischen Praxis. Folgebände 1 und 2. Drogen A-Z. Springer. Berlin, Heidelberg 1998.

Cocoa

Theobroma cacao

DESCRIPTION

Medicinal Parts: The medicinal parts are the seed skins that remain after making cocoa and cocoa butter; the seeds which have been partly freed from their skins and lightly roasted; and the raw, dried, unroasted seeds.

Flower and Fruit: The inflorescences are on the main trunk and thicker branches on a so-called "flower cup." The cymelike branchlets are short, nodded, and persistent. There are 5 sepals, which are narrow. The petals are cap-shaped and stemmed with flaglike laminas. The stamen tube, with 5 fertile stamens and 5 awl-shaped staminoids, is short. The fruit is a 15 to 25 cm long and 10 cm thick, large berry. It is oblong or obovate, thick-skinned, yellow or reddish, grooved and sometimes bumpy and cucumberlike. The 20 to 50 seeds are arranged in rows and embedded in a pink, fruity, sweetish-sour pulp. They are pressed flat, almond-shaped, reddish-brown and without endosperm.

Leaves, Stem and Root: The plant is a 4 to 6 m, occasionally up to 13 m, tall tree with an irregular knotty trunk and a broad crown. The young branches are rounded. The leaves are coriaceous or paperlike, alternate and in 2 rows on the branches. The petiole is downy, cushioned, and 1.5 to 2 cm long. The lamina is oval or elliptical, slightly asymmetrical, rounded at the base with a conspicuous tip. The upper surface is green and pale when dry. The lower surface is paler green, glabrous or has a few, tiny, simple, branched and scattered hairs.

Habitat: The plant is cultivated globally in tropical regions.

Production: Cocoa seeds consist of the seeds of *Theobroma cacao*, which have been removed from their shells, fermented and lightly roasted. Cocoa consists of the testae of *Theobroma cacao*. Cocoa butter is the hard fat obtained from the ripe cocoa seeds of *Theobroma cacao*. After removal of the germ-roots and the shell from the seeds, the seeds are removed from the shell and crushed. The cocoa fat is squeezed out at a temperature of 70° C to 80° C and allowed to cool.

Other Names: Cacao, Chocolate Tree

ACTIONS AND PHARMACOLOGY

COMPOUNDS: COCOA SEED

Purine alkaloids (3 to 4%): main alkaloid theobromine (2.8 to 3.5%), with a lesser amount of caffeine (0.1 to 0.4%)

Fat (50%): chief fatty acids oleic acid (33 to 39%), stearic acid (30 to 37%), palmitic acid (24 to 31%)

Proteic substances (10 to 16%)

Starch (5 to 9%)

Monosaccharides/oligosaccharides (2 to 4%): saccharose, glucose, fructose

Biogenic amines: including phenyl ethyl amine, tyramine, tryptamine, serotonin

Isoquinoline alkaloids: salsolinol

Catechin tannins (10%): including oligomeric proanthocyanidins (8%)

Oxalates (0.6 to 1%)

EFFECTS: COCOA SEED

Cocoa seeds can cause constipation because of the tannin content. The drug contains methylxanthines, mainly theobromin, which have a diuretic, broncholytic, and vasodilatory effect. They also stimulate cardiac muscle performance and act as a muscle relaxant.

COMPOUNDS: COCOA SEED COAT

Purine alkaloids: main alkaloid theobromine (0.4-1.2%) with less caffeine (0.02%)

Fat (5%)

Biogenic amine: including phenyl ethyl amine, tyramine, tryptamine, serotonin

Catechin tannins: among them, proanthocyanidins

EFFECTS: COCOA SEED COAT

Cocoa can cause constipation. Cocoa contains methylxanthines, which have a diuretic, bronchyolitic, and vasodilatory effect. They also improve cardiac muscle performance and act as a muscle relaxant.

COMPOUNDS: COCOA BUTTER

Triglycerides (melting temperature 31 to 35° C): chief fatty acids oleic acid (33 to 39%), stearic acid (30 to 37%), palmitic acid (24 to 31%)

Free fatty acids

Steroids: sterols, including beta-sitosterol

Purine alkaloids (0.001 to 0.1%)

EFFECTS: COCOA BUTTER

The main constituents are triglycerides. High doses of cocoa butter, in contrast to similar saturated fatty acids, do not cause an increase of serum cholesterol and the LDL fraction.

INDICATIONS AND USAGE

COCOA SEED

Unproven Uses: In folk medicine, Cocoa seeds are used for infectious intestinal disease, diarrhea, and as a secretolytic. It is also used to regulate the thyroid and as a mild stimulant (in compound drinks containing caffeine.)

COCOA SEED COAT

Preparations of cocoa seed coat are used for liver, bladder, and kidney ailments, diabetes, as a tonic and general remedy and as an astringent for diarrhea.

COCOA BUTTER

Cocoa Butter is used by the pharmaceutical and cosmetic industries as an inactive ingredient in dermatologic preparations.

PRECAUTIONS AND ADVERSE REACTIONS

COCOA SEED

General: No health hazards or side effects are known in conjunction with either the proper administration of designated therapeutic dosages or the consumption of normal amounts of chocolate products. Large dosages lead to constipation due to the tannin content. Cocoa and cocoa products can cause allergic reactions. The amines can trigger migraine attacks.

Pediatric Use: Large quantities of chocolate products can lead to overexcitability, racing pulse, and sleep disorders in children because of the caffeine content, which can be as high as 0.2% in milk chocolate and 0.4% in bitter chocolate.

COCOA SEED COAT

No health hazards or side effects are known in conjunction with the proper administration of designated therapeutic dosages. Cocoa and cocoa products can cause allergic reactions. Large dosages lead to constipation due to the tannin content. The amines can trigger migraine attacks.

COCOA BUTTER

No health hazards or side effects are known in conjunction with the proper administration of designated therapeutic dosages.

DOSAGE

COCOA BUTTER

Mode of Administration: Cocoa Butter is used as a pharmaceutical base for suppositories and vaginal globules. It is an additive for ointments and cosmetic preparations, such as skin creams and lip balms.

Storage: Store in a cool, dark place.

LITERATURE

Brown JP. A Review of the Genetic Effects of Naturally Occuring Flavonoids, Anthraquinones and Related Compounds. *Mutation Res.* 1980; 75:243-277.

Hänsel R, Keller K, Rimpler H, Schneider G (Hrsg.), Hagers Handbuch der Pharmazeutischen Praxis, 5. Aufl., Bde 4-6 (Drogen): Springer Verlag Berlin, Heidelberg, New York, 1992-1994.

Kaij-a-Kamb M, Amoros M, Girre L. Search for New Antiviral Agents of Plant Origin. *Pharm Acta Helv.* 1992; 67:130-147.

Leung AY, Encyclopedia of Common Natural Ingredients Used in Food Drugs and Cosmetics, John Wiley & Sons Inc., New York 1980.

Lewin L, Gifte und Vergiftungen, 6. Aufl., Nachdruck, Haug Verlag, Heidelberg 1992.

Osawa K, Matsumoto T, Maruyama T, Naito Y, Okuda K, Takazoe I. Inhibitory effects of aqueous extract of cacao bean husk on collagenase of *Bacteroides gingivalis. Bull Tokyo Dent Coll,* 31:125-8, 1990 May.

Roth L, Daunderer M, Kormann K, Giftpflanzen, Pflanzengifte, 4. Aufl., Ecomed Fachverlag Landsberg Lech 1993.

Schröder B, In: Schröder R, Kaffee, Tee und Kardamom, Ulmer-Verlag, Stuttgart. 1991.

Teuscher E, Biogene Arzneimittel, 5. Aufl., Wiss. Verlagsges. Stuttgart 1997.

Teuscher E, Lindequist U, Biogene Gifte - Biologie, Chemie, Pharmakologie, 2. Aufl., Fischer Verlag Stuttgart 1994.

Coconut Palm

Cocos nucifera

DESCRIPTION

Medicinal Parts: The medicinal part of the plant is the fruit.

Flower and Fruit: The flowers are arranged in up to 1.5 m long, spindle-shaped, branching axillary inflorescences, which are surrounded by a woody spathe. On each of the 20 to 40 lateral branches of the inflorescence there is only one 3 to 3.5 cm large, yellowish-green-white female flower. There are 200 to 300 male flowers at the apex of the single branches with their structures arranged in threes. The flowers are up to 1.5 cm wide and yellowish; the ovary is 3-carpeled and fused. The drupe is up to 30 cm long and weighs 1.5 to 2.5 kg. The exocarp is smooth and impervious to water. The mesocarp is fibrous (certain floating ability, coconut fiber) and the endocarp woody and hard. The stone kernel is incorrectly called a nut. The inconspicuous embryo is embedded in the fat rich endosperm (copra). Inside the unripe fruit there is approximately 500 ml of clear, sweet-tasting liquid (coconut milk), which reduces when the fruit ripens. At the side stem insert there are 3 shoot holes, only one of which is covered with a membrane. These allow the embryo to penetrate the surrounding fiber layer.

Leaves, Stem, and Root: Coconut Palm is diclinous and monoecious. The tree grows up to 30 to 35 m high. The frond is up to 5 m long, 1 to 1.7 m wide (up to 15 kg in weight) and clasps the trunk with a wide petiole. The bark is thick and the surface is shaggy with remains of the leaf bases of fallen leaves. The trunk is divided into nodes and internodes. Adventitious roots arise from the base of the trunk.

Characteristics: One palm tree produces up to 70 ripe fruit per year.

Habitat: The native country of this species is disputed, but is believed to be the Pacific regions.

Production: Coconut oil is the fat extracted from the dried solid part of the endosperm of *Cocos nucifera* through cold pressing. Completely ripe fruit is harvested, followed by manual or mechanical opening of the kernel and then followed by the extraction of the endosperm (known as copra). It is dried in the sun, over a fire, or in special drying houses. The pressed oil is refined and cleaned.

ACTIONS AND PHARMACOLOGY

COMPOUNDS

Fatty oil: chief fatty acids lauric acid (45 to 50%), myristic acid (13 to 20%), palmitic acid (7 to 10%), caprylic acid (5 to 10%), including as well stearic acid, linoleic acid, caproic acid.

Free fatty acids (3 to 5%)

Delta-lactones of 5-hydroxy-fatty acids: particularly delta-octalactone (as aroma compounds)

EFFECTS

Coconut oil is characterized by having a large quantity of short-chained fatty acids and a rather small amount of unsaturated fatty acids. It is chiefly used as a dietetic. An immunomodulating effect was observed in animal experiments, as was an inhibiting effect upon the growth of carcinoma cells of the colon in vitro.

INDICATIONS AND USAGE

Unproven Uses: The oil of Coconut Palm has been used for poorly healing wounds and skin infections (Africa). Internally it is used for colds and inflammation of the throat (with salt; Central America) and for tooth decay (southeast Asia).

Indian Medicine: Coconut Palm oil is used for dysuria, coughs, bronchitis, and to stop hair from turning gray.

PRECAUTIONS AND ADVERSE REACTIONS

No health hazards are known in conjunction with the use of the drug as a food or as a pharmaceutical vehicle or raw substance (including its use in the extraction of short- and medium-chained fatty acids and in the manufacture of soaps and solubilizing agents).

DOSAGE

Mode of Administration: Preparations are intended for internal and external use.

Storage: Protect from light in tightly sealed containers at a maximum temperature of 25° C.

LITERATURE

Eghafona NO, Immune responses following cocktails of inactivated measles vaccine and *Arachis hypogaea L.* (groundnut) or *Cocos nucifera L.* (coconut) oils adjuvant. *Vaccine*, 84:1703-6, 1996 Dec.

Jaggi KS, Arora N, Niphadkar PV, Gangal SV, Immunochemical characterization of *Cocos nucifera* pollen. *J Allergy Clin Immunol*, 84:378-85, 1989 Sep.

Karmakar PR, Chatterjee BP, *Cocos nucifera* pollen inducing allergy: sensitivity test and immunological study. *Indian J Exp Biol*, 84:489-96, 1995 Jul.

Kwon K, Park KH, Rhee KC. Fractionation and Characterization of Proteins from Coconut (*Cocos nucifera L.*). *J Agric Food Chem.* 44 (7); 1741-1745 (1996).

Nalini N, Sabitha K, Chitra S, Viswanathan P, Menon VP, Antifungal activity of the alcoholic extract of coconut shell - *Cocos nucifera Linn. J Ethnopharmacol*, 84:291-3, 1980 Sep.

Nalini N, Sabitha K, Chitra S, Viswanathan P, Menon VP, Histopathological and lipid changes in experimental colon cancer: effect of coconut kernel (*Cocos nucifera Linn.*) and (*Capsicum annum Linn.*) red chili powder. *Indian J Exp Biol*, 84:964-71, 1997 Sep.

Cocos nucifera

See Coconut Palm

Coffea arabica

See Coffee

Coffee

Coffea arabica

DESCRIPTION

Medicinal Parts: The medicinal part of the plant is the seed in various forms and stages.

Flower and Fruit: The inflorescences are axillary dense clusters with 10 to 20 flowers. The sessile or very short pedicled partial inflorescences bear dense, overlapping apical leaves. The calyx is 2.5 to 3 mm long with a blunt 5-tipped border. The corolla is white and fragrant. The stamens come from the mouth of the tube and are exserted. The ripe fruit is ellipsoid, 12 to 18 mm long by 12 to 15 mm wide with a 3 to 6 mm long stem. It is initially green, later yellow and dark red when ripe. The exocarp is tough and the mesocarp fleshy and slightly sweet. The endocarp is hard. The seeds are flat-convex with a groove on the flat adaxial side. They are 8 to 12 mm long, 5 to 8 mm wide and 3 to 5 mm thick. When fresh, the seeds are gray-green. They turn brown after roasting.

Leaves, Stem, and Root: Coffea arabica is an evergreen shrub or small tree up to 8 m high with many basal branches. The young branches are glabrous and flattened, and the nodes produce many shoots. The bark of the fruiting branches is ashy-white. The leaves are 6 to 20 cm long, 2.5 to 6 cm wide and live for 2 to 3 years. They are glabrous, slightly coriaceous, dark green, glossy and elliptoid-lanceolate, with a distinct leaf tip. The border is occasionally extensively ribbed.

Habitat: Coffee's area of origin is disputed, but it is now cultivated in many tropical regions of the world, including Brazil, Mexico, Columbia and Ethiopia.

Production: Coffee charcoal is produced by roasting the outer seed parts of the green, dried fruit of *Coffea arabica* (and other *Coffea* species) until almost black, then grinding the carbonized product.

Coffee beans are the seeds of *Coffea arabica*, which are ripe for harvest nine months after flowering. Thereafter, they are processed using one of two methods. In the dry method, the beans are dried for 3 to 4 weeks in the sun, or mechanically with air-stream dryers. In the wet method, the beans are placed in a water-filled tank, where only the ripe ones sink to the bottom. The ripe fruit is then mechanically crushed and subsequently fermented. Fermentation lasts for approximately 48 hours (for arabica varieties). Afterward, the coffee is dried mechanically or in the sun.

Not to be Confused With: Coffee beans are not easily confused with other drugs. However, ground and roasted coffee may contain coffee substitutes such as chicory, dandelion root, figs, sugar beet root, lupin seeds, rye kernels and barleycorn.

Other Names: Arabica Coffee, Arabian Coffee, Caffea

ACTIONS AND PHARMACOLOGY

COMPOUNDS: COFFEE CHARCOAL

Purine alkaloids: main alkaloid caffeine

Trigonelline

Carbonization products of hemicelluloses

EFFECTS: COFFEE CHARCOAL

Coffee charcoal contains purine alkaloids, with caffeine as the man constituent, and is absorbent and astringent.

COMPOUNDS: COFFEE BEANS (SEEDS)

Purine alkaloids: main alkaloid caffeine (0.6 - 2.2%), with it theobromine, theophylline

Caffeic and ferulic acid ester of quinic acid: in particular chlorogenic acid

Trigonelline

Norditerpene glycoside ester: atractylosides

Diterpenes: including the diterpene alcohol fatty acid esters kahweol and cafestol

In roasted coffee beans: numerous aromatic substances yielded from carbohydrates, proteins, fats and aromatic acids through pyrolysis

EFFECTS: COFFEE BEANS

Most of the indicated effects of coffee are due to the presence of caffeine. The primary effects of caffeine can be summarized as follows: Caffeine has a positive inotropic effect. In higher concentrations, it has a positive chronotropic effect on the heart and CNS. It causes a relaxation of the smooth muscles of blood vessels (except for cerebral blood vessels) and the bronchial tubes. Moreover, caffeine works as a short-lived diuretic and produces an increase of gastric secretions and the release of catecholamines.

Caffeine works competitively to block adenosinal receptors that lie on cell surfaces in the brain, fat tissue, liver, kidneys, heart, and erythrocytes.

Heart, circulation, vessels: People who normally do not drink coffee react 1 hour after an intake of 250 gm, with an increase of 10 mm Hg in their systolic blood pressure. Habitual coffee drinkers are tolerant in this regard.

Blood: After 9 weeks of an average daily intake of 5.6 cups of coffee (steeped for 10 min.), the overall and LDL cholesterol increases significantly. The use of coffee filters can reduce this by up to 80%.

Digestive tract: Oral intake of 200 mg of chlorogene acid doubles gastric secretion, as does caffeine alone.

Miscellaneous: In animal studies, a diet consisting of 20% green coffee impedes the growth of DMBA-induced tumors in hamsters by 90%.

Outcome of the stimulating effects of caffeine commence a few minutes subsequent to taking the drug. The maximum plasma concentration of caffeine is reached between 15 and 45 minutes later. The plasma half-life amounts to 4 to 6 hours.

Coffee extracts made from roasted and unroasted seeds are used analogously with other drugs containing caffeine for physical and mental fatigue. The drink can also be used therapeutically in cases of hypotonia, as an analeptic agent, in the treatment of influenza (flu) and migraine and as an additive to analgesia.

INDICATIONS AND USAGE

COFFEE CHARCOAL

Approved by Commission E:

- Diarrhea
- Inflammation of the mouth and pharynx

Unproven Uses: Coffee is used for nonspecific, acute diarrhea, and local therapy of mild inflammation of the oral and pharyngeal mucosa. In folk medicine coffee is also used for festering wounds.

COFFEE BEANS (SEEDS)

Unproven Uses: Coffee is used to treat hypotonia and as a constituent of analgesics. In folk medicine coffee is also used to increase performance capability as well as for anemia, hepatitis and edema.

Homeopathic Uses: Uses in homeopathy include insomnia and neuralgias.

Indian Medicine: Unripe seeds are used in Indian medicine for migraine and fever; ripe seeds for diarrhea; and strong coffee to treat opium and alcohol intoxication.

PRECAUTIONS AND ADVERSE REACTIONS

COFFEE CHARCOAL

General: Health risks or side effects following the proper administration of designated therapeutic dosages are not recorded.

COFFEE BEANS

General: Health risks following the proper administration of designated therapeutic dosages are not recorded. Quantities corresponding to as much as 500 mg caffeine daily (5 cups of coffee) spread out over the day are toxicologically harmless for healthy adults accustomed to drinking coffee. Caution is advised for persons with sensitive cardiovascular systems, kidney diseases, hyperfunction of the thyroid gland, higher disposition to convulsions and certain psychic disorders (for example, panic anxiety states). Side effects of coffee intake, mainly caused by its chlorogenic acid content, can include hyperacidity, stomach irritation, diarrhea and reduced appetite. Nonspecific symptoms such as restlessness, irritability, sleeplessness, palpitations, dizziness, vomiting, diarrhea, loss of appetite, and headache appear with the long-term intake of dosages exceeding 1.5 g caffeine per day. Caffeine can lead to psychic as well as physical dependency (caffeinism). Symptoms of withdrawal can include headache and sleeping disorders.

Pregnancy: Pregnant women should avoid caffeine, under no circumstances exceeding a dosage of 300 mg per day (3 cups of coffee spread out over the day).

Nursing Mothers: Infants nursing from mothers who take drinks containing caffeine may suffer from sleeping disorders.

DRUG INTERACTIONS

POTENTIAL INTERACTIONS

The drug may hinder the resorption of other medicines.

OVERDOSAGE

Dosages exceeding 1.5 g caffeine per day can lead to stiffness, arrhythmic spasms of different muscle groups, opisthotonus, and arrhythmic tachycardia. Fatal poisonings with the drug are not conceivable. The lethal dosage (LD50) for an adult is approximately 150 to 200 mg caffeine per kg body weight (for which 50 kg body weight = 7.5 g = 75 cups of coffee), although there are cases of survival also with 106 g caffeine. The death of a child following the intake of 5.3 g of caffeine has been reported. The first signs of poisonings are vomiting and abdominal spasms. The therapy for caffeine poisoning should begin with the inducement of vomiting or gastric lavage. Afterward, activated charcoal and sorbitol should be given to retard resorption. Spasms are to be treated with diazepam.

DOSAGE

COFFEE CHARCOAL

Mode of Administration: Powdered coffee charcoal and its preparations intended for internal consumption or local application.

Daily Dosage: The average daily dose for internal use is 9 g of ground drug. The average single dose is 3 g of powder.

Storage: Coffee charcoal should be stored in well-sealed containers.

COFFEE BEANS

Mode of Administration: The ground beans are used in different types of infusion, i.e., cooked coffee (filter, espresso, etc.). Caffeine is used in various combinations and preparations for numerous therapeutic uses. Commercial pharmaceutical preparations include tablets, coated tablets, compresses, and diverse compound preparations.

Preparation: The dried seeds are roasted until they procure a deep brown color and a characteristic aroma. This process is usually carried out in the country of consumption. During roasting, the beans float for 1.5 to 3 minutes in hot gas at 220°C to 270°C.

Daily Dosage: 15 g drug

Homeopathic Dosage: 5 drops, 1 tablet, or 10 globules every 30 to 60 minutes (acute) and 1 to 3 times daily (chronic); parenterally: 1 to 2 mL sc acute, 3 times daily; chronic: once a day (HAB1)

Storage: The beans should be stored in sealed containers away from light and moisture.

LITERATURE

COFFEE CHARCOAL

Kuhn A, Schäfer G, (Kaffeekohle). In: Dtsch Med Wochenschr 23:922-923. 1939.

COFFEE BEANS

Ajarem JS, Ahmad M. Teratopharmacological and Behavioral Effects of Coffee in Mice. *Acta Physiol Pharmacol Bulg.* 22; 51-61 (1996)

Bak AA, Grobbee DE. The effect on serum cholesterol levels of cofee brwed by filtering or boiling. *N Engl. J Med* (1989), 321: 1432-1437.

Balduini W, Cattabeni F. Displacement of (3H)-N6-cyclohexyladenosine binding to rat cortical membranes by an hydroalcoholic extract of Valeriana officinalis. Med Sci Res. 17; 639-640 (1989)

Butz S, Nurses'-Health-Studie: Kaffe - kein Risikofaktor für koronare Herzkrankheit? In: *DAZ* 136(19):1680-1582. 1996.

Coffein: Entzugssyndrom bei Kaffeetrinkern. In: *DAZ* 133(6):441. 1993.

Dieudonne S, Forero ME, Llano I, Lipid analysis of *Coffea arabica Linn.* beans and their possible hypercholesterolemic effects. *Int J Food Sci Nutr*, 159:135-9, 1997 Mar.

Fujimori N, Ashihara H. Biosynthesis of Theobromine and Caffeine in Developing Leaves of Coffea arabica. *Phytochemistry* 36; 1359-1361 (1994).

Garattini, Buch. In: Caffeine, Coffee, and Health. Garattini S. Monographs of the Mario Negri Institute for Pharmacological Research, Milan. Raven Press, New York. 1993.

Kokjohn K, Graham M, McGregor M. The effect of coffee consumption on serum cholesterol levels. *J Manipulative Physiol Ther* (1993), 16: 327-335

Martin E, Cholesterolspiegel erhöhender Faktor in Kaffeelipiden. In: *DAZ* 130(42):2376. 1990.

Mensink RP, Lebbink WJ, Lobbezoo IE, Weusten-Van der Wouw MP, Zock PL, Katan MB, Diterpene composition of oils from Arabica and Robusta coffee beans and their effects on serum lipids in man. *J Intern Med,* 237:543-50, 1995 Jun.

Phillips R, Smith D, Characterization of coffea canephora alpha-D-galactosidase blood group B activity. Artif Cells Blood *Substit Immobil Biotechnol*, 103:489-502, 1996 Sep.

Ponepal V, Spielberger U, Riedel-Caspari G, Schmidt FW, Use of *a Coffea arabica* tosta extract for the prevention and therapy of polyfactorial infectious diseases in newborn calves. DTW Dtsch Tierarztl Wochenschr, 103:390-4, 1996 Oct.

Ratnayake WM, Pelletier G, Hollywood R, Malcolm S, Stavric B, Investigation of the effect of coffee lipids on serum cholesterol in hamsters. *Food Chem Toxicol*, 33:195-201, 1995 Mar.

Schröder, Buch. In: Schröder R: Kaffee, Tee und Kardamom, Ulmer-Verlag, Stuttgart. 1991.

Schröder-Rosenstock K, Kaffeegenuβ - ein medizinisches Problem. In: DAZ 130(35):1919. 1990.

Silnermann K et al., (Entzugssymptome nach regelmäβigem Kaffeegenuβ). In: New Engl J Med 327:1109. 1992.

Cola

Cola acuminata

DESCRIPTION

Medicinal Parts: The seeds are the medicinal parts of the plant.

Flower and Fruit: The male flowers with a diameter of 1.5 cm or the androgynous flowers with a diameter of 2.5 cm are axillary or on branches in cymes of few flowers. The 5-part chalice-shaped perigone is white to yellow and marked with red on the inside. The star-shaped fruits have 5 coriaceous, thick, dark brown, unkeeled follicles arranged at right angles to the stem. The fruits grow up to 20 cm long and 5 cm wide. There are up to 14 ovate or square seeds of about 2.5 cm in diameter in 2 rows with a white fleshy seed shell. The seed kernel is usually reddish or red, occasionally white.

Leaves, Stem, and Root: The plant is an evergreen tree 15 to 20 m tall. The trunk is branched down as far as the base. The bark is dark green, rough and breaks off in pieces as it ages. Branches have leaves only at their ends. The tough coriaceous leaves are 15 to 18 cm long and 10 cm wide, elliptoid to ovate, and end in a curled and spiraled tip. Both sides are dark green and glossy.

Habitat: The plant is indigenous to Togo, Sierra Leone, and Angola. It is found today in all tropical regions and is cultivated widely.

Production: The ripe fruit is harvested and the seeds are removed and dried. Cola nut is the endosperm freed from the testa of various Cola species, particularly *Cola nitida.*

Not to be Confused With: Other varieties of Cola, such as Male kola which contains no caffeine.

Other Names: Kola Tree, Guru Nut, Cola Nut, Cola Seeds, Bissy Nut

ACTIONS AND PHARMACOLOGY

COMPOUNDS

Purine alkaloids: main alkaloid caffeine (0.6 - 3.7%), additionally theobromine, theophylline

(+)-catechin, (-)-epicatechin

Catechin tannins

Oligomeric proanthocyanidins

Starch

EFFECTS

Cola's purine (caffeine) content makes it a strong CNS stimulant. In humans it acts as a respiratory analeptic, lipolytic, mildly positively chronotropic, and mild diuretic. In addition, it stimulates gastric acid and increases motility of the gastrointestinal tract. In animal tests, Cola is also analeptic, lipolytic, stimulates production of gastric acid, and increases gastric motility.

INDICATIONS AND USAGE

Approved by Commission E:

- Lack of stamina

Unproven Uses: Cola is used internally to decrease mental and physical fatigue and to suppress hunger. In folk medicine it is chewed to prevent morning sickness and migraine. The powder is used for diarrhea. Externally, it is ground and made into poultices for wounds and inflammations. Cola is also an indigenous cult drug.

CONTRAINDICATIONS

Use of Cola is contraindicated during pregnancy. The drug should not be administered in the presence of stomach or duodenal ulcers, due to the drug's stimulation of gastric juice secretion.

PRECAUTIONS AND ADVERSE REACTIONS

Health risks following the proper administration of designated therapeutic dosages have not been recorded. Side effects that may occur include difficulty falling asleep, hyperexcitability, restlessness, and stomach complaints. Signs of poisoning following the intake of Cola drinks (20 to 60 mg caffeine per glass) or medications or stimulants containing Cola extracts are not expected. Small children should avoid the intake of large quantities of Cola drinks.

DOSAGE

Mode of Administration: Powdered drug and other galenic preparations for internal use.

How Supplied:

Capsules

Tablets

Tonics.

Preparation: Dry extract: from the percolation 1:1 with 45% ethanol; fluid extract: percolation with 70% ethanol (V/V); Cola tincture: 1:5 with 70% ethanol; Cola wine: 50 parts fluid Cola extract with 850 parts Xeres wine and 100 parts sugar syrup.

Daily Dosage: 2 to 6 g of Cola nut drug, usually taken 1 to 3 g, 3 times daily; 0.25 to 0.75 g of Cola extract; 2.5 to 7.5 g of Cola liquid extract; 10 to 30 g of Cola tincture; 60 to 180 g of Cola wine.

Storage: Cola should be protected from light in sealed containers.

LITERATURE

Hänsel R, Keller K, Rimpler H, Schneider G (Hrsg.), Hagers Handbuch der Pharmazeutischen Praxis, 5. Aufl., Bde 4-6 (Drogen): Springer Verlag Berlin, Heidelberg, New York, 1992-1994.

Leung AY, Encyclopedia of Common Natural Ingredients Used in Food Drugs and Cosmetics, John Wiley & Sons Inc., New York 1980.

Lewin L, Gifte und Vergiftungen, 6. Aufl., Nachdruck, Haug Verlag, Heidelberg 1992.

Madaus G, Lehrbuch der Biologischen Arzneimittel, Bde 1-3, Nachdruck, Georg Olms Verlag Hildesheim 1979.

Morton, JF, An Atlas of Medicinal Plants of Middle America, Charles C. Thomas USA 1981.

Oliver-Bever B (Ed.), Medicinal Plants of Tropical West Africa, Cambridge University Press Cambridge, London 1986.

Teuscher E, Lindequist U, Biogene Gifte - Biologie, Chemie, Pharmakologie, 2. Aufl., Fischer Verlag Stuttgart 1994.

Teuscher E, Biogene Arzneimittel, 5. Aufl., Wiss. Verlagsges. mbH Stuttgart 1997.

Cola acuminata

See Cola

Colchicum

Colchicum autumnale

DESCRIPTION

Medicinal Parts: The fresh flowers and the dried ripe seeds, collected in early summer and then sliced, as well as the tubers (fresh and dried) are the medicinal parts of the plant.

Flower and Fruit: The 5 to 20 cm flowers usually bloom in autumn. They are a bright lilac-pink, and appear solitary or in pairs from the corm. The 6 bracts of the involucre are fused into a long, narrow tube. The flower has 6 stamens and 3 threadlike styles. The ovaries are on the side of the corm. The 3-valved capsule is initially green, then turns brown and wrinkled. It contains black seeds with sticky appendages.

Leaves, Stem, and Root: Colchicum can grow to 40 cm in height. The 3 to 4 broadly lanceolate leaves are tuliplike; leaves appear together with the fruit in spring. They are 8 to 25 cm long, 2 to 4 cm wide and overlap at the base to form a tube.

Characteristics: All parts of the plant are very poisonous and have a disgustingly bitter taste.

Not to be Confused With: The tubers are sometimes confused with cooking onions.

Habitat: Colchicum autumnale is primarily a central European plant found in northern Ireland, England, northern Germany, southern Poland, the Ukraine, Bulgaria, Turkey, Albania, and northern Spain. It also grows in central Asia.

Production: Colchicum seeds are the dried seeds of *Colchicum autumnale* harvested in the wild in June or July and air-dried. Colchicum bulbs are the cut and dried tubers of the plant harvested in early summer. After the surrounding leaves have been removed, the tubers are cut into slices and dried at temperatures of 60°C or lower. Colchicum flowers are collected from the wild in late summer and autumn and then air-dried.

Other Names: Meadow Saffron, Meadow Saffran, Autumn Crocus, Naked Ladies, Upstart, Fall Crocus, Tuber-Root

ACTIONS AND PHARMACOLOGY

COMPOUNDS: COLCHICUM BULB

Tropolone alkaloids: colchicine, colchicoside and N-deacetyl-N-formyl-colchicine; companion alkaloids include demecolcine

Starch

COMPOUNDS: COLCHICUM SEEDS

Trupolone alkaloids: colchicine and colchicoside

Fatty oil

COMPOUNDS: COLCHICUM FLOWERS

Tropolone alkaloids: colchicine and N-deacetyl-N-formyl-colchicine, additional alkaloids including demecolcine

EFFECTS: COLCHICUM BULBS, SEEDS AND FLOWERS

Colchicum inhibits mitosis through the inhibition of motility, particularly of the phagocytosing lymphocytes. This is of therapeutic use for blocking the immigration and the autolysis of phagocytes in inflammatory processes and thereby producing an antiphlogistic effect.

INDICATIONS AND USAGE

COLCHICUM BULBS, SEEDS AND FLOWERS

Approved by Commission E:

■ Gout

■ Mediterranean fever (brucellosis)

Unproven Uses: Due to the plant's toxicity, internal application is seldom used with the exception of acute attacks of gout and familial Mediterranean fever (brucellosis). Efficacy for these uses appears plausible. The drug was previously used for skin tumors, condyloma, psoriasis, necrotic vasculitis, tendovaginitis, inflammation of the gastrointestinal tract, Behçet's disease, liver cirrhosis, acute and chronic leukemia; also for lice, asthma, dropsy, and rheumatism.

Homeopathic Uses: In addition to acute and chronic gout, Colchicum is also used for inflammation of the kidney and gastrointestinal tract, bodily secretions, tendovaginitis, and acute joint rheumatism. Efficacy has not been proved.

PRECAUTIONS AND ADVERSE REACTIONS

General: The drugs are severely poisonous. Signs of poisoning, including stomachaches, diarrhea, nausea, vomiting and, less frequently, stomach and intestinal hemorrhages, can occur even with the administration of therapeutic dosages.

Kidney and liver damage, hair loss, peripheral nerve inflammation, myopathia, and bone marrow damage with their resulting symptoms (leukopenia, thrombocytopenia, megaloblastic anemia, and, more rarely, aplastic anemia) have been observed following long-term administration.

Pregnancy: Colchicum is not to be used during pregnancy because of possible teratogenic damage. This also has been noted following intake of the drug by the father before conception.

OVERDOSAGE

Three to 6 hours following intake of acutely toxic dosages, burning of the mouth, difficulty swallowing, and thirst appear. After 12 to 14 hours, the following appear: nausea, severe stomach pains, vomiting, diarrhea, bladder spasms, hematuria, falling blood pressure, and spasms, and later, progressive paralysis. Death follows through exhaustion, asphyxiation, or circulatory collapse. The fatal dosage for an adult is 5 g of the seeds, 1 to 1.5 g for a child. The fatal dosage of an intake of colchicine lies between 7 mg and 200 mg.

The treatment for poisonings, following gastric lavage and the administration of a saline purgative (such as sodium sulfate), proceeds symptomatically (diazepam for convulsion, atropine for intestinal spasm) and includes possible intubation and oxygen respiration.

DOSAGE

COLCHICUM BULBS, SEEDS AND FLOWERS

Mode of Administration: Comminuted drug, freshly pressed juice, and other galenic preparations taken orally.

How Supplied:

Ampules

Tablets

Daily Dosage: For an acute attack of gout, an initial oral dose corresponding to 1 mg colchicine, followed by 0.5 to 1.5 mg every 1 to 2 hours until pain subsides. Total daily dosage must not exceed 8 mg of colchicine. For prophylactic and therapeutic purposes, the dosage should correspond to 0.5 to 1.5 mg of colchicine.

Storage: All forms of the drug should be stored in containers that protect them from light and dampness. In addition, the seeds should be stored over lime.

LITERATURE

Dubois V, Rey N, Constant H, Scherrmann JM, Berthier JC, Aulagner G. Intoxication a la colchicine a propos d'un cas pediatrique. Therapie 49; 339-342. 1994.

Nasreen A, Gundlach H, Zenk MH. Incorporation of phenethylisoquinolines into colchicine in isolated seeds of *Colchicum autumnale. Phytochemistry* 46 (1); 107-115. 1997.

Poulev A, Deus-Neumann B, Bombardelli E, Zenk MH. Immunoassays for the quantitative determination of Colchicine. *Planta Med.* 60; 77-83. 1994.

Santavy F et al., *Coll Czech Chem Comm* 48:2989-2993. 1983.

Sener B, Bingöl F. Screening of Natural Sources for Antiinflammatory Activity (Review). *Int J Crude Drug Res.* 26; 197-207. 1988.

Ulrichovã J et al., Biochemical evaluation of colchicine and related analogs. In: *PM* 59(29):144. 1993.

Colchicum autumnale

See Colchicum

Collinsonia canadensis

See Stone Root

Colombo

Jateorhiza palmata

DESCRIPTION

Medicinal Parts: The medicinal parts of the plant are the roots cut in slices when fresh and then dried.

Flower and Fruit: The plant is dioecious. The male inflorescences are 40 cm long and have green sepals, which are 2.7 to 3.2 mm long and 1.2 to 1.6 mm wide. The stamens are free and are fused at the base with the involuted margins of the petals. The female inflorescence is 8 to 10 cm long and has a 1 to 1.5 mm rust-red, pubescent ovary. The fruit is a 2 to 2.5 cm long and 1.5 to 2 cm wide globose drupe containing a moon-shaped stone.

Leaves, Stem, and Root: The plant is a woody, branched liane, which can climb to tree height. The liane is initially downy, then bristly to villous. The leaves are opposite and have an 18 to 25 cm long petiole. The leaf blades are 15 to 35 cm long and 18 to 40 cm wide. They are bristly haired on both surfaces, broadly rounded, deeply cordate at the base and usually have 5 broad-ovate lobes. The root has a diameter of 3 to 8 cm. It is greenish-black. The root has a floury consistency, an indented center, and a thick bark. The transverse section is yellowish, with vascular bundles in radiating lines.

Characteristics: Colombo's taste is mucilaginous and very bitter; it has a slight odor.

Habitat: Indigenous to Mozambique, east Africa and Madagascar. It is cultivated elsewhere.

Production: Colombo root is the root of *Jateorhiza palmata*, which has been sliced horizontally and dried. The tuber roots, stemming from the rhizome, are dug up in March, washed, thinly sliced, and then dried quickly in the shade to avoid decomposition.

Other Names: Calumba

ACTIONS AND PHARMACOLOGY

COMPOUNDS

Isoquinoline alkaloids: main alkaloid palmatine, additionally jatrorrhizines (jateorhizine), columbamine, and bisjatrorrhizines

Diterpene bitter principles: including palmarin, chasmanthin and their glucosides (palmatoside A and B), columbin, jateorin and their glucosides (palmatoside D and E)

EFFECTS

The drug is no longer used as a bitter (amarum). The alkaloids have a narcotic effect. They act similarly to morphine, increasing resting muscle tone in the smooth muscle of the intestinal tract. Colombo alkaloids are said to act as a CNS paralyzing agent in frogs, and palmatin has the same effect on mammals. No further information is available.

INDICATIONS AND USAGE

Unproven Uses: In folk medicine it is used for digestive disorders accompanied by diarrhea, dyspeptic disorders, chronic diarrhea in patients with lung disease, subacidic gastritis, and chronic entercolitis.

The drug is used in some European countries as an antidiarrheal agent because of its morphinelike side effects.

PRECAUTIONS AND ADVERSE REACTIONS

Health risks or side effects following the proper administration of designated therapeutic dosages are not recorded. Higher dosages of the drug may trigger vomiting and pains in the epigastrium.

OVERDOSAGE

According to older sources, very high dosages can also lead to signs of paralysis and unconsciousness (Lewin).

DOSAGE

Mode of Administration: Due to its morphine-type action, its use as an antidiarrheal agent is limited. Otherwise, the chopped root is used (no preparations known).

Preparation: Colombo liquid extract is prepared with diluted ethanol, according to the German pharmacopoeia. Colombo wine is prepared using 100 parts coarsely powdered drug and 1,000 parts xeres wine. The extract is pressed out after 8 days and filtered.

Daily Dosage: The dose of the decoction is 1 dessertspoonful every 2 hours. The liquid extract standard single dose is 20 drops. Tincture of Colombo standard single dose is 2.5 gm. Colombo wine standard single dose is 5 gm.

Storage: Colombo must be kept dry at all times.

LITERATURE

Chan, EH et al. (Eds), Advances in Chinese Medicinal Materials Research, World Scientific Pub. Co. Singapore 1985.

Fenaroli's Handbook of Flavor Ingredients, Vol. 1, 2nd Ed., CRC Press 1975.

Hänsel R, Keller K, Rimpler H, Schneider G (Hrsg.), Hagers Handbuch der Pharmazeutischen Praxis, 5. Aufl., Bde 4-6 (Drogen), Springer Verlag Berlin, Heidelberg, New York, 1992-1994.

Lewin L, Gifte und Vergiftungen, 6. Aufl., Nachdruck, Haug Verlag, Heidelberg 1992.

Overton KH, Wier NG, Wylie A, *J Chem Soc* 1482-1490. 1966.

Steinegger E, Hänsel R, Pharmakognosie, 5. Aufl., Springer Verlag Heidelberg 1992.

Colt's Foot

Tussilago farfara

DESCRIPTION

Medicinal Parts: The medicinal parts are the dried inflorescences, the dried leaves and the fresh leaves.

Flower and Fruit: The yellow compound flowers are in small, solitary capitula at the end of the scapes. The lateral florets are lingual, narrow, and female. The disc florets are tubular-campanulate, 5-petaled and male. The involucral bracts are almost as long, are linear-lanceolate and have a scarious margin. The fruit is 3 to 11 mm long, cylindrical, brown, glabrous, and stemmed. The pappus is in a number of rows and consists of long, glossy white hairs, which are much longer than the fruit.

Leaves, Stem, and Root: The plant is a perennial, 10 to 30 cm high. It has a broadly branched underground shoot and root system with a thin round, scaly base. There is also a far-reaching, creeping shoot that can grow up to 1.8 m long. The flower stem is a scaly, round, tomentose scape covered with lanceolate, reddish scales, and is 30 cm long when the fruit ripens. The leaves, which appear after flowering, are basal, coriaceous, cordate-round, angular, irregularly dentate, long-petioled, and tomentose beneath. The leaves can reach a diameter of up to 30 cm.

Characteristics: The taste and texture is slimy-sweet and the leaves have a honeylike smell when they are rubbed.

Habitat: The plant grows wild in most of Europe, central, western and northern Asia. It has spread to the mountains of northern Africa and has been introduced into North America.

Production: Colt's Foot flower consists of the fresh or dried flowers of *Tussilago farfara*. Colt's Foot herb consists of the fresh or dried, above-ground parts of *Tussilago farfara*. Colt's

Foot root consists of the fresh or dried, below-ground parts of *Tussilago farfara*.

Not to be Confused With: The leaves of various *Petasites* species, but petasine and flavonoids can be identified using thin layer chromatography.

Other Names: British Tobacco, Bullsfoot, Butterbur, Coughwort, Flower Velure, Foal's-Foot, Horse-Foot, Horsehoof, Hallfoot, Ass's Foot, Foalswort, Fieldhove, Donnhove

ACTIONS AND PHARMACOLOGY

COMPOUNDS: COLT'S FOOT FLOWER

Mucilages (7%): acidic polysaccharides

Tannins

Triterpenes: including beta-amyrin, arnidiol, faradiol

Steroids: including beta-sitosterol

Pyrrolizidine alkaloids (traces, not in plants from all places of origin): tussilagine, isotussilagine, senkirkine, senecionine

Flavonoids

COMPOUNDS: COLT'S FOOT HERB

Mucilages (8%): acidic polysaccharides

Tannins (5%)

Triterpenes: including alpha-amyrin, beta-amyrin

Steroids: including beta-sitosterol, campesterol

Pyrrolizidine alkaloids (not in plants from all places of origin): senkirkine (0.01%), senecionine, tussilagine, isotussilagine

Flavonoids

COMPOUNDS: COLT'S FOOT ROOT

The roots have not been fully investigated. Only the presence of triterpenes and sterols has been established.

EFFECTS: COLT'S FOOT FLOWER, HERB, AND ROOT

The mucin contained in the drug has a sequestering effect and envelopes the mucous membrane with a layer that protects the throat from chemical and physical irritation and thereby reduces cough irritation. The pyrrolizidine alkaloids are antibacterial, carcinogenic, and hepatotoxic.

COMPOUNDS: COLT'S FOOT LEAF

Mucilages (8%): acidic polysaccharides

Tannins (5%)

Pyrrolizidine alkaloids (traces, not from all sources): tussilagine, isotussilagine, senkirkine 0.01%), senecionin

Steroids: including beta-sitosterol, campesterol

Triterpenes: including alpha- and beta-amyrin

Flavonoids

EFFECTS: COLT'S FOOT LEAF

The pyrrolizidine alkaloids are antibacterial, carcinogenic, and hepatotoxic. The mucin polysaccharides cause a demulcent, sequestering, and anti-inflammatory effect. In animal experiments there was evidence of a stimulating effect on the ciliated epithelium.

INDICATIONS AND USAGE

COLT'S FOOT FLOWER, HERB, AND ROOT

Unproven Uses: When added to Colt's Foot leaf, the flower, herb, and root are used to treat rheumatism.

COLT'S FOOT LEAF

Approved by Commission E:

- Cough
- Bronchitis
- Inflammation of the mouth and pharynx

Unproven Uses: Colt's Foot leaf is used for inflammation of the oral and pharyngeal mucosa. In addition, cigarettes made of the leaves are used to help cure smoking addiction.

CONTRAINDICATIONS

COLT'S FOOT FLOWER, HERB, ROOT, AND LEAF

Administration during pregnancy and while nursing is contraindicated.

PRECAUTIONS AND ADVERSE REACTIONS

COLT'S FOOT FLOWER, HERB, AND ROOT

Because of the possible hepatotoxic and carcinogenic pyrrolizidine alkaloid content, the administration of the blossoms should be avoided.

COLT'S FOOT LEAF

Colt's Foot leaves may no longer be brought into circulation in Austria. In Germany, dosages cannot exceed an intake of 10 mcg pyrrolizidine alkaloids with 1.2-unsaturated necic parent substances in the form of tea mixtures, and an intake of 1 mcg in the form of extracts.

Because even traces of the alkaloids present some danger, one should forgo any administration of the drug from the wild species. Varieties have been bred domestically that are free of pyrrolizidine alkaloids. The industrial production of commercial medications that are pyrrolizidine-alkaloid free is possible.

DOSAGE

COLT'S FOOT FLOWER, HERB, AND ROOT

Mode of Administration: The drug is used internally through the use of tea and standardized remedies.

Preparation: To prepare a tea, add 1.5 to 2.5 gm cut drug to boiling water, then strain after 5 to 10 minutes.

Storage: Protect the drug from light and store it tightly sealed.

COLT'S FOOT LEAF

Mode of Administration: Whole, cut, and powdered drug used in teas, infusions, extracts, and tinctures.

Preparation: To make an infusion, pour hot water over 1.5 to 2.5 gm of drug and allow to steep for 10 minutes. Other preparations are made as follows: liquid extract: 1:1 with 20% ethanol; extract: 1.1 with 25% ethanol; tincture: 1:5 with 45% ethanol.

How Supplied:

Liquid Extract

Powder

Daily Dosage: The total daily dose is 4.5 to 6 gm of drug. The maximum daily dosage must not be more than 1 mcg of total pyrrolizidine alkaloids with 1.2 unsaturated necine structure. The drug should not be taken for more than 4 to 6 weeks a year.

The tea is given several times a day. The dosage for the extract is 2 mL 3 times daily; for the tincture, it is 8 mL 3 times daily.

Storage: Protect the drug from light and store it tightly sealed.

LITERATURE

COLT'S FOOT FLOWER, HERB, LEAF, AND ROOT
Bartkowski JPB, Wiedenfeld H, Roeder E. Quantitative Photometric Determination of Senkirkine in *Farfarae Folium. Phytochem* Anal. 8; 1-4. 1997.

Delitheos A, Tiligada E, Yannitsaros A, Bazos I. Antiphage activity in extracts of plants growing in Greece. *Phytomedicine* 4 (2); 117-124. 1997.

Hiller K, Pharmazeutische Bewertung ausgewählter Teedrogen. In: *DAZ* 135(16):1425-1440. 1995.

Hirono I et al., *J Natl Canc Inst* 63(2):469. 1979.

Ihrig M, Pyrrolizidinalkaloidhaltige Drogen im Handverkauf? In: *PZ* 137(40):3128. 1992.

Keller K. Results of the revision of herbal drugs in the Federal Republic of Germany with a special focus on risk aspects. *Z Phytother*. 13; 116-120. 1992.

Masaki H, Sakaki S, Atsumi T, Sakurai H. Active-Oxygen Scavenging Activity of Plant Extracts. *Biol Pharm Bull*. 18 (1); 162-166. 1995.

Paβreiter CM, Co-occurence of 2-pyrrolidineacetic acid with four isomeric tussilaginic acids in Arnica species and *Tussilago farfara*. In: *PM* 58(7):A694. 1992.

Pluta J. Studies on concentration of halogen derivatives in herbal products from various regions of Poland. *Pharmazie* 44; 222-224. 1989.

Ridker PM. Hepatic veno-occlusive disease and herbal teas. *J Pediatr*. 115; 167. 1989.

Röder E, Medicinal plants in Europe containing pyrrolizidine alkaloids. *Pharmazie* 50 (2); 82-98. 1995.

Roulet M, Laurini R, Rivier L, Calame A. Hepatic veno-occlusive disease in newborn infant of a woman drinking herbal tea. *J Pediatr*. 112; 433-436. 1988.

Sommer M, Roulet M, Rivier L. Hepatic veno-occlusive disease and drinking herbal teas Reply. *J Pediatr*. 115; 659-660. 1989.

Wagner H, In: Economic and Medicinal Plant Research, Vol. 1, Academic Press, UK 1985.

Columbine

Aquilegia vulgaris

DESCRIPTION

Medicinal Parts: The medicinal parts are the stems and leaves, the aerial parts gathered and dried in flowering season, and the seeds and preparations of the whole plant, which are also gathered in flowering season.

Flower and Fruit: The long-stemmed flowers are terminal, hanging, and either dark blue, dark violet, pink, or white. The 5 sepals spread like petals. They are broadly ovate, and end in a blunt, green tip. The 5 petals are hood-shaped with long, inwardly hooked spurs. There are numerous stamens and usually 5 ovaries. The follicle is oblong, erect, and glandular-downy. The seeds are glossy black, oval, 2.2 to 2.5 cm long by 1.5 cm wide. They are thick, blunt-tipped, and anatropous. The raphe forms a distinct line on the side of the plant.

Leaves, Stem, and Root: The 30- to 60-cm high plant has a many-headed, light brown, branched rhizome. The stems are erect and are usually branched. They are glabrous or soft-haired. The basal leaves are long-petioled and trifoliate. The leaflets are wedge-shaped to ovoid, irregularly crenate to serrate, and bluntly lobed. The underside of the leaves are usually light green and pubescent. The cauline leaves are smaller than the basal leaves and simpler. The highest leaves are usually made up of a few elongate-ovate, entire-margined lobes.

Habitat: Columbine is indigenous to central and southern Europe and is also found in the eastern U.S. and Asia.

Production: Columbine herb is the complete aerial part of *Aquilegia vulgaris* harvested while in flower and dried.

Other Names: Culverwort, Capon's Feather, Culver Key

ACTIONS AND PHARMACOLOGY

COMPOUNDS

Cyanogenic glycosides: trigloquinine, dhurrin (presumably only traces)

EFFECTS

It is not known which constituents are responsible for the herb's effects. The cyanogenic glycoside trigloquinine could possibly be of toxicological interest but is probably only present in traces. The ethanolic extract has shown in vitro antibacterial effects against *Staphylococcus aureus, Micrococcus luteus, Bacillus subtilus*, and *Candida albicans.*

INDICATIONS AND USAGE

Unproven Uses: Columbine is used internally for scurvy and jaundice; the herb is also used to treat states of agitation due to its supposedly tranquilizing effect.

Homeopathic Uses: The herb is used to treat menopausal vomiting and dysmenorrhea in young women. It is also used to treat the sensation of a lump in the throat (globus hystericus) and nervous shaking.

PRECAUTIONS AND ADVERSE REACTIONS

No health hazards or side effects are known in conjunction with the proper administration of designated therapeutic dosages.

OVERDOSAGE

Poisonings from the leaves because of the cyanogenic glycoside content have not been observed. The amount of hydrocyanic acid that is released from the leaves is apparently too small to cause toxicity.

DOSAGE

Mode of Administration: Columbine is available in tablets and capsules for internal use.

Homeopathic Dosage: 5 to 10 drops, 1 tablet, or 5 to 10 globules 1 to 3 times a day or 1 mL injection solution sc twice a week (HAB1).

LITERATURE

Bylka W, Goslinska O. Determination of isocytisoside and antimicrobial activity of ethanolic extract from *Aquilegia vulgaris L. Acta Pol Pharm.* 58:241-243. 2001.

Bylka W, Matlawaska I. Flavonoids from *Aquilegia vulgaris* . Part I. Isocytisoside and its derivatives. *Acta Pol Pharm.* 54:331-333. 1997.

Bylka W, Matlawaska I. Flavonoids from *Aquilegia vulgaris*. Part II. Derivatives of apigenin and luteolin. *Acta Pol Pharm.* 54:331-333. 1997.

Hänsel R, Keller K, Rimpler H, Schneider G (Hrsg.), Hagers Handbuch der Pharmazeutischen Praxis, 5. Aufl., Bde 4-6 (Drogen). Springer Verlag Berlin, Heidelberg, New York, 1992-1994.

Combretum micranthum

See Opium Antidote

Comfrey

Symphytum officinale

DESCRIPTION

Medicinal Parts: The medicinal parts are the fresh root and the leaves.

Flower and Fruit: The flowers are dull purple or violet. They are arranged in crowded, apical, 2-rayed hanging cymes. The calyx is fused and has 5 tips. The corolla is also fused and is cylindrical-campanulate with a pentangular tube and 5-tipped border. The tips are revolute and there are 5 awl-shaped scales in the mouth of the tube. The scales close together in a clavate form and have a glandular tipped margin. There are 5 stamens and 1 style. The ovary is 4-valved. The fruit consists of 4 smooth, glossy nutlets.

Leaves, Stem, and Root: The plant grows from 30 to 120 cm in height. The root is fusiform, branched, black on the outside and white on the inside. The stem is erect and stiff-haired. The leaves are wrinkly and roughly pubescent; the lower ones and the basal ones are ovate-lanceolate and pulled together in the petiole; the upper ones are lanceolate and broad.

Characteristics: The root is slimy and hornlike when dried.

Habitat: The plant is indigenous to Europe and temperate Asia and is naturalized in the U.S.

Production: Comfrey herb consists of the fresh or dried above-ground parts of *Symphytum officinale*. Comfrey leaf consists of the fresh or dried leaf of *Symphytum officinale*. Comfrey root consists of the fresh or dried root section of *Symphytum officinale*.

Other Names: Ass Ear, Black Root, Blackwort, Boneset, Bruisewort, Consolida, Consound, Gum Plant, Healing Herb, Knitback, Knitbone, Salsify, Slippery Root, Wallwort

ACTIONS AND PHARMACOLOGY

COMPOUNDS

Allantoin

Mucilages (Fructans)

Protein

Triterpene saponins: including symphytoxide A

Tannins

Silicic acid: to some extent water-soluble

Pyrrolizidine alkaloids (0.03% in the leaves): including echinatine, lycopsamine, 7-acetyl lycoposamine, echimidine, lasiocarpine, symphytine, intermedine, symveridine.

EFFECTS

Comfrey exerts anti-inflammatory and antimitotic actions, and furthers the formation of callus. An *in vitro* study found allantoin, found in Comfrey, to accelerate wound healing (Awang, 1987). Anticancer activity also has been demonstrated *in vitro*. Usage for the other areas of administration claimed is plausible.

Anti-inflammatory Effects: A placebo-controlled study documented some anti-inflammatory action in various musculoskeletal disorders, but the effects were not consistent (Peterson et al, 1993). Information on anti-inflammatory actions of Comfrey is sparse, but some positive actions occur. Comfrey suppresses leukocyte infiltration during the inflammation process (Shipochliev, 1981).

Demulcent Effects: The mucilages act as demulcants for a soothing and irritation reduction effect.

Tissue/Nerve Stimulation: The wound-healing effect is thought due to allantoin, a component in Comfrey that stimulates tissue repair and wound healing through cell proliferation (Awang, 1987; Bramwell, 1912; Rieth, 1968). Allantoin has also had significant effect on cellular multiplication in degenerating and regenerating peripheral nerves (Loots, 1979).

CLINICAL TRIALS

Analgesic

A randomized, double-blind, placebo-controlled, clinical trial in 153 women and 67 men found an extract ointment of Comfrey root to be well-suited for the treatment of osteoarthritis of the knee. Topical application of the ointment resulted in significantly reduced pain, improved mobility, and increased quality of life for the treatment groups as compared to the placebo group. The 220 participants included in the final analysis (average age 57.9) reported knee osteoarthritis for 6.5 years. The Comfrey ointment (Kytta Salbe 6 g f (3X2 g) was applied over a 3-week period. The amount of total pain (pain at rest and pain on movement) in the treatment group dropped by 51.6 (54.7%) and in the placebo group by 10.1 (10.7%)—an average difference of 41.5 mm, or 44%. In addition, patients in the treatment group experienced a significant improvement ($p<0.001$) in regard to restriction of movement, which improved an average of 7%. The ointment was well tolerated and did not result in any adverse drug reactions (Grube 2007).

A randomized, placebo-controlled, double blind study of topical Comfrey ointment for unilateral ankle sprain found the treatment to be clinically and significantly superior to placebo in reducing pain ($p<0.0001$) and swelling (ankle edema $p=0.001$), and to be effective in improving ankle mobility and global efficacy. The trial involved 142 individuals (mean age 31.8) at 5 centers, 80 of whom were randomized to apply ointment of Comfrey extract (Kytta-Salbe f) four times daily for 8 days. There were no adverse drug reactions associated with the ointment. The authors attribute Comfrey's effectiveness for ankle sprain treatment to the root's anti-inflammatory and analgesic qualities, as well as its ability to stimulate granulation and tissue regeneration, and callus formation (Koll 2004).

Anti-Inflammatory

The anti-inflammatory effects of Comfrey were studied in musculoskeletal disorders. Forty-one patients with musculoskeletal rheumatism were treated with either a pyrrolizidine alkaloid-free ointment or placebo for 4 weeks. The patient illnesses consisted of epicondylitis, tendovaginitis, and periarthritis. Efficacy was determined by evaluation of different pain parameters (tenderness on pressure, pain at rest, pain on exercise). There was significant improvement with the ointment compared to placebo at weeks 1, 2, and 4 in patients with epicondylitis. There was improvement with tendovaginitis at week 1 and 2, but not at week 4 with the ointment compared to placebo. There was no improvement in the periarthritis patients in either of the two treatment groups (Petersen, 1993).

A Comfrey ointment was effective in alleviating symptoms associated with muscle pain, but was less effective for the pain of degenerative diseases such as osteoporosis in an open, uncontrolled trial. Subjects ($n=105$) with musculoskeletal syndromes including muscle strains, swelling, pain, vertebral syndrome, and osteoporosis-associated pain were given a Symphytum ointment containing 10 g Symphytum concentrate in a 90 g base to apply topically twice daily to the affected area for 14 days. Pain and functional complaints resolved in 57 subjects; 24 had restored function with continued pain, and 21 subjects reported a moderate improvement. Those subjects suffering from muscular disturbances were more likely to see an improvement than those with degenerative locomotor conditions. The maximum effect occurred around 4 hours after application of the ointment, leading the investigators to conclude that it should ideally be applied three times daily (Kucera et al, 2000).

Myalgia

The effectiveness and tolerability of the topical Symphytum product, Traumaplant (10% active ingredient of a 2.5:1 aqueous-ethanolic pressed concentrate of freshly harvested, cultivated comfrey herb, corresponding to 25 g of fresh herb per 100 g of cream), was tested in a randomized, controlled, double-blind clinical study against a 1% reference product (corresponding to 2.5 g of fresh comfrey herb in 100 g of cream) against myalgia. A total of 215 patients were enrolled. With high concentrations of the treatment product, amelioration of pain on active motion ($p<5 \times 10^{-9}$), pain at rest ($p<0.001$), and pain on palpation ($p=5 \times 10^{-5}$) was significantly more pronounced than that attained with the reference treatment product. Tolerability of the highly concentrated study product was good to excellent in all patients (Kucera et al, 2005).

INDICATIONS AND USAGE

Approved by Commission E:

■ Blunt injuries

Externally, Comfrey is used for bruises, sprains, pulled muscles and ligaments, and promotion of bone healing.

Unproven Uses: The root has been used externally as a mouthwash and gargle for gum disease, pharyngitis, and strep throat. Internally, the root has been used for gastritis and gastrointestinal ulcers. In folk medicine, the root of the plant has been used for rheumatism, pleuritis, and as an antidiarrheal agent.

CONTRAINDICATIONS

Comfrey is contraindicated in persons with previous liver or kidney disease.

Alcohol: Concurrent use may result in elevated liver transaminases with or without concomitant hepatic damage. *Clinical management:* Comfrey is a known hepatotoxin and should be avoided.

Pregnancy: Not to be used during pregnancy.

Breastfeeding: Not to be used while breastfeeding.

PRECAUTIONS AND ADVERSE REACTIONS

External administration should only be on areas where the skin is unbroken, and then only with industrially produced, pyrrolizidine alkaloid-free extracts. Despite a long history of oral use, ingestion is not advisable at this time due to its toxic effects (hepatotoxic and carcinogenic).

Liver and possibly kidney disease may occur if taken for more than four weeks or at higher than therapeutic doses. Comfrey should not be used orally for more than four weeks if pyrrolizidine alkaloids might be present (Whitelegg, 1994; Foster, 1993). Comfrey should only be applied to intact skin.

DRUG INTERACTIONS
No information is available.

POTENTIAL INTERACTIONS
Carcinogenic/Mutagenic Effects: Mutagenic effects are associated with aqueous extracts of the alkaloid fractions (Furmanowa, 1983). Hepatocelluar adenomas have been reported in animal models receiving diets containing Comfrey roots and leaves (Hirono, 1978). Comfrey also has chromosome-damaging effects in human lymphocytes (Behninger, 1989). There has been an association between frequent ingestion of tannin-rich plants and gastric cancer. Tannic acid has been oncogenic in animals, and both the roots and leaves have been shown to be carcinogenic in rats (Awang, 1987).

Gastrointestinal/Kidney/Pancreas Effects: Comfrey, through the pyrrolizidine alkaloids, has been shown to produce lesions in the gastrointestinal tract, pancreas, and renal glomeruli in animal models (Winship, 1991).

Hepatotoxicity: Internal administration of the drug, due to the presence of pyrrolizidine alkaloids, has resulted in hepatocyte membrane injury with hemorrhagic necrosis and loss of microvilli (Yeong, 1993; Yeong et al, 1990; Whitelegg, 1994). In July 2001, the Food and Drug Administration released an advisory recommending that Comfrey products be removed from the market due to cases of hepatic veno-occlusive disease (Lewis, 2001). Pyrrolizidine alkaloids are known to cause veno-occulsive disease in man, and have done so via contamination of grain, use in salads, or consumption of herbal teas and medicines (Ridker & McDermott, 1989; Ridker, 1989; Jones & Taylor, 1989). Severe portal hypertension also has been associated with Comfrey ingestion, and in one case report, death resulted by liver failure (Ridker, 1989; Yeong, 1990).

Misidentification: There have been poisonings caused by misidentifying the leaves of Digitalis purpurea for the broad leaves of Comfrey. Bradycardia, nausea, and vomiting have occurred (Bain, 1985; Couper, 1977).

DOSAGE
Mode of Administration: The crushed root, extracts, and pressed juice of the fresh plant are used as semi-solid preparations and poultices for external use. The drug is a component of standardized preparations of analgesics, antirheumatic agents, antiphlogistics, antitussives, and expectorants.

How Supplied:

Cream–1.25 oz., 2 oz.

Capsules–500 mg

Liquid Extract

Preparation: To make an infusion, pour boiling water over 5 to 10 g comminuted or powdered drug, steep 10 to 15 minutes, then strain (1 teaspoonful = 4 g drug). For external application, a decoction of 1:10 is used, or the fresh roots are mashed.

Daily Dosage:

External Use–The daily dosage should not exceed 1 mcg of pyrrolizidine alkaloids for external preparations calculated with 5 to 7% drug, maximum 1 ppm/g for commercial pharmaceutical preparations. The drug should be used for a maximum of 4 weeks.

Despite a long history of oral use, ingestion is not advisable at this time due to its toxic effects (hepatotoxic and carcinogenic).

LITERATURE

Ahmad VU, Noorwala M, Mohammad FV et al. Symphytoxide A, a triterpenoid saponin from the roots of *Symphytum officinale. Phytochemistry* Mar;32(4):1003-1006. 1993

Anderson PC & McLean AEM. Comfrey and liver damage. *Hum Toxicol*; 8:68-69. 1989

Awang DVC. Comfrey. *Can Pharm J*; 120:101-104. 1987

Awang DV & Kindack DG. Atropine as possible contaminant of Comfrey tea (letter). *Lancet*; 2(8653):44. 1989

Bain RJI. Accidental digitalis poisoning due to drinking herbal tea. *BMJ*; 290(6482):1624. 1985

Behninger C, Abel G, Roder E et al. Studies on the effect of an alkaloid extract of *Symphytum officinale* on human lymphocyte cultures. *Planta Med* Dec;55(6):518-522. 1989

Bhandari P. Gray AI. *J Pharm Pharmacol; 37:50P*. 1985

Bramwell W. The new cell proliferant. *BMJ*; 1:12-13. 1912

Branchlij et al. *Experientia;* 38:1085. 1982

Couper L & Grunenfelder G. Poisoning associated with herbal teas - Arizona, Washington. *MMWR*; 26(32):257-258. 1977

Culvenor CJJ et al. Experientia 36:377. 1980

Foster S. Herbal Renaissance. Gibbs-Smith Publisher, Salt Lake City, UT. 1993

Furmanowa M, Guzewska J, Beldowska B. Mutagenic effects of aqueous extracts of Symphytum officinale L. and of its alkaloid fractions. *J Appl Toxicol* Jun;3(3):127-130. 1983

Furuya T & Hikichi M. Alkaloids and triterpenoids of *Symphytum officinale. Phytochemistry*; 10:2217-2220. 1971

Galizia EJ. Clinical curio: hallucinations in elderly tea drinkers. *BMJ*; 287(6397):979. 1983

Garrett BJ, Cheeke PR, Miranda CL et al. Consumption of poisonous plants *(Senecio jacobaea, Symphytum officinale, Pteridium aquilinum, Hypericum perforatum*) by rats: chronic toxicity, mineral metabolism, and hepatic drug-metabolizing enzymes. *Toxicol Lett* Feb;10(2-3):183-188. 1982

Gracza L et al. *Arch Pharm;* 312(12):1090. 1985

Gray AI et al. *J Pharm Pharmacol;* 35:13P. 1983

Grube B, Grunwald J, Krug L., et al. Efficacy of a comfrey root (Symphyti offic. radix) extract ointment in the treatment of patients with painful osteoarthritis of the knee: results of a double-blind, randomised, bicenter, placebo-controlled trial. *Phytomedicine.* 14(1): 2, 10. 2007.

Hansen CE, Stoessel P & Rossi P. Distribution of gamma-linolenic acid in comfrey *(Symphytum officinale)* plant. *J Sci Food Agric*; 54:309-312. 1991

Hirono I, Mori H, Haga M. Carcinogenic activity of *Syphytum officinale. J Natl Cancer Inst* Sep; 61(3):865-869. 1978

Ihrig M, Pyrrolizidinalkaloidhaltige Drogen im Handverkauf? In: *PZ;* 137(40):3128. 1992

Jones JG & Taylor DE: Hepatic veno-occlusive disease and herbal remedies (letter). *Ann Rheum Dis*; 48(9):791. 1989

Koll R, Buhr M, Dieter R, et al. Efficacy and tolerance of comfrey root extract (Extr. Rad. Symphyti) in the treatment of ankle distorsions: results of a multicenter, randomized, placebo-controlled, double-blind study. *Phytomedicine*,11:4707. 2004.

Kucera M, Barna M, Horàcek O, et al. Topical symphytum herb concentrate cream against myalgia: a randomized controlled double-blind clinical trial. *Ad Ther*; 22(6): 681-692. 2005.

Kucera M, Kalal J & Polesna Z. Effects of symphytum ointment on muscular symptoms and functional locomotor disturbances. *Adv Ther*; 17(4):204-210. 2000

Lewis CJ. FDA Advises Dietary Supplement Manufacturers to Remove Comfrey Products from the Market. Jul 6. Available at: http://www.cfsan.fda.gov/dms/dspltr06.html (cited 8/7/2001). 2001

Loots JM, Loots GP, Joubert WS. The effect of allantoin on cellular multiplication in degenerating and regenerating nerves. *S Afr Med J* Jan 13;55(2):53-56. 1979

Makarova GV & Zaraiska KN. Chemical study of the root of common Comfrey (*Symphytum officinale* L). *Chem Abstr*; 66(10):49229h. 1967

Mascolo N et al. *Phytother Res;* 1(1):28. 1987

Mattocks AR. Toxicity of pyrrolizidine alkaloids. *Nature*; 217(130):723-728. 1968

Miskelly FG & Goodyer LI. Hepatic and pulmonary complications of herbal medicines. *Postgrad J*; 68:935-936. 1992

Mohabbat O, Younos MS, Merzad AA et al. An outbreak of hepatic veno-occlusive disease in north-western Afghanistan. *Lancet*; 2(7980):269-271. 1976

Mohammad FV et al. Bisdesmosidic triterpenoidal saponins from the roots of Symphytum officinale. In: *PM;* 61(1):94. 1995

Mütterlein R, Arnold CG, Untersuchungen zum Pyrrolizidingehalt und Pyrrolizidinalkaloidmuster in Symphytum officinale L. In: *PZ-W;* 138(5/6):119. 1993

Noorwala M et al. A bisdesmosidic triterpene glycoside from roots of *Symphytum officinale*. In: *PH*; 36(2):439. 1994

Olinescu A, Manda G, Neagu M et al. Action of some proteic and carbohydrate components of Symphytum officinale upon normal and neoplastic cells. *Roum Arch Microbiol Immunol*; 52(2):73-80. 1993

Panter KE & James LF. Natural plant toxicants in milk: a review. *J Animal Sci*; 68(3):892-904. 1990

Petersen G et al. Anti-inflammatory activity of a pyrrolizidine alkaloid-free extract of roots of *Symphytum officinale*. In: *PM;* 59(7)A703. 1993

Rieth H. Stimulation of tissue reparation with allantoin as adjuvant of the antifungal treatment. *Mykosen;* Jan 1;11(1):93-94. 1968

Ridker PN, McDermont WV. Hepatotoxicity due to Comfrey herb tea. *Am J Med Dec*; 87(6):701. 1989

Ridker PM & McDermott WV. Comfrey herb tea and hepatic veno-occlusive disease. *Lancet*; 1(8639):657-658. 1989

Ridker PM, Ohkuma S, McDermott WV et al: Hepatic venocclusive disease associated with the consumption of pyrrolizidine-containing dietary supplements. *Gastroenterology*; 88(4):1050-1054. 1985

Röder E. Pyrrolizidinhaltige Arzneipflanzen. In: *DAZ;* 132(45):2427-2435. 1992

Roitman JN. Comfrey and liver damage (letter). *Lancet*; 1(8226):944. 1981

Roulet M, Laurini R, Rivier L et al. Hepatic veno-occlusive disease in newborn infant of a woman drinking herbal tea. *J Pediatr*; 112(3):433-436. 1988

Shipochliev T, Dimitrov A, Aleksandrova E. Anti-inflammatory action of a group of plant extracts. *Vet Med Nauki*;18(6):87-94. 1981

Schoental R et al. *Cancer Res;* 30:2127. 1970

Stamford IF, Tavares IA. *J Pharm Pharmacol;* 35:816. 1983

Taylor A, Taylor NC. *Proc Soc Exp Biol Med;* 114:772. 1963

Tyler VE. Herbal medicine in America. *Planta Med*; 53(1):1-4. 1987

Weston CFM, Cooper BT, Davies JD et al, Veno-occlusive disease of the liver secondary to ingestion of Comfrey. *BMJ*(Clin Res Ed); 295(6591):183. 1987

White RD et al. *Toxicol Letters;* 15:25. 1983

Whitelegg M. In defense of comfrey. *Eur J Herbal Med*; 1:11-17. 1994

Winship KA. Toxicity of comfrey. *Adverse Drug React Toxicol Rev*; 10(1):47-59. 1991

Yeong ML, Wakefield SJ, Ford HC. Hepatocyte membrane injury and bleb formation following low dose comfrey toxicity in rats. *Int J Exp Pathol* Apr;74(2):211-217. 1993

Yeong ML, Swinburn B, Kennedy M, Nicholson G. Hepatic veno-occlusive disease associated with comfrey ingestion. *J Gastroenterol Hepatol* Mar-Apr;5(2):211-4. 1990

Commiphora molmol

See Myrrh

Common Kidney Vetch

Anthyllis vulneraria

DESCRIPTION

Medicinal Parts: The medicinal part of the plant is the flower.

Flower and Fruit: The many-floreted capitula are in the upper bract axils. The papilonaceous flowers are almost sessile and have an upright corolla up to 20 mm long. The calyx is membranous and up to 17 mm long. It is tubular/bottle-shaped and shaggy to felt-haired. The color is yellow to white at the bottom, turning violet toward the top. The petals are whitish-yellow to yellow or occasionally crimson. They have a free standard, slightly shorter wings, and an acute, often red, carina. Ten stamens are fused into a tube. The ovaries are stemmed with a thickened style and rounded stigma. The podfruit is enclosed in the dried calyx. It is ovate, reticulate, dark brown, single-seeded, and does not spring open. The seed is ovate, smooth, shiny, and checkered yellow-green.

Leaves, Stem, and Root: Anthyllis vulneraria is a 15 to 30 cm high half-rosette shrub with a sturdy taproot and a short, entire or branched rhizome. The stem is upright, unbranched or branched, and tomentose. The leaves are variously pinnate, depending on where they appear on the stem. All leaves are entire-margined, glabrous or slightly pubescent above, and thickly tomentose beneath. The stipules are small and generally connected to a clasping sheath.

Characteristics: Kidney Vetch has a weak aromatic odor and dry taste.

Habitat: The plant is found all across Europe to the Caucasus and the Middle East. It is found in the south to the Sahara and Ethiopia.

Production: Kidney Vetch are the flowers of *Anthyllis vulneraria* without their stems. Common Kidney Vetch is collected in the wild and then dried quickly in the shade.

Other Names: Ladies' Fingers, Lamb's Toes, Kidney Vetch, Staunchwort, Woundwort

ACTIONS AND PHARMACOLOGY

COMPOUNDS

Tannins

Saponins

Flavonoids

Isoflavonoids

Lectins

EFFECTS

Antiviral activity has been demonstrated with an ethanol extract of the plant. The flavonols quercetin and rhamnetin have a mutagenic effect. The herb's use in the treatment of ulcers and wounds may be due to the tannins (probably of the catechin type).

INDICATIONS AND USAGE

Unproven Uses: Kidney Vetch tea is used in the treatment of ulcers and wounds both internally and externally. The drug is also used in a tea for coughs that also contains ribwort, as an ingredient of blood-purifying teas, and for exposure and vomiting. It is used internally for diseases of the mouth and throat.

PRECAUTIONS AND ADVERSE REACTIONS

No health hazards or side effects are known in conjunction with the proper administration of designated therapeutic dosages.

DOSAGE

Mode of Administration: Preparations are available for internal uses, often as teas, and external uses including poultices, washes and rinses.

Preparation: To prepare tea, use 1 dessertspoonful of the flowers per 250 mL of water.

LITERATURE

Czeczot H, Tudek B, Kusztelak J, Szymczyk T, Dobrowolska B, Glinkowska G, Malinowski J, Strzelecka H, Isolation and studies of the mutagenic activity in the Ames test of flavonoids naturally occurring in medical herbs. *Mutat Res*, 240:209-16, 1990 Mar.

Sile A, Vanaga A, Nauka-Prakt Farm: 82-85. 1974.

Vetter J, Seregelyes-Csomos A, *Magy Allatory Lapja* 43(8):479-482. 1988.

Common Stonecrop

Sedum acre

DESCRIPTION

Medicinal Parts: The medicinal parts are the fresh or dried aerial parts collected during the flowering season.

Flower and Fruit: The flowers are leafy, twining cymes on short pedicles. There are 5 ovate sepals and 5 golden yellow petals that are 7 to 9 mm long, lanceolate and twice as long as the calyx. The fruit is a follicle, which splits after flowering to form a 5-rayed star, which is 3 to 5 mm long and has numerous seeds.

Leaves, Stem, and Root: The perennial plant grows 2 to 15 cm high. It has many heavily branched shoots, which often creep underground and form grass. The leaves are thick, fleshy, almost round, acute, appressed, and knobby-domed. They are rounded at the base and have no spur-like appendage.

Characteristics: The texture is slimy and the taste hot and pepperlike.

Habitat: Common Stonecap is common to all of Europe, western Siberia, the Caucasus region, and North America.

Production: The flowering parts of *Sedum acre* are picked while in bloom and then dried, either in the sun or, preferably, with the use of artificial heat.

Other Names: Wallpepper, Golden Moss, Wall Ginger, Bird Bread, Prick Madam, Gold Chain, Creeping Tom, Mousetail, Jach-of-the-Buttery

ACTIONS AND PHARMACOLOGY

COMPOUNDS

Piperidine alkaloids (0.3%): chief alkaloids are sedinine, sedinon

Flavonoids: including among others, glycosides of isorhamnetin, quercetin, limnocitrin

Tannins (10%)

Hydroquinone glycosides: Arbutin

Mucilages (30%)

EFFECTS

In animal experiments, the drug displayed both motility-inhibiting and motility-stimulating effects. The alkaloids and tannins may make use of the drug in the treatment of wounds plausible, but no reliable documentation is available.

INDICATIONS AND USAGE

Unproven Uses: The drug is used internally for coughs (Spain) and high blood pressure (central Europe), edema, and febrile conditions. Externally, it is used for wounds and ulcers resulting from burns, hemorrhoids, warts, eczema, and oral ulcers.

Homeopathic Uses: In homeopathy, Common Stonecap is used for hemorrhoidal pain and anal fissures.

CONTRAINDICATIONS

The drug should not be administered in the presence of inflammatory diseases of the gastrointestinal tract or of the urinary drainage passages.

PRECAUTIONS AND ADVERSE REACTIONS

No health hazards or side effects are known in conjunction with the proper administration of designated therapeutic dosages.

OVERDOSAGE

Dosages consisting of over 10 g of the juice or 1 to 3.5 g of the dried foliage of the fresh plant result in queasiness, vomiting, and diarrhea. However, cases of poisoning have not been recorded in recent times.

DOSAGE

Mode of Administration: Decoctions or syrups for internal use; poultice of fresh leaves for external use.

Preparation: A decoction is prepared using 1 teaspoonful of the drug in 1 cup of water. Prepare syrup by mixing 100 g of plant juice with 180 g of sugar.

Daily Dosage: The average daily dose of the drug as a decoction is 3 g (approximately 2 teaspoonfuls). Average syrup dosage is 1 dessertspoonful every 3 hours. In external application as a poultice, the fresh plants are crushed and placed on the wart or skin area exhibiting eczema.

Homeopathic Dosage: 5 drops, 1 tablet, or 10 globules every 30 to 60 minutes (acute) or 1 to 3 times daily (chronic); parenterally: 1 to 2 mL sc acute: 3 times daily; chronic: once a day (HAB34).

LITERATURE

Delitheos A, Tiligada E, Yannitsaros A, Bazos. Antiphage activity in extracts of plants growing in Greece. *Phytomedicine* 4 (2); 117-124. 1997.

Malterud KE, Nordal A. Structure Eludication of sedoflorigenin, a flavonoid from Sedum acre. *Acta Pharm Nord.* 3; 99-100. 1991.

Van der Wal R et al., *PM* 43:97. 1981.

Condurango

Marsdenia condurango

DESCRIPTION

Medicinal Parts: The medicinal part is the dried bark of the branches and trunks.

Flower and Fruit: The flowers are in umbel-like inflorescence. The calyx and the campanulate-to-funnel-shaped corolla have 5 sepals and petals. Pollination is only possible by insects. The fruit is a follicle containing the seeds, with a tuft of hair.

Leaves, Stem, and Root: The plant is a climbing shrub with pubescent shoots. The trunk can have a diameter of 10 cm. The transverse section shows granular, yellowish-white, and scattered fine and silky fibers. The outer surface is brownish-gray, often warty, with patches of lichen. The tough, ovate, 8 to 11 cm long and 5 to 8 cm wide leaves are very pubescent. They are crossed opposite.

Characteristics: The taste is bitter and acrid. The odor is faintly aromatic.

Habitat: The plant grows on the western slopes of the Andes in Ecuador, Peru and Columbia.

Production: Condurango bark consists of the dried bark of branches and trunk of *Marsdenia condurango.*

Not to be Confused With: Asclepias umbellata or *Elcomarrhiza amylacea*

Other Names: Eagle Vine

ACTIONS AND PHARMACOLOGY

COMPOUNDS

Pregnane- and pregn-5-ene glycosides (mixture known as condurangin): including condurango glycosides A, A0, A1, B0, C, C1, D0, E0, E2

Caffeic acid derivatives: including chlorogenic acid, neochlorogenic acid

Flavonoids: including trifoliin, hyperoside, quercitrin, rutin, and saponarin

EFFECTS

The drug contains bitter condurango glycosides (condurangin). As with other amaroid drugs, a reflexive increase of saliva and gastric juice secretion is to be expected. The drug stimulates the secretion of saliva and gastric juices. It has an antitumoral effect in animals.

INDICATIONS AND USAGE

Approved by Commission E:

- Dyspeptic complaints
- Loss of appetite

Unproven Uses: Condurango is used for loss of appetite. In folk medicine, it is used for atonia of the stomach, painful nutritional disorders, for stomach cancer to alleviate nausea, as an appetite stimulant, and to increase tolerance of food.

Homeopathic Uses: Condurango is used for cracked skin, constriction of the alimentary canal, and for ulceration of the lips and anus.

PRECAUTIONS AND ADVERSE REACTIONS

Health risks or side effects following the proper administration of designated therapeutic dosages are not recorded.

DOSAGE

Mode of Administration: Comminuted drug for infusions and other bitter-tasting preparations for internal use.

Preparation: An infusion is prepared by adding 1.5 gm comminuted drug to cold water and bringing to a boil; strain when cold. The drug is also added to wine; 50 to 100 g of the drug per liter.

Daily Dosage: The average daily dose of aqueous extract is 0.2 to 0.5 g; tincture, 2 to 5 g; liquid extract, 2 to 4 g; bark, 2 to 4 g; Infusion and wine: 1 cup or 1 liquor glass 30 minutes before meals.

Homeopathic Dosage: 5 drops, 1 tablet, or 10 globules every 30 to 60 minutes (acute) or 1 to 3 times daily (chronic); parenterally: 1 to 2 mL sc acute, 3 times daily; chronic: once a day. Apply ointment 1 to 2 times a day (acute and chronic) (HAB1).

Storage: Condurango should be kept tightly sealed and protected from light.

LITERATURE

Berger S et al., *Arch Pharm* 320:924. 1987.

Berger S et al., *PH* 27:1451. 1988.

Hayashi K et al., (1980) *Chem Pharm Bull* 28:1954.

Hayashi K et al., (1981) *Chem Pharm Bull* 29:2725.

Umehara K, Endoh M, Miyasa T, Kuroyanagi M, Ueno Akira. Studies on Differentiation Inducers. IV. Pregnane Derivatives from Condurango Cortex. *Chem Pharm Bull.* 42; 611-616. 1994.

Yamamoto H MizutantinT, Nomura H. Studies on the mutagenicity of crude drug extracts. *Yakugaku Zasshi,* 102: 596-601. 1982

Congorosa

Maytenus ilicifolia

DESCRIPTION

Medicinal Parts: The medicinal part of the plant is the dried leaf.

Flower and Fruit: The flowers are in clusters in the leaf axils; the bracts have a reddish border. The flowers are radial; their structures are in fives. The calyx is reddish and 5-tipped. The petals are free, oval to elliptical, and yellow. The male flowers have 5 stamens approximately 2 mm long with the ovary covered by a disc. The female flowers have 1 mm long stamens and a 2-carpeled, fused ovary on a thick fleshy disc. The fruit is a reddish, 2-chambered capsule. The seeds are reddish with a thin aril.

Leaves, Stem and Root: Congorosa grows as a dioecious evergreen shrub or tree, reaching up to 5 m high. The leaves are alternate, 2 to 15 cm long and 1 to 7 cm wide. They are elliptical to lanceolate, coriaceous, and covered on both sides with 4 to 7 prickly teeth. Sometimes the leaves are completely entire, with very narrow, dropping stipules.

Habitat: The plant is indigenous to South America.

Production: Congorosa leaves (Argentinean name) are the dried leaves of *Maytenus ilicifolia.*

Not to be Confused With: Congorosa is sometimes confused with (and adulterated with) Yerba Mate.

ACTIONS AND PHARMACOLOGY

COMPOUNDS

Macrocyclic alkaloids (0.00005%): maytansinoides, including maytansine, maytanprine, maytanbutine

EFFECTS

The quinoid triterpene maytenin contained in the drug exhibits antimicrobial and tumor-inhibiting properties, particularly in topical administration for the treatment of basal cell carcinomas. Maytansine exhibits significant cytotoxic and antitumoral efficacy (similar to that of vinca alkaloids). Additionally, an ulcer-preventing effect has been demonstrated in both animal and human studies.

INDICATIONS AND USAGE

Unproven Uses: Congorosa is used mainly in South American folk medicine. In Brazil, external uses focus primarily on skin conditions such as eczema and skin ulcers. Internal uses include skin cancer, gastrointestinal complaints, gastrointestinal ulcers, hyperacidity, flatulence, gastralgia, dyspepsia, pain, states of exhaustion, and anemia.

In Argentina, Congorosa is used for asthma, alcoholism and for wound healing. Other varieties are also used for inflammatory swelling and eye conditions.

PRECAUTIONS

No health hazards are known in conjunction with the proper administration of designated therapeutic dosages. Animal experiments revealed embryotoxic and teratogenic effects of maytansine (no detailed description of dosage or experimental procedure available). Should not be used during pregnancy.

CONTRAINDICATIONS

Congorosa preparations are contraindicated during pregnancy.

DOSAGE

Mode of Administration: Preparations are available for internal and external use.

How Supplied:

Capsules

Daily Dosage:

Infusion/decoction (2 to 5%) - 100 to 400 mL internally. Externally as required.

Powder – 5 to 20 g

Liquid extract – 5 to 20 mL

Extract – 1 to 4 g

Tincture – 25 to 100 mL

Elixir/wine/syrup – 50 to 100 mL

LITERATURE

Itokawa H et al. Antitumor Substances form South American Plants. *J Pharmacobio-Dyn.* 15; S2. 1992.

Lima OG de, Coelho JS, Weigert E, Albuquerque IL d', Lima D de A, Moraes e Souza MA, Antimicrobial substances from higher plants. XXXVI. On the presence of maytenin and pristimerine in the cortical part of the roots of *Maytenus ilicifolia* from the South of Brazil. *Rev Inst Antibiot* (Recife), 11:35-8, 1971 Jun.

Shirota O, Morita H, Takeya K, Itokawa H. Cytotoxic aromatic triterpenes from *Maytenus Ilicifolia* and *Maytenus Chuchuhuasca. J Nat Prod.* 57; 1675-1681. 1994.

Vilegas JHY, Lancas FM, Cervi AC. High Resolution Gas Chromatography Analysis of ''espinheira santa'' (*Maytenus ilicifolia* and *M. aquifolium*): Analysis of Crude Drug Adulterations. *Phytother Res.* 8 (4); 241-244. 1994.

Conium maculatum

See Hemlock

Contrayerva

Dorstenia contrayerva

DESCRIPTION

Medicinal Parts: The medicinal parts are the roots of a number of species.

Flower and Fruit: The plant has long-pedicled, greenish flowers.

Leaves, Stem, and Root: The plant is a perennial, growing to a height of up to 30 cm. It is stemless with palmate leaves. The rhizome is about 2 to 4 cm long and 1 cm thick. It is reddish-brown on the outside, paler on the inside and rough with leaf scars. The rhizome is nearly cylindrical and tapers suddenly at the end into a tail-like root with numerous curled, wiry rootlets.

Characteristics: The taste is slightly aromatic, then acrid.

Habitat: Contrayerva is found in Mexico, Peru and the West Indies.

Production: Contrayerva root is the rhizome of *Dorstenia contrayerva* and related varieties.

ACTIONS AND PHARMACOLOGY

COMPOUNDS

Cardioactive steroids (cardenolides): syriogenin

Furocoumarins

Volatile oil

EFFECTS

Diaphoretic and stimulant.

INDICATIONS AND USAGE

Unproven Uses: Preparations of the root are used as a stimulant and to treat low stamina. It has also been used as an antidote for snakebite (uncertain mechanism).

PRECAUTIONS AND ADVERSE REACTIONS

Health risks or side effects following the proper administration of designated therapeutic dosages are not recorded. The plant can trigger phototoxicosis through skin contact.

DOSAGE

Mode of Administration: Ground root as an infusion.

LITERATURE

Hegnauer R, Chemotaxonomie der Pflanzen, Bde 1-11, Birkhäuser Verlag Basel, Boston, Berlin 1962-1997.

Kanamori H, Sakamoto I, Mizuta M, *Chem Pharm Bull* 34:1826. 1986.

Lewin L, Gifte und Vergiftungen, 6. Aufl., Nachdruck, Haug Verlag, Heidelberg 1992.

Convallaria majalis

See Lily-of-the-Valley

Coolwort

Tiarella cordifolia

DESCRIPTION

Medicinal Parts: The medicinal part is the herb.

Flower and Fruit: The plant has inconspicuous white flowers in racemes. The buds are pink-tinged. The few seeds are somewhat clavate. They have a light acrid taste and are odorless.

Leaves, Stem, and Root: The plant is a 15 to 20 cm high herbaceous perennial, which produces runners. The simple leaves are usually slightly 5-lobed and cordate. The basal leaves are often deep red-orange. The cauline leaves have deep red spots and veins, although the latter are often lacking.

Habitat: The plant is indigenous to North America from Virginia to Canada.

Production: Coolwort is the aerial part of *Tiarella cordifolia*.

Other Names: Foam Flower, Mitrewort

ACTIONS AND PHARMACOLOGY

COMPOUNDS

The effective agents of the plant are unknown.

EFFECTS

The herb is a diuretic and a tonic.

INDICATIONS AND USAGE

Unproven Uses: Coolwort is used for conditions of the urinary tract and digestive disorders.

PRECAUTIONS AND ADVERSE REACTIONS

No health hazards or side effects are known in conjunction with the proper administration of designated therapeutic dosages.

DOSAGE

Mode of Administration: The drug is ground for infusions.

LITERATURE

No literature is available.

Copaiba Balsam

Copaifera langsdorffi

DESCRIPTION

Medicinal Parts: The medicinal parts are the resin oil (containing resin and essential oil) tapped from drillings in the trunk.

Flower and Fruit: The flowers are small and yellow.

Leaves, Stem, and Root: Copaiba is an evergreen tree up to 18 m high with compound leaves.

Characteristics: The resin oil consists of resin and essential oil. The resin oil (oleoresin) ranges in viscosity from very liquid to a resinlike substance, and in color from a pale yellow to a red or fluorescent tint. The taste is unpleasant and there is a characteristic smell. A single tree can yield up to 40 liters.

Habitat: Copaiba Balsam is indigenous to tropical regions of South America and South Africa.

Production: Copaiba Balsam is extracted from *Copaifera reticulata* and other varieties from cavities drilled into the tree trunk.

Other Names: Copaiva

ACTIONS AND PHARMACOLOGY

COMPOUNDS

Volatile oil: chief constituent alpha- and beta-caryophyllene, beta-bisabolene, L-cadinene, (-)-alpha-copaene

Resins: in particular, diterpenoid oleoresins including eperu-8(20)-en-15,18-dicarboxylic acid, (-)-16beta-kaurane-19-carboxylic acid, copaiferic acid, (+)-hardwickiic acid, copalic acid

EFFECTS

Possible bacteriostatic effect on the urinary tract. The sesquiterpenes give the drug an antimicrobial effect.

INDICATIONS AND USAGE

Unproven Uses: This is an obsolete drug. In folk medicine, it was used for infections of the urinary tract.

PRECAUTIONS AND ADVERSE REACTIONS

The drug is irritating to the mucous membranes and toxic in large amounts. Stomach pains appear after the intake of 5 g of the drug. Repeated doses bring about summer cholera, shivers, tremor, pains in the groin and insomnia. Skin contact can lead to contact dermatitis such as erythema, papular or vesicular rash, urticaria, and petechias. Occasionally, the rashes leave brown spots after healing.

LITERATURE

Fenaroli's Handbook of Flavor Ingredients, Vol. 1. 2nd Ed. CRC Press 1975.

Leung AY, Encyclopedia of Common Natural Ingredients Used in Food Drugs and Cosmetics, John Wiley & Sons Inc., New York 1980.

Lewin L, Gifte und Vergiftungen, 6. Aufl., Nachdruck, Haug Verlag, Heidelberg 1992.

Roth L, Daunderer M, Kormann K, Giftpflanzen, Pflanzengifte, 4. Aufl., Ecomed Fachverlag Landsberg Lech 1993.

Steinegger E, Hänsel R, Pharmakognosie, 5. Aufl., Springer Verlag Heidelberg 1992.

Copaifera langsdorffi

See Copaiba Balsam

Coptis trifolia

See Goldthread

Coral Root

Corallorhiza odontorhiza

DESCRIPTION

Medicinal Parts: The medicinal parts are the roots.

Flower and Fruit: The plant has 10 to 20 flowers in terminal panicles. The flower heads are hoodlike, reddish or purplish on the outside, paler and flecked with purple lines on the inside. One petal forms a lip with purple spots and a purple rim. The fruit is a large, bent-back, ribbed, long capsule.

Leaves, Stem, and Root: Coral Root is a perennial found growing around the roots of trees in woodlands. The rhizome is small, brown, and coral-like, about 2 to 3 cm long and 2 mm thick, with minute warts and transverse scars. The fracture is short and horny.

Characteristics: The taste is sweetish, then bitter. The odor is strong and peculiar when fresh.

Habitat: The parasite is indigenous to the U.S.

Production: Coral Root is the rhizome of *Corallorhiza odontorhiza*.

Other Names: Crawley Root, Scaly Dragon's Claw, Chicken Toe, Crawley, Fever Root, Turkey Claw

ACTIONS AND PHARMACOLOGY

COMPOUNDS

Unknown

EFFECTS

Coral Root has diaphoretic, febrifuge and sedative effects.

INDICATIONS AND USAGE

Unproven Uses: Coral Root is used for colds. It is very efficient at inducing perspiration. Its scarcity prevents its wider use.

PRECAUTIONS AND ADVERSE REACTIONS

Health risks or side effects following the proper administration of designated therapeutic dosages are not recorded.

DOSAGE

Mode of Administration: Internally as a liquid extract.

LITERATURE

No references are available

Corallorhiza odontorhiza

See Coral Root

Coriander

Coriandrum sativum

DESCRIPTION

Medicinal Parts: The medicinal parts are the coriander oil and dried ripe fruit.

Flower and Fruit: The flowers are white, compact, 3 to 5 blossomed umbels with no involucre. The floret has a 3-bract epicalyx. The border of the calyx has 5 tips. The corolla of the androgynous lateral florets is splayed. The fruit is globular and has a diameter of 3 cm, is straw yellow to brownish, and drops without dividing.

Leaves, Stem and Root: Coriandrum sativum is a 20 to 70 cm high plant with a bug-like smell. The root is thinly fusiform. The stem is erect, round, glabrous and branched above. The leaves are light green, entire below and double-pinnate above.

Characteristics: The fresh herb and unripe fruit have a bug-like smell. Ripe fruit has a pleasant, tangy smell and taste.

Habitat: The herb is found in the Mediterranean region, central and eastern Europe, eastern Asia, and North and South America.

Production: Coriander consists of the ripe, dried, spherical fruit of Coriandrum sativum and its varieties vulgare A. and microcarpum. The fruit is threshed when it is rust red and is dried in lofts.

Not to be Confused With: Grains and legumes.

Other Names: Cilantro

ACTIONS AND PHARMACOLOGY

COMPOUNDS

Volatile oil (0.4 to 1.7%): chief components D-(+)-linalool (coriandrol, share 60 to 75%), including in addition borneol, p-cymene, camphor, geraniol, limonene, alpha-pinene; the unusual, bug-like smell is caused by the trans-tridec-2-enale content

Fatty oil (13 to 21%): chief fatty acids petroselic acid, oleic acid, linolenic acid

Hydroxycoumarins: including umbelliferone, scopoletin

EFFECTS

The essential oil of coriander stimulates the secretion of gastric juices and is a carminative and spasmolytic; in vitro it has antibacterial and antifungal effects.

INDICATIONS AND USAGE

Approved by Commission E:

- Dyspeptic complaints
- Loss of appetite

Unproven Uses: Coriander is used for dyspeptic complaints, loss of appetite and complaints of the upper abdomen.

In folk medicine, Coriander is also used for digestive and gastric complaints; externally it's used for headaches, oral and pharyngeal disorders, halitosis, postpartum complications; the folk indications have not been proved.

Chinese Medicine: Coriander is used in China for loss of appetite, the pre-eruptive phase of chickenpox and measles, hemorrhoids, and rectal prolapse.

Indian Medicine: In India, Coriander is used to treat nosebleeds, coughs, hemorrhoids, scrofulous, painful urination, edema, bladder complaints, vomiting, amoebic dysentery, and dizziness.

PRECAUTIONS AND ADVERSE REACTIONS

Health risks or side effects following the proper administration of designated therapeutic dosages are not recorded. The drug possesses a weak potential for sensitization.

DOSAGE

Mode of Administration: Crushed and powdered drug, as well as other galenic preparations for internal indication.

Preparations: Coriander extract 1:2 is prepared by percolating 1 weight part of the drug with 45% ethanol so that 2 weights tincture is produced. The infusion is prepared by pouring 150 mL of boiling water over 2 tsp. of crushed drug and straining after 15 minutes.

Daily Dosage: The average daily dose is 3.0 g of drug. The single dose is 1 g.

Infusion – 1 fresh cup between meals.

Tincture – 10 to 20 drops after meals.

Storage: The noncomminuted drug is stored at a maximum temperature of 25°C, protected from light in well-sealed containers.

LITERATURE

Akker TW van den, Roesyanto-Mahadi ID, Toorenenbergen AW van, Joost T van. Contact allergy to spices. *Contact Dermatitis* 22; 267-272. 1990.

Brown JP. A Review of the Genetic Effects of Naturally Occuring Flavonoids, Anthraquinones and Related Compounds. *Mutation Res.* 75; 243-277. 1980.

Chantraine JM, Laurent D, Ballivian C, Saavedra G, Ibanez R, Vilaseca LA. Insecticidal Activity of Essential Oils on *Aedes aegypti* Larvae. *Phytother Res*. 12 (5); 350-354. 1998.

Diedreichsen A et al., Chemotypes of *Coriandrum sativum L.* in the Gatersleben Genebank. In: PM 62, Abstracts of the 44th Ann Congress of GA, 82. 1996.

Formacék, Buch. In: Formacék, V, Kubeczka KH: Essential Oils Analysis by Capillary Gas Chromatography and Carbon-13-NMR Spectroscopy, John Wiley & Sons, Chicester, New York, Brisbane, Toronto, Singapore 1982.

Hethelyi E, Nyaradi-Szabady J. GC/MS Investigation of the Characteristic Compounds of the essential Oil obtained from *Coriandrum sativum. Herba Hung*. 29 (1-2); 69-76. 1990.

Kallio H, Kerrola K. Application of liquid carbon dioxide to the extraction of essential oil of coriander (*Coriandrum sativum L.*) fruits. *Z Lebensm Unters Forsch*. 195; 545-549. 1992.

Kim SW, Park MK, Bae KS, Rhee MS, Liu JR. Production of Petroselinic Acid from Cell Suspension Cultures of *Coriandrum sativum. Phytochemistry* 42 (6); 1581-1582. 1996.

Ochocka RJ, Lamparczyk H. Evaluation of Essential oils from the family *Umbelliferae* using principal component analysis. *Pharmazie* 48; 229-230.1993.

Coriandrum sativum

See Coriander

Corn Cockle

Agrostemma githago

DESCRIPTION

Medicinal Parts: The medicinal part of the herb is the seed.

Flower and Fruit: The flowers are apical or arranged in twos or threes like a curled cyme; the 5 sepals of the calyx have 2 to 4 cm long tips that project above the corolla; the flower tube is 14 to 18 mm. The 5 petals are 30 to 35 mm long, dark purple and occasionally whitish. There are 5 styles and 10 stamens. The ovary is superior, undivided and has a central placenta. The fruit capsule is 15 to 18 mm long with numerous 2.5 to 3.5 mm long, warty seeds.

Leaves, Stem, and Root: Agrostemma githago is an annual herb that grows upright to 100 cm high. The leaves are opposite, linear-lanceolate, acuminate, and grow up to 10 mm wide. The stem is upright, usually unbranched, and shaggy-gray-pubescent. The primary root is spindle-shaped and heavily branched.

Habitat: Europe and Asia

Production: Corn cockle seed is the dried seed of *Agrostemma githago.*

Other Names: Cockle

ACTIONS AND PHARMACOLOGY

COMPOUNDS

Triterpene saponins: chief component is githagoside (0.04%, gypsogenine tetraglycoside), additional components are gypsogenin and quillaic acid gylcosides

Fatty oil: 6%

Steroids: sterols, including alpha-spinasterol

Unusual amino acids: orcyl alanine (0.4%)

EFFECTS

The drug exhibits an antimycotic effect. Cornflower seeds are toxic in higher dosages.

INDICATIONS AND USAGE

Unproven Uses: Folk medicine uses include gastritis, coughs, skin impurities, edema and worm purging.

Homeopathic Uses: Dilutions are used for gastritis.

PRECAUTIONS AND ADVERSE REACTIONS

No health hazards are known in conjunction with the proper administration of designated homeopathic dosages of the drug.

OVERDOSAGE

2 to 3 g of the seeds are considered harmless to humans; poisonous levels are reached between 3 and 5 g due to the toxic triterpene saponin content. Dosages over 5 g are considered lethal. Signs of poisoning include local irritation of mucous membranes (sneezing, lacrimation, conjunctivitis, salivation, nausea, vomiting, colic, diarrhea). The ingestion of toxic levels leads to headache, dizziness, restlessness, circulatory disorders, deliria and possible spasms. Death occurs through asphyxiation. Long-term ingestion of acute nontoxic dosages can cause chronic signs of poisoning. The toxins are not affected by baking or cooking.

Following gastrointestinal emptying (inducement of vomiting, gastric lavage, sodium sulfate) and the instillation of activated charcoal, the treatment for poisoning includes diazepam or barbital (IV) for spasms. In the event of shock, plasma volume expanders should be infused. Monitoring kidney function is necessary. Intubation and oxygen respiration may also be required.

DOSAGE

Mode of Administration: Whole herb preparations for internal, external and parenteral uses.

Homeopathic Dosage: Parenterally: Can be given 1 mL sc., 3 times daily for acute use; and once a day for chronic use but only from D2 (HAB34). Orally: 5 drops, 1 tablet, 10 globules, every 30 to 60 minutes for acute use; and 1 to 3 times daily for chronic use.

LITERATURE

Hänsel R, Keller K, Rimpler H, Schneider G (Ed), Hagers Handbuch der Pharmazeutischen Praxis, 5. Aufl., Bde 4 - 6 (Drogen), Springer Verlag Berlin, Heidelberg, New York, 1992-1994.

Kende H, Shen TC, Nitrate reductase in Agrostemma githago. Comparison of the inductive effects of nitrate and cytokinin. *Biochem Biophys Acta*, 216:118-25, 1972 Nov 24.

Siepmann C, Bader G, Hiller K, Wray V, Domke T, Nimtz M, New saponins from the seeds of *Agrostemma githago* var. *githago*. *Planta Med*, 216:159-64, 1998 Mar.

Smith RA, Miller RE, Lang DG, Presumptive intoxication of cattle by corn cockle, Agrostemma githago (L) Scop. *Vet Hum Toxicol*, 216:250, 1997 Aug.

Stirpe F, Gasperi-Campani A, Barbieri L, Falasca A, Abbondanza A, Stevens WA, Ribosome-inactivating proteins from the seeds of *Saponaria officinalis L.* (soapwort), of *Agrostemma githago L.* (corn cockle) and of *Asparagus officinalis L.* (asparagus), and from the latex of *Hura crepitans L.* (sandbox tree). *Biochem J*, 216:617-25, 1983 D.

Corn Poppy

Papaver rhoeas

DESCRIPTION

Medicinal Parts: The medicinal parts of the plant are the flowers and seeds.

Flower and Fruit: The flowers are solitary, terminal or axillary, and have a diameter of 10 cm. The pedicles are bristly, irregularly curved, and usually axillary. The two sepals are green, bristly, and fall off. The 4 petals are orbicular, usually scarlet or crimson (though occasionally white or violet) with a round, shiny, often white-bordered deep-black mark at the base. The fruit capsule is broad-elliptical, dark brown, and reticulate-pitted.

Leaves, Stem, and Root: Poppy is an annual, occasionally biennial, multiple-stemmed plant 25 to 90 cm high. The stems are erect to semi-erect, simple or branched with stiff, protruding hairs. They have basal rosette lanceolate leaves and deeply indented cauline leaves. The foliage leaves are oblong-lanceolate, pinnatifid to pinnatisect and very bristly.

Habitat: The plant is indigenous to Europe, northern Africa and temperate regions in Asia, and has been introduced in North and South America.

Production: Corn Poppy flower consists of the dried petals of Papaver rhoeas as well as its preparations.

Not to be Confused With: Confusion can occur with *Papaver dibium* and *Papaver argemone*.

Other Names: Copperose, Corn Rose, Cup-Puppy, Headache, Headwark, Red Poppy

ACTIONS AND PHARMACOLOGY

COMPOUNDS

Isoquinoline alkaloids (0.1%): chief alkaloids rhoeadine, isorhoeadine, rhoeagenine, coptisine, isocorydine, stylopine

Anthocyans: including among others mecocyanin (cyanidin-3-isosophoroside), cyanin

Mucilages

EFFECTS

No information is available other than that the drug, which contains alkaloids (not opium alkaloids), is said to be convulsive.

INDICATIONS AND USAGE

Unproven Uses: Corn Poppy flower is used for diseases and disorders of the respiratory tract, for disturbed sleep, as a sedative, and for the relief of pain. In folk medicine, it is used to make a cough syrup for children, as a tea for insomnia, for pain relief, and as a sedative.

Homeopathic Uses: Homeopathy uses Corn Poppy flower for states of agitation and excitation and also for spasms of the hollow organs.

PRECAUTIONS AND ADVERSE REACTIONS

No health hazards or side effects are known in conjunction with the proper administration of designated therapeutic dosages. The drug itself is nontoxic due to the low level of alkaloid content, but reports exist in the scientific literature of children being poisoned by intake of the fresh foliage (with blossoms). Poisoning symptoms include vomiting and stomach pain.

DOSAGE

Mode of Administration: As a component of ''metabolic'' teas.

Preparation: To prepare a tea, use 1 g of the flowers to 1 cup hot water. To make an infusion, scald 2 teaspoonfuls drug, steep for 10 minutes and strain (1 teaspoonful is equal to approximately 8 g drug). A poultice is prepared using 1 to 2 teaspoonfuls of tincture to 250 mL of water. (Prepare tincture in accordance with HAB1 guidelines.)

Daily Dosage: As an expectorant for inflammation of the bronchial mucous membranes, drink 1 cup infusion 2 to 3 times a day. The infusion may be sweetened with honey.

Homeopathic Dosage: Full bath: 2/3 tablespoons tincture in a bath (correspondingly less for partial baths).

Storage: Corn Poppy flower should be thoroughly dried before storing in a tightly sealed container that protects it from light.

LITERATURE

Alcazar MD, Garcia C, Rivera D, Obon C. Lesser-known Herbal Remedies as sold in the Market at Murcia and Cartagena (Spain). *J Ethnopharmacol*. 28; 243-247 (1990)

Frohne D, Pfänder HJ, Giftpflanzen - Ein Handbuch für Apotheker, Toxikologen und Biologen, 4. Aufl., Wiss. Verlags-Ges. Stuttgart 1997.

Lewin L, Gifte und Vergiftungen, 6. Aufl., Nachdruck, Haug Verlag, Heidelberg 1992.

Roth L, Daunderer M, Kormann K, Giftpflanzen, Pflanzengifte, 4. Aufl., Ecomed Fachverlag Landsberg Lech 1993.

Teuscher E, Lindequist U, Biogene Gifte - Biologie, Chemie, Pharmakologie, 2. Aufl., Fischer Verlag Stuttgart 1994.

Wichtl M (Hrsg.), Teedrogen, 4. Aufl., Wiss. Verlagsges. Stuttgart 1997.

Corn Silk

Zea mays

DESCRIPTION

Medicinal Parts: The medicinal part is the seed.

Flower and Fruit: The plant is monoecious. The male flowers form terminal racemes of spikes with two-flowered husks. The female flowers are axillary. The spikes are at varying distances from the ground and are enclosed in a number of thin leaves and the sheathlike maize husk. The spikes consist of a cylindrical substance, the cob, on which the seeds are arranged in 8 rows of 40 or more. Single whitish-green threads of a silky appearance grow from the eyes of the seeds and hang outside the husk, where they catch the pollen. The Maize seeds are usually yellow but can be darker to almost black.

Leaves, Stem, and Root: The plant is 1 to 3 m high and sturdy with a solid stem covered in alternate, over 4 cm wide, linear leaves.

Habitat: The plant is indigenous to America and is cultivated all over the world as green fodder or as a cereal crop.

Production: Corn Silk flowers are the styles and stigmas of *Zea mays*. The styles of the female flowers, as they begin to grow out of the pillow-lace, are gathered for medicinal or therapeutic purposes. They are removed by hand and dried in the shade.

Other Names: Indian Corn, Corn Silk, Stigmata maydis

ACTIONS AND PHARMACOLOGY

COMPOUNDS

Volatile oil (0.2%): including among others carvacrol, alpha-terpineol, menthol, thymol

Flavonoids: including among others maysin, maysin-3′-ethyl ether

Bitter substances

Saponins (2-3%)

Tannins: the main one is probably proanthocyanidins

Sterols: including among others beta-sitosterol, ergosterol

Alkaloids (0.05%)

6-methoxybenzoxazolinone

Fatty oil (2%)

EFFECTS

The active agents are saponin, essential oil, and tannin. Maize stimulates the cardiac muscles, increases blood pressure, acts as a diuretic, and sedates the digestive tract.

INDICATIONS AND USAGE

Unproven Uses: Maize is used for disorders of the urinary tract.

Chinese Medicine: Maize is used in the treatment of liver disorders.

PRECAUTIONS AND ADVERSE REACTIONS

No health hazards or side effects are known in conjunction with the proper administration of designated therapeutic dosages.

DOSAGE

Mode of Administration: Liquid extract, in medicinal preparations and combinations.

Preparation: Prepare an infusion using 2 teaspoons of drug per cup of water. A tincture is prepared by adding 20 gm of drug to 100 ml of 20% alcohol (leave to stand for 5 days).

How Supplied:

Capsules: 450 mg

Liquid Extract

Daily Dosage: Drink 1 cup of infusion every other day. Take 2 to 3 teaspoons of tincture per day.

LITERATURE

Adikwu MU, Onyia CC, Ofokansi KC. Evaluation of the physiochemical properties of Gladiolus actinomorphanthus starch. *Acta Pharm.* 47; 197-202. 1997.

Alcazar MD, Garcia C, Rivera D, Obon C. Lesser-known Herbal Remedies as sold in the Market at Murcia and Cartagena (Spain). *J Ethnopharmacol.* 28; 243-247. 1990.

Bravo HR, Lazo W. Antialgal and Antifungal Activity of Natural Hydroxamic Acids and Related Compounds. *J Agric Food Chem.* 44 (7); 1569-1571. 1996.

Chan H, But P, Pharmacology, Applications of Chinese Materia Medica, Vol 1, World Scientific Singapore 1986.

Devarenne TP, Sen-Michael B, Adler JH. Biosynthesis of Ecdosteroids in *Zea mays. Phytochemistry* 40 (4); 1125-1131. 1995.

Grases F, March JG, Ramis M, Costa-Bauza A. the influence of *Zea mays* on urinary risk factors for kidney stones in rats. *Phytother Res.* 7 (2); 146-149. 1993.

Kern W, List PH, Hörhammer L (Hrsg.), Hagers Handbuch der Pharmazeutisehen Praxis, 4. Aufl., Bde 1-8: Springer Verlag Berlin, Heidelberg, New York, 1969.

Leung AY, Encyclopedia of Common Natural Ingredients Used in Food Drugs, Cosmetics, John Wiley & Sons Inc., New York 1980.

Machuca G, Valencia S, Lacalle JR, Machuca C, Bullon P. A clinical assessment of the effectiveness of a mouthwash based on triclosan and on *Zea mays L* used as supplements to brushing. *Quintessence Int*, 28:329-35, 1997 May.

Shukla K, Narain JP, Puri P, Gupta A, Bijlani RL, Mahapatra SC, Karmarkar MG. Glycaemic Response to Maize, Bajra and Barley. *Indian J Physiol Pharmacol.* 35; 249-254. 1991.

Cornflower

Centaurea cyanus

DESCRIPTION

Medicinal Parts: The medicinal parts are the fast-growing ray flowers and the dried ray florets, which are separated from the receptacle and epicalyx, and to a lesser extent the tubular florets, which have usually are separated from the ovaries.

Flower and Fruit: The 3-cm wide flowers are solitary and terminal. The tubular flowers are blue, the cultivated ones are usually all purple-violet, pale pink, or white. The lateral florets are larger, in rays and funnel-shaped. The oblong gray fruit is an achaene with the remains of a tuft of hair.

Leaves, Stem, and Root: Growing 20 to 70 cm high, the annual or biennial plant contains fusiform, pale tap roots. It has a rosette of basal leaves and an erect, branched, spider-web/pubescent angular stem, covered in alternate, faintly linear-lanceolate leaves. The basal leaves are lyre-shaped, pinnatafid, and long-petioled. The upper leaves are noncompound.

Habitat: The plant is probably indigenous to the Middle East, but is cultivated worldwide because of grain production.

Production: Cornflower consists of the quickly dried flowers of *Centaurea cyanus*. The plant is harvested during the flowering season from June to August.

Other Names: Centaurea, Bachelor's Buttons, Bluebonnet, Bluebottle, Blue Centaury, Cyani, Bluebow, Hurtsickle, Blue Cap, Cyani-flowers. Blue Poppy, Corn Binks

ACTIONS AND PHARMACOLOGY

COMPOUNDS

Anthocyans: chief components succinylcyanin (centaurocyanin, cyanidine-3-O-(6-O-succinyl-beta-D-glucosyl)-5-O-beta -D-glucoside)

Flavonoids

Bitter principles (structure unknown)

EFFECTS

The drug has an antibacterial effect in vitro (centaurocyanin), but only for the aerial parts of the plant without the flowers.

INDICATIONS AND USAGE

Unproven Uses: Cornflowers and their preparations are used internally for fever, constipation, leucorrhea, and menstrual disorders. Externally, Cornflowers are used in preparation of eye washes for eye inflammation and conjunctivitis, and for eczema of the scalp.

PRECAUTIONS AND ADVERSE REACTIONS

Health risks or side effects following the proper administration of designated therapeutic dosages are not recorded. The drug possesses a weak sensitization potential.

DOSAGE

Mode of Administration: Cornflower is rarely used today. Occasionally, it is used as an inactive ingredient in tea mixtures.

Preparation: The infusion is prepared by adding 1 g of drug per cup.

Dosage: The tea should be drunk several times daily.

Storage: Store carefully and protect from light.

LITERATURE

Hänsel R, Keller K, Rimpler H, Schneider G (Hrsg.), Hagers Handbuch der Pharmazeutischen Praxis, 5. Aufl., Bde 4-6 (Drogen), Springer Verlag Berlin, Heidelberg, New York, 1992-1994.

Kakegawa K et al., PH 26:2261-2263. 1987.

Suljok G, Lãszló-Bencsik A, PH 24:1121-1122. 1985.

Takeda K et al., PH 27:1228-1229. 1988.

Cornus florida

See Dogwood

Cornus officinalis

See Asiatic Dogwood

Corydalis (Yan-Hu-Suo)

Corydalis cava

DESCRIPTION

Medicinal Parts: The medicinal parts are the tubers collected and dried when the plant is dormant. The fresh tuber collected just before flowering is also used.

Flower and Fruit: Flowers first appear in the fourth or fifth year. There are 4 to 5 racemes of 6 to 12 blooms, which are symmetrically 2-sided. There are 2 entire-margined bracts under the racemes. The flowers are dull red or yellowish-white, seldom lilac, brown-red or dark blue. The sepals are very small. The upper petal is drawn out into a downward curved spur; the front end is curved upward like a lip. The inner petals form a hood-like protective cover for the 6 stamens fused into 2 bundles. There is one ovary. The fruit is a pale green pod 20 to 25 cm long. The seeds are 3 mm wide, black, round, smooth and glossy.

Leaves, Stem and Root: The plant is perennial and grows to about 15 to 30 cm. A number of erect stems grows from the tuberous rhizome, which quickly becomes hollow. The stems bear the racemes and the 2 leaves. The 2 leaves under the racemes are long-petioled, double trifoliate, sea green above, and whitish green beneath.

Characteristics: The flowers have a slight fragrance of resin.

Habitat: The plant is indigenous to southern and central Europe.

Production: Corydalis tubers are the rhizomes of Corydalis cava. The tubers are dug up in autumn or in spring, once the ground has thawed. They are thoroughly cleaned, the roots and greenery are removed, and the remainder is sliced. The material is dried in a well-aired place, turned regularly and kept in temperatures not exceeding 40°C.

Other Names: Early Fumitory, Turkey Corn, Squirrel Corn, Yan-Hu-Suo

ACTIONS AND PHARMACOLOGY

COMPOUNDS

Isoquinoline alkaloids: very complex, breed-specific mixture of approximately 40 alkaloids, including (+)-bulbocapnine and (+)-corytuberin (aporphine-type) as well as (-)-corydaline (berberine-type)

EFFECTS

The full extract has a mildly sedative, sleep-inducing, spasmolytic, tranquilizing and hallucinogenic effect. It suppresses the CNS, reduces blood pressure and impedes movement of the small intestine.

INDICATIONS AND USAGE

Unproven Uses: Formerly, Corydalis was used for hyperkinetic conditions. Today, it is occasionally used for treat melancholia, pathological neuroses and mild forms of depression, as well as for severe nerve damage, trembling limbs and emotional disturbances.

Folk medicine: Corydalis was used in the past for worm infestation, menstruation disorders, Ménier's disease and Parkinson's. Externally, the plant was used for poorly healing wounds and ulcers.

Homeopathic Uses: Used for inflammations of the respiratory tract and the eyes, rheumatism, hyperorexia, diarrhea and furunculosis.

PRECAUTIONS AND ADVERSE REACTIONS

Health risks or side effects following the proper administration of designated therapeutic dosages are not recorded. Poisonings among humans have not yet been observed.

OVERDOSAGE

Clonic spasms with musculature tremor occur with overdosages.

DOSAGE

Mode of Administration: The drug is available as a full extract in ready-made preparations.

Daily Dosage: Externally: as a compress, 3 to 5 gm of drug to 1/8 Liter of water.

Homeopathic Dosage: Oral: 5 drops, 1 tablet or 10 globules every 30 to 60 minutes (acute) or 1 to 3 times daily (chronic); parenterally: 1 to 2 ml sc acute: 3 times daily; chronic: once a day; eye drops 1 to 3 times daily; liquid dilutions D2 to D6: 20 to 60 drops; D12 to D30: 15 to 45 drops (HAB1).

LITERATURE

Abbasoglu U, Sener B, G,nay Y, Temizer H. Antimicrobial Activity of Some Isoquinoline Alkaloids. *Arch Pharm* (Weinheim) 324; 379-380. 1991.

Boegge SC, Nahrstedt A, Linscheid M, Nigge W. Distribution and Stereochemistry of Hydroxycinnamoylmalic Acids and Free Malic Acids in *Papaveraceae* and *Fumariaceae. Z Naturforsch.* 50c; 608-615. 1995.

Frohne D, Pfänder HJ, Giftpflanzen - Ein Handbuch für Apotheker, Toxikologen und Biologen, 4. Aufl., Wiss. Verlagsges. mbH Stuttgart 1997.

Hänsel R, Keller K, Rimpler H, Schneider G (Hrsg.), Hagers Handbuch der Pharmazeutischen Praxis, 5. Aufl., Bde 4-6 (Drogen), Springer Verlag Berlin, Heidelberg, New York, 1992-1994.

Lewin L, Gifte und Vergiftungen, 6. Aufl., Nachdruck, Haug Verlag, Heidelberg 1992.

Reimeier C, Schneider I, Schneider W, Schäfer H-L, Elstner EF. Effects of Ethanolic Extracts from *Eschscholtzia californica* and Corydalis cava on Dimerization and Oxidation of Enkephalins. *Arzneim Forsch.* 45; 132-136. 1995.

Schäfer HL, Schäfer H, Schneider W, Elstner EF. Sedative Action of Extract Combinations of *Eschscholtzia californica* and *Corydalis cava. Arzneim Forsch.* 45; 124-126. 1995.

Teuscher E, Lindequist U, Biogene Gifte - Biologie, Chemie, Pharmakologie, 2. Aufl., Fischer Verlag Stuttgart 1994.

Corydalis cava

See Corydalis (Yan-Hu-Suo)

Corynanthe pachyceras

See Hwema Bark

Costus

Saussurea costus

DESCRIPTION

Medicinal Parts: The medicinal part of the plant is the root.

Flower and Fruit: The flowers are in tough, orbicular, axillary, or apical capitula, 2.5 to 3.8 cm in diameter and surrounded by an involucre. The epicalyx sepals are in a number of rows, ovate to lanceolate, acuminate, stiff, and revolute. The tubular florets are dark blue to black-violet. The fruit is an achene up to 8 mm long with a brownish, featherlike pappus that is up to 1.7 cm long.

Leaves, Stem, and Root: Saussurea costus is an herbaceous upright perennial growing to a height of up to 2 m. The leaves are alternate, the triangular lamina is simple, irregular dentate, basal, and 0.5 to 1.2 m long. The petiole is lobed-winged. The cauline leaves are smaller, petiolate, or sessile with 2 clasping lobes at the base. The plant has a strong, hard root up to 6 cm thick.

Habitat: The plant is indigenous to India and China.

Production: Indian Costus roots are the dried roots of *Saussurea costus*, which are harvested in September and October when the concentration of essential oils is highest.

Not to be Confused With: Because of the similarity in name, confusion sometimes occurs with Costus speciosus. The plant is also confused with *Inula racemosa*. In the past, confusion existed with many plants such as Byronia or Galanga, which went under the name of Kostus. However, differentiation has been established.

ACTIONS AND PHARMACOLOGY

COMPOUNDS

Volatile oil (1 to 6%): chief components dehydrocostus lactone (35%) and costunolid (15%), including as well alpha-, beta- and gamma-costol, elemol, cyclocostunolide; aroma bearers include acetic acid, 4-ethyl octanoic acid, heptanoic acid, 3-methyl butyric acid, 7-octenoic acid, isopropyliden pentanoic acid

Resins (6%)

Polysaccharides: inulin (18%)

Lignans: including olivil-4″-O-beta-D-glucoside

Sesquiterpenes: saussureamines A to E

Steroids: sterols, including beta-sitosterol, stigmasterol

EFFECTS

The drug contains large quantities of essential oil with the sesquiterpene lactones, costunolid and dehydrocostus lactone. Various drug extracts exhibit antimicrobial and fungistatic efficacy, and have an influence over liver metabolism and liver sugar levels. The saussure amines it contains inhibit the formation of stress-related stomach ulcers. A bronchospasmolytic effect has also been described. A dry extract of the drug administered in 500 mg dosages p.o. 3 times daily over a 3-month period led to a statistically significant reduction of angina pectoris attacks among patients with coronary heart disease.

INDICATIONS AND USAGE

Chinese Medicine: Internal uses include gastric complaints, flatulence, coughs, cholera, loss of appetite and asthma. Externally, it has been used for poorly healing wounds and skin conditions. Efficacy for these indications has not yet been proven.

Indian Medicine: See *Chinese Medicine,* plus the root has been used in India since ancient times as a universal antidote and as a contraceptive. It was also used medicinally as an aromatic and stimulant.

PRECAUTIONS AND ADVERSE REACTIONS

No health hazards are known in conjunction with the proper administration of designated therapeutic dosages. It is conceivable that the plant could cause allergic reactions due to its sesquiterpene lactone content, but no cases of this have as yet been documented.

DOSAGE

Mode of Administration: Whole and powdered drug preparations for internal and external use.

LITERATURE

Cheminat A, Stampf JL, Benezra C, Farrall MJ, Fr chet JM, Allergic contact dermatitis to costus: removal of haptens with polymers. *Acta Derm Venereol*, 61:525-9, 1981.

Hänsel R, Keller K, Rimpler H, Schneider G (Ed), Hagers Handbuch der Pharmazeutischen Praxis, 5. Aufl., Bde 4 - 6 (Drogen), Springer Verlag Berlin, Heidelberg, New York, 1992-1994.

Costus specious

See Cane-Reed

Cotton

Gossypium hirsutum

DESCRIPTION

Medicinal Parts: The medicinal parts are the seeds.

Flower and Fruit: Single axillary, radial flowers are structured in fives. The calyx is approximately 4.5 cm long, fused, divided into 5 sections and surrounded by 3 large, deeply dentate, epicalyx sepals. The 5 petals are 5 to 7 cm long, free, white to cream-yellow. The stamens are numerous, and the filaments are fused into a tube. The ovary is superior, and the carpels are fused. There is 1 style, with 3 to 5 stigmas that project through the stamen tube. The fruit is a walnut-sized capsule that opens on 3 to 5 sides and has 8 to 10 reniform, 3 to 5 mm thick, black seeds. These are covered in single-celled hair up to 46 mm long.

Leaves, Stem, and Root: This evergreen shrub grows up to 2 m high and is typically cultivated as an annual. The leaves are alternate, long-petiolate, 3- to 7-lobed, with serrate margins, a rounded base, and stipules that drop.

Habitat: The plant is indigenous to the U.S., China, Commonwealth of Independent States, India, Pakistan, and Egypt.

Production: Cotton seeds are the ripe seeds of *Gossypium hirsutum, Gossypium oleum,* and *Gossypium herbaceum*, as well as other cultivated *Gossypium* species. Cotton seed oil is the refined, fatty oil from the seeds. The oil is extracted using solvents or pressing followed by refinement with a yield of approximately 19%. Gossypium semen is derived from the industrial extraction of cottonseed oil.

Not to be Confused With: Mistaken identity can occur with sesame and kapok oil, which are sometimes used to adulterate Cotton oil preparations.

Other Names: American Cotton Plant, Cotton Seed

ACTIONS AND PHARMACOLOGY

COMPOUNDS: COTTON OIL

Fatty oil: chief fatty acids include linoleic acid (55%), palmitic acid (22%), oleic acid (15%), myristic acid (5%), as well as stearic acid, eicosanoic acid, di- cyclopropene-fatty acids malvalic acid and sterculiac acid

Lignans: gossypol (traces)

Steroids: sterols, particularly beta-sitosterol, as well as campesterol, stigmasterol, delta7-stigmasterol, 24-methyl cycloartenol

Tocopherols (vitamin E): including 0.04% alpha-tocopherol, 0.04% gamma-tocopherol

EFFECTS: COTTON OIL

The oil contains large amounts of unsaturated fatty acids and is chiefly used as a dietetic.

COMPOUNDS: COTTON SEED

Fatty oil (20 to 30%): chief fatty acids include linoleic acid (55%), palmitic acid (22%), oleic acid (15%), myristic acid (5%), as well as stearic acid, eicosanoic acid, the cyclopropene-fatty acids malvalic acid and sterculic acid

Protein (20 to 25%)

Lignans: (+)-gossypol and (-)-gossypol (0.1 to 6.0%, yellow to red in color); there are also cultivated forms that are low in gossypol (gossypol content

Flavonoids

Monosaccharides/oligosaccharides (7%): saccharose, raffinose, stachyose, glucose, fructose

EFFECTS: COTTON SEED

The pigment substance gossypol contained in the seeds inhibits enzymes of the energy metabolism, decouples the respiratory chain from the oxidative phosphorylation, reduces the cellular ATP concentration, lessens membrane potentials, and inhibits the acrosomal sperm proteinase acrosine (antifertility effect). A cytostatic effect has been demonstrated.

INDICATIONS AND USAGE

COTTON OIL

Unproven Uses: Folk medicine indications for *Gossypii oleum* have included hypercholesterolemia and vitamin E deficiency. It is also used when a nonnitrogenous or parenteral nourishment is required.

INDICATIONS AND USAGE

COTTON SEED

Indian Medicine: Among indications in Indian medicine are headache, coughs, dysentery, constipation, gonorrhea, chronic cystitis, fever, poor lactation, epilepsy, and snake bites. Reference is also made to use as an abortifacient and aphrodisiac. Efficacy for these indications has not yet been proved.

PRECAUTIONS AND ADVERSE REACTIONS

COTTON OIL

No health hazards are known in conjunction with the proper administration of designated therapeutic dosages. Animal experiments over a period of several weeks involving the administration of cyclopropene-fatty acids led to elevated cholesterol and triglyceride blood levels in rabbits and to a delayed sexual development in young female rats.

COTTON SEED

The drug is toxic, due to its gossypol content. Chronic ingestion of Cotton seed will lead to fertility disorders in men. After feeding sheep and cattle a total of 2 to 3 kg of Cotton seed press cakes over a period of 3 to 4 weeks, they exhibited gastroenteritis, kidney damage with hematuria, and icterus. Death occurred 24 to 48 hours after first appearance of symptoms. Eye damage (Cotton-seed blindness) was also noted.

DOSAGE

COTTON OIL

Preparation: Emulsion 10 to 15%: sterilization is carried out at 150° C for 1 hour.

Daily Dosage: Emulsion 40%: 60 ml p.o. in a single dose.

LITERATURE

Bicchi C, Joulain D. Review / Headspace-Gas-Chromatographic Analysis of Medicinal and Aromatic Plants and Flowers. *Flav Fragr J.* 5; 131-145. 1990

Hänsel R, Keller K, Rimpler H, Schneider G (Ed.), Hagers Handbuch der Pharmazeutischen Praxis, 5. Aufl., Bde 4 - 6 (Drogen), Springer Verlag Berlin, Heidelberg, New York, 1992-1994.

Jaroszewski JW, Strom-Hansen T, Hansen SH, Thastrup O, Kofod H. On the Botanical Distribution of Chiral Forms of Gossypol. *Planta Med.* 58; 454-458. 1992

Cotton Tree

Cochlospermum gossypium

DESCRIPTION

Medicinal Parts: The medicinal parts of the plant is the root, which yields a laxative, and the hard exudate of the aromatic bark.

Flower and Fruit: The flowers are in apical, sparsely flowered panicles. Flowers are 11 to 15 cm in diameter with 4 to 5 free silky-haired sepals, 4 to 5 gold-yellow petals, and numerous stamens. The superior ovary has 5 carpels with many ovules attached to the walls. The fruit is an oval, dark-brown, hanging capsule 5 to 10 cm long, 4 cm thick and loculicidal. The seeds are reniform, approximately 7 mm long, 5 mm wide and villous.

Leaves, Stem, and Root: Cotton Tree grows up to 10 m high. The leaves are 10 to 20 cm wide and palmate-lobed. The 3 to 5 lobes are acuminate or digitate; the petioles are 6 to 17 cm long. The young branches are velvet-haired and tinged reddish, the older ones are glabrous and ash gray.

Habitat: The tree is indigenous to India, Southeast Asia, Kenya and Mauritius.

Production: Cotton Tree gum is made up of the irregularly formed, leathery clumps of the exudate from the bark of *Cochlospermum gossypium.*

Other Names: Cotton Shell

ACTIONS AND PHARMACOLOGY

COMPOUNDS

Water-soluble polysaccharides: partially-acetylated, acidic heteroglycans

EFFECTS

The drug (acetylized acid polysaccharide) is laxative in effect.

INDICATIONS AND USAGE

Unproven Uses: The drug is used in folk medicine for constipation and sluggishness of the bowels.

Indian Medicine: Uses include coughs, diarrhea, dysentery, pharyngitis, and venereal disease.

PRECAUTIONS AND ADVERSE REACTIONS

No health hazards are known in conjunction with the proper administration of designated therapeutic dosages, nor with the drug's use as a pharmaceutical vehicle.

DOSAGE

Preparation: There is no information in the literature.

Daily Dose: A single dose of 3 g drug with plenty of liquid

LITERATURE

Blaschek W, Hänsel R, Keller K, Reichling J, Rimpler G, Schneider G (Eds), Hagers Handbuch der Pharmazeutischen Praxis. Folgeb nde 1 und 2. Drogen A-Z. Springer. Berlin, Heidelberg 1998.

Cowhage

Mucuna pruriens

DESCRIPTION

Medicinal Parts: The medicinal parts of the plant are the hairs on the pod and the seeds.

Flower and Fruit: The flowers grow in racemes in twos and threes. They are large and white, with a bluish-purple papilionaceous corolla. The pod is pubescent, thick, and leathery and averages about 10 cm in length. Pods have the shape of the sound opening in a violin. They are dark brown, covered with 0.25-cm long stiff hairs and contain 4 to 6 seeds. The seeds are made up of conical, sharply acuminate cells less than 1 mm in diameter and barbed at the apex. They are extremely irritating to the skin and must be handled with caution.

Leaves, Stem and Root: The plant is a climbing legume with long, thin branches and opposite, lanceolate leaves 15 to 30 cm in length. The petioles are pubescent.

Habitat: The plant is indigenous to tropical regions, especially India and the West Indies.

Production: Cowhage bean pods are the bean pods of *Mucuna pruriens*. The drug is derived from the hair of the pods.

Other Names: Cowitch, Couhage, Kiwach

ACTIONS AND PHARMACOLOGY

COMPOUNDS

Serotonin: 5-methyl-N,N-dimethyl-tryptamine

EFFECTS

Externally, Cowhage is a cutaneous stimulant and rubefacient. Internally, the drug has an anthelmintic effect. Carminative, hypotensive, hypoglycemic, and cholesterol-reducing effects have also been described.

Experiments carried out on frogs demonstrated that prurieninin slowed down the heart rate, lowered blood pressure, and stimulated intestinal peristalisis. The reduction in blood pressure was caused by the release of histamines; the spasmolysis of smooth muscle by indole bases.

INDICATIONS AND USAGE

Unproven Uses: The drug is used externally for rheumatic disorders and muscular pain, and internally for the treatment of worm infestation.

Indian Medicine: Uses in Indian medicine include gonorrhea, sterility, and general debility.

PRECAUTIONS AND ADVERSE REACTIONS

Once in contact with the skin, the stinging hairs lead to extremely aggressive itching and burning, accompanied by long-lasting inflammation, caused by the injection-like introduction of serotonin and proteins (mucunain, proteolytic enzyme). The intake of the hairs for the purpose of fighting intestinal worms should be avoided. Internal administration of the drug in the form of extracts may be harmless due to the difficulty involved in resorbing the active ingredients.

DOSAGE

Mode of Administration: The drug is used internally in extract form and powder form.

LITERATURE

Evans FJ, Schmidt RJ. Plants and Plant Products that Induce Contact Dermatitis. *Planta Med.* 38; 289-316. 1980.

Hegnauer R, Chemotaxonomie der Pflanzen, Bde 1-11, Birkhäuser Verlag Basel, Boston, Berlin 1962-1997.

Infante ME, Perez AM, Simao MR, Manda F, Baquete EF, Fernandes AM, Cliff JL, Outbreak of acute toxic psychosis attributed to *Mucuna pruriens. Lancet*, 29:1129. Nov 3, 1990.

Kern W, List PH, Hörhammer L (Hrsg.), Hagers Handbuch der Pharmazeutischen Praxis, 4. Aufl., Bde. 1-8, Springer Verlag Berlin, Heidelberg, New York, 1969.

Morton JF, An Atlas of Medicinal Plants of Middle America, Charles C Thomas USA.1981.

Nagaraju N, Rao KN. A Survey of Plant Crude Drugs of Rayalaseema, Andrha Pradesh, India. *J Ethnopharmacol.* 29; 137-158. 1990.

Revilleza MJ, Mendoza EM, Raymundo LC, Oligosaccharides in several Philippine indigenous food legumes: determination localization and removal. *Plant Foods Hum Nutr,* 29:83-93. Jan, 1990.

Teuscher E, Lindequist U, Biogene Gifte - Biologie, Chemie, Pharmakologie, 2. Aufl., Fischer Verlag Stuttgart 1994.

Teuscher E, Biogene Arzneimittel, 5. Aufl., Wiss. Verlagsges. Stuttgart 1997.

Woerdenbag HJ, Pras N, Frijlink HW, Lerk CF, Malingre TM, Antidiabetic evaluation of *Mucuna pruriens Linn* seeds. *JPMA J Pak Med Assoc*, 29:147-50. July 1990.

Cowslip

Primula veris

DESCRIPTION

Medicinal Parts: The medicinal parts are the roots and flowers.

Flower and Fruit: The flowers are in richly blossomed umbels with a short peduncle. The flowers are turned to one side and grow in clusters (up to 25) from the center of the leaf rosette. The calyx is cylindrical and appressed with a green margin. The remaining part of the calyx is yellow and is 12 to 15 cm long. The corolla is odorless, usually sulfur yellow, and has a tube with 5 triangular, orange spots. The fruit is an oval capsule with 1.5 to 2.5 mm-long brown, warty seeds.

Leaves, Stem, and Root: This 10 cm high plant is a herbaceous perennial with a short sturdy rhizome. The green plant parts are covered in 2-mm long segmented hairs. The leaves are revolute in the bud. They are wrinkled, ovate or ovate-oblong, and are rounded at the base. They narrow quickly to the winged stems. During the flowering season they are irregularly dentate with blunt teeth. They are 3 to 6 cm long during the flowering season, but grow larger later. The upper side of the leaf is glabrous.

Habitat: The plant is indigenous to all of Central Europe as far as the Southern European mountains. There are many subspecies.

Production: Cowslip flower consists of the dried, whole flowers with calyx of *Primula veris* and/or *Primula elatior* as well as their preparations. Cowslip root consists of the dried rhizome with roots of *Primula veris* and/or *Primula elatior* as well as their preparations. Cowslip root is harvested at best in the third year of growth.

Other Names: Oxlip, True Cowslip, Peagles, English Cowslip, Butter Rose, Herb Peter Paigle, Key Flower, Key of Heaven, Fairy Caps, Petty Mulleins, Buckles, Crewel, Palsywort, Plumrocks, Mayflower, Password, Primrose, Arthritica, Our Lady's Keys

ACTIONS AND PHARMACOLOGY

COMPOUNDS: COWSLIP FLOWER

Flavonoids (3%): including rutin, kaempferol-3-O-rutinoside, isorhamnetin-3-O-glucoside; isorhamnetin rhamnosyl robinoside, isorhamnetin robinoside, isorhamnetin rutinoside, kaempferol robinoside, limocitrin-3-O-glucoside, quercetin gentiobioside, quercetin-3-O-glucoside, quercetin robinoside

Primine

Triterpene saponins

EFFECTS: COWSLIP FLOWER

The drug has an expectorant effect, which is due to the flavonoid and saponin content. An increase of the volume of bronchial secretion has been demonstrated in animal experiments.

COMPOUNDS: COWSLIP ROOT

Phenol glycosides (0.2 to 2.3%, high values in the Spring): primulaverin (3%, 2-hydroxy-5-methoxy- benzoic acid methyl ester-O-xyloglucoside) changing over during dehydration into the characteristic-smelling 5-methoxy-methyl salicylate

Triterpene saponins (5 to 10%): chief components primulic acid A (chief aglycone protoprimulagenin)

EFFECTS: COWSLIP ROOT

The saponin content gives the drug expectorant and diuretic effects. Recent studies on these effects are not available. The mode of action is postulated to be due to vagal stimulation.

INDICATIONS AND USAGE

COWSLIP FLOWER

Approved by Commission E:

■ Cough/Bronchitis

Unproven Uses: Cowslip flower is used internally for catarrh of the respiratory tract. In folk medicine it is used for insomnia, anxiety, and as a cardiac tonic for feelings of dizziness and cardiac insufficiency. It is also used as a nerve tonic for shaking limbs, headaches, and neuralgia.

Homeopathic Uses: Primula veris is used to treat headaches and skin rashes

COWSLIP ROOT

Approved by Commission E:

■ Cough/Bronchitis

Unproven Uses: Cowslip root is used internally for catarrh of the respiratory tract. In folk medicine it is used internally for whooping cough, asthma, gout, rheumatic arthritis, bladder and kidney disease, migraine, dizziness, stomach cramps, scurvy, and neuralgia. Externally it is used for headaches and skin impurities.

CONTRAINDICATIONS

COWSLIP FLOWER

Contraindicated in known allergies to Cowslip.

PRECAUTIONS AND ADVERSE REACTIONS

COWSLIP FLOWER

No health hazards or side effects are known in conjunction with the proper administration of designated therapeutic dosages. The epigeal organs of the *Primula* species possess a very high potential for sensitization due to the primine content. In the cases of *Primula veris* and *Primula* elatior, the primine content is quite low, but sensitizations are nevertheless possible.

COWSLIP ROOT
No health hazards or side effects are known in conjunction with the proper administration of designated therapeutic dosages.

OVERDOSAGE

COWSLIP FLOWER
Overdose could lead to gastric complaints and nausea.

COWSLIP ROOT
Overdose could lead to queasiness, nausea, gastric complaints and diarrhea.

DOSAGE

COWSLIP FLOWER
Mode of Administration: Cowslip preparations are available as solid and liquid pharmaceutical forms for oral intake and also available parenterally for homeopathic use.

Preparations: Tea: boiling water is poured over 2 to 4 gm drug and strained after 10 minutes (1 teaspoon corresponds to approximately 1.3 gm drug).

Liquid extract: drug 1:1 with 25% ethanol (V/V) (BHP83)

Daily Dosage: The average daily dose is 3 gm of drug. The single dose is 1 gm of drug.

Tea: 1 cup several times a day. As a bronchial tea, several cups a day, possibly sweetened with honey

Liquid extract: 1 to 2 ml 3 times a day

Homeopathic Dosage: 5 drops, 1 tablet, or 10 globules every 30 to 60 minutes (acute) or 1 to 3 times daily (chronic); parenterally: 1 to 2 ml sc acute: 3 times daily; chronic: once a day (HAB34); different doses for children.

Storage: Should be protected from light and moisture.

COWSLIP ROOT
Preparations: Tea: 0.2 to 0.5 g finely cut drug are added to cold water and brought to the boil, left to draw for 5 minutes and strained (1 teaspoon corresponds to approximately 3.5 g drug).

Extract: percolation with 50 parts water and 50 parts ethanol, then filtration and vacuum drying. The residue is dissolved in 60 parts ethanol and 40 parts water and neutralized with ammonia. It is then cooled for 24 hours and filtered again. It is finally dehydrated to produce a dry extract under low pressure. (ÖAB90)

Liquid extract: Primula extract is dissolved in a mixture of ethanol (30 parts), glycerol 85% (20 parts) and water (20 parts) and filtered when cool. (ÖAB90)

Tincture: 20 parts root and 100 parts diluted ethanol are processed to a tincture in accordance with the ÖAB VII maceration procedure.

Syrup: 1.5 parts Cowslip are dissolved in 20 parts water while being heated. It is then mixed with 10 parts 85% glycerol and 68.5 parts simple syrup. (ÖAB90)

Daily Dosage: The average daily dose is 1 g of drug. The single dose is 0.5 g of drug.

Tincture: The daily dose is 7.5 g.

Extract: The single dose is 0.1 to 0.2 g.

Liquid extract: The single dose is 0.5 g.

Tea: as an expectorant, 1 cup every 2 to 3 hours, sweetened with honey

Storage: Cowslip should be protected from light.

LITERATURE

COWSLIP FLOWER AND ROOT
Çalis I, Yürüker A, Rüegger H, Wright AD, Sticher O, Triterpene saponins from *Primula veris ssp.* macrocalyx and *Primula elatiro ssp. meyeri*. In: *JNP* 55:1299-1306. 1992.

Ernst E, März R, Sieder C. A controlled multi-centre study of herbal versus synthetic secretolytic drugs for acute bronchitis. *Phytomedicine* 4 (4); 287-293. 1997.

Lepoittevin JP, Benezra C. Allergic contact dermatitis caused by naturally occuring quinones. *Pharm Weekbl Sci Ed.* 13; 119-122. 1991.

Neubauer N, März RW. Placebo-controlled, randomized double-blind clinical trial with Sinupret® sugar coated tablets on the basis of a therapy with antibiotics and decongestant nasal drops in acute sinusitis. *Phytomedicine* 1; 177-181. 1994.

Cranberry

Vaccinium macrocarpon

DESCRIPTION

Medicinal Parts: Fruit

Botanical Description: Cranberries are creeping, evergreen shrubs that spread by rhizomes. Upright shoots form from rhizomes after about 2 years, which produce the flowers and fruit. Uprights may grow 2-4 inches annually, with bases of the stems sagging down as the upright elongates—hence, only the terminal 5 to 8 inches remains in vertical position. Leaves are tiny (1/4′ to ½′ long), evergreen, thick, and oval/oblong in shape with entire margins. Leaves persist for 2 seasons and shed in late summer of the year after development. The plants yield pink flowers, followed by small, red-black edible berries from June to July. The flowers are hermaphrodite.

Habitat: Boreal forests of the world, especially Newfoundland, Nova Scotia, North Carolina, Minnesota, the Great Lakes region, and Scandinavia. In bogs, swamps and along lake shores.

Other Names: American cranberry, Arandano Americano, Arandano trepador, bear berry, black cranberry, bog cranberry, grosse Moosebeere, isokarpalo, Kranbeere, Kronsbeere, large cranberry, low cranberry, marsh apple, mountain cranberry, moosebeere, mossberry, pikkukarpalo, preisselbeere, ronce d'Amerique, trailing swamp cranberry, Tsurukokemomo.

ACTIONS AND PHARMACOLOGY

COMPOUNDS

Cranberry juice contains a variety of constituents. The berries contain about 88% water. The juice contains anthocyanin dyes, catechin, triterpenoids, approximately 10% carbohydrates, and small amounts of protein, fiber, and ascorbic acid (2 to 10 mg). Organic acids present are citric, malic, and quinic acids, with small amounts of benzoic and glucuronic acids. The glycoside leptosine and several related compounds have been isolated along with small amounts of alkaloids. Anthocyanin pigments obtained from cranberry pulp are used in commercial coloring applications.

EFFECTS

The mechanism of action of cranberry has instigated a great deal of scientific debate. Initially, it was assumed that acidification of the urine contributed to an antibacterial effect. The currently proposed mechanism of action focuses primarily on cranberry's ability to prevent bacterial binding to host cell surface membranes. In vitro studies have observed potent inhibition of bacterial adherence of *Escherichia coli* and other gram-negative uropathogens. Cranberry has been found to specifically inhibit hemagglutination of *E. coli* by expression of types 1 and P adhesin through the component compounds, fructose and proanthocyanidins.

CLINICAL TRIALS

Urinary Tract Infections

A prospective, double-blind, placebo-controlled, crossover study was performed to determine the efficacy of cranberry at preventing urinary tract infections (UTIs) in 21 persons with neurogenic bladders secondary to spinal cord injury. Patients were randomly assigned to standardized, 400 mg cranberry tablets or placebo three times a day for 4 weeks. After 4 weeks and an additional 1-week washout period, participants were crossed over to the other groups. There was no statistically significant treatment effect for cranberry supplement, indicating that cranberry tablets were not effective at changing urinary pH or reducing bacterial counts, urinary white blood cell counts, or UTIs in individuals with neurogenic bladders (Linsenmeyer et al, 2004).

Cranberry extract in tablet form was not effective in reducing bacteriuria and pyuria in 48 persons with spinal cord injury. Each patient enrolled in this randomized, double-blind, placebo-controlled study ingested 2 g of concentrated cranberry juice or placebo in capsule form daily for 6 months. There were no differences or trends detected between participants and controls with respect to number of urine specimens with bacterial counts of at least 10(4) colonies per milliliter, types and numbers of different bacterial species, numbers of urinary leukocytes, urinary pH, or episodes of symptomatic urinary tract infection (Waites et al, 2004).

In a randomized, placebo-controlled study, children (mean age 4.3 years) were randomized to receive either cranberry juice (n=171) or a placebo (n=170) for three months to evaluate the effect of cranberry juice on nasopharyngeal and colonic bacterial flora, and to determine how well cranberry juice is accepted by children and whether it affects infectious diseases and related symptoms. Bacterial samples were collected before and after intervention and analyzed for both respiratory bacterial pathogens and enteric fatty acid composition, reflecting changes in the colonic bacterial flora. Cranberry juice was well accepted by the children, but led to no change in either the bacterial flora in the nasopharynx or the bacterial fatty acid composition of stools (Kontiokari et al, 2005).

Infections

A prospective, randomized, double-blind, placebo-controlled trial was conducted with adults suffering from *Helicobacter plyori* infections. Subjects were randomly divided into two groups, one drinking two 250 ml cranberry juice boxes (n=97) and the other drinking matching placebo beverage (n=92) daily for 90 days. The researchers concluded that daily consumption of cranberry juice is capable of suppressing *H. plyori* infection in endemically afflicted populations (Zhang et al, 2005).

Cognitive Performance

In a 6-week, randomized double-blind, placebo-controlled, parallel-group trial, 50 volunteers were randomly assigned to receive either 32 ounces/day of a beverage containing 27% cranberry juice per volume or placebo. Aim was to investigate the efficacy of cranberry juice on the neuropsychologic functioning of cognitively intact older adults. No significant interactions were found between the cranberry and placebo groups and their pretreatment, baseline, and end-of-treatment neuropsychologic assessment. A non-significant trend was noted, however, on a subjective, self-report questionnaire; twice as many participants in the cranberry group rated their overall abilities to remember by treatment end as ''improved'' compared to placebo (Crews et al, 2005).

INDICATIONS AND USAGE

Unproven Uses: Anorexia, blood disorders, cancer treatment, diabetes, diuresis, nephrolithiasis prevention, radiation damage to urinary system, scurvy, stomach ailments, wound care.

Probable Efficacy: Cranberry is widely used to prevent urinary tract infection. There is clinical evidence in support of the use of cranberry juice and cranberry supplements to prevent urinary tract infections. Cranberry has also been investigated for numerous other medicinal uses, including prevention of *H. pylori* infection and dental plaque.

CONTRAINDICATIONS

Aspirin allergy, atrophic gastritis, diabetes (when product is sweetened with sugar), hypochlorhydria, kidney stones.

PRECAUTIONS AND ADVERSE REACTIONS

Generally well tolerated. When consumed in large amounts, gastrointestinal upset and diarrhea may occur.

Pregnancy: Scientific evidence for the safe use of cranberry during pregnancy is not available.

DRUG INTERACTIONS

MAJOR RISK

Warfarin: Concurrent use may result in an increased risk of bleeding. *Clinical Management:* Patients receiving treatment with warfarin should be advised to avoid excessive use of cranberry products.

MODERATE RISK

H2 Blockers: Concurrent use may result in a reduced effectiveness of the H2 blocker. *Clinical Management:* Advise patients to avoid regular use of cranberry juice while taking an H2 blocker. Occasional use of cranberry juice is not likely to have a clinical effect on H2 blocker. The effect of cranberry extract supplements on gastric acid is not known; caution is advised.

Proton Pump Inhibitors: Concurrent use may result in reduced effectiveness of proton pump inhibitors. *Clinical Management:* Advise patients to avoid regular use of cranberry juice while taking a proton pump inhibitor. Occasional use of cranberry juice is not likely to have a clinical effect on proton pump inhibitors. The effect of cranberry extract supplements on gastric acid is not known; caution is advised.

DOSAGE

How Supplied: juice, capsules (spray dried), concentrate

Daily Dose: To prevent urinary tract infections, 30-300g cranberry juice; in children 15mg/kg body weight is recommended. In type 2 diabetes, 200-400mg.

LITERATURE

Ahuja S, Kaack B, Roberts J. Loss of fimbrial adhesion with the addition of Vaccinum macrocarpon to the growth medium of P-fimbriated Escherichia coli. J Urol 1998;159(2):559-562.

Allison DG, Cronin MA, Hawker J, et al. Influence of cranberry juice on attachment of Escherichia coli to glass. J Basic Microbiol 2000;40(1):3-6.

Avorn J, Monane M, Gurwitz J, et al. Reduction of bacteriuria and pyuria using cranberry juice. JAMA 1994;272(8):588-590.

Avorn J, Monane M, Gurwitz JH, et al. Reduction of bacteriuria and pyuria after ingestion of cranberry juice. JAMA 1994;271(10):751-754.

Blatherwick NR, Long ML. Studies of urinary acidity II: The increased acidity produced by eating prunes and cranberries. J Biol Chem 1923;57:815.

Bodel P, Cotran R, Kass E. Cranberry juice and the antibacterial action of hippuric acid. J Lab & Clin Med 1959;54(6):881-888.

Bomser J, Madhavi DL, Singletary K, et al. In vitro anticancer activity of fruit extracts from Vaccinium species. Planta Med 1996;62(3):212-216.

Burger O, Ofek I, Tabak M, et al. A high molecular mass constituent of cranberry juice inhibits helicobacter pylori adhesion to human gastric mucus. FEMS Immunol Med Microbiol 2000;29(4):295-301.

Campbell G, Pickles T, D'yachkova Y. A randomised trial of cranberry versus apple juice in the management of urinary symptoms during external beam radiation therapy for prostate cancer. Clin Oncol (R Coll Radiol) 2003;15(6):322-328.

Chambers BK, Camire ME. Can cranberry supplementation benefit adults with type 2 diabetes? Diabetes Care 2003;26(9):2695-2696.

Crews WD, Harrison DW, Griffin ML, et al. A double-blind, placebo-controlled, randomized trial of the neuropsychologic efficacy of cranberry juice in a sample of cognitively intact older adults: a pilot study findings. J Altern Complement Med; 11(2): 305-309. 2005.

Dignam R, Ahmed M, Denman S, et al. The effect of cranberry juice on UTI rates in a long-term care facility. J Amer Geriat Soc 1997;45(9):S53.

DuGan C, Cardaciotto P. Reduction of ammoniacal urinary odors by the sustained feeding of cranberry juice. J Psych Nurs 1966;4:467-470.

Fleet JC. New support for a folk remedy: cranberry juice reduces bacteriuria and pyuria in elderly women. Nutr Rev 1994;52(5):168-170.

Foda M, Middlebrook PF, Gatfield CT, et al. Efficacy of cranberry in prevention of urinary tract infection in a susceptible pediatric population. Canadian J Urology 1995;2(1):98-102.

Foxman B, Geiger AM, Palin K, et al. First-time urinary tract infection and sexual behavior. Epidemiology 1995;6(2):162-168.

Garcia-Calatayud S, Larreina Cordoba JJ, Lozano De La Torre MJ. [Severe cranberry juice poisoning]. An Esp Pediatr 2002;56(1):72-73.

Gibson L, Pike L, Kilbourne J. Effectiveness of cranberry juice in preventing urinary tract infections in long-term care facility patients. J Naturopath Med 1991;2(1):45-47.

Goodfriend R. Reduction of bacteriuria and pyuria using cranberry juice. JAMA 1994;272(8):588-590.

Habash MB, Van der Mei HC, Busscher HJ, et al. The effect of water, ascorbic acid, and cranberry derived supplementation on human urine and uropathogen adhesion to silicone rubber. Can J Microbiol 1999;45(8):691-694.

Haverkorn MJ, Mandigers J. Reduction of bacteriuria and pyuria using cranberry juice. JAMA 1994;272(8):590.

Hopkins WJ, Heisey DM, Jonler M, et al. Reduction of bacteriuria and pyuria using cranberry juice. JAMA 1994;272(8):588-589.

Howell AB, Foxman B. Cranberry juice and adhesion of antibiotic-resistant uropathogens. JAMA 2002;287(23):3082-3083.

Howell AB, Vorsa N, Der MA, et al. Inhibition of the adherence of P-fimbriated Escherichia coli to uroepithelial-cell surfaces by proanthocyanidin extracts from cranberries. N Engl J Med 1998;339(15):1085-1086.

Hughes BG, Lawson LD. Nutritional content of cranberry products. Am J Hosp Pharm 1989;46(6):1129.

Jepson RG, Mihaljevic L, Craig J. Cranberries for preventing urinary tract infections. Cochrane Database Syst Rev 2000;(2):CD001321.

Kahn HD, Panariello VA, Saeli J, et al. Effect of cranberry juice on urine. J Am Diet Assoc 1967;51(3):251-254.

Kinney AB, Blount M. Effect of cranberry juice on urinary pH. Nurs Res 1979;28(5):287-290.

Konowalchuk J, Speirs JI. Antiviral effect of commercial juices and beverages. Appl Environ Microbiol 1978;35(6):1219-1220.

Kontiokari T, Salo J, Eerola E, Uhari M. Cranberry juice and bacterial colonization in children — a placebo-controlled randomized trial. Clin Nutr; 24(6): 1065-1072. 2005.

Kontiokari T, Sundqvist K, Nuutinen M, et al. Randomised trial of cranberry-lingonberry juice and Lactobacillus GG drink for the prevention of urinary tract infections in women. BMJ 2001;322(7302):1571-1573.

Leaver RB. Cranberry juice. Prof Nurse 1996;11(8):525-526.

Lee YL, Owens J, Thrupp L, et al. Does cranberry juice have antibacterial activity? JAMA 2000;283(13):1691.

Light I, Gursel E, Zinnser HH. Urinary ionized calcium in urolithiasis. Effect of cranberry juice. Urology 1973;1(1):67-70.

Linsenmeyer TA, Harrison B, Oakley A, Kirshblum S, Stock JA, Millis SR. Evaluation of cranberry supplement for reduction of urinary tract infections in individuals with neurogenic bladders secon-dary to spinal cord injury. A prospective, double-blind, placebo-controlled, crossover study. J Spinal Cord Med; 27(1): 29-34. 2004.

Lynch DM. Cranberry for prevention of urinary tract infections. Am Fam Physician. 2005 Sep 15;72(6):1000

McHarg T, Rodgers A, Charlton K. Influence of cranberry juice on the urinary risk factors for calcium oxalate kidney stone formation. BJU Int 2003;92(7):765-768.

Moen DV. Observations on the effectiveness of cranberry juice in urinary infections. Wisconsin Med J 1962;61:282-283.

Nahata MC, Cummins BA, McLeod DC, et al. Effect of urinary acidifiers on formaldehyde concentration and efficacy with methenamine therapy. Eur J Clin Pharmacol 1982;22(3):281-284.

Nahata MC, Cummins BA, McLeod DC, et al. Predictability of methenamine efficacy based on type of urinary pathogen and pH. J Am Geriatr Soc 1981;29(5):236-239.

Ofek I, Goldhar J, Sharon N. Anti-Escherichia coli adhesion activity of cranberry and blueberry juices. Adv Exp Med Biol 1996;408:179-183.

Ofek I, Goldhar J, Zafriri D, et al. Anti-Escherichia coli adhesin activity of cranberry and blueberry juices. N Engl J Med 1991;324(22):1599.

Papas PN, Brusch CA, Ceresia GC. Cranberry juice in the treatment of urinary tract infections. Southwest Med 1966;47(1):17-20.

Pedersen CB, Kyle J, Jenkinson AM, et al. Effects of blueberry and cranberry juice consumption on the plasma antioxidant capacity of healthy female volunteers. Eur J Clin Nutr 2000;54(5):405-408.

Reed J. Cranberry flavonoids, atherosclerosis and cardiovascular health. Crit Rev Food Sci Nutr 2002;42(3 Suppl):301-316.

Saltzman JR, Kemp JA, Golner BB, et al. Effect of hypochlorhydria due to omeprazole treatment or atrophic gastritis on protein-bound vitamin B12 absorption. J Am Coll Nutr 1994;13(6):584-591.

Schlager TA, Anderson S, Trudell J, et al. Effect of cranberry juice on bacteriuria in children with neurogenic bladder receiving intermittent catheterization. J Pediatr 1999;135(6):698-702.

Schmidt DR, Sobota AE. An examination of the anti-adherence activity of cranberry juice on urinary and nonurinary bacterial isolates. Microbios 1988;55(224-225):173-181.

Siciliano AA. Cranberry. Herbalgram 1996;38:51-54.

Sobota AE. Inhibition of bacterial adherence by cranberry juice: potential use for the treatment of urinary tract infections. J Urol 1984;131(5):1013-1016.

Sternlieb P. Cranberry juice in renal disease [letter]. New Engl J Med 1963;268(1):57.

Suvarna R, Pirmohamed M, Henderson L. Possible interaction between warfarin and cranberry juice. BMJ 2003;327(7429):1454.

Swartz JH, Medrek TF. Antifungal properties of cranberry juice. Appl Microbiol 1968;16(10):1524-1527.

Terris MK, Issa MM, Tacker JR. Dietary supplementation with cranberry concentrate tablets may increase the risk of nephrolithiasis. Urology 2001;57(1):26-29.

Tsukada K, Tokunaga K, Iwama T, et al. Cranberry juice and its impact on peri-stomal skin conditions for urostomy patients. Ostomy Wound Manage 1994;40(9):60-68.

Waites KB, Canupp KC, Armstrong S, DeVivo MJ. Effect of cranberry extract on bacteriuria and pyuria in persons with neurogenic bladder secondary to spinal cord injury. J Spinal Cord Med; 27(1): 35-40. 2004.

Walker EB, Barney DP, Mickelsen JN, et al. Cranberry concentrate: UTI prophylaxis. J Fam Pract 1997;45(2):167-168.

Walsh BA. Urostomy and urinary pH. J ET Nurs 1992;19(4):110-113.

Weiss EI, Lev-Dor R, Kashamn Y, et al. Inhibiting interspecies coaggregation of plaque bacteria with a cranberry juice constituent [published erratam appear in J Am Dent Assoc 1999 Jan;130(1):36 and 1999 Mar;130(3):332]. J Am Dent Assoc 1998;129(12):1719-1723.

Wilson T, Porcari JP, Harbin D. Cranberry extract inhibits low density lipoprotein oxidation. Life Sci 1998;62(24):L381-L386.

Yan X, Murphy BT, Hammond GB, et al. Antioxidant activities and antitumor screening of extracts from cranberry fruit (Vaccinium macrocarpon). J Agric Food Chem 2002;50(21):5844-5849.

Zafriri D, Ofek I, Adar R, et al. Inhibitory activity of cranberry juice on adherence of type 1 and type P fimbriated Escherichia coli to eucaryotic cells. Antimicrob Agents Chemother 1989;33(1):92-98.

Zhang L, Ma J, Pan K, et al. Efficacy of cranberry juice on Helicobacter pylori infection: a double-blind, randomized placebo-controlled trial. Helicobacter; 10(2): 139-145. 2005.

Zinsser HH, Seneca H, Light I, et al. Management of infected stones with acidifying agents. NY State J Med 1968;68:3001-3009.

Cranesbill

Geranium maculatum

DESCRIPTION

Medicinal Parts: The medicinal parts are the plant's dried rhizome and the leaves.

Flower and Fruit: The inflorescence is a terminal, cymose umbel. The flowers are radial with the structures arranged in fives with a 2.5 to 4 cm diameter. There are 5 free, pubescent sepals, 5 free purple petals, and 10 stamens. The ovary is formed from 5 carpels, which are fused to the sides of the central column with their long awns. The fruit is a schizocarp, which breaks up into 5 mericarps with beaklike extensions and 1 seed each.

Leaves, Stem, and Root: The herbaceous perennial grows upright, rising to 60 cm high. The leaves are opposite, in fives, with cuneiform lobes and whitish-green spots when older. Leaves growing from the rhizome are large with long, pubescent petioles; those growing from the trunk have short petioles; stipules are visible. The stem is upright, green, pubescent, and dichotomously branched. The rhizome is thick, cylindrical, and branched.

Habitat: The plant is found throughout Europe, but also in North America from Newfoundland to Manitoba and as far south as Georgia and Missouri. It grows in shady and moist ground in mixed and deciduous forests.

Production: American Cranesbill herb is the dried aerial herb of *Geranium maculatum* harvested during the flowering season. American Cranesbill root is the dried rhizome of *Geranium maculatum*, which is collected in late summer and autumn.

Other Names: Alumroot, Crowfoot, Geranium, Spotted Cranesbill, Spotted Geranium, Storksbill, Wild Cranesbill

ACTIONS AND PHARMACOLOGY

COMPOUNDS: CRANESBILL HERB

Tannins (30%): gallotannins

COMPOUNDS: CRANESBILL ROOT

Tannins (10 to 28%): gallotannins

EFFECTS

The tannins give the drug astringent, hemostyptic and tonic properties.

INDICATIONS AND USAGE

Unproven Uses: Folk medicine indications have included hemorrhoids, duodenal ulcers, diarrhea, metrorrhagia, heavy menstruation, and dysmenorrhea. Efficacy for these internal use indications has not yet been proved.

Homeopathic Uses: The root is used for stomach ulcers and bleeding of the mucous membranes, but efficacy for these indications has not yet been proved.

PRECAUTIONS AND ADVERSE REACTIONS

No health hazards are known in conjunction with the proper administration of designated therapeutic dosages. Because of its high tannin content, the intake of preparations of the drug could lead to digestive disorders. Individuals with sensitive stomachs could experience nausea and vomiting.

DOSAGE

CRANESBILL HERB

Daily Dosage: Powder/Infusion: 1 to 2 g, 3 times daily.

Homeopathic Dosage: Literature notes the drug's importance as a homeopathic medicine, but does not state dosage.

CRANESBILL ROOT

Preparation: Liquid extract - drug 1:1 45% ethanol (V/V) percolated (BHP83).

Daily Dosage:

Decoction: 1 to 2 g drug, 3 times daily

Liquid extract: 1 to 2 ml, 3 times daily

Tincture: 2 to 4 ml, 3 times daily.

Homeopathic Dosage: 5 to 10 drops, 1 tablet, or 5 to 10 globules, 1 to 3 times daily, or 1 mL injection solution sc twice weekly (HAB34).

LITERATURE

Hänsel R, Keller K, Rimpler H, Schneider G (Ed.), Hagers Handbuch der harmazeutischen Praxis, 5. Aufl., Bde 4 - 6 (Drogen), Springer Verlag Berlin, Heidelberg, New York, 1992-1994.

Crataegus laevigata

See English Hawthorn

Crithmum maritimum

See Samphire

Crocus sativus

See Saffron

Croton eluteria

See Cascarilla

Croton Seeds

Croton tiglium

DESCRIPTION

Medicinal Parts: The seeds are the medicinal parts. The oil is extracted from the seeds and is toxic; 1 mL can be fatal.

Flower and Fruit: Croton tiglium is a shrub or tree that grows up to 6 m. The leaves are alternate, smooth, ovate, or acuminate. They are dark green above and paler beneath, with an unpleasant smell. There are inconspicuous flowers in terminal racemes. The seeds have a brown, mottled appearance. The outer layer of the seed is easily removed, leaving a hard, black coat.

Characteristics: Croton Seed oil is yellowish or reddish-brown and rather viscid, with an unpleasant odor. It is toxic and should be handled with extreme care.

Habitat: The tree is found throughout Asia and China.

Production: Croton oil is extracted from the seeds of *Croton tiglium.*

Other Names: Tiglium, Tiglium Seeds

ACTIONS AND PHARMACOLOGY

COMPOUNDS

Diterpenes: phorbol ester, including 12-O-tridecane olyphorbol-13-acetate (TPA, myristoylphoarbolacetate, MPA)

Fatty oil

EFFECTS

Croton Seed oil is a laxative, skin irritant, cocarcinogenic, and nephrotoxic. It is a drastic irritant. TPA is a carcinogen, affecting prostaglandin metabolism.

INDICATIONS AND USAGE

Unproven Uses: At present, it is used only in Chinese medicine and in very small doses as a remedy for gall bladder colic, obstruction of the bowels, and malaria. The drug is obsolete in Europe.

Chinese Medicine: In China, Croton Seed oil is used for edema, furuncles, constipation, chest and stomach pain, worm infestation, and sore throat.

Indian Medicine: Indian uses include constipation, abdominal disorders, worm infestation, convulsions, and attacks of dizziness.

PRECAUTIONS AND ADVERSE REACTIONS

The phorbol esters of the oils are severe cocarcinogenics. Therapeutic uses as well as skin or mucous membrane contacts with the drug are to be strictly avoided. The drug possesses acute toxicity. When applied to the skin, it brings about itching, burning and, after a time, blisters. If taken internally, it leads to burning in the mouth, vomiting, dizziness, stupor, painful bowel movements, and ultimately to collapse.

OVERDOSAGE

One to 2 drops are already acutely toxic; the lethal dosage is put at 20 drops. After stomach and intestinal emptying, treatment of poisonings can only proceed symptomatically.

DOSAGE

Mode of Administration: Croton Seed oil is obsolete as drug.

LITERATURE

Benezra C, Ducombs G. Molecular Aspects of Allergic Contact Dermatitis to Plants. *Dermatosen* 35; 4-11. 1987.

Chan EH et al (eds). Advances in Chinese Medicinal Materials Research. World Scientific Pub. Co. Singapore 1985

El Mekkawy S, Meselhy MR, Kusumoto IT, Kadota S, Hattori M, Namba T. Inhibitory Effect of Egyptian Folk Medicines on Human Immunodeficiency Virus (HIV) Reverse Transcriptase. *Chem Pharm Bull.* 43 (4); 641-648. 1995.

Evans FJ (Ed.), Naturally Occurring Phorbol Esters, CRC Press 1986.

Evans FJ, Taylor SE. *Prog Chem Org* Nat Prod 44:1. 1983

Lee TY, Lam TH. Contact dermatitis due to topical treatment with garlic in Hong Kong. *Contact Dermatitis* 24; 193-196. 1991

Croton tiglium

See Croton Seeds

Cubeb

Piper cubeba

DESCRIPTION

Medicinal Parts: The medicinal parts are the dried, not fully ripe fruit.

Flower and Fruit: The male flowering spikes are about 4 cm long and have 2 or 3 stamens. The female spikes are made up of about 50 individual flowers, which mostly consist of the oblong ovary of 4 fused carpels with 4 sessile stigmas. The infructescence is 4 to 5 cm long. When ripe, the base of the ovary grows into a stem-like, cylindrical lower part. The upper portion of the fruit is globular and holds the seed, which contains a tiny embryo in a small cavity at the apex.

Leaves, Stem, and Root: The plant is a 5- to 15-m dioecious climbing shrub. The branches are initially pubescent, later glabrous. The leaves are glabrous, entire-margined, coriaceous, ovate to oblong-elliptical, and up to 15 cm long and 6 cm wide.

Characteristics: The odor is warm and reminiscent of turpentine.

Habitat: The plant is indigenous to Indonesia and is cultivated in Sri Lanka, India and Malaysia.

Production: Cubebs are the fruit of *Piper cubeba*. The fruit is harvested when still green and dried in the sun.

Other Names: Java Pepper, Tailed Cubebs, Tailed Pepper

ACTIONS AND PHARMACOLOGY

COMPOUNDS

Volatile oil (10 to 20%): chief constituents alpha- and beta-cubebenes (11%), copaene (10%), cubebol (10%), delta-cadinene (9%), humulenes

Lignans: chief components (-)-cubebin, additionally (-)-cubebinin, dihydroclusin, (-)-dihydrocubebin, hinokinin

Resins

Fatty oil (12%)

EFFECTS

The sesquiterpene-rich essential oil is said to be expectorant in chronic bronchitis. The resinous acids in the drug are said to have an antiseptic and astringent effect on the urinary tract. There is no information on the mode of action.

INDICATIONS AND USAGE

Unproven Uses: Folk medicine uses include treatment for urinary tract diseases, flatulence and stomach complaints, headaches (dizziness), chronic bronchitis, to increase libido, and for poor memory.

Homeopathic Uses: Piper cubeba is used for inflammation of the mucous membrane of the urogenital tract.

PRECAUTIONS AND ADVERSE REACTIONS

Health risks or side effects following the proper administration of designated therapeutic dosages are not recorded.

OVERDOSAGE

High dosages (over 8 gm) cause irritation of the urinary passages, kidney and bladder pains, albuminuria, and urination problems. Beyond this, vomiting, diarrhea, cardiac pain, and skin rashes can occur. After stomach and intestinal emptying, treatment of poisonings should proceed symptomatically.

DOSAGE

Mode of Administration: Cubeb is contained in medicinal preparations, such as bath additives.

Daily Dosage:

Powder – 2 to 4 g daily for internal administration

Extract (1:1) – daily dose: 2 to 4 mL

Tincture (1:5) – daily dose: 2 to 4 mL

Homeopathic Dosage: 5 to 10 drops, 1 tablet, or 5 to 10 globules 1 to 3 times a day or 1 ml injection solution sc twice weekly (HAB1); children's dosage does not equal adult dose.

LITERATURE

Bicchi C, Manzin V, D'Amato A, Rubiolo P. Cyclodextrin Derivatives in GC Separation of Enantiomers of Essential Oil, Aroma and Flavour Compounds. *Flav Fragr J.* 10; 127-137. 1995.

Koul SK et al., Phenylpropanoids and (-)-ledol from Piper species. In: *PH* 32:478. 1993.

Hänsel R, Keller K, Rimpler H, Schneider G (Hrsg.), Hagers Handbuch der Pharmazeutischen Praxis, 5. Aufl., Bde 4-6 (Drogen), Springer Verlag Berlin, Heidelberg, New York, 1992-1994.

Leung AY, Encyclopedia of Common Natural Ingredients Used in Food Drugs and Cosmetics, John Wiley & Sons Inc., New York 1980.

Lewin L, Gifte und Vergiftungen, 6. Aufl., Nachdruck, Haug Verlag, Heidelberg 1992.

Roth L, Daunderer M, Kormann K, Giftpflanzen, Pflanzengifte, 4. Aufl., Ecomed Fachverlag Landsberg Lech 1993.

Cucurbita pepo

See Pumpkin

Cudweed

Gnaphalium uliginosum

DESCRIPTION

Medicinal Parts: The aerial parts are the medicinal parts of the plant.

Flower and Fruit: The composite flower heads are 3 to 4 mm by 5 mm, sessile and in terminal racemes of 3 to 10. They are shorter than the leaves growing from the leaf axil. The involucral bracts are oblong to linear and brownish. There are 50 to 150 female florets and 5 to 8 hermaphrodite florets. The achaene is 0.5 mm and oblong-cylindrical. The pappus is 1.5 mm.

Leaves, Stem, and Root: The stems are 5 to 20 cm high and branched. The leaves are 10 to 50 mm by 2 to 5 mm, linear-lanceolate to oblong-obovate. They are downy and greenish above; whitish and downy beneath.

Habitat: The plant is native to many parts of Europe, the Caucasus and west Asia. It has been introduced into America.

Production: Cudweed is the aerial part of *Gnaphalium uliginosum.*

Other Names: Cotton Weed, Dysentery Weed, Everlasting, Mouse Ear, Wartwort, Cotton Dawes

ACTIONS AND PHARMACOLOGY

COMPOUNDS

Volatile oil

Tannins

The constituents of the drug have not been extensively investigated.

EFFECTS

Cudweed is an astringent and a stomachic. According to unconfirmed sources, the drug also has antidepressive, aphrodisiac, and hypotensive effects.

INDICATIONS AND USAGE

Unproven Uses: The drug is used as a gargle and rinse in the treatment of diseases of the mouth and throat.

PRECAUTIONS AND ADVERSE REACTIONS

Health risks or side effects following the proper administration of designated therapeutic dosages are not recorded.

DOSAGE

Mode of Administration: Liquid extract used as a gargle and rinse.

LITERATURE

Kern W, List PH, Hörhammer L (Hrsg.), Hagers Handbuch der Pharmazeutischen Praxis, 4. Aufl., Bde. 1-8, Springer Verlag Berlin, Heidelberg, New York, 1969.

Cumin

Cuminum cyminum

DESCRIPTION

Medicinal Parts: The medicinal parts are the Cumin oil extracted from the ripe fruit and the ripe, dried fruit.

Flower and Fruit: The flowers are in umbels radiating in groups of 3 to 5. The petals are white or red, oblong, and deeply bordered with a long indented tip. The involucral bracts are long and simple. The style is short and turned outward at the end. The ovary is inferior and trilocular. The fruit is a schizocarp, about 6 mm long and 1.5 mm wide and crowned with awl-shaped calyx tips. The mericarp is almost round in transverse section, with 5 threadlike, bristly main ribs, and bristly secondary ribs.

Leaves, Stem, and Root: The plant is a delicate, glabrous annual 10 to 50 cm high. The stem is bifurcated at the base and glabrous. The leaves are glabrous and finely pinnatifid with oblong-linear tips, of which the lower are mostly doubly trifoliate.

Habitat: The plant is indigenous to Turkistan (Hager) or northern Egypt (Grieve), but is cultivated today in the whole of the Mediterranean region as well as in Iran, Pakistan, India, China, the U.S., and South America.

Production: Cumin is the dried ripe fruit of *Cuminum cyminum.*

Not to be Confused With: Certain Indian products, such as *Carum carvi* and the fruit of the earth chestnut, *Bunium bulbocastanium* can be mistaken for or confused with Cumin. Synthetic coloring is frequently added to Turkish products.

ACTIONS AND PHARMACOLOGY

COMPOUNDS

Volatile oil (2 to 5%): chief components cuminaldehyde, gamma-terpenes, beta-pinenes, p-cymene, 1,3-p-menthandial

Fatty oil (10 to 15%): chief fatty acids petroselic acid, palmitic acid

Proteic substances (15 to 20%)

EFFECTS

Antimicrobial: The drug contains fatty oil (mainly petroselic acid and oil acid) and has an antimicrobial effect. A powder suspension of the drug has diverse inhibitory effects; it stunts mycelium growth, toxin production or afla-toxin production in *Aspergillus ochraceus*, *C. versicolor*, and *C. flavus*.

Influence on blood-clotting: A dried Cumin ether extract inhibits (in vitro) arachidon acid-induced plate aggregation in platelet-rich human plasma.

Mutagenic effect: In comparison to *Salmonella thyphimurum* TA 100, a mutagenic effect of the polar fractions of chloroform extract and methanol extract of Cumin did appear.

Influence of pharmacological metabolism: An injection of a dried ether extract prolonged the phenobarbituate hypnosis of female albino mice, up to 120%; a higher dose shortened it to 83%.

Estrogenic effect: An acetone extract of cumin, administered to female albino rats (ovariectomised, ovaries have been removed) led, depending on the dosage, to an increase in the weight of the uterus, an increase in the amount of protein in the endometrium and an increase of alkali phosphates.

Other effects (for which there are no experimental results) include the following: obstructive influence on fertility, galactogen, antispasmodic, diuretic. and aphrodisiac.

Cumin also has carminative, stimulant. and analgesic effects.

INDICATIONS AND USAGE

Unproven Uses: In folk medicine, Cumin is used as a carminative for stomach disorders, diarrhea, and colic, particularly in veterinary medicine.

Indian Medicine: In India, Cumin is used as an abortifacient, for kidney and bladder stones, chronic diarrhea, leprosy, and eye disease.

PRECAUTIONS AND ADVERSE REACTIONS

Health risks or side effects following the proper administration of designated therapeutic dosages are not recorded.

DOSAGE

Mode of Administration: Cumin is used both internally and externally in ground form and as a pressed oil.

Daily Dosage: The average single dose is 300 to 600 mg of drug (equivalent to 5 to 10 fruits).

LITERATURE

Aye-Than Kulkarni HJ, Wut-Hmone Tha SJ. Anti-diarrhoeal Efficacy of Some Burmese Indigenous Drug Formulations in Experimental Diarrhoeal Test Models. *Int J Crude Drug Res.* 27; 195-200. 1989.

Garg SC, Siddiqui N. Antifungal activity of some essential oil isolates. *Pharmazie* 47; 467-468. 1992.

Hänsel R, Keller K, Rimpler H, Schneider G (Hrsg.), Hagers Handbuch der Pharmazeutischen Praxis, 5. Aufl., Bde 4-6 (Drogen): Springer Verlag Berlin, Heidelberg, New York, 1992-1994.

Leung AY, Encyclopedia of Common Natural Ingredients Used in Food Drugs and Cosmetics, John Wiley & Sons Inc., New York 1980.

Sathiyamoorthy P, Lugasi-Evgi H, Van-Damme P, Abu-Rabia A, Gopas J, Golan-Goldhirsh A. Larvicidal Activity in Desert Plants of the Negev and Bedouin Market Plant Products. *Int J Pharmacogn.* 35 (4); 265-273. 1997.

Varo PT, Heinz DE, *J Agric Food Chem* 18:234 et 239. 1970.

Cuminum cyminum

See Cumin

Cup Plant

Silphium perfoliatum

DESCRIPTION

Medicinal Parts: The medicinal part is the root.

Flower and Fruit: The flowers are 5 to 8 cm wide, long-pedicled, and clustered. The sepals are overlapping, and the petals are egg-yolk yellow. The disclike flowers are androgynous with long threadlike styles. The lateral flowers are female and lingual. The double-winged fruit is compressed and has a pappus of lateral awns.

Leaves, Stem, and Root: The perennial plant is a 1.25 to 2.5 m high plant with a branched rhizome. The erect, angular, smooth stem is branched higher up and foliated up to the tip. The leaves are opposite, rough, ovate, acuminate, crenate, dark green above, and blue-green beneath. The lower leaves are up to 30 cm long, and the upper ones are oblong-ovate, sessile, and fused at the base to a cup form.

Habitat: The plant is indigenous to the western U.S., Oregon, and Texas.

Other Names: Ragged Cup, Indian Gum, Prairie Dock, Pilot Plant, Polar Plant, Rosinweed, Turpentine Weed

ACTIONS AND PHARMACOLOGY

COMPOUNDS

Triterpene saponins

Sesquiterpenes: including among others silphinene, silphiperfolen, 8-hydroxy-presilphiperfolane

EFFECTS

The drug is a tonic and has a diaphoretic effect.

INDICATIONS AND USAGE

Unproven Uses: Cup Plant has been used for digestive disorders.

PRECAUTIONS AND ADVERSE REACTIONS

No health hazards or side effects are known in conjunction with the proper administration of designated therapeutic dosages.

DOSAGE

Mode of Administration: Cup Root is not used in modern medicine.

LITERATURE

Davidyants ES et al., (1984) Khim Prir Soedin. 5:666.

Hegnauer R, Chemotaxonomie der Pflanzen, Bde 1-11: Birkhäuser Verlag Basel, Boston, Berlin 1962-1997.

Cupmoss

Cladonia pyxidata

DESCRIPTION

Medicinal Parts: The wineglass-shaped scyphi of Cladonia pyxidata are used medicinally.

Flower and Fruit: Cupmoss is a lichen, not a moss as the name suggests. The scyphi are grayish-white, about 2.5 cm long, wineglass-shaped, with hollow stems and terminal cups.

Characteristics: The taste is mucilaginous and slightly sweet. There is no odor.

Habitat: The plant is indigenous to North America and is also common in other areas including Great Britain.

Other Names: Chin Cups

ACTIONS AND PHARMACOLOGY

COMPOUNDS

Lichen acids: including fumaroprotocetraric acid, barbatic acid, psoromic acid

Mucilages

EFFECTS

Cupmoss has the effect of an expectorant and antitussive.

INDICATIONS AND USAGE

Unproven Uses: Cupmoss is used for coughs, bronchitis, and also in the treatment of whooping cough.

PRECAUTIONS AND ADVERSE REACTIONS

Health risks or side effects following the proper administration of designated therapeutic dosages are not recorded.

DOSAGE

Mode of Administration: Cupmoss is used internally as an infusion with honey.

LITERATURE

Hoppe HA, (1975-1987): Drogenkunde, 8. Aufl., Bde 1-3, W. de Gruyter Verlag, Berlin, New York.

Kern W, List PH, Hörhammer L (Hrsg.), Hagers Handbuch der Pharmazeutischen Praxis, 4. Aufl., Bde 1-8, Springer Verlag Berlin, Heidelberg, New York, 1969.

Cupressus sempervirens

See Cypress

Curcuma domestica

See Tumeric

Curcuma

Curcuma xanthorrhizia

DESCRIPTION

Medicinal Parts: The medicinal parts are the dried, tuberous rhizomes cut into slices.

Flower and Fruit: The inflorescence is large; it is purple or crimson. The corolla has a red margin. Otherwise it is very similar to *Curcuma domestica.*

Leaves, Stem and Root: The plant is a 1.75 m high, leafy perennial. The leaves are in long, thin sheaths on the rhizome. The leaf blades are broadly lanceolate or oblong and have a narrow, purple mark on the midrib. The main rhizome is thickened like a tuber, ovate, the size of a fist with numerous roots, and thin lateral rhizomes. The roots terminate partially in ovate tubers.

Habitat: Curcuma is indigenous to the forests of Indonesia and the Malaysian peninsula. It is cultivated mainly on Java, in Malaysia, Thailand, and the Philippines.

Production: Japanese turmeric consists of the sliced, dried, tuberous rhizomes of *Curcuma xanthorrhiza.* Curcuma is cultivated and harvested in the second year of growth. After the rhizome has been washed, the main thick root is isolated, cut and dried at a temperature of 50°C.

Not to be Confused With: The rhizome of *Curcuma domestica.*

Other Names: Tewon Lawa, Temu Lawak

ACTIONS AND PHARMACOLOGY

COMPOUNDS

Volatile oil (3 to 12%): chief components ar-curcumene (alpha-curcumene), xanthorrhizol, beta-curcumene, germacrene, furanodien, furanodienone

Curcuminoids (0.8 to 2%): including curcumin, demethoxycurcumin

Non-phenolic diarylheptanoids: alnustone

Starch (30-40%)

EFFECTS

Curcuma acts in a manner similar to turmeric root but is mainly choleretic and antitumoral (animal testing).

INDICATIONS AND USAGE

Approved by Commission E:

- Dyspeptic complaints
- Loss of appetite

Unproven Uses: Curcuma is used for dyspepsia, particularly feelings of fullness after meals and meteorism.

In Indonesia it has long been used for liver and gallbladder complaints.

PRECAUTIONS AND ADVERSE REACTIONS

Health risks or side effects following the proper administration of designated therapeutic dosages are not recorded. Stomach complaints can occur following extended use or in the case of overdose. Because of the stimulating effect of the drug on the biliary tract, it should not be administered if there is a bile duct blockage. Colic can occur when the patient suffers from gallstones.

DOSAGE

Mode of Administration: Comminuted drug for infusions and other galenic forms for internal use.

Preparation: The infusion is prepared by pouring 1 cup of boiling water over 1/2 teaspoon of drug and straining after 10 minutes.

Daily Dosage: The average daily dose is 2 g of drug; infusion: 2 to 3 times daily between meals.

Storage: It should be protected from light.

LITERATURE

Claeson P et al., Three Non-Phenolic Diarylheptanoids with Anti-Inflammatory Activity from *Curcuma xanthorrhiza. Planta Med.* 59; 451-454. 1993.

Claeson P et al., Non-phenolic linear diarylheptanoids from *Curcuma xanthorrhiza*: a novel type of topical anti-inflammatory agents: Structure-activity relationship. In: PM 62(3):236-240. 1996.

Itokawa H, Hirayama F, Funakoshi K, Takeya K. Studies on the Antitumor Bisabolane Sesquiterpenoids Isolated from *Curcuma xanthorrhiza. Chem Pharm Bull.* 33; 3488-3492. 1985.

Lin SC, Teng CW, Lin CC, Lin Y H, Supriatna S. Protective and Therapeutic Effect of the Indonesian Medicinal Herb *Curcuma xanthorrhiza* on ?-D-Galactosamine-induced Liver Damage. *Phytother Res.* 10; 131-135. 1996.

Reuter HD, Pflanzliche Gallentherapeutika (Teil I) und (Teil II). In: ZPT 16(1):13-20 u. 77-89. 1995.

Siegers CP, Detes M, Strubelt O, Hänsel W. Choleretic properties of different curcuminoids in the rat bile-fistula model. *Pharm Pharmacol Lett.* 7 (2/3); 87-89. 1997.

Suksamrarn A, Eiamong S, Piyachaturawat P, Charoenpiboonsin J. Phenolic Diarylheptanoids from *Curcuma xanthorrhiza. Phytochemistry* 36; 1505-1508. 1994.

Yamazaki M, Maebayashi Y, Iwase N, Kaneko T. Studies on Pharmakologically Active Principles from Indonesian Crude Drugs, I. Principle Prolonging Pentobarbital-Induced Sleeping Time from *Curcuma xanthorrhiza* ROXB. *Chem Pharm Bull.* 36; 2070-2074. 1988).

Curcuma xanthorrhizia

See Curcuma

Curcuma zedoaria

See Zedoary

Cuscuta epithymum

See Dodder

Cyamopsis tetragonoloba

See Guar Gum

Cyclamen

Cyclamen europaeum

DESCRIPTION

Medicinal Parts: The medicinal part is the dried rhizome with the roots.

Flower and Fruit: The flowers are pinkish-red, solitary, and nodding on erect stems. The 5 sepals are ovate, pointed, and dentate. The corolla is a short campanulate tube with 5 revolute tips; it is darker at the base. There are 5 stamens and 1 ovary. The fruit is a capsule, which opens on 5 sides.

Leaves, Stem, and Root: The plant grows from about 5 to 10 cm. The rhizome is a disclike tuber. The leaves are long-petioled, orbicular or cordate, crenate, and glabrous, with a white edge above and red beneath. The petioles and pedicles are roughly glandular.

Characteristics: The flowers are fragrant and poisonous.

Habitat: The plant is found in the Alps and the alpine regions of southern Europe.

Other Names: Groundbread, Sowbread, Swinebread, Ivy-Leafed Cyclamen

ACTIONS AND PHARMACOLOGY

COMPOUNDS

Triterpene saponins: including cyclamine, deglucocyclamine I, deglucocyclamine II

EFFECTS

No information is available.

INDICATIONS AND USAGE

Unproven Uses: The drug is used to treat menstrual complaints, emotional disorders/nervous states, and digestive problems.

Homeopathic Uses: Cyclamen is used for migraine and its accompanying autonomic symptoms, and for the treatment of premenstrual syndrome.

PRECAUTIONS AND ADVERSE REACTIONS

The intake of even small dosages (0.3 g) can lead to nausea, vomiting, diarrhea, and stomach pain.

OVERDOSAGE

High dosages can cause spasm and asphyxiation. Following gastric lavage and the administration of activated charcoal, the treatment for poisoning should proceed symptomatically (e.g., treatment of convulsions with diazepam, treatment of colic with atropine).

DOSAGE

Mode of Administration: Cyclamen is used in homeopathic treatments. It is also used topically and in alcoholic extracts.

LITERATURE

Braccini I, Herve du Penhoat C, Michon V, Goldberg R, Clochard M, Jarvis MC, Huang ZH, Gage DA, Structural analysis of cyclamen seed xyloglucan oligosaccharides using cellulase digestion and spectroscopic methods. *Carbohydr Res*, 276:167-81, Oct 16, 1995.

Calis I, Satana ME, Yrker A, Kelican P, Demirdamar R, Alacam R, Tanker N, Ruegger H, Sticher O, Triterpene saponins from Cyclamen mirabile and their biological activities. *J Nat Prod*, 60:315-8, Mar. 1997

Calis I, Yrker A, Tanker N, Wright AD, Sticher O, Triterpene saponins from Cyclamen coum var. coum. *Planta Med*, 276:166-70, Apr 1997.

Jaspersen-Schib R, Theus L, Guirguis-Oeschger M, Gossweiler B, Meier-Abt PJ, Serious plant poisonings in Switzerland 1966-1994. Case analysis from the Swiss Toxicology Information Center. Schweiz Med Wochenschr, 60:1085-98, 1996 Jun 22.

Cyclamen europaeum

See Cyclamen

Cydonia oblongata

See Quince

Cymbopogon citratus

See Lemongrass

Cynanchum vincetoxicum

See German Ipecac

Cynara scolymus

See Artichoke

Cynoglossum officinale

See Hound's Tongue

Cyperus articulatus

See Adrue

Cypress

Cupressus sempervirens

DESCRIPTION

Medicinal Parts: The medicinal parts are the cones, branches, and oil.

Leaves, Stem, and Root: Cupressus sempervirens is a tree that grows up to 30 m tall. The leaves are 0.5 to 1 mm, dark green, and obtuse. The male cones are 4 to 8 mm, the female cones are 25 to 40 mm. They are elliptical-oblong (rarely globose), green when young and shining yellowish-gray when ripe, with 8 to 14 short and obtusely spiked scales. There are 8 to 20 seeds on each scale.

Habitat: The plant is indigenous to Turkey and is cultivated throughout the Mediterranean region.

ACTIONS AND PHARMACOLOGY

COMPOUNDS

Chief components: alpha-pinene, D-camphene, D-silvestrene, p-cymene, L-cadinene, cedrol, terpinenol-4, terpineol, acetyl- and isovalerianyl esters of monoterpene alcohols

EFFECTS

Cypress acts as an expectorant.

INDICATIONS AND USAGE

Unproven Uses: The drug is used externally for head colds, coughs, and bronchitis.

PRECAUTIONS AND ADVERSE REACTIONS

Health risks or side effects following the proper administration of designated therapeutic dosages are not recorded. Kidney irritation is likely with intake of larger dosages.

DOSAGE

Mode of Administration: Occasionally, Cypress is used externally as an ointment.

LITERATURE

Amouroux P, Jean D, Lamaison JL. Antiviral Activity In Vitro of *Cupressus sempervirens* on Two Human Retrovirus HIV and HTLV. *Phytother Res.* 12 (5); 367-368. 1998

Kern W, List PH, Hörhammer L (Hrsg.), Hagers Handbuch der Pharmazeutischen Praxis, 4. Aufl., Bde 1-8, Springer Verlag Berlin, Heidelberg, New York, 1969.

Vennat B, Gross D, Pourrat A, Pourrat H. Polyphenols from *Cupressus sempervirens*: Qualitative and quantitative assays of Proanthocyanidins and Flavonoids. *Il Farmaco* 46; 685-698. 1991.

Cypress Spurge

Euphorbia cyparissias

DESCRIPTION

Medicinal Parts: The medicinal part of the plant is the flowering plant with the root.

Flower and Fruit: The flowers are in terminal cymes. They are yellow-green but usually red after flowering. What appear to be flowers are in fact inflorescences. Inside each jug-shaped invulucre is 1 hanging pistil with a trivalved ovary and 3 styles each with 2 stigmas and numerous stamens. Four half-moon-shaped nectaries are at the edge. The fruit is covered in small papilla.

Leaves, Stem and Root: The plant is about 15 to 30 cm high. The stem is erect, unbranched, and glabrous. The leaves are alternate, sessile, linear, entire-margined and very narrow on the nonflowering branches.

Characteristics: The entire plant contains white latex, which is poisonous.

Habitat: Indigenous to Europe and Mediterranean.

Production: Cypress Spurge herb and root is the whole plant in flower and root of *Euphorbia cyparissias*.

ACTIONS AND PHARMACOLOGY

COMPOUNDS

Diterpenes: ingenan-di- and triester, for example 13-hydroxy-ingenol-3-(2,3-dimethylbutyryl)-13- dodecanoate, e 113-hydroxy-ingenol-5-(2,3-dimethylbutyryl)-13-dodecanoate, 13-hydroxy-ingenol-3-(2,3-dimethylbutyryl)-13-decanoate

Triterpenes

EFFECTS

The diterpene esters in the drug are severely toxic, a strong irritant, drastically purgative, and encourage growth of tumors.

In animal tests and in vitro there are indications of a cytotoxic, nonspecific immune-stimulating, antiphlogistic, and strongly laxative effect.

INDICATIONS AND USAGE

Unproven Uses: In folk medicine Cypress Spurge is used internally for constipation, toothache, and as a diuretic (macerate). It is used externally for warts and corns (ointment).

Homeopathic Uses: Euphorbia cyparissias is used for diseases of the respiratory organs, diarrhea, and skin diseases.

PRECAUTIONS AND ADVERSE REACTIONS

The Ingenan esters are severely inflammatory in their effect and cocarcinogenic. Administration of the drug should be avoided because of the cocarcinogenic effect.

A particular danger exists with the chyle of the freshly harvested plant, but the ingenan ester retains its efficacy even after drying, which means that the drug also is acutely toxic. If it gets on the skin, the chyle causes reddening, itching, burning, and blisters.

In the eye, the chyle leads to swelling of the lids, conjunctival inflammation, and corneal defects. If taken internally, the chyle in the drug causes burning in the mouth and vomiting. Very high dosages cause pupil enlargement, dizziness, stupor, painful bowel movements, cardiac rhythm disorders, and ultimately collapse. Skin contact with the chyle requires thorough cleaning. Contact with the eye requires thorough rinsing with water. Following stomach and intestinal emptying, the treatment of poisonings is carried out symptomatically.

DOSAGE

Mode of Administration: Cypress Spurge is used only in homeopathic dilutions.

Daily Dosage: Macerate/decoction: 0.5 to 1 gm daily

Homeopathic Dosage: from D4: 5 drops, 1 tablet, or 10 globules every 30 to 60 minutes (acute) or 1 to 3 times daily (chronic); From D6 parenterally: 1 to 2 mL sc acute: 3 times daily; chronic: once a day. Children should be given a weaker dose (HAB1)

LITERATURE

Frohne D, Pfänder HJ, Giftpflanzen - Ein Handbuch für Apotheker, Toxikologen und Biologen, 4. Aufl., Wiss. Verlagsges. mbH Stuttgart 1997.

Lewin L, Gifte und Vergiftungen, 6. Aufl., Nachdruck, Haug Verlag, Heidelberg 1992.

Öksüz S, Gil RR, Chai H, Pezzuto JM, Cordell GA, Ulubelen A. Biologically Active Compounds from the *Euphorbiaceae*; 2. Two Triterpenoids of Euphorbia cyparissias. *Planta Med.* 60; 594-596. 1994

Öksüz S et al., Biological active compounds. In: PM 60(6):594-596. 1994.

Teuscher E, Lindequist U, Biogene Gifte - Biologie, Chemie, Pharmakologie, 2. Aufl., Fischer Verlag Stuttgart 1994.

Cypripedium calceolus

See Nerve Root

Cytisus laburnum

See Laburnum

Cytisus scoparius

See Scotch Broom

Daemonorops draco

See Dragon's Blood (Xue-Jie)

Daffodil

Narcissus pseudonarcissus

DESCRIPTION

Medicinal Parts: The medicinal parts are the bulb, the leaves and the flowers, or the whole flowering plant without the roots.

Flower and Fruit: The pale yellow flowers are solitary and bending on compressed double-edged pedicles. At the base of the flower there is a dry, membranous sheath that is split higher at the side. The perigone is 6-tipped and splayed like a plate. The secondary corolla is egg-yolk yellow and cylindrical, with an undulating, folded, unevenly crenate margin. The stamens are fused to the tube. The ovary is inferior, the style is threadlike and the stigma is obtuse.

Leaves, Stem, and Root: The plant grows from 15 to 30 cm high. The leaves are basal, sprouting from an ovate, brown bulb. They are erect, linear, flatly grooved, and have 2 grooves rather than a keel.

Characteristics: Daffodil has a weak unpleasant odor and is poisonous.

Habitat: The plant is found all over Europe and is cultivated elsewhere.

Production: Daffodil is the flowering plant *Narcissus pseudonarcissus* without the root.

Other Names: Lent Lily

ACTIONS AND PHARMACOLOGY

COMPOUNDS

Amaryllidacae alkaloids (0.08-0.15% in the bulb, with considerably less in the foliage): including, among others, hemanthamine, galanthine, galanthamine, pluviine, masonine, homolycorine

Chelidonic acid

EFFECTS

No information is available.

INDICATIONS AND USAGE

Unproven Uses: Daffodil is used for irritation of the mucous membranes, such as bronchial catarrh, whooping cough, colds, and asthma.

PRECAUTIONS AND ADVERSE REACTIONS

No health hazards or side effects are known in conjunction with the proper administration of designated therapeutic dosages. The plant possesses a weak potential for sensitization, a condition called ''daffodil itch.''

OVERDOSAGE

Overdosage or accidental intake of the bulbs (e.g., confusing them with cooking onions) can lead to poisoning. Symptoms include vomiting, salivation, diarrhea, and central nervous disorders following resorption.

DOSAGE

Mode of Administration: Daffodil is available ground and as an extract. It is also found in homeopathic remedies.

LITERATURE

Goncalo S. Contact Sensitivity to lichenes and compositae in Frullania dermatitis. *Contact Dermatitis* 16; 84-86. 1987

Kreh M, Matusch R. O-Methyloduline and N-Demethylmaronine, Alkaloids from *Narcissus pseudonarcissus. Phytochemistry* 38 (6); 1533-1535. 1995.

Kreh M, Matusch R, Witte L. Acetylated Alkaloids from *Narcissus pseudonarcissus. Phytochemistry* 40 (4); 1303-1306. 1995.

Moraes-Cerdeira RM et al., Alkaloid content of different bulb parts of *Narcissus cv.* Ice follies. In: *PM* 63(1):93-94. 1997.

Suzuki N, Tania S, Furusawa S, Furusawa E, Therapeutic activity of narcissus alkaloids on Rauscher leukemia: Antiviral affect in vitro and rational drug combination in vivo. In: *Proc Soc Expl Biol Med* 145:771-777. 1974.

Tojo E, (+)-Narcidine, a new alkaloid from Narcissus pseudonarcissus. In: JNP 54: 1387. 1991.

Damiana

Turnera diffusa

DESCRIPTION

Medicinal Parts: The medicinal parts are the leaves harvested during the flowering season.

Flower and Fruit: The flowers are yellow, solitary and axillary. The fruit is a small, globular, many-seeded capsule, which breaks up into 3 parts. It is aromatic and resinous.

Leaves, Stem, and Root: The plant is a small shrub that grows up to 60 cm high. The leaves are 1 to 2.5 cm long and up to 6 mm wide. They are smooth and pale green on the upper surface and glabrous with a few scattered hairs on the ribs underneath. The leaves are ovate-lanceolate, short-petioled, and have 2 glands at the base. They have a few serrate teeth and curved margins.

Habitat: The plant is found mainly in the region of the Gulf of Mexico, the Caribbean, and southern Africa.

Production: Damiana leaf and Damiana herb consist of the leaf and herb of *Turnera diffusa* and its variations.

Not to Be Confused With: Biglovia veneta Gray (also called *Haplopappus disoideus) and Chrysactinia mexicana* (False Damiana) have sometimes been represented to be *Turnera diffusa*.

ACTIONS AND PHARMACOLOGY

COMPOUNDS

Volatile oil (0.5-0.9%): chief components 1,8-cineole, alpha- and beta-pinene, p-cymene, as well as thymol, alpha-copene, gamma-cadinene, calamene

Tannins (4%)

Resins (7%)

Hydroquinone glycosides: arbutin (0.2-0.7%)

Cyanogenic glycosides: tetraphylline B (barterin)

EFFECTS

Clinical trials supporting the use of Damiana in humans are lacking. Animal studies have indicated antihyperglycemic, anti-inflammatory, and indomethacin-inhibiting properties. Damiana has demonstrated slight progesterone binding—but not estrogen binding—in vitro. In North America, Damiana is used in patients with nervous depression presenting with poor appetite and vague genitourinary symptoms (Moore, 1996). Damiana is often an ingredient in formulas for menopausal symptoms and in formulas to increase sexual function. There is some evidence to support for its use in impotency and decreased sexual functioning, as well as for use in diabetes and inflammation (Arletti et al, 1999; Alarcon-Aguilara et al, 1998; Antonio & Brito, 1998).

Antihyperglycemic Effects: Damiana had a hypoglycemic effect in healthy rabbits (Alarcon-Aguilara et al, 1998).

Anti-Inflammatory: Damiana had an anti-inflammatory effect in animals (Antonio & Brito, 1998).

Anti-Ulcer Effects: Damiana inhibited gastric lesion formation by indomethacin and ethanol in rats but did not inhibit lesions caused by stress (Antonio MA & Souza Brito ARM). Damiana's anti-ulcerogenic effect may be due to both its anti-inflammatory action as well as its ability in increase gastric mucus secretion.

Effects in Hormone Regulation: In vitro data demonstrated weak estrogen receptor binding activity and increased progesterone binding with Damiana (Zava et al, 1998).

Effects in Sexual Dysfunction: Animal data suggests that Damiana may have some benefit in impotency and in increasing depressed libido; however, Damiana did not increase libido in sexually healthy rats, indicating that it may be ineffective as a general aphrodisiac (Arletti R, Benelli A, Cavazzuti E, 1999).

INDICATIONS AND USAGE

Unproven Uses: Damiana preparations are used as an aphrodisiac and for prophylaxis and treatment of sexual disorders. Damiana is used widely in Mexico and South America for nervous debility, inflammation of the bladder, decreased sexual function, impotence, nephritis, and diabetes (Martinez, 1991).

PRECAUTIONS AND ADVERSE REACTIONS

General: No health hazards or side effects are known in conjunction with the proper administration of designated therapeutic dosages. There is a report of a subject who experienced ''tetanus-like convulsions'' and paroxysms after drinking alcohol and ingesting 8 ounces of Damiana extract (Spencer & Seigler, 1981).

Toxicity: Damiana is a strongly cyanogenic plant, producing tetraphyllin B (Spencer & Seigler, 1981).

DOSAGE

How Supplied:

Capsules – 380 mg, 384 mg, 395 mg, 450 mg

Fluid Extract – 1:1

LITERATURE

Alarcon-Aguilara FJ, Roman-Ramos R, Perez-Gutierrez S et al. Study of anti-hyperglycemic effect of plants used as antidiabetics. *J Ethnopharmacol*; 61:101-110. 1998.

Antonio MA & Souza Brito ARM. Oral anti-inflammatory and anti- ulcerogenic activities of a hydroalcoholic extract and partitioned fractions of *Turnera ulmifolia* (Turneraceae). *J Ethnopharmacol*; 61:215-228. 1998.

Arletti R, Benelli A, Cavazzuti E et al. Stimulating property of *Turnera diffus* and *Pfaffia paniculata* extracts on the sexual behavior of male rats. *Psychopharmacology* (Berl); 143(1):15-19. 1999.

Auterhoff H, Häufel HP. *Arch Pharm* 301:537. 1968.

Dominguez XA. Hinojosa M, *Planta Med* 30:68. 1976.

Foster S. An illustrated guide to 101 medicinal herbs. Interweave Press, Loveland, Colorado: pp. 62-63. 1998.

Jin J. *Lloydia* 29(3):250. 1966.

Martinez M. Las plantas medicinales de Mexico. Ediciones Botas, Justo Sierra 52, Mexico: pp. 119-122. 1991.

Spencer KC & Seigler DS. Tetraphyllin B from *Turnera diffusa. Hippokrates Verlag GmbH*; 43:175-178. 1981.

Steinegger E, Hänsel R, Pharmakognosie, 5. Aufl., Springer Verlag Heidelberg 1992.

Tyler V: Damiana - An Herbal Hoax. Pharmacy in History; 25(2):55-60. 1983.

Zava DT, Dollbaum CM & Blen M. Estrogen and progestin bioactivity of foods, herbs and spices. *Proc Soc Exp Biol Med*; 217(3):369-378. 1998.

Dandelion

Taraxacum officinale

DESCRIPTION

Medicinal Parts: The medicinal parts are the dried leaves harvested before the flowering season, the dried root collected in autumn, the dried aerial parts with the rhizome harvested before the flowering season, and the whole fresh plant.

Flower and Fruit: The flower is a golden yellow composite flower. The composite head is solitary and has a diameter of 3 to 5 cm. All the florets are lingual and androgynous. The epicalyx is oblong-campanulate. The tepals are arranged in 3 imbricate rows, 2 of which are turned back. The inner one is long acuminate with a white margin and erect. The receptacle has no bracts. The fruit is small, long-beaked, light gray-brown, ribbed and has a parachutelike tuft of hair.

Leaves, Stem, and Root: The plant is perennial, hardy, and is found in a number of forms. It grows to about 30 cm tall and has a short rhizome. The rhizome turns into a many-headed, 20 to 50 cm long by 2 cm thick taproot. The hollow stem is erect or ascending. The basal leaves are glabrous or villous, usually deeply notched, lanceolate, and lobed like a saw. They narrow to a red-violet tinged petiole and end in a large deltoid tip.

Characteristics: The flower opens in the morning and closes in the evening remaining closed all night and in dull weather. The plant parts contain bitter latex.

Habitat: Dandelion grows in most temperate regions of Europe and Asia.

Production: Dandelion root with herb consists of the entire *Taraxacum officinale* plant gathered while flowering. It is air-dried.

Not to be Confused With: Cichorium intybus and the leaves of various *Leontodon* species.

Other Names: Blowball, Cankerwort, Irish Daisy, Lion's Tooth, Monk's Head, Priest's Crown, Swine Snout, Wild Endive, Witch Gowan, Yellow Gowan

ACTIONS AND PHARMACOLOGY

COMPOUNDS

Sesquiterpene lactones (bitter substances): including, among others, taraxinacetyl-1'-O-glucosides, 11,13-dihydrotaraxinacetyl-1'-O-glucosides, taraxacolide-1'-O-glucosides, 4alpha,15,11beta,13-tetrahydroridentin B

Triterpenes and sterols: beta-sitosterol, beta-sitosterol-glucosides, taraxasterol, psi-taraxasterol, taraxerol, taraxol

Flavonoids: including among others, apigenin-7-O-glucosides, luteolin-7-O-glucosides

Mucilages

Inulin (2-40%, high values in autumn)

EFFECTS

The amaroids in Dandelion are cholagogic and secretolytic in the upper intestinal tract. The saluretic effect demonstrated in animal experiments requires further investigation.

CLINICAL TRIALS

A 2005 systematic review of the literature on Dandelion reported that while the perennial is widely used in Europe for gastrointestinal ailments and the leaves are a rich source of vitamin A, there are many historical or theoretical uses for which sound evidence is lacking. Data from the test tube and human studies fail to support the common contention that Dandelion simulates the secretion of bile. Clinical trial evidence is sparse or nonexistent overall for Dandelion's reported ability to reduce inflammation, function as an antioxidant, counter cancer or colitis, treat diabetes or work as a diuretic. While one study reported improvements in liver function in patients with hepatitis B following use of Dandelion, the preparation containing the herb also contained multiple other agents which may have been responsible for these effects (Ulbricht, 2005).

INDICATIONS AND USAGE

Approved by Commission E:

- Dyspeptic complaints
- Infections of the urinary tract
- Liver and gallbladder complaints
- Loss of appetite

Unproven Uses: Dandelion is used internally for disturbances in bile flow, inflammatory conditions of the efferent urinary tract, and dyspepsia. It is also used for liver and gallbladder disorders, hemorrhoids, congestion in the portal system, gout, rheumatic disorders, eczema, and other skin disorders. The drug has a diuretic effect and is used for kidney and bladder complaints and kidney stone formation. A diabetic infusion is made from the roots and leaves.

Chinese Medicine: The drug is used for acute mastitis, urinary disorders, and agalactia.

Indian Medicine: The drug is used for chronic ulcers, tuberculosis, flatulence, colic, kidney disease, gout, jaundice, and biliary stones.

CONTRAINDICATIONS

Contraindications include closure of the biliary ducts, gallbladder empyema, and ileus. Consultation with a doctor is necessary in the presence of biliary ailments.

PRECAUTIONS AND ADVERSE REACTIONS

No health hazards are known in conjunction with the proper administration of designated therapeutic dosages. Superacid gastric complaints are possible due to the drug's secretion-stimulating effect. The drug possesses weak potential for sensitization reactions.

DRUG INTERACTIONS

MODERATE RISK

Anticoagulants, Antiplatelet agents, Low molecular weight heparins, and Thrombolytic Agents: Concurrent use with Dandelion root may result in increased risk of bleeding. *Clinical management*: Caution is advised if Dandelion root and these medications are taken concomitantly. Monitor the patient closely for signs and symptoms of bleeding.

Fluoroquinolones: Concurrent use may result in decreased fluoroquinolone effectiveness. *Clinical management:* If possible, avoid concomitant use of Asian dandelion and fluoroquinolones. If Asian dandelion and a fluoroquinolone are taken together, Asian dandelion should be taken either 2 hours before or 4 to 6 hours after the fluoroquinolone.

Potassium: Concurrent use may result in increased risk of hyperkalemia. *Clinical Management:* Avoid Dandelion leaf use during potassium supplementation, since the effect of the leaf may be variable and unpredictable depending on product potassium content. If dandelion and potassium are taken together, frequent monitoring of potassium serum levels is recommended.

DOSAGE

Mode of Administration: Whole, cut, and powdered drug is available in the form of drops, tinctures, juice, and in compound preparations.

How Supplied:

Capsules-140 mg, 425 mg, 475 mg, 515 mg, 520 mg,

Liquid–1:1

Preparation: To make a tea, use 1 to 2 teaspoonfuls finely cut drug with 150 ml rapidly boiled water; strain after 15 minutes and drink warm.

To make a decoction, use 3 to 4 gm cut and powdered drug per cup of water. To make an infusion, use 3 to 4 gm cut drug per 1 cup of water.

For an extract, mix 1 part coarsely powdered Dandelion root with 8 parts of water and 1 part spirit of wine.

Daily Dosage: When using a tincture, the recommended dosage is 10 to 15 drops 3 times daily. A cup of the freshly made tea can be taken mornings and evenings.

Storage: The drug should be protected from light and moisture.

LITERATURE

Atta-Ur-Rahman Zaman K. Medicinal Plants with Hypoglycemic Activity. *J Ethnopharmacol.* 26; 1-55. 1989.

Barnes J, Ernst E. Traditional Herbalist's Prescriptions for Common Clinical Conditions: A Survey of Members of the UK National Institute of Medicinal Herbalists. *Phytother Res.* 12 (5); 369-371. 1998

Bayerl C, Jung EG. Allergic contact dermatitis from Aristochol®, a phytotherapeutic cholagogue. *Contact Dermatitis* 34; 222-223. 1996.

Budzianowski J. Coumarins, caffeoyltartaric acids and their artifactual estres from *Taraxacum officinale*. In: *PM* 63(3):288. 1997.

Caceres A, Cano O, Samayoa B, Aguilar L Plants used in Guatemala for the Treatment of Gastrointestinal Disorders. 1.Screening of 84 Plants against *Enterobacteria. J Ethnopharmacol.* 30; 55-73. 1990

Davies MG, Kersey PJW. Contact allergy to yarrow and dandelion. *Contact Dermatitis* 14; 256-257. 1986

Hausen BM, Osmundsen PE. Contact Allergy to Parthenolide in *Tanacetum parthenium* (L.) Schulz-Bip. (Feverfew, Asteraceae) and Cross-reactions to Related Sesquiterpene Lactone Containing Compositae Species. *Acta Derm Venerol.* 63; 308-314. 1983

Neef H, Declercq P, Laekeman G. Hypoglycaemic Activity of Selected European Plants. *Phytother Res.* 9 (1); 45-48. 1995

Daphne mezereum

See Mezereon

Date Palm

Phoenix dactylifera

DESCRIPTION

Medicinal Parts: The medicinal part is the fruit.

Flower and Fruit: The flowers are androgynous and are in branched, coblike inflorescences. The 3 carpels form 1 ovary. The fruit is a single-seeded berry about 5 cm long (the date with the characteristic seed).

Leaves, Stem, and Root: The Date Palm is a woody plant growing primarily in girth. The leaves form a large long-petioled tuft at the top of the trunk. The lamina are frondlike and pinnatifid.

Habitat: Date Palm is found from India to northern Africa.

Production: Dates are the fruits of *Phoenix dactylifera*.

ACTIONS AND PHARMACOLOGY

COMPOUNDS: IN THE FRUIT PULP

Sugar (50%): saccharose, inverted sugar

Leucoanthocyanidine

Piperidine derivatives: pipecolic acid, 5-hydroxy-pipecolic acid, baikiaine

COMPOUNDS: IN THE SEEDS

Fatty oil (10%)

EFFECTS

No information is available.

INDICATIONS AND USAGE

Indian Medicine: Date Palm is used for bronchitis, clouding of the cornea, headaches, inflamed wounds, kidney disease, and gastric complaints.

PRECAUTIONS AND ADVERSE REACTIONS

No health hazards or side effects are known in conjunction with the proper administration of designated therapeutic dosages.

DOSAGE

Preparation: Honey made from dates is produced in Algeria using juice-rich dates, which are dried in the sun; the leftover liquid results in date honey. Date honey is used to treat chest complaints.

LITERATURE

Gurib-Fakim A, Gueho J, Sewraj-Bisoondoondoyal M. The Medicinal Plants of Mauritius - Part 1. *Int J Pharmacogn.* 35 (4); 237-254. 1997

Hussain HSN, Karatela YY. Traditional Medicinal Plants Used by Hausa Tribe of Kano State of Nigeria. *J Ethnopharmacol.* 27 (4); 211-216. 1989

Magdel-Din-Hussein M, Helmy WA, Salem HM. Biological Activities of Some Galactomannans and Their Sulfated Derivatives. *Phytochemistry* 48 (3); 479-484. 1998

Datura stramonium

See Jimson Weed

Daucus carota

See Wild Carrot

Delphinium consolida

See Larkspur

Delphinium staphisagria

See Stavesacre

Devil's Claw

Harpagophytum procumbens

DESCRIPTION

Medicinal Parts: The medicinal parts are the dried tubular secondary roots and the thick lateral tubers.

Flower and Fruit: The flowers grow on short pedicles in the leaf axils and are solitary, large, and similar to foxgloves. The petals are pale-pink to crimson. The seed capsules are bivalvular, compressed at the sides, and ovate. The capsules are 7 to 20 cm long, 6 cm in diameter, and very woody with longitudinally striped rind. They have a double row of elastic, armlike, branched appendages with an anchorlike hook. The capsules contain about 50 dark oblong seeds with a rough surface.

Leaves, Stem, and Root: The plant is perennial and leafy. It has a branched root system and branched, prostrate shoots 1 to 1.5 m long. The leaves are petiolate and lobed, and may be opposite or alternate. The aerial parts of the plant die back in the dry season. The tuber (storage) roots are formed from the main and lateral roots. The main roots have obtuse, quadrangular, upright collarlike sections, 10 to 20 cm long and 30 to 60 cm thick, which are covered in a fissured cork layer. The nodes of the lateral roots are up to 60 mm thick and 20 cm long, and are light-brown to red-brown on the outside. The roots extend out to an area of about 150 cm around the plant and grow down to a depth of 30 to 60 cm.

Characteristics: The dried, pulverized secondary tubers and roots are yellowish-gray to bright pink and hornlike in their hardness. They have a bitter taste.

Habitat: The plant originated in South Africa and Namibia, and has spread throughout the Savannas and the Kalahari.

Production: Devil's Claw root consists of the dried lateral roots and secondary tubers of *Harpagophytum procumbens*. The lateral roots are cut into slices or pieces, or pulverized immediately after digging because they harden and become very difficult to cut once dry.

Other Names: Grapple Plant, Wood Spider

ACTIONS AND PHARMACOLOGY

COMPOUNDS

Liridoide monoterpenes: including harpagoside (extremely bitter), harpagide, procumbide

Phenylethanol derivatives: including acteoside (verbascoside); isoacteoside

Oligosaccharides: stachyose

Harpagoquinones (traces)

EFFECTS

Devil's Claw stimulates gastric juice secretion and is choleretic. Anti-inflammatory, analgesic (and thus anti-arthritic) effect has been shown in animal experiments. More recent human pharmacological studies indicate that the action mechanism involves the inhibition of eicosanoid biosynthesis. The constituents cinnamic acid and harpagoquinone as well as terpenes could come into question here. No clinical studies on the gastrointestinal effect are available. An improvement in symptoms in rheumatic or arthritic complaints has been demonstrated in controlled studies.

INDICATIONS AND USAGE

Approved by Commission E:

- Dyspeptic complaints
- Loss of appetite
- Rheumatism

Unproven Uses: In folk medicine, Devil's Claw is used as an ointment for skin injuries and disorders. The dried root is used for pain relief; pregnancy discomforts; arthritis; allergies; metabolic disorders; and kidney, bladder, liver and gallbladder disorders. In South Africa it is used for fevers and digestive disorders.

Homeopathic Uses: Chronic rheumatism is the primary use for Devil's Claw in homeopathy.

CONTRAINDICATIONS

The drug should not be used in the presence of stomach or duodenal ulcers, due to the drug's stimulation of gastric juice secretion.

PRECAUTIONS AND ADVERSE REACTIONS

Health risks or side effects following the proper administration of designated therapeutic dosages are not recorded. The drug has a sensitizing effect.

DOSAGE

Mode of Administration: As comminuted drug for infusions and other preparations for internal use, as an ointment for external use.

How Supplied:

Capsules – 405 mg, 480 mg, 510 mg, 520 mg

Tablets - 500 mg

Liquid Extract

Preparation: To make an infusion, use 1 teaspoonful (equivalent to 4.5 g) comminuted drug with 300 ml boiling water. Steep for 8 hours and strain.

Daily Dosage: For loss of appetite, the recommended dosage is 1.5 g of drug; otherwise 4.5 g of drug is used. The infusion can be taken 3 times a day.

Homeopathic Dosage: 5 to 10 drops, 1 tablet or 5 to 10 globules 1 to 3 times a day, or from D3 1 mL injection solution sc twice weekly (HAB1). The ointment is applied 1 to 3 times a day. For external use, 1 dessertspoon of the tincture should be diluted with 250 mL and used for washes or poultices.

Storage: Store Devil's Claw in a container that protects it from light and moisture.

LITERATURE

Baghdikian B et al., An analyticyl study, anti-inflammatory and analgesic effects of *Harpagophytum procumbens* and *Harpagophytum zeyheri*. In: *PM* 63(2):171-176. 1997.

Chrubasik S, Junck H, Breitschwerdt H, Conradt C, Zappe H. Effectiveness of *Harpagophytum* extract WS 1531 in the treatment of exacerbation of low back pain: a randomized, placebo-controlled, double-blind study. *Eur-J-Anaesthesiol.* 16(2); 118-29. 1999

Chrubasik S, Zimpfer C, Sch,tt U, Ziegler R. Effectiveness of Harpagophytum procumbens in treatment of acute low back pain. *Phytomedicine* 3 (1); 1-10. 1996

Ghisalberti EL. Biological and pharmacological activity of naturally occuring iridoids and secoiridoids. *Phytomedicine* 5 (2); 147-163. 1998

Lanhers MC, Fleurentin J, Mortier F, Vinche A, Younos C. Anti-Inflammatory and Analgesic Effects of an Aqueous Extract of *Harpagophytum procumbens. Planta Med.* 58; 117-123. 1992

Moussard C, Alber D, Toubin MM, Thevenon N, Henry JC. A drug used in traditional medicine, *Harpagophytum procumbens*: no evidence for NSAID-like effect on whole blood eicosanoid production in human. Prostaglandins-Leukot-Essent-Fatty-Acids. 46(4); 283-286. 1992

Dicentra cucullaria

See Turkey Corn

Dictamnus albus

See Burning Bush

Digitalis

Digitalis purpurea

DESCRIPTION

Medicinal Parts: The medicinal parts are the dried leaves (in powder form), the ripe dried seeds, the fresh leaves of the 1-year-old plant or the leaves of the 2-year-old plant collected at the beginning of flowering. In the past, the drug of *Digitalis purpurae* was the raw material employed in isolating the cardiac glycosides. Today, *Digitalis lantana* is used.

Flower and Fruit: The flowers are carmine red with white-edged spots on the inside. The flowers appear in long hanging racemes. They have 5 free, short-tipped sepals. The corolla is about 4 cm long, campanulate, bilabiate with an obtuse upper lip and an ovate tip on the lower lip. The flower is glabrous on the outside and has a white awn on the inside. There are 2 long and 2 short stamens, and 1 superior ovary. The fruit is a doublevalved, ovate, glandular, villous capsule.

Leaves, Stem, and Root: The plant is a biennial with a branched tap root. In the first year it develops a leaf rosette. In the second it produces a 2 m high, erect, unbranched, gray, tomentose stem. The leaves are alternate, ovate, tapering upward, and petiolate. Almost all leaves are crenate; only the highest ones are entire-margined.

Characteristics: The plant is very poisonous; it tastes hot-bitter with a slightly unpleasant odor.

Habitat: Digitalis is indigenous to Europe. It was introduced to the east and the American continent.

Production: Digitalis leaves are the leaves of *Digitalis purpurea* or *Digitalis lanata.* The latter corresponds to *Digitalis purpurea* but has a milder effect. The rose leaves are harvested during the first period of vegetation in early autumn. The drying period is decisive for the content of cardenolide glycosides. The temperature for drying is 30° C to 50° C.

Not to be Confused With: Confusion seldom occurs due to cultivation under controlled conditions.

Other Names: Dead Men's Bells, Dog's Finger, Fairy Caps, Fairy Fingers, Fairy Gloves, Fairy Thimbles, Finger Flower, Folks' Glove, Foxglove, Gloves of Our Lady, Ladies' Glove, Lion's Mouth, Virgin's Glove, Witches' Gloves,

ACTIONS AND PHARMACOLOGY

COMPOUNDS

Cardioactive steroid glycosides (cardenolides 0.5 to 1.5%): including ones of the -

□ - *A-sequence (aglycone digitoxigenin):* purpurea glycoside A (primary glycoside), digitoxin (secondary glycoside)

□ - *B-sequence (aglycone gitoxigenin):* purpurea glycoside B (primary glycoside), gitoxin (secondary glycoside), Digitalinum verum

□ - *E-sequence (aglycone gitaloxigenin):* glucoverodoxin, glucogitaloxin, gitaloxin

Pregnane glycosides: including digipurpurin, diginin, digitalonin

Steroid saponin: including desgalactotigonin, digitonine, purpureagitoside

Anthracene derivatives: anthraquinones

EFFECTS

The drug contains cardioactive cardenolide glycosides that are positively inotropic, negatively chronotropic, and improve the contraction power of cardiac muscle.

INDICATIONS AND USAGE

Unproven Uses: In folk medicine, the drug's use originated in Ireland, then came to Scotland and England and finally to central Europe. It was used to treat tumors in the lower abdomen, ulcers, headaches, abscesses, and paralysis. Externally, the drug was used for the granulation of poorly healing wounds and to cure ulcers. Furthermore, the drug was used for cardiac insufficiency, especially high blood pressure.

Use of the raw product has become obsolete because the effect is not reproducible. The use of pure glycosides is recommended instead. Digitoxin is available in mono preparations (extract) and is used as an isolated pure substance.

Homeopathic Uses: Digitalis purpurea is used for cardiac insufficiency and migraine.

PRECAUTIONS AND ADVERSE REACTIONS

General: Because of the narrow therapeutic range of digitalis glycosides, a certain percentage of patients may experience side effects immediately upon administration of therapeutic dosages: hypertonia in gastrointestinal area, loss of appetite, vomiting, diarrhea, and headache.

Contraindicated: Neither the drug nor pure glycosides should be administered in the presence or first- or second-degree AV-block, hypercalcemia, hypokalemia, hypertrophic cardiomyopathy, carotid sinus syndrome, ventricle tachycardia, thoracic aortic aneurysm, or WPW syndrome.

DRUG INTERACTIONS

MAJOR RISK

Thiazide Diuretics: Concurrent use may result in digitalis toxicity (nausea, vomiting, arrhythmias). *Clinical Management:* Patients given diuretics with digitalis should be told to add sources of potassium to their diet or they should be given potassium supplements, even if their serum potassium is normal.

POTENTIAL INTERACTIONS

The simultaneous administration of arrhythmogenic substances (sympathomimetics, methylxanthines, phosphodiesterase inhibitors, quinidine) increases the risk of cardiac arrhythmias.

OVERDOSAGE

With overdosage, in addition to the already-mentioned symptoms, the following can also occur:

Heart: cardiac rhythm disorders, all the way up to life-threatening ventricular tachycardia and atrial tachycardia with atrioventricular block

Central nervous system: stupor, visual disorders, depression, confused states, hallucinations, psychoses

Lethal dosages lead to heart failure or asphyxiation. Administration over extended periods leads in rare cases to gynecomastia. Because of the difficulties in standardizing the drug, the administration of pure glycosides is to be preferred (digitoxin).

The first measures to be taken in case of poisoning are gastric lavage and activated charcoal instillation. All other measures proceed according to the symptoms. For loss of potassium, careful replenishment is necessary. For ectopic irritation buildup in the ventricle, administration of phenytoin as an antiarrhythmatic is recommended. Lidocaine should be used in cases of ventricular extrasystole; atropine is recommended for partial atrioventricular block. The prophylactic installation of a pacemaker is often necessary. Hemoperfusion for the elimination of the glycosides and cholestyramine administration for the interruption of the enterohepatic circulation are possible.

The drugs and pure glycosides should be administered in the following situations (among others): atrioventricular block of the 2nd and 3rd degree, hypercalcaemia, hypocalcaemia, hypertrophic cardiomyopathy, carotid sinus syndrome, ventricular tachycardia, thoracic aortic aneurysm, WPW-syndrome.

DOSAGE

Mode of Administration: Today, the drug is obsolete. Due to the lack of reproductivity of content, the use of appropriate pure glycosides is advisable. Digitoxin is contained in mono preparations (extract) and used as an isolated pure substance.

Preparation: Tincture: shaken for 1 day in 25% ethanol at a ratio of 1:10.

The manufacture of the digoxin and digitoxin is a complicated process that involves fermentation, extraction and evaporation.

Storage: Store carefully away from sources of light.

LITERATURE

Greidziak N, Diettrich B, Luckner M. Batch Cultures of Somatic Embryos of *Digitalis lanata* in Gaslift Fermenters. Development and Cardenolide Accumulation. *Planta Med.* 56; 175-178. 1990

Gurny L, Vuagnat P, Gurny R, Kapetanidis I. Cultures de cals de *Digitalis purpurea L.* / 1re partie: Etude de la croissance par analyse de variance. *Pharm Acta Helv.* 55; 302-306. 1980)

Ikeda Y et al., Quantitative HPLC analysis of cardiac glycosides in *Digitalis purpurea.* In: *JNP* 58(6):897-901. 1995.

Digitalis purpurea

See Digitalis

Dill

Anethum graveolens

DESCRIPTION

Medicinal Parts: The medicinal part is the seed, the fresh or dried leaves, and the upper stem.

Flower and Fruit: The yellow flowers are in large, 20- to 50-rayed umbels. There is no involucre or calyx. The petals have an inward-curving point, which is not indented. The fruit is flattened and oval with a rib on the sharp-edged back. Ribs that appear on the edge have a winged edge.

Leaves, Stem, and Root: The plant is 40 to 120 cm tall. The stem is erect, round, smooth, dark-green, and white-striped. The stem is branched above, with a bluish bloom. The leaves are double and more pinnate, feathery, white-tipped leaflets with a deep groove on the upper surface. The leaf sheath is oblong with a thick-skinned edge.

Characteristics: Dill has an aromatic scent.

Habitat: The plant is indigenous to the Mediterranean region, southern Russia, and cultivated throughout Europe as well as North and South America.

Production: Dill herb consists of the fresh or dried leaf and upper stem of *Anethum graveolens*. Dill seed consists of the dried fruit of *Anethum graveolens.*

Other Names: Dilly

ACTIONS AND PHARMACOLOGY

COMPOUNDS: DILL HERB

Volatile oil (0.5 to 1.5%): chief constituents are carvone, dill apiole, (+) limonene

Phthalides

EFFECTS: DILL HERB

No information is available.

COMPOUNDS: DILL FRUIT

Volatile oil (2.5 to 4.0%): chief constituents are carvone (approximately 50%), dill apiole, (+)- limonene

Phtalides

Fatty oil

Furanocoumarins: including bergaptene

Hydroxycoumarins: including umbelliferone

EFFECTS: DILL FRUIT

The fruit of the Dill plant has an antispasmodic effect on the smooth muscles of the gastrointestinal tract, and a bacteriostatic effect.

INDICATIONS AND USAGE

DILL HERB

Unproven Uses: Dill herb is used for prevention and treatment of diseases and disorders of the gastrointestinal tract, kidney and urinary tract, for sleep disorders and for spasms.

DILL FRUIT

Approved by Commission E:

■ Dyspeptic Complaints

Indian Medicine: Dill is used for halitosis, worm infestation, complaints of the repiratory tract and syphilis.

PRECAUTIONS AND ADVERSE REACTIONS

DILL HERB

No health hazards or side effects are known in conjunction with the proper administration of designated therapeutic dosages.

DILL FRUIT

No health hazards or side effects are known in conjunction with the proper administration of designated therapeutic dosages. Photodermatosis is possible after contact with the juice of the freshly harvested plant.

DOSAGE

DILL FRUIT

Mode of Administration: Whole seeds and crushed fruits are used to make teas and other galenic preparations for internal application.

Daily Dosage: The average daily dosage of the seeds is 3 gm; essential oil daily dose is 0.1 to 0.3 gm.

LITERATURE

DILL HERB AND FRUIT

Badoc A, Contribution à l'étude du genre Anethum. In: Mémoire Diplome supérieur Rech Biol et Physiol, Univ Sci Techn Lille Flandres Artois No. 122, Dec. 1986.

Bouwmeester HJ, Davies JAR, Toxopeus H. Enantiomeric Composition of Carvone, Limonene, and Carveols in Seeds of Dill and Annual and Biennal Caraway Varieties. *J Agric Food Chem.* 43 (12); 3057-3064. 1995

Brown JP. A Review of the Genetic Effects of Naturally Occuring Flavonoids, Anthraquinones and Related Compounds. *Mutation Res.* 75; 243-277.(1980

Hener U, Kreis P, Mosandl A. Enantiomeric Distribution of alpha-Pinene, ?-Pinene and Limonene in Essential Oils and Extracts. Part 3. Oils for Alcoholic Beverages and Seasonings. *Flav Fragr J.* 6; 109-111. 1991

Sathiyamoorthy P et al. Larvicidal Activity in Desert Plants of the Negev and Bedouin Market Plant Products. *Int J Pharmacogn.* 35 (4); 265-273. 1997

Yasukawa K et al. Inhibitory effect of taraxastane-type triterpenes on tumor promotion by 12-O-tetradecanoylphorbol-13-acetate in two-stage carcinogenesis in mouse skin. *Oncology*, 53:341-4, Jul-Aug 1996

Dionaea muscipula

See Venus Flytrap

Dioscorea villosa

See Wild Yam

Dipsacus silvestris

See Teazle

Dipteryx odorata

See Tonka Beans

Divi-Divi

Caesalpinia bonducella

DESCRIPTION

Medicinal Parts: The medicinal part of the plant is seed.

Flower and Fruit: The flowers are dorsiventrally zygomorphous and arranged in dense clusters. The sepals are free or fused at their base, or fused to the base of the petals and stamens to form the corolla. The petals are separate from each other but have an ascending bud covering. There are twice as many stamens as petals, usually 10. The ovary always has only 1 carpel. The fruit is indehiscent or a legume with yellow nuts.

Leaves, Stem, and Root: Divi-Divi is a tree or shrub that grows to a height of 9 m, with alternate entire-margined or double-pinnate thorny leaves.

Habitat: Sri Lanka, Brazil, South America

Production: Nikkar nuts are the seeds of *Caesalpinia bonducella.*

Other Names: Nikkar Nuts, Nichol Seeds, Gray Nicker

ACTIONS AND PHARMACOLOGY

COMPOUNDS

Fatty oil (20 to 25%, bonduc nut oil): chief fatty acids are linoleic acid, oleic acid, palmitic acid, stearic acid

Proteins

Starch

Diterpenes: including, among others, alpha-, beta-, gamma-, eta-caesalpine

Saponins

EFFECTS

Divi-Divi is a febrifuge and tonic.

INDICATIONS AND USAGE

Indian Medicine: The roasted seeds are used in febrile illnesses, the treatment of diabetes, for joint pain, and general inflammation.

PRECAUTIONS AND ADVERSE REACTIONS

No health hazards or side effects are known in conjunction with the proper administration of designated therapeutic dosages.

DOSAGE

Mode of Administration: Seeds are ground and roasted for internal use.

LITERATURE

Biswas TK, Bandyopadhyas S, Mukherjee Bi, Mukherjee Bh, Sengupta BR. Oral Hypoglycemic Effect of *Caesalpinia bonducella. Int J Pharmacogn.* 35 (4); 261-264. 1997

Peter SR, Tinto WF. Caesalpinin, a Rearranged Cassane Furanoditerpene of *Caesalpinia bonducella. Tetrahedron Lett.* 38 (33); 5767-5770. 1997

Kern W, List PH, Hörhammer L (Hrsg.), Hagers Handbuch der Pharmazeutischen Praxis, 4. Aufl., Bde 1-8, Springer Verlag Berlin, Heidelberg, New York, 1969.

Dodder

Cuscuta epithymum

DESCRIPTION

Medicinal Parts: The medicinal parts are the aerial parts of the plant.

Flower and Fruit: The flowers are reddish, wax, or flesh-colored. They are arranged in small clusters. The calyx is divided into 5 and the corolla is fused to a 4 to 5 tipped tube with fringed scales inside. There are 5 stamens and 1 ovary.

Leaves, Stem, and Root: The plant is a leafless parasite up to 150 cm high. The stem is yellow or reddish, threadlike, branched, with sucking roots, and climbing.

Habitat: The plant grows in Europe, Asia and South Africa.

Production: Dodder is the whole plant of *Cuscuta epithymum.*

Other Names: Lesser Dodder, Dodder of Thyme, Devil's Guts, Beggarweed, Hellweed, Strangle Tare, Scaldweed

ACTIONS AND PHARMACOLOGY

COMPOUNDS

Saponins

Tannins

A purgative principle

The drug has been subjected to very little investigation.

EFFECTS

Dodder has hepatic and laxative effects.

INDICATIONS AND USAGE

Unproven Uses: Dodder is used for disorders of the urinary tract, spleen, and liver.

PRECAUTIONS AND ADVERSE REACTIONS

Health risks or side effects following the proper administration of designated therapeutic dosages are not recorded. It is conceivable that the drug triggers intestinal colic in cases of overdosage.

LITERATURE

Kern W, List PH, Hörhammer L (Hrsg.), Hagers Handbuch der Pharmazeutischen Praxis, 4. Aufl., Bde. 1-8, Springer Verlag Berlin, Heidelberg, New York, 1969.

Pagnani F, Ciarallo G, *Boll Chim Farm* 113(1):30. 1974

Dog Rose

Rosa canina

DESCRIPTION

Medicinal Parts: The medicinal parts are the petals, the Rose hips with and without seeds, and the seeds.

Flower and Fruit: The pink flowers are usually solitary or in clusters of 2 or 3. The receptacle deepens to form a cup, the upper edge of which house the 5 pinnatifid sepals, 5 petals, and numerous stamens. There are long white silky hairs in the receptacles and numerous ovaries. The ovaries grow into stiff-haired nuts surrounded by the receptacle and become the scarlet "rosehip."

Leaves, Stem and Root: The plant is an approximately 1 to 3 m high shrub with hanging branches and erect root shoots that are covered in tough, sickle-shaped prickles that are appressed below. The leaves are pinnatifid with 5 to 7 leaflets. They are markedly petiolate, obovate, smooth-margined, glabrous, glossy, and dark green above, lighter and simple-serrate beneath.

Characteristics: The sepals revolute at the end of the flowering period and drop when the fruit ripens.

Habitat: Rosa canina grows in Europe and North Africa and is extensively cultivated.

Production: Dog Rose fruit consist of the ripe, dried fruit (nutlet) of various species of the genus *Rosa* particularly *Rosa moschata.* The fruits are secondary products of Dog Rose shells. Dog Rose shells consist of the ripe, fresh or dried, opened seed receptacle (whole or cut and freed from hairs) of *Rosa canina, Rosa pendulina, Rosa rugosa, Rosa moschata* and other *Rosa* species. The ripe receptacles are harvested by hand and dried in the air, sun, or in drying plants at a maximum temperature of 80° C. The dry Dog Roses are broken up and the fruit and skins are separated by sieving.

Other Names: Brier Hip, Hip, Rose Hip, Sweet Briar, Brier Rose, Eglantine Gall, Hogseed, Dog-Berry, Sweet Brier, Wild Brier, Witches' Brier

ACTIONS AND PHARMACOLOGY

COMPOUNDS: DOG ROSE FRUITS

Fatty oil (8 to 10%)

Tocopherol (vitamin E)

Volatile oil (0.3%)

Proteic substances

EFFECTS: DOG ROSE FRUITS

The pectin and fruit acid content are responsible for the diuretic and laxative effect.

COMPOUNDS: DOG ROSE SHELLS

Carotinoids

Flavonoids

Fruit acids: malic acid, citric acid

Monosaccharides/oligosaccharides (12 to 15%): invert sugar, saccharose

Pectins

Tannins

Vitamins: ascorbic acid (vitamin C, 0.2 to 2.4%)

EFFECTS: DOG ROSE SHELLS

The drug is a vitamin C supplement

INDICATIONS AND USAGE

DOG ROSE FRUITS

Unproven Uses: Dog Rose fruits are used in folk medicine for disorders of the efferent urinary tract and the kidneys, kidney stones, rheumatic conditions such as rheumatism, and gout, colds, scurvy, and febrile conditions.

DOG ROSE SHELLS

Unproven Uses: Dog Rose shells are used in folk medicine for colds and "flu," intestinal conditions, digestive complaints, vitamin-C deficiency, gallstones, subacidic stomach, infectious diseases, conditions of the efferent urinary tract, edema, rheumatism and gout, bleeding, and leukorrhea.

PRECAUTIONS AND ADVERSE REACTIONS

DOG ROSE FRUITS AND SHELLS

No health hazards or side effects are known in conjunction with the proper administration of designated therapeutic dosages.

DOSAGE

DOG ROSE FRUITS

Mode of Administration: Dog Rose fruits are available as whole and powdered drug.

Daily Dosage: The single dose is 2 g drug.

Storage: Dog Rose should be stored in a dry and dark place.

DOG ROSE SHELLS

Mode of Administration: Dog Rose shells are available as whole, crude and powdered drug.

Daily Dosage: Tea: 2 to 5 g drug added to 1 cup and steeped for 10 to 15 minutes

Storage: Should be stored in dark place.

LITERATURE

DOG ROSE FRUIT AND SHELLS

Brantner A, Grein E. Antibacterial activity of plant extracts used externally in traditional medicine. *J Ethnopharmacol.* 44; 35-40. 1994)

Grases F et al. Effect of "*Rosa Canina*" Infusion and Magnesium on the Urinary Risk Factors of Calcium Oxalate Urolithiasis. *Planta Med.* 58; 509-512. 1992

Kurucu S, Coskun M, Kartal M, High pressure liquid chromatographic determination of ascorbic acid in the fruits of some Rosa species growing in Turkey. In: *PM* 58(7):A675. 1992.

Luckner M, Beβler O, PA 21:197. 1966.

Dogwood

Cornus florida

DESCRIPTION

Medicinal Parts: The medicinal part is the dried bark. Fresh bark is also used occasionally.

Flower and Fruit: The flowers are sessile, small, greenish, and in clusters of 12 to 20 at the splayed end of a tough, 3-cm long stem. The bracts are white or pale reddish, ovate to long, and are longer than the inflorescence. The petals are about 4 mm long. The fruit is a scarlet berry.

Leaves, Stem, and Root: The plant is a deciduous shrub or a 4 to 9 m high tree, which is heavily branched and has a dark gray, thick, rough bark. The branches are smooth and covered in leaf scars. The leaves are 7 to 10 cm long, opposite, petiolate, entire, ovate acuminate at both ends, and somewhat rough. The upper surface is dark green. In autumn the upper surface is bright red to violet. The underside is always whitish-green. The leaves are slightly pubescent when young.

Habitat: Cornus florida is indigenous to eastern and southern North America; other varieties are found in Europe.

Production: American Boxwood bark and root-bark are the dried and occasionally fresh bark and root-bark of *Cornus florida*. It is collected in the wild.

Other Names: Dog-Tree, Box Tree, Boxwood, Budwood, False Box, Cornelian Tree, Cornel, Bitter Redberry, Green Ozier, Swamp Dogwood, Silky Cornel, Osier, Rose Willow

ACTIONS AND PHARMACOLOGY

COMPOUNDS

Steroid saponins: including sarsapogenin-O-beta-D-galactoside, sarsapogenin-O-beta-D-xylosyl-(1(2)-beta-D-galactoside

Iridoide monoterpenes: cornin (verbenalin)

Tannins

EFFECTS

Effect on mollusks: The drug destroys the biomphalaria glabratus snails (carrier of bilharziose).

Cardiac effect: Heart activity, at different levels up to the cessation of heartbeat, is examined depending on the concentration of the methanol extract.

Antiplasmodic effect: Induced malaria in chicks and Peking ducks was treated for five days with a water-insoluble fraction. As a result, antiplasmodic activity toward *P cathemerium* could be observed, similar to that deployed by quinine and sulfadiazine. To date, the results cannot be sufficiently assessed.

The bark works as a tonic, an astringent and a stimulant.

INDICATIONS AND USAGE

Unproven Uses: In North America, the dried bark was used in folk medicine for strength, to stimulate appetite, for fever, and chronic diarrhea. It is used externally as an astringent for wounds and boils. Formerly, it was in use as a replacement for quinine. It is still used for headaches and fatigue.

Homeopathic Uses: Uses include for poor digestion and chronic attacks of fever.

PRECAUTIONS AND ADVERSE REACTIONS

Health risks or side effects following the proper administration of designated therapeutic dosages are not recorded.

DOSAGE

Mode of Administration: Formerly the drug was used internally as a tincture as an alternative to quinine and externally as a liquid extract.

How Supplied:

Tablets: 450 mg

Liquid Extract

Homeopathic Dosage: Oral: 5 drops, 1 tablet, or 10 globules every 30 to 60 minutes (acute) or 1 to 3 times a day (chronic); parenterally: 1 to 2 mL sc acute, 3 times daily; chronic: once a day (HAB34).

Preparation: Decoction or infusion (no specifications).

LITERATURE

Caetano-Anolles G, Trigiano RN, Windham MT, Sequence signatures from DNA amplification fingerprints reveal fine population structure of the dogwood pathogen *Discula destructiva*. *FEMS Microbiol Lett*, 145:377-83, Dec 15, 1996

Jacobs, B, In: Jacobs ML, Burlage HM: Index of Plants of North Carolina with Reputed Medicinal Uses, USA. 1958.

Hänsel R, Keller K, Rimpler H, Schneider G (Hrsg.), Hagers Handbuch der Pharmazeutischen Praxis, 5. Aufl., Bde 4-6 (Drogen), Springer Verlag Berlin, Heidelberg, New York, 1992-1994.

Hostettmann K, Hostettmann-Kaldas M, Nakanishi K, *Helv Chim Acta 61*:1990. 1978.

Dong Quai

Angelica sinensis

DESCRIPTION

Medicinal Parts: The medicinal part is the whole root.

Flower and Fruit: The plant bears umbrella-shaped clusters from May to August, each containing one to three dozen greenish-white flowers and winged fruits. Inflorescences are hairless and have five petals with incurvate tips.

Leaves, Stem, and Root: The root tastes bittersweet and spicy. It is divided into 3 parts—the head, body, and tail—and is grayish-brown or dark brown. The root is covered with transverse wrinkles and brown, resinous spots. The smooth, purplish stems grow 0.5 to 1 meter high, and are hollow, fluted, and glabrous. The lower leaves are tripinnate, while the upper leaves are pinnate. Leaflets are oval, dentate-incised, sheathed, and grow 3 to 11 cm long. Bracts are rudimentary.

Habitat: The aromatic herb grows at high altitudes in the cold, damp, mountain regions of China, Korea, and Japan.

Production: The plant must grow for 3 years before the root can be harvested.

Not to be Confused With: Angelica root or *Angelica* seed.

Other Names: Angelica sinensis, Angelica atropurpurea, Angelica dahurica, Chinese angelica, dang-gui, *Radix Angelicae Sinensis,* tang-kuei

ACTIONS AND PHARMACOLOGY

COMPOUNDS

Angelicide

Coumarin derivatives: bergapten, imperatorin, oxypeucedanin, osthol, psoralen, sen-byak-angelicole, and 7-demethylsuberosin

Ferulic acid

Flavonoids

Lactones and lactone derivatives

Sucrose (40%)

Polysaccharides

Sterols: B-sitosterol, phytosterol, stigmasterol

Vitamins: vitamin A, vitamin B12, nicotinic acid, folic acid, folinic acid, biotin, and vitamin E, among others

Volatile oils (0.4% to 0.7%): 45% ligustilide, n-butylphthalide, cadinene, carvacrol, and safrole isosafrol

EFFECTS

Different parts of the roots are said to have different actions. The head of the root purportedly has anticoagulant activity, the main root body serves as a tonic and pain reliever, and the tail of the root eliminates blood stasis (Zhu 1987).

The coumarins in Dong Quai may have anticoagulant and antispasmodic effects, the volatile oil may have analgesic and sedative effects, and the sucrose may have a laxative or diuretic effect. Various fractions have shown, in animals or *in vitro*, antibiotic, anti-anemic, immunomodulatory, and anti-atherosclerotic effects (Zhu 1987; Tyler 1994). Few human studies have been done.

The ferulic acid in Dong Quai inhibits the polymerization of platelets in the blood and retards platelet release of 5-hydroxytryptamine (5-HT) and adenosine diphosphate (ADP). 5-HT and ADP may cause platelets to become more sticky (Zhu 1987). Inhibition of cyclo-oxygenase and thromboxane A2 synthetase also occurs (Lo et al 1995).

Anti-Atherosclerotic Effects: Experimentally induced coronary atherosclerosis was prevented and arterial wall degeneration was reduced after administration of Dong Quai in animals (dose and route unknown). Arterial plaque was also reduced (Zhu 1987).

Anticoagulant Effects: Prothrombin times were significantly longer ($p<0.0001$) in a group receiving intravenous *Radix Angelicae sinensis* solution compared to intravenous placebo (Junjie et al 1984).

Diuretic Effects: Intravenous injection of a Dong Quai water extract produced excitation and contraction of the smooth muscle in the bladder (Zhu 1987).

Immunomsuppressive Effects: Experimentally created immunoglobulin E titers were inhibited by addition of a Dong Quai water extract (Zhu 1987).

Lipolytic Effects: The coumarins were found to activate lipolysis initiated by epinephrine and corticotropin. They also inhibit lipogenesis caused by insulin (Anon 1997).

Sexual Stimulatory Effects: Increased sexual activity has been reported in female animals. No mechanism was proposed (Zhu 1987).

Uterine Effects: The volatile oil content may produce a uterine depressant effect. However, a uterine stimulant effect has also been attributed to an aqueous extract. Some animal experiments have shown increased uterine excitability. Irregular, fast contractions are said to decrease and increase in regularity (Zhu 1987).

Vasodilatory Effects: Various coumarins in Dong Quai are thought to have vasodilating actions (Williamson et al 1997).

CLINICAL TRIALS

Menopausal Symptoms

A major 2005 summary and review of data from studies analyzing efficacy, risks, and benefits of HRT options (and evidence-based clinical guidelines) found that the only complementary therapies studied in any meaningful way for menopausal symptoms were products containing phytoestrogens, such as black cohosh. Clinical trials with Dong Quai for menopausal symptoms showed no benefit greater than placebo, the authors concluded. In addition to the issue of scant safety data, the authors cite the 2004 Position Statement of the North American Menopause Society which indicates that there is insufficient evidence that Dong Quai or any other complementary therapy available is superior to placebo for reducing menopausal vasomotor symptoms (Hickey et al 2005).

Dong Quai was one of several herbs included in a multibotanical treatment whose effectiveness in alleviating menopausal vasomotor symptoms was assessed and compared. The major 1-year, double-blind Herbal Alternatives to Menopause Trial (HALT) completed in September 2004 included both placebo and hormone therapy as benchmark comparison groups to compare with 3 herbal treatment groups: black cohosh 160 mg daily; multibotanical with black cohosh [200 mg daily] plus Dong Quai and eight other ingredients; and multibotanical plus dietary soy counseling. In all, 351 women 45 to 55 years of age with two or more vasomotor symptoms daily were randomized into the groups. None of the 3 herbal treatment groups had clinically meaningful reductions in menopausal symptoms, and at 12 months, symptom intensity was significantly worse for for the group taking multibotanical plus soy ($P=0.016$)—one of the treatment groups that included Dong Quai. (Newton et al 2006).

A 2005 evaluation of the effect of a water extract of Dong Quai on the proliferation of estrogen receptor-positive and negative breast cancer cells determined that it stimulated the growth of MCF-7 cells *in vitro*, possibly dependent of weak estrogen-agnostic activity. The extract also augmented B-20 cell proliferation independent of estrogen receptor-mediated pathway. These data illustrate estrogen-like activity of Dong Quai that might assist in decision-making regarding herbal therapy use by women at risk for breast cancer—both estrogen sensitive and insensitive. Given these findings and the scarcity of clinical data on side effects, caution is warranted for the use of Dong Quai in treating peri- or postmenopausal symptoms in women with breast cancer particularly (Lau et al 2005).

An earlier study shows no statistically significant estrogenic effects in a group of 71 postmenopausal women who took either placebo (maltodextrin) or Dong Quai (4.5 g/day) for 24 weeks. Subjective evaluation by the participants determined it was no better than placebo. No differences in endometrial thickness, vaginal maturation index, number of vasomotor flushes, or Kupperman index scores were detected (Hirata et al 1997).

INDICATIONS AND USAGE

Unproven Uses: Dong Quai is often taken to relieve menopausal symptoms. Dong Quai has also been used for arrhythmia, asthma and bronchitis, cardiovascular disorders, constipation, infertility, infection, insomnia, kidney problems, liver disorders, migraines, neuralgia, menstrual problems, and uterine contractions.

Chinese Medicine: Dong Quai is used to treat amenorrhea and metrorrhagia (standard dose of 5 g 3 times daily), PMS, menopausal symptoms, and fibroid tumors. Additionally, Dong Quai is used for hypertension (antispasmodic effects), rheumatism, ulcers, anemia, allergies, constipation, as a blood tonic, and to strengthen the uterus and aid patients in supportive functions before pregnancy. In Japan, Dong Quai is used as an analgesic, sedative, and nutrient.

CONTRAINDICATIONS

Dong Quai is contraindicated in patients with hemorrhagic disease, hypermenorrhea, chronic diarrhea, abdominal bloating, or acute infections including colds and flu.

Pregnancy: Dong Quai should not be used during pregnancy, particularly in the first trimester.

PRECAUTIONS AND ADVERSE REACTIONS

Possible side effects include fever, gastrointestinal disturbance, and increased bleeding. Because photodermatitis is also a possibility, caution patients to limit sun exposure and use sunscreen. Patients who are taking large doses of Dong Quai, or using it concurrently with blood thinners, should be monitored for increases in prothrombin time and INR (Junjie et al 1984).

DRUG INTERACTIONS

MODERATE RISK

Anticoagulant, low molecular weight heparins, thrombolytic agents: Concurrent use may result in increased risk of bleeding. *Clinical Management*: Caution is advised if Dong Quai and any of these drugs are taken concomitantly. Monitor for signs and symptoms of excessive bleeding.

Benzodiazepines: Concurrent use may result in excessive muscle relaxation and central nervous system depression. *Clinical Management:* Monitor patients taking Dong Quai and benzodiazepines concomitantly for excessive muscle relaxant and sedative effects of benzodiazepines.

Beta-adrenergic blockers: Concurrent use may result in low blood pressure. *Clinical Management*: Monitor blood pressure closely in patients taking beta-adrenergic blockers and dong quai concomitantly.

Nifedipine: Concurrent use may result in low blood pressure. *Clinical Management*: Monitor blood pressure closely in patients taking nifedipine and Dong Quai concomitantly.

Testosterone: Concurrent use may result in increased androgenic and/or adverse effects of testosterone. *Clinical Management*: Monitor for increased androgenic effects of testosterone (such as acne, hirsutism, behavior changes) in patients taking testosterone and dong quai concomitantly.

Tolbutamide: Concurrent use may result in increased risk of hypoglycemia. *Clinical Management*: Monitor blood glucose and signs and symptoms of hypoglycemia in patients taking dong quai and tolbutamide concomitantly.

DOSAGE

Mode of Administration: Oral, subcutaneous in acupuncture therapy; an intravenous form is available in China.

How Supplied: Fluid extract, powdered root, tablet, tea

Daily Dosage:

General Use (fluid extract, tablet): 2 to 3 g 2 to 3 times daily.

Acupuncture: 0.5 to 1 mL of a 5% or 10% solution has been injected into acupuncture points. Do not inject a homemade solution.

General Gynecological Conditions: root extract – 8 to 15 g daily. To make a decoction, combine 100 g of Dong Quai with Chuanxiong Rhizoma Ligustici Chuanxiong (100 g), peony root (100 g), and *Rehmannia* root (100 g). Grind mixture until a powder is formed and boil for 10 minutes in water with 15 mL of red wine. Dose is 9 g (3 g of Dong Quai) two to three times daily (Zhu 1987).

Postpartum Leukostasis: Decoction – Dong Quai, Hong Huai, Safflower, Wahoo (*Euonymus alatus [Thunb.]*) and Quai Gian Yue fine powders are mixed in equal parts, boiled for 10 minutes in wine, then for 20 minutes in water. Dose is 1 cup three times daily (Zhu 1987).

Weakness After Childbirth: soup – 15 g of Dong Quai, 0.5 lb of ginger root, 1 lb of lamb, 15 mL of sweet vinegar, and a little salt are simmered for 3 hours in 4 cups of water. Soup is taken twice daily for 2 weeks (Zhu 1987).

LITERATURE

Anon. Dong Quai. In: *The Review of Natural Products.* Facts and Comparisons, St. Louis, MO; 1997.

Hickey M, Davis SR, Sturdee DW. Treatment of menopausal symptoms: What shall we do now? *Lancet*; 366(9683): 409, 421. 2005.

Hirata JD, Swiersz LM, Zell B et al. Does dong quai have estrogenic effects in postmenopausal women? A double blind, placebo-controlled trial. *Fertility Sterility*; 68(6):981-986. 1997

Junjie T, Huaijun H. Effects of *Radix Angelicae Sinensis* on hemorrheology in patients with acute ischemic stroke. *J Tradit Chin Med*; 4:225-228. 1984

Lau CB, et al. Use of dong quai (Angelica sinensis) to treat peri- or postmenopausal symptoms in women with breast cancer: is it appropriate? *Menopause*; 12(6):734-40. 2005.

Lo ACT, Chan K, Yeung JHK et al. Danggui (*Angelica sinensis*) affects the pharmacodynamics but not the pharmacokinetics of warfarin in rabbits. *Eur J Drug Metab Pharmacokinet*; 20(1):55-60. 23. 1995.

Low Dog T. Menopause: a review of botanical dietary supplements. *Am J Med;* 118 Suppl 12B:98-108. 2005.

McGuffin M, Hobbs C, Upton R et al. *Botanical Safety Handbook.* CRC Press, Boca Raton, FL; 1997.

Newton KM, Reed SD, LaCroix AZ, et al. Treatment of vasomotor symptoms of menopause with black cohosh, multibotanicals, soy, hormone therapy, or placebo: a randomized trial. *Ann Intern Med*; 145 (2):869, 879. 2006.

Tyler VE. Rejuvex for postmenopausal symptoms. *JAMA*; 271(15): 1210. 1994

Williamson JS, Wyandt CM. Herbal therapies: The facts and the fiction. *Drug Topics*; Aug 4: 78-87. 1997

Zhu DPQ. Dong Quai. *Amer J Chin Med*; 15(3-4):117-125. 1987

Dorema ammoniacum

See Ammoniac Gum

Dorstenia contrayerva

See Contrayerva

Dragon's Blood (Xue-Jie)

Daemonorops draco

DESCRIPTION

Medicinal Parts: The medicinal part is the red resin from the fruit, which is extracted from both *Daemonorops draco* and *Daemonorops propinquis*.

Flower and Fruit: The flowers are arranged along the branch. The fruit is a cherry-sized berry ending in a point. When the fruit are ripe, they are covered in a reddish, resinous substance, which is separated in various ways.

Leaves, Stem, and Root: Dragon's Blood is a tree with long, thin, flexible stems, which tend to climb when they are older. The leaves have thorny petioles, which grow into long appendages. The bark is covered in hundreds of flattened thorns.

Habitat: Malaysia, Indonesia.

Production: Dragon's Blood resin is the resin of *Daemonorops draco*.

Other Names: Dracorubin, Draconis Resina, Sanguis Draconis, Xue-Jie

ACTIONS AND PHARMACOLOGY

COMPOUNDS

Ester resins (dracoresin): benzoyl ester of dracoresinotannol

Dracoresen

Flavane quinones: including dracorubin (dracocarmin), dracorhodin, both colored an intense red

EFFECTS

Dragon's Blood has an astringent effect.

INDICATIONS AND USAGE

Unproven Uses: The resin is used for diarrhea, digestive disorders, and as a coloring agent.

PRECAUTIONS AND ADVERSE REACTIONS

Health risks or side effects following the proper administration of designated therapeutic dosages are not recorded.

DOSAGE

Mode of Administration: The resin is used in a powder form.

LITERATURE

Hegnauer R, Chemotaxonomie der Pflanzen, Bde 1-11, Birkhäuser Verlag Basel, Boston, Berlin 1962-1997.

Kern W, List PH, Hörhammer L (Hrsg.), Hagers Handbuch der Pharmazeutischen Praxis, 4. Aufl., Bde 1-8, Springer Verlag Berlin, Heidelberg, New York, 1969.

Merlini L, Gasini G, *J Chem Soc Perkin* I 1976:1570. 1976.

Rao SR et al., *JNP* 45:646. 1982.

Drimys winteri

See Winter's Bark

Drosera ramentacea

See Sundew

Dryas octopetala

See Mountain Avens

Dryopteris filix-mas

See Male Fern

Duckweed

Lemna minor

DESCRIPTION

Medicinal Parts: The medicinal part is the whole fresh plant.

Flower and Fruit: The plant flowers infrequently. The tiny inconspicuous flowers have 2 unevenly sized stamens and 1 pistil. A delicate membranous bract surrounds 3 flowers, which are located on the edge of the stem. The fruit is tubular with 1 ovule. The seeds have longitudinal ribs.

Leaves, Stem, and Root: *Lemna minor* is a water plant with leaflike organs that are 2 to 6 mm long. They are flat, have 3 to 5 ribs, and are sometimes pigmented with red. There are 2 to 6 leaflike shoots that stick together, and each bears a root with a rounded root cover.

Characteristics: The plant has leaflike shoots with 1 root per leaf.

Habitat: The plant is found worldwide in cooler, oceanic climates. The plant is not found in east Asia and South Africa.

Production: Duckweed is the fresh plant *Lemna minor*.

ACTIONS AND PHARMACOLOGY

COMPOUNDS

Flavonoids: in particular C-glucosyl-flavone, including among others orientin, isoorientin, vitexin, isovitexin, lutonarin, vicenin-1; also O-glycosides, including among others apigenin-7-O-glucoside, luteolin-7-O-glycoside

Cyclopentane fatty acids, with structure resembling prostaglandin

Polysaccharides: apiogalacturonans

Cardiac steroids (cardenolides)

EFFECTS

No information is available.

INDICATIONS AND USAGE

Unproven Uses: Duckweed is used internally for inflammation of the upper respiratory tract and externally for gout and rheumatism.

Chinese Medicine: Duckweed is used for measles, edema, joint pain, dysuria, acne, erysipelas, and epilepsy.

Homeopathic Uses: Duckweed is used for chronic colds.

PRECAUTIONS AND ADVERSE REACTIONS

No health hazards or side effects are known in conjunction with the proper administration of designated therapeutic dosages.

DOSAGE

Mode of Administration: The plant is available as fresh or ground herb and as an extract.

Homeopathic Dosage: 5 drops, 1 tablet, or 10 globules every 30 to 60 minutes (acute) or 1 to 3 times daily (chronic); parenterally: 1 to 2 ml s.c., acute: 3 times daily; chronic: once a day (HAB1).

LITERATURE

Hänsel R, Keller K, Rimpler H, Schneider G (Hrsg.), Hagers Handbuch der Pharmazeutischen Praxis, 5. Aufl., Bde 4-6 (Drogen), Springer Verlag Berlin, Heidelberg, New York, 1992-1994.

Madaus G. Lehrbuch der Biologischen Arzneimittel, Bde 1-3, Nachdruck, Georg Olms Verlag Hildesheim 1979.

Dusty Miller

Senecio bicolor

DESCRIPTION

Medicinal Parts: The medicinal parts are the fresh plant harvested before flowering, the herb of the flowering plant, and the whole fresh, flowering plant.

Flower and Fruit: The plant has numerous yellow capitula, 12 to 15 cm in diameter, on short peduncles. The calyx only has a few sepals. There are 10 to 12 lingual florets. The fruit is striped.

Leaves, Stem and Root: Senecio cineraria is a semi-shrub that grows up to 80 cm high. The stem is erect, heavily branched at the base, and sometimes snow-white tomentose. The leaves are densely pubescent beneath and more or less cobwebbed on the upper surface. They may have sparse greenish hairs. The lower leaves are oval to lanceolate, pinnatifid, and the outer lobes are usually longer than they are wide.

Habitat: The plant is indigenous to the Mediterranean region, naturalized in North America and cultivated as an ornamental plant in many countries.

Production: Cineraria juice is the juice of the whole *Senecio cinerarian* plant.

Other Names: Cineraria Maritima

ACTIONS AND PHARMACOLOGY

COMPOUNDS

Pyrrolizidine alkaloids (0.9% in the blossoming foliage): including, among others, jaconine, jacobine, otosenine, retrorsine, senecionine, seneciphylline

Polyynes

EFFECTS

The active agents are the alkaloids jacobin, senecionin, and otosenin. These pyrrolizidine alkaloids are hepatotoxic and carcinogenic.

INDICATIONS AND USAGE

Homeopathic Uses: In homeopathy, the juice is used to treat eyesight problems (for the treatment of spots before the eyes), migraine, and as an emmenagogue.

PRECAUTIONS AND ADVERSE REACTIONS

Dusty Miller should not be taken internally (except in homeopathic dosages) because of the potential hepatotoxicity and carcinogenicity of the pyrrolizidine alkaloids and the 1,2-unsaturated necic parent substances.

DOSAGE

Mode of Administration: The use of the sterilized juice is no longer recommended for internal use, nor is any other preparation of Dusty Miller.

LITERATURE

Roeder E. Medicinal plants in Europe containing pyrrolizidine alkaloids. *Pharmazie* 50 (2); 82-98 (1995)

Pinchon TM, Pinkas M. Les amino-acides libres des capitules de *Senecio bicolor* (Willd.) *Tod ssp. cineraria* (DC) chater. *Pharmazie* 46; 232-233 (1991

Dwarf Elder

Sambucus ebulus

DESCRIPTION

Medicinal Parts: The medicinal parts are the dried leaves, the ripe, dried or fresh fruit, and the dried roots.

Flowers and Fruit: The reddish-white flowers are in a terminal, umbrellalike, richly blossomed, paniculate cyme with 3 main branches. The calyx margin is 5-tipped. The corolla has fused petals and is rotate with 5 acuminate tips. The 5 stamens have dark red anthers and an inferior, 3-valved ovary with 3 stigmas. The fruit is a black, globular, berrylike drupe with at least 3 to 4 ovate seeds. When ripe, the fruit stems are erect and violet or crimson.

Leaves, Stem, and Root: Dwarf Elder is a perennial, herblike plant 0.5 to 2 m high with a sturdy, finger-thick, branched rhizome that creeps deeply and horizontally. The stems are leafy, erect, sturdy, and branched above. They die off in autumn. The leaves are crossed opposite, odd-pinate with 3 to 4 pairs of ovate-lanceolate leaflets and 2 large, ovate-lanceolate, and serrate stipules.

Characteristics: The fragrance is similar to that of sunflowers or almond.

Habitat: The plant is found from southern Sweden throughout central and southern Europe, in northern Africa, in western Asia as far as Iran, and in North America.

Production: Dwarf Elder root is the root of *Sambucus ebulus,* which is collected in the spring or late autumn and then air-dried.

Other Names: Danewort, Walewort, Blood Elder, Blood Hilder

ACTIONS AND PHARMACOLOGY

COMPOUNDS

Iridoides: ebuloside, 6'-0-apiosyl-ebuloside, 7,7-0-dihydroebuloside, secoebuloside, isoswer-oside

Nauseant, purgative resins with unresolved structure

EFFECTS

The drug is said to be a mild diuretic.

INDICATIONS AND USAGE

Unproven Uses: Dwarf Elder is used in folk medicine for constipation, as an emetic, and to treat edema and kidney disease.

PRECAUTIONS AND ADVERSE REACTIONS

Health risks or side effects following the proper administration of designated therapeutic dosages are not recorded.

OVERDOSAGE

According to older scientific reports, large quantities of all parts of the plant, (in particular the raw berries) leads to vomiting, bloody diarrhea, cyanosis, dizziness, headache, and unconsciousness. Cases of death are also mentioned.

DOSAGE

Mode of Administration: Dwarf Elder is obsolete as a drug in most countries. It is found in some tea mixtures, but is not used in medicinal preparations.

LITERATURE

Leporatti ML, Pavesi A. New or uncommon Uses of Several Medicinal Plants in some Areas of Central Italy. J Ethnopharmacol. 29; 213-223. 1990

Hänsel R, Keller K, Rimpler H, Schneider G (Hrsg.), Hagers Handbuch der Pharmazeutischen Praxis, 5. Aufl., Bde 4-6 (Drogen): Springer Verlag Berlin, Heidelberg, New York, 1992-1994.

Lewin L, Gifte und Vergiftungen, 6. Aufl., Nachdruck, Haug Verlag, Heidelberg 1992.

Madaus G, Lehrbuch der Biologischen Arzneimittel, Bde 1-3, Nachdruck, Georg Olms Verlag Hildesheim 1979.

Dyer's Broom

Genista tinctoria

DESCRIPTION

Medicinal Parts: The entire plant has medicinal applications.

Flower and Fruit: The flowers are in short, terminal racemes. They are golden yellow and bean-shaped, 1.5 to 2 cm long and are on pedicles, which are shorter than the calyx. The petal stems of the 4 lower petals are initially straight, but in moments of tension (for example, when touched by an insect) they curl down suddenly and the flower opens. The fruit is a smooth pod 2.5 to 3.5 cm long. It is brown, compressed at the sides, and contains 5 to 10 seeds.

Leaves, Stem, and Root: The plant is a 30 to 60 cm high, always thornless sub-shrub with a creeping, woody rhizome. The florescent green stems are smooth and produce fairly rigid, smooth or pubescent forked branches, which sprout lanceolate leaves. The leaves are alternate, glabrous, entire-margined, 1.25 to 2.5 cm long, nearly sessile, and with a ciliate margin. The stipules are linear-awl shaped.

Habitat: Dyer's Broom is indigenous to the Mediterranean region, the Canary Islands, Europe and western Asia, and cultivated elsewhere, including the eastern U.S.

Production: Dyer's Broom leaves are the green leaves of *Genista tinctoria.*

Other Names: Dyer's Weed, Dyer's Greenwood, Dyer's Whin, Furze, Green Broom, Greenweed, Wood Waxen

ACTIONS AND PHARMACOLOGY

COMPOUNDS

Quinolizidine alkaloids: main alkaloids — cytisine, methylcytisine, anagyrine, as well as isosparteine, lupanine, tinctorin

Flavonoids: in particular luteolin glycosides

Isoflavonoids: genistein, genistin

Lectins

EFFECTS

The drug acts as a purifier, cathartic, diuretic, purgative, and emetic. It increases heart rate, strengthens the walls of blood vessels, stimulates kidney blood circulation, and affects metabolism.

INDICATIONS AND USAGE

Unproven Uses: The drug is used for kidney and bladder stones, digestive disorders, and gout.

PRECAUTIONS AND ADVERSE REACTIONS

General: Health risks or side effects following the proper administration of designated therapeutic dosages are not recorded. Overdosage can lead to diarrhea and to symptoms of a cystine poisoning. Anagyrine has exhibited teratogenic effect in animal experiments.

Pregnancy: Not to be used during pregnancy.

DOSAGE

Mode of Administration: The drug is used internally as an infusion.

Preparations: To prepare a tea, use 1 to 2 g drug per 150 mL boiling water.

Daily Dosage: Drink 1 to 2 cups of infusion daily.

LITERATURE

Chan, EH et al. (Eds), Advances in Chinese Medicinal Materials Research, World Scientific Pub. Co. Singapore 1985.

Kern W, List PH, Hörhammer L (Hrsg.), Hagers Handbuch der Pharmazeutischen Praxis, 4. Aufl., Bde. 1-8, Springer Verlag Berlin, Heidelberg, New York, 1969.

Leung AY, Encyclopedia of Common Natural Ingredients Used in Food Drugs and Cosmetics, John Wiley & Sons Inc., New York 1980.

Lewin L, Gifte und Vergiftungen, 6. Aufl., Nachdruck, Haug Verlag, Heidelberg 1992.

Madaus G, Lehrbuch der Biologischen Arzneimittel, Bde 1-3, Nachdruck, Georg Olms Verlag Hildesheim 1979.

Roth L, Daunderer M, Kormann K, Giftpflanzen, Pflanzengifte, 4. Aufl., Ecomed Fachverlag Landsberg Lech 1993.

Teuscher E, Lindequist U, Biogene Gifte - Biologie, Chemie, Pharmakologie, 2. Aufl., Fischer Verlag Stuttgart 1994.

Wichtl M (Hrsg.), Teedrogen, 4. Aufl., Wiss. Verlagsges. Stuttgart 1997.

Echinacea

Echinaceae species

DESCRIPTION

Medicinal Parts: The medicinal parts are, depending on varieties, the roots, leaves, or the whole plant in various stages of development.

Flower and Fruit: The flower heads are large and solitary on terminal peduncles with spreading ray florets. The bracts are in a number of rows. The bracts are leafy, rigid, thorny tipped, and longer than the conical erect disc florets. The reddish or occasionally white florets are conspicuous. The lingual florets are usually sterile and 3 cm long. The pappus is small or absent.

Leaves, Stem, and Root: Echinacea is usually a perennial herb and grows up to 45 cm in height. The leaves are large, solitary, opposite or alternate, and are smooth-margined. They are 7 to 20 cm long and have a rough surface. The leaves are entire-margined and are on slender petioles. A transverse section of the rhizome shows a thin bark and a yellowish, porous wood, which is flecked with black.

Characteristics: The taste is slightly sweet then bitter leaving a tingling sensation on the tongue. The odor is faintly aromatic.

Habitat: Echinacea purpurea and *Echinaceae pallida* grow in the middle or eastern U.S. and is cultivated in Europe.

Production: Echinacea purpurea herb consists of the fresh, above-ground parts, harvested at flowering time. The root consists of the fresh or dried underground part, gathered in autumn. *Echinacea pallida* herb consists of the fresh or dried above-ground parts, collected at the time of flowering. *Echinacea angustifolia* herb and root consist of the fresh or dried roots, or above-ground parts collected at the time of flowering.

Not to be Confused With: The herbs and roots of *Echinacea purpurea, Echinacea angustifolia,* and *Echinacea pallida* have different medicinal properties. Some Echinacea species may be confused with or adulterated with *Parthenium integrifoium.*

Other Names: Black Sampson, Hedgehog, Purple Coneflower, Red Sunflower, Rudbeckia, Sampson Root

ACTIONS AND PHARMACOLOGY

COMPOUNDS: ECHINACEA PURPUREA HERB

Water-soluble immunostimulating polysaccharides (4-O-methylglucuronylarabinoxylans, acidic arabinorhamnogalactans)

Volatile oil (under 0.08-0.32%): components including germacrene alcohol, borneol, bornylacetate, pentadeca-8-en-2-on, germacrene D, caryophyllene, caryophyllene epoxide

Flavonoids: ferulic acid derivatives including cichoriic acid, cichoriic acid methyl ester, 2-O- caffeoyl-3-O-feruloyl-tartaric acid, 2,3-O-diferuloyl tartaric acid 2-O-caffeoyl tartaric acid

Alkamides: including undeca-2E,4Z-dien-8,10-diin acid- and dodeca-2E,4E-8Z,10E/Z- tetraen acid isobutylamide

Polyenes: trideca-1,11-dien-3,5,7,9,-tetraine, trideca-1-en-3,5,7,9,11-pentaine, trideca-8,10,12-trien-2,4,6-triine, pontica epoxide

COMPOUNDS: ECHINACEA PURPUREA ROOT

Water-soluble immunostimulating polysaccharides

Water-soluble immunostimulating glycoproteins

Volatile oil (0.2%): components including caryophyllene, humules, caryophyllene epoxide, dodeca-2,4-dien-1-yl-isovalerate, germacrene D, palmitic acid, linolenic acid

Caffeic and ferulic acid derivatives (0.6-2.1%): including cichoriic acid, cichoriic acid methyl ester, 2-O- caffeoyl tartaric acid

Alkamides (0.01-0.04%): including undeca-2E,4Z-dien-8,10-diinacetyl- and dodeca-2E,4E-8Z,10E/Z-tetracetyliso-butylamide

Polyynes (0.01mg/%): including trideca-1-en-3,5,7,9,11-pentain, trideca-1,11-dien-3,5,7,9,-tetraine, trideca-8,10,12-trien-2,4,6-triine, pontica epoxide

Effective pyrrolizidine alkaloids: tussilagine, isotussilagine

COMPOUNDS: ECHINACEA PALLIDA HERB

Volatile oil (0.1%): including 1,8-pentadecadien

Flavonoids: in particular rutin

Caffeic acid derivatives: Cichoriic acid, chlorogenic acid, isochlorogenic acid, verbascoside

Alkamides: including dodeca-2E,4E-8Z,10E-tetracetyliso-butylamide

COMPOUNDS: ECHINACEA PALLIDA ROOT

Water-soluble immunostimulating polysaccharides (arabino-rhamnogalactans)

Volatile oil (0.2 - 2%): chief components include pentadeca-8Z-en-2-on, pentadeca-1,8Z-dien, 1-pentadecan

Caffeic acid derivatives: echinacoside

Alkamides: including isomeric dodeca-2E,4E-8Z,10E/Z-tetraenic acid-isobutylamide

Polyynes: including trideca-1-en-3,5,7,9,11-pentain, pontica epoxide

COMPOUNDS: ECHINACEA ANGUSTIFOLIA HERB

Volatile oil (under 0.1%): typical components consist of epishyobunol, beta-farnesene, alpha- and beta-pinenes, myrcene, carvomenthene, caryophyllene

Flavonoids

Caffeic acid derivatives: cichoriic acid, chlorogenic acid, isochlorogenic acid, verbascoside, echinacoside

Alkamides: including dodeca-2E,4E-8Z,10E-tetracetyl-isobutylamide

Polyynes: including trideca-1-en-3,5,7,9,11-pentaine, pontica epoxide

COMPOUNDS: ECHINACEA ANGUSTIFOLIA ROOT

Volatile oil (under 1%): components include dodeca-2,4-dien-1-ylisovalerate, as well as palmitic acid, linolenic acid

Flavonoids

Caffeic acid derivatives (0.3 to 1.3%): echinacoside, cynarin

Alkamides (0.01%): including dodeca-2E,4E-8Z,10E/Z- tetracetyl isobutylamide

Polyynes: including trideca-1-en-3,5,7,9,11-pentaine, pontica epoxide, in dehydrated roots only traces

EFFECTS: ALL VARIETIES

Echinacea activity is directed toward the nonspecific cellular immune system. The herb has demonstrated antibacterial, anti-inflammatory, metabolic, immune-system enhancement, infertility, wound healing, antineoplastic, and antiseptic properties, depending on the type of plant species. The main active principles of the immunostimulating, antibacterial, and virostatic drug are the alkamides, glycoproteins, caffeic acid derivatives (cichoriic acid and echinosides), and polysaccharides. Echinacea preparations are commonly given in Europe for the prophylaxis or treatment of bacterial and viral infections and as an adjunct to treatment of more severe infections. Echinacea extracts are commonly used to treat upper respiratory infections, influenza-like infections, and are reported to significantly reduce the symptoms accompanying the common cold. When taken soon after an exposure, extracts may lessen the severity and lead to earlier resolution (Gruber & DerMarderosian, 1996). The herb is also used as an adjuvant therapy for frequently recurring infections of the urinary tract.

Antibacterial Effects: Echinacea angustifolia, as a part of a combination herbal treatment known as *Mercurius cyanatus* complex, was tested in vitro using serial dilution against 105 clinical microorganisms. The bactericidal activity was approximately that of vancomycin (Vestweber et al, 1995). It is difficult to assess the results since the product was a combination of several herbs. Alcoholic extracts of *Echinacea purpurea* increased phagocytic, metabolic, and bactericidal activities of peritoneal macrophages (Bukovsky et al, 1993; Bukovsky et al, 1993a).

Anti-inflammatory Effects: Polyunsaturated alkamides in *Echinacea angustifolia* exert anti-inflammatory effects through inhibition of cyclooxygenase and 5-lipoxygenase (Muller-Jakic, 1994). The polysaccharide fraction of *Echinacea angustifolia* exerts anti-inflammatory effects (Tubaro, 1987), and the polysaccharide from *Echinacea purpurea* induces an acute phase reaction. The acute phase reaction occurs with enhancing the spontaneous motility of PMN and increasing the ability of these cells to kill bacteria such as staphylococci. (Roesler, 1991). Echinacea extracts have been used to treat arthritis. A few combination products may decrease inflammation and itching after insect bite.

Collagen-Protecting Effects: The caffeic acid derivatives exert a protective effect on the free-radical-induced degradation of Type III collagen. Collagen degradation was inhibited the greatest by echinacoside and chicoriic acid, then cynarine and chlorogenic acid (Facino, 1995). A fibroblast-populated collagen lattice was used to study the influence of Echinacea extracts on the collagen-contracting ability of mouse fibroblasts. Collagen gel contraction was inhibited by herb and root extracts (added at the time of gel preparation) dose dependently. Inhibition of collagen gel contraction parallels the inhibition of morphological changes in the wound (Zoutewelle & van Wijk, 1990).

Cytokine Stimulation Effects: Arabinogalactan, a highly purified polysaccharide from plant cell cultures of *Echinacea purpurea,* is effective in activating macrophage cytotoxicity actions against tumor cells and microorganisms (*Leishmania*

enriettii). This polysaccharide induces macrophages to produce TNF-alpha, interleukin-1 (IL-1), interleukin-6 (IL-6), interleukin-10 (IL-10) and interferon-beta. The component also induces a slight increase in T-cell proliferation (Burger, 1997; Luettig, 1989; Roesler, 1991). Extracts of *Echinacea purpurea* stimulate cell-mediated immunity through the production of lymphokines by lymphocytes (Coeugniet, 1987). *Echinacea purpurea* herb has shown some short-term viral resistance against influenza, herpes, and vesicular stomatitis viruses, which has been credited to an interferon-like effect (Wacker, 1978).

Immunostimulating Effects: Ethanolic root extracts of the *Echinacea purpurea, Echinacea pallida,* and *Echinacea angustifolia* were shown to cause a 23% increase of the phagocytosis rate in granulocyte smears in vitro (Jurcic, 1989; Melchart 1995). Confirmed by the carbon clearance test and granulocyte tests, the ethanolic root extracts significantly enhance phagocytosis (Bauer, 1988). The ethanolic extracts of aerial parts of *Echinacea angustifolia* and *Echinacea purpurea* exert immunostimulatory effects also through metabolic and bactericidal activities of peritoneal macrophages. The ethanolic extracts of both Echinacea plants also increase the total weight of the spleen (Bukovsky, 1993).

Echinacea purpurea extract was tested in vitro. A stimulation of lymphokines by lymphocytes and a stimulation in the transformation test was seen. The potential was for increased cell-mediated immunity (Coeugniet & Elek, 1987). Echinacea extract, at concentrations of greater than or equal to 0.1 mcg/km, significantly enhanced killer cell and peripheral blood mononuclear cells (PBMC) function in vitro. An extract of *Echinacea purpurea* was evaluated on its ability to stimulate cellular immune function by PBMC from normal subjects, patients with chronic fatigue syndrome, and patients with AIDS (See et al, 1997). Extracts of *Echinacea purpurea* increased the in vitro phagocytosis of *Candida albicans* by granulocytes and monocytes from healthy donors by 30% to 45%. Chemotactic granulocyte migration (Boyden Chamber) was increased by 45%. There was no effect on intracellular killing of bacteria and yeasts and in vitro transformation of lymphocytes was not induced (Wildfeuer & Mayerhofer, 1994). Significant immunostimulating actions were demonstrated in water-soluble polysaccharide fractions (heteroglycans) from *Echinacea purpurea* and *Echinacea angustifolia.* (Wagner et al, 1985; Wagner et al, 1984).

Infertility: Echinacea purpurea (8.1 mg/mL) inhibited sperm motility and velocity after 24 hours of contact with 100 donor sperm. Echinacea inhibited the action of hyaluronidase, an enzyme located at the head of the sperm responsible for assisting the sperm to penetrate cumulus cell layers around the oocyte, possibly preventing sperm from successfully fertilizing the oocytes (Ondrizek et al, 1999).

CLINICAL TRIALS

Immunostimulation and Cold/Flu Prevention

A major 2006 Cochrane Collaboration review of the literature on Echinacea analyzed and pooled the results of randomized controlled clinical trials to date that have compared the effectiveness of the herb (mono-preparations as opposed to blends) with a placebo, no treatment, or another treatment for *preventing* or *treating* the common cold. The review found 16 such trials, involving a total of 22 comparisons—19 of Echinacea compared to a placebo, two to no treatment at all, and one to another herbal preparation. All but one trial was double-blind. In terms of preventing the common cold, two trials found no effect in this regard with Echinacea taken for 8 to 12 weeks. And none of the three trials that compared Echinacea's effectiveness over placebo showed benefit from taking Echinacea. Most of the trials, however, looked at whether Echinacea taken *after* cold symptoms begin could shorten the duration of the cold, or decrease the severity of the symptoms any better than a placebo could. In this regard, some Echinacea preparations showed better effectiveness over a placebo for this purpose (in adults). Specifically, a significant effect of Echinacea over placebo was identified in nine of the trials that made this comparison (plus a trend toward effectiveness in one). In terms of actually treating a cold, six of the comparisons showed no effectiveness for Echnicacea over placebo. Echinacea preparations differ widely in the clinical trials—there are more than 200 different ones that use various different types (species) and parts of the plant (root, herb, or both) as well as many methods of extracting the active ingredient. Some, evidence points to effectiveness for early treatment of colds when aerial (above-ground) parts of the herb are used. Rigorous and well-designed clinical trials have yet to be performed that conclusively show that Echinacea has preventive properties (Linde, 2006).

A 2005 structured review of evidence for Echinacea in treating the common cold similarly found little evidence to justify its therapeutic effectiveness. At the time, 322 articles were identified. Nine were placebo-controlled clinical trials, but only two met 11 criteria designed to measure quality (essential elements to provide valid results, such as double-blinding, lack of a quantifiable analysis, compliance testing, and randomized assignment to treatment), and the authors of these two studies themselves deemed the findings for Echinacea to treat the common cold unconvincing (Caruso, 2005).

One 2005 study that set out to test Echinacea in a very controlled setting, using a chemically well-defined preparation, a clearly defined illness, and early exposure to the herb in the development of a cold ultimately did not find the herb to have a clinically significant effect on the infection or course of illness. No statistically significant effects of the chemically defined extracts of *Echinacea angustifolia* root—three different preparations made with either supercritical carbon dioxide, 60% alcohol, or 20% alcohol) from a single lot of the herb root—were observed on rates of infection or severity of symptoms in the volunteers. The participants were given a cold virus (rhinovirus type 39) and kept in a sequestered environment for 5 days. In all, 437 participants (from six different cohorts) were randomly assigned to either a prevention or treatment group with one of the extracts or a placebo, and 399 (mean age 20.8) were actually ''given'' (infected with) the cold virus and then isolated in individual hotel rooms for the rest of the study. In addition to having no significant impact on the participants' clinical course of disease, the Echinacea extract had no significant impact on the amount of virus (quantitative-virus titer in the volunteer's body), the volume of nasal secretions produced, or nasal-lavage specimen measurements of key immune system cells (polymorphonuclear leukocyte or interleukin-8 concentrations) (Turner, 2005).

Somewhat different results were obtained in another 2005 study. Echinilin, a formulation prepared from freshly harvested *Echinacea purpurea* plants and standardized on the basis of three known active components (alkamides, cichoric acid, and polysaccharides) was found to be effective for the treatment of common cold. For a 7-day period, volunteers took either Echinilin or placebo at the onset of their cold, with 8 doses (5 mL/dose) on day 1 and 3 doses on subsequent days. Fasting blood samples were obtained before and during their colds. Those in the Echinacea group experienced a more significant decrease in total daily symptomatic score, suggesting that Echinilin, by enhancing the non-specific immune response and eliciting free radical scavenging properties, may have led to faster resolution of the cold symptoms (Goel et al, 2005).

An earlier study of 282 subjects showed that the same preparation, Echilin, produced lower daily symptom scores than placebo. The subjects, who were aged 18-65 years with a history of two or more colds in the previous year, but otherwise in good health, were randomly assigned to take Echinacea or placebo at the onset of the first symptom related to cold, consuming 10 doses the first day and four doses daily on subsequent days for 7 days. Total daily symptom scores were lower by 23.1% in the Echinacea group than in placebo ($p<0.01$). Throughout the treatment period, the response rate to treatments was greater in patients treated with Echinacea (Goel et al, 2004).

In contrast, symptoms and duration of the common cold were not mitigated in a 2004 randomized, double-blind, placebo-controlled clinical trial. In all, 128 individuals (volunteers from a community) were given either 100 mg *Echinacea purpurea* or a placebo 3 times daily within 24 hours of cold symptoms starting (as reported by the participants), and until cold symptoms ceased or at 14 days—whichever came first. The herb was given in the form of freeze-dried pressed juice from the plant's aerial parts. No statistically significant differences were observed between the Echinacea and placebo groups for the total or mean symptoms scores, which were based on participant-recorded daily record of such symptoms as sneezing, nasal discharge, headache, hoarseness, muscle aches, cough, and sore or scratchy throat. The authors note that relatively few numbers of participants enrolled (Yale, 2004).

Echinacea was deemed ineffective in reducing symptoms or severity of acute upper respiratory tract (URI) infection in children (age 2 to 11 years), but potentially effective in reducing subsequent URI in this treatment-efficacy trial—a secondary analysis of data from a randomized, double-blind, placebo-controlled study. *Echinacea purpurea* (reconstituted dried juice of above-ground portion of the plant) was used. In all, 524 children were monitored for URI over the course of 4 months. In these children, the use of Echinacea for the first URI was linked to a 28% decreased risk of a second URI ($p=0.01$) (Weber, 2005).

The ability of *Echinacea purpurea* to prevent infection with rhinovirus type 39 (RV-39) was tested in a randomized, double-blind, placebo-controlled clinical trial. Forty-eight previously health adults administered Echinacea or placebo, 2.5 mL 3 times per day, for 7 days before and 7 days after intranasal inoculation with RV-39. A total of 92% of the Echinacea recipients and 82% of the placebo recipients were infected. Colds developed in 58% of patients in the Echinacea group and 82% in the placebo group, which was not significantly different ($p=0.114$) (Sperber et al, 2004).

A 2000 study that used Echinacea Plus, an herbal tea preparation containing *Echinacea purpurea* and *Echinacea angustifolia*, decreased the duration of symptoms of cold or flu when taken at early onset of symptoms. The trial was double-blind, placebo-controlled, and involved 95 subjects ages 24 to 62 years. Symptom relief, number of days of symptoms, and number of days before noticeable symptom change were significantly improved in the Echinacea Plus group compared to the placebo group ($p<0.001$ for all 3 results). No significant adverse reactions were reported. Subjects in this study were primarily health care women, thus limiting the ability to generalize these results (Lindenmuth & Lindenmuth, 2000).

Echinacea demonstrated safe and effective symptom relief for viral respiratory tract infections in a double-blind, placebo-controlled, multicenter study. Herbal Echinacea's total efficacy over placebo was significant ($p=0.0497$) with symptom relief response time reduced with treatment ($p=0.022$). Although common colds will resolve spontaneously, the achieved goal was symptom relief (Henneicke-von Zepelin et al, 1999).

Echinacea concentrate and Echinaforce® exhibited low risk, effective, symptomatic relief in a placebo-controlled, double-blind, study involving 246 subjects with the common cold. Subjects were randomized into one of four groups: Echinaforce (n=55), Echinacea concentrate (n=64), *Echinacea purpurea* (n=63), and placebo (n=64) with instructions to take 2 tablets 3 times daily with onset of cold symptoms. Treatment was not to exceed 7 days. Reduction in the complaint index of 12 primary symptoms associated with the common cold was significantly higher in the Echinacea concentrate ($p=0.003$)

and Echinaforce (p=0.02) groups than in the placebo group (Brinkeborn, 1999).

A randomized, placebo-controlled, double-blind trial evaluated the effect of a fluid extract of *Echinacea purpurea* on the incidence and severity of colds and respiratory infections. The fluid extract, given 4 mL twice daily for 8 weeks, did not significantly decrease the incidence, duration, or severity of colds and respiratory infections compared to placebo. (Melchart et al, 1998).

Echinagard® effectively shortened the course of acute, uncomplicated upper respiratory infections (URI) in a double-blind, placebo-controlled study involving 120 patients randomized to either Echinagard (n=60) or placebo (n=60). Significant rapid recovery was demonstrated in the group taking Echinagard versus placebo ($p<0.0001$) with median improvement reported in 4 days versus 8 days. No distinguishing adverse events were reported (Hoheisel et al, 1997).

Overall, a statistically significant decrease in infections was observed when a ''susceptible'' group (members had experienced flu within last 12 months) was compared to the entire population ($p<0.05$) in a placebo-controlled, double-blind clinical trial of Resistan®. The Resistan group experienced 15% fewer primary and 27% fewer secondary infections as compared with the placebo group. In the subgroup of ''susceptible'' subjects, there was a 20% decrease in infections compared to the placebo group. The study also showed that Echinacea products taken at the onset of upper respiratory symptoms may reduce the duration of the illness by 25% to 33%. Evaluation on days 6 to 8 demonstrated a significant reduction in all seven symptoms in the placebo group (Schulz & Haensel, 1996).

Echinacea did not improve symptoms of upper respiratory tract infections (URI) in children in a large, double-blind, placebo-controlled trial. Parents were asked to rate symptoms and adverse events. Complete information existed for a total of 608 URIs that occurred during the 4-month study period. No significant differences were noted between placebo and Echinacea for the primary study outcome (Taylor et al, 2003).

Echinacea did not reduce symptom severity or duration of the common cold in a randomized, double-blind, placebo-controlled community-based trial. One hundred and forty-two participants with early cold symptoms completed this trial. Participants were randomly assigned to receive encapsulated Echinacea or placebo. The mean duration difference was - 0.52 day (95% CI, - 1.09 to 0.22 days) between the placebo group (5.75 days) and Echinacea group (6.27 days). There was no significant difference in symptom severity between the Echinacea and placebo groups. Adverse effects were not different between the two groups (Barrett et al, 2002).

Genital Herpes

Treatment with the plant and root extract of *Echinacea purpurea* had no significant benefit in patients with recurrent genital herpes (Vonau et al, 2001).

INDICATIONS AND USAGE

ECHINACEA PURPUREA HERB

Approved by Commission E:

- Common cold
- Cough/bronchitis
- Fevers and colds
- Infections of the urinary tract
- Inflammation of the mouth and pharynx
- Tendency to infection
- Wounds and burns

Echinacea purpurea herb is used internally as supportive therapy for colds and chronic infections of the respiratory tract and lower urinary tract, and for influenza-like infections. It can also be applied locally to poorly healing superficial wounds.

ECHINACEA PURPUREA ROOT

Unproven Uses: Echinacea purpurea root is used for acute and chronic respiratory tract infections (of viral and bacterial origin); increased susceptibility to infection due to temporarily lowered resistance, treatment of leukopenia following radio and cytostatic therapy and in support of anti-infectious chemotherapy.

ECHINACEA PALLIDA ROOT

Approved by Commission E:

- Fevers and colds

Echinacea pallida root is used as a supportive therapy for influenza-like infections.

ECHINACEA ANGUSTIFOLIA HERB AND ROOT

Unproven Uses: In folk medicine, Native Americans use the drug externally for burns, swelling of the lymph nodes, and insect bites. The drug is used internally for pain associated with headaches and stomach aches, measles, coughs and gonorrhea. The drug has also been used for rattlesnake bites. Today the drug is used for prophylaxis and treatment of ''flu,'' sepsis, and mild to moderate cold infections. Externally, the drug is used for treatment of poorly healing wounds and inflammatory conditions such as abscesses and leg ulcers.

CONTRAINDICATIONS

Because of a possible activation of autoimmune aggressions and other overreactive immune responses, the drug should not be administered in the presence of tuberculosis, multiple sclerosis, leukosis, collagenosis, AIDS or HIV infection, and other autoimmune diseases. Diabetes may worsen in diabetic patient receiving Echinacea intravenously (Bisset, 1994), and parenteral administration should not be used in patients with tendencies to allergies, especially allergies to members of the composite family (Asteraceae).

Pregnancy: Not be used during pregnancy. However, in a prospective study, no statistically significant difference was demonstrated between neonatal malformations in women using Echinacea during pregnancy in comparison with those who did not use the herb. The dosage of Echinacea used by the women varied from 250 to 1000 mg daily for tablet or capsule forms and 5 to 30 drops/day of tincture, with alcohol content between 25% to 45% (Gallo et al, 2000).

PRECAUTIONS AND ADVERSE REACTIONS

ALL VARIETIES AND FORMS

An extensive review of the safety and efficacy of Echinacea found no toxicity in both adults and children in acute as well as long-term administration (Parnham, 1996). When used parenterally, dose-dependent, short-term fever reactions, nausea, and vomiting can occur (Bisset, 1994). Hypersensitivity reactions with anaphylaxis have been reported (Mullins, 1998). Dizziness, headache, skin irritation, or allergic reactions are possible; rashes, itching, occasional swelling of the face, breathing difficulties, dizziness and a drop in blood pressure have been observed after administration of preparations containing Echinacea.

Dermatological: Erythema, exanthema, and pruritus have been reported in isolated cases following topical application of Echinacea (Fachinfo Resistan, 1996; Taylor et al, 2003).

Hypersensitivity: In an analysis of the Australian Adverse Drug Reactions Advisory Committee's database of events of IgE-mediated hypersensitivity reactions, 51 reports were found to be related to Echinacea use. Twenty-six reactions, including urticaria, angioedema, asthma, and anaphylaxis were concluded by the investigators to be IgE-mediated reactions to Echinacea. More than half of the affected patients had a history of asthma, allergic rhinitis, rhinoconjunctivitis, or atopic dermatitis. Four persons required hospitalization due to their reactions and no deaths occurred. In 94% of patients, the symptoms appeared within 24 hours of Echinacea ingestion. Eighty percent of the patients included were female and the median age was 32 years (Mullins & Heddle, 2002).

Fertility: High concentrations of Echinacea had adverse effects on oocytes in animal models (Ondrizek, 1999).

DRUG INTERACTIONS

MAJOR RISK

Basiliximab: Concurrent use may result in decreased effectiveness of basiliximab. *Clinical Management:* Concomitant use of echinacea and basiliximab should be avoided due to the antagonistic effect an immunostimulant such as Echinacea may have on basiliximab, an immunosuppressant.

MODERATE RISK

Azathioprine: Concurrent use may result in decreased effectiveness of azathioprine. *Clinical Management*: Since reduced azathioprine effectiveness may be life-threatening in organ transplantation, avoid concomitant use of Echinacea and azathioprine.

Corticosteroids: Concurrent use may result in decreased effectiveness of corticosteroids. *Clinical Management*: Since reduced corticosteroid effectiveness may be life-threatening, avoid concomitant use of Echinacea and corticosteroids

Cyclosporine: Concurrent use may result in decreased effectiveness of cyclosporine. *Clinical Management*: Since reduced cyclosporine effectiveness may be life-threatening in organ transplantation, avoid concomitant use of Echinacea and cyclosporine.

Daclizumab: Concurrent use may result in decreased effectiveness of daclizumab. *Clinical Management*: Since reduced daclizumab effectiveness may be life-threatening in organ transplantation, avoid concomitant use of Echinacea and daclizumab.

Muromonab: Concurrent use may result in decreased effectiveness of muromonab. *Clinical Management*: Since reduced muromonab effectiveness may be life-threatening in organ transplantation, avoid concomitant use of Echinacea and muromonab.

Mycophenolic acid: Concurrent may result in decreased effectiveness of mycophenolic acid. *Clinical Management*: Echinacea may reduce the effectiveness of mycophenolic acid, and their concomitant use should be avoided.

Mycophenelate mofetil: Concurrent use may result in decreased effectiveness of mycophenolate mofetil. *Clinical Management*: Since reduced mycophenolate mofetil effectiveness may be life-threatening in organ transplantation, avoid concomitant use of Echinacea and mycophenolate mofetil.

Sirolimus: Concurrent use may result in decreased effectiveness of sirolimus. *Clinical Management*: Since reduced sirolimus effectiveness may be life-threatening in organ transplantation, avoid concomitant use of Echinacea and sirolimus.

Tacroliumus: Concurrent use may result in decreased effectiveness of tacrolimus. *Clinical Management*: Since reduced tacrolimus effectiveness may be life-threatening in organ transplantation, avoid concomitant use of Echinacea and tacrolimus.

POTENTIAL INTERACTIONS

Echinacea inhibited cytochrome P450 3A4 in vitro (Budzinski et al, 2000); caution is advised if Echinacea is administered with drugs metabolized by this enzyme.

Drug-Lab Modifications: In one study, using a polysaccharide fraction from *Echinacea purpurea* intravenously, a moderate acceleration in the erythrocyte sedimentation rate was noted (Roesler et al, 1991).

OVERDOSAGE

In tests of *Echinacea purpurea,* toxic cellular effects were seen only at very high, clinically irrelevant concentrations. Administration of very high doses may produce a depressant action (Coeugniet & Elek, 1987).

DOSAGE

ECHINACEA PURPUREA HERB

Mode of Administration: Pressed juice and galenic preparations for internal and external use.

Preparation: The pressed juice is prepared in a concentration of 2.5:1 and is stabilized with 22% alcohol. Other complicated methods of preparation are known.

Daily Dosage: When used internally, the recommended dosage is 6 to 9 ml of the expressed juice. The recommended dosage for parenteral administration should be individualized, depending on the seriousness of the condition as well as the specific nature of the respective preparation. Parenteral application requires a gradation of dosage, especially for children. The manufacturer is required to show this information for the respective preparation. When used externally, semi-solid preparations containing at least 15% pressed juice are used for a maximum of 8 weeks.

ECHINACEA PURPUREA ROOT

Mode of Administration: Comminuted drug for decoctions and galenic preparations.

Daily Dosage: When using the tincture, 30 to 60 drops should be taken three times a day.

Storage: Echinacea should be protected from light sources, and, if possible be uncomminuted.

ECHINACEA PALLIDA HERB AND ROOT

Mode of Administration: As a liquid preparation for oral use.

Preparation: A 1:5 tincture is made using 50% (V/V) ethanol and native dried extract (50% ethanol in a 7 to 11:1 proportion)

Daily Dosage: The daily dose is 900 mg of drug. The drug should be used for a maximum of 8 weeks.

Storage: Protect from light sources. If possible, store uncomminuted.

ECHINACEA ANGUSTIFOLIA HERB AND ROOT

Mode of Administration: Since the efficacy in the claimed areas of application has not been documented, therapeutic application cannot be recommended. Because of the risks, the use of parenteral preparations is not justified.

How Supplied:

Capsule – 100 mg, 125 mg, 167 mg, 200 mg, 250 mg, 380 mg 390 mg, 400 mg, 430 mg, 450 mg, 500 mg

Liquid – 120 mg/5mL

Preparation: The root tea is prepared using 1/2 teaspoonful of comminuted drug with boiling water. Strain after 10 minutes.

Daily Dosage: For colds, drink 1 cup freshly made tea several times daily.

Storage: Protect from light sources. If possible, store uncomminuted.

LITERATURE

Anon: Echinacea vs. the common cold. *Harv Women's Health Watch*; 7(6):1. 2000

Barrett BP, Brown RL, Locken K et al. Treatment of the common cold with unrefined Echinacea. *Ann Intern Med*; 137(12):939-946. 2002

Barrett B, Vohmann M & Calabrese C. Echinacea for upper respiratory infection. *J Fam Pract*; 4(6):628-635. 1999

Bauer R. Arzneipflanzenporträt: Echinacea- welche Inhaltsstoffe wirken immunmodulierend? In: *DAZ;* 132(23):1233. 1992

Bauer R. Echinacea. In: *PM;* 59(6):94. 1992

Bauer R, Jurcic K, Puhlmann J, Wagner H, [Immunologic in vivo and in vitro studies on Echinacea extracts]. German. In: *Arzneim Forsch;* 38(2):276-281. 1988

Bauer R, Neues von. ''immunmodulierenden Drogen'' und ''Drogen mit antiallergischer und antiinflammatorischer Wirkung''. In: *ZPT;* 14(1):23-24. 1993

Bauer R, Remiger P, Jurcic K, Wagner H. Beeinflussung der Phagozytoseaktivität durch Echinacea-Extrakte. In: *ZPT;* 10:43-48. 1989

Bauer R, Remiger P, Wagner H. Echinacea-Vergleichende DC- und HPLC-Analyse der Herba-Drogen von *Echinacea purpurea, Echinacea pallida* und *Echinacea angustifolia*. In: *DAZ;* 128:174-180. 1988

Bauer R, Wagner H. Echinacea - Der Sonnenhut - Stand der Forschung. In: *ZPT;* 9(8):151. 1988

Bauer R, Wagner H. Echinacea-Drogen - Who is who? In: *ZPT;* 9(6):191. 1988

Bauer R, Wagner H. Echinacea. Wissenschaftliche Verlagsgesellschaft mbH, Stuttgart 1990

Bauer, R et al. *Helv Chim Acta;* 68:2355. 1985

Bauer, R et al. *Phytochemistry;* 26(4):1198. 1987

Bendel R, Bendel V, Renner K et al. Additional treatment with Esberitox N in patients with combined chemo-radiotherapy of advanced breast cancer. *Onkologie*; 12(suppl 3):32-38. 1989

Berg AH, Northoff D, Konig C et al. Influence of Echinacin® (EC31) treatment on the exercise-induced immune response in athletes. *J Clin Res*; 1:367-380. 1998

Beuscher N, Scheit KH, Bodinet C, Egert D. Modulation der körpereigenen Immunabwehr durch polymere Substanzen aus Baptisia tinctoria und Echinacea purpurea. In: Immunotherapeutic prospects of infectious diseases, Hrsg. Masihi KN, Lange W. Springer, Heidel.

Beuscher N, Über die medikamentöse Beeinflussung zellulärer Resistenzmechanismen im Tierversuch. Aktivierung von Peritonealmakrophagen der Maus durch pflanzliche Reizkörper. In: *Arzneim Forsch;* 32(I):134-138. 1977

Bodinet C, Beuscher N. Antiviral and immunological activity of glykoproteins from the root of *Echinacea purpurea*. In: PM, Abstracts of the 39th Annual Congress of Medicinal Plant Research. 1991

Bohlmann F, Hoffman H. *Phytochemistry* 22(5):1173. 1983

Bräunig B, Dorn M, Knick E. *Echinaceae purpureae* radix: zur Stärkung der körpereigenen Abwehr bei grippalem Infekten. In: *ZPT;* 13(1):7. 1992

Brinkeborn R, Shah D, Degenring F. Echinaforce and other Echinacea fresh plant preparations in the treatment of the common cold. A randomized, placebo controlled, double-blind clinical trial. *Phytomedicine*. Mar;6(1):1-6. 1999

Budzinski JW, Foster BC, Vandenhoek S et al. An in vitro evaluation of human cytochrome P450 3A4 inhibition by selected commercial herbal extracts and tinctures. *Phytomedicine*; 7(4):273-282. 2000

Bukovsky M, Kostalova D, Magnusova R et al. Testing for immunomodulating effects of ethanol-water extracts of the above-ground parts of the plants echinaceae Moench and Rudbeckia L. *Cesk Farm*; 42(5):228-231. 1993a

Bukovsky M, Vaverkova S, Kostalova D et al. Immunomodulating activity of ethanol-water extracts of the roots of *echinacea gloriosa* L, echinacea angustifolia DC, and Rudbeckia speciosa Wenderoth tested on the immune system in C57BL6 inbred mice. *Cesk Farm*; 42(4):184-187. 1993

Burger RA, Torres AR, Warren RP et al. Echinacea-induced cytokine production by human macrophages. *Int J Immunopharmacol;* Jul;19(7):371-379. 1997

Büsing KH. Hyaluronidasehemmung durch Echinacin. In: *Arzneim Forsch;* 2:467-469. 1952

Coeugniet EG & Elek E. Immunomodulation with Viscum album and *echinacea purpurea* extracts. *Onkologie*; 10(suppl 3):27-33. 1987

Cheminat A, Zawatzky R, Becker H, Brouillard R. Caffeoylconjugates from Echinacea Species: Structure and biological activity. In: *PH;* 27(9):2787-2794. 1988

Caruso TJ, Gwaltney JM. Treatment of the common cold with Echinacea: A structured review. *J Clin Infect Dis;* 40(6):807-10. 2005.

Coeugniet EG & Elek E. Immunomodulation with Viscum album and echinacea purpurea extracts. *Onkologie*; 10(suppl 3):27-33. 1987

Currier NL & Miller SC. *Echinacea purpurea* and melatonin augment natural-killer cells in leukemic mice and prolong life span. *J Altern Complement Med*; 7(3):241-251. 2001

Dorsch W. Klinische Anwendung von Extrakten aus echinacea purpurea oder *echinacea pallida. Z Arztl Fortbild* (Jena); 90(2):117-122. 1996

Fachinformation: Echinacin® -Ampullen, echinaceae purpurea herba. Madaus AG, Koeln, 1994

Fachinformation: Resistan®, echinacea. Lichtixer Pharma GmbH, Berlin. Dr Rentschler. Arzneimittel GmbH & Co, Laupheim, 1996

Facino RM, Carini M, Aldini G et al. Echinacoside and caffeoyl conjugates protect collagen from free radical-induced degradation: a potential use of Echinacea extracts in the prevention of skin photodamage. *Planta Med* Dec;61(6):510-514. 1995

Forth H, Beuscher N, Beeinflussung der Häufigkeit banaler Erkältungsinfekte durch Esberitox. In: *Z Allgemeinmed;* 57:2272-2275. 1981

Gallo M, Sarkar M, Au W et al. Pregnancy outcome following gestational exposure to echinacea. *Arch Intern Med*; 160:3141-3143. 2000

Goel V, Lovlin R, Bartion R, et al. Efficacy of a standardized Echinacea preparation (Echinilin) for the treatment of the common cold: a randomized, double-blind, placebo-controlled trial. *J Clin Pharm Ther*; 29(1): 75-83. 2004.

Goel V, Lovlin R, Chang C, et al. A proprietary extract from the Echinacea plant (Echinacea purpurea) enhances systemic immune response during common cold. *Phytother Res*; 19(8): 689-694. 2005.

Giles JT, Palat CT, Chien SH et al. Evaluation of echinacea for treatment of the common cold. *Pharmacotherapy*; 20(6):690-697. 2000

Grange JM & Davey RW. Detection of antituberculous activity in plant extracts. *J Appl Bacteriol*; 68(6):587-591. 1990

Grimm W, Muller H. A randomized controlled trial of the effect of fluid extract of *Echinacea purpurea* on the incidence and severity of colds and respiratory infections. *Am J Med Fec*; 106(2):138-143. 1999

Gruber JW & DerMarderosian A. An emerging green pharmacy: modern plant medicines and health. *Lab Med*; 27(3):170-176. 1996

Henneicke-von Zepelin HH, Hentschel C, Schnitker J et al. Efficacy and safety of a fixed combination phytomedicine in the treatment of the common cold (acute viral respiratory tract infection): results of a randomized, double-blind, placebo-controlled, multicenter study. *Curr Med Res Op*; 15(3):213-227. 1999

Hill N, Stam C & van Haselen RA. The efficacy of Prikeweg gel in the treatment of insect bites: a double-blind, placebo-controlled clinical trial. *Pharm World Sci*; 18(1):35-41. 1996

Hoheisel O, Sandberg M, Bertram S et al. Echinagard treatment shortens the course of the common cold: a double-blind, placebo-controlled clinical trial. *Eur J Clin Res*; 9:261-268. 1997

Jacobson M. *J Org Chem;* 32:1646. 1967

Jurcic K, Melchart D, Holzmann M, Martin P, Bauer R, Doenecke A, Wagner H, Zwei Probandenstudien zur Stimulierung der Granulozytenphagozytose durch Echinacea-Extrakt-haltige Präparate. In: *ZPT;* 10(2):67-70. 1989

Kinkel HJ, Plate M, Tüllner HU. Objektivierbare Wirkung von Echinacin-Salbe auf die Wundheilung. In: *Med Klinik;* 79:580-583. 1984

Lepik K. Safety of herbal medications in pregnancy. *CPJ/RPC*; April:29-33. 1997

Lersch C, Zeuner M, Bauer A et al. Stimulation of the immune response in outpatients with hepatocellular carcinomas by low doses of cyclophosphamide (LDCY), *echinacea purpurea* extracts (Echinacin) and thymostimulin. *Arch Geschwulstforsch*; 60(5):379-383. 1990

Linde K, Barrett B, Wolkart K, et al. Echinacea for preventing and treating the common cold. *Cochrane Database Syst Rev* 1: CD000530: 2006.

Lindenmuth GF & Lindenmuth EB. The efficacy of Echinacea compound herbal tea preparation on the severity and duration of upper respiratory and flu symptoms: a randomized, double-blind placebo-controlled study. *J Alt Compl Med*; 6(4):327-333. 2000

Luettig B, Steinmuller C, Gifford GE et al. Macrophage activation by the polysaccharide arabinogalactan isolated from plant cell cultures of *Echinacea purpurea. J Natl Cancer Inst* May 3;81(9):669-675. 1989

Melchart D, Clemm C, Weber B et al. Polysaccharides isolated from *Echinacea purpurea* herba cell cultures to counteract undesired effects of chemotherapy - a pilot study. *Phytother Res*; 16:138-142. 2002

Melchart D, Linde K, Worku F, Bauer R, Wagner H. Immunomodulation with Echinacea - a systematic review of controlled clinical trials. *Phytomedicine;* 1:245-254. 1994

Melchart D, Linde K, Worku F et al. Results of five randomized studies on the immunomodulatory activity of preparations of echinacea. *J Altern Complement Med*; 1(2):145-160. 1995

Melchart D, Walther E, Linde K et al. Echinacea root extracts for the prevention of upper respiratory tract infections: a double-blind, placebo-controlled randomized trial. *Arch Fam Med* Nov-Dec;7(6):541-545. 1998

Mengs U, Clare CB, Poiley JA. Toxicity of *echinacea purpurea*: acute, subacute, and genotoxicity studies. *Arzneimittelforschung*; 41(10):1076-1081. 1991

Muller-Jakic B; Breu W; Probstle A et al. In vitro inhibition of cyclooxygenase and 5-lipoxygenase by alkamides from Echinacea and Achillea species. *Planta Med* Feb;60(1):37-40. 1994

Mullins RJ. Echinacea-associated anaphylaxis. *Med J Aust* Feb 16;168(4):170-1. 1998

Mullins RJ & Heddle R. Adverse reactions associated with echinacea: the Australian experience. *Ann Allergy Asthma Immunol*; 88:42-51. 2002

Ondrizek RR, Chan PJ, Patton WC et al. Inhibition of human sperm motility by specific herbs used in alternative medicine. *J Asst Reprod Genet*; 16(2):87-91 1999.

Ondrizek RR, Chan PJ, Patton WC, King A. An alternative medicine study of herbal effects on the penetration of zona-free hamster oocytes and the integrity of sperm deoxyribonucleic acid. *Fertil Steril* Mar;71(3):517-522. 1999

Paranich AV, Pocherniaeva VF, Dubinskaia GM et al. Effect of supposed radioprotectors on oxidation-reduction of vitamin E in the tissues of irradiated rats (Russian). *Radiats Biol Radioecol*; 33(5):653-657. 1993

Parnham MJ. Benefit-risk assessment of the squeezed sap of the purple coneflower *(Echinacea purpurea)* for long-term oral immunostimulation. In: *Phytomedicine;* 3(1):95-102. 1996

Proksch A, Über ein immunstimulierendes Wirkprinzip aus *Echinacea purpurea*. Dissertation, Ludwig-Maximilians-Universität, München. 1982

Rehman J, Dillow JM, Carter SM et al. Increased production of antigen-specific immunoglobulins G and M following in vivo treatment with the medicinal plants *Echinacea angustifolia* and *Hydrastis canadensis. Immunol Lett*; 68:391-395. 1999

Roesler J, Emmendorffer A, Steinmuller C et al. Application of purified polysaccharides from cell cultures of the plant *echinacea purpurea* to test subjects mediates activation of the phagocyte system. *Int J Immunopharmacol*; 13(7):931-941. 1991

Roesler J, Steinmuller C, Kiderlen A et al. Application of purified polysaccharides from cell cultures of the plant *Echinacea purpurea* to mice mediates protection against systemic infections with *Listeria monocytogenes* and *Candida albicans. Int J Immunopharmacol*; 13(1):27-37. 1991a

Schoneberger D. Einflußβ der immunstimulierenden Wirkung von Preβsaft aus herba *Echinaceae purpureae* auf Verlauf und Schweregrad von Erkältungskrankheiten. *Forum Immunologie*;8:18-22. 1992

Schulte KE, Rücker G, Perlick J, Das Vorkommen von Polyacetylen-Verbindungen in *Echinacea purpurea* MOENCH und *Echinacea angustifolia* DC. In: Arzneim-Forsch 17:825-829. 1967

Schulten B, Bulitta M, Ballering-Bruhl B et al. Efficacy of *Echinacea purpurea* in patients with a common cold. *Arzneim Forsch Drug Res*; 51(II):563-568. 2001

Schulz V & Haensel R. Rationale Phytotherapie. Ratgeber fuer die aertzlich Praxis. 3 Aufl. Springer Verlag, Berlin, Germany, 1996

Schumacher A. Echinacea angustifolia und die spezifische und unspezifische zelluläre Immunantwort der Maus. In: Dissertation Heidelberg, 1989

See DM, Broumand N, Sahl L et al. In vitro effects of echinacea and ginseng on natural killer and antibody-dependent cell cytotoxicity in healthy subjects and chronic fatigue syndrome or acquired immunodeficiency syndrome patients. *Immunopharmacology*; 35(3):229-235. 1997

Seidel K & Knobloch H. Nachweis und vergleich der antiphlogistischen wirkung antirheumatischer medikamente. *Z Rheumaforsch*; 16:231-238. 1957

Sperber SJ, Shah LP, Gilbert RD, et al. Echinacea purpurea for prevention of experimental rhinovirus colds. *Clin Infect Dis*; 38(10): 1367-1371. 2004.

Stimpel M, et al. *Infect Immunol;* 46(3):845. 1984

Stimpel M, Proksch A, Wagner H et al. Macrophage activation and induction of macrophage cytotoxicity by purified polysaccaride fractions from the plant *Echinacea purpurea. Infect Immun;* 46:845-849. 1984

Stimpel M, Proksch A, Wagner H, Lohmann-Matthes ML, Macrophage activation and induction of macrophage cytotoxicity by purified polysccharide fraction from plant *Echinacea purpurea*. In: *Infect Immun* 46:845-849. 1984

Taylor JA, et al. Efficacy and safety of echinacea in treating upper respiratory tract infections in children: a randomized controlled trial. *JAMA* Dec 3;290(21):2824-2830. 2003

Tubaro A, Tragni E, Del Negro P et al. Anti-inflammatory activity of a polysaccharidic fraction of *echinacea angustifolia. J Pharm Pharmacol*; 39:576-569. 1987.

Turner RB, Bauer R, Woelkart K, et al. An evaluation of Echinacea angustifolia in experimental rhinovirus infections. *N Engl J Med*; 353:341-348. 2005.

Turner RB, Riker DK & Gangemi JD. Ineffectiveness of Echinacea for prevention of experimental rhinovirus colds. *Antimicrob Agents Chemother*; 44(6):1708-1709. 2000.

Vergin H, Wolter R, Untersuchungen zur Phagozytose-Aktivität der isoliert perfundierten Rattenleber mit *Echinacea purpurea - haltigen* Präparaten. In: *Natur Med;* 1/2:27-29. 1988

Vestweber AM, Beuth J, Ko HL et al. In vitro activity of *Mercurius cyanatus* complex against relevant pathogenic bacterial isolates (German). *Arzneimittelforschung*; 45(9):1018-1020. 1995

Voaden DJ & Jacobson M. Tumor inhibitors. 3. Identification and synthesis of an oncolytic hydrocarbon from American coneflower roots. *J Med Chem*; 15(6):619-623. 1972

Vonau B, Chard S, Mandalia S et al. Does the extract of the plant *Echinacea purpurea* influence the clinical course of recurrent genital herpes? *Int J STD AIDS;* 12:154-158. 2001

Wacker A, Hilbig W. Virushemmung mit *Echinacea purpurea*. In: *PM;* 33:89-102. 1978

Wagner H, Stuppner H, Puhlmann J, Brümmer B, Deppe K, Zenk MH. Gewinnung von immunologisch aktiven Polysacchariden aus Echinacea-Drogen und - Gewebekulturen. In: *ZPT;* 10(2):35. 1989

Weber W, Taylor JA, Stoep A, et al. *Echinacea purpurea for prevention of upper respiratory tract infections in children.* J Alt Comp Med; 11 (6): 1021-1026. 2005.

Wildfeuer A & Mayerhofer D. Untersuchung des Einflusses von Phytopraeparaten auf zellulaere Funktionen der koerpereigenen Abwehr (German). *Arzneimittelforschung*; 44(3):361-366. 1994

Yale SY, Liu K. *Echinacea purpurea* therapy for the treatment of the common cold. *Arch Intern Med*;164:1237-1241. 2004.

Zoutewelle G & van Wijk R. Effects of echinacea purpurea extracts on fibroblast populated collagen lattice contraction. *Phytother Res*; 4(2):77-81. 1990

Echinaceae species

See Echinacea

Elecampane

Inula helenium

DESCRIPTION

Medicinal Parts: The medicinal part is the dried or fresh rhizome.

Flower and Fruit: The inflorescences are yellow composite flowers in loose, terminal, panicled cymes. They are 7 to 8 cm in diameter. The involucre is imbricate and cup-shaped. The inner bracts are dry at the tip and splayed, the outer bracts resemble ovate leaves. The female lateral florets are narrowly linguiform. The androgynous disc florets are tubular. The receptacle is flat, slightly pitted, and glabrous. The flowers are a bright yellow. The achaenes are cylindrical, 4 to 5 mm long, brown, glabrous, and have 4 tips. The pappus is 8 to 10 mm long and consists of brownish, fine, rough, brittle bristles.

Leaves, Stem, and Root: The plant is perennial and 80 to 180 cm high. The rhizome is short with compact branches. It is tuberous and has sturdy, 1 cm thick and 50 cm long roots. The stem is erect, branched above, and villous. The leaves are large, tomentose beneath and irregularly dentate. The cauline leaves are cordate-acute. The basal leaves are oblong and petiolate.

Characteristics: The rhizome has a strong odor and a pungent taste.

Habitat: Indigenous to Europe and temperate Asia, introduced to the U.S. and China.

Production: Elecampane root is the root of *Inula helenium*. It is harvested in autumn. The roots are then cut and hung up to dry or dried artificially at 50° C.

Other Names: Alant, Elfdock, Elfwort, Horse-Elder, Horseheal, Scabwort, Wild Sunflower, Yellow Starwort, Velvet Dock

ACTIONS AND PHARMACOLOGY

COMPOUNDS

Volatile oil: chief components alantolactone, isoalantolactone, 11,13- dihydroisoalantolactone, 11,13- dihydroalantolactone (the mixture of alantolactone derivatives is also known as helenalin or elecampane camphor)

Polyynes

Polysaccharides: above all inulin (fructosan)

EFFECTS

The main active principles are alantolacton, isoalantolacton, and other sesquiterpenlactones. Compounds of this kind have an antiphlogostic and antibiotic effect. Antifungal activity has also been demonstrated.

The antimicrobial and anthelmintic effect results from the sesquiterpene lactones. Alantolactone and isoalantolactone are antitumoral, and helenin shortens clotting time. Alantolactone and helenin lead to complete paralysis of the spontaneous contraction of the intestine in animal studies.

The plant has mild antiseptic and expectorant effect due to the essential oil, which contains sesquiterpene.

INDICATIONS AND USAGE

Unproven Uses: Preparations of the rhizome are used to treat bronchitis, whooping cough, bronchial catarrh, menstrual complaints, urinary tract infections, colds, worm infestation, and headaches. Externally, poultices of the drug are used for skin infections.

Homeopathic Uses: Inula helenium preparations are used for stomach ulcers and chronic cough.

PRECAUTIONS AND ADVERSE REACTIONS

General: The drug is severely irritating to mucous membranes and strongly sensitizing.

Pregnancy: Not to be used during pregnancy.

OVERDOSAGE

Larger administrations of the drug lead to vomiting, diarrhea, spasms, and signs of paralysis. Following gastric lavage, intestinal emptying (sodium sulfate) and the administration of activated charcoal powder, poisoning is treated with the antiemetic trifluopromazine.

DOSAGE

Mode of Administration: The comminuted drug is used in tea mixtures. The extract is used as a constituent in numerous pharmaceutical preparations, including gastrointestinal remedies, alterants, gout remedies, diuretics, and in numerous expectorants.

Preparation: To prepare an infusion, pour boiling water over 1 g of ground drug and steep 10 to 15 minutes, then strain (1 teaspoonful corresponds to about 4 g drug).

Daily Dosage: Average single dose 1 g.

Tea–1 cup is drunk 3 to 4 times daily as an expectorant; may be sweetened with honey.

Helenium Extract–The single dose is 0.5 g.

Homeopathic Dosage: 5 drops, 1 tablet, or 10 globules every 30 to 60 minutes (acute) or 1 to 3 times daily (chronic); parenterally: 1 to 2 ml sc acute, 3 times daily; chronic once a day (HAB34).

Storage: Store in a cool place, protected from light, not in plastic containers.

LITERATURE

Alonso Blasi N, Fraginals R, Lepoittevin JP, Benezra C, A murine in vitro model of allergic contact dermatitis to sesquiterpene alpha-methylene-gamma-butyrolactones. *Arch Dermatol Res*, 284:297-302, 1992

Cantrell CL, Fischer NH, Urbatsch L, McGuire MS, Franzblau SG. Antimycobacterial crude plant extracts from South, Central, and North America. *Phytomedicine* 5 (2); 137-145. 1998

Cantrell CL, Abate L, Fronczek FR, Franzblau SG, Quijano L, Fischer NH. Antimycobacterial eudesmanolides from *Inula helenium* and *Rudbeckia subtomentosa*. *Planta Med*, 1999; 65: 351-355

Fokina GI, Frolova TV, Roikhel VM, Pogodina VV, Experimental phytotherapy of tick-borne encephalitis. Vopr Virusol, 36:18-21, Jan-Feb 1991

Iijima K, Kiyohara H, Tanaka M, Matsumoto T, Cyong JC, Yamada H, Preventive effect of taraxasteryl acetate from *Inula britannica subsp. Japonica* on experimental hepatitis in vivo. *Planta Med*, 61:50-3, Feb 1995

Jiang B, et al. Studies and comparisons on chemical components of essential oils from *Clematis hexapetala Pall.* and *Inula nervosa* Wall. Chung Kuo Chung Yao Tsa Chih, 15:488-90 512, Aug 1990

Pazzaglia M, Venturo N, Borda G, Tosti A, Contact dermatitis due to a massage liniment containing *Inula helenium* extract. *Contact Dermatitis*, 61:267, Oct 1995

Tripathi YB, Chaturvedi P. Assessment of endocrine response of *Inula racemosa* in relation to glucose homeostasis in rats. *Indian J Exp Biol*, 61:686-9, Sep 1995

Wang Q, Zhou BN, Zhang RW, Lin YY, Lin LZ, Gil RR, Cordell GA, Cytotoxicity and NMR spectral assignments of ergolide and bigelovin. Planta Med, 62:166-8, Apr 1996

Woerdenbag HJ, Meijer C, Mulder NH, de Vries EG, Hendriks H, Malingr TM. Evaluation of the vitro cytotoxicity of some sesquiterpene lactones on a human lung carcinoma cell line using the fast green dye exclusion assay. *Planta Med.* 1986; 2: 112-114

Elephant-Ears

Bergenia crassifolia

DESCRIPTION

Medicinal Parts: Whole plant has medicinal properties.

Flower and Fruit: The flowers are arranged in curled cymes. Their structures are arranged in fives and they are radial with the 2 to 3 ovaries joined only at the base. The petals are red or pink-violet and grow up to 1.5 cm long. The ovary is superior, and the fruit has numerous seeds. The seeds are brown to brown-black, edged, up to 2 mm long and 0.5 mm thick.

Leaves, Stem and Root: Bergenia crassifolia is a herbaceous perennial that grows up to 50 cm high. The leaves are basal, oval, up to 20 cm long, over 10 cm wide, orbicular, fleshy, glabrous, with indented glands and slightly dentate. The rhizome is up to 3 cm thick, above ground and covered with the sheaths of the previous year's leaves.

Habitat: Russia, Mongolia

Production: Bergeniae rhizoma are the dried rhizomes of *Bergenia crassifolia*. They are collected in the wild and air-dried for 2 weeks.

Other Names: Leather Bergenia, Siberian Tea

ACTIONS AND PHARMACOLOGY

COMPOUNDS

Hydroquinone glycosides: arbutin (1.8 to 2.3%)

Phenol carboxylic acids: bergenin (6.7 to 10.1%, lactones)

Tannins (28%)

EFFECTS

The watery extracts of the drug have astringent, bacteriostatic, local hemostyptic and antiphlogistic effects, due to the tannin content and that of other phenolic constituents. The arbutin they contain exhibits urine-disinfecting effect (comparable to Uva ursi). A shortening of blood coagulation time could be demonstrated in animal experiments.

INDICATIONS AND USAGE

Unproven Uses: Elephant-Ears have been used for fever, tuberculosis, pneumonia, diarrhea, intestinal disease, and rheumatism. The drug is also used for skin leishmaniosis and as a hemostyptic.

CONTRAINDICATIONS

Preparations are contraindicated in pregnancy, nursing, and for children under 12 years of age.

PRECAUTIONS AND ADVERSE REACTIONS

No health hazards are known in conjunction with the proper administration of designated therapeutic dosages. Because of its high tannin content, the intake of preparations of the drug could lead to digestive disorders; individuals with sensitive stomachs may experience nausea and vomiting.

OVERDOSAGE

Overdose could lead to inflammatory irritation of the mucous membranes of the bladder and urinary tract, accompanied by urgency and blood in the urine. Long-term administration of the drug could lead to liver damage, due to the possible hepatotoxicity of the hydroquinone released, particularly among children.

DOSAGE

Mode of Administration: Whole drug preparations for internal and external use.

LITERATURE

Hänsel R, Keller K, Rimpler H, Schneider G (Ed), Hagers Handbuch der Pharmazeutischen Praxis, 5. Aufl., Bde 4 - 6

(Drogen), Springer Verlag Berlin, Heidelberg, New York, 1992-1994.

Kindl H, Conversion of (4-3H)L-phenylalanine into (4-3H)pyrocatechol and (3-3H)hydroquinone in leaves of Bergenia crassifolia. Hoppe Seylers Z *Physiol Chem,* 350:1289-90, Oct. 1969

Elettaria cardamomum

See Cardamom

Eleutherococcus senticosus

See Siberian Ginseng

Elm Bark

Ulmus minor

DESCRIPTION

Medicinal Parts: The medicinal part is the inner bark of the young branches.

Flower and Fruit: The reddish brown flowers appear before the leaves. They are androgynous, short-pedioled, and appear in globular clusters. The perigone is campanulate/top-shaped and greenish with a purple margin. There are 3 to 4 stamens with dark violet anthers. The tree is wind pollinated. The fruit is a broad-winged, almost circular, oval or elliptical, and glabrous achaene. The reddish nutlet reaches to the front margin of the notch.

Leaves, Stem, and Root: Ulmus minor is a 40 m high tree with black-brown, finely fissured bark. The branches, which develop long grooves, have alternate, petiolate, 6- to 10-cm long leaves with 8 to 12 lateral ribs. The leaves are ovate. The lamina is irregular and the margin double-serrate. The petioles are 8 to 15 mm longer than the buds, which develop in spring on short branches and form into clusters before flowering.

Habitat: The plant is indigenous to Europe as far as the Mediterranean.

Production: Smooth-leaved Elm bark is the bark of *Ulmus minor*. The bark is gathered for therapeutic or medicinal purposes. It is manually cut in circles and the bark is removed from the young (new) twigs (the diameter of the twig should not be more than 1 cm). The long grain and the upper layer of the bark must be removed, then the bark is dried.

ACTIONS AND PHARMACOLOGY

COMPOUNDS

Mucilage: yielding mainly D-galactose, L-rhamnose, D-galacturonic acid after hydrolysis

Tannins (3%)

Caffeic acid derivatives: chlorogenic acid

Sterols: including, among others, beta-sitosterol, stigmasterol

EFFECTS

The drug has diuretic and astringent properties.

INDICATIONS AND USAGE

Unproven Uses: Internally, the drug is used for digestive disorders and severe cases of diarrhea. Externally, it is used to treat open wounds.

PRECAUTIONS AND ADVERSE REACTIONS

No health hazards or side effects are known in conjunction with the proper administration of designated therapeutic dosages.

DOSAGE

Mode of Administration: Elm bark is used both internally and externally in various preparations.

Preparation: The ground bark is used for infusions. A decoction from the bark can be prepared using 2 teaspoons of the drug per cup of water. Externally, a 20% decoction is used, which is diluted 1:1 with water, for the treatment of festering and open wounds.

Daily Dose: The dosage of the decoction prepared from the bark is 1 cup 2 to 3 times daily. In powder form, a dose of 2 to 5 g may be taken daily.

LITERATURE

Hänsel R, Keller K, Rimpler H, Schneider G (Hrsg.), Hagers Handbuch der Pharmazeutischen Praxis, 5. Aufl., Bde 4-6 (Drogen): Springer Verlag Berlin, Heidelberg, New York, 1992-1994.

Kim JP, Kim WG, Koshino H, Jung J, Yoo ID. Sesquiterpene O-naphthoquinones from the root bark of *Ulmus davidiana. Phytochemistry*, 43:425-30, 1996 Sep

English Adder's Tongue

Ophioglossum vulgatum

DESCRIPTION

Medicinal Parts: The medicinal parts of the plant are the root and leaves.

Flower and Fruit: The plant's 12 to 40 ripe yellow sporangia on either side of the middle panicle form an acuminate spike. The tip contains no sporangia.

Leaves, Stem, and Root: This fern grows from 8 to 25 cm high. The stems, covered in the remains of leaves, grow singly from the underground roots. The stems consist of a few sturdy, yellow fibers and are round, hollow and succulent. Each bears a smooth, oblong-oval, acuminate, entire frond.

Characteristics: Though a member of the Fern family, the appearance of English Adder's Tongue is not at all typically fernlike.

Habitat: The plant is indigenous to Britain.

Production: English Adder's Tongue is the aerial part of *Ophioglossum vulgatum*.

Other Names: Serpent's Tongue, Christ's Spear

ACTIONS AND PHARMACOLOGY

COMPOUNDS

Flavonoids: including among others quercetin-3-methyl ether-7-diglucoside-4′ glucoside

The constituents of the drug have not been thoroughly investigated.

EFFECTS

See American Adder's Tongue *(Erythronium americanum).*

INDICATIONS AND USAGE

See American Adder's Tongue *(Erythronium americanum).*

PRECAUTIONS AND ADVERSE REACTIONS

No health hazards or side effects are known in conjunction with the proper administration of designated therapeutic dosages.

DOSAGE

Mode of Administration: See American Adder's Tongue *(Erythronium americanum).*

LITERATURE

Hegnauer R, Chemotaxonomie der Pflanzen, Bde 1-11, Birkhäuser Verlag Basel, Boston, Berlin 1962-1997.

English Chamomile

Chamaemelum nobile

DESCRIPTION

Medicinal Parts: The medicinal parts are the English Chamomile oil extracted from the fresh or dried filled or unfilled flower heads and the dried aerial plant parts; the dried flower heads of the cultivated, filled varieties; and the fresh aerial parts of the flowering plant.

Flower and Fruit: The stems end in 12 to 18 fruit-bearing, white florets, which are about 2 to 2.5 cm wide. The epicalyx is semiglobose. The bracts are in a number of rows and are lanceolate to spatulate with a broad membranous border. The receptacle is clavate, filled with latex, and covered at the edge with slit bracts. The linguiform florets are female and silver-white. The tubular florets are androgynous and yellow. The corolla of every floret has a short appendage at the base, which surrounds the tip of the fruit. The achaenes are 2 mm long, light brown and almost triangular with vertical ribs. The achaenes are smooth and have no pappus.

Leaves, Stem and Root: The 15 to 30 cm high plant has a deeply buried rhizome. The rhizome sprouts numerous, ascending, occasionally upright, simple or branched, rounded, vertically grooved, pubescent stems. The stems are covered in alternating, heavily segmented, gray-green to rich-green leaves that are 2 to 4 cm long.

Habitat: The plant is indigenous to southern and western Europe and northern Africa, and is cultivated all over Europe. The main exporters are Belgium, France, Great Britain and Italy, as well as Poland, the Czech and Slovakian Republics, North America, and Argentina.

Production: English Chamomile consists of the dried flowers of the cultivated double flowered variety of *Chamaemelum nobile*. The plant is harvested in June and July, then dried at temperatures of 35°C.

Other Names: Ground Apple, Whig Plant, Roman Chamomile

ACTIONS AND PHARMACOLOGY

COMPOUNDS

Volatile oil: chief components include ester of angelic- or tiglic acid with isobutanol, isoamyl alcohol or 3-methyl-pentan-1-ol, to some extent present as hydroperoxides

Sesquiterpene lactones: in particular nobilin, besides 3-epinobilin, 1,10-epoxynobilin, 3-dehydronobilin that is present to some extent as hydroperoxides, including 1-beta-hydroperoxy-isonobilin and 4-alpha-hydroperoxy-manolide

Flavonoids: including anthemoside, cosmosioside, luteolin-7-0-glucoside

Caffeic and ferulic acid ester

Polynes: Including cis- and trans-dehydromatricaria ester

EFFECTS

In contrast to true chamomile, few studies are available. The essential oil is active against gram-positive bacteria and dermatomyces. The drug is also cytostatic and acts on the CNS, causing a reduction of aggressive behavior in animal tests. Any efficacy in dyspepsia (including flatulence) may be due to the amaroids.

INDICATIONS AND USAGE

Unproven Uses: In folk medicine, the French use English Chamomile mainly for feelings of fullness, bloating and mild spasmodic gastrointestinal disturbances and sluggishness of the bowels. It is also used for menstrual complaints, nervousness, hysteria, and general debility. It is used topically for inflammation of the mouth and throat, rhinitis, toothache, earache, headache, and influenza. The oil is used in mouthwashes.

Homeopathic Uses: The drug is used in homeopathy to treat nervous gastrointestinal disorders, but efficacy has not been proved.

CONTRAINDICATIONS

Use of the drug is contraindicated during pregnancy.

PRECAUTIONS AND ADVERSE REACTIONS

General: No health hazards or side effects are known in conjunction with the proper administration of designated therapeutic dosages. The drug possesses a small potential for sensitization.

DOSAGE

Mode of Administration: Since the efficacy for the claimed uses is not documented and there is a certain risk involved, a therapeutic application cannot be recommended. English Chamomile is used in folk medicine as a fluid extract, tincture, elixir, wine, syrup, ointment, and powder.

Preparation: To prepare a decoction, add 3 g drug to 100 mL water. An infusion is prepared using 7 to 8 capitula per cup. A liquid rub is prepared using 1 teaspoon diluted in 250 mL water.

Daily Dosage: The average single dose of the drug is 1.5 g at the main meals. The average daily dose of an infusion is 50 mL to 200 mL. When used as a bath additive, add 50 g to 10 liters of water. Liquid rubs are applied as poultices or washes 2 to 3 times daily.

Homeopathic Dosage: 5 drops, 1 tablet, or 10 globules every 30 to 60 minutes for acute conditions. For chronic conditions: 1 to 3 times daily; Parenterally: 1 to 2 ml sc acute 3 times daily; Chronic: once a day (HAB1)

Storage: Store in well-sealed glass or metal containers protected from moisture.

LITERATURE

Damiani P et al., (1983) Fitoterapia 54:213.

Isaac O, Chamaemelum nobile (L.) Allioni - Römische Kamille. In: ZPT 14(4):212. 1993.

English Hawthorn

Crataegus laevigata

DESCRIPTION

Medicinal Parts: The medicinal parts are generally white thorn flowers, leaves, fruit, and various mixtures of different plant parts.

Flowers and Fruit: The white flowers are in richly blossomed cymes. The sepals are usually short, triangular, entire-margined or, particularly the American variety, fairly long with glandular tips. The petals are usually separate, orbicular, crenate, white, or occasionally red. There are 10 to 20 stamens and 1 to 5 carpels, which are more or less fused to the receptacle. There are 2 ovules, the upper one is sterile and covers the lower fertile one like a cap. There is 1 seed in each chamber. The false fruit is ovoid or globose and crowned by the remains of the sepals. It is red, black, or yellow and mealy.

Leaves, Stem, and Root: Hawthorn is a bulky shrub or small tree, 1.5 to 4 m high with hard wood and usually thorny branches. The leaves have many forms. They are shallow, 3 to 5 lobed, with the lobes pointed forward. The leaves are unevenly serrate, obovate, yellowish-green, and glossy.

Characteristics: The flowers have an unpleasant smell and a slightly bitter taste; the fruit has a sour taste.

Habitat: The plant is indigenous to northern temperate zones of Europe, Asia, and North America.

Production: Hawthorn consists of the leaves and flowers of *Crataegus laevigata* and occasionally other species. The medicinal parts of the Hawthorn plant are collected in the wild and dried at room temperature.

Not to be Confused With: Hawthorn is sometimes mistaken for the flowers, leaves, and fruit of *Robinia pseudoacacia, Sorbus aucuparia,* or *Prunus spinosa.*

Other Names: Haw, Hawthorn, May, Whitethorn

ACTIONS AND PHARMACOLOGY

COMPOUNDS

Flavonoides (1.8%): O-glycosides, including hyperoside (0.28%), rutin (0.17%)

6-C- and 8-C-glycosyl compounds, including vitexin (0.02%), vicenin-1, orientin 6-C- and 8-C-glycosyl compounds, linked O-glycosidically as well as with other monosaccharides, including vitexin-2″-O-alpha-L-rhamnoside (0.53%), vitexin-2″-O-alpha-L-rhamnoside-4‴-acetate

Oligomeric proanthocyanidins (2.4%)

Biogenic amines, including tyramine

Triterpenes (0.6%): including oleanolic acid, ursolic acid, 2-alpha-hydroxy oleanolic acid (crataegolic acid)

EFFECTS

Crataegus is a well-studied herb for use in cardiovascular disease. Historically, it has been used for congestive heart failure, commonly in combination with cardiac glycosides as it may potentiate their effects, thereby reducing the dose of cardiac glycoside drugs. The use of Crataegus in hypertension, atherosclerosis, and hyperlipidemia is well-documented. The active principles are procyanidins and flavonoids, which cause an increase in coronary blood flow due to dilatory effects, resulting in an improvement of myocardial blood flow.

The drug is positively inotropic and positively chronotropic. The cardiotropic effect of Crataegus is said to be caused by the increased membrane permeability for calcium as well as the inhibition of phosphodiesterase with an increase of intracellular cylco-AMP concentrations. Increased coronary and myocardial circulatory perfusion and reduction in peripheral vascular resistance were observed. High doses may cause sedation. This effect has been attributed to the oligomeric procyanidins (Anon, 1994).

Crataegus extract has been found to prolong the refractory period and increase the action potential duration in guinea pig papillary muscle. One study demonstrated that a Crataegus extract blocked the repolarizing potassium currents in ventricular myocytes of guinea pigs. This effect is similar to that of class III antiarrhythmic drugs and may explain the antiarrhythmic effect of Hawthorn (Muller et al, 1999).

Crataegus, due to its high flavonoid content, may also be used to decrease inflammation, decrease capillary fragility, and prevent collagen destruction of joints.

Antioxidant Effects: The total number of phenolic groups in catechins and dimeric proanthocyanidins found in Crataegus make it appear promising as an antioxidant plant source. The best antioxidative activities occur in flower buds and leaves. Total and oligomeric proanthocyanidins occur in flowers and fruits while flavonoids act in leaf extracts (Bahorun et al, 1994).

Antiviral Effects: Tested in vitro for activity against HIV-1, certain ethylacetate extracts of the fresh fruits of *Crataegus sinaica boiss* showed activity measured as a ratio of concentrations causing 50% cytotoxicity and 50% inhibition of virus replication (Hammouda et al, 1994). Fractions showing the highest activity included EtOAc and procyanidins A2, B2, and C1 while procyanidin B5 showed relatively little activity. Elsewhere, a comparison of different fractions from fruits and leaves of *Crataegus sinaica* indicated activity toward classical and alternative pathways of the complement system (Shahat et al, 1994).

Cardiovascular Effects: Pharmacologic and biochemical activities of flavonoids include enzyme induction and inhibition, inhibition of platelet aggregation, antioxidant properties, antimicrobial and antiviral activity, and cytotoxic and antimutagenic activity (Schlegelmilch & Heywood, 1994). Dose-dependent increases in coronary flow were the main effect of O-glycosides in guinea pig hearts; effects of C-glycosides were less substantial (Schuessler et al, 1995).

Crataegus has positive inotropic, dromotropic, and chronotropic effects, and negative bathmotropic effects (Siegel et al, 1996; Schuessler et al, 1995; Schuessler et al, 1993; Mang et al, 1997). It causes dilatation of blood vessels, in particular coronary blood vessels, resulting in reduced peripheral resistance and increased coronary circulation (Siegel et al, 1996).

Inhibitory effects on the sodium/potassium ATPase in vitro were most pronounced with application of Crataegus procyandidins, followed by Crataegus flavonoids, and least with Crataegus extracts (Ammon & Kaul, 1994). Compared to cardiac glycosides, the inhibition of sodium/potassium ATPase by Crataegus administration is minimal (Rohr & Meier, 1997).

Inhibition of 3′,5′-cyclic adenosine monophosphate-phosphodiesterase (PDE) in vitro and of the PDE III and IV in enzymes of guinea pig hearts provides evidence that phosphodiesterase inhibition underlies the myocardial action of Crataegus flavonoids (Schuessler et al, 1995). Proanthocyanidins include monomeric catechins and dimeric and oligomeric procyanidins (Rajendran et al, 1996; Bahorun et al, 1994). Oligomeric procyanidins are thought to contribute to vasodilating and positive inotropic effects of the plant (Schuessler et al, 1995).

Antihyperlipidemic Effects: Hawthorn decoction lowered serum cholesterol levels in humans. Hawthorn drink lowered low-density lipoprotein levels, body weight, and body fat in animals (Chen et al, 1995).

Effects on Hypertension: Animal studies, but not human studies, have demonstrated hawthorn extract's hypotensive effect. Larger, controlled human trials are needed.

Effects on Orthostatic Hypotension: Pooled data of two randomized clinical trials demonstrated camphor-Crataegus berry extract attenuated orthostatic hypotension in subjects with orthostatic dysregulation (Belz et al, 2002).

CLINICAL TRIALS

Anxiety Disorders

A double-blind, randomized, placebo-controlled study was performed to evaluate the clinical efficacy of a neurotonic component containing a fixed combination of magnesium and two plant extracts (*Crataegus oxyacantha* and *Eschscholtzia californica*) in patients with mild-to-moderate anxiety disorders with assorted functional disturbances. Subjects (n=264) were divided into two groups: 130 received the study drug (Sympathyl) and 134 received placebo (2 tablets, twice daily for 3 months). The preparation proved safe and more effective than placebo in treating the subjects' anxiety disorders (Hanus et al, 2004).

Congestive Heart Failure

A standardized extract of fresh Crataegus berries (Crataegisan®) enhanced exercise tolerance in patients with congestive heart failure in an 8-week, multicenter, randomized, double-blind, placebo-controlled clinical trial (n=143). Subjects between 44 and 79 years with NYHA Class II heart failure were randomly assigned to oral treatment with 0.75 mL *Crataegus oxyacantha L* extract or an identical placebo 3 times daily 30 minutes prior to meals for 8 weeks. Exercise tolerance, defined as highest wattage sustained on a stationary bicycle over a period of two minutes, was significantly increased in subjects treated with Crataegus extract compared to placebo (p=0.045) (Degenring et al, 2003).

A meta-analysis that included eight double-blind, placebo-controlled, randomized clinical trials concluded that Crataegus (hawthorn) extract was beneficial as an adjunctive treatment for patients with mild chronic heart failure. Most studies evaluated hawthorn as an adjunctive therapy combined with diuretics, ACE inhibitors, or calcium channel blockers. Four of the trials with primary outcome measure of maximal workload reported a significant improvement following hawthorn treatment compared to placebo ($p<0.01$; n=310). Problems identified included a small number of studies and patients and use of concomitant medications, making it difficult to establish efficacy of hawthorn (Pittler et al, 2003).

Crataegus extract (WS 1442, standardized to 18.75% oligomeric procyanidines) significantly enhanced exercise tolerance and symptoms of congestive heart failure compared to placebo in a 16-week randomized, double-blind, placebo-controlled clinical trial of patients with chronic stable NYHA Class III heart failure receiving concomitant treatment with a diuretic (n=209) (Tauchert, 2002).

During a randomized, placebo-controlled study, Crataegus extract improved ergospirometric parameters and subjective assessment in patients with moderately reduced left ventricular ejection fraction (Foerster et al, 1994). In another randomized, double-blind, placebo-controlled, multicenter study, administration of Crataegus extract at a dose of 600 mg daily for 8 weeks resulted in statistically significant improvement in the main confirmatory parameter, bicycle ergometry exercise tolerance, as well as other evaluated parameters (Schmidt et al, 1994).

Hawthorn did not significantly affect pharmacokinetic or pharmacodynamic effects of digoxin in an open-label, randomized, crossover trial of eight healthy subjects (Tankanow et al, 2003).

Hyperlipidemia

One month of ingesting a Hawthorn drink lowered average serum cholesterol levels in study participants clinically diagnosed as hyperlipidemic (Chen et al, 1995). Hawthorn effectively reduced LDL levels ($p<0.001$) but not HDL levels. Similarly, although hawthorn was not effective in raising apo-AI levels, it significantly reduced levels of apo-B, the main component of LDL ($p<0.05$). Average serum lipid peroxidate malonic dialdehyde (MDA) levels decreased from 3.2 nmol/L to 2.5 nmol/mL in the subjects ($p<0.001$) (Chen et al, 1995).

Hypertension

A 2006 study found positive hypotensive effects with Hawthorn for patients with type 2 diabetes (n=79) who were also taking prescription medicines for hypertension. This was the first randomized controlled trial to demonstrate an added hypotensive effect for Hawthorn in such individuals. Seventy-one percent of the participants used blood pressure-lowering medicines. At the end of the 16-week study, the difference in mean diastolic blood pressure reduction between the groups was significant ($P = 0.035$), with the Hawthorn extract group (n=39) showing greater reductions than the placebo group (n=40). However, the difference in systolic blood pressure did not differ (Walker, 2006).

In an earlier randomized, double-blind, placebo-controlled pilot study of mild essential hypertension (n=36) by the same author, Hawthorn extract did not lower blood pressure. At the time, the authors suggested that larger controlled trials evaluating the hypotensive effects of larger doses of hawthorn for a longer duration are warranted (Walker et al, 2002).

In contrast, total peripheral resistance and blood pressure increased with Crataegus in one group. Oral administration of *Crataegus fructi* extracts had cardiostimulating, pressoric, and preload-decreasing effects, the latter possibly because of diuresis (Mang et al, 1997).

Hypotension

A randomized, double-blind, placebo-controlled study with parallel groups showed a preparation of an extract from fresh Crataegus berries plus D-campfor, Korodin Herz-Kreislauf-Tropfen, was efficacious in the treatment of orthostatic hypotension. Only one adverse event, which was unrelated to the medication and was not serious, occurred in the study of 38 patients over age 50 (Kroll et al, 2005).

INDICATIONS AND USAGE

Approved by Commission E:

- Decrease in cardiac output (Stage II NYHA)

Hawthorn is used for senile heart, chronic cor pulmonale, and mild forms of bradycardial arrhythmias.

Unproven Uses: In folk medicine, Hawthorn is also used as a cardiotonic, for hypertension, ischemia of the heart, arrhythmia and as a sedative. Hawthorn has a high flavonoid content and is used to prevent collagen destruction in joints and decrease inflammation and decrease the fragility of capillaries.

Chinese Medicine: In China, Hawthorn is used to reduce food stagnancy and blood stasis.

Homeopathic Uses: Therapeutic dilutions are used for cardiac insufficiency, senile cardiac insufficiency, dysrhythmia, and angina pectoris.

CONTRAINDICATIONS

Pregnancy: Use of Hawthorn during the first trimester of pregnancy is contraindicated.

Pediatrics: Hawthorn is contraindicated in children under 12 years of age.

PRECAUTIONS AND ADVERSE REACTIONS

Infrequent adverse events included palpitations, tachycardia, dizziness, headache, vertigo, hot flashes, gastrointestinal complaints, gastroenteritis, flatulence, and dyspnea (Pittler et al, 2003;Tauchert, 2002).

It is recommended that Hawthorn supplements be prescribed and monitored by a physician. During treatment with Hawthorn, the clinician should monitor heart rate and blood pressure on a regular basis. If the symptoms of the conditions remain unchanged for longer than 6 weeks or if there is edema of the legs, consult a physician. Consult a physician immediately in the case of pains in the area of the heart that spreads to the arms, upper abdomen, or neck region.

DRUG INTERACTIONS

MODERATE RISK

Antiplatelet agents: Concurrent use may result in increased risk of bleeding. *Clinical management:* Caution is advised. Monitor for signs and symptoms of excessive bleeding.

POTENTIAL INTERACTIONS

Cardiac Glycosides: Hawthorn may potentiate the action of these drugs. Coadministration of hawthorn extract and digoxin did not significantly alter pharmacokinetic or pharmacodynamic parameters in an open-label, randomized, crossover trial with eight healthy subjects. This small trial demonstrated a trend toward reduced digoxin bioavailability (Tankanow et al, 2003). *Clinical Management:* Adjust downward the dosage of standard cardiac glycosides.

Antiarrhythmics: Hawthorn has an action similar to Class III antiarrhythmics. *Clinical Management*: Avoid concomitant use.

Cisapride: Hawthorn has been found to inhibit the inward flow of potassium channels resulting in an increased action potential in cardiac ventricular cells. *Clinical Management*: Avoid concomitant use.

OVERDOSAGE

The LD50 via intraperitoneal injection in the mouse model has been reported at a single dose of 1,170 mg/kg and 750 mg/kg in the rat. In both species, signs of overdose included sedation, dyspnea, tremor and piloerection (Schlegelilch & Heywood, 1994). The same authors reported that an oral dose if 3000 mg/kg in mice and rats was well tolerated with no negative clinical signs or death reported in the animal models.

DOSAGE

Mode of Administration: The dried and comminuted drug for decoctions as well as liquid or dry extracts for oral intake.

How Supplied:

Capsules – 80 mg, 100 mg, 200 mg, 300 mg, 450 mg, 455 mg, 480 mg, 500 mg, 510 mg, 565 mg

Liquid – 250 mg/mL

Tablets – 80 mg, 500 mg

Daily Dosage: The average daily dose is 5 g of drug or 160 to 900 mg extract administered in divided doses, 3 times daily, (ethanol 45% V/V or methanol 70% V/V) standardized on procyanidin or flavonoids; single dose: 1 g of drug several times daily. The duration of treatment is minimum 6 weeks.

Homeopathic Dosage: 5 to 10 drops, 1 tablet, or 5 to 10 globules 1 to 3 times a day or 1 ml injection solution sc twice a week; ointment 1 to 2 times a day (HAB1)

Storage: Hawthorn should be protected from light and moisture in well-sealed containers at temperatures below 25° C.

LITERATURE

Ammon VHPT & Kaul R. Crataegus -Teil 1: historisches und wirkstoffe, teil 2: wirkungen auf das herz, teil 3: wirkungen auf den kreislauf. *Dtsch Apoth Z*; 26:33-36, 27:21-35, 28:35-42. 1994

Anon. *Crataegus oxycantha*: common name hawthorne. *Altern Med Rev*; 3(2):138-139. 1998

Anon. Hawthorn monograph, in Olin BR (ed): The Lawrence Review of Natural Products. Facts and Comparisons, St Louis, MO, 1994.

Anon. Behandlung der leichten Herzinsuffiziens: Weiβdornextrakt und ACE-Hemmer im Vergleich. In: *DAZ;* 134(39):3749. 1994

Anon. Phytopharmaka für ältere Menschen: Ginkgo, Kava, Hypericum und Crataegus. In: *DAZ;* 135(5):400-402. 1995

Anon. Weiβdorn bei Herzinsuffiziens und Angina pectoris. In: *Symbiose;* 4(3):16. 1992

Bahorun T et al. Oxygen species scavenging activity of phenolic activities, fresh plant organs and pharmaceutical preparations. In: *Arzneim Forsch;* 46(11):1086-1089. 1996

Bahorun T, Trotin F, Pommery J, Vasseur J, Pinkas M. Antioxydant activities of *Crataegus monogyna* extracts. In: *Planta Med;* 60(4):323-328. 1994

Belz GG, Butzer R, Gaus W et al. Camphor-Crataegus berry extract combination dose-dependently reduces tilt induced fall in blood pressure in orthostatic hypotension. *Phytomedicine*; 9(7):581-588. 2002

Bourin M, Bougerol T, Guitton B et al. A combination of plant extracts in the treatment of outpatients with adjustment disorder with anxious mood: controlled study versus placebo. *Fundam Clin Pharmacol*; 11(2):127-132. 1997

Chen JD, Wu YZ, Tao ZL et al. Hawthorn (shan zha) drink and its lowering effect on blood lipid levels in humans and rats. *World Rev Nutr Diet;* 77:147-154. 1995

Ciplea AG, Richter KD. The protective effect of *Allium sativum* and Crataegus on isoprenaline-induced tissue necroses in rats. *Arzneim Forsch/Drug Res;* 38:1588-1592. 1988

Czygan FC. Crataegus-Arten- Weiβdorn, Portrait einer Arzneipflanze. In: *ZPT;* 15(2):117. 1994

Degenring FH, Suter A, Weber M et al. A randomised double blind placebo controlled clinical trial of a standardised extract of fresh crataegus berries (Crataegisan®) in the treatment of patients with congestive heart failure NYHA II. *Phytomedicine*; 10(5):363-369. 2003

Dingermann T. Phytopharmaka im Alter. Crataegus, Ginkgo, Hypericum und Kava-Kava. In: *PZ;* 140(23):2017-2024. 1995

Eichstädt H, Bäder M, Danne O, Kaiser W, Stein U, Felix R, Crataegus-Extrakt hilft dem Patienten mit NYHA II-*Herzinsuffizien Therapiewoche;* 39: 3288-3296. 1989

Fachinformation Crataezyma®. Weissdornblaetter, -blueten-Trockenextrakt. Zyma GmbH, Muenchen, Germany, 1996.

Fachinformation Cratecor®. Weissdornblaetter, -blueten-Trockenextrakt. Bionorica GmbH, Neumarkt, Germany, 1996.

Fachinformation Cratecor®. Weissdornblaetter, -blueten-Trockenextrakt. Bionorica GmbH, Neumarkt, Germany, 1996.

Fischer K, Jung F, Koscielny J, Kiesewetter H. Crataegus-Extrakt vs. Methyldigoxin. Einfluβ auf Rheologie und Mikrozirkulation bei 12 gesunden Probanden. *Münch Med Wschr;* 136(Suppl 1), 35-38. 1994

Förster A, Förster K, Bühring M, Wolfstädter HD, Crataegus bei mäβig reduzierter linksventrikulärer Auswurffraktion. Ergospirometrische Verlaufsuntersuchung bei 72. Patienten in doppelblindem Vergleich mit Plazebo. *Münch Med Wochenschr;* 136(Suppl 1), 21-26. 1994

Frances D. Crataegus for asthma: case studies. *J Naturopath Med*; 8(2):20-27. 1998

Hammouda FM, Ismail SI, Azzam A et al. Evaluation of the active constituents of *crataegus sinaica Boiss* as inhibitors of human immunodeficiency virus type 1 (HIV-1). *Pharm World Sci*; 16(6)(suppl I):18. 1994

Hanus M, Lavon J, Mathieu M. Double-blind, randomized, placebo-controlled study to evaluate the efficacy and safety of a fixed combination containing two plant extracts (Crataegus oxycantha and Eschscholtzia californica) and magnesium in mild-to-moderate anxiety disorders. *Curr Med Res Opin*; 10(1): 63-71. 2004.

Joseph G, Zhao Y, Klaus W. Pharmakologisches Wirkprofil von Crataegus-Extrakt im Vergleich zu Epinephrin, Amrinon, Milrinon und Digoxin am isoliert perfundierten Meerschweinchenherzen. *Arzneimittelforschung/Drug Res;* 45(12):1261-1265. 1995

Kaul R. Pflanzliche Procyanidine. Vorkommen, Klassifikation und pharmakologische Wirkungen. In: *PUZ;* 25(4):175-185. 1996

Kim SH, Kang KW, Kim KW et al. Procyanidins in crataegus extract evoke endothelium-dependent vasorelaxation in rat aorta. *Life Sciences*; 67(2):121-131. 2000

Klensch O, Nagell A. Die Darreichungsform Tee am Beispiel Weiβdornblätter mit Blüten. In: *DAZ;* 134(32):3005. 1994

Kraft K. Crataegus (common hawthorn) extracts in cardiac failure - are there new promising results and outlooks? *Perfusion*; 13(1):495-498. 2000

Kroll M, Ring C, Gaus W, Hempel B. A randomized trial of Korodin Herz-Kreislauf-Tropfen as add-on treatment in older patients with orthostatic hypotension. *Phytomedicine*; 12(6): 395-402.02005.

Krzeminski T, Chatterjee SS. Ischemia and early reperfusion induced arrhythmias, beneficial effects of an extract of Crataegus oxyacantha L. *Pharm Pharmacol Lett;* 3:45-48. 1993

Kurcok A, Ischemia- and reperfusion-induced cardiac injury; effects of two flavonoids containing plant extracts possessing radical scavenging properties. Naunyn- Schmiedebergs's *Arch Pharmacol*; 345(Suppl RB 81) Abstr 322. 1992

Kurzmann M, Schimmer O. Weiβdorn - Flavonoidmuster und DC-Identitätsprüfung. In: *DAZ;* 136(33):2759-2764. 1996

Leuchtgens H. Cratagus Special Extract WS 1442 in NYHA II heart failure. A placebo controlled randomized double-blind study. In: *Fortschr Med;* 20;111(20021:352-4 Jul 20,1993.

Loew D, Crataegus-Spezialextrakte bei Herzinsuffizien. *Kassenarzt;* 15:43-52. 1994

Loew D, Phytotherapie bei Herzinsuffizienz. In: *ZPT;* 18(2):92-96. 1997

Mang C, Herrmann V, Butzer R et al. Crataegus fructi extract. a placebo-controlled study on haemodynamic effects of single and repetitive doses in normal volunteers. *Eur J Clin Pharmacol*; 52(suppl):A59. 1997

Meier B, Neue Erkenntnisse zur Analytik und Wirksamkeit von Weiβdorn. In. *DAZ;* 136(44):3877-3879. 1996

Meletis CD. Natural approaches to mitigating hypertension. *Alt Comp Ther*; 11(6): 281-284. 2005.

Murray M & Pizzorno J. A Textbook of Natural Medicine, 2nd ed. Batyr University Publications, Seattle, WA, USA, ppV Cratag-1-4. 1996

Muller A, Linke W, Klaus W. Crataegus extract blocks potassium currents in guinea pig ventricular cardiac myocytes. In. *Planta Med;* 65(4). 335-9 May, 1999

Pittler MH, Schmidt K & Ernst E. Hawthorn extract for treating chronic heart failure. Meta-analysis of randomized trials. *Am J Med*; 114(8):665-674. 2003

Pöpping S, Rose H, Ionescu I, Fischer Y, Kammermeier H. Effect of a Hawthorn Extract on Contraction and Energy Turnover of Isolated Rat Cordiomyocytes. *Arzneim Forsch/Drug Res;* 45:1157-1161. 1995

Rajendran S, Deepalakshmi PD, Parasakthy K et al. Effect of tincture of crataegus on the LDL-receptor activity of hepatic plasma membrane of rats fed an atherogenic diet. *Atherosclerosis*; 123(1-2):235-241. 1996

Rehwald A et al. HPLC analysis of the flavonoids of Crataegi folium cum flore. In. *PM;* 59(7)28. 1993

Reuter HD. Crataegus als pflanzliches Kardiakum. In. *ZPT;* 15(2):73. 1994

Rewerski W et al. *Arzneim Forsch;* 21:886. 1971

Rohr G & Meier G. Crataegus. *Dtsch Apoth Z*; 137(42):104-116. 1997

Schlegelmilch R, Heywood R, Toxicity of Crataegus (Hawthorn) Extract (WS 1442). *J Am Coll Toxicol;* 13(2):103-111. 1994

Schmidt U, Kuhn U, Ploch M, Hübner WD. Wirksamkeit des Extraktes LI 132 (600 mg/Tag) bei 8wöchiger Therapie. Plazebokontrollierte Doppelblindstudie mit Weiβdorn an 78 herzinsuffizienten Patienten im Stadium II nach NYHA. *Münch Med Wochenschr;* 136(Suppl 1):S13-S20. 1994

Schüssler M et al. Effect of flavonoids from Crataegus species in Langendorf perfused isolated guinea pig heart. In. *PM;* 58(7)46. 1992

Schuessler M et al. Cardiac effects of flavonoids from Crataegus species. In. *Planta Med;* 59(7)88. 1993

Schussler M, Holzl J, Fricke U. Myocardial effects of flavonoids from Crataegus species. In. *Arzneimittelforschung;* 45(8): 842-845. 1995

Shahat AA, De Bruyne T, Lasure A, et al. Anti-complementary activity of *crataegus sinaica Boiss. Pharm World Sci*; 16(6)(suppl I):18. 1994

Siegel G, Casper U. Crataegi folium cum flore. In, Loew D, Rietbrock N (Hrsg) Phytopharmaka in Forschung und klinischer Anwendung. Steinkopff Verlag, Darmstadt, S. 1-14. 1995.

Siegel G, Casper U, Schnalke F et al. Molecular physiological effector mechanisms of hawthorn extract in cardiac papillary muscle and coronary vascular smooth muscle. *Phytother Res*; 10(suppl):S195-S198. 1996

Siegel G, Casper U, Walter H, Hetzer R, Weiβdorn-Extrakt LI 132. Dosis- Wirkungs-Studie zum Membranpotential und Tonus menschlicher Koronararterien und des Hundepapillarmuskels. *Münch med Wschr;* 136(Suppl 1):45-56. 1994

Steinman H, Lovell C & Cronin E. Immediate-type hypersensitivity to *crataegus monogyna* (hawthorn*). Contact Dermatitis*; 11(5):321-323. 1984

Sticher O, Rehwald A, Meier B, Kriterien der pharmazeutischen Qualität von Crataegus-Extrakten. *Münch Med Wschr;* 136(Suppl 1):69-73. 1994

Tankanow R, Tamer HR, Streetman DS. Interaction study between digoxin and a preparation of hawthorn (*Crataegus oxyacantha). J Clin Pharmacol*; 43(6):637-642. 2003

Tauchert M. Efficacy and safety of crataegus extract WS 1442 in comparison with placebo in patients with chronic stable New York Heart Association class-III heart failure. *Am Heart J*; 143(5):910-915. 2002

Tauchert M, Loew D. Crataegi folium cum flore bei HerzinsuffizienZ In, Loew D, Rietbrock N (Hrsg) Phytopharmaka in Forschung und klinischer Anwendung. Steinkopff Verlag, *Darmstadt, S;* 137-144. 1995

Tauchert M, Ploch M, Hübner WD. Wirksamkeit des Weiβdorn-Extraktes LI 132 im Vergleich mit Captopril. Multizentrische Doppelblindstudie bei 132 Patienten mit Herzinsuffizienz im

Stadium II nach NYHA. *Münch Med Wschr;* 136(Suppl 1):27-34. 1994

Tauchert M, Siegel G, Schulz V. Weiβdorn-Extrakt als pflanzliches Cardiacum (Vorwort). Neubewertung der therapeutischen Wirksamkeit. *Münch Med Wschr;* 136(Suppl 1):3-5. 1994

Trunzler G. Phytotherapeutische Möglichkeiten bei Herz- und arteriellen Gefäβerkrankungen. In. *ZPT;* 10(5):147. 1989

Vibes J, Lasserre B, Gleye J et al. Inhibition of thromboxane A2 biosynthesis in vitro by the main components of Crataegus oxyacantha (Hawthorn) flower heads. *Prostaglandins Leukot Essent Fatty Acids*; 50:173-175. 1994

Walker AF, Marakis G, Simpson E et al. Hypotensive effects of hawthorn for patients with diabetes taking prescription drugs: a randomised controlled trial. *Br J Gen Pract*;56:437-43. 2006.

Walker AF, Marakis G, Morris AP et al. Promising hypotensive effect of hawthorn extract. A randomized double-blind pilot study of mild, essential hypertension. *Phytotherapy Res*; 16:48-54. 2002

Wichtl M. Pflanzliche Geriatrika. In. *DAZ;* 132(30):1576. 1992

Zapfe jun G. Clinical efficacy of crataegus extract WS 1442 in congestive heart failure NYHA class II. *Phytomedicine*; 8(4):262-266. 2001

English Horsemint

Mentha longifolia

DESCRIPTION

Medicinal Parts: The medicinal part is the dried herb.

Flower and Fruit: The flowers are sometimes interrupted lower down by 1 cm thick, gray to white, downy, panicled, false spikes. The false spikes are arranged with linear, villous bracts, which are longer than the flowers. The calyx is fluffy and woolly pubescent with awl-shaped tips. The corolla is lilac to flesh-colored. The fruit is a finely speckled nutlet.

Leaves, Stem and Root: The plant is a perennial. It has a sturdy rhizome with underground runners. The shoots are densely covered in 1- or multicelled tomentose hairs with few glands and a mild odor. The stem is erect, simple or branched, up to 1 m high, tough and obtusely angular. The leaves are sessile, oblong-ovate to lanceolate, and usually acuminate with 6 to 12 pairs of curved pinnate veins. The underside of the leaves are gray to white tomentose.

Production: English Horsemint is the aerial part of *Mentha longifolia*, the dried herb.

Habitat: The plant is common in all of Europe to southern Sweden.

ACTIONS AND PHARMACOLOGY

COMPOUNDS

Volatile oil: chief components piperitone (share 60-80%), furthermore beta- caryophyllene (5-15%), germacren D (5-15%), 1,8-cineole (2-7%), limonene (1-8%), with other chemotypes chief components D-carvone, piperitone, iso-menthone + menthofurane, menthone, piperitol, menthol or linalool

Flavonoids: including among others diosmin, hesperidin, quercitrin, thymonin, apigenine-7-glucuronide

EFFECTS

English Horsemint has carminative and stimulant effects.

INDICATIONS AND USAGE

Unproven Uses: The drug is used for digestive disorders, particularly for flatulence. Historically, it has been used for all kinds of pain, headaches in particular.

PRECAUTIONS AND ADVERSE REACTIONS

No health hazards or side effects are known in conjunction with the proper administration of designated therapeutic dosages.

DOSAGE

Mode of Administration: The ground drug is used internally as an infusion; it is used externally as a bath additive.

LITERATURE

Avato P, Sgarra G, Casadoro G. Chemical composition of the essential oils of *Mentha* species cultivated in Italy. *Sci Pharm.* 63; 223-230. 1995

Hänsel R, Keller K, Rimpler H, Schneider G (Hrsg.), Hagers Handbuch der Pharmazeutischen Praxis, 5. Aufl., Bde 4-6 (Drogen), Springer Verlag Berlin, Heidelberg, New York, 1992-1994.

Kokkini S, Papageorgiou VP. Constituents of Essential Oils from *Mentha longifolia* growing wild in Greece. *Planta Med.* 54; 59-60. 1988

English Ivy

Hedera helix

DESCRIPTION

Medicinal Parts: The medicinal parts are the leaves and berries.

Flower and Fruit: The inflorescences are greenish-yellow umbels, which form dense, semiglobular clusters. The calyx tips are short, almost triangular, tomentose, and drooping. The 5 petals are oblong and slightly involute. There are 5 stamens and 1 inferior ovary with 5 valves. The style is fused into a column. The fruit is a globular, usually 5-valved berry, which becomes black and ripens in spring. It contains 3 to 5 reniform, triangular, acute seeds, which are reddish-violet when young, later dark brown, and finally black.

Leaves, Stem, and Root: The plant is an evergreen perennial, which creeps or, by means of adventitious roots, climbs to a length of 3 to 15 m. The stem is branched, the leaves are alternate, petioled, glabrous, glossy, and coriaceous. Younger leaves are 5-lobed; the leaves of older flowering plants are ovate-rhomboid.

Characteristics: The berries and leaves have a bitter taste.

Habitat: English Ivy is indigenous to the temperate regions of Europe, and also north and central Asia. It is cultivated in the U.S.

Production: English Ivy leaf consists of the dried leaves of *Hedera helix.*

Other Names: Bindwood, Gum Ivy, True Ivy, Woodbind

ACTIONS AND PHARMACOLOGY

COMPOUNDS

Triterpene saponins: aglycone hederagenin, oleanolic acid, bayogenin, chief components hederosaponin C (hederacoside C, slightly transforming into alpha-hederin, aglycone hederagenin), additionally hederosaponin B (hederacoside B)

Volatile oils: including some with methylethylketone, methylisobutylketone

Polyynes: including falcarinol, 11,12-didehydrofalcarinol

Steroids: sterols, including beta-sitosterol, campesterol

Flavonoids: including rutin

EFFECTS

English Ivy is an expectorant and antispasmodic. In animal experiments, the drug is anti-exudative and cytotoxic. Hedera saponin C exhibits an antiviral, antibacterial, antimycotic, anthelmintic and mollusicidal, as well as an antiflagellate, effect. The fresh leaves are an irritant to the skin and mucosa and can have an allergenic effect.

INDICATIONS AND USAGE

Approved by Commission E:

- Cough
- Bronchitis

English Ivy is a respiratory catarrh used for the symptomatic treatment of chronic inflammatory bronchial conditions.

Unproven Uses: In folk medicine, English Ivy is used internally for liver, spleen, and gallbladder disorders and for gout, rheumatism, and scrofulosis. Externally, it is used for burn wounds, calluses, cellulitis, inflammations, neuralgia, parasitic disorders, ulcers, rheumatic complaints, and phlebitis.

Homeopathic Uses: English Ivy is administered in homeopathy for hyperthyroidism, rheumatic disorders, and respiratory tract inflammation.

PRECAUTIONS AND ADVERSE REACTIONS

Health risks or side effects following the proper administration of designated therapeutic dosages are not recorded. The drug has a medium potential for sensitization through skin contact.

DOSAGE

Mode of Administration: English Ivy is available as comminuted drug and other galenic preparations for internal external use.

How Supplied: Forms of commercial pharmaceutical preparations include drops, suppositories, and tablets.

Preparation: Prepare a tea by adding 1 heaped teaspoonful of drug to 1/4 l of hot water and steeping the mixture for 10 minutes. A poultice is prepared by mixing fresh Ivy leaves 1:3 with linseed meal. To make an infusion, add 1 heaping teaspoonful of drug to one-quarter cup boiling water and steep for 10 minutes.

Daily Dosage: Tea and other infusions can be taken internally 3 times daily. The average daily dose is 0.3 to 0.8 g of drug. Fresh leaves may be laid upon festering wounds and burns; a decoction of fresh leaves (200 gm/liter water) may be used externally for rheumatism. The daily dose of a tincture is 40 to 50 drops; single dose: 5 to 10 drops.

Homeopathic Dosage: 5 drops, 1 tablet or 10 globules every 30 to 60 minutes (acute) or 1 to 3 times daily (chronic); parenterally: 1 to 2 ml sc acute, 3 times daily; chronic: once a day (HAB1).

LITERATURE

Boyle J, Harman RMH. Contact dermatitis to *Hedera helix* (Common Ivy). *Contact Dermatitis* 12; 111-112. 1985.

Cioaca C, Margineau C, CuCu V. The Saponins of *Hedera helix* with Antibacterial Activity. Pharmazie 33; 609-610. 1978

Danloy S et al. Effects of alpha-Hederin, a Saponin Extracted from *Hedera helix*, on Cells Cultured in vitro. *Planta Med.* 60; 45-49. 1994

Elias R, Meo Mde Vidal-Ollivier E, Laget M, Balansard G, Dumenik G. Antimutagenic activity of some saponins isolated from *Calendula officinalis L., C.arvensis L.* und *Hedera helix L. Mutagenesis* 5; 327-331. 1990

Facino RM, Carini M, Stefani R, Aldini G, Saibene L. Anti-elastase and anti-hyaluronidase activities of saponins and sapogenins from *Hedera helix, Aesculus hippocastanum,* and *Ruscus aculeatus*: factors contributing to their efficacy in the treatment of venous insufficiency. *Arch-Pharm-Weinheim* 328(10); 720

Gafner F, Epstein W, Reynolds G, Rodriguez E. Human maximization test of falcarinol, the principal contact allergen of English ivy and *Algerinan iva (Hedera helix, H.canariensis). Contact Dermatitis* 19; 125-128. 1988)

Maffei Facino R, Carini M, Bonadeo P. Efficacy of Topically applied *Hedera helix L.* Saponins for Treatment of Liposclerosis (so-called ''Cellulitis''). Acta Therapeut. 16; 337-349. 1990

Mansouri L, Henry M. An ontogenetic study on the sapogenin contents of Ivy. *Pharmazie* 50 (9); 642-643. 1995

Trute A, Gross J, Mutschler E, Nahrstedt A, In vitro antispasmodic compounds of the dry extract obtained from *Hedera helix.* In: *PM* 63(2):125-129. 1997.

Trute A, Nahrstedt A, Identification and quantitative analysis of phenolic dry extracts of *Hedera helix.* In: *PM* 63(2):177-179. 1997.

English Lavender

Lavandula angustifolia

DESCRIPTION

Medicinal Parts: The medicinal parts are the essential oil extracted from the fresh flowers and/or the inflorescences, the flowers collected just before opening and dried, the fresh flowers, and the dried flowers.

Flower and Fruit: The flowers are in false whorls of 6 to 10 blossoms forming interrupted terminal spikes. The pedicles are 10- to 15-cm long downy stems. The bracts are 5 mm long, ovate to broadly triangular, often brown and brown-violet or violet-tinged. The tubular calyx has 5 uneven tips, it is amethyst-colored and tomentose. After flowering it is closed by a lidlike appendage of its upper tip. The corolla is longer with a cylindrically fused base, the lips are flat, and the upper lip is larger with 2 lobes. The lower lip is trilobed with even tips. The stamens are enclosed in the tube. The ovary consists of 4 carpels and has a nectary below it. The fruit is a glossy brown nutlet.

Leaves, Stem, and Root: English Lavender is a 60-cm high subshrub and is heavily branched with leafy, erect, rodlike, gray-green, young branches. The leaves are sessile, oblong-lanceolate, entire-margined, involute, gray, later green with glandular spots beneath.

Characteristics: The flowers have a fresh aromatic fragrance.

Habitat: The plant is indigenous to the Mediterranean region but is common in most of southern Europe and is cultivated extensively.

Production: English Lavender flower consists of the dried flower of *Lavandula angustifolia*, gathered shortly before fully unfolding, as well as its preparations. Flowering shoots are harvested when the middle section of the spike is flowering; it is cut 10 cm beneath the insertion of the spike. The most valuable part is the receptacle.

Not to be Confused With: Other varieties of lavender such as *Lavendula intermedia* (Lavendin) and *Lavendula latifolia.* The varieties are often mixed commercially. When the drug material has a high proportion of stem and leaf material, it is considered less valuable.

Other Names: French Lavender, Garden Lavender, Lavender

ACTIONS AND PHARMACOLOGY

COMPOUNDS

Volatile oil (1-3%): chief components (-)-linalool (making up 20-50%) and linalyl acetate (30-40%), furthermore, including among others, cis-ocimene, terpinene-4-ol, beta-caryophyllene, lavandulyl acetate

Hydroxycoumarins: including among others, umbelliferone, herniarin

Tannins (13%)

Caffeic acid derivatives: including among others, rosmaric acid

EFFECTS

The primary active constituents appear to be monoterpenes, especially (30% to 60%) linalool and linalyl acetate (Schulz et al, 1998; Duke, 1985. Choleretic and cholagogic effects have been described. In addition, an antimicrobial effect has been demonstrated in vitro, and therefore external use on poorly healing wounds is plausible. In animal experiments a neuro-depressive effect was demonstrated (shortening of the falling-asleep period and lengthening of sleep duration) and a reduction of motor activity. Lavender oil inhibits immediate-type allergic reactions by inhibition of mast cell degranulation. The antineoplastic effect of perillyl alcohol is inhibition of isoprenylation of small (21 to 26 kilodaltons) G proteins. Lavender oil is a carminative, thus aiding in reduction of flatulence, colic, and stomach distress (Kim & Cho, 1999; Phillips et al, 1995; Duke, 1985). In humans, after inhalation of the drug, an effect on the limbic cortex (similar to nitrazepam) was demonstrated.

Lavender is one of the most widely used essential oils in aromatherapy. It has a soothing and calming effect and is used therapeutically in a number of disease states. It is used internally and as a bath to ease tension and anxiety. It is also used topically and internally for skin conditions such as acne, rosacea and eczema to help calm the skin and reduce redness and irritation. Lavender has antibacterial qualities that contribute to its effectiveness in treating acne as well as minor cuts and scrapes. Lavender oil can be applied to burns and insect stings. The astringency helps to reduce pain and inflammation. A tea can be taken for headaches or diluted lavender oil can be used to massage the temples or body to ease tension in the muscles. Lavender has also been used for mild depression.

Anti-inflammatory Effects: Animal and in vitro studies suggest lavender oil inhibits immediate-type allergic reactions by inhibition of mast cell degranulation (Kim & Cho, 1999). Lavender oil, in concentrations of 1% or more, showed anti-inflammatory action in mouse inflammation models.

Antilipidemic Effects: D-limonene and perillyl alcohol (minor components of lavender oil) mildly reduce cholesterol by suppressing hepatic 3-hydroxy-3- methylglutaryl-coenzyme A (HMG-CoA) reductase activity. This enzyme is involved in a rate-limiting step of cholesterol synthesis (Elson & Yu, 1994). Perillyl alcohol also inhibited ubiquinone synthesis and blocked conversion of lathosterol to cholesterol (Ren & Gould, 1994).

Antimicrobial Effects: Various components of lavender oil have shown antibacterial, antifungal, and mitocidal activities. Lavender oil has shown promise against methicillin-resistant *Staphlococcus aureus* and vancomycin-resistant strains of *Enterococcus faecium* (Fetrow & Avila, 1999). Lavender oil has been shown to have in vitro antifungal activity against the human pathogens *Malassezia furfur, Trichophyton rubrum,* and *Trichosporon beigelii* (Yamada et al, 1994). Oils of lavender and linalool have been shown to have acaricidal activity against the mite *Psoroptes cuniculi* in vitro. The activity existed both when the oil came in contact with the parasite and when exposed to volatized oil (not direct contact) (Perrucci et al, 1996; Perrucci et al, 1994). In addition, lavender oil has also been shown to be mitocidal at 0.9% to

0.1% against the carmine spider mite *Tetranychus cinnabarinus* (Mansour et al, 1986).

Antineoplastic Effects: The active antineoplastic agents in lavender oil are thought to be attributed to monoterpenes such as d-limonene and perillyl alcohol (Fetrow & Avila, 1999). Perillyl alcohol is hydrogenated d-limonene; limonene has antitumor activity against rodent mammary, liver, lung, pancreatic, stomach, prostate, and skin (Jirtle et al, 1993; Stayrook et al, 1997).

Central Nervous System Effects: Lavender oil is a sedative and hypnotic for humans and animals. Subjects exposed to lavender aromatherapy show EEG changes consistent with drowsiness (Diego et al, 1998). Anticonvulsant activity has been noticed in both mice and rats after induced seizures (Schulz et al, 1998; Atanassova-Shopova & Roussinow, 1970). The oil is a sedative, producing mild drowsiness to coma and convulsions, depending on the amount used (Schulz et al, 1998; Buchbauer et al, 1993).

Gastrointestinal Effects: Lavender oil is a carminative, thus aiding in reduction of flatulence, colic, stomach distress, and tonic (Duke, 1985). Nausea, vomiting, and diarrhea were dose limiting in cancer patients taking up to 0.5 to 12 g/m2/d of d-limonene (Vigushin et al, 1998).

CLINICAL TRIALS

Anxiety

A controlled, prospective trial was performed to evaluate the use of aromatherapy to reduce anxiety in 118 patients prior to a scheduled colonoscopy or esophagogastroduodenoscopy. The control group was given an inert oil (placebo) for inhalation, and the experimental group received the essential oil, Lavender, for inhalation. There was no significant difference in anxiety levels between pre- and post-placebo inhalation in either group (Muzzarelli et al, 2006).

Analgesia

Eight sessions of acupressure enhanced with the use of aromatic essential oil of Lavender effectively resolved short-term, sub-acute and nonspecific neck pain (defined as pain on most days in the 2 weeks previous) in this randomized, controlled clinical trial done at a Hong Kong clinic and community center. Eight sessions of manual acupressure with Lavender oil (3% in olive oil base) used as the lubricant were performed over a 3-week period. One month after treatment had ended, the 14 participants randomized to acupressure with Lavender had 23% reduced pain intensity (p=0.02), 23% reduced neck stiffness (p=0.001), improved lateral neck flexion (p=0.02), and improved neck extension (p=0.001) when compared with the 18 participants in the control group. The regimen (acupressure plus Lavender) has value, the authors conclude, as a complement to conventional medical treatments for sub-acute neck pain (Yip, 2006).

Insomnia

Anecdotal evidence suggests that, unlike conventional insomnia treatments, Lavender oil is not only effective but free of side effects when used for mild insomnia. Ten individuals with insomnia [verified by a score of 5 or more on the the Pittsburgh Sleep Quality Index (PSQI)] took part in a single-blinded, 4-week crossover pilot trial in which half of the individuals were randomized to take Lavender, and half to placebo (sweet almond oil), and then assignments were switched. The Lavender improved the PSQI score by -2.5 points (p=0.07). More notable improvements were seen in females and younger participants, but belief in the power of complementary and alternative medicine therapies did not predict outcome. Milder insomnia also improved more than other intensity levels. Larger trials are needed to draw statistically significant conclusions regarding the positive outcomes for Lavender in this trial (Lewith, 2005).

In a double-blind, randomized, crossover trial, 12 patients receiving lavender extract had increased tiredness after administration. Quantitative EEG analysis and self assessment (tiredness rated on a visual analog scale) were used to determine the sedative effect of oral (1200 mg extract capsule) *Lavandula angustifolia* extract versus a negative, placebo control and a positive, diazepam 10 mg control. A 5 minute EEG (leads Fz-Cz and Oz-T6) was recorded before, and 2 and 3 hours after administration of the products. (Schulz et al, 1998).

Cancer

Treatment with perillyl alcohol resulted in disease stabilization for 6 months or more, but no objective tumor change findings were observed. These patients were treatment failures from chemotherapy, radiation therapy, hormone therapy, or biologic response modifiers. The types of cancers in these patients were prostate, ovarian, sarcoma, renal cell, hepatocellular, chronic myelogenous leukemia, chronic lymphocytic leukemia, and an unknown primary adenocarcinoma (Ripple et al, 1998). Similar stabilization results were seen in a Phase 1 clinical trial of mixed solid tumors (Vigushin et al, 1998).

Antianxiety

A significant ($p<0.05$) difference in anxiety reduction was reported in 36 patients admitted to an intensive care unit who were treated with 1% lavender oil aromatherapy. While anxiety was significantly, but briefly, reduced, mood and coping variables were not significantly changed. The lavender oil was administered via ether inhalation or by application to the skin after determining that none of the patients were allergic to the oil. There were no significant changes in any physiologic values measured (Dunn et al, 1995).

INDICATIONS AND USAGE

Approved by Commission E:

- Loss of appetite
- Nervousness and insomnia
- Circulatory disorders

■ Dyspeptic complaints

Internally, English Lavender is used for mood disturbances such as restlessness or insomnia, functional abdominal complaints (nervous stomach irritations, Roehmheld syndrome, meteorism, nervous intestinal discomfort).

Externally, English Lavender is used for treatment of functional circulatory disorders.

Unproven Uses: In folk medicine, English Lavender is used for migraine, cramps, and bronchial asthma. Externally, it is used for rheumatic conditions (the drug as an extract in liniments), as a sedative in cases of tension, exhaustion; also for poorly healing wounds (lavender baths) and for sleep as aromatherapy (herb pillow).

CONTRAINDICATIONS

English Lavender is contraindicated during pregnancy and lactation (internal use) (Fetrow & Avila, 1999).

PRECAUTIONS AND ADVERSE REACTIONS

Possible adverse effects of English Lavender include drowsiness, gastrointestinal disturbance, and skin irritation. A weak estrogenic and antiandrogenic effect resulting in prepubertal gynecomastia in boys was linked to the use of Lavender, along with tea tree oil, in a 2007 *New England Journal of Medicine* report (Henley, 2007). The volatile oil possesses a weak potential for sensitization. To prevent toxicity, no more than 2 drops of lavender oil should be taken internally (Fetrow & Avila, 1999). Dermatitis, irritation, and phototoxicity may occur after external application of lavender, and possibly limit the concentration of lavender oil that can be applied to the skin.

DRUG INTERACTIONS

No human interaction data available.

OVERDOSE

CNS depression, constipation, respiratory depression, headache, meiosis, vomiting, and convulsions may occur in overdose

DOSAGE

Mode of Administration: The whole drug is used for infusions, as an extract and as a bath additive. Combinations with other sedative and/or carminative herbs may be beneficial.

Preparation: An infusion is prepared by adding 5 to 10 mL of drug per cup of hot water (150 mL), draw for 10 minutes, and strain. For external use as bath additive, 100 g of drug is scalded or boiled with 2 liters of water and added to the bath.

Daily Dosage: A tea prepared as indicated above can be administered 1 cup three times daily.

LITERATURE

Amr A & Yousef M. A natural antioxidant from Lavender *(Lavandula officinalis Chaix.)*. Dirasat Series B Pure and *Applied Sciences*; 22B(5):1271-1288. 1995

Atanassova-Shopova S, Roussinow KS. On certain central neurotropic effects of lavender essential oil. *Bull Inst Physiol;* 8:69-76. 1970

Benito M, Jorro G, Morales C et al. Labiatae allergy: Systemic reactions due to ingestion of oregano and thyme. *Ann Allergy Asthma Immunol*; 76(5):416-418. 1996

Birchall A. A whiff of happiness. *New Scientist*; 127(1731):45-47. 1990

Bouhlal K, Meynadier J, Peyron JL et al. The cutaneous effects of the common concretes and absolutes used in the perfume industry. *J Essent Oil Res*; 1(4):169-195. 1989

Buchbauer G, Jirovet L, Jäger W, Dietrich H, Plank C, Karamat E. Aromatherapy: Evidence for Sedative Effects of the Essential Oil of Lavender after Inhalation. *Z Naturforsch;* 46c:1067-1072. 1991

Cerda S, Wilkinson J & Broitman SA. Enhanced antitumor activity of lovastatin and perillyl alcohol combinations in the colonic adenocarcinoma cell line SW480. *Proceed Amer Assoc Cancer Res*; 35:335. 1994

Dunn C, Sleep J & Collett D. Sensing an improvement: an experimental study to evaluate the use of aromatherapy, message, and periods of rest in an intensive care unit. *J Advanced Nurs*; 21:34-40. 1995

Guillemain J, Rousseau A, Delaveau P. Effets neurodépresseurs de l'huile essentielle de Lavandula angustifolia Mill. *Ann Pharmaceutiques Francaises;* 47:337-343. 1989

Hardy M, Kirk-Smith MD & Stretch DD. Replacement of drug treatment for insomnia by ambient odour. *Lancet*; 346(8976):701. 1995

Henley D, Lipson N, Korach J, et al. Prepubertal gynecomastia linked to lavender and tea tree oils. *N Eng J Med*; 356;479-485. 2007.

Hohl RJ & Lewis K. Differential effects of monotropenes and lovastatin on RAS processing. *J Biol Chem*; 270(29):17508-17512. 1995

Jirtle RL, Haag JD, Ariazi EA et al. Increased mannose 6-phosphate/insulin-like factor II receptor and transforming growth factor beta 1 levels during monoterpene-induced regression of mammary tumors. *Cancer Res*; 53:3849-3852. 1993

Kim HM & Cho SH. Lavender oil inhibits immediate-type allergic reaction in mice and rats. *J Pharm Pharmacol*; 51(2):221-226. 1999

Larrondo JV, Agut M, Calvo-Torras MA. Antimicrobial activity of essences from labiates. *Microbios*; 82:171-172. 1995

Lewith GT, Godfrey AD, Philip P. A single-blinded, randomized pilot study evaluating the aroma of Lavendula angustifolia as a treatment for mild insomnia. *J Alt Comp Med*; 11 (4): 631-637. 2005.

Mansour F, Ravid U & Putievsky E. Studies of the effects of essential oils isolated from 14 species of Labiatae on the carmine spider mite *Tetranychus cinnabarinus. Phytoparasitica*; 14(2):137-142. 1986

Meyer A. Der Duft des Monats: Lavendel. In: *DAZ;* 133(40):3667. 1993

Mukherjee BD, Trenkle RW. *J Agric Food Chem;* 21:298. 1973

Muzzarelli L, Force M, Sebold M. Aromatherapy and reducing preprocedural anxiety: A controlled prospective study. *Gastroenterol Nurs*; 29(6): 466-471. 2006

Perrucci S, Cioni PL, Flamini G et al. Acaricidal agents of natural origin against *Psoroptes cuniculi. Parassitologia* (Rome); 36(3):269-271. 1994

Perrucci S, Macchioni G, Cioni PC et al. The activity of volatile compounds from *Lavandula angustifolia* against *Psoroptes cuniculi. Phytother Res*; 10(1):5-8. 1996

Phillips LR, Malspeis L & Supko JG. Pharmacokinetics of active drug metabolites after oral administration of perillyl alcohol, and investigational antineoplastic agent, to the dog. *Drug Metab Disp*; 23(7):676-680. 1995

Ren Z & Gould MN. Inhibition of ubiquinone and cholesterol synthesis by the monoterpene perillyl alcohol. *Cancer Lett*; 76:185-190. 1994

Ripple GH, Gould MN, Stewart JA et al. Phase 1 clinical trial of perillyl alcohol administration daily. *Clin Cancer Res*; 4:1159-1164. 1998

Ruch RJ & Sigler K. Growth inhibition of rat liver epithelial tumor cells by monotropenes does not involve Ras plasma membrane association. *Carcinogenesis*; 15(4):787-789. 1994

Schilcher H. Pflanzliche Psychopharmaka. Eine neue Klassifizierung nach Indikationsgruppen. In: *DAZ;* 135(20):1811-1822. 1995

Schulz V, Hübner WD, Ploch M. Klinische Studien mit Psycho-Phytopharmaka. In: *ZPT;* 18(3):141-154. 1997

Schulz H, Jobert M & Hubner WD. The quantitative EEG as a screening instrument to identify sedative effects of single doses of plant extracts in comparison with diazepam. *Phytomedicine*; 5(6):449-458. 1998

Shi W & Gould MN. Induction of differentiation in neuro-2A cells by the monotropene perillyl alcohol. *Cancer Lett*; 1-6. 1995

Stayrook KR, McKinzie JH, Burke YD et al. Induction of the apoptosis-promoting protein Bak by perillyl alcohol in pancreatic ductal adenocarcinoma relative to untransformed ductal epithelial cells. *Carcinogenesis*; 18:1655-1658. 1997

Vigushin DM, Poon GK, Boddy A et al. Phase 1 and pharmacokinetic study of d-limonene in patients with advanced cancer. *Cancer Chemother Pharmacol*; 42:111-117. 1998

Yamada K, Mimaki Y & Sashida Y. Anticonvulsant effects of inhaling lavender oil vapour. *Biol Pharm Bull*; 17:359-360. 1994

English Plantain

Plantago lanceolata

DESCRIPTION

Medicinal Parts: The medicinal parts are the dried leaves, the dried herb, and the fresh plant.

Flower and Fruit: The globular or shortly cylindrical spikes are on erect or ascending, 5-grooved, appressed pubescent peduncles. The flowers are small, almost colorless behind scarious, narrow-acuminate bracts. The scarious calyx is deeply divided into 4 parts and has a cylindrical tube and a margin with 4 ovate tips. There are 4 long stamens with yellowish-white filaments and anthers and 1 superior ovary. The fruit is a bivalvular, 3 to 4 mm long capsule. The seeds are oblong, 2 mm long and blackish.

Leaves, Stem, and Root: The plant is perennial and grows from 5 to 50 cm high. It has a very fibrous root. All the leaves are in basal rosettes and are lanceolate or linear-lanceolate, deeply 3 to 5 ribbed, entire-margined or short-dentate.

Habitat: The plant is widespread in the cool temperate regions of the world.

Production: English Plantain herb consists of the fresh or dried above-ground parts of *Plantago lanceolata*, harvested at flowering season (May to September) and dried quickly at 40 to 50° C.

Not to be Confused With: the similar *Digitalis lanata* leaves.

Other Names: Buckhorn, Chimney-Sweeps, Headsman, Narrow-Leaved Plantain, Ribgrass, Ribwort, Ripplegrass, Soldier's Herb

ACTIONS AND PHARMACOLOGY

COMPOUNDS

Iridoide monoterpenes (2-3%): chief components are aucubin (rhinantin) and catalpol as well as asperuloside

Mucilages (2-6%): glucomannans, arabinogalactane, rhamnogalacturonane

Flavonoids: including among other chief components apigenine-6,8-diglucoside, luteolin-7-glucuronide

Caffeic acid esters: chlorogenic acid, neochlorogenic acid, acteoside (verbascoside)

Tannins

Hydroxycoumarins: aesculetin

Saponins (traces)

Silicic acid

EFFECTS

Liquid extract and the pressed juice of fresh Plantain herb have a proven bactericidal effect. The aucubigenin (hydrolised acubin) and an antimicrobial saponin are believed to be responsible for the antibacterial effect. In addition, acceleration of blood clotting has been demonstrated and a possible epithelization effect has been mentioned. The herb has also shown positive effects in respiratory tract infections.

INDICATIONS AND USAGE

Approved by Commission E:

- Common cold
- Cough/bronchitis
- Fevers and colds
- Inflammation of the mouth and pharynx
- Inflammation of the skin

Unproven Uses: In folk medicine, the pressed juice of English Plantain is used internally for conditions of the respiratory tract, cystitis, enuresis, liver disease, stomach cramps, diarrhea, and as a diuretic.

Externally the plant is used for wounds, furuncles, conjunctivitis, and as a hemostyptic.

PRECAUTIONS AND ADVERSE REACTIONS

No health hazards or side effects are known in conjunction with the proper administration of designated therapeutic dosages.

DOSAGE

Mode of Administration: As a comminuted herb and other galenic preparations for internal and external use. It is available as macerations, liquid extracts, lozenges, syrup, and pressed juice of the fresh plant. The drug is available in many standardized preparations of antitussives and expectorants.

Preparation: To make an infusion, pour boiling water over 2 to 4 g cut drug (or put in cold water brought to a boil) and strain after 10 minutes (1 teaspoonful = approximately 0.7 g drug).

Daily Dosage: The average daily dose is 3 to 6 g of herb.

Tea—1 cup of freshly made tea to be drunk several times a day.

LITERATURE

Davini E, The quantitative isolation and antimicrobial activity of aglycone of aucubin. In: *PH* 25:2420. 1986.

Diaz LM, Souto S, Concheiro A, Gomez-Amoza JL, Martinez-Pacheco R. Eudragit RS as major excipient in controlled release tablets for plant dry extracts. *Pharmazie* 52 (6); 466-470. 1997

Handjieva N, Saadi H, Evstatieva L. Iridoid Glucosides from *Plantago altissima L., Plantago lanceolata L., Plantago atrata Hoppe* and *Plantago argentea Chaix.. Z Naturforsch.* 46c; 963-965.(1991

Koedam A, Plantago - history and use. In: *Pharm Weekbl* 112(10):246-252. 1977.

Kraft K. Therapeutisches Profil eines Spitzwegerichkraut-Fluidextraktes bei akuten respiratorischen Erkrankungen im Kindes- und Erwachsenenalter. in: Phytopharmaka III - Forschg. *Und klin. Anwend.* 199-208. 1997

Kurzmann M, Kreis W. A rapid and semiquantitative method for the simultaneous determination of enzyme activities from glycosidases, esterases, peptidases and phosphatases in herbal drugs and other drug preparations using the API ZYM system. Abstraktband 45.*Ann.Congr.Soc.M*

Murai M et al., Phenylethanoids in the herb of Planatago lanceolata and inhibitory effects on arachidonic acid-induced mouse ear edema. In: *PM* 61(5):479-480. 1995.

Wunderer H, Zentral und peripher wirksame Antitussiva: eine kritische Übersicht. In: *PZ* 142(11):847-852. 1997.

Ephedra sinica

See Ma-Huang

Epigae repens

See Trailing Arbutus

Epilobium species

See Willow Herb

Equisetum arvense

See Horsetail

Ergot

Claviceps purpurea

DESCRIPTION

Medicinal Parts: The medicinal part of the fungus is the sclerotium, which grows on rye plants and is later dried.

Flower and Fruit: Ergot is a permanent form of a fungus that is a parasite on ripening rye, wheat, and other grasses. It is black, hard, and much larger than the grains of rye. The cycle of the fungus begins with the infection of the ovary by an ascospore. The spore, usually deposited by a visiting insect, germinates on the stigma, and the hyphae grows down into the ovary where it appropriates food destined for the grain. When the ovary has been completely destroyed, the mycelium grows. Horizontal walls are formed and fat vacuoles become visible. The hyphae of the skin layer store purple pigment three weeks after the infection a long, curved, black sclerotium develops. It reaches a length of up to 8 cm and bears minute condia, which are made up of the remains of the ovary and the style embedded into the loose mycelium. The sclerotium usually falls to the ground before harvest and survives the winter. In the spring, 1 to 3 cm long red-stemmed, capitulalike, pink fruiting bodies grow out of it, which in turn produce 50 to 70 + 1 mm long threadlike ascospores.

Habitat: Claviceps purpurea grows as a parasite on rye (occasionally on other grasses), and is found in all areas of the world where rye is cultivated.

Production: Ergot consists of the sclerotium of *Claviceps purpurea*, a parasitic fungus harvested after it has grown on cultivated rye.

Other Names: Cockspur Rye, Hornseed, Mother of Rye, Smut Rye, Spurred Rye

ACTIONS AND PHARMACOLOGY

COMPOUNDS

Indole alkaloids (ergot alkaloids, varying by variety of ergot)

Chief alkaloid of the lysergic acid amide type: ergometrine (ergobasine) *Chief alkaloid of the lysergic acid ergopeptine type:* ergotamine, ergovaline, ergosine, ergocristine, ergocornine, alpha- and beta-ergocryptine, further alkaloids of the clavine type: including among others agroclavine, elymoclavine, festuclavine

Peptide alkaloids (ergopeptine group): especially ergotamine, as well as ergovaline, ergosine, ergocristine, ergocornine, alpha- and beta-ergocryptine

Xanthone derivatives (ergochromes): including, among others, secalonic acid A to C, ergoflavin

Anthracene derivatives: including, among others, clavorubine, endocrocine

Amines: including, among others, trimethylamine, methylamine

Fatty oil

EFFECTS

The drug contains ergoline alkaloids of which only ergometrin and ergopeptine have a therapeutic and toxic effect. The action of ergot is traceable to its stimulation of the smooth musculature. However, therapeutic use cannot be recommended because of the risks involved.

INDICATIONS AND USAGE

Unproven Uses: Although the risk involved is too high to recommend therapeutic use, ergot and ergot preparations were previously used in gynecology and obstetrics. Uses included hemorrhages, climacteric hemorrhages, menorrhagia and metrorrhagia, before and after miscarriage, for removal of the placenta and shortening of the afterbirth period, for atonia of the uterus, and also for migraine.

Homeopathic Uses: Uses in homeopathy include uterine and muscle spasm, convulsions, paralysis, circulatory problems accompanying arterial disease, and a tendency to bleed. Efficacy has not been proved.

CONTRAINDICATIONS

Ergot is now contraindicated for all therapeutic use, but especially in the presence of peripheral blood flow disorders such as Raynaud's disease, Thrombangitis obliterans, severe arteriosclerotic vascular changes, liver function disorders, severe coronary insufficiency, kidney damage, pregnancy, nursing, infectious diseases, sepsis, hypertonia, and severe hypotonia.

PRECAUTIONS AND ADVERSE REACTIONS

No health hazards are known in conjunction with the proper administration of designated therapeutic dosages, but therapeutic use is not recommended because of the many side effects. Among side effects that may occur are queasiness, vomiting, feeling of weakness in the legs, muscle pain, numbness in the fingers, angina complaints, tachycardia or bradycardia, localized edema, and itching.

OVERDOSAGE

Overdosage or long-term administration can lead to thrombosis, damage to the vessels of the retina (combined with optic atrophy), gangrene of the extremities, hemiplagia, and convulsions.

Symptoms of acute poisonings include queasiness, vomiting, diarrhea, thirst, skin coolness, itching of the skin, rapid and weak pulse, paresthesia, numbness of the extremities, confusion, or unconsciousness.

Chronic poisonings appear as:

Ergotismus gangrenosus: characterized by painful arterial blood flow disorders of the extremities with dry gangrene, angina complaints, field of vision losses, and aphasias.

Ergotismus convulsivus: characterized by muscle twitching, followed by clonic spasm, and ultimately tonic spasms, hemiplagia, loss of consciousness, and death.

Drug overdose is managed by gastrointestinal emptying through inducement of vomiting and gastric lavage with burgundy-colored potassium permanganate solution, sodium sulfate. That is followed by installation of activated charcoal and shock prophylaxis (quiet and warmth). The therapy for poisonings consists of treating angiospasms with Nitrolingual-spray and vascular massage, sedatives for spasm (diazepam or chloral hydrate), administration of blocking agents, electrolyte substitution and treating possible cases of acidosis with sodium bicarbonate infusions. Intubation and oxygen respiration may also be necessary.

DOSAGE

Homeopathic Dosage: 5 drops, 1 tablet, 10 globules every 30 to 60 minutes (acute) or 1 to 3 times a day (chronic); parenterally: 1 to 2 mL sc: acute: 3 times daily; chronic: once a day (HAB1).

Storage: Ergot must be stored in tightly sealed containers and kept in a cool place, protected from light. The powdered form should not be stored.

LITERATURE

Cvak L et al. Ergoladinine, an Ergot Alkaloid. *Phytochemistry* 42 (1); 231-233. 1996

Gaberc-Porekar V, Didek-Brumec M, Socic H. Accumulation of anthranilic acid by *Claviceps purpurea* recombinant strains. *Acta Pharm.* 43; 91-98. 1993

Hänsel R, Keller K, Rimpler H, Schneider G (Hrsg.), Hagers Handbuch der Pharmazeutischen Praxis, 5. Aufl., Bde 4-6 (Drogen): Springer Verlag Berlin, Heidelberg, New York, 1992-1994.

Kobel H, Sanglier JJ, Biotechnology 4:569-609. 1986.

Lewin L, Gifte und Vergiftungen, 6. Aufl., Nachdruck, Haug Verlag, Heidelberg 1992.

Madaus G, Lehrbuch der Biologischen Arzneimittel, Bde 1-3, Nachdruck, Georg Olms Verlag Hildesheim 1979.

Milhahn HC et al., Contributions to the dissociation between antineoplastic and mutagenic activities of the ergot minor alkaloid festucalavine by substitution at C-2. In: PM 59(7):A&83. 1993.

Perellino NC, et al., Identification of ergobine, a new natural peptide ergot alkaloid. In: *JNP* 56(4):489-493. 1993.

Pertz H, Naturally occuring clavines: Antagonism/partial agonism at 5-HT2alpha receptors and antagonism at alpha1-adrenoceptors in blood vessel. In: *PM* 62(5)387-392. 1996.

Teuscher E, Lindequist U, Biogene Gifte - Biologie, Chemie, Pharmakologie, 2. Aufl., Fischer Verlag Stuttgart 1994.

Teuscher E, Biogene Arzneimittel, 5. Aufl., Wiss. Verlagsges. Stuttgart 1997.

Vom Ergolin-Pharmakophor zu selektiven Arzneistoffen. In: DAZ 132(23):1235. 1992.

Wagner H, Wiesenauer M, Phytotherapie. Phytopharmaka und pflanzliche Homöopathika, Fischer-Verlag, Stuttgart, Jena, New York 1995.

Wang BH, Polya GM, The fungal teratogen secalonic acid D is an inhibitor of protein kinase C and of cyclic AMP-dependent protein kinase. In: PM 62(2):111-114. 1997.

Wenzlaff H, Dihydroergotamin. In: DAZ 136(26):2179-2181. 1996.

Erigeron canadensis

See Canadian Fleabane

Eriodictyon californicum

See Yerba Santa

Eryngium campestre

See Eryngo

Eryngo

Eryngium campestre

DESCRIPTION

Medicinal Parts: The medicinal parts are the dried leaves, dried flowers, and dried roots.

Flower and Fruit: The plant bears small terminal cymes on oval to globular capitula on sweeping inflorescences. The linear-lanceolate to awl-shaped bracts terminate in sharp thorns. The sepals are lanceolate, terminate in thorny tips and are twice as long as the white or gray-green petals. The fruit is compressed obovate with lanceolate, pointed scales.

Leaves, Stem, and Root: The plant is 15 to 60 cm high, perennial, with a whitish or yellow-green color. The bifurcated stem is erect, thick, grooved, and spare. The stem forms a round bush with the branches. The leaves are tough, short-petioled, or sessile. The upper leaves are clasping, double pinnatesect and thorny dentate. The root is cylindrical, thick, brown and woody.

Characteristics: The root is spicy.

Habitat: The plant grows in most parts of Europe and northern Africa and has been introduced into North America.

Production: Eryngo root is the root of *Eryngium campestre*, which is gathered and dried in the spring and autumn. It is gathered in uncultivated regions. The roots are halved and air-dried. Eryngo herb is the dried leaves and blossoms of *Eryngium campestre*.

Other Names: Eringo, Sea Holly, Sea Holme, Sea Hulver

ACTIONS AND PHARMACOLOGY

COMPOUNDS: ERYNGO ROOT

Triterpene saponins

Furanocoumarins

Pyranocoumarins: including egelinol and its angeloyl-, senecionyl- or benzyl-esters agasyllin, grandivetin and egelinol benzoate

Monoterpene glycosides of the cyclohexenol type: including 3-(beta-D-glucosyloxymethyl)-2,4,4-trimethyl-2,5-cyclohexadien-1-one

Caffeic acid ester: chlorogenic acid, rosmarinic acid

Oligosaccharides: 1-kestose

EFFECTS: ERYNGO ROOT

The root is said to be mildly expectorant and spasmolytic; however, there is no scientific evidence to support this.

COMPOUNDS: ERYNGO HERB

Triterpene saponins

Caffeic acid ester: chlorogenic acid, rosmarinic acid

Flavonoids

EFFECTS: ERYNGO HERB

The herb is said to be a mild diuretic and an expectorant; however, there is no scientific evidence to support this.

INDICATIONS AND USAGE

ERYNGO ROOT

Unproven Uses: The root is used in the treatment of bladder and kidney stones, renal colic, kidney and urinary tract inflammation, urinary retention, and edema. It is also used for coughs, bronchitis, skin disorders, and respiratory disorders. It also used to aid weaning.

ERYNGO HERB

Unproven Uses: The herb is used in the treatment of urinary tract infections and as an adjuvant to treat inflammation of the efferent urinary tract, prostatitis, and bronchial catarrh.

PRECAUTIONS AND ADVERSE REACTIONS

ERYNGO ROOT AND HERB

Health risks or side effects following the proper administration of designated therapeutic dosages are not recorded.

DOSAGE

ERYNGO ROOT

Mode of Administration: The comminuted root is contained in tea mixtures, extracts, decoctions, liquids and tinctures.

Preparation: To make a tea, use 1 level teaspoonful of the ground root per cup of boiling water (30 to 40 g per liter boiling water). Allow to steep until cold. To make a decoction, boil 4 teaspoonfuls of the ground root in 1 liter of water for 10 minutes and allow to steep for 15 minutes. The tincture is prepared by soaking 20 gm ground drug in 80 g of 60% alcohol for 10 days.

Daily Dosage: The daily dosage is 3 to 4 cups of the tea; 2 to 3 cups of the decoction; 50 to 60 drops of the tincture in 3 or 4 divided doses; or 2 to 3 g of the liquid extract.

ERYNGO HERB

Mode of Administration: The herb is administered as an extract and in homeopathic dilutions (from *E. yuccifolium*).

LITERATURE

Bhargava SK, Dixit VP, (1985) Plant Med Phytother 19(1):29.

Erdelmeier CAJ, Sticher O, (1985) Planta Med 51(5):407.

Gracza L et al., (1985) Arch Pharm 312(12):1090.

Hänsel R, Keller K, Rimpler H, Schneider G (Hrsg.), Hagers Handbuch der Pharmazeutischen Praxis, 5. Aufl., Bde 4-6 (Drogen), Springer Verlag Berlin, Heidelberg, New York, 1992-1994.

Hiller K, In "The Biology and Chemistry of the Umbelliferae". Ed. V. N. Heywood, Academic Press London 1971.

Hiller K, Linzer B, PA 22:321. 1967.

Kartnig T, Wolf J, Flavonoide aus den oberirdischen Teilen von Eryngium campestre. In: PM 59(3):285. 1993.

Lisciani R et al., (1984) J Ethnopharmacol 12(39):263.

Madaus G, Lehrbuch der Biologischen Arzneimittel, Bde 1-3, Nachdruck, Georg Olms Verlag Hildesheim 1979.

Steinegger E, Hänsel R, Pharmakognosie, 5. Aufl., Springer Verlag Heidelberg 1992.

Erysimum diffusum

See Grey Wallflower

Erythronium americanum

See American Adder's Tongue

Erythroxylum coca

See Coca

Eschscholtzia californica

See California Poppy

Eucalyptus

Eucalyptus globulus

DESCRIPTION

Medicinal Parts: The medicinal parts are the oil extracted from the fresh leaves and branch tips as well as the dried leaves.

Flower and Fruit: The flowers are solitary on short pedicles. They have a somewhat pointed, low operculum stretching over the surface of the stamens. There are no sepals, but there are numerous long inward-turning stamens, which open along the whole length in 2 splits. The fruit is 10 to 15 by 15 to 30 mm and is a depressed-globose, somewhat tapering toward the base, with 4 main ribs.

Leaves, Stem, and Root: Eucalyptus is a deciduous tree up to 40 m tall with silver-gray bark, which has scattered warts. The trunk is twisted. The juvenile leaves are 7 to 16 by 4 to 9 cm, ovate to broadly lanceolate, cordate, very glaucous. The mature leaves are 10 to 13 by 3 to 4 cm, lanceolate to falcate-lanceolate, acuminate, asymmetrical rounded, and glossy green.

Habitat: Eucalyptus is indigenous to Australia and Tasmania. It is cultivated today in some subtropical regions of southern Europe, Africa, Asia, and America.

Production: Eucalyptus oil consists of the volatile oil from various cineol-rich species of Eucalyptus, such as *Eucalyptus globulus, Eucalyptus fructicetorum* (syn. *Eucalyptus polybractea*) and/or *Eucalyptus smithii.* The oil is obtained by steam distillation, followed by rectification of the fresh leaves and branch tops. Eucalyptus leaf consists of the dried, mature leaves from older trees of *Eucalyptus globulus*. To harvest eucalyptus, the trees are cut down; drying takes place in the shade.

Not To Be Confused With: Camphor oil and byproducts of turpentine manufacture; the oil is also blended with other expensive oils, such as rosemary and thyme. The properties of Eucalyptus leaves vary from species to species.

Other Names: Blue Gum, Fever Tree, Gum Tree, Red Gum, Stringy Bark Tree

ACTIONS AND PHARMACOLOGY

EFFECTS: GENERAL:

Eucalyptus and its oil have shown antibiotic (antibacterial, antifungal, insecticidal, and anticaries) actions in treatment of wounds, contaminated clothing or blankets, and skin. Although recommended as a decongestant and analgesic, it has not been shown to be effective. It is used primarily for respiratory tract disorders such as colds and bronchitis. Eucalyptus has also demonstrated expectorant activity and possibly some antioxidant, antineoplastic, and anti-inflammatory effects (Yun et al, 2000; Takasaki et al, 2000; Grassmann et al, 2000). Antidiabetic activity has been reported in animals (Gray & Flatt, 1998).

COMPOUNDS: EUCALYPTUS OIL

Chief constituent of the rectified volatile oil: 1,8-cineol (over 80%), furthermore p-cymene, alpha-pinenes, limonene, geraniol, camphene

EFFECTS: EUCALYPTUS OIL

Some of the subsequent properties mentioned refer to isolated cineole. As the standardized commodity, the drug contains 80 to 90% cineole.

In vitro, Eucalyptus oil has an antibacterial (Osawa et al, 1995) and fungicidal effect. The drug inhibits prostaglandin biosynthesis and has a mild hyperemic, expectorant, and secretolytic motor effect when used topically. In animal experiments Eucalyptus was demonstrably cough relieving and displayed a surfactant effect. In vitro, the oil was enzyme inducing and improved pulmonary compliance. It is secretolytic, expectorant, mildly antispasmodic, and a mild local hyperemic.

Antibacterial Effects: Eucalyptus oil was shown to have antibacterial activity when tested against gram-negative bacteria (Harkenthal et al, 1999). Eucalyptus oil (from *Eucalyptus citriodora*) was found to be bactericidal against Escherichia coli (Pattnaik et al, 1995). Eucalyptus oil was shown to have antibacterial activity when tested against gram-negative bacteria using a broth microdilution method. The organisms tested were *Citrobacter freundii, Enterobacter aerogenes, Escherichia coli, Klebsiella pneumoniae, Proteus mirabilis, Pseudomonas aeruginosa, Salmonella cholerae-suis,* and Shigella flexneri (Harkenthal et al, 1999).

Eucalyptus oil was tested and found to possess antifungal properties against 11 of 12 fungi, including 3 that were yeast-like and 9 filamentous species. The minimum inhibitory concentration (MIC) for each species was determined using the broth/agar dilution method. The fungal species used were *Alternaria citrii, Aspergillus fumigatus, Candida albicans, Cryptococcus neoformans, Fusarium oxysporum, Fusarium solani, Helminthosporium compactum, Macrophomina phaseolina, Sclerotium rolfsii, Sporothrix schenkii,* and *Trichophyton mentagrophytes*. Only *Macrophomina phaseolina* was not inhibited by the Eucalyptus oil. The MIC concentrations ranged from 0.25 mcL/mL for *T mentagrophytes* to 10 mcL/mL for *H compactum* (Pattnaik et al, 1996).

Eucalyptus oil (from *Eucalyptus citriodora*) was found to be bactericidal against *Escherichia coli* strain SP-11 at a concentration of 1.66 mcL/mL. The bactericidal effect was noted at both 4° and 37° C. The Eucalyptus oil appeared to produce immediate and irreversible damage to the bacterial cells, since no viable cells were found even if the Eucalyptus oil/bacteria mixture was immediately diluted (Pattnaik et al, 1995).

Anti-inflammatory Effects: During inflammation biochemical reactions generate reactive oxygen species. Eucalyptus oil interacts with OH-radicals and interferes with leukocyte activation. Eucalyptus oil, starting at a concentration of 0.1%, inhibited ethene formation from KMB (alpha-keto-gamma-methiol-butyric acid) driven by the Fenton oxidant (iron 2 and hydrogen peroxide), but did not prevent KMB fragmentation by SIN-1 (3-morpholinosydnonimine). At a concentration of 0.1% or above, ethene formation was strongly inhibited, and at 9.25% of the oil, ACC (1-aminocyclopropane-1- carboxylic acid) fragmentation was almost completely inhibited (Grassmann et al, 2000).

Antioxidant Effects: Twelve agents (including taxifolin, rhamnetin, rhamnazin, quercetin, and eriodictyol) isolated from the stem bark of *Eucalyptus globulus* were shown to have antioxidant capabilities. The listed agents had greater antioxidant activity than vitamin E (IC of 1 mcg/L)(Yun et al, 2000).

Effects Against Mites: Eucalyptus oil washing destroyed over 99% of blankets infested with mites. Mite-infested blankets were treated with a solution containing 100 mL of Eucalyptus oil, 25 mL of a detergent, and 50 liters of warm water (30° C). The percentage of mites that survived on the Eucalyptuss treated blankets was 0.6%, while 97.6% survived after the control washings (Tovey & McDonald, 1997).

COMPOUNDS: EUCALYPTUS LEAF

Volatile oil: chief constituent 1,8-cineol (45-75%), in additions myrtenol, alpha-pinenes, beta-pinenes, pinocarvon, gamma-terpenes, aliphatic aldehydes (butyr-, capron-, valerenaldehyde)

Euglobale: macrocarpale (with acylphloroglucinol-monoterpene or else sesquiterpene- parent substances)

Flavonoids: rutin, hyperoside, quercitrin

EFFECTS: EUCALYPTUS LEAF

The euglobulin is said to have an anti-inflammatory and antiproliferative effect in animal experiments and inhibits in vitro TPA-induced EBV-EA activity.

CLINICAL TRIALS

Cancer

Euglobal G1, derived from *Eucalyptus grandis* leaves, inhibited carcinogenesis in the test of SENCAR mouse skin tumors induced by 7,12-dimethylbenz(a)anthracene (DMBA) (initiator) and fumonisin-B1 (promoter). Euglobal G1 also inhibited tumor promotion on the mouse pulmonary tumor using 4-nitroquinoline-N- oxide (4-DQO) as the initiator, and glycerol as the promoter. In the control group, 86.6% had tumors, while in the euglobal-G1 group 46.6% had tumors (Takasaki et al, 2000).

Dental plaque

A eucalyptus-containing chewing gum reduced plaque formation when compared with placebo in a double-blind, cross-over study. The plaque scores for those using the Eucalyptus gum were significantly less ($p<0.01$) than for those using the control gum (Sato et al, 1998).

Fungal infection

Fifty patients with tinea pedis, tinea corporis, or tinea cruris, diagnosed using KOH-positive results, were treated with a 1% Eucalyptus oil ointment for one week. At the end of the second week, all patients were KOH-negative. The organisms tested were *E floccosum, M audouinii, M canis, M nanum, M gypseum, T mentagrophytes, T rubrum, T tonsurans,* and *T violaceum*. Concentrations of 0.8 mcL/mL was fungicidal for all organisms, 0.2 mcg/mL was fungistatic for all but *E floccosum* and *M audoouinii* (Shahi et al, 2000).

Headache

Headache patients treated with a combination of Eucalyptus oil, peppermint oil, and ethanol experienced improved cognitive performance and a muscle and mental relaxing effect, but did not have significant changes in pain sensitivity. The preparations were applied to forehead and temples using a small sponge (Goebel et al, 1994).

Head and neck ulcers

Twice-daily application of Eucalyptus-based blends of antibacterial essential oils was tested in 30 patients for its value as an additive therapy in local treatments of incurable and malodorous neoplastic ulcers of the head and neck. Patients were treated with a standard course of antibiotics. The blend demonstrated antibacterial and anti-inflammatory effects as well as, in some cases, a small degree of re-epithelization of neoplastic facial ulcers as evidenced by photographic images in this journal article. Benefits also included complete resolution of foul smell by day 3 or 4, significantly improved quality of life due to odor reduction (thereby improving social interactions), and pain relief in some cases. No allergic reactions were observed. (Warnke et al, 2006)

Insect repellant

A lemon Eucalyptus extract (Citrodiol) has previously shown effectiveness in repelling mosquitoes, midges, and stable flies. In the present prospective, crossover field trial, 111 healthy volunteers living in two highly tick-infected areas (*Ixodes ricinus*) were randomly divided into 2 groups. One group applied the Citrodiol spray daily to the lower extremities for 2 weeks; the other group was told not to apply anything. After 2 weeks, the instructions to each group were reversed. Based on evidence written in daily diaries on number and location of ticks, the median number of reported attached ticks decreased to 0.5 from 1.5 during the weeks of Citrodiol use (Gardulf et al, 2004).

Non-purulent rhinositis

Timely treatment with Cineole from Eucalyptus was shown to be effective and safe for acute non-purulent rhinositis in a prospective, randomized, double-blind, and placebo-controlled study in 152 patients. The treatment dosage was 100 mg capsules Cineole three times daily. Differences between the Cineole and placebo groups in terms of symptom scores were clinically relevant and statistically significant after 4 and 7 days (mean values for the symptoms-sum-scores in the Cineole group were 6.9 +/- 2.4 after 4 days and 3.0 +/- 2.8 after 7 days; in the placebo group, 2.2 +/- 2.5 after 4 days and 9.2 +/- 3.0 after 7 days). In conjunction with a decrease in symptom score were lessened headache on bending, sensitivity of pressure points of trigeminal nerve, impairment of general condition, frontal headache, rhinological secretion, and nasal obstruction. Two Cineole-treated patients experienced side effects: heartburn and exanthema (Kehrl et al, 2004).

INDICATIONS AND USAGE

EUCALYPTUS OIL

Approved by Commission E:

- Cough/bronchitis
- Rheumatism

Eucalyptus oil is used internally and externally for catarrh of the respiratory tract and externally for rheumatic complaints.

Unproven Uses: Eucalyptus is primarily used for respiratory conditions including cough suppression, nasal stuffiness, asthma, bronchitis, and emphysema. It is also used as an antiseptic and is found in toothpaste and mouthwash. Eucalyptus is commonly used as an insect repellant, and has been used topically for wounds, burns, ulcers, and rheumatic complaints

EUCALYPTUS LEAF

Approved by Commission E:

- Cough/bronchitis

Eucalyptus leaf is used internally as a catarrh of the respiratory tract.

Unproven Uses: In folk medicine, it is used internally for the treatment of bladder diseases, asthma, fever, flu, whooping cough, liver and gallbladder complaints, loss of appetite and diabetes. It is used externally for wounds, acne, poorly healing ulcers, stomatitis, bleeding gums, pain and rheumatism, neuralgia, gonorrhea and as a gastrointestinal remedy.

CONTRAINDICATIONS

Contraindications for Eucalyptus include hypersensitivity to Eucalyptus or eucalyptol, inflammatory diseases of the gastrointestinal tract or the bile ducts, and serious liver disease.

Pediatrics: Not for use on the face or nose of infants and young children as it may produce laryngeal spasms and subsequent respiratory arrest.

PRECAUTIONS AND ADVERSE REACTIONS

Nausea, vomiting, a burning epigastric pain, esophagitis, and diarrhea may occur occasionally or with concentrated preparations. Erythema, contact urticaria, and pruritus, followed by a micropapular rash, have occurred uncommonly. The use of Eucalyptus may interfere with hypoglycemic control in diabetics. Hypoglycemic activity has been demonstrated in animals, but not in humans. Eucalyptus oil may reduce the effectiveness of drugs metabolized by hepatic microsomal enzymes.

Eucalyptus vapors have been shown to transmit Aspergillus fungus. Proof was demonstrated by observing Aspergillus spores in sputum samples of persons who inhaled the oil (Whitman & Ghazizadeh, 1994).

Hypersensitivity: Topical administration may result in systemic symptoms. One such case involved a 6-year-old with widespread pruritic urticaria who was treated with a folk remedy containing apple cider, vinegar, olive oil, methylated spirits (without menthol), and Eucalyptus oil. The percentage of Eucalyptus oil in the preparation was 7.7%. The remedy was used generally over the entire rash, then a plastic wrap occlusive dressing applied to the truck and limbs. About 400 mL of the solution was applied at each dressing and the dressings were changed every 2 to 4 hours. Two days prior to seeing the dermatologist, the Eucalyptus oil concentration was doubled. The patient developed slurred speech, ataxia, muscle weakness, and finally unconsciousness. Symptoms resolved 6 hours after the removal of the home remedy (Darben et al, 1998).

DRUG INTERACTIONS

MODERATE RISK

Antidiabetic agents: Concurrent use may result in increased risk of hypoglycemia. *Clinical management:* If used together, monitor blood glucose levels and the signs and symptoms of hypoglycemia regularly.

Barbiturates: Concurrent use may result in decreased effectiveness of barbiturates. *Clinical management:* Concomitant use is not recommended. Patients previously on barbiturates who experience a decreased effect should be questioned about the use of Eucalyptus.

POTENTIAL INTERACTIONS

Hepatotoxic Agents: A theoretical interaction has been proposed, in which Eucalyptus may potentiate the toxicity of plants containing pyrrolizidine alkaloids (most notably, comfrey, but also borage, coltsfoot, hound's tooth), which can cause liver damage (White et al, 1983). *Clinical Management*: Concomitant use should be avoided

OVERDOSAGE

EUCALYPTUS OIL

Overdoses can lead to life-threatening poisonings. Severe poisonings are possible for children after a few drops; poisonings have been known in adults with 4 to 5 mL. Symptoms include drop in blood pressure, circulatory disorders, collapse, and asphyxiation. Because of the danger of aspiration, vomiting should not be induced. Following the administration of activated charcoal, therapy consists of diazepam for spasms, atropine for colic, electrolyte replenishment and sodium bicarbonate infusions for any acidosis that may arise. Intubation and oxygen respiration may also be necessary.

DOSAGE

EUCALYPTUS OIL

Mode of Administration: Essential oil and other galenic preparations are available for internal and external application.

Preparation: 1,8-cineole is recovered through a renewed fractional distillation of the oil.

Daily Dosage: For internal use, the average daily dose is 0.3 to 0.6 g Eucalyptus oil.

Inhalation: 2 to 3 drops in boiling water, inhale the steam (single dose: 0.2 g corresponding to 10 drops). Oil: 3 to 6 drops added in 150 ml water, to be taken several times a day.

When used externally, the concentration is 5 to 20% essential oil, in oil and semi-solid preparations and 5 to 10% essential oil, in aqueous-alcoholic preparations. If the essential oil is used, several drops may be rubbed into the skin.

Storage: Eucalyptus must be kept in appropriate, tightly sealed containers protected from light; different consignments must be stored separately.

EUCALYPTUS LEAF

Mode of Administration: Eucalyptus leaf is administered as the comminuted leaf for infusions and other galenic preparations for internal and external application. The drug may also be administered by inhalation.

Preparations:

Eucalyptus tincture: 1:5 70% ethanol (V/V)

Eucalyptus liquid extract: 60% 1:1

Eucalyptus syrup: pour 1500 mL on 100 g cut drug and leave to draw for 6 hours and strain. 180 g sugar is added to 100 mL infusion, brought to a simmer and filtered.

Tea: pour boiling water over 1.5 to 2 g of the finely cut drug, cover and leave to draw for 5 to 10 minutes, strain.

Daily Dosage: The average daily dose is 4 to 6 g of drug, divided up every 3 to 4 hours. Single dose: 1.5 g several times a day

The average dose for the tincture is 3 to 4 g.

Eucalyptus tea: 1 cup up to 3 times a day.

Eucalyptus syrup: 2 to 5 dessertspoons daily.

Eucalyptus powder: daily dose 4 to 16 g; divided over 3 to 4 hours.

Storage: Eucalyptus must be kept in appropriate, tightly-sealed, non-synthetic containers; different consignments must be stored separately.

LITERATURE

Anon. Phytotherapie:Pflanzliche Antirheumatika - was bringen sie? In: *DAZ;* 136(45):4012-4015. 1996

Anpalahan M & Le Couteur DG. Deliberate self-poisoning with eucalyptus oil in an elderly woman. *Aust N Z J Med*; 28:58. 1998

Boland B. In: Eucalyptus leaf oils. Boland DJ, Brophy JJ, House APN (Eds.). Inkata Press, Melbourne, XII + 252 pp. 1992.

Boland DJ, Brophy JJ, House APN. Eucalyptus leave oils. In: Inkata Press Melbourne. 1991

Boukef K, et al. *Plant Med Phytother;* 10:24, 30:119. 1976

Burrow A, Eccles R, Jones AS. The effects of camphor, eucalyptus and menthol vapor on nasal resistance to airflow and nasal sensation. *Acta Otolaryng* (Stockholm); 96(1-2):157-161. 1983

Darben T, Cominos B & Lee CT. Topical eucalyptus oil poisoning. *Aust J Dermatol*; 39(4):265-267. 1998

Day LM, Ozanne-Smith J, Parsons B et al. Eucalyptus oil poisoning among children: mechanisms of access and the potential for prevention. *Aust N Z J Public Health*; 21:297-302. 1997

Fox N. Effect of Camphor, Eucalyptol and Menthol on the vascular state of the mucos membrane. *Arch Otolaryngol;* 6:112-122. 1977

Gardulf A, Wohlfart I, Gustafson R. A prospective crosss-over field trial shows protection of lemon eucalyptus against tick bites. *J Med Entomol*; 41(6):1064-1067. 2004.

Göbel H, Schmidt G. Effekt von Pfefferminz- und Eukalyptusölpräparationen in experimentellen *Kopfschmerzmodellen. Z Phytother;* 16:23-33. 1995a

Göbel H, Schmidt G, Dworschak M, Stolze H, Heuss D. Essential plant oils and headache mechanisms. *Phytomedicine;* 2: 93-102. 1995

Göbel H, Schmidt G, Dworschak M, Stolze H, Heuss D. Essential plant oils and headache mechanisms. *Phytomedicine;* 2: 93-103. 1995.

Göbel H, Schmidt G, Soyka D. Effect of peppermint and eucalyptus oil preparations on neurophysiological and experimental algesimetric headache parameters. *Cephalalgia;* 14: 228-234. 1994

Göbel H, Stolze H, Dworschak M, Heinze A. Oleum menthae piperitae, Wirkmechanismen und klinische Effektivität bei Kopfschmerz vom Spannungstyp. In: Loew D, Rietbrock N (Hrsg) Phytopharmaka in Forschung und klinischer Anwendung. Steinkopff Verlag, Darmstadt, S. 177-184. 1995

Gräfe AK. Besonderheiten der Arzneimitteltherapie im Säuglings- und Kindesalter. In: *PZ;* 140(30):2659-2667. 1995

Grassmann J, Hippeli S, Dornisch K et al. Antioxidant properties of essential oils. *Arzneim-Forsch/Drug Res*; 50(1):135-139. 2000

Gray AM & Flatt PR. Antihyperglycemic actions of Eucalyptus globulus (Eucalyptus) are associated with pancreatic and extra-pancreatic effects in mice. *J Nutr*; 128(12):2319-2323. 1998

Harkenthal M, Reichling J, Geiss H-K et al. Comparative study on the in vitro antibacterial activity of Australian tea tree oil, cajuput oil, niaouli oil, manuka oil, kanuka oil, and eucalyptus oil. *Pharmazie*; 54(6):460-463. 1999

Hindle RC. Eucalyptus oil ingestion. *N Z Med J*; 107(977):185-186. 1994

Ikeda RM et al. *J Food Sci;* 27:455. 1962

Jori A, Bianchetti A & Prestini PE. Effect of essential oils on drug metabolism. *Biochem Pharmacol*; 18(9):2081-2085. 1969

Jori A & Briatico G. Effect of eucalyptol on microsomal enzyme activity of foetal newborn rats. *Biochem Pharmacol*; 22(4):543-544. 1973

Jori A, Di Salle E & Pescador R. On the inducing activity of eucalyptol. *J Pharm Pharmacol*; 24(6):464-469. 1972

Kehrl W, Sonnemann U, Dethlefsen U. Therapy for acute nonpurulent rhinosinusitis with cineole: results of a double-blind, randomized, placebo-controlled trial. *Laryngoscope.* 114 (4):738-742. 2004.

Linsenmann P, Hermat H, Swoboda M. Therapeutischer Wert ätherischer Öle bei chronisch-abstruktiver Bronchitis. *Atemw Lungenkrankh;* 15:152-156. 1989

Linsenmann P, Swoboda M. Therapeutische Wirksamkeit ätherischer Öle bei chronisch-obstruktiver Bronchitis. *Therapiewoche;* 36:1161-1166. 1986

Osawa K et al. Macrocarpals H, I, and J from the leaves of *Eucalyptus globulus*. In: *JNP;* 59(9):824-827. 1996

Osawa K, Yasuda H, Morita H et al. Eucalyptone from *Eucalyptus globulus*. *Phytochemistry*; 40(1):183-184. 1995

Patel S, Wiggins J. Eucalyptus oil poisoning. *Arch Dis Child;* 55(5):405-406. 1980

Pattnaik S, Subramanyam VR & Kole C. Antibacterial and antifungal activity of ten essential oils in vitro. *Microbios*; 86(349):237-246. 1996

Pattnaik S, Subramanyam VR & Rath CC. Effect of essential oils on the viability and morphology of *Escherichia coli* (SP-11). *Microbios*; 84(340):195-199. 1995

Riechelmann H, Brommer C, Hinni M et al. Response of human ciliated respiratory cells to a mixture of menthol, eucalyptus oil and pine needle oil. *Arzneim-Forsch./Drug Res*; 47(9):1034-1039. 1997

Römmelt H, Schnizer W, Swoboda M, Senn E. Pharmakokinetik ätherischer Öle nach Inhalation mit einer terpenhaltigen Salbe. *Z Phytother;* 9:14-16. 1988

Sato S, Yoshinuma N, Ito K et al. The inhibitory effect of funoran and eucalyptus extract-containing chewing gum on plaque formation. *J Oral Sci*; 40(3):115-117. 1998

Shahi SK, Shukla AC, Bajaj AK et al. Broad spectrum herbal therapy against superficial fungal infections. *Skin Pharmacol Appl Skin Physiol*; 13:60-64. 2000

Sharara AL. Lozenge-induced esophagitis. *Gastrointest Endosc*; 51(5):622-623. 2000

Spoerke DG, Vandenberg SA, Smolinske SC, et al. Eucalyptus oil: 14 cases of exposure. *Vet Human Toxicol*; 31(2):166-168. 1989

Takasaki M, Konoshima T, Etoh H et al. Cancer chemoprevention activity of euglobal-G1 from leaves of *Eucalyptus grandis. Cancer Lett*; 155(1):61-655. 2000

Tibballs J. Clinical effects and management of eucalyptus oil ingestion in infants and young children. *Med J Aust;* 163(4):177-180. 1995

Tovey ER & McDonald LG. A simple washing procedure with eucalyptus oil for controlling house dust mites and their allergens in clothing and bedding. *J Allergy Clin Immunol*; 100(4):454-466. 1997

Vidal C & Cabeza N. Contact urticaria due to eucalyptus pollen. *Contact Dermatitis*; 26(4):265. 1992

Warnke PH, et al. Antibacterial essential oils in malodorous cancer patients: Clinical observations in 30 patients. *Phytomed* 13:463-467, 2006.

White RD, Swick RA & Cheeke PR. Effects of microsomal enzyme induction of the toxicity of pyrrolizidine (Senecio) alkaloids. *J Toxicol Environ Health*; 12:633-640. 1983

Whitman BW & Ghazizadeh H. Eucalyptus oil: Therapeutic and toxic aspects of pharmacology in humans and animals. *J Paediatr Child Health*; 30(2):190-191. 1994

Yun B-S, Lee I-K, Kim J-P et al. Lipid peroxidation inhibitory activity of some constituents isolated from the stem bark of *Eucalyptus globulus. Arch Pharm Res;* 23(2):147-150. 2000

Zänker KS, Blümel G. Terpene-induced lowering of surface tension in vitro. In: A rationale for surfactant substitution. *Resp Exp Med;* 182:33-38. 1983

Zänker KS, Blümel G, Probst J, Reiterer W. Theoretical and experimental evidence for the action of terpens as modulators in lung function. *Prog Resp Res;* 18:302-304. 1984

Eucalyptus globulus

See Eucalyptus

Eugenia chequen

See Cheken

Eugenia uniflora

See Surinam Cherry

Euonymus species

See Wahoo

Eupatorium cannabinum

See Hemp Agrimony

Eupatorium perfoliatum

See Boneset

Euphorbia cyparissias

See Cypress Spurge

Euphorbia resinifera

See Spurge

Euphrasia officinalis

See Eyebright

European Elder

Sambucus nigra

DESCRIPTION

Medicinal Parts: The medicinal parts are the bark peeled from the branches in spring and freed from the cork, the air-dried flowers, the fresh and dried leaves, the fresh and dried ripe fruit, the dried roots, and the fresh leaves, and inflorescences in equal parts.

Flower and Fruit: The strongly perfumed, yellowish-white flowers are in large, flat, apical, richly and densely blossomed erect cymes with 5 main branches. The edge of the calyx is small and has 5 tips. The corolla is rotate, deep, and has 5 petals. There are 5 stamens and 1 inferior ovary. The fruit is a black-violet, berrylike drupe with blood-red juice. The seeds are brownish, ovate, and domed on the outside.

Leaves, Stem, and Root: The plant is a shallow-rooted, up to 7-m high tree or bush with spreading branches containing dry white latex. The bark of the trunk is light brown to gray and fissured. The bark on the young branches is green and covered with gray lenticles. The leaves are odd 3 to 7 pinnate. They are matte green above and light blue-green beneath. The leaflets are ovate or oblong acuminate, and densely serrate.

Characteristics: The flowers have a strong, somewhat numbing perfume.

Habitat: European Elder is indigenous to almost all of Europe.

Production: Elder flowers consist of the inflorescence of *Sambucus nigra*, which are collected in the wild, sifted and dried.

Not to be Confused With: Confusion sometimes arises with the flowers of Sambucus ebulus.

Other Names: Black Elder, Black-Berried Alder, Boor Tree, Elder, Bountry, Ellanwood, Ellhorn

ACTIONS AND PHARMACOLOGY

COMPOUNDS

Flavonoids (up to 3%): chief components are rutin, isoquercitrin, quercitrin, hyperoside, astragalin, nicotoflorin

Volatile oil (0.03-0.14%): higher share (65%) of free fatty acids, including among others palmitic acid (share 38%)

Caffeic acid derivatives (3%): chlorogenic acids

EFFECTS

Flowers and berries of *Sambucus nigra* and *Sambucus canadensis* are used to shorten the duration and severity of flu and cold, to treat eczema and other skin disorders, and to reduce pain and inflammation. Animal tests have shown the therapeutic use of Sambucus with colds due to the proven enhancement of bronchial secretion. Human and in vitro studies support the usage of a warm infusion of flowers to increase perspiration and reduce fevers (Zakay-Rones, 1995). While the diaphoretic effect claimed for Elder has not yet been proved experimentally, it can nevertheless be considered documented in view of the empirical data available. *Sambucus nigra* flowers contain water-soluble constituents that directly stimulate muscular glucose metabolism and promote insulin secretion from clonal pancreatic cells in vitro (Gray 2000).

Sambucus is also used to reduce inflammation in hay fever and sinusitis. The cold infusion of the flowers may cause perspiration and diaphoresis and is used both internally and topically for rheumatism and eczema and topically for persistent skin inflammation (Bergner, 1996-1997). Recent studies tend to support its use to relieve pain and inflammation (Ahmahdiani, 1998).

Anti-Inflammatory Effects: Sambucus ebulus and *Sambucus nigra* alleviated inflammation and pain in rat hind paw edema, and inhibited cytokine secretion in vitro. *Sambucus ebulus* and *Sambucus nigra* leaves and flowers showed some in vitro inhibitory effects on interleukin-1alpha (IL-1a), interleukin-1beta (IL-1b), and tumor necrosis factor (TNF), leading the authors to find initial support for folkloric usage of Sambucus in inflammatory disorders (Yesilada, 1997; Ahmahdiani, 1998).

Antimicrobial Effects: Extracts and fractions of the herbaceous parts of *Sambucus ebulus* showed some inhibitory effect by agar dilution method against a standard strain (NCTC 11637) and eight clinical isolates of *Helicobacter pylori*. The chloroform fraction of the ethanolic extract of *Sambucus ebulus* had the most significant anti-*Helicobacter* activities with minimal inhibitory concentrations (MICs) of 31.2 against the standard strain and three of the eight isolates. However, the anti-*Helicobacter* activity of *Sambucus ebulus* was far less than that of amoxicillin and ofloxacin, used as controls (MICs of less than 0.2 and 0.98 respectively against the standard strain and each of the eight isolates) (Yesilada, 1999).

Sambucus mexicana leaves consistently inhibited growth in vitro of *Epidermophyton floccusm, Trichophyton metagrophytes* variety *algodonosa, T mentagrophytes* variety granulare, and *T rubrum* but did not inhibit *Microsporum canis* or *M gypseum*. Powdered Sambucus leaves were boiled in water and evaporated to a concentration of 1 g/mL of dry material. This study provided preliminary scientific validation of the antimycotic activity of many plants used to treat dermatological disorders in Guatemalan folk medicine. Some of the plants studied (such as *Byrsonima crassifolia*) showed broader antimycotic activity than *Sambucus mexicana* (Caceres, 1991).

Sambucus mexicana consistently showed a measurable zone of inhibition in vitro against *Salmonella typhi* and *Shigella dysenteriae* (greater than 8 mm), an intermediate inhibition zone against *Shigella flexneri* (approximately 8 mm), but did not inhibit enteropathogenic *Escherichia coli* and *Salmonella enteritidis*. Powdered Sambucus mexicana leaves were macerated in 50% ethanol for 7 days at room temperature with occasional agitation. Inhibition zones were measured in millimeters and tests were run at least six times. This study provides preliminary scientific validation for the antimicrobial effect of many plants used to treat gastrointestinal disorders in Guatemalan folk medicine. Some plants studied (such as *Tagetes lucida*) showed broader antimicrobial effects than *Sambucus mexicana* (Caceres, 1990).

Effects on Diabetes: Aqueous Sambucus extract increased glucose uptake (70%, $p<0.05$), glucose oxidation (50%, $p<0.01$), and glycogenesis (70%, $p<0.05$) in isolated mouse insulin-sensitive abdominal muscle without significantly changing the stimulatory effect of 10(-8) mol/L of insulin. The lack of potentiation when Sambucus and insulin were combined suggests Sambucus extract acts by the insulin pathways. Test results show that Sambucus' antihyperglycemic component involves smaller heat stable, acetone insoluble, and pH insensitive water-soluble molecules or ions (Gray, 2000).

Osteoporosis: Sambucus Sieboldiana inhibited bone resorption in vivo and in vitro (Li, 1998).

Viral Infections: Elder berry juice decreased the duration and symptoms of flu. Sambucol D (a mixture of Elder berry juice, raspberry extract, and citric acid) reduced hemagglutination and inhibited replication of human influenza viruses in vitro (Zakay-Rones, 1995).

CLINICAL TRIALS

Influenza

The safety and effectiveness of oral Elderberry extract syrup (15 ml) for treating the flu (influenza A and B infections) were tested in a randomized, double-blind, placebo-controlled trial involving 60 patients (18 to 54 years old) who reported experiencing influenza-like symptoms for up to 48 hours. The participants took the Elderberry syrup or placebo syrup 4 times daily for 5 days, and recorded the level and intensity of their flu symptoms with a visual analog scale. Analysis revealed that symptoms subsided, on average, 4 days sooner in those taking the Elderberry syrup. The participants taking the Elderberry syrup were also less likely than those taking placebo to use other symptom-relief medicines. A larger study is needed to confirm these findings, the authors conclude (Zakay-Rones, 2004).

In a study nearly a decade earlier by some of the same researchers, Sambucol® (a syrup of *Sambucus nigra* berry juice, raspberry extract, glucose, citric acid, and honey) decreased the duration of fever and other flu symptoms in a double-blind study of 40 individuals. The sera of patients treated with Sambucol showed higher hemagglutination inhibition titers to influenza B. A complete cure was achieved in 90% of the Sambucol group within 2 to 3 days compared to at least 6 days in the control ($p<0.001$). Convalescent phase serologies showed higher antibody titers to influenza B in the Sambucol group (Zakay-Rones, 1995).

INDICATIONS AND USAGE

Approved by Commission E:

- Cough/bronchitis
- Fevers and colds

The drug is used for colds and coughs. It is a sweat-producing remedy for the treatment of feverish colds.

Unproven Uses: In folk medicine, Elder flowers are used internally as a sudorific tea and for colds and other feverish conditions. Elder is also used as an infusion, as a gargle/mouthwash and for respiratory disorders such as coughs, head colds, laryngitis, flu, and shortness of breath. Elder is used occasionally by nursing mothers to increase lactation. Externally, herbal pillows are used for swelling and inflammation.

Homeopathic Uses: Among uses in homeopathy is inflammation of the respiratory tract.

PRECAUTIONS AND ADVERSE REACTIONS

Only fully ripe purple berries are used, as red berries can be mildly toxic. Leaves, shoots, bark, roots, and raw (red) berries contain a cyanogenic glycoside, sambunigrin, that can cause dizziness, headache, convulsions, gastrointestinal distress, nausea, vomiting, diarrhea and tachycardia (Brinker, 1989). Bark lectins may stimulate hyperplasia of the small intestine. Data suggest Sambucus may be a source of potential harm to diabetic patients and caution should be advised.

DRUG INTERACTIONS:

POTENTIAL INTERACTIONS

Iron: The tannin content of Elder may complex with iron, and may result in adverse sequelae on blood components. *Clinical Management:* Patients who need iron supplementation should separate administration times of iron and Elder by two hours.

DOSAGE

Mode of Administration: Whole herb and other galenic preparations for infusions.

Preparation: To prepare an infusion, brew 2 teaspoonfuls (3 to 4 g) of elder flowers in 150 mL of boiling water and strain after 5 minutes.

Daily Dosage: The average daily dose of the drug is 10 to 15 g. The infusion (tea) should be freshly prepared and drunk in doses of 1 to 2 cups several times–especially in the afternoon and evening.

Homeopathic Dosage: For adults, 5 drops, 1 tablet, or 10 globules every 30 to 60 minutes (acute) or 1 to 3 times daily (chronic); parenterally: 1 to 2 mL sc acute: 3 times daily; chronic once a day (HAB1). Adjust dosages for children.

Storage: Elder should be stored where it is protected from light and moisture.

LITERATURE

Ahmadiani A, Fereidoni M, Semnanian S et al. Antinociceptive and anti-inflammatory effects of Sambucus ebulus rhizome extract in rats. *J Ethnopharm*; 61:229-235. 1998

Bauer R et al. *Helv Chim Acta;* 68:2355. 1985

Bergner P. Elderberry (*Sambucus nigra, canadensis*). *Medical Herbalism*; 8(4):11-12. 1996-1997

Caceres A, Cano O, Samayoa B et al. Plants used in Guatemala for the treatment of gastrointestinal disorders. 1. Screening of 84 plants against enterobacteria. J Ethnopharm; 30:55-73. 1990

Caceres A, Lopez BR, Giron MA et al. Plants used in Guatemala for the treatment of dermatophytic infections. 1. Screening for antimycotic activity of 44 plant extracts. *J Ethnopharm*; 31:263-276. 1991

Czygan FC. Holunder wird wieder gesellschaftsfähig. In: *ZPT;* 15(2):111. 1994

Gray AM, Abdel-Wahab YHA & Flatt PR. The traditional plant treatment, *Sambucus nigra* (elder), exhibits insulin-like and insulin-releasing actions in vitro. *J Nutr;* 130(1):15-20. 2000

Inoue T, Sato K. *Phytochemistry;* 14:1871. 1975

Li H, Li J, Prasain JK et al. Antiosteoporotic activity of the stems of *Sambucus sieboldiana. Biol Pharm Bull*; 21(6):594-598. 1998

Mascolo N et al. *Phytother Res;* 1(1):28. 1987

Paulo E. *Folia Biol;* 24(2):213. 1976

Petitjean-Freytet C et al. *J Pharm Belg;* 46:241. 1991

Richter W, Willuhn G. *DAZ;* 114:947. 1974

Willuhn G, Richter W. *PM;* 31:328. 1977

Yesilada E, Gurbuz I & Shibata H. Screening of Turkish anti-ulcerogenic folk remedies for anti-*Helicobacter pylori* activity. *J Ethnopharmacol*; 66:289-293. 1999

Yesilada E, Ustun O, Sezik E et al. Inhibitory effects of Turkish folk remedies on inflammatory cytokines: interleukin-1alpha, interleukin-1beta and tumor necrosis factor alpha. *J Ethnopharm*; 58:59-73. 1997

Zakay-Rones Z, Thom E, Wollan T, et al. Randomized study of the efficacy and safety of oral Elderberry extract in the treatment of influenza A and B virus infections. *J Int Med Res*; 32(2): 132-140. 2004.

Zakay-Rones Z, Varsano N, Zlotnik M et al. Inhibition of several strains of influenza virus in vitro and reduction of symptoms by an Elderberry extract (*Sambucus Nigra L*) during an outbreak of influenza B in Panama. *J Alt Compl Med*; 1(4):361-369. 1995

European Five-Finger Grass

Potentilla reptans

DESCRIPTION

Medicinal Parts: The medicinal parts are the fresh flowering plant and the roots.

Flower and Fruit: The flowers are solitary or in pairs on long thin pedicles opposite the leaves. The calyx has 5 segments and is 10 to 25 mm across. The golden yellow petals are obcordate and up to twice as long as the calyx. A ringlike swelling at the base of the stamens exudes a kind of honey. The small fruit is oblong-ovate and wrinkled.

Leaves, Stem, and Root: The plant is a herbaceous perennial with a thin, divided rhizome and rosettes of basal leaves. The basal leaves produce 30 cm to 100 cm-long flowering stems from their axils, which are rooted at the nodes. The stems are pubescent or almost glabrous, have no glands and are often tinged red. The cauline leaves are long-petioled and 5 to 7 digitate. The basal stipules are fused to the petiole. The leaflets are obovate, 10 to 70 mm long, dentate to serrate and pubescent or almost glabrous.

Habitat: Europe. The plant is common in Europe, Western Asia, North America, Ethiopia and the Near East. *Potentilla canadensis* is indigenous to Canada and the U.S. and is very similar.

Production: European Five-Finger Grass and root is the complete plant of *Potentilla reptans*.

The drug is a mixture of green and brown in color and has no particular smell or taste. The roots are dug up in September/October and then dried in a sunny, airy place.

Other Names: Cinquefoil, Five Fingers, Five-Finger Blossom, Sunkfield, Synkfoyle

ACTIONS AND PHARMACOLOGY

COMPOUNDS

Tannins (6 to 12%)

Flavonoids: including quercetin-3,7-diglucuronide

EFFECTS

The drug is astringent and has wound healing effect due to the tannin content.

INDICATIONS AND USAGE

Unproven Uses: European Five-Finger Grass is used internally for diarrhea and fever; externally for inflammation of the mucous membranes of mouth and gums, toothache, and heartburn.

PRECAUTIONS AND ADVERSE REACTIONS

No health hazards or side effects are known in conjunction with the proper administration of designated therapeutic dosages. There have been complaints of gastrointestinal upset in conjunction with the drugs use reported in the literature.

DOSAGE

Mode of Administration: Available as crude drug and as an infusion for internal and external use.

Preparation: A decoction for internal use is prepared by adding 3 g of drug per 100 mL of water. A decoction using 6 g of drug per 100 mL of water is used for external application and mouth rinses.

Daily Dosage: Internally, 2 to 3 cups of a decoction prepared according to the formula above are administered daily. Externally, a decoction using the formula above is administered as a gargle, mouthwash or rinse. Moist compresses may be applied to affected areas of the skin.

LITERATURE

Hänsel R, Keller K, Rimpler H, Schneider G (Hrsg.), Hagers Handbuch der Pharmazeutischen Praxis, 5. Aufl., Bde 4-6 (Drogen), Springer Verlag Berlin, Heidelberg, New York, 1992-1994.

European Golden Rod

Solidago virgaurea

DESCRIPTION

Medicinal Parts: The medicinal parts are the dried aerial parts collected during the flowering season, the fresh inflorescences, and the flowering twigs.

Flower and Fruit: The yellow composite flowers are in erect racemes facing all directions and are simple or compound. They are medium-sized. The involucral bracts are imbricate and arranged in numerous rows. The ray florets are narrow, lingual, and female. The disc florets are funnel-shaped, 5-tipped, and androgynous. The fruit is a cylindrical achene with numerous ribs. It is brown, sparsely pubescent, and 3.5 to 4.5 mm long with a tuft of hair.

Leaves, Stem, and Root: The plant is a perennial that ranges in size from a few centimeters to over 1 m. The rhizome is cylindrical, noded, diagonally ascending, and short. The stem is erect, canelike, angularly grooved above, usually red-tinged beneath, and glabrous to loosely appressed pubescent higher up. The basal leaves are long-petioled, elliptical, acuminate, and narrowing to the winged stem. The lower ones are serrate and the upper ones entire-margined.

Habitat: The plant is indigenous to Europe, Asia and North America.

Production: Golden Rod is the aerial part of *Solidago virgaurea*. It occurs in the wild in Hungary, former Yugoslavia, Bulgaria, and Poland

Not to be Confused With: Despite qualitative and quantitative differences in their effects, drugs containing *Solidago gigantea* or *Solidago canadensis* are exchanged with *Solidago virgaurea* on the market; confusions with Senecio species are also conceivable.

Other Names: Aaron's Rod, Woundwort, Goldenrod

ACTIONS AND PHARMACOLOGY

COMPOUNDS

Triterpene saponins (0.2 to 0.3%):

In the European form—3,28-bisdemosidic ester saponins, including acyl-virgaurea saponins 1, 2 and 3; the acid components are acetic acid and beta-hydroxy butyric acid; aglycone is polygalic acid.

In the Asian form—bi- or tridemosidic solidago saponins I to XXIX, acyl-virgaurea saponin 1, acylvirgaurea saponin 2, bellis saponin BA2

Volatile oil (0.4 to 0.5%, in the stored drug less than 0.2%): chief components

In the European form—alpha-pinene, beta-pinene, limonene, delta-elemene, gamma-cadinene, beta-phellandrene, myrcene

In the Asian form—limonene, germacrene-D, germacrene-B and beta-caryophyllene

Polysaccharides (water-soluble, 6 to 8%)

Diterpenes: cis-clerodane-derivatives, presumably only in the Asian variety

Carotinoids (as blossom pigments)

Flavonoids (1.1 to 2%): chief component rutin (0.8%), including as well hyperoside, isoquercitrin, avicularin, quercetin - 3 - O - beta - D - robinoside, astragalin, nicotiflorin, kaempferol - 3 - O - beta - D - galactoside, kaempferol - 3 - O - alpha - arabinoside, kaempferol - 3 - O - beta - D - robinobioside, isorhamnetin - 3 - O - beta - D - galactoside, isorhamnetin - 3 - O - beta - D - glucoside, isorhamnetin - 3 - O - beta - D - rutinoside, rhamnetin - 3 - O - glucorahamnoside

Phenol glucosides (hydroxy benzylbenzoyte diglucosides, 0.2 to 1.0%): leicarposide (0.2 to 1%), virgaureoside A (0.01 to 0.14%), benzyl-2,6-dimethoxy-benzoate

Caffeic acid derivatives (0.2 to 0.4%): including chlorogenic acid, neochlorogenic acid, 3,5-dicaffeoyl quinic acid

Phenol carboxylic acids: salicylic acid (0.1%), as well as vanillic acid, protocatechuic acid, ferulic acid, caffeic acid, sinapineic acid–free, estered or glycosylated

Polyynes (in the roots): 2,8-cis-trans-matricaria ester, 2,8-cis-cis-matricaria ester, cis-lachnophyllum ester, matricaric acid lactone, lachnophyllum lactone

EFFECTS

The drug has a diuretic effect due to the leiocarposide and the phenol glycosides. Golden Rod also inhibits the formation of urinary calculi. Leiocarposide displays an analgesic effect. The saponin is antimicrobial, weakly spasmolytic and anti-exudative. The herb has also exhibited diuretic and spasmolytic effects.

INDICATIONS AND USAGE

Approved by Commission E:

- Infections of the urinary tract
- Kidney and bladder stones

Unproven Uses: In folk medicine, Golden Rod is used internally for rheumatism, gout, diabetes, hemorrhoids, prostatic hypertrophy, nervous bronchial asthma, internal bleeding, enlargement of the liver, acute exacerbation of pulmonary tuberculosis; externally for inflammations of the mouth and throat, as well as festering wounds.

Homeopathic Uses: Solidago virgaurea is used for renal insufficiency and liver disorders.

CONTRAINDICATIONS

Irrigation therapy is contraindicated in cases of edema resulting from reduced cardiac and/or kidney function.

PRECAUTIONS AND ADVERSE REACTIONS

No health hazards or side effects are known in conjunction with the proper administration of designated therapeutic dosages. The drug possesses a weak potential for sensitization. Care must be taken in patients with chronic renal diseases, and the drug should be used in this patient population only under physician supervision.

DOSAGE

Mode of Administration: As chopped drug by itself or in combination preparations.

Preparation: To make an infusion, 1 to 2 teaspoonfuls (3 to 5 g) of drug is scalded with simmering water (150 mL) and strained after 15 minutes.

Daily Dosage: The daily dosage is 6 to 12 g of comminuted drug prepared as an infusion. The infusion dosage is one cupful, 2 to 4 times daily between meals. The recommended dosage for the liquid extract is 0.5 to 2 mL liquid extract (1:1) in 25% ethanol 2 to 3 times daily. A dosage of 0.5 to 1 mL tincture (1:5) in 45% ethanol, 2 to 3 times daily is commonly used. Ample fluid intake should be ensured. In folk medicine, 0.5 to 2 gm drug as an infusion is taken 3 times daily.

Homeopathic Dosage: 5 drops, 1 tablet, or 10 globules every 30 to 60 minutes (acute) or 1 to 3 times daily (chronic); parenterally: 1 to 2 mL sc, acute: 3 times daily; chronic: once a day (HAB1)

Storage: The drug must be protected from light and moisture.

LITERATURE

Bader G, Plohmann B, Franz G, Hiller K, Saponins from *Solidago virgaurea L.* - Possible agent for therapy of cancer? In: PM 62, Abstracts of the 44th Ann Congress of GA, 21. 1996.

Bader G, Wray V, Hiller K, The main saponins from the aerial parts and the roots *of Solidago virgaurea subsp. virgaurea*. In: *PM* 61(2);158-161. 1995.

Budzianowski J, Skrzypczak L, Wesolowska M. Flavonoids and Leiocarposide in Four *Solidago Taxa. Sci Pharm.* 58; 15-23. 1990

Cantrell CL, Fischer NH, Urbatsch L, McGuire MS, Franzblau SG. Antimycobacterial crude plant extracts from South, Central, and North America. *Phytomedicine* 5 (2); 137-145. 1998

El-Ghazaly M, Khayyal MT, Okpanyi SN, Arens-Corell M. Study of the Anti-inflammatory Activity of *Populus tremula, Solidago virgaurea* and *Fraxinus excelsior. Arzneim Forsch.* 42; 333-336. 1992

Hiller K, Bader G, Goldruten-Kraut Portrait einer Arzneipflanze. In: *ZPT* 17(2):123-130. 1996.

Inose Y, Miyase T, Ueno A, Studies on the constituents of *Solidago virga-aurea L.* 1. Structural elucidation of saponins in the herb. In: *Chem Pharm Bull* 39: 2037. 1991.

Kalemba D, Gora J, Kurowska A. Analysis of the Essential Oil of *Solidago canadensis. Planta Med.* 56; 222-223. 1990

Kalemba D, Phenolic acids in four *Solidago* species. In: *PA* 47:471-472. 1992.

Kruedener Sv, Schneider W, Elstner EF. Effects of Extracts from *Populus tremula L., Solidago virgaurea L.* and *Fraxinus excelsior L.* on various Myeloperoxidase Systems. *Arzneim Forsch.* 46 (8); 809-814. 1996

Kruedener Sv, Schneider W, Elstner EF. A Combination of *Populus tremula, Solidago virgaurea* and *Fraxinus excelsior* as an Anti-inflammatory and Antirheumatic Drug. Arzneim Forsch. 45; 169-171. 1995

Lam J, Christensen LP, F..rch T, Thomasen T. Acetylenes from the Roots of *Solidago* Species. Phytochemistry 31; 4159-4161. 1992

Lu T, Menelaou MA, Vargas D, Fronczek FR, Fischer NH. Polyacetylenes and Diterpenes from *Solidago canadensis. Phytochemistry* 32; 1483-1488. 1993

Reznicek G, Freiler M, Schader M, Schmidt U. Determination of the content and the composition of the main saponins from *Solidago gigantea* AIT. Using high-perfomance liquid chromatography. *J Chromatogr* A 755 (1996), 133-37

Vonkruedener S et al., Effects of extracts from *Populus tremula L., Solidago virgaurea L.* and *Fraxinus excelsior L.* on various myeloperoxidase systems. In: *Arzneim Forsch* 46(8):809-814. 1996.

European Mistletoe

Viscum album

DESCRIPTION

Medicinal Parts: The medicinal parts are the leaves and twigs collected before the berries form, the fresh herbs of certain host plants, the fresh leafy twigs with fruit collected in the autumn, the whole fresh plant collected from apple trees, the leaves, and the berries.

Flower and Fruit: The flower is yellowish-green, dioecious, and appears in insignificant, small, 3- to 5-flowered clusters. The perigone of the male flower is 4 tipped. The stamens are fused with the tips. The female flower is smaller and has 4 tepals with a thick stigma sitting on the short style. The fruit is a glossy, white, globular, pea-sized berry with thick sticky flesh. When ripe, it is white to yellowish or orange and has 1 to 2 oval or angular seeds.

Leaves, Stem, and Root: The plant is a semi-parasitic, almost round bush growing on deciduous trees, which are 30 to 80 cm in diameter. The round branches are repeatedly bifurcated and thickened to knots at the joints and are the same yellowish-green as the leaves. The leaves are alternate, sessile, lanceolate or lanceolate-spatulate, coriaceous, and evergreen.

Habitat: European Mistletoe is found mostly in Europe and as far as Iran. It is not found in America or Australia. It is cultivated in central Europe and China.

Production: European Mistletoe berries are the fresh or dried fruit of *Viscum album*. Mistletoe stem is the fresh or dried stem of *Viscum album*. Mistletoe herb consists of fresh or dried younger branches with flowers and fruits of *Viscum album*. The drug is collected in the wild during the spring and is air-dried or put in driers at a maximum temperature of 40° C.

Other Names: All-Heal, Birdlime, Devil's Fuge, Mistletoe, Mystyldene

ACTIONS AND PHARMACOLOGY

COMPOUNDS: EUROPEAN MISTLETOE FRUIT

Mucilage (2%, referred to as Viscin): The mock berries of the Mistletoe have not been fully investigated. Presumably, they lack the toxic lectins and viscotoxins.

COMPOUNDS: EUROPEAN MISTLETOE STEM

The Mistletoe stems contain the same constituents as the Mistletoe foliage (*Visci albi herba*), but because of the high percentage of support elements lacking any effective ingredients, these constituents exist only in very low concentrations.

COMPOUNDS: EUROPEAN MISTLETOE HERB

Lectins (glycoproteins with 11% carbohydrate): Mistletoe lectin I (ML I, VAA 1, viscumin), mistletoe lectin II (ML II), mistletoe lectin III (ML III, VAA II), the lectin fractions named are isolectin mixtures

Polypeptides (built up out of 46 amino acids, 0.05-0.1%): viscotoxins A2, A3, B, Ps 1-

Mucilages (known as viscin, 4-5%): including among others galacturonans, arabino galactans

Sugar alcohols: including among others mannitol, quebrachitol, pinitol, viscumitol

Flavonoids: including glycosides of quercetin, quercetin methyl ethers, isorhamnetin, sakuranetin and homoeriodictyol; in the subspecies V. album ssp. platyspermum: homoeriodictyol - 7 - O - glucoside, isorhamnetin - 3 - O - rutinoside, isorhamnetin - 3 -[apiosyl (1 - 6)] - glucosyl - 7 - O - rhamnoside, 5,7 - dimethoxyflavanone - 4′ - O -glucoside, 3′,5,7 - trimethoxyflavanone - 4′ - O - glucoside

Phenyl alyl alcohols: including among others syringin (syrigenin - 4′ - O - glucosides), coniferyl - 4′ - [apiosyl (1 - 2′)] glucoside

Lignans: including among others syringaresinol and its glycosides

Triterpenes: including among others alpha-amyrin (alpha-viscol), beta-amyrin acetate, betulic acid, oleanolic acid, ursolic acid

EFFECTS

The Mistletoe lectins in the drug are hypotensive, cytotoxic, and immunostimulating. The immunostimulatory action of mistletoe is mainly attributed to a stimulation of the mononuclear phagocytic system and an induction of inflammation by macrophage-derived cytokines (Zarkociv et al, 1998). The antineoplastic activity of mistletoe extracts appears to be due to a stimulation of enzymes that repair damaged DNA by lymphokines (Kovacs et al, 1991).

Mistletoe has also shown anti-inflammatory properties.

Anticancer Effects: Some studies demonstrated benefit in cancer patients (Beuth & Moss, 1999; Heiny et al, 1998a; Friess et al, 1996; Stumpf & Schietzel, 1994; Heiny, 1991); however, they were not well designed. A meta-analysis of ten randomized trials examining the effects of mistletoe failed to demonstrate efficacy as a curative of palliative cancer therapy Ernst et al, 2003). Mistletoe increases DNA repair in lymphocytes. Uncontrolled studies of cancer patients have reported an increased quality of life, well-being, stable physical condition, and a reduction in pain sensitivity. More randomized, controlled clinical trials with specific tumor types are necessary to determine the place of mistletoe therapy in oncology. A concomitant rise in interleukin-1 and interleukin-6, tumor-necrosis factor-alpha, and gamma-interferon has also been reported (Staak et al, 1998; Meyer-Wegener, 1998; Weber et al, 1998; Joller, 1996; Stein & Berg, 1996; Hajto & Lanzrein, 1986; Hajto, 1986).

Cytotoxic Effects: Mistletoe (*Viscum album*) lectin 1 (ML-1) may cause cytotoxicity by inhibition of protein synthesis on a ribosomal level (Franz, 1986; Metzner et al, 1985; Stirpe et al, 1980). Another study demonstrated that viscotoxins 1, 2, 3, and 4b exert a cytotoxic effect by binding to DNA, possibly resulting in impaired replication and replication of target cells (Woynarowski & Konopa, 1980). Natural killer cytotoxicity is enhanced in vitro by a chemical bridging between the effector cell and the tumor cell (Mueller & Anderer, 1990a). An experiment comparing lectin-containing and lectin-free mistletoe preparations gave evidence of mistletoe (*Viscum album*) lectins inducing programmed cell death, or apoptosis, resulting from fragmentation of genomic DNA in susceptible target cells. Several human and murine cell lines were tested in vitro (Janssen et al, 1993).

CLINICAL TRIALS

Cancer

The influence of a perioperative infusion of standardized mistletoe extract (Iscador) on immune function was tested in a prospective, sequential, randomized clinical trial involving 62 patients with colorectal cancer who were undergoing tumor resection. Subjects were randomly assigned to either Mistletoe infusion or no additional therapy. The results revealed that natural killer (NK) cell activity differed significantly between the therapy groups 24 hours after surgery (p=0.027). The absolute number of MHC class II antigen HLA-DR did not differ 7 days after surgery. NK cell activity did not change significantly during the course of the study (-7.9% 24 h after surgery) in patients using mistletoe extract, whereas HLA-DR expression changed significantly (-38.5% at day 7 after surgery). In the control group, both parameters decreased significantly (NK cell activity: -44.4% at 24 h; HLA-DR expression: -32.9% at day 7 after surgery). Results demonstrated that a preoperative infusion of mistletoe extracts prevents a suppression of NK cell activity in cancer patients (Schink et al, 2007).

The efficacy of using the mistletoe preparation Iscador in prolonging the survival of breast cancer patients was reconfirmed in a re-analysis of randomized and non-randomized, controlled cohort studies. The evaluation concluded that previously published data are consistent despite the use of different subsets and analytic methods. Additionally, in the short-term, psychosomatic self-regulation, as a measure of autonomous coping with the disease, rises more under Iscador therapy than under conventional treatment alone (Grossarth-Maticek R, Ziegler R, 2006).

Another clinical trial investigating the impact of Mistletoe extract on patients with breast cancer showed that patients with the disease who received Mistletoe therapy experienced a smaller decrease in immune function than patients who did not receive the therapy. In the study, 352 patients were randomly assigned to two groups and received either the preparation, PS76A2 (15 ng mistletoe lectin/0.5 ml), or matching placebo twice weekly for four to six cycles of CMF (cyclophosphamide, methotrexate, fluorouracil) chemotherapy, followed by 2 months follow-up. The treatment differences were statistically significant. Primary efficacy was the change from baseline of three FACT-G subscales (physical, emotional, and functional well-being) during the fourth CMF cycle. The results demonstrate that PS76A2 is safe and effective in improving quality of life in breast cancer patients during chemotherapy and follow-up (Semiglazov et al, 2006). These results confirm the findings of a previous study with similar objectives and study design (Semiglazov et al, 2004).

A case report of an individual self-injecting Mistletoe (subcutaneously, 20 mg 3 times weekly) for treatment of cancer was published in the *British Medical Journal* (BMJ). Mistletoe is widely used in various parts of the world, including continental Europe, where up to two-thirds of cancer patients reportedly take it. The individual, who for a time did not report using the herb, experienced local subcutaneous inflammation that mimicked metastatic malignancy. The author concluded that rigorous, randomized controlled trials for Mistletoe are lacking and that good communication between provider and patient is necessary for proper oncology care (Finall, 2006).

In addition to the lack of reliable randomized clinical trials showing any benefit in treating cancer with Mistletoe, various reports actually indicate adverse effects, writes the author of a 2006 BMJ editorial titled, ''Mistletoe as a treatment for cancer: Has no proved benefit, and can cause harm.'' This is of concern given the herb's widespread use—at least 30 Mistletoe preparations are available for sale in continental Europe—and the possibility that individuals with cancer may substitute Mistletoe for medicines of more validated and proven effectiveness (Ernst, 2006).

Individuals having undergone transurethral resection of superficial bladder cancer typically follow-up with adjuvant therapy to prevent possible recurrences, and treatment with BCG has shown to be effective for this in patients with pTa nd pT1 tumors. The effectiveness of Mistletoe for generating similar recurrent rate prevention with less toxicity than BCG was explored in a phase I/II clinical trial involving 30 patients. Each was given increasing doses of aqueous Mistletoe extract standardized to Mistletoe lectin and administered intravesically. The 33% recurrence rate within 12 months was comparable to that of adjuvant BCG. Additionally, tolerability of Mistletoe was good at all the concentrations tested, while BCG usually results in severe local and systemic side effects. Future studies may be useful to illustrate optimal dose and clarify Mistletoe's value as an adjuvant treatment for individuals with superficial bladder cancer (Elsasser-Beile, 2005).

A meta-analysis of 10 randomized trials examining the effects of mistletoe failed to demonstrate efficacy as a curative or palliative cancer therapy. Data associated with different types of malignancies was pooled but evidence does not imply that mistletoe extracts are more efficacious for one type of malignancy than another. The authors concluded that most of the trials had weaknesses in reporting or study design or both. Efficacy as it related to quality of life, survival, or other outcome measures was not demonstrated in any of the methodologically stronger trials (Ernst et al, 2003).

In a controlled study of patients with histologically verified breast carcinoma (TNM stages III and IV), 36 patients were assigned to mistletoe lectin-1 therapy and 32 patients to the control group. Twenty-five patients in the mistletoe group responded to the therapy and 11 did not. Among the responders, a statistically significant difference ($p<0.005$) in the beta-endorphin plasma levels compared to basic levels in nonresponders and the control group was found. A relation between plasma beta-endorphin levels and cellular immune parameters was suggested, due to an increased release of interleukin-2, TNF-alpha, and interferon-gamma (Beuth & Moss, 1998).

A randomized clinical study of 47 patients with histologically verified advanced breast cancer demonstrated a significant correlation between natural killer cell and T-cell activity and beta-endorphin plasma levels after mistletoe lectin-1 standardized therapy with Eurixor®. Mistletoe lectin-1 doses ranging between 0.5 to 1 ng/kg were administered subcutaneously twice weekly for 8 weeks followed by a 4-week break. Beta-endorphin plasma levels and immune cell activities were measured after 24 weeks (Heiny et al, 1998). In a randomized study of 79 patients with colorectal carcinoma sturdy, a significant improvement of the quality of life was observed in patients receiving 1 ng/kg of mistletoe lectin-1 standardized extract twice weekly for 8 weeks. The severity of chemotherapy-related side effects, especially leukopenia and mucositis, was significantly reduced with complementary treatment. However, mistletoe therapy did not affect the length of remission, relapse-free intervals, or overall survival (Heiny et al, 1998).

Immunity

A fermented aqueous extract of *Viscum album* (Iscador® M) improved the clinical symptoms and the immunological status of 30 immunocompromised children between 8 and 15 years of age suffering from recurrent respiratory diseases after the Chernobyl accident. Mistletoe therapy produced marked clinical improvement in tiredness, emotional instability, headaches, sweating, and muscle and joint pain. No effects were seen during placebo administration (Chernyshov et al, 1997).

In healthy and allergic individuals, the commercial preparation of Iscador® Pini, derived from mistletoe (*Viscum album*) growing on pine trees, activated specific T-cells and monocytes. Although ML-1 is believed by many groups to be responsible for most of the immunomodulatory activities of mistletoe, Iscador® Pini is lacking ML-1 and has only scarce amounts of ML-2 and ML-3 (Stein & Berg, 1996).

INDICATIONS AND USAGE

EUROPEAN MISTLETOE FRUIT

Unproven Uses: The fruit acts on circulation by regulating blood pressure. It is also an expectorant and a tonic. In addition, the fruit is used to treat internal bleeding, epilepsy, arteriosclerosis, cramps, gout, hysteria and major blood loss.

EUROPEAN MISTLETOE STEM

Unproven Uses: The stem of European Mistletoe is used for its calming effect; in the treatment of mental and physical exhaustion; and as a tranquilizer against nervous conditions such as agitation, anxiety and increased excitability.

EUROPEAN MISTLETOE HERB

Approved by Commission E:

- Rheumatism
- Tumor therapy (adjuvant)

Unproven Uses: For treating degenerative inflammation of the joints and as palliative therapy for malignant tumors through nonspecific stimulation. Other uses include long-term therapy for cases of mild high blood pressure and as an arteriosclerosis prophylactic.

European Mistletoe tea may be used for high blood pressure, epilepsy, whooping cough, asthma, vertiginous attack, amenorrhea, diarrhea, chorea, nervous tachycardia, hysteria, and nervousness.

Chinese Medicine: The drug is used for joint pain, tendon and muscle pain, lumbago, back pain, vaginal bleeding during pregnancy, and agalactia.

Homeopathic Uses: The drug is used for dizziness, high and low blood pressure, cardiac arrhythmia and joint degeneration.

CONTRAINDICATIONS

Contraindications to mistletoe include protein hypersensitivity, chronic-progressive infections (e.g., tuberculosis, AIDS), hyperthyroidism, inflammatory or febrile disorders, tumors of the central nervous system, spinal cord tumors, or intracranial metastasis affecting intracranial pressure.

PRECAUTIONS AND ADVERSE REACTIONS

In 1981, the U.S Food and Drug Administration banned certain commercial preparations of mistletoe from sale in the United Sates and destroyed commercial preparations of this plant. The FDA has classified mistletoe as a food additive that cannot be marketed unless proved safe for consumption. This may not apply to the current suggested use for cancer chemotherapy as found in Europe and suggested by the German Commission E monographs. Consultation with a practitioner familiar with therapeutic use should be obtained prior to use.

All parts of the plant should be considered potentially toxic. The stems, leaves, and berries contain varying amounts, depending on the host tree, of three principal cytotoxic compounds: alkaloids, viscotoxins, and lectins. These compounds are thought to impart the immunomodulatory and cytotoxic effects observed (Tyler, 1993; Khwaja et al, 1986). Other compounds identified are flavonoids, phenol carboxylic acids, phenylpropanes, and lignans (Wagner et al, 1986). These, along with viscotoxins, are thought to be involved in the herb's cardiovascular activity (Hall et al, 1986; Wagner et al, 1986; Rosell & Samuelsson, 1966). Viscumin, a toxic lectin, has been reported in small amounts in mistletoe. The human toxicity of this compound appears to be similar to that of Ricin and Abrin, two extremely toxic compounds (Stirpe, 1983; Olsnes, 1982).

Side effects may include chills, high fever, headaches, angina, orthostatic circulatory disturbances, and allergic reactions. *Viscum album* in oral preparations possesses significant toxicity. Adverse effects at typical dosages can include hypotension and bradycardia. At higher levels, adverse effects can include mydriasis, miosis, hallucinations, delirium, hypertension, gastroenteritis, nausea, vomiting, and diarrhea.

Injectable preparations include slight rise of body temperature, headache, local inflammations and subcutaneous nodes near the injection site, lymph node swelling, and allergic reactions including generalized pruritus, local or generalized urticaria, blisters, exanthema, erythema multiforme, angioneurotic edema, chills, dyspnea, bronchospasms, and shock. A rise of intracranial pressure in patients with brain and spinal cord tumors or intracranial metastasis is possible.

Caution should be used in the geriatric patient. Those consuming mistletoe tea should have their blood pressure checked regularly.

Pregnancy: Not to be used during pregnancy. Mistletoe has been employed in herbal folklore as an abortifacient. American mistletoe is believed to stimulate uterine contractions. These effects have not been studied in humans (Tyler, 1993).

Breastfeeding: Not to be used while breastfeeding.

DRUG INTERACTIONS

No human drug interaction data available.

POTENTIAL INTERACTIONS

Iron: The tannin content in Mistletoe may complex with iron and result in adverse sequelae on blood components. *Clinical Management:* Separate administration of iron and mistletoe by 2 hours.

DOSAGE

EUROPEAN MISTLETOE HERB

Mode of Administration: Whole, cut and powdered herb are available in the forms of juice, coated tablets, drops, oil preparations, ampules and compound preparations.

Preparation: A medicinal tea is prepared using 2.5 g (1 teaspoonful) finely cut drug with 1 cup cold water, steeped for 12 hours at room temperature, then strained. European Mistletoe wine is prepared by adding 40 g drug to 1 liter wine; the preparation is ready for use after 3 days.

A liquid extract is made in the ratio of 1:1 with diluted ethanol; a tincture is made in the ratio of 1:5 with 45% ethanol.

Daily Dosage: dried leaves: 2 to 6 g (or by infusion) 3 times a day; tincture (1:5 preparation in 45% alcohol): 1 to 3 milliliter 3 times a day; fluid extract (1:1 preparation in 25% alcohol): 0.5 mL 3 times a day; dried aqueous extract (4:1 preparation): 100 to 250 mg 3 times a day (Anon, 1983).

The dosage for the treatment of hypertonia and as an arteriosclerotic prophylactic is 2 to 6 g of European Mistletoe powder 3 times daily by mouth.

Storage: European Mistletoe must be stored away from the light over an appropriate drying agent.

LITERATURE

Anon. Die Mistel. In: *DAZ;* 136(48):4330-4332; 1996.

Anon. British Herbal Pharmacopoeia. British Herbal Medicine Association, London, UK; 235-236, 1983.

Anon. FDA Consumer Bulletin. Dec-Jan 1981

Anon. Integrative Konzepte in der Onkologie: Misteltherapie (S. 19). In: *NGM Suppl;* 1/94:1-36; 1994.

Anon. Misteltherapie aus schulmedizinischer Sicht. In: *DAZ;* 131(37):1894. 1991

Anzenberger J. Homoviotensin bei arterieller Hypertonie. *Med Welt*; 49:308-310; 1998.

Becker H, Exner J. *Z Pflanzenphysiol;* 97; 1980.

Berg P, Stein G. Ein Inhaltsstoff allein genügt nicht, s. auch folgenden Artikel. In: *ZPT;* 16(5):282; 1995.

Beuth HJ, Mistel. ''In der Onkologie nur Präparate einsetzen, die auf Mistellektin standardisiert sind!'' In: *ZPT*; 16(1):40-41; 1995.

Beuth J, Ko HL, Gabius HJ, Burrichter H, Oette K, Pulverer G. Behavior of lymphocyte subsets, expression of activation markers in response to immunotherapy with galactoside-specific lectin from Mistletoe in breast cancer. *Clin Invest;* 70:658-661; 1992.

Beuth J, Lenartz D. Uhlenbruck G, Lektionoptimierter Mistelextrakt. In: *ZPT;* 18(2):85-91; 1997.

Beuth J & Moss RW. Immunotherapy with mistletoe lectin-1. *J Oncol;* 30:1-5;1998.

Boecher E, Stumpf C, Buessing A et al. Prospective Bewertung der Toxizitaet hochdosierter Viscum album L.-Infusionen bei Patienten mit progredienten Malignomen. *Z Onkol*; 28:97-106; 1996.

Chernyshov VP, Omelchenko LI, Heusser P. Immunomodulatory actions of Viscum album (Iscador®) in children with recurrent respiratory disease as a result of the Chernobyl nuclear accident. *Complement Ther Med*; 5:141-146; 1997.

Dumont S et al. Lectins from Mistletoe (*Viscum album L.*) induce the production of cytokines by cultured human monocytes. In: *PM*; 61(Abstracts of 43rd Ann Congr):57; 1995.

Elsasser-Beile U, Leiber C, Wolf P, et al. Adjuvant intravesical treatment of superficial bladder cancer with a standardized mistletoe extract. *J Urol*; 174(1):76-9; 2005.

Ernst E. Mistletoe as a treatment for cancer. *BMJ;* 333(7582):1282-1283; 2006.

Ernst E, Schmidt K & Steuer-Vogt M. Mistletoe for cancer? A systematic review of randomised clinical trials. *Int J Cancer;* 107(2):262-267; 2003.

Finall AI, McIntosh SA, Thompson WD. Subcutaneous inflammation mimicking metastatic malignancy induced by injection of mistletoe extract. *BMJ*; 333:1293-1294; 2006.

Fachinformation. Iscador M, mistletoe extract. Weleda AG, Schwaebisch-Gmuend, Germany; 1997.

Fachinformation. Iscador M/Q 5 mg spezial, mistletoe extract. Weleda AG, Schwaebisch-Gmuend, Germany; 1997.

Fachinformation. Iscador P, mistletoe extract. Weleda AG, Schwaebisch-Gmuend, Germany; 1997.

Fachinformation. Iscador Q, mistletoe extract. Weleda AG, Schwaebisch-Gmuend, Germany; 1997.

Fachinformation. Lektinol, standardized mistletoe extract. Madaus AG, Koeln, Germany; 1997.

Franz G. Phytotherapie in der Tumorbehandlung. In: *DAZ;* 130(26):1443. 1990

Franz H. Mistletoe lectins and their A and B chains. *Oncology*; 43(suppl 1):23-34. 1986

Friess H, Beger HG, Kunz J et al. Treatment of advanced pancreatic cancer with mistletoe: results of a pilot trial. *Anticancer Res*; 16:915-920. 1996

Gabius HJ, Gabius S. Die Misteltherapie auf dem naturwissenschaftlichen Prüfstand. In: *PZ*; 139(22):1745. 1994.

Gabius HJ, Gabius S, Joshi SS, Koch B, Schroeder M, Manzke WM, Westerhausen M. From ill-defined extracts to the immunomodulatoty lectin: Will there be a reason for oncological application of Mistletoe? *Planta Med;* 60:2-7. 1994.

Grossarth-Maticek R, Ziegler R. Randomised and non-randomised prospective controlled cohort studies in matched-pair design for the long-term therapy of breast cancer patients with a mistletoe preparation (Iscador): a re-analysis. *Eur J Med Res.* 11(11): 485-495. 2006.

Hajto T. Immunomodulatory effects of Iscador®: a Viscum album preparation. *Oncology;* 1(suppl):51-65. 1986

Hajto T, Hostanka K, Frei K, Rordorf Chr, Gabins H-J. Increased secretion of tumor necrosis factor interleukin 1: und interleukin 6 by Heiman mononuclear cells exposed to galactoside - specific lectin from clinically applied Mistletoe extract. *Canc Res;* 50:3322. 1990a.

Hajto T, Hostanka K, Gabius HI. Modulatory potency of the galactoside-specific lectin from Mistletoe extract (Iscador), the host defense system in vivo in rabbits, patients. *Canc Res;* 49:4803. 1989

Hajto T & Lanzrein C. Natural killer and antibody-dependent cell-mediated cytotoxicity activities and large granular lymphocyte frequencies in Viscum album-treated breast cancer patients. *Oncology*; 43:93-97. 1986

Hall AH, Spoerke DG & Rumack BH. Assessing mistletoe toxicity. *Ann Emerg Med*; 15:1320-1323. 1986

Hamacher H. Mistel (*Viscum album L.*) - Forschung und therapeutische Anwendung. In: *ZPT;* 18(1):34-35. 1997

Hamacher H, Mistel (*Viscum album L.*) - Forschung und therapeutische Anwendung. In: *ZPT;* 18(1):34-35. 1997

Hamacher H, Scheer R. Anthroposophie/Phytotherapie: Mistel-Forschung und therapeutische Anwendung. In: *DAZ;* 136(34):2904-2905. 1996

Harvey J & Colin-Jones DG. Mistletoe hepatitis. *Br Med J;* 282:186-187. 1981.

Hassauer W et al. *Onkologie;* 2(1):28. 1979

Heiny BM. Adjuvant treatment with standardized mistletoe extract reduces leukopenia and improves the quality of life of patients with advanced carcinoma of the breast getting palliative chemotherapy (VEC regimen). *Krebsmedizin*; 12:3-14. 1991

Heiny BM, Albrecht V & Beuth J. Correlation of immune cell activities and beta-endorphin release in breast carcinoma patients treated with galactose-specific lectin standardized mistletoe extract. *Anticancer Res*; 18:583-586. 1998

Heiny BM, Albrecht V & Beuth J. Lebensqualitaetsstabilisierung durch Mistellektin-1 normierten Extrakt beim fortgeschrittenen kolorektalen Karzinom. *Onkologie*; 4(suppl 1):35-39. 1998a

Janssen O, Scheffler A & Kabelitz D. In vitro effects of mistletoe extracts and mistletoe lectins. *Arzneimittelforschung*; 43:1221-1227. 1993

Joller PW, Menrad JM, Schwarz T et al. Stimulation of cytokine production via a special standardized mistletoe preparation in an in vitro human skin bioassay. *Drug Res;* 46(I):649-653. 1996

Kleijnen J, Knopschild P. Mistletoe treatment for cancer. Review of controlled trials in humans. *Phytomedicine;* 1:255-260. 1994

Khwaja TA et al. Isolation of biologically active alkaloids from Korean mistletoe *Viscum album, coloratum. Experientia;* 36(5):599-600. 1980

Khwaja TA, Dias CB & Pentecost S. Recent studies on the anticancer activities of mistletoe (*Viscum album*) and its alkaloids. *Oncology*; 43(suppl 1):42-50. 1986

Konopa J, Woynarowski JM, Lewandowska-Gumieniak M. Isolation of viscotoxins. Cytotoxic basic polypeptides from Viscum album L. *Hoppe-Seylers Z Physiol Chem;* 361(10):1525-1533. 1980

Kovacs E, Hajto T & Hostanska K. Improvement of DNA repair in lymphocytes of breast cancer patients treated with Viscum album extract (Iscador). *Eur J Cancer*; 27(1):1672-1676. 1991

Metzner G, Franz H, Kindt A et al. The in vitro activity of lectin I from mistletoe (ML I) and its isolated A and B chains on functions of macrophages and polymorphonuclear cells. *Immunobiology*; 169:461-471. 1985

Meyer-Wegener J. Mistellektin-1 beguenstigt Vermehrung der Killerzellen. *Fortschr Med;* 116:14-15. 1998

Mueller EA & Anderer AF. Chemical specificity of effector cell/ tumor cell bridging by a *Viscum album* rhamnogalacturonan enhancing cytotoxicity of human NK cells. *Immunopharmacology*; 19:69-77. 1990a

Olsnes S, Stirpe F, Sandvig K et al. Isolation and characterization of viscumin, a toxic lectin from *Viscum album L.* (mistletoe). *J Biol Chem*; 257:13263-13270. 1982

Reynolds JEF (ed). Martindale: The Extra Pharmacopoiea (electronic version). Micromedex, Inc, Englewood, CO; 1997

Rosell S & Samuelsson G. Effect of mistletoe viscotoxin and phoratoxin on blood circulation. *Toxicon*; 4:107-110. 1966

Saenz MT, Ahumada MC, Garcia MD. Extracts from Viscum and Crataegus are cytotoxic against larynx cancer cells. In: Z *Naturforsch;* C 52(1-2):42-44. 1997

Schink M, Troger W, Dabidian A, et al. Mistletoe extract reduces the surgical suppression of natural killer cell activity in cancer patients. A randomized phase III trial. *Forsch Komlementarmed*; 14(1): 9-17. 2007.

Schmidt S Unkonventionelle Heilverfahren in der Tumortherapie. In: *ZPT;* 17(2):115-117. 1996

Schwarz T et al. Stimulation by a stable, standardised Mistletoe preparation of cytokine production in an in vitro human skin bioassay. In: *PM* 62, Abstracts of the 44th Ann Congress of GA, 1996

Semiglazov VF, Stepula VV, Dudov A, et al. Quality of life is improved in breast cancer patients by standardized mistletoe extract PS76A2 during chemotherapy and follow-up: a randomized, placebo-controlled, double-blind, multicenter clinical trial. *Anticancer Res*; 26(2B):1519-1529. 2006.

Semiglazov VF, Stepula VV, Dudov A, et al. The standardized mistletoe extract PS76A2 improvess QoL in patients with breast cancer receiving adjuvant CMF chemotherapy: a randomized, placebo-controlled, double-blind, multicenter clinical trial. *Anticancer Res*; 24(2C):1293-1302. 2004.

Spiller HA, Willias DB, Gorman SE et al. Retrospective study of mistletoe ingestion. *Clin Toxicol*; 34:405-408. 1996

Staak JO, Stoffel B, Wagner H et al. In vitro-Zytotoxicitt der Viscum album-Agglutinine I und II. *Z Onkol*; 30:29-33. 1998

Stein GM & Berg PA. Evaluation of the stimulatory activity of a fermented mistletoe lectin-1 free mistletoes extract on T-helper cells and monocytes in healthy individuals in vitro. *Drug Res*; 46(I):635-639. 1996

Stettin A, Schultze JL, Stechemesser E et al. Anti-mistletoe lectin antibodies are produced in patients during therapy with an aqueous mistletoe extract derived from *Viscum album L.* and neutralize lectin-induced cytotoxicity in vitro. *Klin Wochenschr;* 68:896-900. 1990

Stirpe F. Mistletoe toxicity (letter). *Lancet*; I(8319):295. 1983

Stirpe F, Legg RF, Onyon LJ et al. Inhibition of protein synthesis by a toxic lectin from *Viscum album L.* (mistletoe). *Biochem J*; 190:843-845. 1980

Stirpe F, Sandvig K, Olsnes S, Pihl A. Action of viscumin, a toxic lectin from mistletoe, on cells in culture. *J Biol Chem.* Nov 25;257(22):13271-7. 1982

Timoshenko AV et al. Influence of the galactoside-specific lectin from Viscum album and its subunits on cell aggregation and selected intracellular parameters of rat thymocytes. In: *PM;* 61(2):130-133. 1995

Timoshenko AV & Gabius HJ. Efficient induction of superoxide release from human neutrophils by the galactoside-specific lectin from Viscum album. *Biol Chem;* 374:237-243. 1993

Wagner H. Die Mistel in der Tumortherapie. In: *DAZ;* 132(20):1087/1088. 1992

Wagner H, Jordan E Structure, properties of polysaccarides from *Viscum album* (L). *Oncology;* (Suppl 1):8-15. 1986

Wagner H, Jordan E & Feil B. Studies on the standardization of mistletoe preparations. *Oncology*; 43(suppl 1):16-22. 1986

Weber K, Mengs U, Schwarz T et al. Effects of a standardized mistletoe preparation on metastatic B16 melanoma colonization in murine lungs. *Drug Res*; 48:497-502. 1998

Woynarowski J & Konopa J. Interaction between DNA and viscotoxins. *Hoppe-Seyler's Z Physiol Chem;* 361(10):1535-1545. 1980

Zarkovic N, Kalisnik T, Loncaric I et al: Comparison of the effects of Viscum album lectin ML-1 and fresh plant extract (Isorel) on cell growth in vitro and tumorigenicity of melanoma B16F10. *Cancer Biother Radiopharmacol*; 13:121-131. 1998

European Peony

Paeonia officinalis

DESCRIPTION

Medicinal Parts: The medicinal parts are the dried ripe seeds, the fresh underground parts harvested in spring, and the fresh root.

Flower and Fruit: The large flowers are solitary at the ends of the stems. The calyx consists of 5 green, partly corollalike sepals. The wild species has 5 to 8 ovate red petals 4 to 5 cm long; the cultivated forms have many more. The stamens are light-red with long yellow anthers. The 2 or 3 ovaries have red stigmas and develop into tomentose follicles containing numerous, dark, glossy, pea-sized seeds.

Leaves, Stem, and Root: In its winter state, the plant has a turniplike rhizome and close, gnarled root fibers that are brown on the outside and white inside. The stem is leafy, erect, lightly branched and glabrous, with a stalk about 50 cm high. The leaves are alternate, petiolate, with a dark green glossy upper surface and a light green finely pubescent undersurface.

Habitat: The plant is indigenous to the mountains of southern Europe from Portugal to Albania and Hungary, as far as Asia Minor. It is widely cultivated as a garden plant.

Production: European Peony flower consists of the petals of *Paeonia officinalis* and/or *Paeonia mascula*. European Peony root consists of the dried secondary roots of these. The cultivated Peony roots are dug up in spring, cleaned, and dried in the sun or artificially. The flowers are harvested in dry weather shortly after the end of flowering and dried quickly in the shade or in moderate sunshine.

Other Names: Peony, Piney

ACTIONS AND PHARMACOLOGY

COMPOUNDS: EUROPEAN PEONY FLOWERS

Anthocyans: in particular paeonin (paeonidin-3,5-diglucoside)

Tannins (pentagalloyl glucose)

Flavonoids: in particular kaempferol glycosides

EFFECTS: EUROPEAN PEONY FLOWERS

The plant contains anthocyanin glycosides and tannins (main active principle: paeonidin-3, 5-diglucoside). Animal tests have demonstrated strong uterine contraction, tone reduction in the gastrointestinal tract, and a drop in blood pressure. Anticonvulsive and analgesic effects could not be demonstrated, although hypertonia has been reported in animal tests.

COMPOUNDS: EUROPEAN PEONY ROOT

Monoterpenes: monoterpene ester glucosides of the pinane-type: chief component paeoniflorine (1.5 to 3.5%)

EFFECTS: EUROPEAN PEONY ROOT

The plant contains anthocyanin glycosides and tannins (main active principle: paeonidin-3, 5-diglucoside). Animal tests have demonstrated strong uterine contraction, tone reduction in the gastrointestinal tract, and a drop in blood pressure. Anticonvulsive and analgesic effects could not be demonstrated.

INDICATIONS AND USAGE

EUROPEAN PEONY ROOT

Unproven Uses: In folk medicine, European Peony root is used for neurasthenia and neurasthenia syndrome, neuralgia, migraines, and allergic disorders such as excitability, epilepsy and whooping cough. Additionally, it is used for cramps and rheumatism.

Homeopathic Uses: Among uses in homeopathy are hemorrhoids and other anal conditions.

EUROPEAN PEONY FLOWERS

Unproven Uses: The flowers were formerly used as a folk medicine remedy for epilepsy, as an emetic, emmenagogue, and abortifacient, for diseases of the skin and mucous membranes, fissures, anal fissures associated with hemorrhoids, gout, rheumatoid arthritis, and ailments of the respiratory tract.

Homeopathic Uses: Homeopathic uses include hemorrhoids and other anal conditions.

PRECAUTIONS AND ADVERSE REACTIONS

No health hazards are known in conjunction with the proper administration of designated therapeutic dosages. Side effects that may occur, particularly in cases of overdosages, include gastroenteritis with vomiting, colic, and diarrhea.

DOSAGE

EUROPEAN PEONY FLOWERS

Mode of Administration: Therapeutic use cannot be recommended because efficacy has not been proved.

How Supplied: Forms of commercial pharmaceutical preparations include drops and compound preparations.

Preparation: To make an infusion, use 1 g Tree Peony flowers per cup water.

Daily Dosage: Drink one cup of infusion per day.

Homeopathic Dosage: 5 drops, 1 tablet, or 10 globules every 30 to 60 minutes (acute) or 1 to 3 times daily (chronic). Parenterally: 1 to 2 ml sc acute, 3 times daily; chronic: once a day (HAB1).

Storage: Store protected from light and moisture for no longer than 1 year.

EUROPEAN PEONY ROOT

Mode of Administration: European Peony root is administered as a tincture. European Peony flowers are used as an inactive ingredient in cough and fumigant teas and as a coloring agent in cough syrup.

How Supplied: Forms of commercial pharmaceutical preparations include drops and compound preparations.

Daily Dosage: Tincture: 30 to 50 drops daily.

Storage: Store protected from light and moisture for no longer than 1 year.

LITERATURE

Hänsel R, Keller K, Rimpler H, Schneider G (Hrsg.), Hagers Handbuch der Pharmazeutischen Praxis, 5. Aufl., Bde 4-6 (Drogen), Springer Verlag Berlin, Heidelberg, New York, 1992-1994.

Hikino H, Economic and Medicinal Plant Research, Vol I., Academic Press UK 1985.

Ishida H et al. Studies on the Antihemorrhagic and anticoagulative substances in herbs used for treatments of Bleeding and stagant blood in traditional chinese medicine. *J Pharm Sci.* 76; S200. 1987

Lewin L, Gifte und Vergiftungen, 6. Aufl., Nachdruck, Haug Verlag, Heidelberg 1992.

Roth L, Daunderer M, Kormann K, Giftpflanzen, Pflanzengifte, 4. Aufl., Ecomed Fachverlag Landsberg Lech 1993.

Teuscher E, Lindequist U, Biogene Gifte - Biologie, Chemie, Pharmakologie, 2. Aufl., Fischer Verlag Stuttgart 1994.

Wichtl M (Hrsg.), Teedrogen, 4. Aufl., Wiss. Verlagsges. Stuttgart 1997.

European Sanicle

Sanicula europaea

DESCRIPTION

Medicinal Parts: The medicinal parts are the fresh flowering herb and the basal leaves, which are collected during the flowering season and dried.

Flower and Fruit: The white or reddish inflorescences form a cyme with small headlike umbels with 4 to 6 linear bracts. The calyx is 5-tipped and there are 5 petals. The androgynous florets are in the center of the small umbel surrounded by 10 to 20 male florets. The ribless fruit is densely covered with barbed thorns and almost globular, with long styles that curve downwards. The mericarps are distinctly domed and almost flat at the narrow groove. There are numerous oil lines.

Leaves, Stem, and Root: The perennial plant grows 20 to 40 cm high. The short rhizome is solid, horizontal, multisegmented, broken off, and covered in thick fibers. It has scales formed by leaf stalk remnants at the neck and has a number of segments. The stem is usually undivided, erect, grooved, and has only 1 to 2 sessile leaves. The leaves are basal, long-petioled, and palmate with 5 lobes. The tips are trilobed. The lateral tips are divided in two and are especially glossy underneath.

Characteristics: The taste is slightly salty, bitter and dry.

Habitat: The plant is indigenous to Europe, Asia Minor, the Caucasus, western Siberia, northern Africa, and in the mountains of tropical Africa.

Production: European Sanicle consists of the dried, aboveground parts of *Sanicula europaea*, which is collected in the wild.

Not to be Confused With: Commercially, the herb may be mixed with leaves of *Cardamine enneaphylos*. In some areas, Astrantia major is labeled as sanicle and used accordingly in folk medicine.

Other Names: Black Sanicle, Poolroot, Self-Heal, Sanicle, Wood Sanicle

ACTIONS AND PHARMACOLOGY

COMPOUNDS

Triterpene saponins (up to 13%): including among others, acyl-saniculosides A-D, aglycones including A1-barrigenol, R1-barrigenol, barringtogenol

Caffeic acid derivatives: rosmarinic acid, chlorogenic acid

Flavonoids: chief components rutin, isoquercitrin, astragalin

EFFECTS

The drug has a mild astringent and expectorant effect. It also reduces edema in animal experiments. The saponin complex has been shown to be antimicrobial and antifungal.

INDICATIONS AND USAGE

Approved by Commission E:

■ Cough/bronchitis

European Sanicle is used for mild inflammation of the mucous membranes of the respiratory tract.

Homeopathic Uses: The primary application of European Sanicle in homeopathy is for diarrhea.

PRECAUTIONS AND ADVERSE REACTIONS

No health hazards or side effects are known in conjunction with the proper administration of designated therapeutic dosages.

DOSAGE

Mode of Administration: Comminuted drug for decoctions and other preparations for oral application.

How Supplied: Commercial pharmaceutical preparations include juices, tablets and compound preparations.

Preparation: No information is available.

Daily Dosage: The average daily dose is 4 to 6 g of the herb.

Homeopathic Dosage: 5 drops, 1 tablet, or 10 globules every 30 to 60 minutes (acute) or 1 to 3 times daily (Chronic); parenterally: 1 to 2 mL sc acute: 3 times daily: chronic once a day (HAB34).

Storage: The drug must be kept in sealed containers, protected from light.

LITERATURE

Brantner A, Grein E. Antibacterial activity of plant extracts used externally in traditional medicine. *J Ethnopharmacol*. 44; 35-40. 1994

Engel S, Horn K, Phytodermatosen durch *Dictamnus albus, Sanicula europaea* und *Philodendron consanguineum*. In: *Dermat Mschr* 158(1):22-27. 1972.

Hänsel R, Keller K, Rimpler H, Schneider G (Hrsg.), Hagers Handbuch der Pharmazeutischen Praxis, 5. Aufl., Bde 4-6 (Drogen), Springer Verlag Berlin, Heidelberg, New York, 1992-1994.

European Water Hemlock

Cicuta virosa

DESCRIPTION

Medicinal Parts: The medicinal part is the rhizome with roots.

Flower and Fruit: The flower is a white umbelliferous blossom with distinct calyx tips. The petals have indented tips. The style cushion is flat. The fruit is brown-yellow, 2.5 mm by 3 mm, and has dark-brown stripes.

Leaves, Stem, and Root: The plant grows to a height of 30 to 120 cm. The leaves are 2- to 3-pinnates. The leaflets are lanceolate and sharply serrated. The whole plant is glabrous. The rhizome is tuberous, fleshy, and hollow. The stem is erect, round, hollow, glabrous, branched above, and forms adventitious roots at the nodes.

Characteristics: The rhizome has a bad odor and is extremely poisonous.

Habitat: The plant is indigenous to Europe and Asia.

Other Names: Cowbane

ACTIONS AND PHARMACOLOGY

COMPOUNDS

Polyynes: including cicutoxin (0.07-0.2% in the fresh rhizome tuber), isocicutoxin, cicutol, cicudiole, falcarindiol

Furanocoumarins

Alkyl phthalides

EFFECTS

No information is available.

INDICATIONS AND USAGE

Homeopathic Uses: The drug is used in homeopathic dilutions for migraine, painful menstruation, worm infestation, and inflammation of the skin.

PRECAUTIONS AND ADVERSE REACTIONS

The freshly harvested rootstock is extremely poisonous due to its cicutoxin content. The plant itself is weakly poisonous.

OVERDOSAGE

Two to 3 g of the root stock are said to be fatal for an adult. The toxicity of the drug declines through dehydration and storage. Symptoms of poisoning, following the initial stupor and nausea, include severe tonic-clonic spasms, unconsciousness, canosis, and extremely widened pupils. Death occurs through asphyxiation at the peak of a convulsive attack or through heart failure.

Forced diuresis, hemodialysis, and hemoperfusion are initiated as treatment for poisonings. Gastric lavage should only be carried out under anesthetic because of the danger of convulsion. Benzodiazepine or barbiturates are used to lessen the effects of the spasms.

DOSAGE

Mode of Administration: The drug is used topically and internally as a dilution of the mother tincture.

LITERATURE

Bilia AR, Ctalano S, Fontana C, Morelli I, Palme E, A new saponin from *Potentilla tormentilla*. In: *PM* 58(7):A723. 1992.

Strauss U, Wittstock U, Schubert R, Teuscher E, Jung S, Mix E, Cicutoxin from *Cicuta virosa*–a new and potent potassium channel blocker in T lymphocytes. *Biochem Biophys Res Commun*, 219:332-6. 1996.

Wittstock U, Hadacek F, Wurz G, Teuscher E, Greger H, Polyacetylenes from water hemlock, *Cicura virosa*. In: *PM* 61(5):439-445. 1995.

Wittstock U, Lichtnow KH, Teuscher E, Effects of cicutoxin and related polyacetylenes from *Cicuta virosa* on neuronal action potentials: a comparative study on the mechanism of the convulsive action. In: PM 63(2):120-124. 1997.

Wittstock U, Lichtnow KH, Teuscher E, Effects of polyacetylenes from Cicuta virosa on the electrical activity of molluscan giant neurones. In: PM 61(Abstracts of 43rd Ann Congr):84. 1995.

Evening Primrose

Oenothera biennis

DESCRIPTION

Medicinal Parts: The medicinal parts are the fatty oil extracted from the ripe seeds and the fresh plant gathered at the beginning of the flowering season.

Flower and Fruit: The fragrant flowers are 2 to 3 cm long and are solitary in the leaf axils. The open ones are lower than the buds. The sepals are lanceolate, acuminate, turned down, thin, pale green and smooth on the outside with a few scattered hairs. The petals are obovate. The ovary is inferior. The style has a 4-sectioned stigma. The fruit is a linear-oblong, quadrangular, downy-villous capsule up to 3 cm long. The seeds are 1.5 mm long, dark gray to black with irregular sharp edges.

Leaves, Stem, and Root: This biennial grows up to 1 m and has a spindle-shaped, fleshy, turniplike root, which produces leaf rosettes in the first year. The stem is erect, unbranched, or branched higher up and angular. The ovary is a capsule covered in short glandular hairs, with simple, light hairs on the purple papilla. The cauline leaves are short-petioled or sessile, often hanging, oblong-lanceolate, pointed, irregular, and finely dentate.

Characteristics: The flowers are fragrant and open in the evening.

Habitat: Originally indigenous to North America, it is now naturalized throughout most of Europe and parts of Asia.

Production: Evening Primrose oil is the fatty seed oil of *Oenothera biennis*. The oil is extracted by means of a cold-extraction process, which involves hexane in steel or glass-lined tanks. The extract is washed and the solvent removed using low pressure.

Other Names: Fever Plant, King's Cureall, Night Willow-herb, Scabish, Sun Drop

ACTIONS AND PHARMACOLOGY

COMPOUNDS

Fatty oil: chief fatty acids linoleic acid (65-80%), gamma-linolenic acid (8-14%), oleic acid (6-11%), palmitic acid (7-10%)

EFFECTS

Evening Primrose oil (EPO) is an omega 6 fatty acid that contains approximately 8.9% gamma-linolenic acid (GLA). GLA is converted to dihomo-gamma-linolenic acid and then to prostaglandin E1 (PGE1) in vivo by the enzyme delta-6-desaturase. PGE1 has anti-inflammatory and cell membrane stabilizer activity in the body. Evening Primrose oil supplements provide increased levels of dihomo-gamma-linolenic acid in the blood of people with a deficiency of the enzyme delta-6-desaturase (Newall, 1996; Kershcer & Korting, 1992; Manku et al, 1982). GLA is also a component in breast milk, but is not added to infant formulas. It has been postulated that GLA may be beneficial to neural development in breast-fed infants (Newall, 1996; Makrides et al, 1995). Evening Primrose oil extracts exhibited antioxidant activity in a laboratory analysis (Birch et al, 2001). The oil has also shown positive action against diabetic neuropathy, hypercholesterolemia, hypertension, and irritable bowel syndrome (Keen et al, 1993; Guivernau et al, 1994; Viikari & Lehtonen, 1986; Leeds et al, 1990; Cotterell et al, 1990). Data is lacking, but Evening Primrose oil may prove effective in relieving the physical and psychological symptoms of PMS.

Anticancer Effects: GLA may be a useful adjunct to primary tamoxifen treatment in endocrine-sensitive breast cancer; however, larger trials are needed to fully determine its role. Evening Primrose oil proved ineffective in the treatment of hepatic carcinoma (van der Merwe et al, 1990).

Arthritis Effects: Positive effects of Evening Primrose oil on arthritis are not statistically evident.

Cervical Ripening Effects: Oral Evening Primrose oil was ineffective in reducing incidence of adverse labor outcomes and decreasing overall length of labor in low-risk nulliparous females (Dove D and Johnson P, 1999).

Antimastalgia Effects: Evening Primrose oil can be considered a first-line treatment for cyclical breast pain. Since the response can be slow, treatment should be continued for several months before it is determined whether or not treatment is successful. As a second-line treatment, it does not appear useful (Steinbrunn et al, 1997; Holland & Gateley, 1994).

Pre-eclampsia: Evidence suggests that prostaglandins may have a role in pre-eclampsia. Although one trial indicates the usefulness of Evening Primrose oil to prevent pre-eclampsia, a second trial indicates it is not effective in decreasing existing pre-eclampsia (D'Almeida et al, 1992; Moodley & Norman, 1989).

Skin Conditions: A high dose of Evening Primrose oil and long-term treatment are necessary for anti-inflammatory results to occur in the skin. Evening Primrose oil may supply the appropriate essential fatty acids necessary to maintain cell membranes, as well as act as a precursor to prostaglandins.

Thrombosis: Evening Primrose oil reduced platelet aggregation, thromboxane production, and increased bleeding time in 12 hyperlipidemic males (Guivernau et al, 1994).

CLINICAL TRIALS

Many studies investigating the efficacy of EPO in various diseases lack statistical significance yet report beneficial effects. It is unclear if the lack of statistical significance is due to a true lack of efficacy or an inadequate dose and/or time trial of a particular study.

Arthritis

Evening Primrose oil was able to decrease the use of nonsteroidal anti-inflammatory drugs (NSAIDs) in patients with rheumatoid arthritis. In this double-blind, placebo-controlled trial, 49 patients received either 12 capsules per day of Evening Primrose oil (540 mg of GLA), 12 capsules per day of a combination of Evening Primrose oil and fish oil (450 mg GLA and 240 mg eicosapentaenoic acid), or 12 placebo capsules per day (liquid paraffin). Treatment lasted for 12 months and was followed by three months of placebo for all patients. After three months of treatment, patients were asked to decrease their use of NSAIDs but to maintain their level from 12 to 15 months. There was a significant reduction in the dose of NSAIDS used by both the Evening Primrose oil group ($p<0.003$) and the Evening Primrose oil plus fish oil group ($p<0.002$). No significant changes were seen in clinical or laboratory measurements in the study. The subjective improvement was also higher in the two treatment groups compared to placebo (Belch et al, 1988).

Cancer

Thirty-eight females with locally advanced or metastatic breast cancer receiving 2.8 g of GLA daily in addition to tamoxifen 20 mg once daily experienced significantly ($p=0.016$) quicker initial tumor response at 6 weeks of treatment when compared to patients taking only tamoxifen 20 mg once daily. Change in tumor size, estrogen receptor (ER), and bcl-2 protein expression were used to determine tumor response. Follow-up for the study was not long enough to determine if addition of GLA conferred a longer duration of tumor response to treatment (Kenny et al, 2000).

Diabetic Neuropathy

Evening Primrose oil improved neurophysiological and neurological measures in patients with diabetic polyneuropathy. A one-year, multicenter, randomized, double-blind, placebo-controlled parallel study was conducted with 111 patients who had mild diabetic neuropathy. Patients were randomized to receive 12 capsules daily of Evening Primrose oil, providing 480 mg of GLA per day, or matched placebo capsules of liquid paraffin. Patients were evaluated at baseline and at 3, 6 and 12 months. Evening Primrose oil significantly ($p<0.05$) improved motor nerve conduction velocity, sensory nerve action potential, compound muscle action potential, tendon reflexes, and sensation in both the arm and leg compared to placebo (Keen et al, 1993).

Hypercholesterolemia

In a randomized double-blind crossover study supplementation with Evening Primrose oil daily significantly altered fasting lipid profiles in 12 hyperlipidemic males. A significant reduction in mean serum triglycerides, total cholesterol, and LDL with a significant increase in mean HDL was reported following four months of Evening Primrose oil treatment (Guivernau et al, 1994).

In another study, Evening Primrose oil was not successful in changing serum cholesterol, HDL cholesterol or triglyceride levels in hyperlipidemic patients. (Viikari & Lehtonen, 1986). Supplementation with Evening Primrose oil did not affect serum lipoproteins or platelet function in hypertriglyceridemic patients (Boberg et al, 1986).

Irritable Bowel Syndrome

Fifty three percent of subjects showed improvements in irritable bowel symptoms with Evening Primrose oil. Subjects were given either eight 500 mg capsules of EPO daily (as Efamol®) or eight 500 mg capsules of olive oil as a placebo for 3 menstrual cycles in a placebo-controlled, double-blind, crossover study. Nineteen of 36 patients demonstrated an improvement on Efamol and none improved with placebo. Most subjects demonstrated improvement in the second month of treatment. The irritable bowel syndrome group had significantly lower levels of omega-6 fatty acids and also showed reduced docosapentanoic acid concentrations (Cotterell et al, 1990).

Mastalgia

Fifty females with moderate to severe breast pain were given either Evening Primrose oil (OEP) or a topical non-steroidal anti-inflammatory (NSAID) gel in a one-year, randomized, and open comparative study to determine the relative safety, effectiveness, rapidity of response, cost-effectiveness, and acceptability of each regimen. While 64% of the 25 participants treated with OEP had a clinically significant response following 3 months of treatment, 92% of the 25 participants treated with topical NSAIDs had a clinically significant response. One patient taking OEP reported side effects, in contrast to none with topical NSAIDs. Acceptability rates for OEP and NSAIDs were 68% and 96%, respectively (Qureshi & Sultan, 2005).

More favorable results for Evening Primrose were obtained in a retrospective study covering seven years, in which 556 women with cyclical breast pain (mastalgia) were tracked. Most women were initially treated with Vitamin B-6 (pyridoxine HCL) 100 mg daily for a 3-month period. Those who did not respond were given 3 g of Evening Primrose Oil daily for 1 month followed by 2 g daily for an additional 2 months. Other participants were given the Evening Primrose oil regimen as first-line treatment; 58% of the Vitamin B6/EPO treatment group (71 patients) reported pain relief and 59% of the EPO first-line group (99 patients) reported relief. The author concluded that good responses can be obtained from products devoid of significant side effects, such as EPO and Vitamin B-6 as a first line treatment (McFayden, et al, 1992).

In an older review article, a clinician reported satisfactory treatment of mild mastalgia using three 500-mg doses of Evening Primrose oil twice daily for 1 month. Treatment that was considered successful after this time was continued 1 to 2 months longer. Patients were reported to have long-lasting effects even after the treatment period ended (Steinbrunn et al, 1997). The authors of a review on drug therapy in mastalgia recommended GLA 240 mg to 320 mg daily as a first-line therapy (Holland & Gateley, 1994).

Menopausal Hot Flushes

The effectiveness and safety of one versus two daily doses of a compound containing isoflavones (60 mg), Evening Primrose oil (440 mg), and vitamin E (10 mg) were assessed in an open, multi-center, randomized and group-comparative trial of 1,080 postmenopausal women with moderate to severe hot flushes. At 3 and 6 months, the two study dosages were equally effective in reducing hot flushes, with symptom reduction most significant for both groups in the first 3 months. The authors conclude that higher doses of the blend do not confer better results (Hidalgo et al, 2006).

Premenstrual Syndrome (PMS)

This review of four European studies concluded that Evening Primrose oil is effective in reducing the symptoms of PMS. One study involved 68 women who failed previous treatment for PMS. These women were treated with four Evening Primrose oil capsules daily starting in the luteal phase of the menstrual cycle and increasing to eight capsules daily. Sixty-one percent of these women experienced complete remission of symptoms, both physical and psychological. A second double-blind, placebo controlled study involved 42 patients given Evening Primrose oil for 3 months (dose not indicated). Participants in this study showed improvement in eight categories. The third study was double-blind, placebo controlled, and crossover in design (dose not indicated). Participants had 60% improvement of symptoms with Evening Primrose oil. The fourth study, which is unpublished, determined the value of treatment consisting of four daily capsules of Evening Primrose oil during the luteal phase of the cycle. With this low dose, patients had an improvement in five symptoms (Horrobin, 1983).

In one small study, however, Evening Primrose oil was shown to be ineffective in reducing PMS symptoms. Thirty-eight women took either 8 capsules of Evening Primrose oil or liquid paraffin as placebo on day one of their menstrual cycle through the end of their third cycle. At this time treatment was crossed-over for three more cycles. No differences were seen between the two treatment groups when rated on fluid retention, breast pain or swelling, and mood changes (Khoo et al, 1990).

Skin Conditions

A meta-analysis of nine controlled trials showed oral Evening Primrose oil provided significant ($p<0.0001$) improvement for patients with atopic eczema. All trials were randomized, double-blind, and placebo-controlled. At the first assessment time, Evening Primrose oil gave a significant ($p<0.03$) improvement from baseline on all three scores, while placebo gave significant improvement in none of the categories. At the last assessment time, Evening Primrose oil was still significant ($p<0.0001$) in all three categories and placebo showed significant ($p=0.0001$) improvement only in the clinical global score. The most striking improvement associated with GPO was in relieving itching. The degree of improvement correlated to the dose received, with 12 capsules per day giving the best results (Morse et al, 1989).

A recent, comprehensive follow-up of this meta-analysis concluded that Evening Primrose oil is safe and has a beneficial effect on itching, crusting, redness, and edema. The herb's benefits were shown to be apparent 4 to 8 weeks after the start of treatment. Increased steroid use reduces the magnitude of its beneficial effects, however. The investigators concluded that more research is needed to better comprehend the physiology and potential benefit of fatty acids such as Evening Primrose oil for atopic eczema (Morse & Clough, 2006).

In one older study involving 99 patients, 39 of which were children limited improvement in symptoms of atopic dermatitis with Evening Primrose oil use was demonstrated (Wright & Burton, 1982).

INDICATIONS AND USAGE

Unproven Uses: Evening Primrose oil is used for neurodermatitis, PMS, and as a dietary aid. EPO is also used to treat hyperactivity in children, high cholesterol levels, perimenopausal hot flashes, and cyclic mastalgia. Other common indications include hypertension, rheumatoid arthritis, thrombosis, autoimmune disease such as Multiple Sclerosis, and Raynaud's phenomenon. Capsules containing 500 mg of Evening Primrose oil have been approved for use in Germany, in the treatment of and to relieve the symptoms of atopic eczema.

CONTRAINDICATIONS

Evening Primrose oil is contraindicated in patients with epilepsy.

PRECAUTIONS AND ADVERSE REACTIONS

Evening Primrose oil may cause mild gastrointestinal effects such as nausea, vomiting, diarrhea, flatulence, and bloating. There are case reports of seizures in schizophrenic patients that were being treated with Evening Primrose oil along with phenothiazine medications. Practitioners should be aware that Evening Primrose oil may lower the seizure threshold in patients with seizure disorders or in those being treated with drugs that lower the seizure threshold. In schizophrenic patients and those receiving epileptogenic drugs, Evening Primrose oil may have the potential to manifest temporal lobe epilepsy (Newall, 1996). Evening Primrose oil may potentiate temporal lobe epilepsy.

Blood: A study of 12 hyperlipidemic men taking 3 g Evening Primrose oil daily reported a significant mean 40% increase in bleeding time. A significant reduction in platelet aggregation response stimulated by low concentrations of ADP, adrenaline or collagen was also observed (Guivernau et al, 1993). A probable mechanism of action is inhibition of platelet thromboxane B2 production and increased vascular prostacyclin production leading to a reduction in platelet aggregation response (Guivernau et al, 1994).

Breast Milk: It has been suggested that mothers of children with atopic eczema have an abnormal lipid content of their breast milk. Both studies suggest that supplementation of GLA via Evening Primrose oil can normalize the lipid content of breast milk and thus treat the child's atopic eczema. It seems that there is a greater proportion of linoleic acid and a smaller proportion of dihomo-GLA in total breast milk lipid content of these mothers compared to healthy controls (Melnik & Plewig, 1989; Wright, 1982).

DRUG INTERACTIONS

MODERATE RISK

Anticoagulants, Antiplatelet Agents, Low Molecular Weight Heparins, and Thrombolytic Agents: Concomitant use of Evening Primrose oil and these medications may increase the risk of bleeding. *Clinical Management:* Caution is advised if Evening Primrose oil and anticoagulants, antiplatelet agents, low molecular weight heparins, or thrombolytic agents are used concomitantly. Monitor for signs and symptoms of excessive bleeding.

Anticonvulsants: Theoretically, Evening Primrose oil may reduce the effectiveness of anticonvulsants by lowering the seizure threshold. *Clinical Management:* Avoid concomitant use of Evening Primrose oil with anticonvulsants.

Phenothiazines: Evening Primrose oil may reduce the seizure threshold when taken with phenothiazines. *Clinical Management:* Avoid concomitant use of Evening Primrose oil with phenothiazines.

DOSAGE

Mode of Administration: Evening Primrose oil is available in capsules for oral administration.

How Supplied:

Capsules–500 mg, 1300 mg..

Most commercial products (capsules) are standardized for gamma linolenic acid content of 9%.

Daily Dosage: Treatment with Evening Primrose oil may require up to 3 months duration before positive results are attained for all indications listed below (Newall, 1996).

Atopic eczema

Adult–4 to 8 g daily in divided doses

Pediatric–2 to 4 g daily in divided doses

Mastalgia (breast pain)

3 to 4 g daily in divided doses

Storage: Evening Primrose oil is rinsed in nitrogen and stored in cooled tanks lined with polyethylene. Commercial products should be stored at room temperature in an area that is dry and not in direct sunlight.

LITERATURE

Aman MG, Mitchell EA & Turbott SH. The effects of essential fatty acid supplementation by Efamol in hyperactive children. *J Abnorm Child Psychol*; 15(1):75-90. 1987

Bamford JTM, Gibson RW & Renier CM. Atopic eczema unresponsive to evening primrose oil (linoleic and gamma-linolenic acids). *J Am Acad Dermatol*; 13(6):959-965. 1985

Barber AJ. Evening Primrose oil: a panacea? *Pharm J*; (June 4):723-725. 1998

Belch JJF, Ansell D, Madhok R et al. Effects of altering dietary essential fatty acids on requirements for non-steroidal anti-inflammatory drugs in patients with rheumatoid arthritis: a double blind placebo controlled study. *Ann Rheum Dis*; 47(2):96-104. 1988

Belch JJF & Hill A. Evening Primrose oil and borage oil in rheumatologic conditions. *Am J Clin Nutr*; 71(suppl):352S-356S. 2000

Belch JJF, Shaw B, O'Dowd A et al. Evening Primrose oil (Efamol) in the treatment of Raynaud's phenomenon: a double blind study. *Thromb Haemost*; 54(2):490-494.1985

Berth-Jones & Graham-Brown. Placebo-controlled trial of essential fatty acid supplementation in atopic dermatitis. *Lancet*; 341(8860):1557-1560. 1993

Birch AE, Fenner GP, Watkins R et al. Antioxidant properties of evening primrose seed extracts. *J Agric Food Chem*; 49:4502-4507. 2001

Boberg M, Vessby B & Selinus I. Effects of dietary supplementation with n-6 and n-3 long-chain polyunsaturated fatty acids on serum lipoproteins and platelet function in hypertriglyceridaemic patients. *Acta Med Scand;* 220(2):153-160. 1986

Budeiri D, Li Wan Po A, Dornan JC. Is Evening Primrose oil of value in the treatment of premenstrual syndrome? *Control Clin Trials;* 17:60-68. 1996

Cancelo-Hidalgo M, et al. Effect of a compound containing isoflavones, primrose oil and vitamin E in two different doses on climacteric symptoms. *J Obstet Gynaecol*, 26(4):344-347. 2006.

Chenoy R, Hussain S, Tayob Y et al. Effect of oral gamolenic acid from evening primrose oil on menopausal flushing. *BMJ*; 308:501-503. 1994

Cotterell JC, Lee AJ & Hunter JO. Double blind, cross-over trial of evening Primrose oil in women with menstrually- related irritable bowel syndrome. In Horrobin DF (ed): Omega-6 essential fatty acids, pathophysiology and roles in clinical medicine. Alan R. Liss, Inc: 421-426. 1990

D'Almeida A, Carter JP, Anatol A et al. Effects of a combination of evening Primrose oil (gamma-linolenic acid) and fish oil (eicosapentanoic + docahexanoic acid) versus magnesium, and versus placebo in preventing pre-eclampsia. *Women Health*; 19(2-3):117-131. 1992

Dove D & Johnson P. Oral evening Primrose oil: Its Effect of Length of Pregnancy and Selected Intrapartum Outcomes in Low-Risk Nulliparous Women. *J Nurse Midwifery*; 44(3):320-324. 1999

Ebden P, Bevan C, Banks J et al. A study of evening primrose seed oil in atopic asthma. *Prostaglandins Leukot Essent Fatty Acids*; 35(2):69-72. 1989

Ernst E. Possible interactions between synthetic and herbal medicinal products. Part I: a systematic review of the evidence. *Perfusion*; 13:4-15. 2000

Guivernau M, Meza N, Barja P et al. Clinical and experimental study on the longer-term effect of dietary gamma-linolenic acid on plasma lipids, platelet aggregation, thromboxane formation, and prostacycline production. *Prostaglandins Leukot Essent Fatty Acids*; 51:311-316. 1994

Haslett C, Douglas JG, Chalmers SR et al. A double-blind evaluation of evening Primrose oil as an antiobesity agent. *Int J Obes*; 7(6):549-553. 1983

Holland PA & Gateley CA. Drug therapy of mastalgia: what are the options? *Drugs*; 48(5):709-716. 1994

Holman CP & Bell AFJ. A trial of evening Primrose oil in the treatment of chronic schizophrenia. *J Orthomol Psychiat*; 12:302-304. 1983

Horrobin DF. The role of essential fatty acids and prostaglandins in the premenstrual syndrome. *J Reprod Med*; 28(7):465-468. 1983

Ihrig M, Blume H, Nachtkerzenöl-Präparate. Ein Qualitätsvergleich. In: *PZ;* 139(9):668. 1994

Ippen H. Gamma-Linolensäure besser aus Nachtkerzen- oder aus Borretschöl? In: *ZPT;* 16(3):167-170. 1995

Jenkins AP, Green AT & Thompson RPH. Essential fatty acid supplementation in chronic hepatitis B. *Aliment Pharmacol Ther*; 10(4):665-668. 1996

Keen H, Payan J, Allawi J et al. Treatment of Diabetic Neuropathy With Gamma-Linolenic Acid. *Diabetes Care*; 16(1):8-15. 1993

Kenny FS, Pinder SE, Ellis IO et al. Gamma Linolenic Acid with Tamoxifen as Primary Therapy in Breast Cancer. *Int J Cancer*; 85:643-648. 2000

Kerscher MJ & Korting HC. Treatment of atopic eczema with evening Primrose oil: rationale and clinical results. *Clin Invest*; 70(2):167-171. 1992

Khoo SK, Munro C & Battistutta D. Evening Primrose oil and treatment of premenstrual syndrome. *Med J Aust*; 153(4):189-192. 1990

Makrides M, Neumann MA, Simmer K et al. Erythrocyte fatty acids of term infants fed either breast milk, standard formula, or formula supplemented with long-chain polyunsaturates. *Lipids*; 30(10):941-947. 1995

Manku MS, Horrobin DF, Morse N et al. Reduced levels of prostaglandin precursors in the blood of atopic patients: defective delta-6-desaturase function as a biochemical basis for atopy. *Prostaglandins Leukot Med*; 9(6):615-628. 1982

Manthorpe R, Hagen Petersen S, Prause JU et al. Primary Sjorgren's syndrome treated with Efamol/Efavit. A double-blind crossover investigation. *Rheumatol Int*; 4(4):165-167. 1984

McFayden IJ, Forrest AP & Chetty U. Cyclical breast pain - some observations and the difficulties in treatment. *Br J Clin Pract*; 46(3):161-164. 1992

Melnik BC & Plewig G. Is the origin of atopy linked to deficient conversion of omega-6-fatty acids to prostaglandin E1? *J Am Acad Dermatol*; 21(3 pt 1):557-563. 1989

Midwinter RE, Moore WJ, Soothill JF, Turner MW, Colley JR. Infant feeding and atopy. *Lancet;* Feb 6;1(8267):339. 1982

Moodley J & Norman RJ. Attempts at dietary alteration of prostaglandin pathways in the management of pre-eclampsia. *Prostaglandins Leukot Essent Fatty Acids*; 37(3):145-147. 1989

Morse PF, Horrobin DF, Manku MS et al. Meta-analysis of placebo-controlled studies of the efficacy of Epogam in the treatment of atopic eczema: relationship between plasma essential fatty acid changes and clinical response. *Br J Dermatol*; 121(1):75-90. 1989

Morse NL, Clough PM. A meta-analysis of randomized, placebo-controlled clinical trials of Efamol evening primrose oil in atopic eczema. Where do we go from here in light of more recent discoveries? *Curr Pharm Biotechnol;* 7(6):503-524. 2006.

Norred CL & Brinker F. Potential coagulation effects of preoperative complementary and alternative medicines. *Alt Ther*; 7(6):58-67. 2001

Oxholm P, Manthorpe R, Prause JU et al. Patients with primary Sjogren's Syndrome treated for two months with evening Primrose oil. *Scand J Rheumatol*; 15(2):103-108. 1986

Pye JK, Mansel RE, Hughes LE. Clinical experience of drug treatments for mastalgia. *Lancet* Aug 17;2(8451):373-377. 1985

Qureshi S, Sultan N. Topical nonsteroidal anti-inflammatory drugs versus oil of evening primrose in the treatment of mastalgia. *Surgeon;* 3(1):7-10. 2005.

Seaman GV, Swank RL, Zukoski CF 4th. Red-cell-membrane differences in multiple sclerosis are acquired from plasma. *Lancet* May 26;1(8126):1139. 1979

Steinbrunn BS, Zera RT & Rodriguez JL. Mastalgia, tailoring treatment to type of breast pain. *Postgrad Med*; 102(5):183-198. 1997

Stenius-Aarniala B, Aro A, Hakulinen A et al. Evening Primrose oil and fish oil are ineffective as supplementary treatment of bronchial asthma. *Ann Allergy*; 62(6):534-537. 1989

ten Hoor F. Cardiovascular effects of dietary linoleic acid. *Nutr Metab*; 24 Suppl 1:162-80. 1980

Vaddadi KS. The use of gamma-linolenic acid and linoleic acid to differentiate between temporal lobe epilepsy and schizophrenia. *Prostagl Med*; 6:375-379. 1981

van der Merwe CF, Booyens J, Joubert HF et al. The effect of gamma-linolenic acid, an in vitro cytostatic substance contained in evening Primrose oil, on primary liver cancer: a double-blind placebo controlled trial. *Prostaglandins Leukot Essent Fatty Acids*; 40(3):199-202. 1990

Viikari J & Lehtonen A. Effect of Primrose oil on serum lipids and blood pressure in hyperlipidemic subjects. *Int J Clin Pharmacol Ther Toxicol*; 24(12):668-670. 1986

Willuhn G. Phytopharmaka in der Dermatologie. In: *ZPT* 16(6):325-342. 1995

Wright S & Burton JL. Oral evening-Primrose-seed oil improves atopic eczema. *Lancet*; 2(8308):1120-1122. 1982

Eyebright

Euphrasia officinalis

DESCRIPTION

Medicinal Parts: The medicinal part is the flowering plant.

Flower and Fruit: White, bluish, or reddish-violet flowers are in spikelike inflorescence in the axils of the upper leaves. The calyx has 4 tips and is glabrous to short bristly. The corolla is bilabiate and is 8 to 12 mm long. The upper lip is domed, helmetlike, and revolute at the tips. The lower lip has 9 dark violet long stripes. There are 4 stamens and 1 superior ovary. The fruit is a narrow, oblong capsule with a ciliate edge. The seeds are numerous and grooved.

Leaves, Stem, and Root: The plant is about 30 cm high. It is annual. The stem is rigid, erect, and lightly branched below. The leaves are opposite, sessile, and grass-green. They are ovate or oblong-ovate and twice as long as wide. The involucral bracts have 4 to 7 teeth.

Characteristics: Eyebright is odorless and has a bitter and salty taste. It is semiparasitic.

Habitat: Europe.

Production: Eyebright consists of the whole plant of *Euphrasia officinalis* gathered during flowering season. Eyebright herb consists of the fresh or dried, above-ground parts of *Euphrasia officinalis.*

Other Names: Euphrasia

ACTIONS AND PHARMACOLOGY

COMPOUNDS

Iridoide monoterpenes: aucubin, catalpol, euphroside, ixoroside, veronicoside, verproside, mussaenoside, ladroside

Lignans: dehydrodiconiferyl-4-beta-D-glucoside

Flavonoids: including apigenin-, chrysoeriol- and luteolin-7-O-galactosides and -rhamnogalactosides

Tannins

EFFECTS

The constituent aucubin has anti-inflammatory effects and has shown to be hepatoprotective against poisonings with carbon tetrachloride or alpha-amantitine. Further, aucubin has shown inhibitory effects against hepatitis B virus in vitro.

INDICATIONS AND USAGE

Unproven Uses: Eyebright preparations are used externally as lotions, poultices, and eye-baths, for eye complaints associated with disorders and inflammation of the blood vessels, inflammation of the eyelids and conjunctiva, as a preventive measure against mucus and catarrh of the eyes.

In folk medicine, Eyebright is used for blepharitis, conjunctivitis, styes, eye fatigue symptoms, functional eye disorders of muscular and nervous origin, coughs, and hoarseness.

The efficacy of the herb for its claimed uses is not documented.

PRECAUTIONS AND ADVERSE REACTIONS

Health risks or side effects following the proper administration of designated therapeutic dosages are not recorded.

DOSAGE

Mode of Administration: Since the efficacy of the claimed uses is undocumented, and external eye application is not absolutely hygienic, therapeutic use cannot be recommended.

How Supplied:

Capsules: 470 mg, 500 mg, 750 mg

Preparation: To prepare a tea, add 2 to 3 gm of finely cut drug to boiling water; strain after 5 to 10 minutes.

Decoction: 2%.

Daily Dosage: A decoction is used 3 to 4 times daily for eye rinses.

LITERATURE

Bartholomaeus A, Ahokas J. Inhibition of P-450 by aucubin: is the biological avtivity of aucubin due to its glutaraldehyde-like aglycone? *Toxicol Lett.* 80: 75-83. 1995

Bermejo Benito P, Diaz Lanza AM, Silvan Sen AM, et al. Effects of some iridoids from plant origin on arachidonic acid metabolism in cellular systems. *Planta Med.*, 66: 324-328. 2000

Chang IM, Ryu JC, Park YC, Yun HS, Yang KH. Protective activities of aucubin against carbon tetrachloride-induced liver damage in mice. *Drug Chem Toxicol*; 6:443-453. 1983

Chang IM, Yun HS. Liver-Protective Activities of Plantago asiatica Seeds. *Planta Med.* 39; 246. 1980

Kim DH, Kim BR, Kim JY, Jeong YC. Mechanism of covalent adduct formation of Aucubin to proteins. *Toxicol Lett.*; 114: 181-188. 2000

Fagopyrum esculentum

See Buckwheat

False Schisandra

Kadsura japonica

DESCRIPTION

Medicinal Parts: The fruit of the plant is considered to have medicinal value, but efficacy has not been documented.

Flower and Fruit: Single axillary flowers on up to 4 cm long, purple stems; there are 9 to 15 white, reddish or yellow tepals. Male flowers have numerous stamens; female flowers have numerous carpels and a superior ovary. The fruit is a berrylike, globose aggregate fruit.

Leaves, Stem, and Root: This dioecious climbing shrub has leaves that are 6 to 11 cm long, elliptical to lanceolate, simple, pergamentlike, with a slightly crenate margin.

Habitat: Indigenous to Japan.

Production: False Schisandra fruit are the dried fruits of *Kadsura japonica.* They are collected in the wild.

Not to be Confused With: Schisandra chinensis

Other Names: Kadsura fruit

ACTIONS AND PHARMACOLOGY

COMPOUNDS

Volatile oil: including germacrene C

Lignans: dibenzo[a,c]cyclooctene lignans, including binankadsurin-A-ester

EFFECTS

Although clinically unsubstantiated, False Schisandra fruit is credited in classical Chinese-Tibetan medicine with an efficacy analogous to that of Schisandra fruit. That drug exhibits liver-protective, inflammation- and tumor-inhibiting, neuroleptic, and anticonvulsive effects, as well as a nonspecific enhancement of physical performance ability. Experimental documentation regarding analogous efficacy of kadsura fruit has not been forthcoming, however.

INDICATIONS AND USAGE

Unproven Uses: The fruit is used for chronic coughs and asthma, chronic diarrhea, enuresis, spermatorrhoea, night sweats, and insomnia.

Chinese Medicine: The fruit is used as an analgesic for pain in the bones, ligaments, stomach, and during menstruation, as well as for spontaneous, painful local swellings.

DOSAGE

Preparation: Before being dried and cut, the fruits are simmered in vinegar.

Daily Dosage: drug: 1.5 to 6 g

Chinese Dosage: 9 to 15 g drug daily

PRECAUTIONS AND ADVERSE REACTIONS

No health hazards are known in conjunction with the proper administration of designated therapeutic dosages.

LITERATURE

Hänsel R, Keller K, Rimpler H, Schneider G (Ed), Hagers Handbuch der Pharmazeutischen Praxis, 5. Aufl., Bde 4 - 6 (Drogen), Springer Verlag Berlin, Heidelberg, New York, 1992-1994.

Hikino H, Kiso Y, Taguchi H, Ikeya Y. Antihepatotoxic Actions of Lignoids from *Schizandra chinensis* Fruits. *Planta Med.* 50; 213-218. 1984

False Unicorn Root

Veratrum luteum

DESCRIPTION

Medicinal Parts: The medicinal part is the root.

Flower and Fruit: The flowers are numerous, greenish-white, without covering leaves. They are dioecious and arranged in terminal racemes of 15 cm with nodelike feathers. The petals are narrow and shorter than the stamens, while the filaments taper to a point. The anthers are terminal and double-lobed. The petals of the female flowers are linear, the stamens short, and the ovary ovate, deltoid, and grooved. The stigmas are oblong, have 3 grooves, and open upward. The fruit is numerous and capsulelike, compressed, and acute.

Leaves, Stem, and Root: The plant is a perennial with a strong leafy stem 30 to 90 cm high. The stem is undivided, smooth, and angular. The foliage leaves are alternate; the lower ones spatulate and the upper ones lanceolate. The basal leaves are 20 cm long, 1.25 cm wide, narrow, and whorled at the base. The rhizome is tuberous and stunted. It is approximately 1.25 cm long.

Characteristics: False Unicorn Root has a bitter taste.

Habitat: The plant grows in the Mississippi Delta region.

Production: False Unicorn Root is the rhizome of *Veratrum luteum*.

Other Names: Starwort, Helonias Root, Blazing Star, Fairy-Wand

ACTIONS AND PHARMACOLOGY

COMPOUNDS

Steroid saponins: (mixture is referred to as chamaelirin, ca. 10%), aglycone diosgenin

EFFECTS

Oxytocic, diuretic, anthelmintic

INDICATIONS AND USAGE

Unproven Uses: False Unicorn Root is used for menstrual disturbances, dysmenorrhea, and pregnancy complaints.

PRECAUTIONS AND ADVERSE REACTIONS

General: No health hazards or side effects are known in conjunction with the proper administration of designated therapeutic dosages. The appearance of gastric complaints is conceivable with the drug, due to the high saponin content, particularly in cases of overdosage.

Pregnancy: Not to be used during pregnancy.

DOSAGE

How Supplied: Liquid Extract

LITERATURE

Atta-Ur-Rahman, Ali RA, Choudhary MI, New steroidal alkaloids from rhizomes of Veratrum album. In: *JNP* 55:565-570. 1992.

Hegnauer R, Chemotaxonomie der Pflanzen, Bde 1-11: Birkhäuser Verlag Basel, Boston, Berlin 1962-1997 (unter *Chamaelirium luteum* (L.) GRAY).

Madaus G, Lehrbuch der Biologischen Arzneimittel, Bde 1-3, Nachdruck, Georg Olms Verlag Hildesheim 1979 (unter *Helionas dioica*).

Wagner H, Wiesenauer M, Phytotherapie. Phytopharmaka und pflanzliche Homöopathika, Fischer-Verlag, Stuttgart, Jena, New York 1995.

Fennel

Foeniculum vulgare

DESCRIPTION

Medicinal Parts: The medicinal parts are the Fennel oil extracted from the ripe fruit and the dried ripe fruit and Fennel seeds of *Foeniculum vulgare*.

Flower and Fruit: The inflorescence is fairly large umbels almost 15 cm across on very irregular rays. The flowers are fairly small and usually androgynous. The petals are a rich yellow, broadly ovate, and have an involute lobe at the tip. The style is very short and almost wartlike. The fruit is glabrous, brownish or greenish-gray. They are 6 to 10 mm long, somewhat cylindrical with blunt ribs and strongly domed.

Leaves, Stem, and Fruit: The plant is biennial to perennial, about 80 to 150 cm high, glabrous, sea-green, and has a strong spicy smell. The stem is erect, round, glabrous, smooth and filled with latex. The lower leaves are petiolate and have long sheaths.

Characteristics: Fennel has a spicy aroma.

Habitat: Fennel is indigenous to the Mediterranean region, has spread to England, Germany, South Tyrol, and Argentina. Fennel is also found today in Iran, India, and China.

Production: Fennel oil is the essential oil obtained from the dried, ripe fruits of *Foeniculum vulgare* by steam distillation. Fennel seed consists of the dried, ripe fruits of *Foeniculum vulgare*.

Other Names: Large Fennel, Sweet Fennel, Wild Fennel, Fenkel, Bitter Fennel

ACTIONS AND PHARMACOLOGY

COMPOUNDS: FENNEL OIL

When extracted from bitter fennel the chief components are:

Trans-anethols (50-75%)

Fenchone (12-33%)

Estragole (2-5%)

Additional components are - alpha-pinenes, camphene, p-cymene, myrcene, limonene, alpha- and beta-phellandrene, gamma-terpenes, terpinols, cis-ocimene

When extracted from sweet fennel the chief components are:

Trans-anethole (80-90%)

Fenchone (1-10%)

Estragole (3-10%)

Additional components are - alpha-pinenes, camphene, p-cymene, myrcene, limonene, alpha- and beta-phellandrene, gamma-terpenes, terpinols, gamma-fenchen

EFFECTS: FENNEL OIL

Stimulation of gastrointestinal motility; in higher concentrations, antispasmodic; experimentally, anethole and fenchone have shown a secretolytic action on the respiratory tract. In vitro, the herb is antimicrobial.

COMPOUNDS: FENNEL SEED

Volatile oil

With bitter fennel the chief components are:

Trans-anethole (50-75%)

Fenchon (12-33%)

Estragole (2-5%)

Additional components - alpha-pinenes, camphene, p-cymene, myrcene, limonene, alpha- and beta-phellandrene, gamma-terpenes, terpinols cis-ocimene

With sweet fennel the chief components are:

Trans-anethole (80-90%)

Fenchon (1-10%)

Estragole (3-10%)

Additional components - alpha-pinenes, camphene, p-cymene, myrcene, limonene, alpha- and beta-phellandrene, gamma-terpenes, terpinols, gamma-fenchen

Hydroxycoumarins (traces): umbelliferone, scopoletine, osthenol, scoparin, Furocoumarins traces) including bergapten, columbianetin, psoralen, xanthotoxin

Pyranocoumarins

Flavonoids

Fatty oil

EFFECTS: FENNEL SEED

The seed promotes gastrointestinal motility. In higher concentrations, Fennel has an antispasmodic effect. Experimentally, anethole and fenchone have been shown to have a secretolytic effect in the respiratory tract of frogs. Aqueous Fennel extracts raised the mucociliary activity of the ciliary epithelium.

INDICATIONS AND USAGE

FENNEL OIL AND SEED

Approved by Commission E:

- Cough
- Bronchitis
- Dyspeptic complaints

Peptic discomforts, such as mild, spastic disorders of the gastrointestinal tract, feeling of fullness, flatulence; catarrh of the upper respiratory tract.

Unproven Uses: Fennel honey is used for catarrh of the upper respiratory tract in children. In folk medicine, the herb was used for fish tapeworms, skin conditions, and for various eye complaints, including conjunctivitis.

PRECAUTIONS AND ADVERSE REACTIONS

General: Health risks or side effects following the proper administration of designated therapeutic dosages are not recorded. Allergic reactions following intake of Fennel have been only very rarely observed. Cross Sensitivity among patients with celery allergy appear to be possible.

Pregnancy: Preparations, excluding the drug itself and tea infusions are not to be administered during pregnancy.

Pediatric Use: Preparations, excluding the drug itself and tea infusions are not to be administered to small children.

DOSAGE

FENNEL OIL

Mode of Administration: Essential oil and galenic preparations for internal use.

Note: Diabetics must check the sugar content of available preparations.

Daily Dosage: 0.1 to 0.6 mL of Fennel oil after each meal.

Duration of administration: Maximum of 2 weeks.

FENNEL SEED

Mode of Administration: Crushed or ground seeds for teas, tea-like products, as well as other galenic preparations for internal use.

Daily Dosage: 5 to 7 g of drug; as a tincture, 5 to 7.5 g per day, with a single dose being 2.5 g 2 to 3 times a day.

LITERATURE

Aye-Than Kulkarni HJ, Wut-Hmone Tha SJ. Anti-diarrhoeal Efficacy of Some Burmese Indigenous Drug Formulations in Experimental Diarrhoeal Test Models. *Int J Crude Drug Res.* 27; 195-200. 1989

Chantraine JM, Laurent D, Ballivian C, Saavedra G, Ibanez R, Vilaseca LA. Insecticidal Activity of Essential Oils on *Aedes aegypti* Larvae. *Phytother Res.* 12 (5); 350-354. 1998

Hiller K, Pharmazeutische Bewertung ausgewählter Teedrogen. In: *DAZ* 135(16):1425-1440. 1995.

Kinoshita K, Kawai T, Imaizumi T, Akita Y, Koyama K, Takahashi K. Anti-emetic principles of *Inula linariaefolia* flowers and *Forsythia suspensa* fruits. *Phytomedicine* 3 (1); 51-58. 1996

Masaki H, Sakaki S, Atsumi T, Sakurai H. Active-Oxygen Scavening Activity of Plant Extracts. *Biol Pharm Bull.* 18 (1); 162-166. 1995

Massoud H, Study on the essential oil in seeds of some fennel cultivars under Egyptian environmental conditions. In: *PM* 58(7):A681. 1992.

Pepeljnjak S, Cvetnik Z. Aflatoxigenicity of *Rhizopus nigricans* strains isolated from drug plants. *Acta Pharm.* 48; 139-144. 1998

Fenugreek

Trigonella foenum-graecum

DESCRIPTION

Medicinal Parts: The medicinal parts are the ripe, dried seeds.

Flower and Fruit: The 0.8 to 1.8 cm long flowers are solitary or in pairs in the leaf axils. They are almost sessile. The calyx tube is membranous and usually longer than the lanceolate tips. The corolla is usually pale yellow, occasionally darker or violet, and about double the length of the calyx. The wings are about half as long as the standard and the carina is very obtuse, round, and barely longer than the calyx. The fruit is a 2.5 to 10 cm long and 0.5 to 1 cm wide, erect, leaning, linear and appressed pubescent pod with a long lip. The 4 to 20 seeds are flattened, divided into two uneven halves by a deep groove, ovate, yellow-brown, or brown-red and very hard when dry.

Leaves, Stem, and Root: The plant is an annual, 10 to 50 cm high herb with a long vertical taproot. The stem is sturdy, round, erect, or decumbent and branched. The leaves are trifoliate and the petioles are 0.5 to 2 cm long. The leaflets are 1 to 3 cm long, obovate to oblong-lanceolate, obtusely deltoid to rounded. The stipules are fairly large, membranous, ovate, acute and more or less softly pubescent.

Habitat: The species is common all over the Mediterranean region as far as India and China and southward as far as Ethiopia. The main regions of cultivation are southern France, Turkey, northern Africa, India and China.

Production: Fenugreek consists of the ripe, dried seed of *Trigonella foenum-graecum.*

Other Names: Greek Hay Seed, Bird's Foot

ACTIONS AND PHARMACOLOGY

COMPOUNDS

Mucilages (25-45%, mannogalactans)

Proteins (25-30%)

Proteinase inhibitors

Steroid saponins (1.2-1.5%): including trigofoenosides A to G (to some extent bitter), aglycones including diosgenin, yamogenin, gitogenin, smilagenin, tigogenin, yuccagenin

Steroid saponin-peptide ester: including foenugraecin

Sterols: chief constituents 24xi-ethyl-cholest-5-en-3beta-ole (65%), sterols that are to some extent estered

Flavonoids: including isoorientin, isovitexin, orientin, orientin arabinoside, isoorientin arabinoside, saponaretin, vicenin-1, vincenin-2, vitexin

Trigonelline (coffearin, N-methylbetaine of the nicotinic acid, 0.4%)

Volatile oil (0.01%): aroma bearer 3-hydroxy-4,5-dimethyl-2(5H)-furanone

EFFECTS

Externally, the drug acts as an emollient. Internally, Fenugreek reduces blood sugar, but the mode of action is unclear. In addition, a lipid-lowering effect attributed to the saponin fraction has been proved as well as a hydrogogic effect. There is no indication of a lactation-promoting effect.

INDICATIONS AND USAGE

Approved by Commission E:

- Loss of appetite
- Inflammation of the skin

Unproven Uses: Internal uses include upper respiratory catarrh, diabetes, and to increase milk production. Externally, the drug is used as poultice for local inflammation, ulcers, and eczema.

Chinese Medicine: The drug is used to treat cold pain in the lower abdomen, impotence, and hernia (said to be due to cold "chi").

Indian Medicine: The drug is used for fever, vomiting, anorexia, coughs, bronchitis, and colitis.

CONTRAINDICATIONS

The drug should not be used during pregnancy.

PRECAUTIONS AND ADVERSE REACTIONS

General: Health risks or side effects following the proper administration of designated therapeutic dosages are not recorded. Sensitization is possible through repeated external administration of the drug.

DRUG INTERACTIONS

MODERATE RISK

Anticoagulants, Low Molecular Weight Heparins and Thrombolytic Agents: Concurrent use may result in increased risk of bleeding. *Clinical Management:* Monitor for signs and symptoms of excessive bleeding.

Antidiabetic Agents: Concurrent use may result in increased risk of hypoglycemia. *Clinical Management:* Monitor blood glucose levels for signs and symptoms of hypoglycemia.

DOSAGE

Mode of Administration: Whole and powdered drug is available in the form of teas and compound preparations.

How Supplied:

Capsules — 575 mg, 610 mg, 626 mg

Preparation: To prepare a tea, leave 0.5 gm drug to steep in cold water for 3 hours, then strain; the tea may be sweetened with honey. A poultice is prepared as a thick paste made from the powdered seeds: add 50 gm of powdered drug to 1/4 liter of boiling water for 5 minutes. To make a cold maceration, soak 0.5 g of drug in cold water, then filter.

Daily Dose: The daily internal dose of the drug is 6 g. One cup of the tea may be taken several times a day. For loss of appetite, take 2 g of cut drug with fluid 3 times daily, before meals. The cold maceration can be drunk several times a day.

LITERATURE

Ali L et al., Characterization of the hypoglycemic effect of Trigonella foenum graecum seed. In: PM 61(4):358-360. 1995.

Weder JK, Heuβner K, Z Lebensm Untersuch Forsch 193:242 et 321. 1991.

Ferula foetida

See Asa Foetida

Ferula gummosa

See Galbanum

Ferula sumbul

See Sumbul

Fever Bark

Alstonia constricta

DESCRIPTION

Medicinal Parts: The medicinal parts are the bark of the root and trunk.

Flower and Fruit: The flowers are creamy white and star-shaped.

Leaves, Stem and Root: Alstonia are evergreen trees, which grow to a height of 15 m. The leaves are glossy, oblong, and petiolate. The tree has a 2 to 7 cm rusty-brown, rugose periderm, which is deeply fissured. The inner surface is yellowish brown and coarsely striated longitudinally.

Characteristics: The tree is a protected species in some countries. The taste is very bitter; the odor is slightly aromatic.

Habitat: Alstonia constricta is indigenous to Australia; *Alstonia scholaris* is indigenous to India and the Philippines.

Production: Alstonia bark is the trunk and branch bark of *Alstonia constricta.*

Other Names: Australian Quinine, Australian Febrifuge, Alstonia Bark, Devil Tree, Dita Bark, Pale Mara, Devil's Bit, Australian Fever Bush, Pali-Mara

ACTIONS AND PHARMACOLOGY

COMPOUNDS

Indole alkaloids: including reserpine, deserpidine, alstonine, tetrahydroalstonine, alstonidine, yohimbine

EFFECTS

The drug is said to be a febrifuge, antispasmodic and antihypertensive. The antihypertensive effect is due to the reserpine and echitamin content.

INDICATIONS AND USAGE

Unproven Uses: The drug is used as a febrifuge and stimulant and for its reserpine content. In the past, it was used to treat rheumatism.

Chinese Medicine: In the Far East, Fever Bark is used for diarrhea and malaria. It has also been used as a uterine stimulant.

PRECAUTIONS AND ADVERSE REACTIONS

No health hazards or side effects are known in conjunction with the proper administration of designated therapeutic dosages. Due to the presence of pharmacologically active indole alkaloids of the beta-carbolin type, side effects may resemble those of Rauwolfia. Symptoms of poisoning following the intake of higher dosages are conceivable.

DOSAGE

Mode of Administration: The forms available are powder, liquid extract, infusion, and tincture. Up-to-date information on usage is not available.

Preparation: Fever Bark is available as an infusion, 1:20, a tincture, 1:8 or 1:10 and as a liquid extract, 1:1.

Daily Dosage: The average daily dose of the infusion is 15 to 20 mL; tincture, 2 to 4 mL; liquid extract, 4 to 8 mL.

LITERATURE

Atta-ur-Rahman AM, et al., *Phytochemistry* 24:2771. 1985

Chopra RN, et al., (Eds.) Chopra's Indigeneous Drugs of India, Vol 1, Dhur and Sons Calcutta. 1938.

Gandhi M, Vinayak VK. Preliminary Evaluation of Extracts of *Alstonia scholaris* Bark for in vivo Antimalarial Activity in Mice. *J Ethnopharmacol*. 29; 51-57 1990

Oliver-Bever B (Ed.), Medicinal Plants of Tropical West Africa, Cambridge University Press Cambridge, London 1986.

Feverfew

Tanacetum parthenium

DESCRIPTION

Medicinal Parts: The medicinal parts are the herb of the plant.

Flower and Fruit: The 5 to 20 composite flower heads are in a dense corymb. The epicalyx has a diameter of 6 to 8 mm. The lingual florets are white and female. The ray florets are 2.5 to 7 mm. The achenes are 1.2 to 1.5 mm and 5- to 8-ribbed.

Leaves, Stem, and Root: The plant is a strongly aromatic perennial. The leaves are pinnatisect to pinnatifid and yellowish-green. The basal and lower cauline leaves are more or less ovate with 3 to 7 oblong-elliptical to ovate segments, which are subpinnately divided. They are crenate or entire-margined.

Habitat: The plant originated in southeastern Europe and is now found all over Europe, Australia, and North America.

Production: Feverfew leaves are the leaves of *Tanacetum parthenium*. The plant is cut before full flowering. It is dried in thin layers in the shade, at temperatures not exceeding 35° C.

Other Names: Featherfew, Featherfoil, Midsummer Daisy

ACTIONS AND PHARMACOLOGY

COMPOUNDS

Volatile oil (0.75%): chief constituents are L-camphor, trans-chrysanthyl acetate, including, camphene, p-cymene, gamma-terpinene, D-germacrene, linalool, borneol, terpinenes-4-ol

Sesquiterpene lactones: especially parthenolide, and also 3-beta-hydroxy-parthenolide, costunolid, reynosin, 8-beta-hydroxy-reynosin, tanaparthin-alpha-peroxide, canin, artecanin, secotanapartholide A

Flavonoids: including apigenin-7-0-glucuronide, chrysoeriol-7-0-glucuronide, luteolin-7-0-glucuronide, luteolin-7-0-glucoside, tanetin

Polyynes: presumably only in fresh plants

EFFECTS

Sesquiterpene lactones, especially parthenolide, are the active compounds in Feverfew. Parthenolide, although a key determinant of biological activity for *Tanacetum parthenium* leaf extracts, is not the sole pharmacologically active constituent. Other sesquiterpene lactones such as 3-beta-hydroxyparthenolide, secotanapartholide A, canin and artecanin, contain an alpha-methylene butyrolactone unit responsible for antisecretory (anti-inflammatory) activity (Groenewegen, 1986). Physiochemical methods were used to measure partholide in several purported commercial Feverfew products. The results found a wide variation in partholide content and in some products, partholide was not detected (Heptinstall, 1992).

Crude chloroform extracts of fresh Feverfew leaves (rich in sesquiterpene lactones) and of commercially available powdered leaves (lactone-free) produce a dose-dependent inhibition of thromboxane B2 and leukotriene B4 (eicosanoids) for an anti-inflammatory effect (Sumner, 1992). Anti-inflammatory properties of Feverfew also consist of inhibition of cellular phospholipases, which prevents release of arachidonic acid (Makheja, 1982). Parthenolide and chrysanthenyl acetate have also been shown to inhibit prostaglandin synthetase (Pugh, 1988). Extracts of Feverfew also inhibit granule secretion in blood platelets and polymorphonuclear leukocytes (Heptinstall, 1985).

Major flavonol and flavone methyl ethers (tanetin) of the herb inhibit the major pathways of arachidonate metabolism in leukocytes (Williams, 1999).

Feverfew extract and parthenolide inhibit human blood aggregation and serotonin (5-HT) secretion by platelets (Groenewegen, 1990). The extract does this through neutralizing cellular sulfhydryl-affecting substances, which are properties of monocyte adherence (Krause, 1990). The chloroform extract of the Feverfew leaf contains an unidentified substance capable of producing a selective, open-channel block of voltage-dependent potassium channels, which results in an antispasmodic effect (Barsby, 1993). Feverfew extract inhibited anti-IgE-induced histamine release in a unique way, which concludes that Feverfew extract contains a novel type of mast cell inhibitor (Hayes, 1987).

The actions of Feverfew's components most likely to contribute to its benefit in migraine as shown in vitro or in animal tests are inhibition of prostaglandin synthesis (Sumner et al, 1992; Williams et al, 1995), blocking platelet granule secretion (Marles et al, 1992), and decreasing vascular smooth muscle spasm (Barsby et al, 1992; Barsby et al, 1993a; Barsby et al, 1993b). One preliminary human study has confirmed a platelet granule secretion decreasing action (Biggs et al, 1982). It has also shown antitumor (Hoffmann et al, 1977; Lee et al, 1971) and mast-cell inhibitory activity (Hayes & Foreman, 1987) in preliminary in vitro tests.

Allergen Diagnostic Test: Feverfew has been used successfully to test for allergenicity in other members of the Compositae family. Allergenicity to members of the Compositae occurred in 118 of 3,851 tested individuals (3.1%) in one group. Seventy percent of those reacting to Compositae reacted to Feverfew specifically (Hausen, 1996). Feverfew has been known to cross-react with tansy, yarrow, marguerite, aster, sunflower, laurel, and liverwort (Frullania) (Schmidt, 1986; Hausen & Osmundsen, 1983).

Analgesic Effects (Against Migraine): A Cochrane review is inconclusive to establish efficacy of Feverfew for migraine headache prevention. Dried or freeze-dried leaves, but not ethanolic extracts, reduce the frequency and severity of migraine headaches. Nausea and vomiting were significantly less severe during Feverfew administration compared to placebo (Gerber, 1997). Although parthenolide is considered by some to be the active agent, the actual active component is unknown and parthenolide content may simply represent a portion of the activity, or assurance that a certain percentage of the actual active ingredient is present.

Anti-inflammatory Effects: Findings support a prostaglandin-related anti-inflammatory action for Feverfew. Feverfew has been shown to suppress 86% to 88% of prostaglandin production, but does not inhibit cyclooxygenase (Miller, 1998). Lipophilic extracts rich in sesquiterpene lactones inhibit production of inflammatory prostaglandins in rat and human leukocytes (Sumner et al, 1992; Heptinstall, 1988). Phospholipase inhibition in platelets in vitro has also been directly documented (Makheja & Bailey, 1982). Inhibition of prostaglandin synthetase has been shown in vitro for parthenolide and related lactones (Pugh & Sambo, 1988). The anti-inflammatory effects of Feverfew may be due to a cytotoxic effect (O'Neill et al, 1987).

Antiplatelet Effects: Platelet aggregation was not significantly affected by Feverfew in 10 subjects (Biggs et al, 1982). Parthenolide and Feverfew have been shown to inhibit platelet serotonin (5-HT) secretion in vitro (Marles et al, 1992; Groenewegen & Heptinstall, 1990, Groenwegen et al, 1986). Feverfew may inhibit 5-HT release via sulfhydryl group (SHG) neutralization (Krause et al, 1990). Lactone-rich Feverfew extracts reduced platelet granule secretion in response to several chemical stimulants to a greater extent than high-dose nonsteroidal anti-inflammatory drugs (Heptinstall et al, 1985). Feverfew extract dose-dependently inhibited uptake and release of arachidonic acid (AA) into or from platelet membrane phospholipids (Loesche et al, 1988). Feverfew has been shown to interfere with the initial step of thomboxane synthesis, inhibiting the release of the arachidonic acid substrate from platelet phospholipids, and resulting ultimately in decreased platelet aggregation (Makheja & Bailey, 1981).

Antispasmodic Effects: Feverfew extracts have spasmolytic activity in that they make smooth muscle nonselectively less responsive to agents such as norepinephrine, acetycholine, bradykinin, prostaglandin, histamine, and serotonin (Diamond, 1987).

Antitumor Effects: Parthenolide and similar lactones are cytotoxic to several human cancer cell lines (Hoffmann et al, 1977; Lee et al, 1971). Parthenolide inhibits thymidine incorporation into DNA (Woynarowski et al, 1981; Woynarowski & Konopa, 1981) and inhibits DNA polymerase function in vitro (Hall et al, 1978). Animal and human studies have not been conducted to confirm these results. Parthenolide, the primary active component in Feverfew, exhibited dose-dependent cytostasis and cytotoxicity when tested in human lymphoma line (TK6) and mouse fibrosarcoma cell line (MN-11). It is postulated that cytostasis occurs due to the reversible inhibition of protein kinases (Ross et al, 1999).

Effects Against Rheumatoid Arthritis: Current evidence does not support the traditional use of Feverfew to treat rheumatoid arthritis.

CLINICAL TRIALS

Migraine

A carbon dioxide-based Feverfew extract MIG-00 was found to be safe and effective for migraine prophylaxis when used in a dosage of 6.25 mg 3 times daily for up to 4 months, according to a 2005 randomized, double-blind, placebo-controlled, parallel-group clinical phase III study. The 170 participants (MIG-99, n=89; placebo, n=81) all fulfilled the International Headache criteria for migraine, and were treated for 16 weeks at multiple study centers after a 4-week baseline period. Migraine frequency decreased from 4.76 by 1.9 attacks monthly in the MIG-99 group and by 1.3 attacks in the placebo group, a significant difference (P=0.0456). This was a favorable benefit-risk ratio for the Feverfew treatment, given its effectiveness and adverse event profile (8.4% versus 10.2% for placebo (Diener et al, 2005).

Less promising results were generated by a randomized, placebo-controlled 2004 trial that found a placebo (riboflavin 25 mg) to be comparable in effectiveness for migraine prophylaxis to a combination drug of Feverfew 100 mg, riboflavin 200 mg, and magnesium 300 mg. Forty-nine patients completed the 3-month trial with a 1-month run-in phase, which allowed for 120 patients to be randomized. The authors concluded that the findings only add to the already conflicting evidence for the efficacy of Feverfew and the other substances studied, as there was no significant difference between the two regimens in terms of percentage of migraines reduced, number of migraine days, migraine index, or other parameters measured. The response of placebo (riboflavin) exceeded that of findings in other trials, suggesting a possible role for this substance in migraine prophylaxis (Maizels et al, 2004).

A 2004 Cochrane Collaboration systematic review of evidence from double-blind and randomized controlled trials examining the efficacy of Feverfew in preventing migraine headache found insufficient evidence of superiority over placebo for this purpose. While the review cited studies that showed some efficacy, the authors noted that overall the evidence was mixed and the methodological quality of the trials included in the review was unsatisfying. It appears from the data that with only mild and transient adverse events reported in the trials examined, it can be concluded that Feverfew presents no major safety problems (Pittler 2004).

Among those studies cited in the Cochrane review was a 1997 trial in which dried whole leaf Feverfew capsules were found to be effective in reducing migraine symptoms in a double-blind, placebo-controlled trial of 57 subjects. None of the participants had taken Feverfew prior to entry into the study. Two 50-mg Feverfew capsules were administered during active treatment phases. Pain intensity, vomiting, photophobia, and phonophobia were all significantly lower during Feverfew treatment compared to baseline (in the run-in, uncontrolled period, $p<0.001$ for all symptoms) or placebo (during the double-blind period, $p<0.01$, $p<0.01$ and $p<0.017$, respectively). Adverse effects were not reported (Palevitch et al, 1997).

The efficacy of dried Feverfew leaves for migraine prophylaxis was assessed in another randomized, placebo-controlled, double-blind, crossover study cited by the Cochrane review. The study consisted of 72 patients with classic or common migraine headaches for more than 2 years. The effect of 1 capsule daily of Feverfew was determined by the use of diary cards and visual analog scores. Duration of treatment was 4 months. After this time, Feverfew was associated with a reduction in number and severity of attacks in each 2-month period. The degree of vomiting was also reduced in the Feverfew treatment group. A significant improvement in the visual analog scale was also observed in the Feverfew treatment group (Murphy, 1988).

Also cited by the Cochrane review was a study in which patients already taking Feverfew for migraine prophylaxis were randomized in a double-blind, placebo-controlled trial. The placebo groups had a significant increase in the frequency and severity of headache, nausea, and vomiting with the emergence of untoward effects during the early months of treatment. There was no change in the frequency or severity of symptoms of migraine in the Feverfew treatment group, thus suggesting that Feverfew may be taken prophylactically to prevent attacks of migraines (Johnson, 1985).

Rheumatoid Arthritis

A double-blind, placebo-controlled study evaluated the use of dried chopped Feverfew (70 mg to 86 mg) in patients with symptomatic rheumatoid arthritis. There were 41 patients involved in the study, and they were observed during a 6-week period. Variables assessed in the study included stiffness, pain (visual analog scale), grip strength, articular index, full blood count, erythrocyte sedimentation rate, urea, creatinine, C-reactive protein, complement breakdown products, rheumatoid factor titre, immunoglobulins (IgG, IgA, IgM), functional capacity, and patient and observer global opinions. While grip strength improved significantly in the Feverfew group compared to the placebo group, there were no other important differences in clinical or laboratory variables between the groups during the study period (Pattrick, 1989).

Supplement Form

A placebo-controlled study employing capsules of ethanol extract of Feverfew could not confirm the results of the previous studies using whole leaf. (De Weerdt et al, 1996).

INDICATIONS AND USAGE

Unproven Uses: Feverfew is used mainly for migraine, arthritis, rheumatic diseases, and allergies. Feverfew has also been used in the treatment of tinnitus, vertigo, arthritis, fever, difficulty during labor, toothache, insect bites, and asthma. In folk medicine, Feverfew is used for cramps, as a tonic, a stimulant, a digestive agent, and a blood purifier. Other uses in folk medicine include migraine prophylaxis, digestion problems, intestinal parasites and gynecological disorders. The herb is also used as a wash for inflammation and wounds, as a tranquilizer, an antiseptic, and following tooth extraction as a mouthwash. The infusion is used for dysmenorrhea. In postnatal care, Feverfew is used to reduce lochia. The drug is used externally as an antiseptic and insecticide.

CONTRAINDICATIONS

Pregnancy: Feverfew is not to be used during pregnancy.

Breastfeeding: Not be used during breast-feeding.

Pediatrics: Not to be used in children under two years of age.

PRECAUTIONS AND ADVERSE REACTIONS

Based on questionnaires completed by 300 Feverfew users, the overall incidence of minor side effects is around 20% (Murdoch, 1989). Feverfew inhibits platelet aggregation and caution should be used in patients on other platelet aggregation inhibitors such as aspirin and dipyridamole (Miller, 1998).

The drug has a high potential for sensitization via skin contact. Occupational or direct exposure has caused eczema and allergic dermatitis. Feverfew has been known to cross-react with Tansy, Yarrow, Marguerite, Aster, Sunflower, Laurel, and Liverwort (Schmidt, 1986; Guin & Skidmore, 1987; Paulsen, 1998). Other adverse reactions include abdominal pain, diarrhea, lip swelling, mouth ulcers (from chewing leaf), and glossitis (from chewing leaf) (Klepser & Klepser, 1999; Murdoch, 1989; deSmet & Vulto, 1987).

Cardiovascular: Transient increases in heart rate have occasionally been reported (Murdoch, 1989).

Hypersensitivity: Allergenicity to members of the Compositae family occurred in 118 of 3,851 tested individuals (3.1%) in one group. Seventy percent of those reacting to Compositae reacted to Feverfew specifically (Hausen, 1996). Another study of 686 European patients showed a 4.5% Compositae hypersensitivity (Paulsen et al, 1993).

Musculoskeletal: Feverfew contains sesquiterpenes (parthenolide and cynaropicrin), which have been shown to induce toxic and irreversible inhibition of smooth muscle contractility when there are high concentrations in the tissue (Hay, 1994).

Post-Feverfew Syndrome: About 10% of migraine patients who abruptly stop taking Feverfew may experience rebound headaches, insomnia, muscle stiffness, joint pain, fatigue, nervousness, and tension (Miller, 1998; Murdoch, 1989; Baldwin, 1987).

DRUG INTERACTIONS

MODERATE RISK:

Anticoagulants, low molecular weight heparins, thrombolytic agents: Concurrent use may result in increased risk of bleeding. *Clinical Management*: If Feverfew is taken with any of these drugs, monitor for signs and symptoms of excessive bleeding.

Antiplatelet agents: Concurrent use may result in increased risk of bleeding. *Clinical Management*: If Feverfew is taken with an antiplatelet drug, monitor for signs and symptoms of excessive bleeding to determine if platelet function has been adversely affected by feverfew.

Nonsteroidal Anti-inflammatory Agents: Concurrent use may result in increased risk of adverse effects from the nonsteroidal antiinflammatory agent (i.e., gastrointestinal, renal effects). *Clinical Management*: Avoid concomitant use of Feverfew with nonsteroidal anti-inflammatory agents.

DOSAGE

Mode of Administration: Feverfew preparations are used both internally and externally.

How Supplied:

Capsules – 80 mg, 100 mg, 380 mg, 384 mg, 400 mg, 500 mg, 1000 mg

Tablets – 12 mg (standardized to 600 mcg sesuiterpine lactone content)

Liquid Extract

Fresh leaf: ~25 mg

Preparation: To make an infusion, use 2 teaspoonfuls of the drug per cup, allow to steep for 15 minutes. To make a strong infusion, double the amount and allow to steep for 25 minutes.

Daily Dosage:

Capsules – 200 to 250 mg daily for the treatment of migraines; the usual standardization level is 0.2% parthenolide content (Brown, 1996). Freshly dried powdered Feverfew of 25 mg is approximately equal to 0.1 mg of sesquiterpine lactones (SL) (Mervyn,1986).

Fresh leaf – 1 to 3 leaves (25 to 75 mg) once or twice daily has been recommended (Johnson et al, 1985; O'Hara, 1998).

Unproven uses – 3 cups of the infusion are taken per day. The stronger infusions are used for washes.

Storage: Store the herb in sealed containers.

LITERATURE

Abad MJ, Berjemo P, Villar A. *Phytother Res* 9:79-92. 1995.

Abebe W. Herbal medication: potential for adverse interactions with analgesic drugs. *J Clin Pharm Ther*; 27:391-401. 2002.

Anderson D, Jenkinson PC, Dewdney RS, Blower SD, Johnson ES, Kadam NP. *Human Toxicol* 7:145-152. 1988.

Anonym, Naturmedizin. Mutterkraut gegen Migräne. In: *DAZ* 137(28):2424. 1997.

Awang DVC, Dawson BA, Kindack DG, Crompton CW, Heptinstall S. *JNP* 54:1516-1521. 1991.

Baldwin CA, Anderson LA & Phillpson JD. What pharmacists should know about Feverfew. *J Pharm Pharmacol*; 239:237-238. 1987.

Barsby RW, Knight DW, McFadzean I. A chloroform extract of the herb Feverfew blocks voltage-dependent potassium currents recorded from single smooth muscle cells. *J Pharm Pharmacol* Jul;45(7):641-645. 1993b.

Barsby RWJ, Salan U, Knight DW et al. Feverfew and vascular smooth muscle: extracts from fresh and dried plants show opposing pharmacological profiles, dependent upon sesquiterpene lactone content. *Planta Med*; 59(1):20-25. 1993a.

Barsby RWJ, Salan U, Knight DW et al. Feverfew extracts and parthenolide irreversibly inhibit vascular responses of the rabbit aorta. *J Pharm Pharmacol*; 44(9)737-740.1992.

Biggs MJ, Johnson ES, Persaud NP et al. Platelet aggregation in patients using Feverfew for migraine. *Lancet*; 2:776. 1982.

Biggs MJ, Johnson ES, Persaud NP et al. Platelet aggregation in patients using Feverfew for migraine (letter). *Lancet*; 2(8301):776. 1982.

Bohlmann F, Zdero C. *Phytochemistry* 21(10):2543. 1982.

Brown AMG et al., Inhibition of human neutrophils by aqueous and organic extracts of *Tanacetum ssp*. In: PM 62, Abstracts of the 44th Ann Congress of GA, 66. 1996.

Brown AMG, Edwards CM, Lowe KC et al. Effects of parthenolide and Feverfew (*Tanacetum parthenium*) extracts on human neutrophils in vitro. *Br J Pharmacol*; 119:265P. 1996.

Brown AMG, Edwards CM, Davey MR et al. Pharmacological activity of Feverfew (*Tanacetum parthenium (L.)* Schultz-Bip): assessment by inhibition of human polymorphnuclear leukocyte chemiluminescence in-vitro. *J Pharm Pharmacol* May;49(5):558-61. 1997.

Christensen LP; Jakobsen HB; Paulsen E et al. Airborne Compositae dermatitis: monoterpenes and no parthenolide are released from flowering Tanacetum parthenium (Feverfew) plants. *Arch Dermatol Res* Jul-Aug;291(7-8):425-31. 1999.

Collier HOJ, Butt NM, McDonald-Gibson WJ et al. Extract of Feverfew inhibits prostaglandin biosynthesis. *Lancet*; 1:922-923. 1980.

De Smet PAGM & Vulto AG. Drugs used in nonorthodox medicine. *Side Eff Drugs*; 11:422-431. 1987.

De Weerdt CJ, Bootsma HPR, Hendricks H, Herbal medicines in migraine prevention. In: *Phytomedicine* 3(3):225-230. 1996.

Diamond S. Herbal therapy for migraine: an unconventional approach. *Postgrad Med*; 82(1):197-198. 1987.

Diener H, Pfaffenrath V, Schnitker J et al. Efficacy and safety of 6.25 mg t.i.d. feverfew CO-extract (MIG-99) in migraine prevention - a randomized, double-blind, multicentre, placebo-controlled study. *Cephalalgia*; 25:1031-41. 2005.

Gawel MJ. The use of Feverfew in the prophylaxis of migraine attacks. *J New Dev Clin Med*; 13(2):79-86. 1995.

Goulden V & Wilkinson SM. Patch testing for Compositae allergy. *Br J Dermatol*; 138(6):1018-1021. 1998.

Groenewegen WA, Heptinstall S, A comparison of the effects of an extract of Feverfew and parthenolide, a component of Feverfew, on human platelet activity in-vitro. *J Pharm Pharmacol* Aug;42(8):553-557. 1990.

Groenwegen WA & Heptinstall S. Amounts of Feverfew in commercial preparations of the herb. *Lancet*; 1(8471):44-45. 1986.

Groenewegen WA, Knight DW & Heptinstall S. Compounds extracted from Feverfew that have anti-secretory activity contain an alpha-methylene butyrolactone unit. *J Pharm Pharmacol*; 38(9):709-712.1986.

Groenewegen WA, Knight DW & Heptinstall S. Progress in the medicinal chemistry of the herb Feverfew. *Prog Med Chem*; 29:217-238. 1992.

Guin JD & Skidmore G. Compositae dermatitis in childhood. *Arch Dermatol*; 123(4):500-502. 1987.

Hall IH, Lee KH, Starnes CO et al. Antitumor agents XXX: evaluation of alpha-methylene-gamma-lactone-containing agents for inhibition of tumor growth, respiration, and nucleic acid synthesis. *J Pharm Sci*; 67(9):1235-1239. 1978.

Hausen BM. A 6-year experience with Compositae mix. *Am J Contact Dermatitis*; 7(2):94-99. 1996.

Hausen BM. Berufsbedingte Kontaktallergie auf Mutterkraut (*Tanacetum parthenium* (L) Schultz-Bip.; Asteraceae) (German). *Derm Beruf Umwelt*; 29(1):18-21. 1981.

Hausen BM & Osmundsen PE. Contact allergy to parthenolide in *Tanacetum parthenium* (L.) Schulz-Bip. (Feverfew, Asteraceae) and cross-reactions to related sesquiterpene lactone containing Compositae species. *Acta Derm Venereol*; 63(4):308-314. 1983.

Hay AJ, Hamburger M, Hostettmann K et al. Toxic inhibition of smooth muscle contractility by plant-derived sesquiterpenes caused by their chemically reactive alpha-methylenebutyrolactone functions. *Br J Pharmacol*;112:9-12. 1994.

Hayes NA & Foreman JC. The activity of compounds extracted from Feverfew on histamine release from rat mast cells. *J Pharm Pharmacol*; 39(6):466-470. 1987.

Heptinstall S, Awang DVC, Dawson BA et al. Parthenolide content and bioactivity of Feverfew (*Tanacetum parthenium* (L) Schultz Bip): estimation of commercial and authenticated Feverfew products. *J Pharm Pharmacol*; 44(5):391-395. 1992.

Heptinstall S, Groenewegen P, Spangenberg P et al. Extracts of Feverfew may inhibit platelet behavior via neutralization of sulphydryl groups. *J Pharm Pharmacol*; 39(6):459-465. 1987.

Heptinstall S. Feverfew - an ancient remedy for modern times? *J R Soc Med*; 81(7):373-374. 1988.

Heptinstall S, White A, Williamson L, Mitchell J. Extracts of Feverfew inhibit granule secretion in the blood platelets and polymorphonuclear leukocytes. *Lancet* May 11;1(8437):1071-1074. 1985.

Hoffmann JJ, Torrance SJ, Widehopf RM et al. Cytotoxic agents from *Michelia champaca* and *Talauma ovata:* parthenolide and costunolide. *J Pharm Sci*; 66(6):883-684. 1977.

Hylands PJ, Hylands DM. *Dev Drugs Mod Med* 100-104. 1986.

Hylands DM, Hylands PJ, Johnson ES et al. Efficacy of Feverfew as prophylactic treatment of migraine (letter, reply). *BMJ*; 291(6502):1128. 1985.

Johnson ES, Kadam NP, Hylands DM et al. Efficacy of Feverfew as prophylactic treatment of migraine. *BMJ* Aug 31;291(6495):569-573. 1985.

Klepser TB & Klepser ME. Unsafe and potentially safe herbal therapies. *Am J Health Sys Pharm*; 56(2):125-138. 1999.

Krause S, Arese P, Heptinstall S, Losche W. Influence of substances affecting cell sulfhydryl/disulfide status on ahderence of human monocytes. *Arzneimittelforschung* Jun;40(6):689-92. 1990.

Lamminpaa A, Estlander T, Jolanki R et al. Occupational allergic contact dermatitis caused by decorative plants. *Contact Dermatitis*; 34(5):330-335. 1996.

Lee KH, Huang ES, Piantadosi C et al. Cytotoxicity of sesquiterpene lactones. *Cancer Res*; 31(11):1649-1654. 1971.

Lösche W, Groenewegen WA, Krause S et al. Effects of an extract of Feverfew (*Tanacetum parthenium*) on arachidonic acid metabolism in human blood platelets. *Biomed Biochim Acta*; 47(10-11):S241-S243. 1988.

Lösche W, Mazurov AV et al. An extract of Feverfew inhibits interaction of human platelets with collagen substrates. *Thromb Res.*; 48(5):511-518. 1987.

Lösche W, Mazurov AV, Heptinstall S, Groenewegen WA, Repin VS, Till U. *Throm Res* 48:511-518. 1978.

MacGregor EA. Prescribing for migraine. *Prescrib J*; 33(2):50-58. 1993.

Maizels M, Blumenfeld A, Burchette R. A combination of riboflavin, magnesium, and feverfew for migraine prophylaxis: a randomized trial. *Headache;* 44(9):885-90. 2004

Makheja AN, Bailey JM. *Lancet* II:1054. 1981.

Makheja AN, Bailey JM. A platelet phospholipase inhibitor from the medicinal herb Feverfew (*Tanacetum parthenium*). *Prostaglandins Leukot Med* Jun;8(6):653-660. 1982.

Makheja AN & Bailey JM. The active principle in Feverfew. *Lancet*; 2:1054. 1981.

Makheja AN & Bailey JM. The active principle in Feverfew (letter). *Lancet*; 2(8254):1054. 1981.

Marles RJ, Kaminski J, Arnason JT, et al. A bioassay for inhibition of serotonin release from bovine platelets. *J Nat Prod* Aug;55(8):1044-56. 1992.

Mensing H, Kimmig W & Hausen BJ. Airborne contact dermatitis. *Hautarzt*; 36:398-402. 1985.

Mervyn L. Standardized Feverfew preparations. *Lancet*; 1(8474):209. 1986.

Miller LG, Herbal medicinals. selected clinical considerations focusing on known or potential drug-herb interactions. *Arch Intern Med*; 158(20):2200-2211. 1998.

Mitchell JC, Geissman TA, Dupuis G, Towers GHN. *Invest Dermatol* 56:98-101. 1971.

Murch SJ, Simmons CB & Saxena PK. Melatonin in Feverfew and other medicinal plants. *Lancet*; 350(9091):1598-1599. 1997.

Murdoch JK. Feverfew for migraine prophylaxis. *Can J Hosp Pharm*; 42(5):209-210. 1989.

Murphy JJ, Heptinstall S, Mitchell JRA, Randomized double-blind placebo-controlled trial of Feverfew in migraine prevention. *Lancet* Jul 23;2(8604):189-192. 1988.

Norred CL & Brinker F. Potential coagulation effects of preoperative complementary and alternative medicines. *Alt Ther*; 7(6):58-67. 2001.

O'Hara MA, Kiefer D, Farrell K et al., A review of 12 commonly used medicinal herbs. *Arch Fam Med*; 7(6):523-536. 1998.

O'Neill LAJ, Barrett ML & Lewis GP. Extracts of Feverfew inhibit mitogen-induced human peripheral blood mononumclear cell proliferation and cytokine mediated responses: a cytotoxic effect. *Br J Clin Pharmacol*; 23(1):81-83. 1987.

Pattrick M, Heptinstall S, Doherty M. Feverfew in rheumatoid arthritis: a double-blind, placebo-controlled study. *Ann Rheum Dis* Jul;48(7):547-9. 1989.

Paulsen E. Occupational dermatitis in Danish gardeners and greenhouse workers (II). Etiological factors. *Contact Dermatitis* Jan;38(1):14-9. 1998.

Paulsen E, Andersen E & Hausen BM. Compositae dermatitis in a Danish dermatology department in one year, I: results of routine patch testing with sesquiterpene lactone mix supplemented with aimed patch testing with extracts and sesquiterpene lactones of Compositae plants. *Contact Dermatitis*; 29(1):6-10. 1993.

Pittler MH & Ernst E. Feverfew for preventing migraine (Cochrane review).: In: The Cochrane Library, Issue 1. Chichester, UK: John Wiley & Sons, Ltd. 2004.

Pugh WJ, Sambo K. Prostaglandin synthetase inhibitors in Feverfew. *J Pharm Pharmacol* Oct;40(10):743-5. 1988..

Schmidt RJ, Plant dermatitis. Compositae. *Clin Dermatol* Apr-Jun;4(2):46-61. 1986.

Sumner H, Salan U, Knight D, Hoult J. Inhibition of 5-lipoxygenase and cyclo-oxygenase in leukocytes by Feverfew. Involvement of sesquiterpene lactones and other components. *Biochem Pharmacol* Jun 9;43(11):2313-2320. 1992.

Turner P. Adverse effects to drugs in migraine: some recent reports (editorial). *Hum Toxicol*; 4(5):474-476. 1985.

Voyna-Yasenetskaja TA, Lösche W, Groenewegen WA, Heptintall S, Repin VS, Till U. *J Pharm Pharmacol* 40:501-502. 1988.

Waller PC & Ramsay LE. Efficacy of Feverfew as prophylactic treatment of migraine (letter). *BMJ* (Clin Res Ed); 291(6502):1128. 1985.

Williams CA, Harborne JB, Geiger H, Hoult JR. The flavonoids of *Tanacetum parthenium* and *T. vulgare* and their anti-inflammatory properties. *Phytochemistry* Jun;51(3):417-23. 1999.

Williams CA, Hoult JR, Harborne JB et al., A biologically active lipophilic flavonol from *Tanacetum parthenium. Phytochemistry* Jan;38(1):267-70. 1995..

Woynarowski JM & Konopa J. Inhibition of DNA biosynthesis in HeLa cells by cytotoxic and antitumor sesquiterpene lactones. *Mol Pharmacol*; 19(1):97-102. 1981.

Woynarowski JW, Beerman TA & Konopa J. Induction of deoxyribonucleic acid damage in HeLa S3 cells by cytotoxic and antitumor sesquiterpene lactones. *Biochem Pharmacol*; 30(21):3005-3007. 1981.

Ficus carica

See Figs

Field Scabious

Knautia arvensis

DESCRIPTION

Medicinal Parts: The medicinal parts are the leafy stem including the flower heads and the fresh aerial parts of the flowering plant.

Flower and Fruit: The flat-domed, composite flowers are on long, pubescent, glandular or nonglandular pedicles. The androgynous heads are 2 to 4 cm in diameter and contain 85 to 100 florets. The female capitula are smaller and contain 55 to 60 florets. The florets are blue-lilac, occasionally red-lilac or yellowish-white to pure white. The lateral florets are raylike. The 2- to 3-rowed involucre bracts are lanceolate, compressed, and long-haired. The edge of the calyx has 8 to 16 bristles. The corolla is fused and 4 tipped. There are 4 stamens and 1 inferior ovary. The fruit is a nutlet 5 to 6 mm long and about 2 mm wide. The fruit is thickly covered in vertical hairs.

Leaves, Stem, and Root: The plant is perennial and 30 to 150 cm high. The rhizome is branched and has a strong taproot. The rhizome produces a flowering stem from the leaf rosette, which survives the winter. The stem is erect, lightly branched, and has short gray hairs. The leaves are opposite, gray-green, and matte. The lower ones are petioled, oblong, and entire-margined. The upper leaves are sessile, pinnatisect, and have lanceolate tips.

Habitat: The plant is found all over Europe except the Arctic. It is also found in the Caucasus and western Siberia.

Production: Field Scabious herb consists of the leafy stems and flower heads and also occasionally the root of *Knautia arvensis.*

Other Names: Devil's Bit, Seabridge

ACTIONS AND PHARMACOLOGY

COMPOUNDS

Triterpene saponins: knautioside (1.1-1.7%)

Steroids: sterols, including beta-sitosterol glucoside, knautiosides A and B

Iridoide monoterpenes: including dipsacan

Flavonoids: including leucanthoside, luteoloside

Tannins

EFFECTS

The drug is said to have an astringent, antiseptic, expectorant and even purgative effect. None of these effects have been proven.

INDICATIONS AND USAGE

Unproven Uses: The drug is used for chronic skin diseases, eczema, anal fissures, pruritus ani, urticaria, scabies, favus, and for the cleansing and healing of ulcers. It is also used to treat coughs and throat complaints, as well as cystitis.

Homeopathic Uses: Field Scabious is used in homeopathic remedies to treat respiratory tract inflammations and poor digestion.

PRECAUTIONS AND ADVERSE REACTIONS

No health hazards or side effects are known in conjunction with the proper administration of designated therapeutic dosages.

DOSAGE

Mode of Administration: Decoction and infusion preparations are used both internally and externally.

Preparation: For preparation of the drug, use approximately 30 gm infusion or decoction, add to 1 liter of hot water, strain, and cool.

Daily Dosage: For chronic eczema, add 4 teaspoonfuls to 2 glasses of water, leave to steep for 10 minutes and drink during the course of the day.

Homeopathic Dosage: 5 drops, 1 tablet or 10 globules every 30 to 60 minutes (acute) or 1 to 3 times daily (chronic); parenterally: 1 to 2 mL s.c., acute: 3 times daily; chronic: once a day (HAB1).

LITERATURE

Hänsel R, Keller K, Rimpler H, Schneider G (Hrsg.), Hagers Handbuch der Pharmazeutischen Praxis, 5. Aufl., Bde 4-6 (Drogen), Springer Verlag Berlin, Heidelberg, New York, 1992-1994.

Madaus G, Lehrbuch der Biologischen Arzneimittel, Bde 1-3, Nachdruck, Georg Olms Verlag Hildesheim 1979.

Figs

Ficus carica

DESCRIPTION

Medicinal Parts: The medicinal parts are the fruit and the tree sap latex.

Flower and Fruit: In its known form, the fig is neither a fruit nor a flower. It is a hollow, fleshy receptacle enclosing numerous flowers, which are never exposed to sunlight, but nevertheless develop fully and produce seeds. The inflorescence is hidden in the body of the fruit. The edge of the pear-shaped receptacle is curved inwards forming an almost closed hollow space. The numerous fertile and sterile florets are on the inner surface. When it ripens, the receptacle enlarges and the one-seeded fruit becomes embedded in it. It appears as a single purple-brown fruit.

Leaves, Stem and Root: Ficus carica is a deciduous, heavily branched tree growing to 4 m or more. The leaves are downy beneath and are 10 to 20 cm long, broad-ovate to orbicular with 3 to 5 deep lobes.

Habitat: Indigenous to Asia Minor, Syria, and Iran. It is cultivated or grows wild in many subtropical regions.

Production: Figs consists of the dried fruits of *Ficus carica.*

ACTIONS AND PHARMACOLOGY

COMPOUNDS

Furanocoumarins: including psoralen, bergaptene

Fruit acids: citric acid, malic acid

Monosaccharides/oligosaccharides (approximately 50%), to some extent transformed into inverted sugar

Mucilages

Pectin

Vitamin B and C

EFFECTS

No information is available

INDICATIONS AND USAGE

Unproven Uses: Fig preparations are used as a laxative.

Chinese Medicine: In China, figs are used for dysentery and enteritis.

PRECAUTIONS AND ADVERSE REACTIONS

No health hazards or side effects are known in conjunction with the proper administration of designated therapeutic dosages.

LITERATURE

Ahmed W, Khan AQ, Malik A. Two Triterpenes from the Leaves of *Ficus carica. Planta Med.* 54; 481. 1988

Alwan AH, Al-Bayati ZA. Effects of Milk Latex of Fig (Ficus carica) on 3H-Benzo(alpha)Pyrene Binding to Rat liver Microsomal Protein. *Int J Crude Drug Res.* 26; 209-213. 1988

Al-Bayati ZAF, Alwan AH. Effects of Fig Latex on Lipid Peroxidation and CCl4-induced Lipid Peroxidation in Rat Liver. *J Ethnopharmacol.* 30; 215-221. 1990

Dechamp C, Bessot JC, Pauli G, Deviller P. First report of anaphylactic reaction after fig (*Ficus carica*) ingestion. *Allergy,* 50:514-6, Jun 1995

Gibernau M, Buser HR, Frey JE, Hossaert-McKey M. Volatile Compounds from Extracts of Figs of *Ficus carica. Phytochemistry* 46 (2); 241-244. 1997

Kern W, List PH, Hörhammer L (Hrsg.), Hagers Handbuch der Pharmazeutischen Praxis, 4. Aufl., Bde. 1-8, Springer Verlag Berlin, Heidelberg, New York, 1969.

Siewek F et al. (1985) Z NaturForsch 40 (1/2): 8.

Teuscher E, Biogene Arzneimittel, 5. Aufl., Wiss. Verlagsges. mbH Stuttgart 1997.

Figwort

Scrophularia nodosa

DESCRIPTION

Medicinal Parts: The medicinal parts of the plant are the dried herb harvested before flowering, the herb with the root, and the root alone.

Flower and Fruit: The reddish-brown or greenish-yellow flowers are in terminal panicles. The calyx has 5 segments, with ovate, narrow-tunicate margined cusps. The corolla is a bilabiate, swollen, almost globular tube. The upper lip is divided into 2 and the lower lip is trilobed with revolute lobes. There are 4 stamens and 1 superior ovary. The fruit is an ovate, many-seeded, and pointed green capsule.

Leaves, Stem, and Root: The perennial plant grows from 50 to 100 cm high. The root capitula have ovate, tuberous nodes. The stem is erect, sharply quadrangular, often purple, glabrous, and has a row of hairs at the nodes. The leaves are crossed opposite, dark green, oblong, double serrate and often cordate at the base.

Habitat: The plant is indigenous to Europe, central Asia, and North America.

Other Names: Throatwort, Carpenter's Square, Kernelwort, Heal-All Scrofula Plant, Rosenoble

ACTIONS AND PHARMACOLOGY

COMPOUNDS

Iridoides: including monoterpenes

Flavonoids: including among others, diosmin

Tannins

Saponins

EFFECTS

Figwort has a diuretic and mildly laxative effect. (No new research is available.)

INDICATIONS AND USAGE

Homeopathic Uses: The drug is used for low resistance, chronic tonsillitis, and tonsillar hypertony as well as for lymphedema.

PRECAUTIONS AND ADVERSE REACTIONS

No health hazards or side effects are known in conjunction with the proper administration of designated therapeutic dosages.

DOSAGE

Preparation: Homeopathic preparations of the mother tincture are derived from the whole Figwort plant in dilutions.

Homeopathic Dosage: 15 to 20 drops to be taken orally 3 times daily. *Scrophularia nodosa* can be administered by injection for long-term treatment

LITERATURE

Fernandez MA, Garcia MD, Saenz MT. Antibacterial activity of the phenolic acids fractions of *Scrophularia frutescens* and *Scrophularia sambucifolia. J Ethnopharmacol,* 53:11-4, Jul 26 1996

Fernandez MA, Garcia MD, Saenz MT. Antiinflammatory effects of different extracts and harpagoside isolated from *Scrophularia frutescens L. Farmaco*, 53:443-6, Jun 1996

Fernandez MA, Garcia MD, Saenz MT. Gas chromatographic determination of chlorothalonil in leaves and roots of *Scrophularia* and in soil. *J AOAC Int*, 53:587-8, Mar-Apr 1996

Pauli GF, Ofterdinger-Daegel, S, Teborg D, Digitalis, Scrophularia & Co. In: DAZ 135(2):111. 1995.

Filipendula ulmaria

See Meadowsweet

Fish Berry

Anamirta cocculus

DESCRIPTION

Medicinal Parts: The medicinal part of the plant is the ripe, dried fruit.

Flower and Fruit: The plant's petiolate inflorescences are paniclelike, 16 to 40 cm long, and usually inserted in the stem. Male flowers are occasionally axillary. The two outer petals are smaller and about 1 mm long. The inner petals are imbricate, whitish or yellowish-green, broad-elliptoid, 2 to 3 mm long, and appear in 2 alternating, triple whorls. The synandria are formed from a short-stemmed, globose cluster of about 30 to 35 anthers. The pollen is round and tricolporate. The female flowers have 3 tepals as well as small staminoids. The 3 or 4 carpels are set sideways on a central, erect fruit axis that becomes conically oblong when the fruit ripens. The style is inserted in the side and the stigma is turned back. The drupes are globose to reniform, 9 to 11 mm long, glabrous, and sit on the short, spreading branches of the fruit axis. The fruit is about 1 cm long, blackish, and contains a horseshoe-shaped seed.

Leaves, Stem and Root: Anamirta cocculus are hardy, woody lianas with ash-gray to straw-yellow striped bark. The leaves are ovate to cordate. The leaf blade is 16 to 28 cm long and 10 to 24 cm wide and coriaceous. The main veins are arranged in palmate fashion at the base with parallel secondary veins. The 6 to 18 cm petiole is thickened at both ends.

Characteristics: The fruit shell is tasteless; the seed is bitter and oily.

Habitat: The plant grows in India, Sri Lanka and Malaysia.

Production: Fish Berry seeds are the fruit of the false myrtle *Anamirta cocculus*. They are collected in the wild and sun-dried after harvesting.

Other Names: Levant Nut, Crow Killer, Fish Killer, Indian Berry, Cocculus Indicus

ACTIONS AND PHARMACOLOGY

COMPOUNDS

Sesquiterpens: picrotoxin, a mixture of picrotoxinine and its by product picrotin, picrotoxin acid methyl ester

Isoquinoline alkaloids: menispermine, paramenispermine

Fatty oil

EFFECTS

The effect of the drug is due to the picrotoxin content. Picrotoxin paralyzes presynaptic blocking mechanisms and, like strychnine, has an analeptic effect in low doses. The central ends of the parasympathetic nerves are stimulated, as is the medulla oblongata. Breathing frequency is initially increased and subsequently decreased. The pulse slows due to the stimulation of the vagus and an increase in blood pressure. Central nervous system-stimulated vomiting along with an increase in perspiration and saliva are probably also due to the action of picrotoxin.

INDICATIONS AND USAGE

Unproven Uses: In the past, the drug was used as an insecticide in powder form for scabies. Its use against skin parasites and lice, while not substantiated, seems plausible. It was also used in cases of barbituric acid poisoning. In more recent times, it has been used in the treatment of peripheral and vestibular nystagmus, and in both long- and short-term therapy for peripherally based dizziness as well as travel sickness.

Indian Medicine: The seeds have been used externally in India and on the Malaysian archipelago for gout, skin diseases, and parasites. The tender leaves are used as a contracting agent for the womb after birth.

Homeopathic Uses: The drug is used for nervous exhaustion, attacks of dizziness, cramps, paralysis, dysmenorrhea, and occipital headaches. Efficacy has not been proved.

PRECAUTIONS AND ADVERSE REACTIONS

The drug is very poisonous. Mild poisonings cause headache, dizziness, nausea, coordination disturbances, general depression, and spastic twitching.

OVERDOSAGE

With high dosages, the symptoms above are followed by frequent vomiting, sleepiness and tonic-clonic spasms. Death follows, often not until days later, through asphyxiation and heart failure. Two to three Cocculus kernels can be fatal.

Treatment consists of inducing vomiting and/or gastric lavage, purging with sodium sulphate, instillation of activated charcoal and forced diuresis. The spasms should be suppressed with diazepam, but only as much as is absolutely necessary. In case of fever, the patient should be wrapped in ice packs, administered high-caloric infusions and possibly given oxygen respiration. Phenothiazines and analeptics should be avoided.

DOSAGE

Mode of Administration: In combination preparations.

How Supplied: Commercial preparations include ampules, drops, and tablets.

Preparation: Liquid extract is prepared using a 1:1 ratio of the drug and 90% ethanol A mixture of the extract and coconut oil is prepared using a ratio of 1:8; tincture: 1:10 tincture: 70% ethanol; *unguetum cocculi*: 125 g extract plus 650 g coconut oil plus 50 g beeswax and 250 g paraffin; picrotoxin extraction is made using special procedures; maximum yield 1.5%

Daily Dosage: One to 5 mg can be taken by healthy patients who do not experience side effects. For peripheral states of dizziness: 1 mg to 5 mg (picrotoxin) by slow intravenous infusion. As a long-term treatment: 1 mg suppositories for 3 weeks.

Homeopathic Dosage: 5 drops, 1 tablet, or 10 globules every 30 to 60 minutes (for acute conditions), or 1 ml twice a week sc or ointment 1 or 2 times daily for chronic conditions.

Storage: Because they are poisonous, preparations should be secured in tightly closed containers, protected from light and unauthorized access.

LITERATURE

Frohne D, Pikrotoxin - Renaisssance eines ''obsoleten'' pflanzlichen Arzneistoffes. In: ZPT 10(3):101. 1989.

Hänsel R, Keller K, Rimpler H, Schneider G (Hrsg.), Hagers Handbuch der Pharmazeutischen Praxis, 5. Aufl., Bde 4-6 (Drogen), Springer Verlag Berlin, Heidelberg, New York, 1992-1994.

Lewin L, Gifte und Vergiftungen, 6. Aufl., Nachdruck, Haug Verlag, Heidelberg 1992.

Mahato SB, Sen S. Advances in Triterpenoid Research, 1990-1994. *Phytochemistry* 44 (7); 1185-1236. 1997

Roth L, Daunderer M, Kormann K, Giftpflanzen, Pflanzengifte, 4. Aufl., Ecomed Fachverlag Landsberg Lech 1993.

Steinegger E, Hänsel R, Pharmakognosie, 5. Aufl., Springer Verlag Heidelberg 1992.

Teuscher E, Biogene Arzneimittel, 5. Aufl., Wiss. Verlagsges. mbH Stuttgart 1997.

Teuscher E, Lindequist U, Biogene Gifte - Biologie, Chemie, Pharmakologie, 2. Aufl., Fischer Verlag Stuttgart 1994.

Wagner H, Wiesenauer M, Phytotherapie. Phytopharmaka und pflanzliche Homöopathika, Fischer-Verlag, Stuttgart, Jena, New York 1995.

Flax

Linum usitatissimum

DESCRIPTION

Medicinal Parts: The medicinal parts are the stem as a sterile linen thread, the oil extracted from the seeds, the dry ripe seeds, the linseed cakes and the fresh flowering plant.

Flower and Fruit: The flowers are paniclelike loose cymes on long peduncles in the leaf axils of the upper part of the stem. They have 5 ovate, acuminate, finely ciliate sepals and 5

obovate petals, which are sky blue and longer than the sepals. There are 5 stamens fused at the base and 1 ovary. The fruit is an almost globular, 6- to 8-mm long capsule on an erect or slightly bent stem. The seeds are flat, brown, and glossy.

Leaves, Stem, and Root: The plant is an annual and grows from 20 to 150 cm high. The root is short, fusiform, and light yellow. The stem is unbranched, erect, or ascending in short curves. The leaves are smooth edged, gray-green, sessile, and almost awnlike acuminate.

Characteristics: The plant flowers only in the morning.

Habitat: The plant is cultivated in temperate and tropical regions the world over.

Production: Flaxseed consists of the dried, ripe seed of the collective variations of *Linum usitatissimum* as well as its preparations. The various cultivars of *Linum usitatissimum* are equally acceptable for the indications listed. The plant is cultivated. The ripe seeds are recovered from the capsules by threshing. The oil contained within the seeds is perishable. Processing of the seeds should take place by cold pressing at a temperature below 40° C.

Not to be Confused With: Lolium temulentum and weed seeds.

Other Names: Flaxseed, Linseed, Lint Bells, Winterlien

ACTIONS AND PHARMACOLOGY

COMPOUNDS

Mucilages (3-10%, in the epidermis, high swelling capacity): including arabinoxylans, galactans, rhamnogalacturonans

Cyanogenic glycosides (0.05-0.1%): linustatin and neolinustatin (yielding under optimal conditions 30-50 mg HCN per 100 gm)

Fatty oil (30-45%): chief fatty acids linolenic acid (40-70%), linoleic acid (10-25%), oleic acid (13-30%)

Proteins (20-27%)

Lignans: secoisolariciresinol-diglucoside

Phenylpropane derivatives: including among others, linusitamarine

EFFECTS

Flaxseed oil is the richest known source of omega-3 fatty acids and lignans. Omega-3 fatty acids suppress the production of interleukin, tumor necrosis factor (TNF), and leukotriene B4 from monocytes and polymorphonuclear leukocytes. Flaxseed oil appears beneficial in certain aspects of an insulin-resistant metabolic syndrome (Nestel et al, 1997). Whether or not the composition of platelet lipids is changed with intake of flaxseed is controversial. Several studies have indicated that oral administration of flaxseed oil increases blood levels of alpha-linoleic acid (ALA) and eicosapentaenoic acid (Layne et al, 1996; Allman et al, 1995; Cunnane et al, 1993; Kelley et al, 1993).

Flaxseed has laxative effects arising from increased volume and consequent initiation of intestinal peristalsis from stimulation of stretch receptors (Bisset & Wichtl, 1994). Most studies demonstrate an increase in the omega-3 fatty acid eicosapentaenoic acid (EPA) following ingestion of ALA (Caughey et al, 1996). Flaxseed oil is relatively low in saturated fatty acids, comparable to corn, soy, and canola oils. Compared to canola and olive oils, flaxseed oil is low in oleic acid (Johnston, 1995).

Anti-inflammatory Effects: Metabolites of ALA and linoleic acid (LA) act as substrates for the formation of the anti-inflammatory eicosanoids, comprising prostaglandins, thromboxanes, and leukotrienes (Gerster, 1998).

Anticancer Effects: Flaxseed's lignans have shown antineoplastic effects based on *in vitro* and animal research. Regular consumption may reduce the risk of certain cancers. The antitumoral effect is attributed to the lignans (lignans are antimycotic, anti-oxidative and anti-estrogenic). Dietary supplementation of flaxseed reduced mammary tumor size and number in rats. Several studies have shown an inhibitory effect of dietary ALA on tumor growth and incidence in rodent mammary-tumor models, although one study showed no effect and not all evidence is free of inconsistency (Johnston, 1995). Fiber-rich foods in the human diet contain plant lignans, which promote bacterial synthesis of enterodiol and enterolactone (Shultz et al, 1991).

Cardioprotective: In studies, lowering of serum lipids was similar with ALA and fish-oil supplementation. Prostaglandin precursors did not or were only slightly augmented with ALA supplementation. Coagulation appeared to be inhibited during supplementation with flaxseed and vitamin E. Blood pressure was not affected by ALA.

Digestive Effects: Flaxseed regulates the digestive system by absorbing up to eight times its own weight in water and helping material to move through the intestines (Johnston & Johnston, 1990). High mucilage content protects mucous membranes. Flaxseed may bind to (theoretically) toxic metabolites produced during digestion and may also reduce bloat.

Inhibition of Cytokines: Inhibition of the cytokine TNF-alpha and interleukin-1 beta (IL-1 beta) is one of the therapeutic goals in treating certain inflammatory disorders, such as rheumatoid arthritis (Caughey et al, 1996).

Metabolic Syndrome (Insulin Resistance Syndrome; Syndrome X): Flaxseed showed effects on various aspects of this metabolic syndrome, which consists of obesity, dyslipidemia, insulin resistance, and/or hypertension (Nestel et al, 1997).

Omega-3 Fatty Acid Synthesis: Omega-3 fatty acids are essential for synthesis of components of specialized membranes, such as nervous tissues (Goodnight et al, 1982). ALA is a precursor to certain omega-3 fatty acids contained in marine fish oils and interest in its potential as a substrate for synthesis of these substances runs high.

CLINICAL TRIALS

Breast Cancer

Patients were randomly assigned to daily intake of either a 25 g flaxseed-containing muffin (n=19) or a control (placebo) muffin (n=13). The aim of this randomized, placebo-controlled, double-blind trial was to investigate the effects of dietary flaxseed on tumor biological markers and urinary lignan excretion in postmenopausal patients with newly diagnosed breast cancer. The results suggest that dietary flaxseed has the potential to reduce tumor growth (Thompson et al, 2005).

Cholesterol

In a randomized double-blind clinical trial, 56 participants received 3 g/d of ALA (alpha-linolenic acid) derived from flaxseed oil in capsules (n=31) or olive oil containing placebo capsules (n=25) for 26 weeks. Changes in plasma HDL cholesterol, LDL cholesterol, and triglyceride concentrations did not differ between the two treatment groups. Particle size also was not affected. The results showed that ALA does not seem to decrease CVD risk by altering lipoprotein particle or plasma lipoprotein concentration (Harper et al, 2006).

Flaxseed reduced serum LDL cholesterol levels significantly ($p < 0.02$) compared with sunflower seeds in a double-blind, crossover trial. Both treatments lowered total cholesterol levels compared to baseline but there was no difference between the two; flaxseed alone reduced lipoprotein(a) levels compared to baseline but the difference from sunflower seeds was not significant. HDL cholesterol and triglyceride levels were unaffected by treatment. No weight gain was observed during the study despite an overall increase in caloric intake. Serum estradiol and follicle-stimulating hormone levels were also unaffected (Arjmandi et al, 1998).

Plasma total and LDL cholesterol levels declined significantly ($p<0.05$) compared to baseline in one double-blind, crossover study. Though total and LDL cholesterol levels were significantly lower ($p<0.05$) after 2 weeks of flaxseed consumption compared to controls, by 4 weeks the difference was no longer significant. HDL cholesterol and triglyceride levels were not affected. This study also found no effect of flaxseed on glucose tolerance or lipid peroxidation compared to controls (Cunnane et al, 1995).

In a crossover trial, 16 young male subjects consumed a diet supplemented with 4.3 g/d of flaxseed oil following stabilization on a basal diet. After 55 days of intervention the flaxseed-oil diet did not significantly alter serum triglycerides, cholesterol, LDL-C, HDL-C, apoprotein A-I, or apoprotein B compared with the basal diet of natural foods supplemented, as was the flaxseed-oil diet, with 100 IU of alpha-tocopherol twice weekly. (Kelley et al, 1993).

Coronary Heart Disease

Flaxseed oil as well as other plant sources such as canola oil and walnuts are rich sources of the major dietary (n-3) polyunsaturated fatty acid, Alpha-linolenic Acid (ALA). A 2005 review aimed to determine whether intake of ALA from plants is as effective as ingesting long-chain n-3 polyunsaturated fatty acids from seafood sources—which have been shown to reduce the risk of coronary heart disease through various biological mechanisms including reduction of inflammation and improved endothelial cell function. The authors found that evidence from observational, experimental, and clinical studies, including randomized clinical trials, do point to potential effectiveness in the primary and secondary prevention of coronary heart disease with the consumption of 2 to 3 g of ALA daily (Mozaffarian, 2005).

Cytokines

In one study, levels of TNF-alpha and IL-1 beta were decreased by 30% and 31%, respectively, after 4 weeks of use of flaxseed oil in domestic food preparation in healthy male subjects; levels of the eicosanoids thromboxane B(2) decreased by 29% and of prostaglandin E(2) by 30%. A parallel group of healthy males who ate a sunflower oil-based diet evidenced no change in production of TNF-alpha, IL-1 beta, thromboxane B(2), or prostaglandin E(2) (Caughey et al, 1996).

Endothelial Function

In a randomized study, 22 healthy postmenopausal women consumed a diet containing a muffin enriched with a plant compound (a lignan complex) isolated from Flaxseed—secoisolariciresinol diglucoside (SDG)—hypothesized to be protective to the heart in postmenopausal women as a result of the complex's structural similarity to estrogen. The low-fat muffin provided 500 mg/d of SGD. The 6-week trial was double-blind and placebo-controlled, and included a 6-week washout period followed by a crossover arm in which the participants consumed an identical muffin except for its absence of the contained plant lignan for the next 6 weeks (or vice-versa). Based on plasma and other laboratory tests, as well as ultrasound measurement of endothelial vessels, the authors concluded that daily consumption for 6 weeks of the muffin enriched with the lignan complex had no effect on endothelial function (the health of vessel linings) (Hallund 2006).

Fatty Acids

There are limitations to the body's ability to convert ALA to the cardioprotective elements eicosapentaenoic acid (EPA) and possibly docosahexaenoic acid (DHA). The results of a randomized, double-blind trial in 49 individuals (Flaxseed Oil to Reduce Intermediate Cardiac Endpoints [FORCE]) indicate that 3 g of Flaxseed oil daily versus placebo increases the level of cardioprotective plasma EPA levels at 12 weeks by 60%, and DPA levels by 25%. In contrast, neither EPA nor DPA levels changed in the placebo group. The participants were predominantly African-American and female, and had chronic illnesses such as hypertension and Type II diabetes. Additional clinical trials with ALA are worth pursuing, the authors conclude (Harper, 2006).

Results of earlier studies using supplementary flaxseed oil to affect changes in levels of long-chain fatty acids had mixed results, some of which may have arisen from differences in intervention time, nutritional status of subjects, and analysis methods (i.e., measurement of total lipids versus phospholipids). Although ALA can undergo desaturation and elongation to synthesize eicosapentaenoic acid (EPA) and docosahexaenoic acid (DHA) *in vivo*, most studies of dietary flaxseed supplementation demonstrate moderate increases in EPA and docosapentaenoic acid (DPA). No significant increases or decreases in DHA following supplementation with soy or flaxseed oil were noted while levels of ALA increased (Gerster, 1998; Nestel et al, 1997; Kelley et al, 1993).

Insulin Resistance Syndrome

Systemic arterial compliance (elasticity) increased with flaxseed oil supplementation in 12 overweight subjects showing one or more markers for insulin resistance syndrome (comprising obesity, low HDL cholesterol, raised triglyceride levels, hypertension, or glucose intolerance. Insulin response to flaxseed oil exceeded that of either control period (p=0.16) and of Sunola (nonsignificant). These higher plasma insulin values at 30 and 60 minutes with flaxseed indicate some deterioration in insulin sensitivity, which has also been reported with fish oil supplementation; the importance of this is uncertain (Nestel et al, 1997).

Menopause

To assess the effects of flaxseed incorporation into the diet of healthy menopausal women, 199 women were randomly assigned to consume 40 g flaxseed /d (n=101) or wheat germ placebo (n=98) for 12 months. Dietary supplementation with flaxseed over one year showed favorable, but not clinically significant, effects on blood cholesterol and caused no significant change in bone mineral density or symptoms in healthy menopausal women (Dodin et al, 2005).

Platelet Aggregation

Ingestion of ALA produces changes in the composition of platelet lipids with increases in ALA, eicosapentaenoic acid (EPA), and docosapentaenoic acid (DPA), but not in docosahexaenoic acid (DHA). Long-chain n-3 fatty acids appear to inhibit platelet aggregation by decreasing production of the platelet prostaglandin thromboxane A(2), a potent aggregatory eicosanoid, thereby decreasing the tendency to thrombosis. EPA replaces arachidonic acid, disrupting the substrate for production of thromboxane. Ingestion of an ALA-rich, low-fat diet for 23 days by healthy young men more than doubled levels of EPA in subjects taking 40 g per day of flaxseed oil ($p<0.05$, n=5) while EPA remained unchanged in those taking sunflower seed oil (n=6). As a result, the EPA:arachidonic acid ratio increased in the flaxseed group. The aggregation response induced by collagen decreased in the flaxseed-oil group (p less than 0.05) (Allman et al, 1995).

Rheumatoid Arthritis

Neither flaxseed nor safflower oil improved symptoms of rheumatoid arthritis in a double-blind comparison of the nutrients. Patients (n=22) were randomized to receive either 30 g of flaxseed oil (containing 32 ALA) or 30 g of safflower oil (containing 33% LA), each in the form of powder, for 3 months. Despite increases in ALA in the flaxseed oil group, levels of the long-chain metabolites eicosapentaenoic acid (EPA) and docosahexaenoic acid (DHA) did not increase. The authors cite low serum levels of zinc, as well as a low ALA:LA ratio, in the treatment group as possible reason for absence of change (Nordstrom et al, 1995).

INDICATIONS AND USAGE

Approved by Commission E:

- Constipation
- Inflammation of the skin

Unproven Uses: Internally, Flax is used for constipation, irritable colon, diverticulitis, colons damaged by laxative abuse, and as mucilage for gastritis and enteritis. A decoction is used for bladder catarrh and inflammation, gastritis.

Externally, Flaxseed is used for removing foreign bodies from the eye. A single Flaxseed is moistened and placed under the eyelid, the foreign body should stick to the mucous secretion of the seed. Flaxseed is also used as a cataplasm for local skin inflammation, and for chronic prostatitis (Green, 1991) and mild rectal inflammation.

Indian Medicine: Flax is used in India as a tea for coughs, bronchial conditions, urethritis, diarrhea and gonorrhea; externally for skin infections. The seeds are also used in Indian veterinary medicine.

CONTRAINDICATIONS

Flaxseed is contraindicated in the presence of ileus (intestinal obstruction) of any origin; stricture of the esophagus and in the gastrointestinal area; acute inflammatory illnesses of the intestine, esophagus, and stomach entrance.

PRECAUTIONS AND ADVERSE REACTIONS

No health hazards or side effects are known in conjunction with the proper administration of designated therapeutic dosages and with concomitant administration of sufficient liquid (1:10).

It is recommended that if flaxseed is taken for inflammatory bowel conditions, that the flaxseed be preswollen before use (Bisset & Wichtl, 1994).

Oil contained within the seed is perishable and must be protected not only during processing but also during handling and storing (Johnston & Johnston, 1990). The oil should be kept out of direct light and in refrigeration to preserve it. The oil should never be heated as it becomes mutagenic (Shields et al, 1995).

Due to the considerable caloric content (470 kilocalories per 100 G), overweight people should only use the whole seeds, which, except for swelling of mucilage in the testa, remain intact in the bowel without releasing the fixed oil. Flaxseed differs from other vegetable oils in its high level (45-50%) of ALA.

There is a discussion on the toxic effect of the cyanogenic glycosides in the drug, which may cause prussic acid poisoning in humans. However, neither high single doses nor chronic intake of linseed have caused any signs of poisoning in humans.

DRUG INTERACTIONS

POTENTIAL INTERACTIONS

Flaxseed contains mucilage and cellulose; therefore, the absorption of other drugs taken simultaneously may be delayed.

OVERDOSAGE

The use of large quantities of the drug as a laxative with too little fluid intake can lead to ileus.

DOSAGE

Mode of Administration: Internally, the cracked or coarsely ground seed, in which only the cuticle and mucilage epidermis are damaged is used. Linseed gruel and other galenic preparations are also available for internal use. Externally, as linseed meal or linseed expellant.

The absorption of Flaxseed oil is facilitated when taken with food. A 2005 randomized cross-over study in 12 healthy individuals found that diets supplemented with flaxseeds that had been crushed or milled, as opposed to simply left whole, substantially improved the bioavailability of the seeds' healthful enterolignans (Kuijsten, 2005).

How Supplied:

Capsules – 1000 mg, 1300 mg

Oil

Seeds (whole or crushed)

Powder

Preparation: To prepare a demulcent for use in gastritis and enteritis, allow 5 to 10 g of whole seeds to stand in cold water for 20 to 30 minutes, then pour off the liquid (Bisset & Wichtl, 1994).

Daily Dosage:

Constipation – 1 dessertspoon of whole or bruised (not ground) seed with at least 150 mL of liquid 2 to 3 times daily.

Lower Cholesterol – 35 to 50 g daily of the crushed seeds as a fiber supplement. May be incorporated into muffins or breads (Arjmandi et al, 1998).

Decrease platelet aggregation – 1 to 2 tablespoonfuls flaxseed oil daily (Allman et al, 1995).

Gastritis and enteritis – 2 to 4 tablespoons of milled linseed prepared as recommended above (the seeds should not be taken in the dry state, should be pre-hydrated.)

Topical – 30 to 50 g Flaxseed flour for a hot moist cataplasm or compress.

Storage: Flaxseed oil must be processed and stored properly. Flaxseed meal is less vulnerable to rancidity when exposed to light and heat than the processed oil. The seeds should be protected from light and stored in a sealed container. The oil should also be protected from light and should be refrigerated.

LITERATURE

Allman MA, Pena MM & Pang D. Supplementation with flaxseed oil versus sunflower seed oil in healthy young men consuming a low fat diet: effects on platelet composition and function. In*: Eur J Clin Nutr* 49(3):169-178, 1995.

Anon. Leinöl als diätetisches Adjuvans. In: *DAZ* 135(16):1501. 1995.

Anon. Leinsamen (Semen Lini) ist ungiftig. In: *ZPT* 5:770. 1984.

Anon. Pharmaceutical Care:''Den Mißbrauch von Laxanzien vermeiden helfen.'' In: *DAZ* 135(20):1867-1868. 1995.

Arjmandi BH, Khan DA, Juma S et al. Whole flaxseed consumption lowers serum LDL-cholesterol and lipoprotein(a) concentrations in postmenopausal women. In: *Nutr Res* 18(7):1203-1214, 1998.

Bierenbaum ML, Reichstein R & Watkins TR. Reducing atherogenic risk in hyperlipemic humans with flax seed supplementation: a preliminary report. *J Am Coll Nutr*; 12(5):501-504. 1993.

Bisset NG & Wichtl M (eds). Lini semen. Herbal Drugs and Phytopharmaceuticals: A Handbook for Practice on a Scientific Basis. Medpharm Scientific Publishers, CRC Press, Stuttgart, Germany, pp 298-300, 1994.

Caughey GE, Mantzioris E, Gibson RA et al. The effect on human tumor necrosis factor alpha and interleukin 1-beta production of diets enriched in n-3 fatty acids from vegetable oil or fish oil. *Am J Clin Nutr;* 63(1):116-122. 1996.

Cunnane SC, Ganguli S, Menard C et al. High alpha-linolenic acid flaxseed (Linum-usitatissimum): some nutritional properties in humans. *Br J Nutr*; 69(2):443-453. 1993.

Cunnane SC, Hamadeh MJ, Liede AC et al. Nutritional attributes of traditional flaxseed in healthy young adults. *Am J Clin Nutr*; 61:62-68. 1995.

Curry CE, Laxative products. In: Handbook of Nonprescription Drugs, Am Pharmac Assoc, Washington,S 69-92. 1982.

de Lorgeril M, Renaud S, Mamelle N et al. Mediterranean alpha-linolenic acid-rich diet in secondary prevention of coronary heart disease. *Lancet*; 343(8911):1454-1459. 1994.

Dodin S, Lemay A, Jacques H, et al. The effects of flaxseed dietary supplement on lipid profile, bone mineral density, and symptoms in menopausal women: a randomized, double-blind, wheat germ placebo-controlled clinical trial. *J Clin Endocrinol Metab*; 90(3): 1390-1397. 2005.

Garg ML, Wierzbicki AA, Thomson ABR et al. Dietary saturated fat level alters the competition between alpha-linolenic and linoleic acid. *Lipids*; 24(4):334-339. 1989.

Gemmell HA & Jacobson BH. Effectiveness of flaxseed oil in the symptomatic treatment of rheumatoid arthritis: a single subject experimental design. *Am J Chiropractic Med*; 2(4):151-154. 1989.

Gerster H. Can adults adequately convert alpha-linolenic acid (18:3n-3) to eicosapentaenoic acid (20:5n-3) and docosahexaenoic acid (22:6n-3)? *Int J Vit Nutr Res*; 68(3):159-173. 1998.

Goodnight SH Jr, Harris WS, Connor WE et al. Polyunsaturated fatty acids, hyperlipidemia, and thrombosis. *Arteriosclerosis*; 2:87-113. 1982.

Hallund J, et al. A lignan complex isolated from flaxseed does not affect plasma lipid concentrations or antioxidant capacity in healthy postmenopausal women. *J Nutr*; 136:112-116. 2006.

Harper CR, Edwards MJ, DeFilipis A, et al. Flaxseed oil increases the plasma concentrations of cardioprotective (n-3) fatty acids in humans. *J Nutr*; 136(1):83-88. 2006.

Harper CR, Edwards MC, Jacobson TA. Flaxseed oil supplementation does not affect plasma lipoprotein concentration or particle size in human subjects. *J Nutr*; 136(11): 2844-2848. 2006.

Harris WS. n-3 fatty acids and serum lipoproteins: human studies. *Am J Clin Nutr*; 65(suppl):1645S-1654S. 1997.

Hiller K, Pharmazeutische Bewertung ausgewählter Teedrogen. In: *DAZ* 135(16):1425-1440. 1995.

Hutchins AM, Martini MC, Olson AB et al. Flaxseed influences urinary lignan excretion in a dose-dependent manner in postmenopausal women. *Cancer Epidemiol Biomarkers Prev*; 9(10):1113-1118. 2000.

Johnston IM & Johnston JR. Flaxseed (Linseed) Oil and the Power of Omega-3. Keats Publishing, Inc, New Canaan, CT, USA, 1990.

Johnston PV. Flaxseed oil and cancer: alpha-linolenic acid and carcinogenesis, in Cunnane SC & Thompson LU (eds): Flaxseed in Human Nutrition. AOCS Press, Champaign, IL, USA; pp 207-218. 1995.

Kelley DS, Nelson GJ, Love JE et al. Dietary alpha-linolenic acid alters tissue fatty acid composition, but not blood lipids, lipoproteins or coagulation status in humans. *Lipids*; 28(6):533-537. 1993.

Kuijsten A. The relative bioavailability of enterolignans in humans is enhanced by milling and crushing of flaxseed. *J Nutr*; 135 (12): 2812-2816. 2005.

Layne KS, Goh YK, Jumpsen JA et al. Normal subjects consuming physiological levels of 18:3(n-3) and 20:5(n-3) from flaxseed or fish oils have characteristic differences in plasma lipid and lipoprotein fatty acid levels. *J Nutr*; 126(9):2130-2140. 1996.

Miyazaki M, Takemura N, Watanabe S et al. Dietary docosahexaenoic acid ameliorates, but rapeseed oil and safflower oil accelerate renal injury in stroke-prone spontaneously hypertensive rats as compared with soybean oil, which is associated with expression for renal transforming growth factor-B, fibronectin and renin. *Biochim Biophys Acta*; 1483(1):101-110. 2000.

Mozaffarian D: Does alpha-linolenic acid intake reduce the risk of coronary heart disease? A review of the evidence. *Alt Ther Health Med*; 11 (13): 24-30. 2005.

Nestel PJ, Pomeroy SE, Sasahara T et al. Arterial compliance in obese subjects is improved with dietary plant n-3 fatty acid from flaxseed oil despite increased LDL oxidizability. *Arterioscler Thromb Vasc Biol*; 17(6):1163-1170. 1997.

Nordstrom DCE, Honkanen VEA, Nasu Y et al. Alpha-linolenic acid in the treatment of rheumatoid arthritis: a double- blind, placebo-controlled and randomized study: flaxseed vs safflower seed. *Rheumatol Int*; 14(6):231-234. 1995.

Schiebel-Schlosser G. Leinsamen - die richtige Wahl. In: *PTA* 8(4):300. 1994.

Shields PG, Xu GX, Blot WJ et al. Mutagens from heated Chinese and US cooking oils. *J Natl Cancer* Inst; 87:836-841. 1995.

Shultz TD, Bonorden WR & Seaman WR. Effect of short-term flaxseed consumption on lignan and sex hormone metabolism in men. *Nutr Res*; 11:1089-1100. 1991.

Schulz V. Clinical Pharmacokinetics of Nitroprusside, Cyanide, Thiosulphate and Thiocyanate. *Clinical Pharmacokinetics* 9:239-251. 1984.

Schulz V. Löffler A, Gheorghiu Th, Resorption von Blausäure aus Leinsamen. *Leber Magen Darm* 13:10-14. 1983.

Sewing KFR, Obstipation. In: Fülgraff G, Palm D (Hrsg) Pharmakotherapie, Klinische Pharmakologie, 6. Auflage. Fischer, Stuttgart, S 162-168. 1986.

Singer P, Berger I, Wirth M et al. Slow desaturation and elongation of linoleic and alpha-linolenic acids as a rationale of eicosapentaenoic acid-rich diet to lower blood pressure and serum lipids in normal, hypertensive and hyperlipemic subjects. *Prostaglandins Leukotr Med*; 24:173-193. 1986.

Sprando RL, Collins TFX, Black TN et al. The effect of maternal exposure to flaxseed on spermatogenesis in F1 generation rats. *Food Chem Toxicol*; 38(4):325-334. 2000.

Thompson LU, Chen JM, Li T, et al. Dietary flaxseed alters tumor biological markers in postmenopausal breast cancer. *Clin Cancer Res*; 11(10): 3828-3835. 2005.

Tou JC, Chen J & Thompson LU. Flaxseed and it's lignan precursor, secoisolariciresinol diglycoside, affect pregnancy outcome and reproductive development in rats. *J Nutr*; 128(11):1861-1868. 1998.

Foeniculum vulgare

See Fennel

Fool's Parsley

Aethusa cynapium

DESCRIPTION

Medicinal Parts: The medicinal parts are the entire fresh plant and the dried aerial parts (herb).

Flower and Fruit: The plant has white long-stemmed umbels with many florets and no involucre. The calyx has 5 fused sepals. There are 5 white (sometimes reddish), obcordate, irregular petals. The flowers have 5 stamens and a 2-valved ovate ovary. The fruit is a 3 to 5 mm wide, globose schizocarp, straw yellow when ripe with red-brown stripes; it opens easily. Each section has 5 triangular ribs with 1 or 2 oil grooves in the hollow and 2 in the joints.

Leaves, Stem, and Root: The plant is a leafy, 60 cm high annual or biennial plant. The root is thin, spindle-shaped, and whitish. The stem is erect, round, grooved, hollow, glabrous and usually forked with a bluish bloom, which rubs off when handled. The leaves are glossy, dark green above and light green beneath. Leaflets are serrate with a triangular outline and double to treble pinnatifid. They give off an unpleasant garlic odor when rubbed.

Characteristics: The plant is poisonous. The plant can be mistaken for Parsley because of its similar appearance, but the plant is poisonous and can have fatal consequences. This similarity has resulted in its being given the name Fool's Parsley. It also bears a resemblance to Hemlock, though it is not as poisonous.

Habitat: The plant is indigenous to northern and central Europe, introduced into North America; cultivated and used as an ornamental plant for meadows in southern Germany.

Not to be Confused With: Young garden parsley is very similar. However, it differs in the glossiness of the underside surface of the leaf and pungent, burning, garliclike smell of the leaves when rubbed.

Other Names: Dog Poison, Fool's-Cicely, Small Hemlock, Dog Parsley, Lesser Hemlock

ACTIONS AND PHARMACOLOGY

COMPOUNDS

Polyynes: (only in freshly-harvested leaves) including aethusin, aethusanol A, aethusanol B

Flavone glycosides: including rutoside, narcissine, camphor oil-3-glucorhamnoside

Ascorbic acid

EFFECTS

No information is available.

INDICATIONS AND USAGE

Unproven Uses: Fool's Parsley has been used for gastrointestinal complaints in children, infantile cholera, summer diarrhea, and convulsions.

Homeopathic Uses: Aethusa cynapium is used for milk intolerance in children, pylorus cramp, acute diarrhea with vomiting, and poor concentration (HAB1).

PRECAUTIONS AND ADVERSE REACTIONS

Fool's Parsley is considered a toxic plant. The older literature contains descriptions of poisonings, sometimes fatal, occurring as a result of confusing garden parsley with the freshly harvested drug. Probably, however, these had to do with poisonings by spotted hemlock. Caution should nevertheless be exercised.

DOSAGE

Mode of Administration: The juice of the fresh drug is used in poultices; also available as alcoholic extracts.

Homeopathic Dosage: 5 to 10 drops, 1 tablet, or 5 to 10 globules, 1 to 3 times daily; injection solution 1 ml twice weekly sc (HAB1).

LITERATURE

Frohne D, Pfänder HJ, Giftpflanzen - Ein Handbuch für Apotheker, Toxikologen und Biologen, 4. Aufl., Wiss. Verlags-Ges Stuttgart 1997.

Hänsel R, Keller K, Rimpler H, Schneider G (Hrsg.), Hagers Handbuch der Pharmazeutischen Praxis, 5. Aufl., Bde 4 - 6 (Drogen), Springer Verlag Berlin, Heidelberg, New York, 1992-1994.

Lewin L, Gifte und Vergiftungen, 6. Aufl., Nachdruck, Haug Verlag, Heidelberg 1992.

Madaus G, Lehrbuch der Biologischen Arzneimittel, Bde 1-3, Nachdruck, Georg Olms Verlag Hildesheim 1979.

Roth L, Daunderer M, Kormann K, Giftpflanzen, Pflanzengifte, 4. Aufl., Ecomed Fachverlag Landsberg Lech 1993.

Teuscher E, Lindequist U, Biogene Gifte - Biologie, Chemie, Pharmakologie, 2. Aufl., Fischer Verlag Stuttgart 1994.

Forget-Me-Not

Myosotis arvensis

DESCRIPTION

Medicinal Parts: The medicinal part is the flowering plant.

Flower and Fruit: The blue flowers are in leafless racemes. The calyx is fused and leaflike with 5 tips. The corolla is shaped like a stemmed plate, has 5 tips, and is glabrous with yellow scales in the tube. The tube is enclosed in the calyx. There are 5 stamens and a 4-valvular ovary. The fruit stems are twice as long as the caylx and stand out. The calyx is closed when the fruit ripens. The fruit is composed of 4 nutlets.

Leaves, Stem, and Root: The plant is leafy and grows from 15 to 40 cm high. The stem is erect or ascendent and pubescent. The leaves are alternate. The lower leaves are petiolate and oblong-obovate, the upper ones sessile and lanceolate to lanceolate-oblong.

Habitat: The plant grows in Europe.

Production: Forget-Me-Not is the flowering plant *Myosotis arvensis*.

ACTIONS AND PHARMACOLOGY

COMPOUNDS

Pyrrolizidine alkaloids

Caffeic acid derivatives: rosmarinic acid

EFFECTS

No information is available.

INDICATIONS AND USAGE

Unproven Uses: Forget-Me-Not is used in the treatment of respiratory disorders and nosebleeds.

PRECAUTIONS AND ADVERSE REACTIONS

Hepatotoxicity and carcinogenicity are possible consequences when taken internally, due to the presence of pyrrolizidine alkaloids with 1,2-unsaturated necic parent substances. Therefore, the drug should not be taken internally.

DOSAGE

Mode of Administration: The herb is administered ground and as an extract for external use.

LITERATURE

Kern W, List PH, Hörhammer L (Hrsg.), Hagers Handbuch der Pharmazeutischen Praxis, 4. Aufl., Bde. 1-8, Springer Verlag Berlin, Heidelberg, New York, 1969.

Madaus G. Lehrbuch der Biologischen Arzneimittel, Bde 1-3, Nachdruck, Georg Olms Verlag Hildesheim 1979.

Fragaria vesca

See Strawberry

Frangula

Rhamnus frangula

DESCRIPTION

Medicinal Parts: The medicinal parts are the dried bark of the trunk and branches and the fresh bark of the trunk and branches.

Flower and Fruit: The flowers are in 2 to 10 axillary blossomed cymes on pedicles that are 1 to 3 times as long. The flowers are greenish white, infundibular, 3 to 4 mm long with 5 sepals and 5 petals, which are initially pubescent. The sepals are 3 mm long, oblong-triangular, and acute. The petals are whitish, erect, and stemmed. The petals enclose the stamens. The stamens are somewhat shorter than the petals and have large anthers and short filaments. The fruit is a globular, initially green, later red when ripe. The black-purple drupe is about 8 cm wide containing 2 to 3 seeds. The seeds are wide, flat triangular/lentil shaped with a longer, very narrow groove.

Leaves, Stem, and Root: The plant is a thornless, 1 to 3 m high bush or a 7 m high weedy tree. The branches are piled on the boughs and densely foliated. The bark is initially green later gray-brown and covered in gray-white lenticles. The leaf buds are pubescent. The leaves are thin, soft when young then becoming stiffer. They are broadly elliptical to obovate and about 3.5 to 5 cm long. The leaves are usually entire-margined and pubescent on the ribs of the under surface.

Characteristics: The heartwood is bright yellow-red. The odor is somewhat foul and the taste is disgustingly bitter.

Habitat: The plant is indigenous to all of Europe, Western Asia, Asia Minor, and the Caucasus; it has spread to the wild in North America.

Production: Frangula bark consists of the dried bark of the trunks and branches of *Rhamnus frangula*. The bark is peeled in May and June, then either dried and stored for 1 year to dry or heated for 1 hour at 100° C.

Other Names: Buckthorn, Frangula, Alder Buckthorn, Black Alder, Dog Wood, Black Dogwood, Black Alder Tree, European Black Alder, Black Alder Dogwood, Arrow Wood, European Buckthorn, Persian Berries, Alder Dogwood

ACTIONS AND PHARMACOLOGY

COMPOUNDS

Anthracene derivatives (4 to 6%): anthranoids, chief components glucofrangulin A, glucofrangulin A-diacetate (estered at rhamnose remnant), as well as frangulin A, frangulin C

Naphthalene derivatives: naphthoquinones

Peptide alkaloids (traces): including frangulanine

EFFECTS

The bark contains anthracene derivatives and their aglycones, which have an anti-absorptive and hydrogogic effect. The anthracene derivatives induce active secretion of electrolytes and water in the intestinal lumina and inhibit the absorption of electrolytes and water from the colon by stimulating propulsive contractions. This results in accelerated intestinal passage time. In this manner, the increased water and subsequent volume of the intestinal content raise pressure and stimulate intestinal peristalsis.

INDICATIONS AND USAGE

Approved by Commission E:

- Constipation

Unproven Uses: Frangula bark is used to ease bowel evacuation in the case of anal fissures, hemorrhoids, and after rectal-anal surgery. It may also be used in preparation for exploratory surgery of the gastrointestinal tract.

Homeopathic Uses: Rhamnus frangula is used for weak digestion with a tendency to diarrhea.

CONTRAINDICATIONS

The drug is not to be used with intestinal obstruction, acute inflammatory intestinal diseases, appendicitis or with children under 12 years of age. The drug is not to be administered during pregnancy or while nursing.

PRECAUTIONS AND ADVERSE REACTIONS

General: Long-term use leads to loss of electrolytes, especially potassium ions. This may lead to hyperaldosteronism, inhibition of intestinal motility, and enhancement of the effect of cardioactive steroids, which may lead to arrhythmias. Nephropathies, edema, and accelerated bone deterioration are possible after long-term use.

The question of an increased incidence of carcinoma of the colon following long-term administration of anthracene drugs has not yet been fully clarified. Recent studies show no definite connection between the administration of anthracene drugs and the frequency of carcinoma of the colon.

Do not use this drug in children under 12 years of age.

Pregnancy: Not to be used during pregnancy.

Breastfeeding: Not to be used while nursing.

DRUG INTERACTIONS

MODERATE RISK

Digoxin: Concurrent use may result in hypokalemia leading to digoxin toxicity. *Clinical Management:* If digoxin toxicity occurs, potassium should be monitored and supplemented if necessary while discontinuing frangula.

POTENTIAL INTERACTIONS

Diuretics: Frangula may cause hypokalemia.

Glycosides: Increased effect due to potassium loss with chronic use of drug.

OVERDOSAGE

Vomiting and spasmodic gastrointestinal complaints could occur as side effects to the drug's purgative effect or with overdosages.

DOSAGE

Mode of Administration: Frangula Bark is available in solid pharmaceutical form and in commercial compounded preparations for oral intake. It is also available parenterally for homeopathic use.

Preparations:

Tea — scald 2 g finely cut drug and strain after 15 minutes. The drug may also be left to steep in cold water for 12 hours.

Dry extract — percolation of 100 g bark with methanol, after 1 day 400 g to 500 g percolate are extracted. The liquids (percolate and pressed juice) are left to stand for 8 days at 2 to 8° C before being filtered and dried. The glucofrangulin content must be stabilized at 15 to 17%.

Daily Dosage: 20 mg to 180 mg hydroxyanthracene derivatives

Tea — 1 cup mornings and evenings

The correct dosage for each individual is the smallest dosage necessary to maintain a soft stool. Frangula bark should not be used continuously for more than 1 or 2 weeks.

Homeopathic Dosage: from D3: 5 drops, 1 tablet, or 10 globules every 30 to 60 minutes (acute) or 1 to 3 times daily (chronic); parenterally: 1 to 2 ml sc acute: 3 times daily; chronic: once a day (HAB1)

Storage: Frangula may be stored for at least 1 year if protected from light and moisture.

LITERATURE

Berg AJ van den, Labadie RP. HPLC Separation and quantitative Determination of Aloe-Emodin, Emodin, Chrysophanol and Physcion in Plant Cell Cultures of *Rhamnus frangula* and *Rh.purshiana. Acta Agron Hung. 34; Suppl.; 18.* 1985

Helmholz H, Ruge A, Piasecki A, Schröder S, Westendorf J, Genotoxizität der Faulbaumrinde. In: PZ 138(43):3478. 1993.

Pepeljnjak S, Cvetnik Z. Aflatoxigenicity of *Rhizopus nigricans* strains isolated from drug plants. *Acta Pharm.* 48; 139-144. 1998

Sydiskis RJ, Owen DG, Lohr JL, Rosler KHA, Blosmster RN, Inactivation of enveloped viruses by anthraquinones extracted from plants. In: Antimicrob Agents Chemother 35:2463-2466. 1991.

Frankincense

Boswellia carteri

DESCRIPTION

Medicinal Parts: The medicinal part of the tree is the resin gum exuded when incisions are made in the bark of the trunk.

Flower and Fruit: The flowers are solitary on short stalks and single axillary inflorescences. The calyx is small, has 5 teeth, and is perennial. The corolla has 5 elongated petals, and there are 5 stamens. The long anthers fall early. The fruit is a capsule divided into 3 parts with a seed in each section. A wide membranous leaf surrounds the seeds.

Leaves, Stem, and Root: Boswellia carteri is a richly foliated tree whose leaves alternate unevenly on the branches to the tips. The 10 pairs and one leaflet are short-stalked, elongated, blunt, serrate, finely pubescent, and mostly alternate. The base of the leaf is a fleshy cup-shaped disc that is larger than the corolla. The plant grows on few roots, which appear to be fused with the stony soil via an inert mass.

Habitat: Boswellia carteri is found in Somalia and parts of Saudi Arabia.

Production: (Indian) Frankincense or Olibanum is the hardened gum resin of *Boswellia carteri*, which exudes when incisions are made in the trunk. It is collected after being allowed to harden in the open air for about three weeks.

Not to be Confused With: The exuded gum resin of the trunk of *Boswellia serrata* also is called Frankincense or Olibanum.

Other Names: Olibanum

ACTIONS AND PHARMACOLOGY

COMPOUNDS

Volatile oil (5-9%): chief components 1-octyl acetate (share 60%), 1-octanol (share 12.7%), including as well alpha-pinene (3.5%), incensol (2.7%)

Resins (60%): components including among others alpha-boswellic acid, beta-boswellic acid, methyl ester of 3-acetyl-β-boswellic acid

Mucilages (12-20%)

EFFECTS

Extracts of the gum resin of *Boswellia serrata* have exhibited anti-inflammatory, sedative, and antihyperlipidemic effects and some in vitro antifungal activity. Boswellic acids, found in the gum resin, have inhibited DNA, RNA, and protein synthesis of human leukemic HL-60 cells. The resin has also been reported to have pregnancy interceptive activity.

Extensive *in vitro* and experimental models exist, yet there is a shortage of clinical trials. One double-blind, placebo-controlled trial showed that boswellic acid-containing gum resin was effective in the treatment of bronchial asthma (Gupta et al, 1998). While open and collected case studies demonstrate efficacy in the treatment of osteoarthritis and rheumatoid arthritis (Etzel, 1996), double-blind, placebo-controlled studies have not substantiated its use in (Sander & Herborn, 1998). With regard to inflammatory bowel disease, an extract of the gum resin of *Boswellia serrata* provided symptomatic improvement in patients with ulcerative colitis in a nonrandomized, open trial (Gupta et al, 1997).

Anti-Asthma Effects: Boswellia was effective in treating asthma in one study (Gupta et al, 1998).

Antifungal Effects: The essential oil extracted from *Boswellia serrata* was reported to have some in vitro antifungal activity. The oil demonstrated only weak activity against the human fungal pathogens, but was considered highly effective against plant pathogens (Gangwal & Vardhan, 1995).

Anti-inflammatory Effects: An ethanolic extract of the gum resin of *Boswellia serrata* inhibited the production of leukotriene-type inflammatory mediators in vitro through a direct action on 5-lipoxygenase, the key enzyme of leukotriene production (Ammon et al, 1991). Boswellic acids inhibited the classical pathway of complement activation in vitro through inhibition of C3-convertase, preventing the release of the potent proinflammatory anaphylactic peptides C3a and C5a (Knaus & Wagner, 1996; Kapil & Moza, 1992). Antibody production and cellular response to sheep red blood cells were strongly inhibited by oral administration of an alcoholic extract of the gum resin of *Boswellia serrata* in mice (Sharma et al, 1988).

Antineoplastic Effects: Boswellic acids extracted from *Boswellia serrata* demonstrated dose-dependent inhibitory effects on the DNA, RNA, and protein synthesis of human leukemia HL-60 cells in vitro. The most active of the 4 boswellic acid compounds studied inhibited HL-60 cellular growth. Inhibition is due to interference with cell proliferation rather than a direct cytotoxic effect. Such inhibition can be explained by interference with DNA, RNA, and protein synthesis, all of which are required for cell proliferation (Shao et al, 1998).

Effects on Rheumatoid Arthritis: While some clinical evidence of effectiveness exists, treatment with H15 (boswellia extract) has failed to improve the symptomology of rheumatoid arthritis in double-blind studies. Only combination products with other potentially active ingredients have clinically demonstrated efficacy in the treatment of arthritis (Kulkarni et al, 1992; Kulkarni et al, 1991). Boswellic acids produce a reduction in synovial fluid leukocyte count in animals and have shown positive effects in other experimental models.

CLINICAL TRIALS

Anti-Inflammation

Boswellic acids (BA) demonstrated dose-related anti-inflammatory activity (AIA) in acute tests of carrageenan-, histamine-, and dextran-induced edema in rats and mice. (Singh et al, 1996b; Sailer et al, 1996).

Asthma

Seventy percent of patients treated with Boswellic acid-containing gum resin demonstrated improvement in subjective and objective measures of bronchial asthma in a randomized double-blind, placebo-controlled study of 80 adult patients with bronchial asthma for a mean duration of approximately 9 years. Three outcome criteria were measured: FEV1, PEFR (baseline and after treatment), and number of asthmatic attacks. There were no statistically significant differences between groups in demographics, sputum eosinophil counts, respiratory rates, or eosinophil counts at baseline. There were statistically significant differences in FEV1 and PEFR values indicating that disease was worse in the treatment group compared to the control group at baseline. FEV1 increased by a mean of 0.5 ± 0.5 in the treatment group compared to 0.1 ± 0.2 in the control group ($p=0.0001$). The post-treatment distribution of FEV1 values was slightly smaller in the boswellia group (2.1 compared with 2.2 in the control group) due to the fact that FEV1 values were lower in the boswellia group at baseline. There was also a significant increase in mean PEFR values for the treatment group (76.2 ± 60.3) compared with the controls (31.7 ± 25.3) ($p=0.0001$). The treatment group also had significantly fewer attacks during treatment compared to the controls ($p=0.0001$). Percentage increases in FEV1 were not reported (Gupta et al, 1998).

Collagenous Colitis

A double-blind, multi-center 2005 trial of *Boswellia serrata* extract in 31 individuals was one of several studies selected in a Cochrane Database Review designed to determine therapies of proven effectiveness for collagenous colitis based on quality randomized clinical trials published from 1970 to 2006. While clinical improvement was noted in a significantly larger number of participants in the 6-week *Boswellia serrata* trial who had been randomized to active treatment (7 of 16 [44%]) versus placebo (4 of 15 [27%]), the Cochrane review authors concluded that more research is needed to clarify whether the herb (or other therapies analyzed, such as probiotics) can induce or maintain disease remission of this type of colitis—which is of unknown etiology and pathogenesis and causes chronic diarrhea. The Cochrane reviewers also noted that the small number of participants in the *Boswellia serrata* trial diminished the statistical power of the trial's results. Long-term data for efficacy and safety of *Boswellia serrata* for collagenous colitis are lacking (Chande 2006).

Rheumatoid Arthritis

The effectiveness of H15 was not validated against rheumatoid arthritis in a double-blind, placebo-controlled pilot study (Sander & Herborn, 1998).

Ulcerative Colitis

Patients with ulcerative colitis improved with administration of a gum resin preparation of *Boswellia serrata*. In a nonrandomized, open trial, 42 patients with grade II or III colitis received either a *Boswellia serrata* gum resin preparation in a dose of 350 mg 3 times daily or sulfasalazine 1 g 3 times daily for 6 weeks. There was improvement in abdominal pain in 100% of patients receiving sulfasalazine and 91.7% receiving boswellia. Loose stools improved 100% in sulfasalazine patients and 88.9% in boswellia patients. Disappearance of mucus, blood, and necrotic material was nearly 100% in sulfasalazine-treated patients and 79% to 86% in the boswellia group, with a better response in Grade II patients. No patient experienced deterioration in any of these symptoms during the study. Remissions occurred in 82.4% of boswellia patients, being more frequent for Grade II disease, and in 75% of sulfasalazine patients (Gupta et al, 1997).

INDICATIONS AND USAGE

The primary uses of *Boswellia serrata* are in osteoarthritis, rheumatoid arthritis, and inflammatory bowel disease (ulcerative colitis and Crohn's disease).

PRECAUTIONS AND ADVERSE REACTIONS

Possible adverse reactions include retrosternal burning, nausea, abdominal fullness, epigastric pain, anorexia, and dermatitis. Patients with pre-existing gastritis should be advised to use boswellia with caution as these appear to be the most common side effects associated with the use of boswellia.

Externally, Frankincense can cause mild irritation of the skin. Internally, it is a mild carminative.

DRUG INTERACTIONS

No human interaction data is available.

DOSAGE

Preparation: The Frankincense resin is obtained by tapping the bark and leaving the exudate for about three months, during which time it hardens slightly, allowing the resin to be collected.

For Arthritis: 400 mg 3 times daily.

For Asthma: 300 mg 3 times daily.

LITERATURE

Ammon HPT. Entzündliche Darmerkrankungen: Weihrauch bei Colitis ulcerosa, siehe auch folgenden Artikel. In: *DAZ* 137(3):125. 1997.

Ammon HPT. Hemmstoffe der Leukotrienbiosynthese. In: *DAZ* 137(3):139-40. 1997.

Ammon HPT. Mack T. Singh GB et al. Inhibition of leukotriene B4 formation in rat peritoneal neutrophils by an ethanolic extract of the gum resin exudate of *boswellia serrata. Planta Med*; 57:203-207. 1991.

Ammon HPT. Weihrauch - ein neuer Weg in der Therapie der Entzündungen. In: *DAZ* 132(45).2442. 1991.

Ammon S. Ein pflanzliches Antirheumaticum. In: *DAZ* 131(19):972. 1991.

Anon. Weihrauchtherapie. In: *DAZ* 134(4):324-325. 1995.

Atal CK, Gupta OP, Singh GB. Salai guggal: a promising anti-arthritic and anti-hyperlipidemic agent. Proceedings of the B.P.S., April; pp 203P-204P. 1981.

Chande N, McDonald JW, MacDonald JK. Interventions for treating collagenous colitis. *Cochrane Database Syst Rev* 4:CD003575, Oct 18, 2006.

Etzel R. Special extract of *boswellia serrata* (H15) in the treatment of rheumatoid arthritis. *Phytomedicine*; 3:91-94. 1996.

Gangwal ML & Vardhan DK. Antifungal studies of volatile constituents of *boswellia serrata. Asian J Chem*; 7:675-676. 1995.

Gupta I, Gupta V, Parihar A et al. Effects of Boswellia serrata gum resin in patients with bronchial asthma: results of a double-blind, placebo-controlled, 6-week clinical study. *Eur J Med Res*; 3:511-514. 1998.

Gupta I, Parihar A, Malhotra P et al. Effects of boswellia serrata gum resin in patients with ulcerative colitis. *Eur J Med Res*; 2:37-43. 1997.

Hoernlein RF et al. Die Hemmung der 5-Lipoxygnesae durch Acetyl-11-keto-β-Boswelliasäure (AKBA): Struktur-Wirkungsbeziehungen. In: 8. Frühjahrstagung der DPhG, Salzau, Abstracts, in *PUZ* 25(3):140. 1996.

Kamboj VP. A review of Indian medicinal plants with interceptive activity. *Indian J Med Res*; 87:336-355. 1988.

Kapil A & Moza N. Anticomplementary activity of boswellic acids - an inhibitor of C3-convertase of the classical complement pathway. *Int J Immunopharmacol*; 14:1139-1143. 1992.

Knaus U & Wagner H. Effects of boswellic acid of *boswellia serrata* and other triterpenic acids on the complement system. *Phytomedicine*; 3:77-81. 1996.

Kreymeier J. Rheumatherapie mit Phytopharmaka. In: *DAZ* 137(8):611-613. 1997.

Kulkarni RR, Patki PS, Jog VP et al. Efficacy of an ayurvedic formulation in rheumatoid arthritis: a double-blind, placebo-controlled, cross-over study. *Indian J Pharmacol*; 24:98-101. 1992.

Kulkarni RR, Patki PS, Jog VP et al. Treatment of osteoarthritis with a herbomineral formulation: a double-blind, placebo controlled, cross-over study. *J Ethnopharmacol*; 33:91-95. 1991.

Martinetz D. Der Indische Weihrauch - neue Aspekte eines alten Harzes. In: ZPT 13(4):121. 1992.

McGuffin M, Hobbs C, Upton R et al (eds). Boswellia, in American Herbal Products Association's Botanical Safety Handbook: Guidelines for the Safe Use and Labeling for Herbs in Commerce. CRC Press, Boca Raton, FL, USA; p 21. 1997.

Menon MK & Kar A. Analgesic and psychopharmacological effects of the gum resin of boswellia serrata. *Planta Med*; 19:333-341. 1971.

Müller-Bohn T. Chemie und Pharmakologie des Weihrauchs: Boswelliasäuren gegen chronische Polyarthritis und Colitis ulcerosa. In: *DAZ* 136(48):4324-4325. 1996.

Pfister-Hotz G. Phytotherapie in der Geriatrie. In: *ZPT* 18(3):165-162. 1997.

Rall B et al. Boswellic acids and protease activity (s.auch folgende Abstracts). In: *PM* 61(Abstracts of 43rd Ann Congr):105. 1995.

Sailer ER, Hoernlein RF, Ammon HPT et al. Structure-activity relationships of the nonredox-type non-competitive leukotriene biosynthesis inhibitor acetyl-11-keto-beta-boswellic acid. *Phytomedicine*; 3:73-74. 1996.

Sander O & Herborn G. Is H15 (resin extract of *boswellia serrata*, ''incense'') a useful supplement to established drug therapy of chronic polyarthritis? Results of a double-blind pilot study. *Z Rheumatol*; 57:11-16. 1998.

Shao Y, Ho CT, Chin CK et al. Inhibitory activity of boswellic acids from *boswellia serrata* against human leukemia HL-60 cells in culture. *Planta Med*; 64:328-331. 1998.

Sharma ML, Khajuria A, Kaul A et al. Effect of salai guggal ex-*boswellia serrata* on cellular and humoral immune responses and leucocyte migration. *Agents Actions*; 24:161-164. 1988.

Singh GB, Singh S & Bani S. Anti-inflammatory action of boswellic acids. *Phytomedicine*; 3:81-85. 1996b.

Wasielewski S. Maligne G. Weihrauchextrakt bei bösartigen Hirntumoren. In: *DAZ* 137(26):2250-2251. 1997.

Wildfeuer A, Neu IS, Safayhi H et al. Effects of boswellic acids extracted from a herbal medicine on the biosynthesis of leukotrienes and the course of experimental autoimmune encephalomyelitis. *Arzneimittelforschung*; 48:668-674. 1998.

Fraxinus excelsior

See Ash

Fraxinus ornus

See Manna

French Tarragon

Artemisia dracunculus

DESCRIPTION

Medicinal Parts: The medicinal parts are the dried aerial parts of the plant.

Flower and Fruit: The flowers are drooping, almost globular, and 2 to 3 mm across. They are whitish, later reddish, and clustered in loose panicles. The sepals of the epicalyx are oblong-elliptic and mostly green; the inner sepals are ovate with a broad membranous edge. The ray florets are female. The disc florets are androgynous and infertile. The corolla is yellow with a glabrous receptacle.

Leaves, Stem, and Root: The plant is a glabrous, 60- to 120-cm high herbaceous perennial. There are numerous stems, which are bushily branched with flowering branches at the top. The leaves are simple, lanceolate-linear, 2 to 10 cm by 2 to 10 mm, thorn-tipped, entire or slightly serrate, and somewhat glossy.

Characteristics: The odor is aromatic and intense.

Habitat: The plant is indigenous to Germany, Russia and southern Europe.

Production: French Tarragon leaves or herbs are picked when in bloom and carefully dried.

Other Names: Little Dragon, Mugwort, Estragon

ACTIONS AND PHARMACOLOGY

COMPOUNDS

Volatile oil of complex, variety-specific composition (0.25-3.1%): chavicol methyl ether dominates in German species, accompanied by ocimene, myrcene, alpha-pinene, beta-pinene, camphene, limonene, linalool

Flavonoids: including quercetin and patuletin glycosides

Hydroxycoumarins: including herniarin, scopoletin

Isocoumarins: including artemidin

Polyynes

EFFECTS

The essential oil of the drug is an appetite stimulant.

INDICATIONS AND USAGE

Unproven Uses: French Tarragon is used as an appetite stimulant.

PRECAUTIONS AND ADVERSE REACTIONS

No health hazards or side effects are known in conjunction with the proper administration of designated therapeutic dosages.

DOSAGE

Mode of Administration: Both the fresh and dried plant is used, mostly as a culinary herb.

LITERATURE

Balza F, Jamieson L, Towers GHN, Chemical constituents of the aerial parts of *Artemisia dracunculus*. In: *JNP* 48:339. 1985.

Hänsel R, Keller K, Rimpler H, Schneider G (Hrsg.), Hagers Handbuch der Pharmazeutischen Praxis, 5. Aufl., Bde 4-6 (Drogen). Springer Verlag Berlin, Heidelberg, New York, 1992-1994.

Lakupovic J, Tan RX, Bohlmann F, Jia ZJ, Huneck S, Acetylenes and other constituents from *Artemisia dracunculus*. In: *PM* 57:450. 1992.

Marco JA et al., Sesquiterpenes lactones from *Artemisia* species. In: *PH* 32:460. 1993.

Schormüller B, In: Schormüller J: Alkaloidhaltige Genuβmittel, Gewürze, Kochsalz, Springer Verlag, Berlin, Heidelberg, New York. 1970.

ätherischen Öls aus Estragon (*Artemisia dracunculus L.*). In: *Z Lebensm Untersuch Forsch* 173:365-367. 1981.

Fringetree

Chionanthus virginicus

DESCRIPTION

Medicinal Parts: The medicinal part is the dried root or tree bark.

Flower and Fruit: The tree bears long peduncles of white, snowdrop-shaped flowers with fringed petals the same size as magnolia flowers. The flowers are androgynous, but on some stalks the flowers are almost exclusively male or female. The calyx is short and consists of four parts. The four petals are fused at the base. They are initially green but turn snow white and extend about 2.5 cm. Two stamens are enclosed in the short tube. The fruit is 1.5 to 2 cm across, dark blue to black, and oval and with a hard stone.

Leaves, Stem and Root: Fringetree is a deciduous shrub or tree up to 10 m tall. The leaves are smooth or downy, oblong or oval, 7.5 to 20 cm long, and opposite. The root bark is about 3 mm thick and consists of irregular, quilled pieces up to about 8 cm long. The exterior of the bark is dull brown with concave scars. The inner surface is smooth and buff colored. The fracture is short and dense with projecting bundles of stone cells.

Characteristics: Fringetree is almost odorless and very bitter. The bark is so dense that, unlike most other barks, it sinks in water.

Habitat: Fringetree grows in the central and southern U.S. and also in eastern Asia.

Production: Fringetree root bark is the root bark of *Chionanthus virginicus*.

Other Names: Gray Beard Tree, Old Man's Beard, Poison Ash, Snowflower, White Fringe, Chionanthus, Snowdrop Tree

ACTIONS AND PHARMACOLOGY

COMPOUNDS

Lignane glycosides: phillyrin (chioanthine)

Saponins

EFFECTS

Fringetree, because of its saponin content, is said to have hepatic, cholagogue, diuretic, and tonic effects.

INDICATIONS AND USAGE

Unproven Uses: Fringetree is used in treatment of the liver and gallbladder conditions (including gallstones). North American folk uses included jaundice, hepatatrophy, wounds, and ulcers.

Homeopathic Uses: Although mention is made of significant homeopathic use, no details are given.

PRECAUTIONS AND ADVERSE REACTIONS

No health hazards or side effects are known in conjunction with the proper administration of designated therapeutic dosages.

DOSAGE

Mode of Administration: Liquid extract and preparations are administered internally.

LITERATURE

Kern W, List PH, Hörhammer L (Hrsg.), Hagers Handbuch der Pharmazeutischen Praxis, 4. Aufl., Bde. 1-8, Springer Verlag Berlin, Heidelberg, New York, 1969.

Madaus G, Lehrbuch der Biologischen Arzneimittel, Bde 1-3, Nachdruck, Georg Olms Verlag Hildesheim 1979.

Steinegger E, Jacober H, Pharm Acta Helv 34:585. 1959.

Frostwort

Helianthemum canadense

DESCRIPTION

Medicinal Parts: The medicinal part is the herb.

Flower and Fruit: The plant flowers twice each season, once early and again near the end. The first flowers are flat with large, bright yellow petals. The second flowers are in terminal clusters.

Leaves, Stem, and Root: The plant is a perennial that grows 3 to 6 cm high and has a simple, erect, sparsely branched white stem. The few branches are slender and purplish-green with opposite leaves and leaf scars. The leaves are linear, up to 1.5 cm long, grayish-green and downy.

Characteristics: The taste is astringent and bitter. The plant is odorless.

Habitat: Frostwort is indigenous to the eastern U.S., but is now also found in Europe.

Production: Frostwort is the aerial part of *Helianthemum canadense*.

Other Names: Frost Plant, Frostweed, Rock-Rose, Sun Rose

ACTIONS AND PHARMACOLOGY

COMPOUNDS

Tannins

Glycoside: helianthinin

The constituents of the drug have not been fully investigated.

EFFECTS

Frostwort is astringent and tonic.

INDICATIONS AND USAGE

The herb is used internally for digestive disorders and externally for ulcers.

PRECAUTIONS AND ADVERSE REACTIONS

Health risks or side effects following the proper administration of designated therapeutic dosages are not recorded.

DOSAGE

Mode of Administration: Frostwort is administered as a liquid extract.

LITERATURE

Kern W, List PH, Hörhammer L (Hrsg.), Hagers Handbuch der Pharmazeutischen Praxis, 4. Aufl., Bde. 1-8, Springer Verlag Berlin, Heidelberg, New York, 1969.

Madaus G, Lehrbuch der Biologischen Arzneimittel, Bde 1-3, Nachdruck, Georg Olms Verlag Hildesheim 1979.

Fucus vesiculosus

See Bladderwrack

Fumaria officinalis

See Fumitory

Fumitory

Fumaria officinalis

DESCRIPTION

Medicinal Parts: The medicinal parts are the dried herb and the aerial parts of the fresh flowering plant.

Flower and Fruit: The short-pedioled flowers are in erect, dense, terminal racemes opposite the leaves, and are 5 to 8 mm long. The outer petals are rounded at the front and are crimson to pink. But like the inner petals they are dark-red to black at the tip and have a green keel. The fruit, which appears in the flowering season, is nutlike, globular, slightly flattened at the side, green, and has a dent in the top.

Leaves, Stem, and Root: The plant is 10 to 50 cm high and has a tender, erect, angular, branched, hollow and glabrous stem which, like the leaves, is bluish green. The leaves are alternate and divided into tripinnate sections. They are petiolate, double pinnate, soft with petioled palmate, or pinnatifid pinna.

Characteristics: The herb has a bitter, salty taste.

Habitat: The plant is indigenous to the Mediterranean region to northern Africa and in all of Europe and Siberia. The herb has been introduced into North and South America.

Production: Common Fumitory herb consists of the dried, above ground parts of *Fumaria officinalis*, gathered during the flowering season.

Not to be Confused With: The very similar species *F. vaillanti* and *F. schleicheri*.

Other Names: Earth Smoke, Hedge Fumitory, Beggary, Fumus, Vapor, Wax Dolls

ACTIONS AND PHARMACOLOGY

COMPOUNDS

Flavonoids: including rutin

Hydroxycinnamic acid derivatives: including caffeoylmalic acid

Isoquinoline alkaloids: some of them include -

Protoberberine-type: including (-)-scoulerine

Protopine-type: including protopine; main alkaloid

Spirobenzylisoquinoline-type: fumaricine, (+)-fumariline

Indenobenzazepine-type: including fumaritine, fumarofine

Organic acids: fumaric acid

EFFECTS

Fumitory has a light, antispasmodic effect on the bile ducts and the gastrointestinal tract. It is also amphicholeretic.

INDICATIONS AND USAGE

Approved by Commission E:

- Liver and gallbladder complaints

Spastic discomfort in the area of the gallbladder and bile ducts, as well as the gastrointestinal tract.

Unproven Uses: In folk medicine, the herb has been used for skin diseases, constipation, cystitis, arteriosclerosis, rheumatism, arthritis, as a blood purifier, for hypoglycemia, and infections.

Homeopathic Uses: for chronic, itching eczema resulting from liver disease.

PRECAUTIONS AND ADVERSE REACTIONS

Health risks or side effects following the proper administration of designated therapeutic dosages are not recorded.

DOSAGE

Mode of Administration: Comminuted drug and its galenic preparations for internal use.

Preparation: To prepare an infusion, pour boiling water over 2 to 3 gm drug and strain after 20 minutes.

Daily Dosage: 6 g of drug. Infusions for gallbladder complaints, drink 1 warm cup 30 minutes before meals.

Pressed juice—2 to 3 teaspoons (2.4 to 3.5 g drug) daily as a cold or hot infusion.

Grated fresh plant—1 teaspoon 3 times daily (about 50% plant material).

Homeopathic Dosage: 5 drops, 1 tablet, or 10 globules every 30 to 60 minutes (acute) or 1 to 3 times daily (chronic); parenterally: 1 to 2 mL sc acute: 3 times daily; chronic: once a day (HAB34).

Storage: Protect from light and moisture.

LITERATURE

Boegge SC, Nahrstedt A, Linscheid M, Nigge W. Distribution and Stereochemistry of Hydroxycinnamoylmalic Acids and Free Malic Acids in Papaveraceae and Fumariaceae. *Z Naturforsch*. 50c; 608-615. 1995

Duke JA. Die amphocholeretische Wirkung der Fumaria officinalis. Z Allg Med 34: 1819. 1985

Hahn R, Nahrstedt A. High Content of Hydroxycinnamic Acids Esterified with (+)-D-Malic-Acid in the Upper Parts of *Fumaria officinalis*. In: PM 59(2):189. 1993.

Galanthus nivalis

See Snowdrop

Galbanum

Ferula gummosa

DESCRIPTION

Medicinal Parts: The medicinal part is the oily gum-resin.

Two types of Galbanum are used: Levant or Soft Galbanum is more viscous and often contains small root pieces. Persian or Hard Galbanum sometimes contains pieces of stem and is friable in texture.

Flower and Fruit: The plant bears yellowish-white flowers in a few flat umbels. The fruit is thin and flat. The seeds are glossy.

Leaves, Stem, and Root: Ferula gummosa is a perennial plant with a firm, smooth and hollow stem that grows up to 1.75 m tall. The leaflets are glossy, ovate, wedge-shaped, and have sharply serrate margins.

Characteristics: The gum-resin occurs in translucent yellowish or bluish-green masses of tears. Soft Galbanum (Levant) is more viscous and may contain small pieces of root. Hard Galbanum (Persian) is friable and may contain pieces of stem. The odor is similar to musk or turpentine.

Habitat: The plant is found in central Asia, Iran, the Mediterranean region and also at the Cape of Good Hope.

Production: Galbanum is the resin from the roots and trunk of *Ferula gummosa* and other related varieties. The exuding resin is collected from the pith without wounding the plant.

ACTIONS AND PHARMACOLOGY

COMPOUNDS

Resinous substances (60%): chiefly galbaresenic acid and galbanic acid

Mucilages (40%)

Volatile oil (10-20%): including among others, alpha-pinenes, beta-pinenes, myrcene, cadinenes, guaiazulene, aroma bearer undecatriene

EFFECTS

The drug acts as stimulant, expectorant, and vulnerary. In vitro an antimicrobial effect has been proved.

INDICATIONS AND USAGE

Unproven Uses: Internally, Galbanum is used for digestive disorders and flatulence; externally it is used in the treatment of wounds.

PRECAUTIONS AND ADVERSE REACTIONS

Health risks or side effects following the proper administration of designated therapeutic dosages are not recorded.

DOSAGE

Mode of Administration: Preparations for internal and external use.

LITERATURE

Kern W, List PH, Hörhammer L (Hrsg.), Hagers Handbuch der Pharmazeutischen Praxis, 4. Aufl., Bde 1-8, Springer Verlag Berlin, Heidelberg, New York, 1969.

Galega officinalis

See Goat's Rue

Galeopsis segetum

See Hemp Nettle

Galipea officinalis

See Angostura

Galium aparine

See Cleavers

Galium odoratum

See Sweet Woodruff

Galium verum

See Lady's Bedstraw

Gambir

Uncaria species

DESCRIPTION

Medicinal Parts: The medicinal parts are the leaves and young shoots of the plant.

Flower and Fruit: The flowers are single or in loose, globose inflorescences. The flowers are fused and grow in fives. The corolla is funnel-shaped, the 2-part ovary is inferior. The fruit is a loculicidal capsule opening on two sides. The seeds are long-winged at both ends.

Leaves, Stem, and Root: This woody liana or climbing shrub has leaves that are opposite and short-petiolate. Young branches have four sides and pairs of stipules. Using *Uncaria gambir* as a prototype, the calyx is 5-tipped, the corolla light purple. The leaves are 6 to 11 mm long with a 1 to 2 cm long petiole, coriaceous, lanceolate to oval, entire, pubescent at the veins. After the leaf-axillary flower branches drop, a barbed tendril, which is 1 to 2 cm long and woody, is formed.

Habitat: Indonesia and Malaysia

Production: Yellow catechu is the dried aqueous extract of the leaves and young shoots of *Uncaria gambir*. Cultivated stock is harvested, then the leaves and shoots are boiled with water to form a decoction that is pressed and evaporated to the consistency of syrup. The resulting lumps are dried in the sun.

Not to be Confused With: Acacia

Other Names: Yellow Catechu

ACTIONS AND PHARMACOLOGY

COMPOUNDS

Catechin tannins (20 to 50%): among them gambirines A1 to A3 (astringently active flavanol dimers)

Flavanols (10 to 50%): particularly (+)-catechin, gambirines B1 to B3 (dimers)

Indole alkaloids of the beta-carboline type (presumably only traces in the drug): including gambirtanine, dihydrogambirtanine

EFFECTS

The drug is astringent in effect because of the tannins it contains, which are also said to exhibit antibacterial and algicidal efficacy. The flavonoid fraction (cyanidanol = (+)-catechin) is said to be hepatoprotective in effect.

INDICATIONS AND USAGE

Unproven Uses: Catechu tincture is used in folk medicine for diarrhea, nausea, and gastrointestinal disturbances. Decoction is used for ulcers of the stomach and oral mucosa, and also asthma.

PRECAUTIONS AND ADVERSE REACTIONS

No health hazards are known in conjunction with the proper administration of designated therapeutic dosages.

DOSAGE

Mode of Administration: Whole and powdered drug for internal use.

Preparation: Tincture: 200 g drug (pounded), 50 g cut cinnamon to 1 liter 45% ethanol, macerated (BP88)

Daily Dosage: 0.5 to 2 g drug; Catechu Tincture: 2.5 to 5 ml

LITERATURE

Blaschek W, Hänsel R, Keller K, Reichling J, Rimpler G, Schneider G (Eds), Hagers Handbuch der Pharmazeutischen Praxis. Folgeb nde 1 und 2. Drogen A-Z. Springer. Berlin, Heidelberg 1998.

Haginiwa J, Sakai S, Takahashi K, Taguchi M, Shujiro S, Studies of plants containing indole alkaloids. I. Alkaloids in *Uncaria* genus. *Yakugaku Zasshi*, 25:575-8, 1971 May.

Law KH, Das NP, Initiation and maintenance of callus tissue culture of *Uncaria elliptica* for flavonoid production. *Prog Clin Biol Res*, 25:67-70, 1988.

Lin CC, Lin JM, Chiu HF, Studies on folk medicine "thang-kau-tin" from Taiwan. (I). The anti-inflammatory and liver-protective effect. *Am J Chin Med*, 57:37-50, 1992.

Lin JM, Lin CC, Chen MF, Ujiie T, Takada A, Studies on Taiwan folk medicine, thang-kau-tin (II): Measurement of active oxygen scavenging activity using an ESR technique. *Am J Chin Med*, 57:43-51, 1995.

Mimaki Y, Toshimizu N, Yamada K, Sashida Y, Anti-convulsion effects of choto-san and chotoko (*Uncariae Uncis cam Ramlus*) in mice, and identification of the active principles. *Yakugaku Zasshi*, 57:1011-21, Dec. 1997

Yamanaka E, Kimizuka Y, Aimi N, Sakai S, Haginiwa J, Studies of plants containing indole alkaloids. IX. Quantitative analysis of tertiary alkaloids in various parts of *Uncaria rhynchophylla* MIQ. *Yakugaku Zasshi*, 25:1028-33, Oct 1983.

Zhu M, Bowery NG, Greengrass PM, Phillipson JD, Application of radioligand receptor binding assays in the search for CNS active principles from Chinese medicinal plants. *J Ethnopharmacol*, 57:153-64, Nov. 1996

Gamboge

Garcinia hanburyi

DESCRIPTION

Medicinal Parts: The medicinal part of the tree is the resin extracted from the plant.

Leaves, Stem and Root: The tree grows to about 15 m and has a diameter of about 30 cm. The bark is usually in the form of cylindrical sticks, deep orange-brown, and opaque. The transverse fracture is smooth and almost conchoidal.

Characteristics: The taste is innocuous at first, then becomes very acrid and causes an unpleasant stinging sensation shortly after being placed in the mouth. The powder is highly sternutatory.

Habitat: The plant is indigenous to Indochina and Sri Lanka.

Production: Gamboge is the gum-resin from the trunk of *Garcinia hanburyi* harvested from trees that are at least ten years old.

Other Names: Camboge, Gutta Cambodia, Gutta Gamba, Gummigutta, Tom Rong, Gambodia

ACTIONS AND PHARMACOLOGY

COMPOUNDS

Resins (70-75%): consisting mainly of yellow or red-colored benzophenones and xanthones, including morellic acid, isomorellic acid, alpha-gambogic acid (alpha-guttic acid)

Mucilages (25-30%)

EFFECTS

The drug's mucilage content produces a strong laxative effect. The beta gutteriferine componant acts as a strong irritant to intestinal mucous membranes and also exhibits antimicrobial properties.

INDICATIONS AND USAGE

Unproven Uses: Gamboge is used for the treatment of digestive disorders, in particular constipation, and is used in combination with other laxatives.

PRECAUTIONS AND ADVERSE REACTIONS

As little as 0.2 g of the drug can lead to abdominal pain and vomiting.

OVERDOSAGE

Fatalities have been observed with administration of 4 g.

DOSAGE

No information is available in the literature.

LITERATURE

Hegnauer R, Chemotaxonomie der Pflanzen, Bde 1-11, Birkhäuser Verlag Basel, Boston, Berlin 1962-1997.

Kern W, List PH, Hörhammer L (Hrsg.), Hagers Handbuch der Pharmazeutischen Praxis, 4. Aufl., Bde. 1-8, Springer Verlag Berlin, Heidelberg, New York, 1969.

Lewin L, Gifte und Vergiftungen, 6. Aufl., Nachdruck, Haug Verlag, Heidelberg 1992.

Lu GB et al., Yao Hsueh Husueh Pao 19 (8): 636. 1984

Wagner H, Wiesenauer M, Phytotherapie. Phytopharmaka und pflanzliche Homöopathika, Fischer-Verlag, Stuttgart, Jena, New York 1995.

Garcinia hanburyi

See Gamboge

Garcinia mangostana

See Mangosteen

Garden Cress

Lepidium sativum

DESCRIPTION

Medicinal Parts: The medicinal part is the fresh or dried herb harvested during or shortly after the flowering season.

Flower and Fruit: The racemes are terminal or axillary. The sepals are elliptical, 1 to 1.5 mm long, and bristly-downy. The petals are longer than the calyx, white or reddish, oblong-spatulate, and indistinctly stemmed. The anthers are often violet. The 5- to 6-mm long fruit is a compressed, orbicular-ovate, clearly winged small pod on an erect stem. The seeds are ovate, almost smooth, and red-brown.

Leaves, Stem, and Root: Garden Cress is a 20 to 40 cm high herb with a glabrous bluish bloom. The stem is erect, round, and branched. The leaves are light green and thin. The basal leaves are usually lyrate-pinnatesect. The lower cauline leaves are usually doubly or singly pinnatesect. All leaves have dentate to prickly segments.

Characteristics: Garden Cress has a radishlike taste. The seeds have a slimy skin and swell in water.

Habitat: The herb is grown worldwide.

Production: Garden Cress is the fresh plant (aerial part) of *Lepidium sativum*, harvested during the flowering season or shortly afterward. The fresh herb has a spicy odor. It is rarely dried, either naturally or artificially, since the fresh plant is used most often.

Not to be Confused With: Adulterations rarely occur, since it is usually cultivated.

Other Names: Pepper-gras

ACTIONS AND PHARMACOLOGY

COMPOUNDS: IN THE FRESH FOLIAGE

Glucosinolates: chief components glucotropaeolin, yielding benzyl isothiocyanate (benzyl mustard oil) and its autolysis products (including benzyl cyanide, 3-phenyl propionitrile, benzaldehyde) when the plant is bruised

Ascorbic acid (vitamin C, 37%)

COMPOUNDS: IN THE SEEDS

Glucosinolates (3.5 to 5.3%): glucotropeolin

Cucurbitacins

Cardiac steroids (cardenolides)

EFFECTS

The antibacterial action of Garden Cress has been demonstrated in various tests. It was completely inhibitory in the case of three microorganisms, although the antibacterial characteristics depended largely on the age of the plants used. An antiviral effect against the encephalitis virus *Columbia SH* was demonstrated in tests on mice. Its diuretic action has not been proven through experiments.

INDICATIONS AND USAGE

Unproven Uses: The herb is used for coughs, vitamin C deficiency, constipation, poor immunity, and as a diuretic.

Indian Medicine: Garden Cress is used for vitamin C deficiency, liver disease, asthma, hemorrhoids, and as an abortifacient.

PRECAUTIONS AND ADVERSE REACTIONS

No health hazards or side effects are known in conjunction with the proper administration of designated therapeutic dosages. The mustard oil contained in Garden Cress can cause skin blisters and necrosis in higher concentrations. It is sometimes misused as an abortifacient because the internal administration of mustard oil causes severe anemia of the internal organs.

DOSAGE

Mode of Administration: Garden Cress is administered as a freshly cut herb in oral preparations.

LITERATURE

Al-Yahya MA, Mossa JS, Ageel AM, Rafatullah S. Pharmacological and Safety Evaluation Studies on *Lepidium sativum L.*, Seeds. *Phytomedicine* 1; 155-159. 1994

Hänsel R, Keller K, Rimpler H, Schneider G (Hrsg.), Hagers Handbuch der Pharmazeutischen Praxis, 5. Aufl., Bde 4-6 (Drogen), Springer Verlag Berlin, Heidelberg, New York, 1992-1994.

Iori R, Rollin P, Streicher H, Thiem J, Palmieri S, The myrosinase-glucosinolate interaction mechanism studied using some synthetic competitive inhibitors. *FEBS Lett*, 385:87-90, Apr 29, 1996

Rao KV, Beach JW, Streptonigrin and related compounds. 5. Synthesis and evaluation of some isoquinoline analogs. *J Med Chem*, 19:1871-9, Jun 1991.

Ugazio G et al., co-toxicological study conducted with a battery of biological and phytological tests on sediments carried out on a series of 24 tributaries of the Po in 1994 and 1995. *G Ital Med Lav Ergon*, 19:10-6, Jan-Mar 1997.

Garlic

Allium sativum ingiber officinale

DESCRIPTION

Medicinal Parts: The medicinal parts are the whole fresh bulb, the dried bulb, and the oil of Garlic.

Flower and Fruit: The plant consists of a cluster of long flowers where the floral axis terminates in a single flower and contains few florets (small flowers or buds). There are numerous 1-cm deciduous bulbs capable of producing new plants. The flowers usually remain in bud form and often do not produce any seeds. The petals are reddish or greenish-white and longer than the stamens. The anthers of the middle stamens are spread at the base and have fan-shaped tips.

Leaves, Stem, and Root: Allium sativum is a perennial plant that grows 25 to 70 cm high. The plant contains an erect, rigid or curved stem, which is leafy in the middle. The leaves are flat, 4 to 25 mm, straight and broad, with a wedge-shaped tip; they can be rough or smooth-edged. The sheath, or lower part of the leaf surrounding the stem, is pointed and longer than the flower cluster. The Garlic bulb is usually a compound bulb, and the secondary bulbs are oval in shape. The bulb skin color is either silky white or green.

Habitat: Central to southern Asia is considered the region of origin; Garlic has been introduced to the Mediterranean with cultivation worldwide.

Production: Garlic bulbs, either fresh or carefully dried, consist of the main bulb with several secondary bulbs (cloves). Garlic may be harvested in September and October when the leaves and bulbs are dry.

Other Names: Allium, Clove Garlic, Common Garlic, Poor Man's Treacle, Stinking Rose

ACTIONS AND PHARMACOLOGY

COMPOUNDS

Alliins (alkylcysteine sulfoxides): in particular allylalliin, propenyl alliin and methylalliin (including their gamma-glutamyl conjugates. Once cut, the alliin in the freshly harvested bulbs is converted to allicin (diallyl-disulphide-mono-S-oxide). Bulbs that have been dried and then remoistened ferment into alliaceous oils. These oils are oligosulfides, ajoens (dialkyl-trithiaalkane-monoxides), and vinyl dithiins.

Fructosans (polysaccharides)

Saponins

EFFECTS

Garlic has been recommended for use primarily as a hypolipidemic and antihypertensive agent but also has found use as an antineoplastic. Garlic preparations are used to positively affect blood lipids, fibrinolytic activity, low-density lipoprotein oxidation, blood pressure, and to prevent and treat cardiovascular disease (Murray & Pizzorno, 1999; Lawson, 1998; Orekhov & Grunwald, 1997). Other clinical trials failed to demonstrate a lowering of cholesterol by Garlic (Berthold, 1998; Isaacsohn et al, 1998; Simons et al, 1995).

Garlic-derived compounds in cell and animal systems demonstrated antimicrobial properties (Weber et al, 1992; Hughes & Lawson, 1991). In vitro studies demonstrated antibacterial activities of Garlic (Aydin et al, 1997); ajoene demonstrated antimycotic activity for a number of fungi (Ledezma et al, 1996) while allicin had antifungal activity (Hughes & Lawson, 1991).

Garlic tablets studied in vitro were found to enhance natural killer cells, which are an important part of the immune system in fighting cancers, viruses, and certain bacteria. Antioxidative effects of Garlic, determined by an increase in intracellular glutathione levels, are responsible for decreasing poor cellular function and premature aging. Antiviral activity was also noted *in vitro* with Garlic tablets (See, 1999).

Many studies have demonstrated Garlic to have an inhibitory effect on platelet aggregation, which may cause postoperative bleeding (Petry, 1995). Ajoene is the antithrombotic compound that inhibits fibrinogen receptors on platelets (Robbers, 1996). The allicin and oligosulfides in Garlic oil have antiplatelet activity through inhibition of adenosine diphosphate, collagen and beta-thromboglobulin release after collagen stimulation. The compounds also exert antithrombotic effects through inhibition of platelet thromboxane formation (Bordia, 1998; Legnani 1993).

Antihypertensive Effects: Results of a study of 20 healthy subjects demonstrated that Garlic has an effect on vessels but its mechanism of action has not yet been clarified. Garlic powder significantly increased the diameter of the erythrocyte column of conjunctival vessels. In the venules, the dilation was slightly more pronounced than in the arterioles but no effect on capillaries was observed (Wolf et al, 1990). Garlic may decrease systolic hypertension in the elderly by reducing the amount of cholesterol deposited on the blood vessel linings (Anon, 1998).

Antimicrobial Effects: Studies indicated that Garlic and its components act as a natural antibiotic with broad-spectrum antimicrobial activity against many genera of bacteria, fungi, and even viruses, including antibiotic-resistant organisms (Farbman et al, 1993; Guo et al, 1993). Garlic extracts or powders are antibacterial against *Bacillus, Escherichia, Staphylococcus, Streptococcus, Vibrio, Pseudomonas, Mycobacteria,* and *Enterococcus* organisms in vitro. Garlic and allicin demonstrated bacteriostatic effects on vancomycin-resistant enterococci in vitro. A synergism has also been demonstrated between Garlic and allicin with vancomycin (Jonkers et al, 1999; Aydin et al, 1997).

Garlic oil has been tested in vitro and in vivo against *Helicobacter pylori*, a gram-negative organism that is thought to increase the susceptibility of patients to gastritis, gastric cancer, and peptic ulcers (Aydin et al, 1997). Garlic oil was not effective in the treatment of *H pylori* in dyspeptic patients in a preliminary uncontrolled study (McNulty et al, 2001), nor was it effective in the treatment of *H pylori* infection (Graham et al, 1999). Garlic compounds diallyl sulfide (DAS) and diallyl disulfide (DADS) exhibited concentration-dependent bacteriocidal activity against *H pylori* obtained from peptic ulcer patients. Inhibition of *H pylori* was greater than 90% for some strains with concentrations of 0.25 milligram/milliliter of DAS or DADS (Chung et al, 1998).

Allium sativum and a variety of its components have antiviral activity when tested in vitro against herpes simplex type 1, type 2, parainfluenza type 3, vaccinia, vesicular stomatitis virus, and human rhinovirus. The components of greatest activity, from highest to lowest, were: ajoene, allicin, allyl methyl thiosulfinate, and methyl ally thiosulfinate (Weber et al, 1992). Garlic cloves had antifungal activity against various *Trichophyton, Microsporum, Aspergillus,* and *Candida* species (MIC of 500 to 2000 mcg/mL) (Hughes & Lawson, 1991). Ajoene was antimycotic for a number of fungi, including *Candida albicans, Paracoccidioides brasiliensis,*

Coccidioides immitis, Cladosporium carrionii, Fonseaae pedrosoi, and *Aspergillus niger* (Ledezma et al, 1996).

In vitro studies suggest that allicin and other thiosulfinates from Garlic are responsible for the antimycobacterial activity of Garlic. Those compounds inactivate essential thiol groups, possibly by formation of disulfide or by simple oxidation of adjacent thiols by the labile oxygen of the thiosulfide link (Deshpande et al, 1993). Activity of commercial Garlic extract against meningitis in clinical studies indicated that allicin or other active compounds of commercial Garlic extract may pass the intact or disrupted blood-brain barrier (Davis et al, 1990).

Antineoplastic Effects: The ability of Garlic to inhibit cancers may be due to interference with carcinogens, especially those that require metabolic activation (Milner, 1996). Other studies have shown Garlic to have theoretical protective properties (Munday & Munday, 1999; Milner, 1996; Romano et al, 1997; Ferguson, 1997; Scharfenberg et al, 1994).

Garlic consumption was associated with reduced risk for stomach and colorectal cancer in a meta-analysis of observational epidemiological studies conducted between 1966 and 1999, although other epidemiological studies have not supported the use of Garlic as an anticancer agent. An epidemiological study in China demonstrated a decreased stomach cancer risk with higher Garlic consumption (Met et al, 1982).

A review of a series of animal and *in vitro* studies evaluating the antitumor and immune-enhancing effects of aged Garlic extract suggests potential use in the treatment of bladder cancer. Animal and *in vitro* studies provided evidence that Garlic may inhibit carcinogenesis, inhibit cancer cell growth, and promote chemical carcinogen detoxification. Documented immunological effects of Garlic include increased interleukin-2, TNF-alpha, and interferon-gamma production and stimulation of macrophage infiltration, natural killer cells, and lymphokine-activated killer cells. Based on this review, the authors suggested that clinical trials are warranted (Lamm & Riggs, 2000). A preliminary in vitro study suggested that ajoene may be an effective adjunctive therapy to chemotherapeutic agents, fludarabine, and cytarabine, in treatment-resistant or treatment-relapsed acute myeloid leukemia (Ahmed et al, 2001).

Effects on Cytochrome P450: Various forms of fresh Garlic and Garlic extracts inhibited cytochrome P450 isoenzymes and P-glycoprotein in vitro (Foster et al, 2001). The significance of this in vitro finding is unknown, as Garlic significantly decreased saquinavir levels in humans, suggesting an inductive effect (Piscitelli et al, 2002).

Fibrinolytic Activity: Treatment of 20 hyperlipidemic patients with 200 mg of dried Garlic 3 times daily over a period of 4 weeks demonstrated an increase in fibrinolytic activity. The prothrombin time decreased during medication, but did not reach statistical significance and no significant changes in platelet aggregation and platelet count were observed. Mean cholesterol levels and systolic and diastolic blood pressure were slightly reduced during Garlic therapy (Harenberg et al, 1988).

Hypercholesterolemic Effects: While numerous clinical studies have demonstrated that Garlic and Garlic powder preparations possess hypocholesterolemic action, the mechanism of this effect has not been fully clarified (Gebhardt, 1997). Proposed mechanisms include inhibition of hepatic squalene epoxidase by organic tellurium compounds of Garlic (Larner, 1995), lipid redistribution between tissue and plasma by Garlic-induced membrane effects (Brosche et al, 1990), retarded lipoprotein oxidation (Phelps & Harris, 1993), and improvement of the oxidant resistance of low-density lipoprotein (Lewin & Popov, 1994). These effects are primarily attributed to allicin (Lawson, 1998; Gebhardt, 1997; Holzgartner et al, 1992). Garlic's action in the prevention and treatment of atherosclerosis may involve reduction of excess lipids, lowering of hypertension, and prevention of thrombus formation. Garlic may reduce lipid content in arterial cells and prevent intracellular lipid accumulation (Orekhov & Grunwald, 1997).

Garlic reduces cholesterol, but it is a clinically inefficient means of cholesterol reduction. Numerous double-blind, placebo-controlled studies in patients with high cholesterol levels, demonstrated that Garlic supplements lowered total serum cholesterol levels by 6% to 12%, LDL cholesterol by 4% to 15%, triglyceride levels by 15%, and increased HDL cholesterol levels by 0% to 22%. The majority of studies used Garlic powder in doses of 900 mg to 1200 mg a day (providing a daily dose of at least 10 mg alliin or a total allicin potential of 4000 mcg) (Kanner et al, 2001; Bordia et al, 1998; Lawson, 1998; Orekhov & Grunwald, 1997). A meta-analysis demonstrated a reduction in total cholesterol by 6% (Stevinson et al, 2000). There are data indicating that short-term supplementation of garlic increases resistance of LDL to oxidation, suggesting that suppressed LDL oxidation may be one of the mechanisms that accounts for the heart-healthy benefits of garlic (Lau, 2006).

Platelet Aggregation Effects: Allicin is significantly responsible for the antiplatelet aggregation activity of Garlic, but is only present in the blood for a short time (less than an hour) (Carotenuto et al, 1996). The mechanism by which Garlic influences platelet aggregation has not been fully clarified and there is controversy about the active compounds, but allicin (in vitro) does not affect platelet aggregation via platelet cyclooxygenase, thromboxane synthetase activity, or cyclic AMP levels (Agarwal, 1996). Results of in vitro and ex vivo studies have demonstrated that Garlic preparations possess considerable anti-aggregatory effects on platelets (Rahman & Billington, 2000; Steiner & Li, 2001; Steiner & Lin, 1998; Bordia et al, 1996; Carotenuto et al, 1996).

CLINICAL TRIALS

Atherosclerosis

A pilot trial that evaluated the ability of Aged Garlic Extract (AGE) to retard the progression of calcification in the coronary arteries found incremental benefits for high-risk patients also on stable statin and aspirin therapy, for example. Nineteen of the 23 patients were enrolled in the placebo-controlled, double-blind, one-year trial. Nine were randomized to take 4 mL of AGE (1200 mg), and 10 to take the equivalent amount of placebo. Based on measurements using electron beam tomography (a well-validated tool for tracking atherosclerotic plaque over time), the patients taking AGE experienced a significant slowing of the accumulation of coronary artery calcification over the course of the trial (Budoff, 2006).

In an earlier study, plaque formation in the common carotid and femoral arteries was reduced significantly following treatment with Garlic in 280 subjects with advanced atherosclerotic plaque formation. Subjects received 900 mg Garlic powder or an identical placebo tablet daily for 4 years in a randomized, double-blinded, placebo-controlled study. A regression in plaque volume of 2.6% was observed in subjects treated with Garlic compared to a 15.6% increase in plaque volume in the placebo group, with the difference of 18.3% being significant. The increase in plaque volume was reduced in both men and women from 6% to 18%. Women on placebo showed a 53.1% increase in plaque volume compared to a 4.6% reduction in women taking Garlic. In men, plaque volume increased by 5.5% in those taking placebo compared to 1.1% in those taking Garlic powder (Koscielny et al, 1999).

Cancer

Fresh or cooked Garlic consumption was associated with reduced risk for stomach and colorectal cancer in a meta-analysis of observational epidemiological studies conducted between 1966 and 1999. Subjects who consumed high quantities of fresh or cooked Garlic reduced their relative risk of developing colorectal cancer by approximately 40% and stomach cancer by approximately 47%. In the high Garlic reference group, Garlic intake ranged from any ingestion to 9 to 10 cloves/week vs. 0 to 1 clove/week in the low-intake group, with a mean difference between groups of 5 to 6 cloves/week. For stomach cancer, 4 case-control studies were included in the analysis that compared 2,071 high-intake subjects with 3,193 low-intake controls. For colorectal cancer, 6 case-control and cohort studies were included that compared 1,945 high-intake subjects with more than 50,000 low-intake controls. Epidemiological studies evaluating the effect of commercial Garlic supplements (n=4; 953 active versus 4,836 controls) revealed no protective effect against cancer while the evaluation of all studies on consumption of fresh or cooked Garlic (n=15) reduced cancer (stomach, colon, head, and neck) risk by approximately 46%. This study did not provide details on minimum Garlic intake required to exert an anticarcinogenic effect. Limitations of this analysis include evidence of publication bias, small number of studies, and lack of control for confounding study variables. An analysis of intervention studies is warranted to validate these results (Fleischauer et al, 2000).

More recent results of a preliminary, double-blind, randomized clinical trial of Aged Garlic Extract (AGE) in individuals with precancerous lesions of the large bowels—colorectal adenomas—found that after 12 months of treatment, subjects administered high-dose AGE (2.4mL/d) as an active treatment significantly suppressed both the size and number of colon adenomas after 12 months of treatment (P=0(P=0.04).04) as compared to subjects given low-dose AGE (0.16mL/d) or placebo. In all, 51 patients diagnosed with colorectal adenomas— and following surgical removal of any adenomas larger than 5 mm in diameter—were enrolled in the study and randomly assigned to either the high-dose or low-dose AGE regimen, or placebo. Colonoscopy was used to measure number and size of adenomas immediately before the trial began and at 6 and 12 months. In the control group, the number of adenomas increased linearly over the course of the 12 months. Based on observations made, the authors conclude that AGE may have multiple ways of suppressing cancerous changes and suppressing the growth and proliferation of such shifts in the colorectum (Tanaka, 2006).

Cardiovascular Disease

A series of articles on the significance of Garlic and its constituents in cardiovascular disease (and cancer) was published in 2006 in the American Society for Nutrition's *Journal of Nutrition*. The articles were based on studies presented at an International Research Symposium in Washington DC in April 2005 (Rivlin 2006). One of the critical reviews of in vivo and in vitro studies published in this *Journal of Nutrition* issue concluded that Garlic is promising in terms of reducing the parameters associated with cardiovascular disease, with clinical trials pointing to its capacity to reduce cholesterol and blood pressure, increase antioxidant status, and inhibit platelet aggregation. In vitro studies point to even more cardio-protective properties. Forty-four percent of clinical trials since 1993 indicate that Garlic may reduce total cholesterol. A profound effect on reducing the ability of platelets to aggregate also has been documented. Results for lowering blood pressure and oxidative stress have been less definitive. The authors concluded that more in-depth and appropriate studies are needed before definitive conclusions or recommendations about garlic's cardio-protective powers in humans can be made (Rahman, 2006)

A small trial examining the effects of Aged Garlic Extract (AGE) on endothelial dysfunction in people with cardiovascular risk factors or established vascular disease generated mixed results. The placebo-controlled, blinded, crossover study in 11 healthy subjects (aged 25 to 40) found that pretreatment with AGE for 6 weeks significantly lessened the adverse effects of acute hyperhomocysteinemia on micro- and macro-vessels. The authors hypothesize that AGE exerts this effect in part by preventing a decrease in bioavailable nitric oxide (NO) and endothelium-derived hyperpolarizing factor during acute hyperhomocysteinemia. More research is warranted, the authors conclude (Weiss, 2006)

Common Cold

Garlic was effective in preventing common cold, reducing recovery time, and reducing symptom duration in healthy volunteers in a 3-month randomized, double-blind, placebo-controlled study (n=146). The number of episodes of the common cold during the 3-month study was significantly less in the treatment group compared to the placebo group (24 vs. 65, $p<0.001$), as was the duration of symptoms (1.52 days in treatment group versus 5.01 days in the placebo group; $p<0.001$). Average recovery period for the treatment group was 4.63 days compared to 5.63 days for the placebo group). Common cold reinfection rate in the treatment group was 3% compared to 22% in the placebo group. (Josling, 2001). Further controlled studies that account for some of the flaws in this current study are warranted to verify the results. The current study was based entirely on subjective data and it lacked detailed information on dosing as well as other study details.

Coronary Heart Disease/Coronary Artery Disease

In a double-blind, randomized, placebo-controlled clinical trial, the effects of Allicor, an *Allium sativum* preparation with prolonged activity, was investigated on 10-year prognostic risk for coronary heart disease (CHD), acute myocardial infarction (MI), and sudden death in patients with elevated and high risk of CHD. Prolonged administration (12 months) of Allicor significantly reduced the multifactor risk, which was demonstrated by a 13.2% (p=0.005) reduction of prognostic 10-year risk of CHD in men, and a 7.1% (p=0.040) reduction of the same parameter in women. In men, the main factor of cardiovascular risk reduction was the decrease of cholesterol and low-density lipoprotein concentrations (p=0.004), and, in women, the increase of high-density lipoprotein level (p=0.040). It can be concluded that prolonged Allicor therapy can be applied to patients who are in need of atherosclerosis prevention (Sobenin et al, 2005).

Cytochrome P450 Inhibition

Various forms of fresh Garlic and Garlic extracts inhibited cytochrome P450 isoenzymes and P-glycoprotein *in vitro*. Cytochrome P450 2C9(1), 2C19, 3A4, 3A5, and 3A7 were inhibited by various forms of Garlic. CYP2D6 was unaffected. Garlic had low to moderate effect on P-glycoprotein as compared with verapamil. Three varieties of fresh Garlic (common, Chinese, and elephant) and 10 commercial Garlic products (including aged Garlic, odorless Garlic, Garlic oil, and freeze-dried Garlic) were tested. All types of Garlic inhibited CYP3A4. Fresh Garlic (phosphate buffer extracts) inhibited CYP3A4 by 44% to 59% depending on the variety tested, with common Garlic the most inhibitory. Fresh Garlic (phosphate buffer extracts) had little effect on 2C19 and 2D6 and strongly stimulated 2C9(2) (Foster et al, 2001).

Dementia

With its potential to lower cardiovascular risk factors, the authors of one study note that Garlic may also protect against developments associated with the increased risk for dementia later in life, including high cholesterol, hypertension, inflammation, oxidative stress, and high homocysteine levels. Although additional studies are needed, the authors elucidate these possible links and suggest a possible anti-dementia benefit in tandem with heart disease benefits identified with Aged Garlic Extract (AGE) particularly (Borek 2006).

Hyperlipidemia

Note: There are contradicting results regarding the lipid-lowering effect of Garlic, which may be attributed to lack of manufacturing standardization of the products used in the studies. The fresh Garlic may contain higher amounts of the active ingredient, allicin, which is inactivated upon cooking.

Garlic in various forms failed to have any statistically or clinically significant effects on low-density lipoprotein cholesterol (LDL-C) or other plasma lipid concentrations in a carefully designed, randomized, parallel-design 6-month trial involving 192 adults (169 completed the trial) with moderate hypercholesterolemia. Two types of commercial supplements (powdered Garlic and Aged Garlic Extract) were tested against each other and placebo. The Garlic failed to reduce LDL-C more than 10 mg/dL (0.26 mmol/L) when used for 6 months. In addition, no statistically significant effects were seen with Garlic in terms of HDL-C, triglyceride levels, or the ratio of total cholesterol to HDL-C. Based on various observations made, the authors conclude that Garlic in ''reasonable'' doses in any form is unlikely to generate lipid benefits (Gardner 2007).

The conclusion of Gardner's 2007 study was discussed in an editorial in the same journal entitled, ''Garlic: What We Know and What We Don't Know.'' Arguing that the study's results do not negate Garlic's potential usefulness in preventing cardiovascular disease, the editorial noted that atherosclerosis is a complex phenomenon and that not only dyslipidemia, but inflammation, hypertension, platelet aggregation, diabetes mellitus, and numerous other lifestyle and genetic factors play important roles that Garlic might potentially influence (Charlson, 2007).

Lipid-lowering effects could be found in a double-blind, placebo-controlled study investigating the hypocholesterolemic action of long-acting garlic powder tablets, Allicor. Men with mild hypercholesterolemia received either daily 600 mg Allicor or placebo. Total cholesterol and LDL cholesterol was lowered and HDL cholesterol increased (Andrianova et al, 2004).

In an earlier, randomized, double-blind, placebo-controlled trial, garlic was shown to have a mild cholesterol-lowering effect in moderately hypercholesterolemic adults. Healthy adults (n=53) with fasting LDL levels between 130 to 190 mg/dL were randomly assigned to receive oral treatment with 500 mg dehydrated Garlic, 1000 mg dehydrated Garlic, or placebo daily for 12 weeks. Each 1000 mg of Garlic (equivalent to 1.5 cloves) contained 1500 mcg allicin. A 4% reduction in total cholesterol levels occurred in subjects treated with 1000 mg

Garlic daily compared to an increase of 1.4% in subjects treated with placebo and Garlic 500 mg daily. LDL cholesterol was reduced by 6.1% in subjects treated with 1000 mg Garlic daily compared to an increase of 0.9% in subjects treated with Garlic 500 mg daily. (Gardner et al, 2001).

Similarly, an enteric-coated Garlic supplement reduced cholesterol in subjects with mild to moderate hypercholesterolemia. In the randomized, double-blind, placebo-controlled clinical trial, total cholesterol was reduced by 4.2% and LDL cholesterol was reduced by 6.6% in subjects treated with Garlic ($p<0.05$ compared to placebo), while HDL cholesterol was increased by 9.1% in subjects treated with placebo compared to Garlic ($p<0.05$). Results remained significant after controlling for reductions in dietary fat, carbohydrate, and alcohol intake in subjects treated with Garlic compared to placebo. The authors suggested that positive results observed in this trial may be a result of high allicin content and improved bioavailability due to enteric dosing form (Kannar et al, 2001).

In contrast, Garlic oil failed to positively influence plasma risk factors for coronary heart disease (CHD) in healthy (nonhyperlipidemic) subjects in an 11-week randomized, double-blind, placebo-controlled clinical trial. Garlic oil caused no statistically significant difference in LDL cholesterol, HDL cholesterol, total cholesterol, triglycerides, total antioxidant capacity, or glucose compared to placebo. Significant improvements were observed in HDL cholesterol and the TC/HDL cholesterol ratio in women subjects compared to male subjects ($p=0.004$ and $p=0.003$, respectively). Significant differences in glucose levels were also observed between men and women following Garlic treatment ($p=0.006$), with men exhibiting a reduction in glucose and women exhibiting an increase in glucose. (Zhang et al, 2001).

An earlier meta-analysis of 13 double-blind, placebo-controlled, randomized clinical trials, conducted between 1981 and 1998, suggested that Garlic is an inefficient mechanism for reducing serum total cholesterol levels (n=796). (Stevinson et al, 2000). Garlic powder did not significantly alter plasma lipid measurements in moderately hypercholesterolemic subjects in a 12-week randomized, double-blind, placebo-controlled study (n=50) (Superko & Krauss, 2000).

Administration of Garlic powder (900 mg/d for 12 weeks) was ineffective in lowering cholesterol levels in hypercholesterolemic patients. This was a multicenter, randomized, double-blind, placebo-controlled study of patients with hypercholesterolemia (defined as 160 mg/dL) low density lipoprotein cholesterol or lower, and a triglyceride level of 350 mg/dL or lower) (Isaacsohn et al, 1998).

Administration of Garlic capsules to hyperlipidemic children did not result in statistically significant changes in fasting total cholesterol, LDL cholesterol, HDL cholesterol, triglycerides, apolipoprotein B-100, lipoprotein (a), fibrinogen, homeocysteine, or blood pressure. The study was a randomized, double-blind, placebo-controlled clinical trial of 30 patients (8 to 18 years) with familial hyperlipidemia and cholesterol greater than 4.8 mmol/liter (185 mg/dL). Patients were treated for eight weeks with 300 mg of Garlic extract (0.6 mg of allicin) three times a day (or placebo). Absolute and relative changes in fasting lipid profiles were measured (McCrindle et al, 1998).

Hypertension

Garlic supplementation reduced incidence of hypertension but not incidence of preeclampsia in nulliparous pregnant women at high risk for preeclampsia in a randomized, single-blinded, placebo-controlled clinical trial (n=100). Incidence of hypertension was 36% in women treated with placebo compared to 18% in women treated with Garlic ($p=0.043$) although no significant differences were observed in mean systolic, diastolic, or arterial pressure between groups. (Ziaei et al, 2001).

In a double-blind, placebo-controlled, cross-over evaluation, reduced systolic blood pressure was observed in a Garlic experimental group and a placebo group, but the Garlic experimental group had average systolic pressures 5.5% lower than placebo. Participants were instructed to follow the National Cholesterol Education Program Step I diet during the study. A baseline level was established within a 4-week period that included no treatment other than diet. For testing, patients were randomized and given the Garlic extract or placebo. The first test ran for 180 days and blood pressure was monitored periodically. In the second phase (cross-over), patients received the alternate preparation for 120 days (Steiner et al, 1996).

Peripheral Arterial Occlusive Disease

A meta-analysis of Garlic in the treatment of peripheral arterial occlusive disease concluded that Garlic cannot be recommended as therapy based on negative results reported in the one eligible trial conducted by Kiesewetter et al, 1993. No statistical difference was reported in pain-free walking distance after treatment with Garlic or placebo. Trial inclusion criteria included randomized trials evaluating Garlic in the treatment of peripheral arterial disease. Only one trial was found in the literature. Study flaws included lack of information on method of randomization, failure to conceal allocation, and intention to treat analysis not done. Larger trials of longer duration are recommended (Jepson et al, 2000).

Platelet Aggregation

Epinephrine-, adenosine 5c-diphosphate (ADP)-, and collagen-induced platelet aggregation was inhibited in serum samples obtained from healthy subjects consuming aged Garlic extract (AGE) in a 44-week randomized, double-blind, placebo-controlled crossover study (n=34). Significant reductions in collagen-induced platelet aggregation were observed compared to baseline and placebo at all AGE dose levels ($p<0.05$). Platelet adhesion to collagen was reduced significantly compared to baseline and placebo for doses of 4800 mg to 7200 mg AGE daily while it was not affected at 2400 mg daily. Adhesion to fibrinogen was significantly reduced at all dose levels while an adhesion to von Willebrand factor was only reduced at the highest dose level (Steiner & Li, 2001).

Pregnancy — Pre-eclampsia

A Cochrane Database Review examined available evidence (quality randomized clinical trials) to support the hypothesis that Garlic may have a role to play in preventing pre-eclampsia, a serious complication of pregnancy that occurs in about 2 to 8 of every 100 women. While Garlic's purported ability to lower blood pressure may help with pre-eclampsia, only one quality study was found that examined this—and it showed no difference between dried Garlic tablets and placebo. More research is needed to determine if other Garlic preparations may be effective in treating the dangerous pre-eclampsia of pregnancy (Meher, 2006).

Protease Inhibitors, Concomitant Administration with

Short-term Garlic administration did not significantly alter ritonavir pharmacokinetics in an open-label, randomized, crossover study of 10 healthy subjects. Subjects received Garlic extract 10 mg (equivalent to 1 g of fresh Garlic) daily for 4 days. Ritonavir 400 mg was administered on day 4. The dose and duration of Garlic used in this study were much lower than that used by Piscitelli et al, 2002, in which Garlic reduced saquinavir levels. The authors stated that their results should not be extrapolated to steady-state conditions (Gallicano et al, 2003).

Unstable Angina

An intravenous Garlic infusion exhibited similar efficacy to a nitroglycerin infusion in the treatment of unstable angina pectoris in a randomized, controlled clinical trial (n=34); however, the dose of nitroglycerin was 7- to 10-fold lower than standard doses for angina. Angina symptom control was improved by 82% and 77%, respectively, for Garlic and nitroglycerin treatment. Improvements in electrocardiogram tracings were 62% and 58%, respectively, for Garlic and nitroglycerin treatment. Garlic resulted in significant reductions in systolic and diastolic blood pressure ($p<0.01$ compared to baseline) while no changes were observed in the nitroglycerin treatment group. Plasma endothelium level was reduced significantly compared to baseline and nitroglycerin treatment following treatment with Garlic ($p<0.05$). Reduction in plasma endothelium is suggested as a potential mechanism for Garlic effect in the treatment of spontaneous angina (Li et al, 2000). Study results need to be interpreted with caution due to small sample size, subtherapeutic dose of the comparative drug, and lack of information on study design and results.

INDICATIONS AND USAGE

Approved by Commission E:

- Arteriosclerosis
- Hypertension
- Raised levels of cholesterol

Garlic is used internally as an adjuvant to dietetic measures for elevated lipid levels. The herb is also used for prevention of age-related vascular changes and arteriosclerosis.

Unproven Uses: In folk medicine, Garlic is utilized internally for inflammatory respiratory conditions, whooping cough, and bronchitis. Garlic is also used for gastrointestinal ailments, particularly digestive disorders with flatulence and gastrointestinal spasms. Other uses consist of menstrual pains, treatment of diabetes, and as a tonic for diverse illnesses and debilities. Externally, Garlic is used for corns, warts, calluses, otitis, muscle pain, neuralgia, arthritis, and sciatica.

Indian Medicine: Garlic is used in bronchitis, constipation, joint pain and fever.

Homeopathic Uses: Garlic is used in conditions such as inflammation of the upper respiratory tract, digestive complaints and muscle rheumatism in the lumbar region.

CONTRAINDICATIONS

Garlic may increase the risk of bleeding and should be discontinued at least 10 days before elective surgery (German et al, 1995).

Breastfeeding: Not to be used while breastfeeding.

PRECAUTIONS AND ADVERSE REACTIONS

Anaphylaxis, offensive odor, burns, nausea, and anticoagulation resulting in bleeding have been reported. Adverse effects such as headache, myalgia, fatigue, and vertigo have been seen with therapeutic doses of Garlic (Holzgartner, 1992). Gastrointestinal symptoms, changes to the flora of the intestine, and allergic reactions, including contact dermatitis and asthma (Couturier & Bousquet, 1982), are possible. Garlic may induce cytochrome P450 2E1 and reduce the effectiveness of drugs metabolized through this enzyme (Gurley et al, 2002).

In a meta-analysis of 13 double-blind, placebo-controlled, randomized clinical trials conducted between 1981 and 1998, the severity and nature of adverse events reported were similar between groups with Garlic breath and odor reported most frequently, followed by gastrointestinal complaints (Stevinson et al, 2000). Mild and infrequent adverse reactions, including eructation (belching), flatulence, and constipation were reported in a randomized, double-blind, placebo-controlled trial evaluating the hypocholesterolemic effect of Garlic in moderately hypercholesterolemic adults (n=53). One or more of these adverse events was reported in 11% of placebo subjects, 47% of subjects receiving 500 mg Garlic daily, and 24% of subjects receiving 1000 mg Garlic daily (Gardner et al, 2001).

ALMA Determination: ALMA (N-acetyl-S-allyl-L-cysteine) determination in the urine may be falsely positive or elevated when Garlic is consumed (de Rooij et al, 1996). ALMA is used as a biomarker for exposure to allyl halides, such as allyl chloride. Consumption of Garlic also raises ALMA levels.

Burns: There have been several cases of Garlic associated partial thickness ''burns'' and necrosis reported in the literature. These cases have mostly involved young children who have had the Garlic in contact with the skin for hours to days at a time (Canduela et al, 1995; Parish et al, 1987; Garty, 1993). Burns have also been seen in adults (Roberge et al, 1997; Farrell & Staughton, 1996).

Dermatologic: A pruritic rash was sited as the reason for withdrawal in one subject in a study evaluating oral Garlic in the prevention and treatment of the common cold in healthy volunteers in a 3-month randomized, double-blind, placebo-controlled study (n=146) (Josling, 2001). Local irritation at the injection site following intravenous Garlic infusion was reported in 6 of 34 (18%) subjects during Garlic treatment for unstable angina pectoris in a randomized, controlled, comparative trial with nitroglycerin (Li et al, 2000).

Gastrointestinal: Sixty percent (3 out of 5) of dyspeptic patients subjects with *H pylori* infection reported dyspepsia after ingestion of Garlic oil capsules for total dose of 16 mg daily for 2 weeks in a preliminary uncontrolled study (n=5) (McNulty et al, 2001).

Hepatic: Elevated liver enzymes—alkaline phosphatase (ALP), aspartate aminotransferase (AST), and alanine aminotransferase (ALT)—and urea were found in studies of prolonged high-dose therapy (dose and duration of therapy not specified) with Garlic products (fresh, oil, or powder). These may have been signs of liver toxicity (Kasinath et al, 1997).

Ocular: Lacrimation may occur from crushing Garlic. This effect is due to the action of alliinase on S-propenyl cysteine sulfoxide, forming propene sulfenic acid (Augusti, 1996).

Olfactory Effects: Body odor and halitosis are common side effects of Garlic ingestion.

DRUG INTERACTIONS

MAJOR RISK

Anticoagulants: Concurrent use may result in increased risk of bleeding. *Clinical Management*: Concomitant use of garlic and anticoagulants is not recommended. If garlic is taken with an anticoagulant, monitor bleeding time and signs and symptoms of excessive bleeding. Obtain baseline bleeding times in patients on garlic therapy prior to initiating anticoagulants. Regular ingestion of food products containing small amounts of garlic should not pose a problem. If excessive garlic is consumed with concomitant use of anticoagulants, monitor the INR and/or bleeding time and signs and symptoms of excessive bleeding. Garlic supplements should be discontinued at least 10 days prior to elective surgery (German et al, 1995).

Protease Inhibitors: Concurrent use may result in decreased protease inhibitor concentrations and an increased risk of antiretroviral resistance and treatment failure. *Clinical Management*: Avoid concomitant use of garlic and protease inhibitors. If a patient is using garlic supplements while taking a protease inhibitor, discontinue garlic and monitor blood levels and symptoms of toxicity of the protease inhibitor and adjust the dose of the protease inhibitor as necessary.

MODERATE RISK

Antiplatelet Agents: Concurrent use may result in increased risk of bleeding. *Clinical Management*: Concomitant use of garlic and antiplatelet agents is not recommended. If garlic is taken with an antiplatelet agent, monitor bleeding time and signs and symptoms of excessive bleeding. Obtain baseline bleeding times in patients on garlic therapy prior to initiating antiplatelet agents. Regular ingestion of food products containing garlic should not pose a problem. If garlic extract is taken with concomitant use of antiplatelet agents, monitor bleeding time and signs and symptoms of excessive bleeding. Garlic supplements should be discontinued at least 10 days prior to elective surgery (German et al, 1995).

Coleus forskolii: Concurrent use may result in increased risk of bleeding. *Clinical Management*: Caution is advised in the concomitant use of garlic and Coleus forskolii (forskolin). Regular ingestion of food products containing garlic should not pose a problem. If garlic extract is taken with concomitant use of Coleus forskolii, monitor for signs and symptoms of excessive bleeding. Garlic supplements should be discontinued at least 10 days prior to elective surgery.

Low Molecular Weight Heparins: Concurrent use may result in increased risk of bleeding. *Clinical Management*: Concomitant use of garlic and low molecular weight heparins is not recommended. Regular ingestion of food products containing small amounts of garlic should not pose a problem. If excessive garlic is consumed with concomitant use of low molecular weight heparin, monitor for signs and symptoms of excessive bleeding. Garlic supplements should be discontinued at least 10 days prior to elective surgery.

Indomethacin: Concurrent use may result in increased risk of bleeding. *Clinical Management*: Caution is advised in the concomitant use of garlic and indomethacin. Regular ingestion of food products containing garlic should not pose a problem. If garlic extract is taken with concomitant use of indomethacin, monitor for signs and symptoms of excessive bleeding. Garlic supplements should be discontinued at least 10 days prior to elective surgery.

Thrombolytic agents: Concurrent use may result in increased risk of bleeding. *Clinical Management*: Concomitant use of garlic and thrombolytic agents is not recommended. Regular ingestion of food products containing small amounts of garlic should not pose a problem. If excessive garlic is consumed with concomitant use of thrombolytic agents, monitor for signs and symptoms of excessive bleeding. Garlic supplements should be discontinued at least 10 days prior to elective surgery.

MINOR RISK

Chlorzoxazone: Concurrent use may result in reduced chlorzoxazone effectiveness. *Clinical Management*: Monitor patients for continued effectiveness of chlorzoxazone.

DOSAGE

Mode of Administration: The minced bulb and preparations are for internal use and external treatment. Garlic oil maceration or Garlic oil resulting from steam distillation is widely available.

How Supplied:

Capsules – 3 mg, 100 mg, 270 mg (total allicin 5000 mcg), 300 mg, 500 mg, 580 mg (total allicin 3 mg), 600 mg (total allicin 2500 mcg or standardized to 500 mcg allicin), 1000 mg, 1500 mg, 5000 mg

Dried powder

Oil macerations

Tablets – 300 mg, 400 mg (total allicin 3 mg), 500 mg, 600 mg (total allicin 5000 mcg), 810 mg

Preparation: Garlic oil maceration – Bulbs are homogenized and stirred in fatty oil (1:1) for 48 hours, then filtered.

Solid Garlic extract – An extraction of the chopped bulbs with ethanol or methanol is allowed to evaporate.

Aqueous extract – Fresh bulbs are macerated in cold water (1:1).

Fermented Garlic – The minced drug is soaked over a long duration in a water-ethanol mixture, volatile agents escape, and the Garlic becomes odorless. Steam distillations and tinctures are also possible.

Daily Dosage:

General – The average daily dose is 4 g of fresh Garlic or 8 mg of essential oil. One fresh Garlic clove, 1 to 2 times daily.

Arteriosclerosis – Daily doses of 600-800 mg of Garlic powder and dried Garlic have been shown to be effective (Harenberg, 1988; Kiesewetter, 1991).

Hyperlipidemia – A total daily dose of 600-900 mg of Garlic powder (standardized to 1.3% of alliin content) has been shown effective (Holzgartner, 1992; Isaacsohn, 1998; Mader, 1990; Simons, 1995).

Hypertension – The effective dose is Garlic powder taken 200-300 mg three times daily (Auer, 1990; Sigagy, 1994).

External – Fresh Garlic applied to the skin as an antimicrobial dressing should not be left for more than a few hours due to case reports of burns (Garty, 1993; Parish, 1987; Roberge, 1997).

Homeopathic Dosage: 5 drops, 1 tablet, or 10 globules every 30 to 60 minutes (acute) or 1 to 3 times daily (chronic); parenterally: 1 to 2 times daily sc; ointment 1 to 2 times daily (HAB1)

Storage: Garlic should be hung in plaits in a dry place.

LITERATURE

Agarwal KC. Therapeutic actions of Garlic constituents. *Med Res Rev*; 16(1):111-124. 1996

Ahmed N, Laverick L, Sammons J et al. Ajoene, a Garlic-derived natural compound, enhances chemotherapy-induced apoptosis in human myeloid leukaemia CD34-positive resistant cells. *Anticancer Res*; 21(5):3519-3523. 2001

Andrianova IV, Demidova OM, Medvedeva LA, Latyshev OA. Correction of hyperlipidemia with Allicor. *Klin Med*; 82(4): 56-58. 2004.

Anibarro B, Fontela JL & De La Hoz F. Occupational asthma induced by Garlic dust. *J Allergy Clin Immunol*; 100(6 pt 1):734-738. 1997

Anon. Garlic: can it keep your blood vessels young? *Harvard Heart Lett*; March:6-8. 1998

Anon, Knoblauch. Blockade der Cholesterinsynthese in der Leber. In: *DAZ* 134(45):4468. 1994

Apitz-Castro R, Escalante J, Vargas R et al. Ajoene, the antiplatelet principle of Garlic, synergistically potentiates the antiaggregatory action of prostacyclin, forskolin, indomethacin and dipyridamole on human platelets. Thromb Res; 42(3):303-311. 1986a

Apitz-Castro R, Ledezma E, Escalante J et al. The molecular basis of the antiplatelet action of ajoene: direct interaction with the fibrinogen receptor. *Biochem Biophys Res Commun*; 141(1):145-150. 1986

Apitz-Castro R et al. *Thromb Res* 32:155. 1983

Armentia A & Vega JM. Can inhalation of Garlic dust cause asthma? *Allergy*; 51(2):137-138. 1996

Arora RC & Arora S. Comparative effect of clofibrate, Garlic, and onion on alimentary hyperlipidemia. *Atherosclerosis*; 39(4):447-452. 1981

Arora RC, Arora S & Gupta RK. The long-term use of Garlic in ischemic heart disease - an appraisal. *Atherosclerosis*; 40(2):175-179. 1981

Asero R, Mistrello G, Roncarolo D et al. A case of Garlic allergy. *J Allergy Clin Immunol* Mar;101(3):427-428. 1998

Augusti KT. Therapeutic values of onion (*Allium cepa L.*) and Garlic (*Allium sativum L.*). *Indian J Exp Biol* Jul;34(7):634-640. 1996

Augusti KT. Benaim ME, *Clin Chim Acta* 60:121. 1974

Augusti KT. Mathew PT, *Experientia* 30:468. 1974

Aydin A, Ersoz G, Tekesin O et al. Does Garlic oil have a role in the treatment of Helicobacter pylori infection? *Turk J Gastroenterol*; 8:181-184. 1997

Block E et al. *J Am Chem Soc* 106:8295. 1984

Berthold HK, Sudhop T, von Bergmann K. Effect of Garlic oil preparation on serum lipoproteins and cholesterol metabolism: a randomized controlled trial. *JAMA* Jun 17;279(23):1900-1902. 1998

Bojs G & Svensson A. Contact allergy to Garlic used for wound healing. *Contact Dermatitis*; 18(3):179-181. 1988

Bordia A, Verma SK, Srivastava KC. Effect of Garlic (*Allium sativum*) on blood lipids, blood sugar, fibrinogen and fibrinolytic activity in patients with coronary artery disease. *Prostaglandins Leukot Essent Fatty Acids*. Apr;58(4):257-263. 1998

Borek C. Garlic reduces dementia and heart-disease risk. *J Nutr;* 136;810S-8125. 2006.

Brahmachar MD, Augusti KT. *J Pharm Pharmacol* 14: 254 and 617. 1962

Breithaupt-Grogler K, Ling M et al. Protective effect of chronic Garlic intake on elastic properties of aorta in the elderly. *Circulation*; 96(8):2649-2655. 1997

Brosche T, Platt D & Dorner H. The effect of a Garlic preparation on the composition of plasma lipoproteins and erythrocyte membranes in geriatric subjects. *Br J Clin Pract Symp Suppl*; 69(Aug):12-19. 1990

Budoff M. Aged garlic extract regards progression of coronary artery calcification. *J Nutr*; 136: 741S-744S. 2006.

Burnham BE, Garlic as a possible risk for postoperative bleeding (letter). *Plast Reconstr Surg Jan*;95(1):213. 1995

Canduela V, Mongil I, Carrascosa M et al. Garlic: always good for the health (letter)? *Br J Dermatol*; 132(1):161-162. 1995

Carotenuto A, De Feo V, Fattorusso E et al. The flavonoids of *Allium ursinum. Phytochemistry*; 41(2):531-536. 1996

Charlson M, McFerren M. Editorial: Garlic — What We Know and What We Don't Know. *Arch Intern Med*;167:325-326. 2007

Chaudhuri BN et al. *Biomed Biochim Acta* 41:1045. 1984

Chung JG, Chen GW, Wu LT et al. Effects of Garlic compounds diallyl sulfide and diallyl disulfide on arylamine N-acetyltransferase activity in strains of *Helicobacter pylori* from peptic ulcer patients. *Am J Chin Med*; 26(3-4):353-364. 1998

Couturier P & Bousquet J. Occupational allergy secondary to inhalation of Garlic dust (letter). *J Allergy Clin Immunol*; 70(2):145. 1982

Davis LE, Shen JK & Cai Y. Antifungal activity in human cerebrospinal fluid and plasma after intravenous administration of *Allium sativum. Antimicrob Agents Chemother*; 34(4):651-653. 1990

de Rooij BM, Boogaard PJ, Rijksen DA et al. Urinary excretion of N-acetyl-S-allyl-L-cysteine upon Garlic consumption of human volunteers. Arch Toxicol; 70(10):635-639. 1996

Deshpande RG, Khan MB, Deepashree AB et al. Inhibition of Mycobacterium avium complex isolates from AIDS patients by Garlic (*Allium sativum*). *J Antimicrob Chemother*; 32(4):623-626. 1993

Fachinformation. Kwai® N, Garlic. Lichtwer Pharma GmbH, Berlin, Germany; 1997

Farbman KS, Barnett ED, Bolduc GR et al. Antibacterial activity of Garlic and onions: a historical perspective. *Pediatr Infect Dis J*; 12(7):613-614. 1993

Farrell AM & Staughton RCD. Garlic burns mimicking herpes zoster (letter). *Lancet*; 347(9009):1195. 1996

Ferguson LR. Micronutrients, dietary questionnaires and cancer. *Biomed Pharmacother*; 51(8):337-344. 1997

Fleischauer AT, Poole C & Arab L. Garlic consumption and cancer prevention: meta-analyses of colorectal and stomach cancers. *Am J Clin Nutr*; 72(4):1047-1052. 2000

Foster BC, Foster MS, Vandenhoek S et al. An in vitro evaluation of human cytochrome P450 3A4 and P-glycoprotein inhibition by Garlic. *J Pharm Pharmaceut Sci*; 4(2):176-184. 2001

Gallicano K, Foster B & Choudhri S. Effect of short-term administration of Garlic supplements on single-dose ritonavir pharmacokinetics in healthy volunteers. *Br J Clin Pharmacol*; 55(2):199-202. 2003

Gardner CD, Lawson LD, Bock E, et al. Effect of raw garlic vs commercial garlic supplements on plasma lipid concentrations in adults with moderate hypercholesterolemia. *Arch Intern Med*;167:346-353. 2007.

Gardner CD, Chatterjee LM & Carlson JJ. The effect of a Garlic preparation on plasma lipid levels in moderately hypercholesterolemic adults. *Atherosclerosis*; 154(1):213-220. 2001

Garty BZ, Garlic Burns. *Pediatrics* Mar;91(3):658-659. 1993

Gebhardt R. Garlic: the key to sophisticated lowering of hepatocellular lipid (editorial). *Nutrition*; 13(4):379-380. 1997

Gebhardt R. Multiple inhibitory effects of Garlic extracts on cholesterol biosynthesis in hepatocytes. *Lipids*; 28:613-619. 1993

Gebhardt R, Beck H. Differential inhibitory effects of Garlic-derived organosulfur compounds on cholesterol biosynthesis in primary rat hepatocyte cultures. *Lipids* Dec;31(12):1269-76. 1996

German K, Kumar U, Blackford HN. Garlic and the risk of TURP bleeding. *Br J Urol* Oct;76(4):518. 1995

Graham DY, Anderson AY & Lang R. Garlic or jalapeno peppers for treatment of *Helicobacter pylori* infection. *Am J Gastroenterol*; 94(5):1200-1202. 1999

Guo NL, Lu DP, Woods GL et al. Demonstration of the anti-viral activity of Garlic extract against human cytomegalovirus in vitro. *Chin Med J* (Engl); 106(2):93-96. 1993

Gurley BJ, Gardner SF, Hubbard MA et al. Cytochrome P450 phenotypic ratios for predicting herb-drug interactions in humans. *Clin Pharmacol Ther*; 72(3):276-287. 2002

Harenberg J, Giese C, Zimmermann R. Effect of dried Garlic on blood coagulation, fibrinolysis, platelet aggregation and serum cholesterol levels in patients with hyperlipoproteinemia. *Atherosclerosis* Dec;74(3):247-249. 1988

Holzgartner H, Schmidt U, Kuhn U. Comparison of the efficacy and tolerance of a Garlic preparation vs. bezafibrate. *Arzneimittelforschung* Dec;42(12):1473-1477. 1992

Hughes BG & Lawson LD. Antimicrobial effects of *Allium sativum L* (Garlic), *Allium ampeloprasum L* (elephant Garlic), and *Allium cepa* (onion), Garlic compounds and commercial Garlic supplementation products. *Phytother Res*; 5:154-158. 1991

Ide N et al. Aged Garlic extract and its constituents inhibit Cu+-induced oxidative modification of low-density lipoproteins. *Planta Med* 63(3):263-264. 1997

Imai J et al. Antioxidant and radical scavenging effects of aged Garlic extracts and its constituents. *Planta Med* 60(5):417. 1994

Isaacsohn JL, MoserM, Stein EA et al. Garlic powder and plasma lipids and lipoproteins: a multicenter, randomized, placebo-controlled trial. *Arch Intern Med* Jun 8;158(11):1189-1194. 1998

Jain AK, Vargas R, Gotzkowsky S, McMahon FG. Can Garlic reduce levels of serum lipids? A controlled clinical study. *Am J Med* 94:632-635. 1993

Jain RC, Vyas CR. *BMJ* 2:730. 1974

Jepson RG, Kleijnen J & Leng GC. Garlic for peripheral arterial occlusive disease (Cochrane Review). In: The Cochrane Library; (2):1-8. 2000

Jonkers D, Sluimer J & Stobberingh E. Effect of Garlic on vancomycin-resistant enterococci. *Antimicrob Agents and Chemother;* 43(12):3045. 1999

Josling P. Preventing the common cold with a Garlic supplement: a double-blind, placebo-controlled survey. *Adv Ther*; 18(4):189-193. 2001

Jung EM, Jung F, Mrowietz C et al. Influence of Garlic powder on cutaneous microcirculation. A randomized placebo-controlled double blind cross-over study in apparently healthy subjects. *Arzneimittelforschung* Jun;41(6):626-630. 1991

Jung F, Kiesewetter H, Mrowietz C, Pindur G, Heiden M, Miyashita C, Wenzel E, Akutwirkungen eines zusammengesetzten Knoblauchpräparates auf die Fließfähigkeit des Blutes. ZPT 10(3):87. 1989

Kabelik J. *Pharmazie* 25:266. 1970

Kannar D, Wattanapenpaiboon N, Savige GS et al. Hypocholesterolemic effect of an enteric-coated Garlic supplement. *J Am Coll Nutr*; 20(3):225-231. 2001

Kaplan B, Schewach-Millet M, Yorav S et al. Factitial dermatitis induced by application of Garlic. *Int J Dermatol*; 29:75-76. 1990

Kasinath RT, Joseph PK, Hebron K et al. The effects of Garlic oil upon serum indicators of liver function. Biochem Soc Trans; 25(3):533S. 1997

Kiesewetter H, Jung F, Jung EM et al. Effect of Garlic on platelet aggregation in patients with increased risk of juvenile ischaemic attack. *Eur J Clin Pharmacol*; 45(4):333-336. 1993a

Kiesewetter H, Jung F, Jung EM et al. Effects of Garlic-coated tablets in peripheral arterial occlusive disease. *Clin Investig;* 71(5):383-386. 1993

Kiesewetter H, Jung F, Mrowietz C et al. Effects of Garlic on blood fluidity and fibrinolytic activity: a randomised, placebo-controlled, double-blind study. *Br J Clin Pract Symp Suppl*; 69(Aug):24-29. 1990

Kiesewetter H, Jung F, Pindur G et al. Effect of Garlic on thrombocyte aggregation, microcirculation, and other risk factors. *Int J Clin Pharmacol Ther Toxicol* Apr;29(4):151-5. 1991

Koch HP. Der lange Weg zum "geruchlosen Knoblauch." *PUZ* 25(4):186-191. 1996

Koch HP. Epidemiologie der Knoblauchforschung. *DAZ* 132(40):2103. 1992

Koch HP. Hormonwirkungen bei Allium-Arten. *ZPT* 13(6):177. 1992

Koch HP. Metabolismus und Pharmakokinetik der Inhatsstoffe des Knoblauchs. Was wissen wir darüber? ZPT 13(3):83. 1992

Koch HP. Saponine in Knoblauch und Küchenzwiebel. In: *DAZ* 133(41):3733. 1993

Koch HP. Wie "sicher" ist Knoblauch? Toxische, allergische und andere unerwünschte Nebenwirkungen. *DAZ* 132(27):1419. 1992

Koch B. In: Koch HP, Lawson LD. Garlic - The Science and Therapeutic Application of *Allium sativum L.* and Related Species, Williams & Wilkins, Baltimore. 1996

Koscielny J. Klussendorf D, Latza R et al. The antiatherosclerotic effect of *Allium sativum. Atherosclerosis*; 144(1):237-249. 1999

Kubitschek J. Knoblauch blockiert Cholesterolsynthese in der Leber. *ZPT* 16(2):74, s. auch (3):146. 1995

Lamm DL & Riggs DR. The potential application of *Allium sativum* (Garlic) for the treatment of bladder cancer. *Urol Clin North Am*; 27(1):157-162, xi. 2000

Larner AJ. How does Garlic extract exert its hypocholesterolaemic action? The tellurium hypothesis. Med Hypotheses; 44(4):295-297. 1995

Lau BH. Suppression of LDL oxidation by garlic compounds is a possible mechanism of cardiovascular health benefit. *J Nutr*; 36(3 Suppl):765S-768S. 2006.

Lawson LD. Garlic: a review of its medicinal effects and indicated active compounds, in Lawson LD & Bauer R (eds): Phytomedicines of Europe: Their Chemistry and Biological Activity. American Chemical Society, Washington, DC:176-209. 1998

Lawson LD, Ransom DK & Hughes BG. Inhibition of whole blood platelet-aggregation by compounds in Garlic clove extracts and commercial Garlic products. *Thromb Res*; 65(2):141-156. 1992

Lawson LD, Wang ZJ. Pre-hepatic fate of the organosulfur compounds derived from Garlic (*Allium sativum*). *Planta Med* 59(7):A688. 1993

Lee TY, Lam TH. Contact dermatitis due to topical treatment with Garlic in Hong Kong. *Contact Dermatitis* Mar;24(3):193-6. 1991

Lee TY & Lam TH. Contact dermatitis due to topical treatment with Garlic in Hong Kong. *Contact Dermatitis*; 24(3):193-196. 1991

Legnani C, Frascaro M, Guazzaloca G et al., Effects of a dried Garlic preparation on fibrinolysis and platelet aggregation in healthy subjects. *Arzneimittelforschung* Feb;43(2):119-22. 1993

Lemiere C, Cartier A, Lehrer SB et al. Occupational asthma caused by aromatic herbs. *Allergy*; 51(9):647-649. 1996

Lewin G & Popov I. Antioxidant effects of aqueous Garlic extract: 2nd communication: inhibition of the Cu(2+)-initiated oxication of low density lipoproteins. *Arzneimittelforschung*; 44(51):604-607. 1994

Li G, Shi Z, Jia H et al. A clinical investigation on Garlicin injection for treatment of unstable angina pectoris and its actions on plasma endothelin and blood sugar levels. *J Trad Chin Med*; 20(4):243-246. 2000

Lybarger JA, Gallagher JS, Pulver DW et al. Occupational asthma induced by inhalation and ingestion of Garlic. *J Allergy Clin Immunol* May;69(5):448-454. 1982

Mader FH, Treatment of hyperlipidemia with Garlic-powder tablets. Evidence from the German Association of General Practitioners' multicenter placebo-controlled double-blind study. *Arzneimittelforschung* Oct;40(10):1111-6. 1990

Meher S, Duley L. Garlic for preventing pre-eclampsia and its complications. *Cochrane Database Syst Rev* 3:CD006065, 2006.

McCrindle BW, Helden E & Conner WT. Garlic extract therapy in children with hypercholesterolemia. *Arch Pediatr Adolesc Med*; 152(1):1089-1094. 1998

McGuffin M, Hobbs C, Upton R et al (eds). *Allium sativum L.* The American Herbal Products Associaton's Botanical Safety Handbook. CRC Press, Boca Raton, FL:6-7,183,188. 1997

McNulty CAM, Wilson MP, Havinga W et al. A pilot study to determine the effectiveness of Garlic oil capsules in the treatment of dyspeptic patients with *Helicobacter pylori. Helicobacter*; 6(1): 249-253. 2001

Mei X, Wang ML, Xu HX et al. Garlic and gastric cancer: I. The influence of Garlic on the level of nitrate and nitrite in gastric juice. *Acta Nutrimenta Sinica*; 4:53-56. 1982

Mennella JA, Johnson A & Beauchamp GK. Garlic ingestion by pregnant women alters the odor of amniotic fluid. *Chem Senses*; 20(2):207-209. 1995

Milner JA. Garlic: its anticarcinogenic and antitumorigenic properties. *Nutr Rev*; 54(11 pt 2):S82-S86. 1996

Munday J, James K, Fray L et al. Daily supplementation with aged Garlic extract, but not raw Garlic, protects low density lipoproteins against in vitro oxidation. *Atherosclerosis*; 143:399-404. 1999

Munday R & Munday C. Low doses of diallyl disulfide, a compound derived from Garlic, increase tissue activities of quinone reductase and glutathione transferase in the gastrointestinal tract of the rat. *Nutr and Cancer*; 34(1):42-48. 1999

Murray M & Pizzorno J. A Textbook of Natural Medicine, 2nd ed. Churchill-Livingstone, London, UK; 1999

Mütsch-Eckner M, Erdelmeier CAJ, Sticher O. A novel amino acid glycoside and three amino acids from *Allium sativum. JNP* 56(6):864. 1993

Nagae S et al. Pharmacokinetics of the Garlic compound S-allylcystein. *Planta Med* 60(3):241. 1994

Nakagawa S, Kasuga S & Matsuura H. Prevention of liver damage by aged Garlic extract and its components in mice. *Phytother Res*; 3:50-53. 1989

Newall CA, Anderson LA, Philpson JD, Herbal Medicine: A Guide for Healthcare Professionals. London, UK: The Pharmaceutical Press, 1996

Orekhov AN & Grunwald J. Effects of Garlic on atherosclerosis. *Nutrition*; 13(7-8):656-663. 1997

Parish RA, McIntire S, Heimbach DM, Garlic burns: a naturopathic remedy gone awry. *Pediatr Emerg Care* Dec;3(4):258-60. 1987

Perez-Pimiento AJ, Moneo I, Santaolalla M et al. Anaphylactic reaction to young Garlic. *Allergy*; 54(6):626-629. 1999

Petry JJ. Garlic and postoperative bleeding (letter). *Plast Reconstr Surg*; 96(2):483-484. 1995

Phelps S & Harris WS. Garlic supplementation and lipoprotein oxidation susceptibility. *Lipids*; 28(5):475-477. 1993

Piscitelli SC, Burstein AH, Welden N et al: The effect of Garlic supplements on the pharmacokinetics of saquinavir. *Clin Infect Dis*; 34(2):234-238. 2002

Rahman K, Lowe G. Garlic and cardiovascular disease: a critical review. *J Nutr*; 136:736S-740S. 2006.

Rahman K & Billington D. Dietary supplementation with aged Garlic extract inhibits ADP-induced platelet aggregation in humans. *J Nutr*; 130(11):2662-2265. 2000

Rance F & Dutau G. Labial food challenge in children with food allergy. *Pediatr Allergy Immunol*; 8(1):41-44. 1997

Reuter HD, 6. Kongreβ der Gesellschaft für Phytotherapie:Satelliten-Symposium ''International Garlic Research''. ZPT 17(1):13-25. 1996.

Reuter HD; Chemie, Pharmakologie und medizinische Anwendung von Knoblauch. *ZPT* 10(4):124. 1989

Reuter HD, II. Internationales Knoblauch-Symposium. *ZPT* 12(3):83. 1991

Rivlin R, Budoff M, Amagase H.Preface — Significance of Garlic and its constituents in cancer and cardiovascular disease. *J Nutr;* 136: Preface. 2006.

Robbers JE, Speedie MK, Tyler VE, Pharmacognosy and Pharmacobiotechnology. Baltimore, MD: Williams & Wilkins, 1996

Roberge RJ, Leckey R, Spence R, et al. Garlic burns of the breast (letter). *Am J Emerg Med* Sep;15(5):548. 1997

Romano EL, Montano RF, Brito B et al. Effects of ajoene on lymphocyte and macrophage membrane-dependent functions. *Immunopharmacol Immunotoxicol*; 19(1):15-36. 1997

Rose KD, Croissant PD, Parliament CF, Levin MB. Spontaneous spinal epidural hematoma with associated platelet dysfunction from excessive Garlic consumption: a case report. *Neurosurgery*;26:880-82. 1990

Scharfenberg K, Ryll T, Wagner R et al. Injuries to cultivated BJA-B cells by ajoene, a Garlic-derived natural compound: cell viability, glutathione metabolism, and pools of acidic amino acids. *J Cell Physiol*; 158(1):55-60. 1994

Schiewe FP, Hein T, Knoblauch bei Hyperlipidämie. *ZPT* 16(6):343-348. 1995

Schoetan A et al., *Experientia* 40(3):261. 1984

See, D, Gurnee K, LeClair, M, An in vitro screening study of 196 natural products for toxicity and efficacy. *JANA* Winter;2(1):25-39. 1999

Sendl A, Phytotherapie. Bärlauch und Knoblauch im Vergleich. *DAZ* 133(5):392. 1993

Siegers CP, Neues zur arteriosklerotischen Wirkung des Knoblauchs. *ZPT* 14(1):21. 1993

Silagy C & Neil A. A meta-analysis of the effect of Garlic on blood pressure. *J Hypertens*; 12(4):463-468. 1994a

Simons LA, Balasubramaniam S, von Konigsmark M et al., On the effect of Garlic on plasma lipids and lipoproteins in mild hypercholesterolemia. *Atherosclerosis* Mar;113(2):219-225. 1995

Smeets K, Van Damme EJM, Van Leuven F et al. Isolation and characterization of lectins and lectin-alliinase complexes from bulbs of Garlic (*Allium sativum*) and ramsons (*Allium ursinum*). *Glycoconjugate J*; 14(3):331-343. 1997

Sobenin IA, Prianishnikov VV, Kunnova LM, et al. Reduction of cardiovascular risk in primary prophylaxy of coronary heart disease. *Klin Med*; 83(4): 52-55. 2005.

Srivastava KC & Tyagi OD. Effects of a Garlic-derived principle (ajoene) on aggregation and arachidonic acid metabolism in human blood platelets. *Prostaglandins Leukot Essent Fatty Acids*; 49(2):587-595. 1993

Steiner M, Khan AH, Holbert D et al. A double-blind crossover study in moderately hypercholesterolemic men that compared the effect of aged Garlic extract and placebo administration on blood lipids. *Am J Clin Nutr*; 64(6):866-870. 1996

Steiner M & Li W. Aged Garlic extract, a modulator of cardiovascular risk factors: a dose-finding study on the effects of AGE on platelet functions. *J Nutr*; 131(3s):980S-984S. 2001

Stevinson C, Pittler MH & Ernst E. Garlic for treating hypercholesterolemia. A meta-analysis of randomized clinical trials. *Ann Intern Med*; 133(6):420-429. 2000

Sunter W. Warfarin and Garlic. *Pharm J*; 246:722. 1991

Superko HR & Krauss RM: Garlic powder, effect on plasma lipids, postprandial lipemia, low-density lipoprotein particle size, high-density lipoprotein subclass distribution and lipoprotein(a). *J Am Coll Cardiol*; 35(2):321-326. 2000

Tanaka S, Haruma K, Yoshihara M, et al. Aged Garlic Extrat has potential suppressive effect on colorectal adenomas in humans. *J Nutr*; 136: 821S-826S. 2006.

Tchernychev B, Rabinkov A, Mirelman D et al. Natural antibodies to dietary proteins: the existence of natural antibodies to alliinase (*Alliin lyase*) and mannose-specific lectin from Garlic (*Allium sativum*) in human serum. *Immunol Lett*; 47(1-2):53-57. 1995

Walper A et al., Effizienz einer Diätempfehlung und einer zusätzlichen Phytotherapie mit Allium sativum bei leichter bis mäßiger Hypercholesterinämie. *Medwelt* 45(7/8):327. 1994

Weber ND, Andersen DO, North JA et al. In vitro virucidal effects of *Allium sativum* (Garlic) extract and compounds. *Planta Med*; 58(5):417-423. 1992

Weiss N, et al. Aged Garlic Extract improves homocysteine-induced endothelial dysfunction in macro- and microcirculation. *J Nutr;* 136: 750S-754S. 2006.

Wenkert E et al., *Experientia* 28:377. 1971

Whitaker JR, *Adv Food Res* 22:73. 1976

Wichtl M, Pflanzliche Pille für die ewige Jugend. *DAZ* 131(17):837. 1991

Wolf S, Reim M & Jung F. Effect of Garlic on conjunctival vessels: a randomised, placebo-controlled, double-blind trial. *Br J Clin Pract Symp Suppl*; 69(Aug):36-39. 1990

Zhang XH, Lowe D, Giles P et al. A randomized trial of the effects of Garlic oil upon coronary heart disease risk factors in trained male runners. *Blood Coagul Fibrinolysis*; 11(8):67-74. 2000

Zhang XH, Lowe D, Giles P et al. Gender may affect the action of Garlic oil on plasma cholesterol and glucose levels of normal subjects. *J Nutr*; 131(5):1471-1478. 2001

Ziaei S, Hantoshzadeh S, Rezasoltani P et al. The effect of Garlic tablet on plasma lipids and platelet aggregation in nulliparous pregnants at high risk of preeclampsia. *Eur J Obstet Gynecol Reprod Biol*; 99(2):201-206. 2001

Ziyyat A, Legssyer A, Mekhfi H et al. Phytotherapy of hypertension and diabetes in oriental Morocco. *J Ethnopharmacol*; 58(1):45-54. 1997

Gaultheria procumbens

See Wintergreen

Gelidium amansii

See Agar

Gelsemium sempervirens

See Yellow Jessamine

Genista tinctoria

See Dyer's Broom

Gentiana lutea

See Yellow Gentian

Geranium maculatum

See Cranesbill

Geranium robertianum

See Herb Robert

German Chamomile

Matricaria Recutita

DESCRIPTION

Medicinal Parts: The medicinal parts consist of the entire flowering herb or only the flowers.

Flower and Fruit: The flower heads are terminal and long-pedicled. The flower is white with a yellow center. The margin flowers are obtuse with a tunicate margin. The ray florets are white, linguiform, female, and have 3 teeth. The disc florets are tubular and androgynous, have 5 teeth and a hollow receptacle.

Leaves, Stem, and Root: The plant is a 20 to 40 cm high herb with an erect, glabrous stem, which is branched above. The leaves are 2 to 3 pinnatisect and have a narrow thorny tip.

Characteristic: The receptacle of the compound head of German Chamomile is hollow which distinguishes it from other types of Chamomile.

Habitat: German Chamomile is indigenous to Europe and northwest Asia, naturalized in North America and elsewhere.

Production: German Chamomile consists of the fresh or dried flower heads of *Matricaria recutita* and their preparations.

Other Names: Chamomilla, Chamomile, Hungarian Chamomile, Pin Heads, Single Chamomile

ACTIONS AND PHARMACOLOGY

COMPOUNDS

Volatile oil (0.4-1.5%): chief components (-)-alpha-bisabolol (levomenol), bisabolol oxide A, bisabolol oxide B, bisabolone oxide A, beta-trans-farnesene, trans-en-yne-dicycloether (polyyne spiroether, adjoining cis-en-yn-dicycloether), chamazulene (blue in color, arising from the non-volatile proazulene matricin after steam distillation), spathulenol

Flavonoids: flavone glycosides; aglycones apigenin, luteolin, chrysoeriol, chief glycosides apigenin-7-O-glucoside, apigenin glucoside acetate, - flavonol glycosides, aglycones including quercetin, isorhamnetin, patuletin, for example rutin, hyperoside

Unbound, Highly Methoxylized Flavonoids: jaceidinem chrysospenol, chrysosplenetin

Hydroxycoumarins: including umbelliferone, herniarin

Mucilages: (10% in the mucilage ribs, fructans) including rhamanogalacturonane

EFFECTS

Chamomile has shown wound-healing, antidiarrheal, sedative, and anti-inflammatory properties. Ethanolic extract of *Chamomile matricaria* reduced the symptoms of hemorrhagic cystitis as compared to patients treated with co-trimoxazol (trimethoprim/sulfamethoxazole). Patients receiving Chamomile mouthwash experienced decreased stomatitis.

Anti-Inflammatory Effects: Chamazulene exerts anti-inflammatory effects through inhibition of leukotriene B4 formation (Safayhi, 1994). The en-yne dicycloether inhibits degranulation of mast cells to prevent histamine release (Miller, 1996). Apigenin, a flavonoid, effectively blocks intercellular adhesion molecule-1 upregulation and leukocyte adhesion in response to cytokines. This activity is through a mechanism unrelated to free radical scavenging or leukocyte formation (Panes, 1996).

Anti-Infective Effects: Antibacterial and antiviral effects have been seen in vitro (Rucker et al, 1989; Vilagines et al, 1985; Suganda et al, 1983). Symptoms of hemorrhagic cystitis were improved by Chamomile in another study (Barsom et al, 1993).

Antioxidant Effects: Chamazulene, an extract from *Matricaria chamomilla* and a volatile oil, may have potential antioxidant effects. Chamazulene exerts antioxidant effects through inhibition of lipid peroxidation (Rekka, 1996). Chamazulene also blocks chemical peroxidation of arachidonic acid for antioxidant and anti-inflammatory effects (Safayhi, 1994).

Antineoplastic Effects: Apigenin applied topically has effects on skin tumorigenesis through inhibition of skin papillomas and a tendency to decrease the conversion of papillomas to carcinomas (Li, 1996; Wei, 1990). Apigenin inhibits UV-induced tumorigenesis when applied topically via G2/M and G1 cell-cycle arrest in keratinocytes (Lepley, 1996; Lepley, 1997). The chemoprevention mechanisms occur through inhibition of the mitotic kinase activity, perturbation of cyclin B1 levels, and inhibition of protein kinase C (Lepley, 1996; Lin, 1997). Apigenin suppresses transcriptional activation of cyclooxygenase-2 and inducible nitric oxide synthase in macrophages, which is important for the prevention of carcinogenesis and inflammation (Liang, 1999).

Anxiolytic Effects: Flavonoids are CNS-active molecules and the chemical modification of the flavone nucleus dramatically increases the anxiolytic potency (Paladini, 1999). Apigenin and luteolin are ligands for the central benzodiazepine receptors exerting anxiolytic and slight sedative effects (Viola, 1995).

Dermatological Effects: Chamomile has anti-inflammatory and wound-healing activity associated with both the essential oil and the hydrophilic extract. One double-blind study showed that Chamomile extract decreased the area of wounds significantly when compared to placebo (Glowania et al, 1987). A Chamomile-containing cream was an effective treatment for patients with inflammatory dermatoses of the hands, forearms, and lower legs (Aertgeerts et al, 1985).

Gastrointestinal Effects: The proteolytic activity of pepsin is reduced by (-)-alpha-bisabolol in the gastrointestinal tract (Isaac, 1975). The (-)-alpha-bisabolol exerts a protective effect from gastric toxicity produced by acetylsalicylic acid (Torrado, 1995).

Sedative Effects: German Chamomile's effect on the nervous system is that of an anticonvulsive and sedative. Chamomile acts as anxiolytic and calms conditions due to anxiety (Duke, 1997; Weiner & Weiner, 1994). Sedative effects may be due to the glycosides luteolin and epigenin which aid relaxation and to the antispasmodic effects of the flavonoid content of the plant (Brinker, 1995). Inhalation of Chamomile essential oil can improve mood; the species of Chamomile is thought to be the Roman variety (*Chamaemelun nobile*).

Miscellaneous Effects Apigenin has been associated with an increase in atrial rate as a result of a reduction in noradrenaline uptake and a reduction in monoamine oxidase activity (Lorenzo, 1996). The herb exerts antibacterial and drying effects on weeping wound areas, which increase healing (Glowania, 1987). Chamomile oil has antimicrobial activity against some skin pathogens such as *Staphylococcus* and *Candida* species (Aggag, 1972).

CLINICAL TRIALS

Cancer Therapy, Adjunct to

A Phase III, double-blind, placebo-controlled trial evaluated Chamomile mouthwash for prevention of 5-fluorouracil(5-FU) chemotherapy-induced oral mucositis. There were 164 patients included in the study at the time of their first cycle of 5-FU based chemotherapy. All patients received oral cryotherapy for 30 minutes with each dose of 5-FU. Chamomile mouthwash was administered 3 times daily for 14 days in the treatment group. Stomatitis scores determined by healthcare providers and patients suggested no difference of stomatitis between the Chamomile and placebo-treatment group (Fidler et al, 1996).

Used as aromatherapy, the quality of life was improved for advanced cancer patients who were massaged using essential oil of Chamomile. Fifty-one patients with advanced cancer were randomized to receive a full-body massage with 1% Roman Chamomile essential oil in a carrier oil or massage with the carrier oil alone. Patients were evaluated using 4 questionnaires designed to evaluate quality of life before and after a series of 3 full body massages. Although both groups showed improvement in the top 10 symptoms, this was only statistically significant in the aromatherapy group. When the two groups were compared, several categories indicated Chamomile to be significantly better than oil. These included a decrease in severity of symptoms ($p<0.05$), quality of life ($p<0.01$), and anxiety ($p<0.05$). The aromatherapy patients also had an improvement in physical symptoms, while the massage alone group had a deterioration of physical symptoms (Wilkinson, 1995).

No significant difference in skin-radiation protection was found in a controlled study of 48 patients with breast cancer that compared topical administration of Chamomile and almond oil (Maiche et al, 1991).

Diarrhea

A randomized, placebo-controlled, double-blind study (DIALOG II) assessed the clinical efficacy and tolerability of an apple pectin-chamomile extract (Diarrhoesan) in treating acute diarrhea. A total of 255 children were enrolled. The apple pectin-chamomile extract showed beneficial effects in shortening the course of the disease and relieving associated symptoms. The treatment was well tolerated, with an incidence of adverse effects similar to placebo (Becker et al, 2006).

A pectin/Chamomile preparation decreased the duration of diarrhea when compared to placebo in a double-blind, randomized, multicenter study of 79 children from the ages of 6 months to 5.5 years of age with acute, noncomplicated diarrhea. Patients randomly received both an apple pectin and Chamomile extract (Diarrhoesan®) or placebo for 3 days. At the end of treatment, the diarrhea had ended in significantly ($p<0.05$) more children in the Chamomile group than in the control group (de la Motte et al, 1997).

Eczema

The efficacy of Kamillosan cream (topical Chamomile cream) was compared to steroidal (0.25% hydrocortisone, 0.75% fluocortin butyl ester) and nonsteroidal (5% bufexamac) deramatologic agents for the maintenance therapy of eczematous disease. There were 161 patients suffering from inflammatory dermatoses on hands, forearms, and lower legs included in the study. The patients had initially been treated with 0.1% difluocortolone valerate. The Kamillosan cream was slightly less effective than 0.25% hydrocortisone and superior to 5% bufexamac and 0.75% fluocortin butyl ester (Aertgeerts, 1985).

Hemorrhagic cystitis

Chamomile extract decreased the symptoms of hemorrhagic cystitis in 32 patients randomized to receive either the antibiotic cotrimoxazole (trimethoprim/sulfamethoxazole) alone or with a Chamomile extract administered on day 1 as a bladder instillation, followed by daily hipbath use. Symptoms were evaluated after 10 days and indicated that the Chamomile group experienced more rapid alleviation of symptoms than the group treated with only cotrimoxazole. The product used was Kamillenextrakt, an ethanolic extract of Matricaria flowers (Barsom et al, 1993).

Oral mucositis

A case study of a 76-year-old woman who mistakenly overdosed with methotrexate (MTX) for treatment of her rheumatoid arthritis and developed oral mucositis as a result was successfully treated with Wild Chamomile mouthwashes, highlighting the potential of the herb's mucosa-protective qualities (likely due to anti-inflammatory, antibacterial, and antifungal properties), for prophylaxis or management of this common MTX-associated complication. The authors note that Chamomile is not only readily available but inexpensive, and generally associated with mild side effects (Mazokopakis et al, 2005).

INDICATIONS AND USAGE

Approved by Commission E:

- Cough/bronchitis
- Fevers and colds
- Inflammation of the skin
- Inflammation of the mouth and pharynx
- Tendency to infection
- Wounds and burns

Chamomile is used internally for inflammatory diseases of the gastrointestinal tract associated with gastrointestinal spasms, irritation of the oral pharyngeal mucous membrane and upper respiratory tract. Externally, the drug is used for skin and mucous membrane inflammations, bacterial skin ailments, pulpitis, gingivitis, respiratory catarrh, and anogenital inflammation.

Unproven Uses: In Folk medicine, the herb is used internally for diarrhea and flatulence. The herb is used externally for furuncles, hemorrhoids, abscesses, and acne.

Homeopathic Uses: The herb is used for inflammation and cramps in the gastrointestinal tract, teething symptoms, severe pain, inflammation of the upper respiratory tract, and dysmenorrhea.

CONTRAINDICATIONS

Chamomile should not be taken by anyone with a known allergy to its components or to other members of the Compositae family (e.g., arnica, yarrow, feverfew, tansy, artemesia), or if they have a history of atopic hay fever or asthma.

Pregnancy: Not to be used during pregnancy.

PRECAUTIONS AND ADVERSE REACTIONS

Allergic reactions to Chamomile include emesis in high doses, allergic conjunctivitis, contact dermatitis, and eczema (one case of anaphylactic reaction has been reported).

Allergic Conjunctivitis: Chamomile tea eye washing to treat ocular reactions has induced allergic conjunctivitis with lid angioedema (Subiza et al, 1990).

Anaphylactic Reactions: Ingestion of Chamomile-tea infusion has precipitated an anaphylactic reaction in an 8-year-old male with hay fever and bronchial asthma caused by a variety of pollens (Subiza et al, 1989). A 35-year-old woman in labor was given an enema containing glycerol and Kamillosan, an oily extract of Chamomile flowers. Ten minutes later, the woman developed nausea, urticaria, larynx edema, tachycardia, and hypotension. She required emergency treatment and an emergency cesarean section. The newborn was severely asphyxiated and died the following day; the woman developed paralytic ileus and septic fever postoperatively (Jensen-Jarolim et al, 1998).

Dermatologic: Chamomile, a Compositae plant, is associated with allergic contact dermatitis. Some cases are thought to occur because of contamination of Chamomile flowers with other more allergenic plants (Harris & Lewis, 1994a; Harris & Lewis, 1994b). Acute episodes of eczema following ingestion of Chamomile tea, or application of Chamomile compresses or topical Chamomile preparations, have been reported (Rycroft, 2003; Pereira et al, 1997; McGeorge & Steele, 1991).

DRUG INTERACTIONS

MODERATE RISK:

Anticoagulants: Coumarins present in chamomile may potentiate the effect of anticoagulants and may result in increased risk of bleeding. *Clinical Management:* Caution is advised if used concomitantly. Monitor the patient for signs and symptoms of excessive bleeding.

POTENTIAL INTERACTIONS:

Alcohol/Benzodiazepines: May cause additive effects of alcohol and benzodiazepines. *Clinical Management*: Avoid concomitant use.

OVERDOSAGE

High doses of Roman Chamomile can cause emesis in humans (Bradley, 1992).

DOSAGE

Mode of Administration: Liquid and solid preparations are available for external and internal application.

How Supplied:

Capsule — 125 mg, 345 mg, 350 mg, 354 mg, 360 mg

Liquid — 1:4

Oil — 100%

Tea

Preparation: An infusion for internal use is prepared by pouring boiling water (150 mL) over 3 g of Chamomile, cover for 5 to 10 minutes and strain. (1 teaspoonful = 1 g drug).

An infusion for external poultice application is prepared by pouring 1 1/2 cups of hot water over 2 dessertspoons of the drug, cover, leave to steep for 15 minutes and then strain. Ointments and gels are available in strengths of 3 to 10%.

Daily Dosage: An internal single dose is approximately 3 g as an infusion. Liquid extract 1 to 4 mL or 1 cup of freshly made tea is administered 3 to 4 times daily. Externally as a bath additive, 50 g is added to 1 Liter of water or 6 g of drug for a steam bath. Washes and gargles may be administered several times a day.

Homeopathic Dosage: Internally, the herb is given as 5 to 10 drops, 1 tablet, or 5-10 globules. Externally, dilute 1 dessertspoon with 250 mL water and use 2 to 3 times daily in poultices or washes (HAB1).

LITERATURE

Abebe W. Herbal medication: potential for adverse interactions with analgesic drugs. *J Clin Pharm Ther*; 27:391-401. 2002.

Achterrath-Tuckerman U et al., *Planta Med* 39(1):38. 1980.

Aertgeerts P, Albring M, Klaschka F, Nasemann T, Patzelt-Wenczler R, Rauhut K, Weigl B, Vergleichende Prüfung von Kamillosan(Creme gegenüber steroidalen (0,25 % Hydrocortison, 0,75 % Bluocortinbutylester) und nichtsteroidalen (5 % Bufexamac) Externa in der Erhaltungstherapie von Ekzemerkrankungen. *Z Hautkr* 60:270-277. 1985.

Aggag M, Yousef R. Study of antimicrobial activity of Chamomile oil. *Planta Med* Sep;22(2):140-4. 1972.

Albring M, Albrecht H, Alcorn G, Lücker PW, The measuring of the anti-inflammatory effect of a compound of the skin of volunteers. *Meth Find Exp Clin Pharmacol* 5:75-77. 1983.

Ammon HPT, Kaul R, Pharmakologie der Kamille und ihrer Inhaltsstoffe. Dtsch Apoth Z 132(Suppl 27):3-26. 1992.

Barsom VS, Moosmayr A & Sakka M. Behandlung der hamorrhagischen cystitis (harnblasenschleimhautblutungen) mit kamillenextrakt. *Erfahrungsheilkunde*; 3:138-139. 1993.

Bartle WR & Blakely JA. Potentiation of warfarin anticoagulation by acetaminophen. *JAMA*. Mar 13;265(10):1260. 1991.

Becker B, Kuhn U, Hardewig-Budny B. Double-blind, randomized evaluation of clinical efficacy and tolerability of an apple pectin-chamomile extract in children with unspecific diarrhea. *Arzneimittelforschung*; 56(6): 387-393. 2006.

Budzinski JW, Foster BC, Vandenhoek S et al. An in vitro evaluation of human cytochrome P450 3A4 inhibition by selected commercial herbal extracts and tinctures. *Phytomedicine*; 7(4):273-282. 2000.

de la Motte S, Bose-O'Reilly S, Heinisch M et al. Double-blind comparison of an apple pectin-Chamomile extract preparation with placebo in children with diarrhea. *Arzneimittelforschung*; 47(11):1247-1249. 1997.

Dorsch W, Neues über antientzündliche Drogen. In: *ZPT* 14(1):26. 1993.

Ernst E. Possible interactions between synthetic and herbal medicinial products. Part I: a systematic review of the evidence. *Perfusion*; 13:4-15. 2000.

Fidler R, Loprinzi C, O'Fallon J et al. Prospective evaluation of a Chamomile mouthwash for prevention of 5-FU-induced oral mucositis. *Cancer* Feb 1;77(3):522-5. 1996.

Füller E et al., Anti-inflammatory activity of *Chamomilla* polysaccharides. In: *PM* 59(7):A666. 1993.

Füller E, Franz G, Neues von den Kamillenpolysacchariden. In: *DAZ* 133(45):4224. 1993.

Gasic O et al., *Fitoterapia* 2:51. 1983.

Glowania HJ; Raulin C; Swoboda M. Effect of Chamomile on wound healing–a controlled clinical-experimental double-blind trial (German). *Z Hautkr* Sep 1;62(17):1262-1271. 1987.

Habersang S, *Planta Med* 37(2):115. 1979.

Harris B & Lewis R. Chamomile - Part 1. *Int J Altern Complement Med*; p12. 1994a.

Harris B & Lewis R. Chamomile - Part 2. *Int J Altern Complement Med*; p14. 1994b.

Hausen HM, Busker E, Carle R, Über das Sensibilierungsvermögen von Compositenarten. VII. Experimentelle Untersuchungen mit Auszügen und Inhaltsstoffen von *Chamomilla recutita L. Rauschert* und *Anthemis cotula L. Planta Med* 50:229-234. 1984.

Heck AM, DeWitt BA, Lukes AL. Potential interactions between alternative therapies and warfarin. *Am J Health Syst Pharm*; 57(13):1221-1227. 2000.

Heilmann J, Kamillenflavonoide. Nur Aglyka dringen in die Haut ein. In: *DAZ* 133(37):3296. 1993.

Hylek EM, Heiman H, Skates SJ et al. Acetaminophen and other risk factors for excessive warfarin anticoagulation. *JAMA*. Mar 4;279(9):657-62. 1998.

Isaac D, Die Kamillentherapie - Erfolg und Bestätigung. *Dtsch Apoth Ztg* 120:567-570. 1980.

Isaac O, *Planta Med* 35(2):3, 118. 1979.

Isaac O; Thiemer K. Biochemical studies on camomile components/III. In vitro studies about the antipeptic activity of (-)-alpha-bisabolol. *Arzneimittelforschung* Sep;25(9):1352-4. 1975.

Jakovlev V et al., *Planta Med* 35(2):3. 1979.

Jakovlev V et al., *Planta Med* 49(2):67. 1983.

Jakovlev V, Isaac O, Flaskamp E, Pharmakologische Untersuchungen von Kamillen-Inhaltsstoffen. VI. Untersuchungen zur antiphlogistischen Wirkung von Chamazulen und Matricin. *Planta Med* 49:67-73. 1983.

Jakovlev V, Isaac O, Flaskamp E, Pharmakologische Untersuchungen von Kamilleninhaltsstoffen VI. Untersuchungen zur antiphlogistischen Wirkung von Chamazulen und Matricin. In: *PM* 49:67. 1983.

Jensen-Jarolim E, Redier N, Fritsch R et al. Fatal outcome of anaphylaxis to camomile-containing enema during labor: a case study. *J Allergy Clin Immunol*; 102(6):1041-1042. 1998.

Jenss H, Zur Problematik funktioneller Magen-Darm-Krankheiten am Beispiel des Colon irritabile. In: Oepen I (Hrsg) An den Grenzen der Schulmedizin, eine Analyse umstrittener Methoden. *Deutscher Ärzte-Verlag Köln*, S 197-212. 1985.

Lepley DM; Pelling JC. Induction of p21/WAF1 and G1 cell-cycle arrest by the chemopreventive agent apigenin. *Mol Carcinog* Jun;19(2):74-82. 1997.

Lepley DM; Li B; Birt DF; Pelling JC. The chemopreventive flavonoid apigenin induces G2/M arrest in keratinocytes. *Carcinogenesis* Nov;17(11):2367-75. 1996.

Li B; Pinch H; Birt DF. Influence of vehicle, distant topical delivery, and biotransformation on the chemopreventive activity of apigenin, a plant flavonoid, in mouse skin. *Pharm Res* Oct;13(10):1530-4. 1996.

Liang YC; Huang YT; Tsai SH et al. Suppression of inducible cyclooxygenase and inducible nitric oxide synthase by apigenin and related flavonoids in mouse macrophages. *Carcinogenesis* Oct;20(10):1945-52. 1999.

Lin JK; Chen YC; Huang YT; Lin-Shiau SY. Suppression of protein kinase C and nuclear oncogene expression as possible molecular mechanisms of cancer chemoprevention by apigenin and curcumin. *J Cell Biochem* Suppl;28-29:39-48. 1997.

Lorenzo PS; Rubio MC; Medina JH; Adler-Graschinsky E. Involvement of monoamine oxidase and noradrenaline uptake in the positive chronotropic effects of apigenin in rat atria. *Eur J Pharmacol* Sep 26;312(2):203-7. 1996.

Maiche AG, Gröhn P, Mäki-Hokkonen H, Effect of Chamomile cream and almond ointment on acute radiation skin reaction. *Acta Oncol* 30(3):395-396. 1991.

Maliakal PP & Wanwimolruk S. Effect of herbal teas on hepatic drug metabolizing enzymes in rats. *J Pharm Pharmacol*; 53(10):1323-1329. 2001.

Mazokopakis E, Vrentzos GE, Papadakis JA, et al. Wild chamomile (Matricaria recutita L.) mouthwashes in methotrexate-induced oral mucositis. *Phytomedicine* 12(1-2): 25, 27. 2005.

McGeorge BCL & Steele MC. Allergic contact dermatitis of the nipple from Roman Chamomile ointment. *Contact Dermatitis*; 24:139-140. 1991.

Miller Th, Wittstock U, Lindequist U, Teuscher E, Effects of some components of the essential oil of Chamomile, *Chamomilla recutita*, on histamine release from mast cells. *Planta Med* Feb;62(1):60-61. 1996.

Nissen HP, Blitz H, Kreysel HW, Profilometrie, eine Methode zur Beurteilung der therapeutischen Wirksamkeit von Kamillosan-Salbe. *Z Hautkr* 63:184-190. 1988.

Norred CL & Brinker F. Potential coagulation effects of preoperative complementary and alternative medicines. *Alt Ther*; 7(6):58-67. 2001.

Paladini AC; Marder M; Viola H et al. Flavonoids and the central nervous system: from forgotten factors to potent anxiolytic compounds. *J Pharm Pharmacol* May;51(5): 519-2. 1999.

Panes J; Gerritsen ME; Anderson DC et al. Apigenin inhibits tumor necrosis factor-induced intercellular adhesion molecule-1 upregulation in vivo. *Microcirculation* Sep;3(3):279-86. 1996.

Pereira F; Santos R; Pereira A. Contact dermatitis from Chamomile tea. *Contact Dermatitis* Jun;36(6):307. 1997.

Rekka EA; Kourounakis AP; Kourounakis PN. Investigation of the effect of chamazulene on lipid peroxidation and free radical processes. *Res Commun Mol Pathol Pharmacol* Jun;92(3):361-4. 1996.

Redaelli C et al., *J Chrom*. 209:110. 1981.

Redaelli C et al., *Plant Med* 42:288. 1981.

Rodriguez-Serna M; Sanchez-Motilla JM; Ramon R; Aliaga A. Allergic and systemic contact dermatitis from Matricaria chamomilla tea. *Contact Dermatitis* Oct;39(4):192-3. 1998.

Rucker G, Mayer R & Lee KR. Peroxides as plant constituents: 6 Hydroperoxides from the blossoms of Roman Chamomile, *Anthemis nobilis* L (German). *Arch Pharm* (Weinheim); 322(11):821-826. 1989.

Rycroft RJ. Recurrent facial dermatitis from Chamomile tea. *Contact Dermatitis*. Apr;48(4):229. 2003.

Safayhi H et al., Chamazulene. an antioxidant-type inhibitor of leukotriene B4 formation. In: *PM* 60(5):410. 1994.

Segal R, Pilote L. Warfarin interaction with Matricaria chamomilla. *CMAJ*. 174:1281-2. 2006.

Schilcher H, (1987) Die Kamille. Handbuch für Ärzte, Apotheker und andere Naturwissenschaftler. Wissenschaftliche Verlagsgesellschaft, Stuttgart Ammon HPT, Sabieraj J, Kaul R, Kamille - Mechanismus der antiphlogistischen Wirkung von Kamillenextrakten und -inhaltsstoffen. In: *DAZ* 136(22):1821-1834. 1996.

Sorkin B, Untersuchungen zur Wirksamkeit von Kamille am Menschen. In: Seifen, Öle, Fette, Wachse 108(1):9-10. 1982.

Subiza J; Subiza JL; Hinojosa M et al. Anaphylactic reaction after the ingestion of Chamomile tea: a study of cross-reactivity with other composite pollens. *J Allergy Clin Immunol* Sep;84(3):353-8. 1989.

Subiza J, Subiza JL, Alonso M et al. Allergic conjunctivitis to Chamomile tea. *Ann Allergy* Aug;65(2):127-32. 1990.

Suganda AG, Amoros M, Girre L et al. Inhibitory effects of some crude and semi-purified extracts of indigenous French plants on the multiplication of human herpes virus 1 and poliovirus 2 in cell culture. *J Nat Prod*; 46(5):626-632. 1983.

Szelenyi I et al., *Planta Med* 35(3):218. 1979.

Torrado S; Torrado S; Agis A et al. Effect of dissolution profile and (-)-alpha-bisabolol on the gastrotoxicity of acetylsalicylic acid. *Pharmazie* Feb;50(2):141-3. 1995.

Vilagines P, Delaveau P & Vilagines R. Inhibition of poliovirus replication by an extract of *Matricaria chamomilla. C R Acad Sci III*; 301(6):289-294. 1985.

Viola H; Wasowski C; Levi de Stein M et al. Apigenin, a component of *Matricaria recutita* flowers, is a central benzodiazepine receptors-ligand with anxiolytic effects. *Planta Med* Jun;61(3):213-6. 1995.

Wei H, Tye L, Bresnick E, Birt D. Inhibitory effect of apigenin, a plant flavonoid, on epidermal ornithine decarboxylase and skin tumor promotion in mice. *Cancer Res* Feb 1;50(3):499-502. 1990.

German Ipecac

Cynanchum vincetoxicum

DESCRIPTION

Medicinal Parts: The medicinal parts of the plant are the leaves or rhizome with the attached roots.

Flower and Fruit: The plant has small white flowers in peduncled cymes, 5 sepals, and a wheel-shaped corolla. There is a 5-lobed secondary corolla. There are 5 stamens whose anthers are fused to a 5-sectioned wreath. The two superior ovaries have a common stigma. The 5-cm long fruit is a glabrous, striped, clavate follicle. The seeds have silky tufts of hair.

Leaves, Stem and Root: The plant grows from 30 to 100 cm. The underground creeping rhizome has heavily branched runners. The stem is unbranched, thin, and erect. The leaves are opposite, short petioled, ovate to oblong and entire-margined.

Characteristics: The fresh rhizome has an intensive odor. The taste is sweet, then bitter-hot. It is poisonous.

Habitat: The plant is indigenous to Europe.

Production: German Ipecac herb and rhizome are the leaves and rhizome (including attached roots) of *Cynanchum vincetoxicum.* The subterranean rhizome, including parts of the roots, are dug up in autumn, cleaned and quickly dried at temperatures of up to 50° C.

ACTIONS AND PHARMACOLOGY

COMPOUNDS

Saponin-like 15-oxasteroide glycosides (mixture termed vincetoxin): aglycones including hirundigenin, anhydrohirundigenin, vincetogenin

Isoquinoline alkaloids: including tylophorine

EFFECTS

The drug has diuretic, diaphoretic, digestive, and emmenagogic effects. The alkaloids have an antitumoral effect, and the chloroform extract has an antimicrobial effect.

INDICATIONS AND USAGE

Unproven Uses: The drug was formerly used as a diuretic, diaphoretic, and emetic, and for the treatment of kidney complaints, edema, the plague, snake bites, and dysmenorrhea. Today, it is used in the treatment of digestive and kidney disorders and for dysmenorrhea. The poultices heal swellings and bruising. The drug can also be found in homeopathic preparations.

PRECAUTIONS AND ADVERSE REACTIONS

According to older scientific literature, ''vincetoxin'' in high dosages causes vomiting, apnea and cardiac paralysis in animal experiments. Seed extracts led to advancing paralysis of the central nervous system. Poisonings of humans have not been found in recent reports.

DOSAGE

Mode of Administration: As an infusion, powdered drug, alcoholic extract, and homeopathic dilution.

Preparation: The drug is prepared as an infusion.

Daily Dosage: The infusion should be administered under medical supervision.

LITERATURE

Frohne D, Pfänder HJ, Giftpflanzen - Ein Handbuch für Apotheker, Toxikologen und Biologen, 4. Aufl., Wiss. Verlagsges. mbH Stuttgart 1997.

Hänsel R, Keller K, Rimpler H, Schneider G (Hrsg.), Hagers Handbuch der Pharmazeutischen Praxis, 5. Aufl., Bde 4-6 (Drogen), Springer Verlag Berlin, Heidelberg, New York, 1992-1994.

Lavault M, Richomme P, Bruneton J. New phenatroindolizidine N-oxides alkaloids isolated from Vincetoxicum hirudinaria Medic. *Pharm Acta Helv.* 68; 225-227 1994

Lewin L, Gifte und Vergiftungen, 6. Aufl., Nachdruck, Haug Verlag, Heidelberg 1992.

Roth L, Daunderer M, Kormann K, Giftpflanzen, Pflanzengifte, 4. Aufl., Ecomed Fachverlag Landsberg Lech 1993.

Steinegger E, Hänsel R, Pharmakognosie, 5. Aufl., Springer Verlag Heidelberg 1992.

Teuscher E, Lindequist U, Biogene Gifte - Biologie, Chemie, Pharmakologie, 2. Aufl., Fischer Verlag Stuttgart 1994.

German Sarsaparilla

Carex arenaria

DESCRIPTION

Medicinal Parts: The medicinal part is the dried rhizome.

Flower and Fruit: The inflorescence is somewhat hanging and consists of 6 to 16 ovoid, 1-cm long, terminal, straight, greenish spikes. The lower ones are female; the middle ones are female at the base and male at the tip. The upper ones are only male. These are simple greenish unisexual flowers without a corolla. They have 1 husk with an ovary surrounded by a tubular involucre. The style has 2 stigmas, 3 stamens, and a fruit oval. It is somewhat acute at both ends, and the tube has a winged edge. The flowers form many blossomed spikelets, which in turn form a terminal, oblong ear. The middle spikelets contain male flowers at the tip and female flowers at the base. The upper spikelets are male.

Leaves, Stem and Root: German Sarsaparilla is 15 to 45 cm high with a 2 to 5 mm thick, horizontally creeping rhizome that produces extremely long runners. The plant has black-brown basal leaves, which break up into long fibers. The stem is sturdy, upright, and about 1 mm thick. It is sharply triangular, rough above, and surrounded by brown leaf sheaths at the base. The leaves are linear and usually grooved. The lamina are rigid and gradually taper forward to the involute tip. The roots form such a thick mass that they prevent water from getting in and thus prevent the washing away of dykes and dams.

Characteristics: The rootstock has an aromatic turpentine odor.

Habitat: The plant grows in Europe mainly on the Atlantic, Baltic, and southern Scandinavian coasts as far as central Germany. It was introduced to the American Atlantic coast.

Production: German Sarsaparilla consists of the dried, underground parts of *Carex arenaria*. The root is dug up in March and April, dried, and cut into pieces for sale.

Not to be Confused With: Other Carex varieties

Other Names: Red Sedge, Sand Sedge, Red Couchgrass, Sea Sedge

ACTIONS AND PHARMACOLOGY

COMPOUNDS

Saponins

Volatile oil: contents include methyl salicylate and cineol

Flavonoids: including tricine

Tannin: (8 to 10%, catechin tannins)

EFFECTS

There are no studies available on efficacy. The main constituents, saponins, essential oil and flavones, as well as the tannins, are most likely responsible for the effect.

INDICATIONS AND USAGE

Unproven Uses: In folk medicine, preparations of German Sarsaparilla are used for the prevention of gout, rheumatism, inflammation of the joints, for skin ailments, and as a diaphoretic and diuretic; further, for venereal disease, flatulence, colic, liver disorders, diabetes, edema, lung tuberculosis, and amenorrhea.

PRECAUTIONS AND ADVERSE REACTIONS

No health hazards or side effects are known in conjunction with the proper administration of designated therapeutic dosages.

DOSAGE

Mode of Administration: Since the efficacy for the claimed uses are not documented, a therapeutic application cannot be recommended. The cold maceration and the decoction are used in folk medicine.

Preparation: A decoction is prepared by adding 3 g drug to 1 cup water. A cold maceration is made by adding 2 teaspoonfuls drug to 1/4 liter water.

Daily Dosage: The average daily dose is 3 g drug as a decoction. The cold maceration is dosed 1 cup, 2 to 3 times daily.

LITERATURE

Hänsel R, Keller K, Rimpler H, Schneider G (Hrsg.), Hagers Handbuch der Pharmazeutischen Praxis, 5. Aufl., Bde 4-6 (Drogen), Springer Verlag Berlin, Heidelberg, New York, 1992-1994.

Madaus G, Lehrbuch der Biologischen Arzneimittel, Bde 1-3, Nachdruck, Georg Olms Verlag Hildesheim 1979.

Germander

Teucrium chamaedrys

DESCRIPTION

Medicinal Parts: The medicinal part is the herb collected during the flowering season.

Flower and Fruit: The flowers are 10 to 12 mm long and erect. They are arranged on long pedicles in 1- to 6-blossomed false racemes inclined to one side. The calyx is tubular-campanulate, often tinged with red-violet, and is pubescent. The corolla is usually carmine red, occasionally white. The stamens and styles are exserted. The nutlet is ovoid, 1.5 to 2 cm long, smooth, finely reticulate and has a large, circular, attaching surface.

Leaves, Stem, and Root: The plant is a subshrub with a short-lived main root from which grow long-reaching, branched, thin woody roots and a stem-producing runner. The stems are usually erect and branched. The older branches are decumbent; the younger ones erect, tough, round, and lanate. The branches are occasionally covered in glandular hairs, which are often red-violet. The leaves are in close pairs and are always covered in teeth. They are summer-green and have distinctly protruding pinnatifid ribs.

Habitat: The plant is indigenous to the Mediterranean region as far as Anatolia and the Urals.

Production: Germander is the aerial part of *Teucrium chamaedrys.*

ACTIONS AND PHARMACOLOGY

COMPOUNDS

Volatile oil (0.07%): chief components beta-caryophyllene (20%), humulene (15%)

Iridoide monoterpenes: including among others, harpagide, acetyl harpagide

Diterpenes: including among others, teugin, teuflin, teuflidin, dihydroteugin, teucrin A, B, E, F, G, marrubiin

Caffeic acid derivatives: including among others, teucroside

Flavonoids: including among others, cirsiliol, cirsimaritin, luteolin

EFFECTS

The drug, which contains strong amaroids, is said to have a cholagogic effect, but this has not been scientifically proved. The toxic principle is therefore unknown. Higher doses or poisoning results in hepatitislike symptoms, which may include liver-cell necrosis.

INDICATIONS AND USAGE

Unproven Uses: Germander is used as a digestive aid, as a rinse for gout, as weight-loss aid, and for fever.

CONTRAINDICATIONS

The drug is highly toxic and should not be used (see PRECAUTIONS).

PRECAUTIONS AND ADVERSE REACTIONS

Liver-cell necrosis has been observed following intake of the drug. Symptoms include jaundice and an elevated level of aminotransferase in the blood. One case of death has been recorded. For that reason, the drug is not to be administered.

DOSAGE

Mode of Administration: Germander is occasionally used in tea mixtures (see PRECAUTIONS).

Daily Dosage: Dosages of more than 600 mg daily can cause toxic effects.

LITERATURE

Chialva F et al., *J High Res Chromatogr Chromatogr Commun* 5:182. 1982.

Rodriguez MC et al., PH 23:2960-2961. 1984.

Geum rivale

See Water Avens

Geum urbanum

See Bennet's Root

Giant Milkweed

Calotropis gigantea

DESCRIPTION

Medicinal Parts: The medicinal parts of the plant are the bark and roots.

Flower and Fruit: The flowers are arranged in umbels. The flower structures are arranged in fives. The corolla is fused and campanulate, 3 to 5 cm wide and split up to two-thirds of the length. The lobes are greenish with purple tips. The paracorolla is composed of 5 caplike points. The 5 stamens and the 2 styles are fused to a stemmed gynostegium and the pollen sticks together to form to a pollinium. The sepals are ovate and the ovary superior. The fruit is a swollen follicle, 9 to 10 cm long, and turned back. The seeds have a silky tuft of hair.

Leaves, Stem, and Root: Calotropis gigantea is a shrub, occasionally treelike, which grows up to 3 m high. The leaves are sessile with the base clasping the stem, fleshy, 10 to 20 cm long and 4 to 10 cm wide, elongate-ovate or elliptical. The stem is woody.

Habitat: India, China, and Malaysian archipelago

Other Names: Giant Swallow Root, Swallow Wort, Crown Flower

ACTIONS AND PHARMACOLOGY

COMPOUNDS

Cardioactive steroid glycosides (cardenolids): calotropin, calactin and uscharidin

Steroids: sterols, including beta-sitosterol, taraxasterol

EFFECTS

The drug contains cardioactive cardenolide glycosides and exhibits an emetic-cathartic effect resembling that of Ipecacuanha. In vitro the calotropin demonstrates anti-tumor qualities against human epidermoid carcinoma cells of the nasopharynx,.

INDICATIONS AND USAGE

Unproven Uses: Giant Milkweed has been used for dysentery, vomiting, toothache, syphilis, convulsions, warts, leprosy, and digestion problems.

Indian Medicine: Preparations are used for skin conditions, intestinal worms, coughs, ascites, and anasarca.

Homeopathic Uses: Calotropis gigantea is used for obesity.

PRECAUTIONS AND ADVERSE REACTIONS

No health hazards are known in conjunction with the proper administration of designated therapeutic dosages.

OVERDOSAGE

Higher dosages cause severe mucous membrane irritation, characterized by vomiting and diarrhea, as well as bradycardia and convulsions, sometimes leading to death. It is not known whether those compounds found in the plant that belong chemically to the cardioactive steroid glycoside group are indeed cardioactive, because of their unusual structure (the sugar remnant is bound to the aglycone both as a glycoside and as an ether). Mucilaginous drinks are recommended to treat the symptoms of inflammation; morphine and atrophine for treating pain.

DOSAGE

Mode of Administration: Whole and cut drug preparations for internal use.

Daily Dosage: As an emetic: 2 to 4 g; As a diaphoretic and expectorant: 200 to 600 mg.

Homeopathic Dosage: (from D4) 5 to 10 drops, 1 tablet, 5 to 10 globules, 1 to 3 times daily or from D6 1 mL injection solution sc. twice weekly (HAB1).

LITERATURE

Ali M, Gupta J, Neguerulea MV, Perez-Alonso MJ. New ursan-type triterpenic esters from the roots of *Calotropis gigantea. Pharmazie* 53 (10); 718-721. 1998

Hänsel R, Keller K, Rimpler H, Schneider G (Ed), Hagers Handbuch der Pharmazeutischen Praxis, 5. Aufl., Bde 4 - 6 (Drogen), Springer Verlag Berlin, Heidelberg, New York, 1992-1994.

Kiuchi F, Fukao Y, Maruyama T, Obata T, Tanaka M, Sasaki T, Mikage M, Haque ME, Tsuda Y, Cytotoxic principles of a Bangladeshi crude drug, akond mul (roots of *Calotropis gigantea L.). Chem Pharm Bull* (Tokyo), 46:528-30, Mar. 1998

Sasidharan VK. Search for antibacterial and antifungal Activity of some Plants Kerala. *Acta Pharm.* 47; 47-51. 1997

Sen S, Sahu NP, Mahato SB, Flavonol glycosides from *Calotropis gigantea. Phytochemistry*, 232:2919-21, Aug. 1992

Sengupta A, Bhattacharya D, Pal G, Sinha NK, Comparative studies on calotropins DI and DII from the latex of *Calotropis gigantea. Arch Biochem Biophys,* 232:17-25, Jul. 1984

Gillenia trifoliata

See Indian Physic

Ginger

Zingiber officinale

DESCRIPTION

Medicinal Parts: The medicinal part is the root.

Flower and Fruit: The flower grows directly from the root and terminates in a long, curved spike. A white or yellow flower grows from each spike.

Leaves, Stem, and Root: Ginger is a creeping perennial on a thick tuberous rhizome, which spreads underground. In the first year, a green, erect, reedlike stem about 60 cm high grows from this rhizome. The plant has narrow, lanceolate to linear-lanceolate leaves 15 to 30 cm long, which die off each year.

Characteristics: The fracture is short and fibrous. The odor and taste are characteristic, aromatic, and pungent.

Habitat: The plant is indigenous to southeastern Asia, and is cultivated in the U.S., India, China, the West Indies, and tropical regions.

Production: Ginger root consists of the peeled, finger-long, fresh or dried rhizome of *Zingiber officinale*.

ACTIONS AND PHARMACOLOGY

COMPOUNDS

Volatile oil (2.5-3.0%): chief components vary greatly, depending upon country of origin: (-)-zingiberene and ar-curcumene, beta-bisabolene and ar-curcumene, neral and geranial, D-camphor, beta-phellandrene, geranial, neral and linalool, (E)-alpha-farnesene, important as aroma carrier zingiberol (mixture of cis- and trans-beta-eudesmol)

Aryl alkanes

Gingerols: chief components [6]-Gingerol (pungent substances), [8]-Gingerol, [10]-Gingerol

Shogaols: chief components [6]-shogaol (pungent substane), [8]- shogaol, [10]- shogaol (artifacts formed during storage, arising from the Gingerols)

Gingerdiols

Diarylheptanoids: including among others, Gingerenone A and B

Starch (50%)

EFFECTS

Ginger is primarily used for nausea and vomiting, dyspepsia, and motion sickness. Studies conducted in vitro and in animal models have elicited physiological effects related to a number of the compounds found in the Ginger rhizome. Among these are antiemetic, anti-inflammatory, antimicrobial, antioxidant, antilipid, antitumor, and cardiotonic effects. The root of *Zingiber officinale* has also shown immune-system stimulation and platelet aggregation-inhibitory activity. Other studies show that Ginger root is positively inotropic and antithrombotic, and promotes secretion of saliva, gastric juices and bile.

Antiemetic Effects: Ginger's antiemetic effects are attributed to the Gingerols and shogaols present in the rhizome of Zingiberis officinale. In contrast to most antiemetic medications that act on the CNS, the antiemetic effect of Ginger is thought to be due to local gastrointestinal actions: Ginger stimulates the flow of saliva, bile, and gastric secretions (Mowrey & Clayton, 1982); it suppresses gastric contractions, raises the tone of the intestinal muscles, and increases peristalsis (Bisset, 1994; Iwu, 1993). The mechanism of action is not due to a nystagmus response or vestibular stimulation (Holtmann, 1989). Various fat-soluble components of Ginger, such as galanolactone, have demonstrated antagonism of serotonin receptor sites (Huang, 1991). This latter mechanism may be responsible for some of Ginger's antiemetic effects as well as antispasmodic effects on visceral and vascular smooth muscle. Ginger inhibited serotonin-induced diarrhea (Huang, 1990).

Anti-Inflammatory Effects: The anti-inflammatory effect of Ginger is thought to be due to inhibition of cyclooxygenase and 5-lipoxygenase, resulting in reduced leukotriene and prostaglandin synthesis (Kiuchi, 1992; Srivastava & Mustafa, 1992). A component of Ginger, [6]-Gingerol, caused a significant reduction in 12-0-tetradecanoyl-phorbol-13 acetate (TPA)-induced ear inflammation compared to mice treated with TPA only (Park et al, 1998).

Antilipid Effects: Ginger significantly improved serum lipid parameters and reduced degree of atherosclerosis compared with no treatment in albino rabbits fed a high-cholesterol diet (Bhandari et al, 1998). Significant improvements in serum lipid parameters were observed in albino rats fed a normal diet supplemented with 0.5% Ginger for 4 weeks compared to untreated controls (Ahmed & Sharma, 1997).

Antimicrobial Effects: A sesquiterpene of Ginger may have antirhinoviral efficacy based on in vitro results. Zerumbone, a sesquiterpene isolated from *Zingiber aromaticum* and Z *zerumbet*, demonstrated in vitro inhibitory effects on human immunodeficiency virus (Dai et al, 1997). Two components of Ginger, 8-Gingerol and 10-Gingerol, demonstrated antibacterial activity against *Bacillus subtilis* and *Escherichia coli* K-12 in vitro (Yamada et al, 1992). Ginger has also shown antischistosomal activity. In mice, Gingerol (5 ppm) abolished the infectivity of *Schistosoma mansoni miracidia* and *cercariae* (Adewunmi et al, 1990).

Antimigraine Effects: In a study of phytochemicals, Ginger (*Zingiber officinale*) was rated as possibly useful for the treatment and prophylaxis of headaches. Mechanisms of headache amelioration of Ginger may include its inhibition of thromboxane production and inhibition of free radicals formed in the arachidonic acid cascade. Ginger decreases platelet aggregation and is a potent inhibitor of prostaglandins, which enhance release of substance P from trigeminal fibers (opiates inhibit substance P release) (Laurinaitis, 1995).

Antioxidant Effects: Cassumunin A demonstrated potent antioxidant activity and is a complex curcuminoid isolated from Zingiber cassumunar (Masuda et al, 1997). In rat liver microsomes, zingerone, from Ginger rhizomes, inhibited lipid peroxidation at high concentrations (greater than 150 micromoles) (Reddy & Lokesh, 1992).

Antithrombotic Effects: Preliminary studies have reported an antithrombotic effect for Ginger root, related to a reduction in production of thromboxane A2 and inhibition of platelet aggregation (Verma et al, 1993; Srivastava & Mustafa, 1989a). Subsequent studies of Ginger in therapeutic doses in healthy subjects and patients with coronary heart disease (CHD) were not able to confirm these results (Bordia et al, 1997; Janssen et al, 1996) although a large single dose (10 g) in CHD patients did significantly reduce platelet aggregation induced by adenosine diphosphate and epinephrine (Bordia et al, 1997).

Cardiotonic Effects: Gingerols and shogaols prepared from Zingiber officinale imparted positive inotropic effects on isolated guinea pig atria in an early study (Shoji et al, 1982). In another animal study (guinea pig), 6 and 8-shogaol had approximately equivalent inotropic effects as 8-Gingerol (Yamahara et al, 1995). Gingerol isolated from *Zingiber officinale* accelerated Ca(2+)-pumping rate in a concentration-dependent manner in cardiac sarcoplasmic reticulum (Kobayashi et al, 1987).

Immune System Effects: Increased secretions of interleukin-1 beta, interleukin-6, and granulocyte-macrophage colony-stimulating factor were demonstrated in human peripheral blood mononuclear cells in vitro in the presence of a low concentration of Zingiberis rhizoma extract (Chang et al, 1995).

Motion Sickness Effects: Ginger may have positive effects with motion sickness symptoms although the results of controlled studies are inconsistent. The adverse effects profile of Ginger is more favorable than those of other motion sickness preparations. No significant difference in symptoms occurred when results were tested within 1 hour (or less) of dosing in 1 study; however, in another study, differences between Ginger and placebo were greatest at 4 hours post ingestion (Schmid, 1994).

Postoperative Nausea and Vomiting Effects: Results from randomized, placebo-controlled, double-blind studies are conflicting (Visalyaputra et al, 1998). Comparative studies report statistically significant improvement in symptoms compared to placebo and similar efficacy compared to metoclopramide.

CLINICAL TRIALS

Chemotherapy-Induced Nausea

Forty-eight gynecologic cancer patients were enrolled into a randomized, double-blind crossover study to determine whether ginger has an antiemetic effect in cisplatin-induced emesis. All subjects were randomly allocated to a regimen A or regimen B in their first cycle of the study. All patients received standard antiemetics in the first day of cisplatin administraton. In regimen A, capsules of ginger root powder were given orally 1 g/day for 5 days, starting on the first day of chemotherapy. In regimen B, placebo was given on the first day and metoclopramide was given orally thereafter for 4 days. The patients were then crossed over to receive the other antiemetic regimen during their next cycle of chemotherapy. No significant differences were found between the treatment groups, indicating that the addition of ginger to a standard antiemetic regimen has no advantage in reducing nausea in the acute phase of cisplatin-induced emesis (Manusirivithayaet al, 2004).

Motion Sickness

One double-blind, randomized, non-placebo controlled study compared the effectiveness of Ginger and six other commonly used nonherbal drugs (scopolamine, dimenhydrinate with caffeine, cyclizine, cinnarizine, cinnarizine with domperidone, and meclizine with caffeine) in 1,489 participants during whale-watching voyages off the coast of Norway. About 78% of those who took 500 mg of Ginger root 2 hours prior to a boat trip were symptom-free for the 6-hour duration. The incidence of severe vomiting did not differ in a statistically significant way between Ginger and any of the other test groups (Schmid, 1994).

In an earlier, double-blind, randomized, placebo-controlled study of 80 naval cadets (median age 17 years) unaccustomed to sea travel, powdered Ginger root 1 g produced better control of symptoms (nausea, vomiting, vertigo, cold sweating) than placebo throughout the 4-hour test period. For individual symptoms of vomiting and cold sweating, Ginger was statistically superior to placebo ($p<0.05$); there was no significant difference for nausea and vertigo. The difference in total symptom scores achieved statistical significance four hours post ingestion ($p<0.05$). No adverse effects were attributed to Ginger (Grontved et al, 1988).

Nausea and Vomiting

A comprehensive review of published clinical and experimental data on Medline up to the end of December 2003, in addition to expert consultations, found indications to suggest that Ginger has antiemetic properties, with definitive evidence only for its ability to alleviate pregnancy-induced nausea and vomiting. For all other uses as an antiemetic, including for postoperative nausea and vomiting and for motion sickness, the evidence for Ginger is insufficient, the reviewers concluded. The review also looked at other uses for Ginger (Chrubasik, 2004).

In a study evaluating oral treatment of pregnancy-induced nausea with 125 mg Ginger extract 4 times daily (equivalent to 1.5 g dried Ginger daily) for 4 days compared to placebo (n=120), no differences in birth weight, gestational age, Apgar scores, or congenital abnormalities were observed in infants born from subjects who had consumed Ginger compared to the general population of infants born at the Royal Hospital for Women from 1999 to 2000. Birth defects observed were similar to the general population and were considered minor (Willetts et al, 2003).

Oral Ginger 1 g daily for 4 days was significantly more effective than placebo in the treatment of pregnancy-induced nausea and vomiting in women of less than 17 weeks gestation in a randomized, double-blind, placebo-controlled trial (n=70). Severity of nausea (visual analog and Likert scales) and number of episodes of vomiting was recorded 24 hours prior to treatment and also during treatment. Severity of nausea and episodes of vomiting decreased significantly with supplementation compared to placebo ($p=0.014$ and $p=0.001$, respectively). Patients in the group that received Ginger reported mild abdominal discomfort, diarrhea, and heartburn. No adverse effects on the outcome of the pregnancies were demonstrated in the treatment group (Vutyavanich et al, 2001).

In a double-blind, placebo-controlled study involving 120 females that underwent gynecologic outpatient surgery, the participants were randomly given either 1 g of powdered Ginger root or 10 mg of metoclopramide orally and evaluated for incidence of postoperative nausea and vomiting. Ten percent of the patients in the Ginger group had one or more episodes of vomiting; 17.5% of the metoclopramide arm and 22.5% of the placebo group had one or more episodes of vomiting. Of the Ginger group, 15% required antiemetic treatment compared to 32.5% of the metoclopramide group and 37.5% of the placebo group. The authors concluded that the Ginger group had a statistically significant lower incidence of nausea and vomiting when compared to placebo (Phillips, 1993).

Osteoarthritis and Rheumatoid Arthritis

Evidence for Ginger to treat osteoarthritic or other pain is equivocal, according to a comprehensive review of clinical and experimental data. While there is insufficient evidence to confirm that Ginger actually alleviates clinical osteoarthritis or other pain, constituents in the root clearly do interfere with the inflammatory cascade and certain pain receptors. Further studies may not only provide backup for Ginger's efficacy for osteoarthritis pain but also establish an optimum daily dosage for treating this common ailment (Chrubasik, 2004).

In an earlier study, Ginger proved to be no more effective than placebo in a randomized, placebo-controlled, crossover study comparing Ginger, ibuprofen, and placebo in the treatment of osteoarthritis. Significant improvement was only achieved with ibuprofen (400 mg) as evidenced by the visual analog scale (VAS; $p<0.0001$) and the consumption of rescue medication (acetaminophen; $p<0.01$) (Bliddal et al, 2000).

In a preliminary open study, 74% of patients with rheumatoid arthritis (n=28) and 55% of patients with osteoarthritis (n=18) reported "marked" improvement in pain after taking powdered Ginger 1 to 2 g daily for up to 2.5 years. With regard to swelling, 59% of rheumatoid arthritis and 50% of osteoarthritis patients reported "marked" improvement. Ten patients with myalgias also reported pain relief with Ginger therapy. No adverse effects occurred. The results of this study are based solely on patient questionnaires; controlled, blinded studies are needed (Srivastava & Mustafa, 1992).

Platelet Aggregation

Powdered Ginger significantly inhibited platelet aggregation in a placebo-controlled study of 20 patients with coronary artery disease. Patients received powdered Ginger 10 g as a single dose. Ginger reduced adenosine diphosphate (ADP) and epinephrine-induced platelet aggregation ($p<0.05$). The platelet response appears to be dose dependent, as Ginger 4 g daily for 1.5 and 3 months did not exert any appreciable effect on platelet aggregation, fibrinogen, or fibrinolytic activity. All patients had a history of myocardial infarction greater than 6 months old; all were taking nitrates and aspirin. Aspirin was discontinued 2 weeks prior to the study (Bordia et al, 1997).

Raw Ginger root had no significant effect on platelet function in 18 healthy volunteers in a randomized, placebo-controlled, crossover study. Subjects received either raw Brazilian Ginger root 15 g, cooked stem Ginger 40 g, or placebo for 2 weeks. Subjects discontinued use of any medications for 1 month prior to the study. The mean decrease in thromboxane production was 1 ± 9% for Ginger root and 1 ± 8% for stem Ginger as compared to placebo (p=0.984). Mean thromboxane B2 production was unchanged (Janssen, 1996).

INDICATIONS AND USAGE

Approved by Commission E:

- Loss of appetite
- Travel sickness
- Dyspeptic complaints

Unproven Uses: In folk medicine, Ginger is used as a carminative, expectorant, and astringent.

Chinese Medicine: In China, Ginger is used to treat colds, nausea, vomiting, and shortness of breath.

Indian Medicine: Indian medicine uses include anorexia, dyspeptic symptoms, and pharyngitis.

CONTRAINDICATIONS

Because of its cholagogic effect, the drug should not be taken in the presence of gallstone conditions except after consultation with a physician. Ginger may inhibit thromboxane synthesis and should not be used by patients who are at risk for hemorrhage (Fleming, 2000; Bracken, 1991).

PRECAUTIONS AND ADVERSE REACTIONS

No health hazards or side effects are known in conjunction with the proper administration of designated therapeutic dosages. Adverse reactions include minor gastrointestinal complaints such as gas, bloating, and heartburn.

It has been reported that administration of 6 g of dried powdered Ginger has been shown to increase the exfoliation of gastric surface epithelial cells in human subjects. It is postulated that this action may possibly lead to ulcer formation. Therefore, it is recommended that dosages on an empty stomach be limited to 6 g (Desai, 1990).

There have been reports that Ginger can cause hypersensitivity reactions resulting in dermatitis. Large overdoses can cause central nervous system depression and cardiac arrhythmias.

Pregnancy: Some experts suggest that Ginger should not be used in pregnancy or lactation (McGuffin et al, 1997). The German Commission E lists morning sickness associated with pregnancy as a contraindication, and the American Herbal Products Association lists pregnancy as a contraindication; however, no clinical evidence has been found to substantiate any harmful effects to mother or fetus. Most research provides evidence that Ginger can be used and is effective in the treatment of morning sickness (Vutyavanich et al, 2001; Fischer-Rasmussen et al, 1990). Ginger tea administered to pregnant Sprague-Dawley rats resulted in double the number of fetal losses compared to the control group ($p<0.05$). There were no gross morphologic malformations observed in the fetuses in the treatment group but fetuses in the treatment group were significantly heavier than control fetuses (Wilkinson, 2000).

DRUG INTERACTIONS

MODERATE RISK

Anticoagulants: Concurrent use may result in increased risk of bleeding. *Clinical Management*: The clinical significance of any effect Ginger may have on platelet aggregation is undetermined. Caution is advised if Ginger and an anticoagulant are taken concomitantly. Studies suggest that over 4 grams of dried or 15 grams raw Ginger root daily must be ingested in order to have any effect on blood coagulation.

MINOR RISK

Antiplatelet agents, Low molecular weight heparins, thrombolytic agents: Concurrent use may result in increased risk of bleeding. *Clinical Management*: The clinical significance of any effect Ginger may have on platelet aggregation is undetermined. Caution is advised if Ginger and any of these agents are taken concomitantly. Studies suggest that over 4 grams of dried or 15 grams raw Ginger root daily must be ingested in order to have any effect on blood coagulation.

OVERDOSAGE

According to research, the LD50 of 6-Gingerol and 6-shogaol is set between 250 and 680 mg/kg. (Fulder & Tenne, 1991; Suekawa et al, 1984.) Toxicity tests in mice using a Ginger extract via lavage resulted in no mortality or adverse effects in doses up to 2.5 g/kg over a 7 day period. When the dose was increased to between 3 and 3.5 g/kg, a 10% to 30% mortality rate was reported (Macola, 1989.)

Overdosage may cause cardiac arrhythmia and CNS depression (Iwu, 1993).

DOSAGE

Mode of Administration: Comminuted rhizome and dry extracts for teas and other galenic preparations for internal use. The powdered drug is used in some stomach preparations.

How Supplied:

Capsules – 100 mg, 400 mg, 420 mg, 460 mg, 470 mg, 500 mg, 550 mg, 1000 mg

Chewable Tablets – 67.5 mg

Fluid Extract – 1:1

Liquid – 1:4 Oil – 100%

Tea Bags

Preparation: To prepare an infusion, pour boiling water over 0.5 to 1 g drug and strain after 5 minutes (1 teaspoonful = 3 g drug).

Daily Dosage:

Antiemesis: Capsules/Powder – 0.5 to 2 g (Bisset,1994; Schmid et al, 1994)

Chemotherapy-induced nausea and vomiting: All dosage forms – 1.5 g (Myer et al, 1995).

Dysepsia: Capsules/Powder – 2 to 4 g/day

Motion Sickness: Capsules/Powder – 1 g to be taken 30 minutes before travel; for continuing symptoms, 0.5 to 1 g every 4 hours (Muller & Clauson, 1997).

Rheumatoid Arthritis and Osteoarthritis: Powder – 1 to 2 g/day (Srivastava & Mustafa, 1992).

Storage: Powdered Ginger root should be stored in a cool, dry place protected from light. Powdered Ginger should not be stored in plastic containers.

LITERATURE

ABDA-Datenbank. Zingiberis rhizoma monograph. WuV, Eschborn and Micromedex, Inc, Englewood, CO, 1997.

Adewunmi CO, Oguntimein BO & Furu P. Molluscicidal and antischistosomal activities of *Zingiber officinale. Planta Med*; 56(4):374-376. 1990.

Ahmed RS & Sharma SB. Biochemical studies on combined effects of garlic (*Allium sativum Linn*) and Ginger (*Zingiber officinale Rosc*) in albino rats. *Indian J Exp Biol*; 35(8):841-843. 1997.

Al-Yahya MA, Rafatullah S, Mossa JS et al. Gastroprotective activity of Ginger *Zingiber Officinale Rosc*., in albino rats. *Amer J Chin Med*; 17(1-2):51-56. 1988.

Arfeen Z, Owen H, Plummer JL et al. A double-blind randomized controlled trial of Ginger for the prevention of postoperative nausea and vomiting. *Anaesth Intensive Care*; 23(4):449-452. 1995.

Bhandari U, Sharma JN & Zafar R. The protective action of ethanolic Ginger (*Zingiber officinale*) extract in cholesterol fed rabbits. *J Ethnopharmacol*; 61(2):167-171. 1998.

Bliddal H, Rosetzsky A, Schlichting P et al. A randomized, placebo- controlled, cross-over study of Ginger extracts and ibuprofen in osteoarthritis. *Osteoarthritis & Cartilage*; 8:9-12. 2000.

Bone ME, Wilkinson DJ, Young JR et al., Ginger root- a new antiemetic. The effect of Ginger root on postoperative nausea and vomiting after major gynecological surgery. *Anaesthesia* 45:669-71. 1990.

Bordia A, Verma SK & Srivastava KC. Effect of Ginger (*Zingiber officinale Rosc*.) and fenugreek (*Trigonella foenumgraecum L.*) on blood lipids, blood sugar and platelet aggregation in patients with coronary heart disease. *Prostaglandins Leukot Essent Fatty Acids*; 56(5):379-384. 1997.

Bracken J, Ginger as an antiemetic: possible side effects due to its thromboxane synthetase activity. *Anaesthesia*; 46:705-706. 1991.

Chang CP, Chang JY, Wang FY et al., The effect of Chinese medicinal herb Zingiberis rhizoma extract on cytokine secretion by human peripheral blood mononuclear cells. *J Ethnopharmacol* 48(1):13-19. 1995.

Chen CC, Ho CT, *J Agric Food Chem* 36:322. 1988.

Chrubasik S, et al. Zingiberis rhizome: A comprehensive review on the ginger effect and efficacy profiles. *Phytomedicine* 12: 684-701. 2005.

Dai JR, Cardellina JH II, McMahon JB et al. Zerumbone, an HIV-inhibitory and cytotoxic sesquiterpene of *Zingiber aromaticum* and *Z. zerumbet. Nat Prod Lett*; 10(2):115-118. 1997.

Denyer CV, Jackson P, Loakes DM, Isolation of antirhinoviral sesquiterpenes from Ginger (*Zingiber officinale*). In: *J Natural Products* 57(5):658-662. 1994.

Desai HG, Kalro RH & Choksi AP, Effect of Ginger & garlic on DNA content of gastric aspirate. *Ind J Med Res* 92:139-41, 1990.

Eldershaw TPD, Colquhoun EQ, Dora KA et al. Pungent principles of Ginger (*Zingiber officinale*) are thermogenic in the perfused rat hind limb. *Int J Obesity* 16:755-63, 1992.

Erler J et al., *Z Lebensm Unters Forsch* 186:231. 1988.

Fintelmann V, Phytopharmaka in der Gastroenterologie. In: *ZPT* 15(3):137. 1994.

Fischer-Rasmussen W, Kjaer S, Dahl C et al., Ginger treatment of hyperemesis gravidarum. *Eur J Obstet Gynecol Reprod Biol* 38(1):19-24. 1990.

Fulder S & Tenne M, Ginger as an anti-nausea remedy in pregnancy; the issue of safety. *Herbalgram*; 38(Fall):47-50. 1991.

Gujral S et al., *Nutr Rep Int* 17:183. 1978.

Harvey DJ, *J Chromatogr* 212:75. 1981.

Henry CJK & Piggott SM. Effect of Ginger on metabolic rate. *Human Nutr Clin Nutr*; 41C(1):89-92. 1987.

Hikino H, In: Economic, Medicinal Plant Research, Vol. 1, Acadamic Press UK 1985.

Huang Q, Matsuda H, Sakai K et al. The effect of Ginger on serotonin induced hypothermia and diarrhea. *Yakugaku Zasshi* (Tokyo); 110(12):936-942. 1990.

Huang QR, Iwamoto M, Aoki S et al. Anti-5-hydroxytryptamine3 effect of galanolactone, diterpinod isolated from Ginger. *Chem Pharm Bull* (Tokyo); 39(2):397-399. 1991.

Janssen PLTMK, Meyboom S, van Staveren WA et al. Consumption of Ginger (*Zingiber Officinale Roscoe*) does not affect ex vivo platelet thromboxane production in humans. *Eur J Clin Nutr*; 50(11):772-774. 1996.

Kano Y, Zong QN & Komatsu K. Pharmacological properties of galenical preparation: XIV. Body temperature retaining effect of the Chinese traditional medicine, ''goshuyu-to'' and component crude drugs. *Chem Pharm Bull* (Tokyo); 39(3):690-692. 1991.

Kasahara Y, Hikino H, *Shoyakugaku Zasshi* 37:73. 1983.

Kawai T et al., Anti-emtic principles of Magnolia obovata bark and *Zingiber officinale* rhizome. In: *PM* 60:17. 1994.

Kikuchi F et al., *Chem Pharm Bull* 30. 754. 1982.

Kikuzaki H, Kobayashi M, Nakatani N, Constituents of Zingiberaceae. 4. Diarylheptanoids from Rhizomes of Zingiber officinale. In: *PH* 30: 3947. 1991.

Kikuzaki H, Kobayashi M, Nakatani N, Diarylheptanoids from rhizomes of *Zingiber officinale*. In: *PH* 30(11):3647-3651. 1991.

Kikuzaki H, Tsai SM, Nakatani N, Gingerdiol related compounds from the rhizomes of *Zingiber officinale*. In: *PH* 31(5):1783-1786. 1992.

Kiuchi F, Iwakami S, Shibuya M et al., Inhibition of prostaglandin and leukotriene biosynthesis by Gingerols and diarylheptanoids. *Chem Pharm Bull* 40(2):387-391. 1992.

Kobayashi M, Shoji N, Ohizumi Y. Gingerol, a novel cariotonic agent, activates the Ca+-pumping ATPase in skeletal and cardiac sarcoplasmic reticulum. *Biochim Biophys Acta*; 903(1):96-102. 1987.

Kruth P, Brosi E, Fux R et al. Ginger-associated overanticoagulation by phenprocoumon. *Ann Pharmacother*; 38:257-260. 2004.

Laurinaitis G. Headaches, vascular and non vascular. *Aust J Med Herbalism*; 7(3):69-78. 1995.

Lumb AB. Effect of dried Ginger on human platelet function. *Thromb Haemost*; 71(1):110-111. 1994.

Macolo N, Jain R, Jain SC et al., Ethnopharmacologic investigation of Ginger (Zingiber officinale). *J Ethnopharmacol* 27:129-40, 1989.

Manusirivithaya S, Sripramote M, Tangjitgamol S, et al. Antiemetic effect of ginger in gynecologic patients receiving cisplatin. *Int J Gynecol Cancer*; 14(6): 1063-1069. 2004.

Marles RJ, Kaminski J, Arnason JT, Pazos-Sanou L, Heptinstall S, Fischer NH, Crompton CW, Kindack DG, A bioassay for inhibition of serotonin release from bovine platelets. In: *JNP* 55:1044-1056. 1992.

Masuda T, Jitoe A, Kida A et al. Synthesis of ± cassumunin A, a potent antiinflammatory antioxidant from a medicinal Ginger. *Natural Prod Lett*; 10(1):13-16. 1997.

Mikawa U et al., Delayed-type allergy-controlling agents containing Gingerones. In: *Patent Jap*. 1988.

Mowrey DB & Clayton DE. Motion sickness, Ginger, and psychotropics. *Lancet*; 1(8273):655-657. 1982.

Muller JL & Clauson KA., Pharmaceutical considerations of common herbal medicine. *Am J Managed Care* 1997; 3(11):1753-1770. 1997.

Mustafa T & Srivastava KC. Ginger (*Zingiber officinale*) in migraine headache. *J Ethnopharmacol*; 29(3):267-273. 1990.

Nagabhushan M, Amonkar AJ, Bhide SV, Mutagenicity of Gingerol and shoagol and antimutagenicity in zingerone in Salmonella/microsme assay. In: *Cancer-Lett* (Shannon Irel) 36(2)221-233. 1987.

Nakamura H & Yamamoto T. Mutagen and anti-mutagen in Ginger, Zingiber officinale. *Mutat Res*; 103(2):119-126. 1982.

Narasimhan S, Govinarajan VS, *J Food Tech* 13:31. 1978.

Norred CL & Brinker F. Potential coagulation effects of preoperative complementary and alternative medicines. *Alt Ther*; 7(6):58-67. 2001.

Pace JC. Oral ingestion of encapsulated Ginger and reported self-care actions for the relief of chemotherapy-associated nausea and vomiting. *Diss Abstr Intl*; 47:3297. 1987.

Park KK, Chun KS, Lee JM et al. Inhibitory effects of [6]-Gingerol, a major pungent principle of Ginger, on phorbol ester-induced inflammation, epidermal ornithine decarboxylase activity and skin tumor promotion in ICR mice. *Cancer Lett*; 129(2):139-144. 1998.

Phillips S, Ruggier R & Hutchinson SE., Zingiber officinale (Ginger) - an antiemetic for day case surgery. *Anaesthesia* 48:715-717. 1993.

Reddy AC & Lokesh BR. Studies on spice principles as antioxidants in the inhibition of lipid peroxidation of rat liver microsomes. *Mol Cell Biochem*; 111(1-2):117-124. 1992.

Saller R, Hellenbrecht D, Zingiber officinale. In: *Tägl Praxis* 33(3):629. 1992.

Shoji N, Iwasa A, Takemoto T et al. Cardiotonic principles of Ginger (*Zingiber officinale Roscoe*). *J Pharm Sci*; 71(10):1174-1175. 1982.

Srivastava KC & Mustafa T. Ginger (*Zingiber officinale*) in rheumatism and musculoskeletal disorders. *Med Hypotheses*; 39(4):342-348. 1992.

Srivastava KC & Mustafa T. Spices: antiplatelet activity and prostanoid metabolism. *Prostaglandins Leukot Essent Fatty Acids*; 38(4):255-266. 1989a.

Suekawa M et al., *J Pharmacobio-Dyn* 7 (11):836. 1984.

Sugaya A et al., *Shoyakugaku Zasshi* 29:160. 1975.

Verma SK, Singh J, Khamesra R et al. Effect of Ginger on platelet aggregation in man. *Indian J Med Res*; 98:240-242. 1993.

Visalyaputra S, Petchpaisit N, Somcharoen K et al. The efficacy of Ginger root in the prevention of postoperative nausea and vomiting after outpatient gynaecological laparoscopy. *Anaesthesia*; 53(5):506-510. 1998.

Vutyavanich T, Kraisarin T & Ruangsri R. Ginger for nausea and vomiting in pregnancy: randomized, double-masked, placebo-controlled trial. *Obstet Gynecol*; 97(4):577-582. 2001.

Wilkinson JM. Effect of Ginger tea on the fetal development of Sprague-Dawley rats. *Reprod Toxicol*; 14(6):507-512. 2000.

Willetts KE, Ekangaki A & Eden. Effect of a Ginger extract on pregnancy-induced nausea: a randomised controlled trial. *Aust N Z J Obstet Gynecol*; 43(2):139-144. 2003.

Yamada Y, Kikuzaki H & Nakatani N. Identification of antimicrobial Gingerols from Ginger (*Zingiber officinale* Roscoe). *J Antibact Antifung Agents*; 20(6):309-311. 1992.

Yamahara J, Hatakeyama S, Taniguchi K et al. Stomachic principles in Ginger: II. Pungent and anti-ulcer effects of low polar constituents isolated from Ginger, the dried rhizoma of *Zinigber officinale* Roscoe cultivated in Taiwan (Japanese). *Yakugaka Zasshi*; 112(9):645-655. 1992.

Yamahara J, Matsuda H, Yamaguchi S et al. Pharmacological study on Ginger: processing. I. Antiallergic activity and cardiotonic action of Gingerols and shogaols. *Natural Med*; 49(1):76-83. 1995.

Yamahara J, Mochizuki M, Rong HQ et al. The anti-ulcer effect in rats of Ginger constituents. *J Ethnopharmacol*; 23(2-3):299-304. 1988.

Yoshikawa M, Hatakeyama S, Taniguchi K et al. 6-Gingesulfonic acid, a new anti-ulcer principle, and Gingerly colipids A, B and C, three new monoacyldigalactosylglycerols from zingiberis rhizoma orginating in Taiwan. *Chem Pharm Bull* (Tokyo); 40(8):2239-2241. 1992.

Ginkgo

Ginkgo biloba

DESCRIPTION

Medicinal Parts: The medicinal parts are the fresh or dried leaves, and the seeds separated from their fleshy outer layer.

Flower and Fruit: The tree flowers for the first time when it is between 20 and 30 years old. The flowers are dioecious. They are in the axils of the lower leaves of the current year's short shoots. The male flowering parts are attached to short catkins. The female flowers have longer pedicles and are at the end of a leafless branch. Fertilization occurs months after pollination by spermatozoids, although usually only one ovule is fully formed. The light green or yellowish seeds, incorrectly called fruit, later become fleshy and plumlike. They have a diameter of 2.5 to 3 cm, and each contains a two-edged edible nut.

Leaves, Stem, and Root: Ginkgo biloba is a 30- to 40-m high dioecious tree with a girth of about 4 m. The trees can live for hundreds of years. The bark is light to dark brown with rough grooves and reticulate fissures. The leaves are fan-shaped with bifurcated ribs. They are fresh green to golden yellow in autumn. The female trees are pointed and pyramid-shaped; the male trees are broad and sparer.

Characteristics: The seeds smell like butyric, capric, or valeric acid when ripe.

Habitat: Ginkgo is indigenous to China, Japan and Korea, and is also found in Europe and the U.S.

Production: The leaves are harvested either mechanically or by hand from plantations or in the wild. The leaves are then dried and pressed into balls. A dry extract from the dried leaf of *Ginkgo biloba* is manufactured using acetone/water and subsequent purification steps without addition of concentrates or isolated ingredients.

Other Names: Maidenhair-Tree

ACTIONS AND PHARMACOLOGY

COMPOUNDS

Flavonoids (0.5-1.8%): including monosides, biosides and triosides of quercetin, isorhamnetins, 3-O- methylmyristicins, and kaempferol, to some extent estered with p-coumaric acid

Biflavonoides (0.4-1.9%): for example, amentoflavone, bilobetin, 5-methoxybilobetin, ginkgetin, isoginkgetin

Proanthocyanidins (8-12%)

Trilactonic diterpenes (0.06-0.23%): ginkgolide A, B, C

Trilactonic sesquiterpene bilabolids (0.04-0.2%)

EFFECTS

Ginkgo has shown anti-inflammatory, cognitive-promoting, antioxidant, and vascular effects. Ginkgo has been proved ineffective in the treatment of cocaine-dependency, depression, multiple sclerosis, and ulcerative colitis. Ginkgo has proved effective against peripheral occlusive arterial disease (Schweizer & Hautmann, 1999). One recent study showed Ginkgo improved efficacy of and tolerability of 5-fluorouracil in colon cancer treatment (Hauns et al, 2001); the drug may inhibit some bacteria (Brun-Pascaud et al, 1997; Struillou et al, 1995; Atzori et al, 1993; Mourey et al, 1985). The use of Ginkgo in cardiovascular disease looks promising, but well-controlled trials are needed to determine its effectiveness. Ginkgo has demonstrated antioxidant activity, inhibition of platelet aggregation, enhancement of coronary blood flow, vasodilation, and a decrease in human blood pressure (Mahady, 2002). A small pilot, double blind, placebo-controlled study, demonstrated reductions in frequency of attacks in patients with Raynaud's disease who took *Ginkgo biloba* extract (Muir et al, 2002).

The anti-inflammatory effect of Ginkgo may be related to reduced eosinophil infiltration. Cognitive function may be improved by the antioxidant properties of Ginkgo. Ginkgo may act as a free radical scavenger. Although known to produce symptomatic improvement of dementia, no single mechanism of action has been identified. Glucocorticoid levels may be reduced by Ginkgo. Ginkgo may inhibit several enzymes, including catechol-O-methyl transferase, cytochrome P450 3A4, glycerol-3-phosphate dehydrogenase, and monoamine oxidase, although studies have been contradictory. Ginkgo may improve pancreatic beta cell function and insulin metabolism, and may inhibit serotonin uptake. Several mechanisms have been proposed by which Ginkgo may relax smooth muscle. Ginkgo inhibited platelet-activating factor. Gingko improves hemodynamic parameters, such as blood flow, by decreasing blood viscosity and erythrocyte aggregation.

Anti-inflammatory Effects: Intradermal administration of platelet-activating factor (PAF) induced a biphasic inflammatory response similar to that invoked by antigen challenge in sensitive individuals. Ginkgolides, especially ginkgolide B, antagonized this response. When given orally, ginkgolides reduced eosinophil infiltration in atopic patients given intracutaneous injections of PAF (Rosenblatt & Mindel, 1997; Della-Loggia et al, 1993). Ginkgolide B is a potent inhibitor of platelet-activating factor (PAF), which is important for the induction of arachidonate-independent platelet aggregation. Ginkgolide B blocks the binding of PAF to its receptor resulting in an antagonistic effect (Chung, 1987). This effect will inhibit PAF-induced bronchoconstriction and airway hyperactivity, along with T-lymphocyte proliferation and cytokine production. PAF induces inflammation and changes in vascular permeability (Wada et al, 1988; Braquet, 1987; Anon, 1986).

Antioxidant Effects: *Ginkgo biloba* exerts ischemic protective and antioxidant effects through the flavonoids. This occurs through a free scavenger action and prevention of lipid peroxidation. Lipid peroxidation is involved in producing tissue and vascular damage as well as neuronal loss, which may lead to dementia (Dorman, 1992; Koc, 1995; Otamiri, 1989). The herb also reduces neutrophil infiltration and increases blood flow to prevent the progression of dementia ischemia. The antioxidant and membrane-stabilizing activity increases cerebral hypoxia tolerance (Braquet & Hosford, 1991; Koltringer, 1989; Otamiri, 1989).

Multiple mechanisms of action have been proposed for the action of *Ginkgo biloba* in the treatment of cerebral hypoxia. Ginkgolide B, a potent antagonist of PAF, decreased glycine levels in rats after brain injury, decreased PAF-induced increases in intracellular calcium (2+) levels, attenuated the activation of protein kinase C, and reduced excitatory amino acid receptor function. Other constituents of Ginkgo biloba may protect neurons by acting as oxygen radical scavengers. Ginkgo, acting on the hepatic cytochrome P-450 enzyme system, may also attenuate oxygen-free radical formation and the release of superoxide anions. Ginkgo may also increase the number of H(3)rauwolscine binding sites in the hippocampus as seen in aged rats. This effect could compensate for the declining number of alpha-adrenoreceptors, characteristic of aging. Ginkgo also inhibited catechol-O-methyl transferase and enhanced the vasoregulatory effect of catecholamines (Logani et al, 2000).

Ginkgo may be a free radical scavenger and prevent lipid peroxidation in a dose-dependent manner. This action protects vascular walls (Barth et al, 1991; Pincemail et al, 1989). It may also increase the half-life of endothelium-based relaxing factor by its free radical scavenging action on superoxide anions (thus relaxing contracted blood vessels) (Robak & Gryglewski, 1988). Animal studies demonstrate that Ginkgo also scavenges peroxyl radicals, which are involved in lipid peroxidation (Maitra et al, 1995).

Arteriosclerosis: Ginkgo may reduce arteriosclerotic lesions but human trials are needed. Arteriosclerosis leading to stroke developed more often in untreated rats than in rats treated with Tanakan®, a preparation of *Ginkgo biloba* (Fang et al, 2000). Ginkgo extract (containing 24% ginkgoflavonglycosides) demonstrated a protective effect against oxidation of LDL to oxysterols in a study using human LDL. Oxysterols are highly cytotoxic and through macrophage scavengers create ''foam cells'' which are seen early in atheroma lesions (Rasetti et al, 1997).

Cognitive Function: The majority of studies have demonstrated a benefit with Ginkgo supplementation on cognition. Ginkgo demonstrated a benefit in elderly patients with mild to moderate memory impairment. At least 12 weeks of Ginkgo treatment is necessary before improvement occurs. Ginkgo slowed the rate of deterioration in severe dementia. Noncognitively impaired elderly adults may benefit from Ginkgo. Ginkgo did not enhance memory in young adults.

In dementia due to neuronal loss and impaired neurotransmission, there is a decrease in oxygen and glucose and a release of free radicals and lipid peroxidation (Kleijnen & Knipschild, 1992). The active ingredients in Ginkgo, the flavonoids (ginkgo-flavone glycosides) and terpenoids (ginkgolides and bilobalide), probably affect the progression of dementia in several ways, such as reducing neutrophil infiltration and lipid peroxidation (Otamiri & Tagesson, 1989), increasing blood flow (Koltringer et al, 1989), antagonizing platelet-activating factor (Wada et al, 1988), and changing neuron metabolism (DeFeudis, 1991; Hofferberth, 1991).

Radiolabeled rauwolscine binding to alpha-2-adrenoceptors in the cerebral cortex and hippocampus membranes was enhanced (28%) by Ginkgo extracts in older rats. Alpha-2-adrenoceptor activity was lost as the animals aged (25% to 30% between 4 and 24 months). Ginkgo may alter noradrenergic activity in aged rats (Huguet & Tarrade, 1992). Increased cerebral glucose utilization and conservation of mitochondrial metabolism and adenosine-5′-triphosphate (ATP) production have been associated with improvement in cognitive functions (Duverger et al, 1995).

Enzyme Inhibition: Although antipyrine (the classic model for cytochrome P450 metabolism) was not affected by *Ginkgo biloba* in humans (Duche et al, 1989), in vitro data demonstrated inhibition of P450 3A4 by *Ginkgo biloba* (Budzinski et al, 2000). Four anacardic acids inhibited glycerol-3-phosphate dehydrogenase (an enzyme of synthesis of triacylglycerol) by 50% in concentrations of 1 to 3 micrograms/milliliter (Irie et al, 1996). The potential MAO inhibitory activity of Ginkgo is questionable. A human study did not demonstrate MAO inhibition in the brain following oral consumption (Fowler et al, 2000). Ginkgo biloba extract inhibited MAO-A/MAO-B in the rat brain in vitro (Sloley et al, 2000; White et al, 1996) and MAO-B in human platelets in vitro (White et al, 1996). No significant MAO inhibition was demonstrated in mice following oral consumption (Porsolt et al, 2000).

Insulin Metabolism: Ingestion of *Ginkgo biloba* extract for three months was associated with an increase in pancreatic beta cell function after a 75 g glucose load in an uncontrolled, unblinded study of 20 healthy subjects with normal glucose tolerance blood levels. The authors hypothesized that Ginkgo biloba may increase the rate of insulin metabolic clearance (Kudolo, 2000).

Radiation Exposure: Plasma clastogenic factors found in Chernobyl accident recovery workers were reduced to control levels following supplementation with a Ginkgo extract for 2 months. After the Chernobyl accident, 33 of 47 workers had clastogenic factors in their blood and 30 of these were treated with Ginkgo extract EGb 761 (40 mg three times a day) for 2 months. The patients were followed for one year, and it was found that the anticlastogenic effect persisted for at least 7 months. One-third of workers again had clastogenic factors in their plasma at the end of a year (Emerit et al, 1995).

Vertigo: In a 3-month trial, Ginkgo extract (Egb 761, Rokan®) was significantly more effective than placebo in relieving the intensity, frequency, and duration of vertigo episodes (Haguenauer et al, 1986).

CLINICAL TRIALS

Cancer, Adjunct Therapy

Ginkgo improved efficacy of and tolerability of 5-fluorouracil (5-FU) in colorectal cancer patients in an open-label, prospective, phase II study. Thirty-two patients with progressive advanced colorectal cancer refractory to conventional first line 5-FU therapy were treated with 350 mg of a Ginkgo extract (EGb 761) as a 30-minute IV infusion on days 1 through 6, followed by 5-FU 500 mg/m2/d as a 30-minute infusion on days 2 through 6. Evaluation took place after the second and fourth course of treatment. Progression was observed in 22 patients, no change in 8 patients, and partial response in 2 patients (overall response of 6.3%). Authors claim a good benefit-risk ratio of the combined treatment, citing median survival time of 9.5 months that is similar to other second line combination treatments (Hauns et al, 2001).

Cognitive Performance

Enhancements to a range of cognitive outcomes and basic speed of mental processing and mood (subjective well-being) were detected with 120 mg Ginkgo daily (three 40 mg doses) in a 12-week, double-blind, placebo controlled studying involving 197 healthy adults. Compared with placebo, long-term memory as assessed by associational learning tasks appeared to significantly (p=0.04) improve with Ginkgo when taken by healthy older adults (55-79 years of age). However, no other statistically significant improvements were found in this age range. Nor were significant enhancements as compared to placebo identified in a group of young adults (18 to 43 years old), an age group not previously examined this way at this dosage and for this duration (12 weeks). Overall, side effects were mild or negligible (Burns, 2006).

Benefits to cognition were also limited in a placebo-controlled, double-blind study in healthy postmenopausal women (aged 51 to 67) who were randomly assigned to receive a standardized extract of Ginkgo (n= 45; 120 mg 1ce daily) or a placebo for 6 weeks. At baseline and after 6 weeks of treatment, the only significant effects observed in the Gingko group was in regard to mental flexibility: women in late menopause (mean age 61 years) made fewer errors and needed less time to complete a particular task than they did at the outset of the study (baseline), but those in early menopause (mean age 55 years) showed no benefit from Ginkgo. Other qualities of cognition tested—planning ability, memory, sustained attention, ratings of sleepiness, mood, and bodily and menopausal symptoms—did not change at all with Ginkgo. The authors had earlier seen enhancements in regard to attention, memory, and mental flexibility with 1 week of Ginkgo treatment, but the current study failed to confirm that these benefits persist over 6 weeks (Elsabagh, 2005).

In contrast, a double-blind, placebo-controlled trial demonstrated Ginkgo extract supplementation was ineffective in enhancing memory in healthy male volunteers. Healthy young male subjects (average age 20 years) were supplemented with either two 60-mg tablets of BioGinkgo daily (n=30) or placebo (n=30) for five days. On the fifth day, all subjects were administered a series of 4 memory tests, including the Sternberg Memory Scanning Test (SMST). No significant differences (p > 0.05) in the series of memory test, except for SMST, were noted between the supplemented group and placebo group (Moulton et al, 2001).

Use of Ginkgo in cognitively intact older adults provided a tendency toward improving certain neurocognitive functions. Cognitively intact elderly adults over 55 years (n=40) randomly received Ginkgo biloba extract 60 mg 3 times daily or placebo for 6 weeks. Multiple neuropsychological tests including the Stroop Color and Word Test, Trail-making Test, and the Wechsler Memory Scale-Revised and a follow-up self-report questionnaire were utilized before and after therapy. Although some of the neuropsychological testing demonstrated a trend toward improvement, only on the Stroop Color and Word Test's color-naming task was there significantly more improvement demonstrated in the Ginkgo group as compared to placebo (p<0.03). The patients also perceived their overall ability to remember things either ''somewhat improved'' or ''much improved'' more often in the Ginkgo group as compared to the placebo group (p<0.03). The short-term use and the low number of participants may have limited the significance of these findings (Mix & Crews, 2000).

Dementia

A double-blind trial was performed including 400 patients age 50 and older with Alzheimer's disease (AD) or vascular dementia (VaD). Subjects were randomly assigned to receive the Ginkgo biloba extract, EgB 761, or placebo for 22 weeks. There was a mean -3.2 improvement in the SKT dementia test battery upon treatment with the extract and an average deterioration by +1.3 points on placebo (p<0.001). EGb 761 was significantly superior to placebo on all secondary outcome measures, including the Neuropschiatric Inventory and an activities-of-daily-living scale. Treatment results were essentially similar for AD and VaD subgroups. Adverse events were no more frequent under drug than under placebo treatment (Napryeyenko and Borzenko, 2007).

Clinical evidence is available but limited for Ginkgo's ability to improve cognitive function in individuals with Alzheimer's disease or vascular dementia for up to 52 weeks. In contrast to prescription and formulations typically used in clinical trials, such as high purity Ginkgo extract (EGb 761), nonprescription formulations are often inconsistent in terms of purity and concentration of active ingredients, which means that effectiveness may be blunted. No randomized clinical trials of Ginkgo were identified in individuals with Lewy body dementia (Warner, 2006).

A 24-week, placebo-controlled and double-blind study in 76 men and women 50 to 80 years old with mild to moderate Alzheimer's dementia was carried out in which participants were randomized to one of three treatments: 160 mg Ginkgo biloba daily (special extract EGb 761), 5 mg daily donezepil (a cholinesterase inhibitor), or a placebo. The results indicate that Ginkgo and donezepil are similar in clinical effect for this type of dementia. In all, 60 people completed the trial. Improvements in attention, memory, and cognitive performance as analyzed by the Syndrom Kurz test and other exams were comparable between between the Ginkgo and donezepil groups. Both treatments were also well tolerated (Mazza, 2006).

In a randomized, double-blind, placebo-controlled, parallel-group, multicenter trial, the clinical efficacy of Ginkgo biloba extract in 513 patients with mild-to-moderate dementia of the Alzheimer's type was determined. Subjects with this type of dementia who scored 10 to 24 on the Mini-Mental State Examination and less than 4 on the modified Hachinski Ischemic Score, free of other serious illness and not requiring continuous treatment with any psychoactive drug, were enrolled. Over a period of 26 weeks, the patients received Ginkgo biloba extract at a daily dose of 120 mg, 240 mg, or placebo. Results revealed no efficacy with the Ginkgo extract and no significant differences between groups (Schneider et al, 2005).

Gingko improved cognitive performance and social functioning in a 52-week randomized, double-blind, placebo-controlled, parallel-group, multicenter study in patients with uncomplicated Alzheimer's disease or multi-infarct dementia. These individuals were administered Ginkgo extract (EGb) 40 mg 3 times a day or an unspecified placebo for 52 weeks. Patients were stratified by their Mini-Mental State Examination (MMSE) scores into mild, stratum 1: (MMSE score greater than 23) (n=122), and moderate to severe, stratum 2: (MMSE less than 24) (n=114). Primary outcome measures used were the cognitive subscale of the Alzheimer's Disease Assessment Scale (ADAS-cog) and the Geriatric Evaluation by Relative's Rating Instrument (GERRI). Patients taking Ginkgo in stratum 1 demonstrated significant improvement over baseline on the ADAS-cog ($p<0.001$) and the GERRI ($p=0.04$) although treatment differences compared with placebo were not statistically significant. For stratum 2, the placebo group demonstrated substantial worsening in ADAS-cog ($p=0.0001$) and the GERRI ($p=0.002$) compared with baseline while the Ginkgo-supplemented group demonstrated no difference compared with baseline in ADAS-cog ($p=0.07$) and the GERRI (nonsignificant). A subgroup analysis of patients with severe dementia (MMSE <15)(n=35) demonstrated worsening in the placebo group, ADAS-cog ($p=0.002$) and GERRI ($p=0.035$) while the Ginkgo-supplemented group experienced no statistically significant change. The authors concluded that Ginkgo extract (EGb) induced an improvement in mild to moderate dementia and slowed the deterioration in severe dementia (Le Bars et al, 2002).

In a double blind, two-phase study, no beneficial cognitive effects were demonstrated in a 24-week Ginkgo study given to elderly subjects with dementia (i.e., Alzheimer's dementia, vascular dementia, or a mixed type of dementia) or age-associated memory impairment (vanDongen et al, 2000).

Ginkgo was no more effective than placebo in the performance by noncognitively impaired elderly adults on neuropsychological tests in a 6-week, double-blind, placebo-controlled study (Solomon et al, 2002).

Cocaine Abuse

Ginkgo was ineffective in the prevention of a relapse in cocaine dependent subjects in a 10-week, double-blind, placebo-controlled trial (Kampman et al, 2003).

Intermittent Claudication

A 2004 review of the literature up to March 2002 identified 9 randomized, double-blind, placebo-controlled clinical trials that used oral forms of Ginkgo biloba special extract EGb 761 for people with peripheral arterial occlusive disease rated stage 11 (not higher) and included analysis of such factors as pain-free walking distance. The reviewers concluded that there was enough evidence to confirm a superiority of the extract over placebo as well as clinically important relevance for treatment of the illness, despite the fact that the trials had considerable variations in dosage, length of treatment, and other factors. Six of the 9 studies showed a statistically significant superiority of the extract over placebo. Most showed more cases of pain-free walking of distances as compared to placebo. Four of the studies used 160 mg of the extract while others used 120 mg, for example. The extract also was well tolerated (Horsch, 2004).

An earlier analysis (2000) came to a similar conclusion. In this meta-analysis of 8 randomized, placebo controlled, double-blind trials reported Ginkgo to be superior to placebo in the treatment of intermittent claudication, but clinical relevance was questioned since therapeutic effects were small. An increase of pain-free walking distance of 34 meters was reported during Ginkgo administration. Ginkgo doses ranged from 120 to 160 milligrams daily for up to 24 weeks. Adverse effects were reported in 5 of the 8 trials with abdominal complaints, nausea, and dyspepsia being reported most frequently. Shortcomings of the trials included in this analysis were also mentioned but overall results agreed with those of the largest study performed to date by Peters et al (Pittler & Ernst, 2000).

The clinical efficacy of *Ginkgo biloba* special extract (EGb 761) was demonstrated in 111 patients with peripheral occlusive arterial disease (POAD) in Fontaine stage IIb and intermittent claudication. The mean pain-free walking distances were very similar at the beginning of the treatment period. After 8, 16 and 24 weeks, the EGb treatment group was significantly better than the placebo group with maximum walking distance and relative increases of the pain-free walking distance. The doppler indices remained nearly unchanged during the course of therapy (Peters, 1998).

Ginkgo biloba significantly improved pain-free walking distance and maximum walking distance in patients with peripheral arterial occlusive disease (Fontaine's stage II). Seventy-four patients with unilateral leg pain from PAOD completed this randomized, double- blind, multicenter, dose comparison trial. Patients received either 120 mg (n=38) or 240 mg (n=36) *Ginkgo biloba* extract (Egb 761) daily for 24 weeks. Significant improvement in pain-free walking distance occurred in both groups with a mean improvement of 60.6 meters in the 120 mg/d group and 107 meters in the 240 mg/d group. Superiority of the higher dosage was statistically significant (p=0.0253). Both doses were well tolerated (Schweizer & Hautmann, 1999).

Mountain (Altitude) Sickness

In an attempt to clarify the potential role of Ginkgo in preventing and blunting the severity of acute mountain sickness—previous studies had shown mixed effectiveness for this purpose—a large, prospective, randomized and controlled clinical trial was carried out in 614 healthy western trekkers ascending Mount Everest (approach in the Nepal Himalayas). In all, 487 completed the trial. The climbers took three or four doses of their assigned treatment before continued ascent. Results demonstrated that Ginkgo fails to decrease the incidence or severity of acute mountain sickness. Addition of Ginkgo to acetazolamide—the standard drug—actually decreased the effectiveness of this drug against headache, which is one of the most common symptoms of altitude sickness. The percentage of trekkers developing acute mountain sickness was 34% for placebo, 12% for acetazolamide, and 35% for Ginkgo, and 14% for Ginkgo and acetazolamide combined (Gertsch, 2007).

A previous study by the same author found that ginkgo did not significantly decrease the incidence of acute mountain sickness (AMS) but did significantly decrease the severity of AMS symptoms compared to placebo in a double-blind, placebo-controlled trial (Gertsch et al, 2002). Administration of *Ginkgo biloba* extract (EGb) appeared to prevent the onset of AMS in a randomized, double-blind study (Roncin et al, 1996).

Multiple Sclerosis

An exploratory pilot study (randomized, placebo-controlled, double blind) demonstrated modest beneficial effects of Ginkgo biloba extract EGb 761 (240 mg daily) on fatigue, severity of symptoms, and functionality in some of the 11 individuals with multiple sclerosis (MS) randomized to take the extract daily for 4 weeks. The other 11 individuals with MS in this study were randomized to a placebo. No side effects or adverse reactions were reported. Improvements in four or more measures were seen. The authors recommend that a larger sampling of MS patients be enrolled in a future study so that more meaningful results can be measured following these promising findings (Johnson, 2006).

Schizophrenia, Adjunct Therapy

A double-blind, placebo-controlled trial investigated the effects of Ginkgo biloba extract (EGb 761) administration when added to haloperidol on T-lymphocytes subsets and superoxide dismutase levels in schizophrenia. The researchers concluded that the ginkgo extract resulted in beneficial effects on the immune system and improved symptoms of schizophrenia (Zhang et al, 2006).

Concomitant use of Ginkgo enhanced the effectiveness of haloperidol in a randomized, double-blind, placebo-controlled study. Patients meeting DSM-III-R criteria for schizophrenia received oral haloperidol 0.25 mg/kg/d and either 360 mg a day (in 3 divided doses) of a Ginkgo extract (EGb) (n=56) or placebo (n=53) for 12 weeks. Patients were assessed using the Brief Psychiatric Rating Scale (BPRS), the Scale for the Assessment of Negative Symptoms (SANS), and the Scale for the Assessment of Positive Symptoms (SAPS) at week 6 and 12 and the Treatment Emergent Symptom Scale (TESS) for side effects at week 12. Both the placebo group and Ginkgo group demonstrated significant improvement in BPRS scores following 12 weeks of treatment (p<0.05). Both SAPS and SANS scores were significantly lower compared to baseline in the Ginkgo group (p<0.05) but not the placebo group. After 12 weeks, the SAPS score was significantly better (p=0.26) in the Ginkgo group compared to the placebo group. (Zhang et al, 2001). An earlier study (Zhou et al, 1999) demonstrated the same results.

Seasonal Affective Disorder

Ginkgo had no effect on seasonal depression in a randomized, double-blind, parallel-group study. Patients with seasonal affective disorder (SAD), having had at least one previous episode of winter depression and who were not currently medicated and who scored less than 6 points on the Montgomery-Asberg Depression Rating Scale (MADRS), were enrolled in the study. Patients were supplemented with 2 tablets a day of Gingko extract (N=15) (Bio-Biloba containing 24 mg flavone glycosides and 6 mg terpene lactones/tablet) or a placebo (n=12) for 10 weeks. No significant improvement in MADRS was noted following 10 weeks of supplementation (Lingjaerde et al, 1999).

Sexual Dysfunction

A randomized and placebo-controlled trial of Ginkgo biloba 240 mg daily failed to demonstrate any significant difference in effectiveness between the herb and placebo in people with sexual dysfunction resulting from the use of antidepressant medications. The 12-week study involved 24 individuals with this problem, and analysis was done on 8 males and 5 females on placebo and 6 males and 5 females on Ginkgo. Some notable individual responses were recorded in both groups, but no significant differences in effectiveness or side effects were found. Importantly, neither the participants, the investigators, nor the statisticians were aware of who was taking what (triple-blind study) (Wheatley, 2004).

Sudden Deafness

In a randomized, double-blind comparative study, *Ginkgo biloba* extract (EGb 761) and pentoxifylline (PTX) appeared to be similarly efficacious when used to treat deafness of sudden onset (Reisser & Weidauer, 2001).

Stroke

There is some experimental data to indicate that Ginkgo increases blood flow and glucose uptake into brain tissue. However, the 10 of 14 trials included (792 patients) in this Cochrane Collaboration review of randomized (or quasi-randomized) controlled clinical trials comparing Gingko biloba extract with placebo or open control (no placebo) for promoting recovery following an acute ischaemic stroke found no convincing evidence for use of the herb. Specifically, although such factors as evidence of stroke via confirmation by brain scan was included, the evidence from trials of high quality overall was insufficient. More well-designed and large randomized controlled trials to test the herbs effectiveness for stroke are needed, the authors conclude (Zeng, 2005).

Tinnitus

Results of a randomized, double-blind, placebo-controlled study revealed that administration of Ginkgo biloba extract was not effective in the treatment of patients with tinnitus. In addition to this study, 6 randomized, placebo-controlled, double-blind studies were meta-analyzed. No benefits of Ginkgo biloba were found (Rejali et al, 2004).

Similarly, Ginkgo was found to be no more effective than placebo in the treatment of tinnitus in an earlier, 12-week, double-blind, placebo-controlled trial. Subjects (n=1121) were randomized to receive *Ginkgo biloba* extract LI 1370, 50 mg, 3 times daily or placebo. Of 1,121 subjects, a total of 956 subjects were paired. No significant differences were found between the groups at weeks 4, 12, and 14 as determined by a 21-symptom questionnaire. Audiological measurements were not taken. Adverse effects were similar between groups (Drew & Davies, 2001).

A mini-review of five controlled, randomized trials from 1986 to 1998 demonstrated favorable results in the treatment of tinnitus with Gingko. The studies demonstrating effectiveness used higher doses (typically 120 to 160 mg/d). Authors point to variability of dosing regimens, types of Ginkgo products, and outcome measures as reason for caution for a full recommendation, but consider that Ginkgo has potential for use in the treatment of tinnitus (Ernst & Stevinson, 1999).

Vertigo:

In a 3-month trial, Ginkgo extract (Egb 761, Rokan®) was significantly more effective than placebo in relieving the intensity, frequency, and duration of vertigo episodes (Haguenauer et al, 1986).

Vitiligo

Active progression of depigmentation was halted in subjects with vitiligo treated with *Ginkgo biloba* for 6 months. Forty-seven subjects with progressive vitiligo were enrolled in a double-blind, placebo-controlled trial. Group A (n=25) subjects received Ginkgo extract 40 mg (9.6 mg ginkgoflavonglycosides) orally 3 times daily and group B subjects (n=22) received placebo on the same schedule. Active progression of the disease was halted in 20 patients on Ginkgo compared with 8 patients on placebo (p =0.006). Marked improvement (75% repigmentation of lesions) occurred in 10 patients on Ginkgo compared with 2 patients on placebo (Parsad et al, 2003).

INDICATIONS AND USAGE

Approved by Commission E:

- Symptomatic relief of organic brain dysfunction
- Intermittent claudication
- Vertigo (vascular origin)
- Tinnitus (vascular origin)

The Commission E approvals listed are limited to special standard extracts of Ginkgo.

Unproven Uses: The drug is used for disturbed brain functions that result in dizziness and headache with emotional lability and anxiety. Ginkgo has been demonstrated to improve concentration and memory deficits as a result of peripheral arterial occlusive disease.

Chinese Medicine: Among traditional Chinese uses for *Ginkgo biloba* are asthma, tinnitus, hypertonia, and angina.

Homeopathic Uses: Homeopathy includes tonsillitis and cephalgia among the indications for use of Ginkgo.

CONTRAINDICATIONS

Ginkgo may lower seizure threshold, and caution is recommended in the use of this herb by individuals with a history of convulsive disorders (Kupiec, 2005). Ginkgo or its extracts should not be used in any patient known to be allergic to it or any of its constituents.

PRECAUTIONS AND ADVERSE REACTIONS

General: Mild gastrointestinal complaints could occur as side effects. Also, headaches, blood pressure problems, allergic reactions, and phlebitis have occasionally been documented after parenteral administration. Contact dermatitis has been reported with Ginkgo fruit and/or fruit pulp, which may or may not occur with use of Ginkgo leaves. The possible hypersensitivity reactions consist of occurrence of spasms and cramps and, in cases of acute toxicity, atonia and adynamia. Several cases of bleeding complications have been reported. Palpitations and cardiac arrhythmia have occurred with Ginkgo use. Dizziness, symptomatic hypotension, headache, nausea, and gastrointestinal upset have occurred. Stevens-Johnson syndrome has been reported.

Consider discontinuing Ginkgo prior to elective surgery as it may increase the risk of postoperative bleeding (Fessenden et al, 2001; Norred & Finlayson, 2000).

Central Nervous System Effects: Patients with history of seizures or who are taking medications that are known to lower seizure threshold are advised to avoid Ginkgo leaf and Ginkgo leaf extracts (Gregory, 2001). The United States Food and Drug Administration have reported seven cases of Ginkgo-related seizures (four reports were associated with multi-ingredient products and three with single ingredient products) (Gregory, 2001). Two elderly patients with well-controlled epilepsy relapsed within 2 weeks of consuming gingko leaf extract. Discontinuation of Ginkgo restored effective seizure control (Granger, 2001). Seizures and coma have occurred after ingestion of Ginkgo seeds. Twenty-five percent mortality was experienced by seizure victims. Infants may be more susceptible. No sequelae were noted in those that recovered. The toxin is thought to be the antipyridoxine substance 4-O-methylpyridoxine (Yagi et al, 1993; Wada et al, 1988).

Dermatological Effects: Stevens-Johnson syndrome after oral ingestion of Ginkgo has been reported (Davydov & Stirling, 2001). Contact dermatitis has occurred. Although the intact fruit does not cause dermatitis, the fruit pulp is irritating to mucous membranes and may produce primary irritation and allergic contact dermatitis. Symptoms include intense itching, edema, papules, and pustules. The skin reaction generally subsides within 7 to 10 days (Huh & Staba, 1992; Tomb et al, 1988). Vesicular, pruritic lesions and swollen eyelids were seen in 3 cases of contact dermatitis caused by fruit gathering. Symptoms usually occurred 1 to 4 days after exposure (Tomb et al, 1988).

Hematological Effects: Multiple cases of spontaneous bleeding associated with Ginkgo have been reported (Bent, 2005). Cases of subarachnoid hemorrhage, subdural hematoma, intracerebral hemorrhage, subphrenic hematoma, vitreous hemorrhage, and postoperative bleeding have been reported in patients taking Ginkgo alone (Hauser et al, 2002; Benjamin et al, 2001; Fessenden et al, 2001; Norred & Finlayson, 2000; Vale, 1998; Lewis & Rowin, 1997; Rowin & Lewis, 1996). One report indicates that the cause of bleeding some individuals taking EGb 761 may not, as previously suggested, be due to a platelet-activating factor (PAF) antagonistic effect of ginkgolides but rather to chance factors (Koch, 2005).

Fertility: Ginkgo has adverse effects on oocytes (Ondrizek, 1999).

DRUG INTERACTIONS

MAJOR RISK

Anticoagulants, Antiplatelet Agents: Concomitant use of Ginkgo and these medications may increase the risk of bleeding complications. However, in a randomized, double-blind, crossover study of patients (n=24) receiving stable regimens of warfarin, coadministration of Ginkgo did not affect the International Normalized Ratio (Engelsen et al, 2003). *Clinical Management:* Avoid concomitant use.

Nonsteroidal Anti-inflammatory Agents (NSAIDs): Increased risk of bleeding with concomitant use of Ginkgo; one case report describes a fatal intracerebral hemorrhage associated with concomitant use of Ginkgo and ibuprofen, though definite causality could not be proven (Meisel et al, 2003). *Clinical Management:* Avoid concomitant use of Ginkgo and NSAIDs. If both agents are taken together, monitor bleeding time and signs and symptoms of excessive bleeding frequently to determine if platelet function has been adversely affected by Ginkgo.

Trazodone: Concurrent use may result in excessive sedation and potential coma. *Clinical Management*: A single case report has described a semicomatose state following use of gingko with trazodone. Since no rechallenge of either agent alone or together was performed, it is inconclusive if the reaction was due to the combination or an unusual adverse reaction to either agent alone. Until more is known about this potential interaction, avoid concomitant use of ginkgo and trazodone. If the use of both cannot be avoided, use a low dose of trazodone and monitor the patient carefully for signs of excessive sedation.

MODERATE RISK

Low Molecular Weight Heparins, and Thrombolytic Agents: Concomitant use of Ginkgo and these medications may increase the risk of bleeding complications. However, in a randomized, double-blind, crossover study of patients (n=24) receiving stable regimens of warfarin, coadministration of Ginkgo did not affect the International Normalized Ratio (Engelsen et al, 2003). *Clinical Management:* Avoid concomitant use.

OTHER POSSIBLE INTERACTIONS

Anticonvulsants: Ginkgo may precipitate seizures in epileptic patients. *Clinical Management*: Avoid concomitant use of Ginkgo and anticonvulsants in patients with epilepsy. If seizures occur for the first time or recur in patients previously controlled by anticonvulsant medication, inquire about the use of Ginkgo seed or leaf extract. If possible, an assay should be conducted on the specific product to ascertain if 4′-O-methylpyridoxine is present.

Buspirone: The addition of *Ginkgo biloba* and/or St. John's Wort to therapy with buspirone and fluoxetine may have precipitated a hypomanic episode in a case report (Spinella & Eaton, 2002). *Clinical Management:* Caution patients taking buspirone to discuss the use of nonprescription medicines, herbs, and dietary supplements with their doctor or pharmacist. If a patient presents with hypomanic symptoms when taking buspirone, inquire about the use of nonprescription medicines, herbs, and dietary supplements. It is recommended to avoid Gingko in patients taking buspirone, especially in combination with other psychotropic medicines.

Insulin: Theoretically, Ginkgo may alter insulin requirements. Ginkgo increased fasting insulin levels in healthy subjects, though blood glucose levels were not affected (Kudolo, 2000). *Clinical Management:* Caution is advised if Ginkgo is taken with insulin. Monitor blood glucose frequently and monitor for signs and symptoms of hyperglycemia or hypoglycemia.

Monoamine Oxidase Inhibitors: Theoretically, Ginkgo may potentiate the effect of monoamine oxidase inhibitors (MAOIs) (McGuffin et al, 1997). Animal studies have shown that Ginkgo may inhibit monoamine oxidase (Sloley et al, 2000; White et al, 1996. A human study did not demonstrate MAO inhibition in the brain following oral consumption (Fowler et al, 2000). *Clinical Management:* Avoid concomitant use of Ginkgo and monoamine oxidase inhibitors (MAOIs) until this potential interaction is better understood.

Nicardipine: Ginkgo biloba extract reduced the hypotensive effect of nicardipine in rats, suggested to be due to induction of cytochrome P450 (CYP) 3A2 (Shinozuka et al, 2002). Gingko increased expression of cytochrome P450 enzymes CYP2B1/2, CYP3A1, and CYP3A2 and did not affect CYP1A1, 1A2, 2C11, or 4A1 (Shinozuka et al, 2002). The effect of this interaction in humans is unknown. *Clinical Management:* Caution is advised if patients take Ginkgo with nicardipine. Monitor regularly for continued blood pressure control.

Nifedipine: Ginkgo biloba may increase the mean plasma concentration of nifedipine. *Clinical Management:* Caution is advised if patients take Ginkgo with nifedipine.

Omeprazole: Concurrent use may OMEPRAZOLE result in reduced omeprazole effectiveness. *Clinical Management*: Patients taking ginkgo biloba with omeprazole may require a higher dose of omeprazole to retain effectiveness.

Papaverine: Ginkgo may also increase the incidence of adverse effects when used with papaverine. *Clinical Management:* Caution is advised if Ginkgo is taken concurrently with papaverine. Monitor the patient for increased adverse effects of papaverine.

St. Johns Wort: Concurrent use may result in changes in mental status. *Clinical Management:* If a patient presents with hypomanic symptoms, inquire about the use of nonprescription medicines, herbs, and dietary supplements.

Selective Serotonin Reuptake Inhibitors: The addition of *Ginkgo biloba* and/or St. John's Wort to therapy with buspirone and fluoxetine may have precipitated a hypomanic episode in a case report (Spinella & Eaton, 2002). *Clinical Management:* Monitor patients closely for symptoms of serotonin syndrome if Ginkgo is combined with selective serotonin reuptake inhibitors (SSRIs).

Thiazide Diuretics: A case has been reported involving the combination of *Ginkgo biloba* and a thiazide diuretic that caused increased blood pressure (Shaw et al, 1997). It is not known if this represents a true interaction or an unusual adverse reaction to the thiazide diuretic or *Ginkgo biloba. Clinical Management:* Concomitant use of Ginkgo and thiazide diuretics require cautious monitoring. Patients beginning treatment for hypertension should be questioned regarding herbal medication use. Patients with hypertension who plan to use *Gingko biloba* should monitor their blood pressure frequently. Blood pressure changes should be reported to their physician and a decision to continue treatment with Ginkgo should be made based on risk versus potential benefit.

OVERDOSAGE

Ginkgo biloba can act as a potent inhibitor of platelet-activating factor. Chronic use may be associated with increased bleeding time and the risk of spontaneous hemorrhage.

The fruit and leaf contain the antivitamin B6 neurotoxin 4-methylpyridoxine that causes Ginnan-sitotoxism and can lead to coma, convulsions, and death. Most serious cases have involved eating the raw fruits. Analysis of leaves, commercial food made from Ginkgo, and Ginkgo medications have shown the amount of toxin in these products is unlikely to cause toxicity (Arenz et al, 1996). Previous reports had claimed there was no antivitamin B6 in the leaves (Wada et al, 1993).

Alkylphenols, including anacardic or ginkgolic acids, cardanols, and cardols found in crude Ginkgo, can cause toxicity. These compounds lend no value to the therapeutic effects of Ginkgo. The German Commission E restricts their concentration to 5 parts per million (ppm). When multiple human and animal cell lines were incubated with the standardized Ginkgo extract EGb 761 at varying concentrations (2.2 to 3 ppm ginkgolic acids content), a low toxic potential was found. However, the crude Ginkgo extract SL 180 (2.2% ginkgolic acids content) proved much more toxic. During production, alkylphenol-containing fractions are removed from crude Ginkgo. In this experiment, lipid fractions SL 101 and SL 103 contained 26.6% and 58% ginkgolic acids, respectively, and were the most cytotoxic of all fractions in all cell lines investigated (Siegers, 1999).

DOSAGE

Mode of Administration: Ginkgo is available in liquid or solid pharmaceutical forms for oral intake and parenterally for homeopathic use.

How Supplied:

Capsules–30 mg, 40 mg, 50 mg, 60 mg, 100 mg, 120 mg, 260 mg, 400 mg, 420 mg, 440 mg, 450 mg, 500 mg

Extract–50:1

Liquid–40mg/5mL

Tablets–30 mg, 40 mg, 60 mg, 80 mg, 120 mg, 260 mg

Daily Dosage: *Ginkgo biloba* extract should be standardized to contain 24% flavone and 6% terpene lactones: 40 to 80 mg 3 times a day (van Beek, 1998). Studies have demonstrated efficacy with 120 mg daily in 2 to 3 divided doses for dementia, peripheral arterial occlusive disease, and equilibrium disorders like tinnitus or vertigo (Cesarani, 1998; Le Bar, 1998; Peters, 1998).

Chinese Medicine: In traditional Chinese medicine, the daily dose is 3 to 6 g of leaves as an infusion.

Homeopathic Dosage: 5 drops, 1 tablet, or 10 globules every 30 to 60 minutes (acute) or 1 to 3 times daily (chronic); parenterally: 1 to 2 mL acute, 3 times daily; chronic: once a day (HAB1).

Storage: Ginkgo must be protected from light and moisture.

LITERATURE

Abebe W. Herbal medication: potential for adverse interactions with analgesic drugs. *J Clin Pharm Ther*; 27:391-401. 2002.

Adawadkar PD & ElSohly MA. Isolation, purification and antimicrobial activity of anacardic acids from *Ginkgo biloba* fruits. *Fitoterapia*; 52(3):129-135. 1981.

Amri H, Ogwuegbu SO, Boujrad N et al. In vivo regulation of peripheral-type benzodiazepine receptor and glucocorticoid synthesis by *Ginkgo biloba* extract Egb 761 and isolated Ginkgolides. *Endocrinology*; 137(12):5707-5718. 1996.

Amling R. Phytotherapeutika in der Neurologie. In: *ZPT* 12(1):9. 1991.

Anon. Extract of *Ginkgo biloba* (EGb 761). *Presse Med*; 15:1438-1598. 1986.

Anon. Ginkgo und Crataegus. In: *DAZ* 137(20):1751-1753. 1997.

Anon. Phytopharmaka für ältere Menschen: Ginkgo, Kava, Hypericum und Crataegus. In: *DAZ* 135(5):400-402. 1995.

Anon. Psycho-Phytos: Ginkgo, Johanniskraut und Kava-Kava. In: DAZ 135(18):1632-1634. 1995.

Anon. Therapeutic uses of Ginkgo. Lawrence Review, Facts and Comparison, St. Louis, MO, USA: p. 6. 1985.

Anon. Update: Drugs in Pregnancy and Lactation; 13(2):12-13. 2000.

Anon. Wichtiqe Mitteilungen der Arzneimittel Kommission der Duetschen Apotheker. Vorinformation. Wichtiqe Mitteilungen der Arzneimittel Kommission der Duetschen Apotheker. Vorinformation. Ginkgo-biloba- haltiger Trochenextrakt zur Infusion. *DAZ*; 13:1132-1326. 1994a.

Arenz A, Klein M, Fiehe K et al. Occurrence of neurotoxic 4'-O-methylpyridoxine in *Ginkgo biloba* leaves, Ginkgo medications, and Japanese Ginkgo food. *Planta Med*; 62:548-551. 1996.

Atzori C, Bruno A, Chichino G et al. Activity of bilobalide, a sesquiterpene from *Ginkgo biloba* on Pneumocystis carinii. *Antimicrob Agents Chemother*; 37(7):1492-1496. 1993.

Bach D. Behandlung der benignen Prostatahypertrophie. In: *ZPT* 17(4):209-218. 1996.

Barth SA, Inselmann G, Engemann R et al. Influences of *Ginkgo biloba* on cyclosporin A induced lipid peroxidation in human liver microsomes in comparison to vitamin E, glutathione and N-acetylcysteine. *Biochem Pharmacol*; 4(10)1:1521-1526. 1991.

Bauer R, Zschocke S, Medizinische Anwendung von Ginkgo biloba Geschichtliche Entwicklung. In: *ZPT* 17(5):275-283. 1996.

Becker LE & Skipworth GB. Ginkgo-tree dermatitis, stomatitis, and proctitis. *JAMA*; 231(11):1162-1163. 1975.

Benezra C, Ducombs G, Sell Y et al. Plant Contact Dermatitis. BC Decker Inc, Toronto, Canada:58-59. 1985.

Benjamin J, Muir T, Briggs K et al. A case of cerebral haemorrhage–can *Ginkgo biloba* be implicated? *Postgrad Med J*; 77(904):112-113. 2001.

Bent S, Goldberg H, Padula MS, et al. Spontaneous bleeding associated with Ginkgo biloba. A case report and systematic review of the literature. J Gen Intern Med; 20: 657-61. 2005.

Beske F, Kunczik T, Frühzeitige Therapie kann Milliarden sparen. *Der Kassenarzt* 42:36-42. 1991.

Blaha L. Differential diagnose der zerebralen Insuffizienz in der Praxis. *Geriatrie und Rehabilitation* 2,1:23-28. 1989.

Braquet P. Cedemin, a *Ginkgo biloba* extract should not be considered as a PAF antagonist (letter*). Am J Gastroenterol*; 88(12):2138. 1993.

Braquet P (Ed.), Ginkgolides. Chemistry, Biology, Pharmacology and Clinical Perspectives. Vol I. JR Prous Science, Barcelona 1988.

Braquet P (Ed.), Ginkgolides. Chemistry, Biology, Pharmacology and Clinical Perspectives. Vol II, JR Prous Science, Barcelona 1989.

Braquet P. The Ginkgolides: potent platelet-activating factor antagonists isolated from *Ginkgo biloba L*: chemistry, pharmacology and clinical applications. *Drug Future*; 12:643-649. 1987.

Braquet P & Hosford D. Ethnopharmacology and the development of natural PAF antagonists as therapeutic agents. *J Ethnopharmacol*; 32(1-3):135-139. 1991.

Briggs GG, Freeman RK & Yaffe SK. Ginkgo. In: Drugs in Pregnancy and Lactation, 6th ed; 13(2):12-13. 2002.

Brüchert E, Heinrich SE, Ruf-Kohler P. Wirksamkeit von LI 1370 bei älteren Patienten mit Hirnleistungsschwäche. *Münch Med Wschr* 133(Suppl 1):9-14. 1991.

Brun-Pascaud M, Bertrand G, Chau F et al. Activity of bilobalide *against Pneumocystis carinii, Toxicoplasma gondii,* and *Mycobacterium avium* complex in a rat model of triple infection. *Acta Pathol Microbiol Immunol Scand*; 195:22-23. 1997.

Budzinski JW, Foster BC, Vandenhoek S et al. An in vitro evaluation of human cytochrome P450 3A4 inhibition by selected commercial herbal extracts and tinctures. *Phytomedicine*; 7(4):273-282. 2000.

Bundesgesundheitsamt, Empfehlungen zum Wirksamkeitsnachweis von Nootropika im Indikationsbereich ''Demenz'' (Phase III). *Bundesgesundheitsblatt* 7:342-350. 1991.

Burkard G, Lehrl S. Verhältnis von Demenzen vom Multiinfarkt- und vom Alzheimertyp in ärztlichen Praxen. *Münch Med Wschr* 133(Supp. 1):38-43. 1991.

Burns NR, Bryan J, Nettelbeck T. Ginkgo biloba: no robust effect on cognitive abilities or mood in healthy young or older adults.*Hum Psychopharmacol Clin Exp; 21:27 -37. 2006.*

Caesar W, Alles über Ginkgo. In: *DAZ* 134(44):4363. 1994.

Carrier DJ, Consentino G, Neufeld R et al. Nutritional and hormonal requirements of *Ginkgo biloba* embryo-derived callus and suspension cell cultures. *Plant Cell Reports*; 8:635-638. 1990.

Cesarani A, Meloni F, Alpini D et al., Ginkgo biloba (EGb 761) in the treatment of equilibrium disorders. *Adv Ther* Sep-Oct;15(5):291-304. 1998.

Chung KF, Dent G, McCusker M et al., Effect of a ginkgolide mixture (BN 52063) in antagonising skin and platelet responses to platelet activating factor in man. *Lancet* Jan 31;1(8527):248-251. 1987.

Cianfrocca C, Pelliccia F, Auriti A et al. *Ginkgo biloba*-induced frequent ventricular arrhythmia. *Ital Heart J*; 3(11):689-691. 2002.

Cohen AJ & Bartlick B. *Ginkgo biloba* for antidepressant-induced sexual dysfunction. *J Sex Marital Ther*; 24:139-143. 1998.

Cott J. Medicinal plants and dietary supplements: sources for innovative treatments of adjuncts? *Psychopharm Bull*; 31(1):131-137. 1995.

Davydov L & Stirling AL. Stevens-Johnson syndrome with *Ginkgo biloba. J Herb Pharmacother;* 1:65-69. 2001.

DeFeudis FG. *Ginkgo biloba* Extract (EGb 761): Pharmacological Activities and Clinical Applications. Editions Scientifiques Elsevier, Paris, France:68-73. 1991.

Della Loggia R, Sosa S, Tubaro A, Bombardelli E, Anti-inflammatory activity of *Ginkgo biloba* flavonoids. In: *Planta Med* 59(suppl 1): A588. 1993.

Deutsches Institut für medizinische Dokumentation und Information (Hrsg.), ICD-10. Internationale und statistische Klassifikation der Krankheiten und verwandter Gesundheitsprobleme. 10. Revision. Bd 1. Urban & Schwarzenberg, München Wien Baltimore 1994.

Diamond BJ, Shiflett SC, Feiwel N et al. *Ginkgo biloba* extract: mechanisms and clinical indications. *Arch Phys Med Rehabil*; 81(5):668-678. 2000.

Dingermann T, Phytopharmaka im Alter: Crataegus, Ginkgo, Hypericum und Kava- Kava. In: *PZ* 140(23):2017-2024. 1995.

Dorman D, Cote L, Buck W, Effects of an extract of *Gingko biloba* on bromethalin-induced cerebral lipid peroxidation and edema in rats. *Am J Vet Res* Jan;53(1):138-42. 1992.

Dorn M, Bräunig B, Gross HD, Ginkgo-Dragees bei zerebraler Leistungsschwäche. In: *ZPT* 12(6):180. 1991.

Drew S & Davies E. Effectiveness of *Ginkgo biloba* in treating tinnitus: double-blind, placebo controlled trial. *BMJ*; 322:73-75. 2001.

Duche JC, Barre J, Guinot P et al. Effect of Ginkgo biloba extract on microsomal enzyme induction. *Int J Clin Pharmacol Res*; 9(3):165-168. 1989.

Duverger D, DeFeudis FV & Drieu K. Effects of repeated treatments with an extract of *Ginkgo biloba* (EGb 761) on cerebral glucose utilization in the rat: an autoradiographic study. *Gen Pharmacol*; 26(6):1375-1383. 1995.

Elsabagh S, Hartley DE, File SE. Limited cognitive benefits in stage +2 postmenopausal women after 6 weeks of treatment with Ginkgo biloba. *J Psychopharmacol* 173-181. 2005.

Engelsen J, Nielsen JD & Hansen KF. Effect of coenzyme Q10 and gingko biloba on warfarin dosage in patients on long-term warfarin treatment. A randomized, double-blind, placebo-controlled cross-over trial (Abstract-Article in Danish). *Ugeskr Laeger*; 165(18):1868-1871. 2003.

Ermini-Fünfschilling D, Möglichkeiten und Grenzen eines Gedächtnistrainings mit Patienten bei beginnender Demenz. *Z Moderne Geriatrie* 12:459-456. 1992.

Ernst E & Stevinson C. *Ginkgo biloba* for tinnitus: a review. Clin Otolaryngol; 24(3):164-167. 1999.

Fachinformation. Roekan®, Ginkgo extract. Intersan Gmbh, Ettlingen, 1996.

Fachinformation. Tebonin®, Ginkgo extract. Dr Willmar Schwae Gmbh & Co, Karlsruhe, 1996a.

Fang Y, Huang R, Zhang Y et al. A preliminary investigation of tanakan in the treatment of hypertensive arteriosclerosis and stroke in rats. *CMJ*; 113(5):425-428. 2000.

Fessenden JM, Wittenborn W & Clarke L. *Ginkgo biloba*: A case report of herbal medicine and bleeding postoperatively from a laparoscopic cholescystectomy. *Am Surg*; 67(1):33-35. 2001.

Fowler JS, Wang GJ, Volkow ND et al. Evidence that *Ginkgo biloba* extract does not inhibit MAO A and B in living human brain. *Life Sci*; 66(9):141-146. 2000.

Galluzzi S, Zanetti O, Trabucchi M et al. Coma in a patient with Alzheimer's disease taking low-dose trazodone and Ginkgo biloba. J Neurol Neurosurg Psychiatry; 68(5):679-680. 2000.

Gertsch JH, Basnyat B, Johnson EW, et al. Randomised, double blind, placebo controlled comparison of ginkgo biloba and acetazolamide for prevention of acute mountain sickness among Himalayan trekkers: the prevention of high altitude illness trial (PHAIT). BMJ; 328:797-. 2004.

Gertsch JH, Seto TB, Mor J et al. *Ginkgo biloba* for the prevention of severe acute mountain sickness (AMS) starting one day before rapid ascent (abstract). *High Alt Med Biol*; 3(1):29-37. 2002.

Granger AS. *Ginkgo biloba* precipitating epileptic seizures. *Age Ageing*; 30(6):523-525. 2001.

Gräßel E, Vergleich zweier Personengruppen bezüglich der Auswirkungen des mentalen Trainings (''Gehirn-Jogging'') auf die Selbsteinschätzung der Leistungsfähigkeit in Abhängigkeit von der Trainingszeit (Tageszeit der Trainingsdurchführung*). Geriatrie & Rehabilitation* 2,1:44-46. 1989.

Gregory PJ. Seizure associated with *Ginkgo biloba*? *Ann Intern Med*; 134(4):344. 2001.

Haguenauer JP, Cantenot F, Koskas H et al. Treatment of disturbances of equilibrium with Ginkgo biloba extract: a multicenter double-blind drug vs placebo study. Presse Med; 15(31):1569-1572. 1986.

Halama P. *Ginkgo biloba*: Wirksamkeit eines Speczialextrakts bei Patienten mit zerebraler Insuffizienz. *Muench Med Wochenschr*; 133(12):190-194. 1991.

Hartmann A, Schulz V (Hrsg.), *Ginkgo biloba*, Aktuelle Forschungsergebnisse 1990/91. *Münch Med Wschr* 133:1-64. 1991.

Hauns B, Haring B, Kohler S et al. Phase II study cf combined 5-flourouracil/*Ginkgo biloba* extract (GBE 761 ONC) Therapy in 5-flourouracil pretreated patients with advanced colorectal cancer. *Phytotherapy Res*; 15:34-38. 2001.

Hauser D, Gayowski T & Singh N. Bleeding complications precipitated by unrecognized *Ginkgo biloba* use after liver transplantation. *Transpl Int;* 15(7):377-379. 2002.

Hellegouarch A, Baranes J, Clostre F et al. Comparison of the contractile effects of an extract of *Ginkgo biloba* and some neurotransmitters on rabbit isolated vena cava. *Gen Pharmacol*; 16:129-132. 1985.

Hemmeter U, Annen B, Bischof et al. Polysomnographic effect of adjuvant *Ginkgo biloba* therapy in patients with major depression medicated with trimipramine. *Pharmacopsychiatry*; 34:50-59. 2001.

Hofferberth B. Ginkgo-biloba-Spezialextrakt bei Patienten mit hirnorganischem Psychosyndrom. Pruefung der Wirksamkeit mit neurophysiologischenen und psychometrischen Methoden. *Muench Med Wochenschr*; 1133(suppl 1):S30-S33. 1991.

Hopfenmüller W, Nachweis der therapeutischen Wirksamkeit eines *Ginkgo biloba*-Spezialextraktes. Metaanalyse von 11 klinischen Studien bei Patienten mit Hirnleistungsstörungen im *Alter Arzneim Forsch/Drug Res* 44:1005-1013. 1994.

Horsch S, Walther C. Ginkgo biloba special extract EGb 761 in the treatment of peripheral arterial occlusive disease (PAOD) — a review based on randomized, controlled studies. *Int J Clin Pharmacol Ther* 42 (2): 63-72. 2004.

Huguet F & Tarrade T. alpha-2 adrenoceptor changes during cerebral ageing: the effect of *Ginkgo biloba* extract. *J Pharm Pharmacol*; 44(1):24-27. 1992.

Huh H & Staba EJ. The botany and chemistry of *Ginkgo biloba L. J Herbs Spices Med Plant*; 1:91-124. 1992.

Irie J, Murata M, & Homma S. Glycerol-3-phosphate dehydrogenase inhibitors, anacardic acid, from *Ginkgo biloba. Biosci Biotech Biochem;* 60(2):240-243. 1996.

Israel L, Dell'Accio E, Martin G, Hugonot R, Extrait de Ginkgo biloba et exercices d'entra nement de la memoire. Evaluation comparative chez personnes (gées ambulatoi) *Res Psychologie Médicinale* 19(8):1431-1439. 1987.

Jacobs B & Browner W. *Ginkgo biloba*: A living fossil. *Am J Med*; 108:341-342. 2000.

Johnson SK, Diamond BJ, Rausch S, et al. The effect of Ginkgo biloba on functional measures in multiple sclerosis: A pilot randomized controlled trial. *Explore*;2:19-24. 2006.

Joyeux M et al., Comparative antilipoperoxidant, antinecrotic and scavenging properties of terpenes and biflavones from Ginkgo and some flavonoids. In: *Planta Med* 61(2):126-129. 1995.

Jung F, Schahram R, Kiesewetter H et al. Wirkung von *Ginkgo biloba* auf die kutane Mikrozirkulation. *Muench Med Wochenschr*; 133(suppl 1):S44-S46. 1991.

Kampman K, Majewska MD, Tourian K et al. A pilot trial of piracetam and *ginkgo biloba* for the treatment of cocaine dependence. *Addict Behav*; 28(3):437-448. 2003.

Kang B, Lee S, Kim M et al. A placebo-controlled, double-blind trial of *Ginkgo biloba* for antidepressant-induced sexual dysfunction. *Hum Psychopharm Clin Exp;* 17:279-284. 2002.

Kanowski S, Klinischer Wirksamkeitsnachweis bei Nootropika. *Münch Med Wschr* 133:5-8. 1991.

Kanowski S, Herrmann WM, Stephan K, Wierich W, Hörr R, Proof of efficacy of the *Ginkgo biloba* special extract EGb 761 in outpatients suffering from primary degenerative dementia of the Alzheimer type and multi-infarct dementia. *Pharmacopsychiatry* 4:149-158. 1995.

Kim YS, Pyo MK, Park KM et al. Antiplatelet and antithrombotic effects of a combination of ticlopidine and Ginkgo biloba extract (EGb 761). *Thromb Res*; 91(1):33-38. 1998.

Kleijnen J, Knipschild P, *Ginkgo biloba* for cerebral insufficiency. *Br J Clin Pharmac* 35:352-358. 1992a.

Kleijnen J & Knipschild P. *Ginkgo biloba. Lancet;* 340(8828):1136-1139. 1992.

Koch E. Inhibition of platelet activating factor (PAF)-induced aggregation of human thrombocytes by ginkgolides: considerations on possibly bleeding complications after oral intake of Ginkgo biloba extracts. *Phytomed*; 12: 10-16. 2005.

Koalik F et al., Kombinierte Anwendung von nootroper Therapie und kognitivem Training bei chronischen organischen Psychosyndromen. *Neuropsychiatrie* 6:47-52. 1992.

Koc R, Akdemir H, Kurtsoy A et al., Lipid peroxidation in experimental spinal cord injury. Comparison of treatment with *Ginkgo biloba*, TRH and mehtylprednisolone. *Res Exp Med* (Berl);195(2):117-23. 1995.

Koltringer P, Eber O, Lind P et al., Mikrozirkulation und Viskoelastizitaet des Vollblutes *unter Ginkgo-biloba* extrakt. Eine plazebokonntrollierte, randomisierte Douppelblind-Studie. *Perfusion*; 1:28-30. 1989.

Krieglstein J, Neuroprotective properties of *Ginkgo biloba*-constituents. In: *ZPT* 15(2):92-96. 1994.

Kudolo GB. The effect of 3-month ingestion of *Ginkgo biloba* extract on pancreatic beta-cell function in response to glucose loading in normal glucose tolerant individuals. *J Clin Pharmacol*; 40(6):647-654. 2000.

Kurz A, Ginkgo biloba bei Demenzerkrankungen. In: Loew D, Rietbrock N (Hrsg.), *Phytopharmaka.* Steinkopff Verlag, Darmstadt, S 145-149. 1995.

Lanthony P & Cosson JP. Evolution de la vision des couleurs dans la retinopathie diabetique traitee par extrait de *Ginkgo biloba.* Etude perliminaire a double insu contre placebo (French). *J Fr Ophthamol;* 11(10):671-674. 1988.

Le Bars PL, Katz MM, Berman N et al., A placebo-controlled, double-blind, randomized trial of an extract of *Ginkgo biloba* for dementia. North American EGb Study Group. *JAMA* Oct 22-29;278(16):1327-1332. 1997.

Le Bars P, Velasco F, Ferguson J et al. Influence of the severity of cognitive impairment on the effect of the *Ginkgo biloba* extract Egb 761 in Alzheimer's disease. *Neuropsychobiology*;45:19-26. 2002.

Lebuisson DA, Leroy L & Rigal G. Treatment of senile macular degeneration with *Ginkgo biloba* extract: a preliminary double-blind, drug versus placebo study. *Presse Med*; 15(31):1556-1558. 1986.

Lepoittevin JP, Benezra C & Asakawa Y. Allergic contact dermatitis in *Ginkgo biloba L*: relationship with urushiol. *Arch Dermatol Res*; 281(4):227-230. 1989.

Lewis SL & Rowin J. *Ginkgo biloba. Neurology*; 48:1137. 1997.

Lingjaerde O, Foreland AR & Magnusson A. Can winter depression be prevented by *Ginkgo biloba* extract? Placebo-controlled trial. *Acta Psychiar Scand*; 100:62-66. 1999.

Logani S, Chen MC, Tran T et al. Actions of *Ginkgo biloba* related to potential utility for the treatment of conditions involving cerebral hypoxia. Life Sci; 67(12):1389-1396. 2000.

Mahady G. *Ginkgo biloba* for the prevention and treatment of cardiovascular disease: A review of the literature. *J Cardio Nurs*; 16(4):21-32. 2002.

Maitra I, Marcocci L, Droix-Lefaix MT et al. Peroxyl radical scavenging activity of *Ginkgo biloba* extract EGb 761. *Biochem Pharmacol*; 49(11):1649-1655. 1995.

Matthews MK Jr, Association of *Ginkgo biloba* with intracerebral hemorrhage (letter). *Neurology*;50(6):1933-1934. 1998.

Mazza M, Capuano A, Bria P, et al. Ginkgo biloba and donepezil: a comparison in the treatment of Alzheimer's dementia in a randomized placebo-controlled double-blind study. *Eur J Neurology*; 13: 981-985. 2006.

McGovern TW & Barkley TM. Botanical briefs the ginkgo tree-ginkgo biloba L. *Cutis*; 64:154-156. 1999.

Meisel C, Johne A & Roots I. Fatal intracerebral mass bleeding associated with *Ginkgo biloba* and ibuprofen. *Atherosclerosis*; 167(2):367. 2003.

Mitchell JC, Maibach HI & Guin J: Leaves of *Ginkgo biloba* not allergenic for Toxicodendron-sensitive subjects. *Contact Derm;* 7(1):47-48. 1981.

Mitchell J & Rook A. Botanical Dermatology. Greengrass, Vancouver, BC, Canada; 67:317-318. 1979.

Mix JA & Crews WD. An examination of the efficacy of *Ginkgo biloba* extract EGb 761 on the neuropsychologic functioning of cognitively intact older adults. *J Altern Complement Med*; 6(3):219-229. 2000.

Morgenstern C & Biermann E. The efficacy of Ginkgo special extract Egb 761 in patients with tinnitus. *Int J Clin Pharm*; 40(5):188-197. 2002.

Moulton P, Boyko L, Fitzpatrick J et al. The effect of *Ginkgo biloba* on memory in healthy male volunteers. *Physiol Behav*; 73:659-665. 2001.

Mourey M, Morthier F & Mourey A. Activite' antimicrobienne D'extraits de fueilles de *Ginkgo biloba L* (French). *Plant Med Phytother*; 19(4):270-276. 1985.

Muir A, Robb R, McLaren M et al. The use of *Ginkgo biloba* in Raynaud's disease: a double-blind placebo-controlled trial. *Vasc Med*; 7(4):265-267. 2002.

Napryeyenko O, Borzenko I. Ginkgo biloba special extract in dementia with neuropsychiatric features. A randomized, placebo-controlled, double-blind clinical trial. Arzneimittelforschung; 57(1): 4-11. 2007.

Nieder M, Pharmakokinetik der Ginkgo-Flavonole im Plasma. *Münch Med Wschr* 133:61-62. 1991.

Norred CL & Finlayson CA. Hemorrhage after the preoperative use of complementary and alternative medicines. *AANA J*; 68:217-220. 2000.

Oberpichler-Schwenk H, Krieglstein J, harmakologische Wirkungen von *Ginkgo-biloba*-Extrakt und -Inhaltsstoffen. Pharmazie in unserer Zeit 21:224-235. 1992.

Ondrizek RR, Chan PJ, Patton WC, King A. An alternative medicine study of herbal effects on the penetration of zona-free hamster occytes and the integrity of sperm deoxyribonucleic acid. *Fertil Steril* Mar;71(3):517-22. 1999.

Otamiri T, Tagesson C. *Ginkgo biloba* extract prevents mucosa damage associated with small-intestinal ischaemia. *Scand J Gastroenterol*; 24(6):666-670. 1989.

Paick J-S & Lee JH. An experimental study of the effect of *Ginkgo biloba* extact on the human and rabbit corpus cavernosum tissue. J Urol; 156(5):1876-1880. 1996.

Parsad D, Pandhi R & Juneja A. Effectiveness of oral *Ginkgo biloba* in treating limited, slowly spreading vitiligo. *Clin Exp Dermatol;* 28(3):285-287. 2003.

Peters H, Kieser M, Holscher U. Demonstration of the efficacy of *Ginkgo biloba* special extract EGb 761 on intermittent claudication–a placebo-controlled, double-blind multicenter trial. *Vasa* May;27(2):106-10. 1998.

Pfister-Hotz G, Phytotherapie in der Geriatrie. In: *ZPT* 18(3):165-162. 1997.

Pietri S, Seguin JR, d'Arbigny P et al. *Ginkgo biloba* extract (EGb 761) pretreatment limits free radial-induced oxidative stress in patients undergoing coronary bypass surgery. *Cardiovasc Drugs Ther;* 11(2):121-131. 1997.

Pincemail J, Dupuis M, Nasr C et al. Superoxide anion scavenging effect and superoxide dismutase activity of *Ginkgo biloba* extract. *Experimentia*; 45(8):708-712. 1989.

Pittler M & Ernst E. *Ginkgo biloba* extract for the treatment of intermittent claudication: A meta-analysis of randomized trials. *Am J Med*; 108:276-281. 2000.

Porsolt RD, Roux S & Drieu K. Evaluation of a *Ginkgo biloba* extract (EGb 761) in functional tests for monoamine oxidase inhibition. *Arzneim-Forsch/Drug Res*; 50:232-235. 2000.

Ramassamy C, Clostre F, Christen Y et al. Prevention by a *Ginkgo biloba* extract (GBE 761) of the dopaminergic neurotoxicity of MPTP. *J Pharm Pharmacol*; 42(11):785-789. 1990.

Rasetti MF, Caruso D, Galli G et al. Extracts of *Ginkgo biloba L* leaves and *Vaccinium myrtillus* fruits prevent photo-induced oxidation of low-density lipoprotein cholesterol. *Phytomedicine*; 3(4):335-338. 1997.

Reisser CH & Weidauer H. *Ginkgo biloba* extract EGb 761 or pentoxifylline for the treatment of sudden deafness: a randomized, reference-controlled, double-blind study. *Acta Otolaryngol* (Stockh); 121:579-584. 2001.

Rejali D, Sivakumar A, Balaji N. Ginkgo biloba does not benefit patients with tinnitus: A randomized, placebo-controlled, doubleblind trial and meta-analysis of randomized trials. *Clin Otolaryngol Allied Sci*; 29(3): 226-231. 2004.

Reynolds JEF (ed). Martindale: The Extra Pharmacopoeia (electronic version). MICROMEDEX, Inc, Englewood, CO; 1997.

Riederer P, Laux G, Pöldinger W (Hrsg.), Neuropsychopharmaka. Band 5: Parkinsonmittel und Nootropika. Springer Verlag, Wien Noew York, S. 161-324. 1992.

Robak J & Gryglewski RJ. Flavonoids are scavengers of superoxide anions. *Biochem Pharmacol*; 37(5):837-841. 1988.

Roncin JP, Schwartz F & D'Arbigny P. EGB 761 in control of acute mountain sickness and vascular reactivity to cold exposure. *Aviat Space Environ Med*; 67(5):445-452. 1996.

Rosenblatt M, Mindel J, Spontaneous bilateral hyphema associated with ingestion of *Ginkgo biloba* extract (letter). *N Engl J Med.* Apr 10; 336(15):1108. 1997.

Rowin J, Lewis SL, Spontaneous bilateral subdural hematomas associated with chronic *Ginkgo biloba* ingestion (letter). *Neurology* Jun;46(6):1775-1776. 1996.

Rupalla K, Oberpichler-Schwenk H, Krieglstein J, Neuroprotektive Wirkungen des *Ginkgo-biloba*-Extrakts und seiner Inhaltsstofe. In: Loew D, Rietbrock N (Hrsg.) Phytopharmaka in Forschung und klinischer Anwendung. Steinkopff Verlag, Darmstadt, S 17-27. 1995.

Sasaki K, Hatta S, Haga M et al. Effects of bilobalide on gamma-aminobutyric acid levels and glutamic acid decarboxylase in mouse brain. *Eur J Pharmacol*; 367(2-3):165-173. 1999.

Schilcher H, *Ginkgo biloba L.* In: *ZPT* 9:119. 1998.

Schmid M, Schmoll H (Hrsg.), Ginkgo. Wissenschaftliche Verlagsgesellschaft mbH Stuttgart 1994.

Schmid B, In: Schmid, Schmoll gen. Eisenwert: Ginkgo, Ur-Baum und Arzneipflanze, Mythos, Dichtung und Kunst. 1994.

Schneider LS, DeKosky ST, Farlow MR, et al. A randomized, double-blind, placebo-controlled trial of two doses of Ginkgo biloba extract in dementia of the Alzheimer's type. *Curr Alzheimer Res*; 2(5): 541-551. 2005.

Schwabe U, Paffrath D (Hrsg.), Arzneiverordnungsreport '95. Gustav Fischer Verlag, Stuttgart Jena, S 214-224, 373-374. 1995.

Schweizer J & Hautmann C. Comparison of two dosages of *Ginkgo biloba* extract Egb 761 in patients with peripheral arterial occlusive disease Fontaine's stage IIb. *Arzneim-Forsch/Drug Res*; 49(II):900-904. 1999.

Shaw D, Leon C, Kolev S et al. Traditional remedies and food supplements: A 5-year toxicological study (1991-1995). *Drug Saf*; 17(5):342-356. 1997.

Shinozuka K, Umegaki K, Kubota Y et al. Feeding of *Ginkgo biloba* extract (GBE) enhances gene expression of hepatic cytochrome P-450 and attenuates the hypotensive effect of nicardipine in rats. Life Sci; 70(23):2783-2792. 2002.

Siegers CP. Cytotoxicity of alkylphenols from *Ginkgo biloba. Phytomedicine*; 6(4):281-283. 1999.

Sikora R, Sohn M, Deutz F-J et al. Ginkgo biloba extract in the therapy of erectile dysfunction. *J Urol;* 141:188A. 1989.

Sloley BD, Urichik LJ, Morley P et al. Identification of kaempferol as a monoamine oxidase inhibitor and potential neuroprotectant in extracts of *Ginkgo biloba* leaves. *J Pharm Pharmacol*; 52:451-459. 2000.

Solomon P, Adams F, Silver A et al. Ginkgo for memory enhancement. *JAMA*; 288(7):835-840. 2002.

Sowers S, Weary PE, Collins OD, Cnoley EP. Ginkgo tree dermatitis. In: *Arch Dermatol* 81:452-456. 1965.

Spegg H. *Ginkgo biloba* - ein Baum aus Urzeiten, ein Phytopharmakon mit Zukunft. In: *PTA* 4(12):576. 1990.

Spinella M & Eaton LA. Hypomania induced by herbal and pharmaceutical psychotropic medicines following mild traumatic brain injury. *Brain Injury*; 16(4):359-367. 2002.

Sprecher E, Pflanzliche Geriatrika. In: *ZPT* 9(2):40. 1988.

Sticher O. *Ginkgo biloba* - Ein modernes pflanzliches Arzneimittel. Vierteljahresschrift der Naturforschenden Gesellschaft in Zürich 138/3:125-168. 1993.

Sticher O, Hasler A, Meier B. *Ginkgo biloba* - Eine Standortbestimmung. In: *DAZ* 131(36):1827. 1991.

Sticher O. Quality of Ginkgo preparations. In: *PM* 59(1):2-11. 1993.

Struillou L, Cohen Y, Vilde JL et al. *Ginkgo biloba* extract EGb 761 is not active against Mycobacterium avium infection in C57BL/6 mice. Antimicrob Agents Chemother; 39(4):1013-1014. 1995.

Tamborini A & Taurelle R. Value of standardized Ginkgo biloba extract (EGb 761) in the management of congestive symptoms of premenstrual syndrome (abstract) (French). *Rev Fr Gynecol Obstet*; 88(7-9):447-457. 1993.

Tomb RR, Foussereau J & Sell Y. Mini-epidemic of contact dermatitis from Ginkgo tree fruit *(Ginkgo biloba L). Contact Dermatitis;* 19(4):281-283. 1988.

Vale, S, Subarachnoid hemorrhage associated with *Ginkgo biloba. Lancet* Jul 4;352(9121):36. 1998.

Vesper J, Hänsgen KD. Efficacy of *Ginkgo biloba* in 90 Outpatients with Cerebral Insufficiency Caused by Old Age. *Phytomedicine* 1:9-16. 1994.

Volz HP, Hänsel R. *Ginkgo biloba* - Grundlagen und Anwendung in der Psychiatrie. *Psychopharmakotherapie* 1:70-76. 1994.

Volz HP, Hänsel R, Kava-Kava und Kavain in der Psychopharmakotherapie. *Psychopharmakotherapie* 1:33-39. 1994.

Vorberg G. *Ginkgo biloba* extract: a long term study on chronic cerebral insufficiency in geriatric patients. Clin Trials J; 22(2):149-157. 1985.

Vorberg G, Schenk N, Schmidt U, Wirksamkeit eines neuen *Ginkgo-biloba-* Extraktes bei 100 Patienten mit zerebraler Insuffizien. Z Herz & plus; Gefäβe 9:396-401. 1989.

Wada K, Ishigaki S, Ueda K et al. Studies on the constitution of edible and medicinal plants, I: isolation and identification of 4-O-methylpyridoxine, toxic principle from the seed *of Ginkgo biloba. Chem Pharm Bull;* 36(5):1779-1782. 1988.

Wada K, Sasaki K, Miura K et al. Isolation of bilobalide and gingolide A from *Ginkgo biloba L* shortens the sleeping time induced by anesthetics. *Biol Pharm Bull*; 16(2):210-212.- 1993.

Warner J, Butler R, Wuntakal B. Dementia. *Clinical Evidence*; 14: 1198-1220. 2005.

White HL, Scates PW & Cooper BR. Extracts of *Ginkgo biloba* leaves inhibit monoamine oxidase. *Life Sci;* 58(16):1315-1321. 1996.

Wichtl M, Pflanzliche Geriatrika. In: *DAZ* 132(30):1576. 1992.

Wilkens JH, Wilkens H, Uffmann J et al. Effects of a PAF-antagonist (BN 52063) on bronchoconstriction and platelet activation during exercise induced asthma. *Br J Clin Pharm*; 29:85-91. 1990.

Winther K, Randlov C, Rein E et al. Effects of *Ginkgo biloba* extract in cognitive function and blood pressure in elderly subjects. *Curr Ther Res*; 59(12):881-888. 1998.

Woerdenberg HJ, Van Beek TA. *Ginkgo biloba:* In: DeSmet PAGM, Keller K, Hansel R, Chandler RF ed., Adverse Effects of Herbal Drugs. Springer-Verlag Berlin Heidelberg; 3:51-66. 1997.

Yagi M, Wada K, Sakata M et al. Studies on the constituents of edible and medicinal plants. IV. Determination of 4'-O-methylpyridoxine in serum of the patient with Gin-nan food poisoning. *Yakugaku Zasshi*; 113:596-599. 1993.

Zeng X, Lius M, Tang Y, et al. Ginkgo bilorba for acute ischaemic stroke. Cochrane Database of Systematic Reviews 4: CD003691 2005.

Zhang XY, Zhou DF, Su JM et al. The effect of extract of *Ginkgo biloba* added to haloperidol on superoxide dismutase in inpatients with chronic schizophrenia. *J Clin Psych*; 21:85-88. 2001a.

Zhang X, Zhou D, Zhang P et al. A double-blind, placebo-controlled trial of extract of *Ginkgo biloba* added to haloperidol in treatment-resistant patients with schizophrenia. *J Clin Psych*; 62:878-883. 2001.

Zhang X, Zhou DF, Cao LY, et al. The effects of Ginkgo biloba extract added to haloperidol on peripheral T-cell subsets in drug-free schizophrenia: a double-blind, placebo-controlled trial. *Psychopharmacology*. 188(1): 12-17. 2006.

Zhou D, Zhang X, Su J et al. The effects of classic antipsychotic haloperidol plus the extract of *Ginkgo biloba* on superoxide in patients with chronic refractory schizophrenia. *Chin Med J;* 112(12):1093-1096. 1999.

Ginkgo biloba

See Ginkgo

Ginseng

Panax Ginseng

DESCRIPTION

Medicinal Parts: The medicinal part is the dried root.

Flower and Fruit: The inflorescence is simple or branched with 1 to 3 umbels of 15 to 30 flowers. The flowers are androgynous and have greenish-yellow corollas. The ovary is inferior. The fruit is a pea-sized, globular-to-reniform, scarlet, smooth and glossy drupe, which contains 2 seeds.

Leaves, Stem, and Root: The plant is a perennial, and stands erect from 30 to 80 cm high. It has a smooth, round stem and bears terminal whorls of 3 to 5 palmate leaves. The leaflets are thin, finely serrate, gradually acuminate, 7 to 20 cm long and 2 to 5 cm wide. The rhizome tapers at the ends and is often palmate at the tip, giving it a humanlike form.

Habitat: Panax ginseng is indigenous to China. It is cultivated in China, Korea, Japan and Russia.

Production: Ginseng root consists of the dried main and lateral root and root hairs of *Panax ginseng*.

Other Names: American Ginseng, Chinese Ginseng, Five-fingers, Korean Ginseng, Red Berry, Oriental Ginseng

ACTIONS AND PHARMACOLOGY

COMPOUNDS

Triterpene saponins

Aglycone (20S)-protopanaxadiol: including ginsenoside Ra1, Ra2, Ra3, Rb1, Rb2, Rb3, notoginsenoside R4, Rs1, Rs2, Rs3, Rs4, malonylginsenoside Rb1, Rc, Rd

Aglycone (20S)-protopanaxytriol: including ginsenoside Re, Rf, Rg1, notoginsenoside R1

Aglycone oleanolic acid: including ginsenoside Ro, chikusetsusasaponin-V Rb1, Rb2, Rc, Rd, Re, Rg1

Water-soluble polysaccharides: panaxane A to U

Polyynes: including falcarinol (panaxynol), falcarintriol (panaxytriol), examples estered with acetic acid or linolenic acid

EFFECTS

The anti-inflammatory molecules in Ginseng capable of playing a key role in the inflammation-to-cancer sequence are elucidated in a 2007 *Journal of Nutrition* review, which among other evidence cites Ginseng's apparent induction of apoptosis and inhibition of cell proliferation and DNA damage. The herb's potent effects on the inflammatory cascade are described, and reference made to Ginseng's long, traditional use in countering cancers of the stomach, liver, pharynx, color, and pancreas (Hofseth, 2007).

The main active component in Ginseng consists of the ginsenosides, a diverse group of steroidal saponins. There are 25 ginsenosides that have been separated and detected based on the sugar unit sequences and aglycone moieties (Attele, 1999; Fuzzati, 1999; Wang, 1999). The ginsenosides demonstrate the ability to target a myriad of tissues, producing a variety of pharmaceutical responses quite different from one another. A single ginsenoside may initiate multiple or opposing actions in the same tissue, thus making the overall pharmacology of Ginseng complex (Attele, 1999). Commonly used to enhance physical and mental well-being, *Panax ginseng* has long been employed around the world for its adaptogenic qualities. It is primarily indicated in the treatment of fatigue, weakness, and mild depression, though studies also suggest a beneficial effect on serum glucose (Sotaniemi et al, 1995), cholesterol (Li & Zhang, 1988), and the immune system (Scaglione et al, 1996; Yun & Choi, 1990). Other clinical studies of *Panax ginseng* have examined its use against cancer, immunodepression, hyperlipidemia, for enhancement of cardiovascular status, and alleviating symptoms of climacteric in postmenopausal women. *Panax ginseng* has been used in China for various cardiac conditions including heart failure. Limited human studies showed positive results in the use of *Panax ginseng* to decrease blood glucose and hemoglobin A1c in noninsulin dependent diabetics. German Commission E has recommended a general duration of use of Ginseng of up to 3 months.

Adaptogenic Effects: Ginseng was only slightly more effective than placebo and mostly not as effective as a good night's sleep in improving bodily feelings, mood, and fatigue in 12 fatigued night nurses (Hallstrom et al, 1982). Ginseng administration may have a normalizing effect on the body by increasing its natural resistance to physical, chemical, or biological stress without impairing physiological function. Histamine-like fractions and hormonal content, isolated from the Ginseng root, account for the estrogenic effect (Siegel, 1979).

Antineoplastic Effect: In vitro, ginsenoside Rg3 displayed inhibitory activity against the human prostate carcinoma LNCaP cell line. Suppression occurred of the biomarker genes for prostate specific antigen, the androgen receptor, and 5 alpha reductase. Proliferating cell nuclear antigen was also suppressed (Liu et al, 2000). A protopanaxadiol component of Ginseng was shown to inhibit proliferation of pulmonary adenocarcinoma cells resistant to cisplatin (Lee, 1999). Ginsenoside-Rs4 and -Rs3 elevates protein levels of p53 and p21WAF1, which are associated with the induction of apoptosis in human hepatoma cells (Kim, 1999). Ginsenoside Rh2 induces apoptotic cell death in the glioma cell line through activation of caspase and production of oxygen species (Kim, 1999).

Antioxidant Effects: The antioxidant effects of Ginseng protect against oxidative DNA and protein (globin) damage caused by free radicals (Lee, 1998). Antioxidant activity of the herb also provides a hepatoprotective effect by increasing hepatic gluathione peroxidase activity (Voces, 1999). Antioxidant intervention by Ginseng is exerted by weak radical scavenging activity and stimulation of endothelial nitric oxide synthase in cardiac tissue (Maffei, 1999).

Antiplatelet Effects: The antiplatelet components consist of panaxynol and ginsenosides Ro, Rg1, and Rg2 in the diethyl ether and 1-butanol fractions of the herb. Panaxynol inhibits the aggregation, release reaction, and thromboxane formation in platelets while ginsenosides Ro, Rg1, and Rg2 suppress the release reaction only (Kuo, 1990; Teng, 1989). Compared with aspirin, ginsenoside Rg2 at concentrations of 0.5 mmol and 1 mmol produced strong inhibition of platelet aggregation induced by arachidonic acid, collagen, and endotoxin. The ginsenoside R0 inhibited thrombin-induced fibrinogen conversion to fibrin at 0.1 to 1 mmol (p less than 0.01) (Matsuda et al, 1986).

Cognitive Function Effects: The loss of nicotinic receptor binding has been associated with age-related cognitive impairments. Nicotinic receptor stimulation of the central nervous system is beneficial for neuroprotection against age-associated cognitive disorders. A non-ginsenoside component of the herb has demonstrated affinity for the nicotinic receptor. This binding of the compound to the receptor results in nicotinic activity (Lewis, 1999). Ginsenoside-Rg2 and -Rg3 block nicotinic acetylcholine and gamma-aminobutyric acid receptors. This results in an inhibitory effect of the acetylcholine-evoked secretion of catecholamines. (Tachikawa, 1999). These different effects of *Panax ginseng* contribute to the variety of pharmacological effects.

Decrease in Alcohol Levels: The effect of Ginseng in the reduction of blood ethanol levels may be attributed to different mechanisms. Ginseng increases alcohol dehydrogenase and aldehyde dehydrogenase activity at high concentrations due to an augmented induction of the microsomal ethanol oxidizing system. Ginseng enhances blood alcohol clearance in man (Lee, 1987). The ginsenosides also reduce plasma ethanol by a delay in gastric emptying time (Koo, 1999).

Hypolipidemic/Cardiac Effects: A 2006 review identified 34 studies and mixed results for Ginseng's effect on lipids, with overall inconsistency in findings despite 5 of 9 trials showing improvement over baseline in one or more lipid parameters. Studies were also inconsistent overall in showing Ginseng's ability to lower blood glucose. Heterogeneity and small study size have hampered meta-analyses. The authors conclude that well-designed, controlled, and randomized trials are needed to confirm the cardioprotective actions of Ginseng (Buettner, 2006). Ginseng saponins activate lipoprotein lipase, an enzyme that reduces chylomicrons and very low-density lipoproteins (VLDL), and results in a decrease of triglycerides and cholesterol (Inoue, 1999). The ginsenosides demonstrate negative chronotropic effects and positive and negative inotropic effects on the heart. The mechanism is thought to be similar to verapamil (Wu & Chen, 1988). The anti-arrhythmic properties of Rg1 consist of prolonged ventricular refractoriness and repolarization, and increased ventricular fibrillation threshold (Wu, 1995).

Hemolytic Effects: Ginseng as a whole has shown hemostatic action (Kosuge et al, 1981). The saponin part of Ginseng has no specific action on blood, but individual ginsenosides do. The number of sugars in the ginsenosides, and their sterochemical positions, seems to affect the specific activity (Namba et al, 1974). A study done in vitro and in vivo showed that a methanol extract of *P japonicus* promoted the activation of the fibrinolytic system (Matsuda et al, 1989).

Hepatic Effects: Monitoring of elderly patients with drug or alcohol-induced chronic hepatotoxicity receiving a Ginseng extract showed an increased bromosulphthalein excretion and improved serum-zinc concentrations, suggesting liver detoxification (Zuin et al, 1987). The preparation also included multivitamins and trace elements. Hepatoprotective effects have been observed for various ginsenosides. Hepatotoxicity was reduced in cultured rat hepatocytes by administration of ginsenosides (Nakagawa et al, 1985; Hikino et al, 1985). Higher doses of various ginsenosides in both series actually produced cytotoxic actions (Tsang et al, 1986). In another study, Ginseng was administered orally to hepatotoxic rats. The Ginseng appeared to inhibit the increase of serum glutamic oxaloacetic transaminase levels, and to prevent the connective tissue increases in the liver (Matsuda et al, 1991).

Hypoglycemic Effects: The hypoglycemic activity of Ginseng has been attributed to both the polysaccharide and the saponin (ginsenoside) fractions. Isolated rat pancreatic islets studies demonstrated in vitro that ginsenosides stimulated insulin release. This release was independent of extracellular calcium. It appeared that the mechanism involved was different from that of glucose (Guodong & Zhongqi, 1987). Other in vivo rat studies, utilizing an extract of Ginseng, found the number of insulin receptors to be increased in bone marrow and reduced numbers of glucocorticoid receptors in rat brain homogenate (Yushu & Yuzhen, 1988). Both of these effects are thought to contribute to the hypoglycemic activity of Ginseng. Ginsenosides R(b1) and R(g1) are reported to decrease islet insulin concentrations to an undetectable level (Waki et al, 1982).

Uncharacterized components and glycans (polysaccharides often called panaxans) contributed to the hypoglycemic activity in both normal and alloxan-induced hyperglycemic mice administered Ginseng intraperitoneally (Waki et al, 1982; Kimura et al, 1981). Various researchers have found that ginsenosides increased lipogenesis and decreased the blood glucose levels in rats (Sekiya et al, 1987). Korean red Ginseng powder has been found to contain adenosine and pyro-glutamic acid in vitro. It is suggested that these substances inhibited epinephrine-induced lipolysis and stimulated insulin-mediated lipogenesis from glucose in fat cells (Takaku et al, 1990).

Infertility Effects: The saponin fraction of Panax ginseng enhanced sperm motility and progression at the 1-hour and 2-hour mark. Statistically significant results were obtained at both time intervals for sperm motility and at the 1-hour mark for sperm progression (p at least 0.05). Further study to evaluate the clinical significance of these results was suggested by the investigators (Chen et al, 1998).

CLINICAL TRIALS

Cancer Prevention

Ginseng had a preventative effect against cancer in a prospective, cohort, 5-year study of 4,634 subjects over 40 years old. Seventy percent of the group had consumed Ginseng. There was a decreased relative risk (RR) of 0.48 in Ginseng users versus nonusers. The relative risk for fresh Ginseng extract was 0.23. A significant decrease in relative risk of gastric cancer with fresh Ginseng extract intake (RR=0.19) was noted. There was also a significant positive dose-response relationship (Yun, 1996).

Climacteric Syndrome

A small 2006 clinical trial using Ginseng for menopausal hot flashes failed to find effectiveness for this use, notes a *Journal of the American Medical Association* review of alternatives to estrogen for the prevention of hot flashes (Tice, 2006).

However, use of Korean red Ginseng in postmenopausal women with climacteric syndrome appeared to alleviate some symptoms including fatigue, insomnia, and depression. Postmenopausal women with climacteric syndrome (n=12) received Ginseng 6 g daily for 30 days. Postmenopausal women without climacteric syndrome (n=8) were used as controls. After 30 days, scores on the Cornell Medical Index and the State-Trait Anxiety Inventory (A-state) were significantly reduced ($p<0.001$ as compared to before treatment) and were similar to scores recorded in the postmenopausal women without climacteric syndrome. The women treated had a significant decrease in cortisol and cortisol to dehydroepiandrosterone ratio ($p<0.05$). No adverse effects were noted (Tode et al, 1999).

Cognitive Function

A double-blind, placebo-controlled, crossover study in 27 healthy young adults (17 male and 10 female undergraduates) showed that Ginseng extract (100 mg) and glucose (25 g glucose in a drink) both enhanced performance on a mental arithmetic test by participants during the late stages of the demanding task. The 10-minute, computerized "cognitive demand battery" involved such elements as counting by serial 3s and 7s, subtractions, and a 5-minute rapid visual information processing task. The Ginseng and glucose supplements also blunted the increase in subjective feelings of mental fatigue. Blood glucose levels were monitored. The findings point to possible gluco-regulatory actions of Ginseng, and an ability to enhance cognitive performance (Reay, 2007).

The same authors demonstrated in a double-blind, placebo-controlled, balanced crossover study on 30 healthy adults that treatment with Panax ginseng extract leads to significant reductions in blood glucose levels. The most notable behavioral effects were associated with 200 mg of ginseng and included significantly improved subtraction task performance and reduced subjective mental fatigue. (Reay et al, 2005).

A randomized, double-blind, placebo-controlled study was conducted to evaluate the effect of Ginseng on cognitive function over an 8-week period. There were 112 healthy volunteers over 40 years of age. The primary outcome was the change in score on each cognitive test, evaluated at baseline, and again at 8 weeks. Oral standardized Ginseng 400 mg daily was significantly better compared to placebo with abstract thinking and a tendency toward faster simple reaction times. There was no difference between the groups with regard to concentration, memory, or subjective experience (Sorenson & Sonne, 1996).

Diabetes

The effect on blood glucose with Ginseng was demonstrated in a double-blind, placebo-controlled study including 36 newly diagnosed Type 2 diabetic patients. Ginseng 200 mg daily improved glycated hemoglobin, serum aminoterminal-propetptide concentration, and physical activity after 8 weeks of therapy. A 100-mg and 200-mg daily dose of Ginseng elevated mood, improved psychophysical performance, and reduced fasting blood glucose and weight (Sotaniemi et al, 1995).

Erectile Dysfunction

Panax ginseng was found to be an effective alternative to the invasive approaches for treating erectile dysfunction (ED). This was demonstrated in a double-blind, placebo-controlled study of 60 patients with mild or mild-to-moderate ED in which the efficacy of Panax ginseng (1,000 mg, three times daily) and a placebo were compared (deAndrade et al. 2007).

Immunomodulation

Ginseng at 10 mcg/mL significantly enhanced the in vitro natural killer cell function in healthy subjects and those suffering from chronic fatigue syndrome or AIDS ($p<0.01$). It also significantly increased the in vitro antibody-dependent cellular cytotoxicity of peripheral blood mononuclear cells ($p<0.01$). Subjects could not be using medications with immunomodulating effects concomitantly. Blood samples were collected from subjects and treated with Ginseng extract at varying concentrations (See et al, 1997).

The properties of a standardized extract of Ginseng root for inducing a higher immune response in vaccination against influenza were evaluated in 227 volunteers. The multicenter, placebo-controlled, randomized, double-blind, two-arm study was conducted over a 12-week period. Oral standardized Ginseng extract 100 mg daily was given over the entire 12-

week period, with anti-influenza polyvalent vaccination given to all volunteers at week 4. There were significantly fewer cases of influenza or the common cold in the Ginseng-treatment group, and significantly higher antibody titers and natural killer cell levels at 8 and 12 weeks in the Ginseng treatment group (Scaglione et al, 1996).

Stamina

Aerobic exercise performance did not improve following Ginseng supplementation in a 3-week double blind, randomized, placebo-controlled trial with 28 healthy volunteers. Volunteers received 200 mg standardized to 7% *Panax ginseng* every morning 30 minutes prior to breakfast for 21 days. Exercise performance was measured at baseline and after 21 days via evaluation of heart rate, blood pressure, ventilations and their gas fractions, blood samples, and the Borg rate of perceived exertion self-rating scale following a symptom-limited graded exercise test. Although improvements were seen in peak ventilations and heart rate, and volunteers performed slightly longer after Ginseng supplementation, these parameters did not reach statistical significance (Allen et al, 1998).

Vascular Dysfunction

Korean red Ginseng improved vascular endothelial dysfunction in patients with hypertension. Forearm blood-flow changes were measured with plethysmography in 7 hypertensive patients treated with Ginseng, 10 hypertensive patients without Ginseng, and 10 control patients. Patients received red Ginseng 300 mg 3 times daily for approximately 24 months. Endothelial function was measured while receiving 3 vasodilating substances including acetylcholine, bradykinin, and sodium nitroprusside. Patients in the Ginseng-treated hypertensive group had forearm blood flows significantly higher with high-dose acetylcholine (p=0.0008) and they were higher with high dose bradykinin (p=0.04) than those of the nontreated hypertensive patients, but not significantly different from the control group. No differences were seen between groups with the administration of nitroprusside. The authors hypothesized that Korean red Ginseng improves vascular endothelial dysfunction in patients with hypertension through increasing synthesis of nitric oxide (Sung et al, 2000).

INDICATIONS AND USAGE

Approved by Commission E:

- Lack of stamina

Ginseng is used internally as a tonic and fortification in times of fatigue and debility; for declining performance, capacity for work, and concentration; and during convalescence.

Unproven Uses: In Folk medicine, Ginseng is used for loss of appetite, cachexia, anxiety, impotence and sterility, neuralgia, and insomnia.

Chinese Medicine: In Chinese medicine, Ginseng is used for hemoptysis, gastric disturbances, and vomiting.

Homeopathic Uses: Ginseng is used for rheumatism and debility.

PRECAUTIONS AND ADVERSE REACTIONS

Caution should be taken in patients with cardiovascular disease or diabetes. *Panax ginseng* has lowered blood glucose in diabetic and nondiabetic patients (Sotaniemi et al, 1995). General adverse effects include insomnia, epistaxis, headache, nervousness, and vomiting. Estrogenic effects have been observed with Ginseng products, though the exact type of Ginseng (i.e., American, Panax, Siberian) was not reported.

Note: Caution should be used when attributing adverse effects to Ginseng use, due to the lack of standardization of Ginseng products and the not uncommon practice of adulterating Ginseng with less expensive materials such as *Mandragora officinarum, Rauwolfia serpentina*, and *Cola* species. These adulterants are associated with a plethora of adverse reactions (D'Arcy, 1991). Some formulations have been found to contain aminopyrine and phenylbutazone (Anon, 1980).

Cardiovascular: Both hypertension and hypotension have been reported in patients taking Ginseng for 10 days (Kim et al, 1995). Fourteen of 133 patients developed edema in a 2-year study. The patients used a number of different Ginseng products and forms. Twenty-two of 133 patients developed hypertension the same study. The patients used a number of different Ginseng products and forms (Siegel, 1979).

Central Nervous System: Fourteen of 133 patients, who averaged a 3-gram daily dose, developed symptoms of Ginseng abuse (characterized by hypertension with nervousness, sleeplessness, skin eruptions, and diarrhea) in a 2-year study (Ryu & Chien, 1995; Bahrke & Morgan, 1994; Keji, 1981). Twenty-six of 133 patients enrolled in the same study developed sleeplessness; 25 developed nervousness. The patients used a number of different products and forms.

Dermatologic: Thirty-three of 133 patients involved in a 2-year study developed various skin eruptions. The patients used a number of different products and forms (Siegel, 1979). Skin eruptions are an indicator of Ginseng abuse syndrome (Ryu & Chien, 1995).

Endocrine/Metabolic: Case reports suggest estrogenlike activity of Ginseng (Hopkins et al, 1988; Greenspan, 1983; Punnonen & Lukola, 1980; Palmer et al, 1978). Some authors theorize the saponin content of Ginseng interacts with estrogen receptor proteins in a manner similar to ovarian steroids (Punnonen & Lukola, 1980). A reduction in blood glucose has been shown in nondiabetic patients as well, though these patients have not experienced symptomatic hypoglycemia (Hallstrom et al, 1982). Oral Ginseng and Ginseng face cream have been associated with postmenopausal vaginal bleeding (Greenspan, 1983; Hopkins, 1988).

Gastrointestinal: Forty-seven of 133 patients enrolled in a 2-year study developed morning diarrhea. The patients used a number of different products and forms (Siegel, 1979). Morning diarrhea is an indicator of Ginseng abuse syndrome

(Ryu & Chien, 1995). Gastrointestinal complaints were reported in 9 of 227 patients studied by Scaglione et al (1996) and have been reported as a side effect of both Korean Ginseng and Western Ginseng (Kim et al, 1995).

Teratogenicity

Median total morphological scores of rat embryos exposed to ginsenoside Rb1 at a concentration of 30 mcg/mL were significantly lower ($p<0.05$) compared to control embryos (35 vs 45). A lower morphological score suggests possible teratogenicity. When the concentration of ginsenoside Rb1 was increased to 50 mcg/mL, median total morphological scores further decreased to 28. Ginsenoside Rb1 is the major ginsenoside in North American Ginseng and is one of more than 20 ginsenosides that have been identified in commercially available Ginseng extracts. The authors suggest that further studies are warranted to further evaluate potential teratogenic effects of other ginsenosides on embryogenesis. Ginseng use during the first trimester of pregnancy should be cautiously considered (Chan et al, 2003).

DRUG INTERACTIONS

MODERATE RISK

Anticoagulants: In one case report, *Panax ginseng* was suspected to have caused a decrease in INR in a patient previously stabilized on warfarin (Janetsky & Morreale, 1997). *Clinical Management:* Avoid Ginseng use with anticoagulants if possible. If the patient elects to combine therapy, closely monitor PT/INR.

Diabetic Agents/Insulin: Ginseng has been shown to have hypoglycemic effects. An interaction between Ginseng and antidiabetic agents has not been reported in the literature to date, but is theoretically possible based on the mechanism of action of Ginseng. *Clinical Management:* Monitor blood glucose closely in patients taking Ginseng with antidiabetic agents. In patients having difficulty establishing blood glucose control, it is recommended to avoid concomitant use of Ginseng and antidiabetic agents.

Estrogen: Case reports suggest estrogen-like activity of Ginseng (Greenspan, 1983; Punnonen & Lukola, 1980; Palmer et al, 1978). Concomitant use of Ginseng with conjugated estrogens may result in symptoms of estrogen excess or interference. *Clinical Management:* Since estrogenic effects have been noted with topical and oral estrogen, either dosage form should be treated with the same caution when coadministered with Ginseng. If estrogenic symptoms such as mastalgia and breakthrough menstrual bleeding occur, decrease the Ginseng dosage. Because of the apparent estrogen-like effect, avoid Ginseng in patients with breast cancer, undiagnosed abnormal genital bleeding, active thrombophlebitis or thromboembolic disorders, or if the woman is pregnant.

Loop Diuretics: Concurrent use may result in increased risk of diuretic resistance. *Clinical Management:* Patients should be advised to discontinue use of Ginseng and germanium-supplemented Ginseng products while taking loop diuretics.

Monoamine Oxidase Inhibitors (MAOIs): Two case reports suggest that Ginseng when taken with phenelzine may result in insomnia, tremor, headache, agitation, and worsening of depression suggestive of manic-type symptoms (Jones & Runikis, 1987; Shader & Greenblatt, 1985). *Clinical Management:* Patients should be advised to avoid use of any Ginseng products while taking an MAOI and for several weeks after discontinuation.

Nifedipine: Ginseng increased the mean plasma concentration of nifedipine by 53% at 30 minutes in an open trial of 22 healthy subjects. Effects at other time points were not reported (Smith et al, 2001). *Clinical Management:* Caution is advised if patients take Ginseng with nifedipine.

POTENTIAL INTERACTIONS

Albendazole: Panax ginseng significantly accelerated the intestinal clearance of albendazole sulfoxide (the active metabolite of albendazole) when co-administered to rats. The plasma AUC for albendazole sulfoxide was unchanged, as was the intestinal elimination of the inactive metabolite albendazole sulfone (Merino et al, 2003). *Clinical Management:* Monitor therapeutic efficacy of albendazole.

Drug-Lab Modifications

Digoxin Assay: Asian (Panax) Ginseng provoked digoxinlike immunoreactivity in human serum when digoxin serum concentration was measured by fluorescence polarization immunoassay (FPIA); conversely, false reductions occurred in digoxin concentrations in sera exposed to Ginseng and then measured by the microparticle enzyme immunoassay (MEIA) method (Dasgupta et al, 2003). Similar results occurred in another ex vivo study, where apparent digoxinlike reactivity occurred in digoxin-naïve sera (Chow et al, 2003). Ginseng interferes with digoxin immunoassay because of the molecular structural similarity between *Panax ginseng* and digoxin (Dasgupta et al, 2003; Chow et al, 2003). *Clinical Management:* The clinician should explore the possibility of a false elevation or depression in digoxin concentration due to ingestion of Asian Ginseng. The following digoxin immunoassay instruments may not be falsely altered in the presence of *Panax ginseng*: the Enzyme Multiplied Immunoassay (EMIT: Dade Behring); Chemiluminescent assay (CLIA; Bayer Diagnostics); Randox digoxin assay (Randox Laboratories); Beckman digoxin assay (Beckman).

OVERDOSAGE

Palpitations, insomnia, pruritus, heart pain, decreased sexual potency, vomiting, hemorrhagic diathesis, headache, and epistaxis have all been reported infrequently. Ingestion of large amounts is said to be fatal (Baranov, 1982). Massive overdosages can bring about Ginseng Abuse Syndrome, which is characterized by hypertension, nervousness, insomnia, hypertonia, edema, morning diarrhea, inability to concentrate, and skin eruptions. It may occur after 1 to 3 weeks of ingestion of 3 g/d of Ginseng root (Ryu & Chien, 1995). Weakness and tremor were seen in one patient upon withdrawal. Large doses may cause insomnia, depression, and nervous disorders (Siegel, 1979). About 10% of volunteers taking Ginseng developed this complex (Anon, 1980a).

DOSAGE

Mode of Administration: Comminuted drug infusions, powder and galenic preparations for internal use. Various standardized preparations containing Ginseng root are available.

How Supplied:

Capsules — 50 mg, 100 mg, 150 mg, 200 mg, 250 mg, 404 mg, 405 mg, 410 mg, 424 mg, 470 mg, 500 mg, 505 mg, 520 mg, 535 mg, 560 mg, 648 mg,1000 mg, 1250 mg

Liquid — 300 mg/mL

Tablet — 350 mg, 500 mg

Preparation: To make an infusion, pour boiling water over 3 g comminuted drug and strain after 5 to 10 minutes.

Daily Dosage: The average daily dosage is 1 to 2 g root. The infusion may be taken 3 to 4 times a day over 3 to 4 weeks.

Cognitive Function — Oral standardized Ginseng 400 mg daily was effective in improving cognitive function (Sorenson, 1996).

Hypoglycemic Effects — Dosage of 100 to 200 mg of oral standardized Ginseng has been effective in Type 2 diabetic patients (Sotaniemi, 1995).

Antiviral — Studies have proven efficacy in addition vaccination with 100 to 200 mg daily of oral standardized Ginseng extract (Scaglione, 1996).

Erectile Dysfunction — Korean Red Ginseng given orally as 600 mg three times daily has been effective (Choi, 1995).

Physical and Psychological Performance Capacity (lack of stamina) — Ginsana given 100 mg twice daily has improved oxygen capacity, reduction of maximum stress frequency, increase in ling function parameters and shortened reaction time to visual stimulants after 11 weeks (Forgo, 1985).

Homeopathic Dosage: 5 drops, 1 tablet, 5 to 10 globules or 1 mL injection solution sc twice weekly.

LITERATURE

Abebe W. Herbal medication: potential for adverse interactions with analgesic drugs. *J Clin Pharm Ther.* Dec;27(6):391-401. 2002.

Allen J, McLung J & Nelson A: Ginseng supplementation does not enhance healthy young adults' peak aerobic exercise performance. *J Am Coll Nutr*; 17(5):462-466. 1998.

Anon. Ginseng. Med Lett Drugs Ther; 22(17):72. 1980.

Anon. Ginseng: the root of the problem. Emerg Med; 12:124-126. 1980a.

Anon, Kann Ginseng die Leistungsfähigkeit erhöhen? In: *DAZ* 132(12):XLVIII. 1992.

Anon. Mythos-Tonikum-Arzneimittel. Ginsengextrakt bei Atemwegserkrankungen. In: *DAZ* 134(26):2461. 1994.

Attele AS; Wu JA; Yuan CS. Ginseng pharmacology: multiple constituents and multiple actions. *Biochem Pharmacol* Dec 1;58(11):1685-93. 1999.

Avakian EV et al. *Planta Med* 50:151. 1984.

Awang DV. Maternal use of ginseng and neonatal androgenization. *JAMA* Jul 17;266(3):363. 1991.

Bahrke M. Comments on "Manic episode and ginseng: report of a possible case." *J Clin Psychopharmacol*; 17(2):140-141. 1997.

Bahrke M & Morgan W. Evaluation of the ergogenic properties of ginseng. Sports Med; 18:229-248. 1994.

Baldwin CA et al. *Pharm J* 237:583. 1986.

Baranov AI: Medicinal uses of ginseng and related plants in the Soviet Union: recent trends in the Soviet literature. *J Ethopharmacol;* 6:339-359. 1982.

Bauer R. Neues von "immunmodulierenden Drogen" und "Drogen mit antiallergischer und antiinflammatorischer Wirkung". In: *ZPT* 14(1):23-24. 1993.

Becker BN; Greene J; Evanson J et al. Ginseng-induced diuretic resistance. *JAMA* Aug 28;276(8):606-607. 1996.

Blasius H. Phytotherapie: Adaptogene Wirkung von Ginseng. In: *DAZ* 135(23):2136-2138. 1995.

Buettner C, Yeh GY, Phillips RS, et al. Systematic review of the effects of ginseng on cardiovascular risk factors. *Ann Pharmacother*; 40 (1): 83-96. 2006.

Caesar W. Ginsengwurzel in Europa. Eine alte Geschichte. In: *DAZ* 131(19):935. 1991.

Chan LY, Chiu PY & Lau TK. An in-vitro study of ginsenoside Rb1-induced teratogencity using a whole rat embryo culture model. *Hum Reprod*; 18(10):2166-2168. 2003.

Chang YS, Pezzuto JM, Fong HHS, et al. Evaluation of the mutagenic potential of American ginseng (*Panax quinquefolius*). *Planta Med*; 4:338-339. 1986.

Chen J, Xu M, Chen L et al. Effect of Panax notoginseng saponins on sperm motility and progression in vitro. *Phytomed*; 5(4):289-292. 1998.

Cheng T. Ginseng - is there a use in clinical medicine? (letter). *Postgrad Med J*; 64:427. 1989.

Choi H, Seong D, Rha K. Clinical efficacy of Korean red ginseng for erectile dysfunction. *Int J Impot Res* Sep;7(3):181-6. 1995.

Choi Y, Rha K, Choi H. In vitro and in vivo experimental effect of Korean red ginseng on erection. *J Urol* Oct;162(4):1508-11. 1999.

Chong SKF & Oberholzer VG. Ginseng - is there a use in clinical medicine? *Postgrad Med J*; 64:841-846. 1988.

Chow L, Johnson M, Wells A. Effect of the traditional Chinese medicines Chan Su, Lu-Wan-Shen, and Asian ginseng on serum digoxin measurement by Tina-quant (Roche) and Synchron LX System (Beckman) digoxin immunoassays. *J Clin Lab Anal*; 17:22-27. 2003.

Cui J, Eneroth P & Bjoerkhem I. What do commercial ginseng preparations contain? *Lancet*; 344:134. 1994.

D'Arcy PF. Adverse reactions and interactions with herbal medicines. Part 1. Adverse reactions. *Adverse Drug React Toxicol Rev*; 10:189-208. 1991.

Dasgupta A, Sang W, Actor J et al. Effect of Asian and Siberian ginseng on serum digoxin measurement by five digoxin immunoassays. *Am J Clin Pathol*; 119(2):298-303. 2003.

deAndrade E, de Mesquita AA, Claro Ide A, et al. Study of the efficacy of Korean Red Ginseng in the treatment of erectile dysfunction. Asian J Androl; 9(2): 241-244. 2007.

Dega H, Laporte JL, Frances C et al. Ginseng as a cause for Stevens-Johnson syndrome? *Lancet*; 347:1344. 1996.

Filaretov AA, Bogdanova TS, Podvigina TT et al. Role of pituitary-adrenocortical system in body adaptation abilities. *Exp Clin Endocrinol*; 92:129-136. 1988.

Forgo I, Schimert G. Zur Frage der Wirkungsdauer des standardisierten Ginseng-Extraktes G 115 bei gesunden Leistungssportiern. *Notabene medici* 9:636-649. 1985.

Fulder SJ, *Am J Chin Med* 9:112. 1981.

Fuzzati N; Gabetta B; Jayakar K et al. Liquid chromatography-electrospray mass spectrometric identification of ginsenosides in *Panax ginseng* roots. *J Chromatogr A* Aug 27;854(1-2):69-79. 1999.

Greenspan EM. Ginseng and vaginal bleeding. *JAMA* Apr 15;249(15):2018. 1983.

Guodong L, Zhongqi L. Effects of ginseng saponins on insulin release from isolated pancreatic islets of rats. *Chin J Integr Trad Western Med*;7:326. 1987.

Hah JS, Kang BS, Kand DH. Effect of Panax ginseng alcohol extract on cardiovascular system. *Yonsei Med J*; 19:11-18. 1978.

Halladay A, Yu Y, Palmer J et al. Acute and chronic effects of ginseng total saponin and amphetamine on fixed-interval performance in rats. *Planta Med*; 65:162-164. 1999.

Hallstrom C, Fulder S & Carruthers M. Effects of ginseng on the performance of nurses on night duty. *Comp Med East and West*; 6(4):277-282. 1982.

Hammond T & Whitworth J. Adverse reactions to ginseng (letter). *Med J Aust*; 1:492. 1981.

Hansen L, Boll PM, *Phytochemistry* 25(2):285. 1986.

Hikino H, Kiso Y, Kinouchi J et al. Antihepatoxic actions of ginsenosides from *Panax ginseng* roots. *Planta Med*; 51:62-64. 1985.

Hirakura K, Morita M, Nakajima K, Ikeya Y, Mitsuhashi H, Polyacetylenes from them roots *of Panax ginseng.* In: *PH* 30:3327-3333. 1991.

Hofseth L, Wargovich M. Inflammation, cancer, and targets of Ginseng. *J Nútr*; 137:183S-185S. 2007.

Hopkins M, Androff L, Benninghoff A. Ginseng face cream and unexplained vaginal bleeding. *Am J Obstet Gynecol, 159:1121-*1122. 1988.

Hyo-Won B, Il-Heok K, Sa-Sek H, Byung-Hun H, Mun-Hae H, Ze-Hun K, Nak-Du K, Roter Ginseng. Schriftenreihe des Staatlichen Ginseng-Monopolamtes der Republik Korea. 1987.

Inoue M; Wu CZ; Dou DQ et al. Lipoprotein lipase activation by red ginseng saponins in hyperlipidemia model animals. *Phytomedicine* Oct;6(4):257-65. 1999.

Janetzky K & Morreale AP. Probable interaction between warfarin and ginseng. *Am J Health-Syst Pharm*; 54:692-693. 1997.

Jones BD; Runikis AM. Interaction of ginseng with phenelzine. *J Clin Psychopharmacol* Jun;7(3):201-202. 1987.

Joo CN. Some biochemical effects of saponin fraction of *Panax ginseng* CA Meyer. *Korean J Ginseng Sci*; 16:53-63. 1992.

Keji C. The effect and abuse syndrome of ginseng. J Trad Chin Med; 1:69-72. 1981.

Kim HE, Oh JH, Lee SK, Oh YJ. Ginsenoside RH-2 induces apoptotic cell death in rat C6 glioma via a reactive oxygen and caspase dependent but Bcl-X(L)-independent pathway. *Life Sci*;65(3):PL33-40. 1999.

Kim H-S, Jang C-G & Lee M-Kl. Antinarcotic effects of the standardized ginseng extract G115 on morphine. *Planta Med*; 56:158-163. 1990.

Kim SE; Lee YH; Park JH; Lee SK. Ginsenoside-Rs3, a new diol-type ginseng saponin, selectively elevates protein levels of p53 and p21WAF1 leading to induction of apoptosis in SK-HEP-1 cells. Anticancer Res Jan-Feb;19(1A):487-91. 1999.

Kim SE; Lee YH; Park JH; Lee SK. Ginsenoside-Rs4, a new type of ginseng saponin concurrently induces apoptosis and selectively elevates protein levels of p53 and p21WAF1 in human hepatoma SK-HEP-1 cells. *Eur J Cancer* Mar;35(3):507-11. 1999.

Kim SH, Lee SR, Do JH et al. Effects of Korean red ginseng and western ginseng on body temperature, pulse rate, clinical symptoms and the hematological changes in humans. *Korean J Ginseng Sci*; 19:1-16. 1995.

Kimura M, Waki I, Tanaka O et al. Pharmacological sequential trials for the fractionation of components with hypoglycemic activity in alloxan diabetic mice from Ginseng radix. *J Pharm Dyn*; 4:402-409. 1981.

Kitigawa I, *Yaligali Zasshi* 103:612. 1983.

Kobayashi S et al. Inhibitory actions of phospholipase A(2) and saponins including ginsenoside R(b1) and glycyrrhizin on the formation of nicotinic acetylcholine receptor clusters on cultured mouse myotubes. *Phytother Res*; 4:106-111. 1990.

Konno C, Murakami M, Oshima Y et al. Isolation and hypoglycemic activity of panaxans Q, R, S, T, and U, glycans of Panax ginseng roots. *J Ethopharmacol*; 14:69-74. 1985.

Konno C, Sugiyama K, Kano M et al. Isolation and hypoglycaemic activity of panaxans A, B, C, D, and E, glycans of Panax ginseng roots. Planta Med; 50:434-436. 1984.

Koo MW. Effects of ginseng on ethanol induced sedation in mice. *Life Sci*;64(2):153-60. 1999.

Kuo SC; Teng CM; Lee JC et al. Antiplatelet components in *Panax ginseng. Planta Med* Apr;56(2):164-167. 1990.

Lee FC; Ko JH; Park JK; Lee JS. Effects of *Panax ginseng* on blood alcohol clearance in man. *Clin Exp Pharmacol Physiol* Jun;14(6):543-546. 1987.

Lee BM, Lee SK, Kim HS. Inhibition of oxidative DNA damage, 8-OhdG, and carbonyl contents in smokers treated with antioxidants (vitamin E, vitamin C, beta-carotene and red ginseng). *Cancer Lett Oct* 23;132(1-2):219-27. 1998.

Lee MO, Clifford DH, Kim CY et al. Effects of the first (ether) extract of ginseng on the cardiovascular dynamics of dogs during halothane anesthesia. *Comp Med East West*; 6:115-121. 1978.

Lee SJ; Sung JH; Lee SJ et al. Antitumor activity of a novel ginseng saponin metabolite in human pulmonary adenocarcinoma cells resistant to cisplatin. *Cancer Lett* Sep 20;144(1):39-43. 1999.

Lei XL & Chiou GC. Cardiovascular pharmacology of Panax notoginseng (Burk) F.H. Chen and Salvia militiorrhiza. *Am J Chin Med*; 14:145-152. 1986.

Lewis R; Wake G; Court G et al. Non-ginsenoside nicotinic activity in ginseng species. *Phytother Res* Feb;13(1):59-64. 1999.

Li XJ & Zhang Bh. Studies on the antiarrhythmic effects of panaxatriol saponins (PTS) isolated from Panax notoginseng. *Acta Pharm Sin*; 23:168-173. 1988.

Liu WK, Xu SX & Che CT. Anti-proliferative effect of Ginseng saponins on human prostate cancer cell line. *Life Sci*; 67(11):1297-1306. 2000.

Maffei F, Carini M, Aldini G, et al. *Panax ginseng* administration in the rat prevents myocardial ischemia-reperfusion damage induced by hyperbaric oxygen: evidence for an antioxidant intervention. *Planta Med* Oct;65(7):614-9. 1999.

Matsuda H et al., *Chem Pharm Bull* 34(3):1153. 1986.

Matsuda H, Nambia K, Fukuda S et al. Pharmacological study on *Panax ginseng* C.A. Meyer IV: effect of red ginseng on experimental disseminated intravascular coagulation, (3): effect of ginsenoside-Ro on blood coagulative and fibrinolytic system. *Chem Pharm Bull*; 34:2100-2104. 1986.

Matsuda H, Samukawa K-I, Fukuda S et al. Studies of *Panax japonicus fibrinolysis. Planta Med;* 55:18-21. 1989.

Matsuda H, Samukawa K-I & Kubo M. Anti-hepatic activity of ginsenoside R(o1). *Planta Med*; 57:523-526. 1991.

Merino G, Molina AJ, Garcia JL et al. Ginseng increases intestinal elimination of albendazole sulfoxide in the rat. *Comp Biochem Physiol C Pharmacol Toxicol*; 136(1):9-15. 2003.

Nakagawa S, Yoshida S, Hirao Y et al. Cytoprotective activity of components of garlic, ginseng and ciuwjia on hepatocyte injury induced by carbon tetrachloride in vitro. *Hiroshima J Med Sci*; 34:303-309. 1985.

Newall C, Anderson L & Phillipson J. Ginseng, Panax. Herbal Medicines: A Guide for Health Care Professionals. London. The Pharmaceutical Press:145-150. 1996.

Ng TB, Li WW & Yeung HW. Effects of ginsenosides, lectins and Momordica charantia insulin-like peptide on corticosterone production by isolated rat adrenal cells. *J Ethopharmacol*; 21:21-29. 1987.

Obermeier A, Zur Analytik der Ginseng- und Eteutherococcusdroge. Dissertation Ludwig-Maximilians-Universität München. 1980.

Oh KW, Kim HS & Wagner GC. Ginseng total saponins inhibits the doperaminergic depletions induced by methamphetamines. *Planta Med*; 63:80-81. 1997.

Oshima Y, Sato K & Hikino Hl. Isolation and hypoglycemic activity of quinquefolans A, B, and C, glycans of Panax quinquefolium roots. *J Nat Prod*; 50:188-190. 1987.

Palmer BV, Montgomery ACV & Monteiro JCMP. Gin Seng and mastalgia. *BMJ*;1:1284. 1978.

Peigen X & Keji C. Recent advances in clinical studies of Chinese medicinal herbs, 2: Clinical trials of Chinese herbs in a number of chronic conditions. *Phytother Res*; 2:55-60. 1988.

Petkov VD et al., Memory effect of standardized extracts of *Panax ginseng (*G 115), Ginkgo biloba(GK 501) and their combination Gincosan (PHL-00701). In: *PM* 59(2).106. 1993.

Pfister-Hotz G, Phytotherapie in der Geriatrie. In: *ZPT* 18(3):162-165. 1997.

Phillipson JD & Anderson LA. Ginseng- quality, safety, and efficacy? Pharm J; 232:161-165. 1984.

Porrath SA. Hormonal effects of ginseng tea. *Med Aspects Hum Sexuality*; 117. 1986.

Ploss E, Panax ginseng C. A. Meyer. Wissenschaftlicher Bericht. Kooperation Phytopharmaka, Köln Bonn Frankfurt Bad Homburg. 1988.

Punnonen R; Lukola A. Oestrogen-like effect of ginseng. Br Med J Oct 25;281(6248):1110. 1980. Ramarao P & Bhargava HN: Antagonism of the acute pharmacological actions of morphine by Panax ginseng extract. *Gen Pharmacol*; 21:877-880. 1990.

Reay JL, Kennedy DO, Scholey AB. Single dose of Panax ginseng (G115) reduces blood glucose levels and improve cognitive performance during sustained mental activity. *J Psychopharmacol*; 19(4): 357-365. 2005.

Reay JL, Kennedy DO, Scholey AB. Effects of Panax ginseng, consumed with and without glucose, on blood glucose levels and cognitive performance during sustatained ''mentally demanding'' tasks. *J Psychopharmacol*; 20 (6): 771-781. 2006.

Rhee YH, Ahn JH, Choe J et al. Inhibition of mutagenesis and transformation by root extracts *of Panax ginseng* in vitro. *Planta Med*; 57:125-128. 1991.

Ro JY; Ahn YS; Kim KH. Inhibitory effect of ginsenoside on the mediator release in the guinea pig lung mast cells activated by specific antigen-antibody reactions. *Int J Immunopharmacol* Nov;20(11):625-41. 1998.

Ryu S & Chien Y. Ginseng-associated cerebral arteritis. *Neurology*; 45:829-830. 1995.

Saksena AK et al. Effect of Withania somnifera and *Panax ginseng* on dopaminergic receptors in rat brain during stress. *Planta Med*; 55:95. 1989.

Sanai T, Oochi N, Okuda S, et al. Subacute nephrotoxicity of germanium dioxide in the experimental animal. *Toxicol Appl Pharmacol* Apr;103(2):345-53. 1990.

Scaglione F; Cattaneo G; Alessandria M, et al. Efficacy and safety of the standardised Ginseng extract G115 for potentiating vaccination against the influenza syndrome and protection against the common cold [corrected]. *Drugs Exp Clin Res*;22(2):65-72. 1996.

See DM, Broumand N, Sahl L et al. In vitro effects of Echinacea and ginseng on natural killer and antibody-dependent cell cytology in healthy subjects and chronic fatigue syndrome or acquired immunodeficiency syndrome patients. Immunopharmacology. 35;30:229-235. 1997

Sekiya K, Okuda H, Hotta Y et al. Enhancement of adipose differentiation of mouse 3T3-L1 fibroblasts by ginsenosides. *Phytother Res;* 1:58. 1987.

Shader RI & Greenblatt DJ. Phenelzine and the dream machine – ramblings and reflections (editorial). *J Clin Pharmacol*; 5:65. 1985.

Siegel RK. Ginseng abuse syndrome: problems with the panacea. *JAMA*; 241:1614-1615. 1979.

Siegel RK, Ginseng and the high blood pressure. *JAMA* 243:32. 1980.

Singh VK, George CX, Singh N, et al. Combined treatment of mice with *Panax ginseng* extract and interferon inducer. Amplification of host resistance to Semliki forest virus. *Planta Med.* Apr;47(4):234-6. 1983.

Singh VK, Agarwal SS, Gupta BM. Immunomodulatory activity of *Panax ginseng* extract. Planta Med Dec;50(6):462-5. 1984.

Smith M, Lin KM & Zheng YP. An open trial of nifedipine-herb interactions: nifedipine with St. John's Wort, ginseng, or *Ginkgo biloba* (abstract). *Clin Pharmacol Ther*; 69(2):P86. 2001.

Sonnenborn U, Proppert Y, Ginseng (Panax ginseng C.A. Meyer). *Z Phytotherapie* 11:35-49. 1990.

Sorensen H, Sonne J. A double-masked study of the effects of ginseng on cognitive functions. *Curr Ther Res*;57:959-968. 1996.

Sotaniemi E, Haapakoski E, Rautio A. Ginseng therapy in non-insulin-dependent diabetic patients. *Diabetes Care* Oct;18(10):1373-1375. 1995.

Sprecher E, Pflanzliche Geriatrika. In: *ZPT* 9(2):40. 1988.

Sprecher E, Phytotherapeutika als Wunderdrogen? Versuch einer Bewertung. In. *ZPT* 10(1):1. 1989.

Sung J, Han KH, Zo JH et al. Effect of red ginseng upon vascular endothelial function in patients with essential hypertension. *Am J Chin Med*; 28(2):205-216. 2000.

Sun X-B, Matsumoto T & Yamada H. Purification of an anti-ulcer polysaccharide from the leaves of panax ginseng. *Planta Med*; 58:445-448. 1992.

Tachikawa E; Kudo K; Harada K et al. Effects of ginseng saponins on responses induced by various receptor stimuli. *Eur J Pharmacol* Mar 12;369(1):23-32. 1999.

Takahashi M, Yoshikura M, Yakugaku Zasshi 86:1051 and 1053. 1966.

Takaku T, Kameda K, Matsuura Y et al. Studies on insulin-like substances in Korean red ginseng. *Planta Med*; 56:27-30. 1990.

Teng CM; Kuo SC; Ko FN et al. Antiplatelet actions of panaxynol and ginsenosides isolated from ginseng. *Biochim Biophys Acta* Mar 24;990(3):315-20. 1989.

Tode T, Kikuchi Y, Hirata J et al. Effect of Korean red ginseng on psychological functions in patients with severe climacteric syndromes. Int J Gynecol Obstet; 67:169-174. 1999.

Tsang D, Ho KW, Tse TK et al. Ginensoside modulates K+ stimulated noradrenaline release from rat cerebral cortex slices. *Planta Med*; 52:266-268. 1986.

Voces J, Alvarez A, Vila L, et al. Effects of administration of the standardized *Panax ginseng* extract G115 on hepatic antioxidant function after exhaustive exercise. *Comp Biochem Physiol C Pharmacol Toxicol Endocrino l* Jun;123(2):175-84. 1999.

Vuksan V, Sievenpiper JL, Koo VYY et al. American Ginseng (Panax quinquefolius) reduces postprandial glycemia in nondiabetic subjects and subjects with Type 2 diabetes mellitus. *Arch Intern Med;* 160(7):1009-1013. 2000.

Vuksan V, Stavro SP, Sievenpiper JL et al. Similar postprandial glycemic reductions with escalation of dose and administration time of American ginseng in type 2 diabetes. *Diabetes Care*; 23(9):1221-1226. 2000a.

Waki I, Kyo H, Yasuda M et al. Effects of a hypoglycemic component of Ginseng radix on insulin biosynthesis in normal and diabetic animals. *J Pharm Dyn*; 5:547-554. 1982.

Wang B, Yang M, Jin Y, Liu P. Studies on the mechanism of ginseng polypeptide induced hypoglycemia. *Yao Hsueh Hsueh Pao*;25(10):727-31. 1990.

Wang X; Sakuma T; Asafu-Adjaye E. Determination of ginsenosides in plant extracts from Panax ginseng and Panax quinquefolius L. by LC/MS/MS. *Anal Chem* Apr 15;71(8):1579-84. 1999.

Wichtl M, Pflanzliche Geriatrika. In: *DAZ* 132(30):1576. 1992.

Wu J-X & Chen J-X. Negative chronotropic and inotropic effects of Panax saponins. *Acta Pharmacol Sin*; 9(5):409-412. 1988.

Wu W; Zhang XM; Liu PM et al. Effects of Panax notoginseng saponin Rg1 on cardiac electrophysiological properties and ventricular fibrillation threshold in dogs. *Chung Kuo Yao Li Hsueh Pao* Sep;16(5):459-63. 1995.

Yamamoto M, Uemura T, Nakama S et al. Serum HDL-cholesterol-increasing and fatty liver-improving actions of *Panax ginseng* in high cholesterol diet-fed rats with clinical effect on hyperlipidemia in man. *Am J Chin Med*; 11:96-101. 1983.

Yokozawa T, Kobayashi T, Oura H, Kawashima Y. Studies on the mechanism of the hypoglycemic activity of ginsenoside-Rb2 in streptozotocin-diabetic rats. *Chem Pharm Bull* (Tokyo). Feb;33(2):869-72. 1985.

Youn YS, Analytisch vergleichende Untersuchungen von Ginsengwurzeln verschiedener Provenienzen. Dissertation Freie Universität Berlin. 1987.

Yun T. Experimental and epidemiological evidence of the cancer-preventative effects of Panax ginseng C.A. Meyer. *Nutr Rev*; 54:S71-S81. 1996.

Yun TK & Choi S. A case-control study of ginseng intake and cancer. *Int J Epidemiol*; 19:871-876. 1990.

Yunxiang F & Xiu C. Effects of ginenosides on myocardial lactic acid, cyclic nucleotides and ultrastructural myocardial changes of anoxia on mice. *Chin J Interg Trad Western Med*; 7:326. 1987.

Yushu H & Yuzhen C. The effect of Panax ginseng extract (GS) on insulin and corticosteroid receptors. *J Trad Chin Med*; 8:293-295. 1988.

Zhu M, Chan KW, Ng LS et al. Possible influences of ginseng on the pharmacokinetics and pharmacodynamics of warfarin in rats. *J Pharm Pharmacol*; 51:175-180. 1999.

Glechoma hederacea

See Ground Ivy

Globe Flower

Trollius europaeus

DESCRIPTION

Medicinal Parts: The medicinal part is the whole fresh plant.

Flower and Fruit: Every branch of the stem bears a solitary, terminal flower. They are up to 5 cm in diameter, globular, and have no calyx. The flowers usually have 10 perianth segments. The petals are lemon yellow. The outer petals, which are bent, are occasionally green underneath. The stamens are approximately 12 mm long and have a 0.5- to 5-mm long appendage.

Leaves, Stem, and Root: The plant is 10 to 70 cm high and glabrous. The stem is hollow, smooth, and branched upward. The basal leaves are long-petioled and has 3 to 5 lobes. The lobes are cuneate, deeply indented, and serrate. The cauline leaves are smaller and more or less sessile.

Habitat: The plant is indigenous to northern and central Europe.

Production: Globe flowers are the flowers of *Trollius europaeus*.

Other Names: Globe Ranunculus, Globe Crowfoot, Globe Trollius

ACTIONS AND PHARMACOLOGY

COMPOUNDS

Ranunculin: protoanemonine-forming substance in the freshly harvested plant that changes enzymatically when the plant is cut into small pieces. The pungent, volatile protoanemonine quickly dimerizes to the non-mucous membrane irritating anemonine. When dried, the plant is not capable of protoanemonine formation.

Flavonoids

Carotinoids: including neoxanthine (trollixanthine), xanthophyll epoxide

Ascorbic acid (vitamin C)

EFFECTS

No information is available.

INDICATIONS AND USAGE

Unproven Uses: Formerly, the plant was used to treat scurvy. It loses most of its active properties on drying.

PRECAUTIONS AND ADVERSE REACTIONS

No health hazards or side effects are known in conjunction with the proper administration of designated therapeutic dosages. Extended skin contact with the freshly harvested, bruised plant can lead to blisters and cauterizations due to the resulting protoanemonine formation, which is severely irritating to skin and mucous membranes.

If taken internally, severe irritation to the gastrointestinal tract, combined with colic and diarrhea, as well as irritation of the urinary drainage passages, are possible. Because of the very low level of protoanemonine-forming substances in the plant, the danger of poisoning is quite low.

DOSAGE

Mode of Administration: The drug is obsolete.

LITERATURE

Kern W, List PH, Hörhammer L (Hrsg.), Hagers Handbuch der Pharmazeutischen Praxis, 4. Aufl., Bde. 1-8: Springer Verlag Berlin, Heidelberg, New York, 1969.

Roth L, Daunderer M, Kormann K, Giftpflanzen, Pflanzengifte, 4. Aufl., Ecomed Fachverlag Landsberg Lech 1993.

Glycine soja

See Soybean

Glycyrrhiza glabra

See Licorice

Gnaphalium uliginosum

See Cudweed

Goa Powder

Andira araroba

DESCRIPTION

Medicinal Parts: The medicinal part is the dried and pulverized latex of the trunk and branches.

Flower and Fruit: Andira araroba is a large smooth tree whose yellowish wood has vertically running channels and spaces. The latex collects increasingly in these spaces as the tree ages. The bark forms in long flat pieces about 3 mm thick and is grayish-white with external fissures. The inner surface is brownish and striated. The fracture is laminated with yellow fibers.

Characteristics: The taste is mucilaginous and bitter, and the odor is slight but disagreeable.

Habitat: The tree grows in Brazil.

Production: Goa powder is exuded from the nuclear cavity of *Andira araroba*. The exuded substance is purified by recrystalization in benzol, thus producing raw chrysarobin.

Other Names: Araroba, Bahia Powder, Brazil Powder, Chrysatobine, Crude Chrysarobin, Ringworm Powder

ACTIONS AND PHARMACOLOGY

COMPOUNDS

Anthrone derivatives: in particular chrysophanolanthrone, dehydroemodine anthrone monomethyl ether, emodine anthrone monomethyl ether, dimerics of these compounds

EFFECTS

The powder is a strong reducing agent. It causes severe erythema upon contact with the skin. It inhibits glucose-6-phosphate-dehydrogenization in psoriatic skin conditions. The drug easily absorbs through the skin.

INDICATIONS AND USAGE

Unproven Uses: Goa Powder is used for psoriasis in chrysarobin ointments and for various kinds of dermatomycosis. It has been widely replaced by synthetic anthranol, which is also used in the treatment of psoriasis.

PRECAUTIONS AND ADVERSE REACTIONS

The drug is severely irritating to skin and mucous membranes (redness, swelling, pustules and conjunctivitis, even without eye contact). Internal administration leads to vomiting, diarrhea, and kidney inflammation (with as little as 0.01 g).

External administration on large skin areas could cause resorptive poisonings.

DOSAGE

Mode of Administration: Goa Powder is administered topically in emulsion form, but has largely been replaced by the synthetic anthranol cignolin.

LITERATURE

Anonym, Abwehr von Arzneimittelrisiken, Stufe II. In: DAZ 136(38):3253-2354. 1996.

Müller K, Wiegrebe W, Psoriasis und Antipsoriatika. In: DAZ 137(22):1893-1902. 1997.

Goat's Rue

Galega officinalis

DESCRIPTION

Medicinal Parts: The medicinal parts are the leaves collected at the beginning of the flowering season and dried, as well as the tips of the flowering branches.

Flower and Fruit: The plant's long-peduncled, axillary racemes are made up of numerous 1 cm long, slightly inclined florets. The petals are bluish-white and short stemmed. The filaments are fused. The fruit is a round, indented pod that grows 2 to 3 cm long and 2 to 3 mm thick, and contains many seeds.

Leaves, Stem, and Root: The strong, bright green shrub has numerous erect, branched, hollow stems that from from 40 cm to 1 m high. It has a divided rhizome with brown fibers sprouting numerous erect, corrugated, round, tall stems. The leaves are odd-pinnate; the leaflets are 1.5 to 4 cm long and 4 to 16 mm wide, elliptical to lanceolate, and thorny-tipped with a rich green upper surface and a lighter undersurface.

Characteristics: The plant is odorless unless bruised, whereupon it emits a disagreeable smell, which probably gave rise to the common name Goat's Rue.

Habitat: Goat's Rue grows wild throughout Europe and Asia.

Production: Goat's Rue herb consists of the dried, above-ground parts of *Galega officinalis*, harvested during the flowering season.

Other Names: Italian Fitch, French Lilac

ACTIONS AND PHARMACOLOGY

COMPOUNDS

Guanidine derivatives: galegine, 4-hydroxygalegine

Quinazoline alkaloids: (+)-peganine

Lectins

Flavonoids: including galuteolin

EFFECTS

The herb contains galegin, which affects blood sugar. In vitro, an inhibiting effect on the glucose transport of human epithelium cells has been demonstrated. The reported blood sugar-lowering effect of Goat's Rue herb on humans has not been documented, nor have the reported aggregation-inhibiting, lactagogic, and diuretic effects.

INDICATIONS AND USAGE

Unproven Uses: Preparations of Goat's Rue herb are used as a diuretic, and also as supportive therapy for diabetes.

PRECAUTIONS AND ADVERSE REACTIONS

General: Health risks or side effects following the proper administration of designated therapeutic dosages have not been recorded.

Poisonings have only been observed in animals, and then only following the intake of large quantities of the plant. Sheep reportedly experienced salivation, spasms, paralyses and death through asphyxiation following ingestion of inordinate amounts.

DRUG INTERACTIONS

POTENTIAL INTERACTIONS

A possible interaction exists with hypoglycemic medication. Goat's Rue should not be used by diabetics currently maintained with commercial pharmaceutical hypoglycemics.

DOSAGE

Mode of Administration: Since the efficacy for the claimed uses is not documented, therapeutic application cannot be recommended. Goat's Rue cannot be recommended for diabetes mellitus because of the severity of the disease and the availability of effective therapeutic alternatives.

Preparation: To prepare an infusion, pour boiling water over 2 g of ground drug and strain after 5 to 10 minutes.

Liquid Extract — Drug 1:1

Tincture — 1:10 45% ethanol

LITERATURE

Atanasov AT. Effect of the Water Extract of *Galega officinalis L.* on Human Platelet Aggregation in vitro. *Phytother Res.* 8 (5); 314-316. 1994

Ivorra MD, Paya M, Villar A A Review of Natural Products and Plants as Potential Antidiabetic Drugs. *J Ethnopharmacol.* 27; 243-275. 1989

Marles RJ, Farnsworth NR. Antidiabetic plants and their active constituents. *Phytomedicine* 2 (2); 137-189. 1995

Neef H, Augustinjs P, Declercq P, Declerck PJ, Laekeman G. Inhibitory effects of *Galega officinalis* on glucose transport across monolayers of human intestinal epithelial cells (CaCo-2). *Pharm Pharmacol Lett.* 6 (2); 86-89. 1996

Golden Ragwort

Senecio aureus

DESCRIPTION

Medicinal Parts: The medicinal parts are the fresh plant harvested during the flowering season and the dried herb.

Flower and Fruit: The few capitula are in a loose, many-blossomed corymb that is up to 2.5 cm wide. They are surrounded by a double involucre and consist of 8 to 12 yellow lingual, female florets. There are also numerous androgynous, tubular ray florets, which are somewhat darker.

Leaves, Stem, and Root: The perennial plant grows up to 60 cm tall. The rhizome is 2 to 5 cm thick, has numerous threadlike roots, and produces an erect or ascending stem. The root bark is hard and blackish. It surrounds a ring of whitish, woody bundles, and a large, dark, central pith. The stem is fluffy-haired when young, later glabrous, and bears alternate leaves. The basal leaves grow up to 15 cm long. They are long-petioled, simple, round, and reniform with a cordate base. The cauline leaves are shorter, incised and pinnatifid, becoming bracts.

Characteristics: The herb has a bitter and astringent taste. The smell is slightly acrid.

Habitat: The plant is indigenous to North America.

Other Names: Squaw Weed, Golden Senecio, Golden Groundsel, Ragwort, Coughweed, Cocash Weed, Grundy Swallow, Life Root

ACTIONS AND PHARMACOLOGY

COMPOUNDS

Pyrrolizidine alkaloids: chief alkaloids are floridanine, florosenine, otosenine

Sesquiterpenes of the eremophilane-type: including among others, ligularenolide, tetrahydroligularenolide, dehydrofukinone, trans-9-oxofuranoeremophilane

Flavonoids: including among others, kaempferol-3-O-glucosyl acetate, quercetin-3-O-glucosyl acetate

EFFECTS

The active agents are seneciionin (aurein), other alkaloids, and resins. The drug has menstruation-stimulating, diuretic, and astringent properties, although the mode of action has not been documented. The pyrrolizidine alkaloids are hepatotoxic and carcinogenic.

INDICATIONS AND USAGE

Unproven Uses: Life Root is used for bleeding and menopausal symptoms.

PRECAUTIONS AND ADVERSE REACTIONS

Life Root should not be taken internally. Hepatotoxicity and carcinogenicity are possible due to the pyrrolizidine alkaloids and 1,2-unsaturated necic parent substances.

DOSAGE

Mode of Administration: Internal use of Life Root is not recommended.

Daily Dosage: The traditional average daily dose of the drug as a liquid extract is 4 g taken 3 to 4 times daily. (See Precautions and Adverse Reactions.)

LITERATURE

Hänsel R, Keller K, Rimpler H, Schneider G (Hrsg.), Hagers Handbuch der Pharmazeutischen Praxis, 5. Aufl., Bde 4-6 (Drogen): Springer Verlag Berlin, Heidelberg, New York, 1992-1994.

Roeder E. Medicinal plants in Europe containing pyrrolizidine alkaloids. *Pharmazie* 50 (2); 82-98. 1995

Zalkow LH et al., *J Chem Soc Perkin Trans.* 1:1542. 1979

Goldenseal

Hydrastis canadensis

DESCRIPTION

Medicinal Parts: The medicinal parts are the air-dried rhizome with the root fibers.

Flower and Fruit: The flower is small, solitary, terminal, and erect. It has 3 small greenish-white petals that drop as soon as they emerge. The fruit is a group of small, fleshy, oblong carmine berries with 1 or 2 hard, black, glossy seeds. The fruit is similar to the raspberry but is not edible.

Leaves, Stem, and Root: The plant is a low herbaceous perennial about 30 cm high. It has a horizontal bright yellow, knotty, twisted rhizome about 0.6 to 1.8 cm thick out of which the root fibers grow. It is folded longitudinally and encircled by old leaf scars. The fracture is short and shows a dark, yellow surface, thick bark, large pith and broad medullary rays. The flowering stem appears in spring and is erect, cylindrical, downward pubescent, 15 to 30 cm tall and has a few short brown scales at the base. It bears 2 clearly ribbed, dark green, pubescent, cauline leaves. The lower one is sessile the upper one petiolate, round and divided into 7 lobes and finely serrate. There is also a root leaf on a long petiole, which is similar to the cauline leaves but larger.

Characteristics: The taste is very bitter, the smell is strong, characteristic and disagreeable.

Habitat: Indigenous to the U.S., cultivated elsewhere.

Production: Goldenseal root is the rhizome of *Hydrastis canadensis*. The root is dug up in the autumn and dried.

Not to be Confused With: Goldenseal is often adulterated with Bloodroot.

Other Names: Eye Balm, Eye Root, Ground Raspberry, Indian Dye, Indian Paint, Indian Plant, Jaundice Root, Orange Root, Turmeric Root, Warnera, Wild Curcuma, Yellow Puccoon, Yellow Root

ACTIONS AND PHARMACOLOGY

COMPOUNDS

Isoquinoline alkaloids: chief alkaloids hydrastine (1.5 to 4%), berberine (0.5 to 6%), (-)-canadine (0.5%)

Starch

EFFECTS

Many of the studies that have been conducted focus on the berberine and hydrastine components that are found not only in Goldenseal, but also in numerous other herbs commonly used in Chinese and Indian medicine. The effects reported here focus on these components and not necessarily Goldenseal in its raw form.

Berberine's broad-spectrum antibiotic activity, as well as its anti-infective and immune-enhancing properties, make it a popular recommendation for virtually all types of infections involving the upper respiratory tract, gastrointestinal tract (particularly infectious diarrhea), and genitourinary tract. Goldenseal is also helpful in cirrhosis of the liver, and as an adjunct to standard cancer therapy. Goldenseal has shown some vasoconstriction, antispasmodic, and anticoagulant properties (Leone et al, 1996; Nishino et al, 1986; Leung, 1980; Preininger, 1975)

Antibiotic: Berberine has shown antimicrobial activity against bacteria, protozoa, and fungi, including *Staph sp, Strep sp, Chlamydia sp, Corynebacterium diphtheria, Escherichia coli, Salmonella typhi, Vibrio cholerae, Diplococcus pneumonia, Pseudomonas sp, Shigella dysenteriae, Entamoeba histolytica, Trichomonas vaginalis, Neisseria gonorrhoeae and N meningitidiss, Treponema pallidum, Giardia lamblia, Leishmania donovani,* and *Candida albicans* (Kaneda et al, 1991; (Sun, 1988; Chang & But, 1987; Ghosh, 1983; Majahan et al, 1982). Berberine has also been shown to activate macrophages, via both enhanced priming and triggering (Kumazawa et al, 1984). Berberine, a constituent of goldenseal, when used to treat urinary infections, is known to reduce synthesis of *Escherichia coli* fimbriae, thus preventing adhesion to the bladder lining. At a concentration lower than necessary to kill the bacteria, berberine also blocks *Streptococcus pyogenes* adhesion and interferes with lipotechoic acid complexes that allow the Streptococcus to adhere to fibronectin (Yarnell, 1997).

Berberine was found to be the active constituent in an extract of *Hydrastis canadensis* root that demonstrated activity against a multiple-drug-resistant strain of *Mycobacterium tuberculosis* (Gentry, 1998). Berberine also inhibits *Helicobacter pylori* (Bae, 1998).

Antisecretory Effects: Berberine has hypotensive, antisecretory, and sedative effects. The mechanism for these effects may be explained by the fact that berberine has platelet alpha 2 adrenoceptor agonist activity that is similar to that of clonidine (Hui, 1984). Berberine blocks the secretory effects of the toxins produced by several pathogenic bacteria (Tai et al, 1981; Swabb et al, 1981; Akhter et al, 1979). The toxin-blocking effect is most evident in diarrhea caused by enterotoxins (e.g., Vibrio cholerae and E coli, cholera and traveler's diarrhea respectively) (Rabbani et al, 1987; Khin-Maung et al, 1985).

Antipyretic Effects: Berberine produced an antipyretic effect 3 times as potent as aspirin in a pyretic model in rats (Nishino et al, 1986). However, while aspirin suppresses fever through its action on prostaglandins, berberine appears to lower fever by increasing the immune system's handling of fever-producing compounds from microorganisms.

Anti-inflammatory Effects: The anti-inflammatory activity of berberine sulfate has been postulated as a factor, which is associated with the antitumor promoting activity (Nishino et al, 1986; Preininger, 1975). Inhibition of cyclic AMP phosphodiesterase in vitro is used as a marker for some type of biologic activity (nonspecific). A hot-water extract of goldenseal aerial parts showed greater than 30% inhibition, hinting at potential biologic activity (Thein et al, 1995).

Antineoplastic: There is evidence that berberine also has a direct tumor-killing effect and has the ability to stimulate production of white blood cells (Zhang, 1990; Liu, 1991). Canadine-like alkaloids (similar to those in goldenseal) have displayed cytotoxicity in vitro against KB cells derived from human epidermoid carcinoma (Cushman et al, 1979).

Astringent: Hydrastine (not the whole herb goldenseal) is an astringent for mucous membranes (Tyler et al, 1976). This may be the basis for its use on sore throats, mouth sores, cankers, ulcers, skin lesions, and wounds (Rollins, 1997).

Uterine Bleeding: Goldenseal was previously used to stop uterine bleeding and cause uterine contractions. Its value for these purposes is doubtful. Both hydrastine and berberine (in goldenseal) increase the tonus and stimulate uterine contractions in low doses, but higher doses relax uterine muscle (Duke, 1985).

CLINICAL TRIALS

Cancer, Adjunctive Therapy

Berbamine has been used in China since 1972 in the treatment of depressed white blood cell (WBC) counts due to chemotherapy and/or radiation. In one study, 405 patients with WBC counts below 4,000 were given 150 mg of berbamine daily (50 mg orally 3 times daily) for 1 to 4 weeks. The overall results for the 405 patients: significantly effective in 163 cases (40.2%), effective in 125 cases (38.8%) and ineffective in 117 cases (29%). The total effective rate was 71%. However, WBC before therapy was related to overall effectiveness. The effective rate was only 54.8% in 31 cases where WBC was below 1,000 and 82.7% in cases where WBC count was between 3,100 and 3,800 (Liu et al, 1991).

Cholesterol

Beberine from Goldenseal lowered levels of total cholesterol by 29%, low-density lipoprotein cholesterol by 25%, and triglycerides by 35% in 32 hypercholesterolemic patients who took berberine alone (no other herbs or medications) orally (0.5 g twice daily) for 3 months. Subjects who took placebo (n=11) experienced no significant changes in cholesterol levels. Berberine was well tolerated and produced no reported side effects aside from one case of mild constipation. Analysis of berberine's mechanism of action in hamsters and human hepatoma cells indicated that it works in a way distinct from statin medications—apparently by up-regulating LDLR expression through a post-transcriptional mechanism that stablizes mRNA. The authors say these findings strongly suggest berberine has promise as a new hypolipidemic drug, either alone or in combination with statins (Kong, 2004).

Diarrhea

In one study, patients with traveler's diarrhea randomly received berberine sulfate 400 mg in a single dose or served as controls. In treated patients, the mean stool volumes were significantly less than those of controls during 3 consecutive 8-hour periods after treatment. At 24 hours after treatment, significantly more treated patients stopped having diarrhea as compared to controls (42% versus 20%) (Rabbani et al, 1987).

Organ Transplantation

In a randomized, controlled clinical trial, 52 renal-transplant recipients treated with the key transplant immunosuppressive drug, cyclosporine A, were also given berberine 3 times daily for 3 months. Another group of 52 renal-transplant patients were given the same amount of cyclosporine without berberine. Over time, the first group had elevated blood concentrations of cyclosporine, suggesting that berberine potentiated the therapeutic effect of the drug. The authors conclude that berberine may therefore allow a reduction in the amount of cyclosporine needed in such patients—a valuable finding given the side effects and cost of cyclosporine (Wu, 2005).

Tumors

Berberine demonstrates antitumor activity against human and rat malignant brain tumors. In vitro studies were performed on a series of 6 human malignant brain tumor cell lines and rat 9L brain tumor cells. Berberine used alone at a dose of 150 mcg/mL showed an average cancer cell kill of 91%. This kill rate was over twice that of 1,3-bis(2-chloro- ethyl)-1-nitrosourea (BCNU), the standard chemotherapeutic agent for brain tumors, which had a cell kill rate of 43%. Studies in rats harboring solid 9L brain tumors also showed berberine has antitumor effects. Rats treated with berberine, 10 mg/kg, had a 81% cell kill. However, the combination treatment, berberine and BCNU, exhibited additive effects on killing cancer cells. These results indicate that berberine may prove to be more effective than BCNU or, at the very least, a valuable therapeutic addition in the treatment of difficult brain cancers (Zhang et al, 1990).

INDICATIONS AND USAGE

Unproven Uses: Goldenseal is used as an antiseptic externally on wounds and *herpes labialis.* It is also used for gastritis and as an astringent. The berberine component is used to treat acute diarrhea caused by numerous gastrointestinal pathogens. Berberine is also used as an adjunct treatment in various cancers and in neutropenia resulting from radiation and chemotherapy. Berberine has been used to treat trachoma, gastric ulcers, and gallbladder disease.

Homeopathic Uses: In homeopathic dilutions, *Hydrastis canadensis* is used for the treatment of irregular menstruation, digestive problems, and bronchitis.

CONTRAINDICATIONS

Goldenseal is contraindicated in people with glucose-6-phosphate-dehydrogenase deficiency (Chan, 1993).

Pregnancy: Not to be used during pregnancy and in women with a history of miscarriage.

Breastfeeding: Not to be used while breastfeeding.

PRECAUTIONS AND ADVERSE REACTIONS

If taken over an extended period, the drug can bring about digestive disorders, mucous membrane irritation, constipation, excitatory states, hallucinations, and occasionally deliria. Adverse reactions may include irritation of the mouth, stomach, and mucous membrane in high doses; higher doses may be toxic. Jaundice and hemolytic anemia may occur in people with glucose-6-phosphate-dehydrogenase deficiency. Goldenseal should not be used as a douche due to potential for mucous membrane irritation (Newall et al, 1996).

Cardiovascular Effects: Hydrastine, in higher doses, will produce hypertension based on animal studies (Newall et al, 1996). High doses of berberine inhibit coronary activity; lower doses increase coronary blood flow (Newall et al, 1996).

DRUG INTERACTIONS

POTENTIAL INTERACTIONS

Cytochrome P450 3A4-metabolized drugs: Caution is advised if goldenseal is administered with drugs metabolized by this enzyme (Budzinski et al, 2000).

Vitamin B: There have been reports of decreased vitamin-B absorption with higher doses of Goldenseal (Newall et al, 1996; Tierra, 1980).

OVERDOSAGE

The LD50 for berberine in rats was found to be greater than 1,000 mg/kg of body weight, making the toxicity of this component in Goldenseal very low (Haldon, 1975). The hydrastine component appears to be the toxic compound in Goldenseal. High doses result in strychnine-like convulsions and gastrointestinal relaxation (Osol & Garrar, 1955). Other effects of overdose that have been reported include difficulty in breathing, bradycardia and central paralysis.

Following stomach and intestinal emptying (inducement of vomiting, gastric lavage with burgundy-colored potassium permanganate solution, sodium sulfate) the treatment for poisonings consists of the instillation of activated charcoal and shock prophylaxis (quiet, warmth). The treatment of spasms with diazepam (I.V.), electrolyte substitution and the countering of any acidosis imbalance that may appear with sodium bicarbonate infusions may be necessary. In the event of shock, plasma volume expanders should be infused. Intubation and oxygen respiration may also be required.

DOSAGE

How Supplied:

Capsules: 400 mg, 404 mg, 470 mg, 535 mg, 528 mg, 540 mg

Tea

Daily Dosage:

Extract – Standardized extract (5% hydrastine) 250 to 500 mg 3 times daily (Werbach & Murray, 1994)

Fluid extract – 1/4 to 1 teaspoonful (1.25 to 5 mL) (Grieve, 1971)

Solid extract - 325 to 520 mg (Grieve, 1971)

Local antiseptic – 1 teaspoonful powder steeped in 1 cup boiling water for 15 minutes. Swish around the mouth or gargle for mouth or throat sores (Tyler, 1997).

Traveler's diarrhea – One capsule (500 to 1000 mg root) 3 times daily (Tyler, 1997)

Storage: Store at room temperature. Avoid moisture, high temperatures and direct light.

LITERATURE

Akhter MH, Sabir M & Bhide NK. Possible mechanism of antidiarrhoeal effect of berberine. *Indian J Med Res;* 70(Aug):233-241. 1979.

Babbar OP, Chhatwal VK, Ray IB et al. Effect of berberine chloride eye drops on clinically positive trachoma patients. *Ind J Med Res* 76(suppl):83-88. 1982.

Bae EA, Han MJ, Kim NJ et al. Anti-*helicobacter pylori* activity of herbal medicines. *Biol Pharmaceut Bull* 21(9):990-992. 1998.

Budzinski JW, Foster BC, Vandenhoek S et al. An in vitro evaluation of human cytochrome P450 3A4 inhibition by selected commercial herbal extracts and tinctures. *Phytomedicine*; 7(4):273-282. 2000.

Chan E. Displacement of bilirubin from albumin by berberine. *Biol Neonate*; 63(4):201-208. 1993.

Chang HM & But PPH. Pharmacology and Applications of Chinese Materia Medica, vol 2. World Scientific, Teaneck, NJ, USA:1029-1240. 1987.

Chan MY. The effect of berberine on bilirubin excretion in the rat. *Comp Med East West* 5:161-168. 1977.

Galefi C et al., Canadinic acid: an alkaloid from Hydrastis canadensis. In: *PM* 63(2):194. 1997.

Gentry EJ, Jampani HB, Keshavarz-Shokri A et al. Antitubercular natural products: berberine from the roots of commercial *Hydrastis canadensis* powder. *J Nat Prod* 61(10):1187-1193. 1998.

Ghosh AK, Rakshit MM & Ghosh DK. Effect of berberine chloride on *Leishmania donovani. Indian J Med Res*; 78(Sept):407-416. 1983.

Gleye J et al., *Phytochemistry* 13:675. 1974.

Haginiwa J, Harada M, Yakugaku Zasshi 82:726. 1962.

Haldon B. Toxicity of berberine sulfate. *Acta Pol Pharm* 32:113-120. 1975.

Hui K, Yu J, Chan W, Tse E. Interaction of berberine with human platelet alpha 2 adrenoceptors. *Life Sci* 49(4): 315-24. 1991.

Kaneda Y, Torii M & Tanaka T. In vitro effects of berberine sulfate on the growth of *Entamoeba histolytica, Giardia lamblia* and *Tricomonas vaginalis. Ann Trop Med Parasitol* 85:417-425. 1991.

Khin-Maung-U, Myo-Khin, Nyunt-Nyunt-Wai et al. Clinical trial of berberine in acute watery diarrhoea. *BMJ* (Clin Res Ed); 291(6509):1601-1605. 1985.

Kong W, Wei J, Abidi P, et al. Berberine is a novel cholesterol-lowering drug working through a unique mechanism distinct from statins. *Nature Med* 10 (12): 1344-1351. 2004.

Kowalewski Z, Mrozikiewicz A, Bobkiewicz T et al. Toxicity of berberine sulfate. *Acta Pol Pharm*; 32(1):113-120. 1975.

Kumazawa Y, Itagaki A, Fukumoto M et al. Activation of peritoneal macrophages by berberine alkaloids in terms of induction of cytostatic activity. *Int J Immunopharmacol*; 6(6):587-592. 1984.

Leone MG, Cometa MF, Palmery M et al. HPLC determination of the major alkaloids extracted from *Hydrastis canadensis L. Phytother Res*; 10(suppl 1):S43-S46. 1996.

Liu CX et al. Studies on plant resources, pharmacology and clinical treatment with berbamine. Phytother Res 5:228-230. 1991.

Majahan VM, Sharma A & Rattan A. Antimycotic activity of berberine sulphate: an alkaloid from an Indian medicinal herb. *Sabouraudia*; 20(1):79-81. 1982.

Mikkelsen SL & Ash KO. Adulterants causing false negatives in illicit drug testing. *Clin Chem* 34:2333-2336. 1988.

Mohan M, Pant CR, Angra SK et al. Berberine in trachoma. *Ind J Opthalmol* 30:69-75. 1982.

Nishino H, Kitagawa K, Fujiki H et al. Berberine sulfate inhibits tumor-promoting activity of teleocidin in two stage carcinogenesis on mouse skin. *Oncology* 43(2):131-134. 1986.

Palmery M, Cometa MF, Leone MG. Further studies of the adrenolytic activity of the major alkaloids from Hydrastis canadensis L on isolated rabbit aorta. *Phytother Res;* 10(suppl 1):S47-S49. 1996.

Palmery M, Leone MG, Pimpinella G et al. Effects of *Hydrastis canadensis L* and the two major alkaloids berberine and hydrastine on rabbit aorta. *Pharmacological Res*; 27(suppl 1):73-74. 1993.

Preininger V. The pharmacology and toxicology of the papaveraceae alkaloids. *Alkaloids*; 15:207-251. 1975.

Preininger V. The pharmacology and toxicology of the Papaveraceae alkaloids, in Manske RHF & Holmes HL (eds): The Alkaloids, Vol. 15. Academic Press, p 239. 1975.

Rabbani GH, Butler T, Knight J et al. Randomized controlled trial of berberine sulfate therapy for diarrhea due to enterotoxigenic *Escherichia coli* and *Vibrio cholerae. J Infect Dis*; 155(5):979-984. 1987.

Rollins C. More about goldenseal. Internet aol.com: To Your Health 9/22/1997.

Sack RB & Froehlich JL. Berberine inhibits intestinal secretory response of *Vibrio cholerae* toxins and *Escherichia coli* enterotoxins. *Infect Immun* 35(2):471-475. 1982.

Sun D, Courtney HS & Beachey EH. Berberine sulfate blocks adherence of *Streptococcus pyogenes* to epithelial cells, fibronectin, and hexadecane. *Antimicrob Agents Chemother* 32:1370-1374. 1988.

Swabb EA, Tai YH & Jordan L. Reversal of cholera toxin-induced secretion in rat ileum by luminal berberine. *Am J Physiol*; 241(3):G248-252. 1981.

Tai YH, Feser JF, Marnane WG et al. Antisecretory effects of berberine in rat ileum. *Am J Physiol*; 241(3):G253-258. 1981.

Thein K, Myint W, Myint MM et al. Preliminary screening of medicinal plants for biological activity based on inhibition of cyclic AMP phosphodiesterase. *Int J Pharmacognosy*; 33(4):330-333. 1995.

Tyler VE, Brady LR & Robbers JE. Alkaloids. In: Pharmacognosy, 7th ed. Lea & Febiger, Philadelphia, PA, USA:258. 1976.

Tyler VE. Golden Seal: can this herb boost immunity? *Prevention* July:68-70. 1997.

Watanabe A, Obata T & Nagashima H. Berberine therapy of hypertyraminemia in patients with liver cirrhosis. *Acta Med Okayama*; 36(4):277-281. 1982.

Wu X, Li Q, Xin H, et al. Effects of berberine on the blood concentrations of cyclosporine A in renal transplanted recipients: clinical and pharmacokinetic study. *Eur J Clin Pharmacol*; 61:567-572. 2005.

Yarnell E. Botanical medicine for cystitis. *Alt Complement Ther*; Aug:269-275. 1997.

Zhang RX, Dougherty DV & Rosenblum ML. Laboratory studies of berberine used alone and in combination with 1,3-bis(2-chloroethyl)-1-nitrosourea to treat malignant brain tumors. *Chinese Med J* (Engl) 103(8):658-665. 1990.

Golden Shower Tree

Cassia fistula

DESCRIPTION

Medicinal Parts: The medicinal parts of the plant are the bark, fruit, and seeds.

Flower and Fruit: The flowers are in loose, hanging, 30 to 50 cm long racemes. There are 5 pale yellow, ovate petals. The diameter of the corolla is approximately 3:8 cm. The calyx is deeply divided and has 5 teeth. There are 10 stamens. The 30 to 60 cm long fruit is a hanging, indehiscent legume.

Leaves, Stem, and Root: Cassia fistula is a tree, that grows up to 9 m high. The leaves are 20 to 40 cm long, 4- to 8-paired pinnate. The leaf spindle is hairy and the leaflet is petiolate, ovate to oval, acuminate, 5 to 12 cm long, 4 to 9 cm wide, and silvery haired underneath. The young bark is smooth and greenish-gray. Older bark is dark brown and rough.

Habitat: India, Africa and South America

Production: Cassia pods are the dried ripe fruit of *Cassia fistula*.

Not to be Confused With: Very occasionally the tree has been confused with South American Cassia species.

Other Names: Indian Laburnum, Pudding Pipe Tree, Purging Cassia

ACTIONS AND PHARMACOLOGY

COMPOUNDS

Anthracene derivatives (1% in the mesocarp): sennosides, fistulinic acid

Monosaccharides/oligosaccharides (50%): particularly saccharose

Fruit acids: citric acid

Steroids: sterols (in the seeds), including beta-sitosterol

Fatty oil (in the seeds)

EFFECTS

The anthracene derivatives have a laxative effect. Preparations from the fruit have demonstrated antimicrobial and antiviral effects in vitro.

INDICATIONS AND USAGE

Indian Medicine: Golden Shower Tree is used for flatulence, constipation, fever, anorexia, gout, jaundice, itching, and skin conditions. Efficacy for constipation is plausible because of the anthranoid content; the other indications have not been proved.

CONTRAINDICATIONS

The drug is contraindicated with ileum, acute-inflammatory diseases of the intestine and appendicitis. It is also contraindicated for children under 12 years of age and for women during pregnancy or while nursing.

PRECAUTIONS AND ADVERSE REACTIONS

No health hazards are known in conjunction with the proper administration of designated therapeutic dosages. The question of the increase in probability of the appearance of carcinomas in the colon following long-term administration of Anthracene drugs has not yet been fully clarified. Recent studies, however, have revealed no connection between the administration of Anthracene drugs and the frequency of carcinomas of the colon.

OVERDOSAGE

In the case of overdose, cramplike gastrointestinal complaints could occur as a side effect of the laxative effect of the drug. Prolonged administration leads to loss of electrolytes, particularly of potassium ions, which in turn leads to aldosteronism, albuminuria, hematuria, inhibition of intestinal motility, muscle weakness, enhancement of the effect of cardioactive steroids, and an influence upon the effect of antiarrhythmics. In rare cases, administration of the drug may lead to cardiac arrhythmia, nephropathy, edema, and accelerated osteoclasis.

DOSAGE

Mode of Administration: Whole drug preparations are for internal use.

Preparation: To prepare an extract, use pulp and distilled water in a 1:1 ratio, macerate, then exhaustively percolate with distilled water and filter. Evaporate to a soft extract.

Daily Dosage: 4 to 8 g of fruit pulp

LITERATURE

Asseleih LM, Hernandez OH, Sanchez JR. Seasonal Variations in the Content of Sennosides in Leaves and Pods of Two *Cassia fistula* populations. *Phytochemistry* 29; 3095-3099. 1990 el-Saadany SS, el-Massry RA, Labib SM, Sitohy MZ, The biochemical role and hypocholesterolaemic potential of the legume *Cassia fistula* in hypercholesterolaemic rats. *Nahrung*, 35:807-15, 1991.

Espósito Avella M, Díaz A, de Gracia I, de Tello R, Gupta MP, Evaluation of traditional medicine: effects of *Cajanus cajan L.* and of *Cassia fistula L.* on carbohydrate metabolism in mice. *Rev Med Panama*, 16:39-45, Jan. 1991

Espósito Avella M, Díaz A, de Gracia I, de Tello R, Gupta MP, Studies on the possibilities to infect the cells of callus of *Cassia fistula* by an animal virus & induce production of interferon-like antiviral factor(s). *Indian J Exp Biol*, 16:349-55, Apr. 1981

Hänsel R, Keller K, Rimpler H, Schneider G (Ed), Hagers Handbuch der Pharmazeutischen Praxis, 5. Aufl., Bde 4 - 6 (Drogen), Springer Verlag Berlin, Heidelberg, New York, 1992-1994.

Schukla SC, Das SR. Cure of Amoebiasis by Seed Powder of *Cassia fistula*. *Int J Crude Drug Res*. 26; 141-144. 1988

Goldthread

Coptis trifolia

DESCRIPTION

Medicinal Parts: The medicinal parts are the rhizome and sometimes the stems and leaves.

Flower and Fruit: The solitary flowers are small and white, and arranged on leafless scapes.

Leaves, Stem, and Root: Goldthread is a perennial plant in bushes of up to 15 cm with yellowish, scaly leaves at the base and long-petioled, obovate, evergreen leaves. The rhizome is threadlike, golden yellow with a matte surface and very small roots.

Characteristics: Goldthread has a very bitter taste and slight odor.

Habitat: Coptis trifolia is indigenous to India and *Coptis groenlandica*, which is also used, is indigenous to Greenland and Iceland.

Production: Goldthread rhizome is the rhizome of *Coptis trifolia*.

Other Names: Mouth Root, Cankerroot, Yellowroot, Coptis, Coptide, Coptis Groenlandica

ACTIONS AND PHARMACOLOGY

COMPOUNDS

Isoquinoline alkaloids (6 to 9%): including coptin, berberine

EFFECTS

The herb is a bitter tonic.

INDICATIONS AND USAGE

Unproven Uses: Goldthread is used in digestive disorders.

PRECAUTIONS AND ADVERSE REACTIONS

General: Health risks or side effects following the proper administration of designated therapeutic dosages are not recorded.

Berberine has a mutagenic effect upon yeast cells and in the Ames test (intercalation into the DNA), although that does not necessarily mean a mutagenic effect for the drug when administered to humans.

Pregnancy: Not to be used during pregnancy.

DOSAGE

Mode of Administration: Internally as a powdered drug or a liquid extract.

LITERATURE

Hegnauer R Chemotaxonomie der Pflanzen. Bde 1-11, Birkhäuser Verlag Basel, Boston, Berlin 1962-1997.

Kern W, List PH, Hörhammer L (Ed), Hagers Handbuch der Pharmazeutischen Praxis. 4. Aufl., Bde. 1-8, Springer Verlag Berlin, Heidelberg, New York 1969.

Gossypium herbaceum

See Levant Cotton

Gossypium hirsutum

See Cotton

Gotu Kola

Centella asiatica

DESCRIPTION

Medicinal Parts: The medicinal parts are the dried above-ground parts, the fresh and dried leaves, and stem.

Flower and Fruit: The pedicles are 1.2 to 4 cm long. The sepals of the epicalyx are oval to circular, with a membranous border. They are about 2.5 to 3 mm long and 1.5 to 2.5 mm wide. The umbels have 2 or 3 sessile or short-pedicled florets. The petals are white, purple, or pink. The calyx is not generally dentate. The fruit is oval to globular in shape, and has a diameter of 2 to 5 mm. The mericarps are clearly flattened at the sides and usually have 7 to 9 ribs and are raised rugose.

Leaves, Stem, and Root: Centella asiatica is a tender umbel plant, which has numerous creeping stems. The stems have roots at the nodes, which are smooth. The circular-reniform leaves are 2 to 6 cm long and 1.5 to 5 wide, with a crenate margin and 5 to 9 ribs. The petioles are 3 to 30 cm long.

Characteristics: Gotu Kola is almost tasteless and odorless.

Habitat: The plant is indigenous to southeast Asia, India, Sri Lanka, parts of China, the western South Sea Islands, Madagascar, South Africa, southeast U.S., Mexico, Venezuela, Colombia, and eastern South America.

Production: Hydrocotyle herb is the aerial part of *Centella asiatica*. The plant is gathered throughout the year and dried in the sun.

Other Names: Hydrocotyle, Indian Hydrocotyle, Indian Pennywort, Marsh Penny, Thick-leaved Pennywort, White Rot,

ACTIONS AND PHARMACOLOGY

COMPOUNDS

Triterpene acids: including asiatic acid, madecassic acid (6-hydroxy asiatic acid), terminolic acid

Triterpene acid ester from oligosaccharides (pseudosaponins): including asiaticoside, asiaticoside A, asiaticoside B

Volatile oil (0.1%)

EFFECTS

The main constituents of the drug are triterpene acids and their sugar residues (asiaticoside and madecassoside). Gotu kola is thought to have action as an antimicrobial, antineoplastic, central nervous system depressant, and wound-healing agent (Chatterjee et al, 1992; Tenni et al, 1985; Chaudhuri et al, 1976). Asiaticoside, a component of Gotu kola, facilitates wound healing through an increase in peptidic hydroxyproline content, tensile strength, collagen synthesis, angiogenesis and epithelialization, as shown in animal models (Bonte, 1994; Maquart, 1990; Shukla, 1999).

Animal experiments have demonstrated anti-inflammatory actions, anti-anxiety, and antidepressant effects, and reduced stress ulcer rates. In vitro studies have shown antimicrobial effects. In studies with rats, Gotu kola has exhibited similar sedative effects to chlorpromazine and diazepam and was effective against stress ulcers as compared with famotidine.

Anti-Inflammatory Effects: Asiaticoside and madecassoside have both been shown to have anti-inflammatory actions (Jacker et al, 1982). Anti-inflammatory effects exerted by extracts *of Centella asiatica* were demonstrated by a reduction of acute radiation reaction in rats (Chen, 1999). A diminished growth rate, stimulation of hyaluronic acid, and increased chondroitin sulfate was seen after incorporation of the total triterpenic fraction of *Centella asiatica* into human embryonic fibroblasts (Del Vecchio et al, 1984).

Antineoplastic Effects: The fresh plant juice has moderate cytotoxic actions on human ascites tumor cells, but little, if any other antitumor effects (Jacker et al, 1982). Cytotoxic and antitumor effects of *Centella asiatica* involve direct action on DNA synthesis. The development of solid and ascites tumors was decreased by the herb (Babu, 1985).

Central Nervous System Effects: In a rodent study where an extract of Gotu kola was given orally to produce protection from convulsions and to prolong pentobarbital sleeping time, the mechanism of the antidepressant effect noted was thought to be via D-2 receptors and a cholinergic mechanism (Sakina & Dandiya, 1990). A dose of 25 mg/kg of Gotu kola extract given intraperitoneally to mice decreased spontaneous motor activity, delayed pentylenetetrazol-induced convulsion, and potentiated pentobarbitone-induced sleep, but did not affect immobility time in a swimming test. Authors concluded the extract had an anti-anxiety effect comparable to diazepam (4 mg/kg) but did not affect behavioral despair (Diwan et al, 1991).

Antibacterial Effects: In a placebo-controlled study of Gotu kola extract, 16 patients were tested against ampicillin and placebo for treatment of acute Shigellosis. Compared to the ampicillin, the extract did not show any clinical improvement or bacterial clearing (Haider et al, 1991).

Cognitive Effects: General mental ability, academics, and several tests showed improvement in 8 of 12 educable mentally retarded children (8 to 12 years old). Treatment was given for 6 months; the children were followed up to a year. Tests used for evaluation included Malin's Intelligence Scale for Indian Children, Bender GestaLt Test for Children, and Raven's Color Progressive Matrices (Sharma et al, 1985). An antistress effect of an ethanolic extract of Gotu kola equal to 2.5 mg/kg/d was noted in rats given 100 mg/kg of the extract (Sarma et al, 1996). Significantly better 24-hour mental retention was reported in rats taking an extract of Gotu kola (doses ranged from 0.1 to 16 g/kg of the fresh leaves) compared to saline controls (Nalini et al, 1992).

Antipruritic Effects: Pruritus caused by prickly heat has been relieved by the fresh juice from the leaves of Gotu kola in adults and children (Newall et al, 1996).

Ulcer-protective Effects: Gotu kola may improve blood circulation in the lower legs by the stimulation of collagen synthesis in the vein wall, resulting in greater vein tonicity and decreased vein distention (Newall et al, 1996). The anti-ulcerogenic effect of an ethanolic extract of Gotu kola used to prevent restraint-stress ulcers in rats was equivalent to that of diazepam. The rats were given 100 mg of the extract once a day by lavage for 16 days. The diazepam rats received 2.5 mg/kg/d for the same 16 days (Sarma et al, 1995).

Vascular/Venous Tone Effects: Ethanol extracts of *Centella asiatica,* in vitro, had a remarkable enhancement of fibroblast cell attachment and tissue plasminogen activator (Kim, 1993). Gotu kola was indirectly shown to affect the metabolism of connective tissue of vascular walls. The total tripenic fraction from *Centella asiatica* (60 mg/d for 3 months) was given to 20 patients with varicose veins. The original values of uronic acid and lysosomal enzymes was elevated, but dropped significantly ($p<0.01$) by the end of the treatment period (Arpaia et al, 1990).

A triterpenic fraction of Gotu kola lowered circulating endothelial cells to near normal in patients with postphlebitic syndrome. These patients with vascular insufficiency have an increased number of circulating endothelial cells compared to normal subjects (3.8 cells vs 1.5 cells/counting chamber). After Gotu kola treatment of patients for 3 weeks, the count was reduced to 1.8 cells/counting chamber. Reducing the number of circulating endothelial cells may alter the progression of the vascular disease (Montecchio et al, 1991).

Wound-Healing Effects: Improved wound healing was reported in 19 of 25 wounds treated with a Gotu kola-containing aerosol (Morisset et al, 1987). Asiatic acid and madecassic have also demonstrated an increase in peptidic hydroxyproline, showing an increased remodeling of the collagen matrix (collagen synthesis) in wounds (Bonte, 1994; Maquart, 1999). Asiaticoside also induces enzymatic and non-enzymatic antioxidants, namely superoxide dismutase, catalase, glutathione peroxidase, vitamin E, and ascorbic acid in newly formed tissue (initial stage of wound healing) (Shukla, 1999).

CLINICAL TRIALS

Central Nervous System Depression

An ethanol extract of Gotu kola significantly increased ($p<0.05$) pentobarbital sleeping time, showed significant analgesic effect, protected against induced convulsion, significantly potentiated haloperidol catatonia, reduced immobility time in forced swimming, and reduced behavioral despair. Rodents were dosed orally at 0.2 to 0.5 mL of a 100 mg/mL or 150 to 200 mg/mL crude plant material suspension in gum acacia (Sakina & Dandiya, 1990).

Periodontal Therapy

The efficacy of a combined herbal preparation containing *Centella asiatica* and *Punica granatum* was tested in the treatment of 15 patients who had completed conventional periodontal therapy with remaining probing pocket depths of 5-8 mm. The herbal preparation was administered in the form of biodegradable chips as a subgingival adjunct. Patients in the control group received standard supportive periodontal therapy. The results showed significant improvements of probing pocket depth, attachment level, and gingival index at 3 and 6 months and of bleeding index at 6 months in the test group compared to the control group. In plaque index, no significant differences could be found at all visits. The test group treated with the herbal preparation showed greater reduction of IL-1beta at both 3 and 6 months and lower IL-6 concentration, which almost reached the level of significance at 6 months. The results indicate that adjunctive local delivery of *Centella asiatica* combined with *Punica granatum* significantly improved clinical signs of chronic periodontitis (Sastravaha et al, 2005).

Ulcer Protection

A dose of 500 mg/kg of an aqueous leaf extract of Gotu kola provided cytoprotection for rats given 1 mL of an hydrochloric acid (HCl)/ethanol solution to induce ulcers. The rats were given the HCl solution one hour after receiving the plant extract and were killed one hour later for examination of mucosal surfaces. A control group developed characteristic lesions, while the Gotu kola group showed 100% prevention (Tan et al, 1997).

Venous Insufficiency (Chronic)

A Cochrane Collaboration Review of evidence from randomized, controlled clinical trials of drugs for improving blood flow for people with poor leg vein circulation (chronic venous insufficiency) identified 13 studies involving 1,245 people, but reported overall insufficient evidence to support the "phlebotonics" analyzed. Two trials used *Centella asiatica* (Gotu Kola). In one, a 1981 trial involving 80 patients in Italy, a portion were randomized to take two 10 mg *Centella asiatica* tablets 3 times daily, and the other to take a placebo for 30 days. In a 1987 French study, 94 patients were randomized to take placebo or 120 mg *Centella asiatica* daily. In one study, patients overall assessed Gotu Kola as effective in relieving the sensation of leg "heaviness," a symptom of chronic venous insufficiency. The other study showed insignificant results compared with placebo in terms of relieving leg heaviness, (Martinez, 2007).

Venous Hypertension

The effect of an extract of *Centella asiatica* with capillary filtration and ankle edema was evaluated in patients with venous hypertension. Sixty-two patients were included in the study and administered either placebo or the extract as 60 mg or 30 mg 3 times daily. Capillary filtration rate and ankle edema both significantly improved in a dose-dependent manner in the extract-treatment groups. The subjective symptoms (swelling, sensation, restless lower extremity, pain and cramps, and tiredness) were significantly improved in the extract-treatment groups, with no change in the placebo-treatment group (Belcaro, 1990).

INDICATIONS AND USAGE

Unproven Uses: The drug is used internally for rheumatism and skin diseases. Externally, the drug is used for poorly healing wounds, leprosy sores, and postoperative scarring.

Chinese Medicine: The herb is used for dysentery and summer diarrhea, vomiting, jaundice, urinary calculi, epistaxis, and scabies.

Indian Medicine: The drug is used for skin diseases, syphilis, rheumatism, and leprosy. Gotu kola is also used for the treatment of mental illness, epilepsy, hysteria, and for dehydration.

Homeopathic Uses: Gotu Kola is used for skin diseases associated with itching and swelling and inflammation of the uterus.

CONTRAINDICATIONS

Pregnancy: Not to be used during pregnancy.

PRECAUTIONS AND ADVERSE REACTIONS

Potential adverse effects of Gotu kola include skin irritation (topical), photosensitization, and infertility. Use with caution in patients with diabetes or hyperlipidemia, as Gotu kola may increase blood glucose and lipids (Newall et al, 1996).

Allergic Contact Dermatitis: Although there have been case reports of allergic contact dermatitis due to *Centella asiatica,* the plant's sensitizing capacity is considered low (Bilbao, 1995; Danese, 1994; Gonzalo, 1996; Hausen, 1993). Four cases of contact dermatitis were reported when a Gotu kola ointment was used to treat keloids, burn scarring, or hypertrophic scarring. The rashes appeared in 4 days to 2 weeks and consisted of pruritic, oozing, papular, eczematous lesions. Positive patch tests were obtained in all 4 cases (Eun & Lee, 1985).

Eczema was reported on the fingers of a woman's hand after treating a keloid with Madecassol® for 3 months. Patch testing showed allergic contact dermatitis (Hausen, 1993). A red, vesicular reaction with exudation and intense pruritus appeared after 20 days of treatment with a Gotu kola containing cream (Centelase®). The reaction started at the point of application of the cream and later spread to the trunk and limbs. The rash cleared after treatment with prednisone 25 milligrams/day for a week. Patch testing to Centelase cream was positive (++plus;) (Danese et al, 1994).

Fertility: Infertility is a possible adverse effect. The total saponin fraction (containing brahmic acid and its triand tetraglycosides) has shown antifertility activity in human and rat sperm (Singh & Rastogi, 1969). The fertility of female mice was also negatively affected by oral administration (Newall et al, 1996). In vitro experiments on human sperm did not show spermicidal activity at concentrations up to 2% of a concentrated extract (Setty et al, 1976).

DRUG INTERACTIONS

No drug interaction data available.

DOSAGE

Mode of Administration: Gotu kola is available in liquid or solid pharmaceutical forms, for oral intake. Gotu Kola is also available parenterally for homeopathic use.

How Supplied:

Capsules – 400 mg, 435 mg, 439 mg, 440 mg, 450 mg, 500 mg

Tablets—250 mg

Liquid Extract- 1:1; 250 mg/mL

Tea

Daily Dosage: 0.6 g of dried leaves or infusion taken 3 times daily; normal single dose is 0.33 to 0.68 gm.

Varicose Veins – *Centella asiatica* extract administered as 60 mg daily has shown improvement (Arpaia, 1990).

Venous Hypertension – Total triterpenic fraction of *Centella asiatica* (TTFCA) tablets have demonstrated improvement of venous hypertension at doses of 30 mg or 60 mg given 3 times daily (Belcaro, 1990).

Chronic Venous Insufficiency – Titrated extract of *Centella asiatica* (TECA) administered as 120 mg daily and 60 mg daily have demonstrated efficacy in chronic venous insufficiency (Pointel, 1987).

Homeopathic Dosage: 5 to 10 drops, 1 tablet, 5 to 10 globules or 1 mL injection solution sc twice weekly; ointment 1 to 2 times daily (HAB1).

Storage: Store in a cool, dry place and in well-sealed containers.

LITERATURE

Allegra G et al. *Clin Terap*. 99:507. 1981.

Arpaia MR, Ferrone R, Amitrano M et al. Effects of *Centella asiatica* extract on mucopolysaccharide metabolism in subjects with varicose veins. *Int J Clin Pharmacol Res*; 10(4):229-233. 1990.

Asakawa Y et al., Phytochemistry 21(10):2590. 1982.

Babu TD, Kuttan G, Padikkala J, Cytotoxic and anti-tumour properties of certain taxa of Umbelliferae with special reference to *Centella asiatica* (L.) Urban. *J Ethnopharmacol,* 48:53-7, Aug 11. 1995.

Belcaro GV; Rulo A; Grimaldi R. Capillary filtration and ankle edema in patients with venous hypertension treated with TTFCA. *Angiology* Jan;41(1):12-8. 1990.

Belcaro GV; Grimaldi R; Guidi G. Improvement of capillary permeability in patients with venous hypertension after treatment with TTFCA. *Angiology* Jul;41(7):533-40. 1990.

Bilbao I; Aguirre A; Zabala R et al. Allergic contact dermatitis from butoxyethyl nicotinic acid and *Centella asiatica* extract. *Contact Dermatitis* Dec;33(6):435-6. 1995.

Bonte F; Dumas M; Chaudagne C; Meybeck A, Influence of asiatic acid, madecassic acid, and asiaticoside on human collagen I synthesis. *Planta Med* Apr;60(2):133-5. 1994.

Bossé JP et al. Clinical study of a new antikeloid agent. *Ann Plast Surg*; 3:13-21. 1979.

Brevoort P, Der Heilpflanzenmarkt der USA - Ein Überblick. In: *ZPT* 18(3):155-162. 1997.

Castellani C et al., *Boll Chim Farm* 120:570-605. 1981.

Chatterjee TK; Chakraborty A; Pathak M; Sengupta GC. Effects of plant extract *Centella asiatica* (Linn.) on cold restraint stress ulcer in rats. Indian J Exp Biol Oct;30(10):889-891. 1992.

Chaudhuri S, Ghosh S, Chakraborty T et al. Common Indian herb Mandukaparni in the treatment of Leprosy. *J Indian Med Assoc*; 70:177-180. 1980.

Chen YJ; Dai YS; Chen BF et al. The effect of tetrandrine and extracts of *Centella asiatica* on acute radiation dermatitis in rats. *Biol Pharm Bull* Jul;22(7):703-6. 1999.

Danese P; Carnevali C; Bertazzoni MG. Allergic contact dermatitis due to *Centella asiatica* extract. *Contact Dermatitis* Sep;31(3):201. 1994.

Del Vecchio AD, Senni I, Cossu G et al. Effetti della *Centella asiatica* sull'attivita biosintetica di fibroblasti in coltura. *Farm Ed Prat*; 39:355-364. 1984.

Deshpande S, Gupta SS, Shinde S et al. Psychotropic effect of Centella asiatica. Indian J Pharmacol; 12:64B. 1980.

Di Carlo FI et al., *J Reticuloendothelial* Soc 1:224. 1964.

Diwan PV, Karwande I, Singh AK. Anti-anxiety profile of Manduk Parni (*Centella asiatica*) in animals. *Fitoterapia*; 62:253-257. 1991.

Dutta T, Basu UP, *Ind J Exp Biol* 6(3):181. 1968.

Dutta T, Basu UP, *Ind J Chem* 5:586. 1967.

Dutta T, Basu UP, *Bull Nat Inst Sci India* 37:178-184. 1968.

Eun HC & Lee AY. Contact dermatitis due to Madecassol. *Contact Dermatitis*; 13:310-313. 1985.

Gonzalo Garijo MA, Revenga Arranz F, Bobadilla Gonzalez P, Allergic contact dermatitis due to *Centella asiatica*: a new case. *Allergol Immunopathol* (Madr), 24:132-4, May-Jun 1996.

Grimaldi R et al., Pharmacokinetics of the total triterpenic fraction of *Centella asiatica* after single and multiple administrations to healthy volunteers. A new assay for asiatic acid. *J Ethnopharmacol*, 24:235-41, Feb 1990.

Haider K, Khan BKA, Aziz KMS et al. Evaluation of indigenous plants in the treatment of acute shigellosis. *Trop Geograph Med*; 43:266-270. 1991.

Hausen BM. *Centella asiatica* (Indian pennywort), an effective therapeutic but a weak sensitizer. *Contact Dermatitis* Oct;29(4):175-179. 1993.

Jacker H-J et al. Zum antiexsudativen Verhalten einiger Triterpensaponine. *Pharmazie*; 37:380-382. 1982.

Kamboj VP. A review of Indian medicinal plants with interceptive activity. *Indian J Med Res*; 4:336-355. 1988.

Kim YN; Park YS; Kim HK et al. Enhancement of the attachment on microcarriers and tPA production by fibroblast cells in a serum-free medium by the addition of the extracts *of Centella asiatica. Cytotechnology*;13(3):221-6. 1993.

Maquart FX, Bellon G, Gillery P, Wegrowski Y, Borel JP, Stimulation of collagen synthesis in fibroblast cultures by a triterpene extracted from *Centella asiatica. Connect Tissue Res*, 24:107-20, 1990.

Maquart FX; Chastang F; Simeon A et al., Triterpenes from *Centella asiatica* stimulate extracellular matrix accumulation in rat experimental wounds. *Eur J Dermatol* Ju*n*;9(4):289-96. 1999.

Martinez M, Bonfill X, Moreno R, et al. Phlebotonics for venous insufficiency. *Cochrane Database Syst Rev* 3: CD003229, 2005.

Montecchio GP, Samaden A, Carbone S, et al. *Centella asiatica* Triterpenic Fraction (CATTF) reduces the number of circulating endothelial cells in subjects with post phlebitic syndrome. *Haematologica*, 76(3):256-259, May-Jun 1991.

Morisset R, Cote NG, Panisset JC et al. Evaluation of the healing activity of Hydrocotyle tincture in the treatment of wounds. *Phytother Res;* 1:117-121. 1987.

Nalini K, Aroor AR, Karanth KS et al. Effect of *Centella asiatica* fresh leaf aqueous extract on learning and memory and biogenic amine turnover in albino rats. *Fitoterapia*; 46:330-335. 1992.

Pointel JP; Boccalon H; Cloarec M et al., Titrated extract of *Centella asiatica* (TECA) in the treatment of venous-insufficiency of the lower limbs. *Angiology* Jan;38(1 Pt 1):46-5. 1987.

Rao PS, Seshardri TR, Curr. Sci 38:77. 1969.

Ramaswamy AS, Perityasamy SM & Basu NK. Pharmacological studies *on Centella asiatica. J Res Indian Med*; 4:160-175. 1970.

Ravokatra A; Loiseau A; Ratsimamanga-Urverg S et al., Action of asiaticoside (pentacyclic triterpene) extracted from Hydrocotyle madagascariensis on duodenal ulcers induced with mercaptoethylamine in male Wistar rats. *C R Acad Sci Hebd Seances Acad Sci* D Apr 29;278(18):2317-2321. 1974.

Sakina MR & Dandiya PC. A psycho-neuropharmacological profile of *Centella asiatica* extract. *Fitoterapia*; 61:291-296. 1990.

Sarma DNK, Khosa RL, Chansauria JPN et al. Antiulcer activity of *Tinospora cordifolia* and *Centella asiatica* extracts. *Phytother Res*; 9:589-590. 1995.

Sastravaha G, Gassmann G, Sangtherapitikul P, Grimm WD. Adjunctive periodontal treatment with Centella asiatica and Punica granatum extracts in supportive periodontal therapy. *J Int Acad Periodontol*; 7(3): 70-79. 2005.

Setty BS, Kamboj VP, Garg HS et al. Spermicidal potential of saponins isolated from Indian medicinal plants. *Contraception*; 14:571-578. 1976.

Sharma R, Jaiswal AN, Kumar S et al. Role of Bhrahmi (*Centella asiatica*) in educable mentally retarded children. *J Res Edu Ind Med*; 4:55-57. 1985.

Shukla A; Rasik AM; Jain GK et al. In vitro and in vivo wound healing activity of asiaticoside isolated from *Centella asiatica. J Ethnopharmacol* Apr;65(1):1-11. 1999.

Shukla A; Rasik AM; Dhawan BN. Asiaticoside-induced elevation of antioxidant levels in healing wounds. Phytother Res Feb;13(1):50-4. 1999.

Siegel RK. Herb intoxication. psychoactive effects from herbal cigarettes, tea, and capsules. *JAMA*; 236:473-476. 1976.

Singh B & Rastogi RP. A reinvestigation of the triterpenes of *Centella asiatica. Phytochemistry*; 8:917. 1969.

Suguna L, Sivakumar P, Chandrakasan G, Effects of *Centella asiatica* extract on dermal wound healing in rats. *Indian J Exp Biol*, 24:1208-11, Dec 1996.

Tan PV, Njimi CK & Ayafor JF. Screening of some African medicinal plants for antiulcerogenic activity, part 1. *Phytother Res*; 11:45-47. 1997.

Tang W, Eisenbrand G, Chinese Drugs of Plant Origin, Springer Verlag Heidelberg 1992.

Tenni R, Zanaboni G, De Agostini MP et al. Effect of the triterpenoid fraction of *Centella asiatica* on macromolecules of the connective matrix in human skin fibroblast cultures. *Ital J Biochem*; 37:69-77. 1988.

Vecchaio AD et al., Farm Ed Prat 39(10):355. 1984.

Goutweed

Aegopodium podagraria

DESCRIPTION

Flower and Fruit: The flowers range from 50 to 100 cm. They have large white or reddish double umbels that are usually androgynous. The flowers have no involucre and no calyx. The petals are white or pink, about 1.5 mm long, obcordate and cuneate at the base. The fruit is oblong and brownish with pale veins. The fruit is slightly pressed in at the sides, unwinged, unstriped, with a 3-mm mericarp.

Leaves, Stem, and Root: The stem is erect, angular, grooved, hollow, glabrous, and branched. The lower leaves are double trifoliate, and the upper leaves trifoliate. The leaflets are ovate and crenate-serrate.

Characteristics: Propagates via underground runners.

Habitat: Indigenous to Europe (not Spain), West Asia.

Production: Goutweed is the aerial part of *Aegopodium podagraria*.

Other Names: Goutwort, Ground Elder, Gout Herb, Herb Gerard(e), Jack-Jump-About, Goatweed, Ashweed, Achweed,

English Masterwort, Pigweed, Eltroot, Bishop's Elder, Weyl Ash, White Ash, Bishopsweed, Bishopswort.

ACTIONS AND PHARMACOLOGY

COMPOUNDS

Volatile oil

Polyynes: only in freshly-harvested leaves

Flavonol glycosides: including hyperoside, isoquercitrin

Caffeic acid derivatives: including chlorogenic acid

Ascorbic acid

EFFECTS

No information available.

INDICATIONS AND USAGE

Unproven Uses: The herb is used internally as an infusion for gout and rheumatic diseases. It is used externally in macerations for poultices and baths for hemorrhoids, gout, and rheumatic diseases, as well as for kidney and bladder disorders and intestinal disorders.

PRECAUTIONS AND ADVERSE REACTIONS

No health hazards or side effects are known in conjunction with the proper administration of designated therapeutic dosages.

DOSAGE

Mode of Administration: Internally as a tea; externally, the fresh herb is squeezed for poultices.

Daily Dosage: There is no exact dosage. A daily recommended dose consists of 1 to 2 teaspoonfuls (30 mL) of the juice of the fresh plant.

LITERATURE

Battelli MG et al. Ribosome-inactivating lectins with polynucleotideenosine glycosidase activity. *FEBS Lett,* 408:355-9, May 26 1997.

Hänsel R, Keller K, Rimpler H, Schneider G (Hrsg.), Hagers Handbuch der Pharmazeutischen Praxis, 5. Aufl., Bde 4-6 (Drogen), Springer Verlag Berlin, Heidelberg, New York, 1992-1994.

Schneider V, Ernähr-Umschau 31(2):54-57. 1984.

Grains-of-Paradise

Aframomum melegueta

DESCRIPTION

Medicinal Parts: The medicinal parts are the ripe seeds.

Flower and Fruit: The flowers are solitary, mauve, and waxlike. The fruit is 10 cm long, pear-shaped, and scarlet. The seeds are small, hard, shiny, reddish-brown, and oyster-shaped. They have an aromatic and pungent taste and smell.

Leaves, Stem and Root: Aframomum melegueta is a reedlike plant, 1 to 2.5 m high. The leaves are long and narrow.

Habitat: The plant is indigenous to tropical West Africa.

Not to be Confused With: The seeds can be mistaken for peppercorns.

Other Names: Guinea Grains, Melegueta Pepper, Mallaguetta Pepper

ACTIONS AND PHARMACOLOGY

COMPOUNDS

Volatile oil

Pungent substances: including hydroxyphenylalkanones and hydroxyphenylalkanoles

Tannins

Starch

Fatty oil

EFFECTS

The seed is a stimulant.

INDICATIONS AND USAGE

Unproven Uses: Grains-of-Paradise was used as a stimulant. Now it is obsolete as a drug.

PRECAUTIONS AND ADVERSE REACTIONS

No health hazards or side effects are known in conjunction with the proper administration of designated therapeutic dosages.

OVERDOSAGE

Due to the constituent pungent substances, the intake of larger dosages may lead to irritation of the stomach and the urinary tract.

LITERATURE

Escoubas P, Lajide L, Mizutani J. Termite Antifeedant Activity in *Aframomum melegueta. Phytochemistry* 40 (4); 1097-1099. 1995

Hoppe HA, (1975-1987) Drogenkunde, 8. Aufl., Bde 1-3, W. de Gruyter Verlag, Berlin, New York.

Kern W, List PH, Hörhammer L (Hrsg.), Hagers Handbuch der Pharmazeutischen Praxis, 4. Aufl., Bde. 1-8, Springer Verlag Berlin, Heidelberg, New York, 1969.

Grape

Vitis vinifera

DESCRIPTION

Medicinal Parts: The medicinal parts are the leaves, the fruit, and the juice.

Flower and Fruit: The flowers are in compound compact panicles. The petals are about 5 mm long and droop like the sepals. The fruit is oblong to globular, 6 to 22 mm long, dark blue-violet, red, green or yellow, juicy, sweet or sour. The seeds are pear-shaped, with hard skin and two long dimples on the side.

Leaves, Stem, and Root: The vine is a 30-cm high climber with deep, heavily branched roots and a woody trunk. The trunk has striped, loose bark. The brown-red to brown-yellow branches are glabrous or slightly downy and finely grooved.

The leaves are orbicular, generally in 3 to 5 lobes or blades. They are deeply notched at the stem. The upper surface of the leaves is glabrous, the under surface is lanate.

Habitat: The plant is indigenous to southern Europe and western Asia and is cultivated today in all temperate regions of the world.

Production: Vine leaves are the foliage leaves of *Vitis vinifera.*

ACTIONS AND PHARMACOLOGY

COMPOUNDS

Flavonoids (4 to 5%): including, kaempferol-3-O-glucosides, quercetin-3-O-glucosides

Tannins: procyanidolic oligomers (proanthocyanidins), including constituent monomers of catechin epicatechin

Non-flavonoids (Stilbenes): resveratrol and viniferins

Fruit acids: including, tartaric acid, malic acid, succinic acid, citric acid, oxalic acid

Phenylacrylic acid derivatives: p-cumaroyl acid, caffeoyl acid, feruloylsuccinic acid

EFFECTS

Grape Seed extract has shown positive effects against peripheral venous insufficiency, as an antioxidant, in varicose veins, capillary fragility, disorders of the retina including diabetic retinopathy, edema, ocular stress, and premenstrual syndrome. In vitro and animal trials have demonstrated antioxidant, vascular, cytotoxic, chemopreventive, and cytoprotective effects. In addition, the excellent antioxidant effects of Grape Seed extract may offer protection against atherosclerosis and other chronic degenerative diseases, such as cancer. Grape Seed extract may also support collagen stabilization. Results of an in vitro study demonstrated that procyanidins (from *Vitis vinifera* seeds) are highly effective scavengers of hydrophilic and lipophilic radicals. Procyanidins exhibited remarkable, dose-dependent, anti-lipoperoxidant activity. Furthermore, they can protect liposomal membranes from lipid peroxidation through a radical scavenging action and by a chelation mechanism (Facino et al, 1994).

Antiatherosclerotic Effects: The oxidation of low-density lipoproteins (LDL) by free radicals is associated with the initiation of atherosclerosis. Proanthocyanidin decreases the number of LDL-positive macrophage-derived foam cells in atherosclerotic lesions. The compound also inhibits the oxidation of cholesteryl linoleate in LDL to exert a reduction in atherosclerosis of the aorta (Nuttall, 1998, Yamakoshi, 1999).

Anticarcinogenic/Antitumor Effects: Chemoprotective properties of proanthocyanidins include activity against free radicals and oxidative stress (Ye, 1999). The antitumor-promoting activity due to strong antioxidant effects of the compound has been demonstrated in animal models (Zhao, 1999).

Antioxidant Effects: Proanthocyanidin from Grape Seed extract exerts a concentration-dependent inhibition of oxygen free radicals. In one study, the antioxidant effect of proanthocyanidin was more potent compared to vitamin C and vitamin E succinate (Bagchi, 1999, 1997). The compound also inhibits peroxidation of phosphatidylcholine liposomes (Plumb, 1998). In one study, Grape Seed extract trapped free radicals and inhibited their production, markedly delayed the onset of lipid peroxidation, and inhibited the damaging effects of the enzymes that can degrade connective tissue structures. The antioxidant activity of PCOs from Grape Seed extract were much greater (approximately 50 times) than that of vitamin C and vitamin E, providing a strong rationale for using these compounds in the therapeutic management of microvascular disorders (Facino et al, 1994).

Another in vitro study demonstrated a protective effect of Grape Seed proanthocyanidins against peroxidation of polyunsaturated fatty acids (PUFA) by UV-C irradiation (Bouhamidi et al, 1998). Mice fed Grape Seed proanthocyanidin extract (GSPE) had a decrease in 12-O-tetradecanoylphorbol-13-acetate (TPA) induced production of reactive oxygen species, DNA fragmentation in hepatic and brain tissues and lipid peroxidation. GSPE was a better scavenger of free radicals and inhibitor of oxidative tissue damage than vitamin C, vitamin E succinate, or a combination of these vitamins and beta-carotene in the doses studied (Bagchi et al, 1998).]

Cardioprotective Effects: Dietary polyphenols from Grapes have multiple cardio-protective properties that were initially described through the "French Paradox," in which it was observed that despite a diet high in saturated fat, people who regularly consume red wine are also less likely to develop coronary heart disease. Recent research demonstrates that this effect may be due not only to possible inhibitory effects of polyphenols on LDL oxidation, but to other effects as well: the action of the Grape polyphenols on altering hepatic cholesterol absorption, effects on triglyceride assembly and secretion, and changes in the processing of lipoproteins in plasma. Both in vitro and in vivo models have shown these positive cardio-protective effects on lipid metabolism and inflammation (Zern, 2005).

Collagen Stabilization: Procyanidolic oligomers effectively caused cross-linking in collagen in vitro. An in vitro study determined that procyanidins inhibit the activities of some proteolytic enzymes (collagenase, elastase) involved in the degradation of the main structural components of the extravascular matrix, collagen, elastin, and hyaluronic acid (Facino et al, 1994).

Cytotoxic Effects: One study reported a Grape Seed extract exhibited cytotoxicity toward some cancer cells (Joshi et al, 1998). An abstract reported that Grape Seed extract exerted a chemopreventive effect on adenomas polyposis coli gene mutation-associated intestinal adenoma formation. Tumor multiplicity was significantly reduced ($p<0.01$) from a mean of 78.3 in control mice to 43.5 in mice fed Grape Seed extract.

The number of small polyps was also significantly reduced in the Grape Seed extract group (p value not indicated) (Arii et al, 1998).

Cytoprotective Effects: Various abstracts reported that Grape Seed extract has in vitro effects that may ameliorate the toxic effects of chemotherapeutic agents (Joshi et al, 1998); that it provides some protection against radiation damage to spermatogonial cells in the testes (Lanka et al, 1998); and that it may attenuate acetaminophen induced hepatic DNA damage, apoptopic cell death, and influence gene expression (Ray et al, 1998). Grape Seed extract inhibited stomach mucosal injury in mice induced by 60 percent ethanol (EtOH) containing 150 millimolar hydrochloric acid (HCl) (Saito et al, 1998).

Hair Growth: Proanthocyanidins extracted from Grape Seeds promote proliferation of hair follicle cells, and possess hair-cycle converting activity from the telogen phase to the anagen phase. Epicatechin and catechin are the constitutive monomers inducing the degree of polymerization inducing hair growth (Takahashi, 1998).

Hepatoprotective Effects: Proanthocyanidin has been shown to significantly attenuate acetaminophen-induced hepatic DNA damage, apoptopic and necrotic cell death of liver cells. The component also antagonizes acetaminophen induced changes in bcl-X1 expression (Ray, 1999).

Ischemia Preventive Effects: Maintenance of microvascular injury by procyanidins occurs through the scavenger effect of reactive oxygen species (Maffei Facino, 1994). Procyanidins also reduce ventricular contraction in a dose-dependent fashion. Procyandins decrease coronary perfusion pressure and improve cardiac mechanical performance. (Maffei Facino R, 1996).

Ocular Stress: Grape Seed extract may improve resistance to glare, recovery from exposure to bright light, night vision, and ocular stress. In a 90-day double-blind study in 75 patients with ocular stress caused by their activity in front of a computer screen, Grape Seed extract (300 mg/day) was shown to significantly improve objective (contrast sensitivity) and subjective symptoms of eye strain (Bombardelli & Morazzoni, 1995).

Premenstrual Syndrome: Administration of Grape Seed extract may be beneficial in treating symptoms of premenstrual syndrome. Concomitant use of Grape Seed extract may decrease some of the negative side effects of hormone therapy in women (Henriet, 1993).

Vascular Effects: An abstract reported polymeric phenolic compounds found in Grape Seed extracts to have effects on vascular tone in vitro, which are unlikely associated with antioxidant activity (Karim et al, 1998). PCOs reduced the incidence of atherosclerotic lesions in rabbits fed a high-cholesterol diet. After 8 weeks on a high-cholesterol diet, rabbits fed procyanidins did not exhibit the increased aortic plaque that the other experimental group did (Sevanian, 1998). PCOs also protect against free radical damage with their potent antioxidant and free radical scavenging action; and inhibit enzymatic cleavage of collagen by enzymes secreted by leukocytes during inflammation and microbes during infection (Facino et al, 1994; Meunier et al, 1989).

Procyanidins isolated from Grape Seed stabilizes capillary walls and prevents increases in permeability that inhibits edema (Robert, 1990; Zafirov, 1990). Overproduction of hyaluronan content associated with pathologic venous walls, in particular vein-lymphatic edema, is decreased by procyanidolic oligomers (Drubaix, 1997). Procyanidolic oligomers cross-link collagen fibers, resulting in reinforcement of the natural cross-linking of collagen that forms the collagen matrix of vascular connective tissue (Tixier et al, 1984). The vascular activity of procyanidin has positive effects on diabetic retinopathy, night vision and ocular stress (Boissin, 1988; Corbe, 1988; Soyeux, 1987).

CLINICAL TRIALS

Breast Induration

The efficacy of IH636 Grape seed proanthocyanadin extract (GSPE) for breast induration (tissue hardening) following radiation therapy was tested in a randomized, double-blind, placebo-controlled study of 66 patients with the condition after undergoing high-dose radiotherapy for early breast cancer. Participants, who reported moderate or marked breast induration at a mean 10.8 years since radiotherapy, were randomly assigned to active drug (n=44) or placebo treatment (n=22). All patients were given GSPE 100 mg, 3 times a day orally, or corresponding placebo capsules, for 6 months. No significant differences between the two treatment groups were found in terms of external assessments of tissue hardness or breast appearance, or patient self-assessments of breast hardness, pain, or tenderness (Brooker et al, 2006).

Coronary Artery Disease

A number of lifestyle modifications are likely beneficial for women after menopause to compensate for the loss of estrogen—which has profound effects in increasing lipids and other risk factors for coronary heart disease. In this single-blind, crossover trial, Grape polyphenols delivered in the form of lypholized grape powder (LGP) was shown to have a number of key significant cardio-protective effects in both pre- and postmenopausal women. Twenty women were randomly assigned to consume 36 g of the LGP or a placebo for 4 weeks. After a 3-week washout period, the subjects were assigned to a different treatment for 4 weeks. A number of beneficial effects on plasma lipids were observed. After taking LGP, plasma triglyceride concentrations were reduced by 15% in pre-menopausal women and by 6% in post-menopausal women ($P<0.01$). Plasma LDL cholesterol and apolipoproteins B and E also were significantly lower ($P<0.05$). Whole-body oxidative stress was significantly reduced, and markers of inflammation were likewise lowered (Zern 2005).

Antioxidant

In a double-blind, placebo-controlled study researchers sought to determine the antioxidant effects of PCO Phytosome® in 20 young volunteers. The Phytosome process binds one part of the Grape Seed PCO extract with two parts of phosphatidylcholine. The result is a completely new molecule composed of a central molecule of PCO encased by two phosphatidylcholine molecules. Subjects were given 2 capsules containing 300 mg of PCO Phytosome or a placebo for 5 days. Blood samples were taken at the start of the study and at the end of the study and assayed for antioxidant activity as well as vitamins C and E levels. After a washout period of at least 2 weeks, the study was crossed over. While the PCO Phytosome had no effect on serum vitamins C and E levels, it increased the serum total antioxidant activity (TAC) considerably. On day 5, TAC increased from 408 to 453 βmol/l trolox equivalents one hour after dosage (Nutall et al, 1998).

Energy Intake

A randomized, double-blind, placebo-controlled crossover study of 51 normal to overweight subjects found Grape seed extract effective in reducing 24-hour energy intake (EI) in certain individuals. For 3 days, subjects ate an ad libitum lunch and dinner. Standard breakfast and snacks were provided. Supplements were taken 30-60 minutes prior to each meal. In the total study population, no differences in 24-hour energy intake were found between the two treatment groups. However, in the subgroup of 23 subjects with an energy requirement greater than or equal to the median of 7.5 MJ/day, EI was reduced by 4% (p=0.05) while taking Grape seed extract compared to placebo. The extract had no effects on satiety, mood, or tolerance (Vogels et al, 2004).

Edema

The efficacy of Grape Seed extract (Endotelon) was evaluated in 165 women suffering from edema due to premenstrual syndrome. The multicenter, open study included women ages 18-50 years. Each woman received 4 tablets Grape Seed extract per day (exact dose not mentioned) from day 14 through day 28 of their menstrual cycle, for a total of 4 cycles. Mammary symptoms, abdominal swelling, pelvic pains, weight variations, and venous problems of the legs disappeared or improved in 60.8% of the cases after 2 cycles of treatment and in 78.8% of the cases after 4 cycles of treatment (Amsellem et al, 1987).

The effect of PCO from Grape Seed extract was shown to have protective effects on the postoperative edema compared to placebo in a double-blind, placebo-controlled study. Thirty-two female patients undergoing a facelift were administered either 300 mg Grape Seed extract or placebo daily over the 5 days preceding the operation, and postoperatively from days 2 to 6. Prophylactic decrease in postoperative facial edema was the main efficacy criteria. The Grape Seed extract cohort scored significantly better than placebo against postoperative facial swelling (Baruch, 1984).

Pancreatitis

Three patients with chronic pancreatitis (2 with history of alcohol excess and 1 idiopathic) experienced a decrease in frequency and intensity of abdominal pain and resolution of vomiting (in 1 patient) when taking Grape Seed proanthocyanidin extract ActiVin®, a potent antioxidant. Medical treatments had failed in all patients while invasive procedures were either not indicated or were refused by the patients. ActiVin 200 mg daily orally provided some symptom relief while 300 mg daily was used when there was a worsening of symptoms. ActiVin was well tolerated and may be useful in the management of chronic or relapsing pancreatitis (Banerjee & Bagchi, 2001).

Peripheral Venous Insufficiency

The efficacy of Grape Seed extract was evaluated for the treatment of venous insufficiency and symptoms due to hormonal supplementation. Grape Seed extract (150 mg twice daily) was administered to 4,729 patients in an open-label study. Peripheral venous insufficiency was evaluated 45 and 90 days after treatment. The efficacy score was based on symptoms of nocturnal cramps, paresthesias, sensation of warmth, cyanosis, and edema. The sensation of heaviness in the legs decreased in 57% of cases by day 45 and 89.4% by day 90. In addition, the improvement of symptoms occurred in 66% of cases by day 45 and 79-83% of cases by day 90 (Henriet, 1993).

Vision Improvement

A lower resistance to glare and alteration of scotopic vision are associated with retinal pathology related to age, fatigue, and stress. The effect of procyanidolic oligomers (PCO) on light vision and chorioretinal circulation was determined in 100 subjects. PCO (Endotelon®) was administered in tablets of 50 mg 4 times daily for 5 weeks. Improvements in visual adaptation to low luminance and visual performances after glare, as measured by a nyctometer, were significant (Boissin et al, 1988; Corbe et al, 1988).

INDICATIONS AND USAGE

Unproven Uses: In Folk medicine, Grape preparations are used in venous diseases and blood circulation disorders.

Indian Medicine: Grape is used for headache, dysuria, scabies, skin diseases, gonorrhea, hemorrhoids, and vomiting.

PRECAUTIONS AND ADVERSE REACTIONS

No health hazards or side effects are known in conjunction with the proper administration of designated therapeutic dosages. A reversible inhibition of intestinal enzyme activity (alkaline phosphatase, sucrase and dipeptidyl peptidase) was demonstrated in animal models (Tebib, 1994).

DRUG INTERACTIONS

No human interaction data available.

DOSAGE

How Supplied:

Capsule—25 mg, 30 mg, 50 mg, 60 mg, 500 mg

Tablet—50 mg

Daily Dosage: Grape Seed extract has been used for preventive therapy with 50 mg daily and treatment doses of 150 to 600 mg daily in divided doses (Arne, 1982; Baruch, 1984; Corbe; 1988; Delacroix, 1981; Henriet, 1993; Nuttall, 1998; Soyeux, 1987).

LITERATURE

Amsellem M, Masson JM, Negui B et al. Endotelon in the treatment of venolymphatic problems in premenstrual syndrome - multicenter study on 165 patients. *Tempo Med*; 282:46-51. 1987.

Arii M, Miki R, Hosoyama H et al. Chemopreventive effect of Grape Seed extract on intestinal carcinogenesis in the apc mouse. *Proc Am Assoc Cancer Res*; 39:20. 1998.

Arne JL. Contribution to the study of procyanidolic oligomers: Endotelon in diabetic retinopathy. *Gaz Med France*; 89(30):3610-3614. 1982.

Bagchi D; Garg A; Krohn RL et al. Oxygen free radical scavenging abilities of vitamins C and E, and a Grape Seed proanthocyanidin extract in vitro. *Res Commun Mol Pathol Pharmacol* Feb;95(2):179-89. 1997.

Bagchi D, Garg A, Krohn RL et al. Protective effect of Grape Seed proanthocyanidins and selected antioxidants against TPA-induced hepatic and brain lipid peroxidation and DNA fragmentation, and peritoneal macrophage activation in mice. *Gen Pharmacol*; 30(5):771-776. 1998.

Bagchi M, Balmoori J, Bagchi D et al. Smokeless tobacco, oxidative stress, apoptosis, and antioxidants in human oral keratinocytes. *Free Radic Biol Med*; 26(7-8):992-1000. 1999.

Banerjee B & Bagchi D. Beneficial effects of a novel IH636 Grape Seed proanthocyanidin extract in the treatment of chronic pancreatitis. *Digestion*; 63(3):203-206. 2001.

Baruch. the effects of Endotelon in postoperative edema. Results of a double-blind study versus placebo in 32 female patients. *Ann Chir Plast Esthet*;29(4):393-395. 1984.

Bavaresco L; Fregoni C; Cantu E; Trevisan M. Stilbene compounds: from the grapevine to wine. *Drugs Exp Clin Res*; 25(2-3):57-63. 1999.

Boissin JP; Corbe C; Siou A. Chorioretinal circulation and dazzling: use of procyanidol oligomers (Endotelon). *Bull Soc Ophtalmol Fr* Feb;88(2):173-4, 177-9. 1988.

Bombardelli E & Morrazzoni P. *Vitis vinifera L. Fitoterapia*; 66:291-317. 1995.

Bouhamidi R, Prevost V & Nouvelot A. High protection by Grape Seed proanthocyanidins (GSPC) of polyunsaturated fatty acids against UV-C induced peroxidation. *C R Acad Sci III*; 321(1):31-38. 1998.

Brooker S, Martin S, Pearson A, et al. Double-blind, placebo-controlled, randomised phase II trial of IH636 grape seed proanthocyanadin extract (GSPE) in patients with radiation-induced breast induration. *Radiother Oncol*; 79(1):45-51. 2006.

Corbe C; Boissin JP; Siou A. Light vision and chorioretinal circulation. Study of the effect of procyanidolic oligomers (Endotelon). *J Fr Ophtalmol*;11(5):453-60. 1988.

Delacroix P. Double-blind trial of endotelon in chronic venous insufficiency. *Rev Med*; 27-28:1793-1802. 1981.

Drubaix I; Maraval M; Robert L; Robert AM. Hyaluronic acid (hyaluronan) levels in pathological human saphenous veins. Effects of procyanidol oligomers. *Pathol Biol* (Paris) Jan;45(1):86-91. 1997.

Facino MR, Carini M, Aldini G, et al. Free radicals scavenging action and anti-enzyme activities of procyanidines from *Vitis vinifera*: a mechanism for their capillary protective action (German). *Arzneimittelforschung*; 44(5):592-601. 1994.

Frankel EN, Kanner J, German JB et al. Inhibition of oxidation of human low-density lipoprotein by phenolic substances in red wine. *Lancet*; 34(8843)1:454-457. 1993.

Henriet JP. Veno-lymphatic insufficiency. 4,729 patients undergoing hormonal and procyanidol oligomer therapy. *Phlebologie* Apr-Jun;46(2):313-25. 1993.

Joshi SS, Benner EJ, Balmoori J et al. Amelioration of cytotoxic effects of idarubicin and 4HC on Chang liver cells by a novel Grape Seed proanthocyanidin extract (abstract 4484). *FASEB J*; 12(5):A774. 1998a.

Joshi SS, Ye X, Liu W et al. The cytotoxic effects of a novel Grape Seed proanthocyanidin extract on cultured human cancer cells (abstract 1549). *Proc Am Assoc Cancer Res*; 39:227. 1998.

Karim M, Kappagoda T & German B. Endothelium dependent vasorelaxing activity of polymeric phenolics (flavonoids) present in Grape Seed extract (abstract 2218). *FASEB J*; 12(4):A382. 1998.

Kern W, List PH, Hörhammer L (Hrsg.), Hagers Handbuch der Pharmazeutischen Praxis, 4. Aufl., Bde 1-8: Springer Verlag Berlin, Heidelberg, New York, 1969.

Lagrue G, Oliver-Martin F & Grillot A. A study of the effects of procyanidol oligomers on capillary resistance in hypertension and in certain nephropathies. *Sem Hop Paris*; 57(33-36):1399-1401. 1981.

Lanka VK, Goddu MS, Howell RW et al. Radiation protection with Grape Seed extract (abstract P.31). *Health Phys*; 74(6 suppl):S12. 1998.

Maffei Facino R, Carini M, Aldini G, et al. Free radicals scavenging action and anti-enzyme activities of procyanidines from Vitis vinifera. A mechanism for their capillary protective action. *Arzneimittelforschung* May;44(5):592-601. 1994.

Maffei Facino R, Carini M, Aldini G, et al. Procyanidines from *Vitis vinifera* seeds protect rabbit heart from ischemia/reperfusion injury: antioxidant intervention and/or iron and copper sequestering ability. *Planta Med* Dec;62(6):495-502. 1996.

Meunier MT, Duroux E & Bastide P. Antioxidant activity of procyanidolic oligomers vis a vis the superoxide anion and vis a vis lipid peroxidation. *Planta Med*; 4:267-274. 1989.

Nutall SL, Kendall MJ, Bombardelli E et al. An evaluation of the antioxidant activity of a standardized Grape Seed extract, Leucoselect®. *J Clin Pharm Ther*; 23(5):385-389. 1998.

Plumb GW; De Pascual-Teresa S; Santos-Buelga C et al. Antioxidant properties of catechins and proanthocyanidins: effect of polymerisation, galloylation and glycosylation. *Free Radic Res* Oct;29(4):351-8. 1998.

Ray SD, Kumar MA & Bagchi D. In vivo abrogation of acetaminophen-induced hepatic genomic DNA fragmentation and apoptopic cell death by a novel Grape Seed extract (GSPE) (abstract 4516). *FASEB J*; 12(5):A779. 1998.

Ray SD, Kumar MA, Bagchi D. A novel proanthocyanidin IH636 Grape Seed extract increases in vivo Bcl-XL expression and prevents acetaminophen-induced programmed and unprogrammed cell death in mouse liver. *Arch Biochem Biophy s* Sep 1;369(1):42-58. 1999.

Robert L; Godeau G; Gavignet-Jeannin C et al. The effect of procyanidolic oligomers on vascular permeability. A study using quantitative morphology. *Pathol Biol* (Paris) Jun;38(6):608-16. 1990.

Saito M, Hosoyama H, Ariga T et al. Antiulcer activity of Grape Seed extract and procyanidins. *J Agric Food Chem*; 46:1460-1464. 1998.

Sevanian A & Ursini F. Grape Seed significantly increases antioxidant activity and human health: natural polyphenols and carotenoids: highlights of the Scientific Conference on Aging. Tufts University, May 12, 1998.

Soyeux A; Seguin JP; Le Devehat C; Bertrand A. Endotelon. Diabetic retinopathy and hemorheology (preliminary study). *Bull Soc Ophtalmol* Fr Dec;87(12):1441-4. 1987.

Takahashi T; Kamiya T; Yokoo Y. Proanthocyanidins from Grape Seeds promote proliferation of mouse hair follicle cells in vitro and convert hair cycle in vivo. *Acta Derm Venereol* Nov;78(6):428-32. 1998.

Tebib K, Rouanet JM, Besancon P. Effect of Grape Seed tannins on the activity of some rat intestinal enzyme actfvities. *Enzyme Protein*;48(1):51-60. 1994-95.

Thebaut JF, Thebaut P & Vin F. Study of Endotelon in functional manifestations of peripheral venous insufficiency (French). *Gazette Medicale* 1985;92:96-100.

Tixier JM; Godeau G; Robert AM; Hornebeck W. Evidence by in vivo and in vitro studies that binding of procyagenols to elastin affects its rate of degradation by elastases. *Biochem Pharmacol* Dec 15;33(24):3933-9. 1984.

Vogels N, Nijs IM, Westerterp-Plantega MS. The effect of grape-seed extract on 24 h energy intake in humans. *Eur J Clin Nutr*; 58(4):667-673. 2004.

Yamakoshi J; Kataoka S; Koga T; Ariga T. Proanthocyanidin-rich extract from Grape Seeds attenuates the development of aortic atherosclerosis in cholesterol-fed rabbits. *Atherosclerosis* Jan;142(1):139-49. 1999.

Ye X; Krohn RL; Liu W et al. The cytotoxic effects of a novel IH636 Grape Seed proanthocyanidin extract on cultured human cancer cells. *Mol Cell Biochem* Jun;196(1-2):99-108. 1999.

Zern TL, Fernandez ML. Cardioprotective effects of dietary polyphenols. *J Nutr*; 135: 2291-2294. 2005.

Zern TL, Wood RJ, Greene C, et al. Grape polyphenols exert a cardioprotective effect in pre- and postmenopausal women by lowering plasma lipids and reducing oxidative stress. *J Nutr*; 135: 1911-1917. 2005.

Zafirov D; Bredy-Dobreva G; Litchev V et al. Antiexudative and capillaritonic effects of procyanidines isolated from Grape Seeds (*V. Vinifera*). *Acta Physiol Pharmacol* Bulg;16(3):50-4. 1990.

Zhao J, Wang J, Chen Y, Agarwal R. Anti-tumor-promoting activity of a polyphenolic fraction isolated from Grape Seeds in the mouse skin two-stage initiation-promotion protocol and identification of procyanidin B5-3′-gallate as the most effective antioxidant constituent. *Carcinogenesis* Sep;20(9):1737-4. 1999.

Gratiola officinalis

See Hedge-Hyssop

Great Burnet

Sanguisorba officinalis

DESCRIPTION

Medicinal Parts: The medicinal parts of the plant are the fresh aerial parts, the dried herb, the rhizomes, and roots.

Flower and Fruit: The composite heads are ovate-oblong, approximately 1 to 2 cm long, and consist of 5 to 10 usually androgynous flowers. The calyx has 4 dark red-brown tips, 4 stamens with stiffly patent red filaments and yellow anthers. The smooth, spikelike, quadrangular fruit calyx has 1 carpel and 1 style and is narrowly winged. The fruit is a nut enclosed in the perigone tube.

Leaves, Stem, and Root: Great Burnet is a semi-rosette shrub with a strong dark brown root that produces thick fibers and a short rhizome. The stems are erect, angular, glabrous, and bifurcated. The rosette leaves are 20 to 40 cm long and consist of 7 to 15 ovate leaflets, which are cordate at the base and blue-green beneath. There are only a few cauline leaves, which taper towards the top.

Characteristics: The brown-red composite head is characteristic for this plant.

Habitat: The plant is widespread in the northern, temperate regions of Europe, temperate Asia, and North America.

Production: Great Burnet is the *Sanguisorba officinalis* plant in flower. The fresh aerial parts are collected in the wild during the flowering season. The rhizomes and roots are harvested in autumn, then washed and dried.

Other Names: Garden Burnet, Greater Burnet

ACTIONS AND PHARMACOLOGY

COMPOUNDS

Flavonoids: including among others, rutin, flavonoid sulfates

Tannins: including ellagitannins, sanguinarine H-11, casuarinin

Triterpene glycosides: aglycones pomolic acid, tormentolic acid, including among others, ziyuglycosides I and II (sanguisorbin), betulinic acid, ursolic acid

Sterols: including beta-sitosterol

EFFECTS

The drug has been credited with decongestant, astringent and diuretic properties, but no investigation into effects has been carried out.

INDICATIONS AND USAGE

Unproven Uses: The drug is used internally for female disorders, menorrhagia during menopause, dysentery, enteritis, diarrhea, bladder restraint, hemorrhoids, phlebitis, and varicose veins. Externally, Great Burnet is used in plaster for wounds and ulcers.

Chinese Medicine: The Chinese use Great Burnet for dysentery, reptile bites, bloody coughs, and as an astringent and hemostyptic for nosebleeds.

Homeopathic Uses: Among uses in homeopathy are uterine bleeding, varicose veins, and diarrhea.

PRECAUTIONS AND ADVERSE REACTIONS

No health hazards or side effects are known in conjunction with the proper administration of designated therapeutic dosages.

DOSAGE

Mode of Administration: The drug is used internally and externally. It is available in ground form and is used as an extract, juice, or tea. A plaster is used externally.

Homeopathic Dosage: 5 drops, 1 tablet or 10 globules every 30 to 60 minutes (acute) or 1 to 3 times a day (chronic); parenterally: 1 to 2 mL sc acute: 3 times daily; chronic: once a day (HAB34).

LITERATURE

Bastow KF et al., Inhibition of DNA topoisomerase by sanguiin H-6, a cytotoxic dimeric ellagitannin from *Sanguisorba officinalis*. In: *PM* 59(3):240. 1993.

Chang, EH et al. (Eds), Advances in Chinese Medicinal Materials Research, World Scientific Pub. Co. Singapore 1985.

Hänsel R, Keller K, Rimpler H, Schneider G (Hrsg.), Hagers Handbuch der Pharmazeutischen Praxis, 5. Aufl., Bde 4-6 (Drogen), Springer Verlag Berlin, Heidelberg, New York, 1992-1994.

Iida K, Hase K, Shimomura K, Sudo S, Kadota S, Namba T. Potent Inhibitors of Tyrosinase Activity and Melanin Biosynthesis from *Rheum fficinale. Planta Med.* 61 (5); 425-428. 1995

Inaoka Y et al. Studies on Active Substances in Herbs Used for Hair Treatment. I. Effects of Herb Extracts on Hair Growth and Isolation of an Active Substance from *Polyporus umbellatus F. Chem Pharm Bull.* 42; 530-533. 1994

Ishida H et al. Studies on the Antihemorrhagic and anticoagulative substances in herbs used for treatments of Bleeding and stagnant blood in traditional Chinese medicine. *J Pharm Sci.* 76; S200. 1987

Kashiwada Y, Nonaka GI, Niskioka I, Chang JJ, Lee KH, Antitumor agents, 129. Tannins and related compounds as selective cytotoxic agents. In: *JNP* 55:1033-1043. 1992.

Greater Bindweed

Calystegia sepium

DESCRIPTION

Medicinal Parts: The medicinal parts are the whole flowering plant and the root.

Flower and Fruit: The solitary white flowers are about 5 cm long; the pedicle is quadrangular. Under the calyx there are 2 cordate, pointed, red-bordered bracts, which extend to cover the calyx. There are 5 sepals. The corolla is fused and conical. There are 5 stamens and 1 superior ovary. The fruit is a capsule.

Leaves, Stem, and Root: The plant is about 10 to 30 cm high and has a creeping rhizome. The stem is angular, glabrous, and twining. The leaves are alternate, petiolate, cordate or arrow-shaped. The base of the leaves are acuminate, and they often have dentate lobes. Most twining plants seem to follow the course of the sun and bind round a support from left to right. But the Bindweed will always twine against the sun, confounding all attempts to train it, even dying in the process.

Characteristics: The flowers close in damp weather.

Habitat: The plant is indigenous to Europe and eastern U.S.

Production: The upper part of the herb is harvested during the flowering season and dried at temperatures of no more than 40° C in a well-ventilated place.

Other Names: Devil's Vine, Hedge Lily, Lady's Nightcap, Rutland Beauty, Hedge Convolvulus, Old Man's Night Cap, Bearbind

ACTIONS AND PHARMACOLOGY

COMPOUNDS

Glycoretines: polymeric, resinous glycosides of hydroxy fatty acids (C12-C16) with oligosaccharides; the hydroxyl groups have been esterified with acetic, propionic, isobutyric and valeric acids, among others

Tannins

EFFECTS

The drug has a powerful effect; activity in the smooth muscle area is stimulated, intestinal peristalsis is increased, and there is an increase in bile production.

INDICATIONS AND USAGE

Unproven Uses: Greater Bindweed is used for fevers, urinary tract diseases, as a purgative for constipation, and to increase the production of bile.

PRECAUTIONS AND ADVERSE REACTIONS

No health hazards or side effects are known in conjunction with the proper administration of designated therapeutic dosages. It is conceivable that an overdose of the drug would trigger intestinal colic.

DOSAGE

Mode of Administration: The pressed juice, powdered root and an infusion are used internally. The drug is rarely used anymore due to its strong intestinal effects.

Preparation: An infusion is prepared by adding 1 to 2 teaspoons of cut drug per cup of water.

LITERATURE

Asano N, Kato A, Oseki K, Kizu H, Matsui K, Calystegins of *Physalis alkekengi var. francheti* (Solanaceae). Structure determination and their glycosidase inhibitory activities. *Eur J Biochem*, 14:369-76, 1995.

Damme EJ van, Barre A, Verhaert P, Rouge P, Peumans WJ. Molecular cloning of the mitogenic mannose/maltose-specific rhizome lectin from *Calystegia sepium. FEBS Lett*, 14:352-6, Nov 18 1996

Goldmann A et al. Biological Activities of the Nortropane Alkaloid, Calystegine B2, and Analogs: Structure-Function Relationships. *J Nat Prod.* 59 (12); 1137-1142. 1996

Kern W, List PH, Hörhammer L (Hrsg.), Hagers Handbuch der Pharmazeutischen Praxis, 4. Aufl., Bde 1-8, Springer Verlag Berlin, Heidelberg, New York, 1969.

Peumans WJ, Winter HC, Bemer V, Van Leuven F, Goldstein IJ, Truffa-Bachi P, Van Damme EJ, Isolation of a novel plant lectin with an unusual specificity from *Calystegia sepium. Glycocon J,* 14:259-65, 1997.

Roth L, Daunderer M, Kormann K Giftpflanzen, Pflanzengifte. 4. Aufl., Ecomed Fachverlag Landsberg / Lech 1993.

Van Damme EJ, Barre A, Verhaert P, Rouge P, Peumans WJ, Molecular cloning of the mitogenic mannose/maltose-specific rhizome lectin from *Calystegia sepium. FEBS Lett,* 14:352-6, 1996.

Greek Sage

Salvia triloba

DESCRIPTION

Medicinal Parts: The medicinal part of the plant is the leaf.

Flower and Fruit: The flowers are in false whorls of 2 to 6 blossoms. The calyx is campanulate, dentate, 5 to 8 mm long, often purple and pubescent. The corolla is 16 to 25 mm long, typically lilac or pink but occasionally white.

Leaves, Stem, and Root: Salvia triloba grows as a semi-shrub, up to 1.2 m high. The leaves are petiolate and tomentose. The lamina is simple or pinnatifid with 1 to 2 pairs of lateral leaf sections and a large elongate-ovate end section. The stem is square, appressed pubescent, grayish-white beneath and green above.

Habitat: The plant is indigenous to Greece, the Commonwealth of Independent States, Albania, Turkey, and Cyprus. Various species are particularly widespread in the Mediterranean region.

Production: Greek Sage leaves are the dried leaves of *Salvia triloba,* which are harvested once a year if collected in the wild and three times a year when cultivated.

Other Names: Three-Lobed Sage, Turkish Sage

ACTIONS AND PHARMACOLOGY

COMPOUNDS

Volatile oil (1.5 to 3.5%): chief component 1.8-cineole (40 to 67%), camphor (2 to 25%), thujone (5 to 6%), including as well camphene, beta-caryophyllene, myrcene, alpha-pinene, beta-pinene

Flavonoids: including 7-O-glucosides and 7-O-glucuronides of apigenin, chrysoeriol, hispidulin, luteolin, 6-methyl luteolin, as well as salvigenin, jaceosidin

Caffeic acid derivatives: rosmarinic acid (1.0 to 2.5%)

Diterpenes: including carnosol (0.5%)

Triterpenes (8%): ursolic acid, oleanolic acid

EFFECTS

The chief active ingredient (cineole) of the drug's essential oil has an antimicrobial effect. The combined action of the essential oil and the tannins is antiseptic and anti-inflammatory, particularly in the region of the mouth and throat. Decoctions and infusions of the leaves exhibit antihypertensive, spasmolytic, and blood sugar-reducing effects in animal experiments, during which the plasma insulin levels remain unchanged. The hypoglycemic effect is traced to the inhibition of intestinal glucose resorption. A sedative effect has also been described.

INDICATIONS AND USAGE

Unproven Uses: Salvia triloba is used internally for diabetes in Israel and Cyprus, and elsewhere for cardiac symptoms, lung complaints, colds, coughs, nervousness, and digestion problems. Externally it is used to treat skin damage.

PRECAUTIONS AND ADVERSE REACTIONS

No health hazards are known in conjunction with the proper administration of designated therapeutic dosages.

DOSAGE

Mode of Administration: Aqueous decoctions and infusions prepared from the whole, cut and powdered drug are used internally. The fresh cut leaves are applied topically.

Preparation: For tea, pour 150 mL water over 3 g (3 to 4 teaspoons) of drug. Allow to steep for 10 to 15 minutes.

Storage: Store tightly sealed and protected from light.

LITERATURE

Hänsel R, Keller K, Rimpler H, Schneider G (Ed), Hagers Handbuch der Pharmazeutischen Praxis, 5. Aufl., Bde 4 - 6 (Drogen), Springer Verlag Berlin, Heidelberg, New York, 1992-1994.

Länger R, Mechtler C, Tanzler HO, Jurenitsch J. Differences of the composition of the essential oil within an individium of *Salva officinalis. Planta Med* 59, A635 1993

Liu J, Zapp J, Becker H. Comparative Phytochemical Investigation of *Salvia miltiorrhiza* and *Salvia triloba. Planta Med.* 61 (5); 453-455. 1995

Green Hellebore

Helleborus viridis

DESCRIPTION

Medicinal Parts: The drug derived from the plant's rhizome and roots is obsolete in medicine today.

Flower and Fruit: There are 2 to 3 flowers with a diameter of 4 to 7 cm and 5 ovate, grass-green, broad flower bracts. The petals are in the form of petaloid honey glands, and there are numerous stamens. The ovary is superior with the carpels only fused at the base. The fruit is a 25- to 28-mm long follicle with beak. The seeds have a narrow longitudinal strip with a ring at the end.

Leaves, Stem and Root: This herbaceous perennial grows upright, up to 40 cm high. There are 2 basal, long-petioled leaves; the lamina is divided like a foot into 7 to 13 sections that are narrow-lanceolate, serrate, and dark green. The stem is upright, branching higher up and leafless to that point. The cauline leaves are similar to the basal ones but sessile and smaller. The rhizome is usually branched.

Habitat: The various species of Hellebore grow mainly in mountainous regions of Europe and North America. The plant is most commonly found in the Alps; *Helleborus viridis* is found growing as far north as northwest France.

Production: Green Hellebore root is the dried rhizome with roots of *Helleborus viridis*.

Not to be Confused With: Adulteration and mistaken identity can occur with *Hellebori nigri rhizoma, Actaea spicata, Adonis vernalis, Trollius europaeus* and *Eupatorium cannabium.*

Other Names: Bear's Foot

ACTIONS AND PHARMACOLOGY

COMPOUNDS

Cardioactive steroid glycosides (bufadienolids, 0.5 to 1.5%): chief component hellebrin, including deglucohellebrin

Alkaloids of unknown structure: celliamine, sprintillamine, sprintilline

Steroid saponins

EFFECTS

The steroid saponin mixture helleborin is severely toxic and irritating to mucous membranes (ptarmic). It exhibits digitalis-like effects through the cardioactive glycosides it contains (hellebrin). The alkaloids it contains produce an excitation of the motor centers, eventually leading to convulsions and respiratory failure and triggering bradycardia and a negatively inotropic effect.

INDICATIONS AND USAGE

Unproven Uses: The drug is obsolete today because the risks of use are considered too high, given that efficacy for previously accepted indications has not yet been proved. Previous uses in folk medicine included nausea, constipation, and worm infestation. Root preparations were used also for heart failure and as a diuretic. *Helleborus viridis* was employed as a laxative according to Hager (around 1930) and was important in homeopathic medicine.

Homeopathic Uses: Helleborus viridis is used for diarrhea.

PRECAUTIONS AND ADVERSE REACTIONS

The drug is not to be administered in allopathic medicine. No risks are known in connection with the administration of homeopathic dosages of the drug.

OVERDOSAGE

The mucous membrane-irritating effect of the saponins appears to play the largest role in poisonings with the drug, resulting in scratchiness in mouth and throat, salivation, nausea, vomiting, diarrhea, dizziness, shortness of breath, and possible convulsions and asphyxiation. The ingestion of very large dosages leads to disorders of cardiac function (cardiac arrhythmia).

Following gastrointestinal emptying (gastric lavage, sodium sulfate) and the administration of activated charcoal, the treatment for poisonings consists of the treatment of spasms with diazepam (i.v.), electrolyte substitution and the countering of any acidosis that may appear through sodium bicarbonate infusions. Intubation and oxygen respiration may also be required.

Cases of fatal poisonings are known among animals that fed on the leaves of the plant.

DOSAGE

Mode of Administration: Whole, cut and powdered drug.

Daily Dosage: 1 g drug; maximum single dosage: 0.2 g drug.

Homeopathic Dosage: 5 drops, 1 tablet, or 10 globules every to 30 to 60 minutes (acute) and 1 to 3 times daily (chronic); parenterally: 1 to mL sc acute, 3 times daily; chronic: once a day (HAB34).

Storage: Store securely.

LITERATURE

Colombo ML, Tome F, Servettaz O, Bugatti C. Phytochemical evaluation of *Helleborus* Species Growing in Northern Italy. *Int J Crude Drug Res.* 28 (3); 219-223. 1990

Hänsel R, Keller K, Rimpler H, Schneider G (Ed.), Hagers Handbuch der Pharmazeutischen Praxis, 5. Aufl., Bde 4 - 6 (Drogen), Springer Verlag Berlin, Heidelberg, New York, 1992-1994.

Johnson CT, Routledge JK, Suspected *helleborus viridis* poisoning of cattle. Vet Rec, 89:202, Aug 14, 1971

Green Tea

Camellia sinensis

DESCRIPTION

Medicinal Parts: The medicinal parts are the very young downy leaves, from which green or black tea is prepared according to the treatment being given.

Flower and Fruit: The flowers grow short-pedicled and singly or in clusters of a few flowers in the leaf axils. They are white or pale pink and have a diameter of 3 to 5 cm. The flowers have between 5 and 7 sepals and petals at a time. The petals are fused at the base with the numerous stamens. The ovary has 3 chambers. The fruit is a greenish-brown, woody capsule with a diameter of 1 to 1.5 cm and contains 1 to 3 smooth brown seeds.

Leaves, Stem, and Root: The plant is an evergreen, heavily branched shrub. The leaves are glossy dark green, alternate, short-petiolate, coreacious, lanceolate or elongate-ovate, and roughly serrate. The young leaves appear silver because of the covering of downy hairs on the surface.

Habitat: The plant does not originate in the wild. It was originally cultivated in China and is grown as a tea plant today in India, China, Sri Lanka, Japan, Indonesia, Kenya, Turkey, Pakistan, Malawi, and Argentina.

Production: Tea leaves are the fermented and/or dried leaves of *Camellia sinensis*. Harvesting takes place under stringent quality control. Green Tea is produced by steaming the fresh-cut leaf. Black Tea is produced by allowing the leaves to oxidize. During oxidation, enzymes present in the tea convert many of the polyphenolic therapeutic substances to less active compounds. Oxidation does not occur with Green Tea because the steaming process inactivates the enzymes responsible for oxidation. The anti-oxidant activity of Green Tea is six times greater than that of Black Tea.

ACTIONS AND PHARMACOLOGY

COMPOUNDS

Purine alkaloids (methyl xanthines): caffeine (previously referred to as theine or teine; depending upon the development stage of the leaves, 2.9-4.2%, content declining with age), theobromine (0.15-0.2%), theophylline (0.02-0.04%)

Triterpene saponins (theafolia saponins): aglycones including, among others, barringtogenol C, R1-barringenol

Catechins: in unfermented (green) tea 10-25%, with fermentation partially changing over into oligomeric quinones with tannin character, into theaflavine, theaflavin acid, thearubigene, or into non-water soluble polymeric flavonoids including, among others, quercetin, kaempferol, myrecetin

Flavonoids: including quercetin, kaempferol, myricetin

Caffeic acid derivatives: including among others, chlorogenic acid, theogallin

Anorganic ions: high fluoride content (130-160 mg/kg), potassium and aluminum ions

Volatile oil: chief components linalool, in fermented tea also 2-methyl-hept-2-en-6-on, alpha-ionon and beta-ionon, more than 300 volatile compounds are involved in tea aroma

EFFECTS

The primary clinical application for Green Tea is in the prevention of cancer and heart disease. Cohort and case-control studies indicate Green Tea exerts anticancer properties on cancers of the gastrointestinal tract, stomach, small intestine, pancreas, colon, lung, and estrogen-related cancers, including most breast cancers. Mouthwashes made with Green Tea have been shown to decrease dental plaque formation and inhibit the growth of caries-producing bacteria (Yamamoto et al, 1997). Green Tea displays thermogenic and fat-oxidizing properties and may thus be a useful adjunct in the treatment of obesity. Green Tea may be helpful in the prevention and treatment of Clostridial diarrhea disease and in helping to promote the growth of ''friendly'' bacteria (e.g., *Lactobacillus* and *Bidifobacter* species) in the gut microflora. Animal studies have demonstrated anti-inflammatory action in the treatment of colitis and cholesterol lowering effects.

The polyphenols in Green Tea are believed to be responsible for the majority of the chemoprotective, antiproliferative, and antioxidant activity of Green Tea. Recent studies on nonpolyphenolic constituents of Green Tea have demonstrated that pheophytins A and B have antigenotoxic and anti-inflammatory activities. Several mechanisms for antiproliferative activity and proapoptotic activity related to cancer and vascular disease chemoprevention have been proposed. The caffeine in the drug has a centrally stimulating and antidepressive effect (adenosine antagonism.) Adenosine antagonism leads to dilation of the renal vessels with a consecutive increase of the rate of filtration (diuresis). Caffeine is positively inotropic, promotes the secretion of gastric juices, glycolysis, and lipolysis. In animal tests, bradykinin and prostaglandin antagonism caused a capillary sealing and anti-inflammatory effect.

Activities of nonpolypyenol constituents in Green Tea: Pheophytins A and B extracted from the nonpolyphenolic fraction of Green Tea demonstrated potent suppressive activity against DNA (Okai & Higashi-Okai, 1997). Pheophytins A and B, extracted from the nonpolyphenolic fraction of Green Tea, demonstrated potent suppressive activity against the activation of polymorphonuclear neutrophils (PMNs) function (Higashi-Okai et al, 1998).

Anticancer Effects: There is clinical evidence that Green Tea has cancer preventative effects. The types of cancer that Green Tea has been shown to prevent as demonstrated in well-controlled clinical studies include cancers of the pancreas, colon, small intestine, stomach, breast, and lung. Several in vitro studies have demonstrated a dose-dependent decreased proliferation and/or increased apoptosis in a variety of cancer cell lines (lung, epidermoid, keratinocyte, prostate, Ehrlich ascites, colon, stomach, oral, and breast). This occurs when exposed to Green Tea polyphenols or the specific polyphenol constituents, epigallocatechin-3-gallate (EGCG) and epigallocatechin (EGC) (Chen et al, 1998; Khafif et al, 1998; Mukhtar, 1998; Kennedy et al, 1998; Khafif et al, 1998a; Yang et al, 1998; Fujiki et al, 1998; Gotoh, 1998; Ahmad et al, 1997).

Other mechanisms of action have been proposed, such as stimulation of transcription of phase II detoxifying enzymes, blockade of growth factor associated signal transduction pathways, inhibition of protein expression of inducible nitric oxide, inhibition of nitric oxide production, and inhibition of activator protein-1 activity (Ahmad & Mukhtar, 1999). Two studies demonstrated that Green Tea caused growth arrest or apoptosis specifically in cancer cells and not in normal cells (Chen et al, 1998; Ahmad et al, 1997). Growth arrest of tumor cells by tea polyphenols occurred during the G1 phase of the cell cycle (Khafif et al, 1998; Khafif et al, 1998a; Ahmad et al, 1997).

Green Tea powder (1 g/kg/d for 4 days, administered orally) enhanced the antitumor activity of the chemotherapeutic agent doxorubicin (DOX) (2 mg/kg/d for 4 days, administered intraperitoneally) in mice transplanted with Ehrlich ascites carcinoma or M5076 ovarian sarcoma cells (Sadzuka et al, 1998). A decrease in total cholesterol, but not triglycerides or HDL, has been associated with drinking 9 cups of Green Tea per day (Kono et al, 1992).

Anticaries Activity: Ethylacetate extracts of Green Tea were potent inhibitors of cavity-associated bacteria such as *Escherichia coli, Streptococcus salivarius,* and *Streptococcus mutans* that were isolated from the saliva and dental plaque of carious teeth of cariogenic patients (Rasheed & Haider, 1998). Green Tea had weak inhibitory activity on the growth of *Proteus rettgeri* and *Proteus mirabilis* bacteria using a bulk acoustic wave bacterial growth sensor (Yao et al, 1998). Green Tea was demonstrated to be a weak inhibitor of salivary amylase due to tannins and not catechins that are present in the tea (Zhang & Kashket, 1998). Green Tea polyphenols inhibit the growth of *Porphyromonas gingivalis* and its adherence to oral epithelial cells (Yamamoto et al, 1997).

Anti-inflammatory Effects: In vitro pretreatment of cells with the Green Tea extract epigallocatechin gallate significantly inhibited neutrophil adhesion to and migration through endothelial cell monolayers in a dose-dependent manner ($p<0.05$). Neutrophils play an important part in the inflammatory process. By adhering to the vascular endothelium and migrating into the tissue, invading microorganisms such as bacteria are eliminated (Hofbauer et al, 1999).

Antioxidant Effects: Several in vitro studies demonstrate that Green Tea polyphenols and the specific catechins in Green Tea polyphenols, catechin, and epicatechin inhibit LDL oxidation (Lotito & Fraga, 1998; Pearson et al, 1998; Vinson & Babbgh, 1998; Kaneko et al, 1998; Kannar et al, 1997). This activity may help to prevent the development of cardiovascular pathologies, such as atherosclerosis. Two human studies, one in smokers and one in nonsmokers, found no effect of Green Tea consumption (6 cups of Green Tea daily for 4 weeks) on LDL oxidation ex vivo or on plasma levels of antioxidants (vitamins C, E and B-carotene) and lipids (HDL and LDL cholesterol and triglycerides) (Princen et al, 1998; van het Hof et al, 1997).

Epigallocatechin-3-gallate (EGCG) was effective at inhibiting ultraviolet B exposure (Chen, 1998) and preventing ultraviolet-induced skin damage that correlated with reduced lipid peroxidation (Kim, 1998). In humans, pretreatment of skin with Green Tea extracts 30 minutes prior to ultraviolet B (UVB) exposure resulted in a dose-dependent protection against acute erythema formation (Zhao, 1998).

Cancer Preventative Effects: The results of a case control study for breast cancer in Japanese women suggest that increased consumption of Green Tea prior to clinical cancer onset is associated with improved prognosis in stage I and II breast cancer; this may be related to the modifying effects of Green Tea on the clinical characteristics of the cancer (Nakachi et al, 1998).

The consumption of Green Tea was investigated in a case control study on the risk of digestive tract cancers (esophagus, stomach, colon, and rectal). A lower risk for stomach cancer was associated with a high consumption of Green Tea (7+ cups/day) (Inoue et al, 1998). A case-control study in Shanghai, China, found a strong inverse association between Green Tea consumption and various cancers (Ji et al, 1997).

Chemopreventive effects of Green Tea were examined in cigarette smokers by assessing the levels of sister chromatid exchange in peripheral lymphocytes in nonsmokers, smokers, and smokers who consumed 2 to 3 cups of Green Tea daily for 6 months. Green Tea appeared to block the "smoking-induced" increase in sister chromatid exchange (Lee et al, 1997; Shim et al, 1995).

Effects on Gut Microflora and Diarrheal Disease: Green Tea extract (400 mg polyphenols 3 times daily) promoted the growth of Lactobacillus and Bifidobacter species while inhibiting the growth of *Clostridium perfringens* and *C difficile*. This effect is significant not only in preventing Clostridial diarrhea diseases but also in colon cancer (Yamamoto et al, 1997). Green Tea polyphenols exhibit significant antiviral activity against rotavirus, a common cause of viral gastroenteritis in children (Yamamoto et al, 1997). Extracts of Green Tea inhibited the growth of various bacteria-causing diarrheal diseases including *Vibrio cholerae, Salmonella typhimurium,* and *Salmonella typhi* (Shetty et al, 1994).

Hepatoprotective Effects: Fraction analysis of Green Tea showed that Fraction III, IV, and V had relatively strong effects on D-Galactosamine-induced liver injury. Fraction III contained tea saponins and flavonoids. Fraction IV contained water-soluble compounds of low molecular weights such as free sugars, amino acids, and oligosaccharides. Fraction V was relatively pure and consisted of soluble dietary fibers (polysaccharides) (Sugiyama et al, 1999).

Inhibition of Xanthine Oxidase: Green Tea may be indicated in the treatment of gout as Green Tea polyphenols showed levels of inhibition of the enzyme xanthine oxidase (involved in the conversion of purines to uric acid). This was similar to those achieved by the drug allopurinol in an in vitro model (Aucamp, 1997).

CLINICAL TRIALS

Antioxidant Activity

Green Tea demonstrated significant increased plasma antioxidant activity in vivo in 21 volunteers in a crossover study. Experimentation consisted of 6 treatments on 6 different dates with at least 2 days separating treatments. After overnight fasting, subjects were given either: 300 mL of green or black tea, 240 mL of green or black tea supplemented with 60 mL of full fat milk, 300 mL of mineral water with 60 mL of full fat milk, or 240 mL of mineral water with 60 mL of full fat milk. Blood samples were obtained at baseline and at 30, 60, 90, and 120 minute intervals. Green Tea resulted in a significant increase in plasma antioxidant activity ($p<0.001$) for all timed blood samples. Plasma antioxidant activity was increased about 1.5 times with Green Tea ingestion and the rise in plasma catechins was about 5 times higher (Leenen et al, 2000).

The antioxidant activity of Green Tea was tested on two groups of 5 healthy adults. Each group ingested 300 mL of black or Green Tea after an overnight fast. The experiment was repeated on a separate day, adding 100 mL whole milk to the tea (ratio 1:4). Five subjects acted as controls. The human plasma antioxidant capacity (TRAP) was measured before and 30, 50, and 80 minutes from the ingestion of tea. Both teas inhibited the in vitro peroxidation in a dose-dependent manner. Green Tea was sixfold more potent than black tea. The addition of milk to either tea did not appreciably modify their in vitro antioxidant potential. In vivo, the ingestion of tea produced a significant increase of TRAP ($p<0.05$), similar in both teas, which peaked at 30 to 50 minutes. When tea was consumed with milk, the in vivo activity was totally inhibited. The inhibition of this effect by milk is thought to occur due to the complexity of tea polyphenols by milk proteins (Serafini et al, 1996).

Cancer Treatment/Prevention

Human population studies point to anticancer activities for tea, with early research showing an inverse association between consumption of tea and development of cancers of the stomach, urinary bladder, color, esophagus, lung, and pancreas. An empirical link between Green Tea consumption and cancer-fighting effects was established in the late 1980s. A 2005 review cites the tea's unique set of catechins, with antioxidant, antiangiogenesis, and antiproliferative elements, as explanation for the anticancer actions of Green Tea. The major tea catechin, (-)-epigallocatechin, has anticancer and medicinal properties that are examined. Researchers working with cancer cell lines have linked Green tea's anticancer activity to growth inhibition—a possible explanation for its antitumor activity. Several animal studies point to tea catechins as aids to cancer therapy. Studies on people with severe head and neck cancers indicated a positive role for an herbal mixture containing a blend of decaffeinated green tea and red pepper (*Capsicum* sp). Overall, more research is needed to clearly elucidate Green Tea's promising potential role in preventing and treating cancer (Cooper, 2005).

A proof-of-principle clinical study was conducted to assess the efficacy and safety of green tea catechins (GTCs) for the prevention of prostate cancer in men with high-grade prostate intraepithelial neoplasia. In this double-blind, placebo-controlled study, daily treatment consisted of 3 GTC capsules, 200 mg each, or placebo. After one year, 1 tumor was diagnosed among the 30 GTC-treated men, whereas 9 cancers were found among the 30 placebo-treated men. GTC was found to be safe and effective for treating premalignant lesions before prostate cancer develops. The researchers also observed that GTCs also reduced lower urinary track symptoms (Bettzi et al, 2006).

In an earlier study, Green Tea demonstrated no improvement in subjects with androgen-dependent prostate cancer in a multi-institutional, phase II clinical trial. Forty-two males with progressive prostate specific antigen (PSA) elevation with hormone therapy received 1 g Green Tea orally, mixed in warm or cold water, 6 times daily. Subjects were able to continue use of LH-releasing hormone agonist and visited their oncologist monthly for PSA measurement. After 4 months of treatment, only one patient experienced a tumor response, demonstrated by a 50% decrease in PSA level from baseline (from 229 ng/dL to 105 ng/dL). The response was not maintained beyond 2 months (Jatoi et al, 2003).

Components in Green Tea appear to have effective biochemical modulators for resistant tumors. Ehrlich ascites carcinoma cells were transplanted intraperitoneally into 6-week-old mice. Ascitic fluid was collected 7 days later and Doxorubicin (DOX), an antitumor medium, was introduced to the Ehrlich cancer cells. Theanine, an amino acid and (-)-epigallocatechin gallate (EGCG), both found in Green Tea, affected DOX tumor-cell activity. Theanine and EGCG inhibited DOX cellular efflux by 30.5% ($p<0.05$) and 19.5% ($p<0.05$), respectively. Combining theanine with DOX in P388 leukemia tumor treatment reduced tumor weight by 63% ($p<0.01$). It is believed that Green Tea exhibits few side effects when taken with an antitumor agent and appears to improve cancer chemotherapy (Sadzuka et al, 2000).

The consumption of Green Tea was investigated in a case control study for breast cancer in Japanese women. In stage I and II breast cancer, increased consumption of Green Tea was closely associated with decreased numbers of metastasized axillary lymph nodes among premenopausal patients and increased expression of PgR and ER among postmenopausal women. Long-term consumption of Green Tea (>5 cups daily) prior to clinical cancer onset was associated with significantly lower recurrence in stage I and II breast cancer. These results suggest that increased consumption of Green Tea prior to clinical cancer onset is associated with improved prognosis in stage I and II breast cancer and this may be related to the modifying effects of Green Tea on the clinical characteristics of the cancer (Nakachi et al, 1998).

A large (n = 2226) case-control study was conducted in China where recently diagnosed cancer cases (pancreatic, colon, and rectum) among residents between the ages of 30 and 74 years were included. Controls (n = 1552) were selected and matched to cases by age and gender and adjustments were made for age, income, education and cigarette smoking. As tea consumption increased, the incidence of all three cancers decreased. Women with the highest tea consumption (or = 200 g/month) had a 33% reduced risk for colon cancer, 43% reduced risk of rectal cancer and 47% reduction in the risk for pancreatic cancer (p= 0.07, 0.001, and 0.008 respectively). For men who consumed ≥ 300 g/month of Green Tea, the risk of colon cancer was reduced by 18%, for rectal cancer there was a 28% reduction of risk, and for pancreatic cancer the risk reduction was 37% (p= 0.38, 0.04, and 0.04, respectively) (Ji, 1997).

Colitis

Catechins from Green Tea extract demonstrated anti-inflammatory action in Trinitrobenzene sulfonic acid (TNBS)-induced colitis in Sprague-Dawley rats. Experimentally induced TNBS colitis is histopathologically similar to Crohn's disease in humans. A significant reduction in macroscopic damage of the colon was observed in rats supplemented with catechins; no perforations of the distal colon or adhesions were found, suggesting inhibition of inflammatory processes (Sato et al, 1998).

Dental Caries Prevention

In a double-blind study, 26 adult males (mean age 26.5 years) demonstrated an inhibition rate on plaque development of 30% to 43% when given a solution containing 0.05%, 0.1%, 0.2%, and 0.5% of Green Tea polyphenols as a mouthwash compared to controls. The concentration of caries-promoting bacteria and lactic acid were also reduced (Yamamoto et al, 1997). An extract of oolong tea (semifermented tea leaves of *Camellia sinensis*) containing polymerized polyphenols in 0.2% ethanol was administered to 35 volunteers between 18 and 29 years of age to test the inhibitory effect of the extract on dental plaque deposition. The study was repeated 1 week after the first trial using 0.2% ethanol without the tea extract. The oolong tea cohort showed significant inhibition of plaque deposition (Ooshima, 1994).

Diabetes, Type 2

A retrospective 5-year cohort study in 6,277 men and 10, 686 women from 25 communities in Japan was done to examine the relationship between consumption of tea (Green Tea, black tea, and oolong tea) and risk of developing Type 2 diabetes. The participants were 40 to 65 years old and healthy at study start. Analysis revealed that people who (according to questionnaire answers) frequently drank green tea (more than 6 cups daily) or coffee (more than 3 cups daily) were less likely to develop Type 2 diabetes than people who drank less than 1 cup of either beverage per week (33% lower risk for diabetes with Green Tea and 42% lower risk with coffee). This association was particularly strong for women and overweight men. Consumption of black and oolong teas did not appear to reduce diabetes risk, however. The authors conclude that while it is possible that other factors influenced these results, the higher intake of caffeine—whether from Green Tea or coffee—was significantly associated with a lower risk of developing Type 2 diabetes (Iso, 2006).

To study the effects of the intake of green tea and polyphenols on insulin resistance and systemic inflammation, a randomized, controlled trial was conducted on 66 patients with borderline diabetes or diabetes over a period of two months. Subjects in the intervention group were asked to take a packet of green tea extracts/powder containing 544 mg polyphenols (456 mg catechins) daily, and to divide the green tea extracts/powder in a packet into 3 or 4 portions, each to be dissolved in hot water. Daily supplementary intake of approximately 500 mg green tea polyphenols did not show a clear effect on blood glucose levels, HbA1c levels, insulin resistance, or inflammation markers. However, a positive correlation between the level of polyphenols intake and insulin level was demonstrated, warranting further investigation (Fukino et al, 2006).

Genital Warts

In October 2006, the Food and Drug Administration approved the use of kunecatechins (Veregen) from Green Tea for the treatment of external genital and perianal warts based on the pooled results of two randomized, double-blind, phase III clinical trials that involved 1,000 individuals who were immunocompromised. The participants applied the ointment 3 times daily for up to 16 weeks, or until the warts completely cleared. Of the participants treated with the Green Tea compound in the 2 studies, 53.6% had complete clearance of the warts by week 16, while only 35.3% of those who applied a placebo did (Centerwatch, 2006).

Heart Disease

To clarify the effect of Green Tea consumption on cardiovascular disease and cancer, a large, population-based cohort study was conducted as part of the Ohsaki National Health Insurance Cohort Study in Japan. The cause of mortalities was tracked in these participants for up to 11 years (and for up to 7 years for cause-specific mortalities). In this time frame, 4,209 people died. Analysis revealed that consumption of Green Tea was associated with a lower risk of death from cardiovascular disease, as well as from other causes with the exception of cancer. The strongest inverse association between Green Tea intake and reduced risk of death was for death caused by stroke. Specifically, compared with women who consumed less than 1 cup daily of Green Tea, those who drank 5 or more cups daily had a 42% lower risk of death due to stroke and a 62% lower risk of death due to this cause. The authors attribute the cardioprotective-effects of Green Tea to a threshold effect rather than a dose-response relationship, meaning that a person who typically consumed at least 1 cup of Green Tea daily did accrue some benefit. Future clinical trials will need to be done to confirm GreenTea's apparent protective effect against death from cardiovascular disease and other causes (Kuriyama, 2006).

Hypercholesterolemia

Green Tea extract enriched with theaflavin reduced serum total cholesterol and LDL-C in adults with mild to moderate hypercholesterolemia in a 12-week double-blind trial. Two hundred twenty subjects were randomized to receive 1 capsule orally daily that contained either a theaflavin-enriched Green Tea extract (75 mg theaflavins, 150 mg Green Tea catechins, and 150 mg other tea polyphenols) or placebo. Subjects were asked to maintain their traditional Chinese diet and tea intake. Dietary intake was assessed using 3-day food records. Lipid and lipoprotein concentrations were evaluated at week -2, week 0, week 4, and week 12. The theaflavin-enriched Green Tea extract decreased serum total cholesterol and LDL-C by 11.3% (p=0.01) and 16.4% (p=0.01), respectively. There was no statistical difference for nutrient intake between the treatment and placebo groups at baseline or at 8 weeks for any dietary variable (Maron et al, 2003).

Green Tea may decrease the risk of coronary heart disease by inhibiting the development of atherosclerosis, protecting LDL against oxidation and foam cell formation. Cholesterol was dose-dependently reduced by Green Tea in human umbilical cord vascular endothelial cells (HUVEC). Cellular content of cholesterol in HUVEC treated with 5 and 10 mcg/mL of Green Tea was lower than control oxidized LDL ($p<0.001$ and $p<0.01$, respectively). Catechins found in Green Tea suppressed endothelial cellular LDL oxidation, suggesting catechins may be the primary antioxidant (Yang & Koo, 2000a).

Obesity

Thirty-four obese women with polycystic ovary syndrome (PCOS), an endocrine disorder, were randomized into treatment with Green Tea capsules (Lung Chen tea powder prepared by brewing tea leaves of 2% weight/volume in freshly boiled water for 30 minutes and then filtered and freeze-dried) or placebo over the course of 3 months. During this time, numerous measurements of hormonal, biochemical, and anthropomorphic condition were taken and compared. The group receiving Green Tea showed a nonsignificant drop in body weight (2.4%), while the body mass index and body fat content for the women taking placebo became significantly higher. Analysis revealed that the Green Tea supplement failed to significantly reduce body weight in these obese individuals with PCOS. Nor did the Green Tea change glucose or lipid metabolism, hormone levels, or menstrual regularity (Chan, 2005).

In contrast, moderate weight loss after ingestion of green tea (GT) was found in a double-blind, placebo-controlled study. Forty-six female subjects were fed in energy balance from day 1 to 3, followed by a low-energy diet (LED) with GT or placebo from day 4 to 87. The LED-period consisted of a 4-week phase I, followed by an 8-week phase II. No significant differences were observed between blood parameters of the two groups; however, modest weight loss improved HDL cholesterol and blood pressure (Diepvens et al, 2006).

A randomized, parallel, placebo-controlled study was performed to investigate whether Green Tea improves weight maintenances by preventing or limiting weight regain after weight loss of 5 to 10% in overweight and moderately obese subjects. A total of 104 participants received a 4-week, very low-energy diet intervention, followed by a weight-maintenance period of 13 weeks including either Green Tea or placebo. Body weight regain was not significantly different between the two groups. In the Green Tea group treatment, habitual high caffeine consumption was in fact associated with a higher weight regain compared with habitual low caffeine consumption (Kovacs et al, 2004).

An earlier double-blind trial demonstrated thermogenic properties of Green Tea and its fat oxidizing capabilities. Ten healthy male subjects received Green Tea extract (90 mg epigallocatechin gallate and 50 mg caffeine), 50 mg caffeine, or placebo 3 times daily on 3 separate 24-hour stays in a respiratory chamber. Green Tea extract produced a significantly higher diurnal ($p<0.01$) and total 24-hour energy expenditure (EE; $p<0.01$) compared to caffeine and placebo; nocturnal EE was not significantly affected. The respiratory quotients decreased significantly more during treatment with Green Tea during diurnal, nocturnal, and total 24-hour periods compared to caffeine and placebo ($p<0.01$ in 8/10 subjects compared to placebo). This effect was attributed to an increase in thermogenesis and in fat oxidation since urinary nitrogen losses did not differ between the 3 groups. Compared to placebo, carbohydrate oxidation significantly decreased ($p<0.001$) and fat oxidation significantly increased (41.5% vs 31.6% for placebo; $p<0.001$) with the consumption of Green Tea extract. Investigators concluded that these metabolic effects resulted from Green Tea components other than caffeine (Dulloo et al, 1999).

Skin Protection

The combination regimen of topical and oral Green Tea supplementation on the clinical and histologic characteristic of photoaging was evaluated using 10% green tea cream and 300 mg twice-daily Green Tea oral supplementation or a placebo for 8 weeks. Forty women with moderate photoaging were enrolled into the double-blind, placebo-controlled study. No significant differences in clinical grading were found between the treatment groups. Histologic grading of skin biopsies did show significant improvement in the elastic tissue content of treated specimens in the Green Tea group ($p<0.05$) (Chiu et al, 2005).

INDICATIONS AND USAGE

Though no Commission E monograph exists for Green Tea, there is clinical evidence that it is likely to be useful as a cancer preventive and as a preventive for dental caries.

Unproven Uses: Internal application: Green Tea is used for stomach disorders, migraine, symptoms of fatigue, vomiting and diarrhea when taken as a beverage. It can be used to increase performance (stimulant effect).

Homeopathic Uses: Camellia sinensis is used for cardiac and circulatory conditions, headaches, states of agitation, states of depression, and stomach complaints.

Indian Medicine: In India, tea preparations are used for diarrhea, loss of appetite, hyperdypsia, migraine, cardiac pain, fever, and fatigue.

Chinese Medicine: In China Green Tea is used to treat migraine, nausea, diarrhea resulting from malaria, and digestion problems. It is also used as a cancer preventive.

PRECAUTIONS AND ADVERSE REACTIONS

Side effects of tea consumption are possible with persons who have sensitive stomachs, chiefly due to the chlorogenic acid and tannin content. Hyperacidity, gastric irritation, reduction of appetite, as well as obstipation or diarrhea, could be the result of intense tea consumption. These side effects can be generally avoided by the addition of milk (reduction of the chlorogenic acid and other tannins).

Care should be taken with patients that have weakened cardiovascular systems, renal diseases, thyroid hyperfunction, elevated susceptibility to spasm and certain psychic disorders, such as panicky states of anxiety. With long-term intake of dosages above 1.5 g caffeine per day, nonspecific symptoms occur, such as restlessness, irritability, sleeplessness, palpitations, vertigo, vomiting, diarrhea, loss of appetite, and headache.

Endocrine/Metabolic: Green Tea caused reduction of blood testosterone, estradiol, leptin, insulin, insulin-like growth factor I, and LH levels in Sprague-Dawley rats injected intraperitoneally with (-)-epigallocatechin gallate (EGCG). Food consumption and body weight were reduced as well as glucose, cholesterol, and triglyceride levels. Organ weight of accessory sexual organs (prostate, uterus, and ovaries) also decreased (Kao Yung-Hsi et al, 2000).

Hematologic: Reports of mycrocytic anemia in infants consuming an average of 250 mL of Green Tea per day have been reported. This effect may be due to impaired iron metabolism (Dombek, 1993; Merhav et al, 1985).

Pregnancy: It is recommended that women who are pregnant avoid consumption of Green Tea due to the caffeine content (10 to 50 mg per cup depending on variety and method of preparation), or at least avoid large quantities of Green Tea (Yamamoto et al, 1997).

Breastfeeding: Infants whose nursing mothers consume beverages containing caffeine could suffer from sleep disorders.

DRUG INTERACTIONS

MODERATE RISK

Anticoagulants: Concurrent use may result in reduced anticoagulant effectiveness. *Clinical Management:* It appears that the quantity of Green Tea consumed and the method of production affect the amount of vitamin K in Green Tea. Patients who choose to drink Green Tea should be advised to consume a consistent amount and use a consistent brand and method of brewing.

POTENTIAL INTERACTIONS

Alkaline medications: Reabsorption can be delayed because of chemical bonding with the tannins in tea.

OVERDOSAGE

Overdosage (quantities corresponding to more than 300 mg caffeine, or 5 cups of tea as a beverage) can lead to restlessness, tremor, and elevated reflex excitability. The first signs of poisoning are vomiting and abdominal spasm. Fatal poisonings are not possible with tea beverages.

DOSAGE

Mode of Administration: Green Tea is administered as an infusion or in capsule form for internal use.

How Supplied: The usual concentration of total polyphenols in dried Green Tea leaf is around 8% to 12%. One cup of Green Tea normally contains 50 to 100 mg polyphenols (Murray & Pizzorno, 1998; Yamamoto, 1997).

Capsules – 100 mg, 150 mg, 175 mg, 333 mg, 383 mg, 500 mg

Liquid – 1:1

Tablets – 100 mg

Dried extract (instant tea) — Processed using steam extraction followed by drying

Filter tea bags — Available commercially containing 1.8 to 2.2 g tea

Preparation: To prepare a tea, boiling water is poured over a heaped teaspoon of leaf tea, a level teaspoon of crushed leaves or a tea bag and left to steep for 3 to 10 minutes as required. The caffeine is almost completely drawn after approximately 3 minutes. The tannin-containing substance (and with it the antidiarrheal action) increases when the tea is left to brew.

Daily Dosage: A daily dose of 300 to 400 mg of polyphenols is typical. The amount of polyphenols in 3 cups of Green Tea is between 240 and 320 mg.

Homeopathic Dosage: 5 to 10 drops, 1 tablet, or 5 to 10 globules 1 to 3 times daily or 1 mL injection solution sc twice weekly (HAB1).

Storage: Store tightly sealed and dried; store separately from other chemicals and aromatic substances.

LITERATURE

Ahmad N, Feyes DK, Nieminen AL et al. Green Tea constituent epigallocatechin-3-gallate and induction of apoptosis and cell cycle arrest in human carcinoma cells. *J Natl Cancer Inst*; 89:1881-1886. 1997.

Ahmad N & Mukthar H. Green Tea polyphenols and cancer: Biologic mechanisms and practical implications. *Nutr Rev*; 57(3):78-83. 1999.

Anon, Grüner Tee schützt vor Krebs. In: *DAZ* 137(24):2045. 1997.

Aucamp J. Inhibition of xanthine oxidase by catechins from tea (*Camellia sinensis*). *Anticancer Res*; 17:4381-4386. 1997.

Bettuzzi S, Brausi M, Rizzi F, et al. Chemoprovention of human prostate cancer by oral administration of green tea catechins in volunteers with high-grade prostate intraepithelial neoplasia: a preliminary report from a one-year proof-of-principle study. Cancer Res; 66(2);1234-1240. 2006.

Booth SL, Madabushi HT, Davidson KKW et al. Tea and coffee brews are not significant dietary sources of vitamin K1 (phylloquinone*). J Am Diet Assoc*; 95:82-83. 1995.

Büechi S, Antivirale Saponine, pharmakologische und klinische Untersuchungen. In: *DAZ* 136(2):89-98. 1996.

Centerwatch: Drugs Approved by the FDA. Drug Name: Veregen (kunecatechins). Available at: http://www.centerwatch.com/patient/drugs/dru938.html. Accessed June 18, 2007.

Chan C, Koo MS, Ng EH, et al. Effects of a Chinese Green Tea on weight, and hormonal and biochemical profiles in obese patients with polycystic ovary syndrome—a randomized placebo-controlled trial. *J Soc Gynecol Investig*; 13: 63-68. 2006.

Chen W. EGCG inhibits UVB induced AP-1 activation and c-fos gene expression in a human keratinocyte cell line (abstract 2663). *AACR*; 39:391. 1998.

Chiu AE, Chan JL, Kern DG, et al. Double-blinded, placebo-controlled trial of green tea extracts in the clinical and histologic appearance of photoaging skin. *Dermatol Surg*. 31(7 Pt 2);855-860. 2005.

Cooper R, Morre DJ, Morre DM. Medicinal benefits of Green Tea: Part II. Review of anticancer properties. *J Alt Comp Med*; 11(4): 639-653. 2005.

Diepvens K, Kovacs EM, Vogels N. Westerterp-Plantenga MS. Metabolic effects of green tea and of phases of weight loss. *Physiolo Behav*. 87(1):185-191. 2006.

Dombek C. The Lawrence Review Of Natural Products. Wolters Kluwer Company, St Louis, MO, USA; p 1-2. 1993.

Dulloo A, Duret C, Rohrer D et al. Efficacy of a Green Tea extract rich in catechin polyphenols and caffeine in increasing 24-h energy expenditure and fat oxidation in humans. *Am J Clin Nutr*; 70:1040-1045. 1999.

Finsterer J. Earl gray tea intoxication. *Lancet*; 359:1484. 2002.

Fujiki H, Suganuma M, Okabe S et al. Cancer Inhibition by Green Tea. *Mutat Res*; 402:307-310. 1998.

Fukino Y, Shimbo M, Aoki N, et al. Randomized controlled trial for an effect of green tea consumption on insulin resistance and inflammation markers. *J Nutr Sci Vitaminol*; 51(5); 335-342. 2005.

Gotoh A. Inhibitory effects of Green Tea extract on human prostatic cancer cell lines (abstract 2671). *AACR*; 39:392. 1998.

Graham B, In: Graham HN. Tea: The Plant and Its Manufacture, Chemistry, and Consumption of the Beverage. In: The Methylxanthine Beverages and Foods: Chemistry, Consumption, and Heath Effects, Alan R. Liss, New York, S.29-74. 1984.

Gupta S, Ahmad N, Nieminen AL et al. Growth inhibition, cell-cycle dysregulation, and induction of apoptosis by Green Tea constituent (-)- epigallocatechin-3-gallate in androgen-sensitive and androgen insensitive human prostate carcinoma cells. *Toxicol Appl Pharmacol*; 164(1):82-90. 2000.

Hakim IA, Harris RB & Weisgerber UM. Tea intake and squamous cell carcinoma of the skin: influence of type of tea beverages. *Cancer Epidemiol Biomarkers Prev*; 9:727-731. 2000.

Haslam E. Natural polyphenols (vegetable tannins) as drugs: possible modes of action. In: *JNP* 59(2):205-215. 1996.

Higashi-Okai K, Taniguchi M & Okai Y. Potent suppressive activity of pheophytin a and b from non-polyphenolic fraction of Green Tea (Camellia sinensis) against the activation of oxygen radical generation, cytokine release and chemotaxis of human polymorphonuclear neutrophils (PMNs). *J Fermentat Bioeng*; 85:555-558. 1998.

Hofbauer R, Frass M, Gmeiner B et al. The Green Tea extract epigallocatechin gallate is able to reduce neutrophil transmigration through monolayers of endothelial cells. *Wien Klin Wochenschr*; 111(7):278-282. 1999.

Hosoda K, Wang MF, Liao ML et al. Antihyperglycemia effect of oolong tea in type 2 diabetes. *Diabetes Care*; 26(6):1714-1718. 2003.

Imai K, Nakachi K. Cross sectional study of effects of drinking Green Tea on cardiovascular and liver disease. In: *BMJ* 310:693-696. 1995.

Inoue M, Tajima K, Hirose K et al. Tea and coffee consumption and the risk of digestive tract cancers: data from a comparative case-referent study in Japan. *Cancer Causes Control*; 9:209-216. 1998.

Iso H, Date C, Kenji W, et al. The relationship between Green Tea and total caffeine intake and risk for self-reported type 2 diabetes among Japanese adults. *Ann Intern Med*; 144 (8): 554-562. 2006.

Jain AK, Shimoi K, Nakamura Y, Kada T, Hana Y, Tomita J. Crude tea extracts decrease the mutagenic activity of N-methyl-N'-nitro-N-nitrosoguanidine in-vitro and in gastric tract of rats. In: *Mutat Res* 210(1)1-8. 1989.

Jatoi A, Ellson N, Burch P et al. A phase II trial of Green Tea in the treatment of patients with androgen independent metastatic prostate carcinoma. *Cancer*; 97(6):2-6. 2003.

Ji BT, Chow WH, Hsing AW et al. Green Tea consumption and the risk of pancreatic and colorectal cancer. *Int J Cancer* 70(3):255-258. 1997.

John TJ, Mukundan P. Antiviral property of tea. In: *Curr Sci* 47:159. 1978.

Kaneko T, Mitsuyoshi M & Baba N. Inhibition of linoleic acid hydroperoxide-induced toxicity in cultured human umbilical vein endothelial cells by catechins. *Chemi Biol Interact*; 114:109-119. 1998.

Kannar ML, Wahlqvist ML & O'Brien RC. Inhibition of LDL-oxidation by Green Tea extract. *Lancet*; 349:360-361. 1997.

Kao YH, Hiipakka RA & Liao S. Modulation of endocrine systems and food intake by Green Tea epigallocatechin gallate. *Endocrinology*; 141(3):980-987. 2000.

Kennedy DO, Nishimura S, Hasuma T et al. Involvement of protein tyrosine phosphorylation in the effect of Green Tea polyphenols on ehrlich ascites tumor cells in vitro. *Chem Biol Interact*; 110:159-172. 1998.

Khafif A, Schantz SP, Al-Rawi M et al. Green Tea regulates cell cycle progression in oral leukoplakia. *Head Neck*; 20:528-534. 1998.

Khafif A, Schantz SP, Chou TC et al. Quantitation of chemopreventive synergism between ?(-) epigallocatechin-3-gallate and curcumin in normal, premalignant and malignant human oral epithelial cells. *Carcinogenesis*; 19:419-424. 1998a.

Kim J. Protective effect of Green Tea polyphenols on the ultraviolet-induced dermal extracellular damage (abstract 762). *J Invest Dermatol*; 110:599. 1998.

Kono S, Shinchi K, Ikeda N et al. Green Tea consumption and serum lipid profiles: a cross sectional study in northern Kyushu, Japan. *Prev Med*; 21(4):526-531. 1992.

Kovacs EM, Lejeune MP, Nijs I, et al. Effects of green tea on weight maintenance after body weight loss. *Br J Nutr*; 91(3);431-437. 2004.

Kuriyama S, Taichi S, Kaori O, et al. Green Tea consumption and mortality due to cardiovascular disease, cancer, and all causes in Japan: the Ohsaki study. *JAMA*; 296 (10): 1255-1265. 2006.

Lee IP, Kim YH, Kang MH et al. Chemopreventive effect of Green Tea (*Camellia sinensis*) against cigarette smoke-induced mutations (SCE) in humans. *J Cell Biochem Suppl*; 27:68-75. 1997.

Leenen R, Roodenburg AJC, Tijburg LBM et al. A single dose of tea with or without milk increases plasma antioxidant activity in humans. *Eur J Clin Nutr*; 54:87-92. 2000.

Lotito SB & Fraga CG. (+)-Catechin prevents human plasma oxidation. *Free Radic Biol Med*; 24:435-441. 1998.

Ludewig R. Schwarzer und Grüner Tee als Genuβ- und Heilmittel. *Dtsch Apoth Z* 135:2203-2218. 1995.

Maron DJ, Lu GP, Cai NS, et al. Cholesterol-lowering effect of a theaflavin-enriched Green Tea extract: a randomized controlled trial. *Arch Intern Med*. Jun 23;163(12):1448-1453. 2003.

Merhav H, Amitai Y, Palti H et al. Tea drinking and microcytic anemia in infants. *Am J Clin Nutr*; 41(6):1210-1213. 1985.

Mukhtar H. Inhibition of nuclear transcription factor NFkB by Green Tea constituent epigallocatechin-3-gallate in human epidermoid carcinoma cells A431 (abstract 0296). *ESDR/JSID/SID* Abstracts; 16:S50. 1998.

Murray MT & Pizzorno. *Camellia Sinensis* (Green Tea), in A Textbook of Natural Medicine. Churchill Livingstone, pp 625-627. 1998.

Nakachi K, Suemasu K, Suga K, Takeo T, Imai K, Higashi Y. Influence of drinking Green Tea on breast cancer malignancy among Japanese patients. In: *Jpn J Cancer Res* 89(3): 254-261. 1998.

Okai Y & Higashi-Okai K. Potent suppressing activity of the non-polyphenolic fraction of Green Tea (Camellia sinensis) against genotoxin-induced umu C gene expression in Salmonella typhimurium (TA 1535/pSK) 1002)-association with pheophytins a and b. *Cancer Lett*; 120:117-123. 1997.

Pearson DA, Frankel EN, Aeschbach R et al. Inhibition of endothelial cell mediated low-density lipoprotein oxidation by Green Tea extracts. *J Agric Food Chem*; 46:1445-1449. 1998.

Princen HM, Duyvenvoorde WV, Buytenhek R et al. No effect of consumption of green and black tea on plasma lipid and antioxidant levels and on LDL oxidation in smokers. *Arterioscler Thromb Vasc Biol*; 18:833-841. 1998.

Rasheed A & Haider M, Antibacterial activity of *Camellia sinensis* extracts against dental caries. *Arch Pharm Res* 21:348-352. 1998.

Sadzuka Y, Sugiyama T & Hirota S. Modulation of cancer chemotherapy by Green Tea. *Clin Cancer Res*; 4:153-156. 1998.

Sadzuka Y, Sugiyama T & Sonobe T. Efficacies of tea components on doxorubicin induced antitumor activity and reversal of multidrug resistance (letter). *Toxicology*; 114:155-162. 2000.

Sato K, Kanazawa A, Ota N et al. Dietary supplementation of catechins and alpha-tocopherol accelerates the healing of trinitrobenzene sulfonic acid-induced ulcerative colitis in rats. *J Nutr Sci Vitaminol*; 44:769-778. 1998.

Scholz E, *Camellia sinensis* (L.) O. KUNTZE. Der Teestrauch. In: *ZPT* 16(4):231-250. 1995.

Schröder B. In: Schröder R: Kaffee, Tee und Kardamom, Ulmer-Verlag, Stuttgart. 1991.

Serafini M, Ghiselli A & Ferro-Luzzi A. In vivo antioxidant effect of green and black tea in man. *Eur J Clin Nutr*; 50:28-32. 1996.

Shetty M, Subbannayya K & Shivananda PG. Antibacterial activity of tea (*Camellia sinensis*) and coffee (Coffee arabica) with special reference to Salmonella typhimurium. *J Commun Dis*; 26(3):147-150. 1994.

Shim JS, Kang MH, Kim YH et al. Chemopreventive effect of Green Tea (Camellia Sinensis) among cigarette smokers. *Cancer Epidemiol Biomarkers Prev*; 4:387-391. 1995.

Sugiyama K, Puming H, Wada S et al. Teas and other beverages suppress D-Galactosamine-induced liver injury in rats. J Nutr; 129(7):1361-1367. 1999.

Sur P, Ganguly DK. Tea root extract (TRE) as an antineoplastic agent. In: *PM* 60(2):106. 1994.

van het Hof KH, Boer HS, Wiseman SA et al. Consumption of green or black tea does not increase resistance of low-density lipoproteins to oxidation in humans. *Am J Clin Nutr*; 66:1125-1132. 1997.

Vinson JA & Babbgh YA. Tea phenols: antioxidant effectiveness of teas, tea components, tea fractions and their binding with lipoproteins. *Nutr Res*; 18:1067-1075. 1998.

Yamamoto T, Juneja LR, Chu DC et al., Chemistry and Applications of Green Tea. CRC Press, Boca Raton, FL, USA, 1997.

Yang G, Liao J, Kim K et al. Inhibition of growth and induction of apoptosis in human cancer cell lines by tea polyphenols. *Carcinogenesis*; 19:611-616. 1998.

Yang TTC & Koo MWL. Chinese Green Tea lowers cholesterol level through an increase in fecal lipid excretion. Life Sci; 66(5):411-423. 2000.

Yang TTC & Koo MWL. Inhibitory effect of Chinese Green Tea on endothelial cell-induced LDL oxidation. *Atherosclerosis*; 148:67-73. 2000a.

Yao S, Tan H, Zhang H et al. Bulk acoustic wave bacterial growth sensor applied to analysis of antimicrobial properties of tea. Biotechnol Prog; 4:639-644. 1998.

Yoshizawa S et al. *Phytother Res* 1(1):44. 1987.

Zhang J & Kashket S. Inhibition of salivary amylase by black and Green Teas and their effects on the intraoral hydrolysis of starch. *Caries Res;* 32:233-238. 1998.

Zhao JF. Photoprotection in human skin by Green Tea and black tea (abstract 2666). *AACR*; 39:392. 1998.

Grey Wallflower

Erysimum diffusum

DESCRIPTION

Medicinal Parts: The medicinal part is the plant's radish.

Flower and Fruit: The flowers are in densely flowered racemes. The 4 sepals are upright and gray-haired, the 4 petals are yellow, long-petiolate, pubescent on the lower surface, and 8 to 14 mm long. There are 2 short and 4 long stamens; the ovary is superior with 4 fused carpels. The fruit is a 3.5 to 8 cm long, approximately 1 mm wide, 4-sided, appressed pubescent, dehiscent pod that opens on two sides. The seeds are elongate with a diameter of approximately 1 to 1.5 mm.

Leaves, Stem, and Root: Grey Wallflower is a herbaceous biennial or perennial upright that grows up to 1.2 m high. The leaves are alternate. The lower ones are petiolate, 1 to 8 mm wide, gray-haired, narrow, linear-lanceolate, entire or dentate; the middle and upper ones are sessile. The stem is edged, covered in jointed hairs, and branched in larger plants. The root is thin, spindle-shaped, and branched.

Habitat: The plant is indigenous to the Commonwealth of Independent States and Hungary.

Production: The grey-leaved wild radish is collected during the flowering season of the two-year-old plants of *Erysimum diffusum* and dried after harvesting at a maximum temperature of 40° C.

ACTIONS AND PHARMACOLOGY

COMPOUNDS

Cardioactive steroid glycosides (cardenolids, 1 to 3%): chief component erysimoside (primary glycoside, aglycone k-strophanthidin, 0.6%)

Helveticoside (secondary glycoside)

Canescine

Cheirotoxin

Erycanoside

EFFECTS

The drug contains cardioactive glycosides of the cardenolide type with k-strophantidin as the aglycone. It is accordingly positively inotropic and negatively chronotropic in its effect.

INDICATIONS AND USAGE

Unproven Uses: The drug was used in the past for cardiac insufficiency (NYHA I and II), but can no longer be recommended.

PRECAUTIONS AND ADVERSE REACTIONS

No health hazards are known in conjunction with the proper administration of designated therapeutic dosages.

Although poisonings among humans are both unknown and unlikely, due to the difficulties accompanying resorption of the glycosides, the possibility of a poisoning resulting from either high dosages of the drug or its glycosides through peroral administration is not to be completely ruled out.

DOSAGE

How Supplied:

Capsules

Tablets.

Storage: Drug should be stored in a tightly sealed, secure container.

LITERATURE

Hänsel R, Keller K, Rimpler H, Schneider G (Ed.), Hagers Handbuch der Pharmazeutischen Praxis, 5. Aufl., Bde 4 - 6 (Drogen), Springer Verlag Berlin, Heidelberg, New York, 1992-1994.

Griffonia simplicifolia

See 5HTP

Grindelia camporum

See Gumweed

Ground Ivy

Glechoma hederacea

DESCRIPTION

Medicinal Parts: The medicinal parts are the herb collected during the flowering season and dried, the fresh aerial parts collected during the flowering season, and the whole plant.

Flower and Fruit: The flowers are in 2- to 6-blossomed false whorls in the axils of the foliage leaves. The individual flowers are 1 to 2 cm long with distinct pedicles and bracteoles that are 1 to 1.5 mm long. The calyx is bilabiate and tubular, with 5 tips. The bilabiate corolla is 15 to 22 mm long, usually blue-violet but occasionally red-violet or white. The fruit is a nut of about 2 mm.

Leaves, Stem, and Root: This perennial herb grows 15 to 60 cm high and has a creeping main stem, which roots at the lower nodes and keeps its leaves in winter. The quadrangular stem is up to 2 mm thick and often tinged with blue-violet, as are the petioles. The leaves are crossed opposite, long-petioled, reniform to broadly cordate, and crenate; they are dark green above and paler green beneath.

Characteristics: The plant has a mild unpleasant smell; the taste is hot and bitter.

Habitat: Ground Ivy is a common wild plant in Europe.

Production: Ground Ivy is the aboveground part of *Glechoma hederacea*, gathered when in flower (from April to June). It is air-dried in the shade to keep loss of the essential oil to a minimum.

Other Names: Alehoof, Gill-Go-over-the-Ground, Lizzy-Run-up-the-Hedge, Gill-to-by-the-Hedge, Robin-Run-in-the-Hedge, Catsfoot, Hedgemaids, Tun-Hoof, Haymaids, Turnhoof, Creeping Charlie, Cat's-Paw

ACTIONS AND PHARMACOLOGY

COMPOUNDS

Volatile oil (traces): chief components (-)-pinocarvone, (-)-menthone, (+)-pulegone, also including germacran D, germacran B, cis-ocimene

Sesquiterpenes: glechomafuran, glechomanolide

Hydroxy fatty acid: 9-hydroxy-10-trans, 12-cis-octadecadiendic acid

Caffeic acid derivatives: rosmaric acid

Flavonoids: including cymaroside, cosmosyin, hypersoside isoquercitrin

EFFECTS

The drug is said to be an anti-inflammatory, which is believed to be due to the tripterpen content. No detailed information is available.

INDICATIONS AND USAGE

Unproven Uses: In folk medicine, the drug is used internally for inflammation of gastrointestinal mucous membranes and diarrhea. Ground Ivy is also used for mild respiratory complaints of the upper bronchia; in the symptomatic treatment of coughs; and as a diuretic in cases of bladder and kidney stones. Externally, the drug is used for the treatment of poorly healing wounds, ulcers, and skin diseases. In Italy, it is used for arthritis and rheumatism.

Chinese Medicine: Ground Ivy is used to treat carbuncles, erysipelas, lower abdominal pain, scabies, scrofulous, irregular menstruation, coughs, dysentery, and jaundice. Efficacy has not, however, been proved for these indications.

Homeopathic Uses: Uses in homeopathy include diarrhea and hemorrhoids.

PRECAUTIONS AND ADVERSE REACTIONS

Health risks or side effects following the proper administration of designated therapeutic dosages are not recorded. Fatal poisonings were observed among horses following intake of large quantities of the fresh plant. Mice who were fed solely on the plant died after 3 to 4 days.

DOSAGE

Mode of Administration: The drug is used internally as well as externally.

Preparations: The liquid extract (1:1) is prepared by using 25% ethanol.

Daily Dosage: The normal single daily dose of the dried drug is 2 to 4 g internally; externally, crushed leaves are placed on the affected areas.

Homeopathic Dosage: 5 drops, 1 tablet or 10 globules every 30 to 60 minutes (acute) or 1 to 3 times daily (chronic); parenterally: 1 to 2 mL sc acute, 3 times daily; chronic: once a day; suppositories: 1 suppository 2 to 3 times daily (chronic and acute) (HAB34)

Storage: Ground Ivy should be stored where it is not exposed to light.

LITERATURE

Bohinc P, Korbar-Smid J, Cicerov-Cergol M, Über die kardiotonischen Substanzen des Gnadenkrautes - Gratiola officinalis. In: Sci Pharm 47:108-113. 1979.

Hänsel R, Keller K, Rimpler H, Schneider G (Hrsg.), Hagers Handbuch der Pharmazeutischen Praxis, 5. Aufl., Bde 4-6 (Drogen), Springer Verlag Berlin, Heidelberg, New York, 1992-1994.

Lewin L, Gifte und Vergiftungen, 6. Aufl., Nachdruck, Haug Verlag, Heidelberg 1992.

Milovanovic M, Stefanovic M, Dermanovic V. Flavonoids *from Glechoma hederacea L. J Serb Chem Soc*. 60 (6); 467-469. 1995

Sattar AA et al. Chemical composition and biological activity of leaf exudates from some *Lamiaceae plants. Pharmazie* 50; 62-65. 1995

Sevenet T, Looking for new drugs: what criteria? *J Ethnopharmacol*, 32:83-90, Apr 1991.

Ground Pine

Ajuga chamaepitys

DESCRIPTION

Flower and Fruit: The plant has 2 to 4 flowers at each node. The petals are 4 to 6 mm long. The tips of the petals are as long as or shorter than the tube. The corolla is yellow with red or purple markings, rarely entirely purple. The lower lip is entire, and the stamens are exerted. The filaments are hairy. The mericarps are 2 to 5 mm long, obovate, and reticulate-wrinkled with a pitted surface.

Leaves, Stem, and Root: Ground Pine is an annual or short-lived perennial. The stem is 5 to 30 cm long. It is usually heavily branched, glabrous to densely villous. The leaves are tripartite with linear segments. They are 0.5 to 4 mm wide. The segments are sometimes tripinnatifid. The bracts are similar to the leaves.

Habitat: Sandy, stony areas of southern Britain and parts of Europe.

Other Names: Yellow Bugle

ACTIONS AND PHARMACOLOGY

COMPOUNDS

Volatile oil

Diterpene bitter principles

Caffeic acid derivatives: including rosemary acid

EFFECTS

Emmenagogue (stimulates menstrual flow), stimulant, diuretic.

INDICATIONS AND USAGE

Unproven Uses: Ground Pine is used for gout, rheumatism, and gynecological disorders.

PRECAUTIONS AND ADVERSE REACTIONS

No health hazards or side effects are known in conjunction with the proper administration of designated therapeutic dosages.

DOSAGE

Mode of Administration: Ground Pine is available in compounded preparations as a liquid extract for internal use.

LITERATURE

Camps F, et al., *An Quim* 81C(1):74-75. 1985

Kooiman P, *Acta Bot Nederl* 21(4):417. 1972

Groundsel

Senecio vulgaris

DESCRIPTION

Medicinal Parts: The medicinal part is the herb collected during the flowering season.

Flower and Fruit: The yellow composite flowers are in compact cymes. The small capitula have tubular florets but no lingual ones. The bract calyx is globose. The involucre and the very short outer bracts have black tips. The fruit is 1.2 to 2 mm long and densely downy. The pappus, which is three times as long as the fruit, is silky and pure white.

Leaves, Stem, and Root: Groundsel grows from about 10 to 30 cm high. It is annual, biennial, or occasionally perennial. The plant has a thin, fusiform, pale root, which is densely covered in lateral roots. The stem is erect, simple, or branched. The leaves are glabrous or cobweb-lanate and pinnatisect. The lower leaves narrow to the petiole; the upper ones are slit at the base and clasping. The tips are detached, oblong, obtuse, and unevenly acute dentate.

Habitat: The plant is common in all of Europe, northern and central Asia, northern Africa and has been introduced into various other parts of Africa as well as Australia and the Americas.

Production: Groundsel is the flowering plant of *Senecio vulgaris*. The herb is gathered in uncultivated regions and dried in the shade.

Other Names: Bidseed, Chickenweed, Grounsel, Grundy Swallow, Ground Glutton, Simson

ACTIONS AND PHARMACOLOGY

COMPOUNDS

Pyrrolizidine alkaloids (up to 0.16% in the fresh foliage): chief alkaloids are senecionine, seneciphylline

Flavonoids: including among others, isorhamnetin-3-O-glucosides, isorhamnetin-3-O-rutinosides, isorhamnetin-3-monosulphate

Volatile oil (traces)

EFFECTS

The toxic principles of the drug are the pyrrolizidine alkaloids, which are hepatotoxic and carcinogenic. Use of Groundsel for worm infestation can be explained by the high toxicity of the drug.

INDICATIONS AND USAGE

Unproven Uses: Internal use of Groundsel is not recommended because, similar to *S jacoboeae*, it contains toxic and carcinogenic pyrrolizidine alkaloids. Prior uses have included the treatment of worm infestations, colic, and epilepsy. The pressed juice has been used for dysmenorrhea, epilepsy, and as a styptic in dentistry.

PRECAUTIONS AND ADVERSE REACTIONS

Groundsel should not be taken internally because hepatotoxicity and carcinogenicity are possible due to the pyrrolizidine alkaloids with 1,2-unsaturated necic parent substances in its makeup.

DOSAGE

Mode of Administration: Internal use of Groundsel is not advised.

LITERATURE

Borstel Kv, Witte L, Hartmann T. Pyrrolizidine Alkaloid Patterns in Populations of *Senecio vulgaris, S vernalis* and their hybrids. *Phytochemistry* 28; 1635-1638. 1989

Bull LB et al. in: The Pyrrolizidine Alkaloids, Pub. Wiley NY 1968.

Ingolfsdottir K, Hylands PJ. Pyrrolizidine alkaloids in *Senecio vulgaris L.* growing in Iceland. *Acta Pharm Nord.* 2; 343-348. 1990

Pieters LA, Vlietinck AJ. Spartioidine and Usaramine, Two Pyrrolizidine Alkaloids from *Senecio vulgaris. Planta Med.* 54; 178-179. 1988

Van Borstel K et al., PH 28:1635-1638. 1989.

Van Dooren Bos R et al., Planta Med 42:385. 1981

Guaiac

Guaiacum officinale

DESCRIPTION

Medicinal Parts: The primary medicinal part is the resin of the heartwood, which is used for various preparations. The wood also has some medicinal properties.

Flower and Fruit: The pale blue star-shaped flowers are in false umbels with 6 to 10 blooms that have 2-cm pedicles. There are 5 sepals, 5 petals, 10 stamens and a bilocular ovary. The fruit is a bilocular, cordate capsule that is compressed at the side and contains a long and hard seed, in each chamber.

Leaves, Stem, and Root: Guaiacum officinale is an evergreen tree that grows to 13 m high and has a greenish-brown, usually twisted trunk covered in furrowed bark. The heartwood is greenish brown and heavier than water, with an aromatic taste. The opposite leaves are short-petioled, coriaceous and dipinnate to tripinnate. The leaflets are ovate or oblong, obtuse, and entire-margined.

Characteristics: The shavings turn green on exposure to the air and blue-green in the presence of nitrogen.

Habitat: The plant grows in Florida, on the Antilles, in Guayana, Venezuela, and Columbia. It is closely related to *Guaiacum sanctum,* which grows in the Bahamas and southern Florida.

Production: Guaiac wood consists of the heartwood and sapwood of *Guaiacum officinale* and/or *Guaiacum sanctum.*

Other Names: Guaiacum, Lignum Vitae, Pockwood

ACTIONS AND PHARMACOLOGY

COMPOUNDS

Triterpene saponins: aglycone oleanolic acid

Resin: containing, among others, the lignans (-)-guaiaretic acid, dihydroguajaretic acid, guaiacin

Isoguajacin: alpha-guaiaconic acid, tetrofuroguaiacine A and B

Volatile oil: chief components sesquiterpene alcohols; such as guaiole, which changes into quaiazulene with steam distillation

EFFECTS

Guaiacum officinale is fungistatic because of its saponin content.

INDICATIONS AND USAGE

Commission E Approved:

■ Rheumatism

Unproven Uses: Although folk medicine use has declined, it is used for respiratory complaints, skin disorders, and syphilis in the Caribbean.

PRECAUTIONS AND ADVERSE REACTIONS

Health risks or side effects following the proper administration of designated therapeutic dosages are not recorded. High dosages of the drug can lead to diarrhea, gastroenteritis, and intestinal colic. Skin rashes have also been observed following intake of the drug.

DOSAGE

Mode of Administration: The comminuted wood is used for decoctions and other galenic preparations for internal use. The essential oil, known as guaiac wood oil, must be evaluated separately.

How Supplied: Forms of commercial pharmaceutical preparations include drops, ointments and compound preparations.

Preparation: To make an infusion, use 1.5 g drug in 1 cup cold water (150 mL). Slowly bring to a boil, remove from heat and let steep, then strain after 15 minutes.

Daily Dosage: The average daily dose is 4 to 5 g of the drug. When using a tincture (*Guajaci Ligni* Tinctura), 20 to 40 drops make a single dose.

LITERATURE

Ahmad VU, Bano N, Bano S, PH 23:2612-2616. 1984.

Ahmad VU, Bano N, Bano S, PH 25:951-952. 1986.

King FE, Wilson JG, (1964) J Chem Soc:4011-4024.

Guaiacum officinale

See Guaiac

Guarana

Paullinia cupana

DESCRIPTION

Medicinal Parts: The medicinal parts are the peeled, dried, roasted, and pulverized seeds, formed into a thick paste with water.

Flower and Fruit: The usually unisexual flowers are inconspicuous, yellow to whitish, and fragrant. They are in 30 long panicles, which only produce female or male flowers at any one time. The fruit is a hazelnut-sized, deep yellow to red-orange, trisectioned capsule, which bursts open when ripe and releases 1 purple-brown to black seed in a cuplike aril.

Leaves, Stem, and Root: The plant is a woody, evergreen perennial vine up to 10 m long, which climbs through the jungle. It is bushier in its cultivated form. The leaves are large, palmate, coriaceous, distinctly ribbed, and roughly crenate-serrate.

Characteristics: A paste is formed from the pulverized and roasted seeds, formed into rolls or bars, and dried. The taste is astringent, bitter then sweet, and the odor is reminiscent of chocolate.

Habitat: The plant is indigenous to the Amazon basin and has been introduced into other rain forests. The main area of cultivation is between Maues and Manau in Brazil.

Production: Guarana seeds are the seeds of *Paullinia cupana.* A preparation is also made from the ground seeds. Over a period of approximately 75 days, the pollinated flower develops a ''ripe'' guarana raceme, which is harvested by hand from October to December. Seeds (up to 80 per raceme) are taken out of the capsule shells, soaked for a time in water and then finally separated from the arillus. Subsequent to being dried in the sun, the seeds are roasted for 2 to 3 hours in special clay ovens. Once they have cooled, the parchmentlike shell is removed and the seeds are ground down. Following this, the resulting paste is smoked over aromatic charcoal. The final product is dark brown in color and in stick form.

Other Names: Brazilian Cocoa, Guarana Bread, Paullinia

ACTIONS AND PHARMACOLOGY

COMPOUNDS

Purine alkaloids: chief alkaloid caffeine (3.6-5.8%), in addition, small amounts of theophylline and theobromine

Tannins (12%): oligomeric proanthocyanidins, condensed tannins

Cyanolipides: including among others, 2,4-dihydroxy-3-methylene-butyronitrile

Saponins

Starch (30%)

Proteins (15%)

EFFECTS

Guarana produces a stimulating effect, due to the presence of purines (caffeine, theobromine, theophylline). Caffeine is centrally stimulating, has a positive inotropic and, in high concentrations, has a positive chronotropic cardiac effect. It relaxes the vascular muscles (with the exception of cerebral vessels that constrict) and the bronchial tube.

Caffeine works as a short-term diuretic and increases gastric secretion. Furthermore, it increases the release of catecholamines. Inhibition of blood platelet aggregation has been observed.

CLINICAL TRIALS

Weight Loss

A double-blind, parallel, placebo-controlled trial of yerba mate, guarana, and damiana (YGD) was conducted on 47 healthy volunteers, aged 20 to 60, to evaluate the effects on gastric emptying and weight loss. Subjects, who had body weight taken and ultrasound performed, were instructed to fast for 8 hours prior to the study start. They were then given three YGD capsules, each containing 112 mg yerba mate, 95 mg guarana, and 36 mg damiana extract, to ingest with 20mL of apple juice, and 15 minutes later, with 400mL of apple juice. The subjects were evaluated at 10 and 45 days. The mean gastric emptying times were 38 +/- 7.6 minutes following placebo capsules and 58 +/- 15 minutes after YGD capsules (a mean 53% increase). Subjects in the treatment group showed an increased weight loss (mean decrease of 5.1 +/- 0.5kg after 45 days on YGD vs. 0.3 +/- 0.08kg with placebo). The active treatment was a combination product with each constituent having its own potential to cause weight loss (Andersen, 2001).

An herbal supplement containing principally 600 mg black tea extract (60 percent polyphenols, 20 percent caffeine) and 442 mg guarana extract (36 percent caffeine) was tested for stimulation of thermogenesis. A double-blind, placebo-controlled, crossover study was conducted on 16 healthy, weight-stable, non-smoking subjects, aged 21-55 years, with body mass index (BMI) of 20-30 kg/m2, and not taking any medications other than oral contraceptives or hormone replacement therapy. Subjects had no caffeine for 48 hours, no exercise for 24 hours, and no food for 12 hours before each visit. Area under the curve (AUC) for resting metabolic rate (RMR), respiratory quotient (RQ), blood pressure, pulse rate, and temperature were measured. At each visit RMR was measured at baseline and at one and two hours following oral administration of supplement or placebo. The RMR and systolic blood pressure (SBP) AUCs increased significantly ($p<0.02$ and $p<0.01$, respectively) in the herbal supplement group compared to placebo. The AUC increase in RMR over the two-hour test period was 77.19 kcal/24 hr2 +/- 120.10 kcal/24 hr2 with an average rise of 52.38 +/- 29.52 kcal/24 hrs. The AUC rise in SBP over two hours was 10.3 mm Hg/hr +/- 14 mm Hg/hr. The average rise in SBP over two hours was 3.7 mm Hg +/- 4.4 mm Hg. The herbal supplement increased metabolic rate without changing substrate oxidation. The rise in SBP was consistent with the amount of caffeine the supplement contained (Roberts, 2005).

The effect of a mixture of green tea and guarana extracts containing a fixed dose of caffeine and variable doses of epigallocatechin-3-gallate (EGCG) on 24-hour energy expenditure and fat oxidation was examined. Fourteen subjects took part in this randomized, placebo-controlled, double-blind, cross-over study. Each subject was tested 5 times in a metabolic chamber to measure 24-hour energy expenditure, substrate oxidation, and blood pressure. During each stay, the subjects ingested a capsule of placebo or capsules containing 200 mg caffeine and a variable dose of EGCG (90, 200, 300 or 400 mg) three times daily, 30 min before standardized meals. Twenty-four hour energy expenditure increased significantly by about 750 kJ with all EGCG-caffeine mixtures compared with placebo. No effect of the EGCG-caffeine mixture was observed on lipid oxidation. Systolic and diastolic blood pressure increased by about 7 and 5 mmHg, respectively, with the EGCG-caffeine mixtures compared with placebo. This increase was significant only for 24-hour diastolic blood pressure. The increase in 24-hour energy expenditure with the EGCG-caffeine preparation was similar with all doses of EGCG in the mixtures (Berube-Parent et al, 2005).

Cognitive Enhancement

In a double-blind, counterbalanced, placebo-controlled study of 28 healthy participants aged 18 to 24, the cognitive and mood effects of single doses of guarana, ginseng, a combination of the two, and placebo were assessed. Each sibject received 150 mg guarana dry extract, standardized to 11-13% alkaloid concentration, or 400 mg ginseng extract G115, or a guarana/ginseng combination, or placebo per day. Compared to placebo, the three treatment groups showed improved task performance throughout the day. Guarana showed significant improvements across ''attention'' tasks and on sentence verification, but with some degree of reduced accuracy.

Guarana and the ginseng/guarana combination, and ginseng to a lesser extent, showed improvements in serial subtraction task performance. The ginseng and ginseng/guarana combination enhanced the speed of memory task performance without significant accuracy deficiencies. The effects of the guarana are believed to not be attributed to the caffeine content (Kennedy, 2004).

Mood Enhancement

Euphytose (EUP), a combination of Crataegus, Ballota, Passiflora, Valeriana, Cola, and Paullinia, was examined in a multicenter, double-blind, placebo-controlled general practice study on outpatients with adjustment disorder with anxious mood. Ninety-one patients were included in the EUP group and 91 patients in the placebo group. All received two tablets, three times a day, over 28 days. Evaluation using the Hamilton-anxiety (HAM-A) rating scale were carried out on days 0, 7, 14, and 28. Comparing the two groups, 42.9% of the patients (EUP group) had a HAM-A score of less than 10 at day 28 versus 25.3% in the placebo group (P = 0.012). From day 7 to day 28, there was a statistically significant difference (P = 0.042) between the two treatments, indicating that EUP is better than placebo in the treatment of adjustment disorder with anxious mood (Bourin, 1997).

INDICATIONS AND USAGE

Unproven Uses: Guarana is used as a tonic for fatigue and to quell hunger and thirst, for headache and dysmenorrhoea, digestion problems, fever, and as a diuretic. Its effect in stimulating the circulation, heart, and diuresis can be explained by the caffeine content.

Homeopathic Uses: Headache

PRECAUTIONS AND ADVERSE REACTIONS

General: No health hazards or side effects are known in conjunction with the proper administration of designated therapeutic dosages. Quantities corresponding to up to 400 mg caffeine per day (7 to 11 g of the herb), spread out over the day, are toxicologically harmless to a healthy adult habituated to caffeine through regular consumption of coffee or black tea. The quantities of caffeine considered harmless are calculated to include all of the foodstuffs and beverages containing the substance (including coffee, tea, cola, etc.). Caution is advised for patients with sensitive cardiovascular systems, renal diseases, hyperthyroidism, increased tendency to spasms, and certain psychic disorders such as panic anxiety.

With excessive use, however, the diuretic action of Guarana may lead to hypokalemia. Hypokalemia may increase digoxin toxicity.

When taken concomitantly with other drugs, the caffeine in Guarana may result in unwanted outcomes, such as enhanced CNS stimulation or a reduction of the effectiveness or the bioavailability of the drug.

Pregnancy: Pregnant women should avoid caffeine, and under no circumstances exceed a dosage of over 300 mg per day.

Nursing Mothers: Infants whose nursing mothers consume caffeine products may suffer from sleeping disorders.

OVERDOSAGE

The first symptoms of poisoning are dysuria, vomiting and abdominal spasms.

DOSAGE

Mode of Administration: The seeds of *Paullinia cupana* are grated and taken directly as powder or diluted in water or juice as a drink. It is not in use as a drug. It is available in various medicinal preparations.

How Supplied:

Capsules – 200 mg

Liquid – 1:1

Tablets – 800 mg, 1000 mg

Daily Dosage: Average single dose: 1 g of the powder

Homeopathic Dosage: 5 drops, 10 globules every 30 to 60 minutes (acute) or 1 to 3 times a day (chronic); parenterally: 1 to 2 mL sc, acute: 3 times daily; chronic: once a day (HAB34)

LITERATURE

Andersen T, Fogh J. Weight loss and delayed gastric emptying following a South American herbal preparation in overweight patients. *J Hum Nutr Diet* 2001 Jun;14(3):243-50.

Baumann TW, Schulthess BH, Hänni K. Guaran (*Paullinia cupana*) rewards Seed Dispersers without intoxicating them by caffaine. *Phytochemistry* 39 (5); 1063-1070. 1995

Berube-Parent S, Pelletier C, Dore J, Tremblay A. Effects of encapsulated green tea and Guarana extracts containing a mixture of epigallocatechin-3-gallate and caffeine on 24 h energy expenditure and fat oxidation in men. *Br J Nutr*. 2005 Sep;94(3):432-6.

Bourin M, Bougerol T, Guitton B, Broutin E. A combination of plant extracts in the treatment of outpatients with adjustment disorder with anxious mood: controlled study versus placebo. *Fundam Clin Pharmacol* 1997; 11:127-32

Frohne D, Guaraná; - der neue Muntermacher. In: DAZ 133(3):218. 1993.

Hänsel R, Keller K, Rimpler H, Schneider G (Ed.), Hagers Handbuch der Pharmazeutischen Praxis, 5. Aufl., Bde 4-6 (Drogen), Springer Verlag Berlin, Heidelberg, New York, 1992-1994.

Kennedy DO, Haskell CF, Wesnes KA, Scholey AB. Improved cognitive performance in human volunteers following administration of guarana (Paullinia cupana) extract: comparison and interaction with Panax ginseng. Pharmacol Biochem Behav 2004 Nov;79(3):401-11.

Moraes VL, et al. Inhibition of lymphocyte activation by extracts and franctions of *Kalanchoe, Alternanthera, Paullinia* and *Mikania* species. *Phytomedicine* 1; 199-204. 1994

Leung AY, Encyclopedia of Common Natural Ingredients Used in Food, Drugs and Cosmetics, John Wiley & Sons Inc., New York, 1980.

Roberts AT, de Jonge-Levitan L, Parker CC, Greenway F. The effect of an herbal supplement containing black tea and caffeine on metabolic parameters in humans. *Altern Med Rev*. 2005 Dec;10(4):321-5.

Teuscher E, Biogene Arzneimittel, 5. Aufl., Wiss. Verlagsges. Stuttgart 1997.

Valli M, Paubert-Braquet M, Picot S, Fabre R, Lefrancois G, Rod D. Euphytose (R), an Association of Plant Extracts with Anxiolytic Activity: Investigation of its Mechanism of Action by an In Vitro Binding Study. *Phytother Res*. 5; 241-244. 1991

Wichtl M (Ed.), Teedrogen, 4. Aufl., Wiss. Verlagsges. Stuttgart 1997.

Guar Gum

Cyamopsis tetragonoloba

DESCRIPTION

Medicinal Parts: The whole plant has medicinal properties.

Flower and Fruit: The flowers are in axillary, 6- to 30-flowered racemes. The structures of the flowers are arranged in groups of five. The sepals are fused and hairy on the outside; the lower calyx teeth are longer than the upper ones. The corolla is butterfly-shaped (flag, 2 wings, keel formed from 2 fused petals), small and reddish; there are 10 stamens. The fruit developing from a carpel is a legume that is upright, 3.8 to 5 cm long, and sparsely haired with 5 to 6 seeds; these have a very well-developed, slimy endosperm.

Leaves, Stem, and Root: Cyamopsis tetragonoloba is an annual herb, which grows up to 60 cm high. The leaves are alternate and tripinnate; the leaflets are broad-elliptical, acuminate, dentate, and pubescent on both surfaces. They measure 3.8 to 7.5 cm long and 1.2 to 5 cm wide. The petiole is 2.5 to 3.8 cm long, while the stipules are 6 to 10 mm long. The root and root tuber have symbiotic bacteria, which bonds nitrogen from the air.

Habitat: The plant is native to the Indian subcontinent. It originated from India, Australia, South Africa and the U.S.

Production: Guar Gum is the powder extracted by milling from the endosperm of *Cyamopsis tetragonoloba*. A dry or wet milling process separates the endosperm from the seed shell.

Other Names: Aconite Bean, Calcutta Lucerne, Guar, Clusterbean

ACTIONS AND PHARMACOLOGY

COMPOUNDS

Water-soluble polysaccharides: galactomannans (85%)

Proteins (2 to 5%)

Saponins (0.1%)

EFFECTS

Guar Gum causes a lowering of postprandial serum glucose values through (among other things) the influence of the hydrocolloid guar upon glucose resorption (delaying of stomach emptying into the duodenum), a reduction of glucosuria, improvement of the HBA1 value and leveling of the blood sugar profile. A lipid-lowering effect has also been demonstrated.

INDICATIONS AND USAGE

Unproven Uses: Internal application: Guar Gum has been used for diabetes mellitus, for postprandial hyperglycemia and glucosuria, and for hyperlipoproteinemia. It has also been used to regulate digestion.

Indian Medicine: Night blindness, dyspeptic complaints, anorexia, constipation, and agalactia have all been treated with Guar Gum.

CONTRAINDICATIONS

Contraindicated in diseases of esophagus, stomach, and intestine, which might hinder passage of the chyme.

PRECAUTIONS AND ADVERSE REACTIONS

No health hazards are known in conjunction with the proper administration of designated therapeutic dosages of the drug, nor with its use as a pharmaceutical vehicle. Possible side effects, particularly at the beginning of treatment, might include feelings of fullness, nausea, wind, and diarrhea. Symptoms of hypoglycemia (outbreaks of sweating, vertigo, ravenous hunger) and resorption difficulties involving vitamins, minerals and medications (such as contraceptives) have been observed, although rarely. Inadequate intake of fluids could lead to the danger of bolus formation.

DOSAGE

Mode of Administration: Powdered drug, granules and tablets for internal use.

Daily Dosage: Commercial pharmaceutical preparation with one dose of 5 g per tablet or granules, 3 times daily.

Storage: Keep Guar Gum sealed tightly.

LITERATURE

Atta-Ur-Rahman Zaman K. Medicinal Plants with Hypoglycemic Activity. *J Ethnopharmacol*. 26; 1-55. 1989

Hänsel R, Keller K, Rimpler H, Schneider G (Ed.), Hagers Handbuch der Pharmazeutischen Praxis, 5. Aufl., Bde 4 - 6 (Drogen), Springer Verlag Berlin, Heidelberg, New York, 1992-1994.

Xili L et al. Safety Evaluation Studies of SGF Gum–a potential Food Additive from the seed of *Sesbania cannabina*. *Food Chem Toxic*. 26; 935-946. 1988

Gum Arabic

Acacia senegal

DESCRIPTION

Medicinal Parts: The latex from the trunk and branches is the medicinal part of the plant.

Flower and Fruit: The inflorescences, which grow from the leaf axils, are up to 10 cm long. The flowers are white and grow in cylindrical, dense spikes. The calyx is cup-shaped with 5 sepals. The 5 petals are lanceolate. The numerous stamens are long and fused at the base. The pods are about 10 cm long and contain 5 to 6 shiny brown seeds.

Leaves, Stem, and Root: Acacia senegal is up to 6 m tall with a 12- to 25-cm thick, slightly leaning trunk, which has knotty branches and a thin crown. The sapwood is white and the heartwood is black. The bark is fibrous, gray on the outside, and rust-colored on the inside. The leaves are double abruptly pinnate. The leaflets are in 10 to 15 pairs, narrow, gray-green, up to 5 mm long, opposite and very short-petioled. There are 2 to 3 stipules, which have formed into thorns, and are covered on the upper surface with yellow, fleshy glands.

Habitat: Acacia senegal is found in the tropical Savannah belt of Africa, in the southern Sahara (Senegal, Gambia), in Arabia, Beludschistan, and Sind. It is also grown in forestlike conditions in the western and southwestern Sahara region (Senegal, Gambia, Ivory Coast, northern Dahomey and northern Nigeria).

Production: Acacia gummi, the latex, is the result of a wound infection of the tree, which has occurred naturally or has been induced. The incised bark is removed in strips of approximately 4 cm by 60 cm. The liquid discharge dries to form a hard, glazed substance, which is collected on a weekly basis. The latex is harvested from trees, ranging from 3 to 12 years old.

Not to be Confused With: According to DAB 10 (EUR), USP XXII, only latex from *Acacia senegal* or other African varieties are officially recognized. In other words, Asian, Australian, and American latex are not official.

Other Names: Acacia, Cape Gum, Egyptian Thorn, Gum Acacia, Gum Senegal

ACTIONS AND PHARMACOLOGY

COMPOUNDS

Colloidally soluble polysaccharides: especially Arabic acid (acidic arabinogalactan)

Glycoproteins

EFFECTS

No information is available.

INDICATIONS AND USAGE

Unproven Uses: Acacia gummi is used in the preparation of emulsions. The drug is used as a mild stimulant and to impede absorption. It is also used for the treatment of catarrh and diarrhea. Acacia is often a constituent of cough drops. It is also used in veterinary medicine for mild diarrhea in small animals, foals, and calves.

PRECAUTIONS AND ADVERSE REACTIONS

No health hazards or side effects are known in conjunction with the proper administration of designated therapeutic dosages.

DOSAGE

Mode of Administration: Acacia is used as a pharmaceutical aid and is also administered internally in combination preparations.

Storage: The drug should be stored in tightly closed containers.

LITERATURE

Anderson DM. Evidence for the safety of gum arabic (*Acacia senegal (L.) Willd.*) as a food additive—a brief review. *Food Addit Contam,* 64:225-30, Jul-Sepn 1986

Anderson DM et al. Gum arabic: unambiguous identification by 13C-NMR spectroscopy as an adjunct to the Revised JECFA Specification and the application of 13C-NMR spectra for regulatory/legislative purposes. *Food Addit Contam,* 8:405-21, Jul-Aug 1991

Beuscher N, Bodinet C, Willigmann I, Harnischfeger G, Biological activity of *Baptisia tinctoria* extracts. In: Inst. für Angew. Botanik der Univ. Hamburg, Angewandte Botanik, Berichte 6, 46-61. 1997.

Haukka K, Lindstr om K, Young JP. Three phylogenetic groups of nodA and nifH genes in Sinorhizobium and Mesorhizobium isolates from leguminous trees growing in Africa and Latin America. *Appl Environ Microbiol*, 64:419-26, Feb 1998

Menzies AR, Osman ME, Malik AA, Baldwin TC. A comparison of the physicochemical and immunological properties of the plant gum exudates of *Acacia senegal* (gum arabic) and *Acacia seyal* (gum tahla). *Food Addit Contam*, 13:991-9, Nov-Dec 1996

Gumweed

Grindelia camporum

DESCRIPTION

Medicinal Parts: The medicinal parts are the flowering branches and the dried leaves.

Flower and Fruit: Gumweed has a number of individual composite heads, each with a diameter of 2 to 3 cm, at the end of leafy stems. The involucral bracts are 3 to 8 mm by 0.5 to 1 mm, with very viscid, cylindrical, deflected apexes. If present, the ligules are 7 to 15 mm long and yellow to orange-yellow. The inner florets are yellow. The achaenes are 2 to 3 mm, oblong, and brown. The 2 to 8 pappus-awns are 3 to 5 mm long and usually finely serrulate.

Leaves, Stem, and Root: The plant is an erect biennial or perennial herb or small bush that grows up to 1 m high, often branched above. The alternate leaves are 3 to 7 cm long, triangular to ovate-oblong, clasping, resinous-punctate, serrate-crenate, or entire-margined, and light green. The leaves break off easily when dry.

Habitat: The plant grows in the Southwestern U.S. and in Mexico.

Production: Gumweed herb consists of the dried tops and leaves of *Grindelia robusta* and/or *Grindelia squarrosa*, which are gathered during flowering season.

Other Names: August Flower, California Gum Plant, Grindelia, Resin-Weed, Rosin Weed, Scaly Grindelia, Tar Weed

ACTIONS AND PHARMACOLOGY

COMPOUNDS

Diterpene acids: grindelic acid, hydroxygrindelic acid, 6-oxogrindelic acid. 7alpha,8alpha-epoxygrindelic acid

Volatile oil: including, among others, borneol, bornyl acetate, camphene, camphor, myrcene, alpha- and beta-pinene

Polyynes: including matricarianol, matricarianolacetate

Saponins

Tannins

Flavonoids: including kaempferol-3,7-dimethyl ether, kaempferol-3-dimethyl ether, luteolin, quercetin, quercetin-3,3′-dimethyl ether

EFFECTS

In vitro, the drug has an antimicrobial, fungistatic, and spasmolytic effect caused by the resin, which contains diterpenes, and the phenol carbolic acids. An antibacterial effect has also been demonstrated in vitro. In addition, an inflammation-inhibiting effect has been proved.

INDICATIONS AND USAGE

Approved by Commission E:

- Cough
- Bronchitis

Unproven Uses: Gumweed is also used for infections in the mucous membranes of the upper respiratory tract.

PRECAUTIONS AND ADVERSE REACTIONS

Health risks following the proper administration of designated therapeutic dosages are not recorded. Side effects listed in older scientific literature (Lewin) include gastric irritation and diarrhea. Large dosages, however, are said to have a poisonous effect.

DOSAGE

Mode of Administration: Comminuted herb for teas and other galenic preparations for internal use.

Preparation: The tincture is prepared in a 1:10 or 1:5 concentration with 60% to 80% ethanol (v/v).

How Supplied: Liquid extract

Daily Dosage: The recommended dosage is 4 to 6 g of drug or 3 to 6 g Gumweed liquid extract. If using the tincture, the dosage is 1.5 to 3 mL.

LITERATURE

Hegnauer R, Chemotaxonomie der Pflanzen, Bde 1-11, Birkhäuser Verlag Basel, Boston, Berlin 1962-1997.

Kern W, List PH, Hörhammer L (Hrsg.), Hagers Handbuch der Pharmazeutischen Praxis, 4. Aufl., Bde. 1-8, Springer Verlag Berlin, Heidelberg, New York, 1969.

Lewin L, Gifte und Vergiftungen, 6. Aufl., Nachdruck, Haug Verlag, Heidelberg 1992.

Schimmer O, Egersdörfer S, Grindelia-Arten - Die Grindelie. In: ZPT 9(3):86. 1988.

Wagner H, Wiesenauer M, Phytotherapie. Phytopharmaka und pflanzliche Homöopathika, Fischer-Verlag, Stuttgart, Jena, New York 1995.

Guraea rusbyi

See Cocillana Tree

Haematoxylon campechianum

See Logwood

Hagenia abyssinica

See Kousso

Hamamelis virginiana

See Witch Hazel

Haronga

Haronga madagascariensis

DESCRIPTION

Medicinal Parts: The medicinal parts of the tree are the leaves and bark.

Flower and Fruit: The inflorescences are richly blossomed, terminal, and umbel-like, with a diameter of about 20 cm. The flowers are small and white; they have 5 sepals, 5 petals, 4 stamens, and a fanned ovary with 2 ovules per section. The fruit is a roundish, reddish drupe. The seeds (approximately 10) are cylindrical and have black glandular hairs and a reticulate surface structure.

Leaves, Stem, and Root: Haronga madagascariensis is a small evergreen tree that grows up to 8 m high with a heavily branched crown. It has opposite, elliptical-oval leaves, which are rounded to cordate at the base and dotted black. The upper surface is dark green. The lower surface has red-brown hairs.

Habitat: The plant originated in Madagascar and east Africa; it grows in many areas throughout tropical Africa.

Production: Haronga is a collective term for extracts from the leaves and bark of the trunk and branches of *Haronga madagascariensis,* as well preparations made from those components. The leaves are collected and then air-dried whole; the bark is peeled and also air-dried.

ACTIONS AND PHARMACOLOGY

COMPOUNDS

Anthracene derivatives: including harunganin, madagascin, madagascinanthrone, haronginanthrone, chrysophanol, physcione, hypericin, pseudohypericin, madagascarine

Volatile oil (traces)

Oligomeric procyanidins

Flavonoids (in the leaves): including quercetin-3-O-arabinsoide, quercetin-3-O-xyloside, quercitrin

EFFECTS

Haronga has a digestion regulatory effect through stimulation of the excretory function of the pancreas and gastric juice secretion. In animal experiments, it has demonstrated a choleretic, cholecystokinetic, and antihepatoxic effect. An antimicrobial effect has also been observed.

INDICATIONS AND USAGE

Approved by Commission E:

- Dyspeptic complaints
- Pancreatic insufficiency

Unproven Uses: Internal uses of the bark and leaves in folk medicine include constipation, diarrhea, liver and gallbladder conditions, worm infestations, gonorrhea, hemorrhoids, menstrual disturbances, and puerperal fever. The bark is used externally for eczema. The effect for the external application seems plausible because of the drug's antibacterial effect.

CONTRAINDICATIONS

The drug is not to be used in patients with acute pancreatitis, severe liver function disorders, gallstone illnesses, obstruction of the biliary ducts, gallbladder empyema, or ileus.

PRECAUTIONS AND ADVERSE REACTIONS

Health risks or side effects following the proper administration of designated therapeutic dosages are not recorded. Photosensitization in fair-skinned people can be caused by hypericin and pseudohypericin, but is unlikely due to the small size of therapeutic dosages.

DOSAGE

Mode of Administration: As comminuted Haronga bark with leaves for decoctions, extracts, and other preparations.

How Supplied: Forms of commercial pharmaceutical reparations include drops, tablets, and compound preparations.

Preparation: Extracts are standardized to 0.1% chrysophanic acid derivatives; tinctures are standardized to 0.01% chrysophanic acid derivatives.

Daily Dosage: The average daily dose is 7.5 to 15 mg of an aqueous-alcoholic dry extract corresponding to 25 to 50 mg drug.

LITERATURE

Baldi A et al., Polyphenols from *Harungana madagascarienis*. In: *PM* 58(7):A691. 1992.

Gehrmann B, Analytische Studie an Harungana madagascariensis Lam. ex Poir. In: Dissertation Universität Hamburg. 1989.

Hänsel R, Keller K, Rimpler H, Schneider G (Hrsg.), Hagers Handbuch der Pharmazeutischen Praxis, 5. Aufl., Bde 4-6 (Drogen), Springer Verlag Berlin, Heidelberg, New York, 1992-1994.

Nwodo OFC. Antibiotic and Anti-inflammatory Analgesic Activities of *Harungana madagascariensis Stem Bark. Int J Crude Drug Res.* 27 (3); 137-140. 1989

Steinegger E, Hänsel R, Pharmakognosie, 5. Aufl., Springer Verlag Heidelberg 1992.

Haronga madagascariensis

See Haronga

Harpagophytum procumbens

See Devil's Claw

Hartstongue

Scolopendrium vulgare

DESCRIPTION

Medicinal Parts: The medicinal part is the frond.

Flower and Fruit: Two rows of large sporangia lie almost horizontally on the under surface of the fronds, with a long film stretching toward the margin.

Leaves, Stem, and Root: The evergreen plant is a fern with long, wide, simple, short-petioled dark-green fronds. They are arranged in clusters and are broad linear-lanceolate, double-lobed cordate at the base, and acuminate higher up, with a sinuate margin. The stem is covered in brown, almost hairlike scales. The root is bushy, short, and sturdy.

Habitat: The plant is indigenous to almost all of Europe, North America, northern Africa, and eastern Asia.

Production: Hartstongue is the aerial part of *Scolopendrium vulgare.*

Other Names: Hind's Tongue, Horse Tongue, Buttonhole, God's-Hair

ACTIONS AND PHARMACOLOGY

COMPOUNDS

Tannins

Mucilages

Flavonoids: including among others, kaempferol-7-rhamnoside-3-coffeoyl-7-diglucoside

Thiaminase (probably present only in the fresh plant)

Monosaccharides/oligosaccharides: saccharose, invert sugar

EFFECTS

Hartstongue is a diuretic and has a mild laxative effect.

INDICATIONS AND USAGE

Unproven Uses: Hartstongue is used in folk medicine for digestive disorders and urinary tract diseases.

PRECAUTIONS AND ADVERSE REACTIONS

No health hazards or side effects are known in conjunction with the proper administration of designated therapeutic dosages.

DOSAGE

Mode of Administration: Hartstongue is used internally as an infusion.

LITERATURE

Hegnauer R, Chemotaxonomie der Pflanzen, Bde 1-11: Birkhäuser Verlag Basel, Boston, Berlin 1962-1997.

Kern W, List PH, Hörhammer L (Hrsg.), Hagers Handbuch der Pharmazeutischen Praxis, 4. Aufl., Bde 1-8: Springer Verlag Berlin, Heidelberg, New York, 1969 (unter Phyllitis scolopendrium).

Madaus G, Lehrbuch der Biologischen Arzneimittel, Bde 1-3, Nachdruck, Georg Olms Verlag Hildesheim 1979.

Heartsease

Viola tricolor

DESCRIPTION

Medicinal Parts: The medicinal parts are the dried aerial parts, the fresh aerial parts of the flowering plant, and the whole plant.

Flower and Fruit: The solitary, long-pedicled flower is yellow or tricolored. It has 5 lanceolate, acute, and uneven sepals with an appendage and 5 uneven petals, the largest of which is spurred. The 5 stamens also have an appendage at the tip. There are 3 fused superior ovaries. The fruit is an ellipsoid, obtusely angular capsule, which bursts open at 3 points. The seeds are pear-shaped and yellow.

Leaves, Stem, and Root: Heartsease is annual to perennial and grows about 30 cm high. The shoots are usually yellowish green, glabrous, or covered in scattered hairs. The stem is erect, angular, unbranched or branched, glabrous or short-haired. It has short internodes below and longer ones above. The leaves are alternate, glabrous, or short-haired. The lower leaves are cordate; the upper ones are oblong-elliptical. The stipules are lyrate-pinnatesect and have a large, crenate terminal tip.

Characteristics: The plant is odorless and the taste slimy-sweetish.

Habitat: The plant is indigenous to temperate Eurasia, from the Mediterranean to India and as far as Ireland. It is cultivated in Holland and France.

Production: Viola herb consists of the dried, above-ground parts of *Viola tricolor,* mainly of the subspecies *vulgaris* and subspecies *arvensis*, harvested at flowering season. The herb is cultivated predominantly in central Europe. The flowering above-ground parts are harvested in the summer months and carefully dried on a well-ventilated floor or at 45° C to 50° C. Two to three harvests per year are possible.

Other Names: Biddy's Eyes, Cat's Face, European Wild Pansy, Jack-Behind-the-Garden-Gate, Johnny-Jump-Up, Look-Up-and-Kiss-Me, Love-and-Idle, Pansy Viscum, Wild Pansy

ACTIONS AND PHARMACOLOGY

COMPOUNDS

Flavonoids (0.2-0.4%): including among others rutin (violaquercitrin, 23%), luteolin-7-O-glucosides, scoparin, saponarine, violanthin, vicinein-2, vitexin

Phenol carboxylic acid: salicylic acid (0.06-0.3%), violutoside (violutin, glucoarabinoside of the methyl salicylate)

Mucilage (10%)

Tannins (2-5%)

Hydroxycoumarins: umbelliferone

Triterpene saponins (speculated)

EFFECTS

The drug has soothing, salvelike effects due to its mucin content; in animal experiments, oral administration brought about an improvement of eczemalike skin conditions after long-term use. The antisporiatic effect attributed to the drug may be explained by the saponin content, as can its use for catarrh of the upper respiratory tract. In vitro the drug is hemolytic and increases chloride elimination in the urine.

INDICATIONS AND USAGE

Approved by Commission E:

- Inflammation of the skin

Unproven Uses: External uses include mild seborrheic skin diseases, cradle cap in children, and various skin disorders, including wet and dry exanthema, eczema, *Crusta lactea*, acne, impetigo, and *Pruritus vulvae*. The plant is used internally as a mild laxative for constipation and as an auxiliary agent to promote metabolism.

Homeopathic Uses: The drug is used for eczema and inflammation of the urinary tract.

PRECAUTIONS AND ADVERSE REACTIONS

No health hazards or side effects are known in conjunction with the proper administration of designated therapeutic dosages.

DOSAGE

Mode of Administration: Whole, cut and powdered drug is available for infusions, decoctions, and other galenic preparations. It is also available in ointments and shampoos for external use.

Preparation: To make a tea, pour 1 cup of scalding water over 1 dessertspoonful of drug. An infusion for internal use is prepared using 5 to 10 g drug per 1 liter of water. A decoction for internal use is prepared by adding 1.5 g drug to 1 cup water. The drug is also used as a bath additive.

Daily Dosage: A cup of tea should be taken 3 times daily after meals. The dose for the infusion is 1 dessertspoonful 3 times daily. The dose for the powdered drug is 1/2 teaspoonful in hot sugar water 3 times daily.

Homeopathic Dosage: 5 drops, 1 tablet, or 10 globules every 30 to 60 minutes (acute) or 1 to 3 times daily (chronic); parenterally: 1 to 2 mL sc, acute: 3 times daily; chronic: once a day (HAB1).

Storage: Heartsease must be kept stored away form light sources, and if possible, from moisture in well-sealed containers.

LITERATURE

Baerheim-Svendsen A, Tonnesen HH, Karlsen J. Occurence and prevention of artefact formation during isolation and analysis of plant constituents / Some Alkaloids, essential oil constituents, coumarins and curcuminoids. *Sci Pharm.* 61; 265-275. 1993

Brantner A, Lücke W. Influence of physical parameters on the germ-reducing effect of microwave irridation on medicinal plants. *Pharm Ind.* 50 (11); 762-765. 1995

Molnar P, Szabolcs J, Radics L. Naturally occuring Di-cis-Violaxanthins from Viola tricolor: Isolation and Identification by 1H-NMR Spectroscopy of four Di-cis-Isomers. Phytochemistry 25; 195-199. 1986

Toker G, Türköz S, Erdemoglu N. High performance liquid chromatographic analysis of rutin in plants. *Pharmazie* 53 (7); 494-495.1998

Heather

Calluna vulgaris

DESCRIPTION

Medicinal Parts: The medicinal parts are the complete herb with leaves, the flowers, and the growing shoots of the plant that are collected and dried when the plant is in bloom, as well as the fresh aerial parts collected at the same time.

Flowers and Fruit: The inflorescence is turned to one side, and is dense and hanging. The short-pedicled flowers are nodding, pale-violet-pink but occasionally white; they have 4 small, oval, fringed bracts. The calyx has 4 violet-pink, glossy and petaloid sepals, which have the consistency of straw. The 8 stamens form a brown-red club. The superior ovary has 4 sections, and the style is larger than the calyx. The style has a thick, buttonlike, 4-knobbed stigma. The fruit capsule is globose, 1.5 mm long, and 4 sectioned. The fruit is covered in thick white bristles and is many-seeded. The dividing walls break off easily.

Leaves, Stem, and Root: Calluna vulgaris is a dwarf shrub, 0.2 to 1 m high with decumbent, rooting shoots and ascending branches. The small stems are thin, gray-brown, heavily branched, and have numerous upright branches. The leaves are linear-lanceolate, in groups of 4 rows. They are imbricate, 1 to 3.5 mm long, revolute, sessile, and have 2-mm long points at the base. The margins are glandular with downward-pointing spurs.

Habitat: With the exception of a few Mediterranean islands, the plant is distributed throughout most of Europe, Russia and Asia Minor, as well as on the Atlantic coast of North America.

Production: The herb is harvested from July to October and dried.

Not to be Confused With: Erica tetralix.

Other Names: Ling, Scotch Heather, White Heather

ACTIONS AND PHARMACOLOGY

COMPOUNDS

Flavonoids: including kempferol, quercetin, myricetin, taxifolin, and the glycosides of each, as well as callunin

Catechin tannins (3-7%): (+)-catechin, (-)-epicatechin

Oligomeric proanthocyanidins

Caffeic acid derivatives: including chlorogenic acid

Phenols: orcin, orcinol

Triterpenes: including ursolic acid (2.5%)

Steroids: beta-sitosterol

Hydroquinone glycosides: including arbutin

EFFECTS

Heather is said to be diuretic, antimicrobial, cholagogic, and antirheumatic. It is also used as an agent for wound healing. However, these effects have not yet been documented.

INDICATIONS AND USAGE

Unproven Uses: Preparations of Heather and/or Heather flowers are used as a diuretic for diseases and ailments of the kidneys and the lower urinary tract, and for enlargement of the prostate. They are also used for gastrointestinal disorders, colic, liver and gallbladder disease, gout, rheumatism, respiratory complaints, insomnia, agitation, and wounds.

The efficacy for the claimed uses is not documented.

PRECAUTIONS AND ADVERSE REACTIONS

No health hazards or side effects are known in conjunction with the proper administration of designated therapeutic dosages.

DOSAGE

Mode of Administration: Whole, cut and powdered forms are available for internal and external use.

Preparation: A decoction is prepared by adding 1.5 g of the drug to 1/4 liter of water and then boiling for 3 minutes. For a bath additive, 500 g of the drug is first boiled in a few liters of water then strained. A liquid extract (1:1) is also used.

Daily Dosage: The average daily dose of the decoction is 3 cups daily between meals; the dose for the liquid extract is 1 to 2 teaspoonfuls daily. Externally, the drug is added to full baths.

Storage: Heather should be stored in well-dried, sealed containers.

LITERATURE

Allais DP, Chulia AJ, Kaouadji M, Simon A, Delage C. 3-Desoxycallunin and 2″-Acetylcallunin, Two minor 2,3-Dihydroflavonoid Glukosides from *Calluna vulgaris. Phytochemistry* 39 (2); 427-430. 1995

Brantner A, Grein E. Antibacterial activity of plant extracts used externally in traditional medicine. *J Ethnopharmacol.* 44; 35-40. 1994

Hänsel R, Keller K, Rimpler H, Schneider G (Hrsg.), Hagers Handbuch der Pharmazeutischen Praxis, 5. Aufl., Bde 4-6

(Drogen): Springer Verlag Berlin, Heidelberg, New York, 1992-1994.

Jaläl MAF, Read DJ, Haslam E, Phenolic composition and its seasonal variation in *Calluna vulgaris*. In: *PH* 21(6):1397. 1982.

Madaus G, Lehrbuch der Biologischen Arzneimittel, Bde 1-3, Nachdruck, Georg Olms Verlag Hildesheim 1979.

Simon A, Chulia AJ, Kaoudi M, Delage C. Quercetin 3-[Triacetylarabinosyl(1–>6)Galactoside] and Chromosomes from Calluna vulgaris. Phytochemistry 36; 1043-1045. 1994

Simon A et al., Further flavonoid glycosides from *Calluna vulgaris*. In: PH 32:1045. 1993.

Simon A et al., Two flavonol 3-[triacetylarabinosyl(1-6) glucosides] from *Calluna vulgaris*. In: PH 33:1237. 1993.

Hedera helix

See English Ivy

Hedge Mustard

Sisymbrium officinale

DESCRIPTION

Medicinal Parts: The medicinal parts are the fresh, flowering herb and the fresh aerial parts of the flowering plant.

Flower and Fruit: The inflorescences at the end of the stems and branches have no bracts and are initially umbelliferous-racemous, later stretching into spikes. The pedicles are thin and approximately 1.5 cm long, bearing the small flowers. The 4 sepals are 1.5 to 2.5 mm long, erect, pubescent, and narrowly elliptical. The petals are pale yellow and 3 to 4 mm long. The stamens have 0.5- to 0.5-mm long anthers. The fruit is a pubescent pod appressed to the axis of the infructescence. The fruits are 1 to 1.5 cm long and 1 to 1.5 mm thick. The almost-smooth seeds are about 1 mm long, ovate, compressed, and unwinged with reddish, yellow-brown seed-skins.

Leaves, Stem, and Root: The plant is an annual or biennial, 30 to 60 cm high, and has a thin taproot. The stem is branched, round, leafy, and covered in scattered patent hairs. The basal leaves and lower cauline leaves are petiolate-pinnatifid with 3 to 9 segments. The upper leaves are oblong-lanceolate, simple or with 2 to 4 lateral segments, and often hastate and pubescent.

Habitat: The herb is found mainly in temperate Europe, but it also grows as far as northern Africa and eastern Siberia.

Production: Hedge Mustard is the fresh flowering herb of *Sisymbrium officinale*.

Other Names: Bank Cress, Bank Mustard, Irio, Singer's Plant, St. Barbara's Hedge Mustard, English Watercress, Erysimum, Thalictroc

ACTIONS AND PHARMACOLOGY

COMPOUNDS

Cardioactive steroid glycosides (cardenolides, 0.05% in the tips of the foliage): including among others corchorosid A and helveticosid

Glucosinolates: chiefly sinigrin (allylglucosinolates) and gluconapin (3-butenylglucosinolates), releasing through cell destruction the volatile mustard oil allylisothiocyanate and 3-butenylisothiocyanate

Vitamins: ascorbic acid (vitamin C, up to 0.2 % in the fresh foliage)

EFFECTS

Hedge mustard contains cardio-active steroids (cardenolides) and is said to be spasmolytic and analgesic. Its use for pharyngitis and laryngitis as well as severe hoarseness may be due to the mustard oils.

INDICATIONS AND USAGE

Unproven Uses: In folk medicine, the drug is used for laryngitis and pharyngitis, severe hoarseness including loss of voice, chronic bronchitis, and inflammation of the gallbladder.

PRECAUTIONS AND ADVERSE REACTIONS

No health hazards or side effects are known in conjunction with the proper administration of designated therapeutic dosages.

OVERDOSAGE

It is conceivable that overdosage would have digitalis-like effects. These include queasiness, vomiting, diarrhea, headache, and cardiac rhythm disorders. Cases of poisonings have not, however, been recorded.

DOSAGE

Daily Dosage: The average daily internal dose of the drug is 0.5 to 1.0 g, which would be equal to 3 to 4 cups daily of an infusion. It takes between 6 and 8 g of drug to make 1 g extract. Externally, the infusion is used as a gargle or mouthwash, several times daily.

LITERATURE

Delitheos A, Tiligada E, Yannitsaros A, Bazos I. Antiphage activity in extracts of plants growing in Greece. Phytomedicine 4 (2); 117-124. 1997

Hänsel R, Keller K, Rimpler H, Schneider G (Hrsg.), Hagers Handbuch der Pharmazeutischen Praxis, 5. Aufl., Bde 4-6 (Drogen): Springer Verlag Berlin, Heidelberg, New York, 1992-1994.

Roth L, Daunderer M, Kormann K, Giftpflanzen, Pflanzengifte, 4. Aufl., Ecomed Fachverlag Landsberg Lech 1993.

Teuscher E, Lindequist U, Biogene Gifte - Biologie, Chemie, Pharmakologie, 2. Aufl., Fischer Verlag Stuttgart 1994.

Hedge-Hyssop

Gratiola officinalis

DESCRIPTION

Medicinal Parts: The medicinal parts are the herb and roots. (In contrast to what its name suggests, Hedge-Hyssop is not a member of the Hyssop family, even though it has a similarly bitter taste.)

Flower and Fruit: The pedicled flowers are arranged singly in the axils of the upper leaf pairs and are a pale red or yellowish-white. The calyx is only fused at the base and has 5 tips. The corolla has a distinct tube and a bilabiate border. The upper lip is margined, and the lower lip is divided into 3. There are 4 stamens, 2 sterile and 2 fertile, and 1 superior ovary. The fruit has 4 lids, which burst open.

Leaves, Stem, and Root: The plant is a perennial that grows 15 to 30 cm high. The stem grows from a creeping scaly rhizome. It is erect and becomes glabrous and quadrangular higher up. The leaves are opposite, lanceolate, weakly serrate, smooth, and pale green.

Characteristics: The plant is poisonous and has a bitter taste.

Habitat: The herb is indigenous to western and central Asia, as well as southern Europe.

Production: Hedge-Hyssop is the herb of *Gratiola officinalis*, which is harvested shortly before flowering. The upper portion of the stem is cut down, then dried in thin layers in the shade at temperatures not exceeding 45° C.

Other Names: Gratiola

ACTIONS AND PHARMACOLOGY

COMPOUNDS

Cucurbitacins: gratiogenin, 16-hydroxygratiogenin, cucurbitacins E, I, the glycosides gratiogenin-3beta-D-glucoside, gratioside (gratiolin, gratiogenindiglucoside), elaterinide, desacetylelaterinide

Saponins

Lignans

Flavonoids

EFFECTS

The cucurbaticins, especially elaterinide, cause a reduction of the contraction power of cardiac muscle, a lowering of cardiac frequency and a distinct increase in coronary flow. Elaterinide has a laxative effect. The drug is a strong purgative; it eliminates intestinal parasites and increases micturation.

INDICATIONS AND USAGE

Unproven Uses: The herb was formerly used as a purgative and for treating the liver. In folk medicine, it is used as purgative and emetic for gout, liver complaints and constipation, as well as for chronic skin conditions. The drug is only to be taken under medical supervision of a doctor because of its toxicity.

Homeopathic Uses: Uses in homeopathy include stomach colic and bladder and kidney conditions.

PRECAUTIONS AND ADVERSE REACTIONS

Health risks or side effects following the proper administration of designated therapeutic dosages are not recorded. Nonetheless, the drug is extremely poisonous. It is severely irritating to mucous membranes due to the cucurbitacin and cucurbitacin glycosides content, out of which cucurbitacins are released in watery environments.

OVERDOSAGE

The intake of toxic dosages leads to vomiting, bloody diarrhea, colic, kidney irritation and initially to elevated diuresis, then to anuria. Very high dosages lead to spasm, paralysis and circulatory collapse. Fatalities are seen only rarely. Following gastric lavage, the treatment for poisonings should proceed symptomatically.

DOSAGE

Mode of Administration: Hedge-Hyssop is most effective in alcoholic extracts, but it also is used in infusions and in homeopathic dilutions. Today, it is rarely used in folk medicine.

Daily Dosage: A single dose of tea is noted as containing 0.3 g drug.

Homeopathic Dosage: 5 drops, 1 tablet, or 10 globules every 30 to 60 minutes (acute) or 1 to 3 times daily (chronic); parenterally: 1 to 2 ml sc acute, 3 times daily; chronic: once a day (HAB1).

LITERATURE

Kern W, List PH, Hörhammer L (Hrsg.), Hagers Handbuch der Pharmazeutischen Praxis, 4. Aufl., Bde. 1-8, Springer Verlag Berlin, Heidelberg, New York, 1969.

Lewin L, Gifte und Vergiftungen, 6. Aufl., Nachdruck, Haug Verlag, Heidelberg 1992.

Madaus G, Lehrbuch der Biologischen Arzneimittel, Bde 1-3, Nachdruck, Georg Olms Verlag Hildesheim 1979.

Müller A, Wichtl M, Herzwirsamkeit des Gnadenkrautes (*Gratiola officinalis*). In: Pharm Ztg 124(37):1761-1766. 1979.

Roth L, Daunderer M, Kormann K, Giftpflanzen, Pflanzengifte, 4. Aufl., Ecomed Fachverlag Landsberg Lech 1993.

Teuscher E, Lindequist U, Biogene Gifte - Biologie, Chemie, Pharmakologie, 2. Aufl., Fischer Verlag Stuttgart 1994.

Helianthemum canadense

See Frostwort

Helianthus annuus

See Sunflower

Helichrysum arenarium

See Immortelle

Helleborus niger

See Black Hellebore

Helleborus viridis

See Green Hellebore

Hemlock

Conium maculatum

DESCRIPTION

Medicinal Parts: The medicinal parts of the plant are the fresh flowering foliage, the branches, and the dried leaves.

Flower and Fruit: The plant has white flowers in 10 to 20 rayed umbels. The 3 to 5 triangular to lanceolate bracts are acuminate; 3 to 6 small bracts appear on the outside of the small umbels. The blossoms have 1.5-mm white petals. The fruit is ovate with undulating veins. Deep indentations on the mericarp on the seam side—with no oil marks in the indentations—are a unique feature.

Leaves, Stem, and Root: The plant can be annual or perennial; it grows up to 2 m high. The stem is erect, tubular, hollow, round, and finely grooved. It is branched above, glabrous, with brownish-red marks below. The leaves are a glossy dark green, tripinnate. The root is whitish and fusiform or branched.

Characteristics: When wilting, the highly poisonous herb smells of mice. It tastes disgustingly salty and pungent. The stem has distinctive red marks.

Habitat: The plant is indigenous to Europe and the temperate zones of Asia, North Africa, and North and South America.

Production: Hemlock is the fresh or dried leaves and the flowering branch tips of *Conium maculatum*. They are gathered from June to September in the second year of grown and air-dried in a shaded, open location.

Not to be Confused With: Hemlock may be confused with water hemlock, canine parsley, wild chervil, and with tuberous chervil.

Other Names: Beaver Poison, California Fern, Cicuta, Herb Bennet, Kecksies, Kex, Musquash Root, Poison Parsley, Poison Root, Poison Snakeweed, Spotted Crowbane, Spotted Hemlock, Spotted Parsley, Water Parsley, Winter Fern, Spotted Corobane

ACTIONS AND PHARMACOLOGY

COMPOUNDS

Piperidin alkaloids: main alkaloid coniine, including, among others, N-methyl coniine, gamma-coniceine

The piperidin alkaloids are volatile and are likely to be present in toxicologically harmful quantities only in the freshly harvested plant, particularly in its berries, and in the freshly dried plant.

Polyynes: including falcarinol, falcarindiol

Furanocoumarins: including bergaptene, xanthotoxin

EFFECTS

The plant is poisonous. The effects of the drug are caused by coniine in particular. Toxic doses given to mice, rats, guinea pigs, and cats provoked the autonomous ganglion, clonic, and tonal contractions of individual limbs, cramps, and eventually, paralysis. Small doses given to mice led to blood pressure reduction in the short term. Higher doses resulted in a rise in blood pressure. Smaller doses stimulated respiration in cats, while higher doses impeded or slowed down the initial stimulus. In isolated guinea pig ileum, coniine brought on contractions. In isolated perfused rabbit hearts, coniine was negatively inotropic while a stable heartbeat was maintained. With anesthetized cats, a suppression of the muscle contraction reflex took place. Feeding or injecting lethal doses of coniine into cows, horses, pigs, sheep, and hamsters was initially stimulating, producing twitching of the eyes and ears, which was followed by muscular debility, collapse, limpness and death through paralysis. Coniine absorbed through the skin and mucous membranes is stimulating at first, then causes gradual paralysis of the spinal cord and blockage of the medulla oblongata. Nicotine-like receptors are at first activated, then paralyzed.

INDICATIONS AND USAGE

Unproven Uses: Use is inadvisable due to the uncontrollable amounts of coniine. Formerly, in folk medicine, the drug was used internally for neuralgia, rheumatism of the muscles and joints, stiffness of the neck, tetanic and epileptic cramps, bronchial spasms, and pylori spasms. Externally, the drug was used as an ointment for coughs, asthma, sciatica, backache, and neuralgia.

Homeopathic Uses: Swollen glands, paresis, calcification of cerebral vessels, and depressive moods are considered to be indications for use in homeopathy.

PRECAUTIONS AND ADVERSE REACTIONS

General: The drug is severely poisonous and use is not advised.

Pregnancy: The drug has a teratogenic effect with chronic intake.

OVERDOSAGE

Symptoms of poisoning following intake of toxic quantities (corresponding to 150 mg coniine, approximately 10 g of the freshly dried berries, approximately 30 g of the freshly dried leaves) include burning of the mouth, scratchy throat, salivation, rolling of the eyes, visual disorders, and weakness in the legs. Lethal dosages (corresponding to approximately 500 mg coniine) cause glossoplegia, mydriasis, pressure in the head, dizziness, nausea, vomiting, diarrhea, loss of orientation, rising central paralysis, dyspepsia, and cyanosis. Death ultimately results through central asphyxiation, in the cases of very high dosages, and also through curarelike paralysis of the breathing musculature.

Following stomach and intestinal emptying (gastric lavage, sodium sulfate) and the administration of activated charcoal, plasma volume expanders and sodium bicarbonate infusions should be given in case of shock or to restore acidosis balance. If necessary, intubation and respiration should be carried out.

DOSAGE

Mode of Administration: Hemlock is obsolete and strongly advised against as an internal drug because of the danger of poisoning. Homeopathic dilutions and ointments containing hemlock are used externally.

How Supplied: Liquid rubs, ointments.

Daily Dosage: Use is discouraged, but the maximum single dose mentioned for internal use is 0.3 g, not to exceed 1.5 g, per day. The standard single dose is 0.1 g.

Homeopathic Dosage: 5 drops, 1 tablet, or 10 globules every 30 to 60 minutes (acute) or 1 to 3 times daily (chronic); parenterally: 1 to 2 mL sc acute, 3 times daily; chronic: once a day; ointment 1 to 2 times daily (HAB34).

Storage: Hemlock should be stored above caustic lime, well dried, in closed containers and kept for no more than one year..

LITERATURE

Roberts MF, *Phytochemistry* 14:2395. 1975

Roberts MF, *Planta Med* 39:216. 1980

Seeger R, Neumann HG, DAZ-Giftlexikon Coniin. In: *DAZ* 131(13):720. 1991.

Hemp Agrimony

Eupatorium cannabinum

DESCRIPTION

Medicinal Parts: The medicinal part is the flowering herb.

Flower and Fruit: The flowers are in compact, terminal, umbrellalike umbels. They are small dull-pink tubular androgynous flowers whose corolla tube has a 5-tipped edge. The epicalyx is cylindrical and consists of a few bracts. The edge of the calyx consists of yellowish hairs. The style is divided in two parts and shows above the flower. The corolla is covered in resinous spots. The angular fruit bears a crown of hair and is dirty white.

Leaves, Stem and Root: The plant is a small perennial herb 75 to 150 cm high. The rhizome is woody and has stems growing from it, which have short axillary branches. The stems are erect, reddish, pubescent, and resinous below. The root leaves are long-petioled. The opposite cauline leaves are short-petioled, trifoliate, serrate, and covered in resinous spots.

Habitat: Hemp Agrimony grows in damp regions of Europe.

Production: Hemp Agrimony is the flowering herb of *Eupatorium cannabium.*

Other Names: Holy Rope, St. John's Herb, Sweet-Smelling Trefoil, Water Maudlin

ACTIONS AND PHARMACOLOGY

COMPOUNDS

Caffeic acid ester: chlorogenic acid

Immunostimulating polysaccharides (heteroxylans)

Pyrrolizidine alkaloids: including echinatine, supinine, eucanecine, amabiline, lycopsamin, intermedin

Sesquiterpene lactones: including eupatoriopicrin, eupatolid

EFFECTS

Eupatorin is said to be cytotoxic and has an immune-stimulating effect. It is also a bitter tonic.

INDICATIONS AND USAGE

Unproven Uses: The herb is used for disorders of the liver and gallbladder and for fevers.

Homeopathic Uses: Eupatorium cannabinum is used to treat illnesses of the respiratory organs.

PRECAUTIONS AND ADVERSE REACTIONS

Because of the pyrrolizidine alkaloid content with 1,2-unsaturated necic parent substances, hepatotoxicity and carcinogenicity are likely consequences of internal use. Therefore the drug should not be taken internally. Sensitization after skin contact with the plant has been reported.

DOSAGE

Mode of Administration: The herb is used topically as an alcoholic extract, as a tea, and as an inhalation for the treatment of colds.

LITERATURE

Elsässer-Beile U, Willenbacher W, Bartsch HH, Gallati H, Schulte Mönting J, Kleist von S et al., Cytokine production in leukocyte cultures during therapy with echinacea extract. In: *J Clin Lab Analysis* 10(6):441-445. 1996.

Lexa A, Fleurentin J, Lehr PR, Mortier F, Pruvost M, Pelt JM. Choleretic and Hepatoprotective Properties of *Eupatorium cannabinum* in the Rat. Planta Med. 55; 127-132. 1989

Linde Jcc et al. Role of Membrane Lipid Composition in the Cytotoxicity of the Sesquiterpene Lactone Eupatoriopicrin. *Phytother Res.* 7 (2); 128-133. 1993

Vollmar A, Schäfer W, Wagner H. Immunologically active Polysaccharides of *Eupatorium cannabinum* and *Eupatorium perfoliatum. Phytochemistry* 25; 377-381. 1986

Woerdenbag HJ, Moskal TA, Pras N, MalingreTM, El-Feraly FS. Cytotoxicity of Artemisinin-related Endoperoxides to Ehrlich-Ascites Tumor Cells. *J Nat Prod.* 56; 849-856. 1993

Hemp Nettle

Galeopsis segetum

DESCRIPTION

Medicinal Parts: The medicinal part is the flowering herb.

Flower and Fruit: The large, pale yellow, bilabiate flowers are in false whorls on the branch ends. The calyx is evenly 5-dentate and covered in patent glandular hairs. The upper lip of the corolla is domed, finely dentate, and pubescent. The lateral tips of the trilobed lower lip are wide, obtuse, and have one hollow erect tooth at either side of the base. The stamen halves are horizontal. The fruit is smooth.

Leaves, Stem and Root: The herb grows 15 to 100 cm high. The stem is erect, heavily branched and downy, with unthickened nodes. The leaves are ovate and serrate. The lower ones are long petioled, the upper are short petioled.

Habitat: Hemp Nettle is found in southern and central Europe.

Production: Hemp Nettle consists of the aboveground parts of *Galeopsis segetum Necker* (synonym *Galeopsis ochroleuca Lamarck*) and is gathered in the wild during the flowering season.

ACTIONS AND PHARMACOLOGY

COMPOUNDS

Iridoide monoterpenes: including harpagide, 8-O-acetylharpagide, antirrinoside, 5-O-glucosylantirrinoside

Silicic acid (to some extent water-soluble)

Tannins

Flavonoids

EFFECTS

The herb acts as expectorant, due to its saponin content, and as an astringent because of the tannins, silicic acid, iridoids, and antirrhinoside.

INDICATIONS AND USAGE

Approved by Commission E:

- Cough
- Bronchitis

Unproven Uses: In folk medicine, the herb is used for pulmonary afflictions and as a diuretic.

PRECAUTIONS AND ADVERSE REACTIONS

Health risks or side effects following the proper administration of designated therapeutic dosages are not recorded.

DOSAGE

Mode of Administration: Ground and cut herb for teas and other galenic preparations for internal use.

Preparation: To prepare an infusion, pour boiling water over 2 g of comminuted drug, strain after 5 minutes.

Daily Dosage: Average daily dose: 6 g drug. One cup of the infusion may be taken several times daily and, if preferred, sweetened with honey.

LITERATURE

Junod-Busch U, Dissertation ETH Zürich. 1976.

Kern W, List PH, Hörhammer L (Hrsg.), Hagers Handbuch der Pharmazeutischen Praxis, 4. Aufl., Bde. 1-8, Springer Verlag Berlin, Heidelberg, New York, 1969.

Madaus G, Lehrbuch der Biologischen Arzneimittel, Bde 1-3, Nachdruck, Georg Olms Verlag Hildesheim 1979.

Tomas-Barberan FA et al., PH 30:3311. 1991.

Steinegger E, Hänsel R, Pharmakognosie, 5. Aufl., Springer Verlag Heidelberg 1992.

Wichtl M (Hrsg.), Teedrogen, 4. Aufl., Wiss. Verlagsges. Stuttgart 1997.

Henbane

Hyoscyamus niger

DESCRIPTION

Medicinal Parts: The medicinal parts are the dried leaves or the dried leaves with the flowering branches, the dried seeds, and the whole fresh flowering plant.

Flower and Fruit: The flowers are in terminal, almost-sessile, one-sided leafy and revolute spikes. The calyx is jug-shaped, 5-tipped, and does not drop. The corolla is funnel-shaped, 5-lobed, dirty yellow with violet veins and dark violet in the tube. The flower has 1 superior ovary and 5 stamens. The fruit is a swollen pixidium with up to 200 seeds. The seeds are gray-brown, pitted, slightly reniform, compressed, 1 to 1.3 mm long and 1 mm wide.

Leaves, Stem, and Root: The plant is erect and grows up to 80 cm high. It is an herb with simple leaves. The root is fusiform and turniplike at the top. The stem is erect and sticky-villous. The leaves are oblong, roughly crenate-dentate, and gray-green. The basal leaves are petiolate, and the cauline leaves are stem clasping.

Characteristics: Henbane has a strong, distinctive odor. The plant is poisonous.

Habitat: The plant is indigenous to Europe, western and northern Asia, and northern Africa. It has been introduced to eastern Asia, North America and Australia.

Production: Henbane leaf consists of the dried leaves or the dried leaves and flowering tops of *Hyoscyamus niger,* harvested from cultures or in the wild when in bloom and dried mechanically or in the sun. Henbane seeds are the seeds of *Hyoscyamus niger.*

Other Names: Black Henbane, Devil's Eye, Fetid Nightshade, Stinking Nightshade, Hen Bell, Hogbean, Jupiter's Bean and Poison Tobacco

ACTIONS AND PHARMACOLOGY

COMPOUNDS: HENBANE LEAF

Tropane alkaloids (0.05- 0.28%): chief alkaloid (-)-hyoscyamine, under storage conditions changing over to some extent into atropine, and scopolamine

Flavonoids: including, among others, rutin

COMPOUNDS: HENBANE SEED

Tropane alkaloids (0.05-0.3%): chief alkaloid (-)-hyoscyamine, under storage conditions changing to some extent into atropine, and scopolamine

Fatty oil

EFFECTS: HENBANE LEAF AND SEED

Main active agents: Alkaloids, flavonids. Henbane preparations produce a parasympatholytic or anticholinergic effect by competitive inhibition of acetylcholine. This inhibition affects the muscarinic action of acetylcholine but not its nicotine-like effects on ganglia and motor end plates.

Henbane preparations exert peripheral actions on the autonomic nervous system and on smooth muscle, as well as the central nervous system. Because of their parasympatholytic properties, they cause relaxation of organs containing smooth muscle, particularly in the region of the gastrointestinal tract. Furthermore, they relieve muscular tremors of central nervous origin.

The spectrum of actions of *Hyoscyamus niger* additionally includes a sedative effect.

INDICATIONS AND USAGE

HENBANE LEAF

Approved by Commission E:

■ Dyspeptic complaints, spasms

Unproven Uses: Preparations of henbane oil are used for the treatment of scar tissue.

In folk medicine, Henbane is used internally for various pain syndromes, in particular toothache and facial pain, painful ulcers and tumors, stomach cramps, and lower abdominal pain. Externally, henbane oil is used for the treatment of scar tissue.

The herb has been used for hundreds of years in so-called witches' ointments, as a repellent against mice and rats, as stunning agent for fish, and to increase the narcotic effect of beer.

Indian Medicine: Used for toothache, bleeding gums and nose, orchitis, dysmenorrhea, worm infestation, bloody vomit, asthma, diverse pain syndromes, and meningitis.

HENBANE SEED

Unproven Uses: See Henbane Leaf. In folk medicine, Henbane was formerly used as a fumigant for asthma and toothache.

Chinese Medicine: Used for convulsions, psychoses, joint pains, stomach pains, asthma, chronic dysentery, and diarrhea.

CONTRAINDICATIONS

HENBANE LEAF AND SEED

Tachycardiac arrhythmias, prostatic adenoma, angle-closure glaucoma, acute pulmonary edema, mechanical stenoses in the area of the gastrointestinal tract, and megacolon.

PRECAUTIONS AND ADVERSE REACTIONS

HENBANE LEAF AND SEED

General: No health hazards are known in conjunction with the proper administration of designated therapeutic dosages. Skin reddening, dryness of the mouth, tachycardiac arrhythmias, mydriasis (the four early warning symptoms of a poisoning), accommodation disorders, heat buildup through decline in sweat secretion, micturition disorders, and obstipation can occur as side effects, particularly with overdoses.

DRUG INTERACTIONS

POTENTIAL INTERACTIONS

Enhancement of anticholinergic action caused by tricyclic antidepressants, amantadine, antihistamines, phenothiazines, procainamide, and quinidine with concomitant use.

OVERDOSAGE

HENBANE LEAF AND SEED

Because of the high content of scopolamine in the drug, poisonings lead at first to somnolence, then after the intake of very high dosages, to central excitation (restlessness, hallucinations, deliria, and manic episodes), followed by exhaustion, and sleep. Lethal dosages carry with them the danger of asphyxiation (for adults starting at 100 mg atropine, with an alkaloid-rich drug at 30 mg, considerably less for children). Severe poisonings are particularly conceivable in connection with the misuse of the drug as an intoxicant. Treatment for poisonings include gastric lavage, temperature-lowering measures with wet cloths (no antipyretics), oxygen respiration for respiratory distress, intubation, parenteral physostigmine salts as an antidote, diazepam for spasms, and chlorpromazine for severe excitation.

DOSAGE

HENBANE LEAF

Mode of Administration: Standardized Henbane powder and galenic preparations for internal application.

Daily Dosage: The average single dose is 0.5 g of standardized Henbane powder corresponding to 0.25 to 0.35 mg total alkaloid. Maximum daily dose is 3.0 g of standardized Henbane powder corresponding to 1.5 to 2.1 mg total alkaloid, calculated as hyoscyamine.

Storage: Keep protected from light in tightly sealed containers.

HENBANE SEED

Mode of Administration: The drug is available as an emulsion or powder.

Storage: Should be stored separate from other medicines.

LITERATURE

HENBANE LEAF AND SEED

Dräger B, Almsick Av, Mrachatz G. Distribution of Calystegines in Several Solanaceae. *Planta Med.* 61 (6); 577-579. 1995

Frohne D, Pfänder HJ, Giftpflanzen - Ein Handbuch für Apotheker, Toxikologen und Biologen, 4. Aufl., Wiss. Verlags-Ges. Stuttgart 1997.

Hänsel R, Keller K, Rimpler H, Schneider G (Hrsg.), Hagers Handbuch der Pharmazeutischen Praxis, 5. Aufl., Bde 4-6 (Drogen), Springer Verlag Berlin, Heidelberg, New York, 1992-1994.

Kc SK, Müller K. Antiproliferative activity of selected Nepalese medicinal plants against the growth of human keratinocytes. *Pharm Pharmacol Lett.* 7 (2/3); 63-65. 1997

Lewin L, Gifte und Vergiftungen, 6. Aufl., Nachdruck, Haug Verlag, Heidelberg 1992.

Madaus G, Lehrbuch der Biologischen Arzneimittel, Bde 1-3, Nachdruck, Georg Olms Verlag Hildesheim 1979.

Tattje DHE et al., Zusammensetzung der etherischen Öle von *Laurus nobilis, L. nobilis var. angustifolia* und *L. azorica*. In: *PM* 44:116-119. 1982.

Teuscher E, Lindequist U, Biogene Gifte - Biologie, Chemie, Pharmakologie, 2. Aufl., Fischer Verlag Stuttgart 1994.

Teuscher E, Biogene Arzneimittel, 5. Aufl., Wiss. Verlagsges. Stuttgart 1997.

Wagner H, Wiesenauer M, Phytotherapie. Phytopharmaka und pflanzliche Homöopathika, Fischer-Verlag, Stuttgart, Jena, New York 1995.

Wellen BJ, Zur Geschichte des Bilsenkrautes. Eine pharmaziehistorische Untersuchung besonders zu Hyoscyamus niger L. In: Dissertation Universität Marburg. 1986.

Henna

Lawsonia inermis

DESCRIPTION

Medicinal Parts: The medicinal parts are the pulverized leaves, the fruit, and the bark.

Flower and Fruit: The flowers are in small groups of 4 panicles and yellowy-white to brick-red. The calyx is top-shaped, then later bowl-shaped without appendages. The petals are thick, very wrinkled, yellowish-white to brick-red. The stamens are arranged in pairs. The fruit is an indehiscent or a fibrously torn berry. The seeds are small and angular, and the seed skin is spongy at the tip.

Leaves, Stem and Root: Henna is a deciduous, 2 to 6 m high shrub with partly thorny, short shoots and opposite paired, narrowly acuminate lanceolate leaves.

Habitat: Found in Egypt, India, the Middle East, Kurdistan, and Iran.

Production: Henna is the aerial part of *Lawsonia inermis*.

Other Names: Alcanna, Egyptian Privet, Jamaica Mignonette, Mignonette Tree, Reseda, Henne, Mehndi, Mendee, Smooth Lawsonia

ACTIONS AND PHARMACOLOGY

COMPOUNDS

Naphthalene derivatives (1,4-naphthaquinones): in particular lawsone (2-hydroxy-1,4-naphthaquinone), arising during dehydration of the leaves out of the precursor 1,2,4-trihydroxy-naphthalen-4-beta-D-glucoside

Tannins

EFFECTS

The drug is an astringent and a diuretic, and has an antibacterial effect.

INDICATIONS AND USAGE

Unproven Uses: The drug is used externally for eczema, scabies, fungal infections, and ulcers. It is also used for amebic dysentery and gastrointestinal ulcers. In African folk medicine, it is used as an abortifacient. The drug is also contained in facial and hair lotions and is used to treat dandruff.

Indian Medicine: Henna root preparations are used to treat leprosy, skin diseases, amenorrhea, and dysmenorrhea. Henna leaves are used to treat wounds, ulcers, dysuria, coughs, bronchitis, one-sided headache, rheumatism, and anemia. The flowers are used for headache, fever, and acute psychosis. Henna seeds are used to treat intermittent fever, diarrhea, and dysentery.

PRECAUTIONS AND ADVERSE REACTIONS

Health risks or side effects following the proper administration of designated therapeutic dosages are not recorded. Stomach complaints are possible due to the tannin content.

DOSAGE

Mode of Administration: Henna is used rarely for internal use in ground form or as an infusion. Henna is applied externally as an ingredient in hair and skin lotions.

Daily Dosage: For internal use, 3 g of powder leaves to be taken daily, for amebiasis and ulcers.

LITERATURE

Aguwa AN. Toxic effects of the methanolic extract of *Lawsonia inermis* roots. *Int J Crude Drug Res.* 25; 241-245. 1987

Ali NAA, Jülich WD, Kusnick C, Lindequist U. Screening of Yemeni medicinal plants for antibacterial and cytotoxic activities. *J Ethnopharmacol* 74(2); 173-179. 2001

Anand KK, Singh B, Chand D, Chandan BK. An evaluation of *Lawsonia alba* extract as hepatoprotective agent. *Planta Med.* 58; 22-25. 1992

Babich H, Stern A, Munday R. In vitro cytotoxicity of 1,4-Naphthoquinone derivatives to replicating cells. *Toxicol Lett.* 69; 69-75. 1993

Etienne A, Piletta P, Hauser C, Pasche-Koo F. Ectopic contact dermatitis from henna. *Contact Dermatitis* 37; 183. 1997

Guerrier CJ, Abdulwahab A, Basri N, Revill S. Henna as an antimicrobial agent. *Int J Cosmet Sci.* 10; 131-136. 1988

Kern W, List PH, Hörhammer L (Hrsg.), Hagers Handbuch der Pharmazeutischen Praxis, 4. Aufl., Bde. 1-8, Springer Verlag Berlin, Heidelberg, New York, 1969.

Majoie IML, Bruynzeel DP. Occupational immediate-type hypersensitivity to henna in a hairdresser. *Am J Contact Dermatitis* 7 (1); 38-40. 1996

Teuscher E, Biogene Arzneimittel, 5. Aufl., Wiss. Verlagsges. mbH Stuttgart 1997.

Wichtl M (Hrsg.), Teedrogen, 4. Aufl., Wiss. Verlagsges. mbH Stuttgart 1997.

Hepatica nubilis

See American Liverwort

Heracleum sphondylium

See Hogweed

Herb Paris

Paris quadrifolia

DESCRIPTION

Medicinal Parts: The medicinal part is the whole fresh plant when the fruit begins to ripen.

Flower and Fruit: The flowers are solitary and terminal. The sepals are lanceolate, acuminate, triple-veined and four times as wide as the linear/awl-shaped petals. The stamens are threadlike to awl-shaped and bear linear anthers in the middle. The ovary has 5 threadlike stigmas, both of which are purple-brown. The fruit is a blue-black globular berry the size of a small cherry.

Leaves, Stem, and Root: The 15 to 30 cm high plant is a perennial herb with a creeping, fleshy rhizome. The stem is erect, round, unbranched, and crowned by 4 acuminate leaves. The leaves are whorled, almost obovate, acute, entire-margined, and glabrous. The leaves have 3 to 5 ribs. They are dark green and matte above, pale and slightly glossy beneath.

Characteristics: The plant has an unpleasant smell and is poisonous.

Habitat: The plant is indigenous to Europe and Asian Russia.

Production: Herb Paris is the fresh plant of *Paris quadrifolia*, when the fruit is ripe.

Not to be Confused With: Poisoning can occur in children when they confuse the fruit of the Herb Paris plant with that of blueberries.

Other Names: One Berry

ACTIONS AND PHARMACOLOGY

COMPOUNDS

Steroid saponins: chief components are pennogenin triglycoside, pennogenin tetraglycoside, and their bisdemosidic precursors (26-O-glucosides), including 1-dehydrotrillenoge-nin

EFFECTS

The active agents are the saponins (which irritate mucous membranes), paristyphnin, paridin, citric acid, and pectin. The parissaponins are local irritants as well as absorptive when taken orally. The main toxin is paristyphnin, which, when taken orally, leads to miosis and can consequently cause paralysis of the respiratory system.

INDICATIONS AND USAGE

Homeopathic Uses: Herb Paris is used as a homeopathic remedy for headaches, neuralgia, nervous tension, dizziness, palpitations, and migraine.

PRECAUTIONS AND ADVERSE REACTIONS

The drug is considered poisonous. Symptoms of poisoning following intake of the berries include nausea, vomiting, diarrhea, miosis, and headache. However, no serious poisonings have been recorded in this century.

DOSAGE

Mode of Administration: Herb Paris is available in homeopathic dilutions.

LITERATURE

Frohne D, Pfänder HJ, Giftpflanzen - Ein Handbuch für Apotheker, Toxikologen und Biologen, 4. Aufl., Wiss. Verlags-Ges. Stuttgart 1997.

Kern W, List PH, Hörhammer L (Hrsg.), Hagers Handbuch der Pharmazeutischen Praxis, 4. Aufl., Bde. 1-8, Springer Verlag Berlin, Heidelberg, New York, 1969.

Lewin L, Gifte und Vergiftungen, 6. Aufl., Nachdruck, Haug Verlag, Heidelberg 1992.

Roth L, Daunderer M, Kormann K, Giftpflanzen, Pflanzengifte, 4. Aufl., Ecomed Fachverlag Landsberg Lech 1993.

Teuscher E, Lindequist U, Biogene Gifte - Biologie, Chemie, Pharmakologie, 2. Aufl., Fischer Verlag Stuttgart 1994.

Herb Robert

Geranium robertianum

DESCRIPTION

Medicinal Parts: The medicinal parts of the plant are the fresh or dried aerial parts collected during the flowering season, as well as the whole fresh or dried plant.

Flower and Fruit: The peduncles are usually distinctly longer than the bracts and the permanently erect pedicles, which are 2.2 to 7 mm long. The flowers are longer than their pedicles. There are 5 separate sepals and 5 petals. The sepals are erect when they first bloom then hang when the fruit matures. The petals have long stems. There are 10 stamens and 5 ovaries with long styles, which form an upward curve when mature. The fruit is circular and 2 cm long, with 3 mm long protruding, reticulate, glabrous, or pubescent fruit lobes, which are wrinkled horizontally in an upward direction. These permanently enclose the smooth, finely spotted seeds. The fruit lobes burst off from the central column without the awn.

Leaves, Stem, and Root: Geranium robertianum is a 20 to 40 cm high annual or hardy annual with a weak, branched tap root and a long hypocotyl. The stems are heavily branched, usually red, and glandular-haired. The leaves are 3- to 5-sectioned compound leaves with petiolate, entire-margined to double-pinnasect leaflets.

Characteristics: Herb Robert has an unpleasant smell often associated with goats or bugs.

Habitat: The plant is indigenous to the area stretching from Europe to China and Japan; to Africa southward as far as Uganda; to the Atlantic seaboard of North America; and the temperate areas of South America.

Production: Herb Robert is the aerial parts of *Geranium robertianum*, which are gathered between May and October in uncultivated regions, then dried in the open air in the shade.

Not to be Confused With: The herbs of *Geranium palustre* and *Geranium pratense* are frequently used as an adulteration.

Other Names: Dragon's Blood, Herb Robin, Red Shank, Storkbill, Wild Crane's-Bill

ACTIONS AND PHARMACOLOGY

COMPOUNDS

Flavonoids: including rutin, quercetin-3-O-rhamnogalactoside, kaempferol-3-O-rhamnoglucoside, hyperoside

Tannins: geraniin, isogeraniin, beta-penta-O-galloylglucose

EFFECTS

The drug has the following effects:

Antiviral: The extract of the fresh herb, including rhizome, has been shown to have a mild antiviral effect against the vesicular stomatitis virus. In another study, however, the aqueous solution of the ethanol extract was not shown to have an antiviral effect against the polio virus Type 1, measles, coxsachie-B2, adeno- or Semliki forest virus.

Antimicrobial: The fraction of an extract produced with 80% ethanol was shown to have an inhibitory effect on the growth of *Escherichia coli, Pseudomonas aeruginosa* and *Staphylococcus aureus*. In the serial dilution test, growth of *Microsporum canis* and *Trichophyton mentagrophytes* was completely stunted.

Hypotensive effect: Effects have only been described in general reviews.

INDICATIONS AND USAGE

Unproven Uses: The drug is used in folk medicine internally for diarrhea, functional impairment of the liver and gallbladder, inflammatory conditions of gallbladder and its ducts, kidney and bladder, and calculosis. In addition, washed fresh leaves are chewed or prepared as an infusion or decoction used as a mouthwash or gargle for inflammatory conditions of the oral mucous membrane. External application is used to treat poorly healing wounds and mild rashes. These uses appear plausible because of the tannins.

PRECAUTIONS AND ADVERSE REACTIONS

Health risks or side effects following the proper administration of designated therapeutic dosages are not recorded.

DOSAGE

Mode of Administration: The drug is used internally as well as externally.

Preparation: To prepare an infusion, add 1 dessertspoonful of drug to 1/2 liter of cold water. Bring to a boil and leave to steep.

Daily Dosage: Internally, the average single dose of the drug is 1.5 g; drink 2 to 3 cups of the infusion daily, between meals.

LITERATURE

Chang YC, Maibach HI. Pseudo flautist's lip: allergic contact cheilitis from geraniol. *Contact Dermatitis* 37; 39 (1997)

Hänsel R, Keller K, Rimpler H, Schneider G (Hrsg.), Hagers Handbuch der Pharmazeutischen Praxis, 5. Aufl., Bde 4-6 (Drogen), Springer Verlag Berlin, Heidelberg, New York, 1992-1994.

Kartnig T, Bucar-Stachel J. Flavonoide aus den oberirdischen Teilen von *Geranium robertianum. Planta Med.* 57; 292-293. 1991

Madaus G, Lehrbuch der Biologischen Arzneimittel, Bde 1-3, Nachdruck, Georg Olms Verlag Hildesheim 1979.

Herniaria glabra

See Rupturewort

Hibiscus

Hibiscus sabdariffa

DESCRIPTION

Medicinal Parts: The medicinal parts of the plant are the flowers.

Flower and Fruit: The flowers are solitary, axillary, and almost sessile. The calyx is red, the corolla is yellow, and the anthers are blood red. The fruit is a 2-cm long, ovoid, many-seeded capsule.

Leaves, Stem, and Root: Hibiscus is a bushy annual that is 0.15 to 1 m high and branched from the base. The stems are reddish, almost glabrous. The basal leaves are undivided and ovate; the cauline leaves have 3 lobes that are 7.5 to 10 cm wide. The lobes are 2.5 cm wide and crenate.

Habitat: Hibiscus sabdariffa originally came from the area around the source of the Niger. It grows worldwide in the tropics and is cultivated in Europe.

Production: Hibiscus flowers consist of the calyces of *Hibiscus sabdariffa* (*sabdariffa ruber* variety).

Other Names: Guinea Sorrel, Jamaica Sorrel, Red Sorrel, Roselle

ACTIONS AND PHARMACOLOGY

COMPOUNDS

Fruit acids (15-30%): in particular hibiscus ((+)-allohydroxy citric acid lacton), additionally lemons, malic acid, tartaric acid

Anthocyans (intensive red): including delphinidin-3-xyloglucoside, delphinidin-3-glucoside, cyanidin-3-xyloglucoside

Flavonoids: including gossypetin

Mucilages: rhamnogalacturonans, arabinogalactans, arabinans

EFFECTS

Hibiscus tea has a laxative effect due to the high content of poorly absorbable fruit acids.

Aqueous extracts of hibiscus leaves have a relaxant effect on the uterus musculature. The drug also has a hypotensive effect.

INDICATIONS AND USAGE

Unproven Uses: Hibiscus flowers are used for loss of appetite, and for colds that affect the respiratory tract and stomach.

Chinese Medicine: Preparations of the plant are used to treat carbuncles, swelling and inflammation of the skin, scalding, conjunctivitis, and *herpes zoster*.

PRECAUTIONS AND ADVERSE REACTIONS

Health risks or side effects following the proper administration of designated therapeutic dosages are not recorded.

DOSAGE

Mode of Administration: Hibiscus sabdariffa is available as a tea preparation.

Preparation: To make a tea, pour boiling water over 1.5 g comminuted drug and strain after 5 to 10 minutes.

LITERATURE

Franz M, Franz G, *Hibiscus sabdariffa* - Hibiscusblüten. In: ZPT 9(2):63. 1988.

Kern W, List PH, Hörhammer L (Hrsg.), Hagers Handbuch der Pharmazeutischen Praxis, 4. Aufl., Bde. 1-8, Springer Verlag Berlin, Heidelberg, New York, 1969.

Müller BM, Franz G. Chemical Structure and Biological Activity of Polysaccharides from *Hibiscus sabdariffa. Planta Med.* 58; 60-67. 1992

Steinegger E, Hänsel R, Pharmakognosie, 5. Aufl., Springer Verlag Heidelberg 1992.

Teuscher E, Biogene Arzneimittel, 5. Aufl., Wiss. Verlagsges. mbH Stuttgart 1997.

Wichtl M (Hrsg.), Teedrogen, 4. Aufl., Wiss. Verlagsges. Stuttgart 1997.

Hibiscus sabdariffa

See Hibiscus

High Mallow

Malva sylvestris

DESCRIPTION

Medicinal Parts: The medicinal parts are the dried flowers, the dried leaves and the whole of the flowering fresh plant.

Flower and Fruit: The bright purple flowers with long dark stripes are clustered in leaf axils. They have 3 epicalyx leaves, 5 sepals and 5 petals that are much longer than the calyx and have a deep margin. The numerous stamens are fused to a 10 to 12 mm column. The fruit stems are erect or slanted to one side. The ovaries are made up of a ring of 9 to 11 carpels. The fruit is a 7 to 9 mm wide and 2 mm thick disc, which breaks up into mericarps. These are glabrous or covered in a few scattered hairs, sharply angular and punctate.

Leaves, Stem and Root: Malva sylvestris is a biennial or perennial leafy herb 0.3 to 1.2 m high. The stems are branched, prostrate to curved, ascending, slightly woody and roughly pubescent. The leaves are alternate, long-petioled, reniform-orbicular, 5-lobed and crenate-serrate.

Characteristics: High Mallow has a 3-leaved epicalyx (compare with Althaea officinalis).

Habitat: The plant probably originated in the southern European-Asia region. Today the tree can be found in subtropical and temperate latitudes of both hemispheres.

Production: Blue Mallow flower and leaves consist of the dried flowers of Malva sylvestris and/or Malva sylvestris sps. Mauritiana, Ascherson and Graebner, as well as its preparations. High Mallow leaves are harvested from June to the beginning of September and dried in thin layers in the shade. High Mallow flowers are harvested without the pedicles from the end of June to October and are dried in layers in the shade.

Not to be Confused With: Other varieties of Malvae, the leaves of Althaea officinalis.

Other Names: Blue Mallow, Common Mallow, Mallow, Mauls, Cheeseflower

ACTIONS AND PHARMACOLOGY

COMPOUNDS: MALVA LEAF

Flavonoids: including among others hypolaetin-3-glucoside, gossypetin-3-glucoside; also flavonoid sulfates including among others gossypetin-8-O-beta-D-glucuronide-3-sulfate

Mucilages: 6-8% (galacturonorhamane and arabinogalactans)

COMPOUNDS: MALVA FLOWER

Anthocyans: including among others malvin

Mucilages: 6% to 10% (galacturonorhamane and arabinogalactane)

EFFECTS: MALVA LEAF AND FLOWER

Leaf: Main active principles - polysaccharides, flavonoids, tannins; Flower: Main active principles - polysaccharides, flavonoids.

The drug has a mucous membrane-protective effect; it relieves irritation because of the high level of mucilaginous material.

INDICATIONS AND USAGE

MALVA FLOWER AND LEAF

Approved by Commission E:

- Cough
- Bronchitis
- Inflammation of the mouth and pharynx

Unproven Uses: In folk medicine, the flower is used internally for bronchial catarrh, gastroenteritis, and bladder complaints. Both the flower and leaf are used externally as a bath additive for wound treatment.

PRECAUTIONS AND ADVERSE REACTIONS

MALVA LEAF AND FLOWER

No health hazards or side effects are known in conjunction with the proper administration of designated therapeutic dosages.

DOSAGE

MALVA FLOWER

Mode of Administration: High Mallow flowers are in various tea mixtures as an inactive ingredient.

Preparation: To prepare an infusion, 1.5 to 2 g of comminuted drug is added to cold water and boiled or scalded and strained after 10 minutes.

Daily Dosage: The average daily dose is 5 g of the drug. Tea: Drink 2 to 3 times a day.

Storage: The drug should be protected from light, moisture and insects.

MALVA LEAF

Mode of Administration: Comminuted herb for teas and other preparations are for internal use.

Daily Dosage: The average daily dose is 5 gm of the drug. Tea: drink 2 to 3 times a day.

Preparation: To prepare an infusion, pour 150 mL of boiling water over 3 to 5 g of the drug (about 2 teaspoonfuls) and leave to draw for 2 to 3 hours; stir occasionally.

Storage: The drug should be protected from light, moisture and insects.

LITERATURE

MALVA LEAF AND FLOWER

Classen B, Amelunxen F, Blaschek W, Analytical and structural investigations of the mucilage of Malva species. In: *PM* 59(7):A614. 1993.

Classen B, Amelunxen F, Blaschek W, Malva sylvestris - Mikroskopische Untersuchungen zur Entstehung von Schleimbehältern. In: DAZ 134(38):3597. 1994.

Hänsel R, Keller K, Rimpler H, Schneider G (Hrsg.), Hagers Handbuch der Pharmazeutischen Praxis, 5. Aufl., Bde 4-6 (Drogen), Springer Verlag Berlin, Heidelberg, New York, 1992-1994.

Teuscher E, Biogene Arzneimittel, 5. Aufl., Wiss. Verlagsges. Stuttgart 1997.

Wagner H, Wiesenauer M, Phytotherapie. Phytopharmaka und pflanzliche Homöopathika, Fischer-Verlag, Stuttgart, Jena, New York, 1995.

Wichtl M (Hrsg.), Teedrogen, 4. Aufl., Wiss. Verlagsges. Stuttgart 1997.

Hippophaë rhamnoides

See Sea Buckthorn

Hogweed

Heracleum sphondylium

DESCRIPTION

Medicinal Parts: The medicinal parts are the dried roots, the herb collected in the flowering season and dried, the fruit, the fresh herb, and the whole fresh flowering plant.

Flower and Fruit: The flowers have 15 to 30 rayed, flat umbels with no involucre. The numerous epicalyx leaves are lanceolate and densely pubescent. The petals have a cordate margin with indented lobes. They are irregular, often pubescent on the outside, whitish or greenish, green-yellow or yellowish and sometimes pink. The fruit is compressed, flat, 8 mm long and 5 mm wide, roundish-ova, and brownish yellow. The fruit has 10 ribs and oil grooves.

Leaves, Stem, and Root: The plant grows from 80 to 150 cm high, can be biennial or perennial, and has a strong tuberous, whitish-yellow root. The stem is erect, angular, grooved, hollow, stiff-haired, and branched above. The leaves are large and odd-pinnate, with 1 to 3 pairs of leaflets. The leaflets are large, ovate, and lobed to pinnate. There is a trilobed terminal leaflet. The basal leaves are very large and have grooved petioles, which gradually merge into leaf sheaths. The basal and stem foliage are clasping.

Characteristics: There is hot, yellow latex in the stem. The leaf umbel is fragrant.

Habitat: Heracleum sphondylium is found in most of Europe and in western and northern Asia. Subspecies are found mainly in northwestern Europe, eastern and central Europe, and in the Mediterranean region.

Production: Hogweed is the aerial part of *Heracleum sphondylium* collected between June and August and dried.

Other Names: Masterwort

ACTIONS AND PHARMACOLOGY

COMPOUNDS

Furocoumarins (0.5-0.6%): in particular bergaptene, isopimpinellin, pimpinellin, isobergaptene, sphondin

Volatile oil: including those containing n-octylacetate

EFFECTS

Hogweed is considered a mild expectorant; however, this has not been scientifically proved. A phototoxic effect should be expected after administration.

INDICATIONS AND USAGE

Unproven Uses: The drug is obsolete. In folk medicine, it was used to relieve muscle cramps, stomach disorders, digestion problems, diarrhea, gastrointestinal catarrh, and diarrhea following a cold. The furocoumarin methoxsalin is used in the treatment of psoriasis.

PRECAUTIONS AND ADVERSE REACTIONS

Phototoxic effects must be avoided following intake of the drug due to its furocoumarin content. For that reason, UV-radiation and solaria should be avoided after its administration. The same danger exists following contact with the freshly bruised plant.

DOSAGE

Mode of Administration: An infusion is used internally.

Preparation: To make an infusion, add 3 teaspoonfuls of herb to 2 glasses of cold water and allow to steep for 8 hours.

Daily Dosage: The preparation should be drunk throughout the day.

LITERATURE

Erdelmeier CA, Meier B, Sticher O. Reversed-phase high-performance chromatographic separation of closely related furocoumarins. *J Chromatogr.* 346; 456-460. 1985

Frohne D, Pfänder HJ: Giftpflanzen - EinHandbuch für Apotheker, Toxikologen und Biologen, 4. Aufl., Wiss. Verlagsges. mbH Stuttgart 1997.

Hänsel R, Keller K, Rimpler H, Schneider G (Hrsg.), Hagers Handbuch der Pharmazeutischen Praxis, 5. Aufl., Bde 4-6 (Drogen), Springer Verlag Berlin, Heidelberg, New York, 1992-1994.

Roth L, Daunderer M, Kormann K: Giftpflanzen, Pflanzengifte, 4.Aufl., Ecomed Fachverlag Landsberg Lech 1993.

Teuscher E, Lindequist U: Biogene Gifte - Biologie, Chemie, Pharmakologie, 2. Aufl., Fischer Verlag Stuttgart 1994.

Holly

Ilex aquifolium

DESCRIPTION

Medicinal Parts: The medicinal parts are the dried foliage leaves, the fresh leaves, the young leafy branches with the ripe berries, and the flowers of the branch tips with the leaves.

Flower and Fruit: Because of the shrinking of the one sex, the flowers are usually dioecious. The inflorescence is a white, 1- to 3-flowered axillary cyme. The calyx is small and has 4 to 5 tips. The corolla is rotate with 5 petals. The ovary is superior and there are 4 to 5 stamens. The coral red fruit is a 4-sectioned, sessile, berrylike, pea-sized drupe with 4 to 5 seeds.

Leaves, Stem, and Root: The plant is a 10 m high evergreen bush or tree with smooth, dark, gray-brown bark. The bark on the younger branches is green and glossy. The branches and foliage are glabrous. The leaves are alternate, coriaceous, stiff, ovate or elliptical, and acute. The lower leaves are thorny denate, the upper ones entire-margined.

Characteristics: The flowers have a weak pleasant scent. The berries are poisonous to children.

Habitat: The plant is found in central Europe, North America and eastern Asia.

Production: Holly leaves and fruits are the leaves and fruits of *Ilex aquifolium.*

Other Names: Christ's Thorn, Holm, Holme Chase, Holy Tree, Hulm, Hulver Bush, Hulver Tree, Mountain Holly

ACTIONS AND PHARMACOLOGY

COMPOUNDS

Saponins

Nitrile glycosides: menisdaurin, not cyanogenic

Flavonoids: including, among others, rutin, kaempferol and quercetin glycosides

Caffeic acid derivatives: chlorogenic acid

Sterols: beta-sitosterol, stigmasterol

Triterpenes: alpha-amyrin, alpha-amyrinester, beta-amyrin, ursolic acid

Purine alkaloids: only traces of theobromine

EFFECTS

No information is available.

INDICATIONS AND USAGE

Unproven Uses: Holly is used as a diuretic, for constipation, fevers, gout, rheumatism, and bronchitis and coughs.

In folk medicine, Holly is used for fever, chronic bronchitis, constipation, rheumatism and gout.

Homeopathic Uses: Ilex aquifolium is used for conjunctivitis.

PRECAUTIONS AND ADVERSE REACTIONS

No health hazards or side effects are known in conjunction with the proper administration of designated therapeutic dosages.

OVERDOSAGE

The intake of more than 5 berries can lead to nausea, vomiting and diarrhea. Fatal gastrointestinal inflammation is said to have taken place following the ingestion of very large quantities (20 to 30 berries; Lewin). Stomach emptying and the administration of activated charcoal should therefore be carried out with the intake of more than 10 berries. Further treatment should proceed according to symptoms. Poisonings have not been reported in recent times.

DOSAGE

Mode of Administration: As a tea and alcoholic extract for internal use.

Homeopathic Dosage: 5 drops, 1 tablet, or 10 globules every 30 to 60 minutes (acute) or 1 to 3 times daily (chronic); parenterally: 1 to 2 mlLsc acute, 3 times daily; chronic: once a day (HAB34).

LITERATURE

Catalano S, Marsili A, Morelli J, Pistelli L, Constituents of the leaves of *Ilex aquifolium.* In: *PM* 33:416. 1978.

Hänsel R, Keller K, Rimpler H, Schneider G (Hrsg.), Hagers Handbuch der Pharmazeutischen Praxis, 5. Aufl., Bde 4-6 (Drogen), Springer Verlag Berlin, Heidelberg, New York, 1992-1994 (unter Ilex paraguariensis).

Knights BA, Smith AR. Sterols and Triterpenes of *Ilex aquifolium. Phytochemistry* 16; 139-140. 1977

Ministry of Agriculture Fisheries and Food (Ed). Poisonous Plants in Britain and their effects on Animals and Man, HMSO, UK 1984

Lewin L, Gifte und Vergiftungen, 6. Aufl., Nachdruck, Haug Verlag, Heidelberg 1992.

Willems M, Quantitative Determination and Distribution of a Cyanogenic Glucoside in *Ilex aquifolium. Planta Med.* 55; 195. 1989

Willems M. Quantification and Distribution of a Novel Cyanogenic Glucoside in *Ilex aquifolium. Planta Med.* 55; 114. 1989

Teuscher E, Lindequist U, Biogene Gifte - Biologie, Chemie, Pharmakologie, 2. Aufl., Fischer Verlag Stuttgart 1994.

Hollyhock

Alcea rosea

DESCRIPTION

Medicinal Parts: The medicinal parts are the dried flowers of plants bearing dark purple flowers.

Flower and Fruit: Flowers of 6 to 10 cm in size sit in the axils of the cauline leaves singly or in groups of 2 or 4, with the upper ones forming long spikes. Sepals of the epicalyx are broadly triangular and sharp-edged. The epicalyx is significantly shorter than the calyx and both are gray-green haired.

Leaves, Stem, and Root: Hollyhock is a biennial plant. In the second year it produces a spirelike, hairy stem up to 3 m tall. The leaves are cordate-orbicular to rhomboid, weakly 3- to 5-lobed and slightly scabrid-setulose. The sepals are epiclyx-subacute and triangular. The flowers are found in the leaf axils with short peduncles. The petals are 30 to 50 mm, contiguous, usually pink but sometimes white or violet. The mericarps are 7 mm long. The dorsal face has a deep, narrow furrow with rugose angles produced into parallel wings. The lateral faces are appressed-setose.

Habitat: The plant was originally indigenous to southwest and central Asia. A few species were probably introduced into southeast central Europe as ornamental plants and then spread in the wild. Hollyhock is now widely cultivated in Europe and temperate regions of Asia. The main suppliers of the drug are Belgium, Hungary, Bulgaria, the former Yugoslavia, Rumania, Albania.

Production: Hollyhock flower consists of the flowers of *Alcea rosea* as well as their preparations. The flowers are harvested when not quite in full bloom on plants with over 2 to 3 years of growth, then air-dried at 35°C.

Other Names: Althea Rose, Malva Flowers, Rose Mallow

ACTIONS AND PHARMACOLOGY

COMPOUNDS

Mucilages (acetylated galacturonorhamane)

Anthocyans (termed althaein): delphinidine- and malvidine-mono glycosides

EFFECTS

No information is available.

INDICATIONS AND USAGE

Unproven Uses: The drug has been used internally for respiratory-, gastrointestinal-, and urinary-tract disorders, and to relieve fever, thirst, and dysmenorrhea. Infusions and decoctions made with the flowers have been used as a gargle for oral and pharyngeal inflammation.

PRECAUTIONS AND ADVERSE REACTIONS

No health hazards or side effects are known in conjunction with the proper administration of designated therapeutic dosages.

DOSAGE

Mode of Administration: As a tea and mouthwash.

How Supplied: Whole, cut, and powdered drug.

Preparation: To prepare as a tea, use 1 to 2 g of the drug per teacup. For a mouthwash, boil 1.5 g drug with 100 mL water.

LITERATURE

Hänsel R, Keller K, Rimpler H, Schneider G (Hrsg.), Hagers Handbuch der Pharmazeutischen Praxis, 5. Aufl., Bde 4-6 (Drogen), Springer Verlag Berlin, Heidelberg, New York, 1992-1994 (unter Alcea rosea).

Steinegger E, Hänsel R, Pharmakognosie, 5. Aufl., Springer Verlag Heidelberg 1992 (unter Alcea rosea).

Teuscher E, Biogene Arzneimittel, 5. Aufl., Wiss. Verlagsges. Stuttgart 1997.

Honeysuckle

Lonicera caprifolium

DESCRIPTION

Medicinal Parts: The medicinal parts are the flowers, seeds, and leaves.

Flower and Fruit: The flowers are in groups of 6 directly on the upper leaf pair. There are sometimes whorls of 6 in the next 1 or 2 leaf pairs. The corolla has a tight, 25- to 28-mm long tube and a bilabiate margin. It is yellowish-white, often red-tinged, glabrous inside, and glandular outside. The ovary is jug-shaped. The fruit is a berry. They are ellipsoid, 8 mm long, and coral red. The seeds are ellipsoid, flattened, longitudinally grooved, and 4 mm long.

Leaves, Stem, and Root: Honeysuckle is an up to 4 m high, deciduous, clockwise-climbing shrub. The foliage leaves are short-petioled, elliptical or obovate, blunt, entire, glabrous, blue-green beneath, and 4 to 10 cm by 3.5 to 6 cm. The leaves are shortly fused in pairs, but the upper ones are fused to an oval or circular leaf through which the stem grows. They are short-petioled and elliptical. The lower leaves are paired.

Habitat: The plant grows in the northern temperate zones as far as the northern edges of the subtropics and is cultivated extensively.

Production: Honeysuckle flowers and leaves are from *Lonicera caprifolium.*

Other Names: Goat's Leaf, Woodbine

ACTIONS AND PHARMACOLOGY

COMPOUNDS

Saponins

Further constituents are largely unknown; iridoide monoterpenes have been demonstrated in the rind including among others loganin (extremely bitter), that possibly also occurs in the drug.

EFFECTS

The main active principles are saponin and luteolin. The drug has a laxative and diaphoretic effect.

INDICATIONS AND USAGE

Unproven Uses: The drug is used for digestive disorders and as a diaphoretic agent. It is rarely used today.

PRECAUTIONS AND ADVERSE REACTIONS

No health hazards or side effects are known in conjunction with the proper administration of designated therapeutic dosages.

OVERDOSAGE

Because of the saponin content, irritation of the gastrointestinal tract and possibly of the kidneys, urinary passages, and urinary bladder are possible in the event of overdosage. Case studies are not known. (The berries of the red honeysuckle are considered poisonous. Intakes above 10 berries are said to trigger nausea, vomiting, and tachycardia, elevated body temperature, exanthemas, and cyanosis.)

DOSAGE

Mode of Administration: The drug is obsolete.

LITERATURE

Frohne D, Pfänder HJ, Giftpflanzen - Ein Handbuch für Apotheker, Toxikologen und Biologen, 4. Aufl., Wiss. Verlags-Ges Stuttgart 1997.

Kern W, List PH, Hörhammer L (Hrsg.), Hagers Handbuch der Pharmazeutischen Praxis, 4. Aufl., Bde. 1-8, Springer Verlag Berlin, Heidelberg, New York, 1969.

Roth L, Daunderer M, Kormann K, Giftpflanzen, Pflanzengifte, 4. Aufl., Ecomed Fachverlag Landsberg Lech 1993.

Teuscher E, Lindequist U, Biogene Gifte - Biologie, Chemie, Pharmakologie, 2. Aufl., Fischer Verlag Stuttgart 1994.

Hoodia

Hoodia gordonii

DESCRIPTION

Medicinal Parts: Aerial parts

Botanical Description: Leafless succulents, within thick, fleshy, finger-like stems, which branch near the ground. Rows of small thorns present along the stems. Flower is flesh-colored, smelling strongly of decaying meat.

Habitat: South Africa, Namibia.

Other Names: Bitterghaap, Ghaap, Kalahari cactus, P57

ACTIONS AND PHARMACOLOGY

COMPOUNDS

Ten new C(21)-steroidal derivatives, namely gordonosides A-L were isolated from a chloroform extract of the aerial parts of *Hoodia gordonii*. Compounds are based on 3beta,14beta-dihydroxy-pregn-5-en-17-betaone aglycone. Hoodigosides A-K (1-11), 11 new oxypregnane glycosides and a previously reported oxypregnane glycoside P57AS3 were isolated from the aerial parts of *Hoodia gordonii*. The structures of these 12-O-beta-tigloyl isoramanone glycosides were determined. A steroidal glycoside with anorectic activity in animals, termed P57AS3 (P57), was isolated from *Hoodia gordonii* and found to have homologies to the steroidal core of cardiac glycosides.

EFFECTS

Hoodigosides A-K were tested for cytotoxicity and antioxidant activities in cell-based assays where they were found to be inactive. P57AS3 (P57), an oxypregnane steroidal glycoside, is the only reported active constituent from this plant as an appetite suppressant. Intracerebroventricular (i.c.v.) injections of the purified P57AS3 demonstrated that the compound has a likely central (CNS) mechanism of action. There is no evidence of P57AS3 binding to or altering activity of known receptors or proteins, including Na/K-ATPase, the putative target of cardiac glycosides. The compound increases the content of ATP by 50-150% in hypothalamic neurons. In addition, third ventricle (i.c.v.) administration of P57, which reduces subsequent 24-h food intake by 40-60%, also increases ATP content in hypothalamic slice punches removed at 24 h following the i.c.v. injections. In related studies, in pair fed rats fed a low-calorie diet for 4 days, the content of ATP in the hypothalami of control i.c.v. injected animals fell by 30-50%, which was blocked by i.c.v. injections of P57AS3.

INDICATIONS AND USAGE

Unproven Uses: Hoodia gordonii is traditionally used in South Africa for its appetite suppressant properties. Paradoxically, it is also used as appetite stimulant. *Hoodia*is also used for indigestion, hypertension, diabetes, stomachache, abdominal pain, and peptic ulceration.

CONTRAINDICATIONS

None are known.

PRECAUTIONS AND ADVERSE REACTIONS

No reliable information is available. Safety in pregnancy and nursing has not been established.

DRUG INTERACTIONS

No human drug information is available.

DOSAGE

No information is available.

LITERATURE

Avula B, Wang YH, Pawar RS, Shukla YJ, Schaneberg B, Khan IA. Determination of the appetite suppressant P57 in Hoodia gordonii plant extracts and dietary supplements by liquid chromatography/electrospray ionization mass spectrometry (LC-MSD-TOF) and LC-UV methods. J AOAC Int. 2006 May-Jun;89(3):606-11.

Dall'acqua S, Innocenti G. Steroidal glycosides from Hoodia gordonii. Steroids. 2007 Jun;72(6-7):559-68. Epub 2007 Mar 27.

MacLean DB, Luo LG. Increased ATP content/production in the hypothalamus may be a signal for energy-sensing of satiety: studies of the anorectic mechanism of a plant steroidal glycoside. Brain Res. 2004 Sep 10;1020(1-2):1-11.

Pawar RS, Shukla YJ, Khan SI, Avula B, Khan IA. New oxypregnane glycosides from appetite suppressant herbal supplement Hoodia gordonii. Steroids. 2007 Jun;72(6-7):524-34.

Rader JI, Delmonte P, Trucksess MW. Recent studies on selected botanical dietary supplement ingredients. Anal Bioanal Chem. 2007 Mar 28.

Van Wyk B-E, Gericke N (2000) People's Plants: a guide to useful plants of southern Africa. Briza Publications, Pretoria.

Hoodia gordonii

See Hoodia

Hops

Humulus lupulus

DESCRIPTION

Medicinal Parts: The medicinal parts are the glandular hairs separated from the infructescence, the whole dried female flowers, the fresh cones (preferably with few seeds) collected before the seeds ripen, and the fresh or dried female inflorescence.

Flower and Fruit: The male flowers are yellowish-greenish, inconspicuous, and about 5 mm in diameter. The female flowers are in richly blossomed, heavily branched inflorescence. The ovary, which has 2 long, downy stigmas, is surrounded at the base by a round compressed nutlet. A yellowish fruit cone grows from the female flower. The inside of the bracts is covered with small, glossy, light yellow glandular scales, which contain hop bitter (Lupulin).

Leaves, Stem, and Root: The hop plant is a perennial. The annual shoots reach a height of 6 m (12 m when cultivated). The stems are pencil-thick, green, and do not turn woody. They are covered in 6 rows of climbing barbs. The leaves are 3 to 5 lobed, serrate, and opposite.

Characteristics: Lupulin has a very strong odor and an extremely bitter taste.

Habitat: Indigenous to Europe, cultivated in Asia, U.S., and elsewhere.

Production: Hop cones consist of the whole dried female inflorescence of *Humulus lupulus*. After the harvest, the hops are dried on racks at temperatures of 30 to 60° C.

ACTIONS AND PHARMACOLOGY

COMPOUNDS

Acylphloroglucinols (10%)

Alpha-bitter acids: including, among others, humulone, cohumulone, adhumulone

Beta-bitter acids: including, among others, lupulone, colupulone, adlupulone

Volatile oil (0.3-1.0%): very complex in makeup, chief components myrcene, humulene, beta-caryophyllene, undecane-2-on, furthermore 2-methyl-but-3-en-ol (particularly following storage, as breakdown product of the acylphloroglucinols)

Resins (oxidation products of the bitter acids)

Phenolic acid: including, among others, ferulic acid, caffeic acid and their derivatives, for example, chlorogenic acid

Tannins: oligomeric proanthocyanidines

Flavonoids: including, among others, xanthohumole

EFFECTS

Neurosedative, antibacterial, antifungal, diuretic, antitumor, and estrogenic activities have been established. Many of the effects are thought to be due to the volatile oil (2- methyl-3-butene-2-ol), flavonoids, and/or estrogenic activity of the plant (Stephan et al, 1998; Salvador, 1994; Okamoto & Kumai, 1992; Tyler, 1988). Hops is primarily used for its mild sedative effects and for treating the gastrointestinal system. Hops in combination with valerian, balm leaf, and motherwort produced sedative effects in one human study. This effect, however, strongly depends on the quality of the extract used.

Hops is a bitter, an astringent, and a smooth-muscle relaxant with antibacterial properties. This makes it useful in the treatment of indigestion, nervous gastropathies, colitis, and irritable bowel syndrome as well as a preventive for individuals prone to ulcers.

Research has substantiated the phytoestrogenic properties of hops (Milligan et al, 1999). Animal and in vitro studies found that hops also has significant cancer-cell growth inhibition. The use of hops and phytoestrogens in general in cancer prevention is currently controversial due to an apparent concentration-dependent proliferative effect on human cell lines. Hops also caused preferential inhibition of diacylglycerol acyltransferase (DGAT) inhibition in one in vitro study. The effect of hops on blood glucose levels is unclear.

Hops has been used historically for reproductive conditions including premature ejaculation, as an anaphrodisiac in men, and for dysmenorrhea in women, but clinical evidence to support its use as a phytoestrogen is limited. Externally, an infusion or poultice of hops can be used to treat bruises, boils, and painful swellings. It is often combined with chamomile or poppy for this purpose.

Antibacterial Effects: Lupulone and humulone exhibit gram-positive and gram-negative antibacterial properties. Hexahydrocolupulone (HHC) (a semisynthetic derivative of colupulone and a beta acid congener of lupulone) was active against gram-positive bacteria and mycobacteria (Stephan et al, 1998). One variety and a wild type of the essential oil and solvent extract of hops were found to be active against *Bacillus subtilis* and *Staphylococcus aureus* in an in vitro study evaluating 11 hops cultivars. There was no activity against *Escherichia coli.* The antibacterial effect of weak acids from hops increased with decreasing pH. The essential oil was found to have antifungal effects against *Trichophyton mentagrophytes var. interdigitale* but no activity was seen against *Candida albicans* (Langezaal et al, 1992).

Antitumor Effects: Theoretically, hops may inhibit tumor cell growth via the estrogenic effect of its phytoestrogen components. There is currently minimal clinical data to support this role but initial reports are suggestive (Milligan et al, 1999; Zava et al, 1998).

In an in vitro assessment of six flavonoids found in hops, xanthohumol was found to be the most effective antiproliferative agent in human breast, colon, and ovarian cancer cells. When compared to the flavonoid genistein, which is currently in clinical trials as a chemopreventive agent for breast cancer in humans, xanthohumol was found to be several-fold more potent. Hops flavonoids may inhibit cancer growth at more than one stage of the cell cycle. Inhibition of DNA synthesis may be one of the mechanisms by which some of the hop flavonoids exert their antiproliferative activity on MCF-7 cells (Miranda et al, 1999).

Hexahydrocolupulone (HHC) (a semisynthetic derivative of colupulone that is a beta-acid congener of lupulone) inhibited human tumor cell growth in vitro by a mechanism that may involve the precursor metabolism and transport, macromolecular synthesis, and/or cell-cycle or cell cycle-dependent pathways. HHC had a wide spectrum of activity against solid tumors and leukemias as well as against cells that have been resistant to chemotherapeutic agents. HHC did not damage DNA, interfere with topoisomerase, or generate free radicals (Stephan et al, 1998). Humulone, an alpha acid of hops, was found to inhibit the growth of monoblastic leukemia U937 cells in vitro while enhancing the differentiation-inducing action of vitamin D3 (Honma et al, 1998).

DGAT Inhibition Effects: Two chalcones isolated from hops extract, xanthohumol and xanthohumol B, have been shown to inhibit diacylglycerol acyltransferase (DGAT) activity preferentially. Over accumulation of triacylglycerol in certain organs and tissues has been associated with increased risk for conditions including fatty liver, obesity, and hypertriglyceridemia. DGAT has been found to be exclusively involved in the formation of triacylglycerol (Tabata et al, 1997).

Glucose Tolerance Effect: Colupulone, a beta acid of hops, was shown to produce a small but significant decrease in serum glucose in nondiabetic outbred Swiss-Webster mice 30 minutes after the administration of a test dose of glucose. In a second experiment, it caused a small but significant increase in blood glucose in C57BI/KSJ-db/db diabetic mice but had no effect on nondiabetic C57BI/KSJ-db/db mice. Further research is required to explain these effects (Mannering et al, 1994).

Hormonal Effects: Estrogenic activity is thought to be due to the combined effect of many of the constituents in hops. The hormonal properties may account for its use in skin softening creams (Salvador, 1994). In vitro bioassays using a human endometrial cell line led to the identification of a potent phytoestrogen in hops, 8- prenylnaringenin, which showed equal or greater estrogenic activity than other established plant estrogens. The authors indicated that previous discrepancies over the potential estrogenic activity of hops were probably due to the variable nature of the extracts and the variety of assays used (Milligan et al, 1999). The effective use in hyperexcitable males is thought to be due to estrogenic, antiandrogenic, and antigonadotropic activity (Salvador, 1994).

Using both in vitro bioassays and saliva from human volunteers to assess in vivo bioavailability of exogenous phytoestrogens and phytoprogesterones, hops was found to be one of the six highest estradiol-binding substances out of over 150 herbs and spices. The study confirmed that an ethanol extract of hops contains a significant amount of phytoestrogens with moderate estrogenic bioactivity (Zava et al, 1998). Preliminary data suggests that phytoestrogens can have a positive impact on menopausal symptoms, cardiovascular disease, and osteoporosis (Murkies, 1998; Kurzer & Xu, 1997).

An in vitro study has shown that hop extracts antagonize the stimulatory effect of exogenous gonadotropin (PMSG) on estradiol secretion from ovarian cells via the adenylate cylcase system. (Okamoto & Kumai, 1992).

Analysis of beer extracts utilizing gas chromatography and mass spectrometry identified two phytoestrogenic substances: genistein and daidzein. These authors note that the amount of isoflavones ingested in human beer consumption would not be expected to elicit an estrogenic effect, but patients with advanced liver disease or those with insufficient metabolism of nonsteroidal estrogenic substances may result in significant accumulation resulting in an estrogenic effect (Rosenblum et al, 1992).

Sedative Effects: Hops has been shown to improve sleep in alcohol-dependent males in one study. Hops has been shown to exhibit anticonvulsant, antinociceptive, hypothermic, hypnotic, and sedative effects in mice. Hops extract at doses of 100, 250, or 500 mg/kg were administered intraperitoneally to mice 30 minutes prior to several behavioral tests (Lee et al, 1993). Neurosedative effects are due in part to 2-methyl-3-butene-2-ol in the fresh plant (Salvador, 1994). The 2-methyl-3-butene-2-ol content increases during storage (up to 0.15% in two years) suggesting that lupulone and humulone break down oxidatively generating the sedative principle (Salvador, 1994; Tyler, 1988). The sedative effect of hops is undisputed but the basis for it is not fully known (Bradley, 1992).

CLINICAL TRIALS

Antigonadotropic Activity

Water-soluble extracts of hops (Fractions 1 and 2) caused significant antigonadotropic activity including inhibition of the rise of estradiol and serum luteinizing hormone (LH) levels, which resulted in decreased release of progesterone, decreased uterine thymidine kinase (TK) activity, and decreased ovulation in Sprague-Dawley rats (Okamoto & Kumai, 1992).

Insomnia

A combination of valerian and hops was tested in the treatment of insomnia in a multicenter, randomized, placebo-controlled, parallel group study of 184 adults with mild insomnia. Subjects received either: (1) two tablets of standardized extracts of a valerian and hops combination for 28 days; (2) placebo for 28 days, or; (3) two tablets of diphenhydramine for 14 days followed by placebo for 14 days. The results show a modest hypnotic effect for the valerian-hops combination and diphenhydramine relative to placebo. Sleep improvements with the herbal combination were associated with improved quality of life. Both treatments appeared safe and did not produce rebound insomnia upon discontinuation during the study (Morin et al, 2005).

Menopausal Symptoms

The sedative and estrogenic components of Hops extract (8-PN,or hopein) have potential for prevention or treatment of menopausal symptoms that the authors of this exhaustive literature review elucidate. However, they identify only two clinical trials designed to evaluate the effect of Hops on menopausal symptoms, and neither is a randomized, double blind, placebo-controlled trial that could support the internal use of Hops for benefit of its estrogenic properties. The authors conclude that a consistent dosage form would need to be developed to justify further trials and acceptance of Hops in modern medicine (Chadwick, 2006).

In a prospective, double-blind, placebo-controlled study, a Hops extract standardized to 8-prenylnaringenin (8-PN) content—possibly the first such trial of its kind to use this standardized form—was conducted to examine whether its daily intake might positively affect menopausal discomforts. Healthy women (average age 52.1 years) were enrolled in the study and given either a placebo (n=26; 19 included in final analysis) or Hop extract equivalent to daily intake of 100 u*g* (n=20; 19 in final analysis) or 250 u*g* (n=21; 17 in final analysis) of 8-PN, respectively. Participants randomized to the Hops extract standardized to 100 u*g* 8-PN experienced reduced menopause-related discomforts and complaints, with rapid improvement on incidence of hot flushes in particular. No dose-dependent benefit was identified for the higher 8-PN dosage (Heyerick, 2006).

Sedation

A combination herbal sedative containing hops significantly improved sleep in 50 male alcohol-dependent patients in a 2-day nonparametric study. Subjects were used as their own control. Antistress tablets containing 170 mg valerian, 50 mg hops, 50 mg balm leaf, and 50 mg motherwort were administered one night and placebo containing valerian 5 mg the other night. Subjects' self-report questionnaires indicated improved sleep quality ($p<0.001$), reduced sleepiness the next morning ($p<0.01$), decrease in recall of bad dreams ($p<0.001$), and decrease in frequency of night waking ($p<0.001$). There were no differences found in the group that took the herbal supplement versus the placebo first (Widy-Tyszkiewicz & Schminda, 1997).

Skin Tumors

Topical application of humulon, a constituent in hops, suppressed the promotion of skin tumors induced by 7,12-dimethylbenz[a]anthracene (DBMA) and tetradecanoylphorbol-13- acetate (TPA) in mice. Humulon treatment resulted in a 99% reduction of the average number of tumors per mouse. Treatment with DBMA and TPA resulted in 10.3 tumors per mouse and treatment with DBMA, TPA, and Humulon resulted in 0.1 tumors per mouse. Humulon (1, 0.5 and 0.2 mg/ear) reduced arachidonic acid induced ear inflammation dose dependently. It was not as effective as indomethacin but more effective than quercetin (Yasukawa et al, 1995).

INDICATIONS AND USAGE

Approved by Commission E:

- Mood disturbances such as agitation, anxiety, nervousness, and restlessness
- Sleep disturbances such as insomnia

Unproven Uses: Used as a bitter and stomachic to stimulate the appetite and increase the secretion of gastric juices.

In folk medicine, Hops has been used internally for nerve pain, priapism, inflammation of the intestinal mucous membrane, and tension headaches and used externally for ulcus cruris, ulcers and skin abrasions.

Homeopathic Uses: Humulus lupulus is found in preparations for treating nervousness and insomnia.

CONTRAINDICATIONS

Use in women with estrogen-dependent breast cancer is controversial; some authors report that it is contraindicated (Anon, 1998).

Hops are contraindicated in the presence of depression.

Pregnancy: Not to be used during pregnancy.

PRECAUTIONS AND ADVERSE REACTIONS

Hops should be used with caution when given in conjunction with other central nervous system depressants, antipsychotics, or alcohol due to its sedative effect (Newall, 1996). Excessive use over a long period may cause dizziness, cognitive changes, and mild jaundice symptoms in some individuals. Hops may cause adverse effects when used during periods of menstrual disturbances, nervousness, dermatitis, hypersensitivity reactions, and respiratory allergies. The fresh plant has a sensitizing effect (hops-picker's disease), which may occur, more rarely, with the dust of the drug as well.

Hematologic Effects: Acute limited intravascular hemolysis has been reported after ingestions of a tea made from hops (Ridker, 1987).

Hypersensitivity Reaction: Hops was identified as the agent that provoked anaphylaxis in seven patients with an initial diagnosis of idiopathic anaphylaxis in a study of 102 patients (Stricker et al, 1986).

Musculoskeletal Effects: Malignant hyperthermia, a life threatening disorder of the skeletal muscles, was reported in five dogs after ingestion of large amounts of hops (Duncan et al, 1997).

DRUG INTERACTIONS

MODERATE RISK

Barbiturates: Data available to date suggest that hops may potentiate the sedative-hypnotic effect or increase the risk of central nervous system depression experienced with barbiturates. *Clinical Management:* Until the clinical significance of this potential interaction has been determined, patients should be advised to avoid concomitant use of hops and barbiturates. If patients elect to combine agents despite this advice, they should be advised to avoid activities that require mental alertness, as these agents may result in excessive sedation, psychomotor retardation, and impaired reaction time.

POTENTIAL INTERACTIONS

Estrogens: Theoretically, patients with reduced ability to metabolize nonsteroidal estrogenic substances, such as those with liver disease, may accumulate enough to result in estrogenic activity (Rosenblum et al, 1992). *Clinical Management:* It is unlikely that hops will cause an additive estrogenic effect if taken with estrogens.

DOSAGE

Mode of Administration: Comminuted drug, powdered drug or dry extract powder for infusions or decoctions or other preparations; liquid and solid preparations for internal use and externally for bath additives.

Hops is often found in combination with other sedatives.

How Supplied:

Liquid extract — drug: 1:1 45% ethanol (V/V) (BHP83).

Tincture — drug 1:5 60% ethanol (V/V) (BHP83)

Preparation: To prepare an infusion, boiling water is poured over the ground hop cones and left to steep for 10 to 15 minutes (1 teaspoonful is equal to 0.4 g drug).

Daily Dosage: For most indications, a single dose of 0.5 g is given.

To promote sleep, a single dose of 1 to 2 g drug is given; liquid extract: single dose: 0.5 to 2 mL; tincture: single dose: 1 to 2 mL.

Tea: 1 cup before bedtime for 2 to 3 days.

Homeopathic Dosage: 5 drops, 1 tablet, or 10 globules every 30 to 60 minutes (acute) or 1 to 3 times daily (chronic); parenterally: 1 to 2 mL sc acute, 3 times daily; chronic: once a day (HAB1).

Storage: Protect from light and moisture in well-sealed containers.

LITERATURE

Bravo L et al. *Boll Chim Farm*: 306. 1974.

Caujolle F et al. *Agressologie* 10:405. 1969.

Chadwick LR, Pauli GF, Farnsworth NR. The pharmacognosy of Humulus lupulus L. (hops) with an emphasis on estrogenic properties. *Phytomedicine*; 13(1-2): 119, 131. 2006.

Chappel CI, Smith SY, & Chagnon M. Subchronic toxicity study of tetrahydroisohumulone and hexahydroisohumulone in the beagle dog. *Food Chem Toxicol*; 36(11):915-922. 1998.

Duncan KL, Hare WR, & Buck WB. Malignant hyperthermia-like reaction secondary to ingestion of hops in five dogs. *J Am Vet med Assoc*; 210(1):51-54. 1997.

Field JA et al. Determination of essential oils in hops by headspace solid- phase microextraktion. In*: J Agric Food Chem* 44(7):1768-1772. 1996.

Fintelmann V. Klinisch-ärztliche Bedeutung des Hopfens. In: *ZPT* 13(5):165. 1992.

Ganzer BM. Hopfen: nicht nur für die Bierbrauerei. In: *PZ* 137(38):2824. 1992.

Hansel R, Wohlfart R & Schmidt H. The sedative-hypnotic principle of hops 3. Communication: contents of 2-methyl-e-butene-2-ol in hops and hops preparations. *Planta Medica*; 45(4):224-228. 1982.

Hänsel R. Pflanzliche Beruhigungsmittel Möglichkeiten und Grenzen der Selbstmedikation. In: *DAZ* 135(32):2935-2943. 1995.

Hänsel R, Wagener HH. Versuche, sedativ-hypnotische Wirkstoffe im Hopfen nachzuweisen. *Arzneim Forsch/Drug Res* 17:79-81. 1967.

Hartley RD. *Phytochemistry* 7:1641. 1968.

Hartley RD. Fawcett CH, *Phytochemistry* 7:1395. 1968.

Heyerick A, Vervarcke S, Depypere H, et al. The first prospective, randomized, double-blind, placebo-controlled study on the use of a standardized hops extract to alleviate menopausal discomforts. *Maturitas*; 54(2):164-75. 2006.

Hölzl J. Inhaltsstoffe des Hopfens (*Humulus lupulus L.*). In: *ZPT* 13(5):155. 1992.

Honma Y, Tobe H, Makishima M et al. Induction of differentiation of myelogenous leukemia cells by humulone, a bitter in hop. *Leuk Res*; 22(7):605-610. 1998.

Kumai A & Okamoto R. Extraction of the hormonal substance from hop. *Toxicol Lett*; 21(2):203-207. 1984.

Kurzer M & Xu X. Dietary phytoestrogens. *Ann Rev Nutr*; 17:353-381. 1997.

Langezaal CR, Chandra A & Scheffer JJC. Antimicrobial screening of essential oils and extracts of some *Humulus lupulus L.* cultivars. *Pharm Weekbl Sci*; 14(6):353-356. 1992.

Lee KM, Jung JS, Song DK et al. Effects of *Humulus lupulus* extract on the central nervous system in mice. *Planta Med*; 59(Suppl A):691. 1993.

Mannering GJ, Shoeman JA, & Shoeman DW. Effects of colupulone, a component of hops and brewers yeast, and chromium on glucose tolerance and hepatic cytochrome P450 in nondiabetic and spontaneously diabetic mice. *Biochem Biophys Res Commun*; 200(3): 1455-1462. 1994.

Milligan SR, De Keukeleire D, De Cooman L et al. Do hops contain oestrogens? *J Reprod Fert*; (18):8. 1996.

Milligan SR, Kalita JC, Heyerick A et al. Identification of a potent phytoestrogen in hops (*Hops lupulus L.*) and beer. *J Clin Endocrinol Metab*; 84(6):2249-2252. 1999.

Miranda CL, Stevens JF, Helmrich A et al. Antiproliferative and cytotoxic effects of prenylated flavonoids from hops (*Hops lupulus*) in human cancer cell lines. *Food Chem Toxicol*; 37(4):271-285. 1999.

Moir M et al. *Phytochemistry* 19(10):2201. 1980.

Morin CM, Koetter U, Bastien C, et al. Valerian-hops combination and diphenhydramine for treating insomnia: a randomized, placebo-controlled clinical trial. *Sleep*; 28(11): 1465-1471. 2005.

Murkies A, Wilcox G & Davis S. Clinical review 92: Phytoestrogens. *J Clin Endocrinol Metab*; 83(2):297-303. 1998.

Newmark FM. Hops allergy and terpene sensitivity: an occupational disease. *Ann Allergy*; 41(5):311-312. 1978.

Okamoto R & Kumai A. Antigonadotropic activity of hop extract. *Acta Endocrinol*; 127(4):371-7. 1992.

Orth-Wagner S, Ressin WJ, Friedrich I. Phytosedativum gegen Schlafstörungen. In: *ZPT* 16(3):147-156. 1995.

Ridker PM. Toxic effects of herbal teas. Arch Environ Health. May-Jun;42(3):133-6. 1987.

Rosenblum ER, Campbell IM, Van Thiel DV et al. Isolation and identification of phytoestrogens from beer. *Alcohol Clin Exp Res*; 16(5):843-845. 1992.

Salvador RL. Hops. *Can Pharm J*; 5:203-205. 1994.

Schmalreck AF, Tueber M, Reininger W et al. Structural features determining the antibiotic potencies of natural and synthetic hop bitter resins, their precursors and derivatives. *Can J Microbiol;* 21(2):205-212. 1975.

Schulz V, Hübner WD, Ploch M. Klinische Studien mit Psycho-Phytopharmaka. In: *ZPT* 18(3):141-154. 1997.

Simpson WJ & Smith ARW. Factors affecting antibacterial activity of hop compounds and their derivatives. *J Appl Bacteriol*; 72(4):327-34. 1992.

Stephan T, Ngo E & Nutter L. Hexahydrocolupulone and its antitumor cell proliferation activity in vitro. *Biochem Pharmacol*; 55(4):505-515. 1998.

Stevens JF, Ivancic M, Hsu VL, Deinzer ML. Prenylflavonoids from *Humulus lupulus*. In: *PH* 44(8):1575-1585. 1997.

Stocker HR. Sedative und hypnogene Wirkung des Hopfens. Schweizer Brauerei Rundschau 78:80-89. 1967

Stricker WE, Anorve-Lopez E & Reed CE. Food skin testing in patients with idiopathic anaphylaxis. J *Allergy Clin Immunol*; 77(3):516-519. 1986.

Tabata N, Ito M, Tomoda H et al. Xanthohumols, diacylglycerol acytransferase inhibitors, from *Humulus lupulus*. *Phytochemistry*; 46(4):683-687. 1997.

Tobe H et al. Bone resorption inhibitors from hope extract. In: *Biosc Biotech Biochem* 61(1):158-159. 1997.

Widy-Tyszkiewica E & Schminda R. A randomized double blind study of sedative effects of phytotherapeutic containing valerian, hops, balm and motherwort versus placebo. *Herba Pol*; XLIII(2):154-159. 1997.

Wohlfart R. *Dtsch Apoth Ztg* 123:1637. 1983.

Wohlfart R, Hänsel R, Schmidt H. Nachweis sedativ-hypnotischer Wirkstoffe im Hopfen. 4. Mittlg. Die Pharmakologie des Hopfeninhaltsstoffes 2-Methyl-3-buten-2-ol. *Planta Med* 48:120-123. 1983.

Wohlfart R, Wurm G, Hänsel R, Schmidt H. Der Abbau der Bittersäuren zum 2-Methyl-3-buten-2-ol, einem Hopfeninhaltsstoff mit sedativ-hypnotischer Wirkung. *Arch Pharmaz* 315:132-137. 1983.

Yasukawa K, Takeuchi M & Takido M. Humulon, a bitter in the hop, inhibits tumor promotion by 12-0-tetradecanoylphorbol-13-acetate in two-stage carcinogenesis in mouse skin. *Oncology*; 52(2):156-158. 1995.

Zava D, Dollbaum C & Blen M. Estrogen and progestin bioactivity of foods, herbs, and spices. *Proc Soc Exp Biol Med;* 217(3):369-378. 1998.

Hordeum distichon

See Barley

Horehound

Marrubium vulgare

DESCRIPTION

Medicinal Parts: The medicinal parts are the dried flowering branches, the fresh aerial parts of the flowering plant, and the whole plant.

Flower and Fruit: The small, white, 5- to 7-mm long, labiate globular flowers are sessile. There are 6 to 8 richly flowered false whorls that are 1.5 to 2 cm long on each stem. The calyx is tubular, white, and tomentose with 10 awl-shaped tips, which are curved back in a hook. The corolla is white and downy. The fruit is an ovate, 1.5- to 2-mm long, obtusely triangular, smooth, light brown nut (possibly gray-brown with darker marbling).

Leaves, Stem, and Root: The plant is a perennial herb with a fusiform root and a multiheaded, often woody, root crown. The stems are erect, branched, obtusely quadrangular, and about 40 to 60 cm high and 7 mm thick at the base. The branches are curved, spread out, obtusely quadrangular, and loosely downy, like the leaves. The leaves are tomentose-downy, petiolate, orbicular, and unevenly crenate. They have distinct veins on the underside and are wrinkled.

Characteristics: The leaves smell tangy when rubbed and contain musk juice, which taste bitter and hot.

Habitat: The plant is indigenous to the Mediterranean region to central Asia. It has become established in central Europe; introduced to America, South Africa, and Australia.

Production: Horehound herb consists of the fresh or dried, above-ground parts of *Marrubium vulgare* as well as their preparations. The plant is harvested during the flowering season from June to August. Fast drying is recommended.

Other Names: Houndsbane, Marrubium, Marvel, White Horehound

ACTIONS AND PHARMACOLOGY

COMPOUNDS

Diterpene bitter principles: chief components marrubiin (0.1-1.0%), premarrubiin (0.1%)

Caffeic acid derivatives: including among others chlorogenic acid, cryptochlorogenic acid

Flavonoids: including among others chrysoeriol, vicenin II, lactoyl flavones, for example luteolin-7-lactate, apigenin-7-lactate

Volatile oil (traces): including among others camphene, p-cymene, fenchene

EFFECTS

The bitter ingredients act as a gastric juice stimulant; marrubinic acid acts as a choleretic. In animal experiments, a significant increase of bile secretion was observed after administration of marrubinic acid and its salt. The main active principles, essential oil, diterpene-amaroids, tannins, and flavonoids indicate that the drug would probably stimulate gastric juice secretion.

INDICATIONS AND USAGE

Approved by Commission E:

- Dyspeptic complaints
- Loss of appetite

Unproven Uses: The drug is used for dyspepsia, loss of appetite, bloating and flatulence, and respiratory catarrh. In folk medicine, it is used internally for acute and chronic bronchitis, whooping cough, asthma, tuberculosis, pulmonary catarrh, respiratory infections, diarrhea, jaundice, debility and painful menstruation, and as a laxative in higher doses. Externally it is used for skin damage, ulcers and wounds, and as a gargle for mouth and throat infections.

Homeopathic Uses: Inflammation of the respiratory tract.

PRECAUTIONS AND ADVERSE REACTIONS

General: No health hazards or side effects are known in conjunction with the proper administration of designated therapeutic dosages.

Pregnancy: Not to be used during pregnancy.

DOSAGE

Mode of Administration: Comminuted herb, freshly pressed plant juice, and other galenic preparations for internal use.

Preparation: To prepare an infusion, pour boiling water over 1 to 2 g of the drug; strain after 10 minutes. For a liquid extract, prepare as a (1:1) dilution with ethanol (20%).

Daily Dosage: The average daily dose is 4.5 g of the drug; 30 to 60 mL pressed juice.

The infusion dosage is 1 to 2 g of the drug taken up to 3 times daily. The liquid extract dosage is 2 to 4 mL 3 times daily.

Homeopathic Dosage: 5 drops, 1 tablet, or 10 globules every 30 to 60 minutes (acute) or 1 to 3 times daily (chronic); parenterally: 1 to 2 mL sc acute, 3 times daily; chronic: once a day (HAB1).

LITERATURE

Lamaison JL, Petitjean-Freytet C, Duke JA, Walker J. Hydroxycinnamic Derivative Levels and antioxidant Activity in North American Laminaceae. *Plant med et phyt.* 26; 143-148. 1993

Mascolo N et al., *Phytother Res* 1(1):28. 1987

Schlemper V, Ribas A, Nicolau M, Cechinel-Filho V. Antispasmodic effects of hydroalcoholic extract of *Marrubium vulgare* on isolated tissues. *Phytomedicine* 3 (2); 211-216. 1996

Souza MMde Jesus RAPde Cechinel-Filho V, Schlemper V. Analgesic profile of hydroalcoholic extract obtained from *Marrubium vulgare. Phytomedicine* 5 (2); 103-107. 1998

Tomas-Barberan FA, Gil MI, Ferreres F, Tomas-Lorante F. Flavonoid p-Coumaroylglucosides and 8-Hydroxyflavone allosylglucosides in some Labiatae. *Phytochemistry* 31; 3097-3107. 1992

Horse Chestnut

Aesculus hippocastanum

DESCRIPTION

Medicinal Parts: The medicinal parts are the dried Horse Chestnut leaves, the oil extracted from the peeled fruit capsules (seeds) and dried chestnut seeds.

Flower and Fruit: The white flowers are in stiffly upright panicles gradually thickening near the distal end. Most of the flowers are male, but a few are female or androgynous. The calyx is fused and bell-shaped with 5 irregular tips. The petals are 10 to 15 mm long with a yellow spot, which turns red. There are 3 upward petals and 2 downward, which are folded at the edge. The flower is ciliate and cordate (heart shaped) at the base and contains 7 S-shaped, bending stamens with red anthers that are longer than the petals. The ovary is trivalved, superior, and velvety. The fruit capsules are green and globular with soft spines and fine hairs. There are 1 to 3 red-brown seeds (Chestnuts) within the capsules, which are shiny brown with a yellowish gray-brown navel and a tough shell.

Leaves, Stem, and Root: The seasonal tree is up to 35 m high; it includes a large regular crown and widely spread roots. The trunk is initially smooth but later has thinly scaled, peeling, and fissured bark. The young twigs are yellowish to red-brown and are initially covered with brown hairs. The buds gradually thicken near the distal end and are extremely sticky with dark red bud scales to protect the seed plant bud. The leaves are long, 5 to 7 palmate, with a 20-cm long grooved petiole. The leaflets are initially red-haired, 20 cm long, cuneate-obovate, acute, and dentate. The leaflets are rich green above and beneath are light green.

Habitat: Although the herb is indigenous to the mountains of Greece, Bulgaria, the Caucasus, northern Iran and the Himalayas, it is cultivated elsewhere, especially in northern Europe, including the British Isles, Denmark, Scandinavia, and Russia (Narva and St. Petersburg).

Production: Horse Chestnut leaf consists of the fresh or dried leaf of *Aesculus hippocastanum.* A dry extract is manufactured from Horse Chestnut seeds standardized to a content of

16-20% triterpene glycosides (calculated as anhydrous aescin).

Not to be Confused With: The leaves of the Horse Chestnut are commonly confused with those of Sweet Chestnut.

Other Names: Buckeye, Common Horse Chestnut, Conqueror Tree, Spanish Chestnut

ACTIONS AND PHARMACOLOGY

COMPOUNDS: HORSE CHESTNUT LEAF

Triterpene saponins

Hydroxycoumarins: chief component is aesculin, in addition, fraxin and scopolin

Flavonoids: including rutin, quercitrin, and isoquercitrin

Tannins

EFFECTS: HORSE CHESTNUT LEAF

The main active principles of the anti-exudative effect and improvement of venous tone are hydroxycoumarins (aesculin and fraxin), triterpene saponins in the petioles and leaf veins, flavonoids, and a rich supply of tannins. Although the drug is said to have an anti-exudative effect and improve venous tone, there is a lack of clinical data to support the efficacy.

COMPOUNDS: HORSE CHESTNUT SEEDS

Triterpene saponins (3-5%): The triterpene saponine mixture known as aescin (also escin) consists of diacylated tetra-and pentahydroxy-beta-amyrin compounds. The compounds bear a glucuronic acid remnant substituted with 2 monosaccharide remnants in position 3 at the OH-group. Aglycones, protoescigenin and barringtogenol C, are bonded like esters onto the OH-group at position 21 with either angelic or tiglic acid, or with either alpha-methyl butyric or isobutyric acid remnants. The OH-group in position 22 (beta-escin) or 28 (cryptoescin) is acetylated, and both positional isomeric compounds remain in equilibrium though migration of the acetyl remnant.

Flavonoids: in particular biosides and triosides of the quercetins

Oligosaccharides: including 1-kestose, 2-kestose, stachyose

Polysaccharides: starch (50%)

Oligomeric proanthocyanidins, condensed tannins: (only in the seed-coat)

Fatty oil (2-3%)

EFFECTS: HORSE CHESTNUT SEEDS

As found in different animal tests and preclincal investigations, the principal ingredient of Horse Chestnut seed extract, triterpene glycoside mixture (aescin), has an anti-exudative, vascular tightening effect, and reduction of vascular permeability which result in an antiedemic effect. The vein-toning properties of the Horse Chestnut extract also demonstrated improvement of venous return flow. A significant reduction of transcapillary filtration was seen in a placebo-controlled human pharmacological trial (Bisler, 1986). Significant improvement in the symptoms of chronic venous insufficiency was demonstrated in diverse, randomized, double-blind and cross-over studies (Calabrese, 1993; Steiner, 1990).

There are indications that Horse Chestnut seed extract reduces the activity of lysosomal enzymes, which increases in chronic pathological conditions of the veins. The enzymes will break down glycoacalyx (mucopolysaccharides) in the region of the capillary walls, allowing proteins to leak into the interstitium. The activity of the enzymes is reduced by the aescin and so the breakdown of glycoacalyx is also inhibited. The transcapillary filtration of low-molecular proteins, electrolytes, and water into the interstitium is inhibited through a reduction of vascular permeability by the aescin.

CLINICAL TRIALS

Chronic venous insufficiency and ulceration

A meta-analysis of 17 randomized clinical trials of oral Horse Chestnut seed extract for the treatment of chronic venous insufficiency indicated that, compared to placebo or reference therapy, the extract is effective for short-term treatment, improving signs and symptoms such as leg pain and swelling. Adverse events were mild and infrequent. The authors recommended further trials to confirm apparent benefits (Pittler, 2007).

Researchers conducted a prospective and randomized, placebo-controlled, triple-blind study to determine the clinical efficacy of orally administered Horse Chestnut seed extract in treating venous ulceration. Ulcer assessments at weeks 0, 4, 8, and 12 revealed no statistical difference between the groups taking the Horse Chestnut seed extract (n=27) or placebo (n=27) in regard to the number of healed leg ulcers, or changes in wound surface area, depth, volume, pain, or exudate. The Horse Chestnut seed extract did, however, have a significant effect on the number of dressing changes at week 12 and the percentage of wound slough over time, indicating to the authors a potential value in managing venous leg ulcers (Leach, 2006)

The efficacy and safety of Horse Chestnut seed extract, given as Venostasin retard (50 mg aescin) twice daily, was compared to mechanical compression involving bandages and stockings in a randomized, placebo-controlled clinical study. The 12-week study consisted of 240 patients with chronic venous insufficiency. The results determined a similar decrease of lower leg volume of approximately 25% and noted compression treatment is uncomfortable, inconvenient, and subject to poor compliance (Diehm, 1996).

In another study using Venostasin retard, the extract was administered to 52 pregnant women with edema due to venous insufficiency. The placebo-controlled, double-blind, crossover study showed a significant reduction of edema and greater resistance to edema provocation in the Venostasin retard group. There were also less severe symptoms of pain, fatigue, swelling, and itching with patients receiving Venostasin retard therapy (Steiner, 1990).

A randomized, placebo-controlled, double-blind study was conducted on 40 patients with venous edema in chronic deep vein incompetence to determine the edema-reducing effect of Horse Chestnut seed extract. The edema reduction effect and reduction of leg volume with edema provocation of the Horse Chestnut seed extract were both statistically significant (Diehm, 1992).

Hemorrhoids

Endoscopic examination revealed a notable reduction in bleeding and swelling of acute symptomatic hemorrhoids as compared to placebo in 80 patients taking part in a double-blind, placebo-controlled study of Horse Chestnut Seed extract (40 mg aescin). The extract was administered 3 times daily for up to 2 months. Endoscopy indicated improvement after 2 weeks. Symptoms typically subsided after 6 days (Abascal 2005).

INDICATIONS AND USAGE

HORSE CHESTNUT LEAF

Unproven Uses: Eczema, superficial and deep varicose veins, leg pains, phlebitis, hemorrhoids, pains before and during menstruation. In folk medicine, the leaves are used as a cough remedy, as well as for arthritis and rheumatism.

HORSE CHESTNUT SEEDS

Approved by Commission E:

- Venous conditions (chronic venous insufficiency)

Treatment of symptoms found in pathological conditions of the veins of the legs (chronic venous insufficiency), for example pain and a sensation of heaviness in the legs, nocturnal cramps in the calves, pruritis, and swelling of the legs.

Unproven uses: Horse Chestnut seeds are used for symptoms of post-traumatic and post-operative soft tissue swelling. Further indications are painful injuries, sprains, bruising, pain syndrome of the spine, edema, rheumatic disease, chronic prostatitis, and varicose veins.

Homeopathic Uses: Homeopathic treatments include hemorrhoids, lumbar and low back pain, venous back pressure.

PRECAUTIONS AND ADVERSE REACTIONS

HORSE CHESTNUT LEAF

General: Health risks or side effects following the proper administration of designated therapeutic dosages are not recorded. One case of liver damage following intramuscular administration of an extract of the drug (origin details of the drug uncertain) is known.

DRUG INTERACTIONS

POTENTIAL INTERACTIONS

Horse Chestnut leaf has a coumarin component and may interact with warfarin, salicylates, and other drugs with anticoagulant properties.

HORSE CHESTNUT SEEDS

Health risks following the proper administration of designated therapeutic dosages are not recorded. Susceptible patients may nevertheless experience mucous membrane irritations of the gastrointestinal tract (e.g. nausea) following intake of the drug; decrease in kidney function with pre-existing renal insufficiency and acute nephrotoxicity. Hepatotoxicity and urticaria have also been observed. I.V administration of aescin can lead to anaphylactic reactions.

OVERDOSAGE

HORSE CHESTNUT SEEDS

The intake of larger quantities of Horse Chestnut seeds (in one case of a child with 5 seeds) can bring about vomiting, diarrhea, severe thirst, reddening of the face, enlargement of pupils, vision and consciousness disorders. Following stomach and intestinal emptying (gastric lavage, sodium sulfate) and the administration of activated charcoal, therapy for poisonings consists of diazepam for spasms, atropine for colic, electrolyte replenishment, and sodium bicarbonate infusions for any acidosis that may arise. Intubation and oxygen respiration may also be necessary.

DOSAGE

HORSE CHESTNUT LEAF

Mode of Administration: Extracts of the drug are contained in ''vein teas'' or ''hemorrhoid teas,'' as well as in pharmaceutical preparations for the treatment of venous symptoms.

Preparation: One ampule corresponds to 4 mg flavones in 0.9% NaCl.

Daily Dosage:

Infusion (as a tea)–Pour boiling water over 1 tsp. of finely cut drug and strain after 5 to 10 minutes (1 tsp = 1 g drug).

Intravenously–1 to 2 ampules daily.

Intramuscularly– 1 ampule daily.

HORSE CHESTNUT SEEDS

Mode of Administration: Available in liquid and solid preparations for internal use; semi-solid preparations for external use; and parenterally for homeopathic use.

How Supplied:

Ampules

Capsules – 250 mg, 300 mg, 375 mg, 485 mg

Drops

Liquid extract

Ointment/Gels

Tablets

Tincture

Preparation: Stabilized extract of Horse Chestnut (5:1) is standardized for aescin; tincture of Horse Chestnut 1:1 with 75% ethanol; isolated aescin.

Daily Dosage:

Intravenous—Doses of 5 mg once or twice daily of aescin as the sodium salt has been used for treatment or prevention of post-traumatic edema and potoperative edema. The maximum daily dose is 20 mg.

Oral—Aescin from encapsulated standardized extracts are initially given at doses of 10 mg. The encapsulated standardized extract has been used for the treatment of postoperative or traumatic edema, hemorrhoids or symptoms due to varicose veins in doses providing 40 to 120 mg of aescin per day. Aescin (escin) 100 mg corresponding to 250-312.5 mg extract may be administered twice daily in delayed-release form.

Tincture—For the treatment of painful hemorrhoids, a dose of 1:10 tincture is 0.6 mL

Topical—A 1 to 2% gel is applied topically several times daily for soft tissue injuries, bruises and symptomatic relief of varicose veins.

Homeopathic Dosage: 5 drops, 1 tablet, or 10 globules every 30 to 60 minutes (acute) and 1 to 3 times daily (chronic); parenterally: 1 to 2 mL 3 times daily sc; ointment 1 to 2 times daily (HAB1).

Storage: The herb should be stored in a dry and dark place.

LITERATURE

Abascal, K, Yarnell, E Botanical treatments for hemorrhoids. *Alt Comp Ther;* 11(6); 285, 289. 2005

Acar AM, Paksoy S. Derivative spectrophotometric determination of aescin in *Aesculus hippocastanum L.* seeds. *Pharmazie* 48; 65-66 (1993)

Aizawa X, Fukui, Yamada K, Kogo H, Aescin, antiinflammatory action of Aescin (1, intravenous injection). In: *Pharmacometrics* (Tokyo) 8:211. 1974.

Annoni F, Mauri A, Marincola Resele LF, (1979) Venotonic activity of Escin on the human saphenous vein. Arzneim Forsch/ Drug Res 29:672.

Beck M. Horse chestnut seed extract. *Lancet* 335; 1467 (1990)

Bisler H, Pfeifer R, Kl,ken N, Pauschinger P. Wirkung von Ro bkastaniensamenextrakt auf die transkapilläre Filtration bei chronischer venöser Insuffizien. *Z Dtsch Med Wschr* 111, 1321-1328 1986

Brandt D (ed.): Reparil (R) -Ampoules. In: MDR, MIMS Desk Reference Vol 28. *MIMS*, Pretoria, 1992/93.

Büechi S, Antivirale Saponine, pharmakologische und klinische Untersuchungen. In: *DAZ* 136(2):89-98. 1996.

Calabrese C, Preston P, Report of the results of a double-blind, randomized, single-dose trial of a topical 2% escon gel versus placebo in the acute treatment of experimentally-induced hematoma volunteers. *Planta Med* 59:394-397. 1993.

Chandler RF, Herbal Medicine: Horse Chestnut. *Can Pharm J.*126:297-306. 1993

Comaish JS, Kersey PJ, Contact dermatitis to extract of horse chestnut (esculin). *Contact Dermatitis* Jan;6(2):150-1. 1980

De Smet PA, Van den E, Lesterhuis W, Hepatotoxicity associated with herbal tablets. *BJM*; July 13, 313:92. 1996

Deli J et al. Aesculaxanthin, a New Carotenoid Isolated from Pollens of *Aesculus hippocastanum. Helv Chim Acta* 81; 1815-1820.(1998

Diehm C, Vollbrecht D, Amendt K, Comberg HU, Medical edema protection-clinical benefit in patients with chronic deep vein incompetence. A placebo controlled double blind study. *Vasa* 21 (2):199-92.1992.

Diehm C, Trampisch HJ, Lange S, Schmidt C, Comparison of leg compression stocking and oral horse-chestnut seed extract in patients with chronic venous insufficiency. *Lancet* Feb 3;347:292-294. 1996.

Escribano MM, Munoz-Bellido FJ, Velazquez E et al., Contact urticaria due to aescin. *Contact Dermatitis* Nov:37(5):233. 1997

Felix W, Schneider E, Schmidt A, Grimm G, Vasoaktive Wirkung von alpha-Aescin. In: Fischer H (Hrsg) Ergebnisse der Angiologie: Chronische Veneninsuffizienz. Pathogenese und medikamentöse Therapie, Schattauer, Stuttgart, 30:93-105. 1984.

Fink Serralde C, Dreyfus Cortes GO, Colo Hernandesz, Marquez Zacarias LA, (1975) Valoracion de la escina pura en el tratamiento del sindrome des estasis venosa cronica. Münch Med Wschr (mex. Ausgabe) 117(1):41-46.

Girerd I, DiPasquale, Steinetz G, Beach BG, Pearl VLW, The anti-edema properties of aescin. In: Arch internat Pharmacodyn Thér, Bruxelles 133:127-137. 1961.

Guillaume M, Padioleau F. Veinotonic Effect, Vascular Protection, Antiinflammatory and Free Radical Scavening Properties of Horse Chestnut Extract. *Arzneim Forsch* 44; 25-35. 1994

Hübner G, Wray V, Nahrstedt A, Flavonolglycosides in *Aesculus hippocastanum L.*: Isolation, structure elucidation and quantification. In: *PM* 62, Abstracts of the 44th Ann Congress of GA, 139. 1996.

Karuza-Stojakovic L, Petricic J, Smit Z. The Quantity of Aescin in Various Stages of Development of Horsechestnut Seeds (*Aesculus hippocastanum*). *Planta Med.* 55; 624-625. 1989

Karuza-Stojakovic L, Petricic J, Smit Z. The total Triterpene content expressed as aescin in horse chestnut seeds (*Aesculus hippocastanum L.*) during vegetation. *Pharmazie* 46; 303. 1991

Kreysel HW, Nissen HP, Enghofer E, A possible role of lysosomal enzymes in the pathogenesis of varicosis and the reduction in their serum activity by Venostasin. Vasa 12(4):377-82. 1983.

Leach MJ, Pincombe J, Foster G. Clinical efficacy of horsechestnut seed extract in the treatment of venous ulceration. *J Wound Care.* 15(4):159-67. 2006.

Longiave D, Omini C, Nicosia S, Berti F, The Mode of Action of Escin on Isolated Veins, Relationship with PGF2. Pharmacol Res 10:145. 1978

Maffei Facino R, Carini M, Stefani R, Aldini G, Saibene L. Anti-Elastase and Anti-Hyaluronidase Activities of Saponins and Sapogenins from Hedera helix, Aesculus hippocastanum, and Ruscus aculeatus: Factors contributing to their Efficacy in the Treatment of Venous Insufficiency. *Arch Pharm* (Weinheim) 328; 720-72

Matsuda H, Li Y, Murakami T, Ninomiya K, Yamahara J, Yoshikawa M. Effects of escins Ia, Ib, IIa, and IIb from horse chestnut, the seeds of Aesculus hippocastanum L., on acute inflammation in animals. *Biol-Pharm-Bull.* 20(10); 1092-1095. 1997

Pittler, MH, Ernst E, Horse chestnut seed extract for chronic venous insufficiency. *Cochrane database of systematic reviews (Online)* 1, CD003230; 2006

Rehn D, Unkauf M, Klein P, Jost V, L,cker PW. Comparative Clinical Efficacy and Tolerability of Oxerutins and Horse Chestnut Extract in Patients with Chronic Venous Insufficiency. *Arzneim Forsch.* 46 (5); 483-487. 1996

Rothkopf M, Vogel G, Lang W, Leng E, Animal experiments on the question of the renal toleration of the horse chestnut saponin aescin. *Arzneimittelforschung*; 27(3):598-605. 1977

Rudofsky G, Nei b A, Otto K, Seibel K, Ödemprotektive Wirkung und klinische Wirksamkeit von Ro b kastaniensamenextrakt im Doppelblindversuch. *Phlebol Proktol* 15:47-54. 1986

Simini B, Horse-chestnut seed extract for chronic venous insufficiency (letter;comment). *Lancet* Apr 27;347 (9009):1182-3. 1996

Steiner M, Hillemanns HG, Venostasin retard in the management of venous problems during pregnancy. *Phlebology* 5:41-44. 1990.

Vayssairat M et al., Horse-chestnut seed extract for chronic venous insufficiency. In: *Lancet* 347(9009):182-183. 1996.

Yarnell E, Abascal K, Natural approaches to treating chronic prostatitis and chronic pelvic pain syndromes. *Alt Comp Ther*; Vol 11(5); 246-251. 2005

Horsemint

Monarda Punctata

DESCRIPTION

Medicinal Parts: The medicinal part is the herb.

Flower and Fruit: The flowers grow in axillary whorls. They are bilabiate. The corolla is yellow with red spots. The 2 stamens and the sessile bracts are yellow and purple.

Leaves, Stem, and Root: The plant is a perennial and grows up to 90 cm high with a branched, round stem. The leaves are opposite, lanceolate, and downy.

Characteristics: The taste is pungent and bitter; the odor reminiscent of thyme.

Habitat: The plant is indigenous to the eastern and central U.S.

Other Names: Spotted Monarda, Monarda Lutea, Wild Bergamot

ACTIONS AND PHARMACOLOGY

COMPOUNDS

Volatile oil: including among others thymol (20%), thymol methyl ether, thymol hydroquinone; in Monarda punctata varieties, maritima including also gamma-terpinene, geranylformate, nerylformate

EFFECTS

The drug has carminative, stimulant and emmenagogic effects.

CONTRAINDICATIONS

The drug is not to be used during pregnancy.

INDICATIONS AND USAGE

Unproven Uses: The drug is used for digestive disorders, flatulence, and dysmenorrhea.

PRECAUTIONS AND ADVERSE REACTIONS

No health hazards or side effects are known in conjunction with the proper administration of designated therapeutic dosages. (Oil from the plant, however, is only to be administered externally. Even then, because it raises blisters in its pure form, it should be diluted with olive oil before application.)

DOSAGE

Mode of Administration: Ground drug used as an infusion.

LITERATURE

Kern W, List PH, Hörhammer L (Hrsg.), Hagers Handbuch der Pharmazeutischen Praxis, 4. Aufl., Bde. 1-8, Springer Verlag Berlin, Heidelberg, New York, 1969.

Horseradish

Armoracia rusticana

DESCRIPTION

Medicinal Parts: The medicinal part of the plant is the fresh or dried horseradish root.

Flower and Fruit: The inflorescence is made up of numerous, richly flowered racemes (cymes). The fragrant flowers are on 5- to 7-mm long, upright pedicles. The sepals are 2.5 to 3 mm long, broadly ovate, with a membranous white margin. The white petals are 5 to 7 mm long and broadly obovate. The inner stamens are 2.5 mm long; the outer ones 1.5 mm long. The stigma is broad, round, and gently double-lobed. The small pods are on 20 mm long, upright spreading stems. They are globose to obovate and 4 to 6 mm long. The seeds are smooth.

Leaves, Stem, and Root: The plant is 40 to 120 cm high. It is a sturdy and glabrous perennial. The root is quite thick and woody. In cultivated varieties, it is thick and fleshy with numerous root heads, which are light yellowish-white and have horizontal underground runners. The sometimes solitary stems are upright, branched above, grooved, and hollow. The leaves are long-petioled, oblong-ovate, cordate at the base, 30 to 100 cm long, and unevenly crenate. The lower cauline leaves have shorter petioles and are lobed or comb-shaped pinnate with linear-oblong, entire-margined or serrate sections. The upper cauline leaves with narrowed bases are sessile, oblong or lanceolate, unevenly crenate to serrate, and obtuse. The uppermost leaves are linear or almost entire-margined.

Characteristics: The rootstock has an odor that is strong and irritating, and a sharp, burning taste.

Habitat: The plant is indigenous to the Volga-Don region but has spread to almost all of Europe and other parts of the world.

Production: Horseradish consists of the fresh or dried, peeled or unpeeled roots of *Armoracia rusticana*.

Other Names: Great Raifort, Mountain Radish, Red Cole

ACTIONS AND PHARMACOLOGY

COMPOUNDS

Glucosinolates sinigrin and gluconasturtin: The freshly harvested root contains the glucosinolates sinigrin (0.3%) and gluconasturtin, which release enzymatically triggered (myrosinase) allyl mustard oil (up to 90%) and a little 2-phenyl mustard when the root is cut up. The dehydrated root contains both of these mustard oils.

EFFECTS

Horseradish works antimicrobially against gram-positive and gram-negative pathogens, is hyperemic on skin and mucous membranes, and is carcinostatic (due to the mustard oils). Horseradish demonstrated an antispasmodic effect in animal experiments.

INDICATIONS AND USAGE

Approved by Commission E:

- Cough/Bronchitis
- Infections of the urinary tract

Unproven Uses: Internally, Horseradish is used to treat inflammation of the respiratory tract and as supportive therapy for infections of the urinary tract. Externally, the drug is used for inflammation of the respiratory tract and for hyperemic treatment for minor muscle aches. In folk medicine, horseradish is administered for influenza, respiratory ailments, digestion, gout, rheumatism, and liver and gallbladder disorders.

Homeopathic Uses: Uses in homeopathy include eye inflammations, upper respiratory tract inflammations, and upper abdominal colic.

CONTRAINDICATIONS

Because of the mucous membrane-irritating effect of the mustard oils, the intake of the drug should not be carried out in the presence of stomach or intestinal ulcers or in patients with a history of kidney disease.

PRECAUTIONS AND ADVERSE REACTIONS

General: No health hazards or side effects are known in conjunction with the proper administration of designated therapeutic dosages.

Pediatric Use: Preparations of horseradish should not be administered to children under 4 years of age.

DOSAGE

Mode of Administration: Fresh or dried root that has been cut or ground, freshly pressed juice, or other galenic preparations for internal or external applications.

Daily Dose: The average dose for internal use is 20 g of fresh root; for external use, ointments and gels with a maximum of 2% mustard oils may be used.

Homeopathic Dosage: 5 drops, 1 tablet, or 10 globules every 30 to 60 minutes (acute) or 1 to 3 times daily (chronic); parenterally: 1 to 2 mL 3 times daily sc (HAB34). The mother tincture and first decimal dilution to be taken diluted with water.

Storage: Fresh roots should be buried in soil or sand.

LITERATURE

Hänsel R, Keller K, Rimpler H, Schneider G (Hrsg.), Hagers Handbuch der Pharmazeutischen

Praxis, 5. Aufl., Bde 4-6 (Drogen), Springer Verlag Berlin, Heidelberg, New York, 1992-1994.

Lewin L, Gifte und Vergiftungen, 6. Aufl., Nachdruck, Haug Verlag, Heidelberg 1992.

Simon JE, Chadwick AF, Craker LE (Eds), Herbs. An Indexed Bibliography 1971-80. Archon Books, USA 1984.

Teuscher E, Lindequist U, Biogene Gifte - Biologie, Chemie, Pharmakologie, 2. Aufl., Fischer Verlag Stuttgart 1994.

Teuscher E, Biogene Arzneimittel, 5. Aufl., Wiss. Verlagsges. Stuttgart 1997.

Wagner H, Wiesenauer M, Phytotherapie. Phytopharmaka und pflanzliche Homöopathika, Fischer-Verlag, Stuttgart, Jena, New York, 1995.

Horsetail

Equisetum arvense

DESCRIPTION

Medicinal Parts: The medicinal parts are the dried green, sterile shoots, and fresh sterile shoots.

Flower and Fruit: Horsetail appears in two forms during the year. From March to April the red-brown to straw yellow simple stem develops with leaves arranged in a number of levels on the stem in whorls. The leaves are brown, fused to a sheath at the lower level with black-tipped, dry sporangia cones at the tip sprinkling greenish spore powder. In May and June there is a sterile summer form with 10 to 14 cm high stems and numerous branches that are arranged in whorls at the nodes. The stem and branches are deeply grooved, usually square and rough.

Habitat: Horsetail grows throughout Europe. It grows in Asia as far south as Turkey and Iran. The plant is also found in the Himalayas, central and north China, and Japan.

Production: Horsetail consists of the fresh or dried, green, sterile stems of *Equisetum arvense* harvested in the summer. The herb is collected in the wild and air-dried.

Not to be Confused With: Other Equisetum species.

Other Names: Bottle-Brush, Corn Horsetail, Dutch Rushes, Field Horsetail, Horse Willow, Horsetail Grass, Horsetail Rush, Paddock-Pipes, Pewterwort, Scouring Rush, Shave Grass, Toadpipe

ACTIONS AND PHARMACOLOGY

COMPOUNDS

Flavonoids: (0.6 to 0-9%): apigenin-5-0-glucoside, genkwanin-5-O-glucoside, kaempferol-3,7-di-O-glucoside, kaempferol-3-O-(6′-O-malonyl-glucoside)-7-O-glucoside, kaempferol-3-O-sophoroside, luteolin-5-O-glucoside, quercetin-3-O-glucoside

Caffeic acid ester (up to 1%): including chlorogenic acid, dicoffeoyl-meso-tartaric acid

Silicic acid (5 to 7.7%): to some extent water-soluble

Pyridine alkaloids: nicotine (traces), palustrine (in the gamatophytes and in the rhizome styrolpyrone glucosides, including equisetumpyrone)

EFFECTS

Horsetail has a mild diuretic and spasmolytic action in animal tests. The flavonoids and silicic acid contribute to the astringent effect. The drug has shown to increase diuresis and reduce uric acid content in the blood by increasing uric acid clearing and excretion rates. Plasma composition was improved, as well as excretion of calcium and anorganic phosphorus.

INDICATIONS AND USAGE

Approved by Commission E:

- Infections of the urinary tract
- Kidney and bladder stones
- Wounds and burns

Internal preparations are used for post-traumatic and static edema, flushing-out therapy for bacterial and inflammatory diseases of the lower urinary tract, and renal stones. It is used externally as a supportive treatment for poorly healing wounds.

Unproven Uses: In folk medicine, *Equisetum arvense* is used for tuberculosis, as a catarrh in the kidney and bladder regions, as a hematostatic for profuse menstruation, nasal, pulmonary and gastric hemorrhages, for brittle fingernails and loss of hair, for rheumatic diseases, gout, poorly healing wounds and ulcers, swelling and fractures, and for frostbite.

Homeopathic Uses: The drug is used for urinary tract and kidney disorders.

CONTRAINDICATIONS

Horsetail is contraindicated in patients who have edema due to impaired heart or kidney function.

PRECAUTIONS AND ADVERSE REACTIONS

Health risks or side effects following the proper administration of designated therapeutic dosages are not recorded.

A doctor should be consulted when the drug is utilized as a bath additive in cases of major skin lesions, acute skin lesions of unknown origin, major feverish and infectious diseases, cardiac insufficiency, and hypertonia.

DOSAGE

Mode of Administration: Comminuted herb for infusions and other galenic preparations are available for oral administration. Comminuted herb for decoctions and other galenic preparations are used externally.

Preparation: To make a tea, pour 200 mL boiling water over 2 to 3 g drug and boil for 5 minutes; strain after 10 to 15 minutes. To make an infusion, use 1.5 g drug per 1 cup water. A liquid extract is prepared in a 1:1 ratio in 25% alcohol.

Daily Dosage: Daily dose of Horsetail is 6 g drug. The drug should be administered with plenty of fluids.

The internal dosages are as follows:

Infusion – 2 to 4 g

Liquid extract – 1 to 4 mL 3 times daily

Tea – 2-3 g per cup repeatedly during the day between mealtimes

External use:

Compresses: 10 g drug to 1 liter

Homeopathic Dosage: 5 drops, 1 tablet, or 10 globules every 30 to 60 minutes (acute) or 1 to 3 times a day (chronic); parenterally: 1 to 2 ml sc 3 times daily (HAB1).

Storage: Horsetail must be protected from light in well-sealed containers.

LITERATURE

Carnat A, Lamaison JL, Duband F. Teneurs en pricipaux Constituants de la feuille de frene, *Fraxinus excelsior L. Plant med et phyt.* 24; 145-151. 1990

Fabre B, Beaufils P. Thiaminase Activity in *Equisetum arvense* and its Extracts. *Plant med et phyt.* 26; 190-197. 1993

Hederich M, Beckert C, Veit M. Establishing Styrylpyrone Synthase Activity in Cell Free Extracts Obtained from Gametophytes of *Equisetum arvense L.* by High Performance Liquid Chromatography-Tandem Mass Spectrometry. *Phytochem Anal.* 8; 194-197. 1997

Sökeland J, Phytotherapie in der Urologie. In: *ZPT* 10(1):8. 1989.

Veit M, Problem bei der Bewertung pflanzlicher Diuretika. Als Beispiel Schachtelhalmkraut DAB 10 (Equiseti herba). In: *ZPT* 15(6):331-341. 1994.

Veit M et al., Flavonoids of the Equisetum hybrids in the subgenus Equisetum. In: *PM* 58(7):A697. 1992.

Hound's Tongue

Cynoglossum officinale

DESCRIPTION

Medicinal Parts: The medicinal parts are the aerial and root of the herb.

Flower and Fruit: The flowers are on short, bent pedicles, which grow to 1 cm after flowering. The corolla is cup-shaped and larger than the calyx. The corolla is initially dark violet, then dull brown. It is occasionally white with thickened, velvety purple or light red, tubular scales. The nutlets are flat, ovoid and light brown. They are 5 to 7 mm wide, thickened at the edge, and covered with barbs.

Leaves, Stem, and Root: The plant is a biennial. The taproot is 10 to 30 cm long and up to 1.5 cm thick. It is reddish colored with a few fibers. The shoots are gray-green and smell of mice. The stems are usually rigidly erect, angular, hairy, and heavily foliated. They are 30 to 80 cm high and up to 1 cm thick. The lower leaves are in rosettes, which form a tough, coriaceous sheath at the base. The upper leaves are sessile and clasping.

Habitat: Especially common in Germany and Switzerland, now also found in the U.S. in areas where Germans and Swiss settled.

Production: Hound's Tongue herb consists of the above-ground parts of *Cynoglossum officinale*. Hound's Tongue root is the root of *Cynoglossum officinale*. The root is gathered in the second spring and then dried.

Other Names: Dog's Tongue, Dog-Bur, Gypsy Flower, Sheep-Lice, Woolmat

ACTIONS AND PHARMACOLOGY

COMPOUNDS: HOUND'S TONGUE HERB

Pyrrolizidine alkaloids (0.7 to 1.5%): main alkaloids heliosupine, echinatine, also 7-angeloylheliotridine, acetylheliosupine

EFFECTS

No information is available.

COMPOUNDS: HOUND'S TONGUE ROOT

Pyrrolizidine alkaloids: main alkaloids presumably, as in the plant, are heliosupine and echinatine

Tannins

EFFECTS: HOUND'S TONGUE ROOT

The root has antidiarrheal and wound-healing effects. It is both toxic and carcinogenic.

According to previous reports, cynoglossin has a paralyzing effect on the peripheral nerve ends of frogs. The substances consolicin and consolidin have a paralyzing effect on the CNS, which is 3 times stronger than the effect of cynoglossin. The toxicity should disappear with storage.

INDICATIONS AND USAGE

HOUND'S TONGUE HERB

Unproven Uses: Hound's Tongue's use as an antidiarrheal is considered obsolete. Externally, it is used as an expectorant. The effectiveness of the herb for the claimed applications is not documented.

CYNOGLOSSUM ROOT

Unproven Uses: The root is used externally in the treatment of wounds.

PRECAUTIONS AND ADVERSE REACTIONS

HOUND'S TONGUE HERB AND ROOT

Warning: The traditional folk medicinal preparations should not be used.

Because of its high pyrrolizidine alkaloid content with 1,2-unsaturated necine parent substances, the drug is both hepatotoxic and hepatocarcinogenic in effect. The drug should under no circumstances be taken internally.

DOSAGE

HOUND'S TONGUE HERB AND ROOT

See Warning above regarding internal use.

Storage: The herb should be protected from light and kept dry above annealed calcium chloride in air-tight, sealed glass or chalk containers, with the possible addition of a few drops of chloroform or carbon tetrachloride as an insecticide. It should be renewed annually.

LITERATURE

HOUND'S TONGUE HERB AND ROOT

Frohne D, Pfänder HJ: Giftpflanzen - Ein Handbuch für Apotheker, Toxikologen und Biologen, 4. Aufl., Wiss. Verlagsges. mbH Stuttgart 1997.

Kern W, List PH, Hörhammer L (Hrsg.), Hagers Handbuch der Pharmazeutischen Praxis, 4. Aufl., Bde 1-8, Springer Verlag Berlin, Heidelberg, New York, 1969.

Knight AP, Kimberling CV, Stermitz FR, Roby MR, Cynoglossum officinale (hounds-tongue) - a cause of pyrrolizidine-alkaloid poisoning in horse. In: J Am Vet Med Assoc 185(6):647-650. 1984.

Lewin L, Gifte und Vergiftungen, 6. Aufl., Nachdruck, Haug Verlag, Heidelberg 1992.

Mattocks AR, Pigott CD, Pyrrolizidine lakloids from Cynoglossum germanicum. In: PH 29(9):2871. 1990.

Steinegger E, Hänsel R, Pharmakognosie, 5. Aufl., Springer Verlag Heidelberg 1992.

Teuscher E, Lindequist U, Biogene Gifte - Biologie, Chemie, Pharmakologie, 2. Aufl., Fischer Verlag Stuttgart 1994.

Houseleek

Sempervivum tectorum

DESCRIPTION

Medicinal Parts: The medicinal parts are the fresh leaves before flowering and their juice.

Flower and Fruit: The pink or red flowers are in cymes on their own peduncles, which are about 22 cm high. The individual flowers are short-pedicled and splayed in a star shape. The 12 sepals and petals are twice as long as the calyx. The 24 stamens are in 2 circles. There are 24 ovaries. The small fruit is many-seeded and fused at the base.

Leaves, Stem, and Root: The green succulent leaves grow directly from the perennial fibrous root and form a dense, obovate, basal rosette 5 to 10 cm in diameter. They are fleshy and juicy, flat, and 2.5 to 5 cm long. The purple leaves are sessile-oblong with a ciliate margin and are often in carpets of tufts.

Habitat: The plant is indigenous to central and southern Europe and now grows wild in northern Europe, northern Africa, and western Asia.

Other Names: Aaron's Rod, Ayegreen, Ayron, Bullock's Eye, Hens and Chickens, Jupiter's Eye, Jupiter's Beard, Liveforever, Sengreen, Thor's Beard, Thunder Plant

ACTIONS AND PHARMACOLOGY

COMPOUNDS

Fruit acids: L(-)-malic acid, isocitric acid, succinic acid

Tannins

Mucilage

EFFECTS

The active agents are the leaves containing tannin, bitter substances, sugar, and mucous. Results of research carried out to date point to a possible liver-protective and anti-oxidative effect. There are no studies available for the astringent, diuretic and antiseptic effects attributed to the drug.

INDICATIONS AND USAGE

Unproven Uses: Houseleek is used internally to relieve severe diarrhea. Folk medicine uses include dysentery, dysmenorrhea and amenorrhea, impairment of hearing and fever, worm infestation, uterine neuralgia, tonsillitis, headache, and toothache. Externally, the drug is used for burns, wounds, ulcers and swelling caused by insect bites, open wounds, sore nipples, corns, inflammation of the throat; hemorrhoids, eczema, stomatitis, oral fungal infections and inflammation of mucous membranes, and for the treatment of itchy and burning skin parts. A gargle of diluted juice made from the leaves is used for stomatitis.

PRECAUTIONS AND ADVERSE REACTIONS

No health hazards or side effects are known in conjunction with the proper administration of designated therapeutic dosages.

DOSAGE

Mode of Administration: Houseleek is used internally as a decoction. Freshly pressed leaves and their juice is used externally.

Preparation: To prepare an infusion, allow 15 g of the drug to steep in 1000 mL water for 10 minutes. Poultices are prepared using crushed fresh leaves. A compress is made by soaking a cloth in plant juice that has been diluted with water. Gargles are prepared using plant juice diluted with water and sweetened with honey. The pure plant juice is used for ear drops.

Daily Dosage: Infusion dosage is 1 cup every 3 hours.

LITERATURE

Blazovics A, Lugasi A, Kemeny T, Hagymasi K, Kery. Membrane stabilising effects of natural polyphenols and flavonoids from Sempervivum tectorum on hepatic microsomal mixed-function oxidase system in hyperlipidemic rats. *J Ethnopharmacol* 73(3); 479-485. 2000

Blazovics A, Pronai L, Feher J, Kery A, Petri G. A Natural Antitoxidant Extract from *Sempervivum tectorum. Phytother Res.* 7 (1); 95-97. 1993Blazovics A, Feher J, Feher E, Kery A, Petri G. Liver Protecting and Lipid Lowering Effects of *Sempervivum tectorum* Extract in the Rat. *Phytother Res.* 7 (1); 98-100. 1993

Kern W, List PH, Hörhammer L (Hrsg.), Hagers Handbuch der Pharmazeutischen Praxis, 4. Aufl., Bde 1-8: Springer Verlag Berlin, Heidelberg, New York, 1969.

Madaus G, Lehrbuch der Biologischen Arzneimittel, Bde 1-3, Nachdruck, Georg Olms Verlag Hildesheim 1979.

Humulus lupulus

See Hops

Hwema Bark

Corynanthe pachyceras

DESCRIPTION

Medicinal Parts: The medicinal part of the plant is the bark.

Flower and Fruit: The inflorescence is an apical, up to 10-cm long panicle. The calyx has 4 short tips. The corolla tube is white and urn-shaped with 4 narrow, approximately 2-mm long lobes. The lobes have globular appendages, with 4 stamens, and a 2-chambered ovary. The fruit is 7 to 10 mm long and 2 to 4 mm wide, a loculicidal capsule, which is black when ripe, with numerous double slit winged seeds.

Leaves and Trunk: Corynanthe pachyceras is a tree that grows up to 20 m high. The leaves paperlike are opposite, with simple lamina. The lamina grow from 15 to 25 cm long and 5 to 7 cm wide. They are elongate-ovate with approximately 12 mm long stipules. The branches are glabrous and the trunk bark is dark green to reddish brown.

Habitat: Tropical Africa

Production: Hwema bark is the dried bark of *Corynanthe pachyceras*. It is dried in the sun or drying cupboard with circulating air at temperatures less than 70° C after harvesting.

Not to be Confused With: Incorrect identification can occur with *Cinchonae cortex* and sometimes with Yohimbe Cortex.

ACTIONS AND PHARMACOLOGY

COMPOUNDS

Indole alkaloids of the beta-carboline and oxindole type: chief alkaloids corynanthine (1.2%) and corynantheidine, including as well, corynanthidine (alpha-yohimbine), beta-yohimbine, corynantheine, dihydrocorynantheine, corynoxine, corynoxeine

EFFECTS

The alkaloid-containing drug (yohimbine-corynantheine type) affects the CNS by inhibiting motility in animal experiments. The drug is spasmolytic, hypotensive, and also mildly analgesic and locally anesthetic in effect.

INDICATIONS AND USAGE

Unproven Uses: In folk medicine, Hwema Bark preparations are used for fever and malaria (infusion), leprosy (decoction), colds, and to lower blood pressure (dry extract).

PRECAUTIONS AND ADVERSE REACTIONS

No health hazards are known in conjunction with the proper administration of designated therapeutic dosages. The LD50 in mice was determined to be 4.9 mg dry extract/kg body weight, I.V. The symptoms observed included convulsions and dyspnea.

OVERDOSAGE

Overdoses among humans could conceivably lead to signs of poisoning.

DOSAGE

Mode of Administration: Whole and cut drug, liquid and solid preparations for internal use; solid preparations for external use.

Preparation: To prepare a dry extract (10:1), the bark powder is succussed for 30 minutes at 95°C with a 10-fold amount of isotonic Nacl solution. It is filtered after cooling and the solution is concentrated to double the weight of the drug. Freeze-drying follows a 48-hour clarification period. This produces a brown powder. Drug:native dry extract is 10:1.

Daily Dosage: Dry extract — 200 mg 1 to 4 times daily.

How Supplied: Tablets, capsules, suppositories, and drink ampules.

Storage: Hwema Bark should be stored in a dry place.

LITERATURE

Hänsel R, Keller K, Rimpler H, Schneider G (Ed) Hagers Handbuch der Pharmazeutischen Praxis. 5. Aufl., Bde 4 - 6 (Drogen), Springer Verlag Berlin, Heidelberg, New York, 1992-1994

Hydnocarpus species

See Chaulmoogra

Hydrangea

Hydrangea arborescens

DESCRIPTION

Medicinal Parts: The medicinal parts are the dried rhizome and the roots.

Flower and Fruit: The inflorescence is flat cymes of umbels with creamy white flowers. They are androgynous or completely sexless and have inferior ovaries. The fruit is a schizocarp or capsule.

Leaves, Stem, and Root: Hydrangea is a marsh plant, a bush up to 3 m high whose leaves are only pubescent on the veins of the undersides. The petiole is 2 to 5 cm long. The leaves are simple or lobed and opposite. There are no stipules. The bark is rough and tends to peel off. The roots are of various lengths and widths. They are pale gray on the outside and solid with a slight splitting structure.

Habitat: Indigenous to the eastern U.S. as far south as Florida.

Production: Hydrangea root is the root of *Hydrangea arborescens*.

Other Names: Seven Barks

ACTIONS AND PHARMACOLOGY

COMPOUNDS

Saponins

Flavonolids: including, among others, rutin

Volatile oil

Isocoumarin derivatives: including, among others, hydrangenol

EFFECTS

The drug has a diuretic effect.

INDICATIONS AND USAGE

Unproven Uses: Hydrangea is used in the treatment of conditions of the urinary tract, particularly bladder and kidney stones.

PRECAUTIONS AND ADVERSE REACTIONS

No health hazards or side effects are known in conjunction with the proper administration of designated therapeutic dosages. According to information in older medical literature, the intake of larger dosages can lead to dizziness, feelings of constriction in the chest, and central nervous system disorders. The plant has a weak potential for sensitization (chief allergen hydrangenol).

DOSAGE

Mode of Administration: As a liquid extract, in compounded preparations.

LITERATURE

Frohne D, Pfänder HJ, Giftpflanzen - Ein Handbuch für Apotheker, Toxikologen und Biologen, 4. Aufl., Wiss. Verlags-Ges. Stuttgart 1997.

Hausen B, Allergiepflanzen, Pflanzenallergene, ecomed Verlagsgesellsch. mbH, Landsberg 1988.

Kern W, List PH, Hörhammer L (Hrsg.), Hagers Handbuch der Pharmazeutischen Praxis, 4. Aufl., Bde 1-8, Springer Verlag Berlin, Heidelberg, New York, 1969.

Leung AY, Encyclopedia of Common Natural Ingredients Used in Food, Drugs and Cosmetics, John Wiley & Sons Inc., New York 1980.

Lewin L, Gifte und Vergiftungen, 6. Aufl., Nachdruck, Haug Verlag, Heidelberg 1992.

Madaus G, Lehrbuch der Biologischen Arzneimittel, Bde 1-3, Nachdruck, Georg Olms Verlag Hildesheim 1979.

Roth L, Daunderer M, Kormann K, Giftpflanzen, Pflanzengifte, 4. Aufl., Ecomed Fachverlag Landsberg Lech 1993.

Hydrangea arborescens

See Hydrangea

Hydrastis canadensis

See Goldenseal

Hyoscyamus niger

See Henbane

Hypericum perforatum

See St. John's Wort

Hypoxis rooperi

See African Potato

Hyssop

Hyssopus officinalis

DESCRIPTION

Medicinal Parts: The medicinal parts are the leaves, the flower tips, and the essential oil.

Flower and Fruit: The dark-blue bilabiate flowers are medium-sized false whorls in one-sided, terminal, leafy racemes. The calyx is downy, with 5 tips, and glabrous inside. There are 4 stamens, which are turned away from each other and extend far above the perianth. The style is very long.

Leaves, Stem, and Root: The plant is an evergreen subshrub about 60 cm high. The stem is erect, quadrangular, shrubby, and branched. The leaves are sessile, lanceolate, acute, entire-margined, punctate, glabrous, dark green, and paler beneath.

Characteristics: The plant has a weak sweetish smell. The taste is bitter.

Habitat: The plant is indigenous to southern Europe and grows wild in the Mediterranean region. It is cultivated elsewhere.

Production: Hyssop herb consists of the fresh or dried aboveground parts of *Hyssopus officinalis*. Hyssop oil consists of the essential oil of *Hyssopus officinalis*, obtained by steam distillation.

ACTIONS AND PHARMACOLOGY

COMPOUNDS

In the foliage:

Volatile oil

Tannins

Bitter principles: including, among others, marubiin

Flavonoids: glycosides of hesperidin and diosmetin

In the volatile oil:

Chief components: 1-pinocamphone, isocamphone, pinocarvone, alpha- and beta-pinene

EFFECTS

1-pinocamphone and isopinocamphone are the toxically active constituents of the drug. The oil has an antimicrobial and anthelmintic effect. Extracts of the leaves are antimicrobial, antiviral (*herpes simplex*) and mildly spasmolytic.

INDICATIONS AND USAGE

Unproven Uses: Preparations of Hyssop herb are used for the gentle stimulation of circulation, for intestinal catarrhs, for diseases of the respiratory tract, and colds.

PRECAUTIONS AND ADVERSE REACTIONS

General: No health hazards are known in conjunction with the proper administration of designated therapeutic dosages. Isolated cases of tonic-clonic spasms have been observed among adults after intake of 10 to 30 drops of the volatile oil over a number of days (2 to 3 drops for children).

Pregnancy: Not to be used during pregnancy.

DOSAGE

Mode of Administration: Hyssop herb preparations are available as capsules for internal use.

How Supplied:

Capsules – 445 mg

Liquid extract

LITERATURE

Kern W, List PH, Hörhammer L (Hrsg.), Hagers Handbuch der Pharmazeutischen Praxis, 4. Aufl., Bde. 1-8, Springer Verlag Berlin, Heidelberg, New York, 1969.

Leung AY, Encyclopedia of Common Natural Ingredients Used in Food, Drugs and Cosmetics, John Wiley & Sons Inc., New York 1980.

Opdyke DLJ, *Food Cosmet Toxicol* 16 (Suppl. 1):787. 1978

Sattar AA et al. Chemical composition and biological activity of leaf exudates from some Lamiaceae plants. *Pharmazie* 50; 62-65. 1995

Hyssopus officinalis

See Hyssop

Iberis amara

See Bitter Candytuft

Iceland Moss

Cetraria islandica

DESCRIPTION

Medicinal Parts: The medicinal part is the dried thallus commonly known as Iceland Moss.

Flower and Fruit: Cetraria islandica is a lichen that grows on the ground and has a stiff, curling thallus. The thallus is from 2 to 6 cm high, erect, dichotomously branched, with a 1- to 10-cm wide section. The upper surface is olive-green or brown, the underside is whitish to light brownish. The margins are covered in 0.5 mm long papilla, which contain the reproductive parts.

Characteristics: Iceland Moss tastes bitter, and when wet, has a smell reminiscent of seaweed.

Habitat: Grows in the boreal, alpine and Arctic regions of the Northern Hemisphere and in some regions of the Southern Hemisphere.

Production: Iceland Moss consists of the dried thallus of *Cetraria islandica* as well as its preparations. It is collected in the wild, then air-dried, moistened, cut and redried.

Other Names: Cetraria, Eryngo-Leaved Liverwort, Iceland Lichen

ACTIONS AND PHARMACOLOGY

COMPOUNDS

Mucilages, glucans (50%): lichenan (lichenan), isolichenan (isolichenan)

Aromatic lichen acids (2-3%): fumarprototcetraric acid, protocetraric acid, cetraric acid

Aliphatic lichen acids (1.0-1.5%): esp. protolichesteric acid

EFFECTS

The bitter organic acids have an antibiotic effect. It is also a demulcent and a mild antimicrobial.

The drug has an demulcent effect due to the sesquitering action of the polysaccharides. An ethanol precipitation of the aqueous extract containing lichenan and isolichenan demonstrated an antitumoural effect in animal tests.

INDICATIONS AND USAGE

Approved by Commission E:

- Cough/bronchitis
- Dyspeptic complaints
- Inflammation of the mouth and pharynx
- Loss of appetite

Unproven Uses: Iceland Moss is also used for irritation of the oral and pharyngeal mucous membranes; loss of appetite and gastroenteritis (the bitter organic acids). In folk medicine, the drug has been used for kidney and bladder complaints, gastric conditions, nausea and vomiting (in particular in pregnancy and with migraine), bronchitis, whooping cough, and diarrhea. It is also used externally for poorly healing wounds.

Homeopathic Uses: Cetraria islandica is used to treat bronchitis.

PRECAUTIONS AND ADVERSE REACTIONS

No health hazards or side effects are known in conjunction with the proper administration of designated therapeutic dosages. In rare cases, external administration of the drug led to sensitization.

DOSAGE

Mode of Administration: Comminuted thallus for infusions and other galenic formulations for internal use; comminuted thallus preferably for cold maceration and other bitter-tasting preparations for internal use.

Preparation: To prepare an infusion, pour boiling water over 1.5 to 2.5 g of comminuted drug and strain after 10 minutes (1 teaspoonful = 1.3 g of drug); infusion may be sweetened.

Daily Dosage: The average daily dose is 4 to 6 g. Single dose: 1.5 g drug in a teacup.

Homeopathic Dosage: 5 drops, 1 tablet, 10 globules every 30 to 60 minutes (acute) or 1 to 3 times daily (chronic); parenterally: 1 to 2 mL sc acute: 3 times daily; chronic: once daily (HAB1).

Storage: Store in the dark and well-sealed containers.

LITERATURE

Ingolfsdottir K, Breu W, Huneck S, Gudjonsdottir GA, M,ller-Jakic B, Wagner H. In vitro inhibition of 5-Lipoxygenase by protolichsternic acid from *Cetraria islandica. Phytomedicine* 1; 187-191. 1994

Ingolfsdottir K, Jurcic K, Fischer B, Wagner H. Immunologically Active Polysaccharide from *Cetraria islandica. Planta Med.* 60; 527-531. 1994

Krämer P, Wincierz U, Grübler G, Tschakert J, Voelter W, Mayer H. Rational Approach to Fractionation, Isolation, and Characterization of Polysaccharides from Lichen *Cetraria islandica. Arzneim Forsch.* 45 (6); 726-731. 1995

Nagell A, Grün TA. Reinheitspr, fung an pflanzlichen Rohstoffen und daraus hergestellten Zubereitungen. *Pharm Ind.* 59 (8); 706-711. 1997

Pengsuparp Th, et al., Mechanistic evaluation of new plant-derived compounds that inhibit HIV-1 reverse transcriptase. In: *JNP* 58(7):1024-1031. 1995.

Wunderer H, Zentral und peripher wirksame Antitussiva: eine kritische Übersicht. In: *PZ* 142(11):847-852. 1997.

Ignatius Beans

Strychnos ignatii

DESCRIPTION

Medicinal Parts: The medicinal parts are the ripe seeds and the dried root bark.

Flower and Fruit: The flowers are in dense, axillary thyrses. Their parts are arranged in fives. They are greenish-white, pubescent, and have a 2-valved superior ovary. The fruit is a golden-yellow berry. The berry is up to 13 cm wide and has a hard exocarp. The fruit pulp is yellow and contains up to 40 seeds. The seeds are 2 to 3 cm long by 2 cm wide, oval or rounded-angular, obtuse, and very hard.

Leaves, Stem, and Root: The plant is a climbing shrub with hooked stems that are up to 20 m long. It is occasionally a small tree. The trunk is up to 10 cm thick. It bears leaves that are up to 25 cm long, broad-ovate, opposite, and short-petioled.

Habitat: The plant is common all over southeastern Asia and is cultivated there; especially in Vietnam and the Philippines.

Production: Ignatius beans are the seeds of *Strychnos ignatii*.

Not to be Confused With: The seeds of *S lanata* and *S multiflora* were once treated in the same manner as Ignatii seeds.

ACTIONS AND PHARMACOLOGY

COMPOUNDS

Indole alkaloids (2.5-5.6%): chief alkaloid strychnine (share 45-60%), in addition, above all, brucine, further including, among others, 12-hydroxystrychnine, alpha-colubrine, icajine, vomicine, novacine. There are also chemical strains for which brucine predominates, and others in which strychnine occurs only in traces.

Fatty oil

EFFECTS

The drug, which contains strychnine and brucine, is psychoanaleptic (see Nux Vomica).

INDICATIONS AND USAGE

Unproven Uses: Preparations made of the Ignatius Bean are used to treat faintness. Therapeutic use as a bitter or tonic is not recommended.

Homeopathic Uses: The drug is used for nervous disorders, cramps in hollow organs and muscles, and depressive states.

PRECAUTIONS AND ADVERSE REACTIONS

The drug is severely toxic due to the strychnine content and should not be administered in allopathic medicine.

OVERDOSAGE

Symptoms of poisoning can occur after ingestion of one bean. Strychnine doses of as little as 1.5 mg (30-50 mg of the drug) initially cause restlessness, feelings of anxiety, heightening of sense perception, enhanced reflexes, equilibrium disorders and painful stiffness of the neck and back musculature. Later, twitching, tonic spasms of the masseter and neck musculature, and finally, painful convulsions of the entire body are triggered by visual or tactile stimulation. Dyspnea comes following spasm of the breathing musculature. Death occurs through suffocation or exhaustion. The lethal dosage for an adult is approximately 50 mg strychnine (1-2 gm of the drug). Chronic intake of subconvulsive dosages can also lead to death under similar conditions after a period of weeks. This is due to an accumulation of drug in the body, particularly in those who have liver damage.

Following the administration of a watery suspension of activated charcoal, the therapy for poisoning consists of keeping external stimulation to a minimum through placement in a quiet, warm, darkened room. Convulsions should be treated with dosages of diazepam or barbital (IV). High-calorie glucose infusions should also be given. Intubation and oxygen respiration may also be required. Gastric lavage should be avoided, due to the danger of triggering convulsions. Analeptics or phenothiazines should not be administered. Because of the possibility of unwanted effects occurring in conjunction with the administration of therapeutic dosages, one should forgo any administration of the drug.

DOSAGE

Mode of Administration: It is used in the manufacture of strychnine and brucine.

Daily Dosage: If the drug is taken internally, the maximum single dose is 0.1 gm; the maximum daily dosage is 0.3 gm.

Homeopathic Dosage: from D4: 5 drops, 1 tablet, or 10 globules every 30 to 60 minutes (acute) or 1 to 3 times daily (chronic); parenterally: 1 to 2 mL sc, acute: 3 times daily; chronic: once a day (HAB1).

Storage: Mark the container as ''poisonous'' and keep tightly sealed; protect the drug from cool air and light.

LITERATURE

Hänsel R, Keller K, Rimpler H, Schneider G (Hrsg.), Hagers Handbuch der Pharmazeutischen Praxis, 5. Aufl., Bde 4-6 (Drogen): Springer Verlag Berlin, Heidelberg, New York, 1992-1994.

Lewin L, Gifte und Vergiftungen, 6. Aufl., Nachdruck, Haug Verlag, Heidelberg 1992.

Madaus G, Lehrbuch der Biologischen Arzneimittel, Bde 1-3, Nachdruck, Georg Olms Verlag Hildesheim 1979.

Marini-Bettolo GB, Advances in the research of curare and Strychnos. In: *Rend Accad Naz* 40:1975-1976, 1-2, 61-76. 1977.

Roth L, Daunderer M, Kormann K, Giftpflanzen, Pflanzengifte, 4. Aufl., Ecomed Fachverlag Landsberg Lech 1993.

Teuscher E, Lindequist U, Biogene Gifte - Biologie, Chemie, Pharmakologie, 2. Aufl., Fischer Verlag Stuttgart 1994.

Wagner H, Wiesenauer M, Phytotherapie. Phytopharmaka und pflanzliche Homöopathika, Fischer-Verlag, Stuttgart, Jena, New York 1995.

Ilex aquifolium

See Holly

Ilex paraguariensis

See Maté

Illicium verum

See Star Anise

Immortelle

Helichrysum arenarium

DESCRIPTION

Medicinal Parts: The medicinal parts are the composite heads and the whole of the flowering plant.

Flower and Fruit: The small orange flowers are in dense clustered cymes. The bracts are dry-membranous and usually lemon yellow. All the florets are tubular and funnel-shaped. The fruit is pentangular with a tuft of hair.

Leaves, Stem, and Root: The plant grows from 10 to 30 cm high. The stem is erect, unbranched, and gray-tomentose. The leaves are alternate. The lower leaves are spatulate and the upper ones lanceolate, acute and the same color as the stem.

Characteristics: Immortelle has a weak aroma.

Habitat: The plant grows in Europe and the U.S.

Production: Immortelle consists of the dried flowers of *Helichrysum arenarium* gathered shortly before fully unfolding.

Not to be Confused With: Confusion can arise with the capitula of *Helichrysum stoechas* and *Helichrysum augustifolium.*

Other Names: Common Shrubby Everlasting, Eternal Flower, Goldilocks, Sandy Immortelles, Yellow Chaste Weed

ACTIONS AND PHARMACOLOGY

COMPOUNDS

Flavonoids: in particular isosalipurposide (intensive yellow chalcone glycoside), naringenin-5-glucosyl-glucoside, helichrysin A and B (C-2-enantiomeric narigenin-5-O-glucosides, B-salipurposide)

Phthalides: including 5-methoxy-7-hydroxy-phthalides and their monoglucoside

Alpha-pyrone derivatives: arenole, homoarenole

Sesquiterpene bitter principles

Volatile oil (traces)

Caffeic acid derivatives

EFFECTS

The drug has antibacterial principles, and is mildly choleretic and mildly spasmolytic.

INDICATIONS AND USAGE

Approved by Commission E:

- Dyspeptic complaints

Unproven Uses: The drug is used as an adjunct in the treatment of chronic cholecystitis and gallbladder complaints with accompanying cramps. In folk medicine, it is used as a diuretic.

CONTRAINDICATIONS

Because of the bile-stimulating effect of the drug, it is not to be administered when there is biliary obstruction. The presence of gallstone illnesses can lead to colic.

PRECAUTIONS AND ADVERSE REACTIONS

Health risks or side effects following the proper administration of designated therapeutic dosages are not recorded.

DOSAGE

Mode of Administration: Immortelle is used as a comminuted herb for infusions and other galenic preparations for internal use. Pharmaceutical cholagogues contain extracts of the drug. It is an inactive ingredient in many tea specialties.

How Supplied: Forms of commercial pharmaceutical preparations include teas, drops and compound preparations.

Preparation: To make an infusion, pour boiling water over 2 teaspoonfuls of the drug (3 to 4 g). Allow to stand for 10 minutes and then strain. Drink throughout the day and make a fresh batch daily.

Daily Dosage: The average daily dose is 3 g of drug.

Storage: Store Immortelle protected from light and moisture.

LITERATURE

Bayerl C, Jung EG. Allergic contact dermatitis from Aristochol®, a phytotherapeutic cholagogue. *Contact Dermatitis* 34; 222-223. 1996

Dombrowicz E, Swiatek L, Kopycki W. Phenolic acids in Inflorescentia Helichrysi and Herba Hieracii pilosellae. *Pharmazie* 47; 469-370. 1992

Kern W, List PH, Hörhammer L (Hrsg.), Hagers Handbuch der Pharmazeutischen Praxis, 4. Aufl., Bde. 1-8, Springer Verlag Berlin, Heidelberg, New York, 1969.

Leung AY, Encyclopedia of Common Natural Ingredients Used in Food, Drugs and Cosmetics, John Wiley & Sons Inc., New York 1980.

Madaus G, Lehrbuch der Biologischen Arzneimittel, Bde 1-3, Nachdruck, Georg Olms Verlag Hildesheim 1979.

Teuscher E, Biogene Arzneimittel, 5. Aufl., Wiss. Verlagsges. mbH Stuttgart 1997.

Wichtl M (Hrsg.), Teedrogen, 4. Aufl., Wiss. Verlagsges. Stuttgart 1997.

Impatiens biflora

See Jewel Weed

Indian Hemp

Apocynum cannabinum

DESCRIPTION

Medicinal Parts: The medicinal parts are the root and the juice obtained from the fresh plant.

Flower and Fruit: The small whitish-green, occasionally pink to violet flowers are on pods that grow to 2 to 4 mm in length. The calyx is deeply lobed and half as long as the corolla. The petals are oblong-lanceolate. The tufts of hair on the seeds are 2 to 3 cm long.

Leaves, Stem, and Root: Indian Hemp is a perennial that grows up to 2 m tall. It has an erect stem, which branches at the top. The whole plant is glabrous or downy. The short-petioled leaves are 5 to 11 cm long, yellowish-green and oblong or oblong-ovoid. The tips of the leaves are initially rounded and then terminate abruptly in a thorny tip.

Characteristics: The plant has an acrid taste and is to a certain degree poisonous.

Habitat: The plant is found mostly in the U.S. and Canada.

Not to be Confused With: Indian Hemp (*Cannabis indica*), though both species contain latex and their tough, fibrous bark can be used as a substitute for hemp, hence the name.

Production: Indian Hemp root is the root of *Apocynum cannabinum*, which is gathered (and sometimes dried) in autumn. The plant is cultivated as a crop in Germany and Russia.

Other Names: Bitterroot, Catchfly, Dogbane, Fly-Trap, Honeybloom, Milk Ipecac, Milkweed, Mountain Hemp, Wallflower, Wild Cotton, Canadian Hemp

ACTIONS AND PHARMACOLOGY

COMPOUNDS

Cardioactive steroid glycosides (cardenolids): in particular cymarin, k-strophantoside, apocannoside, cynocannoside

EFFECTS

The high content of cardenolide glycosides causes bradycardia and increased contraction of the heart. Hypotention and rebound vagotonia hypertension can occur. The drug increases diuresis and stimulation of the vasomotor centers. It causes more severe irritation of the intestinal mucous membrane than digitalis and strophantus preparations. It has a lower therapeutic effect on atrial fibrillation than digitalis.

Cardenollide glycoside cymine has an effect that is similar but generally weaker than glycoside strophantine, with the exception of the stronger diuretic effect in edema. It is less cumulative.

INDICATIONS AND USAGE

Unproven Uses: The juice of the fresh plant is used in the treatment of condylomatosis and warts. American Indians use the roots for asthma, dropsy, coughs, syphilis, and rheumatism. In folk medicine, the root is used to strengthen weak heart muscles following pneumonia, valvular insufficiency, and senile heart. It is also used as a diuretic.

Homeopathic Uses: Homeopathic uses include cardiac insufficiency, renal inflammation with edema, and vomiting with diarrhea.

PRECAUTIONS AND ADVERSE REACTIONS

The drug should be administered only by someone who is expert in its use. Topical irritation of the mucous membrane of the alimentary canal, accompanied by nausea and vomiting, is more common than in other drugs containing cardenolid glycosides. Vomiting and gastrointestinal irritations can occur, even with the administration of therapeutic doses of the drug because of the mucous membrane-irritating resin fraction.

OVERDOSAGE

For possible symptoms of overdose and treatment of poisonings see Digitalis folium. Despite the strong efficacy of the drug's cardioactive steroid glycosides in parenteral application, serious poisoning in the course of peroral administration is unlikely, due to the low resorption rate.

DOSAGE

Daily Dosage: The average daily dose of the liquid extract is 10 to 30 drops to be taken 3 times daily or 0.3 to 0.6 mL of a 1:10 tincture.

Homeopathic Dosage: 5 drops, 1 tablet, or 10 globules every 30 to 60 minutes (acute) or every 1 to 3 days (chronic); Parenterally: 1 to 2 mL 3 times daily sc (HAB1).

Storage: Store in secure area as the drug is poisonous.

LITERATURE

Abe F, Yamauchi T. Cardenoliide Glycosides from the Roots of *Apocynum cannabinum. Chem Pharm Bull.* 42 (10); 2028-2031. 1994

Hänsel R, Keller K, Rimpler H, Schneider G (Hrsg.), Hagers Handbuch der Pharmazeutischen Praxis, 5. Aufl., Bde 4-6 (Drogen): Springer Verlag Berlin, Heidelberg, New York, 1992-1994.

Lewin L, Gifte und Vergiftungen, 6. Aufl., Nachdruck, Haug Verlag, Heidelberg 1992.

Madaus G, Lehrbuch der Biologischen Arzneimittel, Bde 1-3, Nachdruck, Georg Olms Verlag Hildesheim 1979.

Roth L, Daunderer M, Kormann K, Giftpflanzen, Pflanzengifte, 4. Aufl., Ecomed Fachverlag Landsberg Lech 1993.

Teuscher E, Lindequist U, Biogene Gifte - Biologie, Chemie, Pharmakologie, 2. Aufl., Fischer Verlag Stuttgart 1994.

Teuscher E, Biogene Arzneimittel, 5. Aufl., Wiss. Verlagsges. Stuttgart 1997.

Wagner H, Wiesenauer M, Phytotherapie. Phytopharmaka und pflanzliche Homöopathika, Fischer-Verlag, Stuttgart, Jena, New York 1995.

Indian Nettle

Acalypha indica

DESCRIPTION

Medicinal Parts: The medicinal part of the plant is the whole flowering plant.

Flower and Fruit: The inflorescence is spikelike, with 3 to 7 female flowers below, which consist only of a tricarpeled ovary with 3 styles. The male flowers are above these with 4 sepals and 8 stamens. On the tips of the young flower shoots are T-shaped, hairy structures approximately 2 mm wide with 2 side openings. The fruit is a 3-chambered capsule with 3 gray-brown seeds of approximately 1 mm diameter.

Leaves, Stem, and Root: Indian nettle is an annual, upright, nettlelike diclinous, monoecious herb, which grows up to 60 cm high. The leaves are alternate, long-petiolate, round to rhomboid, 2 to 6 cm long, 1.5 to 5 cm wide narrowing to the petiole. They are matte above, glossy beneath with strongly protruding ribs, dentate at the front and smooth toward the base. The margin, petiole and ribs are weakly pubescent with 2 awl-like stipules. The stem is usually unbranched and pubescent. The main root is unbranched with thin secondary roots.

Habitat: The plant comes from India, Indochina and Ethiopia.

Other Names: Cat's Nettle

Production: Indian nettle is the whole fresh plant of *Acalypha indica* collected during the flowering season and dried.

ACTIONS AND PHARMACOLOGY

COMPOUNDS

Cyanogenic glycosides: acalyphin (0.3%, 3-cyanopyridone derivative)

Tannins: including tri-O-methyl ellagic acid

Volatile oil

EFFECTS

The drug is hemostyptic and antibacterial in effect (cyanogenic glucoside acalyphine). In vitro, proof of an acceleration of blood coagulation exists, which is due to the high levels of calcium salts. The leaf latex is said to have emetic and expectorant effects upon children. When administered as a suppository for constipation, it is said to immediately relax the contracted anal sphincter.

INDICATIONS AND USAGE

Unproven Uses: Internally used for worm infestation and constipation, for pregnant women, also for upset stomach and bronchitis. Externally used for eczema and skin rashes, ear ache (decoction), tumors (juice), as well as for cuts and other wounds, and also for inflammation of the joints (cut leaves and stems).

Indian Medicine: Preparations are used for skin ulcers, bronchitis, constipation, and arthralgia.

PRECAUTIONS AND ADVERSE REACTIONS

No health hazards or side effects other than possible gastric irritation are known in conjunction with the proper administration of designated therapeutic dosages. Dermatitis has been observed following skin contact with the latex of the fresh plant. Cyanide poisonings from the drug are unlikely, due to the relatively low levels of cyanogenic glycoside content and the lack of stimuli leading to ingestion.

OVERDOSAGE

In animal experiments (rabbits), administration of large quantities of the drug led to gastrointestinal inflammation and to a change in blood color to chocolate-brown, indicating the presence of additional toxic substances.

DOSAGE

Mode of Administration: Liquid preparations and other galenic preparations for internal use and liquid preparations for external use.

Preparation:

Decoction: 100 g drug to 1 liter water
Extract: 1000 g drug to 1000 ml 90% ethanol (V/V)
Infusion: 50 g drug to 1 liter water
Juice: 800 g drug to 800 ml water and 200 mL ethanol 90%
Tincture: 125 g drug to 1000 mL ethanol 90% (V/V)

Daily Dosage:

Decoction – single dose: 15 to 30 mL
Extract – single dose: 0.3 to 2 mL
Infusion – single dose: 15 to 30 mL
Juice – single dose: 0.3 to 2 mL
Tincture – single dose: 2 to 4 mL

LITERATURE

Blaschek W, Hänsel R, Keller K, Reichling J, Rimpler G, Schneider G (Eds), Hagers Handbuch der Pharmazeutischen Praxis. Folgebände 1 und 2. Drogen A-Z. Springer. Berlin, Heidelberg 1998.

Senanayake N, Sanmuganathan PS, *Acalypha indica* induced haemolysis in G6PD deficiency. *Ceylon Med* J, 26: Jan. 1996

Senanayake N, Sanmuganathan PS, Acute intravascular haemolysis in glucose-6-phosphate dehydrogenase deficient patients following ingestion of herbal broth containing *Acalypha indica. Trop Doct*, 26:32, Jan. 1996

Shanmugasundaram KR, Seethapathy PG, Shanmugasundaram ER, Anna Pavala Sindhooram - an antiatherosclerotic Indian drug. *J Ethnopharmacol*, 7:247-65, May. 1983

Indian Physic

Gillenia trifoliata

DESCRIPTION

Medicinal Parts: The medicinal part is the dried and pulverized root bark.

Flower and Fruit: The flowers are white and tinged with red. They are arranged in a few loose, terminal panicles.

Leaves, Stem, and Root: This perennial herb has irregular, cylindrical roots, which are usually transversely grooved and up to 15 cm long. The external surface is blackish, and the transverse section shows a thick, reddish bark, which easily separates from the white woody center. Sprouting from the root are multiple stems 60 to 90 cm high. The leaves and leaflets have various forms.

Characteristics: Indian Physic is odorless, but the plant has a pleasantly bitter taste.

Habitat: The plant is indigenous to the eastern U.S., and is cultivated in Europe and elsewhere.

Production: Indian Physic is the root bark *of Gillenia trifoliata.*

Other Names: Indian Hippo, Bowman's Root, American Ipecacuanha, Gillenia

ACTIONS AND PHARMACOLOGY

COMPOUNDS

Resins

Gillein (Gillenin)

The constituents of the drug have not been fully investigated.

EFFECTS

The drug is an expectorant, emetic and a ''blood purifier.''

INDICATIONS AND USAGE

Unproven Uses: The drug is used in the treatment of digestive disorders, particularly in cases in which a safe and reliable emetic is required.

PRECAUTIONS AND ADVERSE REACTIONS

Health risks or side effects following the proper administration of designated therapeutic dosages are not recorded.

DOSAGE

Mode of Administration: The drug is available as a powder, an infusion or a tonic for internal use.

LITERATURE

Kern W, List PH, Hörhammer L (Hrsg.), Hagers Handbuch der Pharmazeutischen Praxis, 4. Aufl., Bde 1-8, Springer Verlag Berlin, Heidelberg, New York, 1969.

Indian Squill

Urginea indica

DESCRIPTION

Medicinal Parts: The parts used medicinally are the horizontal and vertically cut strips of the dried, middle, fleshy onion layers of the white flowering variety (which are collected after flowering) as well as the fresh, fleshy onion layers of the white and red varieties.

Flower and Fruit: The inflorescence is a 10 to 60 cm long, loose raceme with 4 to 30 flowers in the axils of the bracts, which usually drop before the flower. The peduncle is upright, up to 1 m high, cylindrical, ribbed, glabrous, and reddish-brown. The pedicle is up to 3.5 cm long, splayed when in flower and upright when the fruit is ripe. The flowers are radial with 6 corollalike tepals, which are 5 to 12 mm long, campanulate, and reddish-green. There are 6 stamens, 3 fused carpels, and a 3-chambered, superior ovary. The fruit is a capsule, 10 to 25 cm long, with 12 to 30 seeds. The seeds are clavate to elliptical with a diameter of 4 to 10 mm, dark brown to black, with orbicular, translucent wings.

Leaves, Stem, and Root: Indian squill is a herbaceous perennial bulb plant that reaches up to 35 cm. The flowering varieties might reach up to 1 m high. The leaves are basal, in 2 rows, 13 to 35 cm long, 6 to 30 mm wide, linear to lanceolate or sword-shaped, flat, parallel-veined, glabrous, and whorled at the base. The bulb is whitish, globose to ovoid with a diameter of 3 to 7 cm. The outer layer is membranous, the inner one fleshy.

Characteristics: The bulb tastes bitter; slimy.

Habitat: India and Sri Lanka

Production: Indian squill is the dried and cut bulb of *Urginea indica* freed from the outer layers shortly after harvesting. The bulbs are dug up, cleaned and cut into quarters. Then the core is removed and the remaining pieces are dried in the sun or over a fire until the weight is reduced by 80%.

Not to be Confused With: Because of the similarity in name, it can be confused with *Scilla indica*.

Other Names: South Indian Squill

ACTIONS AND PHARMACOLOGY

COMPOUNDS

Cardioactive steroid glycosides (bufadienolids, 0.1 to 1.5%): chief components proscillaridin A and scillaren A, including as well scillipheoside, scillarenine-bis-alpha-rhamnoside, scillicyanogenine glucoside, scillicyanosidine glucoside, scilliglaucosidine glucoside

Mucilages (50%, glucomannoxylans)

Steroids: sterols, including beta-sitosterol, campesterol, stigmasterol

EFFECTS

The drug's content levels of cardioactive glycosides explain the administration in the presence of cardiac insufficiency and cardio-conditioned edema formation. The expectorant may be due the drug's effect as a mild irritant of the gastrointestinal tract combined with an increase in secretions of the bronchial system. The drug's administration as an antirheumatic appears plausible, due to the skin-irritating effect of the oxalate raphides it contains.

INDICATIONS AND USAGE

Unproven Uses: For chronic bronchitis, asthma, and cardiac insufficiency as a treatment of second choice in the case of hypersensitivity to digitalis.

Indian Medicine: For edema, digestion disturbances, menstruation disorders, worm infestation, chronic bronchitis, asthma, rheumatism, and skin conditions.

CONTRAINDICATIONS

Neither the drug nor pure glycosides should be administered in the presence of first- and second-degree AV-Block, hypercalcemia, hypokalemia, hypertrophic cardiomyopathy, carotid sinus syndrome, ventricle tachycardia, thoracic aortic aneurysm, WPW syndrome.

PRECAUTIONS AND ADVERSE REACTIONS

General: No health hazards are known in conjunction with the proper administration of designated therapeutic dosages. Because of the limited therapeutic range of the cardioactive steroid glycosides, a number of patients receiving no more than therapeutic dosages might experience the following side effects: hypertonia in gastrointestinal area, loss of appetite, vomiting, diarrhea, headache, and irregular pulse. Contact with the latex of the fresh bulbs can lead to skin inflammation (Scilla dermatitis).

DRUG INTERACTIONS

POTENTIAL INTERACTIONS

The simultaneous administration of arrhythmogenic substances (sympathomimetics, methylxanthines, phosphodiesterase inhibitors, quinidine) increases the risk of cardiac arrhythmias.

OVERDOSAGE

Overdose could lead to hypertonia in gastrointestinal area, loss of appetite, vomiting, diarrhea, headache and irregular pulse along with the following:

— Heart: cardiac rhythm disorders as serious as life-threatening ventricular tachycardias or atrial tachycardias with AV block.

— CNS: dizziness, vision disorders, depressions, states of confusion, hallucinations, psychoses.

Lethal dosages lead to cardiac arrest or to asphyxiation. Because of the difficulties involved in standardizing the drug, the administration of pure glycosides is to be preferred (proscillaridin A).

The first-aid measures to be taken with poisonings are gastric lavage and instillation of activated charcoal. All other measures proceed according to the symptoms: careful potassium replacement for potassium loss; phenytoin as an antiarrhythmic for ectopic stimulation formation in the ventricle; lidocaine for ventricular extrasystole; atropine or orciprenaline for pronounced bradycardia. The prophylactic insertion of a cardiac pacemaker is recommended. Hemoperfusion for the elimination of the glycosides or cholestyramine administration for the interruption of the enterohepatic circulation are possible.

DOSAGE

Mode of Administration: Whole herb, cut drug, powdered drug and other galenic preparations for internal and external use.

Preparation: Liquid extract: 100 g drug are percolated with 70% ethanol and then evaporated to 850 mL; the rest is filled to 1000 ml again with 70% ethanol and filtered (BPC79).

Tincture: 100 g drug is macerated with 1000 mL 60% ethanol (BPC79).

Acetic acid maceration: 100 g drug is macerated with 1000 mL acetic acid in a closed vessel and then filtered. Finally the filtrate is heated and re-filtered after 7 days (BPC79).

Daily Dosage:

Drug: single dose: 60 to 200 mg; Tincture: 0.3 to 2 mL; Liquid extract: 0.06 to 0.2 mL; Acetic acid essence: 0.6 to 2 mL.

Storage: Store in a dry place and below 25°C.

LITERATURE

Hakim FS, Evans FJ. The potency and phytochemistry of Indian squill soft extract. *Pharm Acta Helv.* 51; 117-118. 1976

Hänsel R, Keller K, Rimpler H, Schneider G (Ed), Hagers Handbuch der Pharmazeutischen Praxis, 5. Aufl., Bde 4 - 6 (Drogen), Springer Verlag Berlin, Heidelberg, New York, 1992-1994

Inula britannica

See British Elecampane (Xuan-Fu-Hua)

Inula helenium

See Elecampane

Ipecac

Cephaelis ipecacuanha

DESCRIPTION

Medicinal Parts: The medicinal parts are the roots.

Flower and Fruit: The flowers are in terminal, capitulum-shaped inflorescences surrounded by 4 to 6 bracts. The individual florets have a 5-tipped calyx, ciliated at the tips with a white campanulate-conical, 5-tipped corolla. A bitter, dark purple, fleshy drupe develops from the 2-carpeled ovary.

Leaves, Stem, and Root: Cephaelis ipecacuanha is a perennial, evergreen, leafy plant about 40 cm high with a 2 to 4 mm thick rhizome from which sprout numerous 20 cm long fibrous roots. Some of these roots develop into tubers. The green stem may be creeping or ascending, simple or branched. It is somewhat quadrangular, occasionally bears adventitious roots. The opposite leaves are entire-margined, and the leaf blade, narrows into the short petiole. There are stipules at the base of the leaf, which are slit like awls and fused together with the petiole-like leaf sheath.

Habitat: Indigenous to the sparser woods of Brazil; cultivated in India and on the Malaysian archipelago.

Production: Ipecac is the root of *Cephaelis ipecacuanha*. The subterranean parts of the 3- t -4-year-old plants are quickly dried in the sun and then cut into pieces of 5 to 10 cm in length.

Other Names: Brazilian Ipecac, Ipecacuanha, Ipecacuanha Rio, Matto Grosso, Rio Ipecac

ACTIONS AND PHARMACOLOGY

COMPOUNDS

Isoquinoline alkaloids of the emetine type (2-4%): chief alkaloids emetine and cephaelin

Starch (30 to 40%)

EFFECTS

Emetine hydrochloride and cephaelin hydrochloride, alkaloids contained in the drug, have a locally irritating effect on the gastric mucous membrane and are thus responsible for the reflex increase of bronchial secretions and the expectorant effect. The saponins probably support this effect. The drug affects the sensory stomach nerves; it is secretory in small doses and emetic in larger doses. It is also spasmolytic and expectorant. It is partially effective in amoebic dysentery due to the action of the alkaloid emetin on the magna-form of the pathogen.

INDICATIONS AND USAGE

Unproven Uses: Ipecac is contained in expectorants and secretory preparations; it is used for amoebic dysentery, as a bronchial treatment and as an emetic in cases of poisoning. It is also used as an expectorant and to soothe and assist in coughing up of thick phlegm and in the treatment of croup or bronchitis in children.

Homeopathic Uses: Ipecae is used to treat bronchitis, asthma, whooping cough, gastrointestinal inflammations, disorders in blood pressure and bleeding of the mucous membranes.

PRECAUTIONS AND ADVERSE REACTIONS

General: No health hazards or side effects are known in conjunction with the proper administration of designated therapeutic dosages as an expectorant. Administration over extended periods can lead to myopathias. Frequent contact with the drug can trigger allergic reactions of the skin and the mucous membranes (''druggist's asthma,'' the allergen is a glycoprotein).

Pregnancy: Not to be used during pregnancy.

OVERDOSAGE

Higher dosages of the drug (1 to 2 g) have a nauseate effect (therapeutically used as an emetic). Toxic dosages can lead to mucous membrane erosion in the gastrointestinal tract, tachycardia, drop in blood pressure and cardiac rhythm disorders, as well as disorders in respiratory function and possibly to convulsions, shock, and coma.

Following intestinal emptying (sodium sulfate), the treatment for poisonings consists of the administration of generous amounts of liquids (warm tea), instillation of activated charcoal and shock prophylaxis (quiet, warmth), the treatment of spasms with diazepam (IV), electrolyte substitution and the countering of any acidosis imbalance that may appear through sodium bicarbonate infusions. In the event of shock, plasma volume expanders should be infused. Monitoring of kidney function is necessary. Intubation and oxygen respiration may also be required.

DOSAGE

Mode of Administration: Ipecac is used orally as a tincture, extract and fluid extract, and in medicinal preparations with a standardized alkaloid content.

Preparation: Ipecac extract: After the alkaloids have been determined the powder is stabilized with lactose or dextrin (DAB10).

Tincture: 1 part root powder with 8 to 12 parts 70% ethanol (DAB10).

These preparations are stabilized to a standardized alkaloid content.

Dosage: Infusion 0.5%: 10 mL (adults)

Homeopathic Dosage: 5 drops, 1 tablet, 10 globules every 30 to 60 minutes (acute) or 1 to 3 times daily (chronic); parenterally: 1 to 2 mL sc acute: 3 times daily; chronic: once a day; suppositories: 2 to 3 times daily (chronic) (HAB1).

Storage: Store carefully in the dark in tightly sealed containers.

LITERATURE

Garrettson LK, Ipecac home use- we need hope replaced with data- editorial comment. In: *J Toxicol Clin Toxicol* 29(4):515. 1991.

Kleinschartz W, Litovitz T, Overda GM, Bailey KM, Kuba A, The effect of milk on Ipecac-induced emesis. In: *J Toxicol Clini Toxicol* 29(4):505. 1991.

Nagakura N et al., Four tetrahydroisoquinoline-monoterpene glucosides from Cephaelis ipecacuanha. In: PH 32:761. 1993.

Wiegrebe W, Kramer WJ, Shamma M, The emetine alkaloids. In: JNP 47(3):397. 1984.

Ipomoea hederacea

See Morning Glory

Ipomoea orizabensis

See Mexican Scammony Root

Ipomoea purga

See Jalap

Iporuru

Alchornea floribunda

DESCRIPTION

Medicinal Parts: The medicinal part of the plant is the bark.

Flower and Fruit: The female inflorescence is apical and up to 25 cm long; the male inflorescence is axillary and 10 to 25 cm long with pale green flowers. The ovary is tricarpeled and fused. The fruit is a trichambered capsule with glossy brownish seeds.

Leaves, Stem, and Root: Alchornea floribunda is a tree or shrub that grow from 4.5 m to occasionally 10 m high. The leaves are clustered at the end of the glabrous branches. They are short-petiolate, lanceolate to spatulate, 15 to 35 cm long, 6 to 13 cm wide, glabrous above, and slightly downy beneath. The stipules are 3 to 9 mm long and downy.

Habitat: Tropical Africa, Amazon region

Production: Niando root is the fresh or dried root of *Alchornea floribunda* collected in the wild.

Other Names: Macochihua, Niando, Malan

ACTIONS AND PHARMACOLOGY

COMPOUNDS

Imidazole alkaloids (0.6 to 1.2%): alchornein (0.4%), isoalchornein (0.005%)

Tannins

EFFECTS

The drug has stimulating and hallucinogenic effect upon humans, due to the alkaloids it contains (chief active ingredient alchornein). An elevation in the sensitivity of the sympaticus to adrenaline was demonstrated in animal experiments. In comparison to atropine, alchorneine tartrate has a strong anticholinergic, vagolytic, and peristalsis-inhibiting effect; in addition, it exhibits the action of a weak local anesthetic.

INDICATIONS AND USAGE

Unproven Uses: The drug can be used for respiratory and urinary tract infections, and conditions of the gastrointestinal tract. In Africa the drug is used frequently as an aphrodisiac and hallucinogen.

PRECAUTIONS AND ADVERSE REACTIONS

Nothing has been documented regarding side effects in connection with therapeutic administration.

OVERDOSAGE

The drug is considered severely toxic. High dosages in animal experiments led to severe excitation and spasms. Cases of death through exhaustion have been observed among humans following overstimulation and hallucination.

DOSAGE

Mode of Administration: Whole herb and cut drug preparations for internal use.

Preparation: There are traditional preparations in the form of macerates or palm wine with the appropriate dosage.

LITERATURE

de Smet PA, Some ethnopharmacological notes on African hallucinogens. *J Ethnopharmacol*, 261:Drug Information Center, Royal Dutch Association for the Advancement of Pharmacy, The Hague, The Netherlands, 96.

Duke J, and Vasquez R, Amazonian Ethnobotanical Dictionary, CRC Press Inc., Boca Raton, FL, 1994.

Hänsel R, Keller K, Rimpler H, Schneider G (Ed), Hagers Handbuch der Pharmazeutischen Praxis, 5. Aufl., Bde 4 - 6 (Drogen), Springer Verlag Berlin, Heidelberg, New York, 1992-1994.

Iris species

See Orris

Jaborandi

Pilocarpus microphyllus

DESCRIPTION

Medicinal Parts: The medicinal parts are the dried leaves.

Flower and Fruit: The numerous flowers are in terminal or axillary racemes that are up to 30 cm long and 0.5 cm wide. The pedicles are 0.1 to 1.5 mm long and have alternate bracts. The flowers have a diameter of 4 to 5 cm and are glabrous. The 5 sepals are free, broadly triangular to orbicular and coriaceous. The petals have forward-bending tips and are thinly coriaceous and somewhat translucent. The oval anthers have an oblong gland. The disc is 0.5 mm high and 1.3 to 1.5 mm in diameter. The ovary is 0.5 mm and extends past the disc with a headlike stigma. The mericarp has roundish, flattened, black-brown seeds.

Leaves, Stem, and Root: The plant is a tree or shrub 3 to 7 m high with a trunk diameter of 3 to 7.5 cm. The branches are pubescent when young and glabrous when older. The leaves are alternate to opposite, odd-pinnate with 1 to 5 pairs of pinna. The pinna are sessile, elliptical, distinctly asymmetrical at the base and have an indented tip. The leaflets are dull green, up to 5 cm long and 3 cm wide, with entire, slightly recurved margins, and an uneven base. The ribs are prominent on the upper surface and have visible oil cells.

Characteristics: The taste is bitter and the odor slightly aromatic.

Habitat: The plant grows in the northeastern part of Brazil.

Production: Jaborandi leaves are the dried leaves of *Pilocarpus microphyllus.*

Other Names: Arruda Brava, Arruda do Mato, Jamguarandi, Juarandi

ACTIONS AND PHARMACOLOGY

COMPOUNDS

Imidazole alkaloids (0.5-1.0%): chief alkaloid is (+)-pilocarpine, through drying and under storage conditions changing over to some extent into isopilocarpine, companion alkaloids including pilocarpidine, pilosine and others

Volatile oil (0.5%): chief components are limonene and undecanone

EFFECTS

The drug affects the parasympathetic system. It increases the secretion of saliva, sweat, gastric juices and tears, and stimulates the smooth muscle of the gastrointestinal tract, bronchi, bile duct, and bladder.

INDICATIONS AND USAGE

Unproven Uses: Jaborandi is considered an obsolete drug, used now only in the treatment of glaucoma. In folk medicine, it was used for epilepsy, convulsions, gonorrhea, ischuria, as an anesthetic for mucous membranes, for fever, influenza, pneumonia, gastrointestinal inflammations, kidney disease, psoriasis, neurosis and poisoning.

PRECAUTIONS AND ADVERSE REACTIONS

General: No health hazards or side effects are known in conjunction with the proper administration of designated therapeutic dosages. The drug is used today as an industrial agent for the manufacture of pilocarpine, but is used medicinally only for homeopathic applications.

The incorrect administration of pilocarpine eyedrops can lead to poisoning through leakage into the nose or mouth. Symptoms include bradycardia, bronchial spasms, colics, collapse and possible cardiac arrest, convulsions, hypotenstion, dyspnea, nausea, severe salivation, strong secretion of sweat and vomiting.

Pregnancy: Jaborandi should not be used during pregnancy.

OVERDOSAGE

The lethal dose is approximately 60 mg of pilocarpine, corresponding to 5 to 10 g of the drug. Individuals with cardiac and circulatory illnesses are particularly susceptible. Following stomach and intestinal emptying (gastric lavage, sodium sulphate), the treatment for poisonings consists of the instillation of activated charcoal with atropine and the use of diazepam in the case of spasms. Forced dialysis and the administration of plasma volume expanders can also be useful.

DOSAGE

Mode of Administration: Jaborandi is obsolete by itself as a drug.

LITERATURE

Hänsel R, Keller K, Rimpler H, Schneider G (Hrsg.), Hagers Handbuch der Pharmazeutischen Praxis, 5. Aufl., Bde 4-6 (Drogen), Springer Verlag Berlin, Heidelberg, New York, 1992-1994.

Lewin L, Gifte und Vergiftungen, 6. Aufl., Nachdruck, Haug Verlag, Heidelberg 1992.

Madaus G, Lehrbuch der Biologischen Arzneimittel, Bde 1-3, Nachdruck, Georg Olms Verlag Hildesheim 1979.

Roth L, Daunderer M, Kormann K, Giftpflanzen, Pflanzengifte, 4. Aufl., Ecomed Fachverlag Landsberg Lech 1993.

Steinegger E, Hänsel R, Pharmakognosie, 5. Aufl., Springer Verlag Heidelberg 1992.

Tedeschi E, Kamionsky J, Fackler S, Sarel S, Isr J Chem 11:731-733. 1973.

Teuscher E, Lindequist U, Biogene Gifte - Biologie, Chemie, Pharmakologie, 2. Aufl., Fischer Verlag Stuttgart 1994.

Teuscher E, Biogene Arzneimittel, 5. Aufl., Wiss. Verlagsges. Stuttgart 1997.

Wagner H, Wiesenauer M, Phytotherapie. Phytopharmaka und pflanzliche Homöopathika, Fischer-Verlag, Stuttgart, Jena, New York, 1995.

Jack-in-the-Pulpit

Arisaema triphyllum

DESCRIPTION

Medicinal Parts: The medicinal part of the plant is the rhizome.

Flower and Fruit: The inflorescence (spadix) is yellowish-white, later brown, club-shaped, and surrounded by a larger spathe. The spathe is greenish on the outside and white-striped with a weak purple-violet tinge on the inside. The fruit is a scarlet berry.

Leaves, Stem, and Root: Jack-in-the-Pulpit is a herbaceous perennial rhizome, which extends up to 30 cm high. The leaves are basal and trifoliolate-digitate. The leaflets are ovoid, acuminate and entire. The rhizome is tuberous with hairlike roots at the top, shaped into a wreath.

Habitat: The plant is found in North America and China.

Production: Arisaema root is the fresh rhizome of *Arisaema atrorubens*.

ACTIONS AND PHARMACOLOGY

COMPOUNDS

Polysaccharides: starch

Pungent substances: structures are unknown (only in the fresh root)

EFFECTS

The pungent substances contained in the fresh drug are severely irritating to skin and mucous membranes, as well as being toxic. This toxicity is eliminated through dehydration and/or extended cooking. The dried or cooked root serves as a source of starch.

INDICATIONS AND USAGE

Unproven Uses: Preparations have been used for chronic bronchitis, asthma, colic, gastrointestinal disturbances, inflammation of the oral mucosa, rheumatism, for bumps, eye inflammations and abscesses (as a poultice) and as a contraceptive by the Hopi Indians.

PRECAUTIONS AND ADVERSE REACTIONS

General: No health hazards are known in conjunction with the proper administration of designated therapeutic dosages. The fresh rhizome is considered toxic. Internal administration leads to severe mucous membrane irritation and acute gastrointestinal inflammations, and skin inflammation.

Pregnancy: Contraindicated in pregnancy (used as a contraceptive in folk medicine).

DOSAGE

No information is available.

LITERATURE

Blaschek W, Hänsel R, Keller K, Reichling J, Rimpler G, Schneider G (Eds), Hagers Handbuch der Pharmazeutischen Praxis. Folgebände 1 und 2. Drogen A-Z. Springer. Berlin, Heidelberg 1998.

Jacob's Ladder

Polemonium caeruleum

DESCRIPTION

Medicinal Parts: The medicinal part is the herb.

Flower and Fruit: The numerous flowers grow in clusters at the end of the lateral branches. They are open, slightly hanging and have 5 sepals and 5 petals. The corolla is 2 to 2.5 cm, deep blue, and has a short pollen tube. The stamens are enclosed in the tube and have yellow anthers.

Leaves, Stem, and Root: The plant is a perennial. The plant is bright green and smooth. The upper section is covered in short glandular hairs. The rhizome is short and creeping, and the stem is 45 to 90 cm high, hollow, and quadrangular. The leaves with numerous pairs of leaflets are 1.25 to 2.5 cm long. These are pinnate and alternate.

Habitat: The plant is indigenous to central and northern Europe.

Production: Jacob's Ladder is the aerial part of *Polemonium caeruleum*.

Other Names: Charity, English Greek Valerian, Greek Valerian

ACTIONS AND PHARMACOLOGY

COMPOUNDS

Triterpene saponins

Flavonoids

EFFECTS

All parts of the plant contain saponin, which has astringent, diaphoretic and hemolytic effects.

INDICATIONS AND USAGE

Unproven Uses: Jacob's Ladder is used for febrile and inflammatory conditions.

PRECAUTIONS AND ADVERSE REACTIONS

No health hazards or side effects are known in conjunction with the proper administration of designated therapeutic dosages.

DOSAGE

Mode of Administration: The ground drug is used as an infusion.

LITERATURE

Reznicek G et al., A new ester saponine from *Polemonium caeruleum*. In: *PM* 59(7):A612. 1993.

Jalap

Ipomoea purga

DESCRIPTION

Medicinal Parts: The medicinal part is the root tuber.

Flower and Fruit: The flowers are single or in twos (occasionally in threes or fours), radial, with their structures grouped in fives. There are 5 narrow-lanceolate, purple-punctate sepals. The petals are fused to a 7 cm wide, funnel-shaped red corolla, and there are 5 stamens. The superior ovary is 2-chambered. The fruit is a capsule with 4 seeds.

Leaves, Stem, and Root: This winding herb grows up to 4 m high. The leaves are alternate, up to 9 cm long and 5 cm wide, cordate, acuminate, and entire. The stem is purple-tinged and glabrous. The rhizome is tuberously thickened, milky, approximately 5 cm long, with tuberous, thickened, secondary roots.

Habitat: Ipomoea purga grows in South and Central America, Mexico and Jamaica.

Production: Jalap resin (also known as jalap or *Jalapae resina*) is the resin of *Ipomoea purga* derived from alcoholic extraction of the jalap root powder. The tuberous, thickened secondary roots (black rhubarb tubers) of *Ipomoea jalapae* tuber are harvested from May to autumn and dried in the sun, on hot ash or over an open fire

Not to be Confused With: Jalap resin may be confused with Brazil jalap, Aloe, Orizaba jalap, colophonium, starch, dextrin and guaiac resin. Confusion can arise between Jalap tuber and Ipomoea orizabensis, Ipomoea operculata, Operculina turpethum, Convolvulus scammonia and Mirabilis jalapa.

Other Names; Ipomoea, Jalap Bindweed, Mexican Jalap, Orizaba Jalap, Vera Cruz Jalap

ACTIONS AND PHARMACOLOGY

Ipomoea purga is a centuries-old purgative and vermifuge. It has also been used as an anthelmintic.

COMPOUNDS: JALAP RESIN

Glycoretines: convulvin (55%, non-ether-soluble), jalapin (7%, ether-soluble), convulvin and jalapin are mixtures made up of resinous glycosides of hydroxy-fatty acids (C12 to C16) with oligosaccharides, their hydroxyl groups estered to the fatty acid esters with, among others, acetic acid, propionic acid, iso-butyric acid, alpha-methylbutyric acid, tiglic acid and iso-valeric acid or n-valeric acid.

EFFECTS: JALAP RESIN

The drug has a drastic laxative effect due to the glycoretines it contains.

COMPOUNDS: JALAP TUBER

Resins (5 to 20%): glycoretines (see Jalap resin)

Polysaccharides: starch

EFFECTS: JALAP TUBER

The drug has a drastic laxative effect due to the glycoretines it contains.

INDICATIONS AND USAGE

JALAP RESIN

Unproven Uses: Used for constipation.

JALAP TUBER

Unproven Uses: Jalap tuber is considered to be obsolete. In the past, it was used as a laxative and purgative.

PRECAUTIONS AND ADVERSE REACTIONS

JALAP RESIN

General: The drug's laxative effect frequently produces nausea, cramplike pains, and gastroenteritis.

Pregnancy: Administration is not advisable during pregnancy, particularly because of the possible teratogenic effect.

JALAP TUBER

General: Jalap tuber is to be used only under the supervision of an expert qualified in the appropriate use of this substance. The drug's laxative effect is frequently accompanied by nausea, cramplike pains, and gastroenteritis.

Pregnancy: The administration of jalap tuber is not to be used during pregnancy, particularly because of the possible teratogenic effect.

DOSAGE

JALAP RESIN

Preparation: There is no information in the literature.

Daily Dosage: 1.5 g drug; maximum single dosage: 0.1 to 0.3 g drug

Homeopathic Dosage: from D4: 5 drops, 1 tablet, 10 globules, every to 30 to 60 minutes (acute) and 1 to 3 times daily (chronic); parenterally: 1 to ml sc acute: 3 times daily; chronic once a day (HAB34).

Storage: Store securely in a tightly sealed container, protected from light.

JALAP TUBER

Mode of Administration: Whole, cut and powdered drug

Preparation: There is no information in the literature.

Daily Dosage: maximum 4.5 g drug; single dosage: maximum 1.5 g drug

Storage: Store protected from light in a secure, tightly sealed container.

LITERATURE

Hänsel R, Keller K, Rimpler H, Schneider G (Ed), Hagers Handbuch der Pharmazeutischen Praxis, 5. Aufl., Bde 4 - 6 (Drogen), Springer Verlag Berlin, Heidelberg, New York, 1992-1994.

Jamaica Dogwood

Piscidia piscipula

DESCRIPTION

Medicinal Parts: The medicinal part is the bark.

Flower and Fruit: The plant has blue to white flowers with white stripes out of which 4 pods with 4 longitudinal wings develop.

Leaves, Stem, and Root: The plant is a tree or shrub up to 15 m high with compound leaves. The bark is 3 to 6 mm thick and dark gray-brown with thin, longitudinal and transverse ridges. It is roughish and wrinkled, and somewhat fissured. The fracture is tough, fibrous, showing blue-green or brownish-green patches.

Characteristics: The taste is bitter and acrid and the odor characteristic.

Habitat: The tree is indigenous to Central America and the northern parts of South America.

Production: Jamaica Dogwood is the root bark of *Piscidia piscipula.*

Other Names: Dogwood, Fish Poison Tree

ACTIONS AND PHARMACOLOGY

COMPOUNDS

Isoflavonoids: including among others jamaicine, ichthynone, the rotenoids rotenone, milleton, isomilletone

Tannins

EFFECTS

Research indicates that Jamaica Dogwood is mildly sedative and spasmolytic.

INDICATIONS AND USAGE

Unproven Uses: The drug is used for states of anxiety and fear and as a daytime sedative.

PRECAUTIONS AND ADVERSE REACTIONS

No health hazards or side effects are known in conjunction with the proper administration of designated therapeutic dosages.

DOSAGE

Mode of Administration: The drug and liquid extract are no longer in use. It has been used in some medicinal preparations.

How Supplied: Liquid extract

LITERATURE

Pietta P, Zio C, (1983) J Chrom. 260:497.

Kern W, List PH, Hörhammer L (Hrsg.), Hagers Handbuch der Pharmazeutischen Praxis, 4. Aufl., Bde. 1-8, Springer Verlag Berlin, Heidelberg, New York, 1969.

Leung AY, Encyclopedia of Common Natural Ingredients Used in Food, Drugs and Cosmetics, John Wiley & Sons Inc., New York 1980.

Madaus G, Lehrbuch der Biologischen Arzneimittel, Bde. 1-3, Nachdruck, Georg Olms Verlag Hildesheim 1979.

Steinegger E, Hänsel R, Pharmakognosie, 5. Aufl., Springer Verlag Heidelberg 1992.

Wagner H, Wiesenauer M, Phytotherapie. Phytopharmaka und pflanzliche Homöopathika, Fischer-Verlag, Stuttgart, Jena, New York 1995.

Jambol

Syzygium cumini

DESCRIPTION

Medicinal Parts: The medicinal parts are the dried bark, dried seed kernels, disintegrated kernels, dried trunk bark, and macerated seeds.

Flower and Fruit: The flowers are in compound, triple panicles. They are sessile, whitish, fragrant, and are usually on older branches behind the leaves. The calyx tube is 4 to 6 mm long and twisted. The petals are hoodlike. There are approximately 60 stamens, which are as long as the calyx tube. The drupe is initially pink, becoming black when ripe. The drupe is 1.2 to 3 cm long, globular to ovate, 1-valved, 1-seeded and edible. The seeds are subcylindrical, about 6 mm long and rather less in diameter. One end of the seed is truncated and has a central depression. Externally, they are hard, tough and blackish-brown; internally they are pinkish-brown.

Characteristics: The taste of the seeds is faintly astringent and aromatic; the odor is slight.

Habitat: The plant is indigenous to the east Indian Malayian region. It has spread as far as China and Australia and is cultivated on the Antilles.

Production: Jambolan seed consists of the dried seed of *Syzygium cumini* (syn. *Syzygium jambolana*). Because the commodity consists mostly of the dried, fallen apart cotyledons, they must be broken apart in order to produce the drug. Jambolan bark consists of the dried bark from the trunk of *Syzygium cumini* (syn *Syzygium jambolana*).

Other Names: Black Plum, Jambul, Jamum, Java Plum, Rose Apple

ACTIONS AND PHARMACOLOGY

COMPOUNDS: JAMBOL SEED

Fatty oil (3-5%): containing oleic acid, myristic acid, palmitic acid and linoleic acid, sterculiac acid and malvalic acid (cyclopropylidenic acids), among others, as well as vernolic acid (epoxy fatty acid)

Tannins (6%): including corilagin, 3,3′-Di-O-methyl ellagic acid, galloyl glucose

EFFECTS: JAMBOL SEED

Anti-inflammatory actions were demonstrated in animal experiments. Results of hypoglycemic and CNS experiments were not conclusive.

COMPOUNDS: JAMBOL BARK

Tannins: gallic and ellagic acid derivatives including 3,3′-Di-O-methyl ellagic acid

Steroids: sterols, including beta-sitosterol, beta-sitosterol glucoside

Triterpenes: betulinic acid, friedelin, friedelan-3-alpha-ole, epi-friedelanol, eugenin

Flavonoids: including myricetin, kempferol, quercetin, astragalin

EFFECTS: JAMBOL BARK

The bark has astringent effects because of the tannin content.

INDICATIONS AND USAGE

JAMBOL SEED

Unproven Uses: Jambola seed is used for diabetes and in combination preparations for atonic and spastic constipation, diseases of the pancreas, gastric and pancreatic complaints, and nervous disorders.

JAMBOLAN BARK

Approved by Commission E:

- Diarrhea
- Inflammation of the mouth and pharynx
- Inflammation of the skin

Unproven Uses: Preparations are used internally for bronchitis, asthma, and dysentery, and externally for ulcers.

Indian Medicine: The drug is used for diabetes, leukorrhea, stomachache, fever, dysuria, and inflammation of the skin.

Homeopathic Uses: Syzygium cumini is used for diabetes.

PRECAUTIONS AND ADVERSE REACTIONS

JAMBOL SEED

No health hazards or side effects are known in conjunction with the proper administration of designated therapeutic dosages. Administration in the presence of diabetes mellitus is not recommended, due to the fact that the blood sugar-reducing effect is unproved.

JAMBOL BARK

No health hazards or side effects are known in conjunction with the proper administration of designated therapeutic dosages.

DOSAGE

JAMBOL SEED

Daily Dosage: A single dose is made up of 30 seeds (1.9 g) in powdered form.

JAMBOL BARK

Mode of Administration: As a comminuted herb for decoctions and other galenic preparations for internal use (gargle, infusion) and local application (compresses).

Preparation: To make a decoction for internal and external use, place 1 to 2 teaspoonfuls of comminuted drug in about 150 mL cold water, bring to a boil, simmer for 5 to 10 minutes and strain.

Daily Dosage: The average daily dosage is 3 to 6 g drug.

Homeopathic Dosage: 5 drops, 1 tablet, or 10 globules every 30 to 60 minutes (acute) or 1 to 3 times a day (chronic); parenterally: 1 to 2 mL sc, acute: 3 times a day; chronic: once a day (HAB1).

LITERATURE

JAMBOL BARK AND SEED

Bhatia IS et al., *PM* 28:346. 1975

Bhatia IS et al., *PH* 10:219. 1971

Desai HK et al., *Ind J Chem* 13:97-98. 1975.

Kopanski L, Schnelle G, *PM* 54:572. 1988.

Linde H, *Arch Pharm* 316(11):971. 1983

Saeed MT et al., *J Oil Technol Assoc India* 19:86-88. 1991.

Japanese Atractylodes

Atractylodes japonica

DESCRIPTION

Medicinal Parts: The medicinal parts of the plant are the whole plant and roots.

Flower and Fruit: The composite flowers are surrounded by bracts. The capitulas are apical and upright, with a diameter of 1.5 to 2 cm. The calyx is double-rowed and double-pinnate. The lingual florets are in 7 or 8 rows, whitish and 1 to 1.2 cm long. The fruit is an achaene. The pappus is brownish and 8 to 9 mm long.

Leaves, Stem, and Root: The plant is an upright, herbaceous perennial with a rhizome that extends up to 1 m high. The basal leaves wilt rapidly; the upper cauline leaves are alternate, small, usually simple and sessile. The lower leaves are long-petiolate, 8 to 10 cm long. The lamina is pergament-like, single pinnate with 3 to 5 elongate-elliptical leaflets. The apical leaflet is larger with short thorns on the margin. The rhizome is elongate, gnarled, 2 to 3 cm thick, and up to 8 cm long.

Habitat: Japan.

Production: Japanese Atractylodes rhizome is the dried rhizome of *Atractylodes japonica.*

ACTIONS AND PHARMACOLOGY

COMPOUNDS

Volatile oil (1.5%): constituents not investigated

Sesquiterpenes: atractylon, atractylenolids I to III, eudesma-4 (14), 7(11)-dien-8-one

Polyynes: including diacetylatractylodiol, (4E, 6E, 12E)-tetradecatrien-8, 10-diin-1, 3-diolacetate

Water-soluble polysaccharides: atractan A, atractan B

EFFECTS

The furanosesquiterpenes isolated from the essential oil of the drug exhibit antimicrobial, hepatoprotective, mildly analgesic, antiphlogistic, tumor-inhibiting and antioxidative effects.

INDICATIONS AND USAGE

Unproven Uses: Japanese Atractylodes has been used for gastric complaints, inflammations, heavy sweating, and as a diuretic.

Chinese Medicine: Preparations are used for loss of appetite, physical and mental exhaustion, diarrhea, edema, nausea, and vomiting.

PRECAUTIONS AND ADVERSE REACTIONS

No health hazards are known in conjunction with the proper administration of designated therapeutic dosages.

DOSAGE

Mode of Administration: Whole herb, cut drug, powdered drug and liquid preparations for internal use.

Preparation: The powder is prepared in accordance with Jap XI. There is no information available on the preparation of the infusion.

Daily Dosage: Internally: single dose: 0.5 to 1.0 g of powder; daily dose: 1.5 to 3.0 g of powder

Infusion: single dose: 1 to 1.5 g; daily dose: 3 to 5 g

Storage: Should be tightly sealed.

LITERATURE

Blaschek W, Hänsel R, Keller K, Reichling J, Rimpler G, Schneider G (Eds), Hagers Handbuch der Pharmazeutischen Praxis. Folgebände 1 und 2. Drogen A-Z. Springer. Berlin, Heidelberg 1998.

Chen ZL. The Acetylenes from *Atractylodes macrocephala. Planta Med.* 53; 493-494. 1987

Hatano K, Shoyama Y, Nishioka I. Clonal Propagation of *Atractylodes japonica* and *A. ovata* by Tip Tissue Culture and the Atractylon Content of Clonally Propagated Plants. *Planta Med.* 56; 131-132. 1990

Konno C, Suzuki YOishi K, Munakata E, Hikino H. Islation and Hypoglykemic Activity of Atractans A, B and C, Glycans of *Atractylodes japonica* Rhizomes. Planta Med. 51; 102-103. 1985

Satoh K, Nagai F, Ushiyama K, Kano I, Specific inhibition of Na+,K(+)-ATPase activity by atractylon, a major component of byaku-Jutsu, by interaction with enzyme in the E2 state. *Biochem Pharmacol* Feb 21 53(4):611-4. 1997

Japanese Mint

Mentha arvensis var. piperascens

DESCRIPTION

Medicinal Parts: The medicinal parts are the dried aerial parts of the plant and the essential oil, which is extracted by steam distillation followed by partial removal of menthol and rectification.

Flower and Fruit: The flowers are in densely globular, sessile, 8- to 12-blossomed false whorls with small linear-lanceolate bracts. The inflorescence is leafy at the apex. The bracts are like the leaves, smaller above. The tepals are 1.5 by 2.5 mm, broadly campanulate, and hairy. The corolla is lilac, white or, rarely, pink. The nutlets are pale brown.

Leaves, Stem, and Root: Japanese Mint is a pubescent, fragrant perennial or occasionally annual that grows up to 60 cm. The stems are ascending or erect. The leaves are 15 to 70 mm by 10 to 40 mm, and are elliptic-lanceolate to broadly ovate, usually elliptical with the base narrowing to a petiole, and shallowly dentate.

Habitat: The plant is found in Europe as far north as the 65th latitude, in Asia (particularly in Siberia), the Caucasus, the Himalayas, China, Mongolia, Korea, and Japan. It was probably introduced to North America.

Production: Mint oil consists of essential oil recovered from *Mentha arvensis var. piperascens.* The oil is obtained by steam distillation of the fresh, flowering herb, followed by partial removal of menthol and rectification.

Menthol is obtained from various species of Mentha, chiefly *M. arvensis var. piperascens* (from Japan), *M. arvensis var. glabrata* (from China) and *M. piperata* (from America). The product extracted from the first two is less valuable than the third, even though it contains a higher proportion of menthol.

Other Names: Cornmint, Field Mint

ACTIONS AND PHARMACOLOGY

COMPOUNDS

Chief components: menthol (25-40%), menthone (15-30%), isomenthone (7-12%), limonene (7-12%), neomenthol (2-4%), menthyl acetate (1-5%), beta-caryophyllene (2-5%), piperitone (0.5-4%), alpha- and beta-pinene (2-4% each). The composition does not reflect the relationship of the components to one another in the plant. The volatile oil gained through steam distillation loses 30 to 50% of the menthol through winterization and rectification.

EFFECTS

Japanese Mint has carminative, cholagogic, antimicrobial and, possibly, secretolytic effects on the bronchial mucosa. It is also cooling to the skin.

INDICATIONS AND USAGE

Approved by Commission E:

- Common cold
- Cough/bronchitis
- Fevers and colds
- Inflammation of the mouth and pharynx
- Liver and gallbladder complaints
- Pain
- Tendency to infection

Unproven Uses: Internally, the herb is used for sensitivity to weather changes, breathing difficulties, flatulence, functional gastrointestinal and gallbladder disorders, and catarrhs of the upper respiratory tract. Externally, it is used for headaches, myalgia and neuralgic ailments. It is used both externally and internally for functional cardiac complaints.

Chinese Medicine: The herb is used for headaches, dyspeptic complaints, diarrhea and vomiting, toothaches, and skin rashes.

Indian Medicine: The herb is used for joint pains, dyspeptic complaints, diarrhea and vomiting, coughs and asthma, headaches and toothaches, as well as general debility.

CONTRAINDICATIONS

Contraindications for the internal administration of the drug include occlusion of the biliary ducts, gallbladder inflammation, and severe liver damage. Gallstone sufferers could experience colic due to the cholagogic effect.

PRECAUTIONS AND ADVERSE REACTIONS

General: No health hazards are known in conjunction with the proper administration of designated therapeutic dosages. The intake can lead to gastric complaints in susceptible patients. Volatile oils containing menthol can worsen the spasms of bronchial asthma. The volatile oil possesses a weak potential for sensitization due to its menthol content.

Pediatric Use: Preparations containing the oil should not be applied to the faces of infants or small children, particularly not in the nasal area (glottal spasm, bronchial spasm, asthma-like attacks, or even possible respiratory failure could occur).

OVERDOSAGE

Cases of poisoning are not recorded. The minimal lethal dosage of menthol is estimated to be 2 g, although individuals have survived higher dosages (8 to 9 g).

DOSAGE

Mode of Administration: The essential oil and other galenic preparations are available for internal and external application. Varieties are commercially available as Brazilian, Chinese, Indian, and Japanese mint oil.

Daily Dosage: For internal use, the average daily dosage is 3 to 6 drops. When used as inhalation therapy, 3 to 4 drops are placed in hot water. To use externally, rub a few drops on the affected area.

In folk medicine, 2 drops are placed in a glass of water, tea or juice and taken once or twice a day. To make a heart poultice, 10 to 20 drops are placed on a compress, which is applied externally for 10 to 15 minutes. For headaches, 1 to 2 drops can be rubbed on the temples.

Storage: Store in air-tight containers protected from light; oils of different batches should not be mixed.

LITERATURE

Hänsel R, Keller K, Rimpler H, Schneider G (Hrsg.), Hagers Handbuch der Pharmazeutischen Praxis, 5. Aufl., Bde 4-6 (Drogen), Springer Verlag Berlin, Heidelberg, New York, 1992-1994.

Teuscher E, Biogene Arzneimittel, 5. Aufl., Wiss. Verlagsges. Stuttgart 1997.

Jasmine

Jasminum officinale

DESCRIPTION

Medicinal Parts: The medicinal parts of the plant are the fresh and dried flowers.

Flower and Fruit: The flowers are single or in 2 to 12 flowered, axillary cymes. The sepals are fused, with 5 awl-shaped, 6- to 8-mm long tips. The corolla is white. The corolla tube is 15 to 18 mm long with 8 to 9 mm long, ovate tips, which broaden like plates. There are 2 stamens. The fruit is a black berry.

Leaves, Stem, and Root: Common jasmine is a procumbent or climbing shrub, that grows up to 5 m high. The leaves are opposite and 5 to 7 pinnatifid. The leaflets are elongate-lanceolate, acute, narrowing at the base, weakly pubescent on both surfaces with a ciliate margin. The branches are initially lightly pubescent, later becoming glabrous, slightly edged, green and canelike.

Characteristics: The flowers are very fragrant.

Habitat: France, Italy, China, Japan, India, Morocco, and Egypt

Production: Common jasmine flowers are the dried, fresh flowers of *Jasminum officinale var. grandiflorum*

Other Names: Catalonian Jasmine, Italian Jasmine, Poet's Jasmine, Royal Jasmine

ACTIONS AND PHARMACOLOGY

COMPOUNDS

Volatile oil

Pyrridine alkaloids: jasminine (presumably an artifact)

EFFECTS

No definitive data are available.

INDICATIONS AND USAGE

Chinese Medicine: Jasmine is used for hepatitis and abdominal pain in liver cirrhosis or dysentery.

Indian Medicine: Preparations are used for pain symptoms of the stomach, head, teeth and eyes, for leprosy, itching, skin disease, and dysmenorrhea.

PRECAUTIONS AND ADVERSE REACTIONS

No health hazards are known in conjunction with the proper administration of designated therapeutic dosages.

DOSAGE

Preparation: Jasmine is available as a tea blend or oil.

LITERATURE

Elisha EE, Al-Maliki SJ, Ibrahem DK. Effects of *Jasminum officinale* Flowers on the Central Nervous System of the Mouse. *Int J Crude Drug Res.* 26; 221-227. 1988

Iqbal M, Ghosh AKM, Saluja AK. Antifertility Activity of the Floral Buds of *Jasminum officinale Var. grandiflorum* in Rats. Phytother Res. 7 (1); 5-8. 1993

Twaij HA, Elisha EE, Khalid RM, Paul NJ. Analgesic Studies on some Iraqi Medicinal Plants. *Int J Crude Drug Res.* 25; 251-254. 1988

Jasminum officinale

See Jasmine

Jatamansi

Nardostachys jatamansi

DESCRIPTION

Medicinal Parts: The medicinal part of the plant is the rhizome.

Flower and Fruit: The flowers are in 1 to 5 capitula, which are usually surrounded by bracts. Their structures are in fives, the petals fused, the corolla tube 6 mm long and lightly pubescent on the inside. The fruit is crowned by pointed ovate calyx tips, which are covered in splayed white hairs.

Leaves, Stem and Root: This upright herbaceous perennial grows to a height reaching up to 60 cm high. The leaves are opposite, grow from the rhizome, are 15 to 20 cm long, 2.5 cm wide, spatulate and narrow toward the petiole. The cauline leaves are sessile, opposite, 2.5 to 7.5 cm long and narrow-ovate. The finger-thick, woody rhizome is covered with reddish brown fibers from the remains of the petioles.

Habitat: Nardostachys jatamansi is indigenous to China, India and Nepal.

Production: Jatamansi roots are the dried roots and rhizome of Nardostachys jatamansi. An essential oil is extracted from the rhizome.

Not to be Confused With: Selinum vaginatum

Other Names: Indian Nard, Indian Spikenard, Spikenard, Nard, Narrow-Leaved-Echinacea

ACTION AND PHARMACOLOGY

COMPOUNDS

Volatile oil (0.3 to 0.4%): including valeranone (jatamansone), nardosinone, calarene, beta-maaliene, maaliol, beta-ionone, 1(10)-aristelonone-(2), nardol, valerenal

EFFECTS

In rat studies, the drug has shown to have a hepatoprotective effect (Ali 2000). It has also show to act against the peroxidation of lipids in rat liver cells (Tripathi 1996). An increase in the neurotransmitters norepinephrin, dopamine, serotonin, 5-hydroyindol acetic acid, GABA, and taurin were demonstrated following a 15-day administration of an ethanol extract to male Albino Wistar rats so a centrally acting effect can be implied (Prabhy 1994).

INDICATIONS AND USAGE

Unproven Uses: The drug is used to treat insomnia and headache, as well as liver problems, jaundice and kidney complaints.

Indian Medicine: Jatamansi is used for nervous headache, excitement, menopausal symptoms, flatulence, epilepsy, and for pain in the intestinal region.

CONTRAINDICATIONS

Use of the drug is contraindicated during pregnancy.

PRECAUTIONS AND ADVERSE REACTIONS

No health hazards are known in conjunction with the proper administration of designated therapeutic dosages.

DOSAGE

Mode of Administration: Jatamansi root is used in the forms of a whole, cut or powdered drug for internal and external use.

How Supplied: Forms of commercial pharmaceutical preparations include capsules and compound preparations.

Daily Dosage:

Powder – 0.6 to 1.3 g drug as a single dose

Pure drug – 5 g of the drug 3 times daily with a cup of water

Liquid extract/tincture (1:10) – 1 wineglassful, 3 times daily (corresponds to approximately 2 g drug per single dose)

Infusion (1:40) – 1 wineglassful, 3 times daily (corresponds to approximately 2 g drug per single dose)

Storage: Seal tightly and store in a cool, dry place.

LITERATURE

Ali S, Ansari KA, Jafry MA, Kabeer H, Diwakar G. *Nardostachys jatamansi* protects against liver damage induced by thioacetamide in rats. *J Ethnopharmacol* 71: 359-363 2000

Dixit VP, Jain P, Joshi SC, Hypolipidaemic effects of Curcuma longa L and *Nardostachys jatamansi,* DC in triton-induced hyperlipidaemic rats. *Indian J Physiol Pharmacol,* 32:299-304, Oct-Dec. 1988

Hänsel R, Keller K, Rimpler H, Schneider G (Ed), Hagers Handbuch der Pharmazeutischen Praxis, 5. Aufl., Bde 4 - 6 (Drogen), Springer Verlag Berlin, Heidelberg, New York, 1992-1994.

Prabhu V, Karanth KS, Rao A. Effects of *Nardostachys jatamansi* on biogenic amines and inhibitory amino acids in the rat brain. *Planta Med* 60: 114-117. 1994

Rucker G, Tautges J, Sieck A, Wenzl H, Graf E, Isolation and pharmacodynamic activity of the sesquiterpene valeranone from *Nardostachys jatamansi. DC Arzneimittelforschung, 28:7-13, 1978.*

Rucker G, Tautges J, Sieck A, Wenzl H, Graf E, *Nardostachys jatamansi*: a chemical, pharmacological and clinical appraisal. *Spec Rep Ser Indian Counc Med Res,* 28:1-117, 1978.

Tripathi YB, Tripathy E, Upadhyay A. Antilipid peroxidative property of *Nardostachys jatamanasi. Indian J Exp Biol*, 34: 1150-1151. 1996

Jateorhiza palmata

See Colombo

Java Tea

Orthosiphon spicatus

DESCRIPTION

Medicinal Parts: The medicinal parts are the leaves and stem tips collected during the flowering season.

Flower and Fruit: The flowers usually are arranged in a whorl of 6 (occasionally 10) blooms. The calyx tube is short with an upright-curved upper lip. The corolla is blue to light violet. The corolla tube is about 2 cm long with a broad upper lip that has 3 indentations. The lower lip is narrow and ovate-lanceolate. The 4 stamens are blue and 2.5 to 3 cm long. The style is as long as the stamen, and the ovary has a disk. The fruit breaks up into 4 oval-oblong nutlets with bumpy surfaces.

Leaves, Stem, and Root: The plant is a 40 to 80 cm high herb. The stem is quadrangular and glabrous to pubescent with crossed, opposite leaves. The leaves are about 75 mm long, usually short-petioled, ovate-lanceolate with an irregularly coarse, roughly serrate to dentate (or occasionally crenate) margin. The upper surface is brownish-green, the lower surface gray-green with strong, protruding ribs and glandular punctate markings. The plant resembles Peppermint.

Characteristics: The herb has a weak, unusual smell reminiscent of a cattle pen. The taste is salty, bitter and astringent.

Habitat: The plant is found in an area extending from tropical Asia to tropical Australia and is cultivated in those areas and elsewhere.

Production: Java Tea consists of the dried leaf and stem tips of *Orthosiphon spicatus*, which is harvested shortly before flowering. The leaves are then dried in a well-ventilated location.

Not to be Confused With: Confusion can arise with other *Orthosiphon* varieties and *Eupatorium* varieties from Java.

ACTIONS AND PHARMACOLOGY

COMPOUNDS

Volatile oil (0.02-0.06%): including among others beta-caryophyllene, alpha-humulene, caryophyllene-epoxide

Flavonoids: in particular more highly methoxylized examples (0.2%) including eupatorin, sinensetin, scutellarine tetramethyl ethers, salvigenin

Caffeic acid derivatives: including among others 2,3-dicoffeoyltartrate, rosmaric acid, 2-caffeoyl tartrate.

Diterpene ester: orthosiphole A to E, (diterpene dibenzoyl diacetyl ester of primarane type)

Triterpene saponins: (up to 4.5%): aglycone hederagenin

EFFECTS

Java Tea has been shown in human and animal tests to be a mild diuretic. The essential oil of the drug, which contains sesquiterpenes, is antimicrobial, antiphlogistic and possibly antitumoral.

INDICATIONS AND USAGE

Approved by Commission E:

- Infections of the urinary tract
- Kidney and bladder stones

Unproven Uses: In folk medicine, it is used for the above conditions and also for gout, rheumatism, hematuria, and albuminuria.

CONTRAINDICATIONS

Use of the drug for irrigation therapy is contraindicated in the presence of edema resulting from reduced cardiac or renal activity.

PRECAUTIONS AND ADVERSE REACTIONS

No health hazards or side effects are known in conjunction with the proper administration of designated therapeutic dosages.

DOSAGE

Mode of Administration: Comminuted herb for infusions and other galenic preparations for internal use.

How Supplied: Forms of commercial pharmaceutical preparations include:

Capsules

Drops

Tablets

Preparation: To make an infusion (tea), pour 150 mL hot water over the drug and strain after 10 minutes.

Daily Dosage: The daily dosage ranges from 6 to12 g drug. Adequate fluid intake (at least 2 liters per day) is essential.

Storage: Java Tea should be stored in a tightly sealed container that protects it from light and moisture.

LITERATURE

Hänsel R, Keller K, Rimpler H, Schneider G (Hrsg.), Hagers Handbuch der Pharmazeutischen Praxis, 5. Aufl., Bde 4-6 (Drogen), Springer Verlag Berlin, Heidelberg, New York, 1992-1994.

Proksch P, *Orthosiphon aristatus* (Blume) Miquel - der Katzenbart. In: ZPT 13(2):63. 1992.

Schut GA, Zwaving JH. Content and Composition of the Essential Oil of *Orthosiphon aristatus. Planta Med.* 52; 240-241. 1986

Sumaryono W, Proksch P, Wray V, Witte V, Hartmann T. Qualitative and Quantitative Analysis of the Phenolic Constituents from Orthosiphon aristatus. Planta Med. 57; 176-180. 1991

Takeda Y et al., Orthosiphol D and E, minor diterpenes from *Orthosiphon stamineus*. In: PH 33:411. 1993.

Teuber R, Neue Naturstoffe aus *Orthosiphon stamineus* Bentham. In: Dissertation Universität Marburg. 1986.

Teuscher E, Biogene Arzneimittel, 5. Aufl., Wiss. Verlagsges. Stuttgart 1997.

Wichtl M (Hrsg.), Teedrogen, 4. Aufl., Wiss. Verlagsges. Stuttgart 1997.

Jequirity

Abrus precatorius

DESCRIPTION

Medicinal Parts: The medicinal parts are the leaves, roots and seeds.

Flower and Fruit: The flowers are racemes of pink blossoms. The fruit is a pod with oval seeds, which are rounded at the ends. They are about 3 mm in diameter, hard, red and glossy, with a large black dot at one end. One variety has white seeds.

Leaves, Stem, and Root: This deciduous climbing plant with compound leaves grows to about 4 m.

Characteristics: The plant is a protected species in some countries.

Habitat: The plant originated in India and is found today in all tropical regions of the world.

Other Names: Crab's Eyes, Gunga, Goonteh, Indian Licorice, Prayer Beads, Rati, Wild Licorice

ACTIONS AND PHARMACOLOGY

COMPOUNDS

Toxic lectins: abrine and isolectins.

EFFECTS

Jequirity is an irritant and abortifacient.

INDICATIONS AND USAGE

Unproven Uses: Jequirity was used for chronic conjunctivitis and as a contraceptive in folk medicine, but is no longer used for these purposes.

Indian Medicine: Jequirity is used for coughs as well as inflammations and conditions of the upper respiratory tract and lungs.

Chinese Medicine: The drug is used in hepatitis and bronchitis.

PRECAUTIONS AND ADVERSE REACTIONS

The drug is very poisonous because it contains the toxic lectin abrine and isolectins.

OVERDOSAGE

Severe poisonings among adults following the intake of one half to two seeds, as well as cases of death among children following the consumption of two seeds, have been recorded. Besides gastrointestinal emptying, counter-measures include, administration of large amounts of fluid, monitoring of the circulatory system, administration of anti-epileptic drugs and possibly artificial respiration.

LITERATURE

Barri ME, el Dirdiri NI, Abu Damir H, Idris OF. Toxicity of *Abrus precatorius* in Nubian goats. *Vet Hum Toxicol*, 267:541-5, Dec1990

Cambie RC, Brewis AA. Anti-fertility Plants of the Pacific. CSIRO, 1997

Genest K, Lavalle A, Nera E. Comparative Acute Toxicity of *Abrus precatorius* and *Ormosia* Seeds in Animals. *Arzneim Forsch*. 21; 888-889. 1971

Hegde R, Podder SK. A- and B-subunit variant distribution in the holoprotein variants of protein toxin abrin: variants of abrins I and III have constant toxic A subunits and variant lectin B subunits. *Arch Biochem Biophys*, 344:75-84, Aug 1 1997

Kuo SC, Chen SC, Chen LH, Wu JB, Wang JP, Teng CM. Potent antiplatelet anti-inflammatory and antiallergic isoflavanquinones from the roots of Abrus precatorius. Planta Med, 61:307-12, Aug 1995

Jewel Weed

Impatiens biflora

DESCRIPTION

Medicinal Parts: The medicinal part is the herb.

Flower and Fruit: The axillary flowers are orange-yellow with large reddish-brown spots. They have an irregular form. The sepal sac abruptly contracts to a spur of about 5 to 9 mm. The spur is bent 180 degrees to lie parallel with the sac. The fruit is an oblong capsule which, when ripe, bursts open at the slightest touch and spreads the seeds over large distances.

Leaves, Stem and Root: The plant is a glabrous, fleshy annual 20 to 180 cm high. The stems are simple or branched and have swollen nodes. The leaves are thin, ovate, with 5 to 12 (up to 14) teeth on each side and are often undulate. They are rich green.

Habitat: Impatiens is common in the temperate regions and in South Africa, but it grows mostly in the mountainous, tropical regions of Asia and Africa.

Production: Jewel Weed is the aerial part of Impatiens biflora.

Other Names: Wild Balsam, Balsam-Weed, Spotted Touch-Me-Not, Slipperweed, Silverweed, Wild Lady's Slipper, Speckled Jewels, Wild Celandine, Quick-in-the-Hand

ACTIONS AND PHARMACOLOGY

COMPOUNDS

Naphthalene derivatives: 1.4-naphthoquinone, in particular lawsone (2-hydroxy-1, 4- naphthoquinone), yielding from the precursor through drying of the leaves 1,2,4-trihydroxy-naphthalene-4-beta-D-glucoside

EFFECTS

Jewel Weed is a digestive, appetite stimulant and diuretic.

INDICATIONS AND USAGE

Unproven Uses: Jewel Weed is used for mild digestive disorders. In folk medicine the fresh plant is used as an ointment for hemorrhoids and the juice is used for removing warts.

PRECAUTIONS AND ADVERSE REACTIONS

No health hazards or side effects are known in conjunction with the proper administration of designated therapeutic dosages.

DOSAGE

Mode of Administration: Administered as the ground drug and as an infusion.

LITERATURE

Hegnauer R, Chemotaxonomie der Pflanzen, Bde 1-11, Birkhäuser Verlag Basel, Boston, Berlin 1962-1997.

Long D, Ballentine NH, Marks jr, JG. Treatment of Poison Ivy/ Oak Allergic Contact Dermatitis With an Extract of Jewelweed. *Am J Contact Dermatitis* 8 (3); 150-153. 1997

Jimson Weed

Datura stramonium

DESCRIPTION

Medicinal Parts: The medicinal parts are the dried leaves or the dried leaves with the tips of the flowering branches. Occasionally the fruit, the ripe seeds, and the fresh, aerial parts of the plant are used. Parts of the plant are regarded as poisonous.

Flower and Fruit: The flowers are large, white, solitary, terminal or in branch bifurcations. The calyx has a long 5-edged and short, 5-tipped tube. The corolla is funnel-shaped and folded with a short 5-sectioned border. There are 5 free stamens and 1 superior ovary. The fruit is a 5-cm long, 4-valved capsule, which is densely thorny and walnut-sized. The numerous seeds are 3.5 mm long, flat, reniform, and black.

Leaves, Stem, and Root: The plant is an annual and grows to 1.2 m high. It has a simple or bifurcated, round, erect glabrous stem. The leaves are 20 cm long, long-petioled, ovate, dentate, glabrous, and dark green.

Characteristics: The foliage has an unpleasant smell; the flowers are fragrant and poisonous.

Habitat: Jimson Weed is found in most temperate and subtropical parts of the world, probably originated in Central America.

Production: Jimson Weed leaf consists of the dried leaf, or the dried leaves and flowering tops of *Datura stramonium*. Jimson Weed seed consists of the ripe seed of *Datura stramonium*.

Other Names: Datura, Devil's Apple, Devil's Trumpet, Jamestown Weed, Mad-Apple, Nightshade, Peru-Apple, Stinkweed, Stinkwort, Stramonium, Thorn-Apple

ACTIONS AND PHARMACOLOGY

COMPOUNDS: JIMSON WEED LEAF

Tropane alkaloids (0.1-0.65%): chief alkaloids (-)-hyoscyamine, under drying conditions changing over to some extent into atropine and scopolamine (ratio 4:1), furthermore including, among others, apoatropine, belladonnine, tigloylmeteloidin

Flavonoids

Hydroxycoumarins: including, among others, umbelliferone, scopolin, scopoletin

Withanolide: including, among others, withastramonolide

COMPOUNDS: JIMSON WEED SEED

Tropane alkaloids (0.4-0.6%): chief alkaloids (-)-hyoscyamine, under drying conditions changing over to some extent into atropine, and scopolamine (ratio 4:1).

Indole alkaloids (β-carboline type): including, among others, fluorodaturin (very fluorescent).

Lectins

Fatty oil (15-45%)

Proteins (12-25%)

EFFECTS: JIMSON WEED LEAF AND SEED

The drug contains alkaloids (hyoscyamine, scopolamine) in extremely varying concentrations. The effect is anticholinergic and parasympatholytic (see Belladonna); the scopolamine fraction is more responsible for this effect.

INDICATIONS AND USAGE

JIMSON WEED LEAF AND SEED

Due to the inconsistent alkaloid content of the raw herb, the use of nonstandardized Jimson Weed products is not recommended.

Unproven Uses: In folk medicine, Jimson Weed preparations have been used for asthma, convulsive cough, pertussis during bronchitis and influenza, for severe catarrh and as an expectorant. It was also used as a basic therapy for diseases of the autonomic nervous system.

Homeopathic Uses: Used for infection with high temperatures, cramps, and inflammations of the eyes.

Chinese Medicine: Used in Chinese medicine for general states of pain. It is smoked for asthma, dyspnea and coughs; externally it is used for rheumatism.

CONTRAINDICATIONS

JIMSON WEED LEAF AND SEED

Not to be used in the presence of glaucoma, suspicion of glaucoma, paralytic ileus, pyloric stenosis, enlarged prostate, tachycardic arrhythmias, and acute pulmonary edema.

PRECAUTIONS AND ADVERSE REACTIONS

JIMSON WEED LEAF AND SEED

General: Patients with urine retention or coronoary sclerosis should not use Jimson Weed.

DRUG INTERACTIONS

MODERATE RISK

Succinylcholine: Concurrent use may result in increased neuromuscular blockade. *Clinical Management:* Succinylcholine should generally be avoided during anesthesia in patients receiving cholinesterase inhibitors. The use of succinycholine in these situations will lead to prolonged paralysis, which will require ventilation and supportive care until muscle function returns.

OVERDOSAGE

JIMSON WEED LEAF AND SEED

The intake of very high dosages leads to central excitation (restlessness, compulsive speech, hallucinations, delirium, manic episodes), followed by exhaustion and sleep.

The 4 early warning symptoms of poisoning are skin reddening, dryness of the mouth, tachycardic arrhythmia, and mydriasis. Accommodation disorders, heat build-up through decline in sweat secretion, micturtion disorders, and severe constipation can occur as side effects, particularly with overdosages.

Lethal dosages (for adults starting at 100 mg atropine, depending upon atropine content, 15 to 100 g of the leaf drug, 15 to 25 g of the seed drug, considerably less for children) carry with them the danger of asphyxiation. Treatment for poisonings include stomach emptying, temperature-lowering measures with wet cloths (no antipyretics), oxygen respiration for respiratory distress, intubation, parenteral physostigmine salts as antidote, diazepam for spasms and chlorpromazine for severe excitation.

DOSAGE

JIMSON WEED LEAF

Daily Dosage: Stabilized leaf powder: 0.05 to 0.1 g drug as a single dose up to 3 times a day; daily dose: 0.6 g drug (ÖAB90); as a narcotic: 1 g drug.

Homeopathic Dosage: from D4: 5 to 10 drops, 1 tablet, or 5 to 10 globules 1 to 3 times a day or 1 mL injection solution sc twice weekly; eye drops 1 to 3 times a day (HAB1).

Storage: Keep carefully stored and protected from light.

JIMSON WEED SEED

Daily Dosage: Seeds: single oral dose: 0.05 g; daily dose: 0.6 g drug (EB6); seed tincture: single oral dose: 0.3 g; daily dose: 3.0 g (EB6).

Homeopathic Dosage: from D4: 5 to 10 drops, 1 tablet, or 5 to 10 globules 1 to 3 times a day or 1 mL injection solution sc twice weekly; eye drops 1 to 3 times a day (HAB1).

Storage: Keep carefully stored and protected from light.

LITERATURE

JIMSON WEED LEAF AND SEED

Dugan GM, Gumbmann MR, Friedman M. Toxicological Evaluation of Jimson Weed (*Datura stramonium*) Seed. *Food Chem Toxic.* 27; 501-510. 1989

El Mekkawy S, Meselhy MR, Kusumoto IT, Kadota S, Hattori M, Namba T. Inhibitory Effect of Egyptian Folk Medicines on Human Immunodeficiency Virus (HIV) Reverse Transcriptase. *Chem Pharm Bull.* 43 (4); 641-648. 1995

Ford YY, Ratcliffe RG, Robins RJ. In Vivo NMR Analysis of Tropane Alkaloid Metabolism in Transformed Roots and De-Differentiated Cultures of *Datura stramonium. Phytochemistry* 43 (1); 115-120. 1996

Hilton MG, Rhodes MJ. Factors Affecting the Growth and Hyoscyamine Production during Batch cluture of Transformed Roots of *Datura stramonium. Planta Med.* 59; 340-344. 1993

Hilton MG, Wilson PDG. Growth and the Uptake of Sucrose and Mineral Ions by Transformed Root Cultures of *Datura stramonium, Datura candida X aurea, Datura wrightii, Hyoscyamus muticus* and *Atropa belladonna. Planta Med.* 61 (4); 345-350. 1995

Kraft K, Europäische Rauschdrogen. In: *ZPT* 17(6):343-355. 1996.

Jojoba

Simmondsia chinesis

DESCRIPTION

Medicinal Parts: The medicinal part is the liquid Jojoba wax.

Flower and Fruit: The flowers are axillary. The male flowers are small and yellow and have no petals. The female flowers are usually solitary, inconspicuous and pale green. There may also be inflorescences in the form of panicles, umbels and cymes. Pollination is by wind. The fruit capsules contain 1 to 3 seeds although 1-seeded capsules are the most common. The seeds are approximately 2 cm long.

Leaves, Stem and Root: The plant is a heavily branched, evergreen dioecious bush. The male plants are larger, taller and less compact than the female. The desert variety develop taproots up to 3.6 m in length. The horizontal root branches reach from 60 to 90 cm in depth. The leaves are thick, coriaceous, blue-green, entire-margined and oblong. They are in pairs and depending on the dampness of the soil the leaves may remain on the bush for 2 to 3 periods of growth.

Characteristics: The oil from the fruit has a pleasant scent and taste.

Habitat: The plant is indigenous to areas extending from the Sonora dessert of the U.S. to northwest Mexico. It is cultivated in India and Israel.

Production: From the cultivation (of plants) in Mexico and in South America. Liquid Jojoba wax is a clear, light yellow, oily liquid, that is extracted from the seeds of Simmondsia chinesis.

Other Names: Bush Nut, Goat Nut

ACTIONS AND PHARMACOLOGY

COMPOUNDS

Liquid wax exters: esters in position 9-10 simple unsaturated C20- and C22-fatty acids, chiefly gadolenic acid (20:1(9), make up 70% of the fatty acids) with the corresponding alcohols, chiefly eicosanol (20:1 (9)-OH) and docosenol (22:1 (9) OH)

EFFECTS

Active agents are the simple unsaturated C20/22 - fatty acids and alcohol.

Jojoba oil has a robust and stable constitution. It is used in skin care products as a carrier (substance) for oxidation sensitive substances (Vitamin A).

INDICATIONS AND USAGE

Folk Medicine: Native Americans used the was for wound care, acne, and psoriasis.

PRECAUTIONS AND ADVERSE REACTIONS

No health hazards or side effects are known in conjunction with the proper external administration of designated therapeutic dosages. Jojoba wax is not suitable for internal use.

DOSAGE

Mode of Administration: In ointments and creams as a medium (or vehicle) for oxidation sensitive substances.

LITERATURE

Knoepfler NB et al., *Agr Food Chem* 6:118. 1958.

Miwa TK, *J Am Oil Chem Soc* 48:259. 1971.

Hänsel R, Keller K, Rimpler H, Schneider G (Hrsg.), Hagers Handbuch der Pharmazeutischen Praxis, 5. Aufl., Bde 4-6 (Drogen): Springer Verlag Berlin, Heidelberg, New York, 1992-1994.

Steinegger E, Hänsel R, Pharmakognosie, 5. Aufl., Springer Verlag Heidelberg 1992.

Teuscher E, Biogene Arzneimittel, 5. Aufl., Wiss. Verlagsges. Stuttgart 1997.

Juglans cinerea

See Butternut

Juglans regia

See Walnut

Jujube (Da-Zao)

Zyzyphus jujube

DESCRIPTION

Medicinal Parts: The medicinal part is the fruit. The Jujube berry is classed with raisins, dates and figs, and can be eaten fresh or dried.

Flower and Fruit: The flowers are small, pale yellow and solitary. The fruit is of variable size, depending on the origin, but is usually up to 3 cm long and 1.5 cm in diameter. The fruit is red, smooth and shiny when fresh, brownish-red and grooved when dried. It is pulpy and contains 1 or 2 acute, oblong seeds.

Characteristics: The taste of the fruit is sweet and mucilaginous.

Habitat: The plant grows in southern Europe, Africa, Middle East, and the Far East.

Production: Jujube berries are the fruit of *Zyzyphus jujube*; *Zyzyphus vulgaris* is also used.

ACTIONS AND PHARMACOLOGY

COMPOUNDS

Triterpene saponins: zyzyphus saponins I, II and III, jujuboside-B, in the seeds jujuboside-A and -B, aglycone jujubogenine

Mucilage

Tannins (10%)

Flavonoids: including among others naringenin-6,8-di-C-glucosides, in the seeds spinosin (C-glycoflavone)

Isoquinoline alkaloids: oxonuciferin, nornuciferin

Peptide alkaloids: daechucyclopeptide, daechualkaloid-A

Triterpenes: betulinic acid, betulonic acid, maslinic acid, alphitolic acid and oleanolic acid

Hydroxycoumarins

Sugars: including among others saccharose, glucose, fructose, galactose

Fruit acids: including among others malic acid, tartaric acid

EFFECTS

Jujube is emollient, anti-allergenic, and sedative. *Zyzyphus vulgaris* also has a hypotensive effect.

INDICATIONS AND USAGE

Unproven Uses: Jujube is used as a nutrient and tonic. It is also used as a prophylactic against liver disease and stress ulcers.

PRECAUTIONS AND ADVERSE REACTIONS

No health hazards or side effects are known in conjunction with the proper administration of designated therapeutic dosages.

LITERATURE

Ahn YS et al., Korean J Pharmacol 18 (1):17. 1982

Cyong J, Takahashi M, Chem Pharm Bull 30:1081. 1982

Hikino H, In: Economic, Medicinal Plant Research, Vol. 1, Acadamic Press UK 1985.

Okamura N et al., Chem Pharm Bull 29:676, 3507. 1981

Juniper

Juniperus communis

DESCRIPTION

Medicinal Parts: The medicinal parts are the essential oil from the berry cones; the ripe, dried berry cones; the ripe fresh berry cones; the fresh or dried pseudo fruit or berry; and the ripe berry.

Flower and Fruit: The plant is usually dioecious, occasionally monoecious and bearing androgynous flowers. The yellowish male flowers are in elliptical catkins consisting of numerous stamens in 3-segmented whorls in the leaf axils of young shoots. The greenish female flowers are almost ovoid and consist of 3 carpels. The carpels become fleshy and in the second year when ripe form pea-sized, globular, and dark-brown to violet, blue-frosted Juniper berries. The berries ripen over 2 or 3 years so that blue (ripe) and green (unripe) berries are found on the same tree. The seeds are light brown, oblong-triangular. They are somewhat warty between the edges and have a hard shell.

Leaves, Stem, and Root: Juniperus communis is a tree or shrub found in varying forms from 2 to 10 m in height. The bark is smooth and yellow-brown at first, later fissured, gray-black, and peeling. The buds are covered in scalelike needles, which can be distinguished from the foliage needles by their length. The leaves are needles in whorls of 3 spreading from the branchlets. They are evergreen, stiff, pointed, prickly, and sea green. The outer and inner membranes have thickened cell walls.

Characteristics: The berries have a tangy smell. The taste is tangy-sweet, then resinous and bitter.

Habitat: Europe, northern Africa, north Asia, and North America.

Production: Juniper Berry is the ripe, fresh, or dried berry of *Juniper communis* as well as its preparations. The ripe berries are harvested from the end of August to the middle of September and then dried at room temperature and sorted.

Other Names: Enebro, Ginepro, Juniper Berry

ACTIONS AND PHARMACOLOGY

COMPOUNDS

Volatile oil (1-2%): make-up is very dependent upon the source of the drug, chief components monoterpene hydrocarbons, for example alpha-pinene, beta-myrcene, gamma-muurolen, sabinene, additionally including among others limonene, beta-elemene, beta-caryophyllene, beta-pinene, gamma-cadinene, terpinene-4-ol

Diterpenes

Catechin tannins

Flavonoids

Monosaccharides: inverted sugar (20 to 30%)

Oligomeric proanthocyanidins

EFFECTS

Juniper has been primarily noted for its anti-inflammatory, diuretic, and dyspeptic effects. Because of its ability to inhibit cyclooxygenase, it is useful in inflammatory conditions, such as arthritis. Juniper is used to treat chronic urinary tract, bladder, and kidney infections as well as herpes and flu infections. The diuretic effect is primarily due to the volatile oil Terpinen-4-ol. In addition, the drug works to lower blood pressure and may regulate hyperglycemia. In animal experiments a hypotensive, and antiexudative effect was proved. In vitro, an antiviral effect was also demonstrated.

Well-controlled clinical trials on the therapeutic effects of various Juniper preparations are not available. Promising results have been obtained when Juniper was used to treat rheumatoid arthritis and neurasthenic neurosis. Although Juniper tar is used as a keratoplastic and antipruritic agent in formulations intended for the treatment of seborrhea, eczema, and psoriasis, clinical trials supporting the use of Juniper tar for these indications are largely lacking. In animal and in vitro studies, Juniper has demonstrated activity against herpes simplex virus, and Chinese Juniper has shown antitumor activities.

Antigingival Effects: Herbal mouthwash was ineffective in improving gingivitis and plaque formation (Van der Weijden et al, 1998).

Anti-inflammatory Effects: Juniper berry oil is rich in 5,11,14-eicosatrienoic acid, a polyunsaturated fatty acid similar to one found in fish oil, yet less prone to peroxidation. As with fish oil, Juniper berry oil has been shown to effectively reduce hepatic reperfusion injury in rats. Juniper berry reduced cell death by 75%, improved microcirculation, and blunted increases in intracellular calcium and release of the inflammatory prostaglandin E2 (PGE2) by cultured Kupffer cells stimulated by endotoxin. These results seem consistent with the theory that Juniper berry oil reduces reperfusion injury by inhibiting activation of Kupffer cells, thus reducing vasoactive eicosanoid release and improving the hepatic microcirculation in livers undergoing oxidant stress (Jones et al, 1998). A therapeutic bath oil containing Juniper reduced pain and increased circulation

Antitumor Effects: Chinese Juniper extract demonstrated antitumor effects in mice. Alzoon®, an herbal syrup containing extracts of Juniper and other herbs, is ineffective in the treatment of cancer (Ali et al, 1996; Hauser, 1997).

Dermatologic Effects: Juniper tar is noted as an active ingredient by the FDA in certain OTC preparations. Juniper tar has long been used as a keratoplastic and antipruritic agent for the treatment of seborrhea, eczema, and psoriasis (Parfitt, 1999). Juniper may be used along or in combination with other agents such as sulfur, salicylic acid, pine tar; and coal tar.

Herpes Simplex Infection (HSV-1): Isolates from Juniper berry extract have demonstrated activity against HSV-1 (Markkanen, 1981).

Neurasthenic Neurosis: Juniper bath treatment resulted in considerable clinical improvement of emotional disturbances, visceral innervation, and vegetative-vascular disorders associated with neurasthenic neurosis (Jonkov & Naidenov, 1974).

CLINICAL TRIALS

Anti-Inflammatory

Juniper oil contains the nonmethylene interrupted fatty acids (NMIFA) that displace arachidonic acid (AA: 20:4omega6 -5,8,11,14) in the membrane phospholipids. Unlike eicosapentaenoic acid (EPA: 20:5omega3 -5,8,11,14,17), the NMIFA (20:3omega6 -5,11,14 and 20:4omega3 -5,11,14,17) lacking the delta-8 double bond are not substrates for the formation of eicosanoids. Mice fed diets high in EPA (from fish oil) or NMIFA (from Juniper oil) or linoleic acid (from safflower oil and the major precursor of AA) were compared for production of inflammatory eicosanoids and cytokines produced in response to an intraperitoneal injection of endotoxin. The levels of inflammatory eicosanoids, such as PGE2, were markedly lower ($p<0.01$) in mice on the high EPA or high NMIFA diets. These data suggest that effects of NMIFA of Juniper oil, despite their inability to form eicosanoids, are similar to the effects of EPA which decreases formation of inflammatory eicosanoids (Chavali et al, 1998).

Cancer

Alzoon®, an herbal syrup containing extracts of petasites, Juniper, fern, brunellia, and dandelion, was shown to be ineffective in the treatment of cancer in humans. Rat studies have shown it to stimulate the growth of sarcomas. It is purported to aid in the treatment of cachexia, severe pain, anemia due to malignancy, stomach and duodenal ulcers, and to support end-stage cancer patients. A dose of 1 to 2 tablespoons 2 to 3 times daily long-term is recommended by the Swiss manufacturer. In a 1965 trial of 42 cancer patients, Alzoon® had no effect on tumor growth. A laxative effect was observed and 6 patients reported an improvement in well being after 2 to 3 weeks of treatment, including appetite stimulation. Other patients discontinued treatment due to intolerable adverse effects. The company literature does not speculate on any mechanism of action but mentions that petasites is the most important ingredient in its formulation. Available literature on this trial is scarce and no further clinical trials with Alzoon ® have been undertaken (Hauser, 1997).

Diabetes

A decoction from Juniper berries (*Juniperus communis*) decreased glycemic levels in normoglycemic rats at a dose of 250 milligram/kilogram (mg/kg) by increasing peripheral glucose consumption and potentiating glucose-induced insulin secretion. When the same decoction (125 mg total "berries"/kg) was given to streptozotocin-diabetic rats for 24 days, a significant decrease was seen in blood glucose levels and mortality index (Sanchez de Medina et al, 1994).

Gingivitis

A mouth rinse consisting of a 1:1:1 combination of herbal extracts from Juniper (*Juniperus communis*), nettle (*Urtica dioca*), and yarrow (*Achillaea millefolium)* had no effect on plaque growth or gingivitis (Van der Weijden et al, 1998).

Pain Control

A reduction in pain and increase in circulation resulted from the addition of a combination of Juniper oil and wintergreen oil to therapeutic baths in a double-blind, placebo-controlled, crossover study. 30 mL of Kneipp-Rheumabad® (18% Juniper wood oil, 14% wintergreen oil [96% to 99% methylsalicylate]) was added to 300 liters of water starting at 38° C. The placebo group received baths without the therapeutic bath oil. Pressure pain was significantly more reduced in the treatment group following the 2-bath set compared with placebo. The skin was significantly more erythematous in the treatment than in the placebo group, indicating a significant increase in circulation in the former group. Subjective patient evaluation and global assessment by the physician both reported a significant therapeutic effect during the treatment phase compared to placebo. None of the patients experienced adverse effects (Uehleke, 1996).

Tumors

The crude extract of Chinese Juniper (*Juniperus chinensis*) demonstrates antitumor-promoting and antitumor properties in mice. Tumor production was initiated in DC1 mice by the application of DMBA and promoted with twice-weekly application of TPA (tumor promoting substance) for 20 weeks. Until 14 weeks, the number of tumor-bearing mice was less in the Juniper-treated groups. At 20 weeks, a 51% (1 mg group) and 26% (0.5 mg group) reduction in the number of skin tumors per mouse was observed as compared to the nontreated group. Juniper treatment did not retard mouse growth and did not trigger a skin inflammatory response (Ali et al, 1996).

INDICATIONS AND USAGE

Approved by Commission E:

■ Dyspeptic complaints

Unproven Uses: Juniper is used externally for rheumatic symptoms (as a bath additive). In folk medicine it is used internally to regulate menstruation and to relieve menstrual pain, irrigation therapy for inflammatory diseases of the lower urinary tract, gout, arteriosclerosis, for severe irritation resulting from bronchitis and diabetes (ground Juniper berries). It is often chewed for halitosis.

Homeopathic Uses: Juniperus communis is used for discharge disturbances of the efferent urinary tract and dyspeptic complaints.

CONTRAINDICATIONS

Contraindicated in inflammatory renal diseases.

Pregnancy: Not to be used during pregnancy.

Breastfeeding: Not to be used while breastfeeding.

PRECAUTIONS AND ADVERSE REACTIONS

Caution should be used with increased blood glucose levels in diabetics (Anon, 1997), and during periods of prolonged use with hypokalemia (Newall et al, 1996). External administration for large skin wounds, acute skin diseases, feverish diseases, cardiac insufficiency, or hypertonia should only take place under the supervision of a doctor.

Juniper tar is a mild to moderate irritant, less so than phenol. Juniper tar may also have carcinogenic potential. The alpha and beta-pinene (monoterpenes) content in Juniper berry oil is associated with renal toxicity.

Carcinogenic Effects: Juniper tar has been investigated in human skin explants from biopsy samples and skin and lungs of mice. Direct evidence of formation of potentially carcinogenic DNA damage was seen in both human and mouse tissue (Schoket et al, 1990; Phillips, 1989).

Ocular Effects: Juniper tar may be irritating to the eyes and cause conjunctivitis (Gosselin et al, 1984).

Renal Toxicity: Prolonged use or overdose may result in renal damage. Alpha and beta-pinene (monoterpenes) content in Juniper berry oils is associated with renal toxicity. 4-Terpineol is the therapeutic aquaretic component and is not associated with adverse renal effects. In an evaluation of 50 commercially available Juniper oil preparations, concentrations of kidney toxic monoterpenes to therapeutic 4-terpineol were found to vary from 4:1 to 55:1. The concentration of toxic monoterpenes increases when unripe, green berries, needles, and wood are added to the ripe, blue berries before distillation. Two independent toxicologic studies in rats showed no renal toxicity associated with pharmaceutical grade Juniper oil (monoterpenes to 4-terpineol 1:3 and 1:5) at doses of 1000 milligrams/kilogram (Schilcher, 1995). Other animal studies document the renal toxicity as well (Schilcher & Heil, 1994).

DRUG INTERACTIONS

No human drug interaction data available.

OVERDOSAGE

Overdose from external application results in burning, erythema, inflammation with blisters, and edema. Signs of overdose from internal administration are pain in or near the kidneys, heavy diuresis, albuminuria, hematuria, purplish urine, tachycardia, hypertension, and infrequently, convulsions, metrorrhagia, and abortion (Newall et al, 1996).

DOSAGE

Mode of Administration: Whole, crushed, or powdered drug for infusions and decoctions, alcohol extracts, and in wine. Essential oil is used for oral application in liquid and solid medicinal forms. Combinations with other plant drugs in bladder and kidney teas and similar preparations may be useful. Juniper berry is also used as bath salts in the treatment of rheumatism.

How Supplied:

Capsules – 515 mg

Liquid – 1:1

Oil – 100%

Daily Dosage: The daily dose is 2 to 10 g of the drug, corresponding to 20 to 100 mg of the essential oil. The duration of use should be limited to a maximum of 6 weeks. A 1:20 dilution infusion (0.5 g in 1 teacup) may be taken 3 times daily. Tincture (1:5): 1 to 2 mL 3 times daily. Liquid extract: 2 to 4 mL 3 times daily.

Homeopathic Uses: 5 drops, 1 tablet, or 10 globules every 30 to 60 minutes (acute) or 1 to 3 times daily (chronic); parenterally: 1 to 2 mL sc acute, 3 times daily; chronic: once daily (HAB1).

Storage: Juniper should be protected from light.

LITERATURE

Ali AM, Mackeen MM, Intan-Safinar I et al. Antitumor-promoting activities of the crude extract from the leaves of *Juniperus chinensis. J Ethnopharmacol*; 53(3):165-169. 1996.

Anon. *Juniperi Fructus* (Juniper berry). In: European Scientific Cooperative on Phytoptherapy (ESCOP) Monographs on the Medicinal uses of Plant Drugs. European Scientific Cooperative on Phytotherapy, Exeter, England, July, 1997.

Chatzopoulou PS, Katsiotis ST. Study of the Essential Oil from *Juniperus communis* ''Berries'' (Cones)Growing in Greece. In: *PM* 59(6):554. 1993.

Chavali SR, Weeks CE, Zhong WW et al. Increased production of TNF-alpha and decreased levels of dienoic eicosanoids, IL-6 and IL-10 in mice fed menhaden oil and Juniper oil diets in response to an intraperitoneal lethal dose of LPS. *Prostaglandins Leukot Essent Fatty Acids;* 59(2):89-93. 1998.

Cuncliffe WJ & Dodman B. A comparison of tar liquid and cetrimide shampoo in the management of psoriasis of the scalp. *Br J Clin Practice;* 28(9):314-316. 1974.

De Pascuale Teresa J. *An Quim.* 73(3):463. 1977.

Eichler I. Cryptic illness from self-medication with herbal remedy. *Lancet* ; 1:356. 1983.

Freidrich H, Engelshowe R. *Planta Med* 33:251. 1978.

Gardner DR, Panter KE, James LF et al. Abortifacient effects of lodgepole pine (*Pinus contorta*) and common Juniper (*Juniperus communis*) on cattle. *Vet Hum Toxicol*; 40(5):260-263. 1998.

Hauser SP. Alzoon - Krebsheilmittel oder Medizinalsirup? *Praxis* ; 86:1113-1115. 1997.

Jones SM, Zhong Z, Enomoto N et al. Dietary Juniper berry oil minimizes hepatic reperfusion injury in the rat. *Hepatology*; 28(4):1042-1050. 1998.

Jonkov S & Naidenov G. Juniper bath treatment of the neuroasthenic neurosis. *Folia Medica*; 16(5/6):291-296. 1974.

Lamer-Zarawska E. Phytochemical studies on flavonoids and other compounds of Juniper fruits (*Juniperus communsi L.*). In: *Pol J Chem* 54(2):213-219. 1980.

Markkanen T. Antiherpetic agent(s) from Juniper tree (*Juniperus communis*) preliminary communication. *Drugs Exptl Clin Res*; 7(1):69-74. 1981.

Markkanen T, Makinen ML, Nikoskelainen J et al. Antiherpetic agent from Juniper tree (*Juniperus communis*), its purification, identification, and testing in primary human amnion cell cultures. *Drugs Exptl Clin Res*; 7(5):691-697. 1981.

Mascolo N et al. *Phytother Res* 1(1):28. 1987.

O'Muliane NM, Joyce P, Kamath SV et al. Adverse CNS effects of menthol-containing Olbas oil. *Lancet* ; 1:1121. 1982.

Phillips DH. Human adducts due to smoking and other carcinogen exposures. *Environ Mol Mutagen;* 14(15):153. 1989.

Ramic S, Murko D. Chemical composition of fruit of *Juniperus* species. In: *Archiv Farm* 33(1):15-20. 1983.

Sanchez de Medina F, Gamez MJ, Jimenez I et al. Hypoglycemic activity of Juniper ''berries.'' *Planta Med;* 60(3):197-200. 1994.

Schilcher H. Wacholderbeeroel bei Erkrankungen der ableitenden Harnwege? *MMP* ; 18(7):198-199. 1995.

Schilcher H, Boesel R, Effenberger ST Segebrecht S. Neuere Untersuchungsergebnisse mit aquaretisch, antibakteriell und prostatotrop wirksamen Arzneipflanzen. In: *ZPT* 10(3):77. 1989.

Schilcher H, Emmrich D, Koehler C. Gaschromatographischer Vergleich von ätherischen Wacholderölen und deren toxikologische Bedeutung. In: *PZW* 138(3/4)85. 1993.

Schilcher H & Heil BM. Nierentoxicitaet von Wacholderbeerzubereitungen. *Z Phytother*; 15(4):205-213. 1994.

Schmidt M. Wacholderzubereitungen. Muβ die Monographie umgeschrieben werden? In: *DAZ* 135(14):1260-1264. 1995.

Schoket B, Horkay I, Kosa A et al. Formation of DNA adducts in the skin of psoriasis patients, in human skin in organ culture, and in mouse skin and lung following topical application of coal-tar and Juniper tar. *J Invest Dermatol*; 94(2): 241-246. 1990.

Sökeland J. Phytotherapie in der Urologie. In: *ZPT* 10(1):8. 1989.

Thomas AF. *Helv Chim Acta* 55:2429. 1972.

Thomas AF. *Helv Chim. Acta* 56:1800. 1972.

Uehleke B. Phytobalneologie. *Z Phytother*; 17(1):26-43. 1996.

Van der Weijden GA, Timmer C, Timmerman MF et al. The effect of herbal extracts in an experimental mouthrinse on established plaque and gingivitis. *J Clin Peridontol*; 25(5):399-403. 1998.

Juniperus communis

See Juniper

Juniperus sabina

See Savin Tops

Justicia adhatoda

See Malabar Nut

Kadsura japonica

See False Schisandra

Kalmia latifolia

See Mountain Laurel

Kamala

Mallotus philippinensis

DESCRIPTION

Medicinal Parts: The medicinal parts are the glands and hairs covering the fruit.

Flower and Fruit: The tree has dioecious flowers. The male flowers are in threes in the axils of the bracts, while the female flowers are on longer, heavily branched, lateral boughs. Both flowers are covered by rust-red matted hairs. The fruit is a trilobed, pea-sized capsule from which a red, mealy powder is obtained, which consists of minute glands and hairs.

Leaves, Stem, and Root: Mallotus philippinensis is an 8- to 10-m high tree with a diameter of 90 to 120 cm. The bark of the slender branches is pale, and the younger ones are covered in rust-red matted hairs. The leaves are alternate and have articulate petioles, which are 2.5 to 5 cm long. The leaf blade is rusty tomentose, 8 to 15 cm long, ovate with two inconspicuous basal glands. It is entire-margined, coriaceous, and glabrous above with very prominent ribs below.

Habitat: The plant is indigenous to India, Ethiopia, Saudi Arabia, China and Australia.

Production: Kamala fruit skins are from the fruits of *Mallotus philippinensis*, covered in hairs and glands. The fruit is collected in the uncultivated regions and cleaned.

Other Names: Kameela, Kamcela, Spoonwood

ACTIONS AND PHARMACOLOGY

COMPOUNDS

Phloroglucinol derivatives (red to yellow, 47 to 80%): chief constituents include rottlerin (ca. 1%), isorottlerin (ca. 0.1%), 3-hydroxyrottlerin, 3,4-dihydroxyrottlerin, methylene-bis-methyl phloroacetophenone and their resinous polymers, that arise through auto-oxidation

Bergenin

Tannins

EFFECTS

The drug has an anthelmintic and purgative effect.

INDICATIONS AND USAGE

Indian Medicine: Internally, Kamala is used to treat tape worm infestations (ascarides, rectal worms), constipation, kidney and bladder stones, leprosy lesions and as a contraceptive; externally for parasitic skin diseases and wound infections of the ear.

PRECAUTIONS AND ADVERSE REACTIONS

No health hazards or side effects are known in conjunction with the proper administration of designated therapeutic dosages.

DOSAGE

Mode of Administration: The drug is used orally as a powder or liquid extract.

Daily Dosage: For worms: adults: 6 to 12 g drug in 2 to 3 portions at 30 minute intervals; young children: 1.5 g drug; school children: 3 g drug. Preparations can be sweetened with honey prior to administration.

Storage: Keep tightly sealed, dry and protected from light

LITERATURE

Kern W, List PH, Hörhammer L (Hrsg.), Hagers Handbuch der Pharmazeutischen Praxis, 4. Aufl., Bde. 1-8, Springer Verlag Berlin, Heidelberg, New York, 1969.

Ram A, Upadhyaya BB, Pandey HP, Singh RH. Evaluation of some Indian plants for their antibacterial activity. *Alternative Medicine* 3; 173-177. 1990

Widen CF, Puri HS, Planta Med 40:284. 1980

Kava Kava

Piper methysticum

DESCRIPTION

Medicinal Parts: The medicinal parts are the peeled, dried, cut rhizome, which has normally been freed from the roots, and the fresh rhizome with the roots.

Flower and Fruit: The plant has numerous small flowers in spikelike inflorescences 3 to 9 cm long.

Leaves, Stem, and Root: The plant is a 2- to 3-m high, erect dioecious bush. The leaves are very large, measuring 13 to 28 cm by 10 to 22 cm. They have a deeply cordate base and 9 to 13 main ribs that are slightly soft on the undersurface. The stipules are large. The plant has a massive, 2- to 10-kg, branched and very juicy rhizome with many roots. They are blackish-gray on the outside and whitish on the inside. The fracture is mealy and somewhat splintery. The central portion is porous with irregularly twisted thin woody bundles, separated by broad medullary rays, forming meshes beneath the bark.

Characteristics: The taste is pungent and numbing, and the odor is reminiscent of lilac.

Habitat: The plant is indigenous to the South Sea Islands and is mainly cultivated there.

Production: Kava Kava rhizome consists of the dried rhizomes of *Piper methysticum.*

Other Names: Ava, Ava Pepper, Intoxicating Pepper, Kawa, Kawa Pepper, Tonga, Kew

ACTIONS AND PHARMACOLOGY

COMPOUNDS

Kava lactones (kava pyrones, 5-12%): chief components include (+)-kavain, dihydrokavain (marindinine), (+)-methysticin, dihydromethysticin, yangonine, desmethoxy- yangonin

Chalcones: including flavokavin A and B

EFFECTS

The Kava pyrones in the drug have centrally muscle-relaxing, anticonvulsive, and antispasmodic effects. The herb also contains hypnotic/sedative, analgesic, and psychotropic properties contributing to its use for anxiety and insomnia. Kava pyrones are lipophilic and are better absorbed with food. The absorption and activity are enhanced when they are given as part of the whole root or mixtures of Kava pyrones rather than as single pyrones (Fachinfo Antares 120, 1996; Jamieson et al, 1989; Keledjian et al, 1988). Kava has animal or *in vitro* data supporting its use in bacterial infection (limited), cerebral artery occlusion, fungal infection, muscle tension, pain, and seizures. Kava is ineffective in the treatment of menopausal symptoms.

The mechanism of action for various pharmacological effects of Kava remain unclear and research has demonstrated that several factors, including concentration, type of preparation, Kava lactone content, and Kava cultivar used may impact pharmacologic activity. Kava lactones exhibited several effects on ion channels that may result in an overall effect of reduced excitability. These effects may be involved as mechanisms for the anxiolytic, sedative, muscle relaxant, mood stabilization, and anticonvulsant properties of kava.

Analgesic Effects: Kava's analgesic effect is due to inhibition on cyclooxygenase (COX) enzyme-II (Wu et al, 2002; Wu et al, 2002a). The analgesic action of kavain, dihydrokavain, methysticin, and dihydromethysticin is due to antinociceptive activities. Nalaxone (an opiate antagonist) is ineffective in reversing the antinociceptive activities, thus indicating the analgesia produced from the compounds occurs via nonopiate pathways (Jamieson & Duffield, 1990b). Kava lactones may have an analgesic effect on the lining of the urinary tubules and the bladder (Chavallier, 1996). Animal and *in vitro* experiments support certain analgesic actions of Kava (Gleitz et al, 1995). Both the aqueous and the lipid soluble extracts of Kava were tested for analgesia in mice. Both extracts demonstrated an analgesic response (Jamieson & Duffield, 1990b).

Antibacterial Effects: Kava pyrones have demonstrated limited antibacterial activity in vitro. No antibacterial action occurred in laboratory cultures of various bacteria treated with an aqueous extract of Kava (Locher et al, 1995).

Anticonvulsant Effects: Kava pyrones demonstrated an anticonvulsant effect in animals, inhibiting tonic seizures and lengthening and intensifying clonic seizures (Gleitz et al, 1995). Anticonvulsant properties are generally demonstrated in animals in doses up to 30 mg/kg of methysticin and dihydromethysticin, the most potent of the anticonvulsive agents in kava (Backhauss & Krieglstein, 1992).

Antifungal Effects: Animal and *in vitro* studies support certain antifungal actions of Kava (Gleitz et al, 1995; Jamieson & Duffield, 1990b) and Kava aqueous extract (Guerin & Reveillere, 1984).

Anti-inflammatory Effects: Several compounds isolated from a methanol extract of Kava root exhibited less inhibitory activity against COX-II enzymes in vitro than ibuprofen, naproxen, aspirin, celecoxib, and rofecoxib. These Kava compounds exhibited mild to moderate inhibitory activity against COX-II enzymes. Kava has mild anti-inflammatory actions (Wu et al, 2002). Comparable results were reported in a similar analysis. The compounds, dihydrokawain and yangonin, isolated from Kava roots exhibited the strongest inhibitory effects against COX-I and COX-2. Yangonin and another constituent, methysticin exhibited moderate antioxidant effects when compared to vitamin C and E (Wu et al, 2002a).

Kava pyrone (+)-Kavain isolated from *Piper methysticum* dose-dependently inhibited arachidonic acid (AA)-induced human platelet aggregation in vitro, primarily by inhibiting cyclooxygenase (COX). The ability of (+)-Kavain to inhibit cyclooxygenase and thus the formation of prostaglandin E2 provides a plausible mechanism of action for its antithrombotic and anti-inflammatory effects. The inhibitory effect of (+)-Kavain on COX results in the suppression of thromboxane A2 (TXA2) production and resultant platelet aggregation and release of adenosine 5c-triphosphate (ATP) (Gleitz et al, 1997).

Antithrombotic Effects: A recent study investigated the antithrombotic activity of kava pyrones. Kavain exerts antithrombotic action on human platelets through the inhibition of cyclooxygenase (COX) as a primary target. This suppresses the generation of thromboxane (TXA2), which normally induces aggregation of platelets and exocytosis of ATP by its binding on TXA2 receptors (Gleitz, 1997).

Anxiolytic Effects: Kava is approved by the German Commission E for the treatment of nervous anxiety and appears to be effective for mild anxiety of nonpsychotic origin. Mild generalized anxiety disorder may respond to Kava but moderate to severe anxiety does not. The limbic system is inhibited by Kava pyrones. This is associated with suppression of emotional excitability and mood enhancement (Fachinfo Antares 120, 1996). Kava pyrones demonstrated serotonergic and additive effects with serotonin-1A agonist ipsapirone in vitro. These effects may play a role in anxiolytic and sedative effects of kava (Grunze et al, 2001).

Central Nervous System Effects: (±) Kavain exhibited only weak GABA-ergic action in vitro when tested at concentrations required to maintain in vivo plasma concentrations at levels sufficient to produce pharmacological effects in humans (Grunze et al, 2001). Another study reported that kava lactones and dihydrokavain decreased nucleus tractus solitarius release in a rat gastric brainstem preparation in vitro similar to GABA-A receptor agonist, muscimol, but to a lesser extent. Results suggest that regulation of GABA-A receptor neurotransmission is a potential mechanism for the pharmacologic activity of kava (Yuan et al, 2002).

A recent study suggests that kava leaf extracts are more potent GABA-A receptor binders compared to root extracts. Kava lactone content in leaf extracts was less than root extracts, indicating that other constituents may impact GABA-ergic responses. This study also reported that root extracts of kava exhibited weak binding to benzodiazepine, dopamine D2, opioid, and histamine receptors, suggesting that these receptors are not involved as mechanisms for the pharmacological effects of kava root extracts. Results do suggest that dopamine D2, opioid, and histamine receptors may play a more active role in the pharmacologic effects of leaf extracts of Kava. Different cultivars of Kava also exhibited varying GABA-ergic responses (Dinh et al, 2001), providing some explanation for the varying responses observed in different studies.

Kava pyrones have demonstrated serotonergic and additive effects with serotonin-1A agonist ipsapirone in vitro. These effects may play a role in kava's anxiolytic and sedative effects (Grunze et al, 2001). Kava pyrones exhibited weak sodium antagonistic effects, which may, in part, explain the observed anticonvulsant properties of kava (Grunze et al, 2001).

The lipid soluble components of kava do not interact with benzodiazepine binding sites, but do seem to potentiate the activity of GABA-A in the brain center for sedative effects (Davies, 1992; Jussofie, 1994). The psychotropic properties of Kava have been demonstrated by the inhibition of norepinephrine uptake by kavain, dihydromethysticin and the racemate (±) kavain (Seitz, 1997). One study did find that desmethoxyyangonin, methysticin, yangonin, dihydromethysticin, kihydrokavain, and kavain reversibly inhibit MAO-B (Uebelhack, 1998). An increase of dopamine and serotonin by activation of neurons results in central nervous system effects (Fachinfo Antares 120, 1996).

Cerebrovascular Effects: The Kava pyrones methysticin and dihydromethysticin decreased infarct size and protected mouse and rat brains from damage after middle cerebral artery occlusion. The artery was occluded and either 150 mg Kava extract orally or 10 to 30 mg methysticin and dihydromethysticin were given intraperitoneally (Backhauss & Krieglstein, 1992; Backhauss & Krieglstein, 1992a).

Sleep-Inducing Effects: Kava has demonstrated improved sleep quality in patients with stress-induced insomnia in a small, open, uncontrolled trial. Kava demonstrated improved sleep quality in humans, increasing deep sleep but with no effects on rapid eye movement (REM) sleep (Fachinfo Antares 120, 1996).

Effects on Menopausal Symptoms: Kava was not significantly different than placebo in the treatment of menopausal symptoms (Cagnacci et al, 2003).

Muscle Relaxing Effects: Muscle relaxant effects of Kava may be explained by its ability to inhibit sodium ion currents (Grunze et al, 2001). The centrally muscle-relaxing, analgesic, and anticonvulsive actions of the Kava pyrones, kavain, dihydrokavain, dihydromethysticin and (±) kavain (synthetic Kava pyrone) are attributed to the interaction with ion channels. The interaction consists of fast and specific inhibition of voltage-dependent sodium channels and reduction of currents through voltage-activated sodium and calcium channels (Friese, 1998; Gleitz, 1995; Gleitz, 1996; Schirrmacher, 1999). The paralysis effect of Kava on neuromuscular transmission and muscle contractility is similar to that of local anesthetics (Jameison, 1989; Singh, 1983).

Vascular Effects: Kavain demonstrated dose dependently the inhibition of vascular smooth muscle contraction in rat thoracic aorta *ex vivo*, independent of endothelial factors. It has not been determined if Kava will also affect arterial blood pressure and vascular resistance (Martin et al, 2002).

CLINICAL TRIALS

Anxiety and Stress

A major systematic review of controlled clinical trials on herbal remedies for anxiety reported a lack of rigorous studies. Only for Kava was there convincing quality research found, along with clear evidence for effectiveness similar to benzodiazepines for anxiety (Ernst, 2006).

In contrast, a review of results from three placebo-controlled trials that used somewhat different dosages and measures for anxiety failed to confirm any benefit from Kava for generalized anxiety disorder as defined in the widely recognized *Diagnostic and Statistical Manual of Mental Disorders 4th Edition*. In this review, which pooled results involving 64 individuals (kava n=28; placebo n=30, venlafaxine n=6), no significant differences in anxiety symptoms were identified between the treatment groups in any of the trials. No evidence of toxic effects on the liver were found either, a recent concern. All treatments were well tolerated (Connor, 2006)

Reviewers were unable to conclude whether or not azapirone drugs such as buspirone are superior to Kava (or antidepressants or psychotherapy) in treating generalized anxiety disorder in a Cochrane Collaboration Review. The review, which identified 36 trials involving more than 5,000 participants in well-designed research, assessed the effectiveness and acceptability of azapirone drugs (which work at the body's 5-HT1A receptor) for generalized anxiety disorder. The review found azapriones to be superior to placebo (based on studies of four to nine weeks) but no likely superiority to standard benzodiazepines. The Kava study included was from 2003, and results were inconclusive. A limitation of the study was that buspirone was used at a lower than usual dose (Chessick, 2007).

A meta-analysis of six double-blind, placebo-controlled, randomized clinical trials concluded that Kava extract was an effective short-term treatment for symptomatic anxiety. Subjects with nonpsychotic and neurotic anxiety received doses ranging from 105 mg to 210 mg Kava lactones (extract WS1490, standardized to 70% Kava lactone content) daily for 3 to 4 weeks. A significant reduction in the Hamilton Anxiety (HAM-A) Scale score was observed in subjects treated with kava extract compared to placebo (p=0.01; n=345). Observed adverse events, including tiredness, symptom aggravation, and gastrointestinal upset, were reported to be temporary and mild and unrelated to dose; 2 studies reported no adverse events (Pittler & Ernst, 2003).

Kava was no better than placebo in patients with generalized anxiety disorder in a randomized, double-blind, placebo-controlled trial; however, patients with mild anxiety showed some benefit. Patients (n=35) received placebo or Kava (KavaPure®) with 140 mg Kava lactones daily for 1 week and then 280 mg Kava lactones for 3 weeks. Similar response rates between groups were observed on the primary outcome measures. Post hoc analysis of patients with low anxiety versus high anxiety demonstrated that Kava was more effective in reducing anxiety in patients with low anxiety as measured by the Self Assessment of Resilience and Anxiety (p<0.01) (Conner & Davidson, 2002). Two earlier randomized, double-blind, placebo-controlled studies of subjects with anxiety of nonpsychotic origin showed improvement with Kava therapy (Volz, 1997; Lehmann, 1996).

Kava treatment for 7 days was minimally effective in reducing physiological reactivity in healthy subjects in response to a laboratory-induced stressful situation in a randomized, non-placebo-controlled clinical trial (n=54) (Cropley et al, 2002).

The addition of a Kava extract to hormone replacement therapy caused significant reductions in anxiety in postmenopausal women. Forty menopausal women (either physiological or surgical) for 1 to 12 years were assigned to one of 4 treatment groups: combination estrogen and progestin (HRT) with Kava extract (55% kavain) 100 mg daily (n=13); HRT plus a matching placebo (n=9); estrogen alone plus Kava extract 100 mg daily (n=11); or estrogen plus placebo (n=7) for 6 months. Significant reductions HAM-A scores from baseline were demonstrated at 3- and 6-month follow-up in all groups (p<0.05). Significant differences were also observed between the Kava-supplemented groups and those given placebo (p<0.05). After 6 months, reductions in HAM-A from baseline for the HRT groups were: 55.5% for HRT with Kava, 23% for HRT alone (p<0.05 for HRT groups), 53.3% for estrogen with Kava and 25.8% with estrogen, and placebo (p<0.05). All women met DSM-IV diagnostic criteria for generalized anxiety, with a HAM-A score of at least 19 (De Leo et al, 2001).

Insomnia

The Kava special extract WS® 1490was found to be particularly effective in alleviating anxiety-related sleep disturbances (non-psychotic) in a multi-center, double-blind, 4-week clinical study involving 61 individuals randomized to receive either daily doses of 200 mg WS®1490 or placebo. Statistically significant improvement over placebo was found for the Kava extract for sleep questionnaire responses (using a validated self-rating scale) to ''recuperative effect after sleep'' and ''quality of sleep.'' The self-rating of ''well-being'' and the clinical evaluation also pointed to better efficacy for the Kava extract. The formula was well tolerated and no drug-related adverse events or laboratory changes were reported (Lehrl, 2004).

In a placebo-controlled, double-blind outpatient trial, the dosage range and efficacy of the kava special extract WS 1490 was investigated in patients with non-psychotic anxiety. Fifty patients received a daily dose of 3 x 50 mg WS 1490 during a 4-week treatment period followed by a 2-week safety observation phase. WS 1490 was well-tolerated and produced no drug-related adverse events or post-study withdrawal symptoms. The special kava extract was found to be effective and safe in the treatment of non-psychotic anxiety syndromes in a daily dose of 150 mg (Geier & Konstantinowicz, 2004).

Six-week treatment with Kava reduced insomnia in subjects with stress-induced insomnia (23 to 65 years) in an open-label, uncontrolled clinical trial. Subjects (n=24) received 120 mg of oral Kava daily for 6 weeks. Mean insomnia severity scores as measured by time to fall asleep, hours slept, and mood on final wakening decreased from 138 to 107.1 after Kava treatment ($p<0.05$ compared to baseline) (Wheatley, 2001). The validity of the results of this study should be interpreted with caution due to methodological flaws, including uncontrolled study design, lack of a placebo control group, and use of only self-administered rating scales.

Mood

Twenty healthy (11 female and nine male college students) were enrolled in a double-blind, randomized, placebo-controlled trial in which a single dose of standardized Kava root extract (300 mg, containing 90 mg Kava pyrones) was given to half the group. Kava enhanced increased positive affect related to exhilaration in individuals disposed to cheerful mood, but did not alter bad mood or a state of ''seriousness.'' It also enhanced cognitive performance, particularly visual attention and short-term memory retrieval. The authors point to Kava's anxiolytic properties that can facilitate cognition rather than compromise it as conventional benzodiazepine-type anxiolytics tend to do (Thompson, 2004).

INDICATIONS AND USAGE

Approved by Commission E:

- Nervous anxiety and stress
- Restlessness, tension, and agitation

Kava Kava is used for nervous tension, stress, and agitation.

Unproven Uses: In folk medicine, the herb is used as a sleeping agent and sedative; for asthma, rheumatism, dyspeptic symptoms, chronic cystitis, syphilis, gonorrhea, and weight reduction.

Homeopathic Uses: Kava Kava is used for states of excitement and exhaustion. It is also used for gastritis and pain in the urethra.

CONTRAINDICATIONS

Kava is contraindicated in patients with endogenous depression because it may increase the danger of suicide (Fachinfo Antares 120, 1996). Due to case reports of Kava-related dyskinesia, it has been suggested that Kava should be contraindicated in patients with neurological disorders (Stevinson et al, 2002).

Pregnancy: Not to be used during pregnancy.

Breastfeeding: Not to be used while breastfeeding.

PRECAUTIONS AND ADVERSE REACTIONS

NOTE: The United States Food and Drug Administration advised consumers of the potential risk of severe liver injury associated with the consumption of Kava (FDA, 2003) and asked healthcare professionals to review cases of liver toxicity to determine if any may be related to the use of Kava-containing dietary supplements. Consumers and healthcare providers are requested to report any adverse events associated with Kava use to the FDA's MedWatch program (FDA, 2003).

Kava has also been reported to cause mild and reversible gastrointestinal complaints, central nervous system complaints, including dizziness and headache, and various hypersensitivity/dermatological reactions. Pupil dilatation, near-vision abnormalities, and eye movement coordination abnormalities have been reported. Kava dermopathy (a reversible darkening or yellowing of the skin with whitish scaling and flaking) has been reported with long-term use of higher doses. Regular administration of Kava for longer than 3 months is not recommended (Fachinfo Kavosporal Forte 1996; Fachinfo Antares 120, 1996).

Alcohol: Concomitant use of Kava with alcohol may increase the risk of adverse hepatic effects and excessive sedation. Case reports of severe liver toxicity including hepatitis, cirrhosis, and liver failure requiring liver transplant have been reported related to the use of Kava-containing herbal products (Escher et al, 2001; Kraft et al, 2001; Lewis-Taylor, 2001; Strahl et al, 1998). *Clinical Management:* Advise patients of the sedative and hepatotoxic potential of Kava. Patients should be advised to avoid alcohol during Kava use. If Kava and alcohol are taken together, activities requiring mental alertness such as driving and operating heavy machinery should be avoided. For patients who elect to use Kava despite this advice, liver function tests should be closely monitored.

Central Nervous System: Three cases of meningism (meningismus) were reported following the consumption of Kava (Wheatley, 2001). Dyskinesia was reported in four patients who developed clinical signs of central dopaminergic antagonism after Kava use (Schelosky et al, 1995). Choreoathetosis of the limbs, trunk, neck and facial musculature has been reported secondary to the administration of Kava (Schelosky, 1995; Spillane, 1997). Kava intensifies the effects of alcohol (see *Drug Interactions* below).

Gastrointestinal: Two large post-marketing surveillance studies reported good to very good tolerability of Kava in 93% to 96% of subjects. Gastrointestinal complaints were considered mild and reversible (Stevinson et al, 2002).

Hepatotoxicity: See Note above. See following references for case reports of hepatotoxicity (Russman & Helbling, 2001; Escher et al, 2001; Kraft et al, 2001; Strahl, 1998).

Hypersensitivity: Pruritus and a generalized rash with erythema and papules in conjunction with Kava administration have been reported (Stevinson et al, 2002; Schmidt & Boehncke, 2000).

Musculoskeletal: Minor inhibition of movement and impaired motor reflexes have been observed with the use of Kava (Fachinfo Antares 120, 1996; Fachinfo Kavosporal Forte, 1996; Jamieson & Duffield, 1990; Jamieson & Duffield, 1990a).

Ocular: Visual disturbances such as eye movement disorders, near vision abnormalities, and mydriasis have been reported. Increase in pupil diameter, reduction of the near point of accommodation and near point of convergence, and disturbance to the oculomotor balance have been reported with Kava (Garner, 1985). Eye irritation has been reported with the heavy consumption of Kava (Ruze, 1990).

DRUG INTERACTIONS

Kava inhibited cytochrome P450 (CYP) enzymes 1A2, 2C9, 2C19, 2D6, 3A4, and 4A9/11 *in vitro*. Caution is advised when kava is used with drugs metabolized by these enzymes.

MAJOR RISK

Hepatotoxic Drugs: See Note under Precautions and Adverse Reactions. Concomitant use of Kava with other drugs with known potential for hepatotoxicity may increase the risk of adverse hepatic effects. Similarly, Kava should not be combined with other herbs with the potential to cause hepatotoxicity. These include but are not limited to chaparral (*Larrea tridentata*), Russian comfrey (*Symphytum x uplandicum*), coltsfoot (*Tussilago farfara*), germander (*Teucrium chamaedrys*), jin bu huan, pennyroyal (*Mentha pulegium, Hedeoma pulegoides*), and petasites (*Petasites japonicus*). *Clinical Management:* Patients should be advised of the risk of hepatotoxicity associated with Kava. Patients should specifically avoid Kava while taking other drugs with hepatotoxic potential. For those patients who elect to use Kava despite this advice, liver function tests should be closely monitored.

MODERATE RISK

Anticoagulants, Antiplatelet Agents, Low Molecular Weight Heparins, Thrombolytic Agents: Concurrent use of Kava with any of these agents may result in an increased risk of bleeding. *Clinical Management:* Caution is advised. Monitor the patient closely for signs and symptoms of bleeding. Adjust the dose only if the patient is consistently taking kava with a consistent and standardized product.

Amantadine: Concurrent use may result in decreased effectiveness of amantadine. *Clinical Management:* Avoid concomitant use of Kava with amantadine. The dopaminergic effect may be diminished or variable depending on the time of administration of kava and the quality of the kava product (i.e., whether it consistently contains a standardized amount of kava).

Barbiturates: Concurrent use may result in in creased central nervous system depression. *Clinical Management:* Avoid concomitant use of Kava and barbiturates. For patients who choose to use the combination despite this advice, monitor closely for sedation, drowsiness, slowed reflexes, and other indicators of central nervous system depression. Advise against activities that require mental and psychomotor acuity (e.g., handling of heavy machinery).

Benzodiazepines: Concomitant use of Kava and a benzodiazepine may result in increased central nervous system depression. *Clinical Management:* Avoid concomitant use of kava and benzodiazepines. For patients who choose to use the combination despite this advice, monitor closely for sedation, drowsiness, slowed reflexes, and other indicators of central nervous system depression. Advise against activities that require mental and psychomotor acuity (e.g., handling of heavy machinery).

Bromocriptine: Concurrent use may result in decreased effectiveness of bromocriptine. *Clinical Management*: Avoid concomitant use of Kava and bromocriptine. The dopaminergic effect may be diminished or variable depending on the time of administration of kava and the quality of the Kava product (i.e., whether it consistently contains a standardized amount of Kava).

Centrally Acting Muscle Relaxants and Opioid Analgesics: Concurrent use with Kava may result in increased central nervous system. *Clinical Management:* Avoid concomitant use of kava and centrally acting muscle relaxants or opioid analgesics. For patients who choose to use the combination despite this advice, monitor closely for sedation, drowsiness, slowed reflexes, and other indicators of central nervous system depression. Advise against activities that require mental and psychomotor acuity (e.g., handling of heavy machinery).

Dopamine Agonists: Kava may oppose the dopaminergic effect of dopamine agonists, decreasing their effectiveness. *Clinical Management:* Avoid concomitant use of Kava with dopamine agonists. The dopaminergic effect may be reduced or variable depending on the time of administration of Kava and the quality of the Kava product (i.e., whether it consistently contains a standardized amount of Kava).

Dopamine-2 Antagonists and Phenothiazines: Concurrent use of Kava and these medications may result in additive dopamine antagonistic effects, increasing the risk for adverse effects. *Clinical Management:* Avoid concomitant use. The desired effect and/or adverse effects of these agents may be increased or variable depending on the time of administration of Kava and the quality of the Kava product (i.e., whether it contains a standardized amount of Kava).

Monoamine Oxidase Inhibitors: Patients taking Kava with MAOIs may be at risk of increased toxicity associated with excessive inhibition of monoamine amine oxidase. *Clinical Management:* Avoid concomitant use of Kava with MAOIs until this potential drug-herb interaction is better characterized. If Kava and an MAOI are used concomitantly, monitor for early symptoms of MAOI toxicity such as irritability, hyperactivity, anxiety, hypotension, vascular collapse, insomnia, restlessness, dizziness, faintness, drowsiness, hallucinations, trismus, flushing, sweating, tachypnea, tachycardia, movement disorders (e.g., grimacing, opisthotonus), and severe headache.

POTENTIAL INTERACTIONS

Psychoactive Agents: The intensity of psychoactive agents may be intensified with kava (Jamieson, 1990). *Clinical Management:* Monitor carefully.

OVERDOSAGE

The overdose potential for Kava appears to be low. Overdosage can result in disorders of complex movement, accompanied by undisturbed consciousness, later tiredness and tendency to sleep.

DOSAGE

Mode of Administration: Comminuted rhizome and other galenic preparations for oral use.

How Supplied:

Capsules – 100 mg, 125 mg, 128 mg, 150 mg, 250 mg, 390 mg, 400 mg, 425 mg, 455 mg, 500 mg

Liquid – 1:1, 1:2

Tea

Preparation: There are a number of different extraction recipes depending on the pharmaceutical companies.

Daily Dosage:

Capsules – The root extract is taken 150 mg to 300 mg twice daily, with a daily dosage of Kava pyrones 50 to 240 mg (Herberg, 1996; Lehmann, 1996).

Tincture – The tincture is taken as 30 drops with water 3 times daily (Chavallier, 1996).

Infusion – Take 1/2 cup twice daily (Chavallier, 1996).

Note: The drug should be administered with food or liquid due to its lipid solubility (Fachinfo Antares 120, 1996). The activity of the herb is enhanced when mixtures of the kava pyrones are taken instead of a single pyrone (Jamieson, 1989).

Homeopathic Dosage: The herb is taken as 5 to 10 drops, 1 tablet, or 5 to 10 globules 1 to 3 times daily, or 1 ml injection solution sc twice weekly (HAB1).

Storage: The herb should be stored away from direct light, moisture and heat at room temperature.

LITERATURE

Almeida JC & Grimsley EW, Coma from the health food store: interaction between kava and alprazolam (letter). *Ann Intern Med*; 125:940-941. 1996.

Anon. Germany may ban kava-kava herbal supplement. November 19, 2001. Accessed at: http://pharmacists.medscape.com/reuters/prof/2001/11/ 11.20/ 20011119rglt010.html (Cited 12/20/2001).

Anon. Germany's Merck pulls two kava drugs over possible safety worries. November 28, 2001a. Accessed at: http://pharmacists.medscape.com/reuters/prof/2001/11/ 11.29/ 20011128inds003.html (Cited 12/20/2001).

Anon. Warnings/advisories: Kava and liver toxicity: frequently asked questions. Health Canada Online, August, 2002. http://www.hc- sc.gc.ca/english/protection/warnings/2002/200256e.htm (cited 07/03/2003).

Backhauss C & Krieglstein J. Extract of kava (*Piper methysticum*) and its methysticin constituents protect brain tissue against ischemic damage in rodents. *Eur J Phamacol*; 215:265-269. 1992.

Backhauss C & Krieglstein J. Neuroprotective activity of kava extract (*Piper methysticum*) and its methysticin constituents in vivo and in vitro. *Pharmacol Cereb Ischemia; Int Symposium* 4(2-3):501-507. 1992a.

Baum SS, Hill R, Rommelspacher H. Effect of kava extract and individual kavapyrones on neurotransmitter levels in the nucleus accumbens of rats. *Prog Neuropsychopharmacol Biol Psychiatry* Oct;22(7):1105-20. 1998.

Bhate H, Gerster G, Fracza E. Orale Prämedikation mit Zubereitungen aus Piper methysticum bei operativen Eingriffen in Epiduralanästhesie. *Erfahrungsheilkunde* 6:339-345. 1989.

Bhate H, Gerster G. Behandlung mit Phytotranquilizern vor der Narkose. *Therapeutikon* 5:214-222. 1992.

Cagnacci A, Arangino S, Renzi A et al. Kava-Kava administration reduces anxiety in perimenopausal women. *Maturitas*; 44(2):103-109. 2003.

Chessick CA, Allen MH, Thrase M, et al. Azapirones for generalized anxiety disorders. *Cochrane Database Syst Rev* 3: CD006115. 2006.

Connor KM, Payne V, Davidson JR. Kava in generalized anxiety disorder: three placebo-controlled trials. *Int Clin Psychopharmacol;* 21(5):249-53. 2006.

Connor KM & Davidson JRT. A placebo-controlled study of Kava kava in generalized anxiety disorder. *Int Clin Psychopharmacol*; 17(4):185-188. 2002.

Cropley M, Cave Z, Ellis J et al. Effect of kava and valerian on human physiological and psychological responses to mental stress assessed under laboratory conditions. *Phytother Res*; 16(1):23-27. 2002.

Cupp MJ, Herbal remedies: adverse effects and drug interactions. Am Fam Physician Mar 1;59(5):1239-45. 1999.

Davies LP, Drew CA, Duffield P et al., Kava pyrones and resin: studies on GABAA, GABAB and benzodiazepine binding sites in rodent brain. *Pharmacol Toxicol* Aug;71(2):120-6. 1992.

De Leo V. La Marca A, Morgante G et al. Evaluation of combining kava extract with hormone replacement therapy in the treatment of postmenopausal anxiety. *Maturitas*; 39(2):185-188. 2001.

Dingermann T. Phytopharmaka im Alter: Crataegus, Ginkgo, Hypericum und Kava-Kava. In: *PZ* 140(23):2017-2024. 1995.

Dinh LD, Simmen U, Bueter KB et al. Interaction of various Piper methysticum cultivars with CNS receptors in vitro. *Planta Med*; 67(4):306-311. 2001.

Emser W, Bartylla K. Verbesserung der Schlafqualität. *TW Neurol Psychiatr* 5:636-642. 1991.

Ernst E. Herbal remedies for anxiety - a systematic review of controlled clinical trials. *Phytomedicine*; 13(3):205-8. 2006.

Escher M, Desmeules J, Giostra E et al. Hepatitis associated with kava, an herbal remedy for anxiety. *BMJ*; 322(7279):139. 2001.

Fachinformation. Antares® 120, kava-kava extract. Krewel Meuselbach GmbH, Eitorf, 1996.

Fachinformation. Kavosporal® forte, kava-kava extract. Mueller Goeppingen Gmbh & Co KG, Goeppingen, 1996.

FDA. Kava-containing dietary supplements may be associated with severe liver injury. March 25, 2002. Accessed at http://www.cfsan.fda.gov/dms/supplmnt.html (cited 5/17/2003).

FDA. Letter to health-care professionals: FDA issues consumer advisory that kava products may be associated with severe liver injury. Rockville, MD: U.S. Dept of Health and Human Services; 2002.

Friese J, Gleitz J. Kavain, dihydrokavain, and dihydromethysticin non-competitively inhibit the specific binding of [3H]-batrachotoxinin-A 20-alpha-benzoate to receptor site 2 of voltage-gated Na+ channels. *Planta Med* Jun;64(5):458-9. 1998.

Garner LF & Klinger JD. Some visual effects caused by the beverage kava. *J Ethnopharmacol*; 13:307-311. 1985.

Geier FP, Konstaninowicz T. Kava treatment in patients with anxiety. *Phytother Res*; 18(4): 297-300. 2004.

Geβner B, Cnota P. Untersuchung der Vigilanz nach Applikation von Kava-Kava-Extrakt, Diazepam oder Placebo. *Z Phytother* 15:30-37. 1994.

Gleitz J, Beile A, Wilkens P et al., Antithrombotic action of the kava pyrone (+)-kavain prepared from Piper methysticum on human platelets. *Planta Med* Feb;63(1):27-30. 1997.

Gleitz J et al. Kavain inhibits non-stereospecifically veratridine-activated Na+; channels. *Planta Med* 62(6):580-581. 1996.

Gleitz J, Friese J, Beile A et al. Anticonvulsive action of (±)-kavain estimated from its properties on stimulated synaptosomes and Na+ channel receptor sites. Eur J Pharmacol Nov 7;315(1):89-97. 1996.

Gleitz J, Beile A, Peters T et al. (±)-Kavain inhibits veratridine-activated voltage-dependent Na(+)-channels in synaptosomes prepared from rat cerebral cortex. *Neuropharmacology* Sep;34(9):1133-1138. 1995.

Grunze H, Langosch J, Schirrmacher K et al. Kava pyrones exert effects on neuronal transmission and transmembraneous cation currents similar to established mood stabilizers-a review. *Prog Neuropsychopharmacol Biol Psychiatry*; 25(8):1555-1570. 2001.

Guerin JC & Reveillere HP. Activite antifongique d'extracts vegetaux a usage therapeutique: I. Etude de 41 extraits sur 9 souches fonigues (French). *Ann Pharm Fr*; 42(6):553-559. 1984.

Hänsel R, Beiersdorff HU. *Arzneim Forsch* 9:581. 1955.

Hänsel R, Kava-Kava (*Piper methysticum* G. Forster), in der modernen Arzneimittelforschung Portarit einer Arzneipflanze. In: *ZPT* 17(3):180-195. 1996.

Hänsel R. Pflanzliche Sedativa. In: *ZPT* 11(1):14. 1990.

Hänsel R, Woelk H. Spektrum Kava-Kava. 2. Auflage. Aesopus Verlag GmbH, Basel. 1995.

Herberg KW. Alltagssicherheit unter Kava-Kava-Extrakt, Bromazepam und deren Kombination. Z Allge Med;72:973-977. 1996.

Herberg KW. Fahrtüchtigkeit nach Einnahme von Kava-Spezial-Extrakt WS 1490. Z Allge Med 67:842-846. 1991.

Jamieson DD, Duffield PH. The antinociceptive actions of kava components in mice. *Clin Exp Pharmacol Physiol* Jul;17(7):495-508. 1990b.

Jamieson DD & Duffield PH. Interaction of kava and ethanol in mice. *Eur J Pharmacol*; 183(2):559. 1990.

Jamieson DD, Duffield PH, Cheng D et al. Comparison of the central nervous system activity of the aqueous and lipid extract of kava (*Piper methysticum*). *Arch Int Pharmacodyn Ther* Sep-Oct;301:66-80. 1989.

Jamieson DD, Duffield PH. Positive interaction of ethanol and kava resin in mice. *Clin Exp Pharmacol Physiol* Jul;17(7):509-14. 1990a.

Jappe U, Franke I, Reinhold D et al. Sebotrophic drug reaction from kava-kava extract therapy: a new entity? *J Am Acad Dermatol*; 38(1):104-106. 1998.

Johnson E, Frauendorf A, Stecker K, Stein U. Neurophysiologisches Wirkprofil und Verträglichkeit von Kava-Extrakt WS 1490. *TW Neurol Psychiatr* 5:349-354. 1991.

Jussofie A, Schmiz A & Hiemke C. Kavapyrone enriched extract from Piper methysticum as modulator of the GABA binding site in different regions of rat brain. *Psychopharmacology* (Berl). Dec;116(4):469-474. 1994.

Keledjian J, Duffield PH, Jamieson DD et al. Uptake into mouse brain of four compounds present in the psychoactive beverage kava. *J Pharm Sci*; 77(12):1003-1006. 1988.

Kinzler E, Krömer J, Lehmann. Wirksamkeit eines Kava-Spezial-Extraktes bei Patienten mit Angst-, Spannungs- und Erregungszuständen nicht-psychotischer Genese. *Arzneim Forsch/ Drug Res* 41:584-588. 1991.

Kraft M, Spahn TW, Menzel J et al. Fulminant liver failure after administration of the herbal antidepressant kava-kava (Abstract). Dtsch Med Wochenschr; 126(36):970-972. 2001.

Lehmann E, Kinzler E, Friedemann J. Efficacy of a special Kava extract (piper methysticum) in patients with states of anxiety, tension and excitedness of non-mental origin - A double-blind placebo-controlled study of four weeks treatment. *Phytomedicine*;2:113-119. 1996.

Lehrl S. Clinical efficacy of kava extract WS1490 in sleep disturbances associated with anxiety disorders. Results of a multicenter, randomized, placebo-controlled, double-blind clinical trial. *J Affect Disord; 78:101*-10. 2004.

Lewis-Taylor C. FDA Letter to Healthcare Professionals. Dec 19, 2001. Accessed at: http://www.fda.gov/medwatch/safety/2001/safety01.htm kava (cited 12/20/2001).

Locher CP, Burch MT, Mower HF et al. Antimicrobial activity and anti-complement activity of extracts obtained from selected Hawaiian medicinal plants. *J Ethnopharmacol*; 49(1):23-32. 1995.

Martin HB, McCallum M, Stofer WD et al. Kavain attenuates vascular contractility through inhibition of calcium channels. Planta Med; 68(9):784-789. 2002.

Mathews JD, Riley MD, Fejo L et al. Effects of the heavy usage of kava on physical health: summary of a pilot survey in an Aboriginal community. *Med J Aust*; 148:548-555. 1988.

Mathews JM, Etheridge AS & Black SR. Inhibition of human cytochrome P450 activities by kava extract and kavalactones. *Drug Metab Dispos*; 30(11):1153-1157. 2002.

Münte TF, Heinze HJ, Matzke M, Steitz J. Effects of oxacepam and an extract of Kava roots *(Piper methysticum)* on event-related potentials in a word recognition task. *Neuropsychobiology* 27:46-53. 1993.

Norton SA & Ruze P. Kava dermopathy. *J Am Acad Dermatol*; 31(1):89-97. 1994.

Pittler ME & Ernst E. Efficacy of kava extract for treating anxiety: systematic review and meta-analysis. *J Clin Psycholpharmacol*; 20(1):84-89. 2000.

Pittler MH & Ernst E. Kava extract for treating anxiety (Cochrane Review) In: The Cochrane Library, Issue 1. Oxford: Update Software. 2003.

Russman S & Helbling A. Kava hepatotoxicity. Ann Intern Med; 135(1):68-69. 2001.

Ruze P, Kava-induced dermopathy: a niacin deficiency? *Lancet* Jun 16:335(8703):1442-1445. 1990.

Schelosky L, Raffauf C, Jendroska K et al. Kava and dopamine antagonism (letter). *J Neurol Neurosurg Psychiatry* May;58(5):639-640. 1995.

Schirrmacher K, Busselberg D, Langosch JM et al. Effects of (±)-kavain on voltage-activated inward currents of dorsal root ganglion cells from neonatal rats. *Eur Neuropsychopharmacol* Jan;9(1-2):171-6. 1999.

Schmidt M, Kava-Kava. In: *PTA* 8(5):374. 1994.

Schmidt P & Boehncke WH. Delayed-type hypersensitivity reaction to kava-kava extract. *Contact Dermatitis*; 42(6):363-364. 2000.

Seitz U, Schule A, Gleitz J. [3H]-monoamine uptake inhibition properties of kava pyrones. *Planta Med* Dec;63(6):548-549. 1997.

Sibon I, Rosier E & Orgogozo J. Syndrome meninge apres absorption de kava-kava. *Rev Neurol*; 158(12):1205-1206. 2002.

Siegel RK, Herbal intoxication. Psychoactive effects from herbal cigarettes, tea and capsules. *JAMA* 236:473-476. 1976.

Singh YN. Effects of kava on neuromuscular transmission and muscle contractility. *J Ethnopharmacol.* May;7(3):267-76. 1983.

Smith LW, Culvenor CC. Plant sources of hepatotoxic pyrrolizidine alkaloids. *J Nat Prod. Mar*-Apr;44(2):129-52. 1981.

Smith RM. *Tetrahedron* 35(3):437. 1979.

Som UK, Dutta CP, Sarkar GM et al. Antibacterial studies with the compounds isolated from *Piper methysticum* Forst. *Nat Acad Sci Letters*; 8(4):109-110. 1985.

Spillane PK, Fisher DA & Currie BJ. Neurological manifestations of kava intoxication (letter*). Med J Aust;* 167(3):172-173. 1997.

Spree MH, Croy HH. Antares - ein standardisiertes Kava-Kava-Präparat mit dem Spezialextrakt KW 1491. *Der Kassenarzt*;17:44-51. 1992.

Stahl S, Ehret V, Dahm HH et al. Necrotizing hepatitis after taking herbal remedies. Dtsch Med Wochenschr; 123(47):1410-1414. 1998.

Stevinson C, Huntley A & Ernst E. A systematic review of the safety of kava extract in the treatment of anxiety. Drug Saf; 25(4):251-261. 2002.

Strahl S, Ehret V, Dahm HH et al. Necrotizing hepatitis after taking herbal remedies (abstract). Dtsch Med Wochenschr; 123(47):1410-1410. 1998.

Thompson R, Ruch W, Hasenohrl RU. Enhanced cognitive performance and cheerful mood by standardized extracts of *Piper methysticum* (Kava-kava). *Hum Psychopharmacol*;19:243-50. 2004.

Uebelhack R, Franke L, Schewe H-J. Inhibition of platelet MAO-B by kava pyrone-enriched extract from Piper methysticum Forster (kava-kava). *Pharmacopsychiatry* Sep;31(5):187-192. 1998.

Volz HP, Kieser M. Kava-Kava Extract WS 1490 versus Placebo in Anxiety Disorders - A Randomized Placebo-controlled 25-week Outpatients Trial. *Pharmacopsychiatry* Jan;30(1):1-5. 1997.

Volz HP. Die anxiolytische Wirksamkeit von Kava-Spezialextrakt WS 1490 unter Langzeittherapie - eine randomisierte Doppelblindstudie. *Z Phytother Abstractband*, S 9. 1995.

Volz HP, Hänsel R. Kava-Kava und Kavain in der Psychopharmakotherapie. *Psychopharmakotherapie* 1:33-39. 1994.

Warnecke G, Pfaender H, Gerster G, Gracza E. Wirksamkeit von Kawa-Kawa-Extrakt beim klimakterischen Syndrom. *Z Phytother* 11:81-86. 1990.

Wheatley D. Kava and valerian in the treatment of stress-induced insomnia. *Phytother Res*; 15(6):549-551. 2001.

Woelk H et al. Behandlung von Angst-Patienten. *Z Allgemeinmed*;10:271-277. 1993.

Wu D, Nair MG & DeWitt DL. Novel compounds from *Piper methysticum* Forst (Kava Kava) roots and their effect on cyclooxygenase enzyme. *J Agric Food Chem*; 50(4):701-705. 2002.

Wu D, Yu L, Nair MG et al. Cyclooxygenase enzyme inhibitory compounds with antioxidant activities from *Piper methysticum* (kava kava) roots. *Phytomedicine*; 9(1):41-47. 2002a.

Yuan CS, Dey L, Wang A et al. Kavalactones and dihydrokavain modulate GABAergic activity in a rat gastric-brainstem preparation. *Planta Med*; 68(12):1092-1096. 2002.

Kelp

Laminaria hyperborea

DESCRIPTION

Medicinal Parts: The medicinal part is the stemlike part of the thallus.

Flower and Fruit: The plant fits the general description of brown algae. It is unsegmented to heavily segmented and can grow into plants many meters in length. The thallus is reminiscent of root, leaf or stem-like organs (in the case of *L hyperborea* stemlike). The color is greenish-brown to reddish.

Habitat: The plant grows on the North Atlantic coast.

Production: Kelp consists of the dried, stem-like parts of the thallus of *Laminaria hyperborea* (syn. *Laminaria cloustonii*).

ACTIONS AND PHARMACOLOGY

COMPOUNDS

Salts of alginic acid (laminaric acid, 25%)

Iodine (to some extent organically bound, 0.3-0.45%)

Reserve carbohydrates: laminarin (47%), mannitol (5-6%), fucoidin, mannitol glucoside

EFFECTS

No information is available.

INDICATIONS AND USAGE

Unproven Uses: Preparations of kelp are used for the regulation of thyroid function.

PRECAUTIONS AND ADVERSE REACTIONS

No health hazards or side effects are known in conjunction with the proper administration of designated therapeutic dosages. The danger of induction or worsening of hyperthyroidism following internal administration of the drug exists with dosages above 150 mcg iodide per day. In rare cases, it can lead to severe allergic reactions.

DOSAGE

No information is available.

LITERATURE

Chen FP, Soong YK, Hui YL, Successful treatment of severe uterine synechiae with transcervical resectoscopy combined with *laminaria tent. Hum Reprod,* 75:943-7, May. 1997

Chiu KW, Fung AY, The cardiovascular effects of green beans (Phaseolus aureus) common rue (*Ruta graveolens*) and kelp (*Laminaria Japonica*) in rats. *Gen Pharmacol,* 75:859-62, Nov. 1997

Drozhzhina VA, Petrishchev NN, Fedorov IuA, The enhancement of the physiological resistance of the periodontal tissues in white rats under the action of biologically active substances from *Laminaria. Fiziol Zh Im I M Sechenova,* 75:126-33, Dec. 1995

Glatstein IZ, Pang SC, McShane PM, Successful pregnancies with the use of laminaria tents before embryo transfer for refractory cervical stenosis. *Fertil Steril,* 75:1172-4, Jun. 1997

Jain JK, Mishell DR Jr, A comparison of misoprostol with and without *laminaria tents* for induction of second-trimester abortion. *Am J Obstet Gynecol,* 75:173-7, Jul. 1996

Kern W, List PH, Hörhammer L (Hrsg.), Hagers Handbuch der Pharmazeutischen Praxis, 4. Aufl., Bde. 1-8, Springer Verlag Berlin, Heidelberg, New York, 1969.

Lin A, Kupferminc M, Dooley SL, A randomized trial of extra-amniotic saline infusion versus *laminaria* for cervical ripening. *Obstet Gynecol,* 75:545-9, Oct. 1995

Nguyen MT, Hoffman DR, Anaphylaxis to *Laminaria. J Allergy Clin Immunol,* 75:138-9, Jan. 1995

Read SM, Currie G, Bacic A, Analysis of the structural heterogeneity of laminaria by electrospray-ionisation-mass spectrometry. *Carbohydr Res,* 75:187-201, Feb 23. 1996

Schneider D, Halperin R, Langer R, Caspi E, Bukovsky I, Abortion at 18-22 weeks by laminaria dilation and evacuation. *Obstet Gynecol,* 75:412-4, Sep. 1996

Khat

Catha edulis

DESCRIPTION

Medicinal Parts: The medicinal parts of the tree are the leaves.

Flower and Fruit: The inflorescence is a cyme growing from the leaf axil. The flowers are radial and inconspicuous, with a fleshy disk and their structures are in fives. The calyx is 5-lobed and there are 5 elongate-oval, white-yellowish petals, 5 stamens, and 3 blunt stigmas. The fruit is three-sided capsule with chamber containing 1, occasionally 2, seeds. The brownish seeds have a winglike, whitish aril.

Leaves: Khat is an evergreen shrub or tree that reaches about 2 to 25 m high. The leaves are opposite on flowering branches. They are alternate, coriaceous, 3 to 12 cm long, oval to ovate, and crenate or dentate. The upper surface of the leaves is waxlike glossy and olive green. The older leaves are occasionally red-violet.

Habitat: Ethiopia, Kenya, North Yemen, and northern Madagascar

Production: Khat or Arabian tea is the fresh leaves or shoots of *Catha edulis.* The leaves are harvested in the early morning, 5 to 8 years after planting. They are kept in banana leaves, paper or plastic to prevent it drying out.

Other Names: Abyssinian Tea, Arabian Tea, Somali Tea

ACTIONS AND PHARMACOLOGY

COMPOUNDS

Phenyl alkyl amines (0.3 to 0.9%): khatamine, in fresh leaves as chief effective agent (S)-(-)-cathinone (50% in young leaves, in fully-developed leaves only 2%), becoming dimers during dehydration, as well as (+)-norpseudoephedrine (cathine), (-)-norephedrine, merucathinone, pseudomerucathinone, (-)-formyl norephedrine

Sesquiterpene polyester alkaloids: cathaedulines K1 to K15

Catechin tannins

Volatile oil

EFFECTS

The alkaloid-containing drug (chief active ingredient cathinone) is centrally stimulating and indirectly sympathomimetic (amphetamine-like effect). In addition, the leaf preparations have ulcer-protective and insecticidal effects, and the drug's high tannin content makes it constipating.

INDICATIONS AND USAGE

The medicinal use of Khat preparations is obsolete today.

Unproven Uses: Khat has been used for centuries in Islamic culture to improve communicative abilities, performance and to suppress feelings of hunger. The leaves can be chewed or administered as an infusion (Yemen) or paste (Ethiopia/Somalia). Khat leaves are said to have an aphrodisiac effect and are used for depression, headache, gonorrhea, gastric complaints, coughs, asthma, and fever.

PRECAUTIONS AND ADVERSE REACTIONS

The fresh shoot tips may lead to central excitation, suppression of appetite, widening of the pupils, increased motor activity, hypertonia, and hyperthermia through the sympathomimetic effect of cathinone (the other constituents account for only approximately 10% of the effect) and its ability to bypass the blood-brain barrier. Moderate dosages (100 to 300 g of the fresh leaves) lead to a state of general well being, mental alertness, and exaggerated self-regard. Physical ability is temporarily enhanced and the need for sleep is reduced. Depression and anxiety states can follow once the effect wears off. Diabetics could experience hyperglycemia. The tannin content of the drug leads to constipation and digestive disorders. Acute poisonings have not been recorded.

Chronic use can lead to such long-term ill effects as emaciation (through appetite suppression), increased susceptibility to infection, nervousness, insomnia, and disturbances of the circadian rhythm. In addition, Khat preparations have been associated with ulcers in the digestive tract and liver and kidney damage. When the drug is used over periods of years, it can lead to personality disorders.

DOSAGE

Mode of Administration: Available as whole herb and powdered drug

Storage: Can be kept for several months deep-frozen

LITERATURE

Al-Ahdal MN, McGarry TJ, Hannan MA Cytotoxicity of Khat (*Catha edulis*) extract on cultured mammalian cells: effects on macromolecule biosynthesis. *Mutat Res*, 204:317-22, Feb 1988

Al-Meshal IA, Tariq M, Parmar NS, Ageel AM Anti-inflammatory activity of the flavonoid fraction of khat (*Catha edulis Forsk*). *Agents Actions*, 19:379-80, Jan 1986

Bálint GS, Bálint E Kath (*Catha edulis*) - a plant containing an amphetamine-like substance Orv Hetil, 136:1063-6, May 14, 1995

Dhadphale M, Mengech A, Chege SW Miraa (*catha edulis*) as a cause of psychosis. *East Afr Med J*, 19:130-5, Feb 1981

Geisshüsler S, Brenneisen R The content of psychoactive phenylpropyl and phenylpentenyl khatamines in *Catha edulis Forsk.* of different origin. *J Ethnopharmacol*, 19:269-77 May, 1987

Geisshüsler S, Brenneisen R The presumed neurotoxic effects of *Catha edulis* - an exotic plant now available in the United Kingdom. *Br J Ophthalmol*, 19:779-81, Oct 1986

Hänsel R, Keller K, Rimpler H, Schneider G (Ed) Hagers Handbuch der Pharmazeutischen Praxis. 5. Aufl., Bde 4 - 6 (Drogen), Springer Verlag Berlin, Heidelberg, New York, 1992-1994

Kalix P Catha edulis, a plant that has amphetamine effects. *Pharm World Sci,* 18:69-73, Apr 1996

Kalix P Hyperthermic response to (-)-cathinone, an alkaloid of *Catha edulis* (khat). *J Pharm Pharmacol,* 11:662-3, Sep 1980

Nabil Z, Saleh M, Mekkawy H, Allah GA Effects of an extract of khat (*Catha edulis*) on the toad heart. *J Ethnopharmacol*, 18:245-56, Dec 1986

Nencini P, Amiconi G, Befani O, Abdullahi MA, Anania MC Possible involvement of amine oxidase inhibition in the sympathetic activation induced by khat (*Catha edulis*) chewing in humans. *J Ethnopharmacol,* 11:79-86, Jun 1984

Tariq M, Al-Meshal I, Al-Saleh A Toxicity studies on *Catha edulis*. *Dev Toxicol Environ Sci,* 11:337-40, 1983

Knautia arvensis

See Field Scabious

Knotweed

Polygonum aviculare

DESCRIPTION

Medicinal Parts: The medicinal parts are the herb, sometimes with the root, collected during the flowering season and dried, as well as the fresh aerial parts collected during the flowering season.

Flower and Fruit: The inflorescences are axillary cymes with 1 or a few flowers. The flowers are very small, short-pedicled, inconspicuous and green or red with white margins. The epicalyx has 5 bracts and is fused at the base. There are 5 stamens, and the superior ovary has 3 styles. The fruit is a nut, which is as long as the epicalyx and is matte brown with wrinkled stripes, ovate to almost elliptical and flattened on 3 sides.

Leaves, Stem, and Root: The plant is a sturdy annual. The main stem is initially erect, up to 1 m high, and heavily branched. It later becomes closely procumbent and spreads along the ground. The leaves are alternate, entire-margined, short-petioled with varying forms on the main and side shoots. They are broadly elliptical to linear-lanceolate, acute or obtuse. At the base of the leaves there is a scarious divided leaf sheath. The thin, fusiform, brownish roots produce a few hair-thin lateral roots.

Characteristics: The appearance depends on the location. It may also have an ascending stem.

Habitat: The plant is found in most temperate regions of the world.

Production: Knotweed herb consists of the dried herb, occasionally containing roots, of Polygonum aviculare, gathered during flowering season.

Other Names: Allseed Nine-Joints, Armstrong, Beggarweed, Bird's Tongue, Birdweed, Centinode, Cow Grass, Crawlgrass, Doorweed, Hogweed, Knotgrass, Ninety-Knot, Pig-rush, Pigweed, Red Robin, Sparrow Tongue, Swine's Grass, Swynel Grass

ACTIONS AND PHARMACOLOGY

COMPOUNDS

Flavonoids (0.1-1%): chief components are avicularin (quercetin-3-arabinoside), hyperoside, quercitrin, quercetin-3-galactoside, additionally including among others vitexin, isovitexin, rhamnazine bisulphate

Silicic acid (1%): partially water-soluble

Tannins (4%) gallo tannins, catechin tannins

Hydroxycoumarins: umbelliferone, scopoletin

Lignans: aviculin

EFFECTS

Knotweed has astringent properties. In vitro, the flavonoid fraction is said to inhibit aggregation of human erythrocytes, probably by an effect on cyclo-oxygenase.

INDICATIONS AND USAGE

Approved by Commission E:

- Cough/bronchitis
- Inflammation of the mouth and pharynx

The herb is used as a mild catarrh of the respiratory tract for inflammatory changes to the oral and pharyngeal mucosa.

Unproven Uses: In folk medicine it is used as a supportive treatment for pulmonary disordersfor cough, bladder and kidney disorders, oliguria, night sweats, gout, and rheumatism. Externally, it is used as a hemostatic in cases of hemorrhage and for skin disorders.

Chinese Medicine: In China, Knotweed is used for gonorrhea, jaundice, skin defects, dysentery (red), itching, and tapeworm in children.

Homeopathic Uses: In homeopathy, *Polygonum aviculare* is used for rheumatism of the fingers.

PRECAUTIONS AND ADVERSE REACTIONS

No health hazards or side effects are known in conjunction with the proper administration of designated therapeutic dosages.

DOSAGE

Mode of Administration: As a ground herb for teas and other galenic preparations for internal use and local application. The drug is a component of various pectoral and bronchial teas. The extract is found in standardized preparations of antitussives and diuretics.

Preparation: To make a tea, place 1.5 g finely cut drug in cold water and bring to a simmer. Strain after 5 to 10 minutes (1 teaspoonful = 1.4 g drug).

Daily Dosage: The daily dosage is 4 to 6 g of drug.

Tea—As a supportive treatment for coughs and bronchial catarrh, drink 1 cup 3 to 5 times a day.

Infusion for external use—The daily dose is 5 g drug.

Homeopathic Dosage: 5 drops, 1 tablet, or 10 globules every 30 to 60 minutes (acute) or 1 to 3 times daily (chronic); parenterally: 1 to 2 mL sc, acute: 3 times daily; chronic: once a day (HAB34)

LITERATURE

Delitheos A, Tiligada E, Yannitsaros A, Bazos I. Antiphage activity in extracts of plants growing in Greece. *Phytomedicine* 4 (2); 117-124. 1997

Hänsel R, Keller K, Rimpler H, Schneider G (Hrsg.), Hagers Handbuch der Pharmazeutischen Praxis, 5. Aufl., Bde 4-6 (Drogen), Springer Verlag Berlin, Heidelberg, New York, 1992-1994.

Karl J. Bronchitis und Phytotherapie. *Naturheilpraxis* 46; 167-173. 1993

Madaus G, Lehrbuch der Biologischen Arzneimittel, Bde 1-3, Nachdruck, Georg Olms Verlag Hildesheim 1979.

Steinegger E, Hänsel R, Pharmakognosie, 5. Aufl., Springer Verlag Heidelberg 1992.

Wichtl M (Hrsg.), Teedrogen, 4. Aufl., Wiss. Verlagsges. Stuttgart 1997.

Kombe Seed

Strophanthus hispidus

DESCRIPTION

Medicinal Parts: The medicinal part of the plant is the ripe seed.

Flower and Fruit: The inflorescence is a many-blossomed, umbelliferous raceme. The flowers are radial and their structures are in fives. The sepals are 1.3 to 1 cm long and 0.1 to 1 cm wide. They are unevenly divided into five, the outer tips ovate, the inner ones lanceolate and densely pubescent. The corolla is tubular, with the upper part broadened into a cup shape. The margin is covered with 10 scales, 1.1 to 2 cm long with a diameter of 0.8 to 1.7 cm. The margin is white or yellow, with a purple spot in the shaft. There are 5 stamens and a double-chambered, semi-inferior ovary. The fruit is a follicle, 24 to 48 cm long, 1.3 to 1.8 cm in diameter, dark brown, hard, grooved and white punctate with lenticles. The seeds are spindle-shaped, flat, 1 to 1.8 cm long, 2 to 3 mm wide, densely pubescent with an upright, 4 to 8 cm long tuft of hair.

Leaves, Stem, and Root: Strophanthus hispidus is either a liana, up to 100 m long, or a shrub, up to 5 m high. The leaves are opposite. The petiole is 1 to 5 mm long, the lamina 15 to 22 cm long, and 8 to 12 cm wide. The leaves are simple, elliptical to obovate, acuminate, rounded at the base, or cordate. The trunk has a diameter of up to 6 m and has dark gray bark. The branches are dark brown or almost black. The young branches are stiffly villous and punctate with lenticles.

Characteristics: The plant contains latex.

Habitat: West and Central Africa

Production: Brown Strophanthus seeds are the ripe seeds of *Strophanthus hispidus* freed from the bushel-like appendage. The seeds are first harvested after 3 years (first flowering). Then the fruit is picked, and the seeds are removed.

Not to be Confused With: Often confused in the past with *Strophanthus kombe, S. sarmentosus* and other *Strophanthus* species. Can also be confused with Alafia, Futumia, Kickxia and *Holrrhena* species.

Other Names: Arrow Poison

ACTIONS AND PHARMACOLOGY

COMPOUNDS

Cardioactive steroid glycosides (cardenolids, 4 to 8%): chief glycoside presumably k-strophanthoside (primary glycoside, strophanthidin glucosyl cymaroside) from which cymarin (strophantidin cymaroside) is formed through fermentation of the seeds

Saponins (0.2%)

Fatty oil (30%): chief fatty acids oleic acid, linoleic acid, palmitic acid and 9-hydroxy-delta12-octadecenoic acid

EFFECTS

The action mechanism of the drug is dependent upon the cardioactive cardenolide glycosides it contains (see S. kombé semen and strophantine effects).

INDICATIONS AND USAGE

Unproven Uses: Preparations of the herb have been used in the past for cardiac complaints.

Homeopathic Uses: In homeopathy, preparations are used for nervous cardiac complaints and cardiac insufficiency.

PRECAUTIONS AND ADVERSE REACTIONS

General: No health hazards are known in conjunction with the proper administration of designated therapeutic dosages.

DRUG INTERACTIONS

POTENTIAL INTERACTIONS

The simultaneous administration of quinidine, calcium salts, saluretics, laxatives and glucocorticoids enhance effects and side effects.

OVERDOSAGE

Nausea, vomiting, headache, stupor and cardiac arrhythmias could occur as side effects with parenteral administration of glycoside mixtures of the drug, particularly with overdoses.

DOSAGE

Mode of Administration: Communited drug, herb powder, and liquid preparations for internal use.

Homeopathic Dosage: (from D4) 5 drops, 1 tablet, 10 globules every to 30 to 60 minutes, maximum 12 times daily (acute) and 1 to 3 times daily (chronic); parenterally: 1 to 2 mL sc., IV, IM, 3 times daily (acute) and once a day (chronic) (HPUS88).

LITERATURE

Hänsel R, Keller K, Rimpler H, Schneider G (Ed), Hagers Handbuch der Pharmazeutischen Praxis, 5. Aufl., Bde 4 - 6 (Drogen), Springer Verlag Berlin, Heidelberg, New York, 1992-1994

Kousso

Hagenia abyssinica

DESCRIPTION

Medicinal Parts: The medicinal parts are the leaves, the unripe fruit, and the dried panicles of female flowers.

Flower and Fruit: The small flowers are large-branched, thickly glandular-haired panicles up to 0.5 m long. They are androgynous, male, or female. The male flowers are greenish and have fertile stamens and hairy bracts. The female flowers are dark-red.

Leaves, Stem and Root: Hagenia abyssinica is tree that grows up to 6 m high with tuftlike, erect, pinnatifid leaves.

Habitat: The plant is indigenous to northeast Africa and is cultivated in Ethiopia.

Production: Kousso flowers are the flowers of *Hagenia abyssinica.*

Other Names: Cossoo, Kooso, Kosso

ACTIONS AND PHARMACOLOGY

COMPOUNDS

Acylphloroglucinols (kosotoxine): monomeric, dimeric, trimeric compounds, such as protocosin (trimeric); acyl residues are isobutyryl- isovaleryl- and alpha-metylbutyryl residues; representatives include, for example, cosin K6 and cosin K8 (monomerous), cusso toxin (dimerous), protocosin (trimerous)

Tannins

EFFECTS

Kousso is a vermifuge because of its complex mixture of aglyphloroglucinols, which has a taeiafugic effect. An antitumoral effect has also been described

INDICATIONS AND USAGE

Unproven Uses: This obsolete drug can no longer be procured; it was formerly was used to treat tapeworm infestation. Its efficacy depended on the composition of the drug.

PRECAUTIONS AND ADVERSE REACTIONS

Side effects include irritation of the gastrointestinal tract, salivation, nausea and diarrhea. A tendency toward fainting spells, headache, and general weakness has been connected with the use of the drug during use as a tapeworm cure. Abortive effects have been described. The drug should no longer be administered in allopathic dosages.

OVERDOSAGE

Conditions of collapse and vision disorders have been observed with overdosages. The treatment for poisoning consists of gastrointestinal emptying (inducement of vomiting, gastric lavage with burgundy-colored potassium pêrmanganate solution, sodium sulfate), installation of activated charcoal and shock prophylaxis (quiet, warmth). Diazepam (IV) should be used to treat spasms. Atropine and electrolyte substitution should be employed. Possible cases of acidosis should be countered with sodium bicarbonate infusions. In case of shock, plasma volume expanders should be administered. Monitoring of kidney function is essential. Intubation and oxygen respiration may also be necessary.

DOSAGE

Mode of Administration: The drug is obsolete in most countries.

LITERATURE

Kern W, List PH, Hörhammer L (Hrsg.), Hagers Handbuch der harmazeutischen Praxis, 4. Aufl., Bde. 1-8, Springer Verlag Berlin, Heidelberg, New York, 1969.

Lewin L, Gifte und Vergiftungen, 6. Aufl., Nachdruck, Haug Verlag, Heidelberg 1992.

Madaus G, Lehrbuch der Biologischen Arzneimittel, Bde 1-3, Nachdruck, Georg Olms Verlag Hildesheim 1979.

Metzner J et al., Antispastische Wirkung von Hagenia abyssinica. In: PM 47(4):240-241. 1983.

Teuscher E, Lindequist U, Biogene Gifte - Biologie, Chemie, Pharmakologie, 2. Aufl., Fischer Verlag Stuttgart 1994. Metzner J et al Antispastische Wirkung von Hagenia abyssinica. Planta Med 47, 240-241 1983

Woldemariam TZ, Fell AF, Linley PA, Chromatographic and spectroscopic studies on the constituents in male and female flowers of Hagenia abyssinica. J Pharm Biomed Anal, 8:859-65, 1990.

Woldemariam TZ, Fell AF, Linley PA, Bibby MC, Phillips RM, Evaluation of the anti-tumour action and acute toxicity of kosins from Hagenia abyssinica. J Pharm Biomed Anal, 10:555-60, Aug 1992

Krameria triandra

See Rhatany

Kudzu

Pueraria lobata

DESCRIPTION

Medicinal Parts: Root.

Botanical Description: Twining or creeping woody vine with a tuberous root. The stems are densely covered with yellow-brown hairs. The leaves are trifoliate, alternate, the rachis is 8-20 cm long. The terminal blade is mostly ovate and lobed, 8-22 cm x 7-15 cm, shortly acuminate at the apex and rounded at the base. The alternate leaflets are similar, but irregularly lobed. The surfaces are softly pubescent. Stipules are above and below their attachment. The inflorescence is a many-flowered axillary raceme 15-40 cm long. The calyx is 9-14 mm long, divided more than halfway into 5 unequal lobes, hairy, subtended by a pair of small bracteoles. The corolla is papilionaceous, 13-20 mm long, violet with the standard, marked with a yellow blotch. There are 10 stamens, diadelphous. The ovary is superior. The fruit is a flat, brown, densely hairy pod 9-12 cm x 0.9-1.2 cm.

Habitat: Southeastern United States, Southeast Asia and potentially throughout the tropical and subtropical regions of the world.

Not to be Confused With: Daidzein, Fen Ke, Ge Gen, Japanese Arrowroot, Kwaao Khruea, Pueraria, Yege.

ACTIONS AND PHARMACOLOGY

COMPOUNDS

Actives include daidzin, daidzein, puerarin, genistin, genistein, tectorigenin, glycitin, tectoridin, 6'-O-xylosyltectoridin, 6'-O-xyloglycitin, biochanin A, and spinasterol. Roots: flavones, daidzin, daidzein, puerarin and D-xylose. Flowers: butyric and glutamic acids, asparagine, adenine, and the isoflavone glycoside irisolidone 7-O-glucoside.

EFFECTS

The isoflavones in kudzu root extract may suppress alcohol intake and alcohol withdrawal symptoms. Antibacterial effects, anti-cancer effects, anti-inflammatory effects, antioxidant effects, antithrombotic effects, cardiovascular effects, estrogenic effects, hepatic effects, hypoglycemic effects, neurologic effects, and osteoporotic effects have been described for Puerarin. Kudzu also inhibits and induces cytochrome P450 isoenzymes.

CLINICAL TRIALS

Alcoholism

To test the efficacy of a kudzu extract, male and female ''heavy'' drinkers were enrolled in a randomized, controlled study and received either a kudzu extract for seven days or placebo, and were then given the opportunity to drink their preferred brand of beer while in a naturalistic laboratory setting. Drinking behavior was monitored by a digital scale that was located in the top of an end table. The administration of kudzu resulted in a significant reduction in the number of beers consumed which was paralleled by an increase in the number of sips and the time to consume each beer and a decrease in the volume of each sip. These changes occurred in the absence of a significant effect on the urge to drink alcohol. No side effects were reported while using kudzu (Lukas et al, 2005).

A randomized, double-blind, placebo-controlled trial was conducted to assess if kudzu root extract influences the drinking habits of veterans who entered a substance abuse treatment program. Thirty-eight patients diagnosed with alcoholism were randomly assigned to receive either kudzu root extract 1.2 g twice daily (n=21) or a matching placebo (n=17). Patients completed questionnaires that focused on craving for alcohol and sobriety status on a monthly basis. Sobriety level and craving for alcohol were assessed on a visual analog scale from 0 to 10. No statistically significance difference in craving and sobriety scores were noted after one month between kudzu and placebo (Shebek & Rindone, 2000).

Angina Pectoris

Seventy-eight patients with angina pectoris who were to receive Percutaneous Transluminal Coronary Angioplasty (PTCA) and stenting treatment were randomly divided, single-blind, into a conventional group and the puerarin injection group. Based on the conventional treatment and pre-operational preparation, the puerarin injection group was given 200 mL of puerarin by intravenous drip once a day, beginning from one week before operation. Normal saline was given to the conventional group. The condition of angina pectoris attack in balloon dilatory stage of PTCA and change of ST segment of ECG detected by a 12-lead ECG monitor were observed. The blood levels of von Willebrand factor (vWF:Ag), nitric oxide (NO) and endothelin-1 (ET-1) were also observed before and after treatment. As compared with those in the conventional group, the number of patients having angina pectoris attack and ST segment change in PTCA process was lessened in the puerarin injection group, with blood levels of vWF:Ag and ET-1 lower, and NO content higher than those in the conventional group (Xie et al, 2003).

Deafness

The effect of kudzu on sudden deafness was observed in 72 patients who were randomly assigned into a therapeutic group (n=40), who received intravenous infusion of puerarin injection, and a control group (n=32), who were given intravenous infusion of anisodamine. The total efficacy rates against sudden deafness and tinnitus in the therapeutic group were 89.68% and 84.37%, respectively, but only 62.5% and 56.52%, respectively, in the control group, showing a significant difference ($p<0.05$) (Liu et al, 2002).

Diabetes

A study to explore the effect of puerarin in improving insulin resistance and its closely related abnormal lipid and fibrinolytic activity in patients with coronary heart disease (CHD) was conducted. Seventy-six patients were randomly divided into two groups, 40 in the puerarin group and 36 in the routine treatment group. Puerarin 500 mg was given to the former in addition to routine therapy by adding to 250 mL of normal saline for intravenous dripping once a day with a therapeutic course of three weeks. Changes in fasting blood glucose, fasting plasma insulin (FINS), plasma total cholesterol (TC), triglyceride (TG), low- and high-density lipoprotein cholesterol (LDL-C and HDL-C) and plasminogen activator inhibitor-1 (PAI-1) activity were measured before and after treatment, and the insulin sensitivity index (ISI) calculated. At the same time, tissue plasminogen activator (tPA) activity before and during venous occlusion test (VOT) was tested. An additional 30 healthy subjects were taken as control. In CHD patients, FINS, TC, TG, LDL-C and PAI-1 levels were higher and ISI, HDL-C and tPA before and during VOT were lower than those in the healthy controls. After puerarin treatment, FINS level lowered and ISI increased significantly ($p<0.01$), while, compared with the routine group, TC, TG, LDL-C and PAI-1 were lower, but HDL-C and tPA activity before and during VOT were higher in the puerarin group ($p<0.05$, $p<0.01$). The results show that puerarin may improve insulin resistance and insulin resistance-related lipid and fibrinolytic activity abnormality in CHD patients (Shi et al, 2002).

INDICATIONS AND USAGE

Unproven Uses: Allergic rhinitis, cancer, circulation, cirrhosis, colds, diarrhea, dysentery, encephalitis, fever, gastroenteritis, headaches, hypertension, influenza, migraine, osteoporosis, psoriasis, trauma, urticaria.

Probable Efficacy: Uses in alcoholism, cardiovascular disease/angina, diabetes, and menopausal symptoms are reasonably well documented.

CONTRAINDICATIONS

None are known.

PRECAUTIONS AND ADVERSE REACTIONS

There are no side effects reported of oral kudzu treatment. Scientific evidence for the safe use of kudzu during pregnancy and nursing is not available.

DRUG INTERACTIONS

POTENTIAL INTERACTIONS

P. lobata may inhibit the effects of estrogen therapy, interfere with antiarrhythmic agents, lower blood glucose levels, and interfere with hypotensive agents

DOSAGE

Oral: for menopausal symptoms kudzu powder containing 100 mg isoflavones, for alcoholism 2.4 g kudzu root extract daily, for cardiovascular complaints puerarin 400 mg daily

Parenteral: 200-500 mg daily, in various compositions.

LITERATURE

Akita H, Sowa J, Makiura M, et al. Maculopapular drug eruption due to the Japanese herbal medicine Kakkonto (kudzu or arrowroot decoction). Contact Dermatitis 2003;48(6):348-349.

Benlhabib E, Baker JI, Keyler DE, et al. Composition, red blood cell uptake, and serum protein binding of phytoestrogens extracted from commercial kudzu-root and soy preparations. J Med Food 2002;5(3):109-123.

Benlhabib E, Baker JI, Keyler DE, et al. Effects of purified puerarin on voluntary alcohol intake and alcohol withdrawal symptoms in P rats receiving free access to water and alcohol. J Med Food 2004;7(2):180-186.

Benlhabib E, Baker JI, Keyler DE, et al. Kudzu root extract suppresses voluntary alcohol intake and alcohol withdrawal symptoms in P rats receiving free access to water and alcohol. J Med Food 2004;7(2):168-179.

Bennetau-Pelissero C, Latonnelle KG, Lamothe V, et al. Screening for oestrogenic activity of plant and food extracts using in vitro trout hepatocyte cultures. Phytochem Anal 2004;15(1):40-45.

Boue SM, Wiese TE, Nehls S, et al. Evaluation of the estrogenic effects of legume extracts containing phytoestrogens. J Agric Food Chem 2003;51(8):2193-2199.

Carai MA, Agabio R, Bombardelli E, et al. Potential use of medicinal plants in the treatment of alcoholism. Fitoterapia 2000;71 Suppl 1:S38-S42.

Cervellati R, Renzulli C, Guerra MC, et al. Evaluation of antioxidant activity of some natural polyphenolic compounds using the Briggs-Rauscher reaction method. J Agric Food Chem 2002;50(26):7504-7509.

Chen J, Xu J, Li J. [Effect of puerarin on fibrinolytic activity and lipid peroxide in patients with coronary heart disease]. Zhongguo Zhong Xi Yi Jie He Za Zhi 1999;19(11):649-650.

Chen L, Chai Q, Zhao A, et al. [Effect of puerarin on cerebral blood flow in dogs]. Zhongguo Zhong Yao Za Zhi 1995;20(9):560-2, inside.

Chen WC, Hayakawa S, Yamamoto T, et al. Mediation of beta-endorphin by the isoflavone puerarin to lower plasma glucose in streptozotocin-induced diabetic rats. Planta Med 2004;70(2):113-116.

Chen X. [The clinical observation of puerarin injection on unstable angina pectoris]. Zhong Yao Cai 2004;27(1):77-78.

Chiang HM, Fang SH, Wen KC, et al. Life-threatening interaction between the root extract of Pueraria lobata and methotrexate in rats. Toxicol Appl Pharmacol 2005;209(3):263-268.

Choo MK, Park EK, Yoon HK, et al. Antithrombotic and antiallergic activities of daidzein, a metabolite of puerarin and daidzin produced by human intestinal microflora. Biol Pharm Bull 2002;25(10):1328-1332.

Chueh FS, Chang CP, Chio CC, et al. Puerarin acts through brain serotonergic mechanisms to induce thermal effects. J Pharmacol Sci 2004;96(4):420-427.

Dong K, Tao QM, Xia Q, et al. [Endothelium-independent vasorelaxant effect of puerarin on rat thoracic aorta]. Zhongguo Zhong Yao Za Zhi 2004;29(10):981-984.

Dong LP, Wang TY. Effects of puerarin against glutamate excitotoxicity on cultured mouse cerebral cortical neurons. Zhongguo Yao Li Xue Bao 1998;19(4):339-342.

Duan HJ, Liu SX, Zhang YJ, et al. [Effects of puerarin on renal function, expressions of MMP-2 and TIMP-2 in diabetic rats]. Yao Xue Xue Bao 2004;39(7):481-485.

Duan S, Li YF, Luo XL. [Effect of puerarin on heart function and serum oxidized-LDL in the patients with chronic cardiac failure]. Hunan Yi Ke Da Xue Xue Bao 2000;25(2):176-178.

Fan LL, Sun LH, Li J, et al. The protective effect of puerarin against myocardial reperfusion injury. Study on cardiac function. Chin Med J (Engl) 1992;105(1):11-17.

Guerra MC, Speroni E, Broccoli M, et al. Comparison between chinese medical herb Pueraria lobata crude extract and its main isoflavone puerarin antioxidant properties and effects on rat liver CYP-catalysed drug metabolism. Life Sci 2000;67(24):2997-3006.

Guo XG, Chen JZ, Zhang X, et al. [Effect of puerarin on L-type calcium channel in isolated rat ventricular myocytes]. Zhongguo Zhong Yao Za Zhi 2004;29(3):248-251.

Hao LN, Ling YL, He SZ, et al. [Peroxynitrite-induced formation of diabetic cataract and its prevention by puerarin in rat]. Zhonghua Yan Ke Za Zhi 2004;40(5):311-316.

Heyman GM, Keung WM, Vallee BL. Daidzin decreases ethanol consumption in rats. Alcohol Clin Exp Res 1996;20(6):1083-1087.

Hsieh MT, Kuo LH, Tsai FH, et al. Effects of puerarin on scopolamine-, mecamylamine-, p-chloroamphetamine- and dizocilpine-induced inhibitory avoidance performance impairment in rats. Planta Med 2002;68(10):901-905.

Hsu FL, Liu IM, Kuo DH, et al. Antihyperglycemic effect of puerarin in streptozotocin-induced diabetic rats. J Nat Prod 2003;66(6):788-792.

Hsu HH, Chang CK, Su HC, et al. Stimulatory effect of puerarin on alpha1A-adrenoceptor to increase glucose uptake into cultured C2C12 cells of mice. Planta Med 2002;68(11):999-1003.

Jang MH, Shin MC, Kim YJ, et al. Protective effects of puerariae flos against ethanol-induced apoptosis on human neuroblastoma cell line SK-N-MC. Jpn J Pharmacol 2001;87(4):338-342.

Jeon GC, Park MS, Yoon DY, et al. Antitumor activity of spinasterol isolated from Pueraria roots. Exp Mol Med 2005;37(2):111-120.

Jiang B, Liu JH, Bao YM, et al. Hydrogen peroxide-induced apoptosis in pc12 cells and the protective effect of puerarin. Cell Biol Int 2003;27(12):1025-1031.

Jiang XL, Xu LN. [Beneficial effect of puerarin on experimental microcirculatory disturbance in mice]. Yao Xue Xue Bao 1989;24(4):251-254.

Jin LH, Liu CF, Zeng Y. [Protective effects of puerarin on radiation injury of experimental rats]. Zhong Xi Yi Jie He Xue Bao 2005;3(1):43-45.

Jin M, Qin J, Wu W. [Clinical study on Tianbaokang injection against oxidative injury of vascular endothelial function in ischemic apoplexy]. Zhong Yao Cai 2003;26(2):148-151.

Jin WS, Tan YY, Chen YG, et al. [Determination of puerarin, daidzin and daidzein in root of Pueraria lobata of different origin by HPLC]. Zhongguo Zhong Yao Za Zhi 2003;28(1):49-51.

Kang RX. [The intraocular pressure depressive effect of puerarin]. Zhonghua Yan Ke Za Zhi 1993;29(6):336-339.

Kaufman PB, Duke JA, Brielmann H, et al. A comparative survey of leguminous plants as sources of the isoflavones, genistein and daidzein: implications for human nutrition and health. J Altern Complement Med 1997;3(1):7-12.

Keung WM, Lazo O, Kunze L, et al. Potentiation of the bioavailability of daidzin by an extract of Radix puerariae. Proc Natl Acad Sci U S A 1996;93(9):4284-4288.

Keung WM, Vallee BL. Daidzin and its antidipsotropic analogs inhibit serotonin and dopamine metabolism in isolated mitochondria. Proc Natl Acad Sci U S A 1998;95(5):2198-2203.

Keung WM, Vallee BL. Kudzu root: an ancient Chinese source of modern antidipsotropic agents. Phytochemistry 1998;47(4):499-506.

Keyler DE, Baker JI, Lee DY, et al. Toxicity study of an antidipsotropic Chinese herbal mixture in rats: NPI-028. J Altern Complement Med 2002;8(2):175-183.

Kim DH, Jung EA, Sohng IS, et al. Intestinal bacterial metabolism of flavonoids and its relation to some biological activities. Arch Pharm Res 1998;21(1):17-23.

Kim DH, Yu KU, Bae EA, et al. Metabolism of puerarin and daidzin by human intestinal bacteria and their relation to in vitro cytotoxicity. Biol Pharm Bull 1998;21(6):628-630.

Kim OS, Choi JH, Soung YH, et al. Establishment of in vitro test system for the evaluation of the estrogenic activities of natural products. Arch Pharm Res 2004;27(9):906-911.

Kim S, Fung DY. Antibacterial effect of crude water-soluble arrowroot (Puerariae radix) tea extracts on food-borne pathogens in liquid medium. Lett Appl Microbiol 2004;39(4):319-325.

Lau CS, Carrier DJ, Beitle RR, et al. A glycoside flavonoid in Kudzu (Pueraria lobata): identification, quantification, and determination of antioxidant activity. Appl Biochem Biotechnol 2005;121-124:783-794.

Lee DS, Kim YS, Ko CN, et al. Fecal metabolic activities of herbal components to bioactive compounds. Arch Pharm Res 2002;25(2):165-169.

Lee JS. Supplementation of Pueraria radix water extract on changes of antioxidant enzymes and lipid profile in ethanol-treated rats. Clin Chim Acta 2004;347(1-2):121-128.

Li B, Yu S. [Effect of puerarin on the bone metabolism in vitro]. Beijing Da Xue Xue Bao 2003;35(1):74-77.

Li SM, Liu B, Chen HF. [Effect of puerarin on plasma endothelin, renin activity and angiotensin II in patients with acute myocardial infarction]. Zhongguo Zhong Xi Yi Jie He Za Zhi 1997;17(6):339-341.

Li X, Sun S, Tong E. Experimental study on the protective effect of puerarin to Parkinson disease. J Huazhong Univ Sci Technolog Med Sci 2003;23(2):148-150.

Lin RC, Guthrie S, Xie CY, et al. Isoflavonoid compounds extracted from Pueraria lobata suppress alcohol preference in a pharmacogenetic rat model of alcoholism. Alcohol Clin Exp Res 1996;20(4):659-663.

Lin RC, Li TK. Effects of isoflavones on alcohol pharmacokinetics and alcohol-drinking behavior in rats. Am J Clin Nutr 1998;68(6 Suppl):1512S-1515S.

Liu JM, Ma L, He WP. Therapeutic effect of puerarin therapy on sudden deafness. Di Yi Jun Yi Da Xue Xue Bao; 22(11): 1044-1045. 2002.

Liu Q, Lu Z, Wang L. Restrictive effect of puerarin on myocardial infarct area in dogs and its possible mechanism. J Tongji Med Univ 2000;20(1):43-45.

Liu Q, Wang L, Lu Z, et al. [Effect of puerarin on coronary collateral circulation in dogs with experimental acute myocardial infarction]. Zhongguo Zhong Yao Za Zhi 1999;24(5):304-6, 320.

Lu XR, Gao E, Xu LZ, et al. [Blocking effect of puerarin on beta-adrenoceptors of isolated organs and the whole animal]. Zhongguo Yao Li Xue Bao 1986;7(6):537-539.

Lu XR, Gao E, Xu LZ, et al. Puerarin beta-adrenergic receptor blocking effect. Chin Med J (Engl) 1987;100(1):25-28.

Lukas SE, Penetar D, Berko J et al. An extract of the Chinese herbal root kudzu reduces alcohol drinking by heavy drinkers in a naturalistic setting. Alcohol Clin Exp Res; 29(5): 756-762. 2005.

Luo ZR, Zheng B. [Effect of Puerarin on platelet activating factors CD63 and CD62P, plasminogen activator inhibitor and C-reactive protein in patients with unstable angia pectoris]. Zhongguo Zhong Xi Yi Jie He Za Zhi 2001;21(1):31-33.

Ma L, Xiao P, Guo B, et al. [Cerebral protective effects of some compounds isolated from traditional Chinese herbs]. Zhongguo Zhong Yao Za Zhi 1999;24(4):238-inside.

Meng P, Zhou D, Hu X. [Clinical observation of the treatment of infantile viral myocarditis with puerarin]. Zhongguo Zhong Xi Yi Jie He Za Zhi 1999;19(11):647-648.

Mercer LD, Kelly BL, Horne MK, et al. Dietary polyphenols protect dopamine neurons from oxidative insults and apoptosis: investigations in primary rat mesencephalic cultures. Biochem Pharmacol 2005;69(2):339-345.

Overstreet DH, Kralic JE, Morrow AL, et al. NPI-031G (puerarin) reduces anxiogenic effects of alcohol withdrawal or benzodiazepine inverse or 5-HT2C agonists. Pharmacol Biochem Behav 2003;75(3):619-625.

Overstreet DH, Lee D Y-W, Chen YT, et al. The Chinese herbal medicine NPI-028 suppresses alcohol intake in alcohol-preferring rats and monkeys without inducing taste aversion. Perfusion 1998;11:381-390.

Pan HP, Mo XL, Yang JZ, et al. [Effect of puerarin on the expression of Hsp70 in the rats with cerebral injury induced by acute local ischemia]. Zhongguo Zhong Yao Za Zhi 2005;30(7):538-540.

Pan HP, Yang JZ, Li LL, et al. [Experimental study of puerarin injection on the hemorheology in acute blood-stasis model rats]. Zhongguo Zhong Yao Za Zhi 2003;28(12):1178-1180.

Prasain JK, Jones K, Brissie N, et al. Identification of puerarin and its metabolites in rats by liquid chromatography-tandem mass spectrometry. J Agric Food Chem 2004;52(12):3708-3712.

Prasain JK, Jones K, Kirk M, et al. Profiling and quantification of isoflavonoids in kudzu dietary supplements by high-performance liquid chromatography and electrospray ionization tandem mass spectrometry. J Agric Food Chem 2003;51(15):4213-4218.

Qi BL, Qi BM. [Effect of the purariae-isofiavones on estrogen level in normal and ovariectomized rats]. Zhongguo Zhong Yao Za Zhi 2002;27(11):850-852.

Qian Y, Li Z, Huang L, et al. Blocking effect of puerarin on calcium channel in isolated guinea pig ventricular myocytes. Chin Med J (Engl) 1999;112(9):787-789.

Ren P, Hu H, Zhang R. [Observation on efficacy of puerarin in treating diabetic retinopathy]. Zhongguo Zhong Xi Yi Jie He Za Zhi 2000;20(8):574-576.

Rezvani AH, Overstreet DH, Perfumi M, et al. Plant derivatives in the treatment of alcohol dependency. Pharmacol Biochem Behav 2003;75(3):593-606.

Sang HF, Mei QB, Xu LX, et al. Effect of puerarin on neural function and histopathological damages after transient spinal cord ischemia in rabbits. Chin J Traumatol 2004;7(3):143-147.

Shebek J, Rindone JP. A pilot study exploring the effect of kudzu root on the drinking habits of patients with chronic alcoholism. J Altern Complement Med; 6(1): 45-48. 2000.

Shen ZF, Xie MZ. [Hypoglycemic effect of the combined use of puerarin and aspirin in mice]. Yao Xue Xue Bao 1985;20(11):863-865.

Shi RL, Zhang JJ. [Protective effect of puerarin on vascular endothelial cell apoptosis induced by chemical hypoxia in vitro]. Yao Xue Xue Bao 2003;38(2):103-107.

Shi WG, Qu L, Wang JW. Study on interventing effect of puerarin on insulin resistance in patients with coronary heart disease. Zhongguo Zhong Xi Yi Jie He Za Zhi; 22(1): 21-24. 2002.

Song CY, Bi HM. [Effects of puerarin on plasma membrane GLUT4 content in skeletal muscle from insulin-resistant Sprague-Dawley rats under insulin stimulation]. Zhongguo Zhong Yao Za Zhi 2004;29(2):172-175.

Song XP, Chen PP, Chai XS. [Effects of puerarin on blood pressure and plasma renin activity in spontaneously hypertensive rats]. Zhongguo Yao Li Xue Bao 1988;9(1):55-58.

Wang C, Song Z. In vitro monitoring of nanogram levels of puerarin in human urine using flow injection chemiluminescence. Bioorg Med Chem Lett 2004;14(16):4127-4130.

Wang CY, Huang HY, Kuo KL, et al. Analysis of Puerariae radix and its medicinal preparations by capillary electrophoresis. J Chromatogr A 1998;802(1):225-231.

Wang LY, Zhao AP, Chai XS. [Effects of puerarin on cat vascular smooth muscle in vitro]. Zhongguo Yao Li Xue Bao 1994;15(2):180-182.

Wang X, Wu J, Chiba H, et al. Puerariae radix prevents bone loss in ovariectomized mice. J Bone Miner Metab 2003;21(5):268-275.

Woo J, Lau E, Ho SC, et al. Comparison of Pueraria lobata with hormone replacement therapy in treating the adverse health consequences of menopause. Menopause 2003;10(4):352-361.

Wu P, Zeng F, Ma HX. [Study on effect of Puerarin on nitric oxide system in rats' tissue and its mechanism]. Zhongguo Zhong Xi Yi Jie He Za Zhi 2001;21(3):196-198.

Xiao LZ, Gao LJ, Ma SC. [Comparative study on effects of puerarin and granulocyte colony-stimulating factor in treating acute myocardial infarction]. Zhongguo Zhong Xi Yi Jie He Za Zhi 2005;25(3):210-213.

Xiao LZ, Huang Z, Ma SC, et al. [Study on the effect and mechanism of puerarin on the size of infarction in patients with acute myocardial infarction]. Zhongguo Zhong Xi Yi Jie He Za Zhi 2004;24(9):790-792.

Xie CI, Lin RC, Antony V, et al. Daidzin, an antioxidant isoflavonoid, decreases blood alcohol levels and shortens sleep time induced by ethanol intoxication. Alcohol Clin Exp Res 1994;18(6):1443-1447.

Xie RQ, Du J, Hao YM. Myocardial protection and mechanism of puerarin injection on patients of coronary heart disease with ischemia/reperfusion. Zhongguo Zhong Xi Yi Jie He Za Zhi; 23(12): 895-897. 2003.

Xu X, Zhang S, Zhang L, et al. The Neuroprotection of puerarin against cerebral ischemia is associated with the prevention of apoptosis in rats. Planta Med 2005;71(7):585-591.

Xu XH, Zhao TQ. Effects of puerarin on D-galactose-induced memory deficits in mice. Acta Pharmacol Sin 2002;23(7):587-590.

Xu XH. [Effects of puerarin on fatty superoxide in aged mice induced by D-galactose]. Zhongguo Zhong Yao Za Zhi 2003;28(1):66-69.

Xue XO, Jin H, Niu JZ, et al. [Effects of extracts of root of kudzu vine on mammary gland and uterus development in rats]. Zhongguo Zhong Yao Za Zhi 2003;28(6):560-562.

Yanagihara K, Ito A, Toge T, et al. Antiproliferative effects of isoflavones on human cancer cell lines established from the gastrointestinal tract. Cancer Res 1993;53(23):5815-5821.

Yang G, Zhang L, Fan L. [Anti-angina effect of puerarin and its effect on plasma thromboxane A2 and prostacyclin]. Zhong Xi Yi Jie He Za Zhi 1990;10(2):82-4, 68.

Ye HY, Qiu F, Zeng J, et al. [Effect of daidzein on antiarrhythmia]. Zhongguo Zhong Yao Za Zhi 2003;28(9):853-856.

Yin ZZ, Zeng GY. [Pharmacology of puerarin. V. Effects of puerarin on platelet aggregation and release of 5-HT from platelets]. Zhongguo Yi Xue Ke Xue Yuan Xue Bao 1981;3 Suppl 1:44-47.

Yu Z, Zhang G, Zhao H. [Effects of Puerariae isoflavone on blood viscosity, thrombosis and platelet function]. Zhong Yao Cai 1997;20(9):468-469.

Zhang G, Fang S. [Antioxidation of Pueraria lobata isoflavones (PLIs)]. Zhong Yao Cai 1997;20(7):358-360.

Zhang GQ, Hao XM, Dai DZ, et al. Puerarin blocks Na+ current in rat ventricular myocytes. Acta Pharmacol Sin 2003;24(12):1212-1216.

Zhang S, Ji G, Liu J. Reversal of chemical-induced liver fibrosis in Wistar rats by puerarin. J Nutr Biochem 2005;View Abstract

Zhang Y, Chen J, Zhang C, et al. Analysis of the estrogenic components in kudzu root by bioassay and high performance liquid chromatography. J Steroid Biochem Mol Biol 2005;94(4):375-381.

Zhao Y, Du GY, Cui HF, et al. [Experimental study of protective effect of pueraria compound on the cerebral ischemic injury]. Zhongguo Zhong Yao Za Zhi 2005;30(7):548-551.

Zhao Z, Yang X, Zhang Y. [Clinical study of puerarin in treatment of patients with unstable angina]. Zhongguo Zhong Xi Yi Jie He Za Zhi 1998;18(5):282-284.

Zheng G, Zhang X, Zheng J, et al. [Estrogen-like effects of puerarin and total isoflavones from Pueraria lobata]. Zhong Yao Cai 2002;25(8):566-568.

Zheng G, Zhang X, Zheng J, et al. [Hypocholesterolemic effect of total isoflavones from Pueraria lobata in ovariectomized rats]. Zhong Yao Cai 2002;25(4):273-275.

Zhou Y, Su X, Cheng B, et al. [Comparative study on pharmacological effects of various species of Pueraria]. Zhongguo Zhong Yao Za Zhi 1995;20(10):619-21, 640.

Zhu JH, Wang XX, Chen JZ, et al. Effects of puerarin on number and activity of endothelial progenitor cells from peripheral blood. Acta Pharmacol Sin 2004;25(8):1045-1051.

Zhu XY, Su GY, Li ZH, et al. [The metabolic fate of the effective components of puerariae. III. The metabolism of puerarin (author's transl)]. Yao Xue Xue Bao 1979;14(6):349-355.

Zhu ZT, Li HQ, Lu Y, et al. [Inhibitive effect of puerarin on increased NO production by neonatal cardiomyocytes during hypoxia/reoxygenation injury]. Zhongguo Zhong Yao Za Zhi 2001;26(12):856-859.

Labrador Tea

Ledum latifolium

DESCRIPTION

Medicinal Parts: The medicinal parts are the leaves and the flowering shoots.

Flower and Fruit: The flowers are in flat, terminal umbels. The calyx is small and has 5 tips. The 5-petalled corolla is white. The 10 stamens grow from the edge of a honey ring. The ovary is superior. The fruit is a 5-valvular capsule.

Leaves, Stem, and Root: The evergreen, branched shrub grows to about 1.5 m. The young branches are gray or rust-colored. The 1.25- to 2.5-cm long leaves are alternate, short-petioled, entire-margined, and linear, with revolute margins. They are stiff, coriaceous, dark green above, and rust-colored and woolly-downy underneath. *L. palustre* is larger, more regularly formed and has larger leaves.

Characteristics: It has a numbing, tangy aroma and is poisonous. It is a protected species.

Habitat: The plant grows in Greenland, Canada and the U.S. The very similar variety *L. palustre* is more common in northern Europe and northern Asia.

Production: Labrador herb is the aerial part of *Ledum latifolium* and *L. palustre*.

Other Names: St. James's Tea, Marsh Tea, Wild Rosemary

ACTIONS AND PHARMACOLOGY

COMPOUNDS

Volatile oil (0.9-2.6%): chief components sesquiterpenes, in particular ledol (ledum camphor, porst camphor) and palustrol, Japanese sources also yield ascaridol

Catechin tannins

Flavonoids: including among others hyperoside

Hydroglycosides: arbutin

EFFECTS

Internally mildly expectorant. Externally antiphlogistic (neither proven).

INDICATIONS AND USAGE

Unproven Uses: Labrador Tea has been used for respiratory conditions. Externally, it has been used for skin inflammation.

CONTRAINDICATIONS

The drug is contraindicated in pregnancy.

PRECAUTIONS AND ADVERSE REACTIONS

General: Initially, the drug causes severe gastrointestinal irritation (vomiting, gastroenteritis, diarrhea), due to its ledol content. Following absorption, the drug causes severe CNS excitation. This effect may lead to spasms and paralysis in some cases.

Pregnancy: Contraindicated. Poisonings in earlier times were seen in connection with its misuse for purposes of abortion.

OVERDOSAGE

Following gastrointestinal emptying (inducement of vomiting, gastric lavage with burgundy-colored potassium permanganate solution, sodium sulfate), and instillation of activated charcoal, the treatment of poisonings consists of treating spasms with diazepam (I.V.) and colic with atropine; electrolyte substitution and treating possible cases of acidosis with sodium bicarbonate infusions. Monitoring of kidney function is essential. Intubation and oxygen respiration may also be necessary.

DOSAGE

Mode of Administration: Labrador Tea is obsolete as a drug. It has been used as an extract in some bath additives and is also contained in homeopathic preparations.

LITERATURE

Belleau F, Collin G. Composition of the essential oil of Ledum groenlandicum. Phytochemistry 33, 117 1993

Frohne D, Pfänder HJ, Giftpflanzen - Ein Handbuch für Apotheker, Toxikologen und Biologen, 4. Aufl., Wiss. Verlags-Ges. Stuttgart 1997.

Kern W, List PH, Hörhammer L (Hrsg.), Hagers Handbuch der Pharmazeutischen Praxis, 4. Aufl., Bde. 1-8, Springer Verlag Berlin, Heidelberg, New York, 1969.

Lewin L, Gifte und Vergiftungen, 6. Aufl., Nachdruck, Haug Verlag, Heidelberg 1992.

Roth L, Daunderer M, Kormann K, Giftpflanzen, Pflanzengifte, 4. Aufl., Ecomed Fachverlag Landsberg Lech 1993.

Teuscher E, Lindequist U, Biogene Gifte - Biologie, Chemie, Pharmakologie, 2. Aufl., Fischer Verlag Stuttgart 1994.

Wagner H, Wiesenauer M, Phytotherapie. Phytopharmaka und pflanzliche Homöopathika, Fischer-Verlag, Stuttgart, Jena, New York 1995.

Laburnum

Cytisus laburnum

DESCRIPTION

Medicinal Parts: The seeds are the medicinal parts.

Flower and Fruit: The flowers bow down in clusters of 10 to 30. There are racemes that are10 to 25 cm long. The calyx is short, campanulate, pubescent, and marked brown at the base. The anthers are orange. The pod is 5 to 8 cm by 8 to 9 cm, flat, lumpy, and silky-haired with wings. The seeds are flat and dark brown.

Leaves, Stem, and Root: Cytisus laburnum is a small shrub or tree that can occasionally grow up to 7 m high. It has light gray branches and smooth, dark green, initially erect branchlets. The alternate leaves are almost in rosettes on short shoots with 2 to 7 cm long petioles. The leaflets are elliptical to ovate, rounded, or thorn tipped. They are glabrous above and light gray pubescent beneath.

Habitat: The plant is indigenous to mountainous regions of Europe. It is also cultivated worldwide.

Other Names: Bean Trifoil, Golden Chain, Pea Tree

ACTIONS AND PHARMACOLOGY

COMPOUNDS

Quinolizidine alkaloids (1-3%): main alkaloids (-)-cytisine (95%), as well as (-)-N-methylcytisine, epibaptifoline

Lectins

EFFECTS
No information is available.

INDICATIONS AND USAGE

Unproven Uses: Experiments in the use of cytisine as a pesticide (lice) have shown that in the necessary concentration the danger of poisoning is too high.

PRECAUTIONS AND ADVERSE REACTIONS

There are no indications for this drug. The drug is severely toxic. See Overdosage section.

OVERDOSAGE

Symptoms of poisoning include nausea, dizziness, salivation, pains in the mouth, in the throat and in the stomach area, outbreaks of sweat, headache as well as extended, severe and sometimes bloody vomiting. If no vomiting occurs, excitatory states can come about from the centrally stimulating effect of the drug, with tonic-clonic spasms that later change into paralyses. Anuria and uremia have also been observed. Death comes through asphyxiation.

Fifteen to 20 seeds or 3 to 4 unripe berries are considered fatal for an adult. While poisonings occur relatively frequently, cases of death have not been recorded in recent times. If no vomiting has occurred, poisonings are treated with gastric lavage, then through the administration of activated charcoal; spasms are to be treated with chlorpromazine or diazepam. In cases of asphyxiation, intubation and oxygen respiration are to be carried out.

LITERATURE

Frohne D, Pfänder HJ, Giftpflanzen - Ein Handbuch für Apotheker, Toxikologen und Biologen, 4. Aufl., Wiss. Verlagsges. mbH Stuttgart 1997.

Gresser G, Der Besenginster - *Cytisus scoparius* (L.) LINK. In: ZPT 17(5):320-330. 1996.

Hänsel R, Keller K, Rimpler H, Schneider G (Hrsg.), Hagers Handbuch der Pharmazeutischen Praxis, 5. Aufl., Bde 4-6 (Drogen), Springer Verlag Berlin, Heidelberg, New York, 1992-1994.

Lewin L, Gifte und Vergiftungen, 6. Aufl., Nachdruck, Haug Verlag, Heidelberg 1992.

Teuscher E, Lindequist U, Biogene Gifte - Biologie, Chemie, Pharmakologie, 2. Aufl., Fischer Verlag Stuttgart 1994.

Teuscher E, Biogene Arzneimittel, 5. Aufl., Wiss. Verlagsges. mbH Stuttgart 1997.

Tschirch C, Kraus L, Goldregen-Alkaloid Cytisin. In: DAZ 132(47):2560. 1992.

Wagner H, Wiesenauer M, Phytotherapie. Phytopharmaka und pflanzliche Homöopathika, Fischer-Verlag, Stuttgart, Jena, New York 1995.

Lactuca virosa

See Lactucarium

Lactucarium

Lactuca virosa

DESCRIPTION

Medicinal Parts: The medicinal parts are the dried latex and the leaves.

Flower and Fruit: The composite flowers are in pyramid-shaped panicles. The capitula have a few florets, which are androgynous, pale yellow, lingual florets. The bracts are imbricate. The fruit is 4-lipped and black with a broad edge. It is glabrous at the tip. It has a whitish beak that is as long as the fruit, making the hair tuft look stemmed.

Leaves, Stem, and Root: The plant is biennial, up to 1.2 m high, with a fusiform, pale root that produces the erect, branched and hollow stem. It is smooth, light green, and sometimes has purple spots. The leaves are oblong to obovate, narrowed at the base, clasping and usually simple. They are thorny-tipped, lie horizontally, and are thorny on the underside of the midrib.

Characteristics: The whole plant contains milky latex.

Habitat: The plant is indigenous to western and southern Europe and is cultivated in Germany, Austria, France, and Scotland.

Production: Lactucarium leaves are the leaves of the aerial part of *Lactuca virosa.* They are gathered when in flower and then dried.

Not to be Confused With: L.sativa, L.serriola, L.quercina and *Sonchus oleraceus.*

Other Names: Acrid Lettuce, Green Endive, Lettuce Opium, Prickly Lettuce, Poison Lettuce, Strong-Scented Lettuce, Wild Lettuce

ACTIONS AND PHARMACOLOGY

COMPOUNDS
Sesquiterpene lactones: lactucin, lactucopicrin (lactupictin, intybin)

Triterpenes: including among others, taraxasterol, beta-amyrin

EFFECTS
The herb is supposed to have a narcotic effect. It is an analgesic and spasmolytic, and is said to act as a tranquilizer.

INDICATIONS AND USAGE

Unproven Uses: Medicines containing Lactucarium are used to treat whooping cough attacks. The drug is used for bronchial catarrh, asthma, and urinary tract diseases. The oil of the seeds is used for arteriosclerosis and was also used as wheat germ oil.

Homeopathic Uses: Lactuca virosa is used for laryngitis, tracheitis with heavy coughing, for swelling of the liver, and for urinary complaints.

PRECAUTIONS AND ADVERSE REACTIONS

No health hazards or side effects are known in conjunction with the proper administration of designated therapeutic dosages. The drug possesses a low potential for sensitization.

OVERDOSAGE

The following signs of poisoning can occur through overdosage or following intake of the fresh leaves, as in salads: outbreaks of sweating, acceleration of breathing, tachycardia, pupil dilation, dizziness, ringing in the ears, vision disorders, pressure in the head, somnolence, on occasion also excitatory states. The toxicity is, however, relatively low. Following gastrointestinal emptying (inducement of vomiting, gastric lavage with burgundy-colored potassium permanganate solution, sodium sulfate), as well as instillation of activated charcoal, the treatment of poisonings should proceed symptomatically.

DOSAGE

Mode of Administration: Due to its poison content, the drug is only administered under medical supervision. It is ground and used as an alcoholic extract and further processed in the pharmaceutical industry.

LITERATURE

Frohne D, Pfänder HJ, Giftpflanzen - Ein Handbuch für Apotheker, Toxikologen und Biologen, 4. Aufl., Wiss. Verlags-Ges Stuttgart 1997.

Gromek D, Kisiel W, Klodzinska A, Chojnacka-Wojcik E. Biologically Active Preparations from *Lactuca virosa* L. Phytother Res. 6 (5); 285-287. 1992

Kern W, List PH, Hörhammer L (Hrsg.), Hagers Handbuch der Pharmazeutischen Praxis, 4. Aufl., Bde. 1-8, Springer Verlag Berlin, Heidelberg, New York, 1969.

Lewin L, Gifte und Vergiftungen, 6. Aufl., Nachdruck, Haug Verlag, Heidelberg 1992.

Madaus G, Lehrbuch der Biologischen Arzneimittel, Bde 1-3, Nachdruck, Georg Olms Verlag Hildesheim 1979.

Roth L, Daunderer M, Kormann K, Giftpflanzen, Pflanzengifte, 4. Aufl., Ecomed Fachverlag Landsberg Lech 1993.

Teuscher E, Lindequist U, Biogene Gifte - Biologie, Chemie, Pharmakologie, 2. Aufl., Fischer Verlag Stuttgart 1994.

Lady Fern

Athyrium filix-femina

DESCRIPTION

Medicinal Parts: The medicinal part is the rhizome when gathered in spring or autumn.

Leaves, Stem and Root: Athyrium filix-femina is a 10- to 40-cm high fern. The pencil-thick, creeping rhizome is densely covered with dark-brown hairs. Numerous tomentose, long, branched, dark-brown root fibers sprout from the rhizome. The sparse leaves are in rigid, upright, double rows. They are coriaceous, glabrous, oblong-lanceolate or oblong, deeply pinnatifid, and evergreen. The petioles are semi-round, smooth, and whitish. On the underside of the leaf tips there are 2 parallel rows of large groups of filmless sporangia, which are initially yellowish and later turn dark brown.

Habitat: Lady Fern is indigenous to Britain, parts of Europe and the U.S.

Other Names: Brake Root, Common Polypody, Oak Fern, Rock Brake, Rock of Polypody, Wall Fern

ACTIONS AND PHARMACOLOGY

COMPOUNDS

Tannins (8%)

C-glucosyl flavones: including mangiferin

Phytoecdysones

Amaroids

Saponin: including the steroid saponin osladin

Essential oil

EFFECTS

The drug is a mild expectorant; a choleretic-type effect is questionable.

INDICATIONS AND USAGE

Unproven Uses: The drug is used for respiratory and gastrointestinal tract illnesses.

PRECAUTIONS AND ADVERSE REACTIONS

No health hazards or side effects are known in conjunction with the proper administration of designated therapeutic dosages.

DOSAGE

Mode of Administration: Lady Fern is still found in commercial preparations as drops and tablets, as well as in preparations used in the religious system of anthroposophy.

Daily Dosage: In anthroposophic medicine, the usual dose to treat gastrointestinal illnesses is 1 to 2 tablets or 10 to 20 drops taken 3 times daily.

LITERATURE

Abraham H, Zucker und Süβstoff. In: *PTA* 7(10):744. 1993.

Hegnauer R, Chemotaxonomie der Pflanzen, Bde 1-11, Birkhäuser Verlag Basel, Boston, Berlin 1962-1997.

Kern W, List PH, Hörhammer L (Hrsg.), Hagers Handbuch der Pharmazeutischen Praxis, 4. Aufl., Bde 1-8, Springer Verlag Berlin, Heidelberg, New York, 1969.

Madaus G, Lehrbuch der Biologischen Arzneimittel, Bde 1-3, Nachdruck, Georg Olms Verlag Hildesheim 1979.

Lady's Bedstraw

Galium verum

DESCRIPTION

Medicinal Parts: The medicinal part is the dried herb.

Flower and Fruit: The small lemon-yellow flowers are in dense terminal panicles. The peduncle is very downy. The corolla is 2 to 3 mm wide, usually golden yellow, and smells strongly of honey. The border of the calyx is pointed, and the ovaries are bivalvular and inferior. The fruit is smooth, indehiscent, 1.5 mm long, glabrous, and eventually black.

Leaves, Stem, and Root: The true plant is 30 to 100 cm high, an herbaceous perennial with a cylindrical, creeping rhizome that sprouts runners. The stem is ascending or erect, bluntly quadrangular with 4 vertical lines, downy or glabrous, and rough. The leaves are in false whorls of 8 to 12. They are linear, dark green above, and gray and short-haired beneath.

Characteristics: The flowers have a strong honey fragrance.

Habitat: The plant grows throughout Europe (with the exception of Lapland and arctic Russia), as well as in Asia Minor, Iran, and Syria.

Production: Lady's Bedstraw is the herb of *Galium verum,* collected during the flowering season and dried.

Other Names:, Cheese Rennet, Cheese Renning, Curdwort, Maid's Hair, Petty Mugget, Yellow Cleavers, Yellow Galium

ACTIONS AND PHARMACOLOGY

COMPOUNDS

Iridoids: asperuloside, monotropein, scandoside, desacetylasperulosidic acid, asperulosidic acid, giniposidic acid, daphylloside

Rennin

Flavonoids: including rutin, isorutin, palustroside, cynaroside, quercetin-3-O-glucoside, quercetin-7-O-glucoside

Anthracene derivatives

Caffeic acid ester: chlorogenic acid

EFFECTS

No information is available.

INDICATIONS AND USAGE

Unproven Uses: Internally, the drug is used in folk medicine for swollen ankles and as a diuretic for bladder and kidney irritation. Externally, it is used for poorly healing wounds. The efficacy of this drug has not been proved.

PRECAUTIONS AND ADVERSE REACTIONS

Health risks or side effects following the proper administration of designated therapeutic dosages are not recorded.

DOSAGE

Mode of Administration: Currently obsolete but formerly the drug was used internally as a tea and topically in alcoholic extracts as a moist poultice.

Preparation: To prepare a tea or infusion, pour 250 mL of cold water over 2 heaping teaspoonfuls of the drug, bring to simmering point, simmer for 2 minutes and then allow to steep.

Daily Dosage: Internally, 2 to 3 cups of tea daily.

LITERATURE

Hänsel R, Keller K, Rimpler H, Schneider G (Hrsg.), Hagers Handbuch der Pharmazeutischen Praxis, 5. Aufl., Bde 4-6 (Drogen), Springer Verlag Berlin, Heidelberg, New York, 1992-1994.

Mathé I et al., (1982) Planta Med 45:158.

Wichtl M (Hrsg.), Teedrogen, 4. Aufl., Wiss. Verlagsges. Stuttgart 1997.

Lady's Mantle

Alchemilla vulgaris

DESCRIPTION

Medicinal Parts: The medicinal part is the herb collected in the flowering season and dried.

Flower and Fruit: The plant has inflorescences of small, insignificant, yellow-green, many-flowered cymes. The perianth has 4 leaves. The flower has 4 stamens, 1 ovary, and an inferior style. The fruit is enclosed in the calyx. The flowers are infertile.

Leaves, Stem, and Root: Alchemilla vulgaris is a hardy, half-rosette shrub, which grows from 30 to 50 cm. It has a branched stem, which is villous to glabrous. The basal leaves are round with 7 to 9 lobes (dew cup); cauline leaves are short-petioled to sessile, 5- to 7-lobed, crenate or serrate and villous. Even the older leaves remain more or less folded.

Characteristics: Lady's Mantle is odorless and has an astringent taste.

Habitat: The plant grows in the Northern Hemisphere from North America, Greenland and Europe to the Mediterranean and Iceland; and Asia from the Caucasus and the Himalayas to Siberia.

Production: Lady's Mantle herb consists of the fresh or dried above-ground parts of *Alchemilla vulgaris* gathered at flowering time, as well as its preparations. It is produced mostly through cultivation.

Other Names: Bear's Foot, Leontopodium, Lion's Foot, Nine Hooks, Stellaria

ACTIONS AND PHARMACOLOGY

COMPOUNDS

Bitter principles

Flavonoids (2%)

Tannins (5% to 8%) ellagitannins

EFFECTS

Lady's Mantle herb has astringent properties, due to the presence of tannins. It has also been shown to inhibit tumor growth. In mice the total retardation of breast neoplasm-induced tumors was achieved using agrimoniin and the average life expectancy of the animals was increased. An extract of the drug hinders the enzymes elastase, trypsin, and a-chymotrysin.

INDICATIONS AND USAGE

Approved by Commission E:

■ Diarrhea

Lady's Mantle is used for mild and non-specific diarrhea.

Unproven Uses: In folk medicine the drug is used internally for menopausal complaints, dysmenorrhea, gastrointestinal disorders, and as a gargle for mouth and throat inflammation. Externally, it is used for ulcers, eczema, skin rashes, and as an additive in baths for the treatment of lower-abdominal ailments.

Homeopathic Uses: Alchemilla vulgaris is used for leukorrhea and for chronic diarrhea resulting from liver disease.

PRECAUTIONS AND ADVERSE REACTIONS

No health hazards or side effects are known in conjunction with the proper administration of designated therapeutic dosages.

DOSAGE

Mode of Administration: Lady's Mantle herb is administered as a cut herb for infusions and decoctions, as well as other galenic preparations for internal use.

Preparation: Tea: 2 to 4 g drug to 150 mL hot water left to draw for 10 minutes. Prepare a fresh batch every day.

Daily Dosage: Lady's Mantle herb is administered in 2 to 4 g single doses as an infusion; the average daily dose is 5 to 10 g of herb. The tea is taken 3 times daily between meals.

Homeopathic Dosage: 5 drops, 1 tablet, 10 globules, every 30 to 60 minutes (acute) and 1 to 3 times daily (chronic); Parenterally: 1 to 2 mL 3 times daily sc; Ointment: Apply 1 to 2 times daily (HAB1).

LITERATURE

Filípek J, The effect of *Alchemilla xanthochlora* on lipid peroxidation and superoxide anion scavenging acticity. In: PA 47:717-718. 1992.

Geiger C, Ellagitannine aus Alchemilla xanthochlora ROTHMALER und Potentilla erecta (L.) RAEUSCHEL. Beiträge zur Analytik und Strukturaufklärung. In: Dissertation Universität Freiburg. 1990.

Schimmer O, Felser C, Alchemilla xanthochlora ROTHM.- Der Frauenmantel. In: *ZPT* 13(6):207. 1993.

Schimmer O, Lindenbaum M, Tannins with antimutagenic properties in the herb of *Alchemilla* species *and Potentilla anserina.* In: PM 61(2):141-145. 1995.

Laminaria hyperborea

See Kelp

Lamium album

See White Nettle

Larch

Larix decidua

DESCRIPTION

Medicinal Parts: The medicinal part is the outer bark separated from its outermost layer.

Flower and Fruit: The female flowers are cone-shaped, erect, 2 cm long, short-pedicled, round-ovate and encircled by scales at the base. The covering scales turn dark red when in bloom. The male catkins are sessile, about 1.5 cm long, sulfur yellow, and ovoid-globular. The seeds are light brown, glossy with 13 mm long and 5 mm wide wings.

Leaves, Stem, and Root: Larch is a deciduous tree that grows up to 54 m high tree (stunted at high altitudes) with a straight trunk, brown-red bark, and pyramid-shaped, sparsely foliated crown. The main branches are horizontal and turned up at the tips. The secondary branches are hanging. The foliage is light green with delicate needles, arranged singly in spiral rows on long shoots and in bushels on short ones. They fall in autumn.

Habitat: The plant is indigenous to central Europe, cultivated in North America. It was first introduced to England in 1639.

Production: The balsam of *Larix decidua* is obtained by drilling into the trunks. The balsam contains up to 20% essential oil.

Other Names: European Larch, Common Larch

ACTIONS AND PHARMACOLOGY

COMPOUNDS

Volatile oil (14-15%): chief components: (-)-alpha-pinene (70%), Delta3-carene (10%) (-)-beta-pinene (6.5%), beta-pyrones (3%)

Resins: including among others oleoresin acids (50-65%): including among others laricinolic acid, alpha- and beta-laricinolic acid

EFFECTS

When used externally the drug has a hyperemic and antiseptic effect due the essential oil content. Its use for catarrhal infections of the upper respiratory tract also seems plausible.

INDICATIONS AND USAGE

Approved by Commission E:

■ Fevers and colds
■ Cough/bronchitis
■ Tendency for infections

Studies on Antigen Specifity of Immunoreactive Arabinogalactan Proteins extracted from Baptisia tinctoria and Echinacea purpurea. Planta Med. 58; 163-165 (1992)

■ Blood pressure problems
■ Inflammation of the mouth and pharynx
■ Rheumatism
■ Common cold

Unproven Uses: The drug has been used to treat neuralgic discomforts and furuncles.

CONTRAINDICATIONS

Inhalation may cause acute inflammation of the airway passages.

PRECAUTIONS AND ADVERSE REACTIONS

No health hazards or side effects are known in conjunction with the proper external administration of designated therapeutic dosages.

OVERDOSAGE

Resorptive poisonings, such as kidney and central nervous system damage, are possible with large-area administration. Kidney damage is conceivable with internal administration.

DOSAGE

Mode of Administration: Available in form of ointments, gels, emulsions and oils.

Preparation: Liquid and semi-solid preparations 10 to 20% for external use.

LITERATURE

Bicchi C, Joulain D. Review / Headspace-Gas-Chromatographic Analysis of Medicinal and Aromatic Plants and Flowers. Flav Fragr J. 5; 131-145. 1990

Egert D, Beuscher N. Studies on Antigen Specifity of Immunoreactive Arabinogalactan Proteins extracted from Baptisia tinctoria and Echinacea purpurea. Planta Med. 58; 163-165. 1992

Kern W, List PH, Hörhammer L (Hrsg.), Hagers Handbuch der Pharmazeutischen Praxis, 4. Aufl., Bde. 1-8: Springer Verlag Berlin, Heidelberg, New York, 1969.

Larix decidua

See Larch

Larkspur

Delphinium consolida

DESCRIPTION

Medicinal Parts: The medicinal parts are the seeds of the plant.

Flower and Fruit: The flowers are in short racemes and are blue, pink or purple. The petals are fused to a helmetlike form with a honey spur at the back, which reaches into the back of the 5 sepals. There is usually only 1 glabrous ovary, but numerous stamens. The fruit is a follicle with black, flattened seeds, which have sharp edges and a scarred surface.

Leaves, Stem, and Root: The plant grows from 15 to 40 cm. Larkspur is an annual and has a thin stem that is sparsely branched from the middle. The leaves are alternate and divided into narrow linear sections. The lowers ones are petioled and the upper ones sessile.

Habitat: Europe, western U.S.

Production: Delphinium flower consists of the flowers of *Delphinium consolida.*

Not to be Confused With: the flowers of Delphinium oriental.

Other Names: Knight's Spur, Lark Heel, Lark's Claw, Lark's Toe, Staggerweed

ACTIONS AND PHARMACOLOGY

COMPOUNDS

Diterpene alkaloids: chief alkaloid delphinine

The presence of alkaloids has sometimes been described in the literature but they cannot always be found.

EFFECTS

No information is available.

INDICATIONS AND USAGE

Unproven Uses: Larkspur is obsolete. It is used only as an inactive ingredient in tea mixtures. Preparations of delphinium flower are sometimes used as a diuretic and vermifuge, as a sedative and an appetite stimulant. In folk medicine, Larkspur is used occasionally as a diuretic. It was formerly used as an anthelmintic.

PRECAUTIONS AND ADVERSE REACTIONS

Health risks or side effects following the proper administration of designated therapeutic dosages are not recorded.

OVERDOSAGE

Although the delphine has a paralyzing effect upon peripheral and motor nerve endings and the central nervous system, poisonings among humans by *Delphinium consolida* have never been observed.

Toxic dosages in animal experiments have led to death through asphyxiation (LD50 rabbits 1.5-3.0 mg/kg body weight, I.V.). Poisonings of animals with fatal results by Delphinium species are particularly frequent in the U.S.

DOSAGE

Mode of Administration: Since the efficacy of Delphinium and its preparations is not documented, a therapeutic administration cannot be recommended.

Preparation: Larkspur is found only in teas, often as an inactive ingredient.

LITERATURE

Alkondon M, Pereira EF, Wonnacott S, Albuquerque EX, Blockade of nicotinic currents in hippocampal neurons defines methyllycaconitine as a potent and specific receptor antagonist. Mol Pharmacol, 41:802-8, 1992 Apr.

Atta-ur-Rahman AM, Nasreen A, Akhtar F, Shekhani MS, Clardy J, Parvez M, Choudhary MI, Antifungal diterpenoid alkaloids from *Delphinium denudatum. J Nat Prod,* 60:472-4, May 1997

Bhandary KK, Ramasubbu N, Joshi BS, Desai HK, Pelletier SW, Structure of delvestine: a norditerpenoid alkaloid from *Delphinium vestitum Wall. Acta Crystallogr C,* 59:1704-7, Sep 15 1990

Ding LS, Chen WX, Diterpenoid alkaloids from *Delphinium kamaonense var. glabrescens. Yao Hsueh Hsueh Pao,* 59:438-40, 1990.

Kern W, List PH, Hörhammer L (Ed), Hagers Handbuch der Pharmazeutischen Praxis. 4. Aufl., Bde. 1-8, Springer Verlag Berlin, Heidelberg, New York 1969.

Manners GD, Panter KE, Pelletier SW, Structure-activity relationships of norditerpenoid alkaloids occurring in toxic larkspur (*Delphinium*) species. *J Nat Prod,* 59:863-9, Jun 1995

Olsen JD, Sisson DV, Toxicity of extracts of tall larkspur (*Delphinium barbeyi*) in mice hamsters rats and sheep. *Toxicol Lett,* 59:33-41, Apr 1991

Park JC, Desai HK, Pelletier SW Two new norditerpenoid alkaloids from *Delphinium elatum* var. ''black night.'' *J Nat Prod,* 59:291-5, Feb. 1995

Ralphs MH, Olsen JD, Comparison of larkspur alkaloid extract and lithium chloride in maintaining cattle aversion to larkspur in the field. *J Anim Sci,* 70:1116-20, Apr. 1992

Siemion RS, Raisbeck MF, Waggoner JW, Tidwell MA, Sanchez DA, In vitro ruminal metabolism of larkspur alkaloids. *Vet Hum Toxicol,* 34:206-8, Jun. 1992

Teuscher E, Lindequist U, Biogene Gifte - Biologie, Chemie, Pharmakologie. 2. Aufl., Fischer Verlag Stuttgart 1994.

Ulubelen A, Desai HK, Srivastava SK, Hart BP, Park JC, Joshi BS, Pelletier SW, Mericli AH, Mericli F, Ilarslan R, Diterpenoid alkaloids from *Delphinium davisii. J Nat Prod,* 59:360-6, Apr. 1996

Yum L, Wolf KM, Chiappinelli VA, Description of a scale for rating the clinical response of cattle poisoned by larkspur. *Am J Vet Res,* 41:488-93, Mar 1991

Yum L, Wolf KM, Chiappinelli VA, Nicotinic acetylcholine receptors in separate brain regions exhibit different affinities for methyllycaconitine. *Neuroscience,* 41:545-55, May 1996

Laurel

Laurus nobilis

DESCRIPTION

Medicinal Parts: The medicinal parts are the leaves, the fruit and the oil.

Flower and Fruit: The flowers are in axillary bushy umbels or short racemous panicles. They are dioecious, whitish-green with 4 petals fused at the base. The male flower usually has 10 to 12 stamens; the female has 4 staminoids. The ovary is short-stemmed with one chamber with a hanging ovule, a short style, and a triangular obtuse stigma. The fruit develops on the stem into deep-black 2-cm long ovate berries.

Leaves, Stem, and Root: Laurel is an evergreen shrub or up to 10 m high tree with smooth, olive green to black bark. The dark-green bay leaves are lanceolate and alternate, about 10 cm long and acuminate at both ends. They are short petioled and their margins are often sinuate and coriaceous.

Habitat: Laurel is indigenous to Mediterranean countries.

Production: Bay leaves are the leaves of *Laurus nobilis.* Bay berries are the fruits of *Laurus nobilis.*

Other Names: Bay, Bay Laurel, Bay Tree, Daphne, Grecian Laurel, Noble Laurel, Roman Laurel, Sweet Bay, True Laurel

ACTIONS AND PHARMACOLOGY

COMPOUNDS: LAUREL LEAF

Volatile oil (1-3%): chief components 1,8-cineol

Sesquiterpene lactones: dehydrocostuslactone, costunolide, furthermore eremanthin, laurenbiolide

Isoquinoline alkaloids: including, among others, reticulin

COMPOUNDS: LAUREL FRUIT

Volatile oil (1-4%): including, among others, 1,8-cineol, alpha- and beta-pinene, citral, methylcinnamat

Sesquiterpene lactones: dehydrocostuslactone, costunolid, furthermore eremanthin, laurenbiolide

Fatty oil (25-55%): chief fatty acids lauric, palmitic, oleic acid The green salve-like laurel oil is gained by pressing or cooking the berries. Besides fatty oil, it contains the components of the volatile oil and a large percentage of sesquiterpene lactones.

EFFECTS

Laurel leaves are externally rubefacient and allergenic because of the essential oil they contain. An antimicrobial, molluscidal and insect repellent effect has been demonstrated.

INDICATIONS AND USAGE

Unproven Uses: Both forms are used as a skin stimulant (rubefacient) and for rheumatic conditions.

PRECAUTIONS AND ADVERSE REACTIONS

No health hazards or side effects are known in conjunction with the proper administration of designated therapeutic dosages. The drug possesses a medium potential for sensitization.

DOSAGE

LAUREL LEAF

Mode of Administration: The essential oil is used in ointments and soaps.

LAUREL FRUIT

Mode of Administration: The mixture of essential and fatty oils, extracted through pressing, was formerly used in the treatment of furuncles; today Laurel is used externally in veterinary medicine, as an udder ointment.

LITERATURE

Biondi D, Cianci P, Geraci C, Rubertom G, Piatelli M. Antimicrobial Activity and Chemical Composition of Essential Oils from Sicilian Aromatic Plants. Flav Fragr J. 8; 331-337. 1993

Hegnauer R, Chemotaxonomie der Pflanzen, Bde 1-11, Birkhäuser Verlag Basel, Boston, Berlin 1962-1997.

Kern W, List PH, Hörhammer L (Hrsg.), Hagers Handbuch der Pharmazeutischen Praxis, 4. Aufl., Bde 1-8, Springer Verlag Berlin, Heidelberg, New York, 1969.

Novak M, Phytochemistry 24(4):585. 1985

Roth L, Daunderer M, Kormann K, Giftpflanzen, Pflanzengifte, 4. Aufl., Ecomed Fachverlag Landsberg Lech 1993.

Steinegger E, Hänsel R, Pharmakognosie, 5. Aufl., Springer Verlag Heidelberg 1992.

Teuscher E, Lindequist U, Biogene Gifte - Biologie, Chemie, Pharmakologie, 2. Aufl., Fischer Verlag Stuttgart 1994.

Laurus nobilis

See Laurel

Lavandula angustifolia

See English Lavender

Lavender Cotton

Santolina chamaecyparissias

DESCRIPTION

Medicinal Parts: The medicinal part of the plant is the herb.

Flower and Fruit: The yellow flower heads are 1 cm wide, almost semi-globular, long-pedicled, homogamous, and lacking lingual florets. The corolla tube is compressed and somewhat winged, with a one-sided appendage. The fruit is glabrous.

Leaves, Stem, and Root: The evergreen plant is a bushy, aromatic subshrub with brittle branches. There are 4 compact rows of small leaves that are narrow, linear, 2 to 3 cm wide, fleshy, obtuse, paired-pinate, gray-tomentose, and occasionally green.

Habitat: The plant is common in the Mediterranean region.

Characteristics: The plant has a strong scent similar to that of chamomile.

Production: Lavender Cotton is the aerial part of *Santolina chamaecyparissias.*

Other Names: Santolina

ACTIONS AND PHARMACOLOGY

COMPOUNDS

Volatile oil (1%): chief components artemisiaketone (3,5,6-trimethyl-1,5-heptadien-4-one, 65%), as well as myrcene, alpha-pinene

Alkaloids

EFFECTS

The drug has anti-inflammatory, digestive, stimulation of menstruation, and anthelmintic effects.

INDICATIONS AND USAGE

Unproven Uses: Lavender Cotton is used for digestive disorders, PMS, worm infestation, stomach complaints, and also to treat jaundice.

PRECAUTIONS AND ADVERSE REACTIONS

No health hazards or side effects are known in conjunction with the proper administration of designated therapeutic dosages.

DOSAGE

Mode of Administration: The herb is used internally as an infusion, but medicinal use has generally ceased.

LITERATURE

Becchi M, Carrier M, Planta Med 38(3):267. 1980

Giner R et al., Planta Med 6:83P. 1986

Kern W, List PH, Hörhammer L (Hrsg.), Hagers Handbuch der Pharmazeutischen Praxis, 4. Aufl., Bde. 1-8: Springer Verlag Berlin, Heidelberg, New York, 1969.

Lawsonia inermis

See Henna

Ledum latifolium

See Labrador Tea

Lemna minor

See Duckweed

Lemon

Citrus limon

DESCRIPTION

Medicinal Parts: The medicinal parts are the juice, peel and oil of the fruit.

Flower and Fruit: Flowers are arranged singly or in short, sparsely flowered racemes, hermaphrodite or functionally male. The petals are suffused with purple on the outer surface. There are 25 to 40 stamens in coherent groups. The fruit is yellow when ripe and grows to 6.5 to 12.5 cm. It is 8- to 10-locular, oblong or ovoid, with a broad, low, mamilliform projection at the apex. The rind is somewhat rough to almost smooth. The pulp is acidic.

Leaves, Stem, and Root: Lemon is a small tree, growing only 3 to 6 m tall with twigs that are angular when young and soon become rounded and glabrous with stout axillary spines. The leaves are pale green, broadly elliptical, acute, and serrate or crenate. The petiole has a flat wing or is merely margined and is distinctly articulated with the lamina.

Habitat: The tree is indigenous to northern India, cultivated in Mediterranean regions and worldwide in subtropical regions.

Production: Lemons are the fruit, lemon peel is the skin of the fruit and lemon oil the essential oil extracted from the skins of *Citrus limon.*

Other Names: Limon

ACTIONS AND PHARMACOLOGY

COMPOUNDS

Volatile oil in the fresh and dehydrated peel: chief components (+)-limonene in addition to citral (as an odor-bearer), n-nonanal, n-decanal, n-dodecanal, linalyl acetate, geranyl acetat, citronellyl acetat, methyl anthranilate; also in pressed oils, lipophilic flavinoids, including sinensetin, nobiletin and furocoumarins

Flavonoids: in particular the bitter neohesperidosides naringin and neohesperidin dyhydro chalcones, furthermore hesperidin, rutin, and ericitrim

EFFECTS

The citroflavonoids in lemon affect vascular permeability and are anti-inflammatory, diuretic, and a source of vitamin C.

INDICATIONS AND USAGE

Unproven Uses: Lemon is used as a source of vitamin C in cases of general low resistance, scurvy, and colds. In folk medicine, lemon juice was recommended as a drink for fever, as a remedy for acute rheumatism, and as an antidote to intoxicants, particularly opium. Additional traditional uses that are still recommended include sunburn, and as a quinine substitute for malaria or to reduce body temperature in typhus patients.

Indian Medicine: Uses in Indian medicine include as a remedy for shaking and heartburn.

PRECAUTIONS AND ADVERSE REACTIONS

No health hazards or side effects are known in conjunction with the proper administration of designated therapeutic dosages. There is a low potential for sensitization through skin contact with volatile oil.

DOSAGE

Mode of Administration: Lemon is used internally in the form of oil, tincture, or fresh fruit.

LITERATURE

Calomme M et al., Inhibition of bacterial mutagenisis by Citrus flavonoids. In: *PM* 62(3):222-226. 1996.

Kern W, List PH, Hörhammer L (Hrsg.), Hagers Handbuch der Pharmazeutischen Praxis, 4. Aufl., Bde. 1-8, Springer Verlag Berlin, Heidelberg, New York, 1969.

Leung AY, Encyclopedia of Common Natural Ingredients Used in Food, Drugs and Cosmetics, John Wiley & Sons Inc., New York 1980.

Oliver-Bever B (Ed.), Medicinal Plants of Tropical West Africa, Cambridge University Press Cambridge, London 1986.

Paris R, *Plant Med Phytother* 11(Suppl):129. 1977

Paris R, Delaveau P, *Plant Med Phytother* 11(Suppl):198. 1977

Roth L, Daunderer M, Kormann K, Giftpflanzen, Pflanzengifte, 4. Aufl., Ecomed Fachverlag Landsberg Lech 1993.

Steinegger E, Hänsel R, Pharmakognosie, 5. Aufl., Springer Verlag Heidelberg 1992.

Tang W, Eisenbrand G, Chinese Drugs of Plant Origin, Springer Verlag Heidelberg 1992.

Teuscher E, Biogene Arzneimittel, 5. Aufl., Wiss. Verlagsges. mbH Stuttgart 1997.

Wichtl M (Hrsg.), Teedrogen, 4. Aufl., Wiss. Verlagsges. Stuttgart 1997.

Lemon Balm

Melissa officinalis

DESCRIPTION

Medicinal Parts: The medicinal parts are the oil extracted by distillation, the dried leaves, the fresh leaves, and the whole plant.

Flower and Fruit: The small white bilabiate flowers are in 6 one-sided false whorls in the axils of the upper leaves. The calyx is campanulate, bilabiate, and it has a shortly dentate upper lip. The corolla tube is curved upward. The upper lip is slightly domed and divided in two parts, the lower lip is trilobed with an extended middle lobe. The flower has 4 stamens. The fruit is an oblong-ovate, 1.5- to 2-mm long, and chestnut brown nutlet.

Leaves, Stem, and Root: The plant is a perennial that grows up to 90 cm high, with an erect, quadrangular, branched, and sparsely haired to glabrous stem. The leaves are petiolate and have an ovate to rhomboid, 2- to 6-cm long by 1.5- to 5-cm wide crenate leaf blade, which is shortly pointed at the end, and stunted or wedge-shaped at the base. It is usually only pubescent above or completely glabrous.

Characteristics: Before flowering, the taste and smell is lemon-like, later becoming astringent to balm-like and warming.

Habitat: The plant is indigenous to the east Mediterranean region and west Asia, and is cultivated in central Europe or established in the wild.

Production: Lemon balm is the fresh or dried leaves of *Melissa officinalis* as well as its preparations. The leaves are collected before flowering or before there is too much branching. Leaves and stem are separated and comminuted and dried quickly at temperatures between 30 to 40° C.

Not to be Confused With: Nepeta cataria. var. citriodora (lemon cat mint).

Other Names: Balm, Bee Balm, Blue Balm, Garden Balm, Sweet Mary, Honey Plant, Cure-All, Dropsy Plant, Melissa

ACTIONS AND PHARMACOLOGY

COMPOUNDS

Volatile oil (0.02-0.8%): chief components geranial (citral a), neral (citral b), citronellal (together 40-75% of the volatile oil, aroma-carrier), furthermore, linalool, geraniol, geranylactetate, methyl citronellate, trans-β-ocimene, 1-Octen-3-ol, 6-methyl-5-heptene-2-on. beta-caryophyllene, caryophyllebepoxide, germacren D, eugenol

Glycosides: of the alcoholic or phenolic components of the volatile oil, for example eugenol glucoside

Caffeic acid derivatives: rosmaric acid (up to 4.7%)

Flavonoids: including among others cynaroside, cosmosiin, rhamnocitrin, isoquercitrin

Triterpene acids: including among others ursolic acid. Only the very fresh drug (maximum 6 months old) is usable as a sedative, because of the low volatile oil content and its high volatility; the requirements of the German-language medication texts do not take this into consideration (no minimum content requirement given).

EFFECTS

The drug has mild sedative and carminative, spasmolytic, antibacterial, antiviral, anti-oxidative and anti-hormonal effects.

INDICATIONS AND USAGE

Approved by Commission E:

■ Nervousness and insomnia

The drug is used for nervous agitation and sleeping problems.

Unproven Uses: In folk medicine, the drug is utilized as decoctions of the flowering shoots for nervous complaints, lower abdominal disorders, meteorism, nervous gastric complaints, hysteria and melancholia, chronic bronchial catarrh, nervous palpitations, vomiting, migraine, nervous debility, headache, and high blood pressure. It is used externally for rheumatism, nerve pains and stiff necks (compress).

Homeopathic Uses: Melissa officinalis is used for menstrual irregularities.

PRECAUTIONS AND ADVERSE REACTIONS

No health hazards or side effects are known in conjunction with the proper administration of designated therapeutic dosages.

DOSAGE

Mode of Administration: Comminuted herb, herb powder, liquid extracts or dry extracts for teas and other galenic preparations; liquid and solid forms for internal and external use; combinations with other sedative and/or carminative herbs may be beneficial.

How Supplied:

Capsules — 395 mg

Dry Extracts - 4:1 to 6:1 with ethanol or purified water.

Preparation: To prepare an infusion pour one cup of hot water over 1.5 to 4.5 g of the drug and strain after 10 minutes. Drink several cups a day.

Homeopathic Dosage: 5 drops, 1 tablet or 10 globules every 30 to 60 minutes (acute) or 1 to 3 times daily (chronic); parenterally: 1 to 2 mL sc acute, 3 times daily; chronic: once a day (HAB34).

Storage: Store in well-sealed, non-plastic containers, protected from light and moisture for up to 1 year.

LITERATURE

Adzet T, Ponz R, Wolf E, Schulte E. Genetic Variability of the Essential Oil Content of *Melissa officinalis. Planta Med.* 58; 558-561. 1992

Agata I, Kusakabe H, Hatano T, Nishibe S, Okuda T. Melitric Acids A and B, New Trimeric Caffeic Acid Derivatives *from Melissa officinalis. Chem Pharm Bull.* 41; 1608-1611. 1993

Berg T van den, Schultze W, Kubeczka KH, Czygan FC. Ontogenetic variation of the essential leaf oil of *Melissa officinalis L. Pharmazie* 52 (3); 247-253. 1997

Cohen RA, Kucera LS, Herrmann EC Jr, Antiviral activity of *Melissa officinalis* (Limon Balm) extract. In: *Proc Soc Exp Biol Med* 117:431-434. 1964.

Hermann EC Jr., Kucera LS, Antiviral substances in plants of the mint family (Labiatae): II. Nontanninia polyphenols of *Melissa officinalis.* In: *Proc soc Exp Bio Med* 124:869. 1967.

Koch-Heitzmann I, Schultze W, 2000 Jahre *Melissa officinalis.* Von der Bienenpflanze zum Virustatikum. In: ZPT 9(3):77. 1988.

Kümel G, Stoll L, Brendel M, Herpes simplex. Therapie mit rezeptfreien Topika. In: DAZ 131(30):1609. 1991.

Macoy-Mokrżynska A, Loniewski I, Drozdzik M. Central Action of *Valerian off.* and *Melissa off. Pol J Pharmacol Pharm.* 44; Suppl.; 176. 1992

Meyer W, Spiteller G. Increase of Caryophyllene Oxide in Ageing Lemon Balm Leaves (*Melissa officinalis L.*) - A Consequence of Lipid Peroxidation?. *Z Naturforsch.* 51c; 651-656. 1996

Mulkens A, Kapetanidis I. Eugenylglucoside, a new natural Phenylpropanoid Heteroside from *Melissa officinalis. J Nat Prod.* 51; 496-498. 1988

Orth-Wagner S, Ressin WJ, Friedrich I, Phytosedativum gegen Schlafstörungen. In: ZPT 16(3):147-156. 1995.

Pertz H, Naturally occuring clavines: Antagonism/partial agonism at 5-HT2alpha receptors and antogonism at alpha1-adrenoceptors in blood vessel. In: PM 62(5)387-392. 1996.

Sarer E, Kokdil G, Constitutents of the essential oil from *Melissa officinalis*. In: *PM* 57:89. 1991.

Uehleke B, Phytobalneologie. In: ZPT 17(1):26-43. 1996.

Vogt HJ, Tausch I, Wöbling RH, Kaiser PM (1991) Melissenextrakt bei Herpes simplex. Allgemeinarzt 14:832-841.

Zitiert nach: Koch- Heitzmann I, Schültze W, *Melissa officinalis.* Eine alte Arzneipflanze mit neue therapeutischen Wirkungen. Dtsch Apoth Z 124:2137-2145. 1984

Lemongrass

Cymbopogon citratus

DESCRIPTION

Medicinal Parts: The medicinal parts are the dried leaves and the oil.

CYMBOPOGON CITRATUS

Flower and Fruit: The flowers are 30 cm long and have false spikes with reddish brown sheaths 15 to 25 mm long. The racemes are 15 to 17 mm long. The sessile spikelet is 6 mm long and the upper spelts are 0.7 mm wide, lanceolate, narrowly winged, flattened at the back, slightly concave, and ribless in the lower part. The stemmed spikelet is 4.5 mm long, and the lower spelt is 0.7 mm wide. Inflorescences are rarely formed on this variety.

Leaves, Stem, and Root: Cymbopogon citratus is a perennial plant with a smooth and glabrous stalk up to 2 m. The leaf blade is linear, acuminate, up to 90 cm long and 5 mm wide and smooth on both sides. The leaf sheaths are round, glabrous, and smooth. The ligule is paperlike and less than 1 mm long.

CYMBOPOGON NARDUS

Flower and Fruit: The inflorescence is very large and consists of a 1-m long spike with numerous racemes up to 20 mm long and arranged in zigzag configuration. The sessile spike is 5 mm long. The lower spelt is oblong-lanceolate, usually flat, narrowly winged with 3 ribs. The awn, if there is one, is 5 mm long. The petiolar spike is 5 mm long, and the lower spelt lanceolate has 7 ribs.

Leaves, Stem, and Root: Cymbopogon nardus is a perennial plant with a stalk that grows up to 2 to 2.5 m. It is smooth and glabrous. The leaf blade is up to 1 m long and 1.5 cm wide and usually light green. The upper surface is smooth, the lower surface and the margin are rough. The leaf sheaths are glabrous and yellowish-green. The basal leaf sheaths are also glabrous but green to reddish. The ligule is paper-like and about 1 mm long.

Characteristics: Cymbopogon species have essential oils in tubelike cells with corked walls.

Habitat: Citronella grass was originally indigenous to the tropics and the subtropics of the Old World. Today it is cultivated in Central and South America and Queensland, Australia.

Production: Lemongrass consists of the above-ground parts of *Cymbopogon citratus*. West Indian Lemongrass oil consists of the essential oil from *Cymbopogon citratus*. Citronella oil consists of the essential oil from *Cymbopogon winterianus*.

Other Names: Citronella, Fevergrass

ACTIONS AND PHARMACOLOGY

COMPOUNDS: LEMONGRASS LEAVES

Volatile oil (0.2-0.4%)

COMPOUNDS: LEMONGRASS LEAVES

Citral (65-86%)

Myrcene (12-20%)

COMPOUNDS: CITRONELLA OIL

Citronellal (32-45%)

Geraniol (12-25%)

Geranyl acetate (3-8%)

Citronellyl acetate (1-4%)

EFFECTS

Lemongrass is used for headache, flu, rheumatism, and muscle cramping. Aromatherapists recommend lemongrass oil, massaged into joints and muscles, to relieve stiffness. It is thought that the oil decreases lactic acid buildup in muscles. Lemongrass is also used as an anticoagulant. Lemongrass oil, diluted in a carrier oil, is used for oily hair, acne, scabies, ringworm, and other skin infections. The fragrance is used for its calming effect. Lemongrass leaf applied directly to the skin is an effective insect repellent.

Human studies show that powdered lemongrass leaf tea does not improve sleep or anxiety. Animal studies have shown that oral doses of lemongrass are inactive. Animal studies have also shown that lemongrass leaf decoction has a weak diuretic effect, has a minimal effect on inflammation as compared to indomethacin, and that the chemosuppressive effect of lemongrass was slightly less than pyrimethamine. In a controlled study of mice, lemongrass exhibited schizontocidal and prophylactic activity. In vitro studies have shown that main components of pure lemongrass oil, citral (neral and geranial) and myrcene have antibacterial, fungistatic, and fungicidal activity; in higher doses, the oil has a sedative/analgesic effect. In rats, IV administration of an infusion caused a drop in arterial pressure and a mild diuretic effect. The oral administration of an imprecise amount of extract caused a drop in temperature and tendency to lengthen intestinal passage time. Because of the small number of experiments carried out, a hypotensive action cannot be considered as conclusively proved. A controlled study of 32 rats showed lemongrass leaf decoction to have a weak diuretic effect (Carbajal et al, 1989).

Antibacterial Effects: The antibacterial activity of lemongrass is primarily due to the constituents' neral and geranial. The essential oil of lemongrass has exhibited antibacterial effects against several different types of bacteria (Hammer et al, 1999; Pattnaik et al, 1996).

Lemongrass essential oil inhibited numerous gram-negative and gram-positive organisms in vitro at concentrations less than or equal to 2.0%(v/v) (Hammer et al, 1999). Gram-positive organisms are more sensitive to lemongrass oil than are gram-negative organisms. Lemongrass oil is rapidly bactericidal against *E coli* and *B subtilis*. The antibacterial activity of lemongrass is impacted by pH and inoculum size. Increased pH values to the alkaline region increased antibacterial activity of lemongrass oil (Onawunmi & Ogunlana, 1986).

Anti-Inflammatory Effects: In a study of twenty rats, carageenan-induced edema was inhibited by 18.6% in rats receiving oral doses of a 20% lemongrass leaf decoction as compared to 58.6% in the control group of rats receiving indomethacin (Carbajal et al, 1989). Myrcene appears to exert a peripheral analgesic effect in rats that is different than aspirin (or related drugs) in mechanism (Lorenzetti et al, 1991).

Antifungal Effects: Lemongrass essential oil inhibited *Candida albicans* in vitro at concentrations of less than or equal to 2.0%(v/v) (Hammer et al, 1999). Lemongrass oil has demonstrated antifungal activity against several different types of fungi (Pattnaik et al, 1996).

Chemoprotective Effects: Lemongrass extract significantly inhibited the formation of DNA adducts and aberrant crypt foci formation (Suaeyun et al, 1997).

CLINICAL TRIALS

Bacterial Infections

Three main components of pure lemongrass oil, citral, neral/geranial, and myrcene, have been shown to have antibacterial activity of varying degrees with *Staphylococcus aureus, Bacillus subtilis*, and *Escherichia coli*. Myrcene showed no significant antibacterial effect on its own; however, it enhanced the antibacterial activity of neral and geranial. Neral and geranial were active *against E coli, Staph aureus,* and *B subtilis. E coli* was most resistant of the three, then *S aureus*, and *B subtilis* were most sensitive. *Pseudomonas aeruginosa* was resistant to pure lemongrass oil and citral (neral and geranial) (Onawunmi et al, 1984).

Chemoprotection

Lemongrass extract (80% ethanol) significantly inhibited the formation of DNA adducts, 7-meG and O6-meG, in the colonic mucosa and muscular layer (but not the liver) of azoxymethane-treated rats. Rats were administered lemongrass, 0.5 g or 5 g/kg body weight, by intragastric gavage for 1 week prior to injection with azoxymethane (AOM). AOM-injected rats were continuously treated with lemongrass extract and sacrificed 3 weeks after the second AOM injection. Lemongrass significantly inhibited aberrant crypt foci formation at a dose of 0.5 g/kg in both initiation ($p<0.0005$) and promotion stages (p less than 0.05) (Suaeyun et al, 1997).

Fungal Infections

In vitro studies have demonstrated that lemongrass oil has fungistatic and fungicidal activity. *Microsporum gypseum* was the most susceptible and *Aspergillus fumigatus* the least susceptible of those organisms studied. *Candida albicans, Candida pseudotropicalis,* and *Trichophyton mentagrophytes* were also susceptible to lemongrass oil. Constituents of lemongrass oil, neral, geranial, and citronellal also showed good antifungal activity. Lemongrass constituents dipentene and myrcene showed no fungistatic or fungicidal activity (Onawunmi, 1989).

Head Lice

A placebo-controlled, double-blind clinical study in 103 children from four different elementary schools randomized half to a slow-release Citronella formula and 95 to a placebo over a period of four months. Upon examination two months after treatment start, a significant difference was observed between the two groups, with 12.0% of those treated with Citronella and 50.5% of those treated with placebo being infested with lice. Side effects for Citronella included unpleasant smell (4.4%) and mild itching/burning sensation (1.0), but overall the herbal formula scored significantly better than placebo in countering head lice (present in 15.5% versus 55.1%, respectively) overall (Mumcuoglu, 2004).

INDICATIONS AND USAGE

Unproven Uses: Externally, Lemongrass is used for lumbago, neuralgic and rheumatic pain, sprains, and as a mild astringent. Internally, the herb is used for gastrointestinal symptoms, and mild states of agitation.

Indian Medicine: Lemongrass is used for intestinal parasites, stomach complaints, flatulence, leprosy, bronchitis, and fever.

CONTRAINDICATIONS

Pregnancy: Not to be used during pregnancy.

PRECAUTIONS AND ADVERSE REACTIONS

No adverse effects have been reported. The application of salves with the volatile oil upon the skin has led in rare cases to signs of allergy. A toxic alveolitis was observed in 2 cases following inhalation of the volatile oil.

DRUG INTERACTIONS

No human interaction data available.

DOSAGE

How Supplied: Tea

Daily Dose: 2 g of dried leaf in 150 mL of water. Dosage equals approximately 2.0 mL/kg of body weight. Two fresh minced leaves or 2 g of powdered dried leaf is used (Carlini et al, 1986, Souza Formigoni et al, 1986).

Storage: Store in airtight containers protected from light.

LITERATURE

De Silva MG. *Mfg Chemist* 30:415-416. 1959.

Hammer KA, Carson CF & Riley TV. Antimicrobial activity of essential oils and other plant extracts. *J Appl Microbiol*; 86(6):985-990. 1999.

Leite JR, Seabra M de L, Maluf E et al. Pharmacology of lemongrass (*Cymbopogon citratus Stapf*). III. Assessment of eventual toxic, hypnotic and anxiolytic effects on humans. *J Ethnopharmacol*;17(1):75-83. 1986.

Lorenzetti BB, Souza GE, Sarti SJ et al. Myrcene mimics the peripheral analgesic activity of lemongrass tea. *J Ethnopharmacol*; 34(1):43-48. 1991.

Mumcuoglu KY, Magdassi S, Miller J, et al. Repellency of citronella for head lice: double-blind randomized trial of efficacy and safety. *Isr Med Assoc J; 6*(12):756-9. 2004.

Onawunmi GO. Evaluation of the antifungal activity of lemon grass oil. *Int J Crude Drug Res*; 27(2):121-126. 1989.

Onawunmi GO & Ogunlana. A study of the antibacterial activity of the essential oil of lemon grass. *Int J Crude Drug Res*; 24(2):64-68. 1986.

Pattnaik S, Subramanyam VR & Kole C. Antibacterial and antifungal activity of ten essential oils in vitro. *Microbios*; 86(349):237-246. 1996.

Paumgarrten F, De-Carvalho R, Souza C et al. Study of the effects of beta-myrcene on rat fertility and general reproductive performance. *Braz J Med Biol Res*; 31(7):955-965. 1998.

Sarer E, Scheffer JJC, Svendsen AB. Composition of the essential oil of *Cymbopogon citratus* (DC.) STAPF cultivated in turkey. In: *Sci Pharm* 51:58. 1983.

Souza Formigoni MLO, Lodder HM, Gianotti Filho O et al. Pharmacology of lemongrass (*Cymbopogon citratus Stapf*). II. Effects of daily two month administration in male and female rats and in offspring exposed "in utero." *J Ethnopharmacol*; 17(1):65-74. 1986.

Suaeyun R, Kinouchi T, Arimochi H et al. Inhibitory effects of lemon grass (*Cymbopogon citratus Stapf*) on formation of azoxymethane-induced DNA adducts and aberrant crypt foci in the rat colon. *Carcinogenesis*; 18(5):949-955. 1997.

Lemon Verbena

Aloysia triphylla

DESCRIPTION

Medicinal Parts: The medicinal part is the oil of vervain as a distillate of the fresh twigs and the dried leaves and stems.

Flower and Fruit: The plant has numerous small flowers in paniclelike spikes. The hairy calyx is about 3 mm long with 4 tips. The petals are white or bluish, and fused to a 4 to 5 mm long funnel at the base. There are 2 short and 2 long stamens in the funnel.

Leaves, Stem, and Root: Aloysia triphylla is a shrub up to 3 m high. The branches are striate and scabrous. They bear leaves in whorls of 3 or 4 on the stem. The leaves are entire-margined, short-petioled, lanceolate, and about 7 to 10 cm long. They have lateral veins almost at right angles to the midrib, and are dotted on the underside with oil-bearing glands.

Characteristics: The leaves have a lemony fragrance.

Habitat: The plant originated in Argentina, Chile and Peru, and is cultivated in most other warmer countries. Main countries of cultivation are Algeria, Chile, Israel, and Morocco.

Production: Lemon Verbena leaves are the leaves and stems, in whole and ground form, of *Aloysia triphylla.* The shrubs are propagated by runners or cuttings. They are cut from the second year of growth, in the month of July, before flowering. The young lateral branches appear in October. They are dried rapidly in thin layers or bundles. The dried leaves are then stripped off. The harvest consists of approximately 10,000 kg of the leaf drug per hectare.

Other Names: Herb Louisa, Lemongrass Verbena, Lemon-Scented Verbena, Verbain

ACTIONS AND PHARMACOLOGY

COMPOUNDS

Volatile oil: main constituents are geraniol and neral

Flavonoids: including apigenin-, diosmetin- and luteolin-7-O-glucosides, in addition to mono-, di- and trimethoxyflavones, including eupatorin. (See Lippiae triphylla aetherolum.)

Iridoids: iridoid glycosides including geniposidic acid

EFFECTS

The leaves are considered to be antispasmodic, sedative, and are a febrifuge. There are no up-to-date studies available.

INDICATIONS AND USAGE

Unproven Uses: In France, Lemon Verbena is used in the symptomatic treatment of digestive disorders, agitation, and insomnia. The drug has also been used in the treatment of febrile hemorrhoids, varicose veins, and impure skin. In Morocco it is also used for chills and constipation. Efficacy has not been proved in any of these areas. The plant is used as an inactive ingredient to improve the flavor in medicinal teas.

PRECAUTIONS AND ADVERSE REACTIONS

No health hazards or side effects are known in conjunction with the proper administration of designated therapeutic dosages.

DOSAGE

Mode of Administration: In France, the infusion is available in various restaurants under the name "Vervaine oderante." Used in various medicinal preparations and tea mixtures.

Preparation: To prepare an infusion, use 5 to 29 g of the leaf per 1 liter of water.

Daily Dosage: Drink 2 to 5 cups of the infusion during the course of the day. In preparations with a high water content (such as instant teas), the daily dose equivalent should not exceed 10 g. The upper limit for daily dosages of powders and tinctures is 5 g.

Storage: The drug must be stored in sealed containers, protected from light and dampness.

LITERATURE

Carnat A, Carnat AP, Chavignon O, Heitz A, Wylde R, Lamaison JL, Luteolin 7-diglucuronide the major flavonoid compound from *Aloysia triphylla* and *Verbena officinalis. Planta Med,* 61:490, 1995 Oct.

Hänsel R, Keller K, Rimpler H, Schneider G (Hrsg.), Hagers Handbuch der Pharmazeutischen Praxis, 5. Aufl., Bde 4-6 (Drogen), Springer Verlag Berlin, Heidelberg, New York, 1992-1994.

Nakamura T, Okuyama E, Tsukada A, Yamazaki M, Satake M, Nishibe S, Deyama T, Moriya A, Maruno M, Nishimura H. Acteoside as the Analgesic Principle of Cedron (*Lippia triphylla*), a Peruvian Medicinal Plant. *Chem Pharm Bull.* 45 (3); 499-504 (1997)

Rimpler H, Sauerbier H, *Biochem Syst Ecol* 14:307-310. 1986.

Skalta H, Shammas G, *PM* 54:265. 1988.

Tomás-Barberán FA, Harborne JB, Self R, PH 26:2281-2284. 1987.

Torrent Marti MT, *Rev R Acad Farm* (Barcelona) 14:39-55. 1976.

Lemon-Wood

Schisandra sphenanthera

DESCRIPTION

Medicinal Parts: Medicinal properties are attributed to the fruit and seed of the plant.

Flower and Fruit: The flowers are in clusters with a few blossoms in the axils of the bracts. There are 5 to 8 tepals. The perigone of the male flowers has 5 to 8 sections and 11 to 19 stamens. The female flowers have a similar perigone and 30 to 50 ovaries. The fruit is elongate-elliptical, slim and hangs in aggregate clusters. The individual fruit is round, fleshy, brown-red to dark brown, and berrylike.

Leaves, Stem, and Root: The dioecious *Schisandra sphenanthera* has leaves that are alternate and arranged like whorls on short shoots. The petiole is 1 to 3 cm long. The lamina is dark green to brown, 5 to 11 cm long, and 3 to 7 cm wide. It is ovate to elliptical, acute at both ends, and serrate to dentate. The young branches are purple.

Habitat: The plant is indigenous to China.

Production: Southern schisandra fruit is the dried, ripe fruit of *Schisandra sphenanthera.*

ACTIONS AND PHARMACOLOGY

COMPOUNDS

Volatile oil

Ascorbic acid (vitamin C)

Lignans (in the seeds 2 to 10%): dibenzo[a,c]cyclooctene derivatives, including schizandrins A and B, schizandrols A and B, schizantherins A to E, additional lignans with other parent substances, including epigalbacin, anwulignan, and ganschisandrin

Fatty oil (in the seeds)

EFFECTS

Various lignans have been isolated from the drug that are also present in *Schisandra chinensis*; some of the action mechanisms described there may also apply to *Schisandra sphenanthera.* (See *Schisandra chinensis.*)

INDICATIONS AND USAGE

Chinese Medicine: The plant is used for dyspnea, coughs caused by disturbance of lung function, dry mouth, thirst, spontaneous or night sweats, nocturia, insomnia, amnesia, and anxiety states. Efficacy for these indications has not yet been proved.

PRECAUTIONS AND ADVERSE REACTIONS

No health hazards are known in conjunction with the proper administration of designated therapeutic dosages.

DOSAGE

Mode of Administration: Whole drug and preparations for internal use.

Preparation: To prepare Cuwuweizi powder, the drug is evaporated in the ratio of 1:5 with vinegar in closed containers until the surface turns black. The product is then ground to a powder.

Daily Dosage: The literature has no information.

LITERATURE

Hänsel R, Keller K, Rimpler H, Schneider G (Ed), Hagers Handbuch der Pharmazeutischen Praxis, 5. Aufl., Bde 4 - 6 (Drogen), Springer Verlag Berlin, Heidelberg, New York, 1992-1994.

Hikino H, Kiso Y, Taguchi H, Ikeya Y. Antihepatotoxic Actions of Lignoids from *Schizandra chinensis* Fruits. *Planta Med.* 50; 213-218. 1984

Liu CS, Fang SD, Huang MF, Kao YL, Hsu JS, Studies on the active principles of Schisandra sphenanthera Rehd. et Wils. The structures of schisantherin A, B, C, D, E and the related compounds. Sci Sin, 21:483-502, Jul-Aug. 1978

Leonurus cardiaca

See Motherwort

Leonurus japonicus

See Chinese Motherwort

Lepidium sativum

See Garden Cress

Leptandra virginica

See Black Root

Lesser Celandine

Ranunculus ficaria

DESCRIPTION

Medicinal Parts: The medicinal part is the fresh herb.

Flower and Fruit: The golden yellow flowers have a diameter of 25 mm. The calyx usually has 3 sepals, the corolla 8 or more petals, which are glossy and spread out in a star-shape. Since the petals are green underneath, the flowers are inconspicuous when closed. There are numerous stamens and ovaries. The fruit is 1-seeded and indehiscent.

Leaves, Stem, and Root: The plant grows from 5 to 15 cm high. The stems are decumbent and bear bulbils in the leaf axils. The leaves, like the stems, are glabrous and fleshy. The lower ones are long-petioled, alternate, and orbicular-cordate. The upper ones have 5 lobes. There are fleshy, cylindrical clavate tubers between the roots.

Characteristics: The herb has a hot, unpleasant taste and is toxic.

Habitat: The plant is found all over Europe, western Asia and northern Africa.

Production: Lesser Celandine is the fresh herb of *Ranunculus ficaria.*

Other Names: Figwort, Pilewort, Smallwort

ACTIONS AND PHARMACOLOGY

COMPOUNDS

The glycoside ranunculin as protoanemonine-forming agent: The freshly harvested plant (0.06%-0.35% of the fresh weight, of which only 3% of the overall content of the plant is contained in the leaves, 68% in the stalks, 25% in the blossoms) changes enzymatically when it is cut into small pieces, and probably also when it is dried, into the pungent, volatile protoanemonine that quickly dimerizes to non-mucus-membrane-irritating anemonine. When dried, the plant is not capable of protoanemonine-formation.

EFFECTS

Active agents are tannin, the alkaloids chelidonin and cholerytrin, the saponin fikarin and large quantities of vitamin C.

INDICATIONS AND USAGE

Unproven Uses: Lesser Celandine is used for scurvy, treatment of bleeding wounds and gums, and swollen joints.

PRECAUTIONS AND ADVERSE REACTIONS

The dangers of irritation of the skin and mucous membranes are relatively low with Lesser Celandine. The consumption of small quantities of the fresh leaf sheaths (before blossoming; the stem should be discarded) as a springtime salad is unproblematic.

No health hazards or side effects are known in conjunction with the proper administration of designated therapeutic dosages of the dehydrated drug. Extended skin contact with the freshly harvested, bruised plant can lead to blister formation and cauterizations which are difficult to heal due to the resulting protoanemonine, that is severely irritating to skin and mucus membranes.

If taken internally, severe irritation to the gastrointestinal tract, combined with colic and diarrhea, as well as irritations of the urinary drainage passages, are possible. Symptomatic treatment for external contact should consist of irrigation with diluted potassium permanganate solution; in case of internal contact, administration of activated charcoal should follow gastric lavage.

OVERDOSAGE

Death by asphyxiation following the intake of large quantities of protoanemonine-forming plants has been observed in animal experiments.

DOSAGE

Mode of Administration: Ground and as an extract. The drug extracts can be added to baths to treat hemorrhoids, warts and scratches.

LITERATURE

Bonora A et al., *PH* 26:2277. 1987.

Texier O et al., Phytochemistry 23(12):2903. 1984

Lesser Galangal

Alpinia officinarum

DESCRIPTION

Medicinal Parts: The medicinal part of the plant is the rhizome.

Flower and Fruit: Galangal is a perennial plant. It is similar in appearance to the sword lily.

Leaves, Stem, and Root: Lesser Galangal has a dark, reddish-brown, cylindrical rhizome about 1 to 2 cm in diameter and 3 to 6 cm long. The stem is marked at short intervals with raised rings, which are the scars of the leaf bases. Stems are up to 1.5 m with long narrow lanceolate leaves bearing racemes of orchid-shaped flowers, white and veined red. A fracture of the rhizome is hard and tough, showing a pale inside with a darker central column.

Characteristics: Lesser Galangal has a pungent and spicy taste. The odor is aromatic, rather like ginger.

Habitat: The plant is indigenous to China and entered Europe via India and Arabia in the Middle Ages.

Production: Lesser Galangal consists of the dried rhizome of *Alpinia officinarum.*

Not to be Confused With: The rhizome of Kaempferia galanga and other Alpina species

Other Names: Catarrh Root, Chinese Ginger, China Root, Colic Root, East India Catarrh Root, East India Root, Galanga, Gargaut, Galangal, India Root

ACTIONS AND PHARMACOLOGY

COMPOUNDS

Volatile oil: chief components-sesquiterpene hydrocarbons, sesquiterpene alcohols

Diarylheptanoids: mixture termed galangol, some of them pungent substances

Gingerole: phenyl alkanones, pungent substances

Starch

Tannin

Flavonoids: including galangin, galangin-3-methylether, kaempferide

EFFECTS

The plant is said to have antispasmodic, antiphlogistic, and antibacterial properties.

INDICATIONS AND USAGE

Approved by Commission E:

- Dyspeptic complaints
- Loss of appetite

Unproven Uses: Folk medicine uses include painful upper abdominal syndrome of the Roemheld complex.

Chinese Medicine: The drug is used for pain, particularly stomach pain.

PRECAUTIONS AND ADVERSE REACTIONS

Health risks or side effects following the proper administration of designated therapeutic dosages are not reported.

DOSAGE

Mode of Administration: Comminuted drug and powder, as well as other galenic preparations for oral administration.

Preparation: Infusion - Pour boiling water over 0.5 to 1 g drug and strain after 10 minutes.

Daily Dosage: 2 to 4 g. The infusion dosage is 1 cup 30 minutes before meals.

LITERATURE

De Pooter HL, et al., PH 24:93. 1985.

Haraguchi H, et al., Antifungal activity from *Alpinia galanga* and the competition for incorporation of unsaturated fatty acids in cell growth. In: *PM* 62(4):308-313. 1996.

Janssen AM, Scheffer JJ. Acetoxychavicol Acetate, an Antifungal Component of *Alpinia galanga. Planta Med.* 51; 507-511. 1985

Levant Cotton

Gossypium herbaceum

DESCRIPTION

Medicinal Parts: The medicinal parts are the root bark, the fresh inner-root bark, and the seeds.

Flower and Fruit: The yellow flowers have a dark red spot at the base of the petals. The calyx is 2 to 2.5 cm long. The bracts are broadly deltate-ovate to semicircular, usually at least as wide as long. Their margins have 6 to 8 acute or shortly acuminate teeth, usually less than 3 times as long as wide. The fruit is beak-shaped, terminally rounded, up to 18 mm long, with 3 to 4 chambers. The seeds, which are embedded in the hairs, are square with gray pubescense.

Leaves, Stem, and Root: Gossypium herbaceum is an evergreen shrub 2 m high and 1 to 1.5 m wide. The few branches are glabrous to sparsely haired and foliated. The leaves are broadly cordate, coriaceous, reticulate, and pubescent with undulate margins. They have a short tip and narrow base.

Habitat: The variety is indigenous to Asia and Africa. Today it is mainly cultivated in Egypt, China, India, Anatolia, and the southern U.S.

Other Names: Cotton Root, Herbaceous Cotton

ACTIONS AND PHARMACOLOGY

COMPOUNDS

Volatile oil (traces): including with beta-bisabolol

Resinous substance: containing, among others, salicylic acid and 2,3-dihydroxybenzoic acid

Dimeric sesquiterpenes: (+)-gossypol, (+) -gossypol, p-hemigossypol in some strains presumably in very low quantities)

The drug has not been investigated in recent times.

EFFECTS

A histamine-releasing effect has been observed in vitro, in the lung tissue of pigs. The drug also appears to have emmenagogic, oxytocic, and contraceptive (male) effects, but constituents have not yet been sufficiently investigated. The oxytocic effect, similar to that of secale, has been observed in animal experiments, making its use as a contraction stimulant seem plausible.

INDICATIONS AND USAGE

Unproven Uses: The drug has many indications in folk medicine, such as amenorrhea, dysmenorrhea, irregular menstruation, nausea, fever, headache, diarrhea and dysentery; as an oxytoxic, to expel the afterbirth, for urethritis, nerve inflammation, poor lactation, metrorrhagia, hemorrhage, menorrhagia and atonic amenorrhea, painful menstruation, and climacteric complaints.

Chinese Medicine: Cotton is used in China as a male contraceptive.

Homeopathic Uses: The drug is used chiefly in gynecology to treat menstrual disturbances, menstrual bleeding, morning sickness, and uterine bleeding.

PRECAUTIONS AND ADVERSE REACTIONS

General: Health risks or side effects following the proper administration of designated therapeutic dosages are not recorded.

Pregnancy: Cotton is not to be administered during pregnancy, except at delivery.

OVERDOSAGE

In animal studies, numerous poisonings, some of them fatal, have been observed following long-term feeding with large quantities of cotton seed press cakes.

DOSAGE

Mode of Administration: The drug is used as a decoction, liquid extract and tincture, as well as in combination with secale, hydrastis, chaemaelirium, and leonurus.

Preparations: Tincture and liquid extract of 2 to 4 mL, liquid extract 20 to 40 drops per single dose.

Daily Dosage: The standard single dose to be taken internally is 2 g of the drug, or 10 g of a 20% decoction, i.e. 1 teaspoonful for a single-dose decoction. The dosage of the liquid extract administered during labor is a single dose of 1 to 2 level teaspoonfuls, with another similar dose given 2 to 4 times daily after the birth as a post-natal styptic.

Homeopathic Dosage: 5 drops, 1 tablet, or 10 globules every 30 to 60 minutes (acute) or 1 to 3 times daily (chronic); parenterally: 1 to 2 mL sc acute, 3 times daily; chronic: once a day (HAB34).

Storage: Store Cotton in well-filled containers, protected from light and heat.

LITERATURE

Byzova MV, Kraev AS, Pozmogova GE, Skriabin KG, Molecular characteristics of chalcone synthase gene families from two cotton species using the polymerase chain reaction. *Mol Biol* (Mosk), 26:432-40, Mar-Apr 1992.

Hamasaki Y, Tae HH, *Biochim Biophys Acta* 843(1):37. 1985

Liu ZQ et al., In: Recent Advances in Fertility Regulation. Beijing 1980, Eds. C. C. Fen et al. Pub. S. A. Atar, Geneva 1981.

Qian SZ et al., Chin Med J 93:477. 1980

Zheng MS, Zhang YZ Anti-HBsAg herbs employing ELISA technique. Chung Hsi I Chieh Ho Tsa Chih, 26:560-2 518, Sep 1990.

Levisticum officinale

See Lovage

Liatris spicata

See Marsh Blazing Star

Licorice

Glycyrrhiza glabra

DESCRIPTION

Medicinal Parts: The medicinal parts are the unpeeled, dried roots and the runners, the peeled dried roots, and the rhizome with the roots.

Flower and Fruit: The axillary inflorescences are upright, spikelike and 10 to 15 cm long. The individual flowers are 1 to 1.5 cm long, bluish to pale violet and short-pedicled. The calyx is short, bell-shaped, and glandular-haired. The pointed, lanceolate tips of the calyx are longer than the tube. The petals are narrow; the pointed carina petals are not fused. The fruit is a pod, 1.5 to 2.5 cm long, and 4 to 6 mm wide. It is erect and splayed, flat with thick sutures, glabrous, somewhat reticulate-pitted, and usually has 3 to 5 brown, reniform seeds.

Leaves, Stem, and Root: The plant is an herbaceous perennial. It is 1 to 2 m high and has a long sturdy primary taproot. The taproot is 15 cm long and subdivides into 3 to 5 subsidiary roots, 1.25 m in length. There are several horizontal woody stolons that may grow to 8 m. New stems are produced every year. They are sturdy, erect, branched either from the base or from further up, and are generally rough at the top. The foliage leaves are alternate, odd pinnate and 10 to 20 cm long. The leaflets are in 3 to 8 pairs. The stipules are very small and drooping.

Habitat: Individual varieties of Glycyrrhiza are found in different regions. *Glycyrrhiza glanulifera* is found in southeastern Europe and western Asia. *Glycyrrhiza pallida* and *Glycyrrhiza violocea* are found in Iraq. *Glycyrrhiza typica* is indigenous to southern Europe and southwest Asia.

Production: Licorice root consists of the peeled and unpeeled, dried roots and stolons of *Glycyrrhiza glabra*. Licorice juice is the extract of *Glycyrrhiza glabra*.

Other Names: Sweet Root, Sweet Wort

ACTIONS AND PHARMACOLOGY

COMPOUNDS: LICORICE EXTRACT

Triterpene saponins (3-15%): (according to DAB 1996, 4-6% in the adjusted Licorice extract, according to DAC 1995, 5-7% in the dry Licorice extract): chief components are glycyrrhetic acid (sweet-tasting, aglycone 18 beta-glycyrrhetic acid, salts termed glycyrrizin)

Flavonoids: aglycones, including liquiritigenin, isoliquiritigenin (its chalcone), isolicoflavonol

Isoflavonoids: aglycones formononetin, glabren, glabridin, glabrol, 3-hydroxyglabrol, glycyrrhisoflavone

Cumestan derivatives: glycyrol, isoglycyrol, liqcoumarin

Hydroxycoumarins: including herniarin, umbelliferone, glycycoumarin, licopyranocumarin

Steroids: sterols, including beta-sitosterol, stigmasterol

The drug contains considerably more free flavonoid and isoflavonoid aglycones than the root drug does, due to the hydrolysis that takes place during the extraction procedure.

COMPOUNDS: LICORICE ROOT

Triterpene saponins (3-15%): chief components glycyrrhetic acid (sweet-tasting, aglycone 18beta-glycyrrhetic acid, salts termed glycyrrhizin), 18-alpha-glycrrhetic acid, glycyrrhetic acid methyl ester, glabric acid, glabrolide, uralenic acid

Flavonoids: aglycones including liquiritigenin, isoliquiritigenin (its chalcone), isolicoflavonol, isoliquiritin, licoricidin

Isoflavonoids: aglycones formononetin, glabren, glabridin, glabrol, 3-hydroxyglabrol, glycyrrhisoflavone

Cumestan derivatives: glycyrol, isoglycyrol, liquocoumarin

Hydroxycoumarins: including herniarin, umbelliferone, glycycoumarin, licopyranocoumarin

Steroids: sterols, including beta-sitosterol, stigmasterol

Volatile oil (very little): with anethole, estragole, eugenol, hexanoic acid

EFFECTS: LICORICE EXTRACT AND ROOT

Licorice has anti-inflammatory, antiulcer, and expectorant properties. It also has antiplatelet, antifungal, and antibacterial properties. Licorice inhibits calcium ions. Licorice has a long history of use for gastric ulcers that continues into present day. Licorice may be effective for a variety of infectious diseases. It is a common component of cold and flu remedies and is used in bronchitis. Modern use also focuses on the use of licorice for hormonal issues, such as menopause and PMS, as well as stimulating endogenous production of and prolongation of cortical hormones. One recent study showed activity against SARS (Cinatl et al, 2003).

Intravenous treatment with a glycyrrhizin solution prevented the development of hepatocellular carcinoma in patients with chronic hepatitis C. Licorice has also demonstrated some promise in the treatment of cancer in animals and *in vitro*. The use of glycyrrhizin for herpes zoster has been supported by a small trial, but more studies are needed to elucidate licorice's role. Licorice appears to benefit peptic ulcerations, but needs more research to support its role as an effective treatment. The use of licorice in viral infections is intriguing, but lacks large clinical trials supporting its use.

Antibacterial/Antifungal/Antiviral Effects: Some Licorice phenolic compounds and many other compounds in Licorice had antibacterial effects on methicillin-resistant *Staphylococcus aureus* (MRSA) and methicillin-sensitive *Staphylococcus aureus* (MSSA) (Hatano et al, 2000). Leaves of the Licorice plant contain several antifungal and antibacterial compounds, including isoflavin phytoalexin isomucronutalal (Saleh et al, 1990). A chalcone, isolated from an ethanol extract of roots *of Glycyrrhiza inflata Bat*, inhibited thymidine uptake of cultured promastigotes of *Leishmania donovani*. This compound has been previously synthesized and may serve as a lead structure for synthesis of an antiprotozoal drug (Christensen et al, 1994).

Glycyrrhizin induces CD4 T cells, which suppress type 2 cytokines produced by burn-associated type 2 T cells. This improves resistance to *Candida albicans* associated with thermal injury (Utsunomiya, 1999). Glycyrrhizin inhibited growth and cytopathology of HSV-1 in human aneuploid HEp2 cells (Van Rossum et al, 1998). Glycyrrhizin suppressed viral antigen expression in human hepatoma cells infected with hepatitis A virus. Glycyrrhizin may cause a decrease in the negative charge on the cell surface and/or decrease membrane fluidity, thus preventing penetration of the virus. Glycyrrhizin may also enhance the immunogenicity of HbsAg by inhibition of the sialyation of HBsAg (van Rossum et al, 1998).

Glycyrrhizin stimulates interferon gamma produced by T-cells for an antiviral effect against influenza virus infection (Utsunomiya, 1997). Glycyrrhizin suppresses the secretion of hepatitis B virus (HBV) surface antigen (HbsAg) in patients with HBV. The compound is thought to bind to hepatocytes at a concentration able to modify the expression of HBV-related antigens on the hepatocytes and suppress sialylation of HbsAg (Sato, 1996). Glycyrrhizin inhibited proliferation of viruses (Ito et al, 1987), modulated T cells (Kimura et al, 1993), augmented NK activity (Itoh & Kumagai, 1983), and inactivated viruses (Baba & Shigeta, 1987). Antiviral action of glycyrrhizin on the human immunodeficiency virus (HIV) occurs by inhibiting replication through interference with virus-cell binding and also suppression of giant cell formation (Ito, 1987; Nakashima, 1987).

Anticancer Effects: Intravenous treatment with a glycyrrhizin solution prevented development of hepatocellular carcinoma in patients with chronic hepatitis C. Derivatives of licorice have demonstrated antitumor activities in animal studies (Shibata, 1994a; Wang, 1994). Licochalcone-A, a flavonoid component of licorice, demonstrated apoptotic activity against acute leukemia, breast, and prostate cancer cell lines. These effects are mediated by licochalcone's ability to lower the levels of bcl-2, a protein that causes resistance to anticancer drugs. This may increase tumor sensitivity to such anticancer drugs (Anon, 2000).

Anti-Inflammatory/Antiplatelet Effects: Licoricidin, a potent compound in the root, has an inhibitory effect on isoPAF (platelet-activating factor) acetyltransferase resulting in anti-inflammatory activity (Nagumo, 1999). Glabridin exerts anti-inflammatory effects through inhibition of tyrosinase activity, superoxide anion production, and cyclooxygenase activity (Yokota, 1998). The anti-inflammatory effect of glycyrrhizin is attributed to its antithrombin action through inhibition of thrombin-induced platelet aggregation (Francischetti, 1997). Topical licochalcone A, a flavonoid isolated from the root of Glycyrrhiza inflata Betal, significantly inhibited inflammation in mice (Shibata, 1994a). The steroidlike action of glycyrrhizin, glycyrrhetic acid, and liquiritin contribute to the anti-inflammatory effects of licorice (Bradley, 1992).

Antioxidant Effects: Seven compounds with antioxidant properties were found in an acetone extract of Licorice root (*Glycyrrhiza glabra*). In an assay of antioxidant activity using an aqueous free-radical generator, vitamin E showed no antioxidant activity, while equimolar amounts of all licorice components except formononetin protected LDL from oxidation 65% to 85% (Vaya et al, 1997). In comparison with placebo, an ethanolic extract of licorice free of glycyrrhizinic acid reduced the rate of ex vivo oxidation of LDL isolated from plasma of healthy men. In vitro analyses demonstrated that 75% to 85% of the glabridin, the dominant isoflavan derivative (11.6%) of the extract, bound to LDL (Fuhrman et al, 1997).

Antiulcer Effects: Licorice root contains several antiulcer components. Original research focused on glycyrrhetinic acid until it was demonstrated that deglycyrrhizinated licorice (DGL) root extracts were actually more effective and without side effects (Wilson, 1972). Licorice has protective effects against gastric ulcers induced by aspirin (Dehpour, 1994). Licorice increased the rate of mucous secretion by gastric mucosa (Bradley, 1992). Licorice has the ability to release endogenous secretin, which is a potential mediator of the antiulcer actions (Shiratori, 1986). Carbenoxolone, a succinate derivative of glycyrrhetic acid, has been shown to accelerate the healing of ulcers (Barbara, 1979; Bianchi, 1985). Deglycyrrhizinated licorice is also effective for healing ulcers and lacks undesirable side effects seen with carbenoxolone (Morgan, 1982).

Effects Against Atherosclerotic Plaque: The incidence of atherosclerotic lesions was lower in apolipoprotein E-deficient mice (E0; prone to LDL oxidation) that were fed an ethanolic extract of licorice free of glyzzyrhinic acid or glabridin (the dominant isoflavan derivative of the extract) than in control mice. Sixty percent of the placebo-treated mice demonstrated well-defined atherosclerotic lesions of the aortic arch, compared to 20% of the licorice-treated mice (Fuhrman et al, 1997).

Hepatitis Effects: Glycyrrhizin can reduce serum transaminases in hepatitis C, but transaminases may rebound upon discontinuation of treatment. Glycyrrhizin does not reduce hepatitis C virus-RNA (Van Rossum et al, 1999). Occurrence of hepatocellular carcinoma over 15 years was less in hepatitis C patients treated with a glycyrrhizin-containing solution.

Hypertensive Effects: Glycyrrhetinic acid inhibited renal 11 B-hydroxysteroid dehydrogenase (B-HSD), the enzyme that converts cortisol to cortisone, which causes an increase in renal cortisol, resulting in a hypermineralocorticoid effect. Mineralocorticoid activity suppresses renin production and subsequent reduction of angiotensin I to aldosterone. This leads to elevated blood pressure, decreased serum potassium concentration, and retention of fluid and sodium (Van Rossum et al, 1998).

Immunological Effects: Carrageenan-induced dysfunction of clearance of immune complexes in mice was reduced by oral treatment with a licorice extract or with intraperitoneal glycyrrhizin (Matsumoto et al, 1996).

Inhibition of Calcium Ions: Licochalcone flavonoids A and B inhibited the elevation of calcium ions induced by thrombin, in a dose dependent manner. Thrombin-induced platelet aggregation in vitro is also inhibited (Kimura et al, 1993).

Mineralocorticoid Effects: Licorice inhibits the enzyme 11-beta-hydroxysteroid dehydrogenase in the kidney, which leads to decreased transformation of cortisol into cortisone. The mineralocorticoid action of cortisol causes a decrease in serum potassium and an increase in serum sodium concentration resulting in retention of water, causing weight increase and hypertension (Palermo, 1996). Glycyrrhetic acid, the hydrolytic metabolite of glycerrhizic acid causes the inhibition of peripheral metabolism of cortisol and produces a pseudo-aldosterone-like effect (Heikens, 1995). Licorice induces high blood pressure also through inhibition of NADPH-dependent short chain dehydrogenase/reductase enzymes in the kidney (Duax, 1998).

CLINICAL TRIALS

Hepatitis/Hepatitis-Related Hepatocellular Carcinoma

Previous Western studies found that glycyrrhizin from Licorice can effectively lower alanine aminotransferase levels (ALT) in people with chronic hepatitis C, but these studies were relatively short and small. This 26-week, randomized, open phase II trial was done to determine the usefulness of glycyrrhizin as the sole treatment in such individuals. Patients with liver cirrhosis who enrolled—most with a high viral load—were unable to take the standard interferon therapy for their illness and had limited treatment options. In all, 121 patients with elevated ALT and liver disease (marked fibrosis or necro-inflammation, or necrosis and inflammation in the liver) underwent 4 weeks of six infusions weekly of glycyrrhizin. Those with an ALT response at the end of this period (n=72) were randomized to continue treatment for 22 more weeks in one of three dose frequency groups—all of which maintained an ALT response (60% at six injections weekly; 24% at three injections weekly, and 9% at one injection weekly). The biochemical responses at three to six injections weekly are potentially relevant to individuals with chronic hepatitis C, and although frequent dosing was needed, it usually was well tolerated. Viremia was unchanged. More research is needed, for a longer period of time and with a larger group of patients, to determine the effectiveness of this Licorice compound on actual liver fibrosis over time (Orlent, 2006).

Similar findings were observed in earlier trials. Intermittent administration of Stronger Neo-Minophagen C (SNMC), an intravenous solution containing 2 mg glycyrrhizin, 1 mg cysteine, and 20 mg glycine/mL physiologic saline, effectively lowered alanine aminotransferase levels in patients with chronic viral hepatitis (n=100) or compensated liver cirrhosis (n=22). The majority of patients were carriers of hepatitis C virus (89%) and the remaining were either hepatitis B carriers or HBV and HCV carriers. (Miyake et al, 2002).

Intermittent administration of glycyrrhizin decreased serum alanine aminotransferase (ALT) in patients with chronic hepatitis C virus (HCV) but did not reduce HCV-RNA levels. Fifty-seven patients were randomly allocated to receive either 240 mg, 160 mg, 80 mg, or 0 mg of intravenous glycyrrhizin 3 times weekly for 4 weeks in a double-blinded manner. Glycyrrhizin was administered SNMC (see above). Outcome was assessed by percentage decrease and number of patients with normalization of ALT. The secondary outcome was the virological response (decrease in plasma HCV-RNA). ALT decreased 15% below baseline ($p<0.02$) within 2 days of start of therapy in the 3 dosage groups and remained significantly lower through treatment. At the 8-week follow-up (4 weeks post-treatment), ALT levels increased; however, ALT values in the 80 mg and 240 mg groups were significantly lower than they were at baseline ($p<0.001$ and $p<0.05$, respectively). During treatment, the percentage decrease in ALT was significantly higher in all treatment groups compared to the placebo group ($p<0.03$). There was no significant difference in ALT normalization and HCV-RNA levels between the 4 groups at the end of treatment and 4 weeks post-treatment (Van Rossum et al, 1999).

A retrospective study evaluated the long-term use of a glycyrrhizin-containing solution for prevention of hepatocellular carcinoma in patients with chronic hepatitis C. One-hundred and ninety-two patients with chronic hepatitis C were included in the study. Stronger SNMC (see above) 100 mL daily was administered to 83 patients over an 8-week period, then followed by 2 to 7 times per week for 2 to 16 years (median 10.1 years). The other 109 patients were treated with other herbal remedies, such as vitamin K, for 1 to 16 years (median, 9.2 years). The 10-year rate occurrence of HCC was 7% in the SNMC treatment group and 12% respectively in the non-SNMC treatment group. The 15-year rate was 12% in the

SNMC treatment group and 25% in the other treatment group (p=0.032). Elevated alanine aminotransferase (ALT), a characteristic of chronic hepatitis and a risk factor for the development of HCC, normalized in 35.7% in the SNMC treatment group, which was significantly better than the 6.4% of the other treatment group (Arase et al, 1997).

Cytomegalovirus

Hepatic dysfunction normalized and cytomegalovirus (CMV) was no longer detected in the urine in three infants who were administered the glycyrrhizin compound SNMC (see study above). SNMC was administered for a minimum of 1 week by continuous intravenous infusion. Two of the infants received a longer duration of SNMC (3 times a week for 2 weeks, twice a week for 1 week and once a week for 1 week). After SNMC therapy, liver function became normal and no CMV was isolated from the urine. Therapy was well tolerated (Numazaki et al, 1994).

SARS

While the clinical significance is unknown, glycyrrhizin demonstrated potent antiviral activity against the severe acute respiratory syndrome (SARS) virus in vitro. The antiviral activity of ribavirin, 6-azauirdine, pyrazofurin, mycophenolic acid, and glycyrrhizin against the SARS-associated coronavirus isolates (FFM-1 and FFM-2) was assessed in culture. The selectivity index was determined as the ratio of the concentration of the compound that reduced cell viability to 50% to the concentration of the compound needed to inhibit the cytopathic effect to 50% of the control value. Glycyrrhizin was the most potent inhibitor of SARS replication with a selectivity index of 67 (during and after virus adsorption), with selectivity indexes for 6-azauridine of 6 and 12 for Pyrazofurin. Mycophenolic acid and ribavirin demonstrated no activity. Timing of administration was important; glycyrrhizin was most effective when given both during and after adsorption. The selectivity index for glycyrrhizin after virus adsorption was 33 and during virus adsorption was 8.3 (Cinatl et al, 2003).

Ulcers, Gastric

A double-blind study involving thirty-four patients was conducted to compare carbenoloxalone and pirenzepine for treatment of a chronic gastric ulcer. Carbenoxalone was administered as 300 mg daily for 1 week followed by 150 mg daily for 5 weeks. Pirnzepine was administered as 150 mg daily for 6 weeks. There was no significant difference between the groups at the end of the treatment period with ulcers healed in 59% of the pirenzepine group and in 52% of the carbenoxolone group. The healing rates in this study do not compare well with reported treatment success rates of H2-receptor antagonists (Bianchi Porro et al, 1985).

INDICATIONS AND USAGE

LICORICE ROOT

Approved by Commission E:

■ Cough/bronchitis

■ Gastritis

Unproven Uses: The drug is used for catarrh of the upper respiratory tract as well as for gastric/duodenal ulcers. In folk medicine, the herb is used for appendicitis, constipation, and to increase milk production and micturation. The drug is also used as a treatment for epilepsy and inflammation of the gastrointestinal and urogenital tract. Externally, the herb is used for dermatoses.

Indian Medicine: Internally, the herb is used for gastric ulcers, headaches, bronchitis, eye diseases, and sore throat. The drug is used externally for wounds and cuts.

Chinese Medicine: The herb is used for sore throats, carbuncles, spleen disorders, dry cough, and dehydration.

LICORICE EXTRACT

Unproven Uses: The drug is used for gastritis, gastric ulcers, ulcer prophylaxis, and viral liver inflammation.

CONTRAINDICATIONS

LICORICE ROOT AND FRUIT

Contraindications for Licorice include chronic hepatitis, cholestatic diseases of the liver, cirrhosis of the liver, severe renal insufficiency, diabetes mellitus, hypertonic neuromuscular disorders, arrhythmias, hypertension, hypertonia, and hypokalemia. Tobacco use has been associated with licorice toxicity (Synhaivsky, 1980).

Pregnancy: Not to be used during pregnancy.

Breastfeeding: Not to be used while breastfeeding.

PRECAUTIONS AND ADVERSE REACTIONS

LICORICE ROOT AND EXTRACT

Licorice should not be used for a prolonged period of time except under the supervision of a qualified health practitioner. Chronic ingestion of the herb may result in hypertension, edema, cardiac complaints, pseudohyperaldosteronism with hypercortisolism, sodium retention or severe electrolyte imbalances, such as hypernatremia and hypokalemia, resulting in hypotonia, muscular weakness, flaccid paralysis, and in rare cases, myoglobinuria

Cardiovascular: Licorice caused a reversible, dose-dependent increase in blood pressure in both normotensive and hypertensive adults (Sigurjonsdottir et al, 2003; Sigurjonsdottir et al, 2001). Licorice elevated blood pressure by increasing renal cortisol with subsequent retention of fluid and sodium (Van Rossum et al, 1998). Arrhythmias and cardiomyopathy have also been reported (Eriksson et al, 1999; Hasegawa et al, 1998).

Central Nervous System: Two cases of hypertension encephalopathy were linked to chronic consumption of licorice. In both cases, symptoms only disappeared after the patient stopped eating licorice (Russo et al, 2000).

Pseudohyperaldosteronism: Licorice can cause pseudohyperaldosteronism, with the biochemical features of primary aldosteronism: sodium retention (peripheral edema, dyspnea, hypertension) and hypokalemia (polyuria, proximal myopathy, lethargy, paresthesias, muscle cramps, headaches, tetany). Glycyrrhetinic acid, a metabolite of the licorice constituent glycyrrhizic acid inhibited 11-beta-hydroxysteroid dehydrogenase, preventing the conversion of cortisol to its inactive metabolite, cortisone. The resulting high concentration of cortisol, particularly in the kidney, stimulated the mineral corticoid receptors, mimicking the consequences of elevated aldosterone (Van Rossum et al, 2001, 1998; vanUum et al, 1998; Armanini et al, 1996; Walker & Edwards, 1994). Glycyrrhetinic acid also suppressed the renin-aldosterone axis (Bernardi et al, 1994; Farese et al, 1991).

Multiple: Life-threatening hypokalemia, severe hypokalemic myopathy, and generalized weakness, elevated liver function test (including elevated bilirubin, creatine kinase, alkaline phosphatase, and alanine transaminase), as well as flulike symptoms (including nausea, vomiting, and diarrhea) were reported in a 56-year-old woman who had been eating approximately 200 to 400 g of ''Pontefract cake'' (15 g of licorice) daily for managing chronic constipation. Liver function tests returned to normal within a few days after cessation of Pontefract cake consumption and treatment of concomitant hypokalemia with intravenous potassium chloride, coinciding with full recovery (Hussain, 2003).

Musculoskeletal: A case report of a Chinese man who presented to the emergency department with muscular weakness that progressed to paralysis of all extremities concluded that his symptoms were caused by severe hypokalemia due to chronic intake of licorice tea. The man had been consuming tea flavored with 100 g of natural licorice root containing 2.3% glycyrrhizic acid daily for three years. In addition to hypokalemia, his blood pressure was high and metabolic alkalosis was present. Treatment included intravenous potassium chloride. Two weeks later, all symptoms resolved (Lin et al, 2003).

Ocular: A case series of five patients who had ingested 0.25 to 2 pounds of licorice each reported visual disturbances. The investigators concluded that licorice may stimulate retinal and occipital vasospasm and vasospasm of vessels supplying the optic nerve, which may be responsible for the visual disturbances (Dobbins & Saul, 2000).

Testosterone Decreased: Serum testosterone decreased and serum 17-hydroxyprogesterone concentrations increased in healthy young men (ages 22 to 24 years) given 7 g licorice (containing 0.5 g glycyrrhizic acid) daily for seven days (Armanini & Palermo, 1999).

Weight Gain: Weight gain occurred in both normotensive and hypertensive subjects following 4 weeks licorice consumption (150 mg of glycyrrhetinic acid daily). Body mass index increased by a mean of 0.38 ± 0.42 in the normotensive and hypertensive subjects combined with a maximum increase after 2 weeks of licorice consumption (Sigurjonsdottir et al, 2003).

DRUG INTERACTIONS

CONTRAINDICATED

Antihypertensive Drugs: Theoretically, licorice may reduce the effectiveness of antihypertensive drugs, including alpha-1 adrenergic blockers, ACE inhibitors, A2 receptor antagonists, beta-adrenergic blockers, calcium channel blockers, clonidine, guanabenz, guanadrel, guanethidine, guanfacine, hydralazine, methyldopa, minoxidil, and reserpine (Kowalak & Mills, 2001). *Clinical Management:* Licorice use is contraindicated in patients with hypertension. Avoid concomitant use of licorice and any antihypertensive drug, including those named above.

MAJOR RISK

Antiarrhythmics (procainamide, quinidine): Theoretically, licorice-induced hypokalemia may interfere with the effectiveness of antiarrhythmics (Kowalak & Mills, 2001) and result in an increased risk of arrhythmia. *Clinical Management:* Avoid concomitant use of licorice and antiarrhythmic agents.

Laxatives: Concurrent use of licorice and laxatives may lead to increased risk of hypokalemia. *Clinical Management:* Avoid concomitant use of licorice and laxatives.

MODERATE RISK

Anticoagulants, Antiplatelet Agents, Low Molecular Weight Heparins, and Thrombolytic Agents: Concurrent use of licorice and any of these agents may result in an increased risk of bleeding. Licorice root may contain coumarins or coumarin derivatives (Heck et al, 2000) and may inhibit platelet aggregation (Norred & Brinker, 2001). Glycyrrhizin, a component of licorice, demonstrated selective thrombin inhibition *in vitro* (Francischetti et al, 1997). *Clinical Management:* Caution is advised if concomitantly administered. Monitor for signs and symptoms of excessive bleeding.

Antidiabetic Agents: Licorice may reduce the effects of antidiabetic agents by causing hyperglycemia. *Clinical Management:* Caution is advised if licorice is used with antidiabetic agents. Advise patients that regular use of even moderate amounts of licorice can result in hypokalemia and interfere with their blood glucose control.

Combination Contraceptives: Elevated blood pressure and fluid retention has been associated with concomitant use of licorice and oral contraceptives in case reports (deKlerk et al, 1997; Bernardi et al, 1994), which may be related to estrogen and/or progesterone. *Clinical Management:* Caution is advised if licorice is used with contraceptives, as the combination may result in increased risk of fluid retention and elevated blood pressure. If the patient develops fluid retention or hypertension, discontinue licorice.

Corticosteroids: Concurrent use of licorice and corticosteroids may result in increased risk of corticosteroid adverse effects. *Clinical Management:* Caution is advised if licorice is used concomitantly with a corticosteroid. A lower corticosteroid dose may be required to avoid adverse effects.

Digoxin: Concurrent use may result in an increased risk of digoxin toxicity. Symptoms of congestive heart failure and hypokalemia occurred in a patient taking licorice, furosemide, and digoxin (Harada et al, 2002). *Clinical Management:* Avoid concurrent use of licorice and digoxin.

Diuretics: Concurrent use may result in increased risk of hypokalemia and/or reduced effectiveness of the diuretic. *Clinical Management:* Avoid concomitant use of licorice and diuretics.

Estrogens: Concurrent use may result in increased risk of fluid retention and elevated blood pressure. *Clinical Management:* Caution is advised if licorice is taken with estrogen. If the patient develops fluid retention and increased blood pressure, discontinue licorice.

Insulin: Concurrent use may result in an increased risk of hypokalemia and sodium retention. *Clinical Management:* Caution is advised if licorice is used with insulin. Advise patients that regular use of even moderate amounts of licorice can result in hypokalemia.

Monoamine Oxidase Inhibitors: Patients taking licorice with monoamine oxidase inhibitors (MAOIs) may be at risk of increased toxicity associated with excessive inhibition of monoamine amine oxidase. Several licorice constituents noncompetitively inhibited MAO *in vitro* (Hatano et al, 1991). *Clinical Management:* Avoid concomitant use of licorice with MAOIs until this potential drug-herb interaction is better characterized. If licorice and an MAOI are used concomitantly, monitor for early symptoms of MAOI toxicity such as irritability, hyperactivity, anxiety, hypotension, vascular collapse, insomnia, restlessness, dizziness, faintness, drowsiness, hallucinations, trismus, flushing, sweating, tachypnea, tachycardia, movement disorders (e.g., grimacing, opisthotonus), and severe headache.

Potassium: Concurrent use may result in reduced effectiveness of potassium. *Clinical Management:* Avoid concomitant use of licorice and potassium. Large amounts of licorice may lead to resistance to potassium supplementation.

Testosterone: Concurrent use of licorice and testosterone may result in decreased testosterone effectiveness. *Clinical Management:* Avoid concomitant use of licorice and testosterone. Patients reporting decreased libido or other sexual dysfunction for which testosterone supplementation is being considered should be questioned regarding licorice use and advised to discontinue licorice.

POTENTIAL INTERACTIONS

Licorice inhibited cytochrome P450 3A4 in vitro (Budzinski et al, 2000); caution is advised if licorice is administered with drugs metabolized by this enzyme.

OVERDOSAGE

LICORICE ROOT AND EXTRACT

The intake of higher dosages (above 20 g per day for the extract and above 50 g per day for the root) over an extended period of time will lead to hypokalemia, hypernatremia, edemas, hypertension, and cardiac complaints. In rare cases, myoglobinemia has resulted due to the mineralcorticoid (aldosterone-like) effect of the saponins (Heikens, 1995; Saito, 1994; Seelen, 1996). Preparations from the drug should not be administered for longer than 6 weeks. The complaints disappear after discontinuing the drug. (SEE PRECAUTIONS AND ADVERSE REACTIONS)

DOSAGE

LICORICE ROOT

Mode of Administration: Comminuted drug, drug powder, dry extracts for infusions, decoctions, liquid or solid forms for internal use. Various teas contain extracts of the drug, for example, bronchial teas, gastric teas, and laxative teas.

Licorice should not be administered for more than 4 to 6 weeks without medical advice (see side effects). During this time, a high potassium diet should be consumed (McGuffin et al, 1997; Bradley, 1992).

How Supplied:

Capsules — 100 mg, 200 mg, 400 mg, 444 mg, 445 mg, 450 mg, 500 mg

Preparation: To prepare an infusion, use 1 to 1.5 g of finely comminuted drug and add cold water. Bring to a boil, or pour the boiling water over the drug and allow to steep for 10 to 15 minutes and then strain (1 teaspoonful = 3 gm drug).

Daily Dosage: The average daily dose is 5 to 15 g of the root, equivalent to 200 to 600 mg of glycyrrhizin. The drug is not to be taken longer than 6 weeks (SEE OVERDOSAGE). Succus liquiritiae: 0.5 to 1 g for catarrhs of the upper respiratory tract and 1.5 to 3.0 g for gastric/duodenal ulcers.

Tea - Drink one cup of tea after meals.

LICORICE EXTRACT

Mode of Administration: The drug is widely available in medicinal preparations, as tea or in drop form; the juice of licorice is found in licorice edible goods and preparations.

Preparation: For preparation of tea, pour a cup of boiling water over 1 teaspoon of juice, leave to steep for 5 minutes.

Daily Dosage: Drink one cup of tea after each meal. The dosage for the drop form is 25 drops to be taken 4 times daily.

LITERATURE

Aida K, Tawata M, Shindo H et al. Isoliquiritigenin: a new aldose reductase inhibitor from glycyrrhizae radix. *Planta Med*; 56:254-258. 1990.

Aikawa Y, Yoshiike T, Ogawa H. Effect of glycyrrhizin pain and HLA-DR antigen expression on DC8-positive cells in peripheral blood of herpes zoster patients in comparsion with other antiviral agents. In: *Skin Pharmacol* 3(4):268-271. 1990.

Amagaya S, Sugishita E, Ogihara Y, Ogawa S, Okada K, Aizawa T. Comparative studies of the stereoisomers of glycyrrhetinic acid on anti-inflammatory activities. *J Pharmacobiodyn.* Dec;7(12):923-8. 1984.

Anderson J, Smith WG. The antitussive activity of glycyrrhetinic acid and its derivatives. *J Pharm Pharmacol.* 1961.

Anon. Licorice root extract shows antitumor activity. *Oncology*; 14(2):164. 2000.

Arase Y, Ikeda K, Murashima N et al. The long term efficacy of glycyrrhizin in chronic hepatitis C patients. *Cancer*; 79:1494-1500. 1997.

Armanini D, Bonanni G & Palermo M. Reduction of serum testosterone in men by licorice. *N Engl J Med;* 341(15):1158. 1999.

Baba M, Shigeta S, Antiviral activity of glycyrrhizin against varicella-zoster virus in vitro. In: *Antiviral Res* 7(2):99-107. 1987.

Barbara L; Belsasso E; Blasi A et al. Pirenzepine and carbenozolone in gastric ulcer. Preliminary results of a multicentre double-blind controlled clinical trial. *Scand J Gastroenterol Suppl*;57:21-4. 1979.

Bardhan KD et al. *Gut* 19:779. 1978.

Baschetti R. Chronic fatigue syndrome and neurally mediated hypotension (letter). *JAMA*; 275:359. 1996.

Bernardi M, D'Intino PE, Trevisani F et al. Effects of prolonged ingestion of graded doses of licorice by healthy volunteers. *Life Sci*; 55(11):863-872. 1994.

Bhardwaj DK et al. *Phytochemistry* 15:352. 1977.

Bhardwaj DK et al. *Phytochemistry* 16:401. 1977.

Bhardwaj DK, Singh R. *Curr Sci* 46:753. 1977.

Bianchi Porro G, Petrillo M, Lazzaroni M et al. Comparison of pirenzepine and carbenoxolone in the treatment of chronic gastric ulcer: a double-blind endoscopic trial. *Hepatogastroenterology*; 32:293-295. 1985.

Blachley JD & Knochel JP. Tobacco chewer's hypokalemia: licorice revisited. *N Engl J Med;* 302(14): 784-785. 1980.

Budzinski JW, Foster BC. Vandenhoek S et al. An in vitro evaluation of human cytochrome P450 3A4 inhibition by selected commercial herbal extracts and tinctures. *Phytomedicine*; 7(4):273-282. 2000.

Chen MF, Shimada F, Kato H et al. Effect of glycyrrhizin on the pharmacokinetics of prednisolone following low dosage of prednisolone hemisuccinate. *Endocrinol Jpn;* 37:331-341. 1990.

Chen MF, Shimada F, Kato H et al. Effect of oral administration of glycyrrhizin on the pharmacokinetics of prednisolone. *Endocrinol Jpn*; 38(2):167-174. 1991.

Christensen SB, Ming C, Andersen L et al. An antileishmanial chalcone from Chinese licorice roots. *Planta Med*; 60(2):121-123. 1994.

Cinatl J, Morgenstern B, Bauer G et al. Glycyrrhizin, an active component of liquorice roots, and replication of SARS-associated coronavirus. *Lancet*; 361(9374):2045-2046. 2003.

Dehpour AR; Zolfaghari ME; Samadian T; Vahedi Y. The protective effect of liquorice components and their derivatives against gastric ulcer induced by aspirin in rats. J Pharm Pharmacol Feb;46(2):148-9. 1994.

deKlerk G, Neiuwenhuis M & Beutler J. Hypokalemia and hypertension associated with use of liquorice flavoured chewing gum. *BMJ*; 314(7082):731-732. 1997.

Dellow EL, Unwin RJ & Honour JW. Pontefract cakes can be bad for you: refractory hypertension and liquorice excess. *Nephrol Dial Transplant*; 14(1):218-220. 1999.

Dezaki K; Kimura I; Miyahara K; Kimura M. Complementary effects of paeoniflorin and glycyrrhizin on intracellular Ca2+ mobilization in the nerve-stimulated skeletal muscle of mice. *Jpn J Pharmacol* Nov;69(3):281-4. 1995.

DiPaola RS, Zhang H, Lambert GH et al. Clinical and biologic activity of an estrogenic herbal combination (PC-SPES) in prostate cancer. *N Engl J Med*; 339(12):785-791. 1998.

Dobbins KRB & Saul RF. Transient visual loss after licorice ingestion. *J Neuroophthalmol*; 20(1):38-41. 2000.

Duax WL; Ghosh D. Structure and mechanism of action and inhibition of steroid dehydrogenase enzymes involved in hypertension. *Endocr Res* Aug-Nov;24(3-4):521-9. 1998.

Eriksson JW; Carlberg B; Hillorn V. Life-threatening ventricular tachycardia due to liquorice-induced hypokalaemia. *J Intern Med* Mar;245(3):307-310. 1999.

Epstein MT et al. *BMJ* 19:488. 1977.

Farese RV Jr, Biglieri EG, Schackleton CHL et al. Licorice-induced hypermineralcorticoidism. *N Engl J Med;* 325:1223-1227. 1991.

Fintelmann V. Moderne Phytotherapie am Beispiel gastroenterologischer Erkrankungen. In: *ZPT* 11(5):161. 1990.

Folkerson L, Knudsen NA & Teglbjaerg PS. Licorice: A basis for precautions one more time! *Ugeskr Laeger;* 158(51):7420-7421. 1996.

Francischetti IM; Monteiro RQ; Guimaraes JA, et al. Identification of glycyrrhizin as a thrombin inhibitor. *Biochem Biophys Res Commun* Jun 9;235(1):259-263. 1997.

Fuhrman B, Buch S, Vaya J et al. Licorice extract and its major polyphenol glabridin protect low-density lipoprotein against lipid peroxidation: in vitro and ex vivo studies in humans and in atherosclerotic apolipoprotein E-deficient mice. *Am J Clin Nutr*; 66:267-275. 1997.

Harada T, Ohtaki E, Misu K et al. Congestive heart failure caused by digitalis toxicity in an elderly man taking a licorice-containing Chinese herbal laxative. *Cardiology*; 98(4):218. 2002.

Hasegawa J, Suyama Y, Kinugawa T et al. Echocardiographic findings of the heart resembling dilated cardiomyopathy during hypokalemic myopathy due to licorice-induced pseudoaldosteronism. *Cardiovasc Drugs Ther*; 12(6):599-600. 1998.

Hatano T, Fukuda T, Miyase T et al. Phenolic constituents of licorice. III. Structures of glicoricone and licofuranone, and inhibitory effects of licorice constituents on monoamine oxidase. *Chem Pharm Bull* (Tokyo); 39(5):1238-1243. 1991.

Hatano T, Shintani Y, Aga Y et al. Phenolic constituents of licorice. VII. Structures of glicophenone and glicoisoflavone, and effects of licorice phenolics on methicillin-resistant *Staphylococcus aureus. Chem Pharm Bull* (Tokyo); 48(9):1286-1292. 2000.

Hayashi H et al. Distribution patterns of saponine in different organs of *Glycyrrhiza glabra.* In: *PM* 59(4):351. 1993.

Hayashi Y et al. Yakuri to Chiryo 7:3861. 1979.

Heck AM, DeWitt BA, Lukes AL. Potential interactions between alternative therapies and warfarin. *Am J Health Syst Pharm*; 57(13):1221-1227. 2000.

Heikens J, Fliers E, Endert E et al. Liquorice-induced hypertension: a new understanding of an old disease:case report and brief review. *Neth J Med*; 47:230-234. 1995.

Homma M, Oka K, Niitsuma T et al. A novel 11-beta-hydroxysteroid dehydrogenase inhibitor contained in Saiboku-To, a herbal remedy for steroid-dependent bronchial asthma. *J Pharm Pharmacol*; 46(4):305-309. 1994.

Hussain RM. The sweet cake that reaches parts other cakes can't! Postgrad Med J; F79(928):115-116. 2003.

Inoue H, Saito K, Koshihara Y, Murota S. Inhibitory effect of glyzyrrhetinic acid derivatives of lipoxygenase and prostaglandin synthetase. *Chem Pharm Bull* 34:897. 1986.

Itoh K, Tsuchikawa K, Awataguchi T, Shiiba K, Kumagai K. A case of chronic lymphocytic leukemia with properties characteristic of natural killer cells. *Blood*. May;61(5):940-8. 1983.

Kageyama K, Watanobe H, Nishie M et al. A case of pseudoaldosteronism induced by a mouth refresher containing licorice. *Endocr J*; 44(4): 631-632. 1997.

Kato H; Kanaoka M; Yano S, et al. 3-Monoglucuronyl-glycyrrhetinic acid is a major metabolite that causes licorice-induced pseudoaldosteronism. *J Clin Endocrinol Metab* Jun;80(6):1929-1933. 1995.

Khaksa G et al. Anti-inflammatory and anti-nociceptive activity of disodium glycyrrhetinic acid hemiphthalate. In: *PM* 62(4):326-328. 1996.

Killacky J et al. *Planta Med* 30:310. 1976.

Kimura Y, Okuda H & Okuda T. Effects of flavonoids isolated from licorice roots (glycyrrhiza inflata bat) on arachidonic acid metabolism and aggregation in human platelets. *Phytother Res*; 7:341-347. 1993.

Kimura Y, Okuda T & Okuda H. Effects of flavonoids isolated from licorice roots (*glycyrrhiza inflata* bat) on degranulation in human polymorphonuclear neutrophils. *Phytother Res*; 7:335-340. 1993a.

Kinoshita T et al, *Chem Pharm Bull* 26: 141 et 135. 1978.

Kiso Y et al. *Planta Med* 50:298. 1984.

Kobayashi S; Miyamoto T; Kimura I; Kimura M. Inhibitory effect of isoliquiritin, a compound in licorice root, on angiogenesis in vivo and tube formation in vitro. *Biol Pharm Bull*. Oct;18(10):1382-6. 1995.

Kumagai A, Takata M. *Proc Symp Wakan-Yaku* 11:73. 1978.

Lin S-H, Yang S-S, Chau T et al. An unusual cause of hypokalemic paralysis: chronic licorice ingestion. *Am J Med Sci*; 325(3):153-156. 2003.

Matsumoto T, Tanaka M, Yamada H et al. Effect of licorice roots on carrageenan-induced decrease in immune complexes clearance in mice. *J Ethnopharmacol*; 53:1-4. 1996.

Miething H, Speicher-Brinker A, Hänsel R, Hochdruckflüssigchromatographische Untersuchungen der Flavonoidfraktion in Süβholzwurzeln und deren pharmazeutischen Zubereitungen. In: *PZW* 135(6):253. 1990.

Miyake K, Tango T, Ota Y et al. Efficacy of stronger Neo-Minophen C compared between two doses administered three times a week on patients with chronic viral hepatitis. *J Gastroenterol Hepatol*; 17(11):1198-1204. 2002.

Morgan AG, McAdam WAF, Pacsoo C et al. Comparison between cimetidine and Caved-S in the treatment of gastric ulceration, and subsequent maintenance therapy. *Gut*; 23:545-551. 1982.

Morris DJ, Davis E & Latif SA. Licorice, tobacco chewing and hypertension. *N Engl J Med*; 322:849-850. 1990.

Nagumo S; Fukuju A; Takayama M et al. Inhibition of lysoPAF acetyltransferase activity by components of licorice root. *Biol Pharm Bull* Oct;22(10):1144-6. 1999.

Nakashima H; Matsui T; Yoshida O et al. A new anti-human immunodeficiency virus substance, glycyrrhizin sulfate; endowment of glycyrrhizin with reverse transcriptase- inhibitory activity by chemical modification. *Jpn J Cancer Res* Aug;78(8):767-71. 1987.

Neilsen I, Pedersen RS, *Lancet* 1:8389. 1984.

Norred CL & Brinker F. Potential coagulation effects of preoperative complementary and alternative medicines. Alt Ther; 7(6):58-67. 2001.

Nose M et al., A comparision of the antihepatotoxic activity between glycyrrhizin and glycerrhetinic acid. In: *PM* 60(2):136. 1994.

Numuzaki K, Umetsu M, Chiba S, Effects of glycyrrhizin in children with liver dysfunction associated with cytomegalovirus infections. In: *Tohoku J Exp Med* 172:147-153. 1994.

Orlent H, Hansen BE, Willems M, et al. Biochemical and histological effects of 26 weeks of glycyrrhizin treatment in chronic hepatitis C: A randomized phase II trial. *J Hepatol;* 45: 539-546. 2006

Palermo M; Shackleton CH; Mantero F; Stewart PM. Urinary free cortisone and the assessment of 11 beta-hydroxysteroid dehydrogenase activity in man. *Clin Endocrinol* (Oxf) Nov;45(5):605-11. 1996.

Rafi MM, Rosen RT, Vassil A et al. Modulation of bcl-2 and cytotoxicity by licochalcone-A, a novel estrogenic flavonoid. *Anticancer Res*; 20(4):2653-2658. 2000.

Raggi MA; Bugamelli F; Nobile L et al. The choleretic effects of licorice. identification and determination of the pharmacologically active components of *Glycyrrhiza glabra. Boll Chim Farm* Dec;134(11):634-8. 1995.

Rees WDW et al., Scand. *J Gastroenterol*. 14:605. 1979.

Russo S, Mastropasqua M, Mosetti MA et al. Low doses of liquorice can induce hypertension encephalopathy. *Am J Nephrol*; 20(2):145-148. 2000.

Saitoh T et al., *Chem Pharm Bull* 24:991. 1976.

Saitoh T et al., Chem Pharm Bull 26:752. 1978.

Saitoh T et al., *Chem Pharm Bull* 24:752 et 1242. 1976.

Sakamoto K & Wakabayashi K. Inhibitory effect of glycyrrhetinic acid on testosterone production in rat gonads. Endocrinol Jpn; 35:333-342. 1988.

Saleh MM, El-Olemy MM, Metawie HM et al. Response of licorice (*glycyrrhiza glabra*) leaves to certain stress factors. *Planta Med*; 56:610. 1990.

Sato H; Goto W; Yamamura J et al. Therapeutic basis of glycyrrhizin on chronic hepatitis B. *Antiviral Res* May;30(2-3):171-7. 1996.

Saito T; Tsuboi Y; Fujisawa G et al. An autopsy case of licorice-induced hypokalemic rhabdomyolysis associated with acute renal failure: special reference to profound calcium deposition in skeletal and cardiac muscle. *Nippon Jinzo Gakkai Shi* Nov;36(11):1308-14. 1994.

Seelen MA; de Meijer PH; Braun J et al. Hypertension caused by licorice consumption. *Ned Tijdschr Geneeskd* Dec 28;140(52):2632-5. 1996.

Segal R et al., *J Pharm Sci* 74 (1):79. 1985.

Shibata S. Antitumor-promoting and anti-inflammatory activities of licorice principles and their modified compounds, in Food Phytochemicals II: Teas, Spices, and Herbs. American Chemical Society; 1994a.

Shintani S, Murase H, Tsukagoshi H et al. Glycyrrhizin (Licorice)-induced hypokalemic myopathy. *Eur Neurol*; 32(1):44-51. 1992.

Sigurjonsdottir HA, Franzson L, Manhem K et al. Liquorice-induced rise in blood pressure: a linear dose-response relationship. *J Hum Hypertens;* 15(8):549-552. 2001.Sigurjonsdottir HA, Manhem K, Axelson M et al. Subjects with essential hypertension are more sensitive to the inhibition of 11 B-HSD by liquorice. *J Hum Hypertens*; 17(2):125-131. 2003.

Steinberg D, Sgan-Cohen HD, Stabholz A et al. The anticarcinogenic activity of glycyrrhizin: Preliminary clinical trials. *Isr J Dent Sci*; 2(3):153-157. 1989.

Synhaivsky A. Licorice, snuff, and hypokalemia. *N Engl J Med* Aug 21;303(8):463. 1980.

Shiratori K; Watanabe S; Takeuchi T. Effect of licorice extract (Fm100) on release of secretin and exocrine pancreatic secretion in humans. *Pancreas*;1(6):483-7. 1986.

Suzuki H, Ohta Y, Takino T, Fujisawa K, Hirayama C, Effect of glycyrrhizin on biochemical test in patients with chronic hepatitis. Double blind trial. In: *Asian Med J* 26:423-438. 1983.

Takahashi K & Kitao M. Effect of TJ-68 (Shakuyaku-Kanzo-To) on polycystic ovarian disease. *Int J Fertil*; 39(2):69-76. 1994.

Takeuchi T, Nishii O, Okamura T et al. Effect of paeoniflorin, glycyrrhizin and glycyrrhetic acid on ovarian androgen production. *Am J Chin Med*; 19(1):73-78. 1991.

Takeuchi T, Nishii O, Okamura T et al. Effect of traditional herbal medicine, shakuyaku-kanzo-to on total and free serum testosterone levels. *Am J Chin Med*; 17(1-2):35-44. 1989.

Takechi M, Tanaka Y, Structure-activity relationships of the synthetic methyl glycyrrhetate glycosides. In: *PH* 32:1173. 1993.

Tamura Y, Nishikawa T, Yamada K, Yamamoto M, Kumagai A, Effects of glyzyrrhetinic acid and ist derivatives on Delta5-reductase in rat liver. *Arzneimittel Forsch/Drug Res* 29: 647. 1979.

Tanaka S et al., *Planta Med* 53 (1):5. 1987.

Tawata M; Aida K; Noguchi T et al. Anti-platelet action of isoliquiritigenin, an aldose reductase inhibitor in licorice. *Eur J Pharmacol* Feb 25;212(1):87-92. 1992.

Teelucksingh S, Mackie ADR, Burt D et al. Potentiation of hydrocortisone activity in skin by glycyrrhetinic acid. *Lancet*; 335:1060-1083. 1990.

Utsunomiya T; Kobayashi M; Herndon DN et al. Effects of glycyrrhizin, an active component of licorice roots, on Candida albicans infection in thermally injured mice. *Clin Exp Immunol* May;116(2):291-8. 1999.

Utsunomiya T; Kobayashi M; Pollard RB; Suzuki F. Glycyrrhizin, an active component of licorice roots, reduces morbidity and mortality of mice infected with lethal doses of influenza virus. *Antimicrob Agents Chemother* Mar;41(3):551-6. 1997.

Van Hulle C, *Pharmazie* 25:620. 1970.

Van Rossum TG, de Jong FH, Hop WC et al. "Pseudo-aldosteronism" induced by intravenous glycyrrhizin treatment of chronic hepatitis C patients. *J Gastroenterol Hepatol*; 16(7):789-795. 2001.

Van Rossum TGJ, Vulto AG, De Man RA et al. Review article: glycyrrhizin as a potential treatment for chronic hepatitis C. *Aliment Pharmacol Ther*; 12(3):199-205. 1998.

Van Rossum TGJ, Vulto AG, Hop WCJ et al. Intravenous glycyrrhizin for the treatment of chronic hepatitis C: a double-blind, randomized, placebo-controlled phase I/II trial. *J Gastroenterol Hepatol*; 14(11):1093-1099. 1999.

Vaya J, Belinky PA & Aviram M. Antioxidant constituents from licorice roots: isolation, structure elucidation and antioxidative capacity toward LDL oxidation. *Free Rad Biol Med*; 23:302-313. 1997.

Veit M, Wirkungen der Glycyrrhetinsäure auf den Steroidstoffwechsel. In: *ZPT* 14(1):43. 1993.

Walker BR & Edwards CRW. Licorice-induced hypertension and syndromes of apparent mineralcorticoid excess. *Endocrinol Metab Clinics N Amer*: 23:359-377. 1994.

Wang ZY. Anticarcinogenesis of licorice and its major triterpenoid constituents, in Food Phytochemicals II: Teas, Spices, and Herbs. American Chemical Society,; 329-334. 1994.

Watanabe Y, Watanabe K, Proc Symp Wakan-Yaku 13:16. 1980.

Wilson JA. A comparison of carbenoxolone sodium and deglycyrrhizinated liquorice in the treatment of gastric ulcer in the ambulant patient. *Br J Clin Pract*; 26(12):563-566. 1972.

Yagura T et al., Proc *Symp Wakan-Yaku* 11:79. 1978.

Yamamura Y, Kawakami J, Santa T, Kotaki H, Uchino K, Sawada Y, Tanaka N, Iga T, Pharmacokinetic profile of glycyrrhizin in healthy volunteers by a new high-performance liquid chromatographic method. In: *J Pharm Sci* 81(10):1042-1046. 1992.

Yokota T; Nishio H; Kubota Y; Mizoguchi M. The inhibitory effect of glabridin from licorice extracts on melanogenesis and inflammation. *Pigment Cell Res* 1998 Dec;11(6):355-61.

Lilium candidum

See White Lily

Lilium martagon

See Martagon

Lily-of-the-Valley

Convallaria majalis

DESCRIPTION

Medicinal Parts: The medicinal parts are the dried flower tips and the dried inflorescence, the Lily-of-the-Valley herb, the dried root rhizome with the roots, the flowering aerial parts, and the whole, fresh, flowering plant.

Flower and Fruit: The flowers are in racemes nodding to one side, usually with a triangular penduncle. The tips are hemispheric, campanulate, 6-petalled with ovoid revolute tips. The perigone is white or pink. The stamens are attached to the base of the perigone. The fruit is a bright red, globular berry with 2 blue seeds. The plant is autosterile.

Leaves, Stem, and Root: The 15 to 20 cm high plant has 2 to 3 leaves at the tip of the runnerlike, branched rhizome. The leaves are elliptoid and acute. They taper to a long, sharp petiole at the base, which is clasped by a membranous sheath.

Characteristics: Fragrant but poisonous (all parts).

Habitat: The plant is native to Europe and has been introduced into the U.S. and northern Asia.

Production: Lily-of-the-Valley herb consists of the dried, above-ground parts of *Convallaria majalis* (or closely related species), collected during the flowering season. The harvested parts of the plant must be dried quickly at a maximum temperature of 60°C.

Not to be Confused With: Lily-of-the-Valley is easily confused with *Polygonatum odoratum.*

Other Names: Convall-Lily, Convallaria, Jacob's Ladder, Ladder-to-Heaven, Lily Constancy, May Lily, May Bells, Muguet, Our Lady's Tears,

ACTIONS AND PHARMACOLOGY

COMPOUNDS

Cardioactive steroid glycosides (cardenolides): varying according to geographical source, chief glycoside convallatoxin (western and northwestern Europe), convalloside (northern and eastern Europe), or convallatoxin + convallatoxol (central Europe)

EFFECTS

Only older studies are available, which indicate the convallara glycosides are qualitatively similar to digitoxin and strophanthin. The studies show Lily-of-the-Valley to have the following effects:

Cardiac: The power and speed of cardiac muscle contraction is increased and there is a reduced relaxation time. The beat frequency is slowed, stimulation transfer is delayed and the ability of the chamber muscles to be stimulated is increased (positively inotropic, negatively chronotropic, negatively dromotropic and positively bathmotropic effect.)

Renal: In animal tests, the effect was natriuretic and diuretic.

Venous: In animal tests, Lily-of-the-Valley demonstrated a dose-dependent, venoconstrictive effect.

INDICATIONS AND USAGE

Approved by Commission E:

- Arrhythmia
- Cardiac insufficiency NYHA I and II
- Nervous heart complaints

Unproven Uses: In folk medicine, Lily-of-the-Valley was used for weak contractions in labor, epilepsy, dropsy, strokes and ensuing paralysis, conjunctivitis, and leprosy. Use for these applications is no longer common because of the drug's toxic effect.

PRECAUTIONS AND ADVERSE REACTIONS

General: Health risks following the proper administration of designated therapeutic dosages are not recorded. Nausea, vomiting, headache, stupor, disorders of color perception, and cardiac arrhythmias can occur as side effects, particularly with an overdosage.

DRUG INTERACTIONS

POTENTIAL INTERACTIONS

The simultaneous administration of quinidine, digoxin, calcium salts, saluretics, laxatives, and glucocorticoids enhances effects and side effects of these drugs.

OVERDOSAGE

For symptoms of an acute poisoning and therapy, see *Digitalis folium.* The dangers of poisoning are relatively low with oral application, due to the poor absorbability of the glycosides.

DOSAGE

Mode of Administration: Comminuted herb, as well as galenic preparations for internal use; no longer considered safe because of the levels of toxins.

How Supplied: All information is based on stabilized Lily-of-the-Valley powder as specified in the German pharmacopoeia. No other forms can be recommended. However, commercial pharmaceutical preparations are available as capsules, drops, solutions and tablets.

Preparation: Tincture 1:10; liquid extract: 1:1; dry extract: 4:1.

Daily Dosage: The average daily dose of the drug: 0.6 g of tincture; 0.6 g of liquid extract; 0.15 g of dried extract. The average single dose: 2 g of tincture; 0.2 g of liquid extract; 0.05 g of dry extract. In intravenous application, the full effective dose of convaltoxin is 0.4 to 0.6 mg, the prepared dose 0.2 to 0.3 mg.

Storage: The preparations should be stored in well-sealed containers and protected from light.

LITERATURE

Krenn L, Schlifelner L, Stimpfl T, Kopp B, HPLC separation and quantitative determination of cardenolides in Herba Convallariae. In: *PM* 58(7)A82. 1992.

Loew D, Phytotherapie bei Herzinsuffizienz. In: *ZPT* 18(2):92-96. 1997. Loew DA, Loew AD, Pharmakokinetik von herzglykosidhaltigen Pflanzenextrakten. In: *ZPT* 15(4):197-202. 1994.

Lime

Citrus aurantifolia

DESCRIPTION

Medicinal Parts: The medicinal component is the bergamot oil extracted from the plant.

Flower and Fruit: The fragrant flowers are small and pure white. The fruit is about half the size of a lemon, with a smoother, thinner peel, a greenish-yellow color, and sweet taste.

Leaves, Stem, and Root: The evergreen tree is small, bent, thorny, and normally only grows to a height of 2.5 m. The leaves are ovate-lanceolate and acuminate.

Habitat: Lime is indigenous to Southern Asia and is cultivated in the West Indies, semi-tropic areas of the U.S., and Central America.

Production: Limes and lemons are the fruit of *Citrus aurantifolia.*

Other Names: Adam's Apple, Italian Limetta, Limette,

ACTIONS AND PHARMACOLOGY

COMPOUNDS

Volatile oil (in the fruit rind): containing, among others, citral, (+)-limonene, pinenes, alkanes, alkanols, alkanals, beta-bisabolene; also, in pressed oils, furocoumarins

Citric acid

Flavonoids: including hesperidine

EFFECTS

Lime acts as an antiscorbutic and refrigerant as well as a vitamin C supplement.

INDICATIONS AND USAGE

Lime is used as a source of vitamin C to treat scurvy and in cases of general low resistance.

PRECAUTIONS AND ADVERSE REACTIONS

No health hazards or side effects are known in conjunction with the proper administration of designated therapeutic dosages. There is a low potential for sensitization through skin contact with the juice of the fruit or with the volatile oil.

DOSAGE

Mode of Administration: Lime is used internally as a liquid extract of the fresh fruit.

LITERATURE

Lund ED, Bryan WL, *J Food Sci* 42:385. 1977

Natarajan S et al., *Econ Bot* 30:38. 1976

Tatum JH, Berry RE, *Phytochemistry* 16:1091. 1977

Wilson W, Shaw PE, *J Agric Food Chem* 25:211. 1977

Linaria vulgaris

See Yellow Toadflax

Linden

Tilia species

DESCRIPTION

Medicinal Parts: The medicinal parts are the fresh and dried flowers.

Flower and Fruit: The yellowish-white flowers are arranged in clusters of 5 to 11. The calyx has 5 sepals, oblong or ovate-lanceolate, acute and deep. The 5 petals are spatulate-lanceolate with crenate tips. There are numerous stamens and 1 superior ovary, which is almost globular and has silky-haired villi. The fruit is a single-seeded, pear-shaped, indistinctly angular, thin-shelled nut. There is a tongue-shaped, parchmentlike, greenish- or yellowish-white bract at the base of the flowers.

Leaves, Stem, and Root: Linden is an impressive tree up to 25 m high with a large, closed crown. The bark is fissured, gray-brown or black-gray. The bark of the branches is smooth. The branchlets are olive-green, brown, or brown-red with white warts. The leaves are long-petioled, uneven at the base, and broadly cordate. They have a dark upper surface and are bluish-green beneath with rust-colored tufts of down in the vein axils.

Characteristics: The flowers have a strong, sweet fragrance and the fruit tastes slightly sweet, slimy, and dry.

Habitat: The tree is common in northern temperate regions.

Production: Linden charcoal consists of the charcoal obtained from the wood of *Tilia cordata* and/or *Tilia platyphyllos*. Linden leaf consists of the dried leaf of *Tilia cordata* and/or *Tilia platyphyllos*. Silver Linden flower consists of the dried flowers of *Tilia tomentosa* (synonym *Tilia argentea*). Linden wood consists of the dried sapwood of *Tilia cordata* and/or *Tilia platyphyllos*. Linden flower consists of the dried flower of *Tilia cordata* and/or *Tilia platyphyllos*.

Not to be Confused With: Linden flower should not be confused with *Tilia tometosa* and *Tilia x euchlora*

Other Names: European Lime, European Linden, Lime, Linn Flowers

ACTIONS AND PHARMACOLOGY

COMPOUNDS: LINDEN CHARCOAL

Extremely adsorbent charcoals

EFFECTS: LINDEN CHARCOAL

No information is available.

COMPOUNDS: LINDEN LEAF

Flavonoids: including tiliroside, kempferol-3,7,-dirhamnoside, kempferol-3-O-glucoside-7-O-rhamnoside, linarine (acacetin-7-rutinoside), quercetin-3,7-di-O-rhamnoside, quercetin-3-O-glucoside-7-O-rhamnoside

Tannins

Mucilages

EFFECTS: LINDEN LEAF

The apparent diaphoretic effect has not been proved.

COMPOUNDS: SILVER LINDEN FLOWER

Flavonoids: including astragalin, isoquercitrin, kempferitrin, quercitrin, tiliroside, quercetin-3-O-glucoside-7-O-rhamnoside, kempferol-3-O-rhamnoside, kempferol-3-O-glucoside-7-O-rhamnoside, quercetin-rhamnoxyloside

Hydroxycoumarins: including, among others, calycanthoside, aesculin

Caffeic acid derivatives: chlorogenic acid

Mucilages

EFFECTS: SILVER LINDEN FLOWER

A possible sedative-anxiolytic effect and an anti-stress effect are under investigation. The flavonelike substances in the drug are thought to be responsible for these effects.

COMPOUNDS: LINDEN WOOD

Mucilages

Sterols: beta-sitosterol, stigmasterol, stigmastenol and their fatty acid esters

Triterpenes: squalene

EFFECTS: LINDEN WOOD

The diuretic, hypotensive, and choleretic effects ascribed to the drug are insufficiently documented. In animal experiments, an increase of bile secretion and a lowering of arterial pressure have been described. Aqueous extracts of the drug are antimicrobial.

COMPOUNDS: LINDEN FLOWER

Flavonoids (1%): including chief constituents astragalin, isoquercitrin, kempferol-3-O-rhamnoside, quercitrin, tiliroside (astragalin-6″-p-cumaroylester), including as well rutin, hyperoside, afzelin, kempferitrin

Mucilages(10%): arabino galactans with uronic acid share

Volatile oil (0.01-0.02%): including linalool, germacrene, geraniol, 1,8-cineole, 2-phenyl ethanol, phenyl ethyl benzoate, alkanes

Caffeic acid derivatives: chlorogenic acid

Tannins

EFFECTS: LINDEN FLOWER

The antitussive, astringent, diaphoretic, diuretic, sedative, and analgesic effects attributed to the drug have not yet been widely supported by experimental data. The toxic principle is unknown.

An alcoholic extract of the flowers is antimicrobial in vitro with the tannins, glycosides, and the essential oil the active components. Tilia flavonoids, which have not been described in detail, are anti-edemic in animal experiments. In addition, various experimental results point to a sedative effect. The diaphoretic effect is controversial. After steam inhalation with a lime flower additive, an improvement of the symptoms of uncomplicated colds was observed in comparison to a control group (only steam).

INDICATIONS AND USAGE

LINDEN CHARCOAL

Unproven Uses: Preparations of Linden charcoal are used internally for intestinal disorders and externally for ulcus cruris (leg ulcers).

LINDEN LEAF

Unproven Uses: Preparations of Linden leaf are used as a diaphoretic.

SILVER LINDEN FLOWER

Unproven Uses: Preparations of Silver Linden flower are used for catarrhs of the respiratory tract and as an antispasmodic, expectorant, diaphoretic, and diuretic.

LINDEN WOOD

Unproven Uses: Preparations of Linden wood are used for diseases and ailments of the liver and gallbladder systems and for cellulitis.

LINDEN FLOWER

Approved by Commission E:

- Cough
- Bronchitis

Unproven Uses: The flowers are used for catarrh of the respiratory tract and as a diaphoretic for feverish colds and infectious diseases, where a sweating cure is needed. It is occasionally used as a diuretic, a stomachic, an antispasmodic, and a sedative.

PRECAUTIONS AND ADVERSE REACTIONS

No health hazards or side effects are known in conjunction with the proper administration of designated therapeutic dosages.

DOSAGE

LINDEN FLOWER

Mode of Administration: The drug is available as a comminuted herb for teas, infusions, and other galenic preparations for internal use. The drug is a component of some standardized urologic, antitussive, and sedative preparations; it is also found in cold remedy tea mixtures.

Preparation: To make a tea, pour boiling water over 2 g drug, or add the drug to cold water and boil briefly; steep 5 to 10 minutes and strain (1 teaspoonful = 1.8 g drug).

Daily Dosage: The recommended daily dosage is 2 to 4 g of drug.

LITERATURE

LINDEN LEAF AND WOOD

Kern W, List PH, Hörhammer L (Hrsg.), Hagers Handbuch der Pharmazeutischen Praxis, 4. Aufl., Bde. 1-8: Springer Verlag Berlin, Heidelberg, New York, 1969.

SILVER LINDEN FLOWER

Buchbauer G, Jirovetz L, Ätherisches Lindenblütenöl - Aromastoffanalyse. In: *DAZ* 132(15):748. 1992.

LINDEN FLOWER
Buchbauer G, Jirovetz L, Ätherisches Lindenblütenöl-Aromastoffanalyse. In: DAZ 132(15):748. 1992.

Hildebrandt G, Engelbrecht P, Hildebrandt-Evers G, (1954) Physiologische Grundlagen für eine tageszeitliche Ordnung der Schwitzprozeduren. Z Klin Med 152:446-468.

Kram G, Franz G, *PA* 49:149. 1985.

Kram G, Franz G, *PM* 49:149. 1983.

Linum catharticum

See Mountain Flax

Linum usitatissimum

See Flax

Liquidambar orientalis

See Storax

Liriodendron tulipifera

See Tulip Tree

Lithospermum erytrorhizon

See Purple Gromwell (Ying Zicao)

Lobaria pulmonaria

See Lungmoss

Lobelia

Lobelia inflata

DESCRIPTION

Medicinal Parts: The medicinal parts are the fresh and dried herb and the seeds.

Flower and Fruit: The flowers are on long pedicles in the leaf axils. They are pale violet-blue and lightly tinged with pale yellow. The fruit consists of an ovoid or flattened bilocular capsule containing numerous small, brown, reticulate seeds.

Leaves, Stem, and Root: The plant is an erect annual or biennial herb 30 to 60 cm high. The stem is pubescent, angular, branching near the top. It contains an acrid latex. The leaves are pale green or yellowish. The lower ones are petiolate, the upper ones are sessile. They are alternate, ovate-lanceolate, 3 to 8 cm long, with a dentate margin and a finely pubescent lamina.

Characteristics: After chewing the leaves, the taste is similar to tobacco. The taste is acrid, the odor faintly irritant.

Habitat: The plant is indigenous to the regions in the north of U.S., Canada, and Kamchatka. It is cultivated elsewhere.

Production: Lobelia is the aerial part *of Lobelia inflata.*

Other Names: Asthma Weed, Bladderpod, Emetic Herb, Emetic Weed, Eyebright, Gagroot, Indian Tobacco, Pukeweed, Vomitwort, Vomitroot, Wild Tobacco

ACTIONS AND PHARMACOLOGY

COMPOUNDS

Piperidine alkaloids (6%): chief alkaloids L-lobeline (alpha-lobeline); companion alkaloids including among others lobelanine, lobelanidine, norlobelanine, and isolobinine

EFFECTS

The main active principle is lobelin. The drug has a stimulating effect on the respiratory center but it is broken down too quickly in the body to be used as a respiratory analeptic.

INDICATIONS AND USAGE

Homeopathic Uses: Lobelia inflata is used only in homeopathy as an asthma treatment and also as an aid in curing addiction to smoking.

PRECAUTIONS AND ADVERSE REACTIONS

General: No health hazards or side effects are known in conjunction with the proper administration of designated therapeutic dosages.

Pregnancy: Not to be used during pregnancy.

OVERDOSAGE

Overdosage leads to dryness of the mouth, nausea, vomiting, diarrhea, abdominal pain, burning in the urinary passages, feelings of anxiety, dizziness, headache, shivering, respiratory difficulties, paraesthesias, outbreak of sweating, bradycardia, cardiac arrhythmias, somnolence, and muscle twitching; death can occur through respiratory failure, accompanied by convulsions. 0.6 to 1 g of the leaves are said to be toxic, 4 g fatal.

Following gastrointestinal emptying (inducement of vomiting, gastric lavage with burgundy-colored potassium permanganate solution, sodium sulfate), instillation of activated charcoal, and shock prophylaxis (quiet, warmth), the therapy for poisonings consists of treating spasms with diazepam (IV); children are treated with chloral hydrate (rectal); monitoring of ECG. Cardiac massage and artificial respiration may also be required.

DOSAGE

Mode of Administration: The drug is no longer used. It is a constituent in some homeopathic preparations.

LITERATURE

Chang, EH et al., (Eds): Advances in Chinese Medicinal Materials Research, World Scientific Pub. Co. Singapore 1985.

Galeffi C. The Contribution of American Plants to pharmaceutical Sciences / Review Article. Il Farmaco 48; 1175-1195. 1993

Kern W, List PH, Hörhammer L (Hrsg.), Hagers Handbuch der Pharmazeutischen Praxis, 4. Aufl., Bde. 1-8, Springer Verlag Berlin, Heidelberg, New York, 1969.

Leung AY, Encyclopedia of Common Natural Ingredients Used in Food, Drugs and Cosmetics, John Wiley & Sons Inc., New York, 1980.

Lewin L, Gifte und Vergiftungen, 6. Aufl., Nachdruck, Haug Verlag, Heidelberg 1992.

Madaus G, Lehrbuch der Biologischen Arzneimittel, Bde 1-3, Nachdruck, Georg Olms Verlag Hildesheim 1979.

Roth L, Daunderer M, Kormann K, Giftpflanzen, Pflanzengifte, 4. Aufl., Ecomed Fachverlag Landsberg Lech 1993.

Schwarz HD, 100 Jahre Lobelin. In: *ZPT* 11(5):159. 1990.

Wagner H, Wiesenauer M, Phytotherapie. Phytopharmaka und pflanzliche Homöopathika, Fischer-Verlag, Stuttgart, Jena, New York, 1995.

Lobelia inflata

See Lobelia

Logwood

Haematoxylon campechianum

DESCRIPTION

Medicinal Parts: The medicinal part of the tree is the unfermented heartwood.

Flower and Fruit: The small yellow flowers grow in axillary racemes. There are 5 petals. The fruit is a flat pod, usually with 1 seed.

Leaves, Stem, and Root: Logwood is a 10 to 12 m high tree. The twisted branches are thorny, while the bark is rough and dark. The leaves have 4 pairs of small, smooth, and cordate stipules whose tips point to the small trunk.

Habitat: The plant originated in the tropical regions of the U.S. and is cultivated in the Caribbean and other regions.

Production: Logwood is the wood from *Haematoxylon campechianum.* The cultivated trees are felled in their eleventh year and the red heartwood is extracted.

Other Names: Bloodwood, H. lignum, Peachwood

ACTIONS AND PHARMACOLOGY

COMPOUNDS

Homoisoflavanes (neoflavane derivatives): to some extent in glycosidic bonds, changing over into the intensively red-colored, quinoide hematein through oxidation

Tannins (10%)

EFFECTS

Logwood has astringent properties, due to the isoflavone hematoxylin. An antiphlogistic effect has been proven in animal experiments and an antimicrobial effect in vitro. Hemateine and hematoxylin are said to inhibit the production of melanin in skin when used topically.

INDICATIONS AND USAGE

Unproven Uses: Folk medicine uses have included diarrhea and hemorrhage.

PRECAUTIONS AND ADVERSE REACTIONS

Health risks or side effects following the proper administration of designated therapeutic dosages are not recorded. However, internal administration of hematoxylin carried out in animal experiments led to elevated body temperature, vomiting, anuria, coma, and death. Reports of these studies provided no information regarding dosage (Lewin).

DOSAGE

Mode of Administration: The drug is administered as an infusion and a liquid extract.

Daily Dosage: A single dose of a decoction equal to 1 g of drug is mentioned, but the number of times it could be taken daily was not specified.

LITERATURE

Gurib-Fakim A, Gueho J, Sewraj-Bisoondoondoyal M. The Medicinal Plants of Mauritius - Part 1. Int J Pharmacogn. 35 (4); 237-254. 1997

Kern W, List PH, Hörhammer L (Hrsg.), Hagers Handbuch der Pharmazeutischen Praxis, 4. Aufl., Bde. 1-8, Springer Verlag Berlin, Heidelberg, New York, 1969.

Lolium temulentum

See Taumelloolch

Lonicera caprifolium

See Honeysuckle

Loosestrife

Lysimachia vulgaris

DESCRIPTION

Medicinal Parts: The medicinal part is the dried herb.

Flower and Fruit: The flowers grow in long-peduncled racemes in the axils of the upper stem and in terminal, panicled inflorescences. The pedicle is about 1 cm long, downy, and glandular-haired. The calyx is split almost to the base. The filaments are glandular-haired, usually fused to the middle with each other, and in a tube containing the ovary. The seeds are triangular, covered thickly in long warts, whitish and 1.5 mm long.

Leaves, Stem, and Root: The plant is a perennial and has underground runners, which produce new buds. The stem is erect, up to 1.5 m tall, branched, obtusely angular, leafy, and thickly downy. The leaves are slightly downy with glandular hairs. The leaves are in whorls or opposite, rarely spiralled, up to 14 cm long and 3.5 cm wide, short petioled, tightly reticulate, and red-glandular punctate.

Habitat: The plant is found in the temperate regions of Europe and Asia.

Production: Loosestrife is the aerial part of *Lysimachia vulgaris.*

Other Names: Yellow Willowherb

ACTIONS AND PHARMACOLOGY

COMPOUNDS

Flavonoids: glycosides of the myricetin, kaempferol, and quercetin, including rutin among others

Steroids: beta-sitosterol, stigmasterol

The constituents of the drug have not been extensively investigated.

EFFECTS

Loosestrife has an astringent effect. The main active principle is rutin.

INDICATIONS AND USAGE

Unproven Uses: Loosestrife is used for scurvy, diarrhea, and dysentery, as well as hemorrhages (nose bleeds and heavy menstrual blood flow) and wounds.

PRECAUTIONS AND ADVERSE REACTIONS

No health hazards or side effects are known in conjunction with the proper administration of designated therapeutic dosages.

DOSAGE

Mode of Administration: The herb is used externally in the powdered form.

LITERATURE

Hänsel R, Keller K, Rimpler H, Schneider G (Hrsg.), Hagers Handbuch der Pharmazeutischen Praxis, 5. Aufl., Bde 4-6 (Drogen), Springer Verlag Berlin, Heidelberg, New York, 1992-1994.

Zhong-fu Y, Xian-sheng W. Combined Traditional Chinese and Western Medicine / Ultrasonic Studies on the Effect of Artemisia Decoction on the Volume and Dynamics of Gallbladder. *Chin Med J.* 106; 145-148. 1993

Lophophora williamsii

See Peyote

Lotus

Nelumbo nucifera

DESCRIPTION

Medicinal Parts: The medicinal parts are the roots, the seeds, and the aerial parts of the flowering plant.

Flower and Fruit: The solitary flowers are 16 to 23 cm across, pink, and scented. They grow above the leaves. The seeds are 1.7 by 1.3 cm and ovoid.

Leaves, Stem, and Root: The rhizome is 10 to 20 cm long, stout, and branching. It bears numerous scalelike leaves as well as foliage leaves. The foliage leaves are peltate and have no sinuses. The petioles are 1 to 2 cm long, the lamina are 30 to 100 cm in diameter and are glossy, impervious to water, and almost circular,.

Habitat: The plant is indigenous to India.

Production: Lotus is the whole plant of *Nelumbo nucifera*.

ACTIONS AND PHARMACOLOGY

COMPOUNDS

Isoquinoline alkaloids: including,

benzyl isoquinoline type: armepavine, n-methyl coclaurine

aporphine type: roemerine (remerine), nuciferine, n-nornuciferine, nornuciferine, anonaine, liriodenine, asimilobin, lirinidin

proaporphine type: prunuciferine

Flavonoids: including hyperoside, isoquercitrin, nelumboside, quercetin glucuronide, camphor glucuronide

Tannins

EFFECTS

Active agents are the alkaloids nelumbin and roemerine in the leaves. The drug is an astringent.

INDICATIONS AND USAGE

Unproven Uses: The powdered beans are used in the treatment of digestive disorders, particularly diarrhea. The flowers are used as an astringent for bleeding.

Indian Medicine: Lotus is used for cholera, diarrhea, worm infestation, vomiting, states of exhaustion, and intermittent fever.

PRECAUTIONS AND ADVERSE REACTIONS

No health hazards or side effects are known in conjunction with the proper administration of designated therapeutic dosages.

DOSAGE

Mode of Administration: Preparations of the plant are available in powder and liquid extract for internal use.

LITERATURE

Chen C, Lin C, Namba T. Screening of Taiwanese Crude Drugs for Antibacterial Activity against *Streptococcus mutans. J Ethnopharmacol.* 22; 285-295. 1989

Hegnauer R: Chemotaxonomie der Pflanzen, Bde 1-11, Birkhäuser Verlag Basel, Boston, Berlin 1962-1997.

Kern W, List PH, Hörhammer L (Hrsg.), Hagers Handbuch der Pharmazeutischen Praxis, 4. Aufl., Bde. 1-8, Springer Verlag Berlin, Heidelberg, New York, 1969.

Mukherjee PK, Saha K, Das J, Pal M, Saha BP. Studies on the Anti-Inflammatory Activity of Rhizomes of *Nelumbo nucifera. Planta Med.* 63 (4); 367-369. 1997

Lovage

Levisticum officinale

DESCRIPTION

Medicinal Parts: The medicinal parts are the dried rhizome and roots, the cut, dried herb, and the dried fruit.

Flower and Fruit: The flowers are in 8 to 20 rayed, compound umbels. There is an involucre and epicalyx. but no calyx. The orbicular petals are pale yellow and involute. The fruit is yellow-brown, 5 to 7 mm long, compressed, and has sharply keeled to winged ribs.

Leaves, Stem, and Root: The plant is a sturdy perennial. It has a thick, spindle-shaped, branched root, which is brownish-yellow on the outside and whitish on the inside. The stem is erect, round, hollow, finely grooved, glabrous, and up to 4 cm thick at the base. The leaves are rich green, glossy, and coriaceous; the lower ones double pinnate, the upper ones simple-pinnate. The leaflets are broad and obovate.

Characteristics: The rubbed leaves give off an aromatic scent. The fruit is very fragrant.

Habitat: Lovage is indigenous to the Mediterranean region. It grows wild in the Balkans and northern Greece and is cultivated elsewhere.

Production: Lovage root consists of the dried rhizomes and roots of *Levisticum officinale,* as well as their preparations. Roots of 2-year-old plants are collected in autumn. It is important that the roots are not damaged during the drying process since this would result in a loss of the essential oil.

Not to be Confused With: Angelicae radix, Pastinacae radix or *Pimpinellae radix.*

Other Names: Bladder Seed, Lavose, Sea Parsley

ACTIONS AND PHARMACOLOGY

COMPOUNDS

Volatile oil (0.35-1.7%): chief components alkylphthalides (ca. 70% aroma-bearers), including 3-butylphthalide, ligusticumlactone (E- and Z-butylidenphthalides), and E- and Z-ligustilide as well as alpha- and beta-pinene, beta-phellandrene, and citronellal

Hydroxycoumarins: umbelliferone

Coumarin

Furocoumarins: bergaptene, apterin

Polyynes: including falcarindiol (probably only in the fresh rhizome)

EFFECTS

Lovage has diuretic, sedative, antimicrobial, and cholinergic properties. The ligustilide-containing essential oil has an antispasmodic effect on smooth muscle. The folk use for gastric complaints is probably based on the specific odor caused by phthalide as well as on the bitter taste, which increases saliva and gastric secretions.

INDICATIONS AND USAGE

Approved by Commission E:

- Infections of the urinary tract
- Kidney and bladder stones

Lovage is used for irrigating therapy for inflammation of the lower urinary tract and irrigating therapy for prevention of kidney gravel.

Unproven Uses: The folk medicine uses include dyspeptic complaints, such as indigestion, heartburn, feelings of fullness, flatulence, and menstrual complaints. Lovage is also used as a secretolytic for respiratory catarrh.

CONTRAINDICATIONS

Because of the irritating effect of the volatile oil, the drug should not be administered in the presence of inflammation of the kidneys or of the urinary drainage passages, nor with reduced kidney function. No irrigation therapy is to be carried out in the presence of edema resulting from reduced cardiac and kidney function.

PRECAUTIONS AND ADVERSE REACTIONS

General: No health hazards or side effects are known in conjunction with the proper administration of designated therapeutic dosages. The drug possesses a low potential for sensitization. An elevation of UV-sensitivity among light-skinned people is possible (phototoxic effect of the furocoumarins).

Pregnancy: Not to be used during pregnancy.

DOSAGE

Mode of Administration: Comminuted herb and other galenic preparations for internal use.

Daily Dosage: 4 to 8 g drug. Ample intake of liquid is essential. Tea: 2 to 4 g drug to 1 cup, several times a day between meals.

Infusion: 1.5 g per cup.

Storage: Protect from light and insects in well-sealed containers. The whole drug should be stored not longer than 18 months; the powdered drug, not longer than 24 hours.

LITERATURE

Ashwood-Smith MJ, Ceska O, Yeoman A, Kenny PG. Photosensitivity from harvesting lovage (*Levisticum officinale*). Contact Dermatitis 26; 356-357. 1992

Broda B, Grzybek J. Preparation of herbal mixtures / Studies on herbs with designed sedative activity. Z Phytother. 14; 307-314. 1993

Hänsel R, Keller K, Rimpler H, Schneider G (Hrsg.), Hagers Handbuch der Pharmazeutischen Praxis, 5. Aufl., Bde 4-6 (Drogen), Springer Verlag Berlin, Heidelberg, New York, 1992-1994.

Leung AY, Encyclopedia of Common Natural Ingredients Used in Food, Drugs and Cosmetics, John Wiley & Sons Inc., New York 1980.

Madaus G, Lehrbuch der Biologischen Arzneimittel, Bde 1-3, Nachdruck, Georg Olms Verlag Hildesheim 1979.

Segebrecht S, Schilcher H. Ligustilide: Guiding Component for Preparations of *Levisticum officinale* Roots. *Planta Med.* 55; 572-573. 1989

Steinegger E, Hänsel R, Pharmakognosie, 5. Aufl., Springer Verlag Heidelberg 1992.

Teuscher E, Biogene Arzneimittel, 5. Aufl., Wiss. Verlagsges. Stuttgart 1997.

Teuscher E, Lindequist U, Biogene Gifte - Biologie, Chemie, Pharmakologie, 2. Aufl., Fischer Verlag Stuttgart 1994.

Vollmann C, *Levisticum officinale* - Der Liebstöckel. In: *ZPT* 9(4):128. 1988.

Wichtl M (Hrsg.), Teedrogen, 4. Aufl., Wiss. Verlagsges. Stuttgart 1997.

Luffa

Luffa aegyptica

DESCRIPTION

Medicinal Parts: The medicinal part is the dried network of vascular bundles of the ripe cucumberlike plant. When dried, the dense vascular network that makes up the fruit becomes the Loofah, which is used to scrub and soften the skin.

Flower and Fruit: The plant bears solitary, yellow, female flowers, which are 5 to 10 cm wide and have an oblong, clavate calyx tube. The fruit is cylindrical or oblong-clavate. It is not ribbed, prickly, or sharp-edged. It is somewhat tomentose, up to 40 cm long and 5 to 15 cm thick. The seeds are blackish, smooth, and winged.

Leaves, Stem, and Root: The plant is an annual climber that grows from 3 to 6 m high. The stems are thin and pentangular. The leaves are cordate-indented, 15 to 30 cm long with 3 to 7 lobes.

Habitat: The plant probably originated in India and was brought to Egypt in the Middle Ages. Today, it is cultivated in the tropical regions of the world.

Production: Luffa sponge consists of the dried fiber structure of the ripe cucumberlike fruits of *Luffa aegyptica*. The ripe fruit is freed of soft material by banging and washing.

Other Names: Bath-Loofah, Dishcloth Gourd, Smooth Loofah, Vegetable Sponge

ACTIONS AND PHARMACOLOGY

COMPOUNDS: LUFFA FRESH FRUIT

Triterpene saponins: including among others lucyoside A-M (aglycones including oleanolic acid, hederagenin 21-hydroxyhederagenin, gypsogenin, arjunolic acid)

Cucurbitacins (the young fruits are eaten as salad)

Sterols: including delta5-sterols, delta7-sterols

Triterpenes (triterpene acids): including bryonolic acid (3%)

The luffa fungus (*Luffa aegyptica*) is likely to be mostly free of soluble constituents and to consist chiefly of cellulose, hemicellulose, and pectins.

EFFECTS

No information is available.

INDICATIONS AND USAGE

Unproven Uses: Preparations of Luffa sponge are used as a preventive for infections or colds, as a remedy for colds and nasal catarrhs, and for sinusitis and suppuration of the sinus.

Chinese Medicine: Luffa is used for coughs, chronic bronchitis, diseases of the spleen, and paralyzing diseases.

Indian Medicine: Luffa is used for splenopathy, leprosy, syphilis, bronchitis, fever, and hematuria.

PRECAUTIONS AND ADVERSE REACTIONS

No health hazards or side effects are known in conjunction with the proper administration of designated therapeutic dosages.

DOSAGE

No information is available.

LITERATURE

Haldar UC, Saha SK, Beavis RC, Sinha NK. Trypsin inhibitors from ridged gourd (*Luffa acutangula Linn.*) seeds: purification properties and amino acid sequences. *J Protein Chem,* 61:177-84, Feb 1996

Hänsel R, Keller K, Rimpler H, Schneider G (Hrsg.), Hagers Handbuch der Pharmazeutischen Praxis, 5. Aufl., Bde 4-6 (Drogen), Springer Verlag Berlin, Heidelberg, New York, 1992-1994.

Ishihara H, Sasagawa T, Sakai R, Nishikawa M, Kimura M, Funatsu G. Isolation and molecular characterization of four arginine/glutamate rich polypeptides from the seeds of sponge gourd (*Luffa cylindrica*). *Biosci Biotechnol Biochem,* 61:168-70, Jan 1997

Lacaille-Dubois MA, Wagner H. A review of the biological and pharmacological activities of saponins. *Phytomedicine* 2 (4); 363-386. 1996

Ng TB, Wong RN, Yeung HW. Two proteins with ribosome-inactivating cytotoxic and abortifacient activities from seeds of *Luffa cylindrica roem* (Cucurbitaceae). *Biochem Int,* 27:197-207, Jul 1992

Yeung HW, Li WW, Ng TB. Effect of *Luffa aegyptiaca* (seeds) and *Carissa edulis* (leaves) extracts on blood glucose level of normal and streptozotocin diabetic rats. *J Ethnopharmacol,* 38:43-7, Jan 1996

Luffa aegyptica

See Luffa

Lungmoss

Lobaria pulmonaria

DESCRIPTION

Medicinal Parts: The medicinal part is the lichen.

Flower and Fruit: *Lobaria pulmonaria* is a lichen, with deeply pinnatisect lobes with indented tips, measuring from 1.5 cm up to the size of a hand. It is found on the trunks of old woodland trees and is browinsh-green or red-brown with a reticulate, punctate structure. It is tomentose and whitish-brown beneath and is covered with glabrous white spots on the margin and on the reticulate ridges.

Habitat: Lungmoss is found throughout Europe.

Production: Lungmoss is the whole lichen tissue of *Lobaria pulmonaria*. The lichen is gathered throughout the entire year. The minute roots in the subterranean part, along with any possible earth, are cleaned off (do not gather dry lichen, as it is mostly found on dead plants, and therefore is no longer effective).

Not to be Confused With: Common Lungwort, which is a plant.

Other Names: Lungwort, Oak Lungs

ACTIONS AND PHARMACOLOGY

COMPOUNDS

Lichen acids: including among others stictictic, norstictic, thelophoric acid, and gyrophoric acid

Mucilages

EFFECTS

The drug has diaphoretic, expectorant, anti-inflammatory, and antimicrobial effects. The active agents exhibiting the antimicrobial effects are unknown.

INDICATIONS AND USAGE

Unproven Uses: As a result of the relaxing effect of Lungmoss on the respiratory tract, the drug is used for all chronic respiratory tract illnesses: bronchitis, coughs and asthma, as well as for irritable coughs and smoker's cough.

PRECAUTIONS AND ADVERSE REACTIONS

No health hazards or side effects are known in conjunction with the proper administration of designated therapeutic dosages.

DOSAGE

Mode of Administration: Lungmoss is available as dried lichen as a liquid extract for internal use. Lichen preparations can be bought as sweets, syrups, or pastilles.

Storage: The drug should be stored in glass or porcelain containers, protected from light.

LITERATURE

Kern W, List PH, Hörhammer L (Hrsg.), Hagers Handbuch der Pharmazeutischen Praxis, 4. Aufl., Bde. 1-8, Springer Verlag Berlin, Heidelberg, New York, 1969.

Madaus G, Lehrbuch der Biologischen Arzneimittel, Bde 1-3, Nachdruck, Georg Olms Verlag Hildesheim 1979.

Rowe JG, Saenz MT, Garcia MD. Contribution a l'etude de l'activite antibacterienne de quelques lichens du sud de l'Espagne. *Ann pharm franc.* 47; 89-94. 1989

Wagner H, Wiesenauer M, Phytotherapie. Phytopharmaka und pflanzliche Homöopathika, Fischer-Verlag, Stuttgart, Jena, New York 1995.

Lungwort

Pulmonaria officinalis

DESCRIPTION

Medicinal Parts: The medicinal parts are the dried herb and the fresh, aerial parts of the flowering plant.

Flower and Fruit: The blue, later blue-violet flowers are in terminal curled cymelike inflorescences on flowering branches. The calyx is fused and has 5 tips. The corolla is fused to a tube and the 5 tips are rotate. There are 5 stamens and a 4-valved ovary with 1 style. There are both long and short-styled flowers. There are 5 tufts of hair at the entrance to the corolla tube. The fruit consists of 4 nuts 3.5 to 4 mm in length, glabrous when ripe, glossy brown to black, mildly keeled with a distinct displaced ring.

Leaves, Stem, and Root: The plant grows from 15 to 30 cm high. The rhizome is quite thin and branched. First it produces flowering shoots and then the leaf rosettes. The shoots are fresh green and covered in glandular hairs. The stems are erect or ascending, slightly angular, and pubescent. The rosettelike basal leaves that form after flowering are long petioled, cordate-ovate, acute, more long than wide with whitish spots. The cauline leaves are alternate, taper to a winged stem, and are sharply pointed; only the lower ones have some pinnatifid ribs.

Characteristics: The taste is slightly bitter and slimy.

Habitat: The plant is common in many parts of Europe.

Production: Lungwort consists of the dried plant section of *Pulmonaria officinalis* and its effective pharmaceutical preparations. Lungwort is collected in uncultivated regions and air-dried.

Not to be Confused With: Lungwort is occasionally adulterated with other *Pulmonaria* species, particularly *Pulmonaria mollis.*

Other Names: Common Lungwort, Dage of Jerusalem

ACTIONS AND PHARMACOLOGY

COMPOUNDS

Allantoin

Caffeic acid derivatives: chlorogenic acid, rosmarinic acid

Flavonoids (0.3 to 0.5%): especially O-glycosides of the kaempferol and quercetin

Mucilages: polygalacturonane, arabinogalactans, rhamnogalacturonane

Silicic acid: more than 2.5% water-soluble silicic acid

Tannins

EFFECTS

The drug has an expectorant, soothing effect due to the mucilaginous polysaccharide and tannin content.

INDICATIONS AND USAGE

Unproven Uses: In folk medicine Lungwort is used internally for illnesses and conditions of the respiratory tract, gastrointestinal tract, kidney and efferent urinary tract; and externally in the treatment of wounds.

PRECAUTIONS AND ADVERSE REACTIONS

No health hazards or side effects are known in conjunction with the proper administration of designated therapeutic dosages.

DOSAGE

Mode of Administration: Lungwort is available as whole, cut and powdered drug for internal and external use. It is also available in commercial forms as syrup, juice, drops, and in compounded preparations.

Preparation: To prepare a tea, 1.5 g finely cut drug is put in cold water that is brought quickly to a boil or it is scalded with boiling water and strained after 5 to 10 minutes (1 teaspoon corresponds to approximately 0.7 g drug).

Liquid extract: 1:1 with 25% ethanol. (V/V)

Daily Dosage: As bronchial tea it is drunk in sips throughout the day. It may be sweetened with honey.

Storage: Should be protected from light

LITERATURE

Brantner A, Grein E. Antibacterial activity of plant extracts used externally in traditional medicine. *J Ethnopharmacol.* 44; 35-40. 1994

Brantner A, Kartnig Th, Flavonoid glycosides from aerial parts of *Pulmonaria officinalis.* In: *PM* 61(6):582. 1995.

Müller BM, Franz G, Polysaccharide aus *Pulmonaria officinalis* - Wertgebende Bestandteile der Droge? In: *PZW* 135(6):243-251. 1990.

Lupinus luteus

See Yellow Lupin

Lycium barbarum

See Lycium Berries (Go-Qi-Zi)

Lycium Bark (Di-Gu-Pi)

Lycium chinense

DESCRIPTION

Medicinal Parts: The medicinal parts of the plant are the fruit and root bark.

Flower and Fruit: The plant has 1 to 3 axillary, radial flowers. The calyx and petals are fused; the calyx is bilabial with a double-toothed upper lip and triple-toothed lower lip. The corolla is funnel-shaped, light purple or violet with a 5-lobed margin. There are 4 stamens, which are hairy at the base. The ovary is double-chambered with 1 style. The fruit is a yellow-orange, elongate, sweet-tasting berry.

Leaves, Stem, and Root: Lycium chinense is a shrub that grows up to 3 m high. The leaves are alternate, ovate-lanceolate to rhomboid, narrowing suddenly to the petiole, and bright green. The branches are canelike, initially upright, then hanging down bowlike and thornless.

Habitat: The plant is native to eastern Asia, particularly to China and Japan.

Production: Lycium bark is the dried root bark of *Lycium chinense* or *Lycium barbarum*. Harvest begins in early spring or in late autumn when the roots are dug up and then peeled. The root bark is then cleaned and dried in the sun. Lycium leaves are the dried leaves of *Lycium chinense*.

Other Names: Chinese Matrimony Vine, Chinese Wolfberry

ACTIONS AND PHARMACOLOGY

COMPOUNDS: LYCIUM ROOT BARK

Polyamines: kukoamine A (spermidin-dihydrocaffeoyl-bisamide)

Dipeptides: Lyciumamide (N-benzoyl-L-phenylalanyl-L-phenylalaninol-acetate)

Cyclopeptides: lyciumin A, lyciumin B

Steroids: sterols, including beta-sitosterol, 5alpha-stigmastan-3,6-dione

Diterpenes: sugiol

EFFECTS: LYCIUM ROOT BARK

The methanolic root extract and the kukoamine A isolated from the plant are reported to have had significant antihypertensive effects in animal experiments. The isolated octapeptides lyciumines A and B are believed to inhibit the activity of renin and the angiotensin-converting enzyme. Experimental data confirming these results are not available.

COMPOUNDS: LYCIUM LEAVES

Steroids: withasteroids (0.1%), including withanolide A, withanolide B

Sterols: including beta-sitosterol and beta-sitosterol glucoside

EFFECTS: LYCIUM LEAVES

No experimental data regarding the pharmacological efficacy of the drug are available. In vitro experimental models have indicated that the steroid withanolide isolated from it may have immunosuppressive effect.

INDICATIONS AND USAGE

LYCIUM ROOT BARK

Unproven Uses: The root of the plant is used in fever and blood pressure-reducing medications. The berries are considered to provide a liver and kidney tonic.

Chinese Medicine: Used internally for fever, hyperhidrosis, thirst, coughs, nosebleeds, pulpitis, diabetes, hypertension, malaria, and for hematemesis. External uses include eczema and rheumatism. Efficacy for these indications has not yet been proved.

LYCIUM LEAVES

Unproven Uses: Preparations from the leave are used in folk medicine for whooping cough and paroxysmal cough (Iberian peninsula), as a mouthwash for toothache (Indonesia).

Chinese Medicine: Lycium leaf is used for inflammatory processes, such as rheumatism, and as a tea taken for pain.

Indian Medicine: Used for rheumatism.

PRECAUTIONS AND ADVERSE REACTIONS

LYCIUM ROOT BARK AND LEAVES

No health hazards are known in conjunction with the proper administration of designated therapeutic dosages.

CONTRAINDICATIONS

LYCIUM ROOT BARK

Contraindications include pregnancy, symptoms of the common cold and diarrhea.

LYCIUM LEAVES

Not to be used during pregnancy.

DOSAGE

LYCIUM ROOT BARK

Mode of Administration: Whole, cut and powdered drug preparations are administered internally and externally.

Daily Dosage: Drug/tea: 9 to 15 g or 6 to 12 g, depending on the literature source.

Storage: Store in a dry place.

LYCIUM LEAVES

Mode of Administration: Lycium leaf is administered as a tea or as an infusion for use as a gargle.

Daily Dosage: For Whooping Cough, 1 cup of tea sipped throughout the day.

LITERATURE

Aubert C, Kapetanidis I. New Flavonoids from *Lycium chinense. Planta Med.* 55; 612. 1989

Funayama S, Zhang GR, Nozoe S. Kukoamine B, a Spermine Alkaloid from *Lycium chinense. Phytochemistry* 38 (6); 1529-1531. 1995

Hänsel R, Keller K, Rimpler H, Schneider G (Ed), Hagers Handbuch der Pharmazeutischen Praxis, 5. Aufl., Bde 4 - 6 (Drogen), Springer Verlag Berlin, Heidelberg, New York, 1992-1994.

Kim HP, Kim SY, Lee EJ, Kim YC, Kim YC, Zeaxanthin dipalmitate from *Lycium chinense* has hepatoprotective activity. *Res Commun Mol Pathol Pharmacol*, 97:301-14, Sep. 1997

Kim SY, Choi YH, Huh H, Kim J, Kim YC, Lee HS, New antihepatotoxic cerebroside from *Lycium chinense* fruits. *J Nat Prod,* 60:274-6, Mar. 1997

Lin CC, Chuang SC, Lin JM, Yang JJ. Evaluation of the antiinflammatory hepatoprotective and antioxidant activities of *Lycium chinense* from Taiwan. *Phytomedicine* 4 (3); 213-220. 1997

Morita H, Yoshida N, Takeya K, Itokawa H, Shirota O. Configurational and Conformational Analyses of a Cyclic Octapeptide, Lyciumin A, from *Lycium chinense* Mill. *Tetrahedron* 52 (8); 2795-2802. 1996

Yahara S, Shigeyama C, Ura T, Wakamatsu K, Yasuhara T, Nohara T. Cyclic Peptides, Acyclic Diterpene Glycosides and Other Compounds from *Lycium chinense* Mill. *Chem Pharm Bull.* 41; 703-709. 1993

Lycium Berries (Go-Qi-Zi)

Lycium barbarum

DESCRIPTION

Medicinal Parts: The medicinal part is the fruit.

Flower and Fruit: There are 1 to 3 axillary, radial flowers. The calyx and petals are fused; the calyx is bilabial with a double-toothed upper lip and triple-toothed lower lip. The corolla is funnel-shaped, light purple or violet with a 5-lobed margin. There are 4 stamens, which are hairy at the base. The ovary is 2-chambered with 1 style. The fruit is a scarlet, elongate, sweet-tasting berry.

Leaves, Stem, and Root: Lycium barbarum is a shrub, growing up to 3 m high. The gray-green leaves are alternate, lanceolate and gradually narrow to the petiole. The branches are canelike, initially upright, then hanging down bowlike and often thorny.

Habitat: The shrub is indigenous to China and Mongolia.

Production: Barbary wolfberry fruits are the dried ripe fruit of *Lycium barbarum.* The fruit is harvested in summer or autumn. The whole fruit, with stem attached, is dried in the sun until the skin is hard and the fruit pulp is soft inside. After drying, the fruit stem is removed.

Other Names: Barbary Wolfberry, Bastard Jasmine, Box Thorne, Common Matrimony Vine, Prickly Box, Tea Plant, Tea Tree

ACTIONS AND PHARMACOLOGY

COMPOUNDS

Water-soluble polysaccharides

Glycoproteins

Carotinoids: particularly physalien (zeaxanthin dipalmitate)

EFFECTS

A possible immunostimulating and hypoglycemic effect has been described. The plant contains a mydriatic acting protein.

INDICATIONS AND USAGE

Unproven Uses: The drug is administered as a nonspecific strengthening agent due to the minerals and vitamins (particularly vitamin C) that it contains. *Lycium barbarum* is also used as a purgative and diuretic.

Chinese Medicine: The plant is used to treat weakness of the lumbar region and knee, liver and kidney disorders, diabetes, tinnitus, impaired hearing, poor sight, anemia, coughs, dizziness, and excessive tear production.

Indian Medicine: Lycium barbarum is used for ascitis, anemia, menstruation disorders, toothache, scabies, and bleeding hemorrhoids.

CONTRAINDICATIONS

Not to be used during pregnancy.

PRECAUTIONS AND ADVERSE REACTIONS

No health hazards are known in conjunction with the proper administration of designated therapeutic dosages.

DOSAGE

Mode of Application: Whole, cut, and powdered drug.

Daily Dosage: Drug/tea: 6 to 12 g or 6 to 15 g, depending on the literature source.

Storage: Store in cool, dry place and in tightly sealed container.

LITERATURE

Hänsel R, Keller K, Rimpler H, Schneider G (Ed), Hagers Handbuch der Pharmazeutischen Praxis, 5. Aufl., Bde 4 - 6 (Drogen), Springer Verlag Berlin, Heidelberg, New York, 1992-1994.

Liu B, Effects of *Lycium barbarum L* and *Drynaria fortunei J Smith* on in vitro attachment and growth of human gingival fibroblasts on root surfaces. *Chung Hua Kou Chiang Hsueh Tsa Chih,* 27:159-61, 190, May 1992

Lu CX, Cheng BQ, Radiosensitizing effects *of Lycium barbarum* polysaccharide for Lewis lung cancer. *Chung Hsi I Chieh Ho Tsa Chih,* 11:611-2, 582, Oct 1991

Ren B, Ma Y, Shen Y, Gao B, Protective action of *Lycium barbarum L.* (LbL) and betaine on lipid peroxidation of erythrocyte membrane induced by H 2 O 2. *Chung Kuo Chung Yao Tsa Chih,* 20:303-4, inside cover, May 1995

Lycium chinense

See Lycium Bark (Di-Gu-Pi)

Lycoperdon species

See Puff Ball

Lycopersicon esculentum

See Tomato

Lycopodium clavatum

See Club Moss

Lycopus virginicus

See Bugleweed

Lysimachia nummularia

See Moneywort

Lysimachia vulgaris

See Loosestrife

Lythrum salicaria

See Purple Loosestrife

Macrocystis pyrifera

See Brown Kelp

Madder

Rubia tinctorum

DESCRIPTION

Medicinal Parts: The medicinal part is the dried root.

Flower and Fruit: The small yellowish-green flowers are in loose, leafy, long-peduncled terminal or axillary cymes. The margin of the calyx is indistinct, 4 to 5 sectioned and has a tip, which is curved inward. There are 5 stamens and an inferior ovary. The fruit is a black, pea-sized glabrous, smooth drupe containing 2 seeds.

Leaves, Stem, and Root: The perennial plant grows from 60 to 100 cm high. The pencil-thick rhizome creeps widely underground. The stem is quadrangular with backward-turning prickles at the edges. The stems are at times so thin that they are more descendent than erect. The leaves are in whorls, in fours below, in sixes above. They are oblong to lanceolate with 1 rib and protrude reticulately beneath.

Habitat: The plant is indigenous to Southern Europe, Western Asia, and North Africa and is cultivated elsewhere.

Production: Madder root consists of the dried root of *Rubia tinctorum* as well as its preparations.

Other Names: Dyer's Madder, Robbia

ACTIONS AND PHARMACOLOGY

COMPOUNDS

Anthracene derivatives (rubiadins, 2 to 4%): chief components alizarin, lucidin, pseudopurpurin (purpurin carboxylic acid), purpurin, rubiadin, and the glucosides and/or the primerosides of these compounds.

EFFECTS

Madder root inhibits calcium oxalate crystallization in the kidney. Lucidin is the toxic principle and is mutagenic.

INDICATIONS AND USAGE

Unproven Uses: Madder root is used to dissolve kidney stones

PRECAUTIONS AND ADVERSE REACTIONS

Because of the possible carcinogenic effect of the rubiadins, the drug should not be administered.

LITERATURE

Anon. Rubiae-tinctorum-radix-haltige Humanarzneimittel, Widerruf der Zulassung. In: *DAZ* 133(11):888. 1993.

Courchesne M, Brassard P. Identification and characterization of naturally occuring rubiadins. In: *JNP* 56(5):722. 1993.

Westendorf J, Pfau W, Schulte A. Carcinogenicity and DNA adduct formation observed in ACI rats after long-term treatment with madder root, *Rubia tinctorum L. Carcinogenesis.* Dec; 19(12):2163-2168. 1998.

Westendorf J, Poginskky B, Marquardt H, Marquardt H. The genotoxicity of Lucidin, a natural component of *Rubia tinctorum L.*, and lucidinmethylether, a component of ethanolic Rubia extracts. In: *Cell Biol Toxicol* Jun; 4(2):225-239. 1988

Magnolia

Magnolia glauca

DESCRIPTION

Medicinal Parts: The bark is the medicinal part.

Leaves, Stem and Root: The inner bark occurs in long, fibrous strips. The outer surface is rough, almost granular and pitted.

The inner surface is striated but almost smooth. The fracture is short with the inner part tough and fibrous.

Habitat: The plant is indigenous to North America.

Production: Magnolia bark is the bark from the trunk and branches of *Magnolia glauca.*

Other Names: Beaver Tree, Holly Bay, Indian Bark, Red Bay, Swamp Laurel, Swamp Sassafras, Sweet Bay, White Bay, White Laurel

ACTIONS AND PHARMACOLOGY

COMPOUNDS

Neolignans: magnolol

Volatile oil

The constituents of the drug have not been widely investigated.

EFFECTS

Magnolia has diaphoretic, anti-inflammatory, and stimulant effects. It is also a tonic.

INDICATIONS AND USAGE

Unproven Uses: The preparations are used for digestive disorders; used rarely, except in Oriental medicine.

PRECAUTIONS AND ADVERSE REACTIONS

No health hazards or side effects are known in conjunction with the proper administration of designated therapeutic dosages.

DOSAGE

Mode of Administration: Magnolia has been used internally as a powder or liquid extract.

LITERATURE

Hegnauer R, Chemotaxonomie der Pflanzen, Bde 1-11, Birkhäuser Verlag Basel, Boston, Berlin 1962-1997.

Kern W, List PH, Hörhammer L (Hrsg.), Hagers Handbuch der Pharmazeutischen Praxis, 4. Aufl., Bde. 1-8, Springer Verlag Berlin, Heidelberg, New York, 1969.

Yajara S, Nishiyori T, Kohda A, Nohra T, Nishioka I. Isolation and characterization of phenolic compounds from Magnolia cortex produced in China. In: *Chem Pharm Bull Tokyo* 39:2024. 1991.

Magnolia glauca

See Magnolia

Mahonia aquifolium

See Mountain Grape

Ma Huang

Ephedra sinica

DESCRIPTION

Medicinal Parts: The medicinal parts are the young canes collected in autumn and the dried rhizome with roots.

Flower and Fruit: The flowers are small and occasionally reduced to acuminate scales. They are fused in pairs at the base. They are unisexual, usually dioecious and sometimes monoecious. The male inflorescences consist of 2 to 24 blooms. The involucre is 2-lobed and fused to a tube. The fruit is a red, berrylike false fruit formed from the upper bract.

Leaves, Stem, and Root: The plant is a 30 cm tall lightly branched subshrub with lengthened, cylindrical branches that are 1 to 2 mm in diameter. It is similar in appearance to Horsetail, and is sometimes twining and often has underground runners. The stem and branches are round with numerous vertical grooves of gray-green or bright green coloring. Very small leaves are occasionally reduced to pointed scales and are almost always fused at the base to form a sheath. They are reddish brown.

Habitat: Ephedra sinica grows mainly in Mongolia and the bordering area of China; *Ephedra gerardiana* is from India.

Production: Ma Huang consists of the dried, young branchlets, harvested in the fall, of *Ephedra sinica, Ephedra shennungiana,* or other equivalent Ephedra species. It is mostly cultivated. The plant is harvested as late as possible after the last rain, but before the winter frost and is air-dried in the sun.

Not to be Confused With: Many similar species

Other Names: Desert Herb, Ephedrine

ACTIONS AND PHARMACOLOGY

COMPOUNDS

Alkaloids of the 2-aminophenylpropane type: main alkaloids L-(-)-ephedrine (1R,2S-(-)- ephedrine) and D-pseudoephedrine (1S,2S-(+)- ephedrine); lesser alkaloids L-norephedrine, D-norpseudoephedrine.

EFFECTS

The primary active constituent of Ma Huang is ephedrine. Ephedrine is a known sympathomimetic alkaloid with alpha-1, beta-1, and beta-2 receptor-agonist properties. It produces vasoconstriction, cardiac stimulation, acute increases in blood pressure, tachycardia, mydriasis, insomnia, vertigo, headache, and nervousness. Pseudoephedrine enhances beta-2-agonist activity including bronchodilation, but also has alpha-agonist activity that helps with nasal constriction (White et al, 1997).

Clinical trials demonstrated efficacy of Ma Huang or ephedrine in the treatment of asthma and obesity; the primary current applications of Ma Huang are in the treatment of asthma and hay fever, the common cold, and as a weight loss aid. The level of the active principles can fluctuate drastically. Ephedrine acts by indirectly stimulating the sympathomimetic and central nervous system. The herb is bacteriostatic, positively inotropic and positively chronotropic. In animal tests ephedrine acts as an antitussive. The effects of ephedrine result from stimulation of both alpha-adrenergic and beta-adrenergic. It exerts a direct effect on adrenergic receptors and an indirect action due to the release of norepinephrine. Ephedrine stimulates the central nervous system and increases blood pressure by vasoconstriction and increasing cardiac output. Stimulation of beta-adrenergic receptors in the lungs results in bronchodilation. Urinary retention occurs because of constriction of the sphincter muscle and relaxation of the urinary bladder wall receptors (Reynolds, 1999; Gilman et al, 1990). Stimulant alkaloids such as ephedrine and pseudoephedrine make up the major active ingredients, although methylephedrine, norephedrine, methylpseudoephedrine, methylbenzylamine, and norpseudoephedrine (also called cathine) may also be present (Gurley et al, 1998, Kalix, 1991).

Note: All dietary supplements containing ephedrine alkaloids (Ma huang, Ephedra, and epitonin) have been banned by the FDA (see Precautions and Adverse Reactions).

Antiviral Effects: Ma Huang has shown mild antiviral activity against polio virus (Kurokawa et al, 1993).

Blood Pressure Effects: In general Ma Huang products increase blood pressure after administration. A 50% methanolic extract derived from materials from the above ground portions of Ma Huang herb (200 mcg/mL) was shown, in vitro, to have a 98% inhibition of kidney angiotensin converting enzyme (ACE). The exact component responsible was thought to be tannins (Inokuchi et al, 1984).

Midodrine has been at least as effective as ephedrine when employed in the treatment of orthostatic hypotension (McTavish & Goa, 1989; Marini et al, 1984). Midodrine increased standing systolic and diastolic blood pressure to a greater degree than did ephedrine or placebo in a small, randomized, double-blind, crossover study (Fouad-Tarazi et al, 1995). Midodrine therapy was usually associated with decreases in heart rate, whereas significant increases in heart rate were seen with ephedrine and dimetofrine (McTavish & Goa, 1989; Marini et al, 1984). A similar efficacy would be expected if Ma Huang were substituted for the ephedrine; no studies exist to verify.

Diabetic Nephropathy Effects: Ephedrine has been effective in the treatment of diabetic neuropathy in several case reports, including diabetic neuropathic foot pain in a 55-year-old man (Wollersheim et al, 1989). Ephedrine was effective in the treatment of neuropathic edema in 4 insulin-dependent diabetic patients (Edmonds et al, 1983).

Ejaculatory Failure: Ephedrine has been reported to produce an increase in volume of ejaculate and an increase in motility of sperm in men with failure of emission secondary to retroperitoneal lymphadenectomy (Lynch & Maxted, 1983; Proctor & Howards, 1983).

Enzyme Inhibition Activity: In vitro experiments have found inhibition of the enzyme dopa oxidase activity of tyrosnase in the stems of *Ephedra sinica*. Mammalian tyrosinase catalyzes the reaction from tyrosine to dopa and oxidation of dopa to dopaquinone used in melanin synthesis. Inhibition may reduce skin darkening. A 100 mcg/mL Ephedra concentration produced a 9% inhibition (Shin et al, 1997).

Motion Sickness Effects: The use of ephedrine for the prevention of motion sickness has yielded mixed results. Ephedrine 25 mg every 6 hours did not improve the symptoms of motion sickness when given with scopolamine 0.3 mg every 6 hours in 28 healthy naval volunteers during 24 hours in life rafts (Tokola et al, 1984).

Respiratory Tract Effects: Ephedrine, in combination with other drugs, is used for the symptomatic relief of cough associated with respiratory tract conditions such as the common cold, bronchial asthma, or acute or chronic bronchitis (Prod Info Rynatuss®, 1997).

Stimulant Effects: Pharmacologic actions of ephedrine include elevation of systolic and diastolic blood pressure and increased pulse rate due to vasoconstriction and cardiac stimulation. Cardiac output and force of contraction is increased (McEvoy, 1999).

Effects on Urinary Hesitancy: Ephedrine stimulates both the alpha and beta-adrenaline-like receptors producing a relaxation of the urinary bladder muscles (Schuckit, 1996).

Weight-Loss Effects: Ephedrine inhibited gastric emptying in a double-blind study of 23 patients not on medication with no gastrointestinal complaints. This effect may increase satiety (Jonderko & Kucio, 1991). The FDA determined that the modest short-term weight loss provided by ephedrine alkaloids does not outweigh the risk of adverse events and therefore, banned all dietary supplements containing ephedrine alkaloids (FDA, 2004). In both human and animal studies, ephedrine has demonstrated an anorectic effect, promoting weight loss. Ma Huang is a significant source of ephedrine and is expected to have the same weight loss effect as ephedrine. Weight loss effects can be greatly enhanced when used in combination with methylxanthines such as caffeine and theophylline, as well as aspirin, which potentiates the action of ephedrine and other Ma Huang compounds; however, the combination of ephedrine and caffeine may cause cardiovascular adverse events and is not recommended.

CLINICAL TRIALS

Ma Huang is the common name for many of the Ephedra species. The primary active constituent of Ma Huang is ephedrine. While most of the pharmacokinetic information presented here came from Ma Huang, many of the clinical trials used ephedrine. Clinical trials that featured dosing other than oral were excluded from this monograph since Ma Huang has not been approved as an injectable. Ephedrine drug interactions were included due to the potential adverse reactions and interactions that may occur with the use of Ma Huang.

Blood Pressure/Heart Rate

A multicomponent dietary supplement containing ephedra and caffeine (DSEC) increased systolic blood pressure in a randomized, double-blind, placebo-controlled, crossover trial. Fifteen healthy subjects (mean age 27 years) were orally supplemented with one capsule Metabolife 356® (containing ephedra 12 mg, caffeine (40 mg), and 17 other unspecified components) or placebo with a 7-day washout period between treatments. Compared to baseline, the mean QTc (Bazetti) interval increased by 22 milliseconds for the DSEC group (p=0.03) and 3 milliseconds for placebo (p=0.69). Study findings should be cautiously interpreted as the actual ingredient or ingredients in Metabolife 345 are not known (McBride et al, 2004).

The effect of a dietary supplement containing herbal caffeine and ephedra (C&E) on metabolic rate, weight loss, body composition and safety parameters was investigated. In phase I, 12 healthy subjects with a BMI of 25 to 35 kg/m^2 had resting metabolic rate (RMR) measured for 2 hours after ingesting C&E or a placebo on two occasions 1 week apart, followed by a 1-week washout phase before phase II. In phase II, these 12 subjects, plus 28 additional subjects, were randomized to a 12-week, double-blind trial comparing C&E (three times/day) to placebo. In phase III, the C&E group was given open-label C&E for 3 months, and the placebo group was given C&E for 6 months. C&E increased the resting metabolic rate (RMR) significantly by 8% compared to placebo. Other parameters such as lipid levels and blood pressure did not change significantly. C&E was well tolerated (Greenway et al, 2004).

A randomized, double-blind cross-over study was designed to determine whether the consumption of an acute dose of caffeine and Ma Huang increases resting energy expenditure (REE), heart rate (HR), and blood pressure (BP) over a period of 3 hours. A total of 8 healthy subjects took part in the study. The combination of caffeine and herbal ephedra at doses of 150 mg and 20 mg, respectively, resulted in significant elevation of REE, HR and BP. Although significant, the increase in energy expenditure was negligible in terms of weight loss (Vukovich et al, 2005).

Short-term metabolic and hemodynamic effects of ephedra and guarana combinations were tested in a randomized, double-blind, three-arm crossover study. Sixteen healthy adults took two doses each of ephedra-guarana alone or placebo 5 hours apart. Compared to placebo the ephedra-guarana combination significantly increased heart rate (p=0.002), blood pressure (p=0.015), postprandial glucose concentration (p<0.0001), and insulin concentration (p=0.005), which could be detrimental in persons with hypertension, atherosclerosis, or glucose intolerance (Haller et al, 2005).

In a randomized, double-blind, 6-month study of safety and efficacy, small yet significant increases in heart rate occurred in healthy yet overweight men and women after the coadministration of an herbal supplement containing ephedra and kola nut extracts. Patients were given a walking program and a usual diet with controlled-fat intake in conjunction with placebo (n=84) or a combination regimen of Ma Huang (ephedra) 90 milligrams (mg) and kola nut (caffeine) 192 mg daily (n=83). Heart rate, but not blood pressure, showed significant increase at 6 months in association with herbal use compared with placebo (p<0.001). However, the number of patient study withdrawals prior to the end of the trial period appears to reduce the overall power of the study to detect significant change in the safety parameters of ventricular arrhythmia incidence, changes in systolic and diastolic blood pressure and changes in mean arterial pressure. Fourteen out of 15 subjects withdrawn from the study did so because of cardiovascular adverse effects. Usefulness of the study data is further impaired by the restriction of participants to a moderate exercise program (walking 30 minutes/day, 3 times weekly), thereby preventing the assessment of safety in the presence of greater cardiovascular stress normally associated with traditional programs of aerobic exercise (Boozer et al, 2002).

In an open-label, single-arm study, coadministration of ephedra and guarana significantly increased mean maximum change in heart rate and systolic blood pressure in healthy subjects (Haller et al, 2002).

Ma Huang increased heart rate and had variable effects on blood pressure in 12 healthy, normotensive subjects. Blood pressure effects varied in the 3 hours after Ma Huang administration. Four patients had statistically significant blood pressure increases, while two had statistically significant decreases. It was recommended that individuals using ephedrine-containing herbal formulas monitor their heart rate (pulse) and blood pressure and discontinue use if there is an increase in blood pressure or pulse above normal (White et al, 1997).

Weight Loss

In a randomized, double-blind, placebo controlled trial, 10 healthy volunteers given ephedrine (50 mg) or placebo 3 times daily demonstrated a 3.5% greater 24-hour total energy expenditure, not due to an increase in physical activity. The study lasted 21 days and energy expenditure was measured by Vanderbilt's Clinical Research Center in their activity-energy measurement system. Seven of the subjects reported adverse effects that included difficulty sleeping (n=5), increased or stronger heartbeat (n=4) or decreased appetite (n=3). Other reported side effects included skin tingling, coldness of hands and feet and mouth dryness. An increase in energy expenditure during the night with ephedrine was observed in all 10 subjects. This study did not address the long-term effect of ephedrine on weight reduction (Shannon et al, 1999).

The combination of ephedrine and caffeine attenuated the weight gain following smoking cessation in a double-blind, randomized, placebo-controlled study of 225 smokers. Subjects initially received ephedrine 20 milligrams (mg) and caffeine 200 mg three times a day for three months. The dose was tapered down to nothing by the last 3 months of the trial. A significantly higher incidence of side effects such as nausea, palpitations, sweating, dizziness, and difficulty falling asleep was seen in the ephedrine and caffeine group during the first three weeks of the trial. After that, the incidence of such side effects was the same between the ephedrine plus caffeine and the placebo groups (Norregaard et al, 1996).

INDICATIONS AND USAGE

Approved by Commission E:

■ Cough/bronchitis

US Food and Drug Administration labeled indications for over-the-counter ephedrine include treatment for asthma, allergies, nasal congestion, and related upper respiratory symptoms.

Unproven Uses: Ma Huang is used for diseases of the respiratory tract with mild bronchospasms in adults and children over the age of six. Various indications include asthma, cardiovascular stimulation, and as a CNS stimulant.

Chinese Medicine: The drug has been used for over 4,000 years for severe febrile illnesses, bronchial asthma, joint symptoms, inability to perspire, coughing with dyspnea, edema, and pains in the bones.

CONTRAINDICATIONS

Contraindications include diabetes, heart disease, high blood pressure, hypersensitivity to ephedrine or other sympathomimetic amines, hyperthyroidism, thyrotoxicosis, individuals younger than 18 years of age, anorexia, bulimia, states of anxiety and restlessness, insomnia, depression, suicidal tendencies, mental, emotional, or behavioral disorders, seizure disorders, stomach ulcers, pheochromocytoma, thyrotoxicosis, angle-closure glaucoma, cerebral perfusions, use before or during strenuous exercise, use with other stimulants, decongestion or diet aid medications containing sympathomimetics or caffeine, prostate adenoma with residual urine volume, and prostatic hypertrophy (FDA, 2003; Briggs et al, 1998; Brinker, 1998; Gurley et al, 1998; McGuffin et al, 1997).

Pregnancy: Not to be used during pregnancy.

Breastfeeding: Not to be used while breastfeeding.

PRECAUTIONS AND ADVERSE REACTIONS

Note: All dietary supplements containing ephedrine alkaloids (Ma Huang, Ephedra, and epitonin) are banned. The US Food and Drug Administration ruled that dietary supplements containing ephedrine alkaloids are adulterated because they present an unreasonable risk of injury. This ruling does not apply to either oral and topical over-the-counter ephedrine products or Ephedra preparations in traditional Asian medicine. The FDA's decision was based on well-known, scientifically established pharmacology of ephedrine alkaloids; peer-reviewed scientific literature on the effects of ephedrine alkaloids; and adverse event reports. FDA weighed their decision on the safety relative to the benefit of ephedra (FDA, 2004).

A number of severe side effects have been reported, though these are mostly in connection with nutritional supplements and not with medications. Common side effects include headache, dizziness, irritability, motor restlessness, sleeplessness, urinary disorders, nausea, vomiting, tachycardia, cardiac arrhythmia, myocardial infarction, hemorrhagic or ischemic stroke, seizures, and possibly death (Anon, 1996). Chronic use may cause an anxiety state.

Urinary retention secondary to ephedrine use is more commonly seen in males with prostatism.

Dependence can develop with extended intake. Because of the danger of the development of tachyphylaxis and of addiction, the drug should only be administered for short periods. A total of 140 adverse events associated with Ma Huang were reported to the United States FDA between June 1, 1997 and March 31, 1999. Hypertension was reported most frequently (17 reports), palpitations, tachycardia, or both were reported 13 times, stroke was reported 10 times, and seizures were reported 7 times. Ten deaths were reported, including 1 neonatal and 1 fetal death. Thirteen events resulted in permanent impairment (26% of the definite, probable, and possible cases). Forty-three cases were rated definitely or probably related (31%), 44 cases were rated possibly related (31%), 24 cases were rated unrelated (17%) and 29 cases did not have enough information to permit rating (21%) (Haller & Benowitz, 2000).

Cardiovascular: Myocardial infarction, myocarditis, severe hypertension, and lethal cardiac arrhythmias have been associated with the use of ephedrine and related alkaloids. The mechanisms of myocardial infarction and myocarditis appear to be those of constriction of coronary arteries and occasionally, vasospasm. Ephedrine can cause a predisposition to hemorrhagic and ischemic stroke (Haller & Benowitz, 2000). General cardiac effects of the ephedrine in Ma Huang include tachycardia, vasoconstriction, and palpitations (Nadir et al, 1996). Myocardial infarction has followed use of Ma Huang (Gurley et al, 1998). Between December 1993 and September 1995, the Department of Health in Texas received over 500 reports of adverse reactions to ephedrine, including deaths (Powell et al, 1998).

Central Nervous System: General central nervous system effects of the ephedrine in Ma Huang include insomnia, nervousness, heightened awareness, anxiety, and headache (Nadir et al, 1996; Schuckit, 1996). Case reports describe episodes of dizziness, acute headache and hypertension, and acute headache with left-sided weakness and numbness associated with ingestion of Ma Huang (Franklin et al, 1996). All symptoms resolved within a few hours.

Dependence: Nine women and 18 men with no drug use history were given doses of 37.5 to 75 mg of ephedrine and asked to score subjective effects. Scores for being "high" and for "euphoria" were given in 5 of the 27 subjects. The effects were less than that of amphetamines (Schuckit, 1996).

Psychosis: There have been over 20 cases of ephedrine psychosis reported, with wide variation in the dose necessary to produce the effect (Doyle & Kargin, 1996; Capwell, 1995). The average dose was 510 mg, range 125 to 2500 mg (Kalix, 1997; Whitehorse & Duncan, 1987). Eighty percent of the patients had taken the drug for at least one year, but the range was 3 days to 25 years. Ninety percent of these patients had auditory hallucinations, about half had visual hallucinations, and 50% to 67% developed delusions. Thirty percent had severe mood disturbances. Hallucinations cleared (in most cases) in 10 to 14 days when ephedrine was withdrawn (Schuckit, 1996).

Stroke: Three cases of stroke have been associated with excessive use of ephedrine (Schuckit, 1996).

DRUG INTERACTIONS:

Note: The drug interactions reported here are based on ephedrine and are included due to the potential ephedrine content present in Ma Huang.

CONTRAINDICATED

Isocarbixazid: Concurrent use may result in hypertensive crisis (headache, hyperpyrexia, hypertension). *Clinical management:* Sympathomimetic use in patients taking monoamine oxidase inhibitors (MAOIs) is contraindicated. If these drugs are used together, monitor blood pressure and ask the patient about frequent headaches or palpitations as these symptoms may be prodromes of a hypertensive crisis. If a hypertensive crisis occurs, discontinue the MAOI and institute therapy to lower blood pressure (5 mg of phentolamine intravenously given slowly).

Cyclopropane: Concurrent use may result in cardiac arrhythmias. *Clinical Management:* The administration of ephedrine to a patient receiving cyclopropane is contraindicated. The use of a pressor drug with less cardiac stimulating effects than ephedrine should be utilized in a patient who is receiving a myocardial sensitizing anesthetic.

Halothane: Concurrent use may result in cardiac arrhythmias. *Clinical Management:* The administration of ephedrine to a patient receiving a halogenated hydrocarbon such as halothane is contraindicated. The use of a pressor drug with less cardiac stimulating effects than ephedrine should be utilized in a patient who is receiving a myocardial sensitizing anesthetic.

Selegiline: Concurrent use may result in severe hypertension, hyperpyrexia, headache. *Clinical Management:* The concurrent use of selegiline and ephedrine is contraindicated. Allow 14 days to elapse between the discontinuation of selegiline and the initiation of ephedrine therapy or allow a minimum of 7 days to elapse between the discontinuation of the ephedrine and the initiation of therapy with selegiline.

Rasagiline: Concurrent use may result in severe hypertension, hyperpyrexia, headache. *Clinical Management*: The concurrent use of rasagiline and ephedrine is contraindicated. Allow 14 days to elapse between the discontinuation of rasagiline and the initiation of ephedrine.

MAJOR RISK

Iproniazid: Concurrent use may result in hypertensive crisis (headache, hyperpyrexia, hypertension). *Clinical Management*: Do not use ephedrine in patients taking monoamine oxidase inhibitors (MAOIs), or for 14 days after the discontinuation of the MAOI. If these drugs are used together, monitor blood pressure and ask the patient about frequent headaches or palpitations as these symptoms may be prodromes of a hypertensive crisis. If a hypertensive crisis occurs discontinue the MAOI and institute therapy to lower blood pressure (5 mg of phentolamine intravenously given slowly).

Monoamine Oxidase Inhibitors (MAOIs): The German Commission E recommends avoiding combining Ma Huang and monoamine oxidase inhibitors (MAOIs). Coadministration of indirect-acting sympathomimetics such as pseudoephedrine and phenylpropanolamine with MAOIs has resulted in severe hypertension (Smookler & Bermudez, 1982) and one case has been reported of severe agitation, tachycardia, hypotension, and fever with concomitant use of ephedrine and a MAOI (Dawson et al, 1995). Patients who take MAOIs with Ma Huang may be predisposed to hypertensive crisis and other symptoms consistent with excessive sympathomimetic amine activity. Other potential reactions include cardiac arrhythmias, chest pain, hyperpyrexia, and death. *Clinical Management:* Avoid concomitant use.

Procarbazine: Concurrent use may result in hypertensive crisis (headache, hyperpyrexia, hypertension). *Clinical Management*: Do not use ephedrine in patients taking monoamine oxidase inhibitors (MAOIs), or for 14 days after the discontinuation of the MAOI. If these drugs are used together, monitor blood pressure and ask the patient about frequent headaches or palpitations as these symptoms may be prodromes of a hypertensive crisis. If a hypertensive crisis occurs discontinue the MAOI and institute therapy to lower blood pressure (5 mg of phentolamine intravenously given slowly).

Pargyline: Concurrent use may result in hypertensive crisis (headache, hyperpyrexia, hypertension). *Clinical Management*: Do not use ephedrine in patients taking monoamine oxidase inhibitors (MAOIs), or for 14 days after the discontinuation of the MAOI. If these drugs are used together, monitor blood pressure and ask the patient about frequent headaches or palpitations as these symptoms may be prodromes of a hypertensive crisis. If a hypertensive crisis occurs, discontinue the MAOI and institute therapy to lower blood pressure (5 mg of phentolamine intravenously given slowly).

Nialamide: Concurrent use may result in severe hypertension, hyperpyrexia, headache. *Clinical Management:* Do not use ephedrine in patients taking monoamine oxidase inhibitors (MAOIs), or for 14 days after the discontinuation of the MAOI. If these drugs are used together, monitor blood pressure and ask the patient about frequent headaches or palpitations as these symptoms may be prodromes of a hypertensive crisis. If a hypertensive crisis occurs discontinue the MAOI and institute therapy to lower blood pressure (5 mg of phentolamine intravenously given slowly).

Furazolidine: Concurrent use may result in hypertensive crisis (headache, hyperpyrexia, hypertension). *Clinical Management*: Avoid concurrent use. If these drugs are used together, monitor blood pressure and ask the patient about frequent headaches or palpitations as these symptoms may be a prodrome of a hypertensive crisis. If a hypertensive crisis occurs discontinue the MAOI and institute therapy to lower blood pressure.

Tranlycypromine: Concurrent use may result in hypertensive crisis (headache, hyperpyrexia, hypertension). *Clinical Management*: Do not use ephedrine in patients taking monoamine oxidase inhibitors (MAOIs), or for 14 days after the discontinuation of the MAOI. If these drugs are used together, monitor blood pressure and ask the patient about frequent headaches or palpitations as these symptoms may be prodromes of a hypertensive crisis. If a hypertensive crisis occurs, discontinue the MAOI and institute therapy to lower blood pressure (5 mg of phentolamine intravenously given slowly).

Midodrine: Concurrent use may result in an enhanced pressor effect of midodrine. *Clinical Management*: Due to a marked increase in pressor response and potential for adverse effects, concomitant use should be done with caution and only with careful monitoring of blood

Phenelzine: Concurrent use may result in hypertensive crisis (headache, hyperpyrexia, hypertension). *Clinical Management*: Do not use ephedrine in patients taking monoamine oxidase inhibitors (MAOIs), or for 14 days after the discontinuation of the MAOI. If these drugs are used together, monitor blood pressure and ask the patient about frequent headaches or palpitations as these symptoms may be prodromes of a hypertensive crisis. If a hypertensive crisis occurs, discontinue the MAOI and institute therapy to lower blood pressure (5 mg of phentolamine intravenously given slowly).

Clorgyline: Concurrent use may result in hypertensive crisis (headache, hyperpyrexia, hypertension). *Clinical Management*: Do not use ephedrine in patients taking monoamine oxidase inhibitors (MAOIs), or for 14 days after the discontinuation of the MAOI. If these drugs are used together, monitor blood pressure and ask the patient about frequent headaches or palpitations as these symptoms may be prodromes of a hypertensive crisis. If a hypertensive crisis occurs, discontinue the MAOI and institute therapy to lower blood pressure (5 mg of phentolamine intravenously given slowly).

MODERATE RISK

Guanethidine: Concurrent use may result in decreased guanethidine effectiveness. *Clinical Management*: Monitor blood pressure for decreased control of hypertension.

Iobenguane 1-131: Concurrent use may result in false-negative results of scintigraphy. *Clinical Management*: Ephedrine should be discontinued prior to any procedures using iobenguane I-131.

Bethanidine: Concurrent use may result in decreased bethanidine effectiveness. *Clinical Management*: If ephedrine is administered concomitantly with bethanidine, monitor blood pressure closely to detect any loss of antihypertensive effect of bethanidine.

Theophylline: Concurrent use may result in an increased risk or severity of side effects (nausea, nervousness, insomnia). *Clinical Management*: Monitor for gastrointestinal and central nervous system adverse effects.

Sodium Bicarbonate and other Antacids: The renal elimination of ephedrine and pseudoephedrine are urinary pH-dependent. By increasing the urinary pH above 7.5 the renal elimination of either drug may decrease by more than 50%. If the urine remains alkaline for more than 1 to 2 days increased ephedrine toxicity may be observed (Brater et al, 1980). Concurrent use may result in ephedrine toxicity (hypertension, tachycardia). *Clinical Management*: Monitor for possible ephedrine toxicity (eg, hypertension and tachycardia) and decrease the dose as needed. Patients on ephedrine who frequently require a urinary alkalinizer may need the dose of both drugs to be decreased.

POTENTIAL INTERACTIONS

Acetazolamide: Acetazolamide may cause increased serum concentrations of ephedrine due to alkalinization of the urine (Wilkinson & Beckett, 1968). *Clinical Management:* The dose of ephedrine may need to be adjusted in patients receiving acetazolamide.

Antihypertensives: Ma Huang may decrease the effectiveness of antihypertensive medications (White et al, 1997). *Clinical Management*: Ephedrine should be avoided by patients with hypertension.

Cardiac heart glycosides or halothane: Potential disturbance of heart rhythm with concomitant use. *Clinical Management*: Avoid concomitant use.

Clonidine: Pretreatment with clonidine augmented the pressor response to ephedrine (Nishikawa et al, 1991). *Clinical Management*: Use caution if Ma Huang and clonidine are used concomitantly.

Corticosteroids: Ephedrine increased the half-life and metabolic clearance rate of dexamethasone in asthmatic patients (Brooks et al, 1977). *Clinical Management:* The ephedrine content of Ma Huang may increase metabolism of corticosteroids, resulting in lower blood levels. Dose requirements of corticosteroids may be increased in patients requiring corticosteroids for asthma control or immunosuppression.

Dichlorphenamide: Dichlorphenamide alkalinizes the urine. Therefore, the elimination of ephedrine will be decreased, which may lead to an enhanced pharmacologic action of this agent. *Clinical Management*: Avoid concomitant use.

Digoxin: Theoretically, ephedrine could lead to cardiac arrhythmia if taken with digoxin. *Clinical Management*: Avoid concomitant use.

Guarana: Hypertension, stroke, seizures, and fatal cardiac arrhythmia have occurred in previously asymptomatic persons following ingestion of dietary supplements containing guarana and ephedra. The primary pharmacologically active ingredient of guarana is caffeine. Caffeine appears to interact with ephedra in additive fashion, rendering vulnerable patients more at risk for cardiovascular adverse effects (FDA, 2003). In an open-label study of healthy adults, coadministration of ephedra and guarana significantly increased mean maximum change in heart rate and systolic blood pressure, compared with baseline (Haller et al, 2002). In a series of three case reports on previously healthy adults, intracranial hemorrhages and fatal cardiac arrhythmia have occurred following the ingestion of dietary supplements containing a combination of ephedra and guarana. Seizure during weight lifting exercise occurred in a fourth patient who ingested ephedra and caffeine; however, he had also ingested a therapeutic regimen of multiple sympathomimetic asthma medications in the days preceding the seizure (Haller & Benowitz, 2000). *Clinical Management:* Patients should be advised to avoid concomitant use of ephedra (Ma Huang) and guarana.

Halogenated Anesthetics: Cyclopropane sensitizes the myocardium and may induce cardiac arrhythmias in the presence of ephedrine (Prod Info Ephedrine, 1997). *Clinical Management*: Avoid concomitant administration. The use of a pressor drug with less cardiac stimulating effects than ephedrine should be utilized in a patient who is receiving a myocardial sensitizing anesthetic.

Nonsteroidal Anti-inflammatory Agents: Data suggests that concurrent use of ephedra with loxoprofen increases the incidence and severity of gastric lesions in mice. Until human studies are performed, caution is advised when using these two substances concomitantly (Cho et al, 2002). *Clinical Management:* Patients using Ma Huang concurrently with nonsteroidal anti-inflammatory agents should be monitored for the development of gastric lesions.

Oxilofrine: Concurrent administration of oxilofrine and other sympathomimetic agents enhances the sympathomimetic effects of oxilofrine in an additive manner. *Clinical Management:* Caution is warranted when oxilofrine and other sympathomimetics are coadministered. Should concomitant use of these agents be needed, closely monitor patient blood pressure and heart rate and adjust doses accordingly.

Phenylpropanolamine: A case of the combination of pseudoephedrine and phenylpropanolamine likely leading to ventricular arrythmia and presyncope has been reported in a pregnant woman (Onuigbo & Alikhan, 1998). *Clinical Management:* Concomitant use of Ma Huang and phenylpropanolomine should be avoided, as it may lead to excessive adrenergic stimulation, which may increase blood pressure, heart rate, and the risk of cardiac arrhythmia.

Pseudoephedrine: Ma Huang is a source of pseudoephedrine and ephedrine. *Clinical Management:* Concomitant use of Ma Huang and pseudoephedrine should be avoided, as it may lead to excessive adrenergic stimulation, which may increase blood pressure, heart rate, and the risk of cardiac arrhythmia.

Reserpine: Concomitant ephedrine and reserpine therapy has been reported to result in a decrease in the effectiveness of ephedrine due to the depletion of norepinephrine by reserpine (Hansten & Horn, 1990). Patients receiving reserpine may have a diminished response to ephedrine.

Secale alkaloid derivatives or oxytocin: Development of high blood pressure. *Clinical Management:* Avoid concomitant use.

DRUG-FOOD INTERACTIONS

Caffeine – Concomitant use of Ma Huang and caffeine may lead to excessive adrenergic stimulation, which may increase blood pressure, heart rate, and risk of cardiac arrhythmia or stroke. *Clinical Management:* Patients should be advised to avoid concomitant use of ephedra and caffeine-containing agents such as kola nut. Close medical supervision is recommended if Ma Huang (ephedra) and caffeine are used together. Baseline assessment of cardiovascular risk is recommended. Patients at risk for, or who currently have cardiovascular or cerebrovascular disease should not use Ma Huang.

DRUG-LAB MODIFICATIONS

Amphetamine Assay: Several over-the-counter and prescription drugs can interfere with the EMIT assay for amphetamines. These include ephedrine, phenylpropanolamine, pseudoephedrine, phenmetrazine, and phentermine (high doses). Their recent use should be ruled out when test results are positive. *Clinical Management:* When screening for amphetamines using the EMIT assay, recent use of ephedrine should be ruled out when test results are positive.

OVERDOSAGE

Life-threatening poisonings are seen with very high dosages of the drug (over 100 g, lethal dosage with oral administration corresponding to approximately 1 to 2 g L-ephedrine). Symptoms of poisoning include severe outbreaks of sweating, enlarged pupils, spasms and elevated body temperature. Death following overdose is due to heart failure and asphyxiation. Following stomach emptying (gastric lavage with burgundy-colored potassium permaganate solution), therapy consists of the administration of activated charcoal and prophylaxis against shock. Spasms should be treated with diazepam, electrolyte substitution should be employed, and sodium bicarbonate infusions should be used to prevent acidosis. Intubation and oxygen respiration are also on occasion necessary.

DOSAGE

Mode of Administration: Ma Huang is administered as a comminuted herb, as well as other galenic preparations for internal use. The optimum dosage of Ma Huang depends on the alkaloid content in the form used. Standardized preparations are often preferred as they have more dependable therapeutic activity. However, even with products containing standardized doses of Ephedra, there are a number of prescribed agents that are safer and more effective. With neither efficacy nor safety advantages, there is currently no logical reason to use Ma Huang-containing products.

LITERATURE

Anon. Bundesverband der Pharmazeutischen Industrie e.V. Rote Liste. Editio Cantor, Aulendorf, Germany, 1994.

Anon. Therapeutic conferences. Drug Interactions. *BMJ*; 1:389. 1971.

Anon. United States Food and Drug Administration (FDA): Dietary supplements containing ephedrine alkaloids; reopening of the comment period. Rockville, Maryland: Docket No. 95N-0304. February 2002. Accessed at http://www.fda.gov/ohrms/dockets/ (cited 01/05/2004).

Anon. Warning issued about street drugs containing botanical sources of ephedrine. *JAMA*; 275:1533-1534. 1996.

Audicana M, Urrutia I, Echechipia S et al. Sensitization to ephedrine in oral anticatarrhal drugs. *Contact Dermatitis*; 24(3):223. 1991.

Ault A. FDA proposes limits on ephedrine supplements. *Lancet*; 349:1753. 1997.

Bierman CW, Pierson WE & Shapiro GG. Exercise-induced asthma: pharmacological assessment of single drugs and drug combinations. *JAMA*; 234:295-298. 1975.

Boozer CN, Daly PA, Homel P et al. Herbal ephedra/caffeine for weight loss: a 6-month randomized safety and efficacy trial. *Int J Obes Relat Metab Disord*; 26(5):593-604. 2002.

Borum ML. Fulminant exacerbation of autoimmune hepatitis after the use of ma huang. *Am J Gastroenterol*; 96(5):1654-6555. 2001.

Brater DC, Kaojarern S, Benet LZ et al. Renal excretion of pseudoephedrine. *Clin Pharmacol Ther*; 28:690-694. 1980.

Capwell RR. Ephedrine-induced mania from an herbal diet supplement. *Am J Psychiatry*; 152:647. 1995.

Cho S, Hong T, Jin GB et al. The combination therapy of ephedra herb and loxoprofen caused gastric lesions in mice. *Am J Chin Med*;30(4):571-7. 2002.

Chua SS & Benrimoj SI. Non-prescription sympathomimetic agents and hypertension. *Med Toxicol Adverse Drug Exp;* 3:387-417. 1988.

Cuthbert MF, Greenberg MP & Morley SW. Cough and cold remedies: a potential danger to patients on monoamine oxidase inhibitors. *BMJ*; 1:404-406. 1969.

Dawson JK, Earnshaw SM & Graham CS. Dangerous monoamine oxidase interactions are still occurring in the 1990s. *J Accid Emerg Med*; 12(1):49-51. 1995.

Doyle H & Kargin M. Herbal stimulant containing ephedrine has also caused psychosis (letter). *BMJ*; 313:756. 1996.

Edmonds ME, Archer AG & Watkins PJ. Ephedrine: a new treatment for diabetic neuropathic oedema. *Lancet*; 1:548-551. 1983.

FDA. Final rule declaring dietary supplements containing ephedrine alkaloids adulterated because they present an unreasonable risk. Federal Register Docket No. 1995N-0304. February 11, 2004. Accessed at http://www.fda.gov/OHRMS/DOCKETS/98fr/1995n-0304-nfr00 1.pdf (cited 02/13/2004).

FDA. Proposed labeling changes. Federal Register Docket No 95N-0304. February 28, 2003. Accessed at http://www.fda.gov/ohrms/dockets/ (cited 01/05/2003).

Fouad-Tarazi FM, Okabe M & Goren H. Alpha sympathomimetic treatment of autonomic insufficiency with orthostatic hypotension. *Am J Med*; 99:604-610. 1995.

Franklin GM, Pace S & Love IA. Acute neurologic events associated with ingestion of Ma Huang (Ephdera). *Neurology*; 46:A282-A283. 1996.

Gazaliev AM, Fazilov SD, Zhurinov MZ, *Khim Prorod Soed* 23:862-864. 1987.

Goldberg LI. Monoamine oxidase inhibitors: adverse reactions and possible mechanisms. *JAMA*; 190:456-462. 1964.

Greenway FL, De Jonge L, Blanchard D, et al. Effect of a dietary herbal supplement containing caffeine and ephedra on weight, metabolic rate, and body compostion. Obes Res; 12(7): 1152-1157. 2004.

Gulati OD, Dave BT, Gokhale SD et al. Antagonism of adrenergic neuron blockade in hypertensive subjects. *Clin Pharmacol Ther*; 7:510-514. 1966.

Gurley BJ, Gardener SF, White LM et al. Ephedrine pharmacokinetics after the ingestion of nutritional supplements containing *Ephedra sinica* (Ma Huang). *Ther Drug Monit;* 20:439-445. 1998a.

Gurley BJ, Wang P & Gardner SF. Ephedrine-type alkaloid content of nutritional supplements containing Ephedra sinica (Ma-huang) as determined by high performance liquid chromatography. *J Pharm Sci*; 87(12):1547-1553. 1998b.

Haller CA, Jacob P, Benowitz NL. Short-term metabolic and hemodynamic effects of ephedra and guarana combinations. Clin Pharmacol Ther; 77(6): 560-571. 2005.

Haller CA & Benowitz NL. Adverse cardiovascular and central nervous system events associated with dietary supplements containing ephedra alkaloids. *N Engl J Med*; 343(25):1833-1838. 2000.

Haller CA, Jacob III, P & Benowitz NL. Pharmacology of ephedra alkaloids and caffeine after single-dose dietary supplement use. *Clin Pharmacol Ther*; 71:421-432. 2002.

Harada M, Nishimura M, *J Pharm Dyn* 4:691-699. 1981.

Herridge CF & a'Brook MF. Ephedrine psychosis. *BMJ*; 2:160. 1968.

Horler AR & Wynne NA. Hypertensive crisis due to pargyline and metaraminol. *BMJ*; 2:460-461. 1965.

Horton TJ & Geissler CA. Aspirin potentiates the effect of ephedrine on the thermogenic response to a meal in obese but not lean women. *Int J Obes*; 15(5):359-66. 1991.

Inokuchi J-I, Okabe H, Yamauchi T et al. Inhibitors of angiotensin converting enzyme in crude drugs. *Chem Pharm Bull*; 32:3615-3619. 1984.

Jonderko K & Kucio C. Effect of anti-obesity drugs promoting energy expenditure, yohimbine and ephedrine, on gastric emptying in obese patient. Aliment Pharmacol Ther; 5(4):413-418. 1991.

Kalix P. The pharmacology of psychoactive alkaloids from Ephedra and Catha species. *J Ethnopharmacol*; 32:201-208. 1991.

Khafagi FA, Shapiro B, Fig LM et al. Labetalol reduces iodine-131 MIGB uptake by pheochromocytoma and normal tissues. *J Nucl Med*; 30:481-489. 1989.

Kurokawa M, Ochiai H, Nagasaka K et al. Antiviral traditional medicines against herpes simplex virus (HSV-1), poliovirus, and measles virus in vitro and their therapeutic efficacies for HSV-1 infection in mice. Antivir Res; 22:175-188. 1993.

Lynch JH & Maxted WC. Use of ephedrine in post-lymphadenectomy ejaculatory failure: a case report. *J Urol;* 129:379. 1983.

Marini U, Cecchi A & Venturini M. Controlled clinical investigation of dimetophrine versus midodrine in the management of moderately decreased arterial blood pressure. *Curr Med Res Opin;* 9:265-274. 1984.

McBride B, Karapanos A, Krudysz A et al. Electrocardiographic and hemodynamic effects of a multicomponent dietary supplement containing ephedra and caffeine. *JAMA*; 291(2):216-221. 2004.

McTavish D & Goa KL. Midodrine: a review of its pharmacological properties and therapeutic use in orthostatic hypotension and secondary hypotensive disorders. *Drugs*; 38:757-777. 1989.

Misage JR & McDonald RH Jr. Antagonism of hypotensive action of bethanidine by ''common cold'' remedy. *BMJ*; 4:347. 1970.

MMWR. Adverse Events Associated with Ephedrine-Containing Products – Texas, December 1993-September 1995. MMWR weekly August 16, 1996 (cited 1/26/99). Accessed at: http://www.cdc.gov/epo/mmwr/preview/mmwrhtml/ 00056277.htm.

Molnar D: Effects of ephedrine and aminophylline on resting energy expenditure in obese adolescents. *Int J Obes*; 17(suppl 1):S49-52. 1993.

Nadir A, Agrawal S, King PD et al: Acute hepatitis associated with the use of a Chinese herbal product, Ma Huang. *Am J Gastroenterol*; 91:1436-1438. 1996.

Nishikawa T, Kimura T, Taguchi N et al. Oral clonidine preanesthetic medication augments the pressor responses to intravenous ephedrine in awake or anesthetized patients. *Anesthesiology*; 74:705-710. 1991.

Norregaard J, Jorgensen S, Mikkelsen K et al. The effect of ephedrine plus caffeine on smoking cessation and postcessation weight gain. *Clin Pharmacol Ther*; 60:679-686. 1996.

Onuigbo M & Alikhan M. Over-the-counter sympathomimetics: A risk factor for cardiac arrhythmias in pregnancy. *South Med J*; 91(12):1153-1155. 1998.

Pentel P. Toxicity of over-the-counter stimulants. *JAMA*; 252:1898-1903. 1984.

Personal Communication. Leslie Hendeles, PharmD. University of Florida, Gainesville, FL, June 1, 1994.

Powell T, Hsu FF, Turk J et al. Ma-huang strikes again: ephedrine nephrolithiasis. *Am J Kidney Dis*; 153-159. 1998.

Proctor KG & Howards SS. The effect of sympathomimetic drugs on post-lymphadenectomy aspermia. *J Urol*; 129:837. 1983.

Product Information. Ephedrine sulfate injection USP. Abbott Hospital Products, North Chicago, IL, USA, 1997.

Product Information. I-131 MIGB®, iobenguane sulfate I-131 injection. CIS-US, Inc, Bedford, MA, USA, 1994.

Product Information. ProAmatine, midodrine tablets. Roberts Laboratories, Inc, Eatontown, NJ, USA, 1996.

Product Information. Rynatuss®, carbapentane, chlorpheniramine, ephedrine, and phenylephrine. Physician's Desk Reference (electronic version), Micromedex, Inc, Englewood, CO, USA, 1997.

Reynolds JEF (ed). Martindale: The Extra Pharmacopoeia (electronic version). Micromedex, Inc, Englewood, CO, USA, 1999.

Schuckit MA. Ma-huang (ephedrine) abuse and dependence. *Drug Abuse Alcohol Newsletter*; 25:1-4. 1996.

Schweinfurth J, Pribitkin E. Sudden hearing loss associated with ephedra use. *Am J Health Syst Pharm.* Feb 15;60(4):375-377. 2003.

Shin N-H, Lee KS, Kang S-H et al. Inhibitory effects of herbal extracts on dopa oxidase activity of tyrosinase. *Nat Prod Sci*; 3:111-121. 1997.

Shucard DW, Spector SL, Euwer RL et al. Central nervous system effects of antiasthma medication - an EEG study. *Ann Allergy*; 54:177-184. 1985.

Sill V, Voelkel N, Lanser K et al. Bronchospasmolysis with atrovent. *Munch Med Wochenschr*; 118:177-180. 1976.

Smookler S & Bermudez AJ. Hypertensive crisis resulting from an MAO inhibitor and an over-the-counter appetite suppressant. *Ann Emerg* Med; 11:482-484. 1982.

Theoharides TC. Sudden death of a healthy college student related to ephedrine toxicity from a ma huang-containing drink. *J Clin Psychopharmacol.* Oct;17(5):437-439. 1997.

Tinkelman DG & Avner SE. Ephedrine therapy in asthmatic children: clinical tolerance and absence of side effects. *JAMA*; 237:553. 1977.

Tokola O, Laitinen LA, Aho J et al: Drug treatment of motion sickness: scopolamine alone and combined with ephedrine in real and simulated situations. *Aviat Space Environ Med*; 55:636-641. 1984.

Tormey WP & Bruzzi A: Acute psychosis due to the interaction of legal compounds - ephedra alkaloids in ''Vigueur Fit'' tablets, caffeine in ''Red Bull'' and alcohol. *Med Sci Law*; 41(4):331-336. 2001.

Toubro S, Astrup A, Breum L et al: Safety and efficacy of long-term treatment with ephedrine, caffeine and an ephedrine/caffeine mixture. Int J Obes; 17(suppl 1):S69-72. 1993.

Tricker AR, Wacker CD & Preussmann R: 2-(N-nitroso-N-methylamino) propiophenone, a direct acting bacterial mutagen found in nitrosated Ephedra altissima tea. *Toxicol Lett*; 38(1-2):45-50. 1987.

Vahedi K, Domigo V, Amerenco P et al: Ischaemic stroke in a sportsman who consumed MA HUANG extract and creatine monohydrate for body building. *J Neurol Neurosurg Psychiatry*; 68(1):112-113. 2000.

Van Mieghem W, Stevens E & Cosemans J: Ephedrine-induced cardiopathy. *BMJ*; 1:816. 1978.

Vukovich MD, Schoorman R, Heilman C, et al. Caffeine-herbal ephedra increases resting energy expenditure, heart rate and blood pressure. Clin Exp Pharmacol Physiol; 32(1-2): 47-53. 2005.

Weinberger M, Bronsky E, Bensch GW et al: Interaction of ephedrine and theophylline. *Clin Pharmacol Ther*; 17:585-592. 1975.

White LM, Gardner SF, Gurley BJ et al: Pharmacokinetics and cardiovascular effects of ma-huang (Ephedra sinica) in normotensive adults. *J Clin Pharmacol*; 37:116-112. 1997.

Wilkinson GR & Beckett AH: Absorption, metabolism and excretion of the ephedrines in man, I. The influence of urinary pH & urine volume output. *J Pharmacol Exp Ther*; 162:139-147. 1968.

Wollersheim H, Netten PM, Lutterman JA et al: Ephedrine improves microcirculation in the diabetic neuropathic foot. *Angiology*; 40:1030-1034. 1989.

Xue-jun Y, De-xiang L, Hechuan W et al: A study on the mutagenicity of 102 raw pharmaceuticals used in Chinese traditional medicine. *Mutat Res*; 260:73-82. 1991.

Zahn KA, Li RL & Purssel RA: Cardiovascular toxicity after ingestion of "herbal ecstacy." *J Emerg Med*; 17:289-291. 1999.

Maidenhair

Adiantum capillus-veneris

DESCRIPTION

Medicinal Parts: The dried fronds (Maidenhair) are used as a drug as well the dried herb with rhizome and roots (Maidenhair with roots).

Flower and Fruit: There are lumps of sporangia without a veil on the underside of the lateral lobes. The sporangia are square to reniform and later, dark brown.

Leaves, Stem, and Root: Maidenhair is a hardy, up to 35 cm high plant with an aromatic lily fragrance. It has a creeping rhizome. The leaves are double-rowed, tender, glabrous, and grow up to 50 cm long. They have a glossy black petiole and are covered with hairs at the base. The leaf-blade is ovate to oblong-ovate. The leaflets are light-green and periolate. The pinnules have hairlike petioles. The veins of the sterile pinna terminate in teeth at the edge of the leaf.

Habitat: Southern Europe, Atlantic coast as far as Ireland, from the south to the southern Alpine valleys (Tessin, southern Tyrol).

Production: Maidenhair fern, which is gathered in June and dried, is the frond of *Adiantum capillus-veneris*.

Not to be Confused With: It has sometimes been observed that the drug has been made impure by an addition of bracken leaf fronds (*Pteridium aquilinum*).

Other Names: Five-Finger Fern, Hair of Venus, Maiden Fern, Rock Fern, Venus Hair

ACTIONS AND PHARMACOLOGY

COMPOUNDS

Flavonoids

Proanthocyanidins

Hydroxycinnamic acid ester

EFFECTS

The drug is an expectorant, beneficial in bringing up phlegm, and a demulcent.

INDICATIONS AND USAGE

Unproven Uses: In the middle ages, the drug was used for various illnesses of the respiratory tract, in the form of so-called pectoral teas and as a syrup for severe coughs. Because of its similarity to hair, the drug was used to treat a lack of hair growth and to promote dark hair color.

It is still taken as an infusion in Spain, Belgium, and the Canary Islands to treat bronchitis, coughs, and whooping cough, and also for painful and excessive menstruation.

PRECAUTIONS AND ADVERSE REACTIONS

General: No health hazards or side effects are known in conjunction with the proper administration of designated therapeutic dosages.

Pregnancy: Not to be used during pregnancy

DOSAGE

Mode of Administration: The drug is taken internally as a tea prepared from the ground or powdered drug.

Daily Dosage: The standard single dose is 1.5 g of the drug to 1 cup of liquid per dose (average single dose)

Storage: Protect from light.

LITERATURE

Alwan AH, Al-Gaillany AS, Naji A. Inhibition of the Binding of 3H-Benzo(alpha)pyrene to Rat Liver Microsomal Protein by Plant Extracts. *Int J Crude Drug Res.* 27; 33-37. 1989

Cooper-Driver G, Swain T. *Bot J Linn Soc* 74:1-21. 1977.

Mahmoud MJ, Jawad ALM, Hussain AM, Al-Omari M, Al-Naib A. In vitro Antimicrobial Activity of *Salsola rosmarinus* and *Adianthum capillus-veneris. Int J Crude Drug Res.* 27 (1); 14-16. 1989

Twaij HAA et al. *Indian J Pharmacol* 17(1):73. 1985

Malabar Nut

Justicia adhatoda

DESCRIPTION

Medicinal Parts: The medicinal parts are the dried foliage leaves, the flower collected in the flowering season, the dried bark of the trunk, branches and roots, and the fresh leaves.

Flower and Fruit: The flowers are in dense, 2.5 to 7.5 cm long peduncled, axillary spikes. The bracts are elliptical, and the bracteoles are oblong-lanceolate. The calyx is 1.5 cm long, glabrous or black pubescent, with 5 sections containing regular lanceolate segments. The corolla is white with red-to-purple bands. The corolla tube is 1.3 cm long and is cylindrical and pubescent inside the lower half. The upper lip is convexly domed. The anthers are arrow-shaped and sometimes spurred at the base. The ovary is bivalvular with a 2-lobed stigma. The fruit is a 4-seeded, short-haired, longitudinally grooved capsule. The seeds are orbicular, glabrous, slightly bumpy-warty, and 5 to 7 mm across.

Leaves, Stem, and Root: The plant is an evergreen, unpleasant-smelling shrub 2.5 m high with numerous, usually opposite, branches. The bark is yellow. The leaves are 8 to 25 cm long, 2.5 to 8 cm wide, short-stalked, opposite, lanceolate-to-elliptical, tapering to an acute apex with entire margins. The leaf blade and petiole are finely pubescent.

Characteristics: The taste is bitter and the odor tea-like.

Habitat: Originally indigenous to northern India, the plant is now found in all the areas of Ayurveda medicine in India, Sri Lanka, and the Maylan archipelago.

Production: Vasaca leaves are the leaves of *Justicia adhatoda.*

Other Names: Arusa, Adulsa

ACTIONS AND PHARMACOLOGY

COMPOUNDS

Quinazoline alkaloids: including vasicine and vasicinone

Volatile oil

EFFECTS

Mildly spasmolytic, bronchodilatory, and expectorant

INDICATIONS AND USAGE

Unproven Uses: For acute and chronic bronchial infections, catarrh of the upper respiratory tract and tuberculosis, as an expectorant and to alleviate coughs.

Homeopathic Uses: Justicia adhatoda preparations are used for hay fever and acute inflammation of the upper respiratory tract.

CONTRAINDICATIONS

The drug is contraindicated in pregnancy.

PRECAUTIONS AND ADVERSE REACTIONS

General: No health hazards or side effects are known in conjunction with the proper administration of designated therapeutic dosages. Because of the vasicin content, the administration of large dosages can lead to excitatory states.

Pregnancy: Administration during pregnancy is to be avoided.

DOSAGE

Mode of Administration: Today, the extract of the leaves is only found in some combination preparations.

Daily Dosage: 1 to 2 g as drug or liquid extract (1:1) with 40% ethanol (V/V)

Homeopathic Dosage: 5 drops, 1 tablet, or 10 globules every 30 to 60 minutes (acute), and 1 to 3 times daily (chronic); Parenterally: 1 to 2 mL sc acute. 3 times daily; Chronic: once a day (HAB1).

LITERATURE

Brain KR, Thapa BB. *J Chromatogr.* 258:183-188. 1988.

Cooper-Driver G, Swain T. *Bot J Linn Soc* 74:1-21. 1977.

Hänsel R, Keller K, Rimpler H, Schneider G (Hrsg.), Hagers Handbuch der Pharmazeutischen Praxis, 5. Aufl., Bde 4-6 (Drogen), Springer Verlag Berlin, Heidelberg, New York, 1992-1994.

Madaus G, Lehrbuch der Biologischen Arzneimittel, Bde 1-3, Nachdruck, Georg Olms Verlag Hildesheim 1979.

Male Fern

Dryopteris filix-mas

DESCRIPTION

Medicinal Parts: The medicinal parts are the dried fronds, the dried rhizome collected in autumn with the leaf bases, the fresh rhizome, and the fresh aerial parts.

Flower and Fruit: On the underside of the leaflets there are 2 rows of sori, covered by kidney-shaped, red-brown film. The spores are dark brown.

Leaves, Stem, and Root: The root is a crooked half-underground fleshy rhizome, covered in the remains of dark brown petioles, which produces long branched root fibers. The remains of the petioles are linear-lanceolate and tomentose with red-brown scales. The foliage grows in a crown, with fronds arranged in spirals, 60 cm to 1.5 m high. There are bipinnate, oblong-lanceolate, alternate, sessile leaflets, subdivided with round segments. The young fronds are rolled in spirals and thickly covered in hairs. They gradually open out as the fronds grow.

Habitat: The plant is found in the temperate zones of Europe, northern Asia, and in North and South America.

Production: Male Fern leaf consists of the fresh or dried leaf of *Dryopteris filix-mas*. Male Fern herb consists of the fresh or dried above-ground parts of *Dryopteris filix-mas*. Male Fern rhizome consists of the fresh or dried rhizomes separated from the attached roots. The rootstock is collected in autumn and gently dried.

Not to be Confused With: The rhizomes of most European Dyopteris species.

Other Names: Aspidium, Bear's Paw Root, Fern, Knotty Brake, Male Shield Fern, Marginal Fern, Sweet Brake

ACTIONS AND PHARMACOLOGY

COMPOUNDS: MALE FERN RHIZOME

Acylphloroglucinoles (2%, mixtures termed raw filicin or filicin): in particular, flavaspidic acids, filicinic acids, paraspidin, desaspidin

Tannins

COMPOUNDS: MALE FERN LEAVES

Acylphloroglucinoles (0.2%, mixtures termed raw filicin or filicin): in particular, flavaspidic acids, filicinic acids, paraspidin, desaspidin

Flavonoids

EFFECTS

Male Fern herb has an anthelmintic effect and is strongly cytotoxic against band worms and liver flukes, although roundworm and oxyuris are resistant. It is also cell toxic, virostatic, and antiviral. The pharmacological effect is largely due to the flavaspidic acid with filicic acids being the main active principle.

INDICATIONS AND USAGE

Unproven Uses: Preparations of Male Fern herb are used externally for rheumatism, sciatica, muscle pain, neuralgia, earache and toothache, for festering and poorly healing wounds, burns, hemorrhoids, for teething in infants, and sleep disorders, as well as internally for tapeworms and flukes.

Homeopathic Uses: Dryopteris filix-mas is used for weak sight and damage to the optic nerve.

CONTRAINDICATIONS

The drug should not be administered in the presence of anemia, cardiac, liver or kidney diseases, or diabetes.

PRECAUTIONS AND ADVERSE REACTIONS

General: The following can occur even with therapeutic dosages: queasiness, nausea, severe headache, vomiting, diarrhea.

Pregnancy: The drug should not be used during pregnancy.

Pediatric Use: The drug should not be administered to children under 4 years.

Use in the Elderly: The drug should not be administered to elderly persons.

OVERDOSAGE

Overdosages in susceptible patients can lead to liver, cardiac, and kidney damage as well as central nervous system disorders, psychoses, and permanent injuries such as paralysis and visual disorders. Cases of death, particularly among children, have been observed following administration of Filmaron oil (10% solution of volatile extracts of the rhizomic drug in cooking oil).

DOSAGE

Mode of Administration: **Warning:** Dosages may be toxic. Due to the risks, internal application is not recommended; if possible, other remedies should be used. Because the efficacy of the claimed applications is not documented, therapeutic usage is not recommended.

Preparation: Filix-mas extract: The percolate is completely freed from ether by steaming (maximum 50° C). It is made into a dried extract in a vacuum. The content is stabilized with high-fat cooking oil (DAB6)

Daily Dosage: The single and daily dose of Filix-mas extract is 6 to 8 g for adults and 4 to 6 g for children. In case of an unsuccessful cure, the treatment may only be repeated after an interim of a few weeks. The single and daily maximum dose of Filix-mas liquid extract is 3 g. The maximum daily dosage of Aspidinolfilicium oil solution is 20 g.

Homeopathic Dosage: 5 drops, 1 tablet, or 10 globules every 30 to 60 minutes (acute) or 1 to 3 times daily (chronic); parenterally: 1 to 2 mL sc acute: 3 times daily; chronic: once a day (HAB1);

Storage: The drug is stored over absorbant calcium for a maximum duration of 1 year, with a relative humidity below 0.05 in sealed containers away from light sources.

LITERATURE

Frohne D, Pfänder HJ, Giftpflanzen - Ein Handbuch für Apotheker, Toxikologen und Biologen, 4. Aufl., Wiss. Verlagsges. mbH Stuttgart 1997.

Hänsel R, Keller K, Rimpler H, Schneider G (Hrsg.), Hagers Handbuch der Pharmazeutischen Praxis, 5. Aufl., Bde 4-6 (Drogen), Springer Verlag Berlin, Heidelberg, New York, 1992-1994.

Karl C, Pedersen PA, Müller G, *Z Naturforsch* 36C:607-610. 1981.

Leung AY, Encyclopedia of Common Natural Ingredients Used in Food, Drugs and Cosmetics, John Wiley & Sons Inc., New York 1980.

Roth L, Daunderer M, Kormann K, Giftpflanzen, Pflanzengifte, 4. Aufl., Ecomed Fachverlag Landsberg Lech 1993.

Teuscher E, Lindequist U, Biogene Gifte - Biologie, Chemie, Pharmakologie, 2. Aufl., Fischer Verlag Stuttgart 1994.

Widén CJ, Sarvela J, Britton OM, On the location and distribution of phloroglucinols (Filicins) in Ferns. In: *Ann Bot Fennici* 20:407. 1983.

Widén CJ, Vida G, Euw JV, Reichenstein T. *Helv Chim Acta* 54:2824-2850. 1971.

Mallotus philippinensis

See Kamala

Malus domestica

See Apple Tree

Malva sylvestris

See High Mallow

Manaca

Brunfelsia hopeana

DESCRIPTION

Medicinal Parts: The medicinal parts of Manaca are the roots and stem.

Flower and Fruit: The blue or white flowers are large, conical, and very fragrant. The calyx is divided into 5 sections, with rounded lobes and 2 lips covering the bud. There are 4 fertile anthers, which fuse together above where they divide into 2 stigmalike lobes. The fruit is a fleshy or leathery capsule with numerous large seeds embedded in it.

Leaves, Stem, and Root: Manaca is a shrub with obovate, deciduous leaves. The tough, woody roots are about 1.5 cm in diameter. They are yellow in the center and have a papery, pale brown epidermis. The stems have a small yellow medulla.

Habitat: Manaca grows in South America, the West Indies and Brazil.

Production: Manaca root is the root of *Brunfelsia hopeana.*

Other Names: Pohl, Vegetable Mercury

ACTIONS AND PHARMACOLOGY

COMPOUNDS

The active ingredients of the drug have not yet been adequately investigated. The spasmogenic brunfelsamidine (pyrrole-3-carboxamidine, identical with Nierembergia toxin) has been demonstrated in the related species *Brunfelsia grandiflora.*

EFFECTS

Diuretic and antirheumatic effects have been attributed to Manaca.

INDICATIONS AND USAGE

Unproven Uses: Manaca is used in the treatment of rheumatic conditions.

PRECAUTIONS AND ADVERSE REACTIONS

No health hazards or side effects are known in conjunction with the proper administration of designated therapeutic dosages. In animal experiments, anxiety states, restlessness, increase in cardiac and pulmonary frequency, elevated salivation, vomiting, muscle tremors and tonic-clonic spasms were observed following intake of plant parts of *Brunfelsia* species, as well as death.

DOSAGE

Mode of Administration: Liquid extract preparations for internal use.

LITERATURE

Frohne D, Pfänder HJ, Giftpflanzen - Ein Handbuch für Apotheker, Toxikologen und Biologen, 4. Aufl., Wiss. Verlags-Ges Stuttgart. 1997.

Kern W, List PH, Hörhammer L (Hrsg.), Hagers Handbuch der Pharmazeutischen Praxis, 4. Aufl., Bde. 1-8, Springer Verlag Berlin, Heidelberg, New York, 1969.

Lloyd HA et al., Brunfeslamidine: A novel convulsant from the medicinal plant *Brunfelsia grandiflora.* In: *Tetrahedron Letters* 26(22):2623-2624. 1985.

Roth L, Daunderer M, Kormann K, Giftpflanzen, Pflanzengifte, 4. Aufl., Ecomed Fachverlag Landsberg Lech 1993.

Mandragora officinarum

See Mandrake

Mandrake

Mandragora officinarum

DESCRIPTION

Medicinal Parts: The medicinal parts are the dried underground part, the fresh herb, and the root.

Flower and Fruit: The numerous flowers are on light green pedicles. They are glabrous on the outside. The corolla is light green to yellow. The calyx is lanceolate with a pointed tip, half as long as the 3-cm corolla. The hairs on the outside of the corolla have heads, which consist of 15 cells and sit on a tiny stem of 2 to 3 cm. The fruit is yellow, globular, and extends with a diameter of 2 to 3 cm well beyond the calyx.

Leaves, Stem, and Root: The plant has a thick, tuberous root and is almost stemless. The root is light brown on the outside, simple or branched, and up to 60 cm deep. The leaves are all the same size, pubescent, short petiolate, ovate-lanceolate. They have a disgusting smell.

Habitat: The plant is indigenous to the Mediterranean region and bordering frost-free regions.

Production: Mandrake root is the dried, underground part of *Mandragora vernalis* or *M officinarum*. The plant is gathered in uncultivated regions.

Not to be Confused With: The roots of *Atropa belladona,* whose alkaloid pattern is similar.

Other Names: Mandragora, Satan's Apple

ACTIONS AND PHARMACOLOGY

COMPOUNDS: MANDRAGORA ROOT

Tropane alkaloids (0.4%): chief alkaloids (-)-hyoscyamine, under storage conditions changing over to some extent into atropine, and scopolamine

COMPOUNDS: MANDRAKE HERB

The leaves have hardly been investigated, but in view of the demonstrated toxicity, the same alkaloid mixture is to be assumed.

EFFECTS: MANDRAKE ROOT AND HERB

The action of the drug is mainly due to the anticholinergic effect of the main alkaloids (atropine, hyoscamin, and scopolamine).

INDICATIONS AND USAGE

Unproven Uses: The drug is obsolete. In folk medicine, a tincture of Mandragora radix was used for stomach ulcers, colic, asthma, hay fever, and whooping cough.

PRECAUTIONS AND ADVERSE REACTIONS

To be used only under the supervision of an expert qualified in the use of this substance. No health hazards are known in conjunction with the proper administration of designated therapeutic dosages. Skin reddening, dryness of the mouth, tachycardiac arrhythmias, mydriasis (the 4 early warning symptoms of a poisoning), accommodation disorders, heat build-up through decline in sweat secretion, micturition disorders and constipation can occur as side effects, particularly with overdoses.

OVERDOSAGE

Because of the high content of scopolamine in the drug, poisonings lead at first to somnolence, but then after the intake of very high dosages, to central excitation (restlessness, hallucinations, delirium, and manic episodes), followed by exhaustion and sleep. Lethal dosages (for adults starting at 100 mg atropine, considerably less for children) carry with them the danger of respiratory failure. Severe poisonings are particularly conceivable in connection with the misuse of the drug as an intoxicant.

The treatment for poisonings include stomach emptying; temperature-lowering measures with wet cloths (no antipyretics); oxygen respiration for respiratory distress; intubation; parenteral physostigmine salts as antidote; diazepam for spasms while monitoring respiratory function; catheter for cystoparalysis.

DOSAGE

Mode of Administration: The drug is now obsolete and is only rarely used in medicinal preparations.

LITERATURE

Al-Khali S, Alkofahi A, The chemical constituents of *Mandragora autumnalis*. In: PM 62, Abstracts of the 44th Ann Congress of GA, 149. 1996.

Dräger B, Almsick Av, Mrachatz G. Distribution of Calystegines in Several Solanaceae. *Planta Med.* 61 (6); 577-579. 1995

Frohne D, Pfänder HJ, Giftpflanzen - Ein Handbuch für Apotheker, Toxikologen und Biologen, 4. Aufl., Wiss. Verlags-Ges. Stuttgart 1997.

Hänsel R, Keller K, Rimpler H, Schneider G (Hrsg.), Hagers Handbuch der Pharmazeutischen Praxis, 5. Aufl., Bde 4-6 (Drogen), Springer Verlag Berlin, Heidelberg, New York, 1992-1994.

Jackson BP, Berry MI, Hydroxytropane tigliates in the roots of *Mandragora* species. In: *PH* 12(5):1165-1166. 1973.

Kraft K, Europäische Rauschdrogen. In: *ZPT* 17(6):343-355. 1996.

Lewin L, Gifte und Vergiftungen, 6. Aufl., Nachdruck, Haug Verlag, Heidelberg 1992.

Roth L, Daunderer M, Kormann K, Giftpflanzen, Pflanzengifte, 4. Aufl., Ecomed Fachverlag Landsberg Lech 1993.

Scholz E, Alraunenfrüchte - ein biblisches Aphrodisiakum. In: *ZPT* 16(2):109-110. 1995.

Teuscher E, Lindequist U, Biogene Gifte - Biologie, Chemie, Pharmakologie, 2. Aufl., Fischer Verlag Stuttgart 1994.

Wagner H, Wiesenauer M, Phytotherapie. Phytopharmaka und pflanzliche Homöopathika, Fischer-Verlag, Stuttgart, Jena, New York, 1995.

Mangosteen

Garcinia mangostana

DESCRIPTION

Medicinal Parts: Fruit, fruit hull, bark and twigs

Botanical Description: Tree, up to 12m. Leaves simple, opposite, ovate or elliptic-oblong, 6-12 cm wide, 15-25 cm long, thick and glabrous, above dark green, underneath dull pale green. Flowers solitary, axilliary, polygamomonecious, yellowish green to entirely red and succulent. Fruit is a berry, dark purple, 1-3 seeded.

Habitat: India, Myanmar, Sri Lanka, and Thailand

Other Names: Amibiasine, Mang Cut, Manggis, Manggistan, Mangosta, Manguita, Queen of Fruits, Sementah, Xango

ACTIONS AND PHARMACOLOGY

COMPOUNDS

The dried fruit rind contains tannins and xanthones, epecially mangostin.

EFFECTS

The major secondary metabolites of mangosteen have been found to be prenylated xanthone derivatives; some members of this compound class isolated from this plant possess antifungal, antimicrobial, antioxidant, and cytotoxic activities, potentially antiplasmodial. Studies on the xanthones obtained from the fruit have been conducted to examine the anticancer properties against colon preneoplastic lesions, DNA topoisomerases I and II, human leukemia (HL60, K562, NB4, U937, P3HR1, and Raji), hepatoma (HCC36, TONG, HA22T, Hep 3B, HEpG2, and SK-HEp-1), lung (NCI-Hut 125, CH27-LC-1, H2981, and Calu-1), and gastric carcinomas (AZ521, NUGC-3, KATO-III, and AGS),7) and human breast cancer SKBR3 cells.

CLINICAL TRIALS

Dental

A clinical trial was conducted to determine the effects of an herbal mouthwash containing the pericarp extract of *Garcinia mangostana* on volatile sulfur compound (VSC) levels, plaque index (PI), and papillary bleeding index (PBI) in gingivitis subjects and recurrence of these parameters after periodontal treatment. Sixty subjects with mild or moderate chronic gingivitis were randomly divided into herbal or placebo mouthwash groups. On day 1, all parameters were recorded. Subjects rinsed with the assigned mouthwash and VSC was measured at 30 min and 3 h post-rinsing. For the following 2 weeks, subjects practiced their usual oral hygiene and rinsed with the assigned mouthwash twice daily after tooth brushing. On day 15, parameters were recorded again. In the 4-week washout period that followed, subjects received scaling and polishing. After another baseline examination, they were re-randomized into the herbal or placebo group and rinsed with mouthwash for 2 weeks. All parameters were re-evaluated on day 15. All parameters were significantly better compared to baseline in both groups at 30 min, 3 h, and day 15 ($p<0.05$). When compared between groups, VSC was significantly different at day 15 ($p<0.05$). After scaling, polishing and rinsing with mouthwash for 2 weeks, PI and PBI were significantly different compared to baseline ($p<0.05$) while VSC was not ($p>0.05$). When compared between groups, VSC was significantly better ($p<0.05$) (Rassameemasmaung et al, 2007).

INDICATIONS AND USAGE

Unproven Uses: Diarrhea and dysentery. The pericarp of mangosteen has been used in Thai indigenous medicine for the treatment of skin infections, wounds, and diarrhea for many years. Recently, products manufactured from *G. man-*

gostana have begun to be used as a botanical dietary supplement because of their potent antioxidant potential.

CONTRAINDICATIONS

None are known.

PRECAUTIONS AND ADVERSE REACTIONS

POTENTIAL INTERACTIONS

Possibly unsafe when used by patients with cardiovascular disease or clotting disorders, or using anticoagulation medicine, antihistamine agents, phosphodiesterase inhibitors, or selective serotonin reuptake inhibitor (SSRI) antidepressant agents.

DRUG INTERACTIONS

No human drug interaction data is available.

DOSAGE

How Supplied: Products standardized to 10% mangostin are currently available.

Daily Dose: No reliable information available.

LITERATURE

Chairungsrilerd N, Furukawa K, Ohta T, Nozoe S, Ohizumi Y. Histaminergic and serotonergic receptor blocking substances from the medicinal plant Garcinia mangostana. Planta Med. 1996 Oct;62(5):471-2.

Chairungsrilerd N, Furukawa K, Tadano T, Kisara K, Ohizumi Y. Effect of gamma-mangostin through the inhibition of 5-hydroxy-tryptamine2A receptors in 5-fluoro-alpha-methyltryptamine-induced head-twitch responses of mice. Br J Pharmacol. 1998 Mar;123(5):855-62.

Chairungsrilerd N, Furukawa KI, Ohta T, Nozoe S, Ohizumi Y. Gamma-mangostin, a novel type of 5-hydroxytryptamine 2A receptor antagonist. Naunyn Schmiedebergs Arch Pharmacol. 1998 Jan;357(1):25-31.

Chanarat P, Chanarat N, Fujihara M, Nagumo T. Immunopharmacological activity of polysaccharide from the pericarpof mangosteen garcinia: phagocytic intracellular killing activities. J Med Assoc Thai. 1997 Sep;80 Suppl 1:S149-54.

Chen SX, Wan M, Loh BN. Active constituents against HIV-1 protease from Garcinia mangostana. Planta Med. 1996 Aug;62(4):381-2.

Chomnawang MT, Surassmo S, Nukoolkarn VS, Gritsanapan W. Antimicrobial effects of Thai medicinal plants against acne-inducing bacteria. J Ethnopharmacol. 2005 Oct 3;101(1-3):330-3.

Dharmaratne HR, Piyasena KG, Tennakoon SB. A geranylated biphenyl derivative from Garcinia malvgostana. Nat Prod Res. 2005 Apr;19(3):239-43.

Ee GC, Daud S, Taufiq-Yap YH, Ismail NH, Rahmani M. Xanthones from Garcinia mangostana (Guttiferae). Nat Prod Res. 2006 Oct;20(12):1067-73.

Gopalakrishnan G, Balaganesan B. Two novel xanthones from Garcinia mangostana. Fitoterapia. 2000 Sep;71(5):607-9.

Gopalakrishnan G, Banumathi B, Suresh G. Evaluation of the antifungal activity of natural xanthones from Garcinia mangostana and their synthetic derivatives. J Nat Prod. 1997 May;60(5):519-24.

Haruenkit R, Poovarodom S, Leontowicz H, Leontowicz M, Sajewicz M, Kowalska T, Delgado-Licon E, Rocha-Guzman NE, Gallegos-Infante JA, Trakhtenberg S, Gorinstein S. Comparative Study of Health Properties and Nutritional Value of Durian, Mangosteen, and Snake Fruit: Experiments In vitro and In vivo. J Agric Food Chem. 2007 Jun 13

Hawkins DJ, Kridl JC. Characterization of acyl-ACP thioesterases of mangosteen (Garcinia mangostana) seed and high levels of stearate production in transgenic canola. Plant J. 1998 Mar;13(6):743-52.

Ho CK, Huang YL, Chen CC. Garcinone E, a xanthone derivative, has potent cytotoxic effect against hepatocellular carcinoma cell lines. Planta Med. 2002 Nov;68(11):975-9.

Huang YL, Chen CC, Chen YJ, Huang RL, Shieh BJ. Three xanthones and a benzophenone from Garcinia mangostana. J Nat Prod. 2001 Jul;64(7):903-6.

Ji X, Avula B, Khan IA. Quantitative and qualitative determination of six xanthones in Garcinia mangostana L. by LC-PDA and LC-ESI-MS. J Pharm Biomed Anal. 2007 Mar 12;43(4):1270-6. Epub 2006 Nov 28.

Jung HA, Su BN, Keller WJ, Mehta RG, Kinghorn AD. Antioxidant xanthones from the pericarp of Garcinia mangostana (Mangosteen). J Agric Food Chem. 2006 Mar 22;54(6):2077-82.

Mahabusarakam W, Kuaha K, Wilairat P, Taylor WC. Prenylated xanthones as potential antiplasmodial substances. Planta Med. 2006 Aug;72(10):912-6. Epub 2006 Aug 10.

Matsumoto K, Akao Y, Kobayashi E, Ohguchi K, Ito T, Tanaka T, Iinuma M, Nozawa Y. Induction of apoptosis by xanthones from mangosteen in human leukemia cell lines. J Nat Prod. 2003 Aug;66(8):1124-7.

Moongkarndi P, Kosem N, Kaslungka S, Luanratana O, Pongpan N, Neungton N. Antiproliferation, antioxidation and induction of apoptosis by Garcinia mangostana (mangosteen) on SKBR3 human breast cancer cell line. J Ethnopharmacol. 2004 Jan;90(1):161-6.

Nabandith V, Suzui M, Morioka T, Kaneshiro T, Kinjo T, Matsumoto K, Akao Y, Iinuma M, Yoshimi N. Inhibitory effects of crude alpha-mangostin, a xanthone derivative, on two different categories of colon preneoplastic lesions induced by 1, 2-dimethylhydrazine in the rat. Asian Pac J Cancer Prev. 2004 Oct-Dec;5(4):433-8.

Nakagawa Y, Iinuma M, Naoe T, Nozawa Y, Akao Y. Characterized mechanism of alpha-mangostin-induced cell death: Caspase-independent apoptosis with release of endonuclease-G from mitochondria and increased miR-143 expression in human colorectal cancer DLD-1 cells. Bioorg Med Chem. 2007 May 18

Nakatani K, Atsumi M, Arakawa T, Oosawa K, Shimura S, Nakahata N, Ohizumi Y. Inhibitions of histamine release and prostaglandin E2 synthesis by mangosteen, a Thai medicinal plant. Biol Pharm Bull. 2002 Sep;25(9):1137-41.

Nakatani K, Nakahata N, Arakawa T, Yasuda H, Ohizumi Y. Inhibition of cyclooxygenase and prostaglandin E2 synthesis by gamma-mangostin, a xanthone derivative in mangosteen, in C6 rat glioma cells. Biochem Pharmacol. 2002 Jan 1;63(1):73-9.

Nakatani K, Yamakuni T, Kondo N, Arakawa T, Oosawa K, Shimura S, Inoue H, Ohizumi Y. gamma-Mangostin inhibits inhibitor-kappaB kinase activity and decreases lipopolysaccharide-induced cyclooxygenase-2 gene expression in C6 rat glioma cells. Mol Pharmacol. 2004 Sep;66(3):667-74.

Nguyen LH, Venkatraman G, Sim KY, Harrison LJ. Xanthones and benzophenones from Garcinia griffithii and Garcinia mangostana. Phytochemistry. 2005 Jul;66(14):1718-23.

Nilar, Harrison LJ. Xanthones from the heartwood of Garcinia mangostana. Phytochemistry. 2002 Jul;60(5):541-8.

Rassameemasmaung S, Sirikulsathean A, Amornchat C, Hirunrat K, Rojanapanthu P, Gritsanapan W. Effects of herbal mouthwash containing the pericarp extract of Garcinia mangostana L on halitosis, plaque and papillary bleeding index. J Int Acad Periodontol. 2007 Jan;9(1):19-25.

Sakagami Y, Iinuma M, Piyasena KG, Dharmaratne HR. Antibacterial activity of alpha-mangostin against vancomycin resistant Enterococci (VRE) and synergism with antibiotics. Phytomedicine. 2005 Mar;12(3):203-8.

Sato A, Fujiwara H, Oku H, Ishiguro K, Ohizumi Y. Alpha-mangostin induces Ca2+-ATPase-dependent apoptosis via mitochondrial pathway in PC12 cells. J Pharmacol Sci. 2004 May;95(1):33-40.

Suksamrarn S, Komutiban O, Ratananukul P, Chimnoi N, Lartpornmatulee N, Suksamrarn A. Cytotoxic prenylated xanthones from the young fruit of Garcinia mangostana. Chem Pharm Bull (Tokyo). 2006 Mar;54(3):301-5.

Suksamrarn S, Suwannapoch N, Phakhodee W, Thanuhiranlert J, Ratananukul P, Chimnoi N, Suksamrarn A. Antimycobacterial activity of prenylated xanthones from the fruits of Garcinia mangostana. Chem Pharm Bull (Tokyo). 2003 Jul;51(7):857-9.

Suksamrarn S, Suwannapoch N, Ratananukul P, Aroonlerk N, Suksamrarn A. Xanthones from the green fruit hulls of Garcinia mangostana. J Nat Prod. 2002 May;65(5):761-3.

Voravuthikunchai SP, Kitpipit L. Activity of medicinal plant extracts against hospital isolates of methicillin-resistant Staphylococcus aureus. Clin Microbiol Infect. 2005 Jun;11(6):510-2.

Weecharangsan W, Opanasopit P, Sukma M, Ngawhirunpat T, Sotanaphun U, Siripong P. Antioxidative and neuroprotective activities of extracts from the fruit hull of mangosteen (Garcinia mangostana Linn.). Med Princ Pract. 2006;15(4):281-7.

Williams P, Ongsakul M, Proudfoot J, Croft K, Beilin L. Mangostin inhibits the oxidative modification of human low density lipoprotein. Free Radic Res. 1995 Aug;23(2):175-84.

Manna

Fraxinus ornus

DESCRIPTION

Medicinal Parts: The medicinal part is the juice extracted from the bark.

Flower and Fruit: The inflorescence is in upright, later hanging, feathery panicles. The sepals are very short. The petals are fused at the base in pairs. They are linear to narrowly linguiform and white. The 2 stamens have very long filaments. The fruit is a nutlet. It is hanging, linguiform, 3 to 4 mm long, and 7 to 10 mm wide. It is rounded at the base or narrowed wedge-shaped, glossy dark brown, flat, and longitudinally striped. The seeds are ovate, 15 to 20 mm by 4 to 5 mm, broad, flat, longitudinally striped and brown.

Leaves, Stem, and Root: Fraxinus ornus is a tree growing up to 8 m tall with gray, crust-embossed bark. The new-year's branchlets are olive-green or browny gray-green, somewhat glossy, with numerous, light-brown lenticels. The long shoots are downy to the tip; the short shoots are awned at the base. The terminal and lateral buds are orbicular and have 4 scales. The leaflets are elliptical-ovate-lanceolate or ovate, tapering to a tip and crenate-serrate. The upper surface is rich green and the underside lighter green with pink veins. The nerves are pink-tomentose.

Habitat: The tree is indigenous to southern Europe, extending to the southern borders of the Alps and as far as European Turkey. The tree is cultivated in Italy.

Production: Manna consists of the dried sap generated from the slit bark of trunk and branches of *Fraxinus ornus,* as well as its preparations in effective dosage. The 8- to 10-year-old trees are incised. The manna flows out of the bark and is collected.

Other Names: Flake Manna, Flowering Ash, Manna Ash,

ACTIONS AND PHARMACOLOGY

COMPOUNDS

Alditols: Mannitol (70-90%)

Oligosaccharides: Stachyose, Mannotriose, Glucose, Fructose

EFFECTS

Manna acts as a laxative.

INDICATIONS AND USAGE

Approved by Commission E:

■ Constipation

Unproven Uses: Manna is also used for ailments where easier elimination and a soft stool is desirable, such as anal fissures, hemorrhoids, and post-rectal/anal surgery.

CONTRAINDICATIONS

The drug is not to be used in the presence of ileus.

PRECAUTIONS AND ADVERSE REACTIONS

No health hazards or side effects are known in conjunction with the proper administration of designated therapeutic dosages. Susceptible persons could experience flatulence and nausea.

DOSAGE

Mode of Administration: Comminuted herb and other galenic preparations for internal use.

Daily Dosage: For adults, 20 to 30 g of drug; For children, 2 to 16 g of drug. Manna, like other laxatives, should not be used for an extended period of time.

LITERATURE

Galabov AS, Iosifova T, Vassileva E, Kostova I. Antiviral Activity of Some Hydroxycoumarin Derivatives. *Z Naturforsch.* 51c; 558-562. 1996

Hänsel R, Keller K, Rimpler H, Schneider G (Hrsg.), Hagers Handbuch der Pharmazeutischen Praxis, 5. Aufl., Bde 4-6 (Drogen), Springer Verlag Berlin, Heidelberg, New York, (unter *Fraxinus ornus*). 1992-1994

Iossifova T, Mikhova B, Kostova I. A Secoiridoid Glucoside and a phenolic Compound from *Fraxinus ornus* bark. Phytochemistry 34; 1373-1376. 1993

Iossifova T, Kujumgiev A, Ignatova A, Vassileva E, Kostova I. Antimicrobial effects of some hydroxycoumarins and secoiridoids from *Fraxinus ornus* bark. *Pharmazie* 49; 298-299. 1994

Maranta arundinacea

See Arrowroot

Marigold

Calendula officinalis

DESCRIPTION

Flower and Fruit: On the tip of each stem there is a 5- to 7-cm composite flower head consisting of an epicalyx of numerous narrow-lanceolate sepals, which are densely covered on both sides with glandular hairs. The inner section of the flower head is made up of orange-yellow tubular florets. The disc florets are pseudohermaphrodites; the female, sterile. The zygomorphic ray florets at the edge are female, their stamens are completely absent, and their inferior ovaries are much more developed than those of the tubular florets. Fruit forms only in the female ray flowers. The heterocarp achenes are sickle-shaped, curved and ringed.

Leaves, Stem, and Root: The plant is usually an annual. It grows to between 30 and 50 cm high and has a 20-cm long taproot and numerous thin, secondary roots. The stem is erect, angular, downy, and branched from the base up or higher. The alternate leaves are almost spatulate at the base, oblong to lanceolate above and are all tomentose.

Characteristics: The plant has a strong, unpleasant smell.

Habitat: Central and southern Europe, western Asia, and the U.S.

Production: Marigold flowers are the ray florets of the completely unfolded, collected, and dried capitula of *Calendula officinalis*. Harvest begins in July. Drying takes place in the shade at a maximum of 45° C. Calendula herb consists of the fresh or dried above-ground parts of *Calendula officinalis* harvested during flowering season.

Not to be Confused With: Other Asteraceae; arnica and saffron are often adulterated with Marigold.

Other Names: Calendula, Goldbloom, Golds, Holigold, Mary Bud, Mary Gowles, Marybud, Ruddes

ACTIONS AND PHARMACOLOGY

COMPOUNDS: MARIGOLD FLOWERS

Triterpene saponins (2 to 10%): glycosides A to F (mono- or bisdemosidic oleanolic acid glycosides)

Triterpene alcohols: tirterpene monooles (0.8%), triterpene dioles (4%) and triterpene trioles, including lupeol, taraxasterol, psi-taraxasterol, faradiol, arnidiol, their mono- and diesters (chiefly acetic acid, lauric, myristic and palmitic acid as acid components)

Flavonoids (0.3 to 0.8%): including isorhamnetin and quercetin glycosides

Hydroxycoumarins: including scopoletin, umbelliferone, esculetin

Carotinoids: chief components lutein, zeaxanthine

Volatile oil (0.2%): chief components alpha-cadinol, T-cadinol, fatty acids

Water-soluble polysaccharides (15%): rhamnoarabinogalactans, arabinogalactans

Polyynes

COMPOUNDS: MARIGOLD HERB

Triterpene saponins

Flavonoids

Carotinoids

Volatile oil

EFFECTS: MARIGOLD HERB

The astringent and granulation-promoting effect may be attributable to the essential oil, saponins, and the amaroid loliolid. Efficacy has not been documented with valid data.

EFFECTS: MARIGOLD FLOWERS

Studies conducted in vitro and in animal models have elicited many potentially useful effects related to compounds present in *Calendula officinalis* and *Calendula arvensis*. Among these are anti-inflammatory, antimicrobial, antiviral, and antilipid effects. The flowers are antimicrobial due to the terpene alkaloids, lactone and flavones contained in the essential oil. Flavonoids isolated from flowers of *Calendula officinalis* demonstrated positive antimicrobial activity against *Staphylococcus aureus* (at a concentration of 1 mg/mL (Dumenil et al., 1980). Other studies have demonstrated the flavones to be effective against *Klebsiella pneumoniae, Sarcina lutea,* and *Candida monosa.*

Antihypotensive Effects: An infusion made from marigold plants (flowers, leaves, stems) is used to treat hypotension, according to Russian and Ukrainian folk medicine of the Soviet Far East (Moskalenko, 1987). No studies have been found relating to potential vasoconstricting properties of this herbal agent.

Anti-Inflammatory Effects: The faradiol monoester was proved to be the most relevant anti-inflammatory principle due to its quantitative prevalence in the flowers. The unesterified faradiol was found to be the most active of all tested compounds, equal to indomethacin in effect (Della Loggia et al., 1994).

Antilipid Effects: Saponosides from *Calendula officinalis* showed antihyperlipidemic effects in *ex vivo* studies (human serum, rat liver homogenate); the lipid balance was not affected when these saponosides were introduced in normolipidemic serum (Lansky, 1993; Wojcicki & Samochowiec, 1980). Animal studies (rat model) showed calendulosides to have antihyperlipidemic activity (Lutomski, 1983; Samochowiec, 1983).

Antiviral Effects: Organic extracts of the dried flowers of *Calendula officinalis* exhibited potent anti-HIV activity in an in-vitro MTT/tetrazolium-based assay. It was also found that the organic extract caused a significant dose- and time-dependent reduction of HIV-1 reverse transcription activity (Kalvatchev et al, 1997). Antiviral tests performed using the oleanolic acid glycosides from the aerial parts of the plant demonstrated an inhibitory effect against *Vesicular stomatitis virus* (VSV). Only one compound (3.MH) significantly affected replication in *Rhinovirus* (HRV) cultures (De Tommasi et al., 1991).

Gastrointestinal Effects: Calendula is thought to ease gastrointestinal problems by reducing spasms (spasmolytic action) and stimulating the production of bile (choleretic action) (Bisset, 1994).

Wound-Healing Effects: Calendula promotes the formation of granulation tissue, an important step in re-epithelization and healing of wounds (Bisset, 1994). It is thought to increase glycoprotein, nucleoprotein, and collagen metabolism at wound sites (Anon, 1995; Klouchek-Popova et al, 1982). An aqueous extract of calendula was shown to induce new blood vessel formation in vitro, suggesting this as a mechanism of action in promoting granulation (Patrick et al, 1996).

CLINICAL TRIALS

Anti-Inflammatory Action

The anti-inflammatory activity of each of the 3 main triterpendiol esters of Marigold was tested against croton oil-induced edema of the ears in mice. Faradiol-3-myristic acid ester and faradiol-3-palmitic acid ester were found to have the same dose-dependent anti-inflammatory activity. The nonesterified faradiol was more active than the esters and had an equivalent effect on inflammation as an equimolar dose of indomethacin (Zitterl-Eglseer, et al., 1997).

Dermatitis, Radiation-Induced

Many women undergoing radiotherapy after breast cancer surgery develop mild- to- severe dermatitis. The effectiveness of Calendula ointment was compared to that of trolamine, a commonly used topical nonsteroidal compound for enhancing skin healing, in preventing radiation-induced dermatitis in a phase III study involving 254 women undergoing radiation treatment after breast cancer surgery. The women were randomly divided into two groups. In one,126 participants were instructed to apply the Calendula to the irradiated area after each session and two other times during the day, or more if dermatitis and pain were felt. The other 128 patients applied the trolamine. Calendula ointment was found to be highly effective, with the incidence of acute dermatitis (grade 2 or higher) significantly lower with Calendula than with trolamine (41% versus 63%; p<.001). Calendula effectively reduced allergy and incidences of treatment interruption. Participant satisfaction and pain relief were also greater in the Calendula group. According to the results, the only inferior aspect to the Calendula was that it was more difficult than the trolamine to apply to the skin (Pommier, 2004)

Wound Treatment/Tissue Repair

Positive effects of Marigold on wound healing are cited in the literature, but most scientific evidence is based on animal and *in vitro* studies (Basch, 2006).

However, in a preliminary open phase III study that involved a small number of patients and was not blinded, positive effects on wound healing with topical Calendula were observed. A statistically significant acceleration of wound healing was seen in 21 patients with lower venous leg ulcers who were treated with an ointment containing Marigold extract twice daily for 3 weeks, as compared to a control group of 13 patients with 22 venous ulcers who had saline solution dressings applied for the same amount of time. The total surface area of all the ulcers, which was 67,544 mm^2 at the start of the Marigold therapy, had shrunk by 41.7%, to 39,373 mm^2 after 3 weeks. In contrast, the total surface area of all the ulcers in the control group was 69,722 mm^2 to begin, and 58,743 mm3 at the end of the third week, a decrease of only 14.52% (Duran 2005).

In an earlier study, surgically induced skin wounds in rats were treated with a 5% Calendula ointment in combination with allantoin. Histological studies of the damaged tissue were performed at 8 hours, 24 hours, and 48 hours after the infliction of the wounds. The drug combination was found to markedly stimulate physiological regeneration and epithelialization. This effect was attributed to more extensive metabolism of glycoproteins, nucleoproteins and collagen protein during the regenerative period in the tissues (Klouchek-Popova et al., 1982).

INDICATIONS AND USAGE

MARIGOLD FLOWERS

Approved by Commission E:

- Inflammation of the mouth and pharynx
- Wounds and burns

Externally, Marigold is used for inflammation of the oral and pharyngeal mucosa, poorly healing wounds, leg ulcers, to clean wounds, and for acute and chronic skin inflammation.

Unproven Uses: Marigold has been used extensively as a folk medicine. Externally it is used for varicosis, vascular disease wounds, inflammatory skin disease, anal eczema, proctitis, and conjunctivitis. It is a constituent in treatments for sore, dry skin, bee stings, and frostbite.

Marigold is used internally for inflammatory conditions of internal organs, gastrointestinal ulcers, constipation, worm infestation, and dysmenorrhea. It is also used as a diuretic and diaphoretic. In the past (19th century), Marigold was used as a cancer therapy but is no longer in use today for this purpose.

Homeopathic Uses: Calendula officinalis is used for frostbite, burns to the skin, and poorly healing wounds. The efficacy of the homeopathic uses has not been proved.

MARIGOLD HERB
Unproven Uses: Preparations are used for circulation, ulcers, spasms, swelling of the glands, jaundice, and for wounds and eczema. The herb is used in Russia for strep throat, on the Canary Islands for coughs and cramps, and in China for irregular menstruation.

PRECAUTIONS AND ADVERSE REACTIONS

MARIGOLD FLOWERS AND HERB
There is a low potential for sensitization after frequent skin contact with the drug. A low rate of contact dermatitis (less than 1%) occurred in patients patch-tested with a tincture of 10% Calendula. Only 2 of 1,032 patients had a positive skin reaction to Calendula (Bruynzeel et al, 1992). Anaphylactic shock occurred in a Russian patient who gargled calendula infusion (tea), according to one report (Anon, 1995).

DRUG INTERACTIONS

No human drug interaction data available.

DOSAGE

MARIGOLD FLOWERS
Mode of Administration: Comminuted drug for decoctions, and other preparations to be applied topically. It is available as tinctures, liquid extracts and infusions.

How Supplied: Powder, gel ointment, ophthalmic solution, tincture (10%), tea (infusion), shampoo and hand cream.

Cream

Gel – 7%, 10%

Ointment – 4%

Ophthalmic solution

Tea

Tincture

Shampoo

Preparation:

Tea — 150 mL of hot water are poured over 1 to 2 teaspoons drug and strained after approximately 10 minutes.

Diaphoretic — 2 to 4 mL tincture to 250 to 500 mL water or 0.5 to 1 mL liquid extract 1:1 ethanol 40%.

Ointment (10 to 20%) — 2 to 5 g drug in 100 g ointment with a fatty base.

Marigold oil — olive oil extraction 1:10 peanut oil; this 1:1 in 40% ethanol or 1:5 in 90% ethanol.

Daily Dosage:

Sore Throat and Inflammation, powder — 1 to 2 g of Calendula powder to 150 mL of water (Bisset, 1994).

Sore Throat and Inflammation, tea — 1 to 2 g in one cup of water, steep 10 to 15 minutes.

Peptic Ulcer, tea — 1 to 4 g in one cup of water, steep 10 to 15 minutes. Take three times daily (Mills, 1991).

Wound Treatment, ointment 2% to 5% — Apply topically to the affected area (Bisset, 1994).

Wound Treatment, compress — Steep one tablespoon herb in 500 mL water for 10 to 15 minutes and apply as a moist compress (Weiss, 1985).

Homeopathic Dosage: 5 to 10 drops, 1 tablet, or 5 to 10 globules 1 to 3 times daily or 1 mL injection solution sc twice weekly (HAB1).

Storage: Protect from light and moisture. May be stored a maximum of 3 years.

MARIGOLD HERB
Mode of Administration: Since efficacy has not been proved, the therapeutic value is uncertain.

LITERATURE

MARIGOLD FLOWERS

Acevedo JGA, Lopez JLM & Cortes GM. In vitro antimicrobial activity of arious plant extracts used by Purepecha against some Enterobacteriaceae. In: *Int J Pharmacog*; 31(1):61-64, 1993.

Ahmed AA et al.. Sesquiterpene glycosides from *Calendula officinalis*. In: *JNP* 56(10):1821, 1993.

Anon. Calendula Monograph. in Olin BR (ed), The Lawrence Review of Natural Products. Facts and Comparisons, St Louis, MO, January 1995.

Antibiotika und Immunabwehr. In: *Symbiose* 4(2):20. 1992.

Basch E, Bent S, Foppa I., et al. Marigold (Calendula officinalis L.): an evidence-based systematic review by the Natural Standard Research Collaboration. *J Herb Pharmacother;* 6(3-4):135-59. 2006.

BAnz (Federal German Gazette) No. 50; published 13 March 1986.

Bezakova L, Masterova I, Paulikova I et al. Inhibitory activity of isorhamnetic glycosides from *Calendula officinalis L.* on the activity of lipoxygenase. In: *Pharmazie*; 51:126-127, 1996.

Bisset NG. Calendulae floss - marigold. In: Herbal Drugs and Phytopharmaceuticals; a Handbook for Practice on a Scientific Basis. Medpharm Scientific Publishers, Stuttgart and CRC Press, Boca Raton, FL, USA, 1994.

Bruynzeel DP, Van Ketel WG, Young E et al. Contact sensitization by alternative topical medicaments containing plant extracts. In: *Contact Dermatitis*; 27:278-279, 1992.

Della Loggia R et al. The role of triterpenoids in the topical antiinflammatory activity *of Calendula officinalis* flowers. In: *PM* 60(6):516-520, 1994.

Dumenil G, Chemli R & Balansard G et al. Evaluation of antibacterial properties of marigold glowers (*Calendula officinalis L.*) and mother homeopathic tinctures of *C. officinalis L.* and *C. arvensis L.* In: *Ann Pharm Fr* 38(6):493-499,1980.

Duran V, Matic M, Jovanovc M, et al. Results of the clinical examination of an ointment with marigold (Calendula officinalis) extract in the treatment of venous leg ulcers. *Int J Tissue React*; 27(3):101-6. 2005.

Gracza L. Oxygen-containing terpene derivatives from *Calendula Officinalis*. In: *Planta Med*; 53:227, 1987.

Isaac O. Calendula officinalis L.- Die Ringelblume, Portrait einer Arzneipflanze. In: *ZPT* 15(6):357-370. 1994.

Isaac O. Die Ringelblume. Botanik, Chemie, Pharmakologie, Toxikologie, Pharmazie und therapeutsche Verwendung, Wissenschaftl. Verlagsges. mbH Stuttgart, 1992.

Kalvatchev Z, Walder R & Garzaro D. Anti-HIV activity of extracts from Calendula officinalis flowers. In: *Biomed Pharmacother*; 51:176-180, 1997.

Kasprzyk Z, Pyrek J. *Phytochemistry* 7:1631, 1968.

Kasprzyk Z, Wilkomyrski B. *Phytochemistry* 13:2299, 1973.

Kloucek-Popova E, Popov A, Pavlova N et al. Influence of the physiological regeneration and epithelization using fractions isolated from *Calendula officinalis*. In: *Acta Physiol Pharmacol Bulg*; 8(4):63-67, 1982.

Lansky PS. Plants that lower cholesterol. In: *Acta Hort*; 332:131-136, 1993.

Lutomski J. New information on the biological properties of various triterpene saponins. In: *Pharm Unserer Zeit*; 12(5):149-153, 1983.

Mennet-von Eiff M, Meier B. Phytotherapie in der Dermatologie. In: *ZPT* 16(4):201-210. 1995.

Mills SY. Out of the Earth: The Essential Book of Herbal Medicine. London: Viking Arkana, 1991.

Moskalenko SA. Slavic ethnomedicine in the Soviet Far East; part I: herbal remedies among Russians/Ukrainians in the Sukhodol Valley, Primorye. In: *J Ethnopharmacol*; 21:231-251,1987.

Patrick KFM, Kumar S, Edwardson PAD et al. Induction of vascularisation by an aqueous extract of the flowers of Calendula officinalis L the European marigold. In: *Phytomedicine*; 3(1):11-18, 1996.

Pommier P, Gomez F, Sunyach MP, et al. Phase III randomized trial of Calendula officinalis compared with Trolamine for the prevention of acute dermatitis during irradiation for breast cancer. *J Clin Oncol*; 22: 1447-1453. 2004.

Pyrek J. *Roczniki Chemii* 51:1141, 2331, 2493, 1977.

Samochowiec E et al. *Wiad Parazytol* 25(1):77, 1977.

Samochowiec L. Pharmacological study of saponosides from Aralia mandshurica Rupr et Maxim and *Calendula officinalis.* In: Herba Pol; 29(2):151-155, 1983.

Vecherko LP et al. Khim Prir Soed 11(3):366, 1975.

Weiss RF. Herbal Medicine. Ab Arcanum, Gothernburg, Sweden, 1985.

Wilkomirski B. Phytochemistry 24(12):3067, 1985.

Willuhn G. Ringenblumenblüten (Calendulablüten). In: Tägl Praxis 33(3):685. 1992.

Wojcicki J & Samochowiec L. Comparative evaluation of Aralia mandshurica Rupr et Maxim and *Calendula officinalis L* saponosides effect on lipid level in blood serum and liver homogenates. *Herba Pol*; 26(4):233-237. 1980.

Zitterl-Eglseer K, Sosa S. Jurenitsch J et al., Anti-oedematous activities of the main triterpendiol esters of Marigold (Calendula officinalis L.). *J Ethnopharmacol*; 57:139-144, 1997.

Marijuana

Cannabis sativa

DESCRIPTION

Medicinal Parts: The medicinal parts are the twig tips of the female flowers, with either flowers or fruit attached, the flower-bearing twigs that have been dried; the ripe hemp fruit and various homeopathic preparations of the fresh dried plant-parts.

Flower and Fruit: Hemp is dioecious. The female flowers are reduced to the perigone with one bract. The complete inflorescences form a leafy, false spike. The male flowers form panicles rich in pollen. Pollination is by wind. The fruit is a gray-green, glossy achene, 3.5 to 5 mm long and 2.5 to 4 mm wide. The seeds have little endosperm, are white, oily-fleshy, and hooked.

Leaves, Stem, and Root: Cannabis is an annual or biennial plant, which is usually branched and grows up to 5 m. The plant has erect, rough-haired, and compressed bristles. The leaves are long-petioled and 3 to 7 pinnate. The leaflets are lanceolate and serrate.

Habitat: The plant probably originated in the Middle East. Today it is grown worldwide in temperate and tropical regions.

Production: Indian hemp is the dried flowering or fruiting branch tips of *Cannabis sativa var. indica.* Production depends on the origin. One method is by striping the leaves. Another method is stripping the resin exuded from the flowers and multiple fruit, which is shaped into balls or sheet forms. The final method involves cutting 5 cm to 10 cm long branch tips, which have just borne fruit, removing the leaves, pressing the shooting tips and gathering them into bundles.

Not to be Confused With: Prior to being used as a narcotic, marijuana was often combined with *Nicotiana tabacum, Lavandula officinalis, Nepeta catarina*, or *Origanum vulgare*. It is possible to confuse Marijuana with varieties of Urtica, Moraceae, Ulmaceae and Boraginaceae.

Other Names: Bhang, Cannabis, Ganja, Grass, Indian Hemp, Kif, Pot, Weed

ACTIONS AND PHARMACOLOGY

COMPOUNDS

Cannabinoids: chief active agent 9-tetrahydrocannabinol (9-THC = 1-THC), in addition to 60 additional cannabinoids

Volatile oil: of a very complex composition, with, among other things beta-caryophyllenes, humules, caryophyllene oxide, alpha-pinenes, beta-pinenes, limonene, myrcene, beta-ocimene

Flavonoids: including canniflavone-1, canniflavone-2

EFFECTS

Human studies have found strong evidence to support the use of THC as an effective antiemetic. Studies also report that it is effective in reducing intraocular pressure, as an analgesic, and as an appetite stimulant. Cannabis has been reported to be possibly effective for the treatment of headaches, anxiety, bronchodilation/asthma, Tourette syndrome, and as a muscle relaxant. Cannabis also has reported sedative effects. Studies on the use of cannabis for the treatment of seizures, depression, and alcoholism have been inconclusive. Animal studies have reported that cannabis may have anti-inflammatory effects but results are inconclusive. In vitro studies have reported antibacterial, antifungal, and antineoplastic activity. The antineoplastic activity was not confirmed in vivo.

Most cannaboids act on the central nervous system. The multiplicity of effects does not point to just one receptor. Possible interaction with cell-wall lipids or effects on prostaglandin biosynthesis is under discussion at present.

Psychotropic action: In most subjects the effect is registered following an oral dose of 20 mg d-9-tetrahydrocannabinol or after inhaling a cigarette with 2% d-9-tetrahydrocannabinol. The symptoms are mood swings, reduction in drive, inability to think clearly, confusion, lack of concentration, and impairment of short-term memory and perception of time. Sensory impressions become heightened or experienced differently. Complex tasks become more difficult, the capacity to understand or empathize is impaired. Negative reactions such as anxiety, panic and psychosis can occur.

It is only possible to describe this effect in animal tests, on the basis of free behavioral and controlled behavioral tests. A stimulating effect has also been observed with lower doses. Not all cannaboids cause the same effect. CBC, CBD and CBG have no psychomimetic effect. Various interactions occur in combination with d-9-tetrahydrocannabinol.

Analgesic Effect: Recent case studies lend support to the probability of cannabis' analgesic effects (Lynch & Clark, 2003).

Antiemetic Effects: The Food and Drug Administration (FDA) approved cannabis for use in AIDS-related anorexia and treatment of nausea and vomiting associated with chemotherapy.

Anti-inflammatory Effects: Canniprene, a dihydrostilbene isolated from *Cannabis sativa,* was shown to be an inhibitor of lipoxygenase and cyclooxygenase. Canniprene was active in the 5-LPO assay in human neutrophils with an inhibitory concentration 50% of 15 micromoles (mcmol). One hundred percent cyclooxygenase inhibition was found at 100 mcmol in human platelets. Canniprene was not effective in the 12-lipoxygenase assay (ElSohly et al, 1990).

Tumor inhibiting effect: Delta-9 tetrahydrocannabinol and II-hydroxy tetrahydrocannabinol suppress the cytolytic activity of natural killer cells in culture, affecting the stage subsequent to the binding of the killer cell to the target cell (Klein et al, 1991).

Platelet activating factor effect: Platelet activating factor (PAF) is a naturally known mediator of asthmatic responses in the lung and it induces blood platelet aggregation. Cannabidiol was significantly more effective than THC as an inhibitor but was less effective than other synthetic inhibitors such as BN52021 (Evans, 1991)

Respiratory Effects: A short-term bronchodilator response was shown in one study (Ziment & Tashkin, 2000).

CLINICAL TRIALS

Bronchial Dilation

A short-term bronchodilator response to cannabis was demonstrated in healthy males by two separate investigational teams. In volunteers given an inhaled concentration of 1.0 to 2.6% delta-9-tetrahydrocannabinol administered by smoking, the bronchodilator response seen was greater than that of a beta agonist. A dose-dependent response was observed in subjects administered 10 to 20 mg of synthetic delta-8-tetrahydrocannabinol (Ziment & Tashkin, 2000).

Nausea and Vomiting

In a series of 809 patients receiving oral THC as an antiemetic, serious toxicity was rare. In this series of patients, severe psychological disturbances were observed in 4 patients, with 2 cases of myoclonic jerking; one patient developed grand mal seizures. More frequent central nervous system symptoms were sedation (53%), elation (32%), confusion (30%), perception distortions (23%) and depression (19%) (Devine et al, 1987). THC was an effective antiemetic agent against various antineoplastic chemotherapeutic agents in a prospective, randomized, and double-blind study. THC's antiemetic effect was equivalent to that of haloperidol when given to cancer patients (n=52) undergoing chemotherapy. About 10% of the patients had complete control of vomiting and about 33% had fewer than 5 episodes. If one of the antiemetics failed the other agent was effective about 50% of the time. Patients received one of the study drugs for two courses and were then switched to the other agent. The chemotherapeutic agents used were doxorubicin, cisplatin, and nitrogen mustard. After undergoing both treatments patients were asked which treatment they preferred. The adverse effects of THC were less tolerated than those of haloperidol (Neidhart et al, 1981).

Cognitive Function

Cannabis use (heavy or light) was not associated with a differential decline in cognitive function over time when compared with cognitive-function decline in nonusers of cannabis. This finding was based on administration of the Mini-Mental State Examination (MMSE) to 1,318 persons under age 65 in the Baltimore, Maryland Epidemiological

Catchment area. Scores on the MMSE in the time period 1993 to 1996 were compared with scores in 1982 on the same exam in the same cohort. There was an overall decline of 1.2 points on the MMSE over the time lapse of 12 years. There were no significant differences in cognitive function decline between heavy users, light users, and nonusers of cannabis; nor were there any differences for men versus women users of cannabis (Lyketsos et al, 1999).

Cytotoxicity

Delta-9 THC and II-hydroxy THC suppress the cytolytic activity of natural killer cells in culture, affecting the stage subsequent to the binding of the killer cell to the target cell. These two compounds also suppressed the cytolytic properties of cytotoxic T lymphocytes generated by co-cultivation with allospecific stimulators or by TNP-modified-self stimulators. If the cytotoxic T lymphocytes were generated in vivo (mice), these two cannabinols still suppressed them when tested in vitro. There are probably two mechanisms involved; suppression occurs at some point beyond the binding to the target cell and there is suppression of the normal development of mature effector cells from the less effective precursor cells (Klein et al, 1991).

INDICATIONS AND USAGE

Unproven Uses: Cannabis was first mentioned in the pharmacopoeia of the Chinese Emperor about 3,000 years ago. Cannabis resin was used for beriberi, constipation, female conditions, gout, malaria, rheumatism and absent-mindedness. In medieval herbals, it was mostly used externally. There are recipes for balms for healing contractures and for cooling poultices for the head and joints and for podagra.

In 1845, the herb tips were mentioned for internal administration for gonorrhea, angina pectoris, and choking fits. It was not until the 19th century that Indian hemp was described as having a euphoric effect; it was used for insomnia, neuralgia, painful rheumatism, painful gastrointestinal disorders, cholera, tetanus, epilepsy, strychnine poisoning, acute bronchitis, whooping cough, asthma, impending abortion and weak contractions. The extract was used as a sedative and mild soporific.

Dronabinol (delta-9-tetrahydrocannabinol, Marinol®) is marketed as an appetite stimulant in the treatment of AIDS-related anorexia and as an antiemetic for chemotherapy-induced emeses.

Indian and Chinese Medicine: In early Indian and Chinese medicine, it was used for nervous depressive states, insomnia, vomiting, tetanus and coughs.

CONTRAINDICATIONS

Hypersensitivity to sesame seed oil if taking dronabinol (Prod Info Marinol, 1999). Use of dronabinol is contraindicated in patients whose nausea and vomiting is due to reasons other than cancer chemotherapy.

Pregnancy: Not to be used during pregnancy (FDA Pregnancy Category C).

Breastfeeding: Not to be used while breastfeeding.

While there is little data in regard to excretion of THC in breast milk, THC has been reported to be concentrated and secreted in human breast milk and absorbed by nursing babies. THC concentrations were determined in the breast milk and fecal samples from the babies (n=2). One of the mothers had a milk level of 60.3 ng/mL of THC and its metabolites compared to a plasma 7.2 ng/mL. This was one hour after administration of THC. The fecal sample from a baby showed 347 ng of THC that was absorbed and metabolized by the neonate (Perez-Reyes & Wall, 1982). Dronabinol is concentrated and secreted in human milk and is absorbed by the nursing infant (Prod Info Marinol, 1999).

PRECAUTIONS AND ADVERSE REACTIONS

Central nervous system effects are the most common adverse drug reactions (ADRs) reported with dronabinol in AIDS patients during clinical trials. The following ADRs were reported in 3% to 10% of patients: dizziness, euphoria, paranoid reaction, somnolence, and thinking abnormal. Less common CNS ADRs (i.e., occurring in 0.3% to 1% of patients) include depression, nightmares, speech difficulties, and tinnitus (Prod Info Marinol, 1999). No health hazards or side effects are known in conjunction with the proper administration of designated therapeutic dosages. The intake of toxic dosages, as is common with the smoking of cannabis, leads almost at once to euphoric states (pronounced gaiety, laughing fits) with exaggerated apprehension of sensual impressions. Alterations in the perception of time and space, as well as acoustical, visual and sensory hallucinations, lasting for 2 to 3 hours are common in higher dosages. Patients who receive THC should not operate machinery or engage in any hazardous activity that requires clear mentation (Anonym, 2000).

Caution is advised if cannabis is used with central nervous system depressant drugs (Benowitz & Jones, 1977). Geriatric patients are usually more sensitive to the CNS effects than are younger patients (Prod Info Marinol, 1999).

Cardiac: Cannabis should be used cautiously in patients with cardiovascular disease (Anonym, 2000). Hypotension is among the most common side effects of THC and of the synthetic cannabinoids nabilone and levonantradol (Gralla & Tyson, 1985). A mild tachycardia was reported in asthmatic patients smoking marijuana with a concentration of 0.9% or 1.9% THC. This effect peaked at about 15 minutes and was significantly greater (p less than 0.001) when the higher concentration was used (Vachon et al, 1976).

Contamination: Non-pharmaceutical cannabis may be contaminated with the fungus *Aspergillus.* This may be hazardous to patients with compromised immune systems or fungal infections (Sillers, 1981).

Fertility: Marijuana decreases spermatogenesis, sperm motility, and increases abnormal forms of sperm (Nahas, 1984; Margolis & Popkin, 1980).

Immunity: Cannabis has been shown to consistently have adverse effects on immunity, producing immunosuppression. Guinea pigs and mice given cannabis had increased susceptibility to herpes simplex virus. Antibodies to delta-9-THC have been found in chronic users of cannabis and in animal studies (Munson & Holsapple, 1985).

Leukemia: In a case-control study, data suggested that maternal marijuana use may play an etiologic role in childhood acute nonlymphoblastic leukemia (ANLL), and may be specific for morphologically defined subgroups. Exposed cases were younger at diagnosis of ANLL, as compared to ANLL cases not exposed to marijuana; and exposed cases were also more often of the myelomonocytic and monocytic subtypes (Robison et al, 1989). In an earlier study by the Children's Cancer Study Group, data demonstrated that the risk of developing ANLL increased 10-fold among children whose mothers use marijuana during gestation (Briggs et al, 1998).

Motor Impairment: Driving ability can be disturbed for as long as 8 hours. Although only rarely reported, acute poisoning symptoms include nausea, vomiting, tear flow, hacking cough, disturbance of cardiac function and numbness of the limbs. Despite its widespread use as a recreational drug, instances of death are very rare. The results of chronic abuse are laryngitis, bronchitis, apathy, psychic decline and disturbances of genital functions.

Psychotropic: In a cohort study in Australia over six years (1992 to 1998) involving students ages 14 to 15 years who were followed for 7 years, young women who used cannabis daily had a greater than fivefold (odds ratio 5.6, 95% confidence interval 2.6 to 12) increase in the likelihood of reporting depression and anxiety, after standardizing for the use of other substances. After adjustment for possible baseline confounders, teenagers who used cannabis weekly or more frequently had a predicted twofold increase in risk for anxiety and depression (Patton et al, 2002). Cannabis use is an independent risk factor for the development of psychosis in psychosis-free persons and an even greater risk factor in persons with an established vulnerability to psychotic disorder (van Os et al, 2002).

Respiratory: Long-term smoking of cannabis has been associated with chronic respiratory symptoms such as sore throat, rhinitis, bronchitis, and deterioration of pulmonary function suggesting airway narrowing (Wu et al, 1988; Bloom et al, 1987; Tilles et al, 1986; Tashkin et al, 1980). Cannabis smoke has a high tar content and it has been estimated that 2 to 3 cannabis cigarettes may carry the same risk of lung damage as a pack of tobacco cigarettes. A prospective study of chronic cannabis smokers compared to tobacco smokers found that inhalation of cannabis smoke was associated with a 4 to 5 fold increase in blood carboxyhemoglobin, a 3 fold increase in inhaled tar, and increased respiratory tract retention of tar (Wu et al, 1988; Tashkin et al, 1988).

DRUG INTERACTIONS

MAJOR RISK

Sildenafil: Concurrent use may result in cardiovascular adverse effects including myocardial infarction. *Clinical Management:* Avoid concomitant use.

MODERATE RISK

Barbiturates: Concurrent use may result in excessive central nervous system depression. *Clinical Management:* Advise patients to avoid operating heavy machinery or perform other tasks which require mental alertness if barbiturates are used with cannabis.

Calamus: Concurrent use may result in increased effect of cannabinoids. Avoid concomitant use.

Cocaine: Concurrent use of cannabis and cocaine may result in increased pharmacologic and toxic effects of cocaine. *Clinical Management:* In patients presenting with cocaine toxicity with a history of relatively low cocaine doses, consider the possibility of concomitant marijuana use.

Disulfiram: Concurrent use may result in a hypomania-like reaction. Avoid concomitant use.

Ethanol: Concurrent use may result in increased intoxication. *Clinical Management:* Avoid concomitant use.

Protease Inhibitors: Concurrent use may result in reduced protease inhibitor effectiveness. *Clinical Management:* Caution is advised if cannabis is used concomitantly with protease inhibitors. Monitor CD4+ cell counts, HIV RNA, and serum p24 antigen regularly to determine continued antiviral effectiveness.

Selective Serotonin Reuptake Inhibitors: Concurrent use of cannabis and selective serotonin reuptake inhibitors may result in manic symptoms. *Clinical Management:* Caution patients taking selective serotonin reuptake inhibitors to avoid concomitant use of marijuana.

Theophylline: Concurrent use may result in decreased effectiveness of theophylline. *Clinical Management:* Patients who smoke cannabis while taking theophylline may require an increased theophylline dose.

Tricyclic Antidepressants: Concurrent use may result in tachycardia and delirium. *Clinical Management:* Caution is advised if patients use cannabis with a tricyclic antidepressant. Monitor heart rate changes closely.

DOSAGE

Mode of Administration: Marijuana is widely used as an illegal recreational drug. It is usually either smoked or eaten to produce mind-altering effects. The extracted or synthetically produced delta-9-tetrahydrocannabinol component is used legally in capsule form for oral administration.

How Supplied:

Capsules – (Marinol®) 2.5 mg, 5 mg, 10 mg

Dried Herb

Daily Dosage: The former average oral single dose of the drug was 0.1 g.

Appetite stimulation – (Marinol®) 2.5 mg to 10 mg twice daily

Antiemetic – (Marinol®) 5 mg/m2 to 15 mg/m2 4 to 6 times daily

Storage: Store with care, protected from light. Studies have shown that 9-tetrahydrocannabinol has a strong affinity with synthetics and rubber and is easily absorbed by them.

LITERATURE

Anon. Facts and Comparisons. Facts and Comparisons, Inc, St Louis, MO, 2000.

Anon. Cannabis: Hanf als Nutzpflanze. In: *DAZ* 135(27):2538-2541,. 1995.

Anon. Rezeptorforschung: Körpereigener Ligand des Cannabis-Rezeptors isoliert. In: *DAZ* 133(24):2214,. 1993.

Bayewitch M, Rhee MH, Avidor-Reiss T, Breuer A, Mechoulam R, Vogel Z. *Cannabis sativa* - deceptive weed? *S Afr Med J,* 271:1269-70, 1995 Dec 1995.

Beaconsfield P, Ginsburb J & Rainsbury R. Marihuana smoking: cardiovascular effects in an and possible mechanisms. In: *N Engl J Med*; 287:209-212, 1972.

Beal JE, Olson R, Laubenstein L et al. Dronabinol as a treatment for anorexia associated with weight loss in patients with AIDS. In: *J Pain Symptom Manage*; 10:89-97, 1995.

Benowitz NL & Jones RT. Effects of delta-9-tetrahydrocannabinol on drug distribution and metabolism. In: *Clin Pharmacol Ther*; 22:259-268,1977.

Bloom JW, Kaltenborn, Paoletti P et al. Respiratory effects of non-tobacco cigarettes. In: *Br Med J Clin Res*; 295:1116-1518, 1987.

Bonnin A et al. Effects of perinatal exposure to delta 9-tetrahydrocannabinol on the fetal and early postnatal development of tyrosine hydroxylase-containing neurons in rat brain. In: *J Mol Neurosci*, 7:291-308, 1996 Winter 1996.

Briggs GG, Freeman RK & Yaffe SJ. Drugs in Pregnancy and Lactation: A Reference Guide to Fetal and Neonatal Risk, 4th ed. Baltimore, MD: Williams and Wilkins, 1994.

Burke MD, Kilgour C & Pertwee RG. Potent but selective inhibition of cytochrome P-450 by cannabidiol. In: *Br J Pharmacol*; 83:445P,1984.

Castle DJ, Ames FR. Cannabis and the brain. In: *Aust N Z J Psychiatry*, 30:179-83, 1996 Apr 1996.

Chopra GS. Studies on psycho-clinical aspects of long-term marijuana use in 124 cases. In: *Int J Addict*; 8:1015-1026, 1973.

Clarke CC. Marijuana botany. In: And/Or Press, Berkeley, California. 1981.

Devine ML et al. Adverse reactions to 9- tetrahydrocannabinol given as an antiemetic in a multicenter study. In: *Clin Pharmacol* 6:319-322,1987.

Drogenmißbrauch. Drogen im Straßenverkehr. In: *DAZ* 134(27):2575. 1994.

Ekert H, Waters KD, Jurk IH et al. Amelioration of cancer chemotherapy-induced nausea and vomiting by delta-9-tetrahydrocannabinol. *Med J Aust* 1979; 2:657-659.

El Sohly H, Little T Jr. & ElSohly M: Canniprene: a prototype anti-inflammatory natural product. *Planta Med;* 56:662-663. 1990

Evans AT et al., *J Pharm Pharmacol.* 1985

Evans AT et al., FEBS 211:119. 1987

Evans AT et al., (1987) Biochem Pharmacol 36:2035.

Evans FJ. Cannabinoids - The separation of central from peripheral effects on a structural basis. In: PM 57:60. 1991.

Fairbairn JW et al., *J Pharm Pharmacol* 28:130.

Fairbairn JW, Pickens JT. *Br. J Pharmacol* 72:401. 1981

Foltin RW, Fischman MW, Pedroso JJ et al. Marijuana and cocaine interactions in humans: cardiovascular consequences. *Pharmacol Biochem Behav*; 28:459-464,1987.

Gil EW et al., *Nature* 228:135. 1970

Goedecke H, Karkos J. Die arzneiliche Verwendung von Cannabisprodukten. In: *DAZ* 136(34):2859-2862,. 1996.

Gralla RJ & Tyson LB. Delta-9-tetrahydrocannabinol as an antiemetic. In: Harvey DJ: Marijuana '84. Proceedings of the Oxford Symposium on Cannabis. IRL Press Ltd, Oxford, England, 1985.

Hillard JR & Vieweg WV. Marked sinus tachycardia resulting from the synergistic effects of marijuana and nortriptyline. In: *Am J Psychiatry*; 140:626-627, 1983.

Jungmayr P, Rauschmittel. Macht Marihuana dumm? In: *DAZ* 136(34):2867-2868. 1996.

Jusko WJ, Gardner MJ, Mangione A et al., Factors affecting theophylline clearances: age, tobacco, marijuana, cirrhosis, congestive heart failure, obesity, oral contraceptives, benzodiazepines, barbiturates and ethanol. In: *J Pharm Sci*; 68:1358-1366, 1979.

Kettenes-van den Bosch JJ & Salemink CA. Biological activity of the tetrahydrocannabinols. In*: J Ethnopharmacol*; 2:197-231, 1980.

Klein TW, Kawakami Y, Newton C et al. Marijuana components suppress induction and cytolytic function of murine cytotoxic T cells in vitro and in vivo. *J Toxicol Environ Health*; 32:465-477. 1991

Kluin-Neleman JC, Neleman FA, Meuwissen OJA et al., Delta-9-tetrahydrocannabinol (THC) as an antiemetic in patients treated with cancer chemotherapy; a double-blind cross- over study against placebo. In: *Vet Human Toxicol*; 21:338-340,1979.

Kosel BW, Aweeka FT, Benowitz NL et al. The effects of cannabinoids on the pharmacokinetics of indinavir and nelfinavir. In: *AIDS*, 16:543-550, 2002.

Kovar KA. Cannabis - was ist das? In: *DAZ* 132(43):2302. 1992.

Lacoursiere RB & Swateck R. Adverse interaction between disulfiram and marijuana. In: *Am J Psychiatry*; 140:243-244, 1983.

Lukas SE, Sholar M, Kouri E et al., Marihuana smoking increases plasma cocaine levels and subjective reports of euphoria in male volunteers. In: *Pharmacol Biochem Behav*; 48:715-721, 1994.

Lynch M & Clark A. Cannabis reduces opioid dose in the treatment of chronic noncancer pain. *J Pain Symptom Manage* 2003; 25(6):496-498.

Margolis R & Popkin N. Marijuana: a review of medical research with implications for adolescents. In: *Personnel Guidance J*; 59:7-14, 1980.

Munson AE & Holsapple MP. Overview of the immunotoxicology of marihuana. In: Harvey DJ: Marijuana '84. Proceedings of the Oxford Symposium on Cannabis. IRL Press Ltd, Oxford, England, 1985.

Nahas, B. In: Marihuana in Science and Medicine. Nahas G (Ed.) Raven Press New York. 1984.

Neidhart JA, Gagen MM, Wilson HE et al. Comparative trial of the antiemetic effects of THC and haloperidol. *J Clin Pharmacol* 1981; 21:38S-42S.

Noyes R Jr, Brunk SF, Baram DA et al., Analgesic effects of delta-9-tetrahydrocannabinol. In: Braude MC & Szara S: The Pharmacology of Marihuana. Raven Press, New York, NY, 1976.

Paris RR et al., *(1976) Plant Med Phytother* 10:144, 1976.

Patton GC, Coffey C, Carlin J et al., Cannabis use and mental health in young people: cohort study. In: *BMJ*; 325(11):1195-1198, 2002.

Ross SA, ElSohly MA. The volatile oil composition of fresh and air-dried buds of Cannabis. In: *JNP* 59(1):49-51. 1996.

Ruh MF, Taylor JA, Howlett AC, Welshons WV. Failure of cannabinoid compounds to stimulate estrogen receptors. *Biochem Pharmacol*, 53:35-41, 1997 Jan 10 1997.

Ruh MF, Taylor JA, Howlett AC, Welshons WV. The volatile oil composition of fresh and air-dried buds of *Cannabis sativa. J Nat Prod*, 53:49-51, 1996 Jan 1996.

Schwartz RH, Gruenewald PJ, Klitzner M et al., Short term memory impairment in cannabis-dependent adolescents. Am J Dis Child; 143:1214-1219, 1989.

Schwartz RH. Heavy marijuana use and recent memory impairment. In: *Psychiatric Annals*; 21:80-82, 1991.

Segelman A et al., (1977) JIn*: Pharm Sci* 66:1358, 1977.

Sweet DL, Miller NJ, Weddington W et al. Delta-9-tetrahydrocannabinol as an antiemetic for patients receiving cancer chemotherapy. A pilot study. *J Clin Pharmacol* 1981; 21:70S-75S.

Täschner KL. Drogen und Straβenverkehr. In: *DAZ* 134(35):3299. 1994.

Taura F, Morimoto S, Shoyama Y. Three acyclic bis-phenylpropane lignanamides from fruits of Cannabis sativa. In: *Phytochemistry*, 271:1003-7, 1995 Mar 1995.

Turner CE et al., (1980)In: *J Nat Prod* 43:169, 1980.

Vachon L, Mikus P, Morrissey W et al., Bronchial effect of marihuana smoke in asthma. In: Braude MC & Szara S (eds): The Pharmacology of Marihuana. Raven Press, New York, NY, 1976.

Van Os J, Bak M, Hanssen M et al., Cannabis use and psychosis: a longitudinal population-based study. In: *Am J Epidemiol*; 156:319-327, 2002.

Vidal C, Fuente R, Iglesias A, Saez A. Bronchial asthma due to *Cannabis sativa* seed. In: *Allergy*, 40:647-9, 1991 Nov

Wilens TE, Biederman J & Spencer TJ. Case study: Adverse effects of smoking marijuana while receiving tricyclic antidepressants. In: *J Am Acad Child Adolesc Psychiatry*; 36(1):45-48, 1997.

Yamamoto I, Matsunaga T, Kobayashi H, Watanabe K, Yoshimura H. Analysis and pharmacotoxicity of feruloyltyramine as a new constituent and p-coumaroyltyramine in *Cannabis sativa* L. In: *Pharmacol Biochem Behav*, 40:465-9, 1991 Nov 1991.

Yamaudi T. *(1975) Phytochemistry* 14:2189, 1975.

Zanoli P, Avallone R, Baraldi M. Sedative and hypothermic effects induced by beta-asarone, a main component of Acorus calamus. *Phytother Res;* 12(Supp 1):S114-S116, 1998.

Ziment I & Tashkin DP. Alternative medicine for allergy and asthma. *J Allergy Clin Immunol* 2000 Oct; 106(4):603-614.

Marrubium vulgare

See Horehound

Marsdenia condurango

See Condurango

Marsh Blazing Star

Liatris spicata

DESCRIPTION

Medicinal Parts: The medicinal parts are the roots.

Flower and Fruit: The inflorescence is compound spikes of carmine red flowers, 4 to 8 mm in diameter.

Leaves, Stem, and Root: The plant is a perennial and has an erect, leafy stem up 2 m. The leaves are opposite, up to 30 cm long, and 1 cm wide. The rhizome is 1 cm or more in diameter. It is gnarled with several cup-shaped scars. The rhizome is brownish and slightly wrinkled on the outside. Inside it is whitish with dark gray spots.

Characteristics: The root is very solid. The taste is bitter, and the odor is faintly aromatic, resembling cedar.

Habitat: U.S., cultivated in parts of Europe.

Production: Marsh Blazing Star is the rhizome of *Liatris spicata.*

Other Names: Backache Root, Button Snakeroot, Colic Root, Devil's Bite, Gay-Feather

ACTIONS AND PHARMACOLOGY

COMPOUNDS

Coumarin

Flavonoids: including rutin, quercetin-3-O-glucoside

EFFECTS

Main active principle: Coumarin. There is no reliable information available.

INDICATIONS AND USAGE

Unproven Uses: Marsh Blazing Star has been used for disorders of the kidney, dysmenorrhea, as a diuretic, and for gonorrhea treatment.

PRECAUTIONS AND ADVERSE REACTIONS

No health hazards or side effects are known in conjunction with the proper administration of designated therapeutic dosages.

DOSAGE

Mode of Administration: Ground drug as an infusion.

LITERATURE

Benezra C, Ducombs G. Molecular Aspects of Allergic Contact Dermatitis to Plants. *Dermatosen* 35; 4-11. 1987

Kern W, List PH, Hörhammer L (Hrsg.), Hagers Handbuch der Pharmazeutischen Praxis, 4. Aufl., Bde. 1-8, Springer Verlag Berlin, Heidelberg, New York, 1969.

Madaus G, Lehrbuch der Biologischen Arzneimittel, Bde 1-3, Nachdruck, Georg Olms Verlag Hildesheim 1979.

Wagner H, Iyengar MA, Herz W. Flavonoids in ten *Liatris* species. *Phytochemistry* 12; 2063-2064. 1973

Marsh Marigold

Caltha palustris

DESCRIPTION

Medicinal Parts: The medicinal part is the dried aerial part of the flowering plant.

Flower and Fruit: The flowers are about 4 cm in diameter. The involucre is simple and has 5 or more yolk-yellow, 12- to 18-mm long ovate bracts that are glossy greenish on the outside. There are numerous stamens and 5 to 8 ovaries. The fruit is a star-shaped follicle with a short beak. The seeds are dark brown to black, measuring about 2.5 cm long by 1.3 cm wide.

Leaves, Stem, and Root: Caltha palustris is a 15- to 30-cm high perennial marsh plant with a sturdy, many-headed rhizome. The glabrous, hollow stem is ascending or decumbent. The leaves are dark green and have an oily-glossy, cordate to reniform, crenate or serrate-margined leaf blade. The petioles are grooved. The cauline leaves have shorter petioles and are smaller, clasping, and often have a membranous leaf sheath.

Characteristics: The plant is highly poisonous.

Habitat: Caltha palustris is found in all temperate regions of the Northern Hemisphere.

Other Names: Bull's Eyes, Cowslip, Kingcups, Horse Blobs, Leopard's Foot, Meadow Routs, Palsy Root, Solsequia, Sponsa Solis, Verrucaria, Water Blobs, Water Dragon

ACTIONS AND PHARMACOLOGY

COMPOUNDS

Protoanemonine-forming agents: In the freshly harvested plant, it is presumably the glycoside ranunculin that changes enzymatically when the plant is cut into small pieces, and probably also when it is dried. It then changes into the pungent, volatile protoanemonine, which is severely irritating to skin and mucous membranes but quickly dimerizes to anemonine; when dried, the plant is not capable of protoanemonine formation

Triterpene saponins: including hederagenin glycosides

Triterpene lactones: caltholid, palustrolid

Isoquinoline alkaloids (aporphine type, very small quantities): including corytuberine, magnoflorine, protopine

EFFECTS

The drug lowers cholesterol levels and raises blood sugar levels in rats subsequent to oral administration (according to unavailable Russian research). There are also reports of anti-inflammatory effects on formaldehyde-induced inflammation. The drug contains alkaloids of the benzylisoquinoline type (magnoflorine, triterpene saponins, and triterpene lactones). In animal tests, magnoflorine temporally lowers blood pressure and induces hypothermia in mice. An effect on the nicotine receptor in the parasympathetic nervous system is under discussion. Insufficient information is available for an authoritative assessment of these effects.

INDICATIONS AND USAGE

Unproven Uses: Marsh Marigold was formerly used for jaundice, liver, and bilious complaints. Some Native American tribes and those practicing Russian folk medicine used the plant for dressing and cleansing skin lesions and sores. When administered internally, it is meant to have a laxative and diuretic effect. Since this has not been sufficiently proved, and the side effects of Marsh Marigold are so dangerous, its internal use is not recommended.

Homeopathic Uses: The drug is used externally for skin rashes.

PRECAUTIONS AND ADVERSE REACTIONS

No health hazards or side effects are known in conjunction with the proper administration of designated therapeutic dosages of the dehydrated drug. Extended skin contact with the freshly harvested, bruised plant can lead to treatment-resistant blisters and cauterizations due to the release of protoanemonine, which is severely irritating to skin and mucous membranes. If taken internally, large quantities could lead to severe irritation of the gastrointestinal tract, combined with colic and diarrhea, as well as with irritation of the urinary drainage passages.

OVERDOSAGE

Symptomatic treatment for external contact should consist of irrigation with diluted potassium permanganate solution followed by mucilage. Ingestion of the drug should be treated with gastric lavage followed by activated charcoal. The toxicity of this plant is less than that of many other Ranunculaceae (Anemones nemorosae) due to the relatively low levels of protoanemonine-forming agents.

DOSAGE

Mode of Administration: Because of the herb's toxicity, its use is not recommended other than topically and as an extract.

LITERATURE

Bhandari P et al., Triterpenoid saponins from *Caltha palsutris*. In: *PM* 53(1):98-100. 1987.

Bhandari P et al., Two nortriterpene lactones from *Caltha palustris*. In: *PH* 23(8):1699-1702. 1984.

Bruni A et al., Protoanemonin detection in *Caltha palustris*. In: *JNP* 49(6):1172-1173. 1986.

Frohne D, Pfänder HJ, Giftpflanzen - Ein Handbuch für Apotheker, Toxikologen und Biologen, 4. Aufl., Wiss. Verlags-Ges Stuttgart 1997.

Hänsel R, Keller K, Rimpler H, Schneider G (Hrsg.), Hagers Handbuch der Pharmazeutischen Praxis, 5. Aufl., Bde 4-6 (Drogen): Springer Verlag Berlin, Heidelberg, New York, 1992-1994.

Lewin L, Gifte und Vergiftungen, 6. Aufl., Nachdruck, Haug Verlag, Heidelberg 1992.

Roth L, Daunderer M, Kormann K, Giftpflanzen, Pflanzengifte, 4. Aufl., Ecomed Fachverlag Landsberg Lech 1993.

Teuscher E, Lindequist U, Biogene Gifte - Biologie, Chemie, Pharmakologie, 2. Aufl., Fischer Verlag Stuttgart 1994.

Marshmallow

Althaea officinalis

DESCRIPTION

Medicinal Parts: The medicinal parts are the mallow flowers, leaves, syrup and roots.

Flower and Fruit: The reddish-white flowers are usually in axillary or terminal clusters. The 6 to 9 sepals of the epicalyx are fused at the base, pointed and 8 to 10 mm long. There are 5 sepals, 5 heart-shaped petals and numerous stamens fused together with the anthers to a column. The ovaries are in a ring. There are numerous styles. The mericarps are smooth and downy. The 5 to 8 mm fruit is disclike and breaks up into the mericarps, which are downy on the outside and often have fine, branched, radiating ribs. The seeds are dark-brown, glabrous, kidney-shaped, and somewhat compressed.

Leaves, Stem, and Root: The 60 to 120 cm high, hardy, velvety plant has a thick erect root up to 50 cm long by a few cm with secondary roots. The erect, succulent stem is usually woody at the base but unbranched. The leaves are short-petioled with an ovate, acute leaf-blade. The secondary leaves are narrow and drooping. The lower leaves are 5-lobed, and the upper cauline leaves are often triangular, wider than they are long, and irregularly and roughly dentate.

Habitat: The plant was originally indigenous to Asia and then spread westward to southeast Europe and eastward to China. In temperate latitudes, Marshmallow is established as a garden plant.

Production: Marshmallow root consists of the dried root, unpeeled or peeled, of *Althaea officinalis*. The root cultures are harvested from October to November, and after cleaning, are carefully dried at a maximum temperature of 35°C. Marshmallow leaves consist of the dried leaves of *Althaea officinalis*. After harvest, the leaves are dried at a temperature of 40°C.

Not to be Confused With: May be confused with other Althea species.

Other Names: Althea, Cheeses, Mallards, Moorish Mallow, Mortification Root, Schloss Tea, Sweet Weed, White Maoow, Wymote,

ACTIONS AND PHARMACOLOGY

COMPOUNDS

Mucilages: mixture of colloidally soluble polysaccharides, particularly galacturonic rhamnans, arabinogalactans, arabans, and glucans

Pectins

Starch

EFFECTS

The drug alleviates local irritation, inhibits mucociliary activity, stimulates phagocytosis, and functions as an anti-inflammatory and anticomplementary agent, immune stimulant and hypoglycemic. Efficacy has been demonstrated when used as a gargle for inflammation of the mucous membrane of the mouth and throat.

INDICATIONS AND USAGE

MARSHMALLOW LEAF

Approved by Commission E:

- Cough/bronchitis

Unproven Uses: Folk medicine uses diarrhea, for insect bites, ulcers.

MARSHMALLOW ROOT

Approved by Commission E:

- Inflammation of gastric mucosa
- Oral and pharyngeal irritation

Unproven Uses: Folk medicine uses diarrhea, for insect bites, ulcers.

PRECAUTIONS AND ADVERSE REACTIONS

General: No health hazards or side effects are known in conjunction with the proper administration of designated therapeutic dosages.

DRUG INTERACTIONS

MINOR RISK

Orally Administered Drugs: Concurrent use may result in impaired drug absorption. *Clinical Management:* Administration of marshmallow should be separated by at least two hours from that of other orally-administered drugs.

DOSAGE

Mode of Administration: Cut leaves for aqueous extracts as well as other galenic preparations for internal use. Cut or ground root for aqueous extracts as well as other galenic preparations for internal use. Marshmallow syrup is to be used only for treatment of dry coughs.

Note: Diabetics need to consider sugar concentration of marshmallow syrup.

How Supplied:

Capsules – 460 mg

Cough mixture

Drops

Liquid – Generally in syrup form, which is also called ''snail juice'': (1:1)

Powder

Tablets (coated and uncoated)

Preparation: To prepare a tea from the root, use 10 to 15 g with 150 mL of cold water and allow to stand for 90 minutes, then warm to drink throughout the day. To prepare tea from leaf, use 1 to 2 g of drug in 150 mL hot water and let steep for 10 minutes. Drink throughout the day.

Daily Dosage: The average daily dose is 5 g of the leaf.

Storage: The drug should be protected from light sources and insects.

LITERATURE

Barnes J, Ernst E. Traditional Herbalist's Prescriptions for Common Clinical Conditions: A Survey of Members of the UK National Institute of Medicinal Herbalists. *Phytother Res.* 12 (5); 369-371. 1998

Franz G, Madaus A, Stabilität von Polysacchariden. Untersuchungen am Beispiel des Eibischschleims. In: DAZ 130(40):2194. 1990.

Gudej J. Flavonoids, Phenolic Acids and Coumarins from the Roots of *Althaea officinalis. Planta Med.* 57; 284-285. 1991.

Hahn-Deinstrop E, Eibischwurzel Identifizierung von Eibischwurzel-Extrakt und Gehaltsbestimmung in einem Instant-Tee. In: DAZ 135(13):1147-1149. 1995.

Madaus A, Blaschek W, Franz G. Althaeae Radix Mucilage Polysaccharides, Isolation, Characterization and Stability. *Pharm Weekbl Sci Ed.* 9. 239. 1987

Nosalova G, Strapkova A, Capek P, Kardosova A. Antitussive activity of an alpha-D-Glucan isolated from the roots of *Althaea officinalis L., var. robusta. Pharm Pharmacol Lett.* 2; 195-197. 1992

Tomoda M, Kaneko S, Ebashi M, Nagakura T. Plant Mucilagines. XVI. Isolation and Characterization of a Mucous Polysaccharide, ''Althaea-mucilage O'', from the Roots of *Althaea officinalis. Chem Pharm Bull.* 25; 1357-1362. 1977

Wunderer H, Zentral und peripher wirksame Antitussiva: eine kritische Übersicht. In: PZ 142(11):847-852. 1997.

Martagon

Lilium martagon

DESCRIPTION

Medicinal Parts: The medicinal parts are the leaves, stem and flowers, which are collected when the plant is completely mature.

Flower and Fruit: The inflorescence is terminal and racemous with 3 to 10 inclined flowers. The flower buds are globose or oblong-ovate. The tepal petals are 3 to 3.5 cm long, involute, and orange with dark spots. They contain a ciliate mauve honey gland. The anthers are red. The fruit is a 2-winged capsule with an erect fruit stem. The seeds are flat, light brown, and 6 to 8 mm long. Since the seeds do not ripen in northern regions, propagation takes place by means of bulbils, which occur at the leaf axils. Flowers are produced during the third year of growth.

Leaves, Stem, and Root: The plant is a perennial, 30 to 60 cm high or higher. The bulb is golden yellow, ovate, and about 5 cm long. The stem is erect, round, glabrous or with short rough hairs on the upper section. The stem is green or spotted red and leafy in the middle. The leaves are 7 to 11 ribbed, oblong-spatulate, shortly ciliated and up to 15 cm long.

Habitat: The plant comes from China and Japan, but is also cultivated in central and southern Europe.

Production: Martagon is the tuber of *Lilium martagon.*

Other Names: Purple Turk's Cap Lily, Turk's Cap

ACTIONS AND PHARMACOLOGY

COMPOUNDS

Soluble polysaccharides

Starch

Gamma-methylene glutamic acid

Tuliposide

The constituents of the drug have not been fully investigated.

EFFECTS

No information is available.

INDICATIONS AND USAGE

Unproven Uses: The drug is used as a diuretic and in the treatment of dysmenorrhea. It is used externally for ulcers.

Homeopathic Uses: All the above uses are also employed in homeopathic medicine.

PRECAUTIONS AND ADVERSE REACTIONS

No health hazards or side effects are known in conjunction with the proper administration of designated therapeutic dosages.

DOSAGE

Mode of Administration: Martagon is available as cut drug for internal use in infusions and external use in poultices. Homeopathic dilutions are also available.

LITERATURE

Satou T, Mimaki Y, Kuroda M, Sashida Y, Hatakeyama Y, A pyrroline glucoside ester and steroidal saponins from *Lilium martagon. Phytochemistry,* 41:1225-30, Mar. 1996

Masterwort

Peucedanum ostruthium

DESCRIPTION

Medicinal Parts: The medicinal part is the dried root.

Flower and Fruit: The white flowers form many-blossomed compound umbels. There is no involucre. The epicalyx has only a few leaves. The calyx is indistinct. The petals have indented, pointed tips.

Leaves, Stem, and Root: The plant grows from 50 to 100 cm high. The rhizome is gray-brown and produces runners. The stem is round, slightly grooved, and glabrous. The basal leaves are doubly trifoliate. The leaflets are ovate to oblong, about 4 cm wide, roughly serrate, and pale green beneath. The lateral leaflets are dipinnate. The terminal leaflet is tripinnate. The cauline leaves are small with a bulbous, membranous sheath.

Characteristics: Masterwort has an aromatic-bitter taste.

Habitat: The plant grows in central Europe.

Production: Masterwort rootstock is the rhizome of *Peucedanum ostruthium*. The thickened rhizomes are harvested. These are dug up in autumn or spring, then cleaned, freed from any root or green residue, cut and dried at a temperature of 35° C.

ACTIONS AND PHARMACOLOGY

COMPOUNDS

Volatile oil: chief components alpha-pinene, (+)-phellandrene, (+)-limonene, esters of isobutyric and isovaleric acid

Furocoumarins: in particular imperatorin, oxypeucedanin, osthrutol gamma-chromones: peucenine

Phthalides

Polyynes

EFFECTS

Masterwort is said to be stomachic and to have a mild sedative effect. Its main action is as a diuretic.

INDICATIONS AND USAGE

Unproven Uses: Masterwort is used for bloating, flatulence, M. Roemheld syndrome, digestive disorders, weak stomach, and intestinal catarrh.

PRECAUTIONS AND ADVERSE REACTIONS

General: No health hazards or side effects are known in conjunction with the proper administration of designated therapeutic dosages. Light-skinned individuals may experience an increase in UV-sensitivity, due to the phototoxic effect of the furocoumarins.

DOSAGE

Mode of Administration: Masterwort is occasionally used as a constituent in medicinal preparations in combination with other bitters. It is administered as a powder or as an infusion.

Preparation: To prepare an infusion, use a cold extraction of 1 teaspoonful of the drug over a period of 8 hours.

Daily Dosage:

Infusion — Can be drunk throughout the day.

Powder — 0.5 g to 2 g can be taken 2 to 3 times daily.

Storage: Store in a dry place, in closed containers.

LITERATURE

Baerheim-Svendsen A, Tonnesen HH, Karlsen J. Occurence and prevention of Artefact Formation during Isolation and Analysis of Plant Constituents / Some Alkaloids, essential oil constituents, coumarins and curcuminoids. *Sci Pharm.* 61; 265-275. 1993

Gijbels MJM et al Phthalides in roots of Apium graveolens, A. graveolens var. rapeceum, Bifora testiculata and *Petroselinum crispum var. tuberosum. Fitoterapia* 61, 17. 1985

Hiermann A, Schantl D, Schubert-Zsilavecz M, Reiner J. Coumarins from *Peucedanum ostruthium. Phytochemistry* 43 (4); 881-883. 1996

Hegnauer R, Chemotaxonomie der Pflanzen, Bde 1-11, Birkhäuser Verlag Basel, Boston, Berlin 1962-1997.

Kern W, List PH, Hörhammer L (Hrsg.), Hagers Handbuch der Pharmazeutischen Praxis, 4. Aufl., Bde. 1-8, Springer Verlag Berlin, Heidelberg, New York, 1969.

Madaus G, Lehrbuch der Biologischen Arzneimittel, Bde 1-3, Nachdruck, Georg Olms Verlag Hildesheim 1979.

Rauwald HW, Brehm O, Odenthal KP. Evaluation of the calcium antagonist activity of *Peucedanum ostruthium* and *Olea europaea constituents. Pharm Pharmacol Lett.* 1; 78-81. 1991

Teuscher E, Lindequist U, Biogene Gifte - Biologie, Chemie, Pharmakologie, 2. Aufl., Fischer Verlag Stuttgart 1994.

Mastic Tree

Pistacia lentiscus

DESCRIPTION

Medicinal Parts: The medicinal part is the resin.

Flower and Fruit: The inflorescence is compact and spike-like. The flowers are yellowish or purplish. The drupe is approximately 4 mm, globose, apiculate and is red, but later turns black.

Leaves, Stem, and Root: The plant is a small evergreen tree or shrub 1 to 8 m high. The trees are said to be exclusively male. The leaves are bipinnate. The 8 to 12 leaflets measure 1 to 5 cm by 0.5 to 1.5 cm. They are lanceolate to ovate-lanceolate, mucronate, and coriaceous. The rhachis is broadly winged. The petioles are glabrous.

Habitat: The tree thrives in the Mediterranean region, Portugal, Turkey, on the Canaries and in tropical Africa.

Production: Mastic resin is the resin from the trunk of *Pistacia lentiscus*.

Other Names: Lentisk

ACTIONS AND PHARMACOLOGY

COMPOUNDS

Resins (90%): chief components are the triterpenes mastic acid, isomastic acid, oleanolic acid, and tirucallol

Volatile oil (1-3%): including alpha-pinene, myrcene, linalool, beta-pinene, and beta-caryophyllene (constituents vary a great deal)

EFFECTS

In animal experiments Mastic is ulcer protective. The amaroids and essential oil are astringent and aromatic.

INDICATIONS AND USAGE

Unproven Uses: Mastic Tree resin was formerly used in dentistry, as a material for fillings. The masticated resin releases substances that freshen the breath and tighten the gums.

PRECAUTIONS AND ADVERSE REACTIONS

General: No health hazards or side effects are known in conjunction with the proper administration of designated therapeutic dosages.

Pediatric Use: There is an occasional risk of diarrhea in small children.

DOSAGE

Mode of Administration: The resin is used for the production of chewing gum and is used in the food and drink industries.

LITERATURE

Al-Said MS et al., Evaluation of Mastic, a crude drug obtained from *Pistacia lentiscus* for gastric and duodenal anti-ulcer activity. In: ETH 15:271. 1986.

Ford RA. Mastic absolute. *Food Chem Toxic*. 30; Suppl.; 71S-72S. 1992

Marner FJ, Freyer A, Lex J, Triterpenoids from gum Mastic, the resin of *Pistacia lentiscus*. In: PH 30(11):3709-3712. 1991.

Sanz MJ, Terencio MC, Paya M. Pharmacological Actions of a new procyanidin polymer from *Pistacia lentiscus L.* Pharmazie 48; 152-153. 1993

Maté

Ilex paraguariensis

DESCRIPTION

Medicinal Parts: The medicinal parts are the dried or roasted leaves.

Flower and Fruit: The white flowers are axillary and are in clusters of 40 to 50. They have a 4- to 5-sepaled calyx and 4- to 5-petalled corolla, are unisexual and dioecious. The fruit is a globoid reddish drupe with 5 to 8 seeds.

Leaves, Stem, and Root: The plant is an evergreen shrub or tree up to 20 m tall with pale bark and an oblong-oval crown. The leaves are alternate, obovate, acuminate with a crenate or serrate margin. They are dark green above and pale green beneath and are tough, coriaceous, and 6 to 20 cm long and 3 to 9 cm wide.

Characteristics: The taste is astringent and bitter. The odor is characteristic and aromatic.

Habitat: The plant is only found in South America between the 20th and 30th parallel.

Production: Maté consists of the dried leaf and leaf stem of *Ilex paraguariensis*. It is harvested every 2 years from May to September, then dried and cut.

Other Names: Jesuit's Brazil Tea, Paraguay Tea, Yerba Maté

ACTIONS AND PHARMACOLOGY

COMPOUNDS

Purine alkaloids: chief alkaloids caffeine (0.4-2.4%) and theobromine (0.3-0.5%)

Caffeic acid derivatives: including among others chlorogenic acid, neochlorogenic acid, cryptochlorogenic acid

Flavonoids: including among others rutin, isoquercitrin, kaempferol glycosides

Triterpene saponins (mate saponins)

Nitrile glycosides: menisdaurin, not cyanogenic

Volatile oil

EFFECTS

The main active principles are caffeine in varying amounts, tannins and small amounts of essential oil. Depending on the caffeine content the drug can display analeptic, diuretic, positively inotropic and positively chronotropic, glycogenolytic, and lipolytic effects.

The centrally stimulating effect of the drug is due to the chlorogenic acids.

INDICATIONS AND USAGE

Approved by Commission E:

■ Lack of stamina

Maté is used for mental and physical fatigue.

Unproven Uses: In folk medicine Maté is used internally for ulcers, rheumatism, anemia, neurasthenia, depression, as a diuretic for oliguria and as a prophylaxis against fever and infections. Externally Maté is used as a poultice for ulcers and inflammation.

Homeopathic Uses: Ilex paraguariensis is used to treat poor digestion.

PRECAUTIONS AND ADVERSE REACTIONS

No health hazards or side effects are known in conjunction with the proper administration of designated therapeutic dosages.

DOSAGE

Mode of Administration: Maté is available as comminuted herb for infusions, herb powder, and as galenic preparations for internal use. The drug is available as filter teas in mono tea form and in various tea combinations such as bladder and kidney teas.

Preparation: To prepare an infusion, pour water that has just been brought to boil over 1 teaspoonful drug (2 g) and leave to draw for 5 to 10 minutes, then strain. The briefly infused drink is more stimulating, less astringent and tastes better (caffeine dissolves more quickly than the tannins).

Roasted leaves: The dried leaves are heated for 20 minutes to 100° C and then rinsed with water. The leaves are stored for 3 to 4 days to allow the taste and aroma to develop (DAC86).

Daily Dosage: 3 gm of drug.

Tea: as required (1 teaspoon corresponds to 2 g drug).

Homeopathic Dosage: 5 drops, 1 tablet, or 10 globules every 30 to 60 minutes (acute) or 1 to 3 times daily (chronic); parenterally: 1 to 2 mL sc acute, 3 times daily; chronic: once a day (HAB34).

LITERATURE

Gosmann G et al., Triterpenoid saponins from *Ilex paraguariensis.* In: JNP 58(3):438-441. 1995.

Gorzalczany S, Filip R, Alonso MR, Mino J, Ferraro GE, Acevide C. Choleretic effect and ntestinal propulsion of ''mate'' (*Ilex paraguariensis*) and its substitutes or adulterants. *J Ethnopahrmacol.* 75: 291-291. 2001

Gugliucci A. Antioxidant effects of *Ilex paraguariensis*: induction of decreased oxidability of human LDL in vivo. *Biochem Biophys Res Commun*, 224: 338-344 1996

Kraemer KH et al. A new polar saponin from *Ilex paraguariensis. Planta Med* 61(Abstracts of 43rd Ann Congr,), 62. 1995

Kraemer KH, Taketa ATC, Schenkel EP, Gosmann G, Guillaume D. Matesaponin 5, a highly polar Saponin from *Ilex paraguariensis. Phytochemistry* 42 (4); 1119-1122. 1996

Schinella GR, Troiana G, Davila V, de Buschiazzo PM, Tournier HA. Antioxidant effects of an aqueous extract of *Ilex paraguariensis. Biochem Biophys Res Commun*, 269: 357-360. 2000

Hänsel R, Keller K, Rimpler H, Schneider G (Hrsg.), Hagers Handbuch der Pharmazeutischen Praxis, 5. Aufl., Bde 4-6 (Drogen), Springer Verlag Berlin, Heidelberg, New York, 1992-1994 (unter *Ilex paraguariensis*).

Teuscher E, Lindequist U, Biogene Gifte - Biologie, Chemie, Pharmakologie, 2. Aufl., Fischer Verlag Stuttgart 1994.

Teuscher E, Biogene Arzneimittel, 5. Aufl., Wiss. Verlagsges. Stuttgart 1997.

Willems M. Quantitative Determination and Distribution of a Cyanogenic Glucoside in *Ilex aquifolium. Planta Med.* 55; 195. 1989

Matico

Piper elongatum

DESCRIPTION

Medicinal Parts: The medicinal part of the plant is the leaf.

Flower and Fruit: The inflorescence is a long spike of up to 20 cm, opposite the leaf. The flowers have no tepals and are very small with 4 stamens, and an obovoid ovary with a very short 3-stigmaed style. The fruit is a very narrow, black, 1-seeded drupe.

Leaves, Stem, and Root: Piper elongatum is a shrub that typically grows to over 2 m high. The leaves are alternate, entire, up to 20 cm long and 4 cm wide, short petiolate, and coriaceous. The lamina is elongate-lanceolate, long acuminate, and punctate with oil glands. The leaf base is unevenly cordate; the petiole is winged and clasps the stem. The stem is round, conspicuously jointed, and pubescent toward the top.

Characteristics: The leaves have an aromatic smell when rubbed and a bitter, mildly astringent taste.

Habitat: The plant is indigenous to Argentina, Colombia, and Tanzania.

Production: Piper elongatum is cultivated as a medicinal plant in the countries of origin. Matico leaves are the dried leaves of *Piper elongatum.* The fresh leaves are also used medicinally.

Not to be Confused With: Confusion can occur with *Piper aduncum.*

ACTIONS AND PHARMACOLOGY

COMPOUNDS

Volatile oil (0.3 to 6.0%): chief component dill apiol, as well as asarone, parsley apiol

Tannins

Sesquiterpene: maticin

EFFECTS

Use as a hemostyptic could possibly be a result of the tannin content.

INDICATIONS AND USAGE

Unproven Uses: The hemostyptic effect of the leaves is used externally for bleeding wounds and in the treatment of ulcers. Internally, it is used for urogenital complaints (primarily bacterial infections), atonic diarrhea, and dysentery. In Peru, Matico is considered to be an aphrodisiac. It has also been used for minor wounds such as leech bites and after tooth extraction.

PRECAUTIONS AND ADVERSE REACTIONS

No health hazards are known in conjunction with the proper administration of designated therapeutic dosages.

DOSAGE

Mode of Administration: The leaves are administered as whole, cut and powdered forms for internal and external use.

Preparation: There is no information in the literature.

Daily Dosage:

Powder — 0.5 to 2 g drug, 3 to 4 times daily

Infusion — single dose: 1 g drug per cup; or 10% infusion: taken 3 or 4 times daily.

LITERATURE

Hänsel R, Keller K, Rimpler H, Schneider G (Ed), Hagers Handbuch der Pharmazeutischen Praxis, 5. Aufl., Bde 4 - 6 (Drogen), Springer Verlag Berlin, Heidelberg, New York, 1992-1994.

Matricaria Recutita

See German Chamomile

Mayapple

Podophyllum peltatum

DESCRIPTION

Medicinal Parts: The medicinal parts are the dried rhizome and the resin extracted from it.

Flower and Fruit: The solitary white flowers are located in the stem bifurcation between 2 leaves. When the flower drops, the developing fruit swells to the size and shape of a 2.5- to 5-cm long rosehip. It is yellow and fleshy.

Leaves, Stem, and Root: The plant is a perennial reaching a height of 40 cm. It has a bifurcated, 45 cm high stem, and deeply indented, umbrellalike, hand-sized leaves. The rhizome is reddish-brown and is 0.5 cm in diameter. Depending on the time of harvesting, the surface of the rhizome may be smooth or wrinkled. Nodes occur at intervals of 3 to 5 cm, and the fracture is whitish.

Characteristics: The odor is unpleasant and acrid.

Habitat: The plant is indigenous to northeast North America.

Production: Mayapple rhizome consists of the dried rhizome and connected roots of *Podophyllum peltatum*. Mayapple resin consists of the resin of the dried and aged rhizome of *Podophyllum peltatum*.

Not to be Confused With: Mayapple should not be confused with English Mandrake or Bryonia dioica.

Other Names: Duck's Foot, Ground Lemon, Hog Apple, Indian Apple, Mandrake, Raccoon Berry, Wild Lemon

ACTIONS AND PHARMACOLOGY

COMPOUNDS: IN THE ROOT

Podophyllin: mixture of ethanol-soluble extractive material from the root

Lignans: chief components podophyllotoxin (20%), including as well, alpha-peltatin (5%), beta-peltatin (10%), 4′-dimethyl podophyllotoxin, dioxypodophyllotoxin

EFFECTS

The drug is antimitotic.

INDICATIONS AND USAGE

Approved by Commission E:

- Warts

Preparations of Mayapple are used externally for removal of pointed condyloma.

CONTRAINDICATIONS

The drug is contraindicated in pregnancy.

PRECAUTIONS AND ADVERSE REACTIONS

General: The drug is severely irritating to skin and mucous membranes. External administration of the drug over large skin areas can also bring about resorptive poisonings. The drug should not be taken internally in allophathic medicine. With external use, the skin area to be treated should not exceed 25 sq. cm. The drug serves as an industrial drug for the extraction of podophyllotoxin and its semi-synthetic derivatives that are used in tumor therapy.

OVERDOSAGE

In dosages >0.2 g, it causes severe abdominal pain, bloody-watery diarrhea, vomiting of liquid bile, dizziness, headache, coordination disorders, spasms, nephritis, later collaps,e and death in coma through respiratory failure.

Following gastrointestinal emptying (inducement of vomiting, gastric lavage with burgundy-colored potassium permanganate solution, sodium sulfate) and instillation of activated charcoal, the therapy for poisonings consists of treating spasms with diazepam (IV), electrolyte substitution and treating possible cases of acidosis with sodium bicarbonate infusions. In case of shock, plasma volume expanders should be used. Monitoring of kidney function is essential. Intubation and oxygen respiration may also be necessary.

DOSAGE

Mode of Administration: The dried rhizome is used for production of resin exclusively for external application.

Daily Dosage: The daily dosage is 1.5 to 3.0 g root, 1.5 to 3.0 g liquid extract or 2.5 to 7.5 g tincture. The treated skin surface must not be larger than 25 sq. cm. Be sure to protect skin adjacent to the treated area.

LITERATURE

Franz G, Biogene Cytostatica. In: *DAZ* 130(35):2003. 1990.

Kletter C, Kriechbaum M, Szambor P, Qusar N, Holzner W, Kubelka W. Documentation of Tibetan Plants / 3rd Communication / ol-mo-se / *Podophyllum hexandrum Royle. Sci Pharm.* 62; 283-297. 1994

Jardine I, In: Anticancer Agents Based on Natural Product Models, Ed. Cassady JM, Douros JD. Academic Press 1980.

MacRae WD, Towers GHN, Biological activities of lignans. In: PH 23(6):1207-1220. 1984.

Maytenus ilicifolia

See Congorosa

Meadowsweet

Filipendula ulmaria

DESCRIPTION

Medicinal Parts: The medicinal parts are the dried flowers, the dried aerial parts of the flowering plant, and the fresh underground and aerial parts of the flowering plant.

Flower and Fruit: The radial flowers are in terminal compound, loose cymes arranged with erect, very irregular branches. The 5 to 6 free sepals are triangular, pointed, 1 mm long, downy on the outside and fused to the flat receptacle at the base. The 5 to 6 petals are obviate, narrowed to a short stem, yellowish white and 2 to 5 mm long. The ovaries are glabrous or downy and have a flattened-stigma-bearing style under 1 mm. The one-seeded indehiscent fruit twine in a spiral.

Leaves, Stem and Root: The plant is perennial and grows to about 50 to 200 cm high. The stem is erect, simple or branched above, woody below, angular, usually glabrous or occasionally tomentose. The leaves are alternate, long- petioled to almost sessile, irregularly odd-pinnate with paired opposite pinna. These are ovate, rounded at the base or short-wedge-shaped, double serrate to dentate. The pinna is dark green and usually glabrous above and gray to white tomentose beneath and only pubescent on the ribs.

Characteristics: The leaves smell very different from the flowers, having a pleasant, almond-like fragrance.

Habitat: The plant is found in northern and southern Europe, North America and northern Asia.

Production: Meadowsweet flower consists of the dried flower of Filipendula ulmaria (syn. Spiraea ulmaria), as well as its preparations. Meadowsweet herb consists of the dried above-ground parts of Filipendula ulmaria, harvested during flowering season, as well as its preparations. The plant is combed off during the flowering season and air-dried in a dark place.

Not to be Confused With: May be confused with elder flowers and Filipendula hexapetala.

Other Names: Bridewort, Dolloff, Meadsweet, Meadow Queen, Meadow-Wort, Queen of the Meadow, Lady of the Meadow, Spireaea ulmaria

ACTIONS AND PHARMACOLOGY

COMPOUNDS: MEADOWSWEET FLOWER

Flavonoids: chief components - spiraeoside (quercetin-4′-O-glucosides, 3-4%), further including among others kaempferol-4′-O-glucosides, hyperoside, rutin

Volatile oil (0.2%): chief components salicylaldehyde and methyl salicylate (yielded through dehydration from monotropitin - salicylaldehyde primveroside - and spiraeine - salicylic acid ester primveroside), further, a little vanillin and heliotropine

Tannins: ellagic tannins

EFFECTS: MEADOWSWEET FLOWER

Meadowsweet has antiphlogistic and astringent effects. The drug, which contains salicylate, has an antimicrobial, antipyretic and diuretic effect. In animal tests the flavonoid fraction had a positive effect on the healing of stomach ulcers and a tone-increasing effect on smooth muscle was observed.

COMPOUNDS: MEADOWSWEET HERB

Etheric oil (traces): including salicylic acid ester

Flavonoids: including rutin, hyperoside, quercetin-3-O-glucuronide, quercetin-3-O-arabinoside

Tannins: ellagic tannins

EFFECTS: MEADOWSWEET HERB

The drug, which contains salicylate, has an antimicrobial, antipyretic and diuretic effect. In animal tests the flavonoid fraction had a positive effect on the healing of stomach ulcers and a tone-increasing effect on smooth muscle was observed.

INDICATIONS AND USAGE

MEADOWSWEET FLOWER

Approved by Commission E:

- Cough
- Bronchitis
- Fever and cold

MEADOWSWEET HERB

Approved by Commission E:

- Cough
- Bronchitis

Meadowsweet is used as supportive therapy for colds, for febrile colds, and as a diuretic.

Unproven Uses: In folk medicine Meadowsweet is used as a diuretic, for rheumatism of the joints and muscles, for gout, for bladder and kidney disease and for headaches. Meadowsweet herb is used for stomach complaints with hyperacidity, prophylaxis, therapy of stomach ulcers, and for diarrhea in children.

Homeopathic Uses: Filipendula ulmaria is used for rheumatism and inflammation of mucous membranes.

CONTRAINDICATIONS

Preparations are contraindicated in presence of salicylate sensitivity.

PRECAUTIONS AND ADVERSE REACTIONS

No health hazards or side effects are known in conjunction with the proper administration of designated therapeutic dosages.

OVERDOSAGE

Overdosage can lead to queasiness and stomach complaints.

DOSAGE

Mode of Administration: Comminuted drug and other galenic preparations for infusions. Meadowsweet flower is contained in various tea mixtures, which are used for the flu, rheumatism, kidney, and bladder inflammations.

Preparation: To prepare an infusion, pour boiling water over 3 to 6 g cut drug, steam for 10 minutes and then strain. Fluid extract (herb): 1:1 in 25% ethanol (BHP83). Tincture (herb): 1:5 in 45% ethanol (BHP83)

Daily Dosage: 2.5 to 3.5 g of Meadowsweet flower or 4 to 5 gm Meadowsweet herb. Infusion dosage is 1 cup several times a day (1 tsp. = 1.4 g drug). Liquid extract (herb) daily dose: 1.5 to 6 mL; Tincture (herb) daily dose: 2 to 4 mL

Homeopathic Dosage: 5 drops, 1 tablet, or 10 globules every 30 to 60 minutes (acute) or 1 to 3 times daily (chronic); from

D6: parenterally: 1 to 2 mL sc acute: 3 times daily; chronic: once a day (HAB1)

Storage: Should be protected from light and moisture.

LITERATURE

Csedö K et al., The antibiotic activity of *Filipendula ulmaria*. In: PM 59(7):A675. 1993.

Gräfe AK, Besonderheiten der Arzneimitteltherapie im Säuglings- und Kindesalter. In: PZ 140(30):2659-2667. 1995.

Halkes SBA et al. A strong complement inhibitor from the flowers of *Filipendula umlamria* (L.) Maxim. *Pharm Pharmacol Lett.* 7 (2/3); 79-82. 1997

Medicago sativa

See Alfalfa

Melaleuca alternifolia

See Tea Tree

Melaleuca leucadendra

See Cajuput

Melaleucaea viridiflora

See Niauli

Melilotus officinalis

See Sweet Clover

Melissa officinalis

See Lemon Balm

Mentha aquatica

See Wild Mint

Mentha arvensis var. piperascens

See Japanese Mint

Mentha longifolia

See English Horsemint

Mentha piperita

See Peppermint

Mentha pulegium

See Pennyroyal

Mentha spicata

See Spearmint

Menyanthes trifoliata

See Bog Bean

Mercurialis annua

See Mercury Herb

Mercury Herb

Mercurialis annua

DESCRIPTION

Medicinal Parts: The drug is the flowering plant.

Flower and Fruit: The plant has yellow-green flowers. The male flowers are in tightly packed, interrupted ears, on thin, hairlike pedicles. They have 12 stamens. The female flowers are short-petioled in twos or threes in the leaf axils. The style is short or nonexistent. There are 2 stigmas. The fruit is a 2-headed capsule.

Leaves, Stem, and Root: The plant is an annual that grows 20 to 50 cm high. The stem is erect, cross-branched, obtuse, quadrangular, glabrous, and segmented. The leaves are opposite, petiolate, ovate to lanceolate, light green, and have a ciliate margin.

Characteristics: The plant has an unpleasant smell when rubbed. The whole plant has no latex.

Habitat: The plant grows in Europe and is naturalized in the eastern U.S.

Production: Mercury Herb is the flowering herb of *Mercurialis annua.*

ACTIONS AND PHARMACOLOGY

COMPOUNDS

Cyanogenic glycosides (small amounts)

Pyridone derivatives (that color the urine red): including among others hermidin

Saponins (1%)

Amines: including among others, methyl amine (mercurialine), ethyl amine, propyl amine, isobutyl amine, isoamyl amine

Flavonoids: including among others, rutin, narcissine, isorhamnetin.

Nothing is known regarding the type of the toxins. The cyanogenic glycosides are probably not responsible for the toxicity.

EFFECTS

The drug is slightly poisonous, and it can lead to diarrhea and an overactive bladder. The root and stock act as strong laxatives.

INDICATIONS AND USAGE

Unproven Uses: The drug is used for suppurating inflammation, as a laxative and diuretic, and as an adjuvant in the treatment of gastrointestinal and urinary tract diseases.

Homeopathic Uses: Mercury Herb is used for rheumatism and colds.

PRECAUTIONS AND ADVERSE REACTIONS

The fresh plant, in particular the root and the rhizome, are considered poisonous. Symptoms of poisoning include diarrhea, nerve paralysis, and liver and kidney damage. Poisonings, including fatal ones, are only known among animals. There are no reports available on the drug's toxicity in humans. The intake of small doses would likely lead to nothing more than diarrhea.

DOSAGE

Mode of Administration: The drug is administered ground, as an extract, in juice and in homeopathic dilutions.

LITERATURE

Frohne D, Pfänder HJ, Giftpflanzen - Ein Handbuch für Apotheker, Toxikologen und Biologen, 4. Aufl., Wiss. Verlags-Ges. Stuttgart 1997.

Kern W, List PH, Hörhammer L (Hrsg.), Hagers Handbuch der Pharmazeutischen Praxis, 4. Aufl., Bde. 1-8, Springer Verlag Berlin, Heidelberg, New York, 1969.

Lewin L, Gifte und Vergiftungen, 6. Aufl., Nachdruck, Haug Verlag, Heidelberg 1992.

Madaus G, Lehrbuch der Biologischen Arzneimittel, Bde 1-3, Nachdruck, Georg Olms Verlag Hildesheim 1979.

Roth L, Daunderer M, Kormann K, Giftpflanzen, Pflanzengifte, 4. Aufl., Ecomed Fachverlag Landsberg Lech 1993.

Teuscher E, Lindequist U, Biogene Gifte - Biologie, Chemie, Pharmakologie, 2. Aufl., Fischer Verlag Stuttgart 1994.

Mexican Scammony Root

Ipomoea orizabensis

DESCRIPTION

Medicinal Parts: The medicinal parts are the dried roots and the steamed ethanol extract from the roots.

Flower and Fruit: The plant has reddish-purple, campanulate flowers.

Leaves, Stem, and Root: Mexican Scammony Root is a twining plant with large cordate leaves. The root tuber is about 18 to 25 cm long, 9 to 10 cm wide, and cylindrical-fusiform. It is grayish-brown to brownish-black and wrinkled externally. Inside the section shows irregular concentric rings and scattered resin glands, resembling jalap.

Characteristics: The taste is acrid and resinous. The odor is slight.

Habitat: Mexico

Production: Mexican Scammony Root is the root extracted from *Ipomoea orizabensis*. Both the root and the yielded resin are effective as drugs.

Other Names: Ipomoea, Jalap, Mexican Jalap

ACTIONS AND PHARMACOLOGY

COMPOUNDS

Glycoretines (12-15%, resinous): polymeric ester glycosides made up of hydroxy- and dihydroxy fatty acids bonded in esterlike fashion (including 11-hydroxy palmitic acid = jalapinolic acid), on the hydroxyl groups of which oligosaccharide remnants are bonded as glycosides. These bear short-chained acyl remnants (acetyl, isobutyryl, isovaleryl, and tigoyl remnants).

EFFECTS

The drug has a strong laxative effect on the small and large intestines caused by resin (Resina Scammoniae) combined with ester glycoside mixtures (glycoretine).

INDICATIONS AND USAGE

Unproven Uses: Preparations have been used as a very drastic purgative for constipation.

CONTRAINDICATIONS

The drug is contraindicated in pregnancy.

PRECAUTIONS AND ADVERSE REACTIONS

General: No health hazards are known in conjunction with the proper administration of designated therapeutic dosages. Intestinal colic occurs frequently as a side effect.

Pregnancy: Mexican Scammony Root is contraindicated in pregnancy.

OVERDOSAGE

Overdosages cause vomiting.

DOSAGE

Mode of Administration: The herb is obsolete as a drug in many countries. Used on rare occasions in combination preparations. The same applies to other Ipomoea varieties e.g., *I. turpethum, I. operculata.*

Daily Dosage: The average single dose is 1 g of drug.

LITERATURE

Hänsel R, Keller K, Rimpler H, Schneider G (Hrsg.), Hagers Handbuch der Pharmazeutischen Praxis, 5. Aufl., Bde 4-6 (Drogen): Springer Verlag Berlin, Heidelberg, New York, 1992-1994.

Lewin L, Gifte und Vergiftungen, 6. Aufl., Nachdruck, Haug Verlag, Heidelberg 1992.

Madaus G, Lehrbuch der Biologischen Arzneimittel, Bde 1-3, Nachdruck, Georg Olms Verlag Hildesheim 1979.

Noda N et al., *Tetrahedron* 43:3889. 1987.

Roth L, Daunderer M, Kormann K, Giftpflanzen, Pflanzengifte, 4. Aufl., Ecomed Fachverlag Landsberg Lech 1993.

Shellard EJ, PM 9:146-152. 1961.

Singh S, Stacey BE, (1973) Phytochemistry 12:1701.

Steinegger E, Hänsel R, Pharmakognosie, 5. Aufl., Springer Verlag Heidelberg 1992.

Wagner H, (1973) In ''Chemistry in Biochemical Classification'', Nobel Symposium (1973).

Mezereon

Daphne mezereum

DESCRIPTION

Medicinal Parts: The medicinal part is the bark, which is collected before the flowering season.

Flower and Fruit: The flowers are dark pink. They appear before the leaves in irregular, sessile clusters usually in threes. There is a 4-tipped calyx with an external silky-haired tube. There are 8 stamens in 2 rows and 1 free ovary. The fruit consists of a bright red, pea-sized, juicy, ovoid, single-seeded berry.

Leaves, Stem, and Root: The plant is a 50- to 150-cm high perennial. It is a deciduous, sparsely branched shrub with reedlike, grayish or yellow-brown branches that are very tough. The leaves are short-petioled, lanceolate, narrowing toward the petiole and entire-margined.

Characteristics: Mezereon has a strong, pleasant fragrance. The plant is poisonous and can be fatal if ingested. It is a protected species.

Habitat: The plant is indigenous to Europe as far as Siberia. It is cultivated in the U.S., Canada and elsewhere.

Production: Mezereon root, root bark and bark are from *Daphne mezereum*. The bark of the trunk and the root are gathered before flowering, dried and rolled up but with the phloem facing outward. Care should be taken not to destroy the plant during the harvest.

Other Names: Camolea, Daphne, Dwarf Bay, Spurge Flax, Spurge Laurel, Spurge Olive, Wild Pepper

ACTIONS AND PHARMACOLOGY

COMPOUNDS

Diterpenes: diterpene esters, daphnane derivatives, including mezerein, daphnetoxin

Hydroxycoumarins: including umbelliferone, daphnetin, daphnoretin (dimerous), triumbellin (trimerous) and hydroxycoumarin glycosides, for example daphnin, daphnorin

Flavonoids

EFFECTS

The drug acts as a powerful skin stimulant, hallucinogenic, and a rubifacient. A possible immunostimulating effect has been observed in vitro. Antitumoral, anticoagulant, and abortifacient effects have been observed in animal tests.

INDICATIONS AND USAGE

Unproven Uses: Use of Mezeron is no longer recommended due to its toxicity.

In the past, Mezeron root was used to relieve headache, toothache, gout, whooping cough, syphilis, constipation, and worm infestation. It was used externally for joint pains and to increase circulation in the case of rheumatic complaints, skin conditions and conjunctivitis. The drug is known in old drug manuals as ''Spanish fly plaster'' or Drouotic plaster and was recommended for various pain symptoms.

Homeopathic Uses: In homeopathic medicine, *Daphne mezereon* is used for skin conditions such as cradle cap, shingles, weeping eczema, and encrusted, weeping blisters, as well as for neuralgia and pains in the bones.

PRECAUTIONS AND ADVERSE REACTIONS

External contact with the severely irritating toxic diterpenes of Daphne mezereon causes erysipeloid reddening of the skin, swelling, blister formation and shedding of the epidermis. Extended exposure leads to the formation of necroses. Contact with the eyes causes severe conjunctivitis. If taken internally, reddening and swelling of the oral mucous membranes, feeling of thirst, salivation, stomach pains, vomiting, and severe diarrhea occur.

Resorption of the drug may cause headache, dizziness, stupor, tachycardia, spasms, and possibly death through circulatory collapse. Cool wrappings and anesthetic salves are recommended for treatment of the skin injuries.

OVERDOSAGE

Poisoning resulting from ingestion of the drug should be treated with gastric lavage and calcium gluconate, IV. Administration of corticosteroids may also be indicated.

DOSAGE

Mode of Administration: The drug is seldom used today. Used in homeopathic dilutions, topically and internally.

Homeopathic Dosage: 5 drops, 1 tablet, or 10 globules every 30 to 60 minutes (acute) or 1 to 3 times daily (chronic); parenterally: 1 to 2 mL sc acute, 3 times daily; chronic: once a day (HAB1).

Storage: The effect fades if it is stored for too long. Therefore, do not store for a period of more than 2 years.

LITERATURE

Evans B, In: Evans FJ:Naturally Occuring Phorbolesters, CRC Press Inc., Boca Raton, Florida. 1986.

Kreher B, Neszmelyi A, Wagner H. Triumbellin, a Tricoumarin Rhamnopyranoside from *Daphne mezereum. Phytochemistry* 29; 3633-3637. 1990

Kupchan SM, Baxter RL, *Science* 187:652. 1974

Nyborg J, La Cour, T, *Nature* 257:824. 1975

Stout GH et al., *J Am Chem Soc* 92:1070. 1970

Milk Thistle

Silybum marianum

DESCRIPTION

Medicinal Parts: The medicinal parts of the plant are the ripe seeds.

Flower and Fruit: The inflorescences are large, solitary and purple. They consist of somewhat nodding, composite flower heads. The perigone is globular. The inner tepals taper to a slender point, and the outer tepals are tough at the base, then spread and terminate at a horny tip. There are only tubular florets. The fruit is brown, spotted and glossy, with a white tuft of hair.

Leaves, Stem and Root: The plant grows from 70 to 150 cm high with an erect stem. The leaves are arranged in different levels with the lower leaves indented-pinnatisect, and the upper ones lanceolate and clasping. There are white spots along the ribs of the leaf and yellow thorns at the margin.

Habitat: The plant is indigenous to Europe.

Other Names: Marian Thistle, Mediterranean Milk Thistle, Mary Thistle

ACTIONS AND PHARMACOLOGY

COMPOUNDS: MILK THISTLE HERB

Flavonoids: in particular, apigenin-, luteolin- and kaempferol-7-0-glycosides, apigenin-4,7 ¢-'-di-0-glucoside, kaempferol-7-0-glucoside-3-sulfate

Steroids: sterols, including beta-sitosterol, beta-sitosterol glucoside

Polyynes

Organic Acids: fumaric acid (3.3%)

(Silymarin is absent; it is localized only in the seed case)

COMPOUNDS: MILK THISTLE SEED

Silymarin (flavonolignan mixture,1.5-3%): chief components silybin A, silybin B (mixture known as silibinin), isosilybin A, isosilybin B, silychristin, silydianin

Flavonoids: apigenin, chrysoeriol, eriodictyol, naringenin, quercetin, taxifolin

Fatty oil (20-30%)

EFFECTS

In clinical studies, Milk Thistle has been shown to have a positive hepatoprotective effect in the treatment of liver cirrhosis associated with chronic alcohol abuse or viruses. In animal, in vitro and clinical studies, the primary action of silymarin as an antioxidant is a protectant for the kidneys and liver. A small number of studies on silymarin's effect on biliary lipid composition in both animals and adults concluded a reduction of biliary cholesterol concentrations. The effectiveness of silymarin is difficult to evaluate due to multiple agent treatment protocols in studies with adults and animals, but the results appear to be positive in the treatment of mushroom poisoning. The cholagogue effect of the drug has not been documented.

Hepatoprotective Effects: The hepatoprotective activity of the seed is from silymarin, in particular, silychristin and silydianin. The compounds seem to inhibit the entrance of toxins and block toxin-binding sites through alteration of the liver cell's outer membrane. (Hikino, 1994; Leng-Peschlow, 1996). The hepatoprotective effect of silibinin also involves different functions of the Kupffer cells. Silibinin decreases production of superoxide anion radicals and nitric oxide (free-radical scavenger or antioxidant) by the Kupffer cells. Silibinin also inhibits leukotriene formation by the Kupffer cells (Dehmlow, 1996). Silymarin increases glutathione production by the liver, intestines and stomach. Glutathione is used for detoxification cells in the liver (Valenzuela, 1989). Silibinin decreases hepatic and mitochondrial glutathione oxidation induced by iron overload and is a mild chelator of iron (Pietrangelo, 1995).

Anti-inflammatory Effects: Silymarin is thought to exert an anti-inflammatory response via inhibition of leukotriene production. This anti-inflammatory effect may be beneficial in treating liver cirrhosis or fibrosis (Leng-Peschlow, 1996).

Liver Regenerative Effects: Silymarin stimulates RNA polymerase I in the cell nucleus of the hepatocytes, resulting in an increase of ribosomal protein synthesis and the regenerative ability of the liver. This mechanism is of particular importance in the antidote effect against death-cap mushroom poisoning since the poison which it contains, alpha-Amanitin, inhibits this enzyme in the cell nucleus.

Protective Effects: Silymarin is an antioxidant free radical scavenger, reducing iron-2+ induced linoleate peroxidation (Vavreckova et al. 1997; Valenzuela et al. 1986). Flavonoids (including silymarin) are good antioxidants due to their phenolic structure (Campos et al. 1989). They also act as plasma membrane stabilizers (Flora et al. 1998).

A renoprotective effect of the herb on kidney cells damaged by acetaminophen, cisplatin and vincristin was demonstrated in a recent study. Silibinin and silychristin demonstrated remarkable stimulatory effects on proliferation rate, biosynthesis of protein and DNA, and activity of the enzyme lactate dehydrogenase in kidney cells (Sonnenbichler, 1999). Silibinin reduces intracellular and secreted forms of prostate-specific antigen (PSA) levels and inhibits cell growth via a G1 arrest in cell cycle progression in hormone-refractory prostate carcinomas. Silibinin-induced G1 arrest decreases the kinase activity of cyclin-dependent kinases (CDKs) and associated cyclins for an anticarcinogenic effect (Zi, 1999; Zi, 1998)

CLINICAL TRIALS

Hepatitis

Twenty-four subjects with chronic hepatitis C were enrolled into a randomized, double-blind, placebo-controlled, cross-over study. They were assigned, over a period of 12 weeks, to either milk thistle (600 mg or 1200 mg/day) or placebo, separated by a 4-week washout interval. Mean changes in HCV RNA titers, serum ALT levels, and Short Form-36 scores in the group were not statistically significant compared to placebo. Adverse events were similar with milk thistle and placebo (Gordon et al, 2006).

A systematic Cochrane Group review and meta-analyses of high quality, randomized clinical trials of determined that Milk Thistle fails to significantly alter the course of patients with alcoholic and/or hepatitis B or C liver diseases. Evidence to support or refute Milk Thistle's value for liver patients remains insufficient. Of the 13 randomized clinical trials that examined patients with these liver ailments (915 patients total), methodological quality was generally low, with only 46% considered properly double-blinded and only 23% reporting adequate allocation concealment. Liver-related mortality was significantly reduced by Milk Thistle in the high-quality trials, but had no significant effect on all-cause mortality. Among the trials reporting adverse drug events, Milk Thistle was reported as well tolerated and safe (Rambaldi, 2005).

Researchers found that there was a statistically significant reduction in the mean concentrations of alanine aminotransferase (ALT), aspartame aminotransferase (AST), gammaglutamyltranspeptidase (gamma-GT), and total bilirubin after silybin treatment. The study involved 20 patients with chronic active hepatitis who were randomly assigned to a group receiving 240 mg twice a day of silybin (n=10), or placebo (n=10). Liver function tests and (MDA) malondialdehyde were done prior to the initial administration and after seven days of treatment. Alkaline phosphatase decreased only slightly, and there was no significant change in MDA serum concentrations. The silybin agent used was silybin phosphatidylcholine complex (Buzzelli et al, 1993).

Silymarin was not clinically useful in one double-blind, 3-month study of 116 patients with histologically proven alcoholic hepatitis, treated with either placebo or silymarin (420 mg/d). Fifty-seven patients received the silymarin, and 59 received the placebo. Parameters assessed were serum levels and histological scores of alcoholic hepatitis and fibrosis obtained from biopsy samples at the start of the study and 3 months later. The results of the study suggested that in the treatment of moderate alcoholic hepatitis, silymarine was not clinically relevant (Trinchet et al, 1989).

Hepatoprotection

The effect of silymarin in 200 alcoholic patients with cirrhosis of the liver was demonstrated in a controlled, double-blind, randomized and multicenter trial. The study compared 450 mg of silymarin (150 mg/3 times per day) with placebo. Patient survival was similar in the silymarin and placebo treatment group after 2 years of therapy. No relevant side effects were observed in either group, and the results indicated that silymarin has no effect on survival and the clinical course in alcoholics with liver cirrhosis (Pares, 1998).

It has also been shown, however, that silymarin may reduce lipoperoxidative liver damage often seen with the chronic use of phenothiazines or butyrophenone. This was concluded in a double-blind, placebo-controlled study of 60 women on chronic (at least 5 years) phenothiazine or butyrophenone therapy. Eligible patients had aspartate aminotransferase (AST) or alanine aminotransferase (ALT) levels more than twice the normal value. These patients were given silymarin 800 mg/d along with their psychotropic drugs, silymarin without the psychotropic drugs, or placebo with the psychotropic drugs. Serum levels of malon-dialdehyde (MDA) (a polyunsaturated fatty acid oxidation product) and liver enzymes (ALT, AST, GGT, MDA) were measured on days 15, 30, 60, and 90 during the silymarin treatment, and 30 days after the silymarin therapy was finished. MDA decreased by about 7.8% in one month in the group taking silymarin combined with the psychotropic drugs and even more so in the group where the psychotropic drugs were not continued. When these patients were placed back on the psychotherapeutic agents, the MDA levels slowly increased (Palasciano et al, 1994).

A double-blind, randomized, placebo-controlled trial was conducted to determine the hepatoprotective effect of silymarin in 170 cirrhosis patients. The patients were given either 140 mg silymarin three times daily or a placebo. After treatment for 2 years, biochemical markers did not change significantly. After a 4-year analysis, treatment was seen most effective in patients with alcoholic cirrhosis and Child's A group classification of portal hypertension. The drug was ineffective in patients with Child's B and C group hypertension (Ferenci, 1989).

Mushroom Poisoning

In a study of 60 patients with severe Amanita mushroom poisoning who were given 20 mg/kg of silybin intravenously, no patients died from the mushrooms (Vogel, 1981). Death rates for this type of mushroom poisoning vary widely but may reach up to 40% or 50%. Hruby reported a 12.8% death rate in 220 cases of Amanita poisonings seen between 1979 and 1982 (Hruby, 1984).

INDICATIONS AND USAGE

MILK THISTLE HERB

Unproven Uses: Preparations of Milk Thistle herb are used as a stimulant, for functional disorders of liver and gallbladder including jaundice, gallbladder colic and diseases of the spleen. The herb was formerly used as a malaria treatment, emmenagogue and for uterine complaints.

MILK THISTLE SEED

Approved by Commission E:

- Dyspeptic complaints
- Liver and gallbladder complaints

The drug is used for dyspepsia (crude drug); toxic liver damage, hepatic cirrhosis, and as a supportive treatment in chronic inflammatory liver disease.

Unproven Uses: The drug is also used as an antidote to death-cap (Amanita) mushroom poisoning.

PRECAUTIONS AND ADVERSE REACTIONS

Episodes of severe sweating, abdominal cramping, nausea, vomiting, diarrhea and weakness were recently reported in Australia, but the reaction was found to be due to a substance in the Milk Thistle product other than silybin (Adverse Drug Reaction Advisory Committee, 1999).

DRUG INTERACTIONS

MODERATE RISK

Metronidazole: May result in reduced metronidazole and active metabolite exposure. *Clinical management:* Concurrent use with silymarin (an active flavonoid of Milk Thistle) is not recommended. If concomitant use is necessary, the dose of metronidazole may need to be increased.

POTENTIAL INTERACTIONS

The concomitant use of silymarin and butyrophenones or phenothiazines results in a reduction of lipid peroxidation (Palasciano, 1994). Silymarin has an antagonistic effect with yohimbine and phentolamine when given simultaneously (Di Carlo, 1993).

DOSAGE

MILK THISTLE HERB

Preparation: An infusion is prepared by pouring boiling water over 1/2 teaspoonful of the drug and then straining after 5 to 10 minutes.

Daily Dosage: The average dose of the infusion is 2 to 3 cups daily.

MILK THISTLE SEED

Mode of Administration: Comminuted drug for infusions and extracts; tinctures for liquids and solid forms.

How Supplied:

Capsules–70 mg, 100 mg, 140 mg, 150 mg, 175 mg, 180 mg, 300 mg, 500 mg, 540 mg, 1000 mg, 1050 mg

Liquid–1:1, 1:2

Tablet–50 mg, 500 mg

Tea

Preparation: To prepare an infusion, add 3 g of the drug to cold water and bring to a boil. Drain after 10 to 20 minutes.

Daily Dosage: For liver dysfunction or ailments, the daily dosage has been effective and well tolerated at 140 to 420 mg divided in 2 to 3 doses (Ferenci, 1989; Frerick, 1990; Pares, 1998; Schuppan, 1998). The average dose of silymarin was approximately 33 mg/kg/d for cyclopeptide mushroom poisoning. Silymarin administered up to 48 hours after mushroom ingestion appears to be effective in preventing severe liver damage in Amanita phalloides poisoning (Hruby, 1983).

Although products are usually standardized to 70% to 80% (not milligrams) of silymarin, the silymarin concentrations may vary without government regulation (Flora et al. 1998).

Storage: Store away from direct light, heat and moisture; keep at room temperature.

LITERATURE

MILK THISTLE HERB AND SEED

Adverse Drug Reactions Advisory Committee. An adverse reaction to the herbal medication milk thistle (Silybum marianum). *Med J Aust*;170(5):218-9, Mar 1,1999.

Ahmed AA et al. *PH* 28:1751. 1989.

Anon. (Adverse Drug Reactions Advisory Committee). An adverse reaction to the herbal medication milk thistle (*Silybum marianum*). In: *MJA*; 170(1):218-219,1999.

Arnone A, Merlini L, Zanarotti A. Constituents of Silybum marianum. Structure of isosilybin and stereochemistry of isosilybin. *J Chem Soc* (Chem Commun):696-697, 1979.

BAnz (Federal German Gazette) No. 49. published 11 March 1992.

Baumann J. Über die Wirkung von Chelidonium, Curcuma, Absinth und Carduus marianus auf die Galle- und Pankreassekretion bei Hepatopathien. *Med Mschr* 29:173, 1975.

Benda I, Zenz W. *Wien Med Wschr* 123:512, 1973.

Benda L, Dittrich H, Ferenzi P, Frank H, Wewalka F. The influence of therapy with silymarin on the survival rate of patients with liver cirrhosis. *Wien Klin Wschr* 92(19):678-683, 1980.

Bode JCh, Arzneimittel für die Indikation ''Lebererkrankungen''. In: Dölle W, Müller-Oerlingshausen B, Schwabe U (Hrsg.), Grundlagen der Arzneimitteltherapie. Entwicklung, Beurteilung und Anwendung von Arzneimitteln. B.I.- Wissenschaftsverlag, *Mannheim Wien Zürich*, S 202-211, 1986.

Bode JCh. Die alkoholische Hepatitis, ein Krankheitsspektrum. *Internist* 220:536-545, 1981.

Buzzelli G, Moscarella S, Giusti A et al. A pilot study on the liver protective effect of silybin-phosphatidylcholine complex (IdB1016) in chronic active hepatitis. *Int J Clin Pharmacol Ther Toxicol* 1993; 31:456-460.

Campos R, Garrido A, Guerra R et al. Silybin dihemisuccinate protects against glutathione depletion and lipid peroxidation induced by acetaminophen on rat liver. In: *Planta Med*; 55:417-419, 1989.

Desplaces A et al. *Arzneim Forsch* 25, 89, 1975.

Dehmlow C, Erhard J, de Groot H. Inhibition of Kupffer cell functions as an explanation for the hepatoprotective properties of silibinin. *Hepatology*;.23(4):749-54, Apr 1996.

Di Carlo G, Autore G, Izzo AA et al. Inhibition of intestinal motility and secretion by flavonoids in mice and rats: structure-activity relationships. In: *J Pharm Pharmacol*; 45:1054-1059, 1993.

Dölle W, Schwabe U. Leber- und Gallenwegstherapeutika. In: Schwabe U, Paffrath D (Hrsg.), Arzneiverordnungsreport 88, Gustav Fischer, Stuttgart New York, S 242-253, 1988.

Feher J, Deak G, Muezes G, Lang I, Niederland V, Nekam K, Karteszi M. Hepatoprotective activity of silymarin legalon therapy in patients with chronic alcoholic liver disease. *Orv Hetil* 130(51):2723-2727, 1989.

Ferenci P, Dragosics B, Dittrich H et al. Randomized controlled trial of silymarin treatment in patients with cirrhosis of the liver. *J. Hepatol.* Jul;9(1):105-113.1989.

Frerick H, Kuhn U. Strenge-Hesse A et al. Silymarin - ein Phytopharmakon zur Behandlung von toxischen Leberschäden. *Der Kassenarzt*;33/34:36-41, 1990. Ferenci P, Dragosics B, Dittrich H, Frank H, Benda L, Lochs H, Meryn S, Base W, Schneider B. Randomized controlled trial of silymarin treatment in patients with cirrhosis of the liver. *J Hepatol* 9(1):105-113, 1989.

Fintelmann V, Albert A. Nachweis der therapeutischen Wirksamkeit von Legalon bei toxischen Lebererkrankungen im *Doppelblindversuch. Therapiewoche* 30(35):5589-5594, 1980.

Flora K, Hahn M, Rosen H et al. Milk Thistle (*Silybum marianum*) for the therapy of liver disease. *Am J Gastroenterol;* 93:139-143, 1998.

Gordon A, Hobbs DA, Bowden DS, Bailey MJ, Mitchell J, Francis AJ, Roberts SK. Effects of Silybum marianum on serum hepatitis C virus RNA, alanine aminotransferase levels and well-being in patients with chronic hepatitis C. *J Gastroenterol Hepatol*; 21(1 Pt 2): 275-280. 2006.

Hahn G, Lehmann HD, Kürten M et al. Zur Pharmakologie und Toxikologie von Silymarin, des antihepatotocischen Wirkprinzips aus Silybum marianum (L.) Gaertn. *Arzneim Forsch/Drug Res* 18:698-704, 1968.

Hruby K, Fuhrmann M, Csomos G, Thaler H. Pharmakotherapie der Knollenblätterpilzvergiftung mit Silibinin. *Wien Klein Wschr* 95(7):225-231, 1983.

Hruby K, Csomos G, Fuhrmann M, Thaler H. Chemotherapy of Amanita phalloides poisoning with intravenous silibinin. *Hum Toxicol*;2(2):183-95, Apr 1983.

Hruby K. Silibinin in the treatment of deathcap fungus poisoning. *Forum* 1984; 6:23-26.

Khafagy SM et al. *Sci Pharm;* 49:157, 1981.

Kalmar L, Kadar J, Somogyi A et al. Silibinin (Legalon-70) enhances the motility of human neutrophils immobilized by formyl-tripeptide, calcium ionophore, lymphokine and by normal human serum. In: *Agents Actions*; 29:239-246, 1990.

Koch H. Leberschutz-Therapeutika. *Pharmazie in unserer Zeit* 9:33-44:65-74, 1980.

Leng-Peschlow E. Properties and medical use of flavonolignans (silymarin) from *Silybum marianum. Phytother Res*; 10(suppl):S25-S26, 1996.

Leng-Peschlow E. Strenge-Hesse A, Die Mariendistel (*Silybum marianum*) und Silymarin als Lebertherapeutikum. *Z Phytother* 12:162-174, 1991.

Lorenz D, Mennicke WH, Behrendt W. Untersuchungen zur Elimination von Silymarin bei cholecystektomierten Patienten. *Planta Med* 45:216-233, 1992.

Martines G, Copponi V, Cagnetta G. Aspetti del danno epatico dopo somministrazione sperimentale di alcuni farmaci. *Arch Sci Med* 137:367-386, 1980.

Martini GA. Hepatozelluläre Erkrankungen, Leberkrankheiten. In: Riecker G (Hrsg.), Therapie innerer Krankheiten, Springer, Berlin Heidelberg New York, S 638-652, 1988.

Marugg D, Reutter FW. Die Amanita-phalloides-Intoxikation. Moderne therapeutische Ma bnahmen und klinischer Verlauf. *Schweiz Rundschau Med* (Praxis) 14(37):972-982, 1985.

Mericli AH. *PM* 54:44. 1988.

Mennicke WH. Zur biologischen Verfügbarkeit und Verstoffwechselung von Silybin.: *Dtsch Apoth Ztg* 115(33):1205-1206, 1975.

Mironets VI. Krasovskaia EA & Polishchuk II, Sluchai krapivnitsy pri lechenii karsilom (A case of urticaria during carsil treatment). *Vrach Delo*; 7:86-87, 1990.

Palasciano G, Portinacasa P, Palmieri V et al. The effect of silymarin on plasma levels of malondialdehyde in patients receiving long-term treatment with psychotropic drugs. *Curr Ther Res*; 55:537-545, 1994.

Pares A, Planas R, Torres M et al. Effects of silymarin in alcoholic patients with cirrhosis of the liver: results of a controlled, double-blind, randomized and multicenter trial. *J Hepatol*; 28(4):615-21, Apr 1998.

Peeters H (Ed.). Phosphatidylcholine. Biochemical and Clinical Aspects of Essential Phospholipids. Springer Verlag, Berlin Heidelberg New York, 1976.

Rambaldi A, Jacobs BP, Iaquinto G, et al. M ilk thistle for alcoholic and/or hepatitis B or C liver diseases—a systematic Cochrane hepato-biliary group review with meta-analyses of randomized clinical trials. *Am J Gastroenterol;* 100(11):2583-2591. 2005.

Rauen HM, Schriewer H. Die antihepatotoxische Wirkung von Silymarin bei experimentellen Leberschäden der Ratte durch Tetrachlorkohlenstoff, D-Galaktosamin und Allylalkohol. *Arzneim Forsch/Drug Res* 21:1194-1201, 1971.

Reuter HD. Spektrum Mariendistel und andere leber- und gallewirksame Phytopharmaka. In: Bundesverband Dtschr Ärzte für Naturheilverfahren (Hrsg.) Arzneimitteltherapie heute. *Aesopus Verlag*, Basel, 1992.

Reyes H & Simon FR, Intrahepatic cholestasis of pregnancy: an estrogen-related disease. *Semin Liver Dis*; 13:289-301, 1993.

Schulz HU, Schürer M, Krumbiegel G, Wächter W, Weyhenmeyer R, Seidel G. Untersuchungen zum Freisetzungsverhalten und zur Bioäquivalenz von Silymarin- Präparaten. *Arzneim Forsch/Drug Res* 45:61-64, 1995.

Schuppan D, Strösser W, Burkard G, Walosek G et al. Verminderung der Fibrosierungsaktivität durch Legalon bei chronischen Lebererkrankungen Z Allgemeinmed;11/12:577-584, 1998.

Sonnenbichler J et al. Proceedings of the International Bioflavonoid Symposium (Munich); 477, 1981.

Sonnebichler J, Zetl I. Untersuchungen zum Wirkungsmechanismus von Silibinin, Einflu b von Silibinin auf die Synthese ribosomaler RNA, mRNA und tRNA in Rattenlebern in vivo. Hoppe-Seyler's Physiol Chem 365:555-556, 1984

Sonnenbichler J, Zetl I. Biochemical effects of the flavonolignane silibinin in RNA, protein and DANN synthesis of rat livers. *Prog Clin Biol Res* 213:319-331, 1986.

Sonnenbichler J, Zetl I. Stimulating influence of a flavonolignane on proliferation, RNA synthesis and protein Synthesis in liver cells. In, Okoliczányi L, Csomós G, Crepaldi G (Eds.), Assessment and management of hepatobiliary disease. Springer, Berlin Heidelberg New York, S 265-272, 1987.

Sonnenbichler J, Zetl I. Specific binding of a flavonolignane to an estradiol receptor. In: Plant flavonoids in Biology and Medicine II, Biochemical, cellular, and medicinal properties. Alan R Liss, New York, S 369-374, 1988.

Sonnenbichler J, Scalera F, Sonnenbichler I et al. Stimulatory effects of silibinin and silicristin from the Milk Thistle *Silybum marianum* on kidney cells. *J Pharmacol Exp Ther*; 290(3):1375-83, Sep 1999.

Varis K, Salmi HA, Siurala M. Die Therapie der Lebererkrankung mit Legalon; eine kontrollierte Doppelblindstudie. In: Aktuelle Hepatologie, III. Internationales Symposium Köln 15.-17. November 1978. Hanseatisches Verlagskontor. *Lübeck*, S 42-43, 1978.

Valenzuela A, Aspillaga M, Vial S, Guerra. Selectivity of silymarin on the increase of the glutathione content in different tissues of the rat. *Planta Med*; 55(5):420-2, Oct 1989.

Valenzuela A, Guerra R & Videla LA. Antioxidant properties of the flavonoids silybin and (+)-cyanidanolo-3: comparison with butylated hydroxyanisole and butylated hydroxytoluene. In: Planta Med; 52:438-440, 1986.

Vavreckova C, Kosina P, Kubisch J et al. Antilipoperoxidation activity of four silybin glycosides. *Chemicke-Listy;* 91:687-689, 1997.

Vogel G. The anti-amanita effect of silymarin. In: Faulstich et al. (Eds.), Amanita toxins and poisoning. Witzstrock, Baden-Baden Köln New York, S 180-187, 1980.

Wagner H, Seligmann O, Seilz M, Abraham D, Sonnenbichler J. Silydianin und Silychristin, zwei isomere Silymarine aus Silybum marianum L. Gaertn. (Mariendistel). *Z Naturforsch* 31b:876-884, 1976.

Zi X, Agarwal R. Silibinin decreases prostate-specific antigen with cell growth inhibition via G1 arrest, leading to differentiation of prostate carcinoma cells: implications for prostate cancer intervention. *Proc Natl Acad Sci USA*; 96(13):7490-5, Jun 22, 1999.

Zi X, Feyes DK, Agarwal R. Anticarcinogenic effect of a flavonoid antioxidant, silymarin, in human breast cancer cells MDA-MB 468: induction of G1 arrest through an increase in Cip1/p21 concomitant with a decrease in kinase activity of cyclin-dependent kinases and associated cyclins. In: *Clin Cancer Res*; 4(4):1055-64, Apr 1998.

Momordica charantia

See Bitter Gourd

Monarda didyma

See Oswego Tea

Monarda Punctata

See Horsemint

Moneywort

Lysimachia nummularia

DESCRIPTION

Medicinal Parts: The medicinal parts are the fresh or dried whole flowering plant.

Fruit and Flower: The flowers are solitary or in pairs. The leaf axils have 5 free, almost cordate sepals. The corolla is rotate, divided into 5, and fused at the base. It is rich yellow and spotted with dark red glands on the inside. There are 5 glandular-haired stamens fused at the base and 1 ovary. The fruit is a 4- to 5-mm long globular capsule. The seeds are triangular, blackish-brown, warty, and 1.5 mm long.

Leaves, Stem, and Root: The plant is a perennial. The stem is a runnerlike creeper, lightly branched, quadrangular, glabrous to slightly pubescent with roots at the nodes. It grows from 10 to 45 cm. The leaves are entire-margined, crossed-opposite, short-petioled, red-glandular punctate, and orbicular elliptical.

Habitat: The plant is indigenous to all of Europe and the Caucasus and has been introduced into America and Japan.

Production: Moneywort is the complete plant of *Lysimachia nummularia.* The whole flowering plant, including the root, is collected, cleaned and dried in the shade.

Other Names: Creeping Jenny, Creeping Joan, Herb Two-pence, Meadow Runagates, Running Jenny, Serpentaria, String of Sovereigns, Twopenny Grass, Wandering Jenny, Wandering Tailor

ACTIONS AND PHARMACOLOGY

COMPOUNDS

Flavonoids: including among others glycosides of myricetins, kempferols and quercetins, including rutin, hyperosides

Tannins

Triterpene saponins

The constituents of the drug have not been fully investigated.

EFFECTS

Moneywort is mildly astringent and expectorant. Extracts of the aerial plant parts are said to be antibacterial in vitro; however, scientific results are not available.

INDICATIONS AND USAGE

Unproven Uses: Moneywort is used externally as a vulnerary and for acute and chronic eczema. It is used internally for diarrhea and excessive salivation, and as an expectorant for coughs.

PRECAUTIONS AND ADVERSE REACTIONS

No health hazards or side effects are known in conjunction with the proper administration of designated therapeutic dosages.

DOSAGE

Preparation: To make a tea, pour 250 mL boiling water over 2 heaping teaspoonfuls drug and leave to steep for 5 minutes. For a wound poultice, dilute the tea preparation with the same amount of chamomile tea.

Daily Dosage: For the treatment of coughs, drink 1 cup of tea, 2 to 3 times daily with honey if desired.

LITERATURE

Hänsel R, Keller K, Rimpler H, Schneider G (Hrsg.), Hagers Handbuch der Pharmazeutischen Praxis, 5. Aufl., Bde 4-6 (Drogen), Springer Verlag Berlin, Heidelberg, New York, 1992-1994.

Madaus G, Lehrbuch der Biologischen Arzneimittel, Bde 1-3, Nachdruck, Georg Olms Verlag Hildesheim 1979.

Monkshood

Aconitum napellus

DESCRIPTION

Medicinal Parts: Deadly poison.

Flower and Fruit: The flowers are 50 to 160 cm long and form violet, bluish, or reddish upright racemes. The calyx has 5 petal-like sepals. The upper sepal is convex and helmet-shaped. There are 2 petals with nectar-releasing spurs under the upper sepal. There are numerous glabrous or ciliate stamens. There are 3 glabrous ovaries with 10 to 14 ovules. The fruit is a 16 to 20 mm long by 5 mm thick follicle. The seeds are glossy black and triangular with narrow wings on the edges.

Leaves, Stem, and Root: Aconitum napellus is a 0.5 to 1.5 m high shrub with a tuberous, thickened, fleshy root and an erect, rigid, undivided stem. The racem axis and petioles are glabrous or hairy. The leaves are dark green, glossy above, and lighter beneath. They are palmate and 5- to 7-pinnatasect. The sections of the leaf are rhomboid in outline and deeply indented with oblong tips.

Characteristics: The plant is extremely poisonous.

Habitat: Aconitum napellus is common to the Alps and the Carpathians and is to be found in all the mountainous regions of Europe. The plant is found as far as Sweden in the north, as far as England and Portugal in the west, as far as the Pyrenees in the south and as far as the Carpathians in the east.

Production: Monkshood tuber consists of the fresh or dried tubers and roots of *Aconitum napellus* harvested in autumn after flowering. Monkshood herb consists of the dried herb of *Aconitum napellus* collected at the beginning of the flowering season. The collected roots are quickly dried at 40° C.

Not to be Confused With: Other blue-flowering Aconitum species.

Other names: Aconite, Auld Wife's Huid, Blue Rocket, Friar's Cap, Helmet Flower, Mousebane, Priest's Pintle, Wolfsbane,

ACTIONS AND PHARMACOLOGY

COMPOUNDS

Nor-diterpene alkaloids: including aconitine, mesaconitine, hypaconitine, N-desethyl aconitine, oxoaconitine

EFFECTS

The efficacy of the drug is based on the di-ester alkaloids aconitin, mesaconitin and hypaconitin. Aconitin raises membrane permeability for sodium ions and retards repolarization. Aconitin is initially stimulating, and then causes paralysis in the motor and sensitive nerve ends, and in the CNS. The other di-ester alkaloids function in a similar fashion. Hypaconitin works more intensely. Aconitin applied in small doses triggers bradycardia and hypotension; in higher doses it has at first, a positive inotropic effect, followed by tachycardia, cardiac arrhythmia and cardiac arrest. Di-ester alkaloids were shown to be analgesic in animal experiments. Applied topically in humans, the drug is initially stimulating, in the form of itchiness or burning, and then anesthetizing. The drug has an anti-febrile effect. Therapeutic doses influence the heart minimally; the heart rate may increase slightly. Given orally, the drug is active after a few minutes.

INDICATIONS AND USAGE

Unproven Uses: The drug is extremely toxic and should only be used in homeopathic doses. In folk medicine, it was used to reduce pain from neuralgia, particularly with trigeminus and intercostal neuralgia. It was also used for myalgia, muscular and articular rheumatism, serous skin inflammation, and migraine. Preparations of blue monkshood were used for pain, facial paralyses, ailments of the joints, arthritis, gout, rheumatic complaints, inflammation, pleurisy, pericarditis sicca, fever, and skin and mucosal diseases, as well as for disinfecting and wound treatment. In experimental pharmacology, Aconitin is used due to its ability to trigger cardiac arrhythmia.

Homeopathic Uses: Aconitum napellus is used for acute inflammatory illnesses, cardiac palpitations with anxiety states and painful peripheral nerve disease.

PRECAUTIONS AND ADVERSE REACTIONS

The drug is highly toxic. Signs of poisoning can appear even with the administration of therapeutic dosages. The first sign of poisoning is a tingling of the mouth, fingers and toes, which then spreads over the entire body surface and changes into a furry sensation. Body temperature decreases quickly and queasiness, vomiting, diarrhea, and urination follow.

OVERDOSAGE

With fatal doses, breathing becomes irregular and the heartbeat slows down and becomes arrythmic. Intense pains are characteristic. Death usually follows within 6 hours due to heart failure or asphyxiation. For adults, the estimated fatal dosage lies between 1 to 2 g. Countermeasures include gastrointestinal emptying, keeping the patient warm, cardiovascular and pulmonary support, magnesium and calcium infusions, administration of atropine to fight bradycardia, lidocaine for relieving the arrythmias, possibly artificial respiration, and pain relief (no opiates).

DOSAGE

Mode of Administration:

The drug is extremely toxic and should only be used in homeopathic doses.

Preparation: Aconiti tinctura: 1:1

Daily Dosage:

Homeopathic Dosage: 5 drops, 1 tablet, or 10 globules every 30 to 60 minutes (acute) and 1 to 3 times per day (chronic); Parenterally: 1 to 2 mL 3 times daily sc; Ointment 1 to 2 times daily (HAB1).

Storage: The herb must be kept in a dry place protected from light and insects.

LITERATURE

Bugatti C, Colombo ML, Tomé F, Extraction and purification of lipoalkaloids from *Aconitum napellus* roots and leaves. In: *PM* 58(7):A695. 1992.

Capitanio M, Cappelletti EM, Filippini R. Traditional antileukodermic herbal Remedies in the Mediterranean Area. *J Ethnopharmacol.* 27; 193-211. 1989

Erhard M, Kellner J, Wild J, Lösch U, Hatiboglu FS. Effect of Echinacea, Aconitum, Lachesis and Apis Extracts, and their Combinations on Phagocytosis of Human Granulocytes. *Phytother Res.* 8 (1); 14-17. 1994

Honerjäger P, Meissner A, Naunyn-Schmiedeberg's Arch Pharmacol 322:49-58. 1983.

Katz A. Detection of Diterpinoid Alkaloids in Aphids feeding on *Aconitum napellus* and *Aconitum paniculatum. J Nat Prod.* 53; 204-206. 1990

Kimura I, Makino M, Matsui T, Takada M, Kimura M. Aconitine-induced Bradycardia, Centrally Acting Muscarinic Effects are Inhibited Peripherally by Higenamine in Conscious Mice. *Phytother Res.* 8 (3); 129-134. 1994

Liu H, Katz A, Norditerpenoid alkaloids from *Aconitum napellus ssp. neomontanum*. In: *PM* 62(2):190-191. 1997.

Olafsson K, Ingolfsdottir K. Aconitine in Nectaries and Other Organs from an Icelandic Population of Aconitum napellus ssp. vulgare. *Planta Med.* 60; 285-286. 1994

Morinda citrifolia

See Noni

Moringa oleifera

See Behen

Morning Glory

Ipomoea hederacea

DESCRIPTION

Medicinal Parts: The medicinal parts are the seeds and root.

Flower and Fruit: The flowering branches bear 1 to 5 radial flowers with structures in fives. The 5 sepals are 1.3 to 2.5 cm long, narrow-lanceolate, acuminate, and rough-haired at the base. The 5 petals are 3.8 to 5 cm long, funnel-shaped, spotted blue-pink, or are fused at the base of the orange corolla. The plant has 5 stamens and a superior 3-chambered ovary. The fruit is a capsule with a diameter of approximately 8 mm containing 4 to 6 smooth seeds.

Leaves, Stem, and Root: This winding herb grows 1 to 3 m high. The leaves are alternate, ovate-cordate and entire, with a diameter of 5 to 12.5 cm. The stem is slightly pubescent.

Habitat: The plant is indigenous to China, India, and Central and South America.

Production: Morning Glory seeds are the dried, ripe seeds of *Ipomoea hederacea.* The plants are harvested in autumn before the seeds open, then dried in the sun. The seeds are then removed and cleaned.

Not to be Confused With: Morning Glory seeds are similar to and sometimes confused with the seeds of other Ipomoea species.

ACTIONS AND PHARMACOLOGY

COMPOUNDS

Indole alkaloids of the ergoline type (0.5%): chief alkaloids lysergol (50%) and chanoclavine (35%). Smaller amounts of penniclavine and elymoclavine

Fatty oil (12 to 14%): chief fatty acids oleic acid, palmitic acid, stearic acid

Resins (15%): glycoretines (macromolecular, resinous glycosides of hydroxy-fatty acids [C12 to C16]) with oligosaccharides, the so-called pharbitinic acids; the latter's hydroxyl groups are estered with (among others) alpha-methylbutyric acid, tiglic acida and valeric acid to the fatty acid remnant

EFFECTS

The drug has a drastic laxative effect due to the glycoretines it contains, which presumably explains its usefulness against ascarid and tapeworm infestations.

INDICATIONS AND USAGE

Unproven Uses: Morning Glory has been used for worm infestation and constipation.

Indian Medicine: Morning Glory is used for constipation, flatulence, parasite infestation, scabies, and dyspepsia.

Chinese Medicine: Uses of Morning Glory include edema, constipation, parasite infestation, and feelings of fullness.

PRECAUTIONS AND ADVERSE REACTIONS

The drug's laxative effect is frequently accompanied by cramplike pains.

CONTRAINDICATIONS

Because of the possible teratogenic effect, the drug should not be used during pregnancy.

DOSAGE

Mode of Administration: Whole, cut, and powdered drug.

Preparation: Resin is made by heating the powdered drug until it melts, then cooling it to form a pale translucent mass.

Daily dose: Drug: 0.5 to 3 g drug; resin: daily dose: 0.3 g; maximum single dose: 0.1 g

Chinese Dosage: Powder: 1.5 to 5 g drug, can be raised to 12 to 15 g

Tea; 24 to 30 g drug

Storage: Store in dry place.

LITERATURE

Dugan GM, Gumbmann MR. Toxicological Evaluation of Morning Glory seed: Subchronic 90-day Feeding study. *Food Chem Toxic.* 28; 553-559. 1990

Hänsel R, Keller K, Rimpler H, Schneider G (Ed), Hagers Handbuch der Pharmazeutischen Praxis, 5. Aufl., Bde 4 - 6 (Drogen), Springer Verlag Berlin, Heidelberg, New York, 1992-1994.

Morus nigra

See Black Mulberry

Motherwort

Leonurus cardiaca

DESCRIPTION

Medicinal Parts: The medicinal parts are the fresh aerial parts collected during the flowering season.

Flower and Fruit: Small, bright red, bilabiate flowers are in dense false whorls in the upper leaf axils. The calyx is funnel-shaped with 5 rigid, awned tips, which are bent outward. The corolla is densely villous on the outside and longer than the calyx. The stamens stretch out longer than the flower. The fruit is a brown, triangular, 2.5- to 3-mm long nutlet with a tuft of hair at the tip.

Leaves, Stem, and Root: The plant is perennial and has a short woody rhizome. It grows to about 120 cm. The stem is erect, quadrangular, grooved, hollow, often red-violet, and usually hairy. The leaves are long-petioled, pubescent, or glabrous. The lower leaves are palmate and cordate at the base. The upper leaves have 3 lobes. The upper surface is dark green, the lower surface light green.

Characteristics: Motherwort has an unpleasant smell.

Habitat: The plant is indigenous to central Europe and Scandinavia through temperate Russia to central Asia. It was introduced to North America and has become established in the wild there.

Production: Motherwort herb consists of the above-ground parts of *Leonurus cardiaca*, gathered during flowering season, as well as their preparations. They are collected in the wild and dried at 35° C.

Other Names: Lion's Tail, Lion's Ear, Throw-Wort

ACTIONS AND PHARMACOLOGY

COMPOUNDS

Diterpene bitter principles: leocardin

Iridoide monoterpenes: ajugoside (leonuride), ajugol, galiridoside, reptoside

Flavonoids: including, among others, rutin, quercitrin, isoquercitrin, hyperoside, genkwanin

Leonurin: (syringa acid esters of 4-guanidino-butane-1-ols)

Betaine: stachydrine (N-dimethyl-L-proline)

Caffeic acid derivatives: caffeic acid-4-O-rutinoside

Tannins

Volatile oil (traces)

EFFECTS

Mildly negatively chronotropic, hypotonic, sedative.

INDICATIONS AND USAGE

Approved by Commission E:

- Nervous heart complaints
- Thyroid dysfunction

Unproven Uses: Flatulence. In folk medicine it is used for bronchial asthma, climacteric symptoms, and amenorrhea.

Homeopathic Uses: Homeopathic treatments include use for cardiac complaints, flatulence, and hyperthyroidism.

PRECAUTIONS AND ADVERSE REACTIONS

General: No health hazards or side effects are known in conjunction with the proper administration of designated therapeutic dosages.

Pregnancy: Not to be used during pregnancy.

DOSAGE

Mode of Administration: Comminuted herb for infusions and other galenic preparations for internal use.

Daily Dosage: 4.5 g herb; infusion: 2 to 4 g drug 3 times daily; liquid extract (1:1): 2 to 4 mL 3 times daily; tincture: daily dose: 2 to 6 mL.

Homeopathic Dosage: Acute states: 5 drops, 1 tablet, or 10 globules every 30 to 60 minutes. Chronic states: 5 drops, 1 tablet, 10 pellets or a knife tip 1 to 3 times daily. Parenterally: Acute: 1 to 2 ml sc., 3 times daily; chronic: 1 to 2 ml once a day (HAB1).

LITERATURE

Barnes J, Ernst E. Traditional Herbalist's Prescriptions for Common Clinical Conditions: A Survey of Members of the UK National Institute of Medicinal Herbalists. *Phytother Res.* 12 (5); 369-371. 1998

Broda B, Grzybek J. Preparation of herbal mixtures / Studies on herbs with designed sedative activity. *Z Phytother.* 14; 307-314. 1993

Buzogany K, Cucu V, Accumulation, distribution and conservation dynamics of iridoids in *Leonurus cardiaca L.* and *L. villosus Desf.* In: *Farmacia* (Bukarest): 34(3):173-176. 1986.

Kartnig T, Gruber A, Menzinger S. Flavonoid-O-Glycosides from the Herbs of *Leonurus cardiaca. J Nat Prod.* 48; 494-507. 1985

Malakov P, Papanov G, Jakupovic J, Grenz M, Bohlmann F. The Structure of Leocardin, two epimers of a Diterpenoid from *Leonurus cardiaca. Phytochemistry* 24; 2341-2343. 1985

Papanov GY, Malakov PY, Rodriguez B, Torre MC de la. A Prefuranic Labdane Diterpene from *Leonurus cardiaca.* Phytochemistry 47 (6); 1149-1151. 1998

Racz G, Racz-Kotilla E. Sedative and Antihypertensive Activity of *Leonurus quinquelobatus.* Abstracts of Short Lect and Poster Present. 30. 1988

Tschesche R et al., (1980) Phytochemistry 19:2783.

Weischer ML, Okpanyi SN, Pharmakologie eines pflanzlichen Schlafmittels. In: *ZPT* 15(5):257-262. 1994.

Xia XX, (1983) J Trad Chin Med 3:185.

Mountain Ash Berry

Sorbus aucuparia

DESCRIPTION

Medicinal Parts: The medicinal parts are the ripe or dried fruit.

Flower and Fruit: The inflorescence is broadly umbelliferous-paniculate, erect, floriferous, loosely tomentose, occasionally completely or almost completely glabrous. The calyx has 5 segments. There are 5 white petals and numerous stamens. The ovary is inferior and has 2 to 4 free styles, which are pubescent in the lower portion. The false fruit is almost globular with a diameter of 9 to 10 mm and is scarlet. There are usually 3 seeds, which are narrow-oblong, acute, and reddish.

Leaves, Stem, and Root: The plant is usually a medium-sized tree up to 16 m high with a round, rather loose crown. The bark is smooth and pale gray, later becoming vertically fissured and blackish. The leaves are odd-pinnate with 5 to 11 almost sessile leaflets. These are oblong-lanceolate, irregularly thorny-tipped and serrate, pubescent, or almost glabrous.

Characteristics: The flowers have an unpleasant smell and the berries are sharp-tasting and sour. *Sorbus moravica* tastes sweet in contrast.

Habitat: The plant is indigenous to almost all of Europe, to Western Siberia and Asia Minor, and is found in North America.

Production: Mountain Ash Berry consists of the fresh or dried fruit, or fruit cooked and dried thereafter, of *Sorbus aucuparia* as well as its preparations. The ripe, shiny red fruit is harvested from August to October

Other Names: European Mountain Ash, Quick-Beam, Rowan Tree, Sorb Apple, Witchen

ACTIONS AND PHARMACOLOGY

COMPOUNDS

Cyanogenic glycosides (0.06%; in the seeds 0.2 to 0.5%; traces in the fruit pulp): in the seeds amygdalin, in the fruit pulp prunasin

Fruit acids: malic acid (3 to 5%), tartaric acid

Monosaccharides/oligosaccharides: saccharose, glucose, fructose, sorbose

Parasorboside (bitter substance): parasorbic acid is formed from it through cell destruction (lactone of the (5S)-Hydroxy-hex-2-en-acid-1, pungent in odor, mucus-membrane-irritating, 0.1 to 0.3% of the fresh weight). Parasorbic acid is destroyed through dehydration or volatilized during cooking. It is present only in traces (less than 0.01%) in the cultivated variety, which contains few bitter substances.

Sugar alcohols: sorbitol

Tannins

Vitamins: ascorbic acid (vitamin C, 0.03 to 0.13%, higher content in the non-bitter fruits)

EFFECTS

The parascorbic acid is weakly laxative and irritating to the mucous membrane. Ascorbic acid is a vitamin C supplement.

INDICATIONS AND USAGE

Unproven uses: Mountain Ash is used in folk medicine for kidney diseases, diabetes, rheumatism, disorders of uric acid metabolism, for dissolution of uric acid deposits, menstruation disturbances, the alkalization of the blood, to improve the metabolism, and for vitamin C deficiency.

PRECAUTIONS AND ADVERSE REACTIONS

No health hazards or side effects are known in conjunction with the proper administration of designated therapeutic dosages of the dehydrated drug or with the consumption of fruit sauces, juices, jellies, jams, etc., produced through cooking.

OVERDOSAGE

Because of the formation of the mucus-membrane-irritating parasorboside that results from cutting up the fruit, the intake of very large quantities of the fresh fruit leads to gastroenteritis, vomiting, queasiness, gastric pain, diarrhea, kidney damage (albuminuria, glycosuria), and to polymorphic exanthemas.

DOSAGE

Mode of Administration: Mountain Ash is available as whole and crude drug forms.

Daily Dosage: A purée is used for diarrhea. Freshly pressed juice (or juice with sugar) is taken by the dessertspoonful for conditions of the lungs and pleura with fever.

LITERATURE

Kokubun T, Harborne JB, Waterman PG. Antifungal Biphenyl Compounds are the Phytoalexins of the Sapwood of *Sorbus aucuparia. Phytochemistry* 40 (1); 57-59. 1995

Mountain Avens

Dryas octopetala

DESCRIPTION

Medicinal Parts: Mountain Avens is the whole dried plant of *Dryas octopetala.*

Flower and Fruit: The flower stalk is upright, 2 to 8 cm long. The diameter of the flowers is 2 to 4 cm; there are 6 to 9 sepals, which are glabrous on the inside and brown, feltlike and glandular on the outside. There are 6 to 9 white petals and numerous stamens. The carpels are numerous, free, and densely haired, with apical styles twisted like screws. The fruit is like a nut.

Leaves, Stem, and Root: This evergreen dwarf shrub grows up to 0.5 m high. The leaves are 0.5 to 4 cm long, up to 2.5 cm wide, coriaceous, crenate, short-petiolate; the lamina is spatulate, obovate or elongate-elliptical, with a cordate base, wrinkled and glabrous above, tomentose beneath; the stipules are dry-membranous and sharply acuminate. The small stem is heavily branched, the leaves on the horizontal branches are double-rowed. The upright stem has leaves all around. The plant has a primary taproot.

Habitat: The shrub grows in the Arctic, subarctic and high mountainous regions.

Production: The plant is collected in the wild, cut and powdered.

ACTIONS AND PHARMACOLOGY

COMPOUNDS

Tannins (2.5 to 5.5% in the root; 7.5 to 14% in the leaves)

Catechin tannins (7 to 14%)

Flavonoids (0.7 to 1.6%): glycosides of quercetin, kaempferol, isorhamnetin, limocitrin, gossypetin, corniculatusin, and sexangularetin

Triterpenes: including tormentoside

EFFECTS

Due to its tannin and flavonoid glycoside content, the drug is astringent in effect.

INDICATIONS AND USAGE

Unproven Uses: Folk medicine uses include stomach pains and diarrhea.

The effect appears to be plausible because of the flavonoid glycoside content, but is unproven.

PRECAUTIONS AND ADVERSE REACTIONS

No health hazards are known in conjunction with the proper administration of designated therapeutic dosages. The ingestion of larger dosages can lead to digestive complaints and constipation, due to the high tannin content. Available data are insufficient to classify the drug's safety.

LITERATURE

Hänsel R, Keller K, Rimpler H, Schneider G (Ed.), Hagers Handbuch der Pharmazeutischen Praxis, 5. Aufl., Bde 4 - 6 (Drogen), Springer Verlag Berlin, Heidelberg, New York, 1992-1994.

Mountain Flax

Linum catharticum

DESCRIPTION

Medicinal Parts: The medicinal parts are the herb, the fresh flowering plant and the whole plant.

Flower and Fruit: The flowers are on loose, panicled, branched, sparsely leafed twining stems on long peduncles in the leaf axils. They hang before flowering. The sepals are elliptically acuminate, 2 to 2.5 mm long with ciliate glands. The 5 white petals are up to 5 mm long, and yellow at the base. There are 5 stamens fused at the base and 1 ovary with 5 headed stigma on long thin styles. The fruit is an erect, globular, 2 to 3 cm long, and incomplete 10-valved capsule with long, pubescent, dividing membranes. The seeds are elliptical, 1 to 1.5 mm long, flat, smooth, and light brown.

Leaves, Stem, and Root: The plant is an inconspicuous annual (occasionally perennial) that grows up to 30 cm. It has a long erect or ascending stem, which is undivided or dividing into the flowering branches. The leaves are opposite or alternate, entire-margined, sessile, and have a partly ciliate margin.

Habitat: Found in central Europe as far as the British Isles and southward as far as the Mediterranean countries, the Caucasus, Iran, and northern Africa.

Production: Mountain Flax is the flowering plant (aerial part) of *Linum catharticum*, collected in the uncultivated regions.

Other Names: Dwarf Flax, Fairy Flax, Mill Mountain, Purging Flax

ACTIONS AND PHARMACOLOGY

COMPOUNDS

Lignans: achromatin (bitter), presumably present in the fresh plant as a glycoside

Tannins

Volatile oil

The constituents of the drug have not been extensively investigated.

EFFECTS

Mountain Flax has a laxative effect in therapeutic doses of up to 0.5 g. High doses cause vomiting and gastroenteritis.

Although the amaroid linin is not laxative, it is probably present in the form of a glycoside, which has a stronger laxative effect.

INDICATIONS AND USAGE

Unproven Uses: Its use as a laxative is obsolete. In folk medicine Mountain Flax is used for constipation, oliguria, edema, worm infestation, catarrh, and rheumatic conditions.

Homeopathic Uses: Used homeopathically for coughs, hemorrhoids, diarrhea, catarrh, rheumatic disorders, dropsy, and worm infestation. Also used as a purgative and emetic.

PRECAUTIONS AND ADVERSE REACTIONS

No health hazards or side effects are known in conjunction with the proper administration of designated therapeutic dosages. The drug can lead to vomiting, inflammations of the gastrointestinal tract and diarrhea. The emetic and laxative effects are used therapeutically.

DOSAGE

Mode of Administration: Ground and as an extract.

Preparation: To prepare an infusion, add 2.5 g to 1 cup of hot water.

Dosage: 2.0 g powder as a single dose.

LITERATURE

Hänsel R, Keller K, Rimpler H, Schneider G (Hrsg.), Hagers Handbuch der Pharmazeutischen Praxis, 5. Aufl., Bde 4-6

(Drogen), Springer Verlag Berlin, Heidelberg, New York, 1992-1994.

Madaus G, Lehrbuch der Biologischen Arzneimittel, Bde 1-3, Nachdruck, Georg Olms Verlag Hildesheim 1979.

Mountain Grape

Mahonia aquifolium

DESCRIPTION

Medicinal Parts: The medicinal parts are the dried rhizome and the roots, the dried branch and twig bark, as well as the root bark.

Flower and Fruit: The heavily scented flowers are either in dense 5 to 10 cm panicles or in groups of 3 to 6 in erect 5 to 8 cm racemes in the leaf axils. The flowers are yellow and have 9 sepals, 6 petals and 6 stamens, which are about 8 cm long. The pedicles are 5 to 10 mm long. The fruit is a globose, purple-black, frosted berry with red juice. The 2 to 5 seeds are glossy brown.

Leaves, Stem, and Root: The plant is a fast-growing, evergreen, stoloniferous shrub about 50 to 150 cm high with stout stems, sparingly branched. The leaves are odd-pinnate, 10 to 20 cm long with 3 to 6 pairs of leaflets. The leaflets are 4 to 8 cm by 2 to 4 cm, ovate, distally spinose dentate, coriaceous, dark and shining green.

Habitat: Indigenous to the Pacific U.S.; ornamental or cultivated in Europe.

Production: Mountain Grape bark consists of the branch and twig bark as well as the twig tips of *Mahonia aquifolium*.

Other Names: Holly-Leaved Berberis, Oregon Grape

ACTIONS AND PHARMACOLOGY

COMPOUNDS

Isoquinoline alkaloids (in the root bark, 7 to 16%, in the stem bark, 2.4-4.5%):

benzyl isoquinoline type: including among others berberine

bisbenzyl isoquinoline type: including among others berbamine, oxyacanthine

aporphine type: including among others isocorydine

EFFECTS

The use of the drug as a tonic for loss of appetite is plausible in view of the alkaloid and amaroid content. The berberine has a mild mutagenic effect. It is an antipsoriatic when used externally.

INDICATIONS AND USAGE

Unproven Uses: The drug is used internally for scaly skin, psoriasis, eczema, bronchitis, gastritis, cholecystitis, and digestion problems.

Homeopathic Uses: Mountain Grape is used for dry skin rashes (e.g., for psoriasis between the acute phases) and for liver and gallbladder conditions.

PRECAUTIONS AND ADVERSE REACTIONS

General: No health hazards or side effects are known in conjunction with the proper administration of designated therapeutic dosages.

Pregnancy: The drug should not be used during pregnancy.

DOSAGE

Mode of Administration: The drug is available in commercial ointments for external use.

Storage: Protect from light.

LITERATURE

Anonym, Ein Lichtblick in der Psoriasistherapie. In: *DAZ* 134(8):646. 1994.

Augustin M, Mahonia aquifolium bei Psoriasis. In: *ZPT* 17(1):44. 1996.

Bezakova L, Misik V, Melakova L, Sivajdlenka E, Kostalova D. Lipoxygenase inhibition and antioxidant properties of bisbenzylisoquinoline alkaloids isolated from *Mahonia aquifolium. Pharmazie* 51 (10); 758-761. 1996

Galle K, Müller-Jakic B, Proebstle A, Jurcic K, Bladt S, Wagner H. Analytical and pharmacological studies on *Mahonia aquifolium. Phytomedicine* 1; 59-62. 1994

Gieler U, Weth Avd, Heger M. *Mahonia aquifolium* - a new type of topical treatment for psoriasis. *J Dermatol Treat.* 6; 31-34. 1995

Lampert ML, Schaffner W. Mahonia aquifolium (Pursh) Nutt.- Antimicrobial Effect against Propionibacterium acnes. *Sci Pharm.* 63 (4); 324. 1995

Mennet-von Eiff M, Meier B, Phytotherapie in der Dermatologie. In: *ZPT* 16(4):201-210. 1995.

Misik V et al., Lipoxygenase inhibition and antioxidant properties of protoberberine and aporphine alkaloids isolated from *Mahonia aquifolium.* In: *PM* 61(4):372-373. 1995.

Müller K, Ziereis K, Gawlik I, The antipsoriatic *Mahonia aquifolium* and its active constituents II: Antiproliferative activity against cell growth of human keratinocytes. In: *PM* 61(1):74-75. 1995.

Müller K, Ziereis K, The antisporiatic *Mahonia aquifolium* and its active constitutents; Pro- and antioxidant properties and inhibition of 5-lipoxygenase. In: *PM* 60(5):421. 1994.

Wiesenauer M, Lüdtke R. *Mahonia aquifolium* in patients with Psoriasis vulgaris - an intraindividual study. *Phytomedicine* 3 (3); 231-235. 1996

Wirth C, Wagner H. Pharmacologically active phenolic compounds from the bark of *Mahonia aquifolium. Phytomedicine* 4 (4); 357-358. 1997

Mountain Laurel

Kalmia latifolia

DESCRIPTION

Medicinal Parts: The medicinal parts are the fresh or dried leaves.

Flower and Fruit: The inflorescence is a compound umbelled-raceme with numerous flowers. The flowers are red, whitish or purple-brown to chocolate brown. They are solitary on long glandular, hairy pedicles in the axils of the bracts and 2 lateral, brown bracteoles. The bud has 10 folds and spreads out in a bowl shape. There are 10 stamens, red anthers without appendages that burst open at irregular holes. The fruit is an erect, orbicular, 5-to 7-valvular capsule. The numerous seeds are flat, oblong, 1 mm long, and fly away easily.

Leaves, Stem, and Root: The plant is a heavily branched shrub or tree about 4 m high with reddish-brown or gray branches. The evergreen, laurel-like, ovate-lanceolate acuminate, glabrous leaves are alternate, 4 to 12 cm long, and have a 1 to 3 cm long petiole. They are red-brown on the lower surface, have numerous glandular hairs, and a distinct midrib. The upper surface is dark green.

Habitat: Eastern U.S.

Production: Mountain Laurel leaves are the leaves (fresh or dried) of *Kalmia latifolia*.

Other Names: American Laurel, Big Ivy, Broad-Leafed Laurel, Calico Bush, Spoonwood, Sheep Laurel, Rose Laurel, Laurel, Lambkill, Mountain Ivy

ACTIONS AND PHARMACOLOGY

COMPOUNDS

Diterpenes (andromedan- derivatives): including among others grayanotoxin I (andromedotoxin, asebotoxin, acetylandromedol, rhodotoxin), grayanotoxin II, III, XVIII, lyonol A, leucothol A, kalmiatoxine

Acylphloroglucinols: including among others 2′,6′-dihydroxy-4′-methoxy-acetophenone, phloretin

Flavonoids: including among others asebotin, hyperoside

EFFECTS

Use of Mountain Laurel is no longer recommended because of the formation of grayanotoxins, which are highly toxic. Efficacy for the recorded indications has not been proved.

According to earlier sources (which are questionable), the drug is antiphlogistic and mildly diuretic.

INDICATIONS AND USAGE

Unproven Uses: Today, the drug is only used in homeopathic dilutions. In the past it was used as a decoction in the treatment of tinea capitis and to treat psoriasis, herpes, and secondary syphilis.

Homeopathic Uses: Uses include rheumatism, shingles, nerve pain, and rheumatic and cardiac pain.

PRECAUTIONS AND ADVERSE REACTIONS

The andromedan derivatives of the drug prevent the closure of the excitable cells of the sodium channels and thereby prevent conduction. Painful mucous membranes in the mouth and in the stomach, increased salivation, cold sweat, nausea, vomiting, diarrhea, and paresthesias are experienced following intake of the drug. Dizziness, headache, fever attacks, as well as intoxicated states with temporary loss of vision, follow later. Muscle weakness, coordination disorders, and spasms can also occur. Bradycardia, cardiac arrhythmias, drops in blood pressure, eventual cardiac arrest and respiratory failure can lead to death.

OVERDOSAGE

Following gastrointestinal emptying, (inducement of vomiting, gastric lavage with burgundy-colored potassium permanganate solution, sodium sulfate) and instillation of activated charcoal, the treatment of poisoning consists of electrolyte replacement, countering of acidosis with sodium bicarbonate, plasma volume expanders if required, diazepam (IV) in case of spasms and oxygen in case of respiratory failure.

DOSAGE

Mode of Administration: Available in homeopathic preparations.

Homeopathic Dosage: 5 drops, 1 tablet, or 10 globules every 30 to 60 minutes (acute) or 1 to 3 times daily (chronic); parenterally: 1 to 2 mL sc acute, 3 times daily; chronic: once a day (HAB1).

LITERATURE

Frohne D, Pfänder HJ, Giftpflanzen - Ein Handbuch für Apotheker, Toxikologen und Biologen, 4. Aufl., Wiss. Verlags-Ges Stuttgart 1997.

Hänsel R, Keller K, Rimpler H, Schneider G (Hrsg.), Hagers Handbuch der Pharmazeutischen Praxis, 5. Aufl., Bde 4-6 (Drogen), Springer Verlag Berlin, Heidelberg, New York, 1992-1994.

Lewin L, Gifte und Vergiftungen, 6. Aufl., Nachdruck, Haug Verlag, Heidelberg 1992.

Madaus G, Lehrbuch der Biologischen Arzneimittel, Bde 1-3, Nachdruck, Georg Olms Verlag Hildesheim 1979.

Roth L, Daunderer M, Kormann K, Giftpflanzen, Pflanzengifte, 4. Aufl., Ecomed Fachverlag Landsberg Lech 1993.

Teuscher E, Lindequist U, Biogene Gifte - Biologie, Chemie, Pharmakologie, 2. Aufl., Fischer Verlag Stuttgart 1994.

Wagner H, Wiesenauer M, Phytotherapie. Phytopharmaka und pflanzliche Homöopathika, Fischer-Verlag, Stuttgart, Jena, New York 1995.

Wolters B, Zierpflanzen aus Nordamerika. In: *DAZ* 137(26):2253-2261. 1997.

Mouse Ear

Pilosella officinarum

DESCRIPTION

Medicinal Parts: The medicinal parts are the flowering aerial parts.

Flower and Fruit: The yellow, composite flowers are solitary at the end of long pedicles. There are bright yellow, lingual florets. The lateral ones are usually striped reddish underneath. The bracts are linear and acute, have a membranous margin, and are covered in star-hairs. They have black glandular hairs at the base. The fruit is cylindrical and has a simple, brittle tuft of hair.

Leaves, Stem, and Root: The plant is a perennial herb, which grows up to 30 cm. Erect, leafless stems grow from the rosette of basal leaves. The plant produces long, leafy runners. The leaves are oblong or obovate-to-lanceolate. They bear long bristles, which are thickened at the base and are star-haired to tomentose beneath.

Habitat: The plant grows in large areas of Europe and temperate Asia. It is also found in North America.

Production: Mouse Ear is the aerial part of *Pilosella officinarum*.

ACTIONS AND PHARMACOLOGY

COMPOUNDS

Flavonoids: including among others luteolin-7-glucoside, isoetin

Hydroxycoumarins: umbelliferone, skimmine

Tannins

EFFECTS

The plant has been shown to have diuretic, spasmolytic, and diaphoretic effects.

INDICATIONS AND USAGE

Unproven Uses: Mouse Ear is used internally in the treatment of asthma, bronchitis, coughs and whooping cough, and externally in the treatment of wounds.

PRECAUTIONS AND ADVERSE REACTIONS

No health hazards or side effects are known in conjunction with the proper administration of designated therapeutic dosages.

DOSAGE

Mode of Administration: The drug is used internally and externally as a liquid extract.

LITERATURE

Guerin JC, Reveillere HP, *Ann Farm Franc* 43(1):77. 1985

Hegnauer R, Chemotaxonomie der Pflanzen, Bde 1-11, Birkhäuser Verlag Basel, Boston, Berlin 1962-1997.

Kern W, List PH, Hörhammer L (Hrsg.), Hagers Handbuch der Pharmazeutischen Praxis, 4. Aufl., Bde. 1-8, Springer Verlag Berlin, Heidelberg, New York, 1969.

Madaus G, Lehrbuch der Biologischen Arzneimittel, Bde 1-3, Nachdruck, Georg Olms Verlag Hildesheim 1979.

Mucuna pruriens

See Cowhage

Mugwort

Artemisia vulgaris

DESCRIPTION

Medicinal Parts: The medicinal parts are the root and the above-ground parts of the plant, particularly the dried branch tips.

Flower and Fruit: The flower heads are ovoid, 3 to 4 mm long by 2 mm wide. The numerous flowers are short-stemmed, erect or slightly drooping. They are in dense, heavily branched panicles with numerous lanceolate bracts. The bracts are downy white with a green midrib. The inner bracts are lanceolate and acuminate. The outside ones are oblong and obtuse with broad membranous margin. The flowers are yellowish or red-brown and almost glabrous. The inner flowers are androgynous and those on the outside are female. The receptacle is glabrous. The fruit has an indistinct margin.

Leaves, Stem, and Root: The plant is a long-stemmed, 70 to 150 cm high shrub with a branched, many-headed and creeping rhizome without runners or rosette. The shoots are slightly pubescent, often red-tinged, and have a weak unpleasant smell. The erect or ascending, edged, and coriaceous stems die off each year. They are in branched panicles and downy. The leaves are 5 to 10 cm long, coriaceous, and the margins are often rolled back. The upper surface is usually dark green and glabrous, occasionally pubescent, and the lower surface is tomentose. The basal leaves are short-petioled and lobed with an end section and 1 to 2 pairs of small side leaflets. The rest of the leaves are sessile or almost sessile with a slit base. The lower leaves are double-pinnate, the middle and upper ones are pinnatifid and lanceolate, acuminate, entire-margined or slightly serrated.

Characteristics: Mugwort has a pleasant tangy taste. The root is sweet and pungent, the herb is aromatic and bitter.

Habitat: The plant is indigenous to Asia and North America, and is also distributed all over Europe except in the south.

Production: Mugwort herb consists of the above-ground parts of *Artemisia vulgaris*. The branch tips are gathered during the flowering season and carefully dried. Other fresh above- and underground parts of the plant are harvested at the beginning of winter, primarily from the wild. Mugwort root consists of the below-ground parts of *Artemisia vulgaris*.

Not to be Confused With: Some confusion can arise with *Asinthii herba*.

Other Names: Bulwand-Wormwood, Felon Herb, St. John's Plant, Wormwood

ACTIONS AND PHARMACOLOGY

COMPOUNDS

Volatile oil (complex composition): chief constituents, according to plant variety, 1,8- cineol, camphor, linalool or thujone

Sesquiterpene lactones: including vulgarin, pilostachyin, pilostachyin C

Lipophilic flavonoids

Polyynes

Hydroxycoumarins: for example, umbelliferone, aesculetin

EFFECTS

The aqueous extract and essential oil show antimicrobial activity in laboratory tests.

CONTRAINDICATIONS

Mugwort is not to be used during pregnancy.

INDICATIONS AND USAGE

Unproven Uses: Mugwort is used in complaints and problems involving the gastrointestinal tract such as stomach ulcers and indigestion. The plant is also used for worm infestations, epilepsy, persistent vomiting, to promote circulation, as a sedative, and for delayed or irregular menstuation. The root is used for asthenic states as a tonic, and in combination with other remedies also for psychoneuroses, neurasthenia, depression, hypochondria, autonomic neuroses, general irritability and restlessness, insomnia, and anxiety states. The efficacy of Mugwort for the listed indications has not been substantiated.

Chinese Medicine: Mugwort is used in China for female complaints as well as for ulcers and burns.

Homeopathic Uses: Homeopathic uses of the root include convulsions and worm infestations.

PRECAUTIONS AND ADVERSE REACTIONS

General: No health hazards or side effects are known in conjunction with the proper administration of designated therapeutic dosages. Sensitization through skin contact has been observed, although very rarely.

Pregnancy: Mugwort is not to be used during pregnancy.

DOSAGE

Mode of Administration: Since the efficacy for the claimed applications is not verified, therapeutic administration is not recommended.

Preparation: ''Moxibustion'' (China, Japan) leaves are ground with water in a mortar and, after removal of the larger remnants, small cones are formed and dried to be later burnt onto the skin of the patient. Tea is prepared by allowing 1 tsp. to steep in 150 to 200 mL boiling water for 10 minutes. A liquid extract is prepared in a 1:1 proportion from a mixture of the drug in 25% ethanol.

Daily Dosage: An infusion (drug 0.5 to 2 g) is given 3 times daily. Usual dosage of tea is one cup 2 or 3 times daily.

Homeopathic Dosage: 5 drops, 1 tablet, 10 globules every 30 to 60 minutes (acute) or 1 to 3 times daily (chronic); Parenterally: 1 to 2 mL 3 times daily sc (HAB1).

LITERATURE

Brandys J, Grimsoen A, Nilsen BM, Smestad Paulsen B, Park HS, Hong CS. Cross-Reactivity Between Pollen Extracts from Six Artemisia Species. *Planta Med.* 59; 221-228. 1993

Kurz G, Rapaport MJ. External/internal allergy to plants (Artemisia). *Contact Dermatitis* 5; 407-408. 1979

Marco JA et al., Sesquiterpenes lactones from Artemisia species. In: *PH* 32:460. 1993.

Marco JA, Sanz JF, Hierro P, Two eudesmane acids from *Artemisia vulgaris*. In: *PH* 30:2403-2404. 1991.

Michaelis K et al., On the essential oil components from blossoms of *Artemisia vulgaris L.* In: *Z Naturfosch* 37(3/4):152. 1982.

Nano GM et al., Composition of some oils from *Artemisia vulgaris*. In: *PM* 30(3):211. 1976.

Wallnöfer B, Hofer O, Greger H, Polyacetylenes from Artemsia ''Vulgares'' Group. In: *PH* 28(10):2687. 1989.

Zhong-fu Y, Xian-sheng W. Combined Traditional Chinese and Western Medicine / Ultrasonic Studies on the Effect of Artemisia Decoction on the Volume and Dynamics of Gallbladder. *Chin Med J.* 106; 145-148. 1993

Muira-Puama

Ptychopetalum olacoides

DESCRIPTION

Medicinal Parts: The medicinal parts are the dried roots and the dried trunk with bark.

Flower and Fruit: The inflorescences are racemous; there are 1 or 2 per axil. They have 5 to 8 flowers and are about 2 cm long. The calyx is narrow and has 5 tips. The corolla is white, oblong, and about 1.3 to 2 mm long. The outside is smooth, and the inside is white pubescent. There are usually 10 stamens with long anthers. The ovary is clavate. The fruit is a long elliptical drupe that is initially green and changes to pink and finally to lilac-black when ripening. The pericarp is thin, and the endocarp is crusty.

Leaves, Stem, and Root: The plant is a 5- to 15-m high tree with a trunk 25 cm in diameter, which is vertically grooved. The leaves are oblong-lanceolate, very tapered, and narrow toward the base. They are sometimes acute, coriaceous, smooth and gray or frosted to blue-green beneath. The dried leaves are matte with a dark green to black upper surface and a dark gray undersurface. The ribs are pinnatifid, curved, becoming distinct at the margin and protruding on the undersurface. The petioles are deeply grooved and do not thicken.

Habitat: The plant is indigenous to Guyana and the Amazon region of Brazil.

Production: Muira-Puama consists of the wood from the trunk and/or roots of *Ptychopetalum olacoides* and/or *Ptychopetalum unicatum.*

ACTIONS AND PHARMACOLOGY

COMPOUNDS

Triterpene acid esters (0.4-0.5%): chief components are behenolic acid esters of lupeol (60%), including, among others, fatty acid esters of beta-sitosterol

Sterols: beta-sitosterol, campesterol, lupeol

Volatile oil: chief components are alpha-pinene (25%), alpha-humulene (10%), beta-pinene (8%), beta-caryophyllene (8%) camphene (7%), camphor (6%),

EFFECTS
No information is available.

INDICATIONS AND USAGE
Unproven Uses: Muira-Puama is used internally for diarrhea, loss of appetite, and for the prevention of sexual disorders. The herb is also used externally for the prevention of sexual disorders.

PRECAUTIONS AND ADVERSE REACTIONS
No health hazards or side effects are known in conjunction with the proper administration of designated therapeutic dosages.

DOSAGE
Mode of Administration: Muira-Puama is administered whole, ground, as a powder, and as an extract.

Preparation: To prepare a liquid extract, mix the powdered herb in a ratio of 10:2:1 with spirit of wine and glycerine. Then percolate the mixture with spirit of wine, yielding 10 parts liquid extract.

Daily Dosage: When used internally, a single dose is 0.5 g drug. The daily dosage for the liquid extract and the decoction is 0.5 to 2 mL 3 times daily. For external use, the herb can be added to baths.

LITERATURE
Auterhoff H, Momberger B, *Arch Pharm* 304:223-228. 1971.

Hänsel R, Keller K, Rimpler H, Schneider G (Hrsg.), Hagers Handbuch der Pharmazeutischen Praxis, 5. Aufl., Bde 4-6 (Drogen), Springer Verlag Berlin, Heidelberg, New York, 1992-1994.

Steinegger E, Hänsel R, Pharmakognosie, 5. Aufl., Springer Verlag Heidelberg 1992.

Mullein

Verbascum densiflorum

DESCRIPTION
Medicinal Parts: The medicinal parts are the herb at the beginning of the flowering season, the flowers, and the root.

Flower and Fruit: The large, yellow flowers with a diameter of 30 to 35 mm are in apical spikelike racemes. The calyx is divided deeply into 5 sections. The corolla is rotate, has a short tube and a 5-lobed, uneven margin. There are 5 stamens of uneven length. The 3 upper ones are lanate and have long anthers. There is 1 superior ovary. The fruit is a 2-lobed capsule.

Leaves, Stem, and Root: The plant is biennial. It has petiolate basal leaves and is up to 2 m high. The stem is erect, undivided, or lightly branched above. It is tomentose like the leaves and calyx. The leaves are alternate, turned downward and finely crenate. The lower ones are lanceolate or oblong lanceolate; the upper ones, ovate.

Characteristics: The flowers have a honeylike fragrance and an almond-like taste. The leaves are slimy and bitter.

Habitat: The plant is widespread in Europe, temperate Asia and North America.

Production: Mullein flower consists of the dried petals of *Verbascum densiflorum* and/or of *Verbascum phlomoides*.

Not to be Confused With: Other Verbascum species.

Other Names: Aaron's Rod, Adam's Flannel, Beggar's Blanket, Blanket Herb, Blanket-Leaf, Candlewick Plant, Clown's Lungwort, Clot-Bur, Cuddy's Lungs, Duffle, Flannelflower, Feltwort, Fluffweed, Golden Rod, Hare's Beard, Hag's Taper, Hedge-Taper, Jacob's Staff, Torches, Our Lady's Flannel, Woollen, Rag Paper, Shepherd's Club, Shepherd's Staff, Torch Weed, Velvet Plant, Wild Ice Leaf

ACTIONS AND PHARMACOLOGY
COMPOUNDS
Mucilage (3%): including among others, arabino galactans, xyloglucans

Triterpene saponins: chief components verbascosaponine (0.007%)

Iridoide monoterpenes: including among others, aucubin, 6beta-xylosylaucubin, catalpol, isocatalpol, methyl catalpol

Caffeic acid derivatives: verbascoside (acteoside)

Flavonoids (0.5-4.0%): including among others, rutin, diosmin, quercetin-7-O-glucoside, hesperidine, apigenin-7-O-glucoside, kempferol-7-O-glucoside

Invert sugar (11%)

EFFECTS
Mullein alleviates irritation and has an expectorant effect due to its mucin and saponin content.

INDICATIONS AND USAGE
Approved by Commission E:

■ Cough/bronchitis

Unproven Uses: Mullein is used internally for catarrh of the respiratory tract, bladder and kidney conditions, enteritis, rheumatism, coughs, flu, intestinal pain caused by colic, asthma, cystitis, hemorrhoids, dermatoses, and painful diarrhea. The plant is used externally for earache, ear furuncles, eczema of the auditory canal, middle ear infection, inflammatory skin diseases with itch, burns, eczema, weeping eczema, dermatitis, insect bites, and itching in the anal and genital regions.

PRECAUTIONS AND ADVERSE REACTIONS
No health hazards or side effects are known in conjunction with the proper administration of designated therapeutic dosages.

DOSAGE
Mode of Administration: Whole, cut, and powdered drug is available in the form of teas and other galenic preparations for internal and external use.

How Supplied:

Liquid — 250 mg/mL, 285 mg/mL

Liquid Extract — 1:1

Preparation: To prepare tea, pour boiling water over 1.5 to 2 g finely cut drug and strain after 10 to 15 minutes (1 teaspoonful is equivalent to 0.5 g drug).

To make an oil preparation, pour 100 g of olive oil over a handful of fresh flowers. Leave the mixture outdoors in the sun, stirring several times a day, then filter after 3 to 4 weeks.

To prepare a tincture, add 20 g cut drug to 80 gm of 70% ethanol and leave to draw for 10 days.

Daily Dose: The daily dose is 3 to 4 g of drug. The tincture dose is 20 to 30 drops taken several times a day.

Storage: Mullein must be protected from light and particularly from moisture to prevent the drug from changing color to brown or dark brown due to the iridoid content.

LITERATURE

Grzybek J, Szewczyk A, Verbascum-Arten - Königskerze oder Wollblume Portrait einer Arzneipflanze. In: ZPT 17(6):389-398. 1996.

Haslinger E, Schröder H, *Sci Pharm* 60:202. 1992.

Klimek B, *PA* 48:51. 1991.

Kraus K, Franz G, *DAZ* 127:665. 1987.

Seifert K et al., *PM* 51:409. 1985.

Swiatek L et al., *PM* 45:153. 1982.

Swiatek L et al., *Pharm Weekbl* (Sci Ed) 9:246. 1987.

Musa paradisiaca

See Plantain

Muskmallow

Abelmoschus moschatus

DESCRIPTION

Medicinal Parts: The medicinal parts are the seeds of the plant and the oil extracted from them.

Flower and Fruit: The flowers are solitary and axillary. They have 5 to 7 pubescent, linear, 1.5-cm long epicalyx leaves. The sepals are about 3 cm long. The corolla has a diameter of 7.5 cm. The petals are sulfur yellow with a crimson spot at the base. The petals are ovate and lightly pubescent. The fruit is a 5- to 8-cm long capsule, which is shaped like a pentagonal pyramid and filled with numerous large seeds. The seeds are kidney-shaped, compressed, and about 3 mm in diameter. They are grayish-brown, with numerous striations that are concentric around the hilum.

Leaves, Stem, and Root: The plant is an annual erect herb about 1 to 2 m high with star-shaped, pubescent stem, stalks, and leaves. The leaves are 15 to 25 cm long, cordate-to-round with 3 to 7 lobes, which taper to a point. The petioles are as long or longer than the leaves. The stipules are oblong and pubescent.

Characteristics: The seeds have a strong, musky smell, and the taste is oily. The seed pods have an aromatic flavor and are used in some parts of the Middle East to mix with and flavor coffee.

Habitat: The plant is indigenous to Africa, India, Java, and South America and is cultivated in all tropical regions.

Production: Muskmallow seeds are the dried seeds of *Hibiscus abelmoschus*. The seeds are dried in the open air.

Not to be Confused With: Foenugraeci semen.

Other Names: Muskseed, Ambrette Seed, Abelmosk, Ambretta, Egyptian Alcée, Target-Leaved Hibiscus, Okra

ACTIONS AND PHARMACOLOGY

COMPOUNDS

Fatty oil and chief fatty acids: palmitic acid, linoleic acid, stearic acid

Volatile oil: ambrette oil, chief components farnesylacetate, macrocyclic lactones as carriers of the musk smell such as hexadec-7-en-16-olide (ambrettolide), tetradec-5-en-14-olide

Sterols: including beta-sitosterin, beta-sitosterin-beta-D-glucoside

EFFECTS

Muskmallow is said to be an aromatic, a stimulant and carminative.

INDICATIONS AND USAGE

Unproven Uses: The various preparations are used internally and externally for stomach and intestinal disorders with cramps, loss of appetite, and headache.

Homeopathic Uses: Muskmallow is used for feelings of tightness in the rib cage area.

PRECAUTIONS AND ADVERSE REACTIONS

Health risks or side effects following the proper administration of designated therapeutic dosages are not recorded.

DOSAGE

Mode of Administration: Muskmallow is used as a tea or tincture, and is administered both internally and externally.

Homeopathic Dosage: 5 to 10 drops, 1 tablet, 5 to 10 globules, 1 to 3 times a day (HAB34).

LITERATURE

Maurer B, Greider A, *Helv Chim Acta* 60:1155. 1977

Srivastava KC, Rastogi SC, *Planta Med* 17:189. 1969

Hänsel R, Keller K, Rimpler H, Schneider G (Hrsg.), Hagers Handbuch der Pharmazeutischen Praxis, 5. Aufl., Bde 4-6 (Drogen), Springer Verlag Berlin, Heidelberg, New York, 1992-1994 (unter Abelmoschus moschatus).

Myosotis arvensis

See Forget-Me-Not

Myrica cerifera

See Southern Bayberry

Myrica gale

See Sweet Gale

Myristica fragrans

See Nutmeg

Myroxylon balsamum

See Tolu Balsam

Myrrh

Commiphora molmol

DESCRIPTION

Medicinal Parts: The resin, which has exuded from the bark and dried in the air, is the medicinal part. Myrrh is the pale yellow granular secretion that is discharged into cavities in the bark when it is wounded. The exudate hardens to a red-brown mass about the size of a walnut.

Flower and Fruit: The yellowish-red inflorescences are panicled. The fruit is brown, about 7 mm long, ovate, and acuminate.

Leaves, Stem, and Root: Commiphora molmol is a thorny shrub or small tree up 3 m high. It has a thick trunk and numerous irregular knotted branches and smaller clustered branchlets. A few trifoliate leaves grow at the end of short branches, with very small lateral leaflets dentate only at the tip. The terminal leaflet is 1 cm long, obovate, and glabrous. The oleo-gum resin exudes from fissures or incisions in the bark and is collected as irregular masses or tears, varying in color from yellowish to reddish-brown, often with white patches.

Characteristics: The surface may be oily or covered with fine dust. The taste is bitter and acrid. The odor is aromatic.

Habitat: The plant is indigenous to eastern Mediterranean countries, Somalia, Ethiopia, Eritrea, Yemen, and South Arabia.

Production: Myrrh is collected in the wild from June to August and consists of oleo-gum resin exuded from the stems of *Commiphora molmol* after incisions have been made in the bark. It is then air-dried. Myrrh can also originate from other Commiphora species if the chemical composition is comparable to the official drug.

Not to be Confused With: Some confusion can arise with ''False myrrh'' or Commiphora mukul.

Other Names: Guggal Gum, Guggal Resin, Didin, Didthin

ACTIONS AND PHARMACOLOGY

COMPOUNDS

Volatile oil (2-10%): chief components are sesquiterpenes including, among others, delta-elemene, beta-eudesmol, alpha-copaene and furosesquiterpenes, especially 5-acetoxy-2-methoxy-4,5-dienone (aroma-bearer), furanoeudesma-1,3-dien, isofuranogermacren (curzeren), curzenenone, 2-methoxy-furanoguaia-9-ene

Triterpenes (30-50%): including 3-epi-alpha-amyrin, alpha-amyrenone

Mucilages (30-60%): chiefly methyl-glucurono-galactans

EFFECTS

Myrrh is stated to possess antimicrobial, astringent, carminative, expectorant, anticatarrhal, antiseptic and vulnerary properties. Traditionally, it has been used for aphthous ulcers, pharyngitis, respiratory catarrh, common cold, furunculosis, wounds and abrasions, and specifically for mouth ulcers, gingivitis and pharyngitis. Myrrh's local astringent, disinfectant and granulation-promoting effects are a result of its essential oil (consisting mainly of sesquiterpenes) and amaroids.

Hypoglycemic activity in both normal and diabetic rats has been reported for a myrrh extract. Together with an aloe gum extract, myrrh was found to be an active component of a multi-plant extract that exhibited antidiabetic activity. The mode of action was thought to involve a decrease in gluconeogenesis and an increase in peripheral utilization of glucose in diabetic rats. (Al-Awadi & Gumaa, 1987; Al-Awadi et al. 1985)

CLINICAL TRIALS

Hyperlipidemia

An evaluation of Guggul for hyperlipidemia produced by the Natural Standard Research Collaboration in 2005 reports that while multiple studies have been published, most were small and of poor quality. One of the better well-designed trials, published in the *Journal of the American Medical Association* (*JAMA*) in 2003, found small but significant increases in low-density lipoprotein cholesterol levels with Guggul compared to placebo, but no significant changes were measured for high-density lipoprotein cholesterol, total cholesterol, or triglycerides. The authors conclude that, overall, scientific evidence for Guggul for hyperlipidemia or any other condition is weak. Side effects and interactions, however, may be serious and include stomach discomfort and allergic rash. Safety beyond 4 months of use also has not been ascertained (Ulbricht, 2005).

Earlier research reinforces the finding that well-designed clinical studies of myrrh are lacking. Guggulipid has been reported to lower the concentration of total serum lipids, serum cholesterol, serum triglycerides, serum phospholipids and beta-lipoproteins in 20 patients. This effect was reported to be comparable to that of two other known lipid-lowering drugs also used in the study (Malhotra & Ahuja, 1971).

INDICATIONS AND USAGE

Approved by Commission E:

■ Inflammation of the mouth and pharynx

Myrrh is used for the topical treatment of mild inflammations of the oral and pharyngeal mucosa.

Unproven Uses: In folk medicine, Myrrh is occasionally used internally as a carminative for nonspecific intestinal infections and also as an expectorant for coughs. Folk medicine uses have also included stimulating the appetite and the flow of digestive juices.

Chinese Medicine: Uses include carbuncles, furuncles, wounds (as a styptic), amenorrhea, and abdominal tumors.

Indian Medicine: Among uses in Indian medicine are menstrual disorders, stomach complaints, wounds, ulcers and inflammations of the skin and mouth.

CONTRAINDICATIONS

Pregnancy: Not to be used during pregnancy.

Breastfeeding: Not to be used while breastfeeding.

PRECAUTIONS AND ADVERSE REACTIONS

No health hazards or side effects are known in conjunction with the proper administration of designated therapeutic dosages. Myrrh has been reported to be nonirritating, nonsensitizing, and nonphototoxic to human and animal skins.

Fertility: Myrrh is reputed to affect the menstrual cycle (Leung, 1980).

DRUG INTERACTIONS

POSSIBLE INTERACTIONS

Antidiabetic Medications: Myrrh may interfere with existing antidiabetic therapy, as hypoglycemic properties have been documented. *Clinical Management:* Monitor blood glucose carefully.

DOSAGE

Mode of Administration: Powdered resin, myrrh tincture and other galenic preparations for topical use.

How Supplied:

Capsules – 657 mg

Dental powders – 10% powdered resin

Liquid – 1:1 (Myrrh gum)

Oil – 100% (Myrrh commiphora)

Preparation: Prepare 1:5 tincture using 90% ethanol (V/V) in accordance with DAB10.

Daily Dosage: Myrrh tincture: Paint an undiluted tincture (1:5) on 2 to 3 times daily for external applications. As a rinse, use 5 to 10 drops in a glass of water; as a gargle, 30 to 60 drops in a glass of water. In dental powders: 10% of powdered resin.

Storage: The herb and its preparations should be stored in sealed containers that protect them from light and moisture. A desiccant should be present because the carbohydrate component of the drug readily absorbs water. For this reason, powdered forms should not be stored.

LITERATURE

Al-Awadi FM et al. On the mechanism of the hypoglycemic effect of a plant extract. In: *Diabetologia*; 28: 432-434, 1985.

Al-Awadi FM, Gumaa KA. Studies on the activity of individual plants of an antidiabetic plant mixture. In: *Acta Diabetol Lat*; 24: 37-41, 1987.

Arora RB et al. *Ind J Med Res* 60(6):929, 1972.

Bajaj AC, Dev S. *Tetrahedron* 38(19):2949, 1982.

BAnz (Federal German Gazette) No. 193; published 15 Oct 1987.

Brieskorn CH. *Tetrahedron Lett* 21(6):1511, 1980.

Brieskorn CH et al. *Phytochemistry* 22:187 et 1207, 1983.

Delaveau P et al. *Planta Med* 40:49, 1980. Kodama M et al. *Tetrahedron Lett* 35:3065, 1975.

Malhotra SC, Ahuja MMS. Comparative hypolipidaemic effectiveness of gum guggulu (*Commiphora mukul*) fraction "A", ethyl-p-chlorophenoxyisobutyrate and Ciba-13437-Su. *Indian J Med Res*; 59: 1621-1632, 1971.

Mester L et al. *Planta Med* 37(4):367, 1979.

Mincione E, Iavarone C. *Chim Ind* 54:424 and 525, 1972.

Pernet R. *Lloydia* 35:280, 1972.

Ruecker G. *Arch Pharm* 305(7):486, 1972.

Srivastava M et al. *J Biosci* 6(3):277, 1984.

Tariq M, et al. Anti-Inflammatory activity of *Commiphora molmol. Agents Actions*; 17:381-382. 1985

Tripathi SN et al. *Ind. J Exp Biol* 13(1):15, 1975.

Ulbricht C, Basch E, Szapary P, et al. Guggul for hyperlipidemia: a review by the Natural Standard Research Collaboration. *Complement Ther Med*; 13(4):279-90. 2005.

Wiendl RM, Franz G. Myrrhe. Neue Chemie einer alten Droge. In: *DAZ* 134(1):25. 1994.

Wylegalla R. Biblische Botanik: Pflanzen und Früchte aus dem gelobten Land. In: *DAZ* 137(11):867-869. 1997.

Myrrhis odorata

See Sweet Cicely

Myrtle

Myrtus communis

DESCRIPTION

Medicinal Parts: The medicinal parts are the leaves (dried and as a source of oil), twigs and the fresh, flowering branches.

Flower and Fruit: The flowers are medium-sized and stiff. They are short, glandular-haired pedicles, which are covered in bracteoles. They grow solitary in the leaf axils. The petals are white with fine glands and a somewhat tomentose margin covered with fine hairs. The anthers are yellow. The berries are pea-sized, orbicular or ovoid-ellipsoid, blue-black, or white. They are crowned by the calyx.

Leaves, Stem, and Root: Myrtle is an evergreen, bushy shrub or a small tree growing up to 5 m high with opposite branches and quadrangular cane-shaped, delicately glandular, downy branches. The dark green leaves are glossy, glabrous, coriaceous, opposite-paired or whorled, ovate-to-lanceolate, entire-margined, acuminate and 1 to 3 cm long.

Characteristics: The berries have a sweet-spicy taste.

Habitat: Myrtle grows from the Mediterranean region to the northwestern Himalayas.

Production: Myrtle leaves are the dried leaves of *Myrtus communis*. Myrtle oil is the essential oil of *Myrtus communis*, which is extracted from the leaves and branches through steam distillation. (The percentage extracted ranges from 0.1 to 0.5%.) May and June are the best months for harvesting, since the plant has the highest concentration of essential oil during this period.

Not to be Confused With: Confusion can arise with the leaves of *Bux semper-virens* and *Vaccinium vitisidaea*, which resemble Myrtle.

ACTIONS AND PHARMACOLOGY

COMPOUNDS: MYRTLE OIL

Chief components: 1,8-cineol (15-45%), alpha-pinene (15-38%), myrtenol (1-5%), myrtenylacetate (4-20%), limonene (4-10%), alpha-terpineol (2-12%), geraniol (0.5-1.5%), geranylacetate (1-5%), myrtol (a myrtle oil fraction that boils between 160-180°C, chief components 1.8-cineole and alpha-pinene)

EFFECTS: MYRTLE OIL

The oil's mono- and sesquiterterpenes display antibacterial, fungicidal and disinfectant activity.

COMPOUNDS: MYRTLE LEAVES

Volatile oil (0.1-0.5%): (see Myrtle Oil compounds listing above for composition)

Tannins (gallotannins, condensed tannins)

Acylphloroglucinols: myrtocommulon A and B

EFFECTS: MYRTLE LEAVES

The leaves, which contain essential oil and tannins, display antimicrobial activity. An antiedemic and hypoglycemic effect was demonstrated in animal experiments. An effect on the central nervous system (an increase in the duration of sleep) was also proved. The efficacy in cold infections may be attributable to the deodorizing and bronchosecretolytic effect of the essential oil. Aqueous extracts of the leaves showed good antibiotic action against *Pseudomonas aeruginosa* and other bacterial strains that colonize burns, as well as against other strains (Al-Saimary, 2002; Appendino 2002).

INDICATIONS AND USAGE

MYRTLE OIL

Unproven Uses: Myrtle oil is used internally in folk medicine for acute and chronic infections of the respiratory tract such as bronchitis, whooping cough, tuberculosis of the lung, as well as for bladder conditions, diarrhea, hemorrhoids, and worm infestation.

MYRTLE LEAVES

Unproven Uses: Folk medicine internal uses include diarrhea, hemorrhoids, prostatitis, bronchitis, sinusitis, tuberculosis and colds. Among external uses are ear infections, fatigue, and leukorrhea.

CONTRAINDICATIONS

No internal administration of the drug should take place in the presence of inflammatory illnesses of the gastrointestinal area or of the biliary ducts, or in the case of severe liver diseases.

PRECAUTIONS AND ADVERSE REACTIONS

General: No health hazards or side effects are known in conjunction with the proper administration of designated therapeutic dosages. In rare cases, the internal administration of Myrtle oil as a drug leads to nausea, vomiting and diarrhea.

Pediatric Use: Preparations containing the oil should not be applied to the faces of infants or small children because of the possibility of triggering glottal spasm, bronchial spasm, asthma-like attacks or even respiratory failure.

OVERDOSAGE

Overdoses of Myrtle oil (more than 10 g) can lead to life-threatening poisoning, due to the high cineole content. Symptoms include, among others, a decrease in or loss of blood pressure, circulatory disorders, collapse and respiratory failure. Do not induce vomiting if poisoning occurs, because of the danger of aspiration. Following administration of activated charcoal, the therapy for poisonings consists of treating spasms with diazepam (IV); treating colic with atropine; and providing electrolyte substitution. Treat possible cases of acidosis with sodium bicarbonate infusions. Intubation and oxygen respiration may also be necessary.

DOSAGE

MYRTLE OIL

Mode of Administration: Myrtle is available in various medicinal/pharmaceutical preparations for internal use.

Preparation: Prepare an infusion by mixing 15 to 30 g of the drug with 1 L water and leave to draw for 15 minutes.

Daily Dosage: Single dose: 0.2 g of drug to be taken internally.

Storage: Protect from light and keep tightly sealed.

MYRTLE LEAVES

Preparation: Prepare an infusion by mixing 15 to 30 g of the drug with 1 L water and leave to draw for 15 minutes. A wash is prepared by adding 30 g of leaves to 1 L of water and letting it stand.

Daily Dosage: The average daily dosage of powder from the leaves is 5 g taken before meals. 3 cups of an infusion may be taken each day. Washes may be used several times daily.

Storage: Store the leaves in a tightly sealed container that blocks exposure to light.

LITERATURE

Al-Saimary IE, Bakr SS, Jaffar T, Al-Saimary AE, Salim H, AL-Musoaqi R. Effects of some plant extracts and antibiotics on *Pseudomonas aeruginosa* from various burn cases. *Saudi Med J.* 23: 802-805. 2002

Appendino G, Bianchi F, Minassi A, Sterner O, Ballero M, Gibbons S. Oligomeric acylphloroglucinols from myrtle (*Myrtus communis*). *J Nat Prod.* 65: 334-338. 2002

Elfella MS, Akhter MH, Khan MT. Anti-hyperglycaimic effect of an extract of *Myrtus communis* in streptozotocin-induced diabetes in mice. *J Ethnopharmacol* 11: 275-281 1984

Hänsel R, Keller K, Rimpler H, Schneider G (Hrsg.), Hagers Handbuch der Pharmazeutischen Praxis, 5. Aufl., Bde 4-6 (Drogen), Springer Verlag Berlin, Heidelberg, New York, 1992-1994.

Madaus G, Lehrbuch der Biologischen Arzneimittel, Bde 1-3, Nachdruck, Georg Olms Verlag Hildesheim 1979.

Morton JF, An Atlas of Medicinal Plants of Middle America, Charles C Thomas USA 1981.

Pichon N, Joseph MI, Raynaud J. Myricetine-3-fl-D-(6″-O-Galloyl-Galactoside) de *Myrtus communis* L. (Myrtaceae). Plant med et phyt. 26; 86-90. 1993

Roth L, Daunderer M, Kormann K, Giftpflanzen, Pflanzengifte, 4. Aufl., Ecomed Fachverlag Landsberg Lech 1993.

Steinegger E, Hänsel R, Pharmakognosie, 5. Aufl., Springer Verlag Heidelberg 1992.

Wagner H, Wiesenauer M, Phytotherapie. Phytopharmaka und pflanzliche Homöopathika, Fischer-Verlag, Stuttgart, Jena, New York 1995.

Myrtus communis

See Myrtle

Narcissus pseudonarcissus

See Daffodil

Nardostachys jatamansi

See Jatamansi

Nasturtium

Tropaeolum majus

DESCRIPTION

Medicinal Parts: The medicinal parts are the fresh herb, the whole fresh flowering plant and the seeds.

Flower and Fruit: The handsome campanulate flowers are orange with flame-red to fiery red stripes. The calyx is bilabiate, colored, and has a spurred upper lip. There are 5 uneven petals. The 2 upper petals are unstemmed, the 3 lower ones are stemmed and fringed at the base. There are 8 stamens and a superior ovary bearing a style with 3 stigmas. The fruit is a trivalved pericarp. It is orbicular-reniform, fleshy, wrinkled when ripe and dirty yellow.

Leaves, Stem, and Root: The plant is an annual, sometimes perennial and often creeping or climbing plant, 0.3 to 5 m long. The main root is thin and forms an underground runner. The stem is round, branched, fleshy and glabrous, like the whole plant. The leaves are alternate, long-petioled, hastate, and almost circular. The leaves are 3 to 5 cm and deeply lobed at the petiole.

Characteristics: The flowers are fragrant and the leafy parts smell and taste like cress.

Habitat: The plant is indigenous to warmer regions of South America and is becoming naturalized in the Mediterranean region, otherwise found as a garden or ornamental plant.

Production: Garden Nasturtium consists of the aerial parts, the seeds or leaves of *Tropaeolum majus.*

Other Names: Indian Cress

ACTIONS AND PHARMACOLOGY

COMPOUNDS

Glucosinolates (0.1%): in the fresh, unbruised plant: chief components are glucotropaeolin, yielding benzyl isothiocyanate after cell destruction

Ascorbic acid (vitamin C, 300 mg/100 gm fresh weight)

Cucurbitacins (in the fruits): including cucurbitacins B and E

Fatty oil (in the seeds, 7.5%): chief fatty acids erucic acid (50%), 11-cis-eiconsenic acid (25%), oleic acid (12%)

Oxalates

Flavonoids: including among others, isoquercetin and quercetin glycosides

Carotinoids (as blossom pigments): lutein, zeaxanthine

EFFECTS

Benzyl mustard oil extracted from Nasturtium is bacteriostatic, virostatic, and antimycotic in vitro. Mustard oils are eliminated mainly via the breath or are collected and eliminated in the urine; used externally, Nasturtium is a rubefacient.

INDICATIONS AND USAGE

Approved by Commission E:

- Infections of the urinary tract
- Cough
- Bronchitis

Nasturtium is used internally for infections of the urinary tract and catarrh of the upper respiratory tract.

Unproven Uses: Nasturtium is used in folk medicine internally for mild muscular pain, skin diseases, scurvy, tuberculosis, conditions of the respiratory and urinary tracts, and menstrual disorders. The herb is used externally for hair loss and for infected and poorly healing wounds.

CONTRAINDICATIONS

Do not administer to patients with gastrointestinal ulcers or kidney diseases.

Do not administer to infants or small children.

PRECAUTIONS AND ADVERSE REACTIONS

General: No health hazards or side effects are known in conjunction with the proper administration of designated therapeutic dosages. Administration of higher dosages of the fresh plant or of its volatile oil can lead to mucous membrane irritation of the gastrointestinal tract. External administration involving long-term intensive contact with the fresh plant can lead to skin irritations. The plant possesses a low potential for sensitization.

Pediatric Use: Not to be administered to infants or small children.

DOSAGE

Mode of Administration: The cut drug is available in the form of coated and filmed tablets and compound preparations.

Preparation: To make an infusion, add 30 g of leaves to 1 liter of water.

Daily Dosage: The dose for the extract is 14.4 mg of benzylisothiocyanate taken 3 times daily. The dose for the infusion is 2 to 3 cups per day; for the pressed juice, 30 g per day.

LITERATURE

Fanutti C, Gidley MJ, Reid JS. Substrate subsite recognition of the xyloglucan endo-transglycosylase or xyloglucan-specific endo-(1->4)-beta-D-glucanase from the cotyledons of germinated nasturtium (*Tropaeolum majus L.*) seeds. *Planta*, 200:221-8, 1996

Fanutti C, Gidley MJ, Reid JS. *Tropaeolum majus* and contact dermatitis. *Br J Dermatol*, 200:221-8, 1996

Frohne D, Pfänder HJ, Giftpflanzen - Ein Handbuch für Apotheker, Toxikologen und Biologen, 4. Aufl., Wiss. Verlags-Ges. Stuttgart 1997.

Hänsel R, Keller K, Rimpler H, Schneider G (Hrsg.), Hagers Handbuch der Pharmazeutischen Praxis, 5. Aufl., Bde 4-6 (Drogen): Springer Verlag Berlin, Heidelberg, New York, 1992-1994.

Madaus G, Lehrbuch der Biologischen Arzneimittel, Bde 1-3, Nachdruck, Georg Olms Verlag Hildesheim 1979.

Pintao AM et al., In vitro and in vivo antitumor activity of benzyl isothiocyanate: a natural product from *Tropaeolum majus*. In: PH 61(3):233-236. 1995.

Rose JK, Brummell DA, Bennett AB. Two divergent xyloglucan endotransglycosylases exhibit mutually exclusive patterns of expression in nasturtium. *Plant Physiol,* 110:493-9, Feb 1996

Steinegger E, Hänsel R, Pharmakognosie, 5. Aufl., Springer Verlag Heidelberg 1992.

Teuscher E, Lindequist U, Biogene Gifte - Biologie, Chemie, Pharmakologie, 2. Aufl., Fischer Verlag Stuttgart 1994.

Wagner H, Wiesenauer M, Phytotherapie. Phytopharmaka und pflanzliche Homöopathika, Fischer-Verlag, Stuttgart, Jena, New York 1995.

Wichtl M (Hrsg.), Teedrogen, 4. Aufl., Wiss. Verlagsges. Stuttgart 1997.

Nasturtium officinale

See Watercress

Neem

Antelaea azadirachta

DESCRIPTION

Medicinal Parts: The medicinal parts of the plant are the bark, the leaves, the branches, the seeds, and the latex.

Flower and Fruit: The plant has small white flowers.

Leaves, Stem and Root: Antelaea azadirachta is a deciduous tree up to 16 m high with leaves that are compound, alternate, oblong, ovate-lanceolate, and pointed. The bark is grayish-brown, externally fissured, and has a buff inner surface and fibrous fracture.

Characteristics: The plant has no odor; the taste is bitter.

Habitat: Indigenous to the woods of India and Sri Lanka. Found today in other tropical regions such as Indonesia, Australia, and western Africa.

Production: Neem tree bark, leaves and seeds are the trunk and branch bark, leaves and seeds of *Azadirachta indica* or of the closely related variety (in the literature often given as a synonym) of *Melia azedarach.*

Other Names: Holy Tree, Nim

ACTIONS AND PHARMACOLOGY

COMPOUNDS: NEEM SEED OIL

Triterpenes and tetranortriterpenes (limonoids and protolimonoids of the gedunin-group): for example nimbolin A and B, nimbin, gedunin

COMPOUNDS: NEEM BARK AND LEAVES

Tannin

Volatile oil

EFFECTS

Azadirachta indica has anti-inflammatory and antipyretic properties. *Melia azedarach* has an anthelmintic effect.

INDICATIONS AND USAGE

Unproven Uses: Azadirachta indica is used in inflammatory and febrile diseases (including malaria, although unconfirmed) as well as dyspepsia. *Melia azedarach* is used for worm infestation.

Indian Medicine: Antelaea azadirachta is used for inflammatory and febrile diseases (including malaria and leprosy, although unconfirmed), dyspeptic complaints and worm infestation.

PRECAUTIONS AND ADVERSE REACTIONS

No health hazards or side effects are known in conjunction with the proper administration of designated therapeutic dosages.

DOSAGE

Mode of Administration: The drug is available as a tincture. A slightly narcotic decoction can be prepared (said to lower a fever). An ointment for killing lice is administered topically.

How Supplied:

Capsules – 475 mg

LITERATURE

Adnrei GM et al., *Experientia 42* (7):843. 1986

Bray DH et al., *Trans Royal Soc Trop Med Hyg* 79: 426. 1985

El Said et al., (1968), Study of certain Nigerian plants used in Fever. Communication at the Inter-Africa Symposium Dakar.

Garg GP, Nigam SK, Ogle CW, The gastric antiulcer effects of the leaves of Neem tree. In: *PM* 59(3):215. 1993.

Godvindachari T et al., JNP 55:596-601. 1992.

Rojatkar SR et al., 1-Tigloyl-3-acteyl-11-hydroxy-4β-methylmeliacarpin from *Azadirachta indica*. In: PH 32:213. 1993.

Rücker G, Malariawirksame Verbindungen aus Pflanzen, insbesondere Peroxide. In: *PUZ* 24(4):189-195. 1995.

Siidiqui S et al., *JNP* 55:303-310. 1992.

Nelumbo nucifera

See Lotus

Nepalese Cardamom

Amomum aromaticum

DESCRIPTION

Medicinal Parts: The medicinal parts of the plant are the bark and fruit.

Flower and Fruit: The flowers are arranged in globose, 4 cm long spikes with single flowers in the axils of the scalelike, stem-clasping bracts. The inner flower bracts are elongate, ribbed, and thorn-tipped. The flowers are pale yellow with a tubular, 3-toothed calyx. The corolla petals are tubular. The flower tube is approximately 2.5 cm long. The petals are 2.5 cm long, lanceolate, blunt, and somewhat cap-shaped. The lip is twice as long as the petals. The lip is round with a cuneiform base and single stamen. The fruit is 3-chambered and narrow-ovoid in shape. It is approximately 3 cm long and has numerous 3 mm long seeds in each chamber.

Leaves, Stem, and Root: Amomum aromaticum is a herbaceous perennial, which grows up to 1 m high. The leaves are lanceolate, up to 25 cm long and 6 cm wide. They are pubescent beneath, with a 2 mm long ligule. The rhizome is up to 5 m long with shoots growing in clusters from it.

Habitat: India

Production: The ripe fruit is harvested in autumn and dried in the sun at low temperatures. Nepalese cardamoms are the dried, ripe fruit of *Amomum aromaticum*.

Not to be Confused With: Amomum aromaticum may be confused with *Amomum subulatum*.

ACTIONS AND PHARMACOLOGY

COMPOUNDS

Volatile oil (1%): chief constituent 1.8-cineole, including as well, alpha- and beta-pinene, limonene, myrcene, terpinene, p-cymol, terpineol, nerolidol, 1H-indene-2,3-dihydro-5-carboxyl aldehyde

EFFECTS

The efficacy of the drug in the context of folk medicine is believed to be traceable to the cineole contained in the essential oil, although scientific data regarding this are not available.

INDICATIONS AND USAGE

Chinese Medicine: Nepalese cardamom is used for malaria, diarrhea, vomiting, and digestive disturbances.

PRECAUTIONS AND ADVERSE REACTIONS

No health hazards are known in conjunction with the proper administration of designated therapeutic dosages.

OVERDOSAGE

Overdoses of the essential oil can lead to life-threatening poisoning, due to the high levels of cineole. Symptoms include reduced blood pressure, circulatory disorders, circulatory collapse, and asphyxiation. Vomiting is not to be induced in the case of poisoning, due to the danger of aspiration. Following instillation of activated charcoal, the therapy for poisoning consists of the treatment of spasms with diazepam, of colic with atropine, electrolyte substitution and the countering of any acidosis that may appear with sodium bicarbonate infusions. Intubation and oxygen respiration may also be required.

DOSAGE

Mode of Administration: Whole herb, cut drug and liquid preparations for internal use.

Daily Dosage: As decoction 3 to 6 g.

Storage: Should be protected from light and moisture.

LITERATURE

Hänsel R, Keller K, Rimpler H, Schneider G (Ed), Hagers Handbuch der Pharmazeutischen Praxis, 5. Aufl., Bde 4 - 6 (Drogen), Springer Verlag Berlin, Heidelberg, New York, 1992-1994.

Nepeta cataria

See Catnip

Nerium oleander

See Oleander

Nerve Root

Cypripedium calceolus

DESCRIPTION

Medicinal Parts: The medicinal parts are the dried rhizome with the roots, the fresh underground parts harvested in autumn and the fresh roots. The roots of several varieties are used as a sedative and antispasmodic.

Flower and Fruit: The plant develops terminal inflorescences with 1 to 2 flowers that have leaflike bracts. The flowers are 4

to 9 cm long by 0.5 to 1 cm wide. They are linear-lanceolate and twisted. The petals are green, green-brown, or yellow. The petals, including the protruding lip or shoe, are splayed. The shoe is 3 to 4 cm long in the shape of an inflated sack. It is lemon yellow to gold with purple spots and veins. The pollen is powdery. The pollen seeds are in 4 groups. The ovary is single-valved and pubescent.

Leaves, Stem, and Root: Nerve Root is a perennial, 15 to 70 cm high. The plant has a horizontal rootstock with scales and thick root fibers. The stem is round with short hairs, and is covered at the base with scaly brown leaves. There are 3 to 4 leaves above these, which are broad, elliptical, sheathlike, folded, and acute. The upper surface is bright green, the underside is paler.

Characteristics: The plant has a scent faintly of gentian and has an irritating effect on the skin.

Habitat: Indigenous to the U.S. and Canada, cultivated in Europe.

Production: Lady's Slipper rhizome is the rhizome of *Cypripedium calceolus.*

Not to be Confused With: Other Cypripedium varieties

Other Names: American Valerian, Bleeding Heart, Lady's Slipper, Moccasin Flower, Monkey Flower, Noah's Ark, Slipper Root, Venus Shoe, Yellows

ACTIONS AND PHARMACOLOGY

COMPOUNDS

Volatile oil

Phenanthrene quinones: including cypripedine (2,8-dimethoxy-7-hydroxy-1,4-phenanthrene quinone

Tannins

EFFECTS

The constituents of the drug have not been investigated. Some species of *Cypripedium* contain allergens and skin-irritating phenanthrene quinones. Nerve Root is astringent and hemostyptic. No additional information is available.

INDICATIONS AND USAGE

Unproven Uses: In folk medicine, the drug is used for insomnia, emotional tension, states of agitation, and nervousness.

PRECAUTIONS AND ADVERSE REACTIONS

Health risks or side effects following the proper administration of designated therapeutic dosages are not recorded. The plant possesses a medium potential for sensitization through skin contact.

DOSAGE

Mode of Administration: The drug is administered in its dry form or as liquid extract. The supply of higher (concentrated) doses should be avoided.

Preparation: Liquid extract: 1:1 in 45% alcohol.

Daily Dosage: To be taken internally, 2 teaspoonfuls (2 to 4 g) of the dried drug as an infusion.

LITERATURE

Hänsel R, Keller K, Rimpler H, Schneider G (Hrsg.), Hagers Handbuch der Pharmazeutischen Praxis, 5. Aufl., Bde 4-6 (Drogen), Springer Verlag Berlin, Heidelberg, New York, 1992-1994.

Hausen B, Allergiepflanzen, Pflanzenallergene, ecomed, Verlagsgesellsch. mbH, Landsberg 1988.

Madaus G, Lehrbuch der Biologischen Arzneimittel, Bde 1-3, Nachdruck, Georg Olms Verlag Hildesheim 1979.

Schmalle HW, Hausen BM, *Naturwissenschaften*: 66:527. 1979.

New Jersey Tea

Ceanothus americanus

DESCRIPTION

Medicinal Parts: The medicinal parts are the dried leaves, the dried root bark, and the fresh leaves.

Flower and Fruit: The inflorescences grow in the axils of the upper leaves and have long peduncles. They are 5 to 15 cm long, panicled, and have numerous cymelike partial inflorescences. The flowers are white, the petals are 2 to 3 mm long and twice as long as the sepals. The fruit is a globose capsule with a diameter of about 7 mm.

Leaves, Stem, and Root: Ceanothus americanus is a low deciduous shrub 40 to 100 cm high with greenish-purple branches. The petioled leaves are alternate, 3 to 10 cm long by 1.5 to 5 cm wide, ovate or oblong-ovate, rounded at the base, lightly pointed at the tip, and with pinnatifid nerves. The upper surface is glabrous or has finely compressed silky hairs. The lower surface is densely gray and pubescent. The leaf blade is finely and irregularly serrated. The root is tough, woody, dark brown, and striated or finely wrinkled longitudinally. The bark is thin, brittle and dark brown.

Characteristics: The taste is astringent; odorless.

Habitat: Indigenous to eastern and central North America. It is also used for breeding garden hybrids.

Production: Red Root is the root of *Ceanothus americanus.* The shrub is cultivated.

Other Names: Jersey Tea, Mountain-Sweet, Red Root, Walpole Tea, Wild Snowball

ACTIONS AND PHARMACOLOGY

COMPOUNDS

Cyclic peptide alkaloids (0.16% in the root cortex): including ceanothines A to E, americine, adouetines X and Y cyclic peptines

Triterpenes: including ceanothusic acid, ceanothenic acid, and betulic acid

EFFECTS

The tannins have an astringent effect. In blood taken from young rats, an aqueous-ethanol extract of the drug reduced blood-clotting time by 25%. However, the results are difficult to assess. The hemostyptic effect is attributed to the acid fraction of the drug. The drug is still useful as an astringent, expectorant, and antispasmodic. There is no valid data on the expectorant and antispasmodic effect.

INDICATIONS AND USAGE

Unproven Uses: Formerly, New Jersey Tea was used as an astringent, in the clotting of the blood, for fever, gonorrhea, and syphilis.

Homeopathic Uses: In homeopathy, *Ceanothus americanus* is used to treat enlarged spleen.

PRECAUTIONS AND ADVERSE REACTIONS

No health hazards or side effects are known in conjunction with the proper administration of designated therapeutic dosages.

DOSAGE

Mode of Administration: Orally as a liquid extract.

Homeopathic Dosage: 5 drops, 1 tablet, or 10 globules every 30 to 60 minutes (acute) or 1 to 3 times daily (chronic); parenterally: 1 to 2 mL sc 3 times daily (HAB1).

LITERATURE

Hänsel R, Keller K, Rimpler H, Schneider G (Hrsg.), Hagers Handbuch der Pharmazeutischen Praxis, 5. Aufl., Bde 4-6 (Drogen), Springer Verlag Berlin, Heidelberg, New York, 1992-1994.

Prum N, Mure C, Raynaud J, Reynaud J. Les agylcones flavoniques et anthocyaniques de *Ceanothus americanus L.* (Rhamnacees). *Pharmazie* 39; 353 (1984)

Niauli

Melaleucaea viridiflora

DESCRIPTION

Medicinal Parts: The medicinal parts are the young or shrubby plants and the oil, which is distilled from the fresh leaves and twigs.

Flower and Fruit: The plant grows up to 15 m.

Characteristics: The presence of traces of copper in the Niauli oil make it slightly greenish. The aromatic odor is reminiscent of camphor.

Habitat: The plant grows in tropical parts of southeast Asia and Australia.

Production: Niauli oil consists of the essential oil from the leaves of *Melaleucaea viridiflora*, obtained by water distillation.

ACTIONS AND PHARMACOLOGY

COMPOUNDS

Chief components: 1,8-cineole (up to 40%), viridiflorol (up to 25%), nerolidol (up to 95%), linalool (up to 30%); (+)-alpha-terpineol and (-)-alpha-terpineol as well as their valeric acid esters, alpha-pinene, limonene

EFFECTS

The drug is antibacterial and stimulates circulation.

INDICATIONS AND USAGE

Approved by Commission E:

- Cough/bronchitis

Unproven Uses: Niauli is used for catarrhs of the upper respiratory tract, rheumatism, neuralgia, and cystitis.

CONTRAINDICATIONS

Contraindications to internal use include inflammatory illnesses of the gastrointestinal area or of the biliary ducts, and severe liver diseases.

PRECAUTIONS AND ADVERSE REACTIONS

General: No health hazards or side effects are known in conjunction with the proper administration of designated therapeutic dosages. The internal administration of Niauli oil as a drug leads, in rare cases, to nausea, vomiting, and diarrhea.

Pediatric Use: Preparations containing the oil should not be applied to the faces of infants or small children, since glottal spasm, bronchial spasm, and asthmalike attacks are possible, as is respiratory failure.

DRUG INTERACTIONS

POTENTIAL INTERACTIONS

Niauli oil contains 35-60% cineole. Cineole causes the induction of the enzymes involved in the detoxification of the liver. The effect of other drugs can therefore be reduced and/or shortened.

OVERDOSAGE

Overdosages of Niauli oil (more than 10 g), can lead to life-threatening poisonings due to the high cineole content. Symptoms include, among others, fall in blood pressure, circulatory disorders, collapse and respiratory failure. In case of poisoning, vomiting should not be induced because of the danger of aspiration. Following administration of activated charcoal, the therapy for poisonings consists of treating spasms with diazepam (IV), treating colics with atropine, electrolyte substitution, and treating possible cases of acidosis with sodium bicarbonate infusions. Intubation and oxygen respiration may also be necessary.

DOSAGE

Mode of Administration: The oil and other galenic preparations are for internal and external application.

Preparation: Oily nose drops are prepared in a 2 to 5% concentration in vegetable oil. For external use, preparations contain 10 to 30% active ingredient in oil.

Daily Dosage: For internal use, the single dose is 0.2 g, with the daily dosage ranging from 0.2 to 2.0 g.

LITERATURE

Kern W, List PH, Hörhammer L (Hrsg.), Hagers Handbuch der Pharmazeutischen Praxis, 4. Aufl., Bde. 1-8, Springer Verlag Berlin, Heidelberg, New York, 1969.

Medici D de, Pieretti S, Salvatore G, Nicoletti M, Rasoanaivo P. Chemical Analysis of Essential Oils of Madagasy Medicinal Plants by Gas Chromatography and NMR Spectroscopy. *Flav Fragr J.* 7; 275-281. 1992

Steinegger E, Hänsel R, Pharmakognosie, 5. Aufl., Springer Verlag Heidelberg 1992.

Teuscher E, Biogene Arzneimittel, 5. Aufl., Wiss. Verlagsges. Stuttgart 1997.

Nicotiana tabacum

See Tobacco

Night-Blooming Cereus

Selenicereus grandiflorus

DESCRIPTION

Medicinal Parts: The medicinal parts are the fresh or dried flowers, the fresh young stems and flowers, and the fresh young shoots and sprouts.

Flower and Fruit: The flowers are 18 to 25 cm long and have a diameter of 15 to 27 cm. They have numerous, long, acute, lanceolate tepals that are arranged in a spiral. The outer tepals are brown; the middle ones are light yellow and the inner ones are spatulate to acute, lanceolate, and snow white. The numerous stamens are white and have yellow anthers. The styles with the 4-rayed stigmas become yellow toward the top. The ovary is globular and bumpy, with triangular scales and many brownish-gray hairs and thorns, which are approximately 10 mm long, dark brown, and bristly.

Leaves, Stem, and Root: The plant has a succulent trunk as well as a 1- to 4-cm thick snakelike, creeping or climbing, branched stem, which can grow to 10 m long or longer. The stem is 4 to 8 sided, green to bluish, has no bumps and is covered in adventitious roots. It has white tomentose axis buds on the protruding vertical ribs with 6 to 11 needlelike thorns that are 4 to 6 mm long.

Characteristics: The plant has sweet-smelling flowers, which only bloom for about 6 hours before dying.

Habitat: The plant is indigenous to Central America and is cultivated in Mexico and also in Europe.

Production: The young shoots and flowers are harvested in June or July and then preserved in alcohol. Some cultivated production is done in greenhouse settings, particularly in Europe.

Not to be Confused With: Confusion can arise with the flowers of *Opuntia maxima, Selenicereus hamatus*, and *Selenicereus pteranthus*. The drug is adulterated commercially with the flowers of *Opuntia vulgaris* and *Opuntia ficus-indica.*

Other Names: Large Blooming Cereus, Sweet-Scented Cactus

ACTIONS AND PHARMACOLOGY

COMPOUNDS

Flavonoids (1.5%): including among others, narcissin, rutin, cacticine, kaempferitine, grandiflorin, hyperoside

Amines: (found only in the shoots) chief components are hordenine (cactine), tyramine, N-methyltyramine, N,N-dimethyl tyramine

Betacyans: (in the blossoms, yellow pigments)

EFFECTS

The drug has an effect similar to digitalis, which includes cardiac stimulation as well as coronary and peripheral vessel dilation. The drug is also said to stimulate the motor neurons of the spinal cord. In addition, the drug may act topically as an antiphlogistic, but this is unproved.

INDICATIONS AND USAGE

Unproven Uses: Preparations of *Selenicereus grandiflorus* are used for nervous cardiac disorders, and urinary ailments. In Mexico and Central America, folk medicine internal uses include hemostasis, menorrhagia, dysmenorrhea, hemorrhage, cardiac complaints, cystitis, and shortness of breath.

PRECAUTIONS AND ADVERSE REACTIONS

No health hazards or side effects are known in conjunction with the proper administration of designated therapeutic dosages. Intake of the fresh juice is said to cause itching and pustules on the skin, burning of the mouth, queasiness, vomiting and diarrhea.

DOSAGE

Mode of Administration: Fluid extracts and tinctures are used internally and externally.

Preparations: Fluid extract (Extractum Cerei liquidum 1:1); Tinctura Cerei (1:4) BPC 34; Tincture in sweetened water (1:10).

Daily Dosage: For the folk medicine dosages, a liquid extract is used in doses up to 0.6 mL, one to 10 times daily. The Tincture Cerei dosage is 0.12 to 2 mL taken 2 to 3 times daily. Dosage for the tincture in sweetened water is 10 drops, 3 to 5 times daily.

LITERATURE

Hänsel R, Keller K, Rimpler H, Schneider G (Hrsg.), Hagers Handbuch der Pharmazeutischen Praxis, 5. Aufl., Bde 4-6 (Drogen): Springer Verlag Berlin, Heidelberg, New York, 1992-1994.

Madaus G: Lehrbuch der Biologischen Arzneimittel, Bde 1-3, Nachdruck, Georg Olms Verlag Hildesheim 1979 (unter Cactus grandiflorus).

Roth L, Daunderer M, Kormann K, Giftpflanzen, Pflanzengifte, 4. Aufl., Ecomed Fachverlag Landsberg Lech 1993.

Wagner H, Wiesenauer M, Phytotherapie. Phytopharmaka und pflanzliche Homöopathika, Fischer-Verlag, Stuttgart, Jena, New York 1995.

Willaman JJ, Schubert BG. Tech. Bull 1234: USDA Washington DC. 1961.

Noni

Morinda citrifolia

DESCRIPTION

Medicinal Parts: The medicinal parts of the plant are the leaf, fruit and root.

Flower and Fruit: The inflorescence is globose. The flowers are radial, their structures in fives with fused yellowish-white tepals. The ovary is inferior with 1 stigma. The fruit is a many-seeded, glassy-white berry the size of a chicken egg.

Leaves, Branches: Morinda citrifolia is a tree that is occasionally shrub-like. It grows up to 10 m high. The leaves are opposite, 10 to 30 cm long. The petiole is approximately 12 mm long. The lamina is coriaceous, glossy, elliptical to elliptical-ovate, acuminate, somewhat crenate and cuneiform at the base with stipules. The branches are square, divided jointed and contain nodes.

Characteristics: The fruit is inedible.

Habitat: Malaysia

Production: Noni fruit and leaves are the fresh ripe fruit and dried leaves of Morinda citrifolia.

Other Names: Mengkudu

ACTIONS AND PHARMACOLOGY

CONSTITUENTS

Numerous components have been identified in the noni plant, such as scopoletin, octoanoic acid, potassium, vitamin C, terpenoids, alkaloids, anthraquinones (such as nordamnacanthal, morindone, rubiadin, and rubiadin-1-methyl ether, anthraquinone glycoside), -sitosterol, carotene, vitamin A, flavone glycosides, linoleic acid, alizarin, amino acids, L-asperuloside, caproic acid, caprylic acid, ursolic acid and rutin.

Volatile oil Iridoids: asperulosid, deacetylasperuloside

EFFECTS

Antiviral, antibacterial, anti-inflammatory, antioxidant, antitumor, anti-atherosclerotic, anthelmintic, analgesic, and hypotensive effects could be shown for Noni. Further, Noni effects gastric emptying, transit, and CCK.

CLINICAL TRIALS

General wellbeing

In a statistical clinical survey of the results of more than 10,000 noni juice users, various efficacious medical properties were investigated. A total of 67% percent of 847 people with cancer experienced improvement of their symptoms; 91% of noni juice users noticed an increase in energy levels; 72% of overweight patients lost weight; and 87% of patients suffering from high blood pressure experienced a significant drop in blood pressure. Nearly 90% of those with chronic pain experienced a significant decrease in pain and 80% of arthritis sufferers reported a lessening of arthritic symptoms. In addition, 80% of patients with heart disease experienced an improvement of their symptoms; 83% of patients with type 1 and 2 diabetes experienced a noticeable change in their condition; and 89% of patients experienced improved digestion. Further, 85% of patients with allergies experienced a decrease in their symptoms and 77% of people with depression experienced lessening of symptoms. Side effects among all participants were minimal or nonexistent (Solomon, 1998; Solomon, 1999; Solomon, 2000; Solomon, 2001; Sharps, 2000).

A small human clinical trial of the effect of Tahitian Noni Juice on auditory function and quality of life in the patients with decreased bone mineral density and auditory function has been conducted This study showed that Tahitian Noni Juice provided a positive benefit on mental health and improved high frequency hearing. Increased amounts or extended duration of Tahitian Noni Juice intake may be required to affect this disorder (Langford, 2004).

Oxidative Damage Induced by Tobacco Smoke

A one-month, double blind, randomized, and placebo-controlled clinical trial was designed to test the protective effect of Tahitian Noni Juice on plasma superoxides (SAR) and lipid peroxides (LPO) in current smokers. The subjects were supplemented daily with two ounces of Tahitian Noni Juice (n=38) or placebo (n=30), twice a day for 30 days. The plasma SAR and LPO levels were determined before and after trial by TNB and LPO assay, respectively. There was no effect observed on plasma SAR (0.23± 0.15 versus 0.21±0.17 μmol/mL) and LPO (0.58±0.22 versus 0.59±0.21 μmol/mL) in the placebo group. The LPO and SAR levels in the Tahitian Noni Juice group showed 23 % reduction (0.59±0.21 μmol/mL versus 0.45±0.20 μmol/ml, P=0.06) and 27 % reduction (0.23±0.18 μmol/mL versus 0.17±0.10 μmol/mL, P<0.05), respectively. These results indicate that Tahitian Noni Juice may protect individuals from oxidative damage induced by tobacco smoke by (Wang, 2002).

Cancer and cancer-related symptoms

Wong reports two clinical cases of adenocarcinoma in which the ingestion of Noni juice may have proved essential to the patient's long-term survival and concludes that Noni should be studied further for its potential use in adjuvant immunotherapy for cancer (Wong, 2004).

Patients with advanced cancer took part in a phase I dose-finding study with capsules containing 500mg ripe Noni fruit extract. First dose level was 4 capsules (2 g) daily, the highest recommended dosing of the commercial product. Subsequent dose levels were increased by 2 g daily up to a maximum dose level of 10 g (20 capsules) daily. A minimum of 5 patients at each dose level were observed for 28 days before new patients were entered at the next higher dose level. In addition to conventional toxicity and response measures, quality of life and symptom status were measured with QLQ C-30, Brief Fatigue Inventory (BFI), and CES-D, depression scale at baseline and every 4 weeks. A total of 29 patients were assessed for toxicity, quality of life/symptom status and pharmacokinetics. The distribution of performance status, extent of disease, and prior treatment did not show any significant variation across the 5 dose levels. There were no adverse events (CTCAE criteria) attributable to Noni. Using a multilevel regression analysis of Noni dose (2, 4, 6, 8, 10 grams) and week of study, there was a statistically significant [t(35)=-2.84, p=.006] decrease in pain interference with activities. Although not reaching statistical significance, consistent dose response effects were found for global health status, physical functioning, and fatigue. There was no dose response relationship found for the BFI and CES-D measures. No measured tumor regressions using RESIST criteria were noted. In a separate study, the same author entered over 40 patients at different dose levels and found no dose-limiting toxicities with doses up to 24 capsules (12 g) daily. In the absence of any dose-limiting effects, the researchers aim to identify a maximum dose which would sustain quality of life to be used for subsequent Phase II efficacy studies with placebo controls (Issel, 2005).

INDICATIONS AND USAGE

Unproven Uses: Noni is used for diabetes, as a blood purifier (for women), for fever, and stomachache (Malaysia).

PRECAUTIONS AND ADVERSE REACTIONS

No health hazards are known in conjunction with the proper administration of designated therapeutic dosages.

DOSAGE

Preparation: The dried leaves are used as hot compresses on the chest and stomach (for fever and stomachache).

LITERATURE

Hirazumi A, Furusawa E, Chou SC, Hokama Y, Immunomodulation contributes to the anticancer activity of morinda citrifolia (noni) fruit juice. *Planta Med*, 39:7-9, 1996.

Issell BF, Gotay C, Pagano I, Franke A. Quality of life measures in a phase I trial of noni. 2005 ASCO Annual Meeting.

Langford J, Doughty A, Wang M, Clayton L, Babich M. Effects of *Morinda citrifolia* on quality of life and auditory function in postmenopausal women. J Altern Complement Med 2004;10(5):737-9.

Sharps J. NONI juice, A prescription for the good health. Integrated Health Service; 2000.

Solomon N. Nature's amazing healer, Noni. Pleasant Grove, Utah: Woodland Publishing; 1998.

Solomon N. The tropical fruit with 101 medicinal uses, Noni juice. 2nd ed. Woodland Publishing; 1999.

Solomon N. The Noni phenomenon. Discover the powerful tropical healer that fights cancer, lowers high blood pressure and relieves chronic pain. Direct Source Publishing; 1999.

Solomon N. Tahitian Noni juice: How much, how often, for what. Direct Source Publishing; 2000.

Solomon N. Tahitian Noni juice: The pain fighter (arthritis/pain). Direct Source Publishing; 2001.

Wang MY, Nowicki D, Anderson G, Su C, Jensen J. Protective effects of *Morinda citrifolia* on plasma superoxides (SAR) and lipid peroxides (LPO) in current smokers. The Proceedings of XIth Biennial Meeting of the Society for Free Radical Research International. 2002. Paris.

Wong DK. Are immune responses pivotal to cancer patient's long term survival? Two clinical case-study reports on the effects of *Morinda citrifolia* (Noni). *Hawaii Med J* 2004; 63(6):182-4.

Younos C, Rolland A, Fleurentin J, Lanhers MC, Misslin R, Mortier F, Analgesic and behavioral effects of Morinda citrifolia. *Planta Med*, 56:430-4, 1990 Oct.

Northern Prickly Ash

Zanthoxylum americanum

DESCRIPTION

Medicinal Parts: The medicinal parts are the root bark and the berries.

Flower and Fruit: The greenish-yellow flowers are in terminal umbels. The fruit is black or deep blue and enclosed in a gray shell.

Leaves, Stem, and Root: The plant is an aromatic shrub or small tree up to 3 m tall. The branches are alternate and the leaves pinnatifid. The bark and the petioles are covered in sharp spines about 5 mm long. The bark is brownish-gray on the outside and faintly furrowed with whitish patches and flattened spines that are about 5 mm long.

Characteristics: The leaves and berries have an aromatic lemonlike fragrance, and the bark has a pungent, acrid taste.

Habitat: The plant grows in North America.

Other Names: Prickly Ash, Suterberry, Toothache Tree, Yellow Wood

ACTIONS AND PHARMACOLOGY

COMPOUNDS

Pyranocoumarins: xanthoxyletin (xanthoxyloin), xanthyletin, alloxanthyletin

Isoquinoline alkaloids: chelerythrine, berberine, N-methylisocorydine, laurifoline, magnoflorine, nitidine

Volatile oil

Resins

EFFECTS

No information is available.

INDICATIONS AND USAGE

Unproven Uses: Northern Prickly Ash is used for low blood pressure, rheumatic disorders, fever, and inflammation.

Indian Medicine: The drug is used for toothache, headache, eye and ear conditions, dyspeptic symptoms, colic, flatulence, worm infestation, diarrhea, fever, coughs, asthma, paralyses, and leprosy.

PRECAUTIONS AND ADVERSE REACTIONS

No health hazards or side effects are known in conjunction with the proper administration of designated therapeutic dosages.

OVERDOSAGE

Overdosage is said to lead to salivation, increased cardiac function and elevated blood pressure. Severe poisonings resulting from intake of the drug have not been recorded.

DOSAGE

Mode of Administration: Liquid extract, in preparations and in combinations.

How Supplied: Liquid extract–1:4

LITERATURE

Fish F, Waterman PG, *J Pharm Pharmac*. 25S, 115. 1973

Kern W, List PH, Hörhammer L (Hrsg.), Hagers Handbuch der Pharmazeutischen Praxis, 4. Aufl., Bde 1-8: Springer Verlag Berlin, Heidelberg, New York, 1969.

Leung AY, Encyclopedia of Common Natural Ingredients Used in Food, Drugs, Cosmetics, John Wiley & Sons Inc., New York 1980.

Madaus G, Lehrbuch der Biologischen Arzneimittel, Bde 1-3, Nachdruck, Georg Olms Verlag Hildesheim 1979.

Oliver-Bever B (Ed.), Medicinal Plants of Tropical West Africa, Cambridge University Press, Cambrigde 1986.

Roth L, Daunderer M, Kormann K, Giftpflanzen, Pflanzengifte, 4. Aufl., Ecomed Fachverlag Landsberg Lech 1993.

Nutmeg

Myristica fragrans

DESCRIPTION

Medicinal Parts: The medicinal parts are the nutmeg seeds, which through various processes yield several therapeutic components. They include the essential oil of the seed; the compressed, dried aril; the mixture of fat, oil and color pigment from the pressed seeds; the dried seed kernels freed from the aril and shell of the nut; calcified seed kernels; and the dried seed kernels.

Flower and Fruit: Myristica fragans is either male or female, although there are male trees with female flowers and fruit. The flowers are unisexual. The male flowers are in sparsely flowered inflorescence; the female ones are solitary and inconspicuous. The flowers have a simple 3-lobed involucre; the filaments are fused to a tube. The fruit ripens 7 to 10 months after flowering. The fruit is fleshy, almost round, acuminate at the stem end, 3 to 6 cm long and 2.5 to 5 cm thick. The fruit is light yellow and about the size of a peach. The fruit flesh bursts open when ripe and exposes the bright red seed's aril that surrounds the dark brown seed. Within the aril, the seed kernel is covered in a hard brown testis that shows the marks of the aril.

Leaves, Stem, and Root: Nutmeg is an evergreen tree up to 15 m in height. The smooth bark is green on the young branches, then turns grayish-brown. The alternate leaves are dark green, entire-margined, sharp edged, short-petioled, ovate-elliptical, and up to 8 cm long.

Habitat: The plant is indigenous to the Molucca Islands and New Guinea and has spread to Indonesia, the West Indies, and other tropical areas, where it also is cultivated.

Production: Nutmeg is the seed of *Myristica fragrans.* After harvesting, the nut is shelled and dried (maximum 45° C), and the seed is opened after 4 to 8 weeks. The lacy, fleshy covering of the nut, which is scarlet when fresh and dark orange when dried, yields Nutmeg and Mace. After being separated, both parts are dried slowly. The nut is ground and then distilled. Nutmeg butter is made by pressing and steaming the nuts to extract the fatty and essential oils from the seeds.

Not to be Confused With: Several other nuts are often given the name nutmeg. Confusion may occur with calabash nutmeg (*Monodora myristica*), Papua nutmeg (*Myristica succedanea*) and *Myristica malabarica, Laurelia sempervirens, Atherosperma moschatum, Ravensara aromatica, Cryptocarya moschata,* and *Torreya californica.* Nutmeg oil is sometimes confused with the oil from the green leaves of *Myristica fragrans.*

Other Names: Mace, Myristica

ACTIONS AND PHARMACOLOGY

COMPOUNDS: NUTMEG

Volatile oil (7-16%)

Fatty oil (30-40%): fatty acids including among others lauric, myristic, pentadecanoic, palmitic, heptadecanoic, stearic, oleic acid

Triterpene saponins

Sterols: including among others beta-sitosterol, campesterol

COMPOUNDS: NUTMEG OIL

Monoterpene hydrocarbons 80%): including sabinene (39%), alpha-pinene (13%), beta-pinene (9%)

monoterpene alcohols (5%): including 1,8-cineole (3.5%)

phenyl propane derivatives (10 to 18%): including myristicin (2 to 5%), elemicin (1 to 2.5%)

Fatty oil (30 to 40%) in the nutmeg oil rendered through pressing

EFFECTS

In animal experiments, the eugenol in the essential oil inhibits, dose-dependently, medicinally induced diarrhea and slows down the transport of active carbon in the gastrointestinal tract. An effect on prostaglandin synthesis and an antimicrobial effect have also been demonstrated. The use of the drug for dysentery and rheumatic complaints seems plausible.

INDICATIONS AND USAGE

Unproven Uses: Internal folk medicine uses of nutmeg include diarrhea and dysentery, inflammation of the stomach membranes, cramps, flatulence and vomiting. Externally, the oil is used for rheumatism, sciatica, neuralgia, and disorders of the upper respiratory tract.

Chinese Medicine: Indications include diarrhea, vomiting, and digestive problems.

Indian Medicine: Indications in Indian medicine include headaches, poor vision, insomnia, fever and malaria, cholera, impotence, and general debility.

Homeopathic Uses: Among uses in homeopathy are nervous physical symptoms, digestive problems with flatulence, and disturbed perception.

CONTRAINDICATIONS
The drug is not to be used during pregnancy.

PRECAUTIONS AND ADVERSE REACTIONS
Should be used only under expert supervision. No health hazards or side effects are known in conjunction with the proper administration of designated therapeutic dosages. However, the drug can trigger allergic contact dermatitis.

OVERDOSAGE: NUTMEG SEED AND OIL
Ingestion of 1 to 3 ''nuts'' (or even fewer) can produce amphetamine derivatives through bioconversion of the phenylpropane derivatives in the human body. This eventually leads to intense thirst, nausea, reddening and swelling of the face, and alterations of consciousness from mild changes, such as anxiety or lethargy, to intensive hallucinations. The stupor can last from 2 to 3 days. The therapy for poisonings consists of gastrointestinal emptying (inducement of vomiting, gastric lavage with burgundy-colored potassium permanganate solution, sodium sulfate), and installation of activated charcoal. That is followed by treating spasms intravenously with diazepam; treating colic with atropine; electrolyte substitution; and treating possible cases of acidosis with sodium bicarbonate infusions. In case of shock, plasma volume expanders should be infused. Monitoring of kidney function is essential. Intubation and oxygen respiration may also be necessary.

DOSAGE
Mode of Administration: Nutmeg oils, extracts, powders, syrups and butters are used internally. The oil also is used externally as a liniment 10%

Preparation: There is no information in the literature.

Daily Dosage:

Infusion/decoction: 1%, 50 to 200 mL daily.

Liquid extract: 1 to 2 times daily.

Oil: 1 to 3 drops internally 2 to 3 times a day.

Powder: 0.3 to 1 g; not to exceed 3 times daily.

Syrup: 10 to 40 mL daily.

Tincture: 2 to 10 mL daily.

Homeopathic Dosage: 5 drops, 1 tablet, or 10 globules every 30 to 60 minutes (acute) or 1 to 3 times daily (chronic); parenterally: 1 to 2 mL sc acute, 3 times daily; chronic: once a day (HAB1).

Storage: Nutmeg should be stored in tightly sealed containers and kept cool and dry. The oil should be protected from light in containers that are tightly sealed, completely filled and kept at a temperature not to exceed 25° C.

LITERATURE: NUTMEG SEED AND OIL
Akker TW van den, Roesyanto-Mahadi ID, Toorenenbergen AW van, Joost T van. Contact allergy to spices. *Contact Dermatitis* 22; 267-272. 1990

Aye-Than Kulkarni HJ, Wut-Hmone Tha SJ. Anti-diarrhoeal Efficacy of Some Burmese Indigenous Drug Formulations in Experimental Diarrhoeal Test Models. *Int J Crude Drug Res.* 27; 195-200. 1989

Bennett A et al., *New Eng J Med* 290:110.

Hattori M, Yang XW, Miyashiro H, Namba T. Inhibitory Effects of Monomeric and Dimeric Phenylpropanoids from Mace on Lipid Peroxidation In Vivo and In Vitro. *Phytother Res.* 7 (6); 395-401.1 993

Kasahara H, Miyazawa M, Kameoka H. Absolute Configuration of 8-O-4'-Neolignans from *Myristica fragrans. Phytochemistry* 40 (5); 1515-1517. 1995

Miller EC et al. Cancer Res 43:1124. 1983

Miyazawa M, Kasahara H, Kameoka H. A New Lignan (+)-Myrisfragransin from *Myristica fragrans. Nat Prod Lett.* 8; 25-26. 1996

Ozaki Y, Soedigdo S, Wattimena YR, Suganda AG. Antiinflammatory Effect of Mace, Aril of Myristica fragrans Houtt., and Its Active Principles. *Jap J Pharmacol.* 49; 155-163. 1989

Pecevski J et al., *Toxicol Lett* 7:739. 1980

Sarath-Kumara SJ et al., *J Sci Food Agric* 36(2):93. 1985

Shafkan I et al., *New Eng J Med* 296:694. 1977

Nux Vomica

Strychnos nux vomica

DESCRIPTION
Medicinal Parts: The medicinal parts are the ripe, dried seeds, and the dried bark.

Flower and Fruit: The inflorescences are terminal and cymelike. The flowers have a 5-tipped calyx and a white to greenish-white plate-shaped corolla with a long tube. There are 5 sessile stamens in the mouth of the corolla tube. The ovary is superior, bivalved and has a long style and a 2-lobed stigma. The fruit, when ripe, is an orange-red, globular berry with a diameter of 4 to 6 cm. The pulp is white, bitter and surrounded by a tough, brittle exocarp about 1.5 mm thick. There are usually 1 to 9 seeds in the pulp, of which 2 to 4 are erect. The seeds are disclike, orbicular, 12 to 25 mm wide, radially striped, appressed pubescent, and exceptionally bitter.

Leaves, Stem, and Root: The plant is a tree up to 25 m high with a trunk circumference of up to 3 m. The branches are obtuse-quadrangular, close together, and repeatedly bifurcated. They are glabrous and they have 1 to 2 leaf pairs, which are thickened at the nodes. The trunk bark is blackish-ash-gray and the branch bark is gray. The twigs are green and glossy. The leaves are petiolate and crossed-opposite. The leaf blade is glabrous, broadly ovate, entire-margined, and has a curved main rib. The broad stipules dry later.

Habitat: The plant grows all over southeast Asia from Pakistan to Vietnam.

Production: Nux Vomica consists of the seeds of *Strychnos nux-vomica*. The berries are picked when ripe. The hard exocarp is removed and the seeds are taken out and washed to remove any pulp residue. They are subsequently dried in the sun.

Not to be Confused With: The seeds of *Strychnos nux-blanda, Strychnos potatorum* and *Strychnos wallichiana*. Nux vomica powder may be confused with the powder of date nuts or olive stones and with by-products of stone-nut processing.

Other Names: Poison Nut, Quaker Button's

ACTIONS AND PHARMACOLOGY

COMPOUNDS

Indole alkaloids (2.0-5.0%): chief alkaloids strychnine and brucine (approximately in a 1:1 ratio), including among others, 12-hydroxystrychnine, 15-hydroxystrychnine, alpha-colubrine, beta-colubrine, icajine

Fatty oil

Polysaccharides as insoluble reserve substances

Iridoide monoterpenes: including among others, loganin

EFFECTS

Nux Vomica increases reflex excitability. Endogenic and exogenic stimuli reach the targeted organ without hindrance and, as a result, possess a strengthened effect that can be attributed to the alkaloid strychnine. The toxic principle strychnine deadens the inhibitory synapse of the CNS and results in overextended musculature reactions.

The strychnine and brucine components act as competitive antagonists of the neurotransmitter glycine. The drug is psychoanaleptic due to an increase in reflex action, i.e., endogenic and exogenic stimuli reach the targeted organ without hindrance and as a result have a strengthened effect. In addition, strychnine is cholinolytic in animal experiments.

In lower doses, the drug causes a reflexive increase of glandular secretion in the gastrointestinal tract through the amaroids.

INDICATIONS AND USAGE

Unproven Uses: Nux Vomica and its preparations are used in combinations for diseases and conditions of the gastrointestinal tract, organic and functional disorders of the heart and circulatory system, diseases of the eye, nervous conditions, depression, migraine, and climacteric complaints. In addition, the herb is used as a tonic, an appetite stimulant, for respiratory complaints, for secondary anemia, and for unspecific geriatric complaints.

Chinese Medicine: The drug is used for general pain, febrile illnesses, sore throat, and abdominal tumors.

Indian Medicine: The drug is used for loss of appetite, anemia, lumbago, asthma, bronchitis, constipation, diabetes, intermittent and malarial fever, skin diseases, paralyses, and muscle weakness; a special procedure is supposed to detoxify the seeds.

Homeopathic Uses: The drug is used for inflammations of the respiratory and gastrointestinal tracts, disorders of the urinary tract, febrile illnesses, hepatocystic disorders, hemorrhoids, dizziness, headache, neuralgia, rheumatic pain, cramps, paralyses, insomnia, and nervous irritability.

PRECAUTIONS AND ADVERSE REACTIONS

The drug is severely toxic due to the strychnine content and is not recommended for use.

OVERDOSAGE

Symptoms of poisoning can occur after ingestion of one bean. Strychnine doses of as little as 1.5 mg (30-50 mg of the drug) initially cause restlessness, feelings of anxiety, heightening of sense perception, enhanced reflexes, equilibrium disorders, and painful stiffness of the neck and back musculature. Later, twitching, tonic spasms of the masseter and neck musculature, and finally painful convulsions of the entire body that are triggered by visual or tactile stimulation occur. Dyspnea comes following spasm of the breathing musculature. Death occurs through suffocation or exhaustion. The lethal dosage for an adult is approximately 50 mg strychnine (1-2 g of the drug). Chronic intake of subconvulsive dosages can also lead to death under similar conditions after a period of weeks. This is due to an accumulation of drug in the body, particularly in those who have liver damage.

Following the administration of a watery suspension of activated charcoal, the therapy for poisoning consists of keeping external stimulation to a minimum through placement in a quiet, warm, darkened room. Convulsions should be treated with dosages of diazepam or barbital (IV). High-calorie glucose infusions should also be given. Intubation and oxygen respiration may also be required. Gastric lavage should be avoided, due to the danger of triggering convulsions. Analeptics or phenothiazines should not be administered. Because of the possibility of unwanted effects occurring in conjunction with the administration of therapeutic dosages, one should forgo any administration of the drug.

DOSAGE

Mode of Administration: Nux Vomica is used almost exclusively in homeopathy. Radioactively tagged strychnine is used in medicine to detect glycinergic receptors. In industry, the drug is used as an active agent for pest control.

Daily Dosage: The average single dose is 0.02 to 0.05 g.

The daily dosages for various preparations are as follows: liquid (0.05 to 2 mL), extract (0.005 g, with a maximun dose of 0.1 g), tincture (0.5 to 2 mL (BP80), or Strychninum nitricum (maximum single dose of 0.005 g).

Homeopathic Dosage: 5 drops, 1 tablet, or 10 globules every 30 to 60 minutes (acute) or 1 to 3 times daily (chronic); parenterally: 1 to 2 mL sc, acute: 3 times daily; chronic: once a day (HAB1).

Storage: Mark the container as ''poisonous'' and keep tightly sealed; protect the drug from cool air and light.

LITERATURE

De B, Datta PC. Alkaloids of *Strychnos nux-vomica* Flower. *Planta Med. 54*; 363. 1988

El-Mekkawy S, Meselhy MR, Kawata Y, Kadota S, Hattori M, Namba T. Metabolism of Stychnine N-Oxide and Brucine N-Oxide by Human Intestinal Bacteria. *Planta Med.* 59; 347-350. 1993

Hänsel R, Keller K, Rimpler H, Schneider G (Hrsg.), Hagers Handbuch der Pharmazeutischen Praxis, 5. Aufl., Bde 4-6 (Drogen): Springer Verlag Berlin, Heidelberg, New York, 1992-1994.

Lewin L, Gifte und Vergiftungen, 6. Aufl., Nachdruck, Haug Verlag, Heidelberg 1992.

Madaus G, Lehrbuch der Biologischen Arzneimittel, Bde 1-3, Nachdruck, Georg Olms Verlag Hildesheim 1979.

Marini-Bettolo GB, Advances in the research of curare and Strychnos. In: *Rend Accad Naz* 40:1975-1976, 1-2, 61-76. 1977.

Roth L, Daunderer M, Kormann K, Giftpflanzen, Pflanzengifte, 4. Aufl., Ecomed Fachverlag Landsberg Lech 1993.

Steinegger E, Hänsel R, Pharmakognosie, 5. Aufl., Springer Verlag Heidelberg 1992.

Teuscher E, Biogene Arzneimittel, 5. Aufl., Wiss. Verlagsges. Stuttgart 1997.

Teuscher E, Lindequist U, Biogene Gifte - Biologie, Chemie, Pharmakologie, 2. Aufl., Fischer Verlag Stuttgart 1994.

Tripathi YB, Chaurasi S. Studies on the inhibitory effect of *Strychnos nux vomica*-alcohol extract on iron induced lipid peroxidation. *Phytomedicine* 3 (2); 175-180. 1996

Wagner H, Wiesenauer M, Phytotherapie. Phytopharmaka und pflanzliche Homöopathika, Fischer-Verlag, Stuttgart, Jena, New York 1995.

Wahbi AM, Abounassif MA, Gad-Kariem EA. High-performance liquid chromatographic determination of strychnine and brucine in nux vomica liquid extract. *Arch Pharm Chem. Sci Ed.;* 15; 87-90. 1987

Withmarsh TE, Coleston-Shields DM, Steiner TJ. Double-blind randomized placebo-controlled study of homoeopathic prophylaxis of migraine. *Cephalgia* 17; 600-604. 1997

Zong YY, Che CT. Determination of Strychnine and Brucine by Capillary Zone Electrophoresis. *Planta Med.* 61 (5); 456-458. 1995

Nymphaea odorata

See American White Pond Lily

Oak

Quercus robur

DESCRIPTION

Medicinal Parts: The medicinal parts are the dried bark of the young branches and the lateral shoots, the dried bark of the trunk and branches, the dried leaves of various oak species, and the seed kernels without the seed coats.

Flower and Fruit: The flowers are reddish brown and monoecious. The male flowers consist of a 5-part perigone with 6 to 10 stamens that appear in small groups in limp, hanging catkins. The female flowers, solitary or in groups of up to 5, appear in an involucre, which clasps the base of the fruit and later becomes bowl-shaped. The fruit is solitary or in groups of up to 5 on a shared glabrous or sparsely pubescent stem. They are oblong-ovate, acuminate, and enclosed in the cupule.

Leaves, Stem, and Root: The tree is about 50 m high with a broad, irregular, heavily branched crown and a trunk which divides into gnarled, strong, bent branches. The bark is deeply fissured, thick, and grey-brown. The leaves are short-petioled, almost sessile, oblong-obovate, almost lobed, usually cordate, or polled at the base.

Habitat: The tree is widespread in Europe, Asia Minor, and the Caucasus region.

Production: Oak bark consists of the dried bark of young branches and saplings of *Quercus robur* and/or *Quercus petraea,* harvested in the spring, as well as their preparations. Oak bark is harvested from March to April. The trees fall every 10 years. The bark is dried rapidly.

Other Names: Common Oak, English Oak, Pedunculate Oak, Tanner's Bark

ACTIONS AND PHARMACOLOGY

COMPOUNDS

Catechin tannins: oligomeric proanthocyanidins

Ellagitannins: (including castalagin, pedunculagin, vesvalagin, 2,3-(S)-hexahydroxy diphenoyl glucose), flavano-ellagitannins (acutissimins A and B, eugenigrandin, guajavacin B, stenophyllanin C)

Gallo tannins

Monomeric and dimeric catechins and leucocyanidins

Tannins (12 to 16%)

EFFECTS

The drug, which contains tannins, is astringent, antiphlogistic, antiviral and anthelmintic.

INDICATIONS AND USAGE

Approved by Commission E:

- Cough/bronchitis
- Diarrhea
- Inflammation of the mouth and pharynx

■ Inflammation of the skin

Oak is used internally for nonspecific diarrhea. In smaller doses it is used as a stomach tonic. The drug is used externally for inflammatory skin diseases and inflammation of the mouth and throat.

Unproven Uses: In folk medicine, Oak is used for inflammation of the genital and anal area, suppurating eczema, hyperhydrosis, intertrigo, and as an adjuvant treatment of chilblains. Oak is also used in folk medicine internally for hemorrhagic stool, nonmenstrual uterine bleeding, hemoptysis, and chronic inflammation of the gastrointestinal tract. External uses include hemorrhoid bleeding, varicose veins, uterine bleeding, vaginal discharge (washes/douches), rashes, chronic, itching, scaly and suppurating eczema, and eye inflammations.

CONTRAINDICATIONS

Whole-body baths are contraindicated with large-area weeping eczemas and skin injuries, with feverish and infectious illnesses, with cardiac insufficiency in stages III and IV (NYHA), and with hypertonia in stage IV (WHO).

PRECAUTIONS AND ADVERSE REACTIONS

General: No health hazards or side effects are known in conjunction with the proper administration of designated therapeutic dosages. Internal administration could lead to digestive complaints because of the secretion-inhibiting effect of the tannins.

DRUG INTERACTIONS

POTENTIAL INTERACTIONS

The absorption of alkaloids and other alkaline drugs may be reduced or inhibited.

DOSAGE

Mode of Administration: Oak is available as whole, crude, and powdered drug form, as a bath additive and in compounded preparations. It is also available in solid pharmaceutical form for oral intake.

Preparation:

Tea – 1 gm finely cut or coarse powdered drug is put in cold water, rapidly boiled and strained after some time (1 teaspoon corresponds to 3 g drug).

Bath additive – 5 g drug is boiled with 1 Liter water and added to the full or hip bath.

Daily Dosage:

Internally – 3 g of drug; Tea: 1 cup 3 times a day.

Externally – Rinses/gargles: boil 2 dessertspoons finely cut drug with 3 cups water.

Bath additive – duration: 20 minutes at 32 to 37° C.

Storage: Should be tightly sealed and protected from light.

LITERATURE

Brantner A, Grein E. Antibacterial activity of plant extracts used externally in traditional medicine. *J Ethnopharmacol.* 44; 35-40. 1994

Las Rivas J, de Milicua JC, Gomez R. Determination of carotinoid pigments in several tree leaves by reversed-phase high-performance liquid chromatography. *J Chromatogr.* 585; 168-172. 1991

König M et al., Ellegitannins and complex tannins from *Quercus petraea* bark. In: *JNP* 57(10):1411-1415. 1994.

Pallenbach E, Scholz E, König M, Rimpler H, Proanthocyanidins from *Quercus petraea* bark. In: *PM* 59(3):264. 1993.

Romussi G, Parodi B, Pizza C, Tommasi Nde. Triterpensaponine und Acylflavonoide aus *Quercus robur var. stenocarpa* Beck. / Inhaltsstoffe von Fagaceae (Cupuliferae), 19. Mitteilung. Arch Pharm (Weinheim) 327; 643-645. 1994

Vivas N, Laguerre M, Glories Y, Bourgeois G, Vitry C. Structure Simulation of Two Ellagitannins from *Quercus robur L. Phytochemistry* 39 (5); 1193-1199. 1995

Willuhn G, Pflanzliche Dermatika. Eine kritische Übersicht. In: DAZ 132(37):1873. 1992.

Oak Gall

Quercus infectoria

DESCRIPTION

Medicinal Parts: The medicinal part of the plant is the leaf.

Flower and Fruit: The male flowers are tangled into hanging, axillary catkins, with a 6- to 8-tepaled perigone and 6 to 10 stamens. The female sessile flowers are single or in small groups in the leaf axils of dropping stipules. The perigone has 6 tips with an inferior 3-chambered ovary surrounded by an initially inconspicuous cupula that later becomes cup-shaped. The fruit is up to 4 cm long, cylindrical, shiny brown, and is 3 times longer than the cupula, which is covered with narrow scales.

Leaves, Stem, and Root: The plant grows as a shrub or small tree, and is diclinous and monoecious. The leaves are alternate, approximately 5 cm long, short-petiolate, elongate, sinuate, and roughly thorny-tipped serrate.

Habitat: The various Quercus species originated in Iran, Iraq, and Turkey, but are now widespread and particularly common in Asia Minor, Europe, and North Africa.

Production: Oak Gall is the gall of *Quercus infectoria* produced by gall wasps (Andricus gallae-tinktoriae) laying their eggs in the leaf buds. The development of the larva probably stimulates the bud as an infection would and produces the gall as a reaction.

Other Names: Blue Galls, Gallinaccia Oak, Nutgalls, Smyrna Galls

ACTIONS AND PHARMACOLOGY

COMPOUNDS

Tannins (60 to 70%): gallotannins, particularly hexa- and heptagalloyl-glucoses

Phenol carboxylic acids: gallic acid (3%), ellagic acid (2%)

EFFECTS

The astringent quality of the drug can be explained by the tannins it contains. The dry extract exhibits analgetic, hypoglycemic, and sedative-hypnotic efficacy.

INDICATIONS AND USAGE

Unproven Uses: External uses include treatment of inflammation of the skin and frostbite and as an adjuvant in the treatment of infectious skin conditions. Oak gall is used externally for chilblains and gingivitis, for which efficacy appears plausible but has not yet been sufficiently documented.

Indian Medicine: Uses include intestinal hemorrhaging, coughing blood, diarrhea, dysentery, ulcerative stomatitis, coughs, bronchitis, dyspepsia, fever, gonorrhea, leukorrhea, menorrhagia, impetigo, eczema, hemorrhoids, pharyngodynia, diabetes, hyperhidrosis, and tonsillitis.

Chinese Medicine: Uses include dysentery, hyperhidrosis, oral ulceration, leukorrhea, hemorrhoids, wounds, and rectal prolapse. Efficacy for these indications has not yet been proved.

PRECAUTIONS AND ADVERSE REACTIONS

No health hazards are known in conjunction with the proper external administration of designated therapeutic dosages.

DOSAGE

Mode of Administration: Preparations of the whole, cut, and powdered drug have internal and external applications.

Preparation: Tincture - Powdered gall apples are mixed roughly 1:5 with spirit of wine.

Storage: The drug should be stored in a tightly sealed container.

LITERATURE

Dar MS, Ikram M, Fakouhi T, Constituents of *Quercus infectoria. Planta Med*, 65:286-7, May 1977

Dar MS, Ikram M, Fakouhi T, Pharmacology of *Quercus infectoria. J Pharm Sci,* 65:1791-4, Dec 1976

Dar MS, Ikram M, Fakouhi T, Studies on *Quercus infectoria*; isolation of syringic acid and determination of its central depressive activity. Planta Med, 65:156-61, Feb 1979

Hänsel R, Keller K, Rimpler H, Schneider G (Ed), Hagers Handbuch der Pharmazeutischen Praxis, 5. Aufl., Bde 4 - 6 (Drogen), Springer Verlag Berlin, Heidelberg, New York, 1992-1994.

Marles RJ, Farnsworth NR. Antidiabetic plants and their active constituents. *Phytomedicine* 2 (2); 137-189. 1995

Oats

Avena sativa

DESCRIPTION

Medicinal Parts: The medicinal parts are the fresh or dried above-ground plant, the ripe, dried fruits, and the dried, threshed leaf and stem.

Flower and Fruit: The spikelet has 2 to 3 flowers. The outer glume has no awn, is 18 to 30 mm long and has 7 to 11 ribs. The top glumes grow from 12 to 24 mm long, have 2 divisions and a dentate tip. They have 7 ribs and can either be awned or unawned. The awn is 15 to 40 mm long, upright, and rough. The double-ribbed husks are 10 to 20 mm long and are thickly ciliate on the short ridge. The 3 stamens are 2.5 to 4 mm long. The ovary has a pinnatifid stigma. The fruit is 7 to 12 mm long, narrowly elliptoid, and pubescent.

Leaves, Stem, and Root: Oat is a light-green annual grass with a bushy root. The stalks are 60 to 100 cm high, smooth, and glabrous. The linear-lanceolate, tapering, flat leaves are in double rows, and the leaf sheath is clasping. The ligula is short and ovate with triangular pointed teeth. The leaf blade is linear-lanceolate and is 45 cm long by 5 to 15 mm wide.

Habitat: Oats originated in England, France, Poland, Germany, and Russia, and are now cultivated worldwide.

Production: Wild oat herb consists of the fresh above-ground parts of *Avena sativa*, which are harvested shortly before the height of the flowering season and then quickly dried. Oats consist of the ripe, dried fruits of *Avena sativa*. Oat bran is taken from the outer layer of the husked fruit. To make rolled oats, the husked fruit is treated with steam, then crushed. Oat straw consists of the dried, threshed leaves and stems of *Avena sativa*, also harvested shortly before the height of the flowering season.

Other Names: Grain, Groats, Oatmeal, Straw

ACTIONS AND PHARMACOLOGY

COMPOUNDS: OAT HERB

Soluble oligo- and polysaccharides: including saccharose, kestose, neokestose, bifurcose, β-glucans, galactoarabinoxylans

Silicic acid (partially water-soluble)

Steroid saponins: avenacoside A and B

Unusual amino acids: avenic acid A and B

Flavonoids: including vitexin-, isovitexin-, apigenin-, isoorientin-, tricinglycosides

EFFECTS: OAT HERB

In one poorly constructed experimental investigation, the drug was said to lower the uric acid level and to display an antihepatoxin effect in animal experiments. The mode of action was not explained.

COMPOUNDS: OAT FRUIT

Starch

Soluble polysaccharides: in particular β-glucans and arabinoxylans

Proteic substances: including gliadin, avenin, avenalin

Peptides: alpha-avenothionine, β-avenothionine

Steroid saponins: avenacoside A and B

Sterols: including β-sitosterol, delta-5-avenasterol

Fatty oil

Vitamins of the B-group

Amines: including gramine

COMPOUNDS: OAT STRAW

Soluble oligo- and polysaccharides: including saccharose, kestose, neokestose, bifurcose, β-glucans, galactoarabinoxylans

Silicic acid (partially water-soluble)

Steroid saponins: avenacoside A and B

Unusual amino acids: avenic acid A and B

Flavonoids: including vitexin-, isovitexin-, apigenin-, isoorientin-, tricinglycosides

EFFECTS: OAT STRAW

A positive monograph has been issued by Commission E (1987) concerning external use of oat straw with inflammatory and seborrheic skin disease, particularly with itching. The efficacy of the drug has not yet been documented in accordance with valid criteria for the clinical testing of medicinal drugs for the other areas of indication claimed.

EFFECTS: OAT FRUIT

Oats limit glycemic and insulin responses to food intake. Dehusked oats are, according to various studies, able to lower blood levels of total and LDL cholesterol in healthy individuals and those with elevated lipid levels. The latest research attributes the cholesterol-lowering effect to the water-soluble polysaccharides, in particular β-glucans. They are also said to hinder prostaglandin biosynthesis. One study has shown Oats to have a positive effect in smoking cessation (Anon, 1997).

Glycemic Control Effects: Providing soluble oat extract in the diet improved glucose and insulin responses to food intake in men and women with moderate hypercholesterolemia (Hallfrisch et al, 1995).

Hyperlipidemic Effects: Studies have demonstrated that the β-glucan content of oat products independently exerted a hypocholesterolemic effect in patients with elevated cholesterol, who follow a National Cholesterol Education Program step 1 diet (Davidson et al, 1991). Taking 40 g of oat bran daily for 14 days enhanced postprandial lipid responses in 6 men with initially normal blood lipid levels. Compared to a low-fiber control diet, 2 weeks on a diet supplemented with oat bran increased plasma levels of free cholesterol, LDL cholesterol, and HDL free cholesterol, and decreased concentrations of plasma esterified cholesterol and HDL esterified cholesterol (Dubois et al, 1995).

CLINICAL TRIALS

Cholesterol

A Cochrane Database review identified 10 randomized placebo-controlled trials of apparent quality that examined the effect of consumption of wholegrain foods on cardiovascular disease risk factors and related illness and death in adults. A meta-analysis of these 10 trials showed lower total cholesterol (-0.20 mmol/L; p= 0.0001) and LDL cholesterol (0.18 mmol/L, p<0.0001) resulting from consumption of oatmeal foods. The authors recommend caution in interpreting these seemingly positive effects, however, which typically accounted for risk factors for coronary heart disease but not actual death or coronary events or illness. Cholesterol-lowering and other coronary risk factors reported in these and other trials were recorded over a relatively short period of time (4 to 8 weeks in most cases), and were often small in size and therefore limited in the statistically significant conclusions they could draw. There is a need for adequate and longer randomized studies involving wholegrain foods and diets including whole grains other than oats (Kelly, 2007).

In this randomized, controlled, crossover study, 40 essentially healthy adults despite mildly elevated cholesterol levels were randomly assigned to receive one of three types of muesli cereal two times daily for four weeks. One provided 5 g control fiber from wheat (the control group). One provided 5 g oat *B*-glucan. The other provided 5 g oat *B*-glucan plus 1.5 g plant stanols (the ''combination muesli'') group. Analysis revealed that consuming muesli enriched with *B*-Glucan effectively and significantly lowered LDL cholesterol concentrations. Importantly, the addition of plant stanol esters to the B-glucan—the combination muesli—significantly lowered LDL cholesterol concentrations as well (by 4.4%), but less than predicted. The authors hypothesize that this blunted effect may have been due to the impact of *B*-glucan or possibly the food matrix (Theuwissen, 2006).

A 2005 review examined the cholesterol-lowering powers of National Cholesterol Education Program-recommended combination therapies, one of which involved supplementing the diet with functional foods such as oat bran, plant sterols, and fish oil. Supplements containing these compounds, combined with exercise, decreased total cholesterol, low-density lipoprotein cholesterol, and triglyceride concentrations by 8-26%, 8-30%, and 12-39%, respectively, while increasing high-density lipoprotein cholesterol levels by 2-18%. The two oat bran studies included in the analysis also included exercise. In one, a four-week trial, 13 individuals ingested less than 30% total fat and the equivalent of 100 g of oat bran daily. In another trial, also four weeks long, 235 people ingested less than 30% in the diet and the equivalent of 35-50 g oat bran daily. Consistent and substantial decreases in plasma lipids were found. The authors note a minimal dose of 3 g of *B*-glucan daily with exercise as the effective regimen for decreasing total cholesterol and low-density lipoprotein cholesterol levels in people with high cholesterol (Varady, 2005).

Oat fiber extract containing a greater amount of β-glucan resulted in significantly lower total cholesterol levels than a low-β-glucan diet in 23 volunteer subjects whose baseline cholesterol levels were between the 50th and 75th percentiles for age and gender. For 7 days the participants received an oat fiber extract containing 1% or 10% soluble β-glucans by weight. This had the effect of replacing 5% of fat energy by an increase in energy from carbohydrate. Both total and LDL cholesterol decreased significantly from baseline levels regardless of the β-glucan content ($p<0.0001$). The total cholesterol was significantly lower after the 10% β-glucan diet than when subjects took the low-β-glucan diet ($p<0.017$). LDL cholesterol levels also were lower with the high-β-glucan diet, but the difference was not significant (Behall et al, 1997).

Celiac Disease

A randomized, double-blind, multicenter study was performed with 116 children with celiac disease who were randomized to one of two groups. One group was given a standard gluten-free diet (GFD). The other group was given a GFD with additional, wheat-free oat products over a one-year period. The results indicate that addition of moderate amounts of oats to a GFD does not interfere with clinical or small bowel mucosal healing, or prevent humoral immunological down-regulation in children with celiac disease, indicating that oats may be safely added to the diets of children with the condition (Hogberg et al, 2004).

Diabetes/Heart Disease Prevention

Consumption of a beverage containing oat β-glucans was shown to improve lipid and glucose metabolism in an 8-week, single-blind, controlled study with 5 parallel groups. 100 hypercholesterolemic subjects were recruited; 89 completed the study. During a three-week run-in period, all subjects consumed a control beverage. Over the following five weeks, four groups consumed a beverage with 5 g or 10 g β-glucans from oats or from barley, and one group continued with the control beverage. Compared to control, 5 g of β-glucans from oats significantly lowered total-cholesterol by 7.4% ($P<0.01$), and postprandial concentrations of glucose (30 min, $P=0.005$) and insulin (30 min, $P=0.025$). When compared to control, no statistically significant effects of the beverages with barley β-glucans were found (Biorklund et al, 2005).

Sixteen women and 7 men ranging in age from 38 to 61 years, received a standard diet for 1 week, followed by two 5-week periods of an oat diet or standard diet, using a crossover design. Oat extracts containing 1% or 10% soluble β-glucans replaced carbohydrate and fat in a variety of foods and contributed 10% of energy. At baseline most of the subjects had exaggerated insulin responses to glucose. Insulin scores were 15% lower after taking the 1% β-glucan diet and 24% lower with the 10% β- glucan diet. Insulin responses decreased as the intake of soluble fiber increased. Glucose responses to food intake were reduced by both extracts in both men and women. In women, the 10% extract provided the lowest responses. Glucagon responses to eating were lower after oat extract use in men only. The investigators believe that oat extract can be usefully substituted for fat energy in those who are at risk of diabetes or heart disease (Hallfrisch et al, 1995).

Hypertension

To examine the effect of dietary fiber intake on blood pressure (BP), a randomized, double-blind, placebo-controlled trial was conducted. Subjects (n=110) were recruited who had untreated, but higher than optimal BP or stage-1 hypertension. Participants were randomly assigned to receive 8 g/day of water-soluble fiber from oat bran or a control intervention. Differences were not significant, although oat fibers demonstrated a moderate BP-lowering effect (He et al, 2004).

Skin Disorders

A topical preparation of oat straw, consisting of dried leaves and stems of *Avena sativa* and containing silicic acid, is used in bath form to relieve itching from inflammatory and seborrheic skin disorders. A dose of 100 g serves for one full bath (Blumenthal, 1998). Severe itching caused by dry skin may be treated symptomatically using a variety of bath products including colloidal oatmeal mixtures, bath soaps and gels, and powders containing oat extracts (Anonym, 1997).

Smoking Cessation

A blinded study suggested that Oats may help smokers to cut down their cigarette use. The 26 smokers participating in the trial received either an alcohol extract of oats or a placebo for 4 weeks. Average daily cigarette use declined from 20 at baseline to 6 at the end of the treatment period, whereas control subjects continued to smoke an average of 17 cigarettes each day. The difference was statistically significant, and responders continued to smoke less, 2 months after treatment ended. These results could not be replicated in a 12-week blinded trial of oat extract (Anonym, 1997).

INDICATIONS AND USAGE

OAT HERB

Unproven Uses: Wild oat herb preparations are used for many purposes, including acute and chronic anxiety, atonia of the bladder and connective tissue, connective tissue deficiencies, excitation, gout, kidney ailments in Kneipp therapy, neurasthenic and pseudoneurasthenic syndromes, old age symptoms, opium and tobacco withdrawal treatment, rheumatism, skin diseases, sleeplessness, stress, weakness of the bladder, and as a tonic and roborant. The efficacy for the claimed applications is not documented.

Homeopathic Uses: Oats are used in homeopathy for exhaustion and insomnia.

OAT FRUIT

Unproven Uses: Oat preparations are used for diseases and complaints of the gastrointestinal tract, gallbladder and kidneys, for cardiovascular disorders, constipation, diabetes, diarrhea, physical fatigue, rheumatism, and as a gruel for chest and throat complaints. The claimed efficacy has not been fully substantiated.

OAT STRAW

Approved by Commission E:

- Inflammation of the skin
- Warts

The drug is employed externally for seborrheic skin disorders, especially those accompanied by itch.

Unproven Uses: Oat straw is used for abdominal fatigue, bladder and rheumatic disorders, eye ailments, frostbite, gout, impetigo, and metabolic diseases. It is used in foot baths for chronically cold or tired feet. It is also used as a tea for flu and coughs.

CONTRAINDICATIONS

Persons with celiac disease should avoid oats.

PRECAUTIONS AND ADVERSE REACTIONS

OAT HERB, FRUIT, AND STRAW

No health hazards or side effects are known in conjunction with the proper administration of designated therapeutic dosages. Oats may pose a risk to the rare individual who is hypersensitive to the gluten they contain. Toxic effects of oats, given in moderate amounts, have not been observed in patients with dermatitis herpetiformis, but it remains possible that only large amounts are harmful. Until toxicity is conclusively ruled out and oat products are labeled as being gluten-free, gluten-sensitive patients should be advised to avoid oats (Parnell et al, 1998). Like most fiber products, oat bran products should be taken with large amounts of water to assure that the fiber is well dispersed in the bowel (Anonym, 1997). Contact dermatitis has been reported in persons consuming oat flour.

Atherogenesis: An increase in triglyceride-rich lipoprotein (TRL) secondary to chronic oat bran intake could pose a risk of increased atherogenesis. Not all TRLs have cholesterol-loading properties, and cholesterol ester enrichment was not observed in either large or small TRLs in this study. The postprandial increase in TRL concentration was transient (Dubois et al, 1995).

DRUG INTERACTIONS

MODERATE RISK

Statins: Oat bran may impair absorption and effectiveness of HMG-CoA reductase inhibitors as illustrated by 2 case reports of patients taking lovastatin with oat bran. Low-density lipoprotein (LDL) cholesterol significantly increased in 2 patients taking lovastatin 80 milligrams and oat bran fiber 50 to 100 grams daily for hypercholesterolemia after 4 weeks. When oat bran was discontinued, LDL decreased to baseline levels (Richter et al, 1991). *Clinical Management*: Administer oat bran two hours before or four to six hours after an HMG CoA reductase inhibitor. If this is not possible, separate administration times as much as possible.

DOSAGE

OAT HERB

Mode of Administration: The herb is used in combination therapy, as a tea for internal use, and in homeopathic mother tinctures and dilutions.

How Supplied:

Liquid – 1000 mg/mL

Preparation: To make a tea, 3 g drug is boiled in 250 mL water, which is strained after cooling.

Daily Dosage: The tea is taken repeatedly throughout the day and shortly before going to bed.

Homeopathic Dosage: 5 to 10 drops, 1 tablet, or 5 to 10 globules 1 to 3 times daily or 1 mL injection solution twice weekly sc (HAB1).

Storage: The herb should be protected from light and moisture.

OAT FRUIT

Mode of Administration: The fruit is used in homeopathy and in combination preparations.

OAT STRAW

Mode of Administration: As a comminuted herb for decoctions and other galenic preparations as teas and bath additives.

Preparation: To make oat straw bath, 100 g chopped drug is boiled with 3 liters water for 20 minutes and the decoction is added to the bath.

Daily Dosage: 100 g of herb is used for one full bath.

LITERATURE

OAT HERB, FRUIT, AND STRAW

Anonym, Oats. In: DerMarderosian (ed): The Review of Natural Products. Facts and Comparisons, St Louis, MO; 1997.

Anand CL, *Nature* 233:496,1971.

BAnz (Federal German Gazette) No. 193; published 15 Oct 1987.

Blumenthal M, Busse WR, Goldberg A et al (eds): The Complete German Commission E Monographs, 1st ed., American Botanical Council, Austin, TX; 1998.

Biorklund M, Van Rees A, Mensink RP, Onning G. Changes in serum lipids and postprandial glucose and insulin concentrations after consumption of beverages with β-glucans from oats or barley: a randomized, dose controlled trial. *Eur J Clin Nutr*; 59(11): 1272-1281. 2005.

Connor J et al., *J Pharm Pharmacol* 27:92, 1975.

Davidson M, Dugan L, Burns J et al., The hypocholesterolemic effects of β- glucan in oatmeal and oat bran: a dose-controlled study. In: *JAMA*; 265:1833-1839, 1991.

Dubois C, Armand M, Senft M et al., Chronic oat bran intake alters postprandial lipemia and lipoproteins in healthy adults. In: *Am J Clin Nutr*; 61:325-333, 1995.

Effertz B et al., *Z Pflanzenphysiol* 92:319, 1979.

Gabrinowicz JW, *Med J Aust Ii*: 306, 1974.

Hallfrisch J, Scholfield D & Behall K, Diets containing soluble oat extracts improve glucose and insulin responses of moderately hypercholesterolemic men and women. In: *Am J Clin Nutr*; 61:379-384, 1995.

Hänsel R, Keller K, Rimpler H, Schneider G (Hrsg.), Hagers Handbuch der Pharmazeutischen Praxis, 5. Aufl., Bde 4-6 (Drogen), Springer Verlag Berlin, Heidelberg, New York, 1992-1994.

He J, Steiffer RH, Muntner P, et al. Effect of dietary fiber intake on blood pressure: a randomized, double-blind, placebo-controlled trial. *J Hypertens*; 22(1): 73-80. 2004.

Hogberg L, Laurin P, Faith-Magnusson K, et al. Oats to children with newly diagnosed coeliac disease: a randomized double-blind study. Gut; 53(5): 649-654. 2004.

Jaspersen-Schib R, Ballaststoffe als Lipidsenker. In: *DAZ* 132(39):1991. 1992.

Keenan J, Wenz J, Myers S et al., Randomized, controlled, crossover trial of oat bran in hypercholesterolemic subjects. In: J Fam Pract; 33:600-608, 1991.

Kelly S, Summerbell C, Brynes A, et al. Wholegrain cereals for coronary heart disease. *Cochrane Database Syst Rev* (2):CD005051. 2007.

Kim et al., *Biochim Biophys Acta* 537:22, 1978.

Madaus G, Lehrbuch der Biologischen Arzneimittel, Bde 1-3, Nachdruck, Georg Olms Verlag Hildesheim 1979.

McGuffin M, Hobbs C, Upton R et al., American Herbal Products Association's Botanical Safety Handbook. CRC Press, Boca Raton, FL; 1997.

Parnell N, Ellis H & Ciclitira P, Absence of toxicity of oats in patients with dermatitis herpetiformis. In: *N Engl J Med*; 338:1470-1471, 1998.

Richter WO, Jacob BG & Schwandt P, Interaction between fibre and lovastatin. In: *Lancet*; 338(8768): 706, 1991.

Schneider E, Lösliche Silikate im grünen Hafer. In: *ZPT* 11(4):129. 1990.

Willuhn G, Pflanzliche Dermatika. Eine kritische Übersicht.. In: *DAZ* 132(37):1873. 1992.

Teuscher E, Lindequist U, Biogene Gifte - Biologie, Chemie, Pharmakologie, 2. Aufl., Fischer Verlag Stuttgart 1994.

Theuwissen E, Mensink RP. Simultaneous intake of zβ-glucan and plant stanol esters affects lipid metabolism in slightly hypercholesterolemic subjects. *J Nutr*;137 (3): 583-588. 2007.

Varady KA, Jones PJH. Combination diet and exercise interventions for the treatment of dyslipidemia: an effecgtive preliminary strategy to lower cholesterol levels? *J Nutr*; 135: 1829-1835. 2005.

Youngs V, Peterson D & Brown C, Oats. In: Pomeranz Y (ed). Advances in Cereal Science and Technology, vol. V. American Association of Cereal Chemists, Inc., St. Paul, MN; 49-105, 1982.

Wichtl M (Hrsg.), Teedrogen, 4. Aufl., Wiss. Verlagsges. Stuttgart 1997.

Ocimum basilicum

See Basil

Oenanthe aquatica

See Water Fennel

Oenanthe crocata

See Water Dropwort

Oenothera biennis

See Evening Primrose

Oilseed Rape

Brassica napus

DESCRIPTION

Medicinal Parts: The medicinal parts of the plant are the roots and seeds.

Flower and Fruit: The flowers are in racemes with 4 upright, splayed sepals. The 4 petals are yellow, 11 to 14 mm long, almost twice as long as the calyx, with an orbicular-elliptical surface. There are 2 short and 4 long stamens. The ovary is superior, with 4 fused carpels. The fruit is 4.5 to 11 cm long and is a dehiscent pod opening on 2 sides with a septum and 20 to 40 seeds. The seeds are globose and approximately 1.5 to 3 mm in diameter.

Leaves, Stem, and Root: Oilseed Rape is an annual or biennial herb that grows up to 1.4 m high. The leaves are alternate with a bluish bloom; the lower ones are petiolate and pinnatisect, with slightly pubescent, relatively large terminal lobes. The middle and upper leaves are sessile, partly clasping, simple, glabrous, dentate, or entire. The stem of larger plants is branched. The root is thin and spindle-shaped.

Habitat: Europe, North Africa, and U.S.

Production: The seeds are cold-pressed and then refined. Rapeseed oil is the cold-pressed and refined oil from the ripe seeds of *Brassica napus*.

Not to be Confused With: Rapeseed oil may be adulterated with resins and mineral oil. *Sinapis arvensis* is a permitted substitute.

Other Names: Colza, Cole, Rape, Rape Seed

ACTIONS AND PHARMACOLOGY

COMPOUNDS

Fatty oil: chief fatty acids: oleic acid (60%), linoleic acid (20%), linolenic acid (10%), as well as palmitic acid, stearic acid, eicosanoic acid, behenic acid. Varieties with high erucic acid content (40 to 50%) are no longer cultivated (reduction of the erucic acid content in the Common Market countries to below 5%)

Sterols: beta-sitosterol, campesterol, brassicasterol, estered to some extent

EFFECTS

Rapeseed oil, when ingested in high dosages over an extended period of time, is cardiotoxic. The drug is chiefly used as a substitute for olive oil and in the manufacture of salves and liniments.

INDICATIONS AND USAGE

No medicinal indications

PRECAUTIONS AND ADVERSE REACTIONS

No health hazards are known in conjunction with the proper administration of designated therapeutic dosages of the oil, which is low on erucic acid.

DOSAGE

Storage: Store in the dark, in well-filled containers.

LITERATURE

Butcher RD, Goodman BA, Deighton N, Smith WH, Evaluation of the allergic/irritant potential of air pollutants: detection of proteins modified by volatile organic compounds from oilseed rape (*Brassica napus ssp. oleifera*) using electrospray ionization-mass spectrometry. *Clin Exp Allergy*, 25. 1995

Förster K, Schuster C, Belter A, Diepenbrock W. Agragökologische Auswirkungen des Anbaus von transgenem herbizidtoleranten Raps (*Brassica napus L.*). Bundesgesundhbl. 41 (12); 547-552. 1998

Gatti GL, Michalek H. Investigations on Rapeseed Oil Toxicology. *Arzneim Forsch.* 25 (1); 1639-1642. 1975

Hänsel R, Keller K, Rimpler H, Schneider G (Ed), Hagers Handbuch der Pharmazeutischen Praxis, 5. Aufl., Bde 4 - 6 (Drogen), Springer Verlag Berlin, Heidelberg, New York, 1992-1994.

Jakobsen HB, Friis P, Nielsen JK, Olsen CE. Emission of Volatiles from Flowers and Leaves of *Brassica napus* in situ. *Phytochemistry* 37; 695-699. 1994

Kull D, Pfander H. Isolation and Identification of Carotenoids from Petals of Rape (*Brassica napus*). *J Agric Food Chem.* 43 (11); 2854-2857. 1995

Meding B. Immediate hypersensitivity to mustard and rape. *Contact Dermatitis* 13; 121-122. 1985

Ninan TK, Milne V, Russell G. Oilseed rape not a potent antigen. *Lancet* 336; 808. 1990

Slabas AR, Cottingham IR, Austin A, Hellyer A, Safford R, Smith CG, Immunological detection of NADH-specific enoyl-ACP reductase from rape seed (*Brassica napus*) - induction, relationship of alpha and beta polypeptides, mRNA translation and interaction with ACP. *Biochim Biophys Acta,* 1039:181-8, Jun 19, 1990

Olea europaea

See Olive

Oleander

Nerium oleander

DESCRIPTION

Medicinal Parts: The leaves are the medicinal part of the plant.

Flower and Fruit: The corolla is 4 to 7 mm in diameter, usually pink to red but sometimes white. The petals are thickly covered in glands. The tube is 2 cm long as are the obtuse and patent lobes. The anther appendages are long, pubescent and twisted. The follicles are 8 to 16 cm by 0.5 to 1 cm, erect, and reddish-brown.

Leaves, Stem, and Root: The evergreen plant can be tree or shrublike. The trunks are up to 4 m high. The leaves are 6 to 12 by 1.2 to 2 cm, linear-lanceolate, sharp-edged, coriaceous, and dark green.

Habitat: Nerium oleander grows mainly in the Mediterranean region but also in parts of Asia. It is cultivated in Europe.

Production: Oleander leaf is the leaf of *Nerium oleander,* collected shortly before flowering and then dried in the shade.

Other Names: Rose Laurel

ACTIONS AND PHARMACOLOGY

COMPOUNDS

Cardiac steroids (cardenolide): chief components are 16-acetyl neogistonin, adynerin, 5alpha-adynerin, gentiobiosyl-adynerin, delta16-dehydroadynerin, digitoxigenin oleandroside, gentibioosyl-odoroside A, gentiobiosyl-oleandrin, glucosyl-oleandrin, oleandrigenin glucoside, kaneroside, neriaside, nerigoside, neriumoside

Pregnanes and pregnane glycosides: including 12beta-hydroxy-16alpha-methoxy-pregna-4,6-dien-3,20-dione

EFFECTS

Oleander is positively inotropic and negatively chronotropic. The cardenolide glycosides of the drug are qualitatively digitoxin-like in their action, but generally weaker, probably due to the lower rate of absorption.

INDICATIONS AND USAGE

Unproven Uses: Folk medicine uses of Oleander leaf include diseases and functional disorders of the heart, as well as skin diseases. Previous internal application for myocardial insufficiency, decompensated hypertonia, and cardiac insufficiency is no longer common.

Indian Medicine: Among uses in Indian medicine are scabies, eye diseases (using only the juice of the leaves), and hemorrhoids.

PRECAUTIONS AND ADVERSE REACTIONS

General: No health hazards are known in conjunction with the proper administration of designated therapeutic dosages. Side effects can include, particularly in the case of overdosages, nausea, vomiting, diarrhea, headache, stupor, and cardiac arrhythmias.

DRUG INTERACTIONS

MAJOR RISK

Digoxin: Concurrent use may result in increased risk of digoxin toxicity. *Clinical Management:* Cardiac glycosides in oleander are detectable by a digoxin radioimmunoassay; however, the digoxin level obtained varies according to the assay used and cannot be used to guide dosing of digoxin-specific Fab antibody fragments. Administration of digoxin-specific Fab antibody fragments has been successful in treating cases of oleander toxicity.

POTENTIAL INTERACTIONS

Quinidine, Calcium Salts, Saluretics, Laxatives, or Glucocorticoids: Concurrent use may result in increases of both efficacy and side effects.

OVERDOSAGE

See Precautions and Adverse Reactions.

DOSAGE

How Supplied: Forms of commercial pharmaceutical preparations include solutions, coated tablets and compound preparations.

Dosage: No information is available.

Storage: Oleander should be stored where it is protected from dampness and light.

LITERATURE

Begum S, Sultana R, Siddiqui BS. Triterpenoids from the Leaves of *Nerium oleander. Phytochemistry* 44 (2); 329-332. 199)

Langford SD, Boor PJ. Oleander toxicity: an examination of human and animal toxic exposures / Review paper. Toxicology 109; 1-13. 1996

Loew D, Phytotherapy in heart failure. *Phytomedicine* 4 (3); 267-271. 1997

Mazumder PK, Rao PVL, Kumar D, Dube SN, Gupta SD. Toxicological Evaluation of *Nerium oleander* on Isolated Preparations. *Phytother Res.* 8 (5); 297-300. 1994

Paper D, Franz G. Glycosylation of Cardenolide Aglycones in the Leaves of *Nerium oleander. Planta Med.* 55; 30-34. 1989

Profumo P, Gastaldo P, Caviglia AM, Riboldi U. Formation of Cardiac Glyco sides in Calli from Leaf Explants of *Nerium oleander L. Plant med et phyt.* 26; 340-346. 1993

Siddiqui BS, Begum S, Siddiqui S, Lichter W. Teo cytotoxic Pentacyclic Triterpenoids from *Nerium oleander. Phytochemistry* 39 (1); 171-174. 1995

Siddiqui BS, Sultana R, Begum S, Zia A, Suria A. Cardenolides from the Methanolic Extract of *Nerium oleander* Leaves Possessing Central Nervous System Depressant Activity in Mice. *J Nat Prod.* 60 (6); 540-544. 1997

Siddiqui S et al., Isolation and structure of two cardiac glycosides from the leaves of *Nerium oleander.* In: *PH* 26(1):237-241. 1985.

Yamauchi T et al., Quantitative variations in the cardiac glycosides of oleander. In: *PH* 22:2211-2214. 1983.

Olive

Olea europaea

DESCRIPTION

Medicinal Parts: The medicinal parts are the dried leaves, the oil extracted from the ripe drupes, and the fresh branches containing leaves and clusters of flowers.

Flower and Fruit: The flowers are in small axillary clustered inflorescence. The calyx has 4 tips. The white corolla has a short tube and 4 lobes. The superior ovary is bilocular, with each side having 2 hanging anatropal ovules. The drupe has 1 to 2 seeds, is fleshy, plumlike, or round. The smooth drupe is initially green, then red, and finally blue-black when ripe. The very hard stone contains oblong compact seeds with many endosperm.

Leaves, Stem, and Root: Olive grows as a medium high shrub or a tree up to 10 m high. The plant has pale bark and canelike, quadrangular to round, initially downy, thorny or thornless branches. The leaves are opposite, entire, stiff, coriaceous, narrow-elliptical to lanceolate, or cordate with thorny tips. The upper surface is dark green, glabrous, or covered with scattered scutiform hairs; the underside shimmers silver with scutiform hairs.

Habitat: The plant grows in almost all of the southern European countries and throughout the entire Mediterranean region as far as Iran and beyond the Caucasus. Olive trees are cultivated in many regions of the world.

Production: Olive leaves consist of the fresh or dried leaves of *Olea europaea*. The leaves are harvested from cultivated trees and dried in the shade. Olive oil is the fatty oil extracted from the drupes of *Olea europaea*, using the cold-press method.

Not to be Confused With: Confusion can arise between Olive leaves and the leaves of Nerium oleander. The oils of *Camellia sasanqua* and other Camellia species can be mistaken for Olive oil.

Other Names: Olivier

ACTIONS AND PHARMACOLOGY

COMPOUNDS: OLIVE OIL

Chief fatty acids: oleic acid (56-83%), palmitic acid (8-20%), linoleic acid (4-20%)

Steroids (0.125 to 0.25%): beta-sitosterol, delta7-stigmasterol, delta5-avenasterol, campesterol, stigmasterol

Tocopherols (0.02%)

COMPOUNDS: OLIVE LEAVES

Iridoide monoterpenes: including among others, oleoropine (6-9%), additionally 6-O-oleoropinesaccharose, ligstroside, oleoroside, oleoside-7,11-dimeth-ylether

Triterpenes: including oleanolic acid, maslinic acid

Flavonoids: luteolin-7-O-glucoside, apigenine-7-O-glucoside

Chalcones: olivin, olivin-4′-O-diglucoside

EFFECTS: OLIVE OIL

Through the presence of polyunsaturated fatty acids, the drug has an antisclerotic effect by positively influencing the serum lipids. A reduction of plasma glucose has also been observed. Contraction of the gallbladder was observed with the increase of cholecystokinin in the plasma.

EFFECTS: OLIVE LEAVES

Olive leaf extract is used to enhance the immune system, as an antimicrobial, as an antioxidant, as a hypoglycemic agent, and in heart disease. Preparations of olive leaves help to control hyperglycemia in experimentally induced diabetes. Some practitioners tout its use in hepatitis. Animal tests have demonstrated hypotensive, antiarrhythmic, and spasmolytic effects on the smooth muscle of the intestine, caused by the terpenes and phenols of the drug.

Antioxidant Effects: Olive leaf contains flavonoids that possess antioxidant activity, and tissue antioxidant status has been proposed as a key factor in the development of diabetic complications. This may help explain why an orally administered preparation of olive leaf substantially diminished tissue damage in the kidneys and liver in rats with streptozotoxin-induced diabetes (Onderoglu et al, 1999).

Anticomplement Effects: Because surveys of traditional medicines in the Mediterranean region have suggested that a decoction of olive leaf has anti-inflammatory activity, in vitro hemolytic assays were undertaken and showed that a methanolic extract of the leaves strongly inhibited the classical complement pathway without activating the alternative pathway. This activity appeared to reside in several flavonoids present in the leaf extracts (Pieroni et al, 1996).

Hypoglycemic Effects: Oral administration of an infusion or decoction of olive leaf exerted a hypoglycemic effect in normoglycemic rats and in animals made diabetic with alloxan (Gonzalez et al. 1992). In another experimental model of diabetes, induced by streptozotocin, olive leaf failed to lower blood glucose levels or prevent glucosuria and ketonuria, but it did reduce circulating levels of liver enzymes and minimized histopathologic abnormalities in both the kidneys and liver (Onderoglu et al, 1999).

Smooth Muscle Relaxant Effects: In experiments demonstrating that a dried extract of olive leaf has relaxant effects on both isolated rat ileal tissue and rat tracheal segments, the effects were not altered in the presence of calcium antagonists including verapamil and nifedipine. It is possible, however, that olive leaf extract alters calcium transport through an increase in the intracellular concentration of cyclic adenomonophosphate (Fehri et al, 1995).

CLINICAL TRIALS

Antioxidation

A study was done to identify the major phenolic compounds present in an extract of olive leaf and estimate their antioxidant activity by their ability to scavenge the radical cation ABTS. Several structural attributes of flavonoids present in olive leaf, including 3-hydroxyl groups, influenced the ability of these compounds to scavenge free radicals. Radical scavenging capacity increased with the number of free hydroxyl groups present in the flavonoid structure. The flavonoid rhamnoglucoside rutin was the most effective compound. The flavonoids, oleuropeosides, and substituted phenols present in olive leaf extract exhibited synergism with respect to antioxidant activity (Benavente-Garcia et al, 2000).

Hypertension

Olive leaf extract had an antihypertensive effect in patients with essential arterial hypertension. Patients were separated into two groups: first timers who had never been previously treated with hypotensive medication (n=12), and a second group who had previously benefited from some sort of antihypertensive therapy such as diuretic or beta-blocker medication (n=18). For the second group, all therapeutic medications were removed 15 days prior to the beginning of the study. Both groups then received placebo gel capsules for 2 weeks. For the 3 months that followed, the placebo was replaced with similar gel capsules, each containing 400 mg olive leaf extract. Patients took 2 capsules daily for total dose of approximately 1.6 g olive leaf extract daily. A significant decrease in blood pressure occurred in all patients ($p<0.001$). No adverse effects were reported during treatment with olive leaf extract and patients especially noted a disappearance of gastric disturbances that they had previously experienced on beta-blocker medication. As a side note, the authors also found a small, but significant decrease of glycemia ($p<0.01$) and calcium ($p<0.001$) in the groups (Cherif et al, 1996).

Triclycerides

Compared with milk fat and safflower oil, olive oil resulted in significantly higher postprandial plasma triglyceride and triacylglycerol remnantlike particle concentrations (p less than 0.05). Eight healthy subjects ingested a fat load in the form of a drink and blood samples were taken at 2, 4, and 6 hours. Blood samples were not measured through the 10 to 12 hours it normally takes to clear chylomicrons. Plasma triglycerides were maximal 4 hours post-dose. None of the fat loads significantly increased total or HDL cholesterol (Higashi et al, 1997).

INDICATIONS AND USAGE

OLIVE LEAVES

Unproven Uses: Folk medicine uses include hypertonia, arteriosclerosis, rheumatism and gout, diabetes mellitus, and fever.

OLIVE OIL

Unproven Uses: Internal uses of the oil in folk medicine include cholangitis, inflammation of the gallbladder, flatulence, constipation, icterus, Roemhel syndrome, gastrointestinal ulcers and kidney stones. Externally, it has been used for psoriasis, eczema, sunburn, mild burns and rheumatism. Its use as a lubricant for constipation and dry skin conditions appears plausible because of the oily characteristics.

CONTRAINDICATIONS

The internal administration of the drug can trigger colic among gallstone sufferers, so its use is contraindicated.

PRECAUTIONS AND ADVERSE REACTIONS

Intraocular use of olive leaf may irritate the surface of the eye (Brinker, 1998). If olive leaf preparations are administered to patients with biliary tract stones, there may be a risk of causing biliary colic through promoting the secretion of bile (Brinker, 1998). Pollinosis, in the form of rhinitis or bronchial asthma, has been reported.

DRUG INTERACTIONS

No human interaction data available.

DOSAGE

OLIVE LEAVES

Mode of Administration: The drug is available for oral use in mono and combination tea mixture preparations.

How Supplied:

Capsules — 580 mg

Tablets — 150 mg

Drops

Preparation: An infusion is prepared by pouring 150 mL of hot water over 7 to 8 g of the dried leaves. Prepare a tea by pouring hot water over 2 teaspoonfuls of the drug and allowing it to steep for 30 minutes.

Daily Dosage: Tea: 3 to 4 cups throughout the day.

OLIVE OIL

Daily Dosage:

Constipation — 100 to 500 mL Olive oil at body temperature applied rectally.

Gastrointestinal ulcers — 15 to 30 mL 3 taken times daily at mealtimes.

LITERATURE

OLIVE LEAVES

Anon. Positive Auswirkungen von Olivenöl auf den Blutdruck. In: *ZPT* 12(1):13. 1991.

Benavente-Garcia O, Castillo J, Lorente J et al. Antioxidant activity of phenolics extracted from *Olea Europaea L.* leaves. In: *Food Chemistry*; 68(4):457-462, 2000.

Bianchi G, Pozzi N. 3,4-Dihydroxyphenylglycol, a major C6-C2 phenolic in *Olea europaea.* In: *PH* 35(5):1335. 1994.

Bianco A et al. Partial synthesis of oleuropein. In: *JNP* 55(6):760-766, 1992.

Cherif S, Rahal N, Haouala M et al. Essai clnique d'un extrait tire de feuilles d'olivier dans le traitment de l'hypertension arterielle essentielle. In: *J Pharm Belg*; 51(2):69-71, 1996.

Duarte J et al. Effects of oleuropeosid in isolated guinea-pig atria. In: *PM* 59(4):318. 1993.

Fehri B, Mrad S, Aiache JM et al. Effects of *Olea europaea L.* extract on the rat isolated ileum and trachea. In: *Phytotherapy Res*; 9(6):435-439, 1995.

Flemming S. Ist Olivenöl erlaubt? In: *DAZ* 131(29):1525. 1991.

Gonzalez M, Zarzuelo A, Gamez MJ et al. Hypoglycemic activity of olive leaf. In: *Planta Med*; 58(6):513-515, 1992.

Higashi K, Ishikawa T, Shige H et al. Olive oil increases the magnitude of postprandial chylomicron remnants compared to milk fat and safflower oil. In: *J Am Coll Nutr*; 16(5):429-434. 1997.

Kuwajima H et al. A secoiridoid glucoside from *Olea europaea.* In: *PH* 27(6):1757. 1988.

Lasser B et al. *Naturwissenschaften* 70:95, 1983.

Onderoglu S, Sozer S, Erbil KM et al. The evaluation of long-term effects of cinnamon bark and olive leaf on toxicity induced by streptozotocin administration to rats. In: *J Pharm Pharmacol*; 51(11):1305-1312, 1999.

Pieroni A, Heimler D, Pieters L et al. In vitro anti-complementary activity of flavonoids from olive (*Olea europaea L.*) leaves. In: *Pharmazie*; 51(10):765-768, 1996.

Zarzuelo A, Duarte J, Jimenez J et al: Vasodilator effect of olive leaf. In: *Planta Med*; 57(5):417-419, 1991.

Onion

Allium cepa

DESCRIPTION

Medicinal Parts: The medicinal part is the bulb.

Flower and Fruit: The peduncles are up to 3 cm long. The flowers are greenish-white, in orbicular umbels, with 6 free flower bracts that are shorter than the 6 stamens. The pedicles are eight times as long as the flowers. The fruit is a thin-skinned capsule. The seeds are black and angular.

The flowers are in globular umbels, before blooming in membranous sheaths.

Leaves, Stem, and Root: The plant is perennial or biennial. There are many varieties and can be compressed-globose, ovate, or oblong. Most varieties have secondary bulbs. Leaves are shorter than the peduncle, tubular or swollen, and blue-green. There is a hollow scape, which is gray-blue, expanded, and bloated below the middle.

Habitat: Central Asia is considered to be the region of origin. Onion was introduced to the Mediterranean and is cultivated worldwide.

Production: Onion consists of the fresh or dried, thick and fleshy leaf sheaths and stipules of *Allium cepa.*

ACTIONS AND PHARMACOLOGY

COMPOUNDS

Alliins (alkylcysteine sulphoxides): in particular allylalliin (allyl-L-(+)-cysteine sulphoxide) and its gamma-glutamyl conjugates, that in the course of cutting up either the freshly harvested bulbs or those that have been already dried and then re-moistened, are transformed into the so-called alliaceous oils.

Fructosans (polysaccharides, 10-40%)

Saccharose and other sugars

Flavonoids: including quercetin-4'-O-beta-D-glucoside (spiraeoside)

Steroid Saponins

EFFECTS

The thiosulphinate exhibits an antimicrobial effect, and is effective against *Bacillus subtilis, Salmonella typhi, Pseudomonas aeroginosa* and *Escherichia coli.*

Lipid and blood pressure-lowering effect: Certain constituents function similarly to those in garlic, although this is not yet clinically proven.

Inhibits thrombocyte aggregation: Dimethyl and diphenylthiosulphinateboth retard thrombocyte biosynthesis using thrombase stimulation.

Antiasthmatic and antiallergic effect: Guinea pigs sensitized using ovalbumin were protected from asthma attack through the oral administration of onion juice. Administration of an ethanol onion extract significantly reduced allergy-induced bronchial constriction in asthma patients.

INDICATIONS AND USAGE

Approved by Commission E:

- Loss of appetite
- Arteriosclerosis
- Dyspeptic complaints
- Fevers and colds
- Cough/bronchitis
- Hypertension
- Tendency to infection
- Inflammation of the mouth and pharynx
- Common cold

Unproven Uses: In folk medicine, the drug is administered internally for whooping cough, asthma, tonsillitis, and angina. Onion has been used to stimulate gallbladder functions, for digestive disorders with bloating, flatulence, and colic pain, for dehydration, as an aid at the introduction of menstruation. Onion is also used for ascariasis, high blood pressure, arteriosclerosis and in the treatment of diabetes. Externally the drug is used for insect bites, wounds, light burns, furuncles, warts, and in the after-care of bruises.

Indian Medicine: Onion preparations are used for dyspeptic conditions, respiratory conditions, wounds, pain, and for malarial fever.

Chinese Medicine: Preparations are used for worm infestation, fungal, and bacterial infections.

Homeopathic Uses: Allium cepa is used for acute inflammatory illnesses, pain syndrome, and flatulent colic.

PRECAUTIONS AND ADVERSE REACTIONS

No health hazards or side effects are known in conjunction with the proper administration of designated therapeutic dosages. The intake of large quantities can lead to stomach complaints. Frequent contact with the drug leads on rare occasion to allergic reactions (hand eczema).

DOSAGE

Mode of Administration: Cut onions, pressed juice from fresh onions and other oral galenic preparations.

Preparation: Onion oil maceration: same as garlic maceration drug extract 1:1.

Old recipe: Siripus Cepae: freshly grated onions 15 g; water 60 ml; ethanol 90% (V/V) 15 mL; saccharose 150 g; the ethanolic extract is boiled with the saccharose.

Popular: pressed juice and onion syrup: made of 500 g onions, 500 g water, 100 g honey, and 350 g sugar.

Onion tincture: 100 g minced onions in 300 g ethanol 70% macerated for 10 days.

Daily Dosage: Raw drug is used therapeutically.

Externally the juice is spread or laid on as a poultice or in slices.

Internally: onion tincture 4 to 5 teaspoonfuls daily; onion syrup 4 to 5 tablespoons daily.

Average daily dose: 50 g of fresh onions or 20 g of dried drug.

Homeopathic Dosage: 5 drops, 1 tablet, 10 globules every 30 to 60 minutes (acute) or 1 to 3 times daily (chronic); Parenterally: 1 to 2 mL 3 times daily sc; Ointment 1 to 2 times daily (HAB1)

LITERATURE

Agarwal RH, Controlled trial of the effect of cycloalliin on the fibrinolytic activity of venous blood. In: *Atherosclerosis* 27:347-351. 1977.

Ahluwalia P, Mohindroo A. Effect of Oral Ingestion of Different Fractions of *Allium cepa* on the Blood and Erythrocyte Membrane Lipids and Certain Membran-Bound Enzymes in Rats. *J Nutr Sci Vitaminol.* 35; 155-161. 1989

Atta-Ur-Rahman Zaman K. Medicinal Plants with Hypoglycemic Activity. *J Ethnopharmacol.* 26; 1-55. 1989

Bayer T, Breu W, Seligmann O, Wray V, Wagner H. Biologically active Thiosulphinates and alpha-Sulphinyl-Disulphides from *Allium cepa. Phytochemistry* 28; 2373-2377. 1989

Bayer T, Wagner H, Wray V, Dorsch W. Inhibitors of Cyclo-Oxygenase and Lipoxygenase in Onions. *Lancet II*; 906. 1988

Breu W. *Allium cepa L.* (Onion) / Part 1: Chemistry and analysis. *Phytomedicine* 3 (3); 293-306. 1996

Breu W, Sendl A, Bürgi C, Rüedi P, Wagner H. In Vitro Inhibition of 5-Lipoxygenase by Extracts and Constituents of *Plectranthus albidus* and *Allium ssp. Planta Med.* 56; A665-A666. 1990

Didry N, Dubreuil L, Pinkas M. Antimicobial Activity of Naphthoquinones and Allium Extracts Combined with Antibiotics. *Pharm Acta Helv.* 67; 148-151. 1992

Dorsch W, Schnneider E, Bayer T, Breu W, Wagner H. Anti-Inflammatory Effects of Onions: Inhibition of Chemotaxis of Human Polymorphonuclear Leukocytes by Thiosulfinates and Cepaenes. *Int Arch Allergy Appl Immunol.* 92; 39-42. 199)

Ernst E. Plants with hypoglycemic activity in humans. *Phytomedicine* 4 (1); 73-78. 1997

Fossen T, Pedersen AT, Andersen OM. Flavonoids from Red Onion (*Allium cepa*). *Phytochemistry* 47 (2); 281-285. 1998

Kumari K, Augusti KT, Antidiabetic effects of S-methylcystein sulphoxide on alloxan diabetes. In: *PM* 61(1):72-74. 1995.

Kupidlowska E, Bieniak B, Ruchirawat A, Zobel AM. Influence of methyl derivatives of coumarin on mitotic activity and ultrastructure of meristemic cells of *Allium cepa* root tips. *Phytomedicine* 2 (3); 275-281. 1996

Lancaster JE, Shaw ML. Gamma-Glutamyl Peptides in the Biosynthesis of S-Alk(en)yl-L-Cysteine Sulphoxides (Flavour Precursors) in Allium. *Phytochemistry* 28; 455-460. 1989

Paradiz J. Assessement of damage to irridated onion (*Allium cepa L.*) by cytogenic analyses. *Acta Pharm.* 48; 167-178. 1998

Sendl A, Elbl G, Steinke B, Redl K, Breu W, Wagner H. Comparative Pharmacological Investigations of Allium ursinum and *Allium sativum. Planta Med.* 58; 1-7. 1992

Tverskoy L, Dmetriev A, Kozlovsky A, Grodzinsky D, Two phytoalexins from *Allium-cepa* bulbs. In: *PH* 30:799. 1991.

Wagner H, Bayer Th, Dorsch W, Das antiasthmatische Wirkprinzip der Zwiebel (*Allium cepa L.*). In: ZPT 9(6):165. 1988.

Ononis spinosa

See Spiny Rest Harrow

Onopordum acanthium

See Scotch Thistle

Ophioglossum vulgatum

See English Adder's Tongue

Opium Antidote

Combretum micranthum

DESCRIPTION

Medicinal Parts: The dry leaves and stems are the medicinal parts of the plant.

Leaves, Stem and Root: The leaves are 10 to 13 cm long and about 6 cm wide, with 8 to 10 lateral spreading veins, transparent in the axils. The surface of the young leaves has small scales.

Characteristics: The taste is astringent and strong.

Habitat: The plant is indigenous to China, Malaysia, and Indonesia.

Production: Combretum leaves are the dried leaves of *Combretum micramthum.*

Other Names: Combretum, Jungle Weed

ACTIONS AND PHARMACOLOGY

COMPOUNDS

Pyrrolidine alkaloid betaines: stachydrines, 4-hydroxystachydrines, combretin-A (betaines drawn from the proline)

Catechin tannins

Flavonoids: including vitexin, saponaretin, orietin

EFFECTS

The drug has mild choleric and astringent effects.

INDICATIONS AND USAGE

Unproven Uses: The drug has been used for cholecystopathy, dyspepsia and liver disease. It is obsolete as a drug and now found only in combination preparations.

PRECAUTIONS AND ADVERSE REACTIONS

Health risks or side effects following the proper administration of designated therapeutic dosages are not recorded.

LITERATURE

Bassène E, *Plantes Med Phytotherapie* 21:173. 1987.

Bassène E et al., *Ann Pharm Franc* 44:491. 1986.

Hegnauer R, Chemotaxonomie der Pflanzen, Bde 1-11, Birkhäuser Verlag Basel, Boston, Berlin 1962-1997.

Kern W, List PH, Hörhammer L (Hrsg.), Hagers Handbuch der Pharmazeutischen Praxis, 4. Aufl., Bde 1-8, Springer Verlag Berlin, Heidelberg, New York, 1969.

Orchis species

See Salep

Oregano

Origanum vulgare

DESCRIPTION

Medicinal Parts: The medicinal parts are the oil extracted from the fresh or dried leaves through a process of steam distillation, the herb picked during the flowering season and freed from the thicker stems and dried, as well as the fresh flowering herb.

Flower and Fruit: The bright purple labiate flowers are in cymelike panicles with elliptical, pointed, and usually dark purple bracts, which are longer than the calyx. The calyx is tubular and has 5 even tips. The upper lip of the corolla is flat. The lower lip has 3 lobes; the middle lobe is the widest. There are 4 stamens, the longer ones extending beyond the lower lip.

Leaves, Stem, and Root: Origanum vulgare is a woody perennial plant, which grows up to 90 cm high. The upper part is branched. The plant has rhizomelike runners and is downy, bristly or velvety. The leaves are 10 to 40 cm long and 4 to 25 mm wide, ovate, entire-margined or slightly crenate, glabrous or pubescent, translucent-punctate and petiolate.

Characteristics: The plant has an aromatic scent, similar to *Origanum majorana.*

Habitat: The plant is common throughout Asia, Europe, and northern Africa.

Production: Oregano consists of the above-ground parts of *Origanum vulgare*. It is harvested 5 cm above the ground during the flowering season and dried carefully on the field or under a roofed loft.

Other Names: Mountain Mint, Origano, Wild Marjoram, Winter Marjoram, Wintersweet

ACTIONS AND PHARMACOLOGY

COMPOUNDS

Volatile oil (0.15-1.0%): chief components carvacrol (share 40-70%), gamma-terpinene (8-10%), p-cymene (5-10%), additionally alpha-pinene, myrcene, thymol. There are also strains with thymol, linalool + terpinene-4-ol, linalool, caryophyllene + germacren D, or germacren D as chief components

Flavonoids: including naringin

Caffeic acid derivatives: in particular, rosmaric acid (5%)

EFFECTS

General: The essential oil, which contains carvacrol, is antimicrobial in vitro.

The antibacterial and antifungal activity of Oregano is thought to be mainly due to the presence of phenolic compounds such as thymol (11.6%) and carvacrol (3.5%) (Stiles et al,1995; Biondi et al, 1993).

AnticancerEffects: Antimutagenic and anticarcinogenic properties have been attributed to rosemaric acid isolated from rosemary and Oregano (Milic & Milic, 1998).

Antimicrobial Effects: The essential oil of Oregano inhibited the following microbes with a minimum inhibitory concentration of <2% (volume/volume): *</Acinetobacter baumanii, Aeromonas sobria, Candida albicans, Enterococcus faecalis, Escherichia coli, Klebsiella pneumonia, Pseudomonas aeruginosa, Salmonella typhimurium, Serratia marcescens,* and *Staphylococcus aureus* (Hammer et al, 1999).

Essential oil of Oregano inhibited *Candida albicans* growth. Zones of inhibition were similar to that of nystatin (22 to 25 mm). Carvacrol was the proposed antifungal component of Oregano and proved to be about twice as potent as the unfractionated oil (Stiles et al, 1995).

Essential oil of Oregano was bactericidal against *Proteus vulgaris* but showed no inhibitory activity against *Pseudomonas aeruginosa.* Bacteriostatic activity was reported against *Streptococcus faecalis, Staphylococcus aureus, Micrococcus luteus, Bacillus subtilis, Escherichia coli,* and *Hafnia alvei.* Oregano also exhibited antifungal properties against *Aspergillus niger, Aspergillus terreus, Candida albicans,* and *Fusarium* species (Biondi et al, 1993).

Antioxidant Effects: The essential oil of Oregano has been demonstrated to be a potent antioxidant. The non-polar fraction of the residue obtained after the essential oil is removed from Oregano also exhibited antioxidant activity. Tocopherols, especially gamma tocopherol, have been identified as the major antioxidative components of the non-polar fraction, accounting for as much as 1% of the constituents of the non-polar fraction (Lagouri & Boskou, 1996).

Antiparasitic Effects: Oil of Oregano inhibited enteric parasites in adults. Thirteen patients were treated for enteric parasites (*Blastocystis hominis,* n=8; *Entamoeba hartmanni,* n=4) in tablet form three times daily for 6 weeks. Following treatment, 10 of 13 (77%) patients were parasite-free. *E hartmanni, Endolimax nana,* and *B hominis* with an initial parasite score of less than 2 were completely eradicated. Those patients with an initial *B hominis* score of more than 2 demonstrated reduced parasite scores but not eradication. By the study's end, patients initially infected with *B hominis* reported amelioration of their symptoms (bloating, gastrointestinal cramping, alternating diarrhea and constipation, and fatigue) (Force et al. 2000).

CLINICAL TRIALS

In a study to determine the antioxidant potential of Oregano extract in vivo, 45 healthy nonsmoking males were randomized to consume mango-orange juice (placebo), mango-orange juice enriched with 300 mg/d Oregano extract phenolic compounds, or mango-orange juice enriched with 600 mg/d Oregano extract phenolic compounds daily for 4 weeks. While the excretion of phenolic compounds was markedly increased in the higher phenolic group as compared to the placebo group, no significant short-term or long-term effects on biomarkers of lipid peroxidation or on serum lipid levels were observed (Nurmi, 2006).

INDICATIONS AND USAGE

Unproven Uses: Oregano herb is used for respiratory disorders such as coughs, inflammation of the bronchial mucous membranes, and as an expectorant. Topical formulations have been used to treat herpes simplex virus outbreaks. In folk medicine, it is used for coughs, dyspepsia, painful menstruation, rheumatoid arthritis, scrofulosis, urinary tract disorders, and as a diaphoretic.

Chinese Medicine: In China, Oregano is used for colds, fever, vomiting, dysentery, jaundice, and malnutrition for children.

Homeopathy Uses: Oregano is used to increase sexual excitability.

PRECAUTIONS AND ADVERSE REACTIONS

No health hazards or side effects are known in conjunction with the proper administration of designated therapeutic dosages.

DRUG INTERACTIONS

No drug interaction data available.

DOSAGE

Mode of Administration: Oregano infusions and powders are used as teas, gargles, and bath additives.

Preparation: For internal use, pour 250 mL boiling water over 1 heaped teaspoonful and strain after 10 minutes; the tea can be sweetened with honey. The unsweetened infusion is used as gargle and mouthwash. To use as a bath additive, pour 1 liter of water over 100 g drug, strain after 10 minutes and add to a full bath.

Daily Dosage: Tea: 1 cup several times a day. Powder: 0.5 to 1 dessertspoon 2 to 3 times daily with food.

Homeopathic Dosage: 5 to 10 drops, 1 tablet, or 5 to 10 globules 1 to 3 times daily or 1 mL injection solution sc twice weekly (HAB34).

Storage: Store Oregano where it is protected from moisture and light.

LITERATURE

Afshaypuor S et al. Volatile constituents of *Origanum vulgare ssp. viride* (syn. *O. heracleoticum*) from Iran. In: *PM* 63(2):179-180. 1997.

Afshaypuor S. Essential oil constituents of wild marjoram from Iran. In: PM 62, Abstracts of the 44th Ann Congress of GA, 133. 1996.

Biondi D, Cianci P, Geraci C et al. Antimicrobial activity and chemical composition of essential oils from Sicilian aromatic plants. In: *J Flav & Frag*; 8(6):331-337, 1993.

Force M, Sparks W & Ronzio R. Inhibition of enteric parasites by emulsified oil of oregano in vivo. In: *Phytother Res*; 14(3):213-214, 2000.

Hammer K, Carson C & Riley T. Antimicrobial activity of essential oils and other plant extracts. *J App Microbiol* 1999; 86(6):985-990.

Lagouri V & Boskou D. Nutrient antioxidants in oregano. In: *Int J Food Sci Nutr*; 47:493-497, 1996.

Nurmi A, Mursu J, Nurmi T, et al. Consumption of juice fortified with oregano extract markedly increases excretion of phenolic acids but lacks short- and long-term effects on lipid peroxidation in healthy nonsmoking men. *J Agric Food Chem;* 54(16):5790-5796, 2006.

Stiles J, Sparks W & Ronzio R. The inhibition of Candida albicans by oregano. In: *J Appl Nutr*; 47:96-102, 1995.

Yarnell, E. & Abascal, K.: Herbs for treating herpes simplex infections. *Alt Compl Ther; 11*(2): 83, 88. 2005.

Oriental Arborvitae

Thuja orientalis

DESCRIPTION

Medicinal Parts: The medicinal parts are the dried leaves and leafy branches.

Flower and Fruit: The inflorescence forms cones with horned cone scales. The male cones are apical and globose with 3 to 6 stamens. The female cones are small, ovoid-to-globose with 3 pairs of scales, the upper one sterile, the middle one with 1 ovule, and the lower one with 3. The seeds are ovoid to elliptical and have no wings.

Leaves, Stem, and Root: Oriental arborvitae is a diclinous, monoecious, evergreen tree, which grows up to 10 m high. The leaves are decussately arranged, scalelike, imbricate, appressed to the branches, thick, and acute. The edge leaves are pressed together and keeled. The surface leaves are ovate-rhomboid, grooved on the back, needlelike when young and acutely splayed. The branches are vertical, flattened and vertically branched. The smaller branches are the same color on both sides.

Habitat: China, Korea, Afghanistan, and Iran

Production: Oriental Aborvitae tops are the dried leaves and leafy branches of *Thuja orientalis*. They are harvested from cultivated stock in late summer or early autumn, followed by drying in the shade.

Not to be Confused With: May be confused with other *Thujae* species.

Other Names: Chinese Arborvitae

ACTIONS AND PHARMACOLOGY

COMPOUNDS

Volatile oil (0.4%): containing alpha-pinene, alpha-thujone (6%)

Flavonoids: including tricetin-3-glucoside

Wax (0.5%, estolides): chief acid juniperic acid

EFFECTS

The terpene-containing drug is severely toxic. The hemostyptic and hair growth-promoting effects with which it is credited have not yet been documented in experimental data.

INDICATIONS AND USAGE

Chinese Medicine: Oriental Arborvitae is used for coughing blood, nose bleeds, dysentery, hematuria, and hair loss.

PRECAUTIONS AND ADVERSE REACTIONS

No health hazards are known in conjunction with the proper administration of designated therapeutic dosages.

DOSAGE

Mode of Administration: Whole herb preparations, cut, and powdered drug for internal and external use.

Preparation: To prepare Biotae Cacumen, the rubbed branches are roasted in an iron pan until the surface blackens.

Daily Dosage: 3 to 18 g of drug

Storage: Should be stored in a dry place and protected from light.

LITERATURE

Banthorpe DV, Davies HF, Gatford C, Williams SR. Monoterpene pattern in Juniperus and Thuja species. *Planta Med.* 23; 64-69. 1973

Baumann I, Flamme D, Harnischfeger G. Thujae occidentalis herba / Pharmakognostische Untersuchungen zur Identifizierung von Lebensbaumblättern. Dtsch Apoth Ztg. 127; 2518-252. 1987

Hänsel R, Keller K, Rimpler H, Schneider G (Ed), Hagers Handbuch der Pharmazeutischen Praxis, 5. Aufl., Bde 4 - 6 (Drogen), Springer Verlag Berlin, Heidelberg, New York, 1992-1994.

Yang HO, Suh DY, Han B H. Isolation and Characterization of Platelet-Activating Factor Receptor Binding Antagonists from *Biota orientalis. Planta Med.* 61 (1); 37-40. 1995

Origanum majorana

See Sweet Marjoram

Origanum vulgare

See Oregano

Orris

Iris species

DESCRIPTION

Medicinal Parts: The medicinal part is the rhizome with the roots.

Flower and Fruit: The flowers are long-pedicled and perfumed. The tepals are white or slightly blue. The outer ones are darker with a yellow beard. The anthers are as big as the filaments. The upper lip of the stigma branch is inclined forward. The fruit is a large capsule with a number of sections in which the brown seeds are lined up like rolls of coins.

Leaves, Stem, and Root: The plants are perennial, 30 to 100 cm high. The rhizome is thick and short. The strong flower-bearing stem is branched from the middle. The leaves are broad, sword-shaped, usually curved, and gray-green.

Habitat: Indigenous to southern Europe.

Production: Orris root is the root *of Iris germanica, Iris versicolor,* and other varieties.

Other Names: Blue Flag, Daggers, Dragon Flower, Flaggon, Flag Lily, Fliggers Florentine Orris, Gladyne, Iris, Jacob's Sword, Liver Lily, Myrtle Flower, Poison Flag, Segg, Sheggs, Snake Lily, Water Flag, White Flag Root, Wild Iris, Yellow Flag, Yellow Iris

ACTIONS AND PHARMACOLOGY

COMPOUNDS

Volatile oil: chief constituent's irone, in particular alpha-, beta- and gamma-irone (odor resembling violets)

Triterpenes: Iridale (mono-, bi- and spirocyclic compounds, precursors of the irones), including among others irigermanal

Isoflavonoids: including, among others, irilon, irisolone, irigenine, tectorigenin and their glycosides including iridine

Flavonoids

Xanthones: C-glucosylxanthones, for example iris xanthone, magniferin

Starch

EFFECTS

Orris root is mildly expectorant. Some of the flavonoids (in particular the isoflavon irigenin) have an inhibitory effect on c-AMP phosphodiesterase. Root extracts are said to have an ulcer-protective, spasmolytic, and serotonin-antagonistic effect.

INDICATIONS AND USAGE

Unproven Uses: Orris has been used for disorders of the respiratory system.

Homeopathic Uses: This species has been used to treat disorders of the respiratory tract or thyroid gland, for digestion complaints, and headaches.

PRECAUTIONS AND ADVERSE REACTIONS

General: No health hazards or side effects are known in conjunction with the proper administration of designated therapeutic dosages. The juice of the fresh plant has a severely irritating effect upon skin and mucous membranes. If taken internally, it can lead to vomiting, abdominal pain, and bloody diarrhea. Severe inflammation occurs following mucous membrane contact.

Pregnancy: Not to be used during pregnancy.

DOSAGE

Mode of Administration: Iris is available in homeopathic dilutions, as a constituent of various combination preparations and in various tea mixtures.

LITERATURE

Bambhole VD, Jiddewar GG, *Sach Ayurveda* 37(9):557. 1985

Duke JA, A Handbook of Medicinal Herbs, Pub. CRC Press Boca Raton. 1985.

El Moghazy AM et al., *Fitoterapia* 5:237. 1980Frohne D, Pfänder HJ, Giftpflanzen - Ein Handbuch für Apotheker, Toxikologen und Biologen, 4. Aufl., Wiss. Verlags-Ges Stuttgart 1997.

Kern W, List PH, Hörhammer L (Hrsg.), Hagers Handbuch der Pharmazeutischen Praxis, 4. Aufl., Bde. 1-8, Springer Verlag Berlin, Heidelberg, New York, 1969.

Lewin L, Gifte und Vergiftungen, 6. Aufl., Nachdruck, Haug Verlag, Heidelberg 1992.

Madaus G, Lehrbuch der Biologischen Arzneimittel, Bde 1-3, Nachdruck, Georg Olms Verlag Hildesheim 1979.

Poisonous Plants in Britain and Their Effects on Animals and Man, Ministry of Agriculture Fisheries and Food, Pub; HMSO UK 1984.

Steinegger E, Hänsel R, Pharmakognosie, 5. Aufl., Springer Verlag Heidelberg 1992.

Teuscher E, Lindequist U, Biogene Gifte - Biologie, Chemie, Pharmakologie, 2. Aufl., Fischer Verlag Stuttgart 1994.

Wagner H, Wiesenauer M, Phytotherapie. Phytopharmaka und pflanzliche Homöopathika, Fischer-Verlag, Stuttgart, Jena, New York 1995.

Wichtl M (Hrsg.), Teedrogen, 4. Aufl., Wiss. Verlagsges. Stuttgart 1997.

Orthosiphon spicatus

See Java Tea

Oryza sativa

See Rice

Oswego Tea

Monarda didyma

DESCRIPTION

Medicinal Parts: The medicinal part of the plant is the herb.

Flower and Fruit: The terminal flowers are in 1 to 3 richly blossomed false whorls supported by bracts. The bracts bear leaflets that are pale green with a reddish tinge. The calyx tips are awl-shaped. The corolla is scarlet and 3.5 to 6 cm in length. The plant is propagated using root cuttings.

Leaves, Stem, and Root: The plant is a bristly haired-to-glabrous, 50- to 90-cm high herbaceous perennial with runners. The stems are erect, acutely quadrangular, grooved, and hard. The leaves are in pairs, ovate-lanceolate, clearly petiolate, crenate, and often rough on both sides.

Characteristics: Monarda didyma has a scent similar to that of the bergamot orange.

Habitat: The plant is indigenous to swampy regions from Georgia and Michigan in the U.S. and to wetlands extending northward to Ontario, Canada.

Other Names: Bee Balm, Bergamot, Blue Balm, High Balm, Low Balm, Mountain Balm, Mountain Mint, Scarlet Monarda

ACTIONS AND PHARMACOLOGY

COMPOUNDS

Volatile oil (0.1-0.3%): including among others carvacrol, thymol, p-cymene, linalool, linalyl acetate, limonene, ocimene, alpha-pinene, camphene, Delta3-carene

Flavonoids: including linarin, didymin (isosakurenatin-7-O-beta-D), isosakuranin, genkwanin

Anthocyans: monardein (triacyliertes pelargonidine-3, 5-di-O-glucoside, 2 malonyl- and 1 p-cumaroyl- residue)

EFFECTS

The drug has antispasmodic, digestive, carminative and diuretic effects; it is also used to regulate menstruation.

CONTRAINDICATIONS

Oswego Tea is not to be used during pregnancy.

INDICATIONS AND USAGE

Unproven Uses: The drug is used for flatulence and other digestive disorders and also menstrual complaints including premenstrual syndrome. In Europe, the herb is sometimes used as an aromatic, carminative, and antipryretic. Former use of the drug as an alternative to quinine is no longer common.

PRECAUTIONS AND ADVERSE REACTIONS

No health hazards or side effects are known in conjunction with the proper administration of designated therapeutic dosages.

DOSAGE

Mode of Administration: Ground drug (powder) prepared as an infusion or tea.

LITERATURE

Hegnauer R, Chemotaxonomie der Pflanzen, Bde 1-11, Birkhäuser Verlag Basel, Boston, Berlin 1962-1997.

Kern W, List PH, Hörhammer L (Hrsg.), Hagers Handbuch der Pharmazeutischen Praxis, 4. Aufl., Bde. 1-8, Springer Verlag Berlin, Heidelberg, New York, 1969.

Nikolaevski VV, Kononova NS, Pertsovski i AI, Shinkarchuk IF, Effect of essential oils on the course of experimental atherosclerosis. *Patol Fiziol Eksp Ter*:52-3, Sep-Oct, 1990.

Shubina LP, Siurin SA, Savchenko VM, Inhalations of essential oils in the combined treatment of patients with chronic bronchitis. *Vrach Delo*:66-7, May 1990.

Ox-Eye Daisy

Chrysanthemum leucanthemum

DESCRIPTION

Flower and Fruit: Long pedicled flowers with a semi-globular calyx. Sepals are imbricate, green and wide, the corolla golden-yellow, and orbicular. The young flowers are white and 1 to 2 cm long. The fruit is 2.5 to 3 mm long and top-shaped.

Leaves, Stem, and Root: Ox-Eye Daisy is a perennial growing 10 to 100 cm high. It is somewhat hairy or glabrous with cylindrical knotted root. The stem is erect, glabrous, simple or divided into numerous oblong single-headed branches. The leaves are tough, compound and glabrous or slightly pubescent. The cauline leaves are petiolate, linear to ovate-oblong, roughly dentate to almost pinnatisect.

Habitat: The plant is found in Britain, Europe, Russia, Asia, and numerous other parts of the world.

Production: Ox-Eye Daisy is the above-ground part of *Chrysanthemum leucanthemum.*

Other Names: Butter Daisy, Dun Daisy, Golden Daisy, Goldenseal, Great Ox-Eye, Herb Margaret, Horse Daisy, Horse Gowan, Marguerite, Maudlin Daisy, Maudlinwort, Moon Daisy, Moon Flower, Moon Penny, Poverty Weed, White Daisy, White Weed

ACTIONS AND PHARMACOLOGY

COMPOUNDS

Cyclitols: including meso-inositol, L(-)-quercitol, meso-inositol, L(-)-quercitol

Polyynes: among them the strongly sensitizing trideca-3,5,7,9,11-pentain-1-ol and its acetate

Flavonoids: including niviaside (a C-glycosyl flavone, containing a cyclitol instead of a sugar), apigenein-7-0-glucuronide

EFFECTS

Ox-Eye Daisy herb and flowers are used similarly to Chamomile as a tonic, although they have a much weaker effect. They are also considered to have an antispasmodic and diuretic effect.

INDICATIONS AND USAGE

Unproven Uses: Internal folk medicine uses include asthma, whooping cough, and nervous agitation. Among external applications are skin ulcers, wounds, and nosebleeds. (Also see Chamomile.)

PRECAUTIONS AND ADVERSE REACTIONS

No health hazards or side effects are known in conjunction with the proper administration of designated therapeutic dosages. There is, however, a strong potential for sensitization resulting from skin contact with the drug.

DOSAGE

Mode of Administration: See Chamomile.

Daily Dosage: Decoction: 1 cup 3 times daily.

LITERATURE

Hausen B, Allergiepflanzen, Pflanzenallergene, ecomed Verlagsgesellsch. mbH, Landsberg 1988.

Hegnauer R, Chemotaxonomie der Pflanzen, Bde 1-11, Birkhäuser Verlag Basel, Boston, Berlin 1962-1997.

Kern W, List PH, Hörhammer L (Hrsg.), Hagers Handbuch der Pharmazeutischen Praxis, 4. Aufl., Bde 1-8, Springer Verlag Berlin, Heidelberg, New York, 1969.

Teuscher E, Lindequist U, Biogene Gifte - Biologie, Chemie, Pharmakologie, 2. Aufl., Fischer Verlag Stuttgart 1994.

Oxalis acetosella

See Wood Sorrel

Paeonia officinalis

See European Peony

Pagoda Tree

Sophora japonica

DESCRIPTION

Medicinal Parts: The medicinal parts are the ripe seeds.

Flower and Fruit: The white flowers are in large, broad, sweeping terminal panicles made up of racemes. The flowers are papilionaceous with a patent standard. The lower edges of the lateral wing petals are bent so that one surrounds the others. The fruit is a round pod tied in around the seeds like a string of pearls.

Leaves, Stem, and Trunk: The tree is reminiscent of the robinia, with a densely branched crown. It grows 12 to 15 m high. It has smooth, green branches. The leaves are odd-pinnate with 11 to 15 leaflets. The leaflets are ovate, acute, dark green above and glaucous beneath. The main leaf petiole is very thick at the base.

Habitat: The plant is indigenous to China and Japan, and is found in Europe as an ornamental and roadside tree.

Production: Pagoda Tree seeds are the ripe seeds of *Sophora japonica.*

ACTIONS AND PHARMACOLOGY

COMPOUNDS

Quinolizidine alkaloids (0-0.04%): including among others cytisine, N-methyl cytisine, matrine, sophocarpine

Flavonoids: including rutin, sophorine

Toxic lectins

Polysaccharides: galactomannans

Fatty oil

Proteins

EFFECTS

The active agent rutin increases the permeability of the capillaries.

INDICATIONS AND USAGE

Homeopathic Uses: Pagoda Tree is used in homeopathy for dysentery.

PRECAUTIONS AND ADVERSE REACTIONS

No health hazards, side effects, or cases of poisoning are known in conjunction with the proper administration of designated therapeutic dosages. Nevertheless, according to older reports, regular consumption of the seed can cause facial edema and even death. Cystine poisonings are possible through the intake of very high dosages.

DOSAGE

Mode of Administration: As a mother tincture in homeopathic dilutions. Sophora is used by the pharmaceutical industry in the production of rutin (a substance that influences the resolution and porousness of the dilation of the capillaries). The drug is contained in medicinal preparations, which are used to stabilize blood circulation and as a cure for nervous disorders and inflammation.

LITERATURE

Gorbacheva LA, Grishkovets VI, Drozd GA, Chirva VYa. Triterpene glycosides from *Sophora japonica L.* seeds. *Adv Exp Med Biol,* 597:501-4. 1996

Kass E, Wink M. Phylogenetic relationships in the Papilionoideae (family Leguminosae) based on nucleotide sequences of cpDNA (rbcL) and ncDNA (ITS 1 and 2). *Mol Phylogenet Evol*, 8:65-88, Aug 1997

Kern W, List PH, Hörhammer L (Hrsg.), Hagers Handbuch der Pharmazeutischen Praxis, 4. Aufl., Bde. 1-8: Springer Verlag Berlin, Heidelberg, New York, 1969.

Narimanov AA, Kuznetsova SM, Miakisheva SN. The modifying action of the Japanese pagoda tree (*Sophora japonica*) and pantocrine in radiation lesions. *Radiobiologiia*, 30:170-4, Mar-Apr 1990

Shirataki Y, Tagaya Y, Yokoe I, Komatsu M. Studies on the Constituents of Sophora Species: Constituents of the Root of *Sophora japonica. J Pharm Sci.* 76; S214. 1987

Tang W, Eisenbrand G, Chinese Drugs of Plant Origin, Springer Verlag Heidelberg 1992.

Teuscher E, Lindequist U, Biogene Gifte - Biologie, Chemie, Pharmakologie, 2. Aufl., Fischer Verlag Stuttgart 1994.

Panax ginseng

See Ginseng

Papaver rhoeas

See Corn Poppy

Papaver somniferum

See Poppyseed

Papaya

Carica papaya

DESCRIPTION

Medicinal Parts: The medicinal parts are the leaves and fruits.

Flower and Fruit: The plant has varying yellow to yellowish-white flowers of both sexes. The male flowers form many-branched, hanging panicles with small flowers. The female flowers are almost sessile in the leaf axils on the trunk. In addition there are androgynous, fertile flowers. The yellow to yellow-green berry fruit is up to 30 cm long, 15 cm thick and weighs 2 to 5 kg. The fruit is clavate and lightly grooved. It contains numerous peppercorn-sized seeds surrounded by orange-yellow and melon-flavored flesh.

Leaves, Stem, and Root: Carica papaya is a 4 to 8 m high bushy tree with an unbranched fleshy-woody trunk that is hollow in the middle. The leaves are long-petioled, very large, and segmented into 5 to 7 palmate lobes, which terminate in sharp tips.

Habitat: Indigenous to tropical America. Cultivated in all tropical regions today.

Production: Papaya leaves consist of the fresh or dried leaves of *Carica papaya* harvested before the fruit appears. Raw papain is the latex from *Carica papaya*, which has been dried using various methods; where necessary the latex is decontaminated mechanically or by filtration.

Other Names: Mamaeire, Melon Tree, Papaw

ACTIONS AND PHARMACOLOGY

COMPOUNDS: PAPAYA LEAVES

Polyketide alkaloids: carpaine, pseudocarpaine

Glucosinolates

Cyanogenic glycosides (traces): including prunasin

Saponins

Proteolytic ferments (ficin)

EFFECTS: PAPAYA LEAVES

No information is available.

COMPOUNDS: RAW PAPAIN

Proteolytic enzymes (proteinases): papain, chymopapain A and B, proteinase A and B, papaya peptidase A

Other enzymes: lysozyme, chitotransferase, glycosidases, callase, pectinesterases, lipases, phosphatases, cycloligases

EFFECTS: RAW PAPAIN

The proteolytic activity of the raw papain enzymes can be used within the parameters of enzyme substitution for digestive complaints, particularly pancreatic conditions. Papain has an antimicrobial, anthelmintic, and anti-ulcerative effect. Papain is commonly used in industry as a meat tenderizer, a clearing agent in beer production, an enzymatic contact lens cleaner, and a pharmaceutical and immunochemical reagent (Blanco et al, 1998; Mansfield, 1995).

The results of the analgesic and anti-inflammatory effects are contradictory. Experiments have shown that papain has an edema-reducing effect. The fibrinogenous effect has not been sufficiently proved.

Wound-Healing Effects: The wound-healing effects of papaya are attributed to its proteolytic enzymes: papain, chymopapain, and leukopapain. The proteolytic action of papain is well known in its function as a meat tenderizer. Chymopapain is thought to be a desloughing agent that promotes growth and improves scar tissue. Carpaines and aglycones have also been isolated from papaya and demonstrate broad antimicrobial activity (Starley et al, 1999). In poor regions of Africa, pediatric full-thickness and infected burns have been successfully treated by applying mashed papaya fruit on gauze to the burn once to twice daily for several weeks. In some cases, this treatment has resulted in wounds clean enough for grafting and the wounds accepting the graft. When partial thickness burns were dressed with papaya, full-thickness wounds sometimes resulted. It is unclear if these wounds were misinterpreted at the outset or if the papaya dressing caused the worsening (Starley et al, 1999).

CLINICAL TRIALS

Scientific evidence for the use of papain for any indication is largely lacking. Anecdotal evidence for the successful use of papaya paste in the topical treatment of full-thickness and infected burns is available, as well as for the use of a polyenzyme preparation as an adjuvant in the treatment of cancer.

Antioxidant Actions

It remains unclear whether antioxidant supplementation is of potential therapeutic value, and how this may potentially vary in individuals with different genetic make-ups; there appears to be genetic susceptibility to oxidative stress for which antioxidants may prove useful. The antioxidant effect of a fermented Papaya preparation (FPP) was measured in a randomized, placebo-controlled, crossover study in which 54 elderly (mean age 72 years) but generally healthy individuals were divided into two groups and given either FPP or placebo. Three months of supplementation (FPP 9 g/day orally,1 hour after breakfast) were followed by a six-week washout period, followed by an additional three-month supplementation period. Based on monthly blood analyses, there was a significant enhancement of antioxidant protection ($P<0.01$ vs. A) and defense, even in those without clear antioxidant deficiency. The glutathione-S transferase MI genotype was also examined in terms of its reaction to the introduction of FPP (Marotta, 2006).

Type-2 diabetes

For two months, 25 subjects with type 2 diabetes and a control group that included 25 clinically healthy subjects received 3 g of a nutriceutical, Fermented Papaya Preparation. The researchers found that the papaya preparation induced a significant decrease in plasma sugar levels in both healthy subjects and those with type 2 diabetes. This hypoglycemic effect enabled patients with diabetes to reduce the dosage of their antidiabetic oral therapy and one patient to suspend his oral therapy altogether (Danese et al, 2006).

Immunomodulation

In a placebo-controlled study, the administration of a polyenzyme preparation (Wobenzyme®) resulted in increased production of reactive oxygen species (ROS) and cytotoxicity in polymorphonuclear leukocytes (PMN). Twenty-eight healthy volunteers received single oral doses of Wobenzyme in a dose ranging from 5 to 20 tablets; 8 volunteers received placebo. Upon measurement of PMN respiratory burst, a dose-dependent increase in ROS production was documented that was significant with the 10- and 20-tablet doses ($p<0.05$ and $p<0.001$, respectively). Peak ROS production occurred at 4 hours following tablet administration and was still documented at 6 hours. Wobenzyme contains per 100 mg: 33 mg panceatin, 830 Units (U) amylase, 790 U lipase, 75 U protease, 20 mg papain, 15 mg bromelain, 8 mg trypsin, 3.3 mg lipase, 3.3 mg amylase, and 0.3 mg chymotrypsin (Zavadova et al, 1995).

INDICATIONS AND USAGE

RAW PAPAIN

Unproven Uses: Papaya is used for gastrointestinal digestion complaints, inflammations and ulcers in the gastro-duodenal area, and pancreas excretion insufficiency.

PAPAYA LEAVES

Unproven Uses: Papaya leaf preparations are used singly or in combinations for prophylaxis and therapy of diseases and disorders of the gastrointestinal tract and for infections with intestinal parasites.

Indian Medicine: Worm infestation, damage to the urinary tract and stones, hemorrhoids, coughs, and bronchitis have been treated with Papaya leaves.

CONTRAINDICATIONS

Pregnancy: Not to be used during pregnancy. Because of the experimentally proven embryotoxic and teratogenic effects, as well as its known abortifacient effect in humans, unripe papain fruit should not be used during pregnancy.

PRECAUTIONS AND ADVERSE REACTIONS

Allergic reactions, including asthma attacks, are possible.

DRUG INTERACTIONS

MAJOR RISK

Anticoagulants: Concurrent use may result in increased risk of bleeding. Papaya extract was shown to increase the international normalized ratio (INR) levels when used in conjunction with warfarin (Shaw et al, 1997). *Clinical Management:* Avoid concomitant use. If taken together, the patient should be monitored closely for symptoms of bleeding and the INR should be closely monitored.

DOSAGE

RAW PAPAIN

Daily Dosage: The dosage depends on the composition of the enzyme substitute preparation.

How Supplied:

Chewable Tablets

Tablets

PAPAYA LEAVES

Daily Dosage: No information is available.

LITERATURE

RAW PAPAIN AND PAPAYA LEAVES

Blanco C, Ortega N, Castillo R et al. *Carica papaya* pollen allergy. In: *Ann Allergy Asthma Immunol*; 81(2):171-175, 1998.

Buttle DJ et al. Affinity purification of the novel cysteine proteinase papaya proteinase IV, and papain from papaya latex. In: *Biochem J* 261(2):469-476, Jul 15, 1989.

Danese C, Esposito D, D'Alfonso V, et al. Plasma glucose level decreases as collateral effect of fermented papaya preparation use. *Clin Ter*; 157(3): 195-198. 2006.

Lohiya NK et al. Antifertility effects of aqueous extract of *Carica papaya* seeds in male rats. In: *PM* 60(5):400. 1994.

Mansfield L, Ting S, Haverly R et al. The incidence and clinical implications of hypersensitivity to papain in an allergic population, confirmed by blinded oral challenge. In: *Ann Allergy*; 55(4):541-543, 1985.

McKee RA, Smith H. Purification of proteinases from Carica papaya. In: *PH* 25:2283. 1986.

Shaw D, Leon C, Kolev S et al., Traditional remedies and food supplements: a 5-year toxicological study. In: *Drug Saf;* 17(5):342-356, 1997.

Starley I, Mohammed P, Schneider G et al. The treatment of paediatric burns using topical papaya. In: *Burns*; 25(7):636-639, 1999.

Zavadova E, Desser L & Mohr T. Stimulation of reactive oxygen species production and cytotoxicity in human neutrophils in vitro and after oral administration of a polyenzyme preparation. In: *Cancer Biother*; 10(2):147-152, 1995.

Zoch E. Über die Inhaltsstoffe des Handelspapains. In: Arzneim Forsch 19:1593. 1969.

Pareira

Chondrodendron tomentosum

DESCRIPTION

Medicinal Parts: The medicinal parts are the curare, which is the extract from the fresh or dried trunk, along with the bark and the dried roots.

Flower and Fruit: The flowers grow in axillary clusters 10 to 15 cm long on stems that are often unbranched. There are 9 outer pubescent sepals about 1 mm long. The inner 6 sepals are about 3.5 mm long and glabrous. The petals are 0.4 mm long. The fruit is a drupe about 12 mm long and 9 mm wide on a stem 4 mm long.

Leaves, Stem, and Root: The plant is a climber that grows up to 30 m in height. The stems are velvety. The petioles are short-haired at the base, have long erect hairs near the leaf blade, and are about 8 to 12 cm long. The leaves are somewhat coriaceous, entire-margined, sparse above and tomentose beneath. They are mildly cordate, triangular-ovate or roundish and obtuse, 10 to 15 cm in length and width. The root is about 2 to 5 cm in diameter, tortuous, black, longitudinally furrowed with transverse ridges and some constrictions. Internally the root is grayish-brown, and the transverse section shows three or four concentric rings traversed by wide medullary rays. The stem pieces are similar but the external surface is grayish and marked with numerous round, warty lenticels.

Characteristics: The taste is at first bitter, then slightly sweet. The plant is odorless.

Habitat: The plant is found in western Bolivia, Peru, Ecuador, central Colombia, and Panama.

Production: Pareira root is the root of *Chondrodendron tomentosum.* Tubocurare is extracted from the fresh or dried trunk with bark of the same plant.

Other Names: Ice Vine, Pereira Brava, Velvet Leaf

ACTIONS AND PHARMACOLOGY

COMPOUNDS

Bibenzyl isoquinoline alkaloids: including, among others, D-tubocurarine, chondrocurarine, (-)-curine, (+)-chondrofoline, chondrocurine, isochondrodendrine

EFFECTS

Tubocurare contains tubocurarine and acts as an emmenagogic and diuretic.

INDICATIONS AND USAGE

Unproven Uses: Only the tubocurarine extracted from the bark and twigs is in use. It is a peripheral muscle relaxant, which inhibits the stimulation of transference in the neuromuscular, hence causing a paralysis of the skeletal muscles. Tubocurare is used in modern anesthetics as tubocurarine.

PRECAUTIONS AND ADVERSE REACTIONS

No health hazards or side effects are known in conjunction with the oral administration of designated therapeutic dosages of the drug. The alkaloids with curarelike effect, such as tubocurarine, are not resorbed with oral administration of the drug.

OVERDOSAGE

Nausea and heavy urine flow have been observed in individuals poisoned with tubocurare.

DOSAGE

Mode of Administration: Use of drug is no longer common.

Storage: The plant is considered poisonous and should be stored in clearly marked containers that are impervious to insects.

LITERATURE

Guha et al., *J Nat Prod* 42:1. 1979

Hänsel R, Keller K, Rimpler H, Schneider G (Hrsg.), Hagers Handbuch der Pharmazeutischen Praxis, 5. Aufl., Bde 4-6 (Drogen), Springer Verlag Berlin, Heidelberg, New York, 1992-1994.

Madaus G, Lehrbuch der Biologischen Arzneimittel, Bde 1-3, Nachdruck, Georg Olms Verlag Hildesheim 1979.

Teuscher E, Lindequist U, Biogene Gifte - Biologie, Chemie, Pharmakologie, 2. Aufl., Fischer Verlag Stuttgart 1994.

Parietaria officinalis

See Pellitory-of-the-Wall

Paris quadrifolia

See Herb Paris

Parsley

Petroselinum crispum

DESCRIPTION

Medicinal Parts: The medicinal parts are the oil extracted from the parsley fruit, the dried, separated schizocarp, the fresh or dried aerial parts, the dried underground parts, and the whole fresh plant at the beginning of the flowering season.

Flower and Fruit: The inflorescences are long pedicled, terminal, occasionally apical, 10 to 20 rayed yellowish umbels. The involucre has 1 to 2 bracts, and the epicalyx has 6 to 8 leaves. The petals are splayed with a curved tip. The style thickening is very developed. The fruit is orbicular-ovate, 2.5 mm long, and greenish-gray.

Leaves, Stem, and Root: The plant is a biennial. It is glabrous, has a characteristic odor and grows from 60 to 100 cm high. The usually numerous stems grow from 1 root and are erect, round, finely grooved, glabrous, and branched. The root is thin or thick fusiform to tuberous, vertical, and almost fiberless. The leaves are ovate and tripinnate. The upper ones are shorter stemmed and less compound. The leaflets are tripinnate.

Characteristics: Parsley has a spicy smell.

Habitat: The plant originated in the Mediterranean region and is cultivated worldwide today.

Production: Parsley consists of the fresh or dried plant section of *Petroselinum crispum.* Parsley root is the dried root of *Petroselinum crispum.* The fresh herb is harvested from cultivations. Parsley seed consists of the dried ripe fruits of *Petroselinum crispum.*

Not to be Confused With: The leaves of *Aethusa cynapium.*

Other Names: Common Parsley, Garden Parsley, Hamburg Parsley, Persely, Petersylinge, Rock Parsley

ACTIONS AND PHARMACOLOGY

COMPOUNDS: PARSLEY HERB

Volatile oil (0.02-0.3%): chief components, according to variety, up to 90%

Apiole

Myristicin

1-allyl-2,3,4,5-tetramethoxybenzole: additionally including among others mentha-1,3,8-triene (up to 50%, aroma-bearer). alpha- and beta-pinene, alpha- and beta-phellandrene; hybrid strains also exist

Furocoumarins: including among others, bergapten, oxypeucedanin, isopimpinellin, psoralen, xanthotoxin, imperatorin

Flavonoids (1.9-5.6%): chief components apiin

Vitamins: in particular ascorbic acid (up to 165 mg per 100 g)

COMPOUNDS: PARSLEY ROOT
Volatile oil (0.05-0.12%): chief components of Petroselinum crispum ssp. crispum apiole, myristicin, terpinolene, tuberosum apiole, beta-pinene, additionally including among others, alpha- and beta-pinene, (+)-limonene, beta-bisabolene

Phthalides: including among others, ligustilide, senkyunolide

Furocoumarins: including among others, bergaptene, oxypeucedanin, isopimpinellin, psoralen, xanthotoxin and imperatorin

Flavonoids (0.2-1.3%): chief components apiin

Polyynes: including among others, falcarinol, falcarindiol

EFFECTS: PARSLEY HERB AND ROOT
Although its mode of action has not been clearly explained, its use for urinary tract complaints seems plausible.

COMPOUNDS: PARSLEY FRUIT
Volatile oil (2-6%): chief components, according to variety

Apiole (58-80%)

Myristicin (49-77%)

1-allyl-2,3,4,5-tetramethoxybenzole (50-60%)

Alpha- and beta-pinene, beta-phellandrene: among others

Furocoumarins: including among others bergapten, oxypeucedanin, isopimpinellin, psoralen, xanthotoxin and imperatorin

Fatty oil: chief fatty acid petroselic acid (60-80%)

EFFECTS: PARSLEY FRUIT
In animal experiments, a diuretic effect, as well as a moderate increase in uterine tone, has been reported with low doses. Higher doses increase contractility of the smooth muscle of the intestine, bladder and especially the uterus and therefore may be abortifacient; this explains its use for menstruation complaints.

INDICATIONS AND USAGE

PARSLEY HERB AND ROOT
Approved by Commission E:

- Infections of the urinary tract
- Kidney and bladder stones

The herb is used for flushing the efferent urinary tract and for the prevention and treatment of kidney gravel.

Unproven Uses: In folk medicine, it is used for gastrointestinal disorders, jaundice, kidney and bladder inflammation, as a diuretic, and an emmenagogue.

Homeopathic Uses: Inflammation of the urinary tract and irritable bladder.

PARSLEY FRUIT
Unproven Uses: In folk medicine, the fruit has been used for menstrual disturbances, disorders of the gastrointestinal tract, the kidneys and lower urinary tract, and as a digestive.

CONTRAINDICATIONS

PARSLEY HERB, ROOT AND FRUIT
The herb is contraindicated in patients allergic to parsley or apiole, those with kidney inflammations and in pregnant women. Irrigation therapy should not be carried out in the presence of edema resulting from reduced cardiac and kidney function.

PRECAUTIONS AND ADVERSE REACTIONS

PARSLEY HERB AND ROOT
General: No health hazards or side effects are known in conjunction with the proper administration of designated therapeutic dosages. The drug leads rarely to contact allergies; photodermatosis is also conceivable following intensive skin contact between freshly harvested plant parts and light-skinned individuals.

Pregnancy: Therapeutic doses are contraindicated in pregnancy.

PARSLEY FRUIT
General: No health hazards or side effects are known in conjunction with the proper administration of designated therapeutic dosages. The drug leads rarely to contact allergies; photodermatoses occur somewhat more frequently following skin contact.

Pregnancy: Parsley fruit preparations are contraindicated in pregnancy; an abortive effect has been observed.

OVERDOSAGE

PARSLEY HERB, ROOT AND FRUIT
The administration of higher dosages of the volatile oil or of preparations with high concentrations of the volatile oil can lead to poisonings. Symptoms include elevated contractility of the smooth musculature, in particular of the urinary bladder, of the intestines, and of the uterus. Other symptoms may include anuria, bloody stools, emaciation, fatty liver, hemolysis, methemoglobinuria, and mucous membrane bleeding.

DOSAGE

PARSLEY HERB AND ROOT
Mode of Administration: Comminuted drug for infusions as well as other galenic preparations with a comparably small proportion of essential oil to be taken orally. Dry extracts are used in pharmaceutical products, such as tablets.

How Supplied:

Capsules — 450 mg, 455 mg, 900 mg, 1,350 mg

Liquid — 1:1

Tea

Preparation: Infusion: Pour boiling water over 2 g finely cut drug and strain after 10 to 15 minutes.

Daily Dosage: A total of 6 g in the appropriate preparations. Infusion: 2 to 3 cups over the course of the day. Adequate intake of liquid is essential for flushing out treatment.

Homeopathic Dosage: 5 drops, 1 tablet, or 10 globules every 30 to 60 minutes (acute) or 1 to 3 times a day (chronic); parenterally: 1 to 2 mL sc, acute: 3 times daily; chronic: once a day (HAB1). The daily dosage is 6 g drug. Adequate intake of liquid is essential for flushing out treatment.

Storage: Protect from light and moisture and tightly sealed.

PARSLEY FRUIT

Mode of Administration: Preparations of the fruit are for internal use.

Preparation: To make an infusion, pour boiling water over 1 gm freshly pressed drug and strain after 10 minutes.

Daily Dosage: The average single dose is 1 g.

Tea — Two to 3 cups of the infusion can be taken daily.

Storage: Protect from light and moisture.

LITERATURE

PARSLEY HERB, ROOT, AND FRUIT

Busse WW et al., *J All Clin. Immunol.* 73:801. 1984

Chaudhary SK et al., *Planta Med* (6):462. 1986

Gijbels MJM et al., Phthalides in roots of *Apium graveolens, A. graveolens var. rapeceum, Bifora testiculata* and *Petroselinum crispum var. tuberosum. Fitoterapia* 61 17. 1985

Hänsel R, Keller K, Rimpler H, Schneider G (Eds.), Hagers Handbuch der Pharmazeutischen Praxis, 5. Aufl., Bde 4-6 (Drogen), Springer Verlag Berlin, Heidelberg, New York, 1992-1994.

Leung AY, Encyclopedia of Common Natural Ingredients Used in Food Drugs and Cosmetics, John Wiley & Sons Inc., New York 1980.

MacLeod AJ, Snyder CH, Subramanian G, Volatile aroma constituents from parsley leafs. In: *PH* 24(11):2623-2627. 1985.

Madaus G, Lehrbuch der Biologischen Arzneimittel, Bde 1-3, Nachdruck, Georg Olms Verlag Hildesheim 1979.

Neuhaus-Carlisle K, Vierling W, Wagner H. Calcium-channel blocking activity of essential oils from *Petroselinum crisp., Apium graveolens* and isolated phenylpropane constituents. *Pharm Pharmacol Lett.* 3; 77-79. 1993

Neuhaus-Carlisle K et al., Calcium-antagonistic activity of extracts and constituents of *Petroselinum crispum* and other phenylpropane derivatives. In: *PM* 59(7):A582. 1992.

Özcelik F et al. Limited effects of parsley (*Petroselinum crispum*) on protein glycation and glutathione in lenses of streptozotocin-induced diabetic rats. *Pharm Biol* 39(3); 230-233. 2001

Porter NG. Composition and Yield of Commercial Essential Oils from Parsley. 1: Herb Oil and Crop Development. Flav Fragr J. 4; 207-219. 1989

Roth L, Daunderer M, Jormann K, Giftpflanzen, Pflanzengifle. 4. Aufl., Ecomed Fachverlag Landsberg/ Lech 1993.

Sökeland J, Phytotherapie in der Urologie. In: *ZPT* 10(1):8. 1989.

Teuscher E, Lindequist U, Biogene Gifte - Biologie, Chemie, Pharmakologie, 2. Aufl., Fischer Verlag Stuttgart 1994.

Teuscher E, Biogene Arzneimittel, 5. Aufl., Wiss. Verlagsges. Stuttgart 1997.

Wagner H, Wiesenauer M, Phytotherapie. Phytopharmaka und pflanzliche Homöopathika, Fischer-Verlag, Stuttgart, Jena, New York, 1995.

Warncke D, *Petroselinum crispum* - Die Gartenpetersilie. In: *ZPT* 15(1):50-58. 1994.

Zheng GQ, Kenney PM, Lam LKT, Myristicin - a potential cancer chemopreventive agent from parsley leaf oil. In: J Agric Food Chem 40(1):107. 1992.

Parsley Piert

Aphanes arvensis

DESCRIPTION

Medicinal Parts: The medicinal part of the plant is the above-ground section.

Flower and Fruit: The flowers are in axillary clusters of 10 to 20. They are encircled by stipules. The sepals are erect, acuminate-ovate and pubescent on the outside and on the margins. They are glabrous on the inside and draw together when the fruit ripens. The fruit is 1 mm long, ovate, keeled, flat, and jug-shaped. The calyx is vertically wrinkled and pubescent.

Leaves, Stem, and Root: The plant is an annual or hardy annual 2 to 30 cm long and dull green in color. The root is thin, branched, and fusiform. The stem is generally branched and decumbent, with short internodes. The leaves have 3 to 5 lobes that are fan- or diamond-shaped. The upper ones are short-petioled. The lower leaves are sessile and usually rough-haired, occasionally only ciliate. The stipules are semi-ovate, indentate-serrate, leafy, and pubescent.

Habitat: Parsley Piert grows in Britain, Europe, northern Africa, and the U.S.

Production: Parsley Piert herb is the above-ground part of *Aphanes arvensis*.

Not to be Confused With: The plants name is a reference to the serrated shape of the leaves; it is not related to the parsley herb.

Other Names: Field Lady's Mantle, Parsley Breakstone, Parsley Piercestone

ACTIONS AND PHARMACOLOGY

COMPOUNDS

Tannin

EFFECTS

The herb is claimed to be effective as a diuretic and a psychostimulant.

INDICATIONS AND USAGE

Unproven Uses: Parsley Piert is used in folk remedies in the treatment of urinary tract disorders, especially kidney and bladder stones, and as a diuretic.

PRECAUTIONS AND ADVERSE REACTIONS

No health hazards or side effects are known in conjunction with the proper administration of designated therapeutic dosages.

DOSAGE

Mode of Administration: The fresh or dried drug and the liquid extract are used.

LITERATURE

Kern W, List PH, Hörhammer L (Hrsg.), Hagers Handbuch der Pharmazeutischen Praxis, 4. Aufl., Bde 1-8, Springer Verlag Berlin, Heidelberg, New York, 1969.

Parsnip

Pastinaca sativa

DESCRIPTION

Medicinal Parts: The medicinal parts are the dried fruit, the dried herb, the dried root, and the fresh, 2-year-old root of cultivated plants.

Flower and Fruit: The golden yellow flowers are in 8- to 12-rayed umbels, which are quite flat and contain androgynous blooms. There is usually no involucre or epicalyx; if present, they consist of 1 or 2 dropping bracts. The petals are even-sized, golden yellow, 0.5 mm long when rolled up and 1 mm wide. The fruit is broad-elliptical, compressed (similar to a lentil), 5 to 7 mm long and 4 to 5.5 mm wide. It is yellow-brownish when ripe. The fruit is marked with oil marks and hollows.

Leaves, Stem, and Root: The plant is a biennial, which grows from 30 to 100 cm. The root is fusiform or tuberous like a carrot or turnip. It is whitish and usually bears only 1 stem. The stem is erect, angular, grooved, short-haired to glabrous, and branched above. The leaves are simple pinnate, glossy above, paler and soft-haired beneath. The cauline leaves are on a long sheath, which is rolled at the edge. The basal leaves are petiolate; the leaflets are ovate-oblong and deeply lobed at the base. The terminal leaflet is 3-lobed and roughly crenate to serrate.

Characteristics: The root tastes like carrot.

Habitat: Parsnip grows wild in most parts of Europe and Asia Minor as far as western Siberia. It is naturalized in the U.S. It is cultivated in Europe, America, Australia, India, China, and southern Africa.

Production: Parsnip root or herb consist of the dried parts of *Pastinaca sativa*.

Not to be Confused With: Other types of root such as Corium, Parsley Roots and the root of Bear's Breech (also known as Hogweed).

Other Names: Bird's Nest, Hart's Eye, Madnep, Queen-Weed

ACTIONS AND PHARMACOLOGY

COMPOUNDS: PARSNIP HERB

Furocoumarins: in particular angelicin, bergaptene, xanthotoxin, imperatorin, psoralen

Volatile oil: chief components cis- and trans-beta-ocimene, trans-beta-farnesene, terpineols, palmitolactone

Flavonoids: including rutin

COMPOUNDS: PARSNIP ROOT

Furocoumarins: in particular angelicin, bergaptene, xanthotoxin, imperatorin, psoralen

Volatile oil (1.9-3.1%): chief components including aliphatic ester, in particular octylbutyrate (29-85%), in certain strains also octylacetate, additionally other esters and some myristicin (depending on strain, 5-65%)

Fatty oil: chief fatty acid petroselic acid (46%)

EFFECTS

No information is available.

INDICATIONS AND USAGE

PARSNIP HERB

Unproven Uses: The herb is used in kidney and gastrointestinal complaints and for digestion problems.

Homeopathic Uses: The herb is used for delirium.

PARSNIP ROOT

Unproven Uses: The root is used for kidney stones, sprains, and fever.

Homeopathic Uses: The root is used for delirium.

PRECAUTIONS AND ADVERSE REACTIONS

No health hazards or side effects are known in conjunction with the proper administration of designated therapeutic dosages. An increase in UV-sensitivity is possible among light-skinned persons (due to phototoxic effect of the furocoumarins).

DOSAGE

PARSNIP HERB

Mode of Administration: Available ground, as a decoction of the dried herb.

Preparation: 1 handful of Parsnip herb cooked in 1 liter of water for 10 minutes.

Daily Dosage: For the first 8 days, drink one wineglassful 3 times daily; during the second week drink one waterglassful. The daily intake can be increased up to 2 liters. The cure takes 4 to 6 weeks.

Homeopathic Dosage: 5 drops, 1 tablet, or 10 globules every 30 to 60 minutes (acute) or 1 to 3 times daily (chronic);

parenterally: 1 to 2 mL sc, acute, 3 times daily; chronic: once daily (HAB34).

PARSNIP ROOT

Daily Dosage: Take 1 teaspoon of freshly grated root, containing 50% plant material, 3 times daily.

Homeopathic Dosage: 5 drops, 1 tablet, or 10 globules every 30 to 60 minutes (acute) or 1 to 3 times daily (chronic); parenterally: 1 to 2 mL sc, acute, 3 times daily; chronic: once daily (HAB34).

LITERATURE

Aberer W. Occupational dermatitis from organically grown parsnip (*Pastinaca sativa L.*). *Contact Dermatitis* 26; 62 1992

Ivie GW, Holt DL, Ivey MC, Natural toxicants in human foods: psoralen an raw and cooked parsnip roots. In: *Science* 213:909. 1981.

Kubeczka KH et al., Über das ätherische Öl der Apiaceae (Umbeliiferae). II. Das ätherische Öl der oberirdischen Teile von *Pastinaca sativa*. In: *PM* 31(2):173-184. 1977.

Stahl E et al., Über das ätherische Öl der Apiaceae (Umbeliiferae). VI.Untersuchungen zum Vorkommen von Chemotypen bei *Pastinaca sativa*. In: *PM* 371(12):49-56. 1979.

Parthenocissus quinquefolia

See American Ivy

Pasque Flower

Pulsatilla pratensis

DESCRIPTION

Medicinal Parts: The medicinal part is the whole fresh plant collected during the flowering season.

Flower and Fruit: The flowers are solitary and almost always nodding. They have 6 campanulate, close, bright-violet tepals. These are usually thickly silky-haired on the outside with revolute tips, and are 1.5 to 3 cm long. The stamens are yellow and numerous; the longer ones are at least two-thirds the length of the tepals. The carpels with the style are as long as the tepals. The ripe fruit is oblong and densely pubescent. The protruding style is up to 6 cm long.

Leaves, Stem, and Root: The plant is a perennial, 7 to 50 cm high with a strong, dark, usually divided, rhizome. The basal leaves usually appear after the flowers and are delicate. They are 3 to 4 pinnate with narrow linear acuminate end sections that, along with the petioles, are thickly white villous. The stems are erect and densely pubescent with 3 whorled high leaves, divided into linear, pubescent tips.

Characteristics: The plant is poisonous.

Habitat: The plant originated in southwestern Europe and now also grows in central and eastern Europe.

Production: Pasque Flower herb consists of the dried, above-ground parts of *Pulsatilla vulgaris* and/or *Pulsatilla pratensis.*

Other Names: Easter Flower, Meadow Anemone, Passe Flower, Pulsatilla, Wind Flower

ACTIONS AND PHARMACOLOGY

COMPOUNDS

Protoanemonine-forming agents: In the freshly harvested plant, presumably the glycoside ranunculin changes enzymatically when the plant is cut into small pieces, and probably also when it is dried, into the pungent, volatile protoanemonine that quickly dimerizes to anemonin. When dried, the plant is not capable of protoanemonine formation.

Triterpene saponins

EFFECTS

In animal experiments, the protoanemonin and anemonin had an antipyretic and motility-inhibiting effect. In the inhibition test, an antibiotic effect was shown. Protoanemonin is a strong local irritant to the mucous membranes and skin.

INDICATIONS AND USAGE

Unproven Uses: Pasque Flower is used for diseases and functional disorders of genital organs; inflammatory and infectious diseases of skin and mucosa; diseases and functional disorders of the gastrointestinal tract and the urinary tract; neuralgia; migraine; and general restlessness. It has also been used to treat iritis, scleritis, cataracts, and glaucoma.

Homeopathic Uses: Homeopathic uses include inflammation of the respiratory tract, digestive organs, female genital organs, bladder, eyes, middle ear, menstruation complaints, problems during pregnancy and nursing, rheumatism, problems with voiding urine, headaches, insomnia, measles, mumps, and depressive states.

CONTRAINDICATIONS

The drug is contraindicated during pregnancy.

PRECAUTIONS AND ADVERSE REACTIONS

General: No health hazards or side effects are known in conjunction with the proper administration of designated therapeutic dosages of the dehydrated drug. Extended skin contact with the freshly harvested, bruised plant (which releases protoanemonine that is severely irritating to skin and mucous membranes) can lead to blister formation and cauterizations that are difficult to heal. If taken internally, severe irritation to the gastrointestinal tract, combined with colic and diarrhea, as well as irritation of the urinary drainage passages, are possible.

OVERDOSAGE

Death by asphyxiation following the intake of large quantities of protoanemonine-forming plants has been observed in animal experiments.

Symptomatic treatment for external contact should consist of mucilaginosa, after irrigation with diluted potassium permanganate solution; in case of internal contact, activated charcoal should follow gastric lavage.

DOSAGE

Mode of Administration: Whole, cut and powdered forms of the drug are used, as are homeopathic forms for internal use.

Daily Dosage: A single dose of a decoction/liquid extract/ infusion is 0.12 to 0.3 g taken 3 times daily. The usual single dose of the drug is 0.2 g; Powder 0.1 to 0.4 g; Tincture: single dose: 0.3 to 1 mL.

Conditions of the inner eye: 1 to 3 pills 3 times daily (from powder and extract at 50 g /75 pills).

Homeopathic Dosage: From D2: 5 to 10 drops, 1 tablet, or 5 to 10 globules 1 to 3 times a day; from D3: 1 suppository 2 to 3 times a day; from D4: 1 mL injection solution sc twice weekly and 3 to 4 nose drops 3 to 5 times a day (HAB1).

LITERATURE

Chan H, But P (Eds.), Pharmacology and Applications of Chinese Materia Medica, Vol 1, World Scientific Singapore 1986.

Frohne D, Pfänder HJ, Giftpflanzen - Ein Handbuch für Apotheker, Toxikologen und Biologen, 4. Aufl., Wiss. Verlags-Ges. Stuttgart 1997.

Hänsel R, Keller K, Rimpler H, Schneider G (Hrsg.), Hagers Handbuch der Pharmazeutischen Praxis, 5. Aufl., Bde 4-6 (Drogen), Springer Verlag Berlin, Heidelberg, New York, 1992-1994.

Madaus G, Lehrbuch der Biologischen Arzneimittel, Bde 1-3, Nachdruck, Georg Olms Verlag Hildesheim 1979.

Pourrat A et al., *Planta Med* 38:289. 1980.

Roth L, Daunderer M, Kormann K, Giftpflanzen, Pflanzengifte, 4. Aufl., Ecomed Fachverlag Landsberg Lech 1993.

Teuscher E, Lindequist U, Biogene Gifte - Biologie, Chemie, Pharmakologie, 2. Aufl., Fischer Verlag Stuttgart 1994.

Wagner H, Wiesenauer M, Phytotherapie. Phytopharmaka und pflanzliche Homöopathika, Fischer-Verlag, Stuttgart, Jena, New York 1995.

Passiflora incarnata

See Passion Flower

Passion Flower

Passiflora incarnata

DESCRIPTION

Medicinal Parts: The medicinal parts are the whole or cut dried herb and the fresh aerial parts. The yellow pulp from the berry is edible. Several other related species also have edible fruits or healing properties.

Flower and Fruit: The axillary pedicle grows up to 8 cm and bears 1 flower. The flowers are androgynous and rayed with a diameter of 5 to 9 cm and have an involucre. The 5 sepals are green on the outside, white on the inside and tough. The 5 petals are white to pale red. There is a secondary corolla inside the petals made up of 4 thread wreaths arranged in rays around the axis of the flower, which are white on the inside and purple on the outside. The ovary has 3 carpels and 3 style branches, which end in a thickened stigma. The 5 stamens are joined at the base and fused to the androgynophor.

Leaves, Stem, and Root: The Passion Flower is a perennial vine on a strong, woody stem reaching up to about 10 m in length. The vine is initially angular, later gray and rounded with longitudinally striated bark. The leaves are alternate, petiolate, serrate, and very finely pubescent. The under surface is hairier than the upper surface. There are bumpy extra-floral nectaries on the leaf blades. Stipules and tendrils grow from the leaf axils.

Habitat: The plant is indigenous to an area from the southeast U.S. to Argentina and Brazil. It is cultivated in Europe as a garden plant.

Production: Passion Flower herb consists of the fresh or dried aerial parts of *Passiflora incarnata*. The flowering shoots are cut 10 to 15 cm above the ground, usually after the formation of the first apple-sized fruit. The harvest is dried in a haydryer or in the air. For a maximum flavonoid content in the flowering shoot, twice yearly harvest is recommended; opinions are not, however, unanimous.

Not to be Confused With: Passiflora caeulea, Passiflora foetida or Passiflora edulis

Other Names: Apricot Vine, Granadilla, Maypop, Passion Vine

ACTIONS AND PHARMACOLOGY

COMPOUNDS

Flavonoids (up to 2.5%): in particular C-glycosyl-flavones, including among others isovitexin-2″-o-glucoside, schaftoside, isoschaftoside, isoorientin, isoorientin-2″-o-glucoside, vicenin-2, lucenin-2

Cyanogenic glycosides: gynocardine (less than 0.1%)

Volatile oil (trace)

The frequently postulated presence of harmaline alkaloids could not be confirmed.

EFFECTS

Passion Flower contains glycosides and in animal tests is hypotensive and stimulates respiration. Sedative or spasmolytic effects could not be definitively proven. The use of the herb for nervous agitation, difficulty falling asleep or nervous gastrointestinal symptoms needs further investigation. A motility-inhibiting effect has been observed in animal tests.

INDICATIONS AND USAGE

Approved by Commission E:

- Nervousness and insomnia

Unproven Uses: Passion Flower is used internally for depressive states such as hysteria, general nervous agitation, insomnia and nervous gastrointestinal complaints. The herb is used externally for hemorrhoids and as a bath additive for nervous agitation.

Homeopathic Uses: Passiflora incarnata is used for insomnia, convulsions, and agitation.

PRECAUTIONS AND ADVERSE REACTIONS

No health hazards or side effects are known in conjunction with the proper administration of designated therapeutic dosages.

DOSAGE

Mode of Administration: As a comminuted herb for tea and other galenic preparations for internal use or as sedative bath additives.

How Supplied:

Capsules – 400 mg

Liquid (alcohol free) – 1:1

Preparation: To make an infusion, pour 150 mL of hot water over 1 teaspoon drug and strain after 10 minutes. To make a rinse for the external treatment of hemorrhoids, put 20 g drug into 200 mL simmering water, strain and use when cooled.

Daily Dosage:

Tea – Pour 150 mL of hot water over 1 teaspoon of the herb and strain after 10 minutes. Drink 2 to 3 times throughout the day and one-half hour before bedtime.

Tincture – 0.5 to 2 mL, 3 times daily.

External use – 20 gm of the herb in 200 mL simmering water. Strain and use when cool as a wash or rinse.

Homeopathic Dosage: 5 drops, 1 tablet, 10 globules every 30 to 60 minutes (acute) or 1 to 3 times daily (chronic); parenterally: 1 to 2 mL SC, acute: 3 times daily; chronic: once a day; ointment: 1 to 2 times daily; 1 suppository 2 to 3 times daily (acute and chronic) (HAB1).

LITERATURE

Anon, Phytotherapeutika: Nachgewiesene Wirkung, aber wirksame Stoffe meist nicht bekannt. In: *DAZ* 137(15):1221-1222. 1997.

Aoyagi N et al., Studies on *Passiflora incarnata* Dry Extract. I. Isolation of Maltol and Pharmacological Action of Maltol and Ethyl Maltol. *Chem Pharm Bull.* 22; 1008-1013. 1974.

Bokstaller S, Schmidt PC. A comparative study on the content of passiflower flavonoids and sesquiterpenes from valerian root extracts in pharmaceutical preparations by HPLC. *Pharmazie* 52 (7); 552-557. 1997

Buchbauer G, Jirovetz L, Jäger W. Passiflora and Lime-blossoms: Motility Effects after Inhalation of the Essential Oils and of Some of the Main Constituents in Animal Experiment. *Arch Pharm* (Weinheim) 325; 247-248. 1992

Buchbauer G, Jirovetz L. Volatile Constituents of the Essential Oil of *Passiflora incarnata L. J Essent Oil* Res. 4; 329-334. 1992

Burkard W et al. Receptor binding studies in the CNS with extracts of *Passiflora incarnata. Pharm Pharmacol Lett.* 7 (1); 25-26. 1997

Caesar W, Passionsblume Kulturhistorische Aspekte einer Arzneipflanze. In: *DAZ* 137(8): 587-93. 1997.

Capasso A, Pinto A. Experimental Investigations of the synergistic-sedative Effect of Passiflora and Kava. *Acta Therapeut.* 21; 127-140. 1995

Chimichi S, Mercati V, Moneti G, Raffaeli A, Toja E. Isolation and Characterization of an Unknown Flavonoide in Dry Extracts from *Passiflora incarnata. Nat Prod Lett.* 11; 225-232. 1998

Eiff MV et al. Hawthorn/Passion Flower Extract and Improvement in physical Exercise Capacity of Patients with Dyspnoe Calss II of the NYHA Functional Classification. *Acta Therapeut.* 20; 47-66. 1994

Hänsel R, Pflanzliche Beruhigungsmittel Möglichkeiten und Grenzen der Selbstmedikation. In: *DAZ* 135(32), 2935-2943. 1995.

Hänsel R, Keller K, Rimpler H, Schneider G (Ed.), Hagers Handbuch der Pharmazeutischen Praxis, 5. Aufl., Bde 4 - 6 (Drogen), Springer Verlag Berlin, Heidelberg, New York, 1992-1994.

Leung AY, Encyclopedia of Common Natural Ingredients Used in Food Drugs and Cosmetics. John Wiley & Sons Inc. New York 1980.

Maluf E, Barros HMT, Frochtengarten ML et al., Assessment of the Hypnotic/Sedative Effects and Toxicity of *Passiflora edulis* Aqueous Extract in Rodents and Humans. *Phytother Res* 5:262-266. 1991

Meier B, *Passiflora incarnata* - Portrait einer Arzneipflanze. Z Phytother 16:115-126. 1995

Meier B, *Passiflorae herba* - pharmazeutische Qualität. Z Phytother 16:90-99. 1995

Moraes M, Vilegas JHY, Lancas FM. Supercritical Fluid Extraction of Glycosylated Flavonoids from Passiflora leaves. Phytochem Anal. 8; 257-260. 1997

Pietta P. Isocratic liquid chromatographic method for the simultaneous determination of *Passiflora incarnata L.* and *Crataegus monogyna* flavonoids in drugs. *J Chromatogr.* 357; 233-238. 1986

Rahman K et al. Flavone-C-Glycosides from *Herba Passiflorae. Sci Pharm.* 65; Suppl.1; S56. 1997

Rahman K et al. Isoscoparin-2'-O-Glucoside from *Passiflora incarnata. Phytochemistry* 45 (5); 1093-1094. 1997

Roth L, Daunderer M, Kormann K, Giftpflanzen, Pflanzengifte. 4. Aufl., Ecomed Fachverlag Landsberg / Lech 1993.

Schulz R, Hänsel R, Rationale Phytotherapie. Springer Verlag Heidelberg 1996.

Speroni E, Minghetti A, Neuropharmacological activity of extracts from *Passiflora incarnata. Planta Med*:488-491. 1988

Steinegger E, Hänsel R, Pharmakognosie. 5. Aufl., Springer Verlag Heidelberg 1992.

Teuscher E, Biogene Arzneimittel. 5. Aufl., Wiss. Verlagsgesellschaft Stuttgart 1997.

Wagner H, Wiesenauer M, Phytotherapie. Phytopharmaka und pflanzliche Homöopathika. Fischer-Verlag, Stuttgart, Jena, New York 1995.

Wichtl M, (Ed) Teedrogen. 4. Aufl., Wiss. Verlagsges. Stuttgart 1997.

Pastinaca sativa

See Parsnip

Patchouli

Pogostemon cablin

DESCRIPTION

Medicinal Parts: The medicinal parts are the young leaves and shoots and the oil extracted from them.

Flower and Fruit: The flowers, which are whitish and often have reddish marks and grow in terminal and axillary spikes.

Leaves, Stem and Root: The plant is a pubescent, perennial herb, which grows from 60 to 90 cm high. The stem is erect and quandrangular, and the leaves are ovate, opposite, and soft.

Characteristics: The ovate leaves have a strong characteristic odor when rubbed. The extracted oil is used in perfumery. The desired characteristics improve with age.

Habitat: The plant is cultivated in tropical and subtropical regions worldwide.

Production: Patchouli oil is extracted from the leaves of *Pogostemon cablin.*

Other Names: Patchouly, Putcha-Pat

ACTIONS AND PHARMACOLOGY

COMPOUNDS

Volatile oil (1.5-4%): chief components are sesquiterpenes, including among others patchouli alcohol (35%), alpha-guaiene (20%), alpha-bulnesen (20%), beta-patchoulen (2%) as well as nordehydropatchoulol (aroma-bearer); Sesquiterpene pyridine alkaloids were isolated from the volatile oil, including patchouli pyridine and epiguai pyridine

EFFECTS

No information is available.

INDICATIONS AND USAGE

There is no known medicinal use. The herb is used in perfumes and cosmetics.

PRECAUTIONS AND ADVERSE REACTIONS

No health hazards or side effects are known in conjunction with the proper administration of designated therapeutic dosages.

DOSAGE

Mode of Administration: It is used only in the perfume and cosmetic industry.

LITERATURE

Kern W, List PH, Hörhammer L (Hrsg.), Hagers Handbuch der Pharmazeutischen Praxis, 4. Aufl., Bde. 1-8, Springer Verlag Berlin, Heidelberg, New York, 1969.

Leung AY, Encyclopedia of Common Natural Ingredients Used in Food Drugs and Cosmetics, John Wiley & Sons Inc., New York 1980.

Paullinia cupana

See Guarana

Pausinystalia yohimbe

See Yohimbe Bark

Peanut

Arachis hypogaea

DESCRIPTION

Medicinal Parts: The oil has medicinal applications.

Flower and Fruit: The flowers are 5 to 7 cm long, monosymmetrical and have a large golden-yellow standard. The flowers have lemon-yellow wings and a pure white carina. They are arranged singularly or in pairs in the leaf axils. They blossom at sunrise and wilt in the same morning, during which time they stretch from 5 to 20 cm and turn down away from the sunlight. After pollination, a meristem develops at the base of the ovary, from which the fruit axis grows. The fruit only starts to grow when the stem is 5 to 10 cm underground, where it grows horizontally. The fruit is a 4 cm long by 1.5 cm thick closed pod with a fibrous, reticulate-wrinkled wall and 1 to 4 large seeds with no endosperm and a thin, red shell.

Leaves, Stem, and Root: The peanut plant is an annual herbaceous 30 to 70 cm high legume, with glabrous, double pinnate leaves, and a decumbent to upright stem.

Habitat: Peanuts were originally indigenous to tropical and subtropical South America. Today, *Arachis hypogaea* is cultivated in all tropical and subtropical regions worldwide except in the rain forests.

Production: Peanut oil is the fatty oil extracted from the husked seeds of *Arachis hypogaea* by means of a ''cold press'' method or by hexane extraction and refining.

Other Names: Arachis, Groundnuts, Monkey Nuts

ACTIONS AND PHARMACOLOGY

COMPOUNDS

Fatty oil: chief fatty acids include oleic acid, linolic acid and palmitin acid. Also present in small quantities are longer-chained fatty acids such as eicosanoic acid and tetracosanoic acid.

EFFECTS

The effect obtained when used as an enema for constipation and in dermatology for dry skin, eczema, and dandruff is achieved primarily from the drug's oiliness, although it has been shown to contain lectines.

INDICATIONS AND USAGE

Unproven Uses: Peanut oil is added to ointments and medicinal oils, and applied rectally in rectal constipation. It is also used in dermatology for crusting and scaling of the scalp (with hair), baby care, and dry skin. Other applications include use as a bath additive for subacute and chronic eczema and for atrophic eczema and ichthyosis.

The pharmaceutical and medical industries use peanut oil as a vehicle for medication in external, enteral, or parenteral preparations; the cosmetics industry uses it in skin, sun, and massage oil. Domestically, it is used as a salad or cooking oil that is said to lower blood cholesterol levels.

Indian Medicine: Peanut oil is used for constipation, neuralgia, and dislocated joints.

PRECAUTIONS AND ADVERSE REACTIONS

No health hazards or side effects are known in conjunction with the proper administration of designated therapeutic dosages.

CONTRAINDICATED

In the presence of peanut allergy.

DOSAGE

Mode of Administration: As an enema, oil, bath additive, and medicinal base component.

Daily Dosage: As a rectal enema, use 130 mL of oil at body temperature. For use in a bath, the recommended concentration is 4 mL per 10 liters of water. Adults should bathe for 15 to 20 minutes 2 to 3 times weekly. Children and babies should bathe for a few minutes 2 to 3 times weekly.

Storage: Protect from light in well-sealed and, if possible, fully filled containers. Oils from different deliveries should not be stored together. Oils with a tocopherol content less than 50 mg/100 mg do not store well.

LITERATURE

Andre F, Andre C, Colin L, Cacaraci F, Cavagna S. Role of new allergens and of allergens consumption in the increased incidence of food sensitizations in France. *Toxicology* 93; 77-83. 1994

Avichezer D, Arnon R, Differential reactivities of the *Arachis hypogaea* (peanut) and Vicia villosa B4 lectins with human ovarian carcinoma cells grown either in vitro or in vivo xenograft model. *FEBS Lett*, 395:103-8, Oct 21, 1996

Bhagya S, Prakash V, Srinivasan KS, Effect of different proteolytic enzymes on the nature of subunit composition of arachins from groundnut (*Arachis hypogaea L.*). *Indian J Biochem Biophys,* 12:154-9, Apr. 1992

Burks AW, et al., Identification and characterization of a second major peanut allergen Ara h II with use of the sera of patients with atopic dermatitis and positive peanut challenge. *J Allergy Clin Immunol*, 90:962-9, Dec. 1992

Calori-Domingues MA, Fonseca H. Laboratory evaluation of chemical control of aflatoxin production in unshelled peanuts (*Arachis hypogaea L.*). *Food Addit Contam,* 12:347-50, May-Jun 1995

Codex Alimentarius Commission, Alinorm 79/17, Report 10th Session. Codex Committee on Fats and Oils, London 1987.

Eghafona NO, Immune responses following cocktails of inactivated measles vaccine and *Arachis hypogaea L.* (groundnut) or *Cocos nucifera L.* (coconut) oils adjuvant. *Vaccine*, 14:1703-6, Dec. 1996

Garcia GM, Stalker HT, Shroeder E, Kochert G, Identification of RAPD SCAR and RFLP markers tightly linked to nematode resistance genes introgressed from *Arachis cardenasii* into *Arachis hypogaea. Genome,* 39:836-45, Oct. 1996

Hänsel R, Keller K, Rimpler H, Schneider G (Hrsg.), Hagers Handbuch der Pharmazeutischen Praxis, 5. Aufl., Bde 4-6 (Drogen): Springer Verlag Berlin, Heidelberg, New York, 1992-1994.

Hourihane JonathanOB Bedwani JB, Dean TP, Warner JO. Randomised, double blind, crossover challenge study of allergenicity of peanut oils in subjects allergic to peanuts. *BMJ.* 314; 1084-1088. 1997

Langkilde NC et al., Human urinary bladder carcinoma glycoconjugates expressing T-(Gal beta(1-3)GalNAc alpha 1-O-R) and T-like antigens: a comparative study using peanut agglutinin, poly- and monoclonal antibodies. *Cancer Res,* 52:5030-6, Sep 15. 1992

Roth L, Daunderer M, Kormann K, Giftpflanzen, Pflanzengifte, 4. Aufl., Ecomed Fachverlag Landsberg Lech 1993.

Sanford GL, Harris-Hooker S, Stimulation of vascular cell proliferation by beta-galactoside specific lectins. *FASEB J,* 52:2912-8, Aug. 1990

Sreenivas A, Sastry PS, A soluble preparation from developing groundnut seeds (*Arachis hypogaea*) catalyzes de novo synthesis of long chain fatty acids. *Indian J Biochem Biophys,* 14:213-7, Aug. 1995

Srivastava R, Rajput YS, Khare SK, Tyagi R, Gupta MN, Purification and characterization of an acid phosphatase from *Arachis hypogaea. Biochem Mol Biol Int,* 224:949-56, Apr 1995.

Steinegger E, Hänsel R, Pharmakognosie, 5. Aufl., Springer Verlag Heidelberg 1992.

Swamy MJ, Gupta D, Mahanta SK, Surolia A, Further characterization of the saccharide specificity of peanut (*Arachis hypogaea*) agglutinin. *Carbohydr Res*, 137:59-67, Jun 25. 1991

Teuscher E, Biogene Arzneimittel, 5. Aufl., Wiss. Verlagsges. Stuttgart 1997.

Urtz BE, Elkan GH, Purification and partial characterization of acyl carrier proteins from developing oil seeds of pisa (*Actinodaphne hookeri*) and ground nut (*Arachis hypogaea*). *Indian J Biochem Biophys,* 224:137-46, Jun. 1995

Zhang X, Ling L, Dai R, Constituents of the seed coat of *Arachis hypogaea L. Chung Kuo Chung Yao Tsa Chih,* 137:356-8 384, Jun. 1990

Pear

Pyrus communis

DESCRIPTION

Medicinal Parts: The medicinal part is the fruit.

Flower and Fruit: The fleshy fruit is typically smaller near the stem and larger at the apical end, with a relatively tough skin. The core has a number of carpels, which are large and edible. The seeds are pointed at one end and rounded at the other. When ripe, they are dark brown to black, glabrous and about 0.5 cm long.

Leaves, Stem, and Root: The pear is a tree, up to 20 m tall, with a long, clavate crown. The bark is dark brown to black and broken into square plates. The glabrous or slightly pubescent branches are glossy brown or thorny. The leaves are 2 to 8 cm long, ovate-round, acuminate, tough, and serrate. The ribs are protruding.

Habitat: The pear tree grows mainly in the temperate regions of the Northern Hemisphere.

Production: Pears are the fruit of *Pyrus communis*.

ACTIONS AND PHARMACOLOGY

COMPOUNDS

Fruit acids: malic acid (0.06-0.1%), additionally citric acid, quinic acid

Cyanogenic glycosides: amygdalin (only in the seeds)

Aromatic substances: including (E,Z)-2,4-deca-dien-(E)-2-octen and -(Z)-4-decenacylethylester, acetic acid hexylester

Caffeic acid derivatives: in particular 5-caffeoyl quinic acid

Pectin

EFFECTS

In folk remedies, Pear is said to be astringent and cooling.

INDICATIONS AND USAGE

Unproven Uses: Pear is used in the treatment of mild digestive disorders, while its syrup is used as a diuretic and laxative.

PRECAUTIONS AND ADVERSE REACTIONS

No health hazards or side effects are known in conjunction with the proper administration of designated therapeutic dosages.

DOSAGE

Mode of Administration: Fresh fruit (as food)

LITERATURE

Belitz HD, Grosch W, Lehrbuch der Lebensmittelchemie, 4. Aufl., Springer Verlag Berlin, Heidelberg, New York 1992.

Kern W, List PH, Hörhammer L (Hrsg.), Hagers Handbuch der Pharmazeutischen Praxis, 4. Aufl., Bde 1-8, Springer Verlag Berlin, Heidelberg, New York, 1969.

Stahly EA, Buchanan EA. High-Performance Liquid Chromatographic Procedure for Separation and Quantification of Zeatin and Zeatin Riboside from Pears, Peaches and Apples. *J Chromatogr*. 235; 453-459. 1982

Pellitory

Anacyclus pyrethrum

DESCRIPTION

Medicinal Parts: The medicinal part of the plant is the root.

Flower and Fruit: Each stem bears a 1-cm wide flower. The bracts are fused. The ray florets are white and tinged purple beneath. The disc florets are pointed. The fruit has transparent wings.

Leaves, Stem, and Root: Pellitory is a perennial grass plant whose thickened, hollow stems grow a short distance along the ground before turning upward. The plant grows to about 45 cm high and has tough double-pinnate leaves. The root is almost cylindrical, easily twisted, tapered, and crowned with a tuft of gray hair. The outside is brown and fissured with shiny black markings.

Habitat: The plant grows in North Africa and is cultivated in the Mediterranean.

Production: Pellitory root is the root of *Anacyclus pyrethrum*.

Other Names: Pellitory of Spain, Pyrethre, Pyrethrum, Roman Pellitory, Spanish Camomile

ACTIONS AND PHARMACOLOGY

COMPOUNDS

Alkamides: including deca-2, 4-dien acid-isobutylamide, anacycline, dehydroanacycline

Lignans: including sesamine

Inulin (fructosan)

Tannins

EFFECTS

Application to the skin stimulates the nerve ends, resulting in redness and irritation (hot, burning sensation). Pellitorin (rather than anacycline) is the local irritant. The drug, which contains alkamides (pellitorin) and tannins, had an inhibitory effect in vitro on cyclo-oxygenase and 5-lipoxygenase (affecting prostaglandin metabolism), and also an antimicrobial, insecticidal and molluscicidal effect. In tests on animals and humans, a local anesthetic effect was observed indicating ptery mandibular block with infiltration of the long buccal nerves after extraction of mandibular molars.

INDICATIONS AND USAGE

Unproven Uses: Pellitory is used externally for rheumatic conditions, the treatment of toothache. Pellitory is used internally as a tonic to aid digestion and as an insecticide.

Indian Medicine: Used as a gargle for toothache and as a powder mixed with honey for epilepsy.

PRECAUTIONS AND ADVERSE REACTIONS

No health hazards or side effects are known in conjunction with the proper administration of designated therapeutic dosages.

OVERDOSAGE

Signs of irritation are possible in connection with overdoses due to the mucous-membrane-stimulating character of the alkamides.

DOSAGE

Mode of Administration: There is mention of use as a gargle and as a powder, but no precise information is available.

LITERATURE

Kern W, List PH, Hörhammer L (Hrsg.), Hagers Handbuch der Pharmazeutischen Praxis, 4. Aufl., Bde 1-8, Springer Verlag Berlin, Heidelberg, New York, 1969.

Patel VK et al. A Clinical Appraisal of *Anacyclus pyrethrum* Root Extract in Dental Patients. *Phytother Res*. 6; 158-159. 1992

Pellitory-of-the-Wall

Parietaria officinalis

DESCRIPTION

Medicinal Parts: The medicinal part is the herb.

Flower and Fruit: The small, green, sessile flowers grow in axillary racemes and bloom throughout the summer. The bracteoles are free and shorter than the calyx. The filaments of the stamens are strangely jointed and so elastic that when they are touched before the flower has opened, they uncoil from their rolled-up position and distribute the pollen. The achaenes are black.

Leaves, Stem, and Root: The plant is a perennial, heavily branched, bushy, and leafy. It grows to 70 cm high. It has a reddish hard stem and narrow petiolate, ovate-lanceolate or elliptical, long-acuminate leaves that are 2.5 to 5 cm long. The leaf stalk is shorter than the leaf blade. The stem and the undersurface of the leaf ribs are pubescent with short, soft hairs. The upper surface of the leaves is almost glabrous and the ribs sunken.

Habitat: The herb is indigenous to Europe.

Production: Pellitory-of-the-Wall is the aerial part of *Parietaria officinalis.*

Other Names: Lichwort

ACTIONS AND PHARMACOLOGY

COMPOUNDS

Flavonoids: including among others kaempferol-, quercetin- and isorhamnetin-3-glucosides, -3-sophoroside, -3-rutinosides, -3-neohesperidosides

Caffeic acid derivatives: including caffeoyl malic acid

Bitter principles

EFFECTS

The drug is a mild diuretic.

INDICATIONS AND USAGE

The herb is used to treat diseases of the urinary tract.

PRECAUTIONS AND ADVERSE REACTIONS

No health hazards or side effects are known in conjunction with the proper administration of designated therapeutic dosages.

DOSAGE

Mode of Administration: The herb is obsolete as a drug, but is occasionally used in commercial medicinal preparations.

LITERATURE

Budzianowski J et al., *J Nat Prod* 48(2):336. 1985

Hegnauer R, Chemotaxonomie der Pflanzen, Bde 1-11, Birkhäuser Verlag Basel, Boston, Berlin 1962-1997.

Kahlert H, Weber B Teppke M, Wahl R, Cromwell O, Fiebig H. Characterization of Major Allergens of Parietaria officinalis. *Int Arch Allergy Immunol.* 109; 141-149. 1996

Kern W, List PH, Hörhammer L (Hrsg.), Hagers Handbuch der Pharmazeutischen Praxis, 4. Aufl., Bde. 1-8, Springer Verlag Berlin, Heidelberg, New York, 1969.

Pennyroyal

Mentha pulegium

DESCRIPTION

Medicinal Parts: The medicinal parts are the essential oil extracted from the fresh plant, the dried aerial parts, and the whole plant.

Flower and Fruit: The flowers are in axillary, loose, and globular false whorls. The calyx is cylindrical/funnel-shaped, grooved, and is awned in the tube. The lower tips are awl-shaped, the upper ones shorter and wider. The upper lip has 3 tips and is curved slightly upward. The straight lower lip is divided in two. The corolla is violet, glabrous or downy. It has a tube, which suddenly widens in a sacklike manner and has a slightly developed ring of hair as well as lobes. These extend well beyond the calyx. The nutlets are glossy brown.

Leaves, Stem, and Root: Pennyroyal is a glabrous-to-downy perennial, which grows from 10 to 40 cm high. The stem is ascendent or decumbent, branched, and slightly downy. The leaves are elliptical to narrow ovate-elliptical, short-petioled, entire-margined, translucently glandular punctate with 1 to 3 pairs of shallow teeth and curved pinnate ribs.

Characteristics: Strongly aromatic.

Habitat: The plant thrives in western, southern and central Europe, in Asia as far as Turkmenistan, Iran, in the Arab countries, and Ethiopia. It is naturalized in America.

Production: Pennyroyal is the flowering herb of *Mentha pulegium.* The plants are harvested during the flowering season and dried.

Other Names: Lurk-in-the-Ditch, Mosquito Plant, Pulegium, Piliolerial, Pudding Grass, Run-by-the-Ground, Squaw Balm, Squawmint, Tickweed

ACTIONS AND PHARMACOLOGY

COMPOUNDS

Volatile oil (1-2%): chief constituents D-pulegone (60-90%), menthone (10-20%), isomenthone (2-10%), additionally including among others piperitone, neoisomenthylacetate

Tannins: presumably rosmaric acid

Flavonoids: including among others diosmin, hesperidin

EFFECTS

Pennyroyal oil (main component pulegone) has an antimicrobial and insecticidal effect. There is no scientific proof of the described effects.

INDICATIONS AND USAGE

Unproven Uses: The drug is used for digestive disorders, liver and gallbladder disorders, amenorrhea, gout, colds, and increased micturation; externally, it is used for skin diseases.

PRECAUTIONS AND ADVERSE REACTIONS

General: European Pennyroyal oil is hepatotoxic in effect. Acute poisonings are not to be feared in conjunction with the proper administration of designated therapeutic dosages of the foliage drug. Still, because of its hepatotoxicity, it is recommended that the drug not be used.

Pregnancy: In high doses, Pennyroyal has been reported to cause abortion. Use in pregnancy is not recommended.

OVERDOSAGE

Severely acute poisonings have been observed following administration of 5 g of the volatile oil. Vomiting, blood-pressure elevation, anesthetic-like paralysis, and death through respiratory failure have been reported following larger dosages. Cases of death have been described following misuse of the volatile oil to induce abortion.

DOSAGE

See: Precautions and Adverse Reactions.

Mode of Administration: Internally as a ground drug, an extract and a tea. The oil is applied topically.

Daily Dosage: The average daily internal dose of the dried drug is 1 to 4 g, taken 3 times daily. Pennyroyal is prepared as an infusion. Drink one cupful at a time during the course of the day. Extract: 1 to 4 mL, 3 times daily.

LITERATURE

Frohne D, Pfänder HJ, Giftpflanzen - Ein Handbuch für Apotheker, Toxikologen und Biologen, 4. Aufl., Wiss. Verlags-Ges. Stuttgart 1997.

Hänsel R, Keller K, Rimpler H, Schneider G (Hrsg.), Hagers Handbuch der Pharmazeutischen Praxis, 5. Aufl., Bde 4-6 (Drogen), Springer Verlag Berlin, Heidelberg, New York, 1992-1994.

Lewin L, Gifte und Vergiftungen, 6. Aufl., Nachdruck, Haug Verlag, Heidelberg 1992.

Madaus G, Lehrbuch der Biologischen Arzneimittel, Bde 1-3, Nachdruck, Georg Olms Verlag Hildesheim 1979.

Miller EC et al., *Cancer Res* 43: 1124. 1983

Roth L, Daunderer M, Kormann K, Giftpflanzen, Pflanzengifte, 4. Aufl., Ecomed Fachverlag Landsberg Lech 1993.

Steinegger E, Hänsel R, Pharmakognosie, 5. Aufl., Springer Verlag Heidelberg 1992.

Peppermint

Mentha piperita

DESCRIPTION

Medicinal Parts: The medicinal parts are the oil extracted from the aerial parts of the flowering plant, the dried leaves and flowering branch tips, the fresh flowering plant, and the whole plant.

Flower and Fruit: The flowers are false spikes with numerous inconspicuous bracts. The calyx is tubular with a ring of hair. The corolla is violet, glabrous inside and has an almost even margin divided into four parts.

Leaves, Stem, and Root: The plant is a perennial that reaches 50 to 90 cm high. The usually branched stems are normally glabrous. They are gray-tomentose and are often tinged violet. The leaves are short-petioled, oblong-ovate, and serrate. The plant has above- and underground runners.

Habitat: Common in Europe and the U.S., usually cultivated.

Production: Peppermint oil consists of the essential oil of *Mentha piperita* obtained by aqueous steam distillation from freshly harvested, flowering springs and preparations of same. Peppermint leaves consist of the fresh or dried leaf of Peppermint as well as its preparations.

Peppermint leaf is harvested several times a year. The maximum leaf harvest and highest oil content is shortly before the flowering season. The harvest is dried mechanically on drying belts at a temperature of 42° C. Peppermint is harvested mechanically shortly after flowering and dried in the field.

Not to be Confused With: Peppermint should not be confused with rectified mint oil. Sometimes adulterated by increasing the ester content with racemic menthol acetate.

Other Names: Brandy Mint, Lamb Mint

ACTIONS AND PHARMACOLOGY

COMPOUNDS: PEPPERMINT LEAVES

Volatile oil: chief components: menthol (35-45%), menthone (15-20%), menthyl acetate (3-5%), neomenthol (2.5-3.5%), isomenthone (2-3%), menthofurane (2-7%), additionally including among others limonene, pulegone, alpha- and beta-pinene, trans-sabinene hydrate

Caffeic acid: including among others, rosmaric acid

Flavonoids: apigenine-, diosmetin- and luteolin glycosides, free lipophile methoxylized flavone including among others, xanthomicrol, gardenine D

COMPOUNDS: PEPPERMINT OIL

Chief components: menthol (35-45%), menthone (15-20%), menthyl acetate (3-5%), neomenthol (2.5-3.5%), isomenthone (2-3%), menthofurane (2-7%), additionally including among others limonene, pulegone, alpha- and beta-pinene, trans-sabinene hydrate

Labiatentannins: including, among others rosmaric acid

Flavonoids: apigenine-, diosmetin- and luteolin glycosides, free lipophile methoxylized flavone including, among others xanthomicrol, gardenine D

EFFECTS: PEPPERMINT LEAVES

The drug has a spasmolytic effect on the smooth muscle of the digestive tract. It also has antiviral, antimicrobial, diuretic, cholagogic, carminative, and mild sedative effects.

EFFECTS: PEPPERMINT OIL

It is a carminative, cholagogue, antibacterial, insecticidal, and secretolytic agent; it also has a cooling effect on the skin.

Human clinical studies have demonstrated enteric-coated Peppermint Oil is possibly effective in reducing the abdominal symptoms of irritable bowel syndrome. Clinical studies demonstrated an effective reduction in spasms during barium enemas and endoscopies, relieving dyspepsia, and alleviating headaches. In comparison studies, Peppermint Oil was equally effective as acetaminophen in relieving headaches and improved symptoms of irritable bowel syndrome (Lui et al, 1997).

Analgesic Effects: Both 5-hydroxytryptamine (serotonin) and substance P play an important role in the nociceptive regulation of the trigemino-vascular system which is the origin of many headaches. Peppermint Oil is therefore believed to act locally at the origin of pain by modifying pain receptor sensitivity, thus exhibiting analgesic activity. Preparations containing Peppermint with or without eucalyptus were superior in pain reduction and overall well-being to preparations containing eucalyptus and ethanol, or ethanol alone (Goebel & Schmidt, 1995; Goebel et al, 1995; Goebel et al, 1994).

Dyspeptic Effects: A combination product of Peppermint and caraway oil showed positive effects in reducing multiple gastrointestinal complaints (May et al, 1996).

Spasmolytic Effects: In a double-blind, placebo-controlled, randomized study, 141 patients using Peppermint experienced fewer spasms when undergoing a barium enema (Sparks et al, 1995).

CLINICAL TRIALS

A 2007 review of evidence reported that while results from clinical trials are somewhat mixed, most evidence points to modest effectiveness of enteric-coated Peppermint Oil in alleviating common symptoms of irritable bowel syndrome. Clinical trials to date also show a trend for mild effectiveness in reducing flatulence, abdominal pain, and distension in particular. Evidence also indicates that Peppermint Oil is ''probably effective'' for tension headache and for non-ulcer dyspepsia when taken in combination with caraway oil. The trials for tension headache used topically applied Peppermint Oil, with a randomized, controlled study showing a 10% reduction in headache intensity after 15 minutes in 41 patients with 164 headaches. Limited data show effectiveness for the herb's ability to reduce spasm during gastrointestinal procedures (given by enema). Caution is merited in following dosage directions carefully given the significant toxicity observed at higher dosage levels (Kliger, 2007).

Antispasmodic Effects

A single-blind, randomized, controlled study evaluated the efficacy of peppermint oil (PO) for double-contrast barium meal examination (DCBM) without other antispasmodics. A total of 255 individuals were randomly chosen to receive PO by mouth in addition to a barium suspension mixture before undergoing DCBM, while 215 sex- and age-matched controls also underwent the procedure. Results revealed PO orally administered reduced spasm of the esophagus, lower stomach, and duodenal bulb, inhibited barium flow to the distal duodenum, and improved diagnostic quality without using other antispasmodics. There was no significant difference in subject acceptance between PO and control groups (Mizuno et al, 2006).

Irritable Bowel Syndrome

Four weeks of treatment with Peppermint Oil (two enteric-coated capsules twice daily) resulted in improvement of abdominal symptoms in people with irritable bowel syndrome in this prospective, randomized, double-blind, and placebo-controlled trial. To rule out the possible distortion of results due to the presence of small intestinal bacterial overgrowth, lactose intolerance, or celiac disease, the 57 patients with irritable bowel syndrome were selected in part because they did not have these issues. Changes in such symptoms as abdominal bloating, pain and discomfort, feeling of incomplete evacuation, constipation, diarrhea, passage of gas or mucus, and urgency at defecation were evaluated. At week four, 75% of the patients randomized to Peppermint oil had a more than 50% reduction in their symptom score total, while 38% of those in the placebo group had such a reduction—a significant difference (P<0.009) (Cappello, 2007).

A literature search was performed evaluating 16 clinical trials that investigated 180-200 mg enteric-coated peppermint oil (PO) in irritable bowel syndrome (IBS) or recurrent abdominal pain in children (one study). A total of 651 patients were enrolled. Nine out of 16 studies were randomized, double-blind, crossover trials with (n=5) or without (n=4) run in and/or washout periods. Five had a randomized, double-blind, parallel group design and two were open label studies. PO was compared to placebo in 12 and to anticholinergics in three studies. Eight out of 12 placebo controlled studies showed statistically significant effects in favor of PO. Adverse effects were generally mild and transient, with PO causing heartburn and anal/perianal burning or discomfort, while anticholinergics caused dry mouth and blurred vision. Results showed anticholinergics and 5HT3/4-ant/agonists did not offer superior improvement rates compared to PO (Grigoleit & Grigoleit, 2005).

Dyspepsia, Nonulcerative

In a double-blind, randomized, placebo-controlled, multicenter, 4-week trial, patients (n=39) with nonulcerative dyspepsia complaining of moderate-to-severe pain were given a combination product of peppermint and caraway oil. Both primary and secondary endpoint analyses concluded the superiority of the peppermint/caraway preparation with respect to pain intensity and pathological picture as well as cardinal symptomology and other subjective gastrointestinal complaints. The dosage was 3 capsules daily for 4 weeks of Enteroplant® (90 mg Peppermint Oil and 50 mg caraway oil). After 2 weeks, 42% of patients receiving active treatment were pain free (1 patient (5%) in the placebo group) (p=0.002). Results were similar after 4 weeks (63.2% versus 25%, respectively). At the end of 4 weeks, moderate-to-severe pain was still reported in

10.6% of the treatment group and 55% of the placebo group. Change in pain intensity (decrease in pain) was significantly greater in the treatment group than the placebo group (84.2% versus 50% at 15 days, p=0.002; 89.9% versus 45% at 29 days, p< 0.015). Overall, 95.7% of actively treated patients reported improvement after 4 weeks, as compared to 55% in the placebo group (May et al, 1996).

Gallbladder Disease

In an uncontrolled study, 19 of 31 patients with common bile duct stones were given a terpene preparation called Rowachol®. All patients initially took up to 7 capsules daily. Patients later took 3 capsules or less. Eight (42%) had total stone disappearance within 3 to 48 months. Rowachol and bile acid were given to 15 (including 3 of the above). Within 18 months, 11 (73%) had total stone resolution (Somerville et al, 1985).

INDICATIONS AND USAGE

PEPPERMINT LEAVES

Approved by Commission E:

- Cramplike complaints of the gastrointestinal tract, as well as the gall bladder and bile ducts
- Symptomatic treatment of digestion problems (e.g., dyspepsia, flatulence, gastritis, enteritis)

The drug is used for convulsive complaints of the gastrointestinal tract as well as gallbladder and bile ducts.

Unproven Uses: In folk use, peppermint is utilized for nausea, vomiting, morning sickness, respiratory infections, dysmenorrhea, and colds.

Homeopathic Uses: The drug is used for colds.

PEPPERMINT OIL

Approved by Commission E (for internal application):

- Cramplike complaints in the upper gastrointestinal tract and the bile ducts
- Irritable bowel
- Catarrh of the upper respiratory tract
- Inflammation of the upper mucosa

Approved by Commission E (for external application):

- Muscle pain and neuralgia

The drug is used internally for cramps of the upper gastrointestinal tract and bile ducts, irritable colon, catarrhs of the respiratory tract, and inflammation of the oral and pharyngeal mucosa.

CONTRAINDICATIONS

PEPPERMINT LEAVES

Contraindicated in cases of gallstones.

PEPPERMINT OIL

Contraindications for the internal administration of the drug include occlusion of the biliary ducts, gallbladder inflammation and severe liver damage. Gallstone carriers could experience colic due to the cholagogic effect.

Pediatric Use: Preparations containing the oil should not be applied to the faces of infants or small children, particularly not in the nasal area (glottal spasm or bronchial spasm up to asthma-like attacks or even possible respiratory failure).

PRECAUTIONS AND ADVERSE REACTIONS

PEPPERMINT LEAVES

No health hazards are known in conjunction with the proper administration of designated therapeutic dosages. Gallstone carriers could experience colic due to the cholagogic effect.

Pregnancy: Excess use contraindicated in early pregnancy due to its emmenagogue effect (Brinker, 1998).

PEPPERMINT OIL

The volatile oil possesses a weak potential for sensitization due to its menthol content. Use is not recommended in the presence of a tendency to gastroesophageal reflux. The intake can lead to gastric complaints in susceptible persons. Hypersensitivity reactions may include skin rash, abdominal pain, heartburn, and perianal burning. Do not apply topical peppermint to open skin areas (Fetrow, 1999).

Pregnancy: Excess use contraindicated in early pregnancy due to its emmenagogue effect (Brinker, 1998).

DRUG INTERACTIONS

MODERATE RISK

Calcium channel blockers: Concurrent use of Peppermint Oil and calcium channel blockers may result in reduced effectiveness of calcium channel blockers. *Clinical Management:* Caution is advised when using Peppermint Oil with calcium channel blockers until this drug-herb interaction has been better characterized.

POTENTIAL INTERACTIONS

Peppermint tea extract inhibited cytochrome P450 1A2 and 2E in rats. Caution is advised if Peppermint is used with other drugs metabolized by these enzymes (Maliakal & Wanwimolruk, 2001).

DOSAGE

PEPPERMINT LEAVES

Mode of Administration: Comminuted herb for infusions, extracts of Peppermint leaves for internal use.

Preparation: To prepare an infusion, pour 150 mL of hot water over 1 teaspoon of the drug, strain after 10 minutes (one study has shown that the maximum level of menthol and methon is present after this time).

Tincture: leave 200 parts leaves in spirit of wine for 10 days (shaken at intervals), which is filtered after this time (EB6).

Daily Dosage: The average daily dose of the drug is 3 to 6 g. The average daily dose of the tincture (1:10) is 5 to 15 g. Tea: 1 cup to be consumed 3 to 4 times a day between meals. Infusion: 2 to 4 g drug, drink slowly in sips while warm.

Homeopathic Dosage: 5 drops, 1 tablet, or 10 globules every 30 to 60 minutes (acute) or 1 to 3 times a day (chronic); parenterally: 1 to 2 mL sc acute, 3 times daily; chronic: once a day (HAB34).

Storage: Peppermint should be stored cool and dry and protected from light in nonplastic containers.

PEPPERMINT OIL

Mode of Administration: The essential oil and the galenic preparations are for internal and external use.

Daily Dosage: Only use at recommended doses. Significant toxicity can occur at higher doses. The average daily internal dose is 6 to 12 drops; inhalation, 3 to 4 drops in hot water; for irritable bowel, daily dose: 0.6 mL; single dose: 0.2 mL in enteric coated form. The therapeutic dosage range studied in most recent clinical trials for irritable bowel syndrome was 0.2 mL to 0.4 mL taken three times a day in enteric-coated capsules (Kliger, 2007).

Externally, a few drops rubbed into the affected skin areas several times a day (2 to 4 times). For young children: Rub 5 to 15 drops on the chest and back. The drug is available as semisolid and oily preparations (5 to 20%); aqueous-ethanol preparations (5 to 10%); nasal ointments with 1 to 5% essential oil.

Storage: Peppermint should be stored cool and dry and protected from light in nonplastic containers.

LITERATURE

BAnz (Federal German Gazette) No. 23; published Nov 30, 1985; revised Mar 13, 1990 and Sep 1, 1990.

BAnz (Federal German Gazette) No. 50; published Mar 13, 1986.

Bowen ICH, Cubbin IJ, *Mentha piperita* and *Mentha spicata*. In: *De Smet PAGM* 1993.

Bromm B, Scharein E, Darsow U, Ring J. Effects of menthol and cold on histamine-induced itch and skin reactions in man. *Neuroscience Lett* 187:157-160, 1995.

Burrow A, Eccles R, Jones AS. The effects of camphor, eucalyptus and menthol vapor on nasal resistance to airflow and nasal sensation. Acta Otolaryng (Stockholm) 96: 157-161, 1983.

Capello G, Spezzaferro M, Grossi L, et al. Peppermint oil (Mintoil®) in the treatment of irritable bowel syndrome: A prospective double blind placebo-controlled randomized trial. *Dig Liver Dis*; 39(6): 530-536. 2007.

Carling L, Svedberg L & Hultsen S. Short-term treatment of the irritable bowel syndrome: a placebo-controlled trial of Peppermint oil against hyoscyamine. Opusc Med; 34:55-57, 1989.

Clark M, *Econ Bot* 35:59, 1981.

Dew MJ, Evans BK, Rhodes J. Peppermint oil for the irritable bowel syndrome: a multicentre trial. *Br J Clin Pract* 38:394-395, 1984.

Eccles R, Jones AS. The effects of menthol on nasal resistance to airflow. *J Laryngology Otology* 97:705-709, 1982.

Eccles R, Lancashire B, Tolley NS. Experimental studies on nasal sensation of airflow. *Acta Otolaryngol* (Stockholm) 103:303-306, 1987.

Eccles R, Morris S, Tolley NS. The effects of nasal anaesthesia upon nasal sensation of airflow. *Acta Otolaryngol* (Stockholm) 106:152-155, 1988.

Fetrow C & Avila J: Professional's Handbook of Complementary and Alternative Medicine. Springhouse, MO: Springhouse Corporation: 433-437, 1999.

Fintelmann V. Möglichkeiten und Grenzen der Phytotherapie bei Magen-Darm- Krankheiten. In: *ZPT* 10(1):29. 1989.

Fintelmann V. Phytopharmaka in der Gastroenterologie. In: *ZPT* 15(3):137. 1994.

Freise J & Kohler S. Peppermint oil-caraway oil fixed combination in non-ulcer dyspepsia– comparison of the effects of enteric preparations. In: *Pharmazie*; 54(3):210-215, 1999.

Friederich HC, Vogelsberg, H, Neiss A. Ein Beitrag zur Bewertung von intern wirksamen Venenpharmaka. *Z Hautkrankheiten* 53 (11):369-374, 1978.

Göbel H, Schmidt G. Effekt von Pfefferminz- und Eukalyptusölpräparationen in experimentellen Kopfschmerzmodellen. Z Phytother 16:23-33, 1995a.

Göbel H, Schmidt G, Dworschak M, Stolze H, Heuss D. Essential plant oils and headache mechanisms. *Phytomedicine* 2:93-102. 1995.

Göbel H, Schmidt G, Dworschak M, Stolze H, Heuss D. Essential plant oils and headache mechanisms. *Phytomedicine* 2:93-103, 1995b.

Göbel H, Schmidt G. Effekt von Pfefferminz- und Eukalyptusölpräparationen in experimentellen *Kopfschmerzmodellen*. In: ZPT 16(1):23-33. 1995.

Göbel H, Schmidt G, Soyka D. Effect of peppermint and eucalyptus oil preparations on neurophysiological and experimental algesimetric headache parameters. In: *Cephalalgia* 14:228-234, 1994.

Gräfe AK. Besonderheiten der Arzneimitteltherapie im Säuglings- und Kindesalter. In: *PZ* 140(30):2659-2667. 1995.

Grigoleit HG, Grigoleit P. Peppermint oil in irritable bowel syndrome. *Phytomedicine*; 12(8) 601-616. 2006.

Hamann KF, Bonkowsky V. Minzölwirkung auf die Nasenschleimhaut von Gesunden. *Dtsch Apoth Z* 125:429-436, 1987.

Harries N et al. *J Clin Pharm* 2:171, 1978.

Hawthorn M, Ferranthe J, Luchowski E, Rutledge A, Wie XY, Triggle DJ. The actions of peppermint oil and menthol on calcium channel dependent processes in intestinal, neuronal and cardiac preparations. *Aliment Pharmacol Therap* 2:101-118, 1988.

Hefendehl FW, Murray MJ. *Planta Med* 23:101, 1973.

Heinze A. Oleum menthae piperitae: Wirkmechanismen und klinische Effektivität bei Kopfschmerz vom Spannungstyp. In: Loew D, Rietbrock N (Hrsg) Phytopharmaka in Forschung und klinischer Anwendung. Steinkopff Verlag, Darmstadt, S 177-184, 1995c.

Herrmann EC Jr., Kucera LS, Antiviral substances in plants of the mint family (Labiatae). III. Peppermint (*Mentha piperita*) and other mint plants. In: *Proc Soc Exp Biol Med* 124:874-878. 1995.

Kantarev N, Peicev P. *Folia Med* 19(1):41, 1977.

Keller K, Hänsel R, Chandler RF, (eds). Adverse Effects of Herbal Drugs 1. Springer Verlag, Berlin Heidelberg New York, S 171-178.

Kligler B, Chaudhary S. Peppermint Oil. *Am Fam Physician*; 75:1027-30. 2007.

Kucera LS, Hermann EC Jr. *Proc Soc Exp Biol Med* 124:865 et 874, 1967.

Leiber B, Dieskussionsbemerkung. In: Dost FH, Leiber B (Hrsg) Menthol and menthol-containing external remedies. *Thieme Stuttgart* 1967, S. 22, 1967.

Leicester RJ, Hunt RH. Peppermint oil to reduce solonic spasm during endoscopy. In: *Lancet*: 989, 1982.

Liu JH, Chen GH, Yeh HZ et al., Enteric-coated peppermint oil capsules in the treatment of irritable bowel syndrome: a prospective, randomized trial. In: *J Gastroenterol*; 32(6):765-768, 1997.

May B, Kuntz H, Keiser M et al. Efficacy of a fixed peppermint oil/caraway oil combination in non-ulcer dyspepsia. In: *Arzneimittelorschung*; 46:1149-1153, 1996.

Mizuno S, Kato K, Ono Y, et al. Oral peppermint oil is a useful antispasmodic for double-contrast barium meal examination. *J Gastroenterol Hepatol*; 21(8): 1297-1301. 2006.

Nash P, Gould SR, Barnardo DE. Peppermint oil does not relieve the pain of irritable bowel syndrome. *Br J Clin Pract* 40:292-293, 1986.

Nöller HG. Elektronische Messungen an der Nasenschleimhaut unter Mentholwirkung. In: Menthol and menthol-containung external remedies. Thieme, Stuttgart, S 146-153, 179, 1967.

Rees WDW, Evans BK, Rhoes J. Treating irritable bowel syndrome with peppermint oil. *BMJ* II:835-838, 1979.

Reuter HD. Pflanzliche Gallentherapeutika (Teil I) und (Teil II). In: *ZPT* 16(1):13-20 u. 77-89. 1995.

Rohmeder J. Menthol: Verum statt Racemicum. In: *PZ* 139(4):300. 1994.

Sommerville KW, Richmond CR, Bell GD. Delayed release peppermint oil capsules (Colpermin) for the spastic colon syndrome: a pharmacokinetic study. In: *Br J Clin Pharmac* 18:638-640, 1984.

Somerville KW, Ellis WR, Whitten BH, et al., Stones in the common bile duct: experience with medical dissolution therapy. In: *Postgrad Med J*; 61:313-316, 1985.

Sparks M, O'Sullivan P, Herrington A et al., Does peppermint oil relieve spasms during barium enema? In: *BRJ Radiol*; 68:841-843, 1995.

Taylor BA, Luscombe DK, Duthie HL. Inhibitory effect of peppermint on gastrointestinal smooth muscle. Gut 24: A 992 (Abstract), 1983.

Weizel A. Colon irritabile. *Therapiewoche* 30:3898-3900, 1980.

White DA, Thompson SP, Wilson CG, Bel JD. A pharmacokinetic comparison of two delayed release peppermint oil preparations, Colpermin and Mintec for treatment of the irritable bowel syndrome. *Int J Pharmaceutics* 40:151-155, 1987.

Wildgrube HJ. Untersuchung zur Wirksamkeit von Pfefferminzöl auf Beschwerdebild und funktionelle Parameter bei Patienten mit Reizdarmsyndrom (Studie). *NaturHeilpraxis* 41:2-5, 1988.

Perilla

Perilla fructescens

DESCRIPTION

Medicinal Parts: The medicinal parts of the plants are the leaf-bearing branches and leaves.

Flower and Fruit: The flowers are in 2-blossomed false whorls in the axils of the triangular bracts in 5 to 15 cm long, spikelike, downy-haired inflorescences. The calyx is campanulate, bilabiate, 3 to 10 mm long, with a triple-toothed upper lip and a divided lower lip divided. The corolla is 4 to 5 mm long, almost radial, with a short tube and a broadened, almost circular section having a whitish, 5-lobed margin. There are 4 stamens of almost equal length and a superior, 2-carpeled, 4-chambered ovary. The fruit is globose, gray-brown, with purple reticulate stripes and a diameter of approximately 1.5 mm. The pericarp is thin and brittle; the seeds yellowish-white.

Leaves, Stem, and Root: The herb, stands up to 1 m high. The leaves are long-petiolate. The lamina is wide-ovate, acuminate, rounded at the base, crenate, curly, dull green with brown-red spots to blackish-purple. The leaves are glossy and downy-haired along the veins. The stem is square, branched and downy.

Habitat: The species is found in India, Burma, Japan, and China.

Production: Perilla leaves are the dried leaves and leaf-bearing branches of *Perilla fructescens*. Harvesting is from July to August, after which the leaves and branches are dried in the sun or shade.

Other Names: Beefsteak Plant

ACTIONS AND PHARMACOLOGY

COMPOUNDS

Volatile oil: constituents vary greatly according to chemotype, with perillaldehyde, L-limonene + perillaldehyde, perilla ketone, myristicin, dill apiole or elsholtzia ketone predominating

Caffeic acid derivatives: rosmarinic acid (0.4 to 1.7%)

Monoterpene glucosides: including perillosides A to D, citrusine C

Flavonoids: apigenin glucoside and luteolin glucoside, estered to some extent with caffeic acid

EFFECTS

Perilla aldehyde (chemotype PA) is sedative and antibacterial in effect; perilla ketone (chemotype PK) acts as a propulsive in the gastrointestinal tract. In addition, a cytotoxic and antitumorous effect was able to be demonstrated. Perilla leaves may trigger allergic skin reactions (Kanzaki & Kimura, 1992.) In at least one study, serum cholesterol and triglyceride levels in rats that were fed Perilla oil were lowered (Sakono et al, 1993.)

INDICATIONS AND USAGE

Chinese Medicine: Perilla is used in traditional Chinese medicine for colds with fever, coughs, shortness of breath, chills, swelling of the nasal mucous membranes, headache, and to treat poisoning from ingestion of fish or crab. Efficacy for these indications has not yet been proved.

CONTRAINDICATIONS

Use during pregnancy is contraindicated because perillaldehyde was demonstrated to have a mutagenic effect in some in vitro studies.

PRECAUTIONS AND ADVERSE REACTIONS

No health hazards are known in conjunction with the proper administration of designated therapeutic dosages. The plant possesses potential for sensitization. In tests with sheep using 15 to 20 mg/kg body weight administration per infusion, Perilla ketone triggered pulmonary edema. Perillaldehyde had mutagenic effect in some in vitro studies.

DOSAGE

Mode of Administration: Whole, cut, powdered drug preparations and oil for internal use.

Daily Dosage: Extract (aqueous): 3 to 10 g

LITERATURE

Blaschek W, Hänsel R, Keller K, Reichling J, Rimpler G, Schneider G (Eds), Hagers Handbuch der Pharmazeutischen Praxis. Folgebände 1 und 2. Drogen A-Z. Springer. Berlin, Heidelberg 1998.

Kanzaki T, Kimura S, Occupational allergic contact dermatitis from Perilla frutescens (shiso). *Contact Dermatitis.* Jan;26(1):55-6. 1992

Sakono M, Yoshida K, Yahiro M, Combined effects of dietary protein and fat on lipid metabolism in rats. J Nutr Sci Vitaminol (Tokyo) Aug;39(4):335-43. 1993

Perilla fructescens

See Perilla

Periwinkle

Vinca minor

DESCRIPTION

Medicinal Parts: The medicinal parts are the dried leaves, the fresh aerial parts of the flowering plant, and the whole fresh flowering plant.

Flower and Fruit: The flowers are solitary, long-pedicled, 40 to 50 mm in diameter and grow in the axils of the upper leaves. The calyx is funnel-shaped with long, narrow-linear, pointed-ciliated tips. The corolla is light blue or violet with a funnel-shaped tube and 5 irregularly terminated tips. The fruit is a follicle. It is oblong, acuminate, 15 to 2 mm long, and has 2 to 3 seeds.

Leaves, Stem, and Root: The plant is a perennial subshrub, 10 to 60 cm high. The nonflowering shoots are prostrate root at the nodes. The flowering shoots are ascending, up to 20 cm high and woody at the base. The leaves are evergreen, ovate, tapering at the front, and distinctly pinnate-ribbed. They are 5 cm by 2 cm, petiolate with finely ciliated margins, which become glabrous later.

Habitat: The plant is indigenous to northern Spain, through western France, eastward via central and southern Europe as far as the Caucasus; it has been naturalized in many regions.

Production: Periwinkle herb consists of the above-ground parts of *Vinca minor*.

ACTIONS AND PHARMACOLOGY

COMPOUNDS

Indole alkaloids (0.15-1.4%): chief alkaloid vincamine (eburnamine-type, 25-65%), including as well vincine, apovincamine, vincadifformin

Flavonoids: including kempferol-3-O-rhamnoside-7-O-glucoside, kempferol-3-O-rhamnoglucoside-3-O-galactoside, kempferol-3-O-rhamnoglucoside-3-O-glucoside, quercetin-3-O-rhamnoglucoside-7-O-glucoside

EFFECTS

The alkaloid vincamine is hypotensive, negatively chronotropic, spasmolytic, hypoglycemic, and sympatholytic. Scientifically validated studies on the hypotensive effect on humans have not yet been carried out. Its use as an amaroid seems plausible.

INDICATIONS AND USAGE

Unproven Uses: Periwinkle is used internally for circulatory disorders, cerebral circulatory impairment and support for the metabolism of the brain. It is also used internally for loss of memory, hypertension, cystitis, gastritis and enteritis, diarrhea, raised blood sugar levels, and to help weaning. Periwinkle is used externally for sore throats, nosebleeds, bruising, abscesses, eczema, and to stop bleeding.

Homeopathic Uses: Periwinkle is used for weeping eczema and bleeding mucous membranes.

PRECAUTIONS AND ADVERSE REACTIONS

No health hazards are known in conjunction with the proper administration of designated therapeutic dosages. Gastrointestinal complaints and skin flushing have been observed as side effects.

OVERDOSAGE

Overdosage will bring about a severe drop in blood pressure. Cases of poisonings have not yet been recorded.

Treatment includes gastrointestinal emptying (inducement of vomiting, gastric lavage with burgundy-coloured potassium permanganate solution, sodium sulphate), instillation of activated charcoal and shock prophylaxis (appropriate body position, quiet, warmth). The therapy for poisonings consists of treating bradycardia with atropine or Alupent, cardiac arrhythmias with lidocaine or phenytoin and treating possible cases of acidosis with sodium bicarbonate infusions. In case of shock, plasma volume expanders should be infused.

DOSAGE

Mode of Administration: Whole, cut and powdered drug is available in the form of capsules, ampules, coated and filmed tablets, and compound preparations.

Preparation: To make a tea, pour 200 mL boiling water over 1 teaspoonful of drug, steep for 10 minutes, then strain. To make a decoction, boil 60 g of drug in 1 liter of water for 2 minutes, steep for 10 minutes, then strain. To make an infusion, boil 15 g of drug in 1/4 liter of water. To make wine, macerate 100 g of drug in 1 liter of wine for 10 days, decant, then press. To make a liquid for gargling, boil 2 dessertspoonfuls of drug for a few minutes in 1/2 liter water.

Daily Dosage: The usual drug dosage is as follows: Tea–2 to 3 cups daily; Decoction–2 to 4 cups between meals; Infusion—drink after meals for diarrhea; Wine–1 dessertspoonful after meals; a gargle or wash can be used externally as needed.

Homeopathic Dosage: 5 drops, 1 tablet, or 10 globules every 30 to 60 minutes (acute) or 1 to 3 times daily (chronic); parenterally: 1 to 2 mL sc, acute: 3 times daily; chronic: once a day (HAB1).

LITERATURE

Behninger C, Abel G, Schneider E, Vinca minor zeigt keine antimitotische Eigenschaften. In: *ZPT* 13(2):35. 1992.

Taylor, B, In: Taylor WI, Farnsworth N (Ed.): The Vinca Alkaloids, Marcel Dekker Inc., New York. 1973.

Trunzler G, Phytotherapeutische Möglichkeiten bei Herz- und arteriellen Gefäßerkrankungen. In: ZPT 10(5):147. 1989.

Vinpocetin. In: ZPT 14(1):11. 1993.

Persea americana

See Avocado

Persicaria bistorta

See Bistort

Persicaria hydropiper

See Smartweed

Petasites

Petasites hybridus

DESCRIPTION

Medicinal Parts: The medicinal parts are the dried or fresh leaves, the underground parts collected in autumn, the dried, the aerial parts collected toward the end of the flowering season, and the whole fresh plant.

Flower and Fruit: The reddish flowers appear before the leaves, immediately after the snow has melted. They grow on flowering shafts from the base of the plant. The shaft is erect, thick, and has purplish scales. The shafts bearing the male flowers are 15 to 20 cm high; those bearing the female flowers are 40 cm high. The capitula of the mainly male flowers are initially in ovate, compact racemes. The flowers are tubular campanulate. The female flowers have a threadlike, tight tube and a bilabiate margin. The involucre is in 1 to 2 rows and is reddish. A prismatic fruit with a yellowish-whitish pappus develops from the flower.

Leaves, Stem, and Root: The short and gnarled rhizome lies vertically or somewhat slanted in the ground. It is about 4 cm thick, brownish, and thickened at the nodes. The root creeps and branches under the surface. The leaves are large, basal, long-petioled, and roundish with a deeply cordate base. It is gray underneath and irregularly dentate.

Characteristics: Petasite has the largest leaves of all indigenous flora and has an unpleasant smell.

Habitat: The species is found in northern Asia, Europe and some areas of North America.

Production: Petasite consists of the whole plant of *Petasites hybridus*. Petasite leaf consists of the leaves of Petasites hybridis. The leaves are harvested before the end of the flowering season and quickly dried. Only leaves that are the size of the palm of the hand are picked, as these are said to have a higher level of active principles than the larger leaves. Petasite root consists of the dried underground parts of *Petasites hybridus*. A distinction is made between androdynamic and gynodynamic varieties. The roots of the former are dug up in autumn; those of the latter are harvested in spring. After being dug up they are washed and dried. If drugs containing petasin are to be extracted, then cultivation must be carried out under laboratory conditions.

Not to be Confused With: Other Petasite varieties and the leaves of *Adenostyles alliariae* or *Tussilago farfara*.

Other Names: Blatterdock, Bog Rhubarb, Bogshorns, Butterbur, Butter-Dock, Butterfly Dock, Capdockin, Flapperdock, Langwort, P. Vulgaris, Umbrella Leaves

ACTIONS AND PHARMACOLOGY

COMPOUNDS: PETASITES LEAF

Sesquiterpene alcohol esters: chief components including among others according to chemotype - petasitine, neopetasitine and isopetasitine, or furanopetasin and 9-hydroxyfuranoeremophilone

Pyrrolizidine alkaloids: senecionine, integerrimine, senkirkine, presumably only in traces

Volatile oil: including, among others, dodecanal (aroma-bearer)

Flavonoids: including among others, isoquercitrin, astragaline

Mucilages

Tannins

EFFECTS: PETASITES LEAF

A spasmolytic effect has been demonstrated in animals.

COMPOUNDS: PETASITES ROOT

Sesquiterpene alcohol esters: including among others, chief components according to chemotype - petasitine, neopetasitine and isopetasitine or furanopetasine and 9-hydroxyfuranoeremophilone

Volatile oil (0.1-0.4%): including among others, 1-nonen, eremophilone, furanoeremophilone

Pyrrolizidine alkaloids: senecionine, integerrimine

EFFECTS: PETASITES ROOT

In animals, the pyrrolizidine alkaloids inhibit leukotriene synthesis and are spasmolytic and spasmoanalgesic as well as cytoprotective. In humans, it provides analgesia for nervous headaches. Its application for psychasthenic symptoms seems plausible.

In higher doses and with chronic use, a hepatotoxic, mutagenic, teratogenic, and carcinogenic effect may be expected.

INDICATIONS AND USAGE

PETASITES LEAF

Unproven Uses: Petasite leaves are used to stimulate the appetite and to treat nervous cramplike states and states associated with pain, colic, and headaches. In folk medicine, the leaves are used internally for respiratory disorders, liver, gallbladder, or pancreas disorders, as a prophylaxis for agitation, and to induce sleep. Externally, the leaves are used to heal wounds and as a poultice for malignant ulcers.

PETASITES ROOT

Approved by Commission E:

■ Kidney and bladder stones

Unproven Uses: The underground stem is used as an adjunct in the treatment of acute spastic pain in the efferent urinary tract, particularly if stones are present. It is also used for respiratory disorders, particularly for coughs, whooping cough, and bronchial asthma. Other uses include gastrointestinal disorders, and migraine and tension headaches.

Homeopathic Uses: Smooth muscle cramps.

CONTRAINDICATIONS

All forms of the drug should not be used during pregnancy or by nursing mothers.

PRECAUTIONS AND ADVERSE REACTIONS

PETASITES LEAF

General: One should entirely forgo any administration of the drug, due to the presence of pyrrolizidine alkaloids with hepatotoxic and carcinogenic effects in the parts of the plant above ground, as even mere traces of the alkaloids present a danger. The industrial manufacture of extracts virtually free of pyrrolizidine alkaloids is possible. The drug should not be used without knowledge of the pyrrolizidine alkaloids content.

Note: Alkaloid-free varieties are cultivated.

Pregnancy: The administration of the drug during pregnancy is absolutely contraindicated.

Nursing Mothers: The drug should not be consumed by nursing mothers.

PETASITES ROOT

One should unconditionally forgo any administration of the drug, due to the presence of pyrrolizidine alkaloids with hepatotoxic and carcinogenic effect. The industrial manufacture of extracts virtually free of pyrrolizidine alkaloids is possible.

DOSAGE

PETASITES LEAF

Preparation: Note: The herb should not be used unless the pyrrolizidine content is known. The maximum daily dose of pyrrolizidine alkaloids is 0.1 mcg. To make an infusion, pour boiling water over 1.2 to 2 g comminuted drug and strain after 10 minutes.

Daily Dosage: Drink 2 to 3 cups of the infusion per day.

PETASITES ROOT

Mode of Administration: Extracts obtained with ethanol or lipophilic solvents and other galenic preparations for internal use.

Daily Dosage: Dosing of herbal preparations is highly dependent on a variety of factors, such as growing and harvesting conditions, plant parts, extraction methods used, and the dosage form chosen by the manufacturer. Standardization to single constituent makers has proved unreliable. Since no official standards have been established to date to regulate production of herbal medicines in the United States, dosage ranges must be employed as guidelines.

Preparations equivalent to 4.5 to 7 g drug may be used. When used internally, the daily dosage must not exceed 0.1 micrograms of pyrrolizidine alkaloids with 1.2 unsaturated necine structure including their N-oxides. When used externally, the maximum daily dosage should not exceed 10 mcg of pyrrolizidine alkaloids with 1.2 unsaturated necine structure including their N-oxides. Teas should not be used.

Homeopathic Uses: 5 drops, 1 tablet, or 10 globules every 30 to 60 minutes (acute) or 1 to 3 times daily (chronic); parenterally: 1 to 2 mL sc, acute: 3 times daily; chronic: once a day (HAB1).

LITERATURE

PETASITES LEAF AND ROOT

Bicket D et al., Identification and characterization of inhibitors of peptide-leukotriene-synthesis from *Petasites hybridus*. In: *PM* 60(4):318. 1994.

Brune K, Bickel D, Peskar BA, Gastro-Protective Effects by Extracts of Petasites hybridus: The Role of Inhibition of Peptido-leukotriene Synthesis. In: *PM* 59(6):494. 1993.

Carle R, Pflanzliche Antiphlogistika und Spasmolytika. In: *ZPT* 9(3):67. 1988.

Chizzola R, Distribution of the pyrrolizidine alkaloids senecionine and intergerrimine within the *Petasites hybridus*. In: *PM* 58(7):A693. 1992.

Dorsch W, Neues über antientzündliche Drogen. In: ZPT 14(1):26. 1993.

Frohne D, Pfänder HJ, Giftpflanzen - Ein Handbuch für Apotheker, Toxikologen und Biologen, 4. Aufl., Wiss. Verlags-Ges. Stuttgart 1997.

Hänsel R, Keller K, Rimpler H, Schneider G (Hrsg.), Hagers Handbuch der Pharmazeutischen Praxis, 5. Aufl., Bde 4-6 (Drogen), Springer Verlag Berlin, Heidelberg, New York, 1992-1994.

Hasler A et al., Trace analysis of pyrrolizidine alkaloids by GC-NPD of extracts from the roots of *Petasites hybridus*. In: *PM* 62, Abstracts of the 44th Ann Congress of GA, 147. 1996.

Madaus G, Lehrbuch der Biologischen Arzneimittel, Bde 1-3, Nachdruck, Georg Olms Verlag Hildesheim 1979.

Roth L, Daunderer M, Kormann K, Giftpflanzen, Pflanzengifte, 4. Aufl., Ecomed Fachverlag Landsberg Lech 1993.

Siegenthaler P, Neuenschwander M. Sesquiterpenes from *Petasites hybridus* (Furanopetasin chemovar): Separation, isolation and quantitation of compounds from fresh plant extracts. *Pharm Acta Helv*. 72; 57-67. 1997

Teuscher E, Lindequist U, Biogene Gifte - Biologie, Chemie, Pharmakologie, 2. Aufl., Fischer Verlag Stuttgart 1994.

Wichtl M (Hrsg.), Teedrogen, 4. Aufl., Wiss. Verlagsges. Stuttgart 1997.

Petasites hybridus

See Petasites

Petroselinum crispum

See Parsley

Peucedanum ostruthium

See Masterwort

Peumus boldo

See Boldo

Peyote

Lophophora williamsii

DESCRIPTION

Medicinal Parts: The medicinal parts are the pincushion-like, aerial, transversely cut and dried, tough-corky shoot, and the fresh plant.

Flower and Fruit: The flowers grow from the center of the cactus head. They are 1 to 2.5 cm long and 1 to 2.2 cm across. The outer petals are green with a darker middle stripe and have green-pink or white margins. The filaments are white with yellow anthers. The ovary is glabrous. The fruit is a 15 to 20 mm long berry, which is 2 to 3.5 mm across, sturdy, clavate, initially fleshy, glabrous, and red. It turns brown-white and dries out when ripe. The seeds are black, rough, 1 to 1.5 mm long and 1 mm wide.

Leaves, Stem, and Root: The plant is a succulent, spineless, globular or top-shaped, bluish-green cactus with up to 13 distinct vertical ribs. It grows to 20 cm. From one rhizome side shoots are produced to create a cactus formation of 1.5 m across. The roots are tuberous and 8 to 11 cm long. The aerial part has a diameter of 4 to 12 cm, and the concave top is filled with gray, woolly bushels of hair. The head is divided into irregular flat warts by horizontal grooves. Roundish aueroles of paintbrush-like yellowish or whitish tufts of hair grow from the tip of the warts.

Habitat: The plant grows in northern Mexico and bordering southern Texas.

Production: Peyote is the cactus *Lophophora willamsii*, cut into slices and dried. The root and hair tuft of the Peyote plant are cut off. Particularly mescaline and chlorophyll-rich center is dried as a slice. This slice is referred to as the Mescal Button.

Other Names: Devil's Root, Diabolic Root, Dumpling Cactus, Mescal Buttons, Pellote, Sacred Mushroom

ACTIONS AND PHARMACOLOGY

COMPOUNDS

Alkaloids phenylethylamine type: chief among them mescaline (up to 7%), hordenine; tetrahydroisoquinoline type: including among others pellotin, anhalonidine, anhalamine

EFFECTS

Peyote has a hallucinogenic effect. The psychotropic effects of Peyote consumption are mainly due to the mescaline content. Controlled pharmacological studies on the Peyote cactus are unknown. Mescal beans cause visual, auditory, taste, and kinesthetic hallucinations.

INDICATIONS AND USAGE

Unproven Uses: Peyote is rarely used as a medicinal preparation. In folk medicine, Peyote is one of the oldest hallucinogens.

PRECAUTIONS AND ADVERSE REACTIONS

Due to its mescaline content, the drug causes chiefly visual, but also aural, kinesthetic, and synesthetic hallucinations when taken in dosages of between 4 and 12 dried slices of the sprout (so-called Mescal Buttons: diameter 3 to 4.5 cm, thickness 0.5 cm).

DOSAGE

Mode of Administration: Peyote is obsolete as a drug; it is often ingested illegally for its hallucinogenic effect.

LITERATURE

Hänsel R, Keller K, Rimpler H, Schneider G (Hrsg.), Hagers Handbuch der Pharmazeutischen Praxis, 5. Aufl., Bde 4-6 (Drogen), Springer Verlag Berlin, Heidelberg, New York, 1992-1994.

Madaus G, Lehrbuch der Biologischen Arzneimittel, Bde 1-3, Nachdruck, Georg Olms Verlag Hildesheim 1979 (unter Anhalonium).

Roth L, Daunderer M, Kormann K, Giftpflanzen, Pflanzengifte, 4. Aufl., Ecomed Fachverlag Landsberg Lech 1993.

Seeger R, Mescalin. In: DAZ 133(2):24. 1993.

Steinegger E, Hänsel R, Pharmakognosie, 5. Aufl., Springer Verlag Heidelberg 1992.

Teuscher E, Lindequist U, Biogene Gifte - Biologie, Chemie, Pharmakologie, 2. Aufl., Fischer Verlag Stuttgart 1994.

Phaseolus vulgaris

See Bean Pod

Phoenix dactylifera

See Date Palm

Phragmites communis

See Reed Herb

Phyllanthus amarus

See Black Catnip

Physalis alkekengi

See Winter Cherry

Physostigma venenosum

See Calabar Bean

Phytolacca americana

See Poke

Picea species

See Spruce

Picrasma excelsa

See Quassia

Picrorhiza

Picrorhiza kurroa

DESCRIPTION

Medicinal Parts: The medicinal part of the plant is the rhizome, which is cut and dried.

Flower and Fruit: The inflorescence is a terminal, dense spike, 5 to 10 cm long, on an upright peduncle over a rosette of dentate leaves (may be absent). The sepals are fused, approximately 6 mm long. The calyx is 5-lobed and pubescent, the corolla 5-lobed, radial, pale blue or reddish-blue. There are 4 stamens, and the ovary is 2-chambered with numerous ovules. The flowers are dimorphic, having either 6 to 8 mm long corollas and 8 mm long filaments or a single 6 mm long corolla and 2 cm long filaments. The fruit is an approximately 1.3 cm long, ovoid, 4-sided capsule. The seeds are ellipsoid with a translucent, thick, blistery aril.

Leaves, Stem, and Roots: The leaves on this herbaceous creeping perennial are alternate, 5 to 15 cm long and 2 to 6 cm wide. The lamina is coriaceous, spatulate to narrow-elliptical with a rounded tip. The margin is dentate and the petiole winged. The rhizome is woody, up to 25 cm long, and covered in the remains of dried leaf bases.

Habitat: The plant is native to the mountains of India, Nepal, Tibet, and Pakistan.

Production: Kharbagehindi (Arabic name) roots are the cut and dried rhizome of *Picrorhiza kurroa*, which are collected in the wild.

Not to be Confused With: Mistaken identity can occur with *Lagotis cashmiriana.*

Other Names: Kharbagehindi

ACTIONS AND PHARMACOLOGY

COMPOUNDS

Iridoids: catalpol derivatives, including picroside I (0.6 to 7.4%, extremely bitter), kutkoside (10-O-vanilloyl catalpol, with picroside I present in a stable state as a mixed crystal: kutkin), picroside II (3 to 5%), minecoside (0.5%), veronicoside and picroside III

Acetophenone derivatives: androsine (0.1 to 0.7%), apocynin (0.1%), picein

Cucurbitacins: chief component 25-acetoxy-2beta-D-glucosyloxy-3,16,20-trihydroxy-9-methyl-19-norlanosta-5,23-dien-22-one (1.0 to 1.5%. extremely bitter)

Glycoproteins

EFFECTS

The acetophenone derivatives androsine and apocynine are bronchospasmolytic and antiasthmatic in effect. In addition, antiphlogistic, immunostimulating, antibacterial and antiviral, hepatoprotective, choleretic, spasmolytic, and insecticidal action mechanisms were able to be demonstrated. The positive influence of Picrorhiza kurroa in the treatment of vitiligo is traceable to the immunomodulating and hepatoprotective characteristics of the drug.

INDICATIONS AND USAGE

Unproven Uses: Folk medicine uses have included menstrual complaints, enteritis, gall bladder complaints, for stomach conditions as an emetic, fever, constipation, chronic dysentery, scabies, leucoderma, joint pain, chronic asthma, infections, inflammations, and coughs.

Chinese Medicine: Picrorhiza is used for fever induced by strain, hyperemia, dysentery, jaundice, carbuncles, hemorrhoids, epilepsy, and malnutrition in children.

PRECAUTIONS AND ADVERSE REACTIONS

No health hazards are known in conjunction with the proper administration of designated therapeutic dosages.

DOSAGE

Mode of Administration: Preparations for internal use.

Preparation: To prepare a tincture, 100 g finely cut and crushed Kharbagehindi root with 37.5 g dried and crushed orange peels, 12.5 g crushed cardamom to 1000 ml 45% ethanol.

Daily Dosage: Powder: 0.6 to 1.2 g drug; as an antiperiodic 3 to 4 g. Tincture: 2 to 4 ml.

LITERATURE

Blaschek W, Hänsel R, Keller K, Reichling J, Rimpler G, Schneider G (Eds), Hagers Handbuch der Pharmazeutischen Praxis. Folgeb nde 1 und 2. Drogen A-Z. Springer. Berlin, Heidelberg 1998.

Chander R, Kapoor NK, Dhawan BN. Picroliv, picroside-I- and kutkoside from Picrorrhiza kurrooa are scavangers of superoxide anions. *Biochem Pharmacol.* 44; 180-183. 1992

Chander R, Dwivedi Y, Rastogi R, Sharma SK, Garg NK, Kapoor NK, Dhawan BN, Effect of different extracts of kutaki (*Picrorhiza kurroa*) on experimentally induced abnormalities in the liver. *Indian J Med Res*, 95:34-7, Feb. 1990

Chander R, Dwivedi Y, Rastogi R, Sharma SK, Garg NK, Kapoor NK, Dhawan BN, Evaluation of hepatoprotective activity of picroliv (from *Picrorhiza kurroa*) in Mastomys natalensis infected with Plasmodium berghei. *Indian J Med Res*, 95:34-7, Feb. 1990

Dorsch W, Stuppner H, Wagner H, Gropp M, Demoulin S, Ring J, Antiasthmatic effects of *Picrorhiza kurroa*: androsin prevents allergen- and PAF-induced bronchial obstruction in guinea pigs. *Int Arch Allergy Appl Immunol*, 95:128-33, 1991.

Mahajani SS, Kulkarni RD, Effect of disodium cromoglycate and *Picrorhiza kurroa* root powder on sensitivity of guinea pigs to histamine and sympathomimetic amines. *Int Arch Allergy Appl Immunol*, 42:137-44, 1977.

Pandey BL, Das PK, Immunopharmacological studies on Picrorhiza kurroa Royle-ex-Benth. Part III: Adrenergic mechanisms of anti-inflammatory action. *Indian J Physiol Pharmacol*, 42:120-5, Apr-Jun. 1988

Pandey BL, Das PK, Immunopharmacological studies on Picrorhiza kurroa Royle-ex-Benth. Part IV: Cellular mechanisms of anti-inflammatory action. *Indian J Physiol Pharmacol,* 42:28-30, Jan-Mar. 1989

Rastogi R et al. Picroliv Protects Against Alcohol-Induced Chronic Hepatotoxicity in Rats. *Planta Med.* 62 (3); 283-285. 1996

Shukla B, Visen PK, Patnaik GK, Dhawan BN, Choleretic effect of picroliv, the hepatoprotective principle *of Picrorhiza kurroa. Planta Med*, 95:29-33, Feb. 1991

Singh GB et al. Antiinflammatory Activity of The Iridoids Kutkin, Picroside-1 and Kutkoside from *Picrorhiza kurrooa. Phytother Res.* 7 (6); 402-407. 1993

Vaidya AB, Antarkar DS, Doshi JC, Bhatt AD, Ramesh V, Vora PV, Perissond D, Baxi AJ, Kale PM, Picrorhiza kurroa (Kutaki) Royle ex Benth as a hepatoprotective agent - experimental & clinical studies. *J Postgrad Med*, 42:105-8, Oct-Dec. 1996

Picrorhiza kurroa

See Picrorhiza

Pilocarpus microphyllus

See Jaborandi

Pilosella officinarum

See Mouse Ear

Pimenta racemosa

See Pimento

Pimento

Pimenta racemosa

DESCRIPTION

Medicinal Parts: The medicinal parts are the berries and the oil extracted from them.

Flower and Fruit: The inflorescences are racemes of white or lilac flowers, which develop very quickly into the infructescence. The fruit is a brown, globular berry, which is about 0.75 cm in diameter. The fruit has a rough surface and the remains of the calyx are present as a toothed ring at the apex. It contains 2 reniform seeds.

Leaves, Stem, and Root: The tree is an evergreen up to 12 m in height. The leaves are oblong and coriaceous.

Characteristics: The odor is aromatic and reminiscent of cloves.

Habitat: The plant is indigenous to the West Indies and is cultivated in South America, Central America, and Jamaica.

Production: Pimento leaves are the foliage leaves of *Pimenta racemosa. Pimentae fructus* is obsolete as a drug.

Other Names: Allspice, Clove Pepper, Jamaica Pepper, Pimenta

ACTIONS AND PHARMACOLOGY

COMPOUNDS

Volatile oil (bay oil, 0.7-1.2%): chief components- eugenol (50-60%), chavicol (20%), additionally including among others eugenol methyl ether, methyl chavicol, myrcene, limonene, (-)-phellandrene, 3- octanon, 1-octen-3-ole, citral

EFFECTS

Pimento is antiseptic and analgesic, and is a skin irritant.

INDICATIONS AND USAGE

Unproven Uses: Pimento is used externally in rubefacient lotions or liniments.

PRECAUTIONS AND ADVERSE REACTIONS

General: No health hazards or side effects are known in conjunction with the proper administration of designated therapeutic dosages. Allergic reactions to eugenol occur rarely.

DOSAGE

Mode of Administration: Pimento preparations are administered externally as lotions or liniments.

LITERATURE

Kern W, List PH, Hörhammer L (Eds.), Hagers Handbuch der Pharmazeutischen Praxis, 4. Aufl., Bde. 1-8, Springer Verlag Berlin, Heidelberg, New York, 1969.

Leung AY, Encyclopedia of Common Natural Ingredients Used in Food Drugs and Cosmetics, John Wiley & Sons Inc., New York 1980.

Steinegger E, Hänsel R, Pharmakognosie, 5. Aufl., Springer Verlag Heidelberg 1992.

Pimpinella

Pimpinella major

DESCRIPTION

Medicinal Parts: The medicinal parts are the dried rhizome, the dried roots and the fresh roots collected in May.

Flower and Fruit: The white flowers are in compound 5- to 15-rayed umbels. There is no involucre or epicalyx. The flowers are small. The petals are uneven with curved lobes. The style is longer than the ovary during the flowering season. The fruit is dark brown to black, oblong-ovate, compressed at the sides, 2 to 3.5 mm long, heavily grooved, and has no beak.

Leaves, Stem, and Root: The 50- to 100-cm high plant is a perennial. During the flowering season, it develops lateral rosettes of leaves for the following year. These are usually glabrous, occasionally finely downy to short-bristly. The root is fusiform or carrot-shaped. The root is 10 to 20 cm long and 1 to 1.5 cm thick, gray-yellow, and somewhat ringed. The stem is erect, angular, grooved, hollow, glabrous, somewhat leafy, and branched from the ground up. The leaves are simple pinnate and glossy. The leaflets of the lower leaves are petiolate. They are ovate or oblong-indented or serrate acuminate.

Characteristics: The fresh root smells rancid, suet or carrot-like. The taste is tangy at first then burning-hot.

Habitat: The plant grows all over Europe with the exception of Scandinavia and the southern Balkans. It has been introduced to North America.

Production: Pimpinella herb consists of the above-ground parts *of Pimpinella saxifrage* and/or *Pimpinella major*. Pimpinella root consists of the dried rhizomes and roots of *Pimpinella saxifrage* and/or *Pimpinella major*. The root is dug up in spring and autumn. The uncut root is dried at temperatures of 40° C to prevent loss of essential oils. The drying process is completed when the roots can be broken.

Not to be Confused With: Pimpinellae radix should not be confused with other Apiaca roots. It is often adulterated with the roots of Heracleum sphondylium, Heracleum mantegazzianum and Pastinaca sativa.

Other Names: Burnet Saxifrage, Lesser Burnet, Pimpernell, Saxifrage,

ACTIONS AND PHARMACOLOGY

COMPOUNDS: PIMPINELLA HERB

Flavonoids

The foliage of the plant has not been fully investigated.

EFFECTS: PIMPINELLA HERB

No information is available.

COMPOUNDS: PIMPINELLA ROOT

Volatile oil (0.05 to 0.7%): chief components- trans-epoxy-pseudo-isoeugenol (20-57%), additionally pregeijeren (10%), geijerene (3%), beta-bisabolene, germacrenes A to D, 1,4-dimethyl azulene

Furocoumarins (1.2-2.3%): including among others bergaptene, isopimpinellin, pimpinellin, isobergapten, sphondine

Hydroxycoumarins: umbelliferone, scopoletin

Caffeic acid esters: including among others, chlorogenic acid

Polyynes: including trideca-2,8,10-trien-4,6-diine; trideca-2,8-dien-4,6-diin-10-ole

EFFECTS: PIMPINELLA ROOT

The drug contains essential oil. The efficacy of the drug as a flushing-out therapy in bacterial infections of the urinary tract seems plausible. The expectorant effect has not been proven.

INDICATIONS AND USAGE

PIMPINELLA HERB

Preparations of Pimpinella herb are used internally for lung ailments and to stimulate gastrointestinal activity. The herb is used externally for varicose veins.

PIMPINELLA ROOT

Approved by Commission E:

- Cough/bronchitis

Preparations of the root are also used for colds, chills and catarrh of the upper respiratory tract.

Unproven Uses: In folk medicine, it is used internally for disorders of the urinary organs, inflammation of the bladder and kidney, bladder and kidney stones, and edema. Externally, it is used for inflammation of the oral and pharyngeal mucous membrane and as a bath additive for poorly healing wounds.

Homeopathic Uses: Homeopathic uses include febrile states and spinal pain.

PRECAUTIONS AND ADVERSE REACTIONS

PIMPINELLA HERB

No health hazards or side effects are known in conjunction with the proper administration of designated therapeutic dosages.

PIMPINELLA ROOT

No health hazards or side effects are known in conjunction with the proper administration of designated therapeutic dosages. Photosensitivity may occur in light-skinned individuals.

DOSAGE

PIMPINELLA ROOT

Mode of Administration: Pimpinella root is administered as a tincture (Tinctura Pimpinellae) and as a comminuted herb for teas and other galenic preparations for internal use.

Daily Dosage: 6 to 12 g drug for infusions or 6 to 15 ml pimpernel tincture (1:5).

Folk medicine – Add freshly cut drug to cold water and bring to the boil, use as a gargle and as a bath additive.

Infusion – 3 to 10 g; 1 cup 3 to 4 times daily (sweetened with honey).

Gargle tincture – 30 drops in a glass of water.

For coughs – 5 to 10 drops on a sugar lump.

Homeopathic Dosage: 5 drops, 1 tablet, or 10 globules every 30 to 60 minutes (acute) or 1 to 3 times daily (chronic); parenterally: 1 to 2 mL sc, acute: 3 times daily; chronic: once a day (HAB1).

LITERATURE

PIMPINELLA HERB AND ROOT

Bohn IU, Pimpinella saxifraga und *Pimpinella major*-Kleine und Große Bibernelle. In: ZPT 12(3):98. 1991.

Kubeczka KH, Formacek V, New Constituents from the Essential Oils of Pimpinella. In: Brunke EJ (Ed.) Progress in Essential Oil Research, Walter de Gruyter & Co, Berlin 1986. 1986.

Martin R et al., Reinvestigation of the Phenylpropanoids from the Roots of Pimpinella Species. *Planta Med.* 51; 198-202. 1985

Reichling J, Martin R, Pseudoisoeugenole - eine Gruppe seltener Phenylpropanoide im Genus Pimpinella: Biosynthese unfd biologische Wirkung. In: PZW 136(5/6)225. 1991.

Pimpinella anisum

See Anise

Pimpinella major

See Pimpinella

Pineapple

Ananas comosus

DESCRIPTION

Medicinal Parts: The medicinal part of the plant is the fruit.

Flower and Fruit: The white, blue, or purple flowers are arranged in approximately 30 cm long spikes. The flowers are in the axils of reddish, thorny bracts. The 3 sepals are free or fused at the base, and the 3 petals form a tube. There are 6 stamens and a trichambered ovary. The fruit is fused with the thickening receptacle to an oval to cylindrical, conelike pseudocarp. The pseudocarp is 10 to 25 cm thick, 15 to 25 cm high, 0.5 to 5 kg in weight, yellow to orange-red with large warts and a hexagonal area bearing a leaf cluster at the tip.

Leaves, Stem, and Root: Pineapple is a leafy rosette perennial plant, which grows up to 1.2 m high. The leaves are narrow-linear, thorny-tipped, up to 0.9 m long and 6 cm wide. They are usually thorny dentate and arranged in rosette. The stem is short.

Characteristics: The fruit is usually parthenocarpic. The cultivated fruits are seedless. The fruit pulp is white to yellow with a sourish-sweet, aromatic smell and taste.

Habitat: Hawaii, Japan, and Taiwan

Production: Bromelain is a mixture of proteolytic enzymes from the main stump of *Ananas comosus.* Bromelain is produced from the main pineapple stumps harvested after 4 years. The main stumps are pressed and put through an extraction process with water. The juice is then precipitated with acetone to produce raw bromelain. The resulting waste product is a soft wax, which is used in the cosmetic industry.

ACTIONS AND PHARMACOLOGY

COMPOUNDS

Proteases: mixture of at least 5 chemically very similar cysteine proteinases, including EC 3.4.22.4 and EC 3.4.22.5, that can be deactivated with oxidizing substances or activated with thiols such as cysteine, as well as small amounts of a phosphatase, a peroxidase, or protease inhibitors.

EFFECTS

Pineapple is antiphlogistic, fibrinolytic, and proteolytic. The proteolytic enzymes promote the healing of wounds. In addition, an inhibition of thrombocyte aggregation and an antineoplastic effect have been observed, as well as an elevation of the serum level of antibiotics when administered concurrently.

INDICATIONS AND USAGE

Approved by Commission E:

- Wounds and burns

Unproven Uses: Internal application: For post traumatic and postoperative swelling to stimulate healing and as an enzyme substitution for digestive symptoms after pancreatic disease. The drug can also be used for edema, digestive complaints, for inflammation, and febrile conditions (Hawaiian Islands, Philippines and South America), for asthmatic conditions in children (Zaire), and as a vermifuge (Brazil). Pineapple bran is used in weight reduction.

Indian Medicine: The fruit is used for dyspeptic symptoms, constipation, amenorrhea, and dysmenorrhea, as well as for black vomiting and fever.

PRECAUTIONS AND ADVERSE REACTIONS

No health hazards are known in conjunction with the proper administration of designated therapeutic dosages. Gastric complaints and diarrhea may occur as side effects of internal administration. Allergic reactions following repeated administration have been observed.

DRUG INTERACTIONS

POTENTIAL INTERACTIONS

There is an increased tendency toward bleeding in connection with the simultaneous administration of Pineapple and anticoagulants or thrombocyte aggregation inhibitors. When bromelain and tetracyclines are taken at the same time, their concentrations in plasma and urine are elevated.

DOSAGE

Mode of Administration: Available as tablets, granules and galenic preparations for internal use; compounded preparations for external use.

Daily Dosage: 500 to 2,000 mg daily; children: 150 to 300 FIP (Federation Internationale Pharmaceutique) units

Storage: Seal tightly and air dry.

LITERATURE

Hänsel R, Keller K, Rimpler H, Schneider G (Ed), Hagers Handbuch der Pharmazeutischen Praxis, 5. Aufl., Bde 4 - 6 (Drogen), Springer Verlag Berlin, Heidelberg, New York, 1992-1994.

Harrach T, Eckert K, Schulze-Forster K, Nuck R, Grunow D, Maurer HR, Isolation and partial characterization of basic proteinases from stem bromelain. *J Protein Chem,* 57:41-52, Jan. 1995

Holtum JA, Summons R, Roeske CA, Comins HN, O'Leary MH, Allergic reactions, including asthma, to the pineapple protease bromelain following occupational exposure. *Clin Allergy*, 57:443-50, Sep. 1979

Hotz G, Frank T, Zöller J, Wiebelt H, Antiphlogistic effect of bromelaine following third molar removal. *Dtsch Zahnarztl Z,* 57:830-2, Nov. 1989

Sripanidkulchai B, Wongpanich V, Laupattarakasem P, Suwansaksri J, Jirakulsomchok D. Diuiretic effects of selected Thai indigenous medicinal plants in rats. *J Ethnopharmacol* 75(2-3); 185-190. 2001

Taussig SJ, Batkin S, Abortifacient effect of steroids from *Ananas comosus* and their analogs on mice. *J Reprod Fertil,* 22:461-2, Mar. 1976

Taussig SJ, Batkin S, Bromelain, the enzyme complex of pineapple (*Ananas comosus*) and its clinical application. An update. *J Ethnopharmacol*, 22:191-203, Feb-Mar. 1988

Taussig SJ, Batkin S, Modulation of pulmonary metastasis (Lewis lung carcinoma) by bromelain, an extract of the pineapple stem (*Ananas comosus*). *Letter Cancer Invest,* 22:241-2, 1988.

Pink Root

Spigelia marilandica

DESCRIPTION

Medicinal Parts: The medicinal parts are the dried rhizomes and roots.

Fruit and Flower: The inflorescences are terminal, sometimes branched spikes that are inclined to one side. The flowers are erect. The high leaves are narrow, tiny, awl-shaped in groups of 5. The 5-petaled corolla is red or yellow. The fruit is a bivalved capsule. The seeds are angular and packed tightly in the fruit.

Leaves, Stem, and Root: The plant is a perennial that grows up to 45 cm high and has fibrous, twisted roots. The stem is quadrangular and glabrous. The foliage leaves are opposite, membranous, ovate to ovate-lanceolate, acuminate, rounded at the base, entire-margined, and sessile. The stipules are small.

Habitat: The plant is indigenous to the U.S.

Production: Pink Root and herb are the rhizome and aerial parts of *Spigelia marilandica*.

Other Names: American Wormgrass, Indian Pink, Maryland Pink, Pinkroot, Starbloom, Wormgrass

ACTIONS AND PHARMACOLOGY

COMPOUNDS

The drug has not been investigated in recent times. Older sources include, among others, references to the presence of acidic resins, volatile oil, tannins, waxes and a volatile base (presumably identical with isoquinoline).

EFFECTS

Pink Root has anthelmintic actions.

INDICATIONS AND USAGE

Unproven Uses: The herb is used for worm infestation, as a febrifuge and for malaria.

Homeopathic Uses: Spigelia marilandica is used as a calmative during states of excitement.

PRECAUTIONS AND ADVERSE REACTIONS

According to older sources, the drug allegedly contains a toxin that paralyzes the spinal marrow and leads to death through asphyxiation.

DOSAGE

Mode of Administration: As a powdered root or herb or as a liquid extract.

LITERATURE

Hänsel R, Keller K, Rimpler H, Schneider G (Hrsg.), Hagers Handbuch der Pharmazeutischen Praxis, 5. Aufl., Bde 4-6 (Drogen): Springer Verlag Berlin, Heidelberg, New York, 1992-1994.

Lewin L, Gifte und Vergiftungen, 6. Aufl., Nachdruck, Haug Verlag, Heidelberg 1992.

Richardson MD, Peterson JR, Clark AM. Bioactivity Screenings of Plants Selected on the Basis of Folkloric Use or Presence of Lignans in a Family. *Phytother Res.* 6 (5); 274-278. 1992

Pinus Bark

Tsuga canadensis

DESCRIPTION

Medicinal Parts: The medicinal parts are the latex, which exudes from the plant and the essential oil.

Flower and Fruit: The pedicle of the male flower is shorter than the scale sheath. The cones are small (1.5 to 2.5 cm long) and light brown. The wood contains no resin.

Leaves, Stem, and Root: The young shoots are villous, becoming pubescent. The leaves have a leaf cushion and are flat, short (1 to 1.5 cm long), and obtuse. The upper surface is dark green and the under surface has 2 blue-white long stripes.

Habitat: The plant is indigenous to North America.

Other Names: Canada Pitch, Hemlock Bark, Hemlock Gum

ACTIONS AND PHARMACOLOGY

COMPOUNDS

Tannins (8-15%)

Flavonoids: hemlock tannin

Stilbene derivatives (8-10%): picea tannols

EFFECTS

The active agents are the tannin, hemlock tannin, and picea tannols. The drug has astringent, anti-inflammatory, diaphoretic, and diuretic properties.

INDICATIONS AND USAGE

Unproven Uses: Pinus Bark is used for digestive disorders, diarrhea, and diseases of the mouth and throat. It was formerly used to treat scurvy.

PRECAUTIONS AND ADVERSE REACTIONS

No health hazards or side effects are known in conjunction with the proper administration of designated therapeutic dosages. Administration in allopathic medicine is not common.

DOSAGE

Mode of Administration: The drug is available as a liquid extract, in medicinal preparations and combinations.

LITERATURE

Richardson MD, Peterson JR, Clark AM. Bioactivity Screenings of Plants Selected on the Basis of Folkloric Use or Presence of Lignans in a Family. Phytother Res. 6 (5); 274-278. 1992

Kern W, List PH, Hörhammer L (Hrsg.), Hagers Handbuch der Pharmazeutischen Praxis, 4. Aufl., Bde 1-8: Springer Verlag Berlin, Heidelberg, New York, 1969.

Pinus species

See Scotch Pine

Piper betle

See Betel Nut

Piper cubeba

See Cubeb

Piper elongatum

See Matico

Piper methysticum

See Kava Kava

Piper nigrum

See Black Pepper

Pipsissewa

Chimaphila umbellata

DESCRIPTION

Medicinal Parts: The medicinal parts are the dried leaves (occasionally mixed with twigs and flowers), the fresh aerial parts of the flowering plant, and the complete dried plant.

Flower and Fruit: The plant has terminal inflorescences 10 cm long with umbels of 2 to 7 flowers. The flowers, which are initially bright pink and then white, are nodding and mildly campanulate. The 5 sepals are obovate, dentate, and about a third as long as the 5 petals, which are broadly ovate, domed, pink, and 5 to 6 mm long. The 10 stamens are thickened at the base, the edges are winged and ciliate. The anthers are short, thick, and red. The style is very short and the stigma broad and shorter than the anthers. The fruit is a 5-grooved capsule with erect stems.

Leaves, Stem, and Root: The plant is a perennial semishrub growing up to 25 cm high with an upright, angular stem and a creeping white rhizome. The evergreen, alternate leaves are short-petioled, coriaceous, ovate-spatulate to linear and wedge-shaped. The leaf margin is sharply serrate.

Habitat: The plant grows extensively in Europe, Asia, Siberia, and North and South America. It is a protected species in Germany.

Production: Pipsissewa is the aerial part of *Chimaphila umbellata*, which is collected in the wild.

Not to be Confused With: Confusion sometimes arises with *Chimaphila maculata*.

Other Names: Butter Winter, Ground Holly, King's Cure, King's Cureall, Love in Winter, Prince's Pine, Rheumatism Weed, Umbellate Wintergreen

ACTIONS AND PHARMACOLOGY

COMPOUNDS

Hydroquinone glycosides: chief component isohomoarbutin, additionally homoarbutin

Naphthacene derivatives (naphthoquinone): chimaphilin (2,7-dimethyl-1,4-naphthoquinone)

Flavonoids: including among others hyperoside, avicularin

Tannins: (4-5%)

EFFECTS

The drug contains quinine, which is said to be a urinary antiseptic. (See Uva Ursi) Alcoholic and aqueous extracts of the plant are said to have antimicrobial properties in vitro.

INDICATIONS AND USAGE

Unproven Uses: Internal applications include acute and chronic cystitis and edema. Pipsissewa is used internally by American Indians for complaints of the kidneys and bladder, and to regulate menstruation, both before and after giving birth. It is also used for rheumatism and cancerous conditions. It is used externally for skin diseases and smallpox.

Homeopathic Uses: Among uses in homeopathy are chronic inflammation of the efferent urinary tracts, prostate gland, and mammary glands.

PRECAUTIONS AND ADVERSE REACTIONS

No health hazards or side effects are known in conjunction with the proper administration of designated therapeutic dosages. The drug possesses a weak sensitizing effect, due to its chimaphilin content. The drug is not suitable for long-term use because of its hydroquinone glycoside content. (See Uva-Ursi leaf.)

DOSAGE

Mode of Administration: Constituent of homeopathic preparations in dilutions or as a mother tincture.

Preparation: A liquid extract is prepared 1:1 with ethanol.

Daily Dosage: The usual single dose is 2 g drug, 1 to 3 g drug in a tea, or 1 to 4 ml of extract.

Homeopathic Dosage: 5 to 10 drops, 1 tablet, 5 to 10 globules 1 to 3 times daily, or 1 mL sc injection solution twice weekly (HAB1).

LITERATURE

Hänsel R, Keller K, Rimpler H, Schneider G (Hrsg.), Hagers Handbuch der Pharmazeutischen Praxis, 5. Aufl., Bde 4-6 (Drogen), Springer Verlag Berlin, Heidelberg, New York, 1992-1994.

Hausen BM, Schiedermair I. The sensitizing capacity of chimaphilin, a naturally-occuring quinone. *Contact Dermatitis* 19; 180-183. 1988

Madaus G, Lehrbuch der Biologischen Arzneimittel, Bde 1-3, Nachdruck, Georg Olms Verlag Hildesheim 1979.

Thomson RH, Naturally Occuring Quinones, 2nd Ed., Academic Press New York 1971.

Zelling K et al. Gehaltsbestimmung von Chimaphilin in Chimaphila umbellata Urtinktur mittels differentieller Pulspolarographie. Pharmazie 52 (6); 451-453. 1997

Piscidia piscipula

See Jamaica Dogwood

Pistacia lentiscus

See Mastic Tree

Pitcher Plant

Sarracenia purpurea

DESCRIPTION

Medicinal Parts: The medicinal parts are the leaves and roots.

Flower and Fruit: The androgynous flowers usually have numerous stamens and a large 3- to 5-valved superior ovary. The style spreads into a wide, stemmed umbrella, which spreads over the stamens. The 5 stigma sit as small conelike structures on the underside of the roof of the tips. The numerous marginal ovules are on individual axillary shafts. The fruit is a valved capsule. The small, membranous, thin-skinned seeds contain an abundance of endosperm.

Leaves, Stem, and Root: Sarracenia purpurea is a strange, perennial plant with leaves that are in a basal rosette and change into a tube formation. The beaker bears a long winglike strip on the side turned towards the stem. These beakers are often very colorful and fill up with rainwater and insects. During hot weather they are closed because of a concentration of fibers. The enclosed rainwater and insects form a mass, which probably acts as a fertilizer and has a strong odor.

Habitat: The plant is indigenous to the U.S.

Production: Pitcher Plant root and leaves are the root and leaves of *Sarracenia purpurea.*

Other Names: Eve's Cups, Fly-Catcher, Fly-Trap, Huntsman's Cup, Purple Side-Saddle Flower, Side-Saddle Plant, Smallpox Plant, Water-Cup

ACTIONS AND PHARMACOLOGY

COMPOUNDS

Piperidine alkaloids: coniine, gamma-conicein (particularly in the trapping fluid of the pitcher leaves)

EFFECTS

The drug has stomachic, diuretic, and laxative effects due to its active agents, which include sarracenia acid, tannin, resin, and the alkaloid sarracenin, which is similar to veratrin.

INDICATIONS AND USAGE

Unproven Uses: Pitcher Plant was formerly used for digestive disorders, particularly constipation, also for urinary tract diseases, and as a cure for smallpox. Indigenous North American Indians believe the drug not only saved lives of smallpox victims, but they also administered it to prevent scar formation.

PRECAUTIONS AND ADVERSE REACTIONS

No health hazards or side effects are known in conjunction with the proper administration of designated therapeutic dosages.

DOSAGE

Mode of Administration: Both the root and leaf preparations are considered completely obsolete.

LITERATURE

Foder GB, Colasenko B, In: Alkaloids, Vol. 3, Ed. SW Pelletier, Pub. John Wiley 1985.

Kern W, List PH, Hörhammer L (Hrsg.), Hagers Handbuch der Pharmazeutischen Praxis, 4. Aufl., Bde. 1-8: Springer Verlag Berlin, Heidelberg, New York, 1969.

Teuscher E, Lindequist U, Biogene Gifte - Biologie, Chemie, Pharmakologie, 2. Aufl., Fischer Verlag Stuttgart 1994.

Plantago afra

See Psyllium Seed

Plantago lanceolata

See English Plantain

Plantago ovata

See Psyllium

Plantain

Musa paradisiaca

DESCRIPTION

Medicinal Parts: The medicinal part of the plant is the fruit.

Flower and Fruit: The inflorescence, growing through the false trunk and curving downward, bears groups of male flowers in the axils of the bracts at the tip, groups of androgynous flowers beneath, and finally female flowers. The flowers are zygomorphic with 5 fused and 1 free tepal. There are 5 stamens and a superior ovary. The fruit is a berry. The 10 to 16 single fruits that develop from the flowers of a bract are called a hand.

Leaves, Stem, and Root: The herbaceous perennial grows up to 6 m high. The leaves are very large, entire, and simple. They are often pinnatifid and grow from an underground rhizome. The leaf sheaths form a hollow false trunk. There are adventitious roots.

Characteristics: A seedless berry fruit develops from the female flowers without pollination.

Habitat: The plant grows in tropical areas.

Production: Plantain banana pulp is the unripened pulp of *Musa paradisiaca*. Plantains are harvested when still green and ripened in special rooms for 3 to 10 days.

Other Names: Banana, Banana Tree

ACTIONS AND PHARMACOLOGY

COMPOUNDS

Polysaccharides: starch (20% of fresh weight)

Protein (1% of fresh weight)

Ascorbic acid (vitamin C): 10 to 20 mg/100 g fresh weight

Amines: serotonin (28 g/g fresh weight), tyramine (7 g/g fresh weight), dopamine (8 g/g fresh weight), noradrenaline (2 g/g fresh weight)

Fruit acids: including malic and citric acid

Aromatic substances: 180 components, including isopentenyl acetate (chief aroma-bearer)

EFFECTS

The starchy fruit has antiulcerogenic and cholesterol-reducing effects, and is a source of potassium. In East Africa and elsewhere, Plantain is used to prepare a narcotic drink.

INDICATIONS AND USAGE

Unproven Uses: The drug is used for dyspepsia, gastrointestinal complaints, diabetes, scurvy, diarrhea, hypertension, and gout.

Indian Medicine: Uses include worm disease, scabies, severe thirst, bronchitis, itching, kidney disease, pharyngalgia, and dysuria. Efficacy for these indications has not yet been proved.

PRECAUTIONS AND ADVERSE REACTIONS

No health hazards are known in conjunction with the proper administration of designated therapeutic dosages. It is conceivable that the amine content could trigger attacks of migraine headache. The frequency of myocardial fibrosis in tropical countries is said to be caused by chronic ingestion of the plant. (Plantain should never be eaten raw; it must be cooked or fried.)

DOSAGE

Mode of Administration: Preparations of the whole, cut and powdered drug are administered orally.

Preparation: Plantain starch is extracted through the elutriation of the ground fruit pulp. Plantain powder is produced by dividing the fruit into slices and air- or chamber-drying them to a water content of only 15%, and then grinding. Plantain powder (or the unripened mashed fruit) is added to milk and drunk or made into bread called Chapatis.

LITERATURE

Chattopadhyay S, Chaudhuri S, Ghosal S, Activation of peritoneal macrophages by sitoindoside-IV, an anti-ulcerogenic acylsterylglycoside from *Musa paradisiaca*. *Planta Med*, 94:16-8, Feb. 1987.

Englyst HN, Cummings JH, Digestion of the carbohydrates of banana (*Musa paradisiaca sapientum*) in the human small intestine. *Am J Clin Nutr*, 44:42-50, Jul. 1986

Goel RK, Gupta S, Shankar R, Sanyal AK, Anti-ulcerogenic effect of banana powder (*Musa sapientum var. paradisiaca*) and its effect on mucosal resistance. *J Ethnopharmacol*, 18:33-44, Oct. 1986

Lyte M, Induction of gram-negative bacterial growth by neurochemical containing banana (*Musa x paradisiaca*) extracts. *FEMS Microbiol Lett*, 44:245-50, Sep 15. 1997

Mukhopadhyaya K, Bhattacharya D, Chakraborty A, Goel RK, Sanyal AK, Effect of banana powder (*Musa sapientum var. paradisiaca*) on gastric mucosal shedding. *J Ethnopharmacol*, 21:11-9, Sep-Oct. 1987

Srivastava A, Raj SK, Haq QM, Srivastava KM, Singh BP, Sane PV, Association of a cucumber mosaic virus strain with mosaic disease of banana, *Musa paradisiaca* - an evidence using immuno/nucleic acid probe. *Indian J Exp Biol,* 94:986-8, Dec. 1995

Usha V, Vijayammal PL, Kurup PA, Aortic/glycosaminoglycans alterations in antiatherogenic action of dietary fiber from unripe banana (*Musa paradisiaca*). *Indian J Med Res,* 94:143-6, Apr. 1991

Usha V, Vijayammal PL, Kurup PA, Effect of dietary fiber from banana (*Musa paradisiaca*) on cholesterol metabolism. *Indian J Exp Biol,* 44:550-4, Oct. 1984

Usha V, Vijayammal PL, Kurup PA, Effect of dietary fiber from banana (*Musa paradisiaca*) on metabolism of carbohydrates in rats fed cholesterol free diet. *Indian J Exp Biol,* 44:445-9, May. 1989

Platycodon grandiflorum

See Balloon-Flower (Jie-Geng)

Pleurisy Root

Asclepias tuberosa

DESCRIPTION

Medicinal Parts: The medicinal part of the plant is the root.

Flower and Fruit: The plant bears panicles of deep yellow and orange petalous flowers on the apex of the stem.

Leaves, Stem, and Root: The plant is perennial, erect, 50 to 100 cm high with a fleshy tuberous root stock bearing a few stout, hairy stems. The leaves are alternate, oblong, glabrous, narrowly lanceolate, and dark green. The under surface of the leaves is somewhat lighter than the upper surface. The rootstock is mildly ring-shaped with a branched crown. The roots are grooved lengthwise, grayish brown on the outside, and whitish on the inside. The tissue is made up of concentric rings, which divide easily. The root is tough, short and starchy. *Asclepias tuberosa* is devoid of the latex typical of the genus (see *Asclepias incarnata*).

Characteristics: Pleurisy Root has a nutty and bitter taste. The odor is faint.

Habitat: Indigenous to America and Canada.

Production: Pleurisy Root is the root of *Asclepias tuberosa.*

Other Names: Butterfly Weed, Canada Root, Flux Root, Orange Milkweed, Orange Swallow-Wort, Swallow-Wort, Tuber Root, White Root, Wind Root,

ACTIONS AND PHARMACOLOGY

COMPOUNDS

Cardioactive steroids (cardenolids): including frugoside, glucofrugoside, coriglaucigenin (aglycone)

EFFECTS

Pleurisy Root is said to act as an expectorant, tonic, diaphoretic, and antispasmodic.

INDICATIONS AND USAGE

Unproven Uses: Pleurisy Root is used for coughs, pleurisy, disorders of the uterus, as an analgesic, and to ease breathing. The plant plays a particularly important role in the medicine of American Indians as a remedy for pleurisy. It is also used as a diaphoretic in treating pneumonia, inflammation of the mucous membranes, local or general atrophy, diarrhea, dysentery, rheumatism and stomach ache. Pleurisy Root is also used as a diaphoretic and expectorant.

CONTRAINDICATIONS

Pleurisy Root is not to be used during pregnancy.

PRECAUTIONS AND ADVERSE REACTIONS

No health hazards or side effects are known in conjunction with the proper administration of designated therapeutic dosages.

OVERDOSAGE

The drug has an emetic effect in higher dosages, and digitalis-like poisonings are possible due to the cardioactive steroid content. For possible symptoms and treatments for poisonings, see *Digitalis purpurea.*

DOSAGE

Mode of Administration: The drug is used internally as a liquid extract and is also available in combination preparations.

LITERATURE

Kern W, List PH, Hörhammer L (Hrsg.), Hagers Handbuch der Pharmazeutischen Praxis, 4. Aufl., Bde. 1-8, Springer Verlag Berlin, Heidelberg, New York, 1969.

Madaus G, Lehrbuch der Biologischen Arzneimittel, Bde. 1-3, Nachdruck, Georg Olms Verlag Hildesheim 1979.

Pagani F, Boll Chim Farm 114(8):450. 1975

Roth L, Daunderer M, Kormann K, Giftpflanzen, Pflanzengifte, 4. Aufl., Ecomed Fachverlag Landsberg Lech 1993.

Plumbago

Plumbago zeylanica

DESCRIPTION

Medicinal Parts: The medicinal parts of the plant are the leaf and root.

Flower and Fruit: The flowers are radial, their structures are arranged in fives with white petals and a superior ovary. The fruit is a single-seeded nut.

Leaves, Stem and Root: Plumbago is a semi-shrub. The leaves are simple and entire.

Habitat: The plant is indigenous to Malaysia and China.

Production: Plumbago herb is the dried aerial part of *Plumbago zeylandica.*

ACTIONS AND PHARMACOLOGY

COMPOUNDS

Naphthalene derivatives: chief component plumbagin (0.04%), including as well 3-chlorplumbagin, isoshinanolone, 3,3′-biplumbagin, elliptinone (6,6′-biplumbagin), droserone,

3,6′-biplumbagin (chitranone), zeylanone, isozey- lanone, maritinone, 2-methyl naphthazarine

EFFECTS

No definitive data available.

INDICATIONS AND USAGE

Chinese Medicine: The herb has been used for rheumatism, intestinal parasites, joint pain, anemia, scabies, and furuncles.

PRECAUTIONS AND ADVERSE REACTIONS

No health hazards are known in conjunction with the proper administration of designated therapeutic dosages.

DOSAGE

Daily Dosage: 9 to 15 g of drug

LITERATURE

No data available.

Plumbago zeylanica

See Plumbago

Podophyllum peltatum

See Mayapple

Pogostemon cablin

See Patchouli

Poison Ivy

Rhus toxicodendron

DESCRIPTION

Medicinal Parts: The medicinal parts are the leaves collected after flowering and dried, the fresh young shoots, the young flowering branches. and the fresh leaves.

Flower and Fruit: The pedicled flowers are in axillary, pubescent panicles. They are dioecious, sometimes androgynous. The stemmed petals are whitish-green with red hearts. The fruit is an almost globular, glabrous, yellow or yellowish-white, 10-grooved drupe. The fruit varies in size and contains a viscous latex in resin channels, which turns black in the air.

Leaves, Stem, and Root: The plant is a dioecious shrub up to 1 m high with ascending, procumbent or climbing rooting branches and underground runners. The branches are initially green and softly pubescent, later brown and glabrous. There are numerous lenticels on the two-year-old shoots. The leaves are trifoliate with 8- to 14-cm long petioles. The leaflets are oblong, acute or obtuse, entire-margined, or roughly serrate in the middle. They have a dark-green upper surface and slightly pubescent lower surface, which is a lighter green.

Habitat: The plant is indigènous to North America; it is also found in east Asia and is cultivated in Germany in botanical and apothecary gardens.

Production: Poison Ivy leaves are the leaves of *Rhus toxicodendron*. Subsequent to the flowering period, the leaves of *R. toxicodendron* are gathered and then well-dried. Gloves should be worn to protect hands while gathering the leaves, as they can cause unpleasant inflammation of the skin.

Not to be Confused With: Although it is sometimes called ''Ampelopsis hoggii,'' *Rhus toxicodendron* actually has nothing in common with the Ampelopsis group of vines.

Other Names: Epright Sumach, Joy Tree, Mercury Vine, Poison Oak, Poison Vine, Three-Leaved Ivy

ACTIONS AND PHARMACOLOGY

COMPOUNDS

Alkyl phenols: urushiol, chiefly cis,cis-3-(n-heptadeca-8′,11″-dienyl)catechol, cis,cis, cis-3-(n-heptadeca-8′,11′,14″-trienyl)catechol, cis-3-(n-heptadec-8′-enyl)catechol

Tannins

Flavonoids

EFFECTS

''Rhus poison,'' even in very small amounts, causes severe irritation to the skin. Following contact it can result in reddening, swelling, and herpes simplex-like blisters. It also has a strong toxic effect if taken internally. The mother tincture (main constituents: gallic acid and urushiol) inhibits in vitro prostaglandin biosynthesis.

INDICATIONS AND USAGE

Homeopathic uses: The drug is used to treat rheumatism in the joints and muscles; overexertion (stress and strain); febrile infections with giddiness; inflammation of the respiratory tract, gastrointestinal tract and the eyes; menstrual disturbances; anxiety and depressive states; and itching skin diseases.

PRECAUTIONS AND ADVERSE REACTIONS

Contact with larger quantities of the allergen can bring about resorption and generalized erythema; in severe cases also fever and unconsciousness. Severe conjunctivitis and corneal inflammations, with possible loss of sight, may result after contact with the eyes. External application of the drug should be avoided. Skin affected by accidental contact should be intensively rinsed with a soapy solution and then cleaned with ether or ethanol. The points of inflammation should be covered with bicarbonate of soda paste (mixed with water). Internal treatment is carried out with systematically effective corticosteroids. Cooling bandages give relief in mild cases.

OVERDOSAGE

Overdoses of homeopathic preparations lead to severe mucous membrane irritation, accompanied by queasiness, vomiting, intestinal colic and diarrhea, as well as signs of resorption, e.g., vertigo, stupor, and kidney damage (nephritis, hematuria).

Following gastrointestinal emptying (gastric lavage with burgundy-colored potassium permanganate solution, sodium sulfate), installation of activated charcoal and shock prophylaxis (quiet, warmth), the therapy for these sorts of poisonings consists of treating spasms with diazepam (IV), electrolyte substitution and treating possible cases of acidosis with sodium bicarbonate infusions. In case of shock, plasma volume expanders should be infused. Monitoring of kidney function is essential. Intubation and oxygen respiration may also be necessary. Furthermore, the leaves possess a very severe potential for sensitization, due to their urushiol content. Following sensitization (which can also occur through contact with decorative art from the Far East, such as wooden chairs that have been treated with toxicodendron lacquers), renewed contact leads within a few hours to itching eczemas and eventual blister formation.

DOSAGE

Mode of Administration: Homeopathic dilutions of the mother tincture.

Homeopathic Dosage: 5 drops, 1 tablet, or 10 globules every 30 to 60 minutes (acute) or 1 to 3 times daily (chronic); parenterally: 1 to 2 mL sc; acute: 3 times daily; chronic: once a day (HAB34); children are given different doses.

Storage: In tightly sealed containers, not to be kept for more than a year.

LITERATURE

Randall RC, Phillips GO, Williams PA, *Food Hydrocolloids* 3:65-75. 1989.

Shobha SV et al., Inhibition of soybean lipoxygenase-1 by anacardic acids, cardols, and cardanols. In: *JNP* 57(12):1755-1757. 1994.

Symes WF, Dawson CR, Nature 171:841. 1953.

Zhai H, Chang YC, Singh M, Maibach HI. Patch testing versus history in poison ivy/oak dermatitis. *Contact Dermatitis* 36; 336. 1997

Poisonous Buttercup

Ranunculus sceleratus

DESCRIPTION

Medicinal Parts: The medicinal part is the fresh herb.

Flower and Fruit: The plant produces numerous flowers. They are small, pale yellow, and 4 to 10 mm in size. The petals are as long as the calyx. The sepals are revolute, ovate, and downy. There are many stamens and numerous ovaries. The fruit consists of an oblong, earlike capitula. The calyx and corolla drop easily.

Leaves, Stem, and Root: The plant grows from 20 to 60 cm high with an annual root. The plant is pale, glossy, yellowish-green, fleshy, and glabrous. The upper part of the stem is occasionally pubescent. The stem is erect, tubular, glabrous, and branched. The leaves are palmate; the lower ones are long-petioled with 2- to 3-lobed segments, and the upper ones are sessile and usually trifoliate.

Characteristics: A bruised leaf coming into contact with the skin creates a blister that heals very slowly.

Habitat: The plant is indigenous to central and northern Europe.

Production: Poisonous Buttercup is the fresh herb of *R. sceleratus*, which is gathered in October.

Other Names: Celery-Leaved Crowfoot, Cursed Crowfoot, Marsh Crowfoot, Water Crowfoot

ACTIONS AND PHARMACOLOGY

COMPOUNDS

Glycoside ranunculin: as protoanemonine-forming agent in the freshly harvested plant (1.4% of the fresh weight) that changes enzymatically when the plant is cut into small pieces, and probably also while it is drying, into the pungent, volatile protoanemonine that quickly dimerizes to non-mucous-membrane-irritating anemonine. When dried, the plant may not be capable of protoanemonine formation.

Saponins

EFFECTS

The active agents are ranunculin, protoanemonin and anemonin and flavoid in the leaves. The plant is highly toxic. The juice contains protoanemonin, which causes pain and burning sensations, increases saliva secretion and causes severe inflammation of the tongue.

INDICATIONS AND USAGE

Unproven Uses: Poisonous Buttercup is used as a skin stimulant for skin diseases (such as scabies) and leukoderma.

Homeopathic Uses: Poisonous Buttercup is used for skin complaints, swollen muscles and joints, and influenza.

PRECAUTIONS AND ADVERSE REACTIONS

Extended skin contact with the freshly harvested, bruised plant can lead to blister formation and cauterizations that are difficult to heal due to the resulting protoanemonine, which is severely irritating to skin and mucous membranes. If taken internally, severe irritation to the gastrointestinal tract, combined with colic and diarrhea, as well as irritation of the urinary drainage passages, may occur. Symptomatic treatment for external contact consists of mucilaginosa after irrigation with diluted potassium permanganate solution. In case of internal contact, administration of activated charcoal should follow gastric lavage.

OVERDOSAGE

Death by asphyxiation following the intake of large quantities of protoanemonine-forming plants has been observed in animal experiments.

DOSAGE

Mode of Administration: The herb is available as a mother tincture and extract in homeopathic dilutions.

LITERATURE

Bonora A et al., *PH* 26:2277. 1987.

Frohne D, Pfänder HJ, Giftpflanzen - Ein Handbuch für Apotheker, Toxikologen und Biologen, 4. Aufl., Wiss. Verlags-Ges. Stuttgart 1997.

Hegnauer R, Chemotaxonomie der Pflanzen, Bde 1-11: Birkhäuser Verlag Basel, Boston, Berlin 1962-1997.

Kern W, List PH, Hörhammer L (Hrsg.), Hagers Handbuch der Pharmazeutischen Praxis, 4. Aufl., Bde. 1-8: Springer Verlag Berlin, Heidelberg, New York, 1969.

Madaus G, Lehrbuch der Biologischen Arzneimittel, Bde 1-3, Nachdruck, Georg Olms Verlag Hildesheim 1979.

Roth L, Daunderer M, Kormann K, Giftpflanzen, Pflanzengifte, 4. Aufl., Ecomed Fachverlag Landsberg Lech 1993.

Teuscher E, Lindequist U, Biogene Gifte - Biologie, Chemie, Pharmakologie, 2. Aufl., Fischer Verlag Stuttgart 1994.

Poke

Phytolacca americana

DESCRIPTION

Medicinal Parts: The medicinal parts are the dried root and the berries.

Flower and Fruit: The racemes are about 10 cm long and more or less erect. The flowers are androgynous. There is a calyx without a corolla. The involucre segments are 2.5 cm, broadly ovate, greenish-white, and turn reddish at the fruit. There are 10 stamens and 10 carpels, which are fused. The fruits are 10 mm depressed-globose, purplish-black berries, which cover the stem like a raceme. They are similar to blueberries.

Leaves, Stem, and Root: The plant is a glabrous, perennial herb, somewhat woody at the base. The root is long and fleshy. The stems are 1 to 3 m high, hollow, bifurcated, and often marked with grooves. The leaves are alternate, entire-margined, unpleasantly scented, 12 to 25 cm by 5 to 10 cm, ovate-lanceolate, and petiolate.

Habitat: The plant is indigenous to the U.S. and has also become common in Mediterranean countries.

Production: Poke Root and berries are the root and fruit of *Phytolacca americana*.

Other Names: American Nightshade, American Spinach, Bear's Grape, Branching Phytolacca, Cancer-Root, Coakum-Chongras, Cokan, Crowberry, Inkberry, Jalap, Phytolacca Berry, Phytolacca Root, Pigeon Berry, Pocan, Poke Root, Poke Berry, Pokeweed, Red Weed, Red-Ink Plant, Scoke, Skoke, Virginian Poke

ACTIONS AND PHARMACOLOGY

COMPOUNDS: POKE FRUIT

Triterpene saponins (mixture termed phytolaccatoxin): phytolaccoside A-G, phytolaccasaponin B, aglycones 28,30-dicarboxy-oleans, including jaligonic acid, esculentic acid, phytolaccagenic acid, pokeberrygenin

Triterpenes: including alpha-amyrin, beta-amyrin, taraxasterol, psi-taraxasterol, tirucallol

Lectins (pokeweed-mitogens)

Ribosome: inactivating proteins (1-RIP), in the seeds

Betacyans (red pigments): including among others phytolaccanin (betanin), particularly in the fruits

Lignans: caffeic acid aldehyde-oligomerics; including among others americanine A, B and D

Histamine: gamma-aminobutyric acid (in the rhizomes)

Saccharose: cyclitols

EFFECTS: POKE FRUIT

An antihepatotoxic and antiviral effect has been demonstrated for the fruit. The saponins have an emetic effect.

COMPOUNDS: POKE ROOT

Triterpene saponins (mixture termed phytolaccatoxin): phytolaccosides A, B, D, D2, E (chief component, aglycone phytolaccagenin), F, G, phytollaccasaponin B, aglycone 28,30-dicarboxy-oleans, including jaligonic acid, jaligonic acid-30-methyl ester, esculentic acid, phytolaccagenic acid

Amines: histamine (0.13 to 0.16%), in the roots

Starch

EFFECTS: POKE ROOT

An antiedemic and immune-stimulating effect has been demonstrated for the root. The saponins have an emetic effect.

INDICATIONS AND USAGE

POKE FRUIT

Unproven Uses: Rheumatism and skin ulcers

POKE ROOT

Unproven Uses: Poke has been used to treat dysmenorrhoea, dyspepsia, catarrh, rheumatism, tonsillitis, pharyngitis, syphilis, mumps, conjunctivitis, scabies, ring worm infestation, ulcers, constipation, and as an emetic.

Homeopathic Uses: Uses in homeopathic medicine include inflammation of the mucous membranes (particularly of the respiratory tract), feverish infections, inflammation of conditions of the mammary glands, and rheumatic conditions.

PRECAUTIONS AND ADVERSE REACTIONS

General: All parts of the plants are poisonous, due to the presence of mucous membrane-irritating saponins and of the toxic, perorally effective lectins. The toxicity is reduced through cooking, since this destroys the lectins.

Pediatric Use: Emergency poison treatment procedures should be instituted in small children who consume even one berry.

OVERDOSAGE

Symptoms of poisoning include diarrhea (sometimes bloody), dizziness, hypotension, severe thirst, somnolence, tachycardia, vomiting, and in severe cases, spasm and death through respiratory failure. Up to 10 berries are considered harmless for an adult, but could be dangerous for a small child. Adults who consume more than 10 berries and small children who consume any berries should be treated for poisoning. This includes stomach and intestinal emptying (inducement of vomiting, gastric lavage with burgundy-colored potassium permanganate solution, sodium sulphate) and instillation of activated charcoal. Electrolyte substitution and the use of sodium bicarbonate to treat possible acidosis may be necessary.

DOSAGE

Mode of Administration: Administered as a powder, liquid extract and tincture.

Daily Dosage: Usual dosage is 60 to 100 mg

Homeopathic Dosage: 5 drops, 1 tablet, or 10 globules every 30 to 60 minutes (acute) or 1 to 3 times daily (chronic); parenterally: 1 to 2 mL SC, IV., IM, acute: 3 times daily; chronic: once a day (HAB1).

Storage: The drug should be stored in paper or sacks made from cloth.

LITERATURE

Aron GM, Irvin JD, *Antimicrob Agents Chem* 17:1032. 1980

Kang SS, Woo WS, Triterpenes from the berries of *Phytolacca americana*. In: *JNP* 43(4):510-513. 1980.

Kern W, List PH, Hörhammer L (Hrsg.), Hagers Handbuch der Pharmazeutischen Praxis, 4. Aufl., Bde. 1-8, Springer Verlag Berlin, Heidelberg, New York, 1969.

Kobayashi A, Hagihara K, Kajiyama SI, Kanzaki H, Kawazu K. Antifungal Compounds Induced in the Dual Culture with *Phytolacca americana* Callus and Botrytis fabae. *Z Naturforsch.* 50c; 398-402. 1995

Lewin L, Gifte und Vergiftungen, 6. Aufl., Nachdruck, Haug Verlag, Heidelberg 1992.

Lewis WH, *JAMA*. Dec. 21; 242(25):2759-60. 1979

Madaus G, Lehrbuch der Biologischen Arzneimittel, Bde 1-3, Nachdruck, Georg Olms Verlag Hildesheim 1979.

MecPherson A, In: Toxic Plants, Ed. AD Kinghorn, Columbia Press 1979.

Roth L, Daunderer M, Kormann K, Giftpflanzen, Pflanzengifte, 4. Aufl., Ecomed Fachverlag Landsberg Lech 1993.

Steinegger E, Hänsel R, Pharmakognosie, 5. Aufl., Springer Verlag Heidelberg 1992.

Tang W, Eisenbrand G, Chinese Drugs of Plant Origin, Springer Verlag Heidelberg 1992.

Teuscher E, Lindequist U, Biogene Gifte - Biologie, Chemie, Pharmakologie, 2. Aufl., Fischer Verlag Stuttgart 1994.

Wagner H, Wiesenauer M, Phytotherapie. Phytopharmaka und pflanzliche Homöopathika, Fischer-Verlag, Stuttgart, Jena, New York 1995.

Polemonium caeruleum

See Jacob's Ladder

Polemonium reptans

See Abscess Root

Poley

Teucrium polium

DESCRIPTION

Medicinal Parts: The medicinal part is the whole herb.

Flower and Fruit: The flowers are axillary forming a capitula. They are fused and sessile, and their structures are in fives. The calyx is turned slightly upward with 5 acuminate tips and is white-gray pubescent. The corolla is reddish-white or yellowish. The upper lip is deeply divided into two and fused to half of the lower lip so that it appears 5-tipped. There are 4 stamens, which are much longer than the corolla, and a 2-carpeled ovary, divided, but not to the base. The fruit is a nutlet.

Leaves, Stem, and Root: Poley is a dwarf shrub that grows up to 45 cm high. The leaves are decussate, obovate to elongate, crenate, involute, and pubescent. The stem is densely covered with white, greenish, or golden hairs.

Habitat: Mediterranean region

Production: Poley herb is the dried aerial part of *Teucrium polium* collected during the flowering season.

ACTIONS AND PHARMACOLOGY

COMPOUNDS

Diterpenes: including picropolin, picropolinol, picropolinon, teucrin A, teucrin P1, teucrin H3, montanines B and C, teupolins I to V, gnaphalidin, the diterpene spectrum varies a great deal according to both the subspecies being investigated and its source.

Volatile oil (0.1 to 1%): the following have been demonstrated to be chief components, varying according to chemical race, alpha-pinene and beta-pinene, alpha-cadinol, alpha-humulene, beta-caryophyllene, caryophyllene oxide, cedrol, gamma-cadinene, delta-cadinene, limonene, linalool, menthofurane, myrcene, ocimene, T-cadinol, terpine-4-ol

Iridoids: iridoid glycosides, including 8-O-acetyl harpagide, harpagide, teucardoside

Flavonoids: including apigenin-7-O-glucoside, luteolin-7-O-glucoside, acacetine, apigenin, cirsiliol, cirsimaritin, eupatorin, luteolin, salvigenin

EFFECTS

The antidiabetic and anti-ulcer efficacy with which the drug has been credited has not yet been documented in definitive clinical studies. A reduction of the ulcer index was described in connection with animal experiments; furthermore, a definite reduction of the blood sugar levels was exhibited following the I.V. administration of a 4% decoction of the dried herb. The drug is additionally antibacterial, antipyretic and possibly antiedemic and antiexudative in effect.

INDICATIONS AND USAGE

Unproven Uses: Poley is used for diabetes (Israel), gastric complaints (North Africa), fever (Italy), and as a vulnerary (Spain).

PRECAUTIONS AND ADVERSE REACTIONS

No health hazards are known in conjunction with the proper administration of designated therapeutic dosages.

DOSAGE

Mode of Administration: Cut drug and liquid extract for internal use.

Daily Dosage: Single dose for infusion: 1.5 g drug per cup

Storage: Should be tightly sealed and protected from light.

LITERATURE

Autore G, Capasso F, De Fusco R, Fasulo MP, Lembo M, Mascolo N, Menghini A, Antipyretic and antibacterial actions of *Teucrium polium (L.). Pharmacol Res Commun, 16*:21-9, Jan. 1984

Capasso F, Cerri R, Morrica P, Senatore F, Chemical composition and anti-inflammatory activity of an alcoholic extract of *Teucrium polium L. Boll Soc Ital Biol Sper,* 59:1639-43, Nov 30. 1983

Gharaibeh MN, Elayan HH, Salhab AS, Hypoglycemic effects of *Teucrium polium. J Ethnopharmacol,* 24:93-9, Sep. 1988

Hänsel R, Keller K, Rimpler H, Schneider G (Ed), Hagers Handbuch der Pharmazeutischen Praxis, 5. Aufl., Bde 4 - 6 (Drogen), Springer Verlag Berlin, Heidelberg, New York, 1992-1994.

Mattéi A, Rucay P, Samuel D, Feray C, Reynes M, Bismuth H, Liver transplantation for severe acute liver failure after herbal medicine (*Teucrium polium*) administration. *J Hepatol*, 22:597, May. 1995

Rizk AM, Hammouda FM, Rimpler H, Kamel A, Chemical composition of the wild Egyptian plant *Teucrium polium L. Pharmazie,* 22:540-1, Aug. 1974

Rizk AM, Hammouda FM, Rimpler H, Kamel A, Iridoids and flavonoids of *Teucrium polium* herb. *Planta Med,* 22:87-8, Apr. 1986

Rizk AM, Hammouda FM, Rimpler H, Kamel A, On the essential oil of *Teucrium polium L. Pharmazie*, 22:351-2, May. 1974

Suleiman MS, Abdul-Ghani AS, Al-Khalil S, Amin R, Effect of *Teucrium polium* boiled leaf extract on intestinal motility and blood pressure. *J Ethnopharmacol,* 22:111-6, Jan. 1988

Polygala amara

See Bitter Milkwort

Polygala senega

See Seneca Snakeroot

Polygonatum multiflorum

See Solomon's Seal

Polygonum aviculare

See Knotweed

Pomegranate

Punica granatum

DESCRIPTION

Medicinal Parts: The medicinal parts are the root, the bark, the fruits, the peel of the fruit, and the flowers.

Flower and Fruit: The flowers are infundibulate or rotate, usually solitary or in pairs of threes at the tips of the branches. The calyx and receptacle are bright coral-red and have a tough margin. There are 5 to 8 bright-red campanulate, nodding petals and numerous stamens. The filaments are orange-red and the anthers yellow-gold. The ovary consists of 2 or 3 layers lying on top of one another. The fruit is an apple-sized, round, 1.6 to 12 cm wide false berry whose skin turns from bright red to leather-brown. The seeds are roughly square and purple, later acquiring a soft red outer skin.

Leaves, Stem, and Root: The plant is an erect, roughly branched shrub up to 1.5 m high or a small, tree 3 to 5 m tall with a curved trunk and glabrous 4- to 6-edged, sometimes spiny-tipped branches. The branches are narrowly winged when young. The trunk later becomes fissured and twisted. The leaves are generally opposite or in clusters on the short shoots. They are deciduous, simple, pinnate-veined, short-petioled, glabrous, hard, oval-lanceolate with a tough middle rib.

Habitat: The plant probably originated in Asia. Today it is widespread in the Mediterranean region as far as South Tyrol, the Near East, South Africa, South Asia, China, Australia, U.S., and South America.

Production: Pomegranate bark is the dried bark of the trunk roots and branches of *Punica granatum*. The roots, trunk, and older branches are collected at the beginning of autumn. Their bark is peeled off and air-dried.

Other Names: Delima, Grenadier

ACTIONS AND PHARMACOLOGY

COMPOUNDS: POMEGRANATE FRUIT PEEL

Tannins (25 to 28%; gallo tannins): including punicalin (granatine D), punicalagin (granatine C), granatine A, granatine B

COMPOUNDS: POMEGRANATE STEMS AND ROOT

Tannins (20 to 25% gallo tannins): including punicalagin, punicacortein C, casuarin

Piperidine alkaloids (0.4% in the rind of the stem, up to 0.8% in the rind of the root): chief alkaloids isopelletierine, N-methylisopelletierine, pseudopelletierine

EFFECTS

The drug, which contains tannins and alkaloids, is anthelmintic and amoeboid. Pelletierin triggers, like strychnine, a raised stimulant reflex, which can escalate to tetanus and is effective against diverse tapeworms, ring worms and nematodes. The tannins in the drug makes it useful as an astringent for sore throats, diarrhea and dysentery.

INDICATIONS AND USAGE

Unproven Uses: In folk medicine Pomegranate is used for infestation with tapeworm and other worms, for diarrhea and dysentery, as an abortifacient and astringent; externally used for hemorrhoids and as a gargle in cases of sore throat.

Chinese Medicine: In China, Pomegranate is used to treat chronic diarrhea and dysentery, blood in the stool, worm infestation, and anal prolapses.

Indian Medicine: In India, uses include diarrhea, dysentery, vomiting, and eye pain.

Homeopathic Uses: Punica granatum is used for gastrointestinal disturbances.

PRECAUTIONS AND ADVERSE REACTIONS

No health hazards are known in conjunction with the proper administration of designated therapeutic dosages. The high levels of tannin content in the drug could lead to gastric irritation.

OVERDOSAGE

Due to the alkaloid content, overdoses with the rind of the stem or the root (above 80 g) lead to vomiting, including the vomiting of blood, later to dizziness, chills, vision disorders, collapse, and possible death through respiratory failure. Total blindness (amaurosis) could occur within a few hours or a few days, then disappear within a few days or weeks.

Following gastrointestinal emptying, (inducement of vomiting, gastric lavage with burgundy-colored potassium permanganate solution, sodium sulfate), installation of medicinal charcoal and shock prophylaxis (quiet, warmth), the therapy for poisonings consists of treating spasms with diazepam (IV), electrolyte substitution and treating possible cases of acidosis with sodium bicarbonate infusions. In case of shock, plasma volume expanders should be infused. Monitoring of kidney function is essential. Intubation and oxygen respiration may also be necessary.

DOSAGE

Mode of Administration: Pomegranate is available as whole, crude and powder forms for internal and external use. It is also available in parenteral form for homeopathic use.

Preparation:

Decoction — 1 part drug and 5 parts water.

Macerations — 60 parts drug and 400 parts water macerated for 12 hours to half the initial volume.

Liquid extract — percolation of 1,000 parts coarse powder and 59% ethanol (V/V). The percolate is evaporated to the initial amount of the drug (EB6).

Decoction — 250 parts bark powder and 1,500 parts water boiled for 30 minutes (Belg IV).

Daily Dosage:

Tapeworm treatment 1 (decoction) — 4 doses of 60 mL with 2 hour intervals between doses accompanied before treatment and after treatment by a laxative.

Tapeworm treatment 2 (maceration) — administration of 3 doses of 65 mL with a duodenal probe at 30 minute intervals; a laxative is administered after an hour.

As pomegranate bark juice extract — single dose: for tapeworm 20 g.

Homeopathic Dosage: 5 drops, 1 tablet, or 10 globules every 30 to 60 minutes (acute) or 1 to 3 times daily (chronic); parenterally: 1 to 2 mL sc acute: 3 times daily; chronic: once a day (HAB1).

Storage: Pomegranate should be sealed in containers and protected from moisture.

LITERATURE

Beckham N, Phyto-oestrogens and compounds that affect oestrogen metabolism. In: *Aust Herbalism* 7:11-16. 1995.

Chauhan D, Chauhan JS. Flavonoid diglycoside from *Punica granatum. Pharm Biol* 39(2); 155-157. 2001

Foder GB, Colasenko B, In: Alkaloids, Vol. 3, Ed. SW. Pelletier, John Wiley 1985.

Gaig P, Botey J, Gutierrez V, Pena M, Eseverri JL, Marin A. Allergy to pomegranate (*Punica granatum). J Investig Allergol Clin Immunol,* 2:216-8, Jul-Aug 1992

Gaig P, Botey J, Gutierrez V, Pena M, Eseverri JL, Marin A. Somatic embryogenesis and plantlet from petal cultures of pomegranate *Punica granatum L. Indian J Exp Biol,* 2:719-21, Jul 1996

Hussein SAM, Barakat HH, Merfort I, Nawwar MAM. Tannins from the Leaves of *Punica granatum. Phytochemistry* 45 (4); 819-823. 1997

Neuhöfer H et al., The occurence of pelletierine derivatives in *Punica granatum.* In: 37. Annual Congr Med Plant Res Braunschweig 1989 P1-13. 1989.

Schilling G, Schick H, On the structure of punicalagin and punicalin. In: *Liebigs Ann Chem* (11):2240. 1985.

Segura JJ, Morales-Ramos LH, Verde-Star J, Guerra D. Growth inhibition of Entamoeba histolytica and E. invadens produced by pomegranate root (*Punica granatum L.) Arch Invest Med* (Mex), 21:235-9, Jul-Sep 1990

Pontian Rhododendron

Rhododendron ponticum

DESCRIPTION

Medicinal Parts: The medicinal part of the plant is its leafy branches.

Flower and Fruit: The inflorescence is an umbelliferous raceme with 8 to 15 single flowers on 3 pubescent pedicles that are up to 3.5 cm long. The flower structures are in fives and fused. The calyx is inconspicuous, up to 3 mm long, and 5-toothed. The corolla is campanulate, 5-lobed, 4 to 5 cm in diameter, violet to pink-violet with green-yellow spots on the upper lobes. There are 10 stamens and a multichambered ovary on sessile disc. The fruit is an elongate-cylindrical capsule. The seeds are small and can fly.

Leaves, Stem, and Root: Rhododendron ponticum is an evergreen shrub typically growing up to 5 m high, occasionally up to a tree height of 8 m. The leaves are 8 to 15 cm long, 3 to 5 cm wide with a 1 to 2 cm long petiole. The lamina is elliptical-elongate, acute at both ends, entire, coriaceous, dark green, smooth and glabrous above, pale green and glabrous beneath. The plant is heavily branched. The branches are glabrous.

Habitat: The plant is indigenous to the Balkan states, the Commonwealth of Independent States, Spain, Portugal, and England.

Production: Pontian rhododendron herb is the dried leafy branches of *Rhododendron ponticum*.

ACTIONS AND PHARMACOLOGY

COMPOUNDS

Diterpenes of the andromedan type: grayanotoxin I (andromedotoxin, acetylandromedol, asebotoxin, rhodotoxin, 0.001 to 0.02%), grayanotoxin II (andromedol), grayanotoxin III (andromedenol)

Flavonoids: myricetin, gossypetin, azaleatin, malvin

Steroids: sterols, including beta-sitosterol, alpha-amyrin, ursolic acid

EFFECTS

The drug has the effect of reducing blood pressure in animal experiments, due to the diterpenes it contains of the andromedan type (grayanotoxins). Historically, effects also have been described as stimulating, narcotic, diaphoretic and diuretic.

INDICATIONS AND USAGE

Therapeutic use is no longer recommended because of the drug's possibly dangerous side effects due to its toxic content.

Unproven Uses: Folk medicine uses have focused on primary hypertension and arthritis. Various species of Rhododendron have been used for rheumatic and gouty conditions and for stones.

PRECAUTIONS AND ADVERSE REACTIONS

All medicinal administration of the drug is discouraged. The observed effect (lowered blood pressure resulting from bradycardia) is the first sign of a toxic reaction.

The plant is toxic because of its andromedan derivative content. The grayanotoxins it contains prevent the closure of the sodium channels and thus inhibit conduction.

OVERDOSAGE

Symptoms of poisoning in case of overdosage could include salivation, cold sweats, paresthesia, vomiting, diarrhea, severe stupor, coordination disorders, spasm, bradycardia, cardiac arrhythmias, hypotension, and eventually death through cardiac failure or apnea. While poisonings among humans have not been documented, poisonings (including fatal ones such as ''goat death'') occur frequently among animals. The presumed explanation is that the leathery leaves are not tempting to humans to eat, and because of the low levels of andromendan derivatives present in medicinal preparations.

Toxic and/or lethal dosage levels cannot be determined with any precision because the plant's andromendan derivative content can vary so wildly. The LD50 for mice amounts to 5.1 mg grayonotoxin I/kg body weight, p.o.

Following gastrointestinal emptying (inducement of vomiting, gastric lavage with burgundy-colored potassium permanganate solution, sodium sulfate), installation of medicinal charcoal and shock prophylaxis (quiet, warmth), the therapy for poisonings consists of treating spasms with diazepam (IV), bradycardia with atropine and electrolyte substitution, and treating possible cases of acidosis with sodium bicarbonate infusions. In case of shock, plasma volume expanders should be infused. It is crucial that no opiates are administered. Monitoring of kidney function is essential. Intubation and oxygen respiration may also be necessary.

DOSAGE

Mode of Administration: Whole drug. Folk medicine modes also include administration as a tea or cigarette.

How Supplied: Forms of commercial pharmaceutical preparations include coated tablets and compound preparations.

Daily Dosage: There are no more exact details available.

LITERATURE

Hänsel R, Keller K, Rimpler H, Schneider G (Ed), Hagers Handbuch der Pharmazeutischen Praxis, 5. Aufl., Bde 4 - 6 (Drogen), Springer Verlag Berlin, Heidelberg, New York, 1992-1994.

Keller S, von Kürten S, Pachaly P, Zymalkowski F, Sterines and triterpenes from *Rhododendron ponticum. Pharmazie*, 25:621-5, Oct. 1970

Thieme H, Walewska E, Winkler HJ, Isolation of salidroside from leaves of *Rhododendron ponticum x catawbiense. Pharmazie*, 24:783, Dec 12. 1969

Poplar

Populus species

DESCRIPTION

Medicinal Parts: The medicinal parts are the bark, leaves, and leaf buds.

Flower and Fruit: The plant is dioecious. The carmine red flowers are in large, cylindrical hanging, thick catkins with carmine anthers. The male flowers have carmine red anthers; the female flowers have carmine stigmas. The flowers appear before the leaves. The seeds, which ripen in May/June, are very small and have a white lanate tuft of hair.

Leaves, Stem, and Root: The tree may grow up to 30 m. The bark is initially yellow brown and later black-gray and fissured. The leaf buds are viscid. The leaves are almost circular with a dark green upper surface and a light grey-green under surface. They are dentate or lobed with obtuse teeth, initially silky-haired, later glabrous. The petioles are long, thin and laterally compressed.

Habitat: There are both European and North American species within the genus that have spread to other temperate zones.

Other Names: Black Poplar, Canadian Poplar, European Aspen, Quaking Aspen Trembling Poplar, White Poplar

Production: Poplar bark consists of the fresh or dried bark of salicin-rich Poplar species as well as their preparations. Poplar leaves consist of the leaves of salicin-rich Poplar species as well as their preparations. Poplar buds consist of the dried, unopened leaf buds of *Populus* species, as well as their preparations.

ACTIONS AND PHARMACOLOGY

COMPOUNDS: POPLAR BARK AND LEAVES

Glycosides and esters yielding salicylic acid:

In Populus alba (leaf 6%, bark 2%) chief components: salicortin, tremulacin, salicin

In Populus nigra (leaf 2%, bark 1.5%) chief components: salicortin, salicin

In Populus tremula (leaf 3%, bark 2%) chief components: salicin, tremulacin, salicortin including as well as salireposide, populin, tremuloidin

EFFECTS

Poplar bark and leaves have antiphlogistic, analgesic, antibacterial, and spasmolytic effects.

The salicylate acid derivatives and flavonoids are responsible for the antiphlogistic, analgesic, spasmolytic, and antibacterial characteristics of the drug. The beneficial effect in micturition complaints due to prostate hypertrophy may be due to the content of zinc lignans in the drug.

COMPOUNDS: POPLAR LEAF BUDS

Flavonoids: (particularly in the glutinous coating of the buds, also yielding propolis) including chrysin, tectochrysin, galengine, izalpinine, galangin-3-methyl ether, kaempferol-3-methyl ether, pinocembrin, pinocembrin-7-methyl ether, apigenin

Glycosides and esters yielding salicylic acid: including salicin, populin

Volatile oil: chief components alpha- and beta-caryophyllene

EFFECTS: POPLAR LEAF BUDS

Poplar buds have antiphlogistic, antibacterial, and wound healing effects.

INDICATIONS

POPLAR BARK AND LEAVES

Unproven Uses: Poplar bark and leaves are used for pain and rheumatism therapy; and in micturition complaints due to prostate hypertrophy.

POPLAR LEAF BUDS

Approved by Commission E:

- Hemorrhoids
- Wounds and burns

Unproven Uses: Poplar buds are used for frostbite and sunburn.

CONTRAINDICATIONS

POPLAR BARK AND LEAVES

Contraindicated in cases of hypersensitivity to salicylates.

POPLAR LEAF BUDS

Contraindicated in cases of hypersensitivity to salicylates, propolis, and balsam of Peru, which may be a component in commercially available ointments.

PRECAUTIONS

POPLAR BARK AND LEAVES

No health hazards or side effects are known in conjunction with the proper administration of designated therapeutic dosages.

POPLAR LEAF BUDS

No health hazards are known in conjunction with the proper administration of designated therapeutic dosages. External administration of the drug occasionally leads to allergic skin reactions.

DOSAGE

POPLAR BARK AND LEAVES

Mode of Administration: Poplar leaves are available in crude form as well as galenic preparations for internal use. Poplar bark is only available in compounded preparations.

Daily Dosage: 10 g of drug

POPLAR LEAF BUDS

Mode of Administration: Poplar buds are available in semi-solid preparations for application to the skin.

How Supplied: Semi-solid preparations equivalent to 20% to 30% of drug.

Daily Dosage: Externally, 5 g drug.

LITERATURE

POPLAR BARK, LEAVES, AND LEAF BUDS

Anonym, Phytotherapie: Pflanzliche Antirheumatika - was bringen sie? In: *DAZ* 136(45):4012-4015. 1996.

Jossang A et al., Cinnamrutinoses A and B, glycosides from *Populus tremula*. In: *PH* 35(2):547. 1994.

Picard S et al., Isolation of a new phenolic compound from leaves of Populus deltoides. In: *JNP* 57(6):808-810. 1994.

Vonkruedener S et al., Effects of extracts from *Populus tremula L., Solidago virgaurea L.* and *Fraxinus excelsior L.* on various myeloperoxidase systems. In: *Arzneim Forsch* 46(8):809-814. 1996.

Poppyseed

Papaver somniferum

DESCRIPTION

Medicinal Parts: The medicinal part is the latex extracted from the seed capsule.

Flower and Fruit: A solitary flower grows on a long, glabrous or pubescent pedicle. The flowers are erect with a diameter of 10 cm. There are 2 green, glabrous, falling sepals and 4 violet-white or red petals with a darker mark at the base. The fruit is round or ellipsoid and often has a very large capsule. The numerous seeds are reniform, pitted, black, and blue-frosted or whitish.

Leaves, Stem, and Root: The opium Poppy is an annual that grows 30 to 150 cm high. It is a single-stemmed, blue-gray frosted plant. The stem is erect, straight or branched, and produces white milky latex, as does the whole plant. The leaves are entire, glabrous, serrated, or crenate at the margin and clasping.

Characteristics: The cultivation of the plant and the extraction and sale of opium is banned in many countries.

Habitat: The plant originated in western Asia. It is cultivated worldwide commercially.

Production: Opium is the thickened latex collected from the outside of immature Poppy capsules that have had incisions made in the fruit capsules. The unripe seed capsules suitable for the production of opium are trimmed. Subsequent to drying, the processed latex is scraped off and formed into pieces of varying size. The obtained material is referred to as raw opium (Rohopium) and is also the basic substance used for the production of heroin.

Other Names: Garden-Poppy, Mawseed, Opium Poppy

ACTIONS AND PHARMACOLOGY

COMPOUNDS

Isoquinoline alkaloids (20-30%): chief alkaloids morphine (3-23%), narcotine (2-10%), codeine (0.2-3.5%), papaverine (0.5-3%), thebaine (0.2-1%).] The alkaloids are present as salts of meconic acid, lactic acid or fumaric acid.

Benzyl isoquinoline type: papaverine (0.5 to 3%)

Phthalide isoehinoline type: narcotine (noscapine, 2 to 10%)

Rubber (5-10%)

Resins

Mucilages

EFFECTS

The main alkaloid is morphine, which is a strong analgesic that, even in small doses, causes euphoria, sedation, then narcotic sleep. It depresses breathing and slows down evacuation of the stomach, causing constipation and urine retention. Codeine has an antitussive effect and papaverine is spasmolytic and vasodilatory.

INDICATIONS AND USAGE

Unproven Uses: Opium is used most frequently as a sedative and/or analgesic. Uses in folk medicine include as a sedative in cases of typhus, intestinal tuberculosis and intestinal ulcers; for spasms of smooth muscle, bile ducts and urinary tract; for peritonitis; for gallstones, kidney stones and bladder colic; as well as for coughs and certain types of depression.

Chinese Medicine: Uses in Chinese medicine include chronic coughs, diarrhea, dysentery, anal prolapse, and abdominal symptoms.

Indian Medicine: Irritable cough, ear and eye inflammation, proctologic symptoms, diarrhea, and dysentery are considered indications for use in Indian medicine.

CONTRAINDICATIONS

Contraindications include pregnancy (alkaloids pass through the placenta barrier), nursing (alkaloids entering the mother's milk), illnesses connected with reduced respiratory function, pancreatitis, colon ulcers, elevated internal cranial pressure, acute hepatitis propheria, and biliary colic. Caution is to be observed when administering in the presence of Addison's disease and hypothyroidism because of opium's centrally depressive effect.

PRECAUTIONS AND ADVERSE REACTIONS

No health hazards are known in conjunction with the proper administration of designated therapeutic dosages. However, the following can occur as side effects: clonic twitching, constipation, dizziness, general weakness, headache, hyperthermia, itchy skin, rashes, and trembling of the hands. Sensitization has been reported, with papaverin the presumed allergen.

OVERDOSAGE

Overdosage leads initially to reduction of mental capacity, reactive euphoria, analgesia, miosis, bradycardia, slowed respiration. That can progress to respiratory failure, cyanosis, tonic-clonic spasms, pylorospasm and sphincterism, intestinal atonia, nausea, vomiting, pulmonary and brain edemas. Following gastrointestinal emptying (inducement of vomiting, gastric lavage with burgundy-colored potassium permanganate solution, sodium sulfate) and instillation of activated charcoal, the therapy for poisoning consists of electrolyte substitution, treating possible cases of acidosis with sodium bicarbonate infusions and administration of plasma volume expanders in the event of shock. Intubation and oxygen respiration may also be necessary. Naloxone (IV) is suitable as an antidote.

DOSAGE

Mode of Administration: Opium is obsolete as a drug. Morphine is administered as a pure substance and in combination with other active substances, although it has been extensively replaced by synthetic analgesia. Codeine is used by itself and in combination with other agents. Numerous cases of death due to opium use are known.

LITERATURE

Amann T, Zenk MH, Endogenes Morphin. In: *DAZ* 136(7):519-527. 1996.

Buch, In: Handbook of Experimental Pharmacology. Volume 104/I und 104/II: Opioids I und II. Springer-Verlag Berlin, Heidelberg, New York, 1993.

Buchbauer G et al., Headspace constituents of opium. In: *PM* 60(2):181. 1994.

Czygan FC, Hellas und Phytopharmaka. In: *DAZ* 135(51/52):4707-4711. 1995.

Freye E, Leopold C, Opiate und Opiatantagonisten. I. Theoretischen Grundlagen der Opioidwirkung. In: DAZ 131(29):1517. 1991.

Gomez-Serranillos MP, Palomino OM, Carretero E, Villar A. Analytical Study and Analgesic Activity of Oripavine from *Papaver somniferum L. Phytother Res.* 12 (5); 346-349. 1998

Lal RK, Sharma JR. Genetics of Alkaloids in *Papaver somniferum. Planta Med.* 57; 271-274. 1991

Paul BD, Dreka C, Knight ES, Smith ML. Gas Chromatographic/Mass Spectrometric Detection of Narcotine, Papaverine, and Thebain in Seeds of *Papaver somniferum. Planta Med.* 62 (6); 544-547. 1996

Pfeifer S, Mohn - eine Arzneipflanze seit mehr als zweitausend Jahren, Teil 1 und 2. In: *PA* 17:467-479 et 536-554. 1962.

Répási J, Hosztafi S, Szabó Z, 5′-O-Demethylnarcotin: A New Alkaloide from *Papaver somniferum*. In: *PM* 59(5):477. 1993.

Stano J, Nemec P, Bezakova L, Kovacs P, Kakoniova D, Liskova D. Invertase in immobilized cells of *Papaver somniferum L. Pharmazie* 52 (3); 242-244. 1997

Stano J et al. Distribution of dipeptidyl peptidase IV in organs and tissue cultures of poppy plants *Papaver somniferum L.cv. Amarin. Pharmazie* 52 (4); 319-321. 1997

Wilhelm R, Zenk MH. Biotransformation of Thebaine by Cell Cultures of *Papaver somniferum* and *Mahonia nervosa. Phytochemistry* 46 (4); 701-708. 1997

Znek MH, Über das Opium, das den Schmerz besiegt und die Sucht weckt. In: PZ 139(48):4185. 1994.

Populus species

See Poplar

Potentilla

Potentilla anserina

DESCRIPTION

Medicinal Parts: The medicinal parts are leaves and flowers, whole or macerated, collected during or shortly before the flowering season and dried.

Flower and Fruit: The flowers are solitary on long pedicles of lateral shoots growing from the stem nodes. They are 1.5 to 3 cm wide. There are 5 epicalyx bracts, 5 sepals, and 5 petals. The last are twice as long as the sepals and are golden yellow, ovate and without a distinct margin. The 20 stamens have ovate anthers. The styles occur laterally, are threadlike, and only thickened at the stigmas. The ripe fruit is glabrous, ovate to almost globular, and grooved on the back.

Leaves, Stem, and Root: The plant is a two-axis herbacious perennial with a short, thick, branched rhizome and rosettes of basal leaves. The stems are 80 cm long, creeping, rooting at the nodes, softly pubescent, and eventually becoming glabrous. The leaves are unevenly paired, pinnate, and glossy with silky white hairs beneath, tomentose and fresh green above.

Characteristics: The plant has an almondlike fragrance and dry taste.

Habitat: The plant is found in temperate and colder regions of the entire Northern Hemisphere.

Production: Potentilla herb consists of the fresh or dried leaf and flowers of *Potentilla anserina* harvested shortly before or during flowering, as well as its preparations.

Other Names: Cinquefoil, Crampweed, Goose Tansy, Goosegrass, Goosewort, Moor Grass, Silver Cinquefoil, Prince's Feathers, Trailing Tansy, Wild Agrimony

ACTIONS AND PHARMACOLOGY

COMPOUNDS

Tannins (5 to 10%): chiefly ellagitannins

Flavonoids: including quercitrin

Hydroxycoumarins: umbelliferone, scopoletin

EFFECTS

The drug is astringent because of the tannin concentration.

On isolated rat uterus a paralyzing effect was proven which is due to the presence of ammonium salts. The empirical evidence of a spasmolytic effect in dysmenorrhea could not be definitively proved.

INDICATIONS

Approved by Commission E:

- Diarrhea
- Inflammation of the mouth and pharynx
- Premenstrual syndrome (PMS)

Internal application is indicated for topical treatment of inflammation of the oral and pharyngeal mucosa, adjuvant treatment of non-specific, acute diarrhea, and dysmenorrhea symptoms.

Unproven Uses: In folk medicine, Potentilla is used externally as a wash for poorly healing wounds.

PRECAUTIONS

No health hazards or side effects are known in conjunction with the proper administration of designated therapeutic dosages. There have been complaints of stomach irritation associated with Potentilla.

DOSAGE

Mode of Administration: Potentilla is available in commercial forms for oral intake. It is also available in crude and powder forms.

Preparation: To prepare a tea, pour boiling water over 2 g finely cut drug, strain after 10 minutes (1 teaspoon corresponds to approximately 0.7 g drug).

Daily Dosage: 4 to 6 g of drug; Tea: 1 cup freshly prepared several times a day between meals.

Storage: Protect from light and moisture.

LITERATURE

Kombal R, Glasl H, Flavan-3-ols and flavonoids from *Potentilla anserina*. In: *PM* 61(5):484-485. 1995.

Schimmer O, Lindenbaum M, Tannins with antimutagenic properties in the herb of Alchemilla species and *Potentilla anserina*. In: *PM* 61(2):141-145. 1995.

Potentilla anserina

See Potentilla

Potentilla erecta

See Cinqefoil

Potentilla reptans

See European Five-Finger Grass

Premorse

Scabiosa succisa

DESCRIPTION

Medicinal Parts: The medicinal part is the dried herb.

Flower and Fruit: The flowers are purple-blue, globular, and long pedicled composite blooms, with a 2- to 3-rowed involucre. The florets are all the same size. The epicalyx has thorn-tipped teeth and the calyx has 5 bristles. The corolla is fused and has 4 tips. There are 4 stamens and 1 inferior ovary. The fruit is a nutlet.

Leaves, Stem, and Root: The plant grows from 15 to 80 cm high. It has a short, finger-thick rhizome, which looks bitten off. In the first year of growth, the root resembles a carrot. Later it becomes woody and dies off except for the upper part, which accounts for its appearance. The remaining upper part then develops lateral roots. The stem is erect, sparsely branched, pubescent, and has few leaves. The basal leaves are petiolate, oblong, and obtuse. The cauline leaves are narrow and acute.

Habitat: Scabiosae succisae is indigenous to all of Europe.

Production: Premorse is the aerial part of *Scabiosa succisa*.

Other Names: Devil's Bit, Ofbit, Premorse Scaboius

ACTIONS AND PHARMACOLOGY

COMPOUNDS

Iridoide monoterpenes: including among others, dipsacan, cephalaroside (structures unknown)

Saponins

Tannins

Flavonoids: including among others, saponarine (C-glycosylflavone)

Triterpenes: including among others, ursolic acid

EFFECTS

Premorse is a febrifuge and a diaphoretic.

INDICATIONS AND USAGE

Unproven Uses: The herb is used for febrile colds and coughs.

PRECAUTIONS AND ADVERSE REACTIONS

No health hazards or side effects are known in conjunction with the proper administration of designated therapeutic dosages.

DOSAGE

Mode of Administration: The herb is ground as a drug for infusion.

LITERATURE

Hegnauer R, Chemotaxonomie der Pflanzen, Bde 1-11: Birkhäuser Verlag Basel, Boston, Berlin 1962-1997.

Kern W, List PH, Hörhammer L (Hrsg.), Hagers Handbuch der Pharmazeutischen Praxis, 4. Aufl., Bde 1-8: Springer Verlag Berlin, Heidelberg, New York, 1969 (unter *Succisa pratensis*).

Madaus G, Lehrbuch der Biologischen Arzneimittel, Bde 1-3, Nachdruck, Georg Olms Verlag Hildesheim 1979.

Primula veris

See Cowslip

Prunella vulgaris

See Self-Heal

Prunus africana

See Pygeum

Prunus laurocerasus

See Cherry Laurel

Prunus serotina

See Wild Cherry

Prunus species

See Almond

Prunus spinosa

See Sloe

Psyllium

Plantago ovata

DESCRIPTION

Medicinal Parts: The medicinal parts are the ripe and dried seeds, the epidermis, the adjacent, broken-down layers of the Indian variety, and the fresh plant.

Flower and Fruit: The flowers are on cylindrical, glabrous, or finely pubescent scapes, which are only slightly longer than the leaves. They form 0.5 to 3.5 cm long spikes. The bracts are about 3 mm, suborbicular to ovate, and sometimes shortly pubescent. The sepals are about 2.5 mm, similarly shaped, almost free, keeled at the apex with wide scarious margins. The anterior ones are usually pubescent. The corolla-tube is 1.5 to 2 mm long and glabrous. The lobes are 2.5 mm, ovate-orbicular, subobtuse to very shortly acuminate. The stamens are exserted up to 1 mm and the capsule is about 3 mm. The seeds are 2.2 to 2.5 mm and cymbiform.

Leaves, Stem, and Root: The plant is an annual almost stemless, softly pubescent plant. The plant may have one or several rosettes. The leaves are 2.5 to 12 cm by 0.1 to 0.8 cm, linear to linear-lanceolate. The leaves are entire-margined or slightly denticulate and sparsely to densely villous-lanate.

Habitat: The plant grows in India, Afghanistan, Iran, Israel, northern Africa, Spain, and the Canary Islands. The plant is cultivated in India and neighboring countries, Arizona, and southern Brazil.

Production: Psyllium consists of the ripe seeds or epidermis of *Plantago ovata* (syn. *Plantago isphagula*).

Other Names: Black Psyllium, Blond Psyllium, Blood Plantago, Indian Plantago, Ispaghula, Sand Plantain, Spogel

ACTIONS AND PHARMACOLOGY

COMPOUNDS: PSYLLIUM SEED

Mucilages (20-30%): chiefly arabinoxylans and glacturonosidorhamnoses

Fatty oil

Iridoids: aucubin

Proteic Substances

COMPOUNDS: PSYLLIUM SEED EPIDERMIS

Mucilages (parent substances arabinoxylans)

EFFECTS

Human studies have demonstrated Psyllium's laxative, cholesterol lowering, anti-hypertensive, and expectorant effects. Animal studies have shown anti-inflammatory, anti-neoplastic, cholesterol lowering, hypoglycemic, and hypotensive effects, as well as growth suppression. An ethanolic extract has also demonstrated ileum stimulation and cholinergic effects (Newall et al, 1996; Nordgaard et al, 1996; Maurai et al, 1995; Turnbull & Thomas, 1995; Tyler et al, 1981).

Antidiarrheal Effects: The mucilage absorbs water from the gastrointestinal tract, adjusting the consistency of the feces (Newall et al, 1996). Plantago major has an antigiardiasic activity that may reduce diarrhea (Ponce-Macotela et al, 1994).

Anti-inflammatory Effects: Five phenylethyanoids were isolated from *Plantago lanceolata* herbage and tested in mice with arachidonic acid induced mouse ear edema. Acetoside and plantamajoside were found to have an anti-edema effect (Murai et al, 1995).

Cholesterol-Lowering Effects: Psyllium increases fecal excretion of bile acids and cholesterol, binds bile acids and cholesterol in the intestines, allows less circulation for reabsorption, and causes the liver to use more cholesterol to make bile acids (Chan & Schroeder, 1995). Psyllium may lower serum cholesterol levels by replacing dietary fats, thereby reducing the amount available for absorption, and not directly affecting cholesterol (Swain, 1990). A decrease in LDL cholesterol levels and total cholesterol with the herb has been seen in many studies (Davidson, 1998; MacMahon, 1998; Rodriguez-Moran, 1998; Romero, 1998). Although one study indicated an increase in HDL cholesterol and a decrease in serum triglycerides (TG) with Psyllium, other studies have reported no change in these parameters (Anderson, 1988; Bell, 1989; Davidson, 1998; Rodriguez-Moran, 1998).

Glucose Controlling Effects: Postprandial glucose and fasting plasma glucose significantly improved in type 2 diabetic patients taking Psyllium (Anderson, 1999; Rodriguez-Moran, 1998).

Gallstones Inhibiting Effects: Psyllium hydrocolloid exerts bile acid sequestrant properties determined by a rise in the cholic/chenodeoxycholic acid ratio. This activity protects against cholesterol gallstone formation (Berman, 1975). Psyllium also protects against cholesterol gallstone formation by reducing biliary cholesterol saturation index. The protective effect is associated with a selective decrease in biliary cholesterol and chenodeoxycholic acid (Schwesinger, 1999).

Effects on Irritable Bowel Syndrome/Ulcerative Colitis: Stool frequency and consistency, abdominal pain, and abdominal distention have shown improvement in IBS patients taking Psyllium (Hotz, 1994; Prior, 1987). A decrease in transit time of bowel content may also be seen with the herb (Prior, 1987).

Laxative Effects: Psyllium decreases the passage time of the bowel content by increasing the volume of the stool, thus exerting a laxative effect. The herb acts as stool softener by increasing stool water content. Psyllium was superior to docusate sodium in subjects with chronic idiopathic constipation (McRorie, 1998).

CLINICAL TRIALS

Cancer

Daily consumption of 7 g of Ispaghula husk (Psyllium) significantly lowered fecal lithocholic and isolithocholic acids. These fecal bile acids are associated with both colorectal cancer and serum cholesterol levels. Eighteen stool samples were taken from each of the 16 healthy volunteers during the study. Stools were analyzed at a rate of 12 samples/week. This was a single center study that took place over a 12-week period that included a 2-week pretreatment phase followed by an 8-week treatment phase and a 2-week post-treatment phase. No adverse reactions were reported by study participants (Chaplin et al, 2000).

Cholesterol/Type 2 diabetes

A randomized, double-blind, placebo-controlled study was conducted to determine the plasma-lowering effects of 5.1g twice daily of psyllium husk fibers, used as an adjunct to dietary and drug therapy on lipid and glucose levels in patients with type 2 diabetes. Forty-nine subjects received either the psyllium preparation, Plantago ovata Forsk, or placebo in combination with their antidiabetic drugs. Results showed psyllium significantly decreased cholesterol levels and improved type 2 diabetes. Psyllium therapy was also safe and well tolerated (Ziai et al, 2005).

Constipation

Forty-three percent of patients had some improvement in a study involving 149 patients suffering from chronic constipation treated with 15 to 30 g/d of *Plantago ovata* seeds for a minimum of 6 weeks. Measurement of effectiveness included oroanal transit time as measured using radiopaque markers, symptom evaluation, and rectoanal evaluation (represented by proctoscopy, manometry, and defecography). Results indicated that 32 (21%) patients became symptom free, 33 (22.1%) were improved, and 84 (56.4%) did not show any effects. When divided on the basis of type of patient disorder, 80% of patients with slow transit times and 63% of patients with defecation disorders did not respond positively. A favorable response was noted in 85% of patients with a pathological finding (Voderholzer et al, 1997).

Hemorrhoids/Hemorrhoidectomy relief

A prospective, randomized study was used to evaluate the effects of laxative Plantago ovata after open hemorrhoidectomy. Sixty patients were divided into two groups. Thirty patients were treated postoperatively with two sachets of bulk agent Laxomucil (3.26 g Plantago ovata) twice daily, for 20 days. Thirty patients were treated with glycerin oil. Patients treated with psyllium had a statistically shorter postoperative hospital stay and pain after stool was significantly more tolerable (Kecmanovic et al, 2004).

Psyllium treatment decreased the number of bleeding episodes in 50 patients with internal bleeding hemorrhoids. The patients were randomized into two groups. The first received a commercially available *Plantago ovata* preparation while the control group received a placebo. Each patient received an endoscopy before and after the treatment. In the first 15 days the number of bleeding episodes was reduced from 6.4 in controls to 4.8 in the study group. In the 15 days after administration of the Psyllium bleeding episodes decreased to 3.1 in the study group and 5.5 in the control group. Examination during the last 10 days of the study showed a further reduction in the study group to 1.1 bleeding episodes while the control group remained at 5.5. Congested hemorrhoidal cushions diminished from 2.6 to 1.6 in the treatment group but did not change in the controls. Fiber treatment produced no changes in the degree of prolapse (Perez-Miranda et al, 1996).

Hyperlipidemia

In a 12-week, double-blind and placebo-controlled trial, 68 individuals were randomized to take either 20 mg of a ''statin'' drug (simvastatin) plus placebo, 10 mg of simvastatin plus placebo, or 10 mg of simvastatin plus Psyllium (15 g) daily. At 8 weeks, the mean LDL-C levels in the group receiving 10 mg of simvastatin plus placebo fell by 55 mg/dL from baseline, compared with 63 mg/dL in the group receiving 10 mg of simvastatin plus Psyllium (p=.03). There were no significant changes for triglyceride or HDL cholesterol levels. All the treatment regimens were well-tolerated. The authors conclude that Psyllium can be viewed as a safe addition to further lowering cholesterol, with Psyllium supplementation along with 10 mg of simvastatin, and appears to function as powerfully in lowering cholesterol as 20 mg of simvastatin alone (Moreyra, 2005).

A study a year earlier was done to test the optimal timing of Psyllium consumption for the purpose of lowering cholesterol, with the hypothesis being that taking it in the morning would have more impact than taking it in the evening. But the timing of Psyllium use was found to have no impact, in fact, on its cholesterol-lowering strength in a randomized crossover study in 16 men and 47 women with normal cholesterol levels. A one-month dietary stabilization period was followed by an average daily dose of 12.7 g of Psyllium (hydrophilic mucilloid; a larger dose than the 10.2 g for which the FDA allows health claims to be made) for 8 weeks in the morning and 8 weeks in the evening. No effect on any measurement of lipids—total cholesterol, LDL, HDL, triglycerides—was found in the group overall or in any sub-group analysis, leading the authors to conclude that recommending Psyllium for lowering these risk factors and preventing heart disease may be altogether premature. Total cholesterol for the ''AM first'' group was 5.76 mmol/L at baseline, 5.77 5.76 mmol/L at 8 weeks, and 5.80 5.76 mmol/L at 16 weeks, while the ''PM first'' group readings were 5.47, 5.61, and 5.57 mmol/L, respectively. Previous meta-analyses indicate that starting cholesterol level may be highly predictive of another substance's cholesterol-lowering ability—that of oat bran—and the authors note that that this may play a role in Psyllium's effectiveness as well; similarly, individuals who have high cholesterol may derive some benefit from Psyllium intake while those with normal cholesterol may not (Van Rosendaal, 2004).

In contrast, serum total cholesterol and LDL cholesterol decreased in patients who consumed 5.1 g Psyllium husk twice daily for 26 weeks. This double-blind, placebo-controlled, parallel, multicenter study included men and women (ages 21 to 70 years) with hypercholesterolemia, but otherwise free of major organic disease. No serious adverse events were reported. Total cholesterol decreased by 4.7% LDL cholesterol decreased by 6.7% in the Psyllium group compared to placebo (Anderson et al, 2000).

A randomized, double-blind, placebo-controlled study was conducted to determine the lipid and glucose-lowering effects of Psyllium in type 2 diabetic patients. One hundred twenty-five subjects were included in the study and received either placebo or Psyllium (5 g 3 times daily) over a 6-week period. Prior to the treatment period, all patients participated in a 6-week period of diet counseling. Fasting plasma glucose, total cholesterol, LDL cholesterol, and TG levels were significantly reduced in the Psyllium treatment group compared to placebo. HDL significantly increased in the Psyllium treatment group compared to the placebo group, suggesting Psyllium as a useful adjunct to diet in Type 2 diabetes (Rodriguez-Moran, 1998).

A reduction in total cholesterol and LDL cholesterol, but not in either HDL cholesterol or TG, was noted in a double-blind crossover trial of 12 weeks' duration in hyperlipidemic men. The men were tested with either a wheat bran diet of 2 g of soluble fiber or a Psyllium diet of 12 g of soluble fiber per day (Roberts et al, 1994).

Irritable Bowel Syndrome

A double-blind, placebo-controlled study of *Plantago ovata* husk (3.6 g per dose, once a day) treatment of 80 patients with IBS showed a global assessment improvement of 82% in the treatment group and 53% in the placebo group. Treatment resulted in less or no bowel movements as compared to controls (p=0.026) and resulted in a better over-all sense of effectiveness (p=0.2). No significant differences in abdominal pain or bloating were recorded (Prior & Whorwell, 1987).

Ulcerative Colitis

The objective of an open label, parallel-group, randomized clinical trial was to assess the efficacy and safety of *Plantago ovata* seeds compared with mesalamine in maintaining remission in ulcerative colitis patients. One hundred and five ulcerative colitis patients who were in remission received oral treatment with *Plantago ovata* seeds (10 g twice daily), mesalamine (500 mg 3 times daily), or *Plantago ovata* seeds plus mesalamine at the same doses. After 12 months, treatment failure rate was 40% in the *Plantago ovata* seed group, 35% in the mesalamine group, and 30% in the *Plantago ovata* plus mesalamine group. The probability of continued remission was similar between all treatment groups (Mantel-Cox test, p = 0.67; intent-to-treat analysis), thus implicating the herb might be as effective as mesalamine to maintain remission in ulcerative colitis (Fernandez-Banares F, 1999).

INDICATIONS AND USAGE

Approved by Commission E:

- Constipation
- Diarrhea
- Raised levels of cholesterol
- Hemorrhoids

Psyllium is used for disorders where easy bowel movements with a loose stool are desirable (e.g., in patients with anal fissures and hemorrhoids; following anal/rectal surgery; and during pregnancy).

Unproven Uses: In Folk medicine, the herb is used internally for inflammation of the mucous membrane of the urogenital tract and gastrointestinal tract, and dysentery. Externally, Psyllium is used for gout, rheumatism, furuncles, and as an analgesic.

Indian Medicine: Psyllium is used for gastritis, chronic diarrhea, constipation, dysentery, dry cough, gout, gonorrhea, nephropathy, dysuria, duodenal ulcers, and hemorrhoids.

CONTRAINDICATIONS

Psyllium is contraindicated in patients who have pathological narrowing in the gastrointestinal tract, intestinal obstruction, obstruction or threatening obstruction of the bowel (ileus), fecal impaction, difficulty swallowing or esophageal narrowing or difficulties in regulating diabetes mellitus.

PRECAUTIONS AND ADVERSE REACTIONS

Gastrointestinal distention and flatulence, potentially severe (but rare) allergic reactions-including sneezing, chest congestion and wheezing-and appetite suppression. Psyllium contains various antigens, and cases of anaphylaxis and asthma have been reported. Incorrect administration procedures (with too little fluid) can cause the product to swell and lead to obstruction of the esophagus or of the intestine, particularly with older people. Patients with exocrine pancreatic insufficiency should avoid use of Psyllium due to inhibitory actions on pancreatic lipase (Hansen, 1987).

DRUG INTERACTIONS

MAJOR RISK

Licorice: Concurrent use of licorice and Laxatives may result in increased risk of hypokalemia. *Clinical management*: Avoid concomitant use.

MODERATE RISK

Antidiabetic Agents: Concurrent use may result in increased risk of hypoglycemia. *Clinical Management*: Closely monitor blood glucose and signs and symptoms of hypoglycemia following antidiabetic agents and meals. Psyllium may delay absorption of glucose from meals, leading to less postprandial hyperglycemia and potentially allowing a reduced dosage of the antidiabetic agent.

Carbamazepine: In healthy volunteers, carbamazepine bioavailability was reduced when Psyllium was administered concomitantly (Etman, 1995). *Clinical Management:* If patients are treated with carbamazepine and Psyllium, their administration times of should be separated as far as possible, and plasma levels of carbamazepine should be monitored.

Lithium: Concurrent use may result in decreased plasma levels and effectiveness of lithium. *Clinical Management*:

Separate administration of lithium and psyllium by at least two hours to reduce the likelihood of this interaction.

DOSAGE

Mode of Administration: The whole or coarsely chopped drug and other galenic preparations are used internally. Sufficient fluid must be taken with the drug (150 mL water per 5 g drug). One study did show a greater effect of Psyllium on cholesterol after mixing with food (Wolever, 1994). The dose should be taken 1/2 hour to 1 hour after taking other medication.

How Supplied:

Capsule – 525 mg, 567 mg, 610 mg, 625 mg

Powder – 2.0 g Psyllium per dose, 3.4 g Psyllium per dose, 6.0 g Psyllium per dose (available in a variety of package sizes)

Daily Dosage: The daily dosage ranges from 12 to 40 g of the drug. The powder products should be administered as 1 teaspoonful (3.4 g to 6.0 g drug) in 8 oz. of fruit juice or cool water. Either stir briskly or shake for 3 to 5 seconds, depending on the specific product. Psyllium may be taken up to 3 times daily

Children: For children 6 to 12 years of age administer 1 teaspoonful (2.0 g of the drug) in an empty glass and add 8 oz. of cool water. Stir briskly for 3 to 5 seconds. The dose may be taken up to 3 times daily

LITERATURE

Anderson JW, Zettwoch N, Tietyen-Clark et al., Cholesterol lowering effects of Psyllium hydrophilic mucilloid for hypercholesterolemic men. In: *Arch Intern Med*; 148:292-296, 1988.

Anderson JW, Allgood LD, Turner J et al., Effects of Psyllium on glucose and serum lipid responses in men with type 2 diabetes and hypercholesterolemia. In: Am *J Clin Nutr*; 70(4):466-73, Oct 1999.

Anon. Pharmaceutical Care: "Den Mißbrauch von Laxanzien vermeiden helfen." In: *DAZ* 135(20):1867-1868. 1995.

BAnz (Federal German Gazette) No. 22a; published 1 Feb 1990; revised 19 April 1991.

Basaran, Ceritogly, Undeger et al., Immunomodulatory activities of some Turkish medicinal plants. In: *Phytother Res*; 11(6):609-611, 1997.

Bell LP, Hectorne K, Reynolds H et al., Cholesterol-lowering effects of Psyllium hydrophilic mucilloid. Adjunct therapy to a prudent diet for patients with mild to moderate hypercholesterolemia. In: *JAMA* 16; 261(23):3419-23, Jun 1989.

Bergman F, van der Linden W. Effect of dietary fibre on gallstone formation in hamsters. In: *Z Ernahrungswiss;* 14(3):217-24, Sep 1975.

Chan EK & Schroeder DJ. Psyllium in hypercholesterolemia. In: *Ann Pharmacother*; 29(6):625-627. 1995.

Chaplin MF, Chaudhury S, Dettmar PW et al., Effect of ispaghula husk on the faecal output of bile acids I healthy volunteers. In: *J Steroid Biochem Mol Biol*; 72(5):283-292, 2000.

Curry CE. Laxative products. In: Handbook of Nonprescription Drugs, Am Pharmac Assoc, Washington, S 69-92, 1982.

Davidson MH, Maki KC, Kong JC et al., Long-term effects of consuming foods containing Psyllium seed husk on serum lipids in subjects with hypercholesterolemia. In: *Am J Clin Nutr*; 67(3):367-76, Mar 1998.

Ershoff BH. *J Food Sci* 41:949, 1976.

Etman MA. Effect of a bulk forming laxative on the bioavailability of carbamazepine in man. In*: Drug Develop Indust Pharm*; 21(16):1901-1906, 1995.

Fernandez-Banares F, Hinojosa J, Sanchez-Lombrana JL. Randomized clinical trial of Plantago ovata seeds (dietary fiber) as compared with mesalamine in maintaining remission in ulcerative colitis. Spanish Group for the Study of Crohn's Disease and Ulcerative Colitis (GETECCU). In: *Am J Gastroenterol*; 94(2):427-33, Feb 1999.

Fintelmann V. Phytopharmaka in der Gastroenterologie. In: *ZPT* 15(3):137, 1994.

Ford MA, Cristea G Jr, Robbins WD et al., Delayed Psyllium allergy in three nurses. In: *Hosp Pharm*; 27(12):1061-2, Dec 1992.

Gelpi E et al., *PH* 8:2077-2081. 1969.

Hansen WE. Effect of dietary fiber on pancreatic lipase activity in vitro. In: *Pancreas*; 2(2):195-8, 1987.

Hansen WE & Schulz G. The effect of dietary fiber on pancreatic amylase activity in vitro. In: *Hepatogastroenterology*; 29(4):157-60, Aug 1982.

Hotz J, Plein K. Effectiveness of plantago seed husks in comparison with wheat bran on stool frequency and manifestations of irritable colon syndrome with constipation. In: *Med Klin*; 89(12):645-51, Dec 15, 1994.

Jaspersen-Schib R. Ballaststoffe als Lipidsenker. In: *DAZ* 132(39):1991. 1992.

Kasper H. Ernährungsmedizin und Diätetik. 5. Aufl. Urban & Schwarzenberg, München Wien. Leng-Peschlow E, 1985.

Kasper H. Ernährungsmedizin und Diätetik. 5. Aufl. Urban & Schwarzenberg, München Wien. Leng-Peschlow E. 1985

Kecmanovic D, Pavlov M, Ceranic M. Plantago ovata (Laxomucil) after hemorrhoidectomy. *Acta Chir Lugosi*; 51(3) 121-123. 2004.

Kennedy JF et al., *Carbohydr Res* 75:265-274. 1979.

Khorana ML et al., *Ind J Pharm* 20:3, 1958.

Koedam A. Plantago - history and use. In: *Pharm Weekbl* 112(10):246-252. 1977. McRorie JW, Daggy BP, Morel JG et al., Psyllium is superior to docusate sodium for treatment of chronic constipation. In: *Aliment Pharmacol Ther*; 12(5):491-7, May 1998.

Maciejko JJ, Brazg R, Shah A et al., Psyllium for the reduction of cholestyramine-associated gastrointestinal symptoms in the treatment of primary hypercholesterolemia. In: *Arch Fam Med*; 3(11):955-60, 1994 Nov.

MacMahon M, Carless J. Ispaghula husk in the treatment of hypercholesterolaemia: a double- blind controlled study. In: *J Cardiovasc Risk*; 5(3):167-72, Jun 1998.

Matev M, Angelova I, Koichev A et al., Clinical trial of a Plantago major preparation in the treatment of chronic bronchitis. (Bulgarian) *Vutr Boles*; 21(2):133-137, 1982.

Mengs U. No renal pigmentation by plantago ovata seeds or husks. In: Med Sci Res 18:37-38, 1990.

Miettinen TA & Tarpila S. Serum lipids and cholesterol metabolism during guar gum, *plantago ovata* and high fibre treatments. In: *Clin Chim Acta*; 183(3):253-62, Aug 31, 1989.

Miller JN. In: Industrial Gums, Ed. R. L. Whistler, Academic Press 1973.

Moreyra AE, Wilson AC, Koraym A. Effect of combining psyllium fiber with simvastatin in lowering cholesterol. Arch Intern Med; 165(1): 1161-1166. 2005.

Murai M, Tamayama Y & Nishibe S. Phenylethanoids in the herb of Plantago lanceolata and inhibitory effect on arachidonic acid-induced mouse ear edema. In: *Planta Med*; 61(5):479-480, 1995.

Nordgaard I, Hove H, Clausen MR et al., Colonic production of butyrate in patients with previous colon cancer during long-term treatment with dietary fiber (Plantago ovata seeds). In: *Scand J Gastroenterol*; 31(10):1011-1020, 1996.

Oshio H, Inouye H. *Planta Med* 44:204, 1982.

Perez-Miranda M, Gomez-Cedernilla A & Leon-Colombo T. Effect of fiber supplements on internal bleeding hemorrhoids. *Hepatogastroenterology* 1996; 43(12):1504-1507.

Perlman BB. Interaction between lithium salts and ispaghula husk. In: *Lancet*; 1:416, 1990.

Ponce-Macotela M, Navarro-Alegria I, Martinez-Gordillo MN et al., Efecto antigiardias in vitro de 14 extractos de plantas. (Spanish) *Rev Invest Clin*; 46(5):343-347, 1994.

Popov S. *IUPAC Int Symp Chem Nat Prod* 11(2):61 (via CA 92:59170), 1978.

Prior A & Whorwell PJ. Double-blind study of ispaghula in irritable bowel syndrome. In: *Gut*; 28:1510-1513, 1987.

Product Information. Metamucil®, Proctor & Gamble, Cincinnati, OH, 1999.

Product Information. Konsyl for Kids®, Konsyl Pharmaceuticals, Inc., Fort Worth, Texas, 1999.

Product Information. Konsyl®, Konsyl Pharmaceuticals, Inc., Fort Worth, Texas, 1999.

Ramos-Ruiz A, De la Torre RA, Alonso N et al., Screening of medicinal plants for induction of somatic segregation activity in *Aspergillus nidulans*. In: *J Ethnopharmacol*; 52(3):123-127, 1996.

Rigaud D, Paycha F, Meulemans A, et al. Effect of Psyllium on gastric emptying, hunger feeling and food intake in normal volunteers: a double blind study. In: *Eur J Clin Nutr*; 52(4):239-45, Apr 1998.

Roberts DCK, Truswell AS, Bencke A et al. The cholesterol-lowering effect of a breakfast cereal containing Psyllium fibre. *Med J Aust* 1994; 161(11-12):660-664.

Rodriguez-Moran M, Guerrero-Romero F, Lazcano-Burciaga G. Lipid- and glucose-lowering efficacy of Plantago Psyllium in type II diabetes. In: J Diabetes Complications; 12(5):273-8, Sep-Oct 1998.

Romero AL, Romero JE, Galaviz S, Fernandez ML. Cookies enriched with Psyllium or oat bran lower plasma LDL cholesterol in normal and hypercholesterolemic men from Northern Mexico. In*: J Am Coll Nutr; 17*(6):601-8, Dec 1998.

Sandhu JS, et al., *Carbohdr Res* 93:247-259. 1981.

Sierra M, Garcia JJ, Fernandez N et al., Effects of ispaghula husk and guar gum on postprandial glucose and insulin concentrations in healthy subjects. In: *Eur J Clin Nutr*; 55(4):235-243, 2001.

Schwartz HJ, Arnold JL, Strohl KP. Occupational allergic rhinitis reaction to Psyllium. In: *J Occup Med*; 31(7):624-6, Jul 1989.

Schwesinger WH, Kurtin WE, Page CP, et al., Soluble dietary fiber protects against cholesterol gallstone formation. In: *Am J Surg*; 177(4):307-10, Apr 1999.

Seggev JS, Ohta K, Tipton WR. IgE mediated anaphylaxis due to a Psyllium-containing drug. In: *Ann Allergy;* 53(4): 325-6, Oct 1984.

Shub HA, Salvati EP & Rubin RJ. Conservative treatment of anal fissures: an unselected, retrospective, and continuous study. In: *Dis Colon Rectum*; 21(8):582-583, 1978.

Spence JD, Huff MW, Heidenheim P et al., Combination therapy with colestipol and Psyllium mucilloid in patients with hyperlipidemia. In: *Ann Intern Med*;123(7):493-9; Oct 1, 1995.

Swain JF, Rouse IL, Curley CB, Sacks FM. Comparison of the effects of oat bran and low-fiber wheat on serum lipoprotein levels and blood pressure. In: *N Engl J Med*;322(3):147-52; Jan 18, 1990.

Tomoda M et al., *Planta Med* 53(1):8, 1987.

Turnbull WH, Thomas HG. The effect of a Plantago ovata seed containing preparation on appetite variables, nutrient and energy intake. In: *Int J Obes Relat Metab Disord*; 19(5):338-42, May 1995.

Tyler VE, Brady LR & Robbers JE. Pharmacognosy, 8th ed. Lea & Febiger, Philadelphia, PA, pg. 50-51, 1981.

Van Rosendaal GMA, Shaffer EA, Edwards AL, et al. Effect of time of administration on cholesterol-lowering by psyllium: a randomized cross-over study in normocholesterolemic or slightly hypercholesterolemic subjects. Nutr J; 3: 17. 2004.

Washington N, Harris M, Mussellwhite A, Spiller RC. Moderation of lactulose-induced diarrhea by Psyllium: effects on motility and fermentation. In: *Am J Clin Nutr*; 67(2):317-21, Feb 1998.

Wolever TM, Jenkins DJ, Mueller S, et al., Method of administration influences the serum cholesterol-lowering effect of Psyllium. In: *Am J Clin Nutr*; 59(5):1055-9, May 1994.

Ziai SA, Larijana B, Akhoondzadeh S, et al. Psyllium decreased serum glucose and glycosylated hemoglobin significantly in diabetic outpatients. *J Ethnopharmacol*; 102(2): 202-207. 2005.

Zumarraga L, Levitt MD, Suarez F. Absence of gaseous symptoms during ingestion of commercial fibre preparations. In: *Aliment Pharmacol Ther*; 11(6):1067-72, Dec 1997.

Psyllium Seed

Plantago afra

DESCRIPTION

Medicinal Parts: The medicinal parts are the ripe seeds.

Flower and Fruit: The inflorescence is a 12-mm long spike with glandular hairs and ovate-lanceolate bracts with a midrib and translucent lateral lamina. The corolla is disc-shaped with 4 translucent petals. The edge of the calyx has 4 acute lobes. The sepals are 3 to 4.5 cm and lanceolate. The ovary is superior, and the fruit is a 2-sectioned, membranous pyxidium. The seeds are dark brown, glossy and narrowly oblong in outline.

Leaves, Stem and Root: The plant is an annual that is erect with stems up to 60 cm high. The stems have ascending, pubescent branches with patent or ascending hairs and are more or less minutely glandular above. The leaves are 3 to 8 by 0.1 to 0.3 cm, linear or linear-lanceolate; they are not fleshy. The bracts are 3.5 to 8 mm and all have a similar shape. They are ovate-lanceolate to lanceolate, sharp-edged or acuminate, with a broad dry membranous margin without lateral ribs.

Habitat: The plant is indigenous to the Mediterranean region and western Asia. Psyllium Seeds are cultivated in Spain, central Europe, Israel, Russia, India, Pakistan, Japan, Cuba, and southern Brazil.

Production: Psyllium Seed (blonde) consists of the dried, ripe seed of *Plantago psyllium* (syn. *Plantago afra*) and of *Plantago indica* (syn. *Plantago arenaria*), with a swell index of at least 10, and its formulations.

Not to be Confused With: The seeds of other Plantago seeds.

Other Names: Plantain, Fleaseed, Flea Wort, Psyllion, Psyllios

ACTIONS AND PHARMACOLOGY

COMPOUNDS

Mucilages (only in the epidermis of the seed coat, 10-12%): chiefly arabinoxylans

Iridoids: aucubin (0.14%)

Pyrridine alkaloids: boschniakines, including plantagonine, indicaine, indicainine

Proteic substances

Fatty oil

EFFECTS

The mucins are laxative and antidiarrheal; they regulate intestinal peristalsis through the swelling effect.

INDICATIONS AND USAGE

Approved by Commission E:

- Diarrhea
- Constipation

Psyllium Seed is used internally for constipation and diarrhea.

Unproven Uses: The drug is used for cystitis and all conditions in which a soft stool is desirable, such as anal fissures, hemorrhoids, anal-rectal surgery, and pregnancy. It is also used externally for furunculosis.

CONTRAINDICATIONS

Psyllium Seed is contraindicated in pathologic constriction of the gastrointestinal tract, inflammatory illnesses of the gastrointestinal tract, the threat or presence of ileus, and in severely variable diabetes mellitus.

PRECAUTIONS AND ADVERSE REACTIONS

General: No health hazards or side effects are known in conjunction with the proper administration of designated therapeutic dosages. Allergic reactions could, however, arise in isolated cases (rhinitis, conjunctivitis, asthma and urticaria). Incorrect administration procedures (with too little fluid) can lead to obstruction (blockage) of the esophagus or the intestine, particularly with older people.

DRUG INTERACTIONS

POTENTIAL INTERACTIONS

Absorption of other drugs taken simultaneously may be delayed.

DOSAGE

Mode of Administration: Internally as whole, cut or powdered drug, and externally as a poultice.

Preparation: The ratio for the liquid extract is 1:1 (25% ethanol).

Daily Dosage: The recommended daily dose is 12 to 40 g drug. The dose for the liquid extract is 2 to 5 mL.

Storage: The cut drug should be protected from light and moisture and used within 24 hours.

LITERATURE

Anonym, Pharmaceutical Care: ''Den Mißbrauch von Laxanzien vermeiden helfen''. In: DAZ 135(20):1867-1868. 1995.

Curry CE, Laxative products. In: Handbook of Nonprescription Drugs, Am Pharmac Assoc, Washington, S 69-92. 1982

Fintelmann V, Phytopharmaka in der Gastroenterologie. In: ZPT 15(3):137. 1994.

Hänsel R, Keller K, Rimpler H, Schneider G (Hrsg.), Hagers Handbuch der Pharmazeutischen Praxis, 5. Aufl., Bde 4-6 (Drogen), Springer Verlag Berlin, Heidelberg, New York, 1992-1994.

Jaspersen-Schib R, Ballaststoffe als Lipidsenker. In: DAZ 132(39):1991. 1992.

Karawya MS et al., *PM* 20:14-35. 1971.

Kennedy JF et al., *Carbohydr Res* 75:265-274, 1979.

Schulz R, Hänsel R, Rationale Phytotherapie, Springer Verlag Heidelberg 1996.

Steinegger E, Hänsel R, Pharmakognosie, 5. Aufl., Springer Verlag Heidelberg 1992.

Teuscher E, Biogene Arzneimittel, 5. Aufl., Wiss. Verlagsges. Stuttgart 1997.

Wagner H, Wiesenauer M, Phytotherapie. Phytopharmaka und pflanzliche Homöopathika, Fischer-Verlag, Stuttgart, Jena, New York 1995.

Wichtl M (Hrsg.), Teedrogen, 4. Aufl., Wiss. Verlagsges. Stuttgart 1997.

Ptelea trifoliata

See Wafer Ash

Pterocarpus santalinus

See Red Sandalwood

Ptychopetalum olacoides

See Muira-Puama

Pueraria lobata

See Kudzu

Puff Ball

Lycoperdon species

DESCRIPTION

Medicinal Parts: The medicinal parts are the aerial parts and the mature spores of the fungus.

Flower and Fruit: The giant form of this fungus attains a diameter of 20 to 50 cm and a weight of 9 kg. The outer covering is at first whitish, smooth and downy. It later turns gray-yellow or ochre, develops grooves and patches, and starts to break off from above. The now-visible inner section bursts at the vertex and disintegrates. The content is composed of a whitish mass, which turns yellow and mushy and finally breaks down into greenish-brown spore dust. A cup-shaped receptacle with torn edges remains.

Habitat: Lycoperdon species are indigenous to Europe.

Production: Puff Ball is the aerial part and the mature spores of Lycoperdon species.

Other Names: Bovista, Deer Balls, Hart's Truffle

ACTIONS AND PHARMACOLOGY

COMPOUNDS

Calvacin (mucoprotein)

Steroids: mycosterols

Urea

EFFECTS

The main active agents are various amino acids, glucosamine, sterol, enzymes and approximately 3% urea.

INDICATIONS AND USAGE

Unproven Uses: The drug is used for dysmenorrhea, nosebleeds, and skin disorders.

Homeopathic Uses: Lycoperdon is used for anemia, skin complaints, and chronic catarrh.

PRECAUTIONS AND ADVERSE REACTIONS

No health hazards or side effects are known in conjunction with the proper administration of designated therapeutic dosages. The young mushroom is edible.

DOSAGE

Mode of Administration: Puff Ball is available ground or in alcoholic extracts.

LITERATURE

Gasco A et al., *Tetrahedron Lett* 38:3431. 974

Kern W, List PH, Hörhammer L (Hrsg.), Hagers Handbuch der Pharmazeutischen Praxis, 4. Aufl., Bde. 1-8, Springer Verlag Berlin, Heidelberg, New York, 1969.

Madaus G, Lehrbuch der Biologischen Arzneimittel, Bde 1-3, Nachdruck, Georg Olms Verlag Hildesheim 1979.

Pulmonaria officinalis

See Lungwort

Pulsatilla pratensis

See Pasque Flower

Pumpkin

Cucurbita pepo

DESCRIPTION

Medicinal Parts: The medicinal parts are the fresh and dried seeds.

Flower and Fruit: The flower is yellow, monoecious, very large, and solitary in the leaf axils. The male flower has a longer pedicle. The calyx is fused to the corolla except for the 5 awl-shaped tips. The corolla is 5-tipped and funnel-shaped. The interior is pubescent. There are 3 stamens fused to the anther. The ovary is inferior and 3-locular. The fruit is very large with many seeds. The flesh is fibrous, yellow-orange to white, and has a viscous placenta. The seeds are 7 to 15 mm long, narrow, broad or narrow-ovate, with a shallow groove and flat ridge around the margin.

Leaves, Stem, and Root: Annual plant 3 to 8 m long. The stem is sharply angular with longitudinal grooves and hairy spines. The leaves are alternate, very large and bristly, petiolate with 5 to 7 lobes from a cordate base.

Characteristics: The seeds taste somewhat like almonds.

Habitat: Pumpkin is indigenous to America and widely cultivated, especially in temperate climates.

Production: Pumpkin seed consists of the ripe, dried seed of *Cucurbita pepo* and cultivated varieties of *Cucurbita pepo.*

Other Names: Field Pumpkin

ACTIONS AND PHARMACOLOGY

COMPOUNDS

Steroids: Delta5-, Delta7- and Delta8-phytosterols (24- alkyl sterols), including clerosterol, isofucosterol, sitosterol, stigmasterol, cholesterol, isoavenasterol, spinasterol

Fatty oil: chief fatty acids are oleic acid and linoleic acid

Proteic substances (25 to 42%)

Unusual amino acids: including cucurbitin (vermifuge)

Gamma-tocopherol

EFFECTS

The efficacy of lipophilic pumpkin seed extracts or pumpkin seed oil for micturation complaints accompanying benign prostatic hyperplasia or irritable bladder has been confirmed by several clinical and experimental studies. As well as amaroids (cucurbitacin), the drug contains delta-7-sterols, which are similar in conformation to the dihydrostesterone. Cucurbitacin has anthelmintic properties. Pumpkin is also antiphlogistic and antioxidative.

Anti-diabetic effects. A review of pharmacological activities of Pumpkin indicates that it has been most widely studied for its antidiabetic actions, with the fruit seeds (and pulp) showing hypoglycemic activity in rat and rabbit studies. Pumpkin is used in China and other parts of the world to reduce blood sugar, increase insulin level, and lower branched chain amino acids. Standardization of Pumpkin's antidiabetic components, with follow-up in clinical trials, is a needed next step (Caili, 2006).

Antihelmintic Effects: The anthelmintic effect is attributed to the constituent curcurbitin, although the concentration of cucurbitin varies widely among species and even within seeds of the same species (Foster & Tyler, 1999).

Urolithiasis Promoting Effects: Pumpkin seed supplementation lowered the occurrence of calcium-oxalate crystals in one study. Oxalate crystalluria was similarly reduced with pumpkin seed supplementation and orthophosphate supplementation. The longer the supplementation period, the lower the calcium-oxalate crystal occurrence (Suphakarn et al, 1987).

Effects on Prostatic Hyperplasia: The prostatic tissue of treatment subjects showed a significant decline in dihydrotestosterone levels compared to the prostatic tissue from an untreated control group (Schulz et al, 1998). Studies using a combination of pumpkin seed and saw palmetto demonstrate significant improvement of symptoms (Grups & Schiebal-Schlosser, 1995).

CLINICAL TRIALS

Chronic Insomnia

In a double-blind, placebo-controlled study, 57 subjects were randomly assigned to one of three groups: (1) protein source tryptophan (de-oiled gourd seed) in combination with carbohydrate; (2) pharmaceutical grade tryptophan in combination with carbohydrate; or (3) carbohydrate alone. Objective and subjective measures of sleep were employed to measure sleep changes. After 3 weeks, researchers found that, in 49 subjects who completed the study, both the tryptophan-rich seed with carbohydrate and the pharmaceutical grade tryptophan with carbohydrate, but not carbohydrate alone, significantly improved insomnia. Therefore, tryptophan derived from pumpkin seed proved comparable to pharmaceutical grade tryptophan in significantly reducing time awake during the night when combined with carbohydrate (Hudson et al, 2005).

Benign Prostatic Hyperplasia

A randomized, double-blind, placebo-controlled, multicenter study assessed whether a combination preparation that contained pumpkin seed was effective in the treatment of symptoms of benign prostatic hyperplasia (BPH). The study included 53 males between the ages of 50 to 80 years with voiding problems attributed to BPH. The preparation Curbicin® contained 80 mg of standardized extract PS6 from *Cucurbita pepo L* and 80 mg of *Sabal serrulata* (saw palmetto). Curbicin or identical placebo tablets were given as 2 tablets 3 times daily for a duration of 3 months. Subjective parameters were difficulties in voiding, frequency of urination during the day, and nocturia. Objective parameters included urinary flow rate in mL/second, voiding time measured in seconds, and residual volume. Significant improvement in subjective and objective improvement occurred with the combination preparation and no change was seen in subjects receiving placebo. The results differed from an earlier pilot study in which only nocturia was significantly improved. The authors concluded that the difference in outcome of their study was attributed to the fact that the pilot study used a combination preparation that contained only 15 mg of less refined Sabal serrulata (Carbin et al, 1990).

An open, multicenter clinical trial assessed the efficacy of a combination preparation of pumpkin seed and sabal fruit (80 mg each) for urinary complaints associated with BPH. A total of 1,305 male patients, aged 50 to 82 years, with BPH stage I and II were included in the study. The dosage was not standardized, but determined by the physician. At the end of the three-month period, the combination product produced significant symptomatic improvement. A total of 68% of patients reported reduced daytime urination frequency, 82% reported reduced nighttime urination, 86% had reduced dribbling, and 86% experienced improvement in symptoms of painful urination. No undesired side effects occurred in 98% of patients (Grups & Schiebal-Schlosser, 1995).

Urolithiasis

A small study investigated the effect of a pumpkin seed snack on inhibitors and promoters of urolithiasis in Thai adolescents. Ten adolescents from a hyperendemic area of Thailand, aged 13 to 16 years, received a prepared pumpkin seed snack supplement (which contained peeled roasted pumpkin seeds, milk powder, roasted sesame seeds and sugar) for 2 days. The amount of pumpkin seed snack supplement received was equivalent to 1200 mg phosphorous per day. Urinary pH was significantly lower in the pumpkin seed group compared to urine samples taken prior to the start of the trial and also during a 2-day period in which subjects received a snack supplement that contained all ingredients except pumpkin seed. There was a significant increase in urinary oxalate among the participants in the pumpkin seed snack group compared to snack without pumpkin seeds. There was a significant decrease in magnesium and pyrophosphate, inhibitors of crystal formation with pumpkin seed snack as compared to before treatment (Suphiphat et al, 1993).

INDICATIONS AND USAGE

Approved by Commission E:

- Irritable bladder
- Prostate complaints

Unproven Uses: Pumpkin is used for irritable bladder, prevention, and treatment of calcium oxalate kidney stones, micturition problems accompanying prostate adenoma stages I to II. This medication relieves only the difficulties associated with an enlarged prostate without reducing the enlargement. Medical supervision is essential.

In folk medicine, it is also used for kidney inflammation, intestinal parasites, particularly tape worm, and vulnary.

PRECAUTIONS AND ADVERSE REACTIONS

Indigestion and diarrhea, which were controlled by treating with sodium bicarbonate or paregorics, were reported by patients in an open trial of 80 g three times daily of powdered pumpkin seed used for treatment of schistosomiasis (Hsueh-Chang & Ming, 1960). There is a case report of intestinal impaction in a 61-year-old female who ingested 1 cup of roasted pumpkin seed (Chandrasekhara, 1983).

DRUG INTERACTIONS

MODERATE RISK

Warfarin: Concurrent use may result in increased risk of bleeding. Two cases of increased INR have been reported in patients taking a combination of pumpkin seed, saw palmetto, and vitamin E (Curbicin®). One of the patients had been stable on warfarin prior to starting Curbicin and one patient was not taking any concomitant anticoagulant therapy (Yue & Jansson, 2001). It is unclear if the increased INR was due to the vitamin E content alone, pumpkin seed or saw palmetto alone, or a combination of all three ingredients. *Clinical Management:* Caution is advised. Monitor the INR and signs and symptoms of excessive bleeding.

DOSAGE

Mode of Administration: Whole and coarsely ground seed and other galenic preparations are for internal use.

Daily Dosage: The average daily dose is 10 g of ground seeds; 1 to 2 heaping dessert spoons with liquid in the mornings and evenings.

Storage: It should be protected from light and moisture.

LITERATURE

Anon. Welche Bedeutung haben pflanzliche Prostatamittel. In: *DAZ* 133(9):720. 1993.

BAnz (Federal German Gazette) No. 223, published 30 Nov 1985; revised 17 Jan 1991.

Buck AC. Phytotherapy for the prostate. *Br J Urol* 78:325-336, 1996.

Caili F, Huan S, Quanhong L. A review on pharmacological activities and utilization technologies of pumpkin. *Plant Foods Hum Nutr*;61(2):73-80. 2006.

Carbin BE, Larsson B & Lindahl O. Treatment of benign prostatic hyperplasia with phytosterols. *Br J Urol* 66(6):639-641, 1999.

Chandrasekhara KL. Pumpkin-seed impaction. *Ann Intern Med*; 98(5 pt 1):675, 1983.

Grups JW & Schiebel-Schlosser G. Therapy of benign prostatic hyperplasia. *Therapiewoche* 8:495-498, 1995.

Hudson C, Hudson SP, Hecht T, MacKenzie. Protein source tryptophan versus pharmaceutical grade tryptophan as an efficacious treatment for chronic insomnia. *Nutr Neurosci*; 8(2);121-127. 2005.

Koch E. Pharmakologie und Wirkmechanismen von Extrakten aus Sabalfrüchten (Sabal fructus), Brennesselwurzeln (Urticae radix) und Kürbissamen (Cucurbitae peponis semen) bei der Behandlung der benignen Prostatahyperplasie. In: Loew D, Rietbrock N (Hrsg.) Phytopharmaka in Forschung und klinischer Anwendung. Steinkopff Verlag, Darmstadt, S 57-79, 1995.

Miersch WDE. Benigne Prostatahyperplasie. In: *DAZ* 133(29):2653. 1993.

Nahrstedt A. Pflanzliche Urologica - eine kritische Übersicht. *Pharm Z* 138:1439-1450, 1993.

Schabort JC. *Phytochemistry* 17:1062, 1978.

Schiebel-Schlosser G. Kürbiskerne stärken die Blasenfunktion. In: *PTA* 4(11):552. 1990.

Schilcher H. Möglichkeiten und Grenzen der Phytotherapie am Beispiel pflanzlicher Urologika. *Urologe* [B] 27, 316-319, 1987.

Schilcher H. (1987a) Pflanzliche Diuretika. Urologe [B] 27:215-222; (1987b)n Möglichkeiten und Grenzen der Phytotherapie am Beispiel pflanzlicher Urologika. *Urologe* [B] 27:316-319.

Schilcher H, Boesel R, Effenberger ST Segebrecht S. Neuere Untersuchungsergebnisse mit aquaretisch, antibakteriell und prostatotrop wirksamen Arzneipflanzen. In: *ZPT* 10(3):77. 1989.

Schilcher H, Dunzendorfer U, Ascali F. Dekta-7-Sterole, das prostatatrope Wirkprinzip des Kürbis? In: *Urologe* (B) 27:316-319. 1987.

Suphakarn VS, Yarnnon C & Ngunboonsri P. The effect of pumpkin seeds on oxalcrystalluria and urinary compositions of children in hyperendemic area. In: *Am J Clin Nutr* 45(1):115-121, 1987.

Suphiphat V et al. The effect of pumpkin seeds snack on inhibitors and promoters of urolithiasis in Thai adolescents. *J Med Assoc Thai. Sep;76*(9):487-493. 1993

Tewary JP, Srivasta MC. *J Pharm Sci* 57:328, 1968.

Yue QY & Jansson K. Herbal drug Curbicin and anticoagulation effect with and without warfarin: possible related to the vitamin E component. In: *J Am Geriatr Soc* 49(6):838, 2001.

Punica granatum

See Pomegranate

Purple Gromwell (Ying Zicao)

Lithospermum erytrorhizon

DESCRIPTION

Medicinal Parts: The medicinal part of the plant is the root, which is dried.

Flower and Fruit: The radial flowers are in axillary or apical racemes. The calyx has up to 5 tips, and the sepals are fused. The petals are white and also fused. The corolla tube is approximately 4 mm long. The diameter of the corolla is approximately 4 mm. There are 5 stamens and 1 superior, 2-

carpeled, 4-chambered ovary. The fruit is a glossy nutlet, approximately 3 mm long, ovoid, and gray-white.

Leaves, Stem, and Root: This herbaceous perennial grows up to 80 cm high. The leaves are alternate, sessile, simple, lanceolate to elongate-lanceolate with acute tips and parallel veins. It has a few upright, roughly pubescent stems and a thick root.

Characteristics: The root becomes purple when dried.

Habitat: This herb is indigenous to Korea, China, and Japan.

Production: Purple Gromwell root or Ying Zicao (Chinese) is the dried root of *Lithospermum erythrorhizon*. The 3-year-old roots are collected in spring or autumn, cleaned, cut in slices, and then dried.

Other Names: Ying Zicao

ACTION AND PHARMACOLOGY

COMPOUNDS

Naphthalene derivatives (0.5 to 3%): isohexenylnaphthazarines, particularly esters of the (R)-(+)-shikonins with short-chained fatty acids, including acetic acid, isobutyric acid, isovaleric acid

Water-soluble polysaccharides: lithospermans A to C

Pyrrolizidine alkaloids: chief alkaloid intermedine, as well as myoscorpine, hydroxymyoscorpine

Hydroquinone derivatives (0.3%): furylhydroquinones and furylquinones, including shikonofurane A to E

Caffeic acid derivatives: rosmarinic acid, lithospermic acid, caffeic acid esters of higher alcohols, for example docosanylcaffeat

EFFECTS

The naphthoquinone derivatives contained in the drug are antimicrobial, antiphlogistic, analgetic, antipyretic, tumor-inhibiting, and immunomodulating in their activity. In addition, a hypoglycemic effect from the glycane fraction has been described.

INDICATIONS AND USAGE

Unproven Uses: Uses in folk medicine include fever, constipation, smallpox, strangury, bacterial skin conditions, and insect bites (Korea).

Chinese Medicine: Uses include constipation, swellings, tumors, and eczema of the skin. Efficacy for these indications has not yet been proved.

PRECAUTIONS AND ADVERSE REACTIONS

The drug is no longer considered safe for internal use. Hepatotoxicity and carcinogenicity are to be assumed for the drug, due to the pyrrolizidine alkaloid content with 1,2-unsaturated necic parent substances.

DOSAGE

Mode of Administration: Whole drug.

Preparation: There is no exact information in the literature.

Daily Dosage: Drug/tea: 3 to 10 g. The traditional daily dose for smallpox is 5 to 8 g drug to taken internally. (The drug is no longer considered safe for internal use.)

LITERATURE

Bechthold A, Berger U, Heide L, Partial purification, properties, and kinetic studies of UDP-glucose:p-hydroxybenzoate glucosyltransferase from cell cultures of *Lithospermum erythrorhizon*. *Arch Biochem Biophys*, 288:39-47, Jul. 1991

Blaschek W, Hänsel R, Keller K, Reichling J, Rimpler G, Schneider G, (Eds) Hagers Handbuch der Pharmazeutischen Praxis. Folgeb nde 1 und 2. Drogen A-Z. Springer. Berlin, Heidelberg 1998.

Hisa T, Kimura Y, Takada K, Suzuki F, Takigawa M, Isolation and hypoglycemic activity of lithospermans A, B and C, glycans of *Lithospermum erythrorhizon* roots. *Planta Med*, 18:157-8, Mar-Apr. 1998

Hisa T, Kimura Y, Takada K, Suzuki F, Takigawa M, Shikonin, an ingredient of *Lithospermum erythrorhizon*, inhibits angiogenesis in vivo and in vitro. *Anticancer Res*, 18:783-90, Mar-Apr. 1998

Purple Loosestrife

Lythrum salicaria

DESCRIPTION

Medicinal Parts: The medicinal parts are the flowering plant without the roots and flowering branch tips.

Flower and Fruit: The purple flowers are in axillary whorls and form terminal spikes. There are 6 small sepals, 6 long thin tips, 6 free petals, 12 stamens, and 1 half-superior ovary. There are flowers with long, short or medium-long styles and similar stamens.

Leaves, Stem, and Root: The plant is an annual and grows from 60 to 120 cm high. It has a creeping rhizome with 4 to 6 unbranched, erect, 6-sided, reddish-brown, pubescent stems. The leaves are simple lanceolate, 7.5 to 15 cm long, sometimes opposite and sometimes clasping whorls.

Habitat: The plant is indigenous to Europe including Russia, central Asia, Australia, and North America.

Production: Purple Loosestrife is the plant in flower, excluding the root, of *Lythrum salicaria*. Before the seeds form, the plants are cut and gathered during the blossoming period, which occurs from June to August. The material is bound into small bundles. It is hung in an open-air, shaded area to dry.

Other Names: Blooming Sally, Flowering Sally, Long Purples, Loosestrife, Lythrum, Milk Willow-Herb, Purple Willow-Herb, Rainbow Weed, Salicaire, Soldiers, Spiked Loosestrife, Spiked, Willow Sage

ACTIONS AND PHARMACOLOGY

COMPOUNDS

Tannins (ellagitannins = lythrartannin, condensed tannins)

Flavonoids: including among others vitexin, orientin

Phthalides: diisobutyl-, butyl-, isobutyl-, dibutylphthalides

Steroids: beta-sitosterol

EFFECTS

The active agents are tannin, pectin, resins, cholin, and salicarin.

The drug has an anti-inflammatory, astringent, and antibiotic effect. The astringent properties of the Purple Loosestrife is attributed not just to the tannin content, but also to the glycoside salcarin, which has a special antimicrobial effect on various bacteria in the intestinal tract.

INDICATIONS AND USAGE

Unproven Uses: The drug is used internally for diarrhea, chronic intestinal catarrh and menstrual complaints; externally, in the treatment of varicose veins, bleeding of the gums, hemorrhoids, and eczema.

PRECAUTIONS AND ADVERSE REACTIONS

No health hazards or side effects are known in conjunction with the proper administration of designated therapeutic dosages.

DOSAGE

Mode of Administration: The drug is used internally as well as externally.

Preparation: For internal use, an infusion is made from 3 g of the drug added to 100 mL of water. To prepare a tincture, add 20 g of the drug to 100 mL of 20% alcohol (leave to set for 5 days).

Daily Dosage: Two to 3 cups of an infusion are to be taken per day. Two to 3 teaspoons of the tincture should be taken per day.

Storage: Keep wrapped in paper or in cloth sacks.

LITERATURE

Kern W, List PH, Hörhammer L (Hrsg.), Hagers Handbuch der Pharmazeutischen Praxis, 4. Aufl., Bde. 1-8, Springer Verlag Berlin, Heidelberg, New York, 1969.

Madaus G, Lehrbuch der Biologischen Arzneimittel, Bde 1-3, Nachdruck, Georg Olms Verlag Hildesheim 1979.

Pygeum

Prunus africana

DESCRIPTION

Medicinal Parts: The drug consists of the dried bark of the trunk of *Prunus africana.*

Botanical Description: An evergreen tree, usually 10-25 m high, with straight, cylindrical trunk and dense, rounded crown. Leaves alternate, 8-12 cm long, long-stalked, simple, elliptic, bluntly pointed at apex, with shallow crenate margins; leathery, deep green, and glossy, with midrib sharply impressed or channelled on upper surface and strongly prominent on underside; smell of almonds when bruised. Leafstalks and young branchlets often reddish. Flowers small, white or cream, fragrant, in axillary racemes 3-8 cm long; corolla lobes up to 2 mm long. Fruits cherry-shaped, red to purplish-brown, 8-12 mm in diameter; very bitter flesh and bony stone. Wood pale red, with strong cyanide smell when freshly cut, darkening to rich dark red or mahogany-brown on exposure to air; straight-grained and even textured, strong and elastic, very hard and very heavy.

Habitat: The tree occurs in tropical and subtropical parts of Africa, including Angola, Cameroon, Ethiopia, Ghana, Kenya, Madagascar, Malawi, Mozambique, Republic of Congo, South Africa, Uganda, United Republic of Tanzania, Zambia and Zimbabwe, Burundi, Equatorial Guinea (Bioko, Sao Tome and Principe), Rwanda, Sudan, and Swaziland.

Production: Wild-crafted. Wild-harvesting of bark is very destructive and some attempts have been made to establish plantations for sustainable bark production. Fresh bark is harvested, dried, crushed, and extract obtained from which a drug is segregated. Bark harvesting occurs year-round.

Other Names: African plum tree, African prune tree, alumty, iluo, kirah, Natal tree, prunier d'afrique, vla, wotangue, armaatet, chati, inkhokhokho, inyangazoma-elimnyama, kiburabura, lemalan migambo, mueri, muiru, murugutu, mutimailu, mweria, mwiritsa, nuwehout, ol-koijuk, oromoti, red stinkwood, rooistinkhout, tenduet, tendwet, twendet, umdumizulu, umkakase, umkhakhazi, umlalume; mwiluti, mfila, mpembati, mdundulu, ligambo, mufubia, gwaami, kondekonde, olkonjuku, mkonde-konde.

ACTIONS AND PHARMACOLOGY

COMPOUNDS

Docosanol (0.6%) and B-sitosterol (15.7%). Other major constituents include alkanols: tetracosanol (0.5%) and trans-ferulic acid esters of docosanol and tetracosanol, fatty acids (62.3%, comprising myristic, palmitic, linoleic, oleic, stearic, arachidic, behenic and lignoceric acids); sterols: sitosterone (2.0%) and daucosterol and triterpenes: ursolic acid (2.9%), friedelin (1.4%), 2-a-hydroxyursolic acid (0.5%), epimaslinic acid (0.8%) and maslinic acid.

EFFECTS

Multiple mechanisms have been proposed for the genitourinary effects of prunus, including 5α-reductase inhibition, estrogenic effects, and anti-inflammatory properties. Genitourinary effects: *P. africana* extract appears to inhibit human prostatic 5α-reductase (IC50 63,000 ng/mL), but much less powerfully than finasteride (IC50 1.0 ng/mL). Reduction of urethral obstruction and improvement of bladder function have been observed. Most studies of *P. africana* extract have addressed outcomes related to the obstructive component. In rats, prunus inhibits dihydrotestosterone-induced prostate hyperplasia, with a mechanism that appears unrelated to androgen receptor blockade. In rats and humans, *P. africana* extract has been found to stimulate secretory activity of the prostate and seminal vesicles. Reduction of contractile dysfunction of the bladder caused by partial outlet obstruction has been observed with pre-treatment of rabbits with *P. africana* extract (Tadenan®, 1-100mg/kg/day oral).

Anti-inflammatory effects: In vitro studies report *P. africana* extract to inhibit production of 5-lipoxygenase metabolites at concentrations of 3mcg/mL when dissolved in DMSO, and 10mcg/mL when dissolved in NaOH/HCl ($p<0.01$). *P. africana* inhibits fibroblast proliferation induced by epidermal growth factor (EGF; IC50=4.5mcg/mL), insulin-like growth factor type I (IGF-I; IC50=7.7mcg/mL), and basic fibroblast growth factor (bFGF; IC50=12.6mcg/mL) in vitro. *P. africana* extract appears to possess phytoestrogenic properties.

CLINICAL TRIALS

Benign prostatic hypertrophy/BPH symptoms

In 2002, Wilt et al conducted a systematic review and meta-analysis to investigate the evidence surrounding the use of prunus in the treatment of BPH. The authors searched for trials in multiple databases, including Medline, Embase, the Cochrane Library, Phytodok, by checking bibliographies, and by contacting relevant manufacturers and researchers. Trials were eligible if they were randomized, included men with BPH, compared preparations of *Prunus africana* (alone or in combination) with placebo or other BPH medications, and if they included clinical outcomes such as urologic symptom scales, symptoms, or urodynamic measurements. The main outcome measure for adverse effects was the number of men reporting adverse effects. A total of 18 randomized controlled trials involving 1562 men met inclusion criteria and were analyzed. Only one of the studies reported a method of treatment allocation concealment, although 17 were double-blinded. There were no studies comparing *Prunus africana* to standard pharmacologic interventions such as alpha-adrenergic blockers or 5-alpha reductase inhibitors. The mean study duration was 64 days (range, 30-122 days). According to the authors, most studies did not report results in a method that permitted meta-analysis. Compared to men receiving placebo, prunus provided a moderately large improvement in the combined outcome of urologic symptoms and flow measures as assessed by an effect size defined by the difference of the mean change for each outcome divided by the pooled standard deviation for each outcome (-0.8 SD [95% confidence interval (CI), -1.4, -0.3 (n=6 studies)]). Men using prunus were more than twice as likely to report an improvement in overall symptoms (RR=2.1, 95% CI = 1.4, 3.1). Nocturia was reduced by 19%, residual urine volume by 24%, and peak urine flow was increased by 23%. Adverse effects due to prunus were mild and comparable to placebo. The overall dropout rate was 12% and was similar between prunus (13%), placebo (11%) and other controls (8%). Although the authors concluded that standardized preparations of prunus may be a useful treatment option for men with lower urinary symptoms consistent with BPH, they noted that further research is necessary, as the reviewed studies overall were small in size, short in duration, used varied doses/preparations, and rarely reported outcomes using standardized validated measures of efficacy (Wilt et al, 2002).

In 2000, Ishani et al. conducted a systematic review and meta-analysis of 18 randomized controlled trials to evaluate the efficacy of prunus extract in the treatment of symptomatic BPH. Out of 31 randomized trials with a duration of 30 days or greater, 18 matched the inclusion criteria for this analysis. All 18 trials were conducted in Europe and included a total of 1562 subjects. Ten trials compared *P. africana* to placebo, two trials evaluated *P. africana* versus an anti-inflammatory drug, one study compared *P. africana* to both placebo and *P. africana* plus medroxyprogesterone, one trial compared once daily versus twice daily dosing of *P. africana*, two trials compared *P. africana* combined with another herbal vs. placebo, one trial compared *P. africana* to another herbal agent, and one trial compared two different doses of *P. africana* plus *Urtica dioica*. The doses of *P. africana* extract used in trials varied from 75mg to 200mg per day. The data were pooled using two methods: First, for summarizing trials with various outcome measures, treatment effect size for continuous variables was assessed by dividing the difference of the mean change for each outcome by the pooled standard deviation for that outcome. Second, effect size was estimated using the most clinically important outcome per study, according to the following preference scale: symptom score > nocturia > peak urine flow > residual urine volume. The summary effect size (difference in mean outcome divided by the pooled standard deviation for that outcome) was then assessed using the following key: 0.8 = large effect, 0.5 = moderate effect, 0.2 = small effect. Among 474 men from six trials comparing *P. africana* to placebo, summary effect size was calculated to be -0.8 (95%CI -1.4 to -0.3), which suggests a large, statistically significant improvement in symptomatic BPH with *P. africana* compared to placebo. Furthermore, men taking *P. africana* were 2.1 (95%CI 1.4 to 3.4) times more likely experience an overall improvement of symptoms than those taking placebo, and also experienced a 19% reduction in nocturia as compared with those taking placebo (weighted mean difference of -0.9). The latter two results, however, were not statistically significant (95%CI -2.0 to 0.1). Peak urine flow, as analyzed from four trials (363 subjects), was significantly increased by 23% as compared to placebo (95% CI 0.3 to 4.7). For none of the effect measures, in none of the analyzed studies, was control treatment superior to *P. africana* extract (Ishani et al, 2000).

INDICATIONS AND USAGE

Unproven Uses: Aphrodisiac, bladder sphincter disorders, fever, impotence, inflammation, kidney disease, malaria, male baldness, partial bladder outlet obstruction, prostate cancer, prostatic adenoma, prostatitis, psychosis, sexual performance, stomach upset, urinary tract health. *Prunus africana* is traditional medicine in Africa used to treat chest pain, malaria, and fevers (Cunningham and Mbenkum 1993). The fresh bark, leaf, and fruits contain amygalin, yielding hydrocyanic acid when crushed; hence, they have an almond flavor. The bark was traditionally powdered and drunk as tea for genitourinary complaints, allergies, inflammation, kidney disease, malaria, stomach ache, and fever, among other uses.

Possible Efficacy: Treatment of lower urinary tract symptoms of benign prostatic hyperplasia (BPH) stages I and II, as defined by Aiken (e.g. nocturia, polyuria and urinary retention), where diagnosis of prostate cancer is negative.

CONTRAINDICATIONS

Pregnancy/lactation: Prunus cannot be recommended during pregnancy or breast-feeding because of a lack of scientific information and possible hormonal effects.

Pediatrics: There is not sufficient scientific information to recommend prunus for use in children.

PRECAUTIONS AND ADVERSE REACTIONS

Caution in taking 5 α-reductase inhibitors or saw palmetto

DRUG INTERACTIONS

POTENTIAL INTERACTIONS

Prunus extract appears to inhibit human prostatic 5α-reductase. In theory, prostate specific antigen (PSA) values in serum may be reduced with the use of 5α-reductase inhibitors, masking otherwise elevated levels. Prunus may interact with estrogen or other hormones. Prunus may interact with herbs/supplements containing chemicals with estrogen-like constituents.

DOSAGE

How Supplied: Lipophilic extract of the crude drug.

Daily Dose: 75-200mg lipidosterolic extract of the crude drug, in divided doses. To minimize gastrointestinal disturbances, take with food or milk.

LITERATURE

Andro M, Riffaud J. Pygeum africanum extract for the treatment of patients with benign prostatic hyperplasia: a review of 25 years of published experience. Curr Ther Res 1995;56(8):796-817.

Anon. [Tadenan (Pygeum africanum extract) in the treatment of patients with benign prostatic hyperplasia]. Urologia 2004 Sep-Oct;(5):70-2.

Anon. Pygeum africanum (Prunus africanus) (African plum tree). Monograph. Altern Med Rev 2002 Feb;7(1):71-4.

Barry M. Review: Pygeum africanum extracts improve symptoms and urodynamics in symptomatic benign prostatic hyperplasia. ACP J Club 2002 Sep-Oct;137(2):61.

Bombardelli E, Morazzoni P. Prunus africana (Hook. f) Kalkm. Fitoterapia, 1997, 68: 205-218.

Buck AC. Is there a scientific basis for the therapeutic effects of serenoa repens in benign prostatic hyperplasia? Mechanisms of action. J Urol 2004 Nov;172(5 Pt 1):1792-9.

Chen MW, Levin RM, Horan P, Buttyan RB. Effects of Unilateral Ischemia on the

Contractile Response of the Bladder: Protective Effect of Tadenan (Pygeum africanum Extract). Mol Urol, 1999, 3(1):5-10.

Choo MS, Bellamy F, Constantinou CE. Functional evaluation of Tadenan on micturition and experimental prostate growth induced with exogenous dihydrotestosterone. Urology 2000 Feb;55(2):292-8.

Cristoni A, Di Pierro F, Bombardelli E. Botanical derivatives for the prostate. Fitoterapia, 2000, 71 Suppl 1:S21-8.

Dreikorn K. The role of phytotherapy in treating lower urinary tract symptoms and benign prostatic hyperplasia. World J Urol 2002 Apr;19(6):426-35.

Dreikorn K. Phytotherapeutic agents in the treatment of benign prostatic hyperplasia. Curr Urol Rep 2000 Aug;1(2):103-9.

Dreikorn K, Berges R, Pientka L, Jonas U. [Phytotherapy of benign prostatic hyperplasia. Current evidence-based evaluation]. Urologe A 2002 Sep;41(5):447-51.

Dutkiewicz S. Usefulness of Cernilton in the treatment of benign prostatic hyperplasia. Int Urol Nephrol 1996;28(1):49-53.

Gathumbi PK, Mwangi JW, Mugera GM, Njiro SM. Toxicity of chloroform extract of prunus africana stem bark in rats: gross and histological lesions. Phytother Res, 2002 May;16(3):244-7.

Gathumbi PK, Mwangi JW, Njiro SM, Mugera GM. Biochemical and haematological changes in rats administered an aqueous extract of Prunus africana stem-bark at various dosage levels. Onderstepoort J Vet Res 2000 Jun;67(2):123-8.

Gerber GS. Phytotherapy for benign prostatic hyperplasia. Curr Urol Rep 2002 Aug;3(4):285-91.

Hartmann RW, Mark M, Soldati F. Inhibition of 5a-reductase and aromatase by PHL00801 (Prostatonin®), a combination of PY 102 (Pygeum africanum) and DR 102 (Urtica dioica) extracts. Phytomedicine, 1996,3:121-128.

Hass MA, Nowak DM, Leonova E, Levin RM, Longhurst PA. Identification of components of Prunus africana extract that inhibit lipid peroxidation. Phytomedicine, 1999 Nov;6(5):379-88.

Ishani A, MacDonald R, Nelson D, Rutks I, Wilt TJ. Pygeum africanum for the treatment of patients with benign prostatic hyperplasia: a systematic review and quantitative meta-analysis. Am J Med 2000 Dec 1;109(8):654-64.

Levin RM, Das AK. A scientific basis for the therapeutic effects of Pygeum africanum and Serenoa repens. Urol Res 2000 Jun;28(3):201-9.

Lowe FC, Ku J. Phytotherapy in the treatment of benign prostatic hyperplasia: a critical review. Urology 1996, 48:12-20.

Mathe G, Hallard M, Bourut CH, Chenu E. A Pygeum africanum extract with so-called phyto-estrogenic action markedly reduces the volume of true and large prostatic hypertrophy. Biomed Pharmacother 1995;49(7-8):341-3.

Mathe G, Orbach-Arbouys S, Bizi E, Court B. The so-called phyto-estrogenic action of Pygeum africanum extract. Biomed Pharmacother 1995;49(7-8):339-40.

McQueen CE, Bryant PJ. Pygeum. Am J Health Syst Pharm 2001;58(2):120-123.

Nieri E et al. New lignans from Prunus africana Hook. Rivista ltaliana Eppos, 1996, 7: 27-31.

Santa Maria Margalef A, Paciucci Barzanti R, Reventos Puigjaner J, Morote Robles J,

Thomson Okatsu TM. [Antimitogenic effect of Pygeum africanum extracts on human prostatic cancer cell lines and explants from benign prostatic hyperplasia]. Arch Esp Urol 2003 May;56(4):369-78.

Stewart KM. The African cherry (Prunus africana): can lessons be learned from an over-exploited medicinal tree? J Ethnopharmacol 2003 Nov;89(1):3-13.

Strong KM. African plum and benign prostatic hypertrophy. J Herb Pharmcother 2004;4(1):41-6.

Szolnoki E, Reichart E, Marchal S, Szegedi G. The effect of Pygeum africanum on fibroblast growth factor (FGF) and transforming growth factor beta (TGF beta 1/LAP) expression in animal model. Acta Microbiol Immunol Hung 2001;48(1):1-9.

Verschaeve L, Kestens V, Taylor JL, Elgorashi EE, Maes A, Van Puyvelde L, De Kimpe N,

Van Staden J. Investigation of the antimutagenic effects of selected South African medicinal plant extracts. Toxicol In Vitro 2004 Feb;18(1):29-35.

Wilt T, Ishani A, Mac Donald R, Rutks I, Stark G. Pygeum africanum for benign prostatic hyperplasia. Cochrane Database Syst Rev 2002;(1):CD001044.

Yablonsky F, Nicolas V, Riffaud JP, Bellamy F. Antiproliferative effect of Pygeum africanum extract on rat prostatic fibroblasts. J Urol 1997 Jun;157(6):2381-7.

Yarnell E. Botanical medicines for the urinary tract. World J Urol 2002 Nov;20(5):285-93. Epub 2002 Oct 17.

Pyrethrum

Chrysanthemum cinerariifolium

DESCRIPTION

Medicinal Parts: The part of the plant used for medicinal purposes (primary as an insecticide) is the flower.

Flower and Fruit: Solitary flower heads are at the end of long slender peduncles, consisting of white lingual florets and yellow tubular florets. The fruit is an achene.

Leaves, Stem, and Root: Pyrethrum is a perennial, 20- to 60-cm high plant with an erect stem covered in alternating, pinnate, roughly serrated leaves. The underside of the leaves is downy.

Characteristics: The entire plant gives off a heavy perfume.

Habitat: Pyrethrum is indigenous to Kenya and the Mediterranean region and is widely cultivated in other parts of the world.

Production: Pyrethrum flowers are the just-opening compound flower heads of 2-to-8-year-old *Chrysanthemum cinerariifolium* and/or *Chrysanthemum coccineum.* The heads are left to wilt and then dried in special drying plants.

Other Names: Dalmatian Insect Flowers, Dalmatian Pellitory

ACTIONS AND PHARMACOLOGY

COMPOUNDS

Pyrethrine (ester of monoterpene acid with alkylcyclopentenolone, 1%): chief components pyrethrines I and II, cinerines I and II, jasmoline I and II

Flavonoids: including apigenin-, luteolin- and quercetin-7-O-glucosides and –glucuronides

Sesquiterpenes: sesquiterpene lactones, including pyrethrosine, cyclopyrethrosine

Lignans: sesamine

Polyynes: thiophenes, including 5-(4-hydroxy-1-butenyl)-2,2′-bithienyl

EFFECTS

Pyrethrum exhibits a neurotoxic effect on the sodium canal of insects with no development of habitual immunity. Pyrethrine and cinerine are contact insecticides that paralyze the nerve center of lower animals.

INDICATIONS AND USAGE

Unproven Uses: Pyrethrum is used as an insecticide for scabies, head lice, crab lice, and their nits.

PRECAUTIONS AND ADVERSE REACTIONS

No health hazards or side effects are known in conjunction with the proper administration of designated therapeutic dosages. The pyrethrines possess only limited toxicity in humans, with dosages up to 2 g of the drug are considered nontoxic.

OVERDOSAGE

Dosages exceeding 2 g of the drug have been observed to produce poisoning symptoms including headache, tinnitus, nausea, paresthesias, respiratory disturbances and other neurotoxic complaints.

Following gastric lavage with burgundy-colored potassium permanganate solution and installation of activated charcoal, the therapy for poisonings consists of treating possible cases of acidosis with sodium bicarbonate infusions. In case of shock, plasma volume expanders should be infused. Monitoring of kidney function is essential. Intubation and oxygen respiration may also be necessary.

DOSAGE

Mode of Administration: Externally as a liquid extract. (Area must be rinsed after use.) Some homeopathic remedies contain Pyrethrum mother tincture and dilutions.

How Supplied: Solutions, sprays, and shampoos.

LITERATURE

Anonym, Bio-Insektensprays: Wirken Pyrethroide als Nervengifte? In: *DAZ* 132(31):1632. 1992.

Garcia-Bravo B, Rodriguez-Pichardo A, Fernandez de Pierola S, Camacho F. Airborne erythema-multiforme-like eruption due to pyrethrum. *Contact Dermatitis* 33; 433. 1995

Kern W, List PH, Hörhammer L (Hrsg.), Hagers Handbuch der Pharmazeutischen Praxis, 4. Aufl., Bde. 1-8, Springer Verlag Berlin, Heidelberg, New York, 1969.

Lewin L, Gifte und Vergiftungen, 6. Aufl., Nachdruck, Haug Verlag, Heidelberg 1992.

Pachaly P, Pflanzenschutzmittel in der Apotheke - Pyrethrum. In: *DAZ* 132(19):1032. 1992.

Roth L, Daunderer M, Kormann K, Giftpflanzen, Pflanzengifte, 4. Aufl., Ecomed Fachverlag Landsberg Lech 1993 (unter Chrysanthemum cinerariifolium).

Stüttgen G, Skabies und Läuse heute. In: DAZ 132(34):1745. 1992.

Teuscher E, Lindequist U, Biogene Gifte - Biologie, Chemie, Pharmakologie, 2. Aufl., Fischer Verlag Stuttgart 1994.

Teuscher E, Biogene Arzneimittel, 5. Aufl., Wiss. Verlagsges. Stuttgart 1997.

Zito SW, Srivastava V, Adebayo-Olojo E. Incorporation of (1-14C)-Isopentenyl Pyrophosphate into Monoterpenes by a Cell-Free Homogenate Prepared from Callus Cultures of *Chrysanthemum cinerariaefolium. Planta Med.* 57; 425-427. 1991

Pyrola rotundifolia

See Round-Leafed Wintergreen

Pyrus communis

See Pear

Quassia

Picrasma excelsa

DESCRIPTION

Medicinal Parts: The medicinal part of the plant is the dried trunk wood.

Flower and Fruit: The flowers are in leaf-axillary, richly blossomed cymose panicles. The flower structures are in fours or fives. There are 5, 0.6 to 0.9 mm long, pubescent sepals, 5 yellow-green (in male flowers approximately 2 mm long, in androgynous flowers 3 mm long) petals, 10 stamens, and 5 carpels surrounded by a disc. The fruit is a single-seeded, orbicular-to-oval, blue-black drupe.

Leaves, Stem, and Root: An evergreen, this tree is usually dioecious and grows to a height of up to 25 m. The leaves are alternate, 15 to 35 cm long, odd pinnate, with 9 to 13 leaflets. The leaflets are 5 to 13 cm long, 20 to 45 cm wide, blunt-acuminate, and glossy. The trunk has gray grooved bark.

Habitat: The tree is indigenous to the Caribbean and northern Venezuela.

Production: Bitterwood is the dried trunk wood of *Picrasma excelsa*, collected in the wild.

Not to be Confused With: Mistaken identity can occur with *Rhus metopium.*

Other Names: Ash, Bitter Ash, Bitterwood

ACTIONS AND PHARMACOLOGY

COMPOUNDS

Triterpenes: decanor-triterpenes (picrasan derivatives, quassinoids, simaroubolides, 0.15 to 0.3%), chief components quassin (nigaki lactone D) and neoquassin (both extremely bitter), and also including isoquassin (picrasmine) and 18-hydroxyquassin

Indole alkaloids: beta-carboline types, including N-methoxy-2-vinyl-beta-carboline and canthinone types, including canthine-6-one, 4-methoxy-5-hydroxycanthine-6-one

EFFECTS

The bitter substances contained in the drug (quassinoids and canthinones) exhibit antimicrobial, antiviral, anthelminthic, and insecticidal effects. Quassia extract is positively inotropic and negatively chronotropic in animal experiment models. An antitumorous activity was demonstrated for various quassionoids. The drug's use to stimulate appetite and promote digestion is traceable to the bitter substances it contains.

INDICATIONS AND USAGE

Unproven Uses: Folk medicine uses include dyspepsia (Mexico and Brazil), loss of appetite, and stimulation of gastric juice and saliva production. These effects are attributed to the amaroid content. Quassia is also used for fever (Costa Rica and Surinam), malaria, dysentery, gonorrhea (Brazil), lice and worm infestations, as an antiseptic wound treatment, for diarrhea (Costa Rica and Brazil), for snake bites (Guyana), for liver disease, edema, and menstrual complaints.

Homeopathic Uses: Uses in homeopathy include poor digestion and liver disease.

CONTRAINDICATIONS

Not to be used during pregnancy.

PRECAUTIONS AND ADVERSE REACTIONS

No health hazards are known in conjunction with the proper administration of designated therapeutic dosages. Internal administration has occasionally led to dizziness and headache, as well as uterine pain.

OVERDOSAGE

Gastric mucous membrane irritation has been observed with cases of overdosage, followed by vomiting. It is said that prolonged use can lead to weakened vision and total blindness.

DOSAGE

Mode of Administration: Preparations are available for internal and external use.

Daily Dosage:

Drug – single dose, 0.3 to 0.6 g, 3 times daily; Tincture: daily dose; 2 to 4 mL; Lice: apply tincture twice weekly to the scalp.

Homeopathic Dosage: 5 drops, 1 tablet, 10 globules, every 30 to 60 minutes (acute), and 1 to 3 times daily (chronic); Parenterally: 1 to 2 ml sc, IV, IF; Acute: 3 times daily; Chronic: 1 to 3 times daily (HA).

Storage: Store protected from light and moisture.

LITERATURE

Dou J, Khan IA, McChesny JD, Burandt jr, CL. Qualitative and Quantitative High Performance Liquid Chromatographic Analysis of Quassinoids in Simaroubaceae Plants. *Phytochem Anal.* 7; 192-200. 1996

Hänsel R, Keller K, Rimpler H, Schneider G (Ed), Hagers Handbuch der Pharmazeutischen Praxis, 5. Aufl., Bde 4 - 6 (Drogen), Springer Verlag Berlin, Heidelberg, New York, 1992-1994.

Wagner H, Nestler T, Neszmelyi A, New constituents of *Picrasma excelsa. Planta Med,* 36:113-8, Jun. 1979

Quassia amara

See Amargo

Quebracho

Aspidosperma quebracho-blanco

DESCRIPTION

Medicinal Parts: The medicinal part of the plant is the bark.

Flower and Fruit: The inflorescences, which grow from the upper leaf axils, are opposite or in threes. They are shaped like a thyrsus and are warty to almost glabrous with numerous flowers. The flowers are 1 to 3 cm long. The bracts, which fall off, are very small and have a 2 to 3 mm stem. The sepals are ovate, obtuse, 1 to 2 mm long, and uneven. The corolla is white, yellow or yellowish-green, smooth or uneven on the outside. The tube is 3 to 5 mm long and has long, narrow, lanceolate petals. The stamens are in the middle of the corolla tube. The anthers are 1 mm long. The follicles are cylindrical to ovoid, 4 to 10 cm long and 1 to 7 cm wide. They are very woody, slightly warty, with or without a midrib, uneven and stemless.

Leaves, Stem, and Root: The tree grows to a height of 20 m and has slim branches. The young branches are warty; the older branches are smooth with thin orange-brown bark. The leaves are opposite or trifoliate, oblong-elliptoid, ovate-lanceolate to lanceolate, acuminate, and gradually narrow at the base. They are 3 to 5 cm long by 0.5 to 1.5 cm wide, coriaceous, often yellow-green, and smooth. The leaves have 20 to 30 pairs of steeply ascending secondary ribs, which are very close to each other and sunk into a thick mesophyll. The exterior of the bark is grayish and deeply fissured. The inner surface is yellowish-brown, often with a reddish tint, and is grooved. The transverse fracture shows a coarsely granular outer layer and a fibrous or splintery, darker inner layer.

Characteristics: The bark has a bitter taste and is odorless.

Habitat: The plant grows in Chile, Argentina, southeast Bolivia and southeast Brazil.

Production: Quebracho bark is the bark of *Aspidosperma quebracho-blanco*.

Not to be Confused With: Confusion can arise with *Aspidosperma horco kebracho*.

ACTIONS AND PHARMACOLOGY

COMPOUNDS

Indole alkaloids (0.5-1.5%): chief alkaloids aspidospermine (30%), yohimbine (quebrachine, 10%), further including, among others, (-)-quebrachamine, akuammidine

Tannins

EFFECTS

Quebracho bark works as an expectorant and stimulates the respiratory center. A respiratory-stimulating effect has been proved for the main alkaloid aspidospermin in animal tests, but there are no studies available on the effect of the whole drug.

INDICATIONS AND USAGE

Unproven Uses: Internal folk medicine uses of Quebracho include bronchial asthma, breathing difficulties, bronchitis, fever, cramps, malaria, and loss of appetite.

Homeopathic Uses: Uses in homeopathy are primarily chronic respiratory tract conditions with accompanying breathing difficulties.

PRECAUTIONS AND ADVERSE REACTIONS

No health hazards are known in conjunction with the proper administration of designated therapeutic dosages. Side effects can include, among others, salivation, headache, outbreaks of sweating, vertigo, stupor, and sleepiness.

OVERDOSAGE

Intakes of larger-than-recommended therapeutic dosages lead to queasiness and vomiting.

DOSAGE

Mode of Administration: The drug is available in extract and powder form, and is often used in combination bronchial preparations. However, it is rarely used as a drug in asthma remedies.

How Supplied: Commercial pharmaceutical preparations include powder, tablets, coated tablets, drops and elixir.

Preparation: Quebracho tincture is a 1:5 (ethanol 70%) combination.

Daily Dosage: A single dose of the drug is 1 to 2 g. (Recommended daily amount not specified.)

Homeopathic Dosage: 5 to 10 drops, 1 tablet, 5 to 10 globules, 1 to 3 times daily or 1 mL injection solution sc twice weekly (HAB1).

Storage: Keep the drug in tightly sealed containers.

LITERATURE

Jemec GB, Hausen BM, Contact dermatitis from Brazilian box tree wood (*Aspidosperma sp.*). *Contact Dermatitis,* 25:58-60, 1991.

Hänsel R, Keller K, Rimpler H, Schneider G (Ed), Hagers Handbuch der Pharmazeutischen Praxis, 5. Aufl., Bde 4 - 6 (Drogen), Springer Verlag Berlin, Heidelberg, New York, 1992-1994.

Wilson E et al., Rev farm (Buenos Aires) 125:9, 1983.

Quercus infectoria

See Oak Gall

Quercus robur

See Oak

Quillaja

Quillaja saponaria

DESCRIPTION

Medicinal Parts: The medicinal part is the inner bark.

Flower and Fruit: The terminal inflorescence consists of white androgynous flowers with a calyx and corolla but no epicalyx. They are arranged in groups of 3 to 5 on the peduncle. The flower head is 5-lobed, splayed flat, and formed into a disc on the upper surface. The many-seeded carpels spread into a star shape in the ripe fruit. The seeds are winged with little or no endosperm.

Leaves, Stem, and Root: The tree is up to 18 m tall. The leaves are smooth, glossy, short petioled, and oval. The bark is thick, dark, and very hard. It is odorless, very bitter, and astringent.

Habitat: The plant is indigenous to Chile, Peru, and is cultivated in India and California.

Production: Quillaja Bark is the bark of *Quillaja saponaria.*

Other Names: Cullay, Panama Bark, Quillai, Quillaja Bark, Soap Tree

ACTIONS AND PHARMACOLOGY

COMPOUNDS

Tannins (10 to 15%)

Triterpene saponins (8.5 to 17%): chief saponins quillajasaponins 17 (QS 17, QS III), 18 (QS 18), 21 (QS 21), chief saponin quillaic acid

EFFECTS

Because of its saponin content the drug is lipid-lowering, antiexudative, and immune-stimulating in animal experiments. The expectorant and purgative effect is also attributed to the saponin content.

INDICATIONS AND USAGE

Unproven Uses: Quillaja is used internally for coughs, chronic bronchitis, and conditions of the respiratory tract. It is used externally for dandruff.

PRECAUTIONS AND ADVERSE REACTIONS

No health hazards or side effects are known in conjunction with the proper administration of designated therapeutic dosages.

OVERDOSAGE

Mucus membrane irritation could occur in the event of overdosage. Overdosage complaints include gastroenteritis, combined with vertigo, stomach pain and diarrhea. The drug possesses a low potential for sensitization.

DOSAGE

Mode of Administration: Quillaja is available as liquid extract and tincture for internal and external use.

LITERATURE

Higuchi R et al., *Phytochemistry* 26 (1):229. 1987

Higuchi R et al., *PH* 27:1165. 1988.

Topping DL et al., *Proc Nutr Soc Aust* 5:195. 1980

Wolters B, Arzneipflanzen und Volksmedizin Chiles. In: DAZ 134(39):3693. 1994.

Quillaja saponaria

See Quillaja

Quince

Cydonia oblongata

DESCRIPTION

Medicinal Parts: The medicinal parts are the fruit and seeds.

Flower and Fruit: The flowers are pink, relatively large, solitary, and perfumed. The fruit is yellow, downy, and apple or pear-shaped.

Leaves, Stem, and Root: Qunice is a 3- to - m high tree or shrub with tomentose branches covered in alternate, ovate leaves. The undersurface of the leaves is grass-green and tomentose..

Habitat: Quince is indigenous to southwest and central Asia, but it has also spread to Europe and in particularly the Mediterranean.

Production: Quince seeds are the seeds of *Cydonia oblongata*. The ripe quinces are picked, stored for a period, then cut and finally dried at temperatures not exceeding 50°C. The seeds are gathered up and used in whole or ground form.

ACTIONS AND PHARMACOLOGY

COMPOUNDS

Cyanogenic glycosides: amygdalin (corresponding to 0.4 to 1.5%, 27 to 75 mg HCN/100 g)

Mucilages

Fatty oil

EFFECTS

The main active principles are mucilage, some tannins and vitamin C. There is no information is available on the mode of action.

INDICATIONS AND USAGE

Unproven Uses: Quince is used as a demulcent in digestive disorders and diarrhea. As a lotion, it is used to soothe the eyes. The seeds are also used to treat coughs and gastrointestinal catarrh. Additionally, the herb is used in compresses or poultices for injuries, inflammation of the joints, injuries of the nipples, and gashed or deeply cut fingers.

PRECAUTIONS AND ADVERSE REACTIONS

Health risks or side effects following the proper administration of designated therapeutic dosages are not recorded. Because quince mucilage is prepared from the whole seeds, and/or the whole seeds are taken internally, the cyanogenic glycosides are credited with a slight toxicological relevance.

DOSAGE

Mode of Administration: The drug is used as a powder, a lotion, a decoction and an extract.

Preparation: Extract/decoction: 1 tsp. of whole seeds per cup of water. A viscous poultice is prepared from the ground seeds.

LITERATURE

De Tommasi N et al., New tetracyclic sesterterpenes from *Cydonia vulgaris*. In: JNP 59(3):267-270. 1996.

Kern W, List PH, Hörhammer L (Hrsg.), Hagers Handbuch der Pharmazeutischen Praxis, 4. Aufl., Bde. 1-8, Springer Verlag Berlin, Heidelberg, New York, 1969.

Reis D, Vian B, Chanzy H, Roland JC, Liquid crystal-type assembly of native cellulose-glucuronoxylans extracted from plant cell wall. Biol Cell, 30:173-8, 1991

Steinegger E, Hänsel R, Pharmakognosie, 5. Aufl., Springer Verlag Heidelberg 1992

Teuscher E, Lindequist U, Biogene Gifte - Biologie, Chemie, Pharmakologie, 2. Aufl., Fischer Verlag Stuttgart 1994.

Quinine

Cinchona pubescens

DESCRIPTION

Medicinal Parts: The medicinal part is the dried bark of 6- to 8-year-old trees.

Flower and Fruit: The 35 cm long inflorescence is panicled, opposite, often leafy and densely blossomed. The flowers are almost sessile, and the tube is thickly covered in silky hairs. The calyx has appressed hairs, and the tips are short and widely acuminate. The corolla is red or pink and 10 to 12 mm long. The fruit is an oblong, glabrous, and longitudinally grooved capsule.

Leaves, Stem, and Root: The plant is an evergreen tree, sometimes a bush, which grows from 5 to 15 m high, with a dense crown. The branches are at right angles to the trunk. The young branches are usually pubescent. The stipules are large, ovate, obtuse or acuminate, silky-haired or glabrous. The leaves have an up to 8 cm long petiole. The leaf blade is 15 to 40 cm long and 7 to 25 cm wide, oblong-elliptoid to roundish with curved side ribs. The bark occurs in quills or flat pieces up to 30 cm long and 3 to 6 mm thick. The external surface is brownish-gray, usually fissured with an exfoliating cork. Lichens and mosses may be seen as grayish-white or greenish patches. The inner surface is yellowish to reddish-brown. The fracture is fibrous.

Characteristics: The bark has an astringent, bitter taste and the odor is slight.

Habitat: The herb is indigenous to mountainous regions of the tropical U.S. and is cultivated elsewhere.

Production: Cinchona bark consists of the dried bark of *Cinchona pubescens* or other varieties. Trees are felled at between 6 and 12 years. They are dried slowly in the sun initially and then artificially dried at maximum temperatures of 70° C.

Not to be Confused With: Yellow factory bark

Other Names: Cinchona, Jesuit's Bark, Peruvian Bark, Yellow Cinchona

ACTIONS AND PHARMACOLOGY

COMPOUNDS

Quinoline alkaloids (5-15%): main alkaloids are quinine (0.8-4%), quinidine (0.02-0.4%), cinchonine (1.5-3%), cinchonidine (1.5-5%)

Triterpenes: bitter acid monoglycosides, in particular chinovic acid-3-O-chinovoside, chinovic acid-3-O-glucoside

Catechin tannins (3-5%)

EFFECTS

Quinine promotes stimulation of the secretion of saliva and gastric juices.

INDICATIONS AND USAGE

Approved by Commission E:

- Loss of appetite
- Dyspeptic complaints

Unproven Uses: Quinine is used internally to correct flatulence with a sense of fullness. The bark is used for malaria, flu, enlarged spleen, muscle cramps, muscle pain, cancer, and gastric disorders. Externally, it is used for scrapes and skin ulcers.

Chinese Medicine: Quinine is used for malaria, fever, and alcohol intoxication.

Indian Medicine: The drug is used to treat intermittent fever, malaria, intercostal neuralgia, sciatica, and neuritis (especially of the arm).

Homeopathic Uses: Quinine is used to treat general poisoning, attacks of fever, inflammation of the respiratory tract, acute diarrhea, anemia, general debility, skin rashes, and neuralgia.

CONTRAINDICATIONS

Quinine should not be used during pregnancy.

PRECAUTIONS AND ADVERSE REACTIONS

General: Sensitization to Quinine and Quinidine have been observed (eczema, itching). Even at therapeutic dosages, an enhanced pseudohemophiliac effect can occur through the triggering of thrombocytopenia.

DRUG INTERACTIONS

MAJOR RISK

Digoxin: Concurrent use may result in digoxin toxicity (nausea, vomiting, cardiac arrhythmias). *Clinical Management:* In patients taking digoxin who require quinine for greater than five to seven days, monitor digoxin levels and adjust dose accordingly.

Pancuronium: Concurrent use may result in pancuronium toxicity (respiratory depression, apnea). *Clinical Management:* Quinine should be avoided if possible in the immediate postoperative period when the effects of neuromuscular blockers may be present. If quinine is used, the need for respiratory support should be anticipated.

MODERATE RISK

Dicumarol: Concurrent use may result in increased risk of bleeding. *Clinical Management:* Adjustment of dicumarol dose may be necessary in order to maintain the desired level of anticoagulation.

Rifampin: Concurrent use may result in an increase in clearance of quinine and a reduction of quinine plasma levels and efficacy. *Clinical Management:* Rifampin should not be combined with quinine for the treatment of malaria, and the doses of quinine should probably be increased in patients what are already receiving rifampin treatment. Rifampin significantly increases the metabolic clearance of quinine and thereby reduces cure rates.

Rifapentine: Concurrent use may result in decreased quinine efficacy. *Clinical Management:* Monitor patients for reduced quinine plasma concentrations and reduced quinine efficacy. Quinine doses may need to be increased when quinine is given concomitantly with rifapentine.

Warfarin: Concurrent use may result in an increased risk of bleeding. *Clinical Management:* Adjustments of the warfarin dose may be necessary in order to maintain the desired level of anticoagulation.

MINOR RISK

Flecainide: Concurrent use may result in flecainide toxicity (cardiac arrhythmias). *Clinical Management:* Monitor flecainide levels and PR interval two to four days after starting or discontinuing quinine. A dosage reduction for flecainide may be required.

POTENTIAL INTERACTIONS

Astemizole: Concurrent use may result in increased astemizole concentrations and potential cardiotoxicity (QT prolongation, torsades de pointes, cardiac arrest). Severe cardiotoxicity, including electrocardiographic abnormalities, torsades de pointes, ventricular arrhythmias, and cardiac arrest, have occurred in cases of high serum concentrations of astemizole.

Clinical Management: Avoid concomitant use.

Ranolazine: Concurrent use may result in an increased risk of QT interval prolongation.

OVERDOSAGE

In cases of overdose (more than 3 cardiac arrhythmias, buzzing in the ears, hearing and visual disorders (all the way to complete deafness and blindness) may occur. Death comes with dosages of 10 to 15 g of Quinine through heart failure and asphyxiation. Following gastric lavage, the symptomatic therapy for acute poisonings includes atropine for bradycardia and phenytoin in the presence of tachycardic heart rhythm disorders. Forced diuresis and hemodialysis are not suitable as therapeutic measures.

DOSAGE

Mode of Administration: Whole, cut, and powdered drug are used in various galenic preparations, including tonics, drops, tablets, compresses, ampules, coated tablets, suppositories and compound preparations.

Preparation: A tea is prepared by pouring 150 ml of boiling water over 1/2 teaspoonful of the drug and allowing it to draw for 10 minutes. A decoction is prepared by adding 0.5 g to 1 teacup of water. A tincture in the proportion of 1:5 in 75% ethanol is also used.

Daily Dosage: Total daily dose is 1 to 3 g of drug. The liquid extract daily dose is 0.6 to 3 g of cinchona liquid extract, which contains 4 to 5% total alkaloids. A daily dose of 0.15 to 0.6 g cinchona extract with 15 to 20% total alkaloids may also be used.

The standard single dose of the extract is 0.2 g. The liquid extract single dose is 0.5 to 1 g.

Homeopathic Dosage: 5 drops, 1 tablet, or 10 globules, every 30 to 60 minutes (acute) or 1 to 3 times a day (chronic); parenterally: 1 to 2 mL sc, acute: 3 times daily; chronic: once a day (HAB1).

Storage: Keep protected from light and moisture.

LITERATURE

Chan, EH et al. (Eds.), Advances in Chinese Medicinal Materials Research, World Scientific Pub. Co. Singapore 1985.

Chinidin: Photoallergische Reaktion. In: *DAZ* 133(30):2765. 1993.

Risdale CE, Hasskarls cinchona barks. 1. Historical review. In: Reinwardtia 10, Teil 2: 245-264. 1985.

Schönfeld, Fleischer K, Eichenlaub D, Die Malariavorbeugung. Mückenschutz und Arzneimittel zur Kurzzeitprophylaxe und Notfallbehandlung. In: DAZ 133(21):1981. 1993.

Hänsel R, Keller K, Rimpler H, Schneider G (Hrsg.), Hagers Handbuch der Pharmazeutischen Praxis, 5. Aufl., Bde 4-6 (Drogen): Springer Verlag Berlin, Heidelberg, New York, 1992-1994.

Leung AY, Encyclopedia of Common Natural Ingredients Used in Food Drugs and Cosmetics, John Wiley & Sons Inc., New York 1980.

Lewin L, Gifte und Vergiftungen, 6. Aufl., Nachdruck, Haug Verlag, Heidelberg 1992.

Madaus G, Lehrbuch der Biologischen Arzneimittel, Bde 1-3, Nachdruck, Georg Olms Verlag Hildesheim 1979.

Manske RHF, Holmes HL, fortgeführt von Rodrigo RGA, Brossi A): The Alkaloids - Chemistry and Physiology, III:1, XIV:181, XXXIV:331, Academic Press New York 1950-1997.

Roth L, Daunderer M, Kormann K, Giftpflanzen, Pflanzengifte, 4. Aufl., Ecomed Fachverlag Landsberg Lech 1993.

Steinegger E, Hänsel R, Pharmakognosie, 5. Aufl., Springer Verlag Heidelberg 1992.

Teuscher E, Lindequist U, Biogene Gifte - Biologie, Chemie, Pharmakologie, 2. Aufl., Fischer Verlag Stuttgart 1994.

uscher E, Biogene Arzneimittel, 5. Aufl., Wiss. Verlagsges. mbH Stuttgart 1997.

Wagner H, Wiesenauer M, Phytotherapie. Phytopharmaka und pflanzliche Homöopathika, Fischer-Verlag, Stuttgart, Jena, New York 1995.

Wichtl M (Hrsg.), Teedrogen, 4. Aufl., Wiss. Verlagsges. Stuttgart 1997.

Radish

Raphanus sativus

DESCRIPTION

Medicinal Parts: The medicinal part is the fresh root. The plant is an important drug in homeopathic medicine.

Flower and Fruit: The raceme is loose and has about 30 flowers. The pedicles are 1 to 2 cm long and are covered in scattered bristles. The sepals are 6.5 to 10 mm long, oblong, acute, glabrous or with scattered bristles, and red or green. The petals are 17 to 22 mm long, obovate, slightly margined, violet or white with dark veins. The fruit is on upright, patent stems. They are upright, cylindrical, and conically acuminate. The upper segment is up to 9 cm long and even or slightly constricted between the seeds, and strawlike on the outside. The seeds are ovate, 4 mm long and 3 mm wide, light brown with a black hilum.

Leaves, Stem, and Root: The root is annual or biennial and thin. The stem is up to 1 m high, bent, canelike, branched, glabrous or covered with bristles, and often violet, particularly in the axils of the lateral branches. The lower leaves are lyrate-pinnatisect with large sweeping crenate end segments and smaller, oblong-ovate, obtuse, dentate lateral lobes. They are light green, often red-veined and covered with scattered, appressed bristles.

Characteristics: The large, thick, tuberous, fleshy root is hot to the taste.

Habitat: The plant is probably indigenous to China and Japan and today is cultivated in most temperate regions of the world.

Production: Radish consists of the fresh roots of *Raphanus sativus* and its preparations. It is a cultivated plant.

Other Names: Common Radish, Garden Radish

ACTIONS AND PHARMACOLOGY

COMPOUNDS

Glucosinolates in the fresh, unbruised rhizome: chief component 4-methylthio-3-butenyl-glucosinolate, glucobrassin, sinigrin, glucoraphanine

EFFECTS

The drug is said to be choleretic and antimicrobial and to increase motility in the upper gastrointestinal tract, an effect caused by the mustard oils. A choleretic effect and an antiviral effect were proved in animal experiments. Radish has a secretolytic effect in patients suffering from chronic bronchitis.

INDICATIONS AND USAGE

Approved by Commission E:

- Cough/Bronchitis
- Dyspeptic complaints

Radish is used internally for respiratory catarrh and dyspeptic disorders, especially those related to dyskinesia of the bile ducts.

Unproven Uses: In folk medicine Radish is used for whooping cough and gallstones.

Chinese Medicine: In China, Radish is used to treat coughs, diarrhea, and abdominal pain.

Indian Medicine: Uses in India include dyspeptic complaints, nausea, flatulence, gallbladder disturbances, headache, neuralgias, and urological conditions.

Homeopathic Uses: Raphanus sativus is used for poor digestion and oily skin.

PRECAUTIONS AND ADVERSE REACTIONS

No health hazards or side effects are known in conjunction with the proper administration of designated therapeutic dosages.

CONTRAINDICATED

Not to be used in the presence of cholelithiasis.

OVERDOSAGE

Administration of higher dosages of the fresh root could lead to mucus membrane irritation of the gastrointestinal tract. Due to the cholagogic effect of the drug, biliary colic could be triggered in patients with gallstones.

DOSAGE

Preparation:

Radish-honey juice — 1 radish is grated and the resulting juice is mixed with honey, then allowed to stand for 10 hours.

Radish plant juice — The Radish is washed, cut and grated and up to 17% of the liquid is pressed out. 1-liter of juice is extracted from 1.3 kg of fresh drug.

Daily Dosage:

Pressed juice — 50 to 100 mL; 1/2 tablespoon several times daily over a 3-day period.

Radish-honey juice — spoonfuls taken over the course of the day for whooping cough.

Homeopathic Dosage: 5 drops, 1 tablet, or 10 globules every 30 to 60 minutes (acute) or 1 to 3 times daily (chronic); parenterally: 1 to 2 mL sc acute: 3 times daily; chronic: once a day (HAB1)

LITERATURE

Han DH, Lee JH. Effects of liming on uptake of lead and cadmium by *Raphanus sativa. Arch Environ Contam* Toxicol, 31:488-93, Nov 1996

Hänsel R, Keller K, Rimpler H, Schneider G (Hrsg.), Hagers Handbuch der Pharmazeutischen Praxis, 5. Aufl., Bde 4-6

(Drogen): Springer Verlag Berlin, Heidelberg, New York, 1992-1994.

Kasjanovova D, Macejka J. The effect of extracts from garden radish (*Raphanus sativus*) and horseradish (*Amoracia rusticana*) on platelet functional activity in vitro. *Pharmazie* 47; 876-877. 1992

Miron A et al. Immunologically active Polysaccharides isolated from Raphani radix. *Sci Pharm.* 43 (4); 333. 1995

Teuscher E, Lindequist U, Biogene Gifte - Biologie, Chemie, Pharmakologie, 2. Aufl., Fischer Verlag Stuttgart 1994.

Ragwort

Senecio jacoboea

DESCRIPTION

Medicinal Parts: The medicinal parts are the dried aerial parts of the flowering plant and the entire fresh plant gathered during the flowering season.

Flower and Fruit: The golden yellow composite flowers grow in dense, terminal, erect, branched cymes. The linguiform ray florets are female. The disc florets are tubular and androgynous. The capitula has a diameter of 15 to 20 mm. The involucre is cylindrical. The bracts are in a single row and are oblong-lanceolate, acuminate, and black at the tip, with a short 1- to 4-leafed epicalyx. The lateral fruit is glabrous and has drooping tufts of hair. The other fruit is covered in thick tufts of loosely attached hair.

Leaves, Stem, and Root: The plant is biennial to perennial and grows 30 to 90 cm high. The stem is erect, branched above, and cobweb-pubescent. The basal leaves are lyrate-pinnatifid. The cauline leaves are pinnatifid with indented pinna. The lateral tips are almost at right angles and have small, 4-sectioned, slit ears that clasp the stem.

Habitat: The plant is indigenous to all of Europe, Asia Minor and northern Africa, and is naturalized in North America.

Production: Ragwort is the flowering plant of *Senecio jacoboea*. The plant is gathered in the wild, usually during the flowering season. The cut drug is dried away from direct sunlight.

Other Names: Cankerwort, Dog Standard, Ragweed, St. James Wort, Staggerwort, Stammerwort, Stinking Nanny, Tansy Ragwort

ACTIONS AND PHARMACOLOGY

COMPOUNDS

Pyrrolizidine alkaloids (0.1-0.9%): the alkaloid spectrum depends upon the chemotype. Jacobine chemotype: chief alkaloid jacobine; erucifoline chemotype: chief alkaloids erucifoline and O-acetylerucifoline

Volatile oil (traces)

EFFECTS

The toxic principles of the drug are the pyrrolizidine alkaloids, which should be assumed to be hepatotoxic and carcinogenic. Countless experiments have shown the plant to be acutely and chronically poisonous in animals.

INDICATIONS AND USAGE

Because of its potential carcinogenic effect, Ragwort should not be used.

PRECAUTIONS AND ADVERSE REACTIONS

Ragwort should not be taken internally since hepatotoxicity and carcinogenicity are possible due to the pyrrolizidine alkaloids with 1,2-unsaturated necic parent substances in its makeup.

DOSAGE

Mode of Administration: The drug is used externally as a component of lotions, but should not be taken internally.

Preparation: The lotion is made using 1 part of the drug and 5 parts of 10% ethanol.

Daily Dosage: The lotion is applied topically for the treatment of rheumatic arthritis.

LITERATURE

Deinzer ML et al., *Science* 195:497. 1977.

Moghaddam MF, Cheeke PR. Effects of dietary pyrrolizidine (Senecio) alkaloids on vitamin A metabolism in rats. *Toxicol Letters* 45; 149-156. 1989

Roeder E. Medicinal plants in Europe containing pyrrolizidine alkaloids. *Pharmazie* 50 (2); 82-98. 1995

Van Dooren, Bos R et al., *Planta Med* 42:385. 1981

Van Dorren B et al., *PM* 42:385. 1981.

Frohne D, Pfänder HJ: Giftpflanzen - Ein Handbuch für Apotheker, Toxikologen und Biologen, 4. Aufl., Wiss. Verlags-Ges. Stuttgart 1997.

Hänsel R, Keller K, Rimpler H, Schneider G (Hrsg.), Hagers Handbuch der Pharmazeutischen Praxis, 5. Aufl., Bde 4-6 (Drogen): Springer Verlag Berlin, Heidelberg, New York, 1992-1994.

Madaus G: Lehrbuch der Biologischen Arzneimittel, Bde 1-3, Nachdruck, Georg Olms Verlag Hildesheim 1979.

Roth L, Daunderer M, Kormann K, Giftpflanzen, Pflanzengifte, 4. Aufl., Ecomed Fachverlag Landsberg Lech 1993.

Teuscher E, Lindequist U, Biogene Gifte - Biologie, Chemie, Pharmakologie, 2. Aufl., Fischer Verlag Stuttgart 1994.

Ranunculus acris

See Buttercup

Ranunculus bulbosus

See Bulbous Buttercup

Ranunculus ficaria

See Lesser Celandine

Ranunculus sceleratus

See Poisonous Buttercup

Raphanus raphanistrum

See Wild Radish

Raphanus sativus

See Radish

Raspberry

Rubus idaeus

DESCRIPTION

Medicinal Parts: The medicinal parts are the leaves and fruit.

Flower and Fruit: The white flowers are in cymes. The calyx has 5 sepals and the corolla is 5-petalled. There are numerous stamens and ovaries. Similar to the blackberry, the small fruit forms a red aggregate fruit, the raspberry.

Leaves, Stem and Root: Raspberry is a 2 m high deciduous bush with erect, woody stems, which are densely covered in tough thorns. The aerial part is usually biennial while the creeping root is perennial. The leaves are pale green. There are 3 leaves that sit atop 7 leaflets.

Habitat: The plant is indigenous to Europe and Asia and is cultivated in temperate climates.

Production: Raspberry leaf consists of the leaf of Rubus idaeus.

Not to be Confused With: Blackberry leaves.

Other Names: Red Raspberry

ACTIONS AND PHARMACOLOGY

COMPOUNDS

Tannins: gallo tannins, ellagic tannins

Flavonoids

EFFECTS

General: The main active agents are tannin, flavonoids, and vitamin C. The tannins give the fruit an astringent effect. In addition to tannins, active constituents of extracts of raspberry leaves include a smooth-muscle stimulant, an anticholinesterase, and a spasmolytic (Newall et al, 1996; Beckett et al, 1954).

Dermatologic

Raspberry leaf's tannin content (between 13% and 15%) is responsible for its astringent properties. Applied topically to mucous membranes or abraded skin, tannins have a local anti-inflammatory effect, produce capillary vasoconstriction, and decrease vascular permeability (Jellin et al, 2000). Astringency of the leaves accounts for its effectiveness in extracts and as a poultice applied to skin wounds. This astringency also contributes to decreasing mucous discharge from the eyes (Briggs & Briggs, 1997).

Uteroactivity

Active constituents in aqueous extracts of raspberry leaves include a smooth muscle stimulant, an anticholinesterase, and an antispasmodic that antagonizes the stimulant action of the two former fractions. The smooth muscle stimulant fraction has greater effect in uterine muscle (Newall et al, 1996). Results of animal studies indicate that raspberry can reduce and initiate uterine contractions (Newall et al, 1996). As incoordination of uterine action is a major problem in obstetrics, it may be that extract of raspberry leaf produces more coordinated labor contractions (Parsons et al, 1999).

Hypoglycemia

A related species, Rubus fructicosus, has hypoglycemic effects in both non-diabetic and diabetic rabbits. This slight hypoglycemic activity is thought to be produced from increased insulin liberation, which may be related to the astringency of raspberry tannins (Newall et al, 1996).

CLINICAL TRIALS

A leaf infusion of raspberry inhibited contractions of uterine strips from pregnant rats and from human uteri at 10 to 16 weeks of pregnancy while having little or no effect on uterine strips from non-pregnant rats and humans. With exposure to the infusion, the intrinsic rhythm of pregnant rat and human uteri became more regular, with less frequent contractions in most cases. After 3 to 4 minutes of inhibition, intrinsic contractions resumed (Bamford et al, 1970).

Results of a retrospective, observational study investigating effects of raspberry-leaf products on labor and birth outcomes in pregnant women indicate no difference between women who took the products and those who did not as to average gestation period, likelihood of medical augmentation of labor, occurrence of meconium liquid in the infant, or need for epidural block. Significant variance between groups in measures of time for first-stage labor necessitated application of an unequal-variance assumption to the t-test of difference between means, which suggests they did not differ significantly, although a tendency toward a decrease in time for first-stage labor in women taking raspberry-leaf products was observed. Records were accessed for 51 women who took no raspberry product and for 57 who did. No attempt was made to control for such variables as timing and amount of raspberry leaf products consumed, parity of the women, or care providers. The products consumed consisted of tea, tablets, or combinations of tea, tablets, and tincture. Groups differed as to maternal age ($p=0.86$) (Parsons et al, 1999).

Some herbal baby drinks, particularly those with a fruit component, may have acidogenic and/or erosive potential. In a two-part study of commonly available herbal baby drinks, all drinks tested had cariogenic potential. In vitro analysis of the inherent acidity of fruit-containing, herbal baby drinks, as well as in vivo assessment of their ability to depress plaque acidity in adult volunteers, revealed that 3 of 6 test drinks had a low pH although most had a low titratable acidity. Next to that of a 10% solution of sucrose used as a positive control, the area under the curve below the resting pH was highest for apple and raspberry herbal drinks. Damage to teeth from fruit drinks is thought to be caused from two properties, erosion of enamel surface from low pH and high titratable acidity and demineralization of enamel from organic acids in the dental plaque generated by plaque micro- organisms during metabolism of fermentable carbohydrates (Duggal et al, 1996).

INDICATIONS AND USAGE

Raspberry is unapproved by the German Commission E because of lack of reliable studies to confirm effectiveness and safety. Raspberry is listed by European authorities as an N1 natural food flavoring and has no restrictions on use.

Unproven Uses: Raspberry leaf is used for disorders of the gastrointestinal tract, the respiratory tract, the cardiovascular system, and the mouth and throat. In folk medicine, Raspberry preparations were used to facilitate childbirth.

CONTRAINDICATIONS

Raspberry leaf should not be used topically during pregnancy as there is insufficient information about its safety. Animal study evidence indicates that raspberry can initiate and reduce uterine contractions (Jellin et al, 2000; Newall et al, 1996). Oral use of raspberry as a food flavoring during pregnancy is possibly safe (Jellin et al, 2000).

PRECAUTIONS AND ADVERSE REACTIONS

General: No health hazards or side effects are known in conjunction with the proper administration of designated therapeutic dosages. Use of raspberry leaf may cause a blood pressure change. In separate human studies a rise in blood pressure as well as a slight fall in systolic blood pressure has been reported (Parsons et al, 1999). Raspberry leaf tea has not been evaluated for carcinogenicity, although some herbal teas, if used chronically, contain tannins that can be carcinogenic, causing esophageal or stomach tumors (Briggs & Briggs, 1997).

Pregnancy: Raspberry should not be used during pregnancy without medical supervision.

Breast Milk: Scientific evidence for the safe use of raspberry during lactation is not available.

DRUG INTERACTIONS

No drug interactions were found.

DOSAGE

Mode of Administration: As a component of purgative and ''blood purifying'' teas, and in fruit tea mixtures.

Preparation: To prepare an infusion, scald 1.5 gm finely cut drug, steep for 5 minutes and then strain. (1 teaspoonful = 0.8 gm drug).

How Supplied:

Capsules: 345 mg

Liquid Extract

Tea

LITERATURE

Bamford DS et al., (1970) Brit J Pharmacol 40(1):161P. Bamford DS, Percival RC & Tothill AU, Raspberry leaf tea: a new aspect to an old problem. *Br J Pharmacol*; 40(1):161P-162P, 1970.

Beckett A et al., (1954) *J Pharm Pharmacol* 6:785, 1954.

Briggs CJ & Briggs K, Raspberry. *Can Pharm J*; 130(3):41-43, 1997.

Czygan FC, Die Himbeere - Rubus idaeus L. In: ZPT 16(6):366-74. 1995.

Duggal MS, Toumba KJ, Pollard MA et al., The acidogenic potential of herbal baby drinks. *Br Dent J*; 180(3):98-103, 1996.

Jellin JM, Gregory P, Batz F, Hitchens K, et al, eds. Pharmacist's Letter/Prescriber's Letter. Natural Medicines Comprehensive Database, 3rd Edition. Stockton CA: Therapeutic Research Facility, 2000.

Henning W, (1981) Lebensm Unters Forsch 173:1, 1981. Henning W, (1981) Lebensm Unters Forsch 173:180.

Marczal G, (1963) Herba Hung 2:343, 1963.

Newall CA, Anderson LA & Phillipson JD, Herbal Medicines: A Guide for Health-Care Professionals. The Pharmaceutical Press, London, England; 1996.

Parsons M, Simpson M & Ponton T, Raspberry leaf and its effect on labour: Safety and efficacy. *J Aust Coll Midwives*; 12(3):20-25, 1999.

Rauwolfia

Rauwolfia serpentina

DESCRIPTION

Medicinal Parts: The medicinal part is the dried root.

Flower and Fruit: The white to pink flowers are in terminal or axillary cymes that have a diameter of 2.5 to 5 cm and are 5 to 13 cm long in main axis. The corolla tube is 11 to 19 cm long and therefore much longer than the tips, which form a platelike margin. The fruit is a bilabiate drupe, which is purple-black when ripe.

Leaves, Stem, and Root: The plant is an erect, glabrous evergreen semishrub 0.5 to 1 m in height. The trunk is pale and unbranched. The leaves are concentrated toward the top of the trunk and are entire-margined. They are in whorls of 3 to 5 and occasionally opposite. The leaves are 7 to 18 cm long, 2.5 to 5 cm wide, oblong-ovate or lanceolate and taper to an irregular base. The petiole is 5 to 15 cm long.

The rhizome is vertical and woody, the root is gray-brown with a wrinkled surface and is 3 to 22 mm in diameter.

Characteristics: The fresh root has a very bitter, unpleasant taste.

Habitat: The plant is indigenous to India, Indochina, Borneo, Sri Lanka, and Sumatra.

The drug is derived from wild collections in India, Pakistan, Thailand, and Indonesia.

Production: Rauwolfia root consists of the dried root of *Rauwolfia serpentina* as well as its preparations. It is collected in the uncultivated regions, mostly from 4-year-old plants. When cultivated, 2-year-old plants are harvested. Roots are air-dried at 60° C.

Not to be Confused With: The roots of other Rauwolfia species and *Withania sonnifera.*

ACTIONS AND PHARMACOLOGY

COMPOUNDS

Ajmalane-type: including ajmaline

Heteroyohimbane-type: including serpentinine, serpentine, raubasine, ajmalicine

Indole alkaloids (1 to 2.5%)

Sarpagan-type: including raupine, sarpagine

Starch

Yohimbine-type: including reserpine, isorauhimbine, rescinnamine, reserpinine

EFFECTS

The drug contains alkaloids of the rauwolfia type. Reserpine and other alkaloids in the root have a sympatholytic effect by releasing noradrenaline and inhibiting its resorption in the vesicles of the noradrenergic nerve ends. This results in a lowering of catecholamine, which causes a hypotensive effect. The ajmalin in the root has an antiarrhythmic effect brought about by membrane stabilization. In animal experiments a centrally generated sedative effect was demonstrated.

INDICATIONS AND USAGE

Approved by Commission E:

- Hypertension
- Nervousness and insomnia

Rauwolfia is used internally for hypertension due to vascular hypertonia. It is also useful for anxiety and tension states and other psychomotoric disorders.

Unproven Uses: Rauwolfia is also used in folk medicine for flatulence, vomiting, insomnia, eclampsia, and liver disease. It is used to encourage uterine contraction during birth, and is used locally in the treatment of wounds.

Indian Medicine: The drug is used as an antidote for snakebites and the poisonous bites of other reptiles; also for hypertension, dysuria, fever, colic, and in the treatment of wounds.

CONTRAINDICATIONS

Rauwolfia is contraindicated in depression, ulceration, pheochromocytoma, pregnancy, and lactation.

PRECAUTIONS AND ADVERSE REACTIONS

General: No health hazards are known in conjunction with the proper administration of designated therapeutic dosages. Side effects could include nasal congestion, states of depression, tiredness erectile dysfunction. The drug may cause drowsiness and care must be taken when operating an automobile or machinery.

Pregnancy: Not to be used during pregnancy.

Breast-Feeding: Not to be used while breast-feeding.

POTENTIAL INTERACTIONS

Alcohol: Combination with alcohol considerably increases the impairment of reactions.

Neuroleptics and Barbiturates: An increase of drug effect occurs with these medications.

Digitalis-Glycosides: Severe bradycardia occurs in combination with digitalis glycosides.

Levodopa: Drug effect is reduced in combination with levodopa along with an increase in the undesired extrapyramidal motor symptoms in combination with sympathomimetics. Cough or ''flu'' remedies and appetite suppressants may cause a significant increase in blood pressure in combination with Rawolfia.

DOSAGE

Mode of Administration: Rauwolfia is available in whole, crude and powder form for internal and external use. It is also available in solid pharmaceutical form and in compounded preparations.

Preparation: Rauwolfia serpentina dry extract contains 7% total alkaloids (DAB10). Various processes are used to isolate reserpine.

Daily Dosage: 600 mg drug/6 mg total alkaloids

Storage: The drug should be protected from light.

LITERATURE

Beim HJ, *Pharmacol Rev* 8:281. 1978.

Cornett GBR, *World Crops* 17:33. 1965.

Lounasmaa M et al., On the structure of the indole alkaloid ajmalicidine. In: *PM* 60(5):480. 1994.

Rauwolfia serpentina

See Rauwolfia

Red Bryony

Bryonia cretica

DESCRIPTION

Medicinal Parts: The medicinal part of the plant is the root.

Flower and Fruit: The female flowers are in short-pedicled clusters; the male flowers are in long-pedicled racemes. The flowers are radial and their structures are arranged in fives. The corolla of the female flowers are up to 10 mm wide. The sepals are half as a long as the petals. The ovary is inferior and trichambered. The corolla of the male flowers is up to 20 mm wide, yellowish and green-veined; the 5 stamens are fused in groups (2+2+1). The fruit is a 1 to 2 seeded, globose berry, 6 to 10 mm thick. They are scarlet when ripe.

Leaves, Stem, and Root: Bryonia cretica is a herbaceous perennial. The stem is dioecious and 2 to 4 m long. It climbs with the aid of simple tendrils. The leaves are alternate, short petiolate, broad-cordate to palmate-5-lobed. The lobes are entire or have blunt teeth. Both surfaces of the leaf are covered in short bristly hairs. Each leaf is positioned opposite a tendril. The root is tuberous, up to 2.5 kg, light yellow, and white and slimy inside.

Habitat: Central and southern Europe

Production: Red Bryony root is the dried root of *Bryonia cretica*. The plant is cultivated.

ACTIONS AND PHARMACOLOGY

COMPOUNDS

Cucurbitacins: cucurbitacins B, D, E, I, J, K, L and S (present in the fresh root as aglycones of the glycosides, presumably the result of decomposition after dehydration), small quantities of intact glycosides, for example bryoamarid, bryoside, bryodiosides A to C

Triterpenes: triterpene acids, including bryonolic acid, bryocoumaric acid, 3alpha-hydroxymultiflora-8-ene-29alpha-acid

Fatty acids (polyhydroxyderivatives, resembling the eicosanoids): for example 9,12,13-trihydroxy-octadeca-10 (E)-15(Z)-dienic acid

Ribosome-inactivating proteins: bryodine-L and bryodine-R

EFFECTS

The protein bryodine has cytotoxic effect in vitro. The drug is used as a laxative and an emetic. The chief active ingredients are the cucurbitacins, which even in low dosages lead to irritation of the mucous membrane of the gastrointestinal tract with subsequent increase of peristalsis. The drug is severely toxic in higher dosages.

INDICATIONS AND USAGE

Unproven Uses: The drug can be used for respiratory tract and rheumatic conditions, gastrointestinal tract, metabolic disorders, liver disease, and acute and chronic infectious conditions.

Homeopathic Uses: Bryonia cretica is used for acute and chronic rheumatism, peritonitis, and inflammation of the respiratory organs and the pleura.

PRECAUTIONS AND ADVERSE REACTIONS

No health hazards are known in conjunction with the proper administration of designated homeopathic therapeutic dosages. Side effects connected with the ingestion of the base tincture and D1 include signs of irritation in the gastrointestinal tract. All parts of the plant are strongly toxic, due to the cucurbitacins content, which is irritating to mucous membranes.

OVERDOSAGE

Symptoms of poisoning include vomiting, bloody diarrhea, colic, kidney irritation, anuria, spasms, palsies and aborted pregnancy. Death occurs through asphyxiation. Forty berries are considered lethal for an adult, 15 for a child. 3.5 g of the drug is considered poisonous; one death has been documented following the ingestion of an infusion made from 30 g of the root.

Following gastrointestinal emptying (in case vomiting has not occurred, gastric lavage with burgundy-colored potassium permanganate solution, sodium sulfate) and installation of activated charcoal, the therapy for poisoning consists of treating spasms with diazepam (IV), electrolyte substitution and treating possible cases of acidosis with sodium bicarbonate infusions. In the event of shock, plasma volume expanders should be infused. Monitoring of kidney function is imperative. Intubation and oxygen respiration may also be necessary.

DOSAGE

Mode of Administration: Liquid and solid preparations for internal use; semi-solid preparations for external use.

Preparation:

Wine – 40 g drug to 1 L white wine, leave to draw for 1 day.

Tincture – 10 g to 90 g ethyl alcohol (60%), leave to draw for 8 days.

Honey decoction – 20 g drug to 250 g honey and 350 g wine vinegar, simmer for 30 minutes at a low temperature, strain when cool and store in a well-sealed bottle.

Ointment – Mix 30 g cut drug with the same amount of Vaseline or wax.

Daily Dosage:

Powder – 0.3 to 0.5 g as a laxative and emetic.

Decoction – 0.5 g to 1 g per cup.

Wine – 1 to 2 dessertspoons daily.

Tincture – 1 to 10 drops per day; maximum 20 drops.

Homeopathic Dosage: 5 to 10 drops, 1 tablet, 5 to 10 globules, 1 to 3 times daily or 1 mL injection solution sc. twice weekly; ointment 1 to 2 times daily; mother tincture D1 diluted to be taken with liquid (HAB1)

Storage: Should be sealed tightly.

LITERATURE

Hänsel R, Keller K, Rimpler H, Schneider G (Ed), Hagers Handbuch der Pharmazeutischen Praxis, 5. Aufl., Bde 4 - 6 (Drogen), Springer Verlag Berlin, Heidelberg, New York, 1992-1994.

Red Clover

Trifolium pratense

DESCRIPTION

Medicinal Parts: The medicinal parts are the dried and the fresh flower heads.

Flower and Fruit: One to 4 globular, ovate flower heads form on the tip of the stem. The calyx is tubular-campanulate. The petals are light carmine to fleshy red, occasionally yellowish-white or pure white. The fruit is a pod, which is ovate, single-seeded and thin-skinned. The seed is oblong-ovate, yellow to brownish or violet.

Leaves, Stem, and Root: The plant is a perennial herb, 15 to 40 cm high with a bushy rhizome and a basal leaf rosette. An erect, angular stem grows from the rhizome. The rhizome is covered in alternate, trifoliate, elliptical or ovate leaves, which have a characteristic arrow-shaped white spot on the upper surface. The leaflets are short-petioled, almost entire-margined, appressed, softly pubescent on both surfaces or only on the upper surface.

Habitat: The plant is indigenous to Europe, central Asia, northern Africa, and is naturalized in many other parts of the world.

Production: Red Clover flowers are the flowers of *Trifolium pratense*. The dried flower buds are used to produce the drug.

Other Names: Purple Clover, Trefoil, Wild Clover

ACTIONS AND PHARMACOLOGY

COMPOUNDS

Volatile oil: including among others, benzyl alcohol, 2-phenyl ethanol, their formates and acetates, methyl salicylate, methyl anthranilate (likely only in the fresh blossoms)

Isoflavonoids: including among others, biochanin A

Coumarin derivatives

Cyanogenic glycosides: presumably lotaustralin, linamarin

EFFECTS

Arterial compliance, an important cardiovascular risk factor, was significantly improved in one small study of women given isoflavones from Red Clover extract. Isoflavones may have a protective effect on lumbar spine in women. Chemoprotective and estrogenic effects of Red Clover have only been studied in vitro and in animals.

Cardioprotective Effects: Isoflavones derived from Red Clover significantly improved arterial compliance in 17 menopausal women. Biological variables that affect arterial compliance, including plasma lipoprotein levels, mean body mass index, and arterial pressures remained unchanged. An isoflavone-induced positive effect on endothelium related arterial relaxation is postulated (Nestel et al, 1999).

Chemoprotective Effects: Biochanin A, a major active compound isolated from Red Clover extract, inhibited carcinogen benzo(a)pyrene activation in cell cultures. Chemoprotective action is attributed to the ability of biochanin A to inhibit the metabolism of the carcinogen and the extent of its binding to DNA (Cassady et al, 1988).

Estrogenic Effects: Red Clover extract stimulated cell proliferation of estrogen receptor-positive breast cancer cells in vitro. Red Clover extract acts as an estrogen agonist by binding to intracellular estradiol receptors. Red Clover was defined as an antiprogestin, due to the extract's inhibition of progesterone induction of alkaline phosphatase, an end product of progestin activity, in vitro (Zava et al, 1998). Red Clover increased uterine weight and teat circumference and decreased cervical mucous viscoelasticity in ewes (Adams, 1995; Nwannenna et al, 1995). An examination of the chemical and biological profile of a (preformulated) clinical phase II Red Clover extract identified both major and minor chemical and active estrogenic components as examined *in vitro*. In all, 22 compounds were identified and 20 quantitatively measured, offering a marked improvement in the characterization of Red Clover supplements—as only four isoflavone components currently are fully described elsewhere (daidzein, genistein, formononetin, and biochanin A) (Booth, 2006).

CLINICAL TRIALS

Bone Mineral Density

The loss of bone mineral density and lumbar spine bone mineral content was significantly decreased in women following a 12-month treatment with an isoflavone supplement in a randomized, double-blind, placebo-controlled trial. Women (n=177, 49 to 65 years) received a Red Clover-derived isoflavone tablet (26 mg biochanin A, 16 mg formononetin, 1 mg genistein, and 0.5 mg daidzein) (n=86) or placebo (n=91) daily for 12 months. In women taking isoflavone, loss of lumbar spine mineral content and bone mineral density was lower (p=0.04 and p=0.03, respectively) compared to placebo. Bone formation markers were significantly increased (p=0.04 and p=0.01 for bone-specific alkaline phosphatase and N-propeptide of collagen type I, respectively) in the treatment group compared to placebo in postmenopausal subjects. Markers and bone turnover were not significantly different between treatment groups (Atkinson et al, 2004).

Cardioprotection

Systemic arterial compliance, a relationship between volumetric blood flow into the aorta and carotid artery pressure as measured by ultrasound, increased by 23% compared with placebo in 13 menopausal women after 5 weeks of oral treatment with a Red Clover proprietary product. Each standardized tablet contained 40 milligrams (mg) total isoflavones, including genistein, daidzein, biochanin and formononetin. The women took two placebo tablets for 5 weeks, followed by one placebo and one 40 mg tablet for 5 weeks, and finally two 40 mg tablets for 5 weeks. Arterial compliance was slightly less improved with the 40 mg dose. The study was double blinded but only three of the five women randomized to placebo completed the trial (Nestel et al, 1999).

Cholesterol

Lipid levels hardly changed in 255 postmenopausal women receiving two dietary supplements derived from red clover (Promensil and Rimostil), when taking them for 12 weeks in a randomized, double-blind, placebo-controlled trial. Only a small decrease could be found for triglycerides (Schult et al, 2004).

Results of a randomized, placebo-controlled trial support the possibility that individual isoflavones affect low-density lipoprotein cholesterol (LDL-C) differently, and could therefore explain the previous inability to show cholesterol-lowering actions with mixed isoflavones in studies involving primarily females. In this trial, plasma lipids were measured in 46 middle-aged men and 34 postmenopausal women. Placebo and two mixtures of Red Clover isoflavones (40 mg/day) enriched in either biochanin (n=40) or formononetin (n=40) were given in blinded fashion for 6 weeks each in a crossover design within two parallel groups. While isolated isoflavones from Red Clover enriched in biochanin (a genistein precursor) significantly lowered LDL-C, it only did so in men. The formononetin-enriched isoflavone (daidzein precursor) was ineffective in lowering LDL-C in both men and women, however (Nestel 2004).

Mammographic Breast Density

A clinical study was designed to determine the effects of a Red Clover-derived isoflavone supplement taken daily for 1 year on mammographic breast density. A total of 205 women with Wolfe P2 or DY mammographic breast patterns were randomly assigned to receive either a Red Clover-derived isoflavone tablet or placebo. Mammographic breast density decreased in both groups but the difference between treatment groups was not statistically significant. Furthermore, there were no effects on estradiol, gonadotrophins, lymphocyte tyrosine kinase activity, or menopausal symptoms (Atkinson et al, 2004).

Menopause

A sweeping systematic review and meta-analysis of randomized, controlled trials including one or more non-hormonal therapies for menopausal hot flushes was conducted. A total of 43 trials from the search of MEDLINE and the Cochrane Controlled Clinical Trials Register Database between 1966 and October 2005, as well as other databases, met inclusion criteria such as English language, double-blind, randomized, and placebo-controlled. There were 10 trials of clonidine, 6 trials of other prescribed medications, and 17 of of isoflavone extracts—six trials of which used Red Clover isoflavone extracts (genistein, daidzein, formononetin, biochanin). A meta-analysis of these Red Clover trials indicated no efficacy for the herb in reducing frequency or other aspects of hot flushes, and only mixed results for soy isoflavones. There was, however, some supportive evidence for efficacy of SSRIs or SNRIs, clonidine, and gabapentin in reducing the frequency and severity of hot flashes (Nelsson, 2006).

In contrast, a systematic literature search of randomized, controlled trials studies to assess the evidence for oral supplements containing Red Clover isoflavones in reducing the frequency of hot flushes in menopausal women identified 17 potentially relevant clinical trials, a meta-analysis of which revealed a marginally significant effect of the extract for hot flush reduction. With Red Clover supplementation over the course of 12 to 16 weeks, the average of 5 to 9 hot flushes daily were reduced by approximately 1 flush daily. Whether the magnitude of this reduction is clinically important remains unclear, the authors conclude. The three trials that included adverse event data indicated no apparent evidence thereof with short-term use (Coon 2006).

In a double-blind, placebo-controlled study, 60 postmenopausal women were randomly assigned to receive either a commercially available red clover isoflavone supplement (80 mg/day) or placebo for 90 days to evaluate the effect of isoflavones contained in Red Clover extracts on menopausal symptoms, lipids, and vaginal cytology. Red Clover isoflavones significantly decreased the rate of menopausal symptoms and had a positive effect on vaginal cytology as expressed by improvement in karyopyknotic, cornification, and basal cell maturation indices. Mean total cholesterol, LDL cholesterol, and triglyceride level also decreased, but only the latter was significantly lower compared to placebo (Hidalgo et al, 2005).

To evaluate the effects of a nonprescription Red Clover extract (MF11 RCE) on selected sex hormones and endometrium in postmenopausal women, 109 women age 40 years and older were randomly assigned to one of two groups receiving either two capsules of Red Clover extract (80 mg isoflavone) per day for a 90-day period or placebo. Combined evaluation demonstrated that supplementation with MF11 RCE, in contrast to placebo, significantly increased plasma testosterone levels and decreased endometrial thickness (Imhof et al, 2006).

Hot flushes were significantly decreased by 44% ($p<0.01$) by a standardized extract of Red Clover in postmenopausal women in a randomized, double-blind, placebo-controlled trial. Women (n=30, 49 to 65 years) experiencing more than 5 hot flashes daily and amenorrheic for more than 12 months were enrolled in the trial. Subjects were asked not to eat legumes and to avoid isoflavone supplements. All subjects received placebo tablets for 4 weeks during the single-blind run-in period. Subjects were then randomized to receive either 2 tablets of a standardized extract of Red Clover isoflavones (Promensil®, 40 mg/tablet) (n=16) or 2 placebo tablets to be taken every morning for 12 weeks. Menopausal symptoms, as scored by the Greene Climacteric Scale (scoring list of 21 symptoms) were slightly decreased in the active group; however, the level of difference between groups was not significant (van de Weijer & Barentsen, 2002).

Postmenopausal Cognitive Function

A randomized, placebo-controlled trial of the effects of dietary supplementation with an extract from Red Clover did not appear to have major short-term effects on cognitive function in the 30 postmenopausal women studied. The participants, all 60 years of age or older, took 2 tablets of an extract of aglycone isoflavones from Red Clover (each contained formononetin 25 mg, biochanin 2.5 mg, and less than 1 mg daidzein and genistein). Tests of cognitive function after 6 months of isoflavone or placebo therapy failed to show significant change from baseline (Howes, 2004).

INDICATIONS AND USAGE

Unproven Uses: Internally, Red Clover is used for coughs and respiratory conditions, particularly whooping cough. Externally, it is used in the treatment of chronic skin conditions such as psoriasis and eczema. Isoflavone extracts of Red Clover are often used to treat menopausal symptoms, such as hot flashes.

CONTRAINDICATIONS

Not to be used in patients with estrogen receptor-positive neoplasias.

Pregnancy: Not to be used during pregnancy.

Breastfeeding: Not to be used while breastfeeding

PRECAUTIONS AND ADVERSE REACTIONS

Use of Red Clover should be avoided in patients taking hormonal medications, as competition for the same hormonal receptor sites may interfere with the effect of the medication and lead to unpredictable results. An isolated case of blistering and inflammation of the eyes, mouth, and penis occurred in a patient within a few days of oral ingestion of an herbal formula containing Red Clover (Monk, 1986). Excessive intake should be avoided due to the estrogenic constituents.

Fertility: Red Clover-fed animals show decreased cervical mucus viscoelasticity, a condition that renders their cervix less accessible to spermatozoa. Reduced fertility may thus result from the excessive use of Red Clover (Adams, 1995; Kallela et al, 1984).

DRUG INTERACTIONS

MAJOR RISK

Tamoxifen: Concurrent use may result in decreased tamoxifen effectiveness. *Clinical management:* Avoid concomitant use.

MODERATE RISK

Anticoagulants, Thrombolytic Agents, and Low Molecular Weight Heparins: Possible increased risk of bleeding. *Clinical Management:* Avoid concomitant use of Red Clover with anticoagulants, thrombolytic agents, and low molecular weight heparins. If Red Clover and any one of these medications are taken together, monitor for signs and symptoms of excessive bleeding.

Contraceptives, Combination: Possible altered contraceptive effectiveness or increased side effects. *Clinical Management:* Caution is advised if Red Clover is taken with hormonal contraceptives. Monitor the patient for symptoms of estrogen excess or loss of efficacy.

Estrogens: See Contraceptives, above.

Progesterone: Possible decreased effectiveness of progesterone. *Clinical Management:* Caution is advised if Red Clover is taken with progesterone. Monitor the patient for symptoms of loss of efficacy.

DOSAGE

Mode of Administration: The drug is used internally and externally as a liquid extract and in medicinal preparations.

Preparation: Liquid extract 1:1 can be prepared in 25% ethanol.

Daily Dosage: The daily dosage is 4 g of drug, taken as an infusion, up to 3 times a day. Alternately, 1.5 to 3 mL of the liquid extract can be taken 3 times daily.

LITERATURE

Adams NR. Organizational and activational effects of phytoestrogens on the reproductive tract of the ewe. *PSEBM*; 208:81-87, 1995.

Atkinson C, Compston J, Day N et al., The effects of phytoestrogen isoflavones on bone density in women: a double-blind, randomized, placebo-controlled trial. *Am J Clin Nutr*; 79(2):326-333, 2004.

Atkinson C, Warren RM, Sala E, et al. Red clover-derived isoflavones and mammographic breast density: double-blind, randomized, placebo-controlled trial. *Breast Cancer Res*; 6(3): R170-179. 2004.

Booth NL, et al. The Chemical and Biologic Profile of a Red Clover (Trifolium pretense L.) Phase II Clinical Extract. *J Alt Comp Med* 12(2):133-139, 2006.

Cassady JM, Zennie TM, Chae Y-H et al., Use of a mammalian cell culture benzo(a)pyrene metabolism assay for the detection of potential anticarcinogens from natural products: inhibition of metabolism by biochanin A, an isoflavone from Trifolium pratense L. In: *Cancer Res*; 48(22):6257-6261, 1988.

Coon JT, Pittler MS, Ernst E. *Trifolium pretense* isoflavones in the treatment of menopausal hot flushes: A systematic review and meta-analysis. *Phytomedicine.* 14:153-159, 2007.

Dewick P. *Phytochemistry* 16:93, 1977.

Guggolz J et al., *Agric Food Chem* 9(4):331, 1961.

Hidalgo LA, Chedraui PA, Morocho N, et al. The effect of red clover isoflavones on menopausal symptoms, lipids and vaginal cytology in menopausal women: a randomized, double-blind, placebo-controlled study. *Gynecol Endocrinol*; 21(5): 257-264. 2005.

Howes JB, et al. The effects of dietary supplementation with isoflavones from red clover on cognitive function in postmenopausal women. *CLIMACTERIC* 7:70-77. 2004.

Imhof M, Gocan A, Reithmayr F, et al. Effects of a red clover extract (MF11RCE) on endometrium and sex hormones in postmenopausal women. *Maturitas*; 55(1): 76-81. 2006.

Kallela K, Heinonen K & Saloniemi H. Plant oestrogens; the cause of decreased fertility in cows: a case report. In: *Nord Vet Med;* 36(3-4):124-129, 1984.

Kattaev NS et al., *Khim Prir Soed* 6:806, 1972.

Monk B. Severe cutaneous reactions to alternative remedies. In: *BMJ*; 293(6548):665-666, 1986.

Nelson HD, Vesco KK, Haney E, et al. Nonhormonal Therapies for Menopausal Hot Flashes, Systematic Review and Meta-analysis. *JAMA* 295(17):2057-2071, 2006.

Nestel P, Cehun M, Chronopoulos A, et al. A biochanin-enriched isoflavone from red clover lowers LDL cholesterol in men. *Eur J Clin Nutr*; 58:403-408, 2004.

Nestel PJ, Pomeroy S, Kay S et al., Isoflavones from Red Clover improves systemic arterial compliance but not plasma lipids in menopausal women. In: *J Clin Endocrinol Metab*; 84(3):895-898, 1999.

Nwannenna AI, Lundh TJ-O, Madej A et al., Clinical changes in ovariectomized ewes exposed to phytoestrogens and 17-estradiol implants. *PSEBM*; 208:92-97, 1995.

Sachse J. *J Chrom* 96(1):123, 1974.

Schult TM, Ensrud KE, Blackwell T, et al. Effect of isoflavones on lipids and bone turnover markers in menopausal women. *Maturitas*; 48(3): 209-218. 2004.

van de Weijer P & Barentsen R. Isoflavones from Red Clover (Promensil® significantly reduce menopausal hot flush symptoms compared with placebo. *Maturitas*; 42(3):187-193, 2002.

Yoshihara T et al., *Agric Biol Chem* 41(9):1679, 1977.

Zava DT, Dollbaum CM & Blen M. Estrogen and progestin bioactivity of foods, herbs, and spices. In: *PSEBM*; 217(3):369-378, 1998.

Red Currant

Ribes rubrum

DESCRIPTION

Medicinal Parts: The medicinal parts are the fruit and leaves.

Flower and Fruit: The flowers are in hanging, many-blossomed racemes. The green flowers are inconspicuous and their structures are in fives. The sepals and petals are fused with the hollowed receptacle. The calyx tips are wide obovate and longer than the petals. The corolla tube is flat with a pentagonal ring swelling. There are 2 carpels fused with the corolla tube to an inferior, single-chambered ovary. The ovary has a concave tip and a disc ring. The fruit is multiseeded red berry. The cultivated forms are pink or white.

Leaves, Stem and Root: Ribes rubrum grows as a shrub, reaching up to 2 m high. The leaves are alternate, over 10 cm wide with a petiole half as long as the lamina, which have 3 to 5 lobes, which are blunt to acute, double crenate, and cordate at the base with an acute indentation.

Habitat: The plant is indigenous to Western Europe.

Production: Red Currants are the fresh ripe berries of *Ribes rubrum*.

ACTIONS AND PHARMACOLOGY

COMPOUNDS

Fruit acids: chief fruit acid is citric acid; other acids include malic acid, isocitric acid and tartartic acid

Monosaccharides/polysaccharides (7%): D-glucose, D-fructose

Pectins (15%)

Fatty oil (in the seeds 20%) with gamma-linolenic acid (6%)

Ascorbic acid (vitamin C, 0.005 to 0.015%)

Caffeic acid derivatives: including caffeoyl glucose, p-cumaric acid-O-glucoside

EFFECTS

Red Currant is a source of vitamin C and exhibits in vitro radical scavenger qualities. The fruit and juice are considered cooling and antiscorbutic and have often been used as a febrifuge. The jelly prepared from the berries has an antiseptic effect and was often used to treat burns to prevent the formation of blisters. The leaves are said to have emmenagogic properties.

INDICATIONS AND USAGE

Unproven Uses: Red currant has been used in folk medicine to treat febrile conditions.

PRECAUTIONS AND CONTRAINDICATIONS

No health hazards are known in conjunction with the proper administration of designated therapeutic dosages.

DOSAGE

No data are available in the literature.

LITERATURE

Hänsel R, Keller K, Rimpler H, Schneider G (Ed), Hagers Handbuch der Pharmazeutischen Praxis, 5. Aufl., Bde 4 - 6 (Drogen), Springer Verlag Berlin, Heidelberg, New York, 1992-1994.

Red Maple

Acer rubrum

DESCRIPTION

Medicinal Parts: The medicinal part is the bark.

Flower and Fruit: The flowers are red and aromatic, forming round bunches. The ovary is formed from 2 simple carpels pressed together at the sides, which are also present in the male flowers in rudimentary form. Each section contains 2 ovules. The fruit is a schizocarp with 2 one-sided or many-sided, often heavily veined wings. There is usually only one seed in each section.

Leaves, Stem, and Root: The Red Maple tree grows to a height of up to 36 m. The leaves are crossed-opposite, petiolate and partially trilobed.

Habitat: Canada and the U.S., introduced into England and Europe around 1650.

Production: Red Acorn bark is the trunk bark of *Acer rubrum*.

Other Names: Bird's Eye Maple, Sugar Maple, Swamp Maple

ACTIONS AND PHARMACOLOGY

COMPOUNDS

Tannins

Triterpenoid saponins

Allantoins

EFFECTS

Red maple has an astringent effect.

INDICATIONS AND USAGE

Unproven Uses: Red Maple is used for eye conditions (folk medicine of the North American Indians).

This product should not be used otherwise.

PRECAUTIONS AND ADVERSE REACTIONS

No health hazards or side effects are known in conjunction with the proper administration of designated therapeutic dosages.

DOSAGE

Mode of Administration: Comminuted drug.

LITERATURE

McConnico RS, Brownie CF. The use of ascorbic acid in the treatment of 2 cases of red maple (Acer rubrum)-poisoned horses. *Cornell Vet,* 82:293-300, Jul 1992

Weber M, Miller RE. Presumptive red maple (*Acer rubrum*) toxicosis in Grevy's zebra (Equus grevyi). J Zoo Wildl Med, 28:105-8, Mar 1997

Red Sandalwood

Pterocarpus santalinus

DESCRIPTION

Medicinal Parts: The medicinal part is the wood.

Flower and Fruit: The tree bears spikes of yellow flowers.

Leaves, Stem and Root: The plant is a 6 to 8 m high tree with red bark.

Habitat: The plant grows in South India, Sri Lanka and the Philippines.

Production: Red Sandalwood consists of the heartwood of the trunk of Pterocarpus santalinus separated from the sapwood, in some regions also obtained from other Pterocarpus species. It is collected in uncultivated regions.

Other Names: Real Sandalwood, Rubywood, Red Saunders, Sanderswood Red, Sappan

ACTIONS AND PHARMACOLOGY

COMPOUNDS

Benzxanthenone derivatives (red pigments): chief components santalins A and B (red), additionally santalin AC and santalin Y (yellow)

Isoflavonoids: santal, pterocarpine, and homopterocarpine

Stilbene derivatives: pterostilbene

Volatile oil (traces): chief components cedrol (cedar camphor, up to 50%), including as well pterocarpol, isopterocarpol, eudesmol

EFFECTS

In animal experiments, extracts of the wood are hypoglycemic. Insecticidal and antidiabetic effects are attributed to the pterostilbene constituent. In addition CNS-suppressive, spasmolytic and antiexudative effects have been described, although detailed information is unavailable.

INDICATIONS AND USAGE

Indian Medicine: Red Sandalwood is used for headaches, toothaches, vomiting, black vomit, diarrhea, fever and conditions of the eye. It is also used to treat stomach ulcers, gallbladder complaints, diabetes, and snakebite poisoning.

PRECAUTIONS AND ADVERSE REACTIONS

No health hazards or side effects are known in conjunction with the proper administration of designated therapeutic dosages.

DOSAGE

Mode of Administration: Red Sandalwood is available as whole, crude and powdered drug forms for internal and external use.

Preparation: To prepare a tincture, 200 parts coarsely powdered drug are mixed with 1,000 parts ethanol (EB6).

Daily Dosage: As a tincture, 5 g.

Storage: Red Sandalwood should be tightly sealed, powdered and protected from light.

LITERATURE

Atta-Ur-Rahman Zaman K. Medicinal Plants with Hypoglycemic Activity. *J Ethnopharmacol.* 26; 1-55. 1989

Nagaraju N, Rao KN. A Survey of Plant Crude Drugs of Rayalaseema, Andrha Pradesh, India. *J Ethnopharmacol.* 29; 137-158. 1990

Sandra A, Shenoi SD, Srinivas CR. Allergic contact dermatitis from red sandalwood (*Pterocarpus santalinus*). *Contact Dermatitis* 34; 69. 1996

Singh S et al., *Fitoterapia* 63:555. 1992.

Singh S et al., *Fitoterapia* 64:84. 1993.

Red-Rooted Sage (Dan-Shen)

Salvia miltiorrhiza

DESCRIPTION

Medicinal Parts: The medicinal parts of the plant are the dried rhizome and root.

Flower and Fruit: The inflorescences are false whorls with 6 to 8 flowers arranged very close together in glandularly haired racemes with a few lanceolate bracts. The calyx is campanulate, dark purple, and glandularly pubescent. The upper lip is simple, the lower lip is longer than the upper lip and thorny-double-dentate with an inner dense ring of white hairs. The petals are violet and glandularly pubescent on the outside. The corolla tube is approximately 1.9 cm long; the upper lip slightly enlarged and turned out. There are 2 long and 2 short stamens and a superior, 2-carpeled, 4-chambered ovary. The fruit breaks up into 4, 1-seeded mericarps.

Leaves, Stem, and Root: Salvia miltiorrhiza is a herbaceous perennial growing upright to a height of up to 80 cm. The lower leaves are cordate to ovate. The upper leaves are trifoliolate, crenate-dentate, pubescent above and along the ribs of the lower surface. The rhizome is thick and short.

Habitat: The plant is found in China and Japan.

Production: Red sage root is the dried rhizome and root of *Salvia miltiorrhiza.* The plant is dug up in spring or autumn, cleaned, cut and dried.

Not to be Confused With: Mistaken identity can occur with *Salvia przewalskii* or *Salvia trijuga.*

Other Names: Dan-Shen, Red Ginseng, Red-Rooted Salvia

ACTIONS AND PHARMACOLOGY

COMPOUNDS

Diterpenes: the so-called tanshinones, including cryptotanshinone, isocryptotanshinone, isotanshinones I and II, tanshinones I and II, miltiron, ferruginol, salviol

Caffeic acid derivatives: including rosmarinic acid, lithospermic acid ethyl ester, salvianolic acids A to E

EFFECTS

Patients with coronary heart disease experienced an improvement in various hemodynamic parameters. At the same time, a significant increase in coronary blood flow due to a reduction of vascular resistance was demonstrated. The drug is antithrombotic, antihypertonic, antimicrobial, antipyretic/anti-inflammatory, and hepatoprotective in its effect; it is also said to possess sedative characteristics.

INDICATIONS AND USAGE

Chinese Medicine: Preparations of the root are used for metrorrhagia, pain following menstruation, amenorrhea, postpartum bleeding and pain, angina pectoris, furuncles, carbuncles, painful swellings, swelling of the liver and spleen, and joint pain. Efficacy for these indications has not yet been proved.

PRECAUTIONS AND ADVERSE REACTIONS

No health hazards are known in conjunction with the proper administration of designated therapeutic dosages.

DOSAGE

Mode of Administration: Whole and cut drug and their preparations are for internal use.

Preparation: Jiudanshen - Slices of the root, to which wine has been added in accordance with the Jiuzhi method, are roasted until dry.

Daily Dosage: The daily dosage of the drug is 9 to 15 g. The daily dosage of tea is an amount prepared from 3 to 15 g of the drug.

Storage: The drug should be stored in a dry place.

LITERATURE

Chang HM, Chui KY, Tan FW, Yang Y, Zhong ZP, Lee CM, Sham HL, Wong HN, Structure-activity relationship of miltirone, an active central benzodiazepine receptor ligand isolated from *Salvia miltiorrhiza Bunge* (Danshen). *J Med Chem,* 56:1675-92, May. 1991

Chen KY, Wen SF, Zhi ZJ, Shao JS, Preliminary observation of 131Cs distribution in experimental acute myocardial infarction and coronary insufficiency treated with root of *Salvia miltiorrhiza*, flower of *Chrysanthemum morifolium* and *Chrysanthemum indicum. J Tradit Chin Med,* 56:265-70, 1983.

Chen WZ, Pharmacology of *Salvia miltiorrhiza Yao Hsueh Hsueh Pao*, 56:876-80, Nov. 1984

Ding Y, Soma S, Takano-Yamamoto T, Matsumoto S, Sakuda M, Effects of *Salvia miltiorrhiza bunge* (SMB) on MC3T3-E1 cells. *J Osaka Univ Dent Sch*, 26:21-7, Dec. 1995

Fu X, Tian H, Sheng Z, Wang D, Multiple organ injuries after abdominal high energy wounding in animals and the protective effect of antioxidants. *Chin Med Sci J,* 56:86-91, Jun. 1992

Hansel R, Keller K, Rimpler H, Schneider G (Ed), Hagers Handbuch der Pharmazeutischen Praxis, 5. Aufl., Bde 4 - 6 (Drogen), Springer Verlag Berlin, Heidelberg, New York, 1992-1994.

Hu L, Yu T, Jia Z, Experimental study of the protective effects of astragalus and *Salvia miltiorrhiza bunge* on glycerol induced acute renal failure in rabbits. *Chung Hua Wai Ko Tsa Chih,* 26:311-4, May. 1996

Huang YS, Zhang JT, Antioxidative effect of three water-soluble components isolated from *Salvia miltiorrhiza* in vitro. *Yao Hsueh Hsueh Pao,* 18:96-100, 1992.

Li W, Zhou CH, Lu QL, Effects of Chinese materia medica in activating blood and stimulating menstrual flow on the endocrine function of ovary-uterus and its mechanisms. *Chung Kuo Chung Hsi I Chieh Ho Tsa Chih,* 56:165-8, 134, Mar. 1992

Liu GT, Zhang TM, Wang BE, Wang YW, Prediction and prevention of hypertension syndrome of pregnancy. *Chung Hsi I Chieh Ho Tsa Chih,* 43:530-2, 516, Jan 22. 1992

Liu GT, Zhang TM, Wang BE, Wang YW, Prognostic factors and treatment of severe acute pancreatitis. *Chung Hua Nei Ko Tsa Chih,* 43:82-5, 125, Feb. 1991

Liu GT, Zhang TM, Wang BE, Wang YW, Protective action of seven natural phenolic compounds against peroxidative damage to biomembranes. *Biochem Pharmacol,* 43:147-52, Jan 22. 1992

Murakami S, Kijima H, Isobe Y, Muramatsu M, Aihara H, Otomo S, Li LN, Ai CB, Effect of salvianolic acid A, a depside from roots of *Salvia miltiorrhiza*, on gastric H+,K(+)-ATPase. Planta Med, 56:360-3, Aug. 1990

Qi XG, Protective mechanism of *Salvia miltiorrhiza* and *Paeonia lactiflora* for experimental liver damage. *Chung Hsi I Chieh Ho Tsa Chih,* 18:102-4, 69, Feb. 1991

Wang L, Huang X, Ding Z, Chen H, Peng R, Yuan G, Zhou D, The effects of *Salvia miltiorrhiza* and polysaccharide sulphate on the adhesion of erythrocytes of the patients with cerebral thrombosis to cultured endothelial cells. *Hua Hsi I Ko Ta Hsueh Hsueh Pao,* 26:381-5, Dec. 1995

Wu YJ, Hong CY, Lin SJ, Wu P, Shiao MS, Effect of *Salvia miltiorrhiza* on serum lipid peroxide, superoxide dismutase of the patients with coronary heart disease. *Chung Kuo Chung Hsi I Chieh Ho Tsa Chih,* 18:287-8, May. 1996

Wu YJ, Hong CY, Lin SJ, Wu P, Shiao MS, Experimental study of *Salvia miltiorrhiza* on prevention of restenosis after angioplasty. *Chung Kuo Chung Hsi I Chieh Ho Tsa Chih, 18*:480-2, Aug. 1996

Wu YJ, Hong CY, Lin SJ, Wu P, Shiao MS, In vitro cytotoxicity of tanshinones from *Salvia miltiorrhiza. Planta Med,* 18:339-42, Aug. 1997

Wu YJ, Hong CY, Lin SJ, Wu P, Shiao MS, Increase of vitamin E content in LDL and reduction of atherosclerosis in cholesterol-fed rabbits by a water-soluble antioxidant-rich fraction of *Salvia miltiorrhiza. Arterioscler Thromb Vasc Biol,* 18:481-6, Mar. 1998

Xie M, Jin ZY, Ye GH, Clinical research of compound salviae miltiorrhizae injection for severe pancreatitis. *Chung Kuo Chung Hsi I Chieh Ho Tsa Chih,* 43:269-70, May. 1995

Zhang FC, Zheng LJ, Effects of different administration of Salvia miltiorrhiza and heparin on antithrombin IIIAg, antithrombin III: A and alpha 2-macroglobulin in patients with cor pulmonale. *Chung Hsi I Chieh Ho Tsa Chih,* 18:589-91, 579, Oct. 1991

Zhao BL, Jiang W, Zhao Y, Hou JW, Xin WJ, Scavenging effects of Salvia miltiorrhiza on free radicals and its protection for myocardial mitochondrial membranes from ischemia-reperfusion injury. *Biochem Mol Biol Int,* 38:1171-82, May. 1996

Red-Spur Valerian

Centranthus ruber

DESCRIPTION

Medicinal Parts: The medicinal part is the root of the plant.

Flower and Fruit: The numerous flowers are in dense cymes, red, pink, or (seldom) white. The corolla is tubular and spurred at the base. Each flower contains 1 stamen. The fruit is small and dry. The margin of the surrounding calyx forms a pinnatifid rosette or a papus.

Leaves, Stem, and Root: The plant grows from about 30 to 80 cm high. The rhizome is perennial and very branched. The stems are tough, bushy at the base, hollow, and smooth. The leaves are 5 to 10 cm long in opposite pairs, somewhat fleshy and entire-margined.

Habitat: The plant is probably indigenous to the Mediterranean region, although it is found in Europe.

Other Names: Bovisand Soldier, Bouncing Bess, Delicate Bess, Drunken Sailor, Pretty Betsy

ACTIONS AND PHARMACOLOGY

COMPOUNDS

Iridoids (iridoid epoxy compounds, 1-3%): valepotriates, including valtrate, acevaltrate, didrovaltrate

EFFECTS

The drug has sedative and equilibratory effects.

INDICATIONS AND USAGE

Unproven Uses: The drug is not in current use. It was previously used as a sedative.

PRECAUTIONS AND ADVERSE REACTIONS

No health hazards or side effects are known in conjunction with the proper administration of designated therapeutic dosages.

DOSAGE

No information is available.

LITERATURE

Handjieva N et al., *PM* 34:203. 1978.

Hegnauer R: Chemotaxonomie der Pflanzen, Bde 1-11, Birkhäuser Verlag Basel, Boston, Berlin 1962-1997.

Kern W, List PH, Hörhammer L (Hrsg.), Hagers Handbuch der Pharmazeutischen Praxis, 4. Aufl., Bde 1-8, Springer Verlag Berlin, Heidelberg, New York, 1969.

Schneider G, Valepotriat-Artefakte aus *Centrantus ruber*. In: *Arch Pharmaz* 318(6):515- 519. 1985.

Reed Herb

Phragmites communis

DESCRIPTION

Medicinal Parts: The medicinal parts are the stem and the rhizome.

Flower and Fruit: The grassy flowers appear in long panicles of up to 30 cm with a thick crown of hair.

Leaves, Stem, and Root: The plant is a sturdy grass with a long, creeping rhizome. It grows up to 3 m and has gray-green leaves.

Habitat: Reed Herb is common worldwide.

Production: Reed Herb and rhizome are the stem (base) and rhizome of *Phragmites communis*.

Other Names: Common Reed

ACTIONS AND PHARMACOLOGY

COMPOUNDS

Flavonoids: including tricine, luteolin, chrysoeriol, rutin, isoquercitrin

Vitamin A (5 mg/100 gm in the fresh foliage)

Ascorbic acid (vitamin C, 100 mg/100 gm in the fresh foliage)

B vitamins

Sugar: in particular saccharose, inverted sugar (relatively high content in the rhizome)

Triterpenes: including beta-amyrin, taraxerol, taraxerone

EFFECTS

The plant has diuretic and diaphoretic effects.

INDICATIONS AND USAGE

Unproven Uses: Reed Herb is used as a diuretic and diaphoretic to treat digestive disorders. The juice is used to soothe insect bites.

Chinese Medicine: Reed Herb is used for diabetes, leukemia, and breast cancer.

PRECAUTIONS AND ADVERSE REACTIONS

No health hazards or side effects are known in conjunction with the proper administration of designated therapeutic dosages.

DOSAGE

Mode of Administration: Preparations are used internally and externally. The fresh and dried forms are used as infusions.

LITERATURE

Hegnauer R, Chemotaxonomie der Pflanzen, Bde 1-11, Birkhäuser Verlag Basel, Boston, Berlin 1962-1997.

Kern W, List PH, Hörhammer L (Hrsg.), Hagers Handbuch der Pharmazeutischen Praxis, 4. Aufl., Bde. 1-8, Springer Verlag Berlin, Heidelberg, New York, 1969.

Tsitsa-Tzardi E, Skaltsa-Diamantidis H, Philianos S, Delitheos A. Chemical and pharmacological study of *Phragmites communis* Trin. *Ann Pharm Fr,* 48:185-91, 1990.

Van Ree R, Driessen MN, Van Leeuwen WA, Stapel SO, Aalberse RC, Variability of crossreactivity of IgE antibodies to group I and V allergens in eight grass pollen species. *Clin Exp Allergy,* 22:611-7, Jun. 1992

Rehmannia (Di-Huang)

Rehmannia glutinosa

DESCRIPTION

Medicinal Parts: The medicinal part of the plant is the root tuber.

Flower and Fruit: The inflorescences are racemes with approximately 10 flowers. The flower structures are in fives; the calyx is approximately 1.5 cm long, 5-tipped and campanulate. The corolla is a tube that broadens higher up, is 3 to 4 cm long, and red-violet. There are 4 stamens and a superior, bichambered ovary. The fruit is a loculicidal capsule.

Leaves, Stem, and Root: This herbaceous perennial grows up to 40 cm high. The leaves are alternate, 3 to 10 cm long, and 1.5 to 4 cm wide. The lamina is obovate to lanceolate and undulating with a crenate margin; the leaves and stem are velvet-pubescent. The roots are partly thickened to tubers.

Habitat: Rehmannia glutinosa is indigenous to China, Japan, and Korea.

Production: Rehmannia glutinosa is harvested in autumn; the root tuber is either cleaned and used as it is (called Shoudihuang or Xiandihuang) or is moistened with steam, cut into slices and dried over a fire until the water is reduced by 80% (Shengdihuang).

ACTIONS AND PHARMACOLOGY

COMPOUNDS

Iridoids: chief component catalpol (0.3 to 0.5%), including ajugol, aucubin, melittoside, rehmaniosides A to D

Monoterpene: rehmapicroside

Ionone glucosides: rehmaionones A and B

Monosaccharides/oligosaccharides: stachyose (10%, based upon the fresh weight), saccharose, raffinose, D-fructose, D-glucose, D-galactose

Steroids: sterols, including beta-sitosterol, campesterol, stigmasterol

EFFECTS

The phenolic glycosides of the drug are antibacterial, immunosuppressive and antihepatotoxic in effect. Verbascoside inhibits the thromboxane synthetase system; its efficacy with rheumatic diseases, among others, is thus plausible.

INDICATIONS AND USAGE

Chinese Medicine: The drug is used in traditional Chinese medicine as a diuretic and for its nourishing and strengthening effect on the liver, kidney and heart. The fresh and dried forms are used differently.

Shoudihuang (fresh root tuber) is used in the liver and kidney meridians for paralysis of the larynx, irregular menstruation, allergic lowered immunity, insomnia, vertigo, tinnitus, impaired hearing, hyperhidrosis, diabetes, and increased frequency of urination.

Shengdihuang (dried root tuber) is used mainly in the heart, kidney and liver meridians for febrile conditions, dry mouth, nosebleeds, internal bleeding, rheumatism, constipation, hepatitis, diabetes, and metrorrhagia.

Efficacy for the indications rheumatism, eczema and viral hepatitis (IV) has been proved in clinical trials with decoctions of the fresh root. Efficacy for the other indications has not yet been proven.

PRECAUTIONS AND ADVERSE REACTIONS

No health hazards are known in conjunction with the proper administration of designated therapeutic dosages.

DOSAGE

Mode of Administration: Whole and powdered drug. Preparations are for internal use.

Preparation: Shoudihuang can be prepared in two ways:

Jiushoudihuang (jiudun method): The drug is simmered in yellow rice wine over a low flame until all of the wine has been absorbed (30 to 50 kg for 100 kg drug). It is then dried in the sun until the outer skin (initially slimy) is dry, and is then cut into 2 to 4 mm thick slices, which are dried.

Zhengshoudihuang (zheng method): Using this method, the drug is steamed until it is smooth and black (80% loss of moisture). It is then cut into 2 to 4 mm thick slices and dried.

Daily Dosage: Decoction - 9 to 15 g drug

Storage: The fresh root is stored in sandy earth, protected from frost. The dried drug is stored dry in areas having good air circulation.

LITERATURE

Graham-Brown R, Rustin M, Atherton D, Perharic-Walton L, Murray V. Toxicity of Chinese herbal remedies. *Lancet* 340; 673-674. 1992

Hänsel R, Keller K, Rimpler H, Schneider G (Ed), Hagers Handbuch der Pharmazeutischen Praxis, 5. Aufl., Bde 4 - 6 (Drogen), Springer Verlag Berlin, Heidelberg, New York, 1992-1994.

Harper J. Traditional Chinese medicine for eczema / Seemingly effective, but caution must prevail. *BMJ.* 308; 489-490. 1994

Harper J. Chinese herbs for eczema. *Lancet* 336; 177. 1990

Kojima S, Hikiami H, Matsumi S, Umeda Y, Terasawa K. Effects of Shimotsu-to on the microcirculation of the bulbar conjunctiva and hemorheological parameters in normal subjects. *Phytomedicine* 5 (1); 19-24. 1998

Kubo M, Asano T, Matsuda H, Yutani S, Honda S, Studies on *Rehmanniae radix*. III. The relation between changes of constituents and improvable effects on hemorheology with the processing of roots of *Rehmannia glutinosa. Yakugaku Zasshi,* 116:158-68, Feb. 1996

Latchman Y, Whittle B, Rustin M, Atherton DJ, Brostoff J. The Efficacy of Traditional Chinese Herbal Therapy in Atopic Eczema. *Int Arch Allergy Immunol.* 104; 222-226. 1994

Lu CS, Effects of *Rehmannia glutinosa* in the treatment of Sheehan's syndrome. *Chung Hsi I Chieh Ho Tsa Chih,* 116:476-8, 451, Aug. 1985

Ni M, Bian B, Wang H, Constituents of the dry roots of *Rehmannia glutinosa. Libosch Chung Kuo Chung Yao Tsa Chih,* 116:297-8, inside backcover, May. 1992

Tomoda M, Miyamoto H, Shimizu N. Structural features and Anti-complementary Activity of Rehmannan SA, a Polysaccharide from the Root of *Rehmannia glutinosa. Chem Pharm Bull.* 42 (8); 1666-1668. 1994

Wei XL, Ru XB. Effects of low-molecular-weight *Rehmannia glutinosa* polysaccharides on p53 gene expression. *Acta Pharmacol Sin.* 18 (5); 471-474. 1997

Yasukawa K, Yu SY, Kakinuma SI, Takido M. Inhibitory Effects of Rikkunshi-To, a Traditional Chinese Herbal Prescription, on Tumor Promotion in Two-Stage Carcinogenesis in Mouse Skin. *Biol Pharm Bull.* 18 (5); 730-733. 1995

Rehmannia glutinosa

See Rehmannia (Di-Huang)

Rhamnus catharticus

See Buckthorn

Rhamnus frangula

See Frangula

Rhamnus purshiana

See Cascara Sagrada

Rhatany

Krameria triandra

DESCRIPTION

Medicinal Parts: The medicinal part is the air-dried root, separated from the rhizome.

Flower and Fruit: The 7- to 12-mm long flowers are spare terminal racemes. The calyx is petaloid. The sepals are splayed, lanceolate, dark red, and silky-haired on the outside. The petals are irregular, with 2 wedge-shaped glands, 3 to 5 mm wide, crimson, and spatulate. The flower has 3 stamens. The ovary is ovate, covered in bristly hairs with a thick glabrous style. The fruit is solitary angular and bristled. It is ovate and has numerous red-black bristly thorns.

Leaves, Stem, and Root: The plant is a 0.3 to 1 m high subshrub whose long, 3-cm root is covered in a brown-red, smooth, peeling bark. The younger branches are dark green, silky to bristly haired, the older ones are black and often gnarled. The leaves are entire-margined, ovate, silver-gray pubescent, 6 to 15 mm long and 2 to 6 mm wide.

Habitat: Rhatany is mostly found in Peru, but there are a few areas in countries bordering Peru and in the central Andes where it is also found.

Production: Rhatany root consists of the dried root of *Krameria triandra Ruiz et Pavon* as well as its preparations collected in the wild, washed and air-dried in the shade.

Not to be Confused With: roots of other *Krameria* species

Other Names: Krameria Root, Mapato, Peruvian Rhatany, Red Rhatany, Rhatania,

ACTIONS AND PHARMACOLOGY

COMPOUNDS

Tannins (10-15%): oligomeric proanthocyanidins

Tanner's reds (phlobaphenes): polymeric, insoluble oxydation products of the tannins

Neolignans: including among others rhatany phenols I-III (0.3%)

EFFECTS

In vitro the drug is antimicrobial, fungitoxic and astringent. Because of the tannin and lignan content, local treatment of oral and pharyngeal mucous membrane inflammation seems reasonable.

INDICATIONS AND USAGE

Approved by Commission E:

- Inflammation of the mouth and pharynx

Unproven Uses: In folk medicine used internally as an antidiarrheal agent for enteritis, inflammation of female genital organs and urinary tract. It is used externally to strengthen gums and clean teeth.

Homeopathic Uses: Krameria triandra is used for bleeding mucous membranes and rectum pain.

PRECAUTIONS AND ADVERSE REACTIONS

No health hazards or side effects are known in conjunction with the proper administration of designated therapeutic dosages. Internal administration can lead to digestive complaints because of the secretion-inhibiting efficacy. Allergic mucus membrane reactions have been observed in rare cases.

DOSAGE

Mode of Administration: Comminuted herb for decoctions and other galenic preparations for topical application, especially in oral and pharyngeal areas.

The drug is a component of various standardized preparations of pharyngeal remedies.

Preparation: 1.5 to 2 gm coarsely powdered drug in boiling water, strain after 10 to 15 minutes (1 teaspoonful = approx. 3 g drug).

Daily Dosage: 1.5 g comminuted drug in 1 cup of water, 3 times daily. Undiluted Rhatany tincture painted on the affected surface 2 to 3 times daily. Tea: freshly prepared as a rinse or gargle 2 to 3 times a day.

Storage: Rhatany should be protected from light.

LITERATURE

Bujan JJG et al. Allergic contact dermatitis from *Krameria triandra* extract. *Contact Dermatitis* 38; 120-121. 1998

Hänsel R, Keller K, Rimpler H, Schneider G (Hrsg.), Hagers Handbuch der Pharmazeutischen Praxis, 5. Aufl., Bde 4-6 (Drogen): Springer Verlag Berlin, Heidelberg, New York, 1992-1994.

Madaus G, Lehrbuch der Biologischen Arzneimittel, Bde 1-3, Nachdruck, Georg Olms Verlag Hildesheim 1979.

Masaki H, Sakaki S, Atsumi T, Sakurai H. Active-Oxygen Scavening Activity of Plant Extracts. *Biol Pharm Bull.* 18 (1); 162-166. 1995

Scholz E, Rimpler H, Proanthocyanidins from *Krameria triandra* Root. *Planta Med.* 55; 379-384. 1989

Steinegger E, Hänsel R, Pharmakognosie, 5. Aufl., Springer Verlag Heidelberg 1992.

Teuscher E, Biogene Arzneimittel, 5. Aufl., Wiss. Verlagsges. Stuttgart 1997.

Wichtl M (Hrsg.), Teedrogen, 4. Aufl., Wiss. Verlagsges. Stuttgart 1997.

Rheum palmatum

See Chinese Rhubarb (Da-Huang)

Rhodiola

Rhodiola rosea

DESCRIPTION

Medicinal Parts: Root.

Botanical Description: The plant reaches a height of 12 to 30 inches (70cm) and produces yellow blossoms. It is a perennial with a thick rhizome, fragrant when cut.

Habitat: China; Kazakhstan; Uzbekistan; Mongolia; Russian Federation; Austria; Bulgaria; Czechoslovakia; Finland; France; Greenland, Iceland; Ireland; Italy; Norway; Poland; Romania; Spain; Sweden; United Kingdom; Canada; United States.

Other Names: Roseroot, Golden Root

ACTIONS AND PHARMACOLOGY

COMPOUNDS

Various compounds have isolated from the root of *Rhodiola rosea.* These include flavonoids (rodiolin, rodionin, rodiosin, acetylrodalgin, tricin), monoterpernes (rosiridol, rosaridin), phenylpropanoids (rosavin, rosin, rosarin), triterpenes (daucosterol, beta-sitosterol), phenolic acids (chlorogenic and hydroxycinnamic, gallic acids), and phenylethanol derivatives (salidroside, rhodioloside, tyrosol).

EFFECTS

Effects upon the central nervous system, adaptogenic, anti-stress, and neuroendocrine effects, antioxidant, anti-carcinogenic, cardioprotective, as well as endocrine and reproductive effects are reported.

CLINICAL TRIALS

Physical/Cognitive Performance

During a 12-week drug monitoring study, efficacy and tolerability of a Rhodiola extract combined with vitamins and minerals (vigodana®) was assessed in 120 adults suffering from physical and cognitive deficiencies. The patients received a daily dose of 2 capsules. A statistically significant improvement ($p<0.001$) was demonstrated for physical and cognitive deficiencies. The preparation was well-tolerated (Gruenwald et al, 2007).

A double-blind, placebo-controlled, randomized study was designed to investigate the effect of acute *Rhodiola rosea* intake on physical capacity, muscle strength, speed of limb movement, reaction time, and attention in healthy volunteers. The participants were randomly assigned to receive either *Rhodiola rosea* (200 mg *Rhodiola rosea* extract) or placebo (700 mg starch) over a period of 4 weeks. The results documented that Rhodiola can improve endurance exercise capacity (De Bock, et al, 2004).

The antifatigue effect of a standardized *Rhodiola rosea* extract (SHR-5) was demonstrated in a randomized, double-blind, placebo-controlled, parallel-group clinical study. A total of 161 cadets, aged 19 to 21 years, received a single dose of Rhodiola extract or placebo. Antifatigue index was significantly different in the Rhodiola group compared to placebo, indicating antifatigue effects of *Rhodiola rosea* (Shetsov et al, 2003).

The objective of a double-blind, placebo-controlled, randomized clinical trial was to investigate the stimulating and normalizing effect of *Rhodiola rosea* extract SHR-5 in 40 foreign students during a stressful examination period. The study medication or placebo was taken for 20 days. The most significant improvement in the SHR-5 group was seen in physical fitness, mental fatigue, and neuromotor tests ($p<0.01$). A self-assessment of general well-being was also significantly better ($p<0.05$) in the Rhodiola group. No significance was found in the correction of text tests or a neuromuscular tapping test (Spasov et al, 2000).

A clinical study was designed to determine the effects of repeated low-dose treatment with a standardized extract derived from *Rhodiola rosea*, SHR-5, on fatigue during night duty among 56 young, healthy physicians. A double-blind, placebo-controlled, crossover design was used. The effect was measured as total mental performance, calculated as Fatigue Index. A statistically significant improvement of test parameters was observed in the Rhodiola group and no side effects were reported. The results suggest that *Rhodiola rosea* extract can reduce general fatigue under certain stressful conditions (Darbinyan et al, 2000).

INDICATIONS AND USAGE

Unproven Uses: Traditional folk medicine used *R. rosea* to increase physical endurance, work productivity, longevity, resistance to high altitude sickness, and to treat fatigue, depression, anemia, impotence, gastrointestinal ailments, infections, and nervous system disorders.

Probable Efficacy: Rhodiola may be helpful in relieving mental and physical fatigue and improving endurance exercise performance and general well-being.

CONTRAINDICATIONS

Rhodiola rosea has demonstrated very low occurrences of side effects, and available clinical evidence suggests it has a low toxicity. There are currently no contraindications with prescription medications. Most users find that it improves their mood, energy level, and mental clarity. *R. rosea* should be taken early in the day because it can interfere with sleep or cause vivid dreams (not nightmares) during the first few weeks. It is contraindicated in excited states.

PRECAUTIONS AND ADVERSE REACTIONS

Because *R. rosea* has an activating, antidepressant effect, it should not be used in individuals with bipolar disorder who are vulnerable to becoming manic when given antidepressants or stimulants.

DRUG INTERACTIONS

POTENTIAL INTERACTIONS

Rhodiola does not appear to interact with other medications, although it may have additive effects when taken with other stimulants.

DOSAGE

Daily Dose: 50 to 200mg per day is recommended for clinical effectiveness.

LITERATURE

Abidov M, Crendal F, Grachev S, Seifulla R, Ziegenfuss T. Effect of extracts from Rhodiola rosea and Rhodiola crenulata (Crassulaceae) roots on ATP content in mitochondria of skeletal muscles. Bull Exp Biol Med. 2003 Dec;136(6):585-7.

Abidov M, Grachev S, Seifulla RD, Ziegenfuss TN. Extract of Rhodiola rosea radix reduces the level of C-reactive protein and creatinine kinase in the blood. Bull Exp Biol Med. 2004 Jul;138(1):63-4.

Afanas'ev SA, Alekseeva ED, Bardamova IB, Maslova LV, Lishmanov IuB. [Cardiac contractile function following acute cooling of the body and the adaptogenic correction of its disorders] Biull Eksp Biol Med. 1993 Nov;116(11):480-3. Russian.

Akgul Y, Ferreira D, Abourashed EA, Khan IA. Lotaustralin from Rhodiola rosea roots. Fitoterapia. 2004 Sep;75(6):612-4.

Anon. Rhodiola rosea. Monograph. Altern Med Rev. 2002 Oct;7(5):421-3.

Battistelli M, De Sanctis R, De Bellis R, Cucchiarini L, Dacha M, Gobbi P. Rhodiola rosea as antioxidant in red blood cells: ultrastructural and hemolytic behaviour. Eur J Histochem. 2005 Jul-Sep;49(3):243-54.

Bocharova OA, Matveev BP, Baryshnikov AIu, Figurin KM, Serebriakova RV, Bodrova NB.[The effect of a Rhodiola rosea extract on the incidence of recurrences of a superficial bladder cancer (experimental clinical research)] Urol Nefrol (Mosk). 1995 Mar-Apr;(2):46-7. Russian.

Brown RP, Gerbarg PL, Ramazanov Z. Rhodiola rosea: A Phytomedicinal Overview. HerbalGram. 2002;56:40-52

Colson SN, Wyatt FB, Johnston DL, Autrey LD, FitzGerald YL, Earnest CP. Cordyceps sinensis- and Rhodiola rosea-based supplementation in male cyclists and its effect on muscle tissue oxygen saturation. J Strength Cond Res. 2005 May;19(2):358-63.

Darbinyan V, Kteyan A, Panossian A, et al. Rhodiola rosea in stress induced fatigue — A double-blind cross-over study of a standardized extract SHR-5 with a repeated low-dose regimen on the mental performance of healthy physicians during night duty. Phytomedicine; 7(5): 365-371. 2000.

De Bock K, Eijnde BO, Ramaekers M, Hespel. Acute Rhodiola rosea intake can improve endurance exercise performance. Int J Sport Nutr Exerc Metab; 14(3): 298-307. 2004.

De Sanctis R, De Bellis R, Scesa C, Mancini U, Cucchiarini L, Dacha M. In vitro protective effect of Rhodiola rosea extract against hypochlorous acid-induced oxidative damage in human erythrocytes. Biofactors. 2004;20(3):147-59.

Dement'eva LA, Iaremenko KV. [Effect of a Rhodiola extract on the tumor process in an experiment] Vopr Onkol. 1987;33(7):57-60. Russian.

Gruenwald J, Busch R, Biller A. Wirksamkeit und Verträglichkeit einer Kombination mit Rhodiola-rosea-Extrakt bei älteren Erwachsenen mit verminderter körperlicher und geistiger Vitalität. Erfahrungsheilkunde; 56: 138-142. 2007.

Iaremii IN, Grigor'eva NF. [Hepatoprotective properties of liquid extract of Rhodiola rosea] Eksp Klin Farmakol. 2002 Nov-Dec;65(6):57-9. Russian.

Kelly GS. Rhodiola rosea: a possible plant adaptogen. Altern Med Rev. 2001 Jun;6(3):293-302. Review.

Kim SH, Hyun SH, Choung SY. Antioxidative effects of Cinnamomi cassiae and Rhodiola rosea extracts in liver of diabetic mice. Biofactors. 2006;26(3):209-19.

Kucinskaite A, Briedis V, Savickas A. [Experimental analysis of therapeutic properties of Rhodiola rosea L. and its possible application in medicine] Medicina (Kaunas). 2004;40(7):614-9. Review. Lithuanian.

Kwon YI, Jang HD, Shetty K. Evaluation of Rhodiola crenulata and Rhodiola rosea for management of type II diabetes and hypertension. Asia Pac J Clin Nutr. 2006;15(3):425-32.

Lishmanov IuB, Maslova LV, Maslov LN, Dan'shina EN. [The anti-arrhythmia effect of Rhodiola rosea and its possible mechanism] Biull Eksp Biol Med. 1993 Aug;116(8):175-6. Russian.

Lishmanov IuB, Naumova AV, Afanas'ev SA, Maslov LN. [Contribution of the opioid system to realization of inotropic effects of Rhodiola rosea extracts in ischemic and reperfusion heart damage in vitro] Eksp Klin Farmakol. 1997 May-Jun;60(3):34-6. Russian.

Ma G, Li W, Dou D, Chang X, Bai H, Satou T, Li J, Sun D, Kang T, Nikaido T, Koike K. Rhodiolosides A-E, monoterpene glycosides from Rhodiola rosea. Chem Pharm Bull (Tokyo). 2006 Aug;54(8):1229-33.

Maimeskulova LA, Maslov LN, Lishmanov IuB, Krasnov EA. [The participation of the mu-, delta- and kappa-opioid receptors in the realization of the anti-arrhythmia effect of Rhodiola rosea] Eksp Klin Farmakol. 1997 Jan-Feb;60(1):38-9. Russian.

Maimeskulova LA, Maslov LN. [The anti-arrhythmia action of an extract of Rhodiola rosea and of n-tyrosol in models of experimental arrhythmias] Eksp Klin Farmakol. 1998 Mar-Apr;61(2):37-40. Russian.

Majewska A, Hoser G, Furmanowa M, Urbanska N, Pietrosiuk A, Zobel A, Kuras M. Antiproliferative and antimitotic effect, S phase accumulation and induction of apoptosis and necrosis after treatment of extract from Rhodiola rosea rhizomes on HL-60 cells. J Ethnopharmacol. 2006 Jan 3;103(1):43-52. Epub 2005 Sep 19.

Maslova LV, Kondrat'ev BIu, Maslov LN, Lishmanov IuB. [The cardioprotective and antiadrenergic activity of an extract of Rhodiola rosea in stress] Eksp Klin Farmakol. 1994 Nov-Dec;57(6):61-3. Russian.

Mattioli L, Perfumi M. Rhodiola rosea L. extract reduces stress- and CRF-induced anorexia in rats. J Psychopharmacol. 2007 Jan 26

Ming DS, Hillhouse BJ, Guns ES, Eberding A, Xie S, Vimalanathan S, Towers GH. Bioactive compounds from Rhodiola rosea (Crassulaceae). Phytother Res. 2005 Sep;19(9):740-3.

Perfumi M, Mattioli L. Adaptogenic and central nervous system effects of single doses of 3% rosavin and 1% salidroside Rhodiola rosea L. extract in mice. Phytother Res. 2007 Jan;21(1):37-43.

Petkov VD, Yonkov D, Mosharoff A, Kambourova T, Alova L, Petkov VV, Todorov I. Effects of alcohol aqueous extract from Rhodiola rosea L. roots on learning and memory. Acta Physiol Pharmacol Bulg. 1986;12(1):3-16.

Pogorelyi VE, Makarova LM. [Rhodiola rosea extract for prophylaxis of ischemic cerebral circulation disorder] Eksp Klin Farmakol. 2002 Jul-Aug;65(4):19-22. Russian.

Rohloff J. Volatiles from rhizomes of Rhodiola rosea L. Phytochemistry. 2002 Mar;59(6):655-61.

Salikhova RA, Aleksandrova IV, Mazurik VK, Mikhailov VF, Ushenkova LN, Poroshenko GG. [Effect of Rhodiola rosea on the yield of mutation alterations and DNA repair in bone marrow cells] Patol Fiziol Eksp Ter. 1997 Oct-Dec;(4):22-4. Russian.

Sarris J. Herbal medicines in the treatment of psychiatric disorders: a systematic review. Phytother Res. 2007 Jun 11; [Epub ahead of print]

Shetsov VA, Zholus BI, Shervarly VI, et al. A randomized trial of two different doses of a SHR-5 Rhodiola rosea extract versus placebo and control of capacity for mental work. Phytomedicine; 10: 95-105. 2003.

Spasov AA, Mandrikov VB, Mironova IA. [The effect of the preparation rodakson on the psychophysiological and physical adaptation of students to an academic load] Eksp Klin Farmakol. 2000 Jan-Feb;63(1):76-8. Russian.

Spasov AA, Wikman GK, Mandrikov VB, et al. A double-blind, placebo-controlled pilot study of the stimulating and adaptogenic effect of Rhodiola rosea SHR-5 extract on the fatigue of students caused by stress during an examination period with repeated low-dose regimen. Phytomedicine; 7(2): 85-89. 2000.

Tolonen A, Pakonen M, Hohtola A, Jalonen J. Phenylpropanoid glycosides from Rhodiola rosea. Chem Pharm Bull (Tokyo). 2003 Apr;51(4):467-70.

Udintsev SN, Shakhov VP. The role of humoral factors of regenerating liver in the development of experimental tumors and the effect of Rhodiola rosea extract on this process.

Neoplasma. 1991;38(3):323-31.

Walker TB, Robergs RA. Does Rhodiola rosea possess ergogenic properties? Int J Sport Nutr Exerc Metab. 2006 Jun;16(3):305-15. Review.

Wiedenfeld H, Dumaa M, Malinowski M, Furmanowa M, Narantuya S. Phytochemical and analytical studies of extracts from Rhodiola rosea and Rhodiola quadrifida. Pharmazie. 2007 Apr;62(4):308-11. Erratum in: Pharmazie. 2007 May;62(5):400.

Yousef GG, Grace MH, Cheng DM, Belolipov IV, Raskin I, Lila MA. Comparative phytochemical characterization of three Rhodiola species. Phytochemistry. 2006 Nov;67(21):2380-91.

Rhodiola rosea

See Golden Root

Rhododendron ferrugineum

See Rust-Red Rhododendron

Rhododendron ponticum

See Pontian Rhododendron

Rhus aromatica

See Sweet Sumach

Rhus toxicodendron

See Poison Ivy

Ribes nigrum

See Black Currant

Ribes rubrum

See Red Currant

Rice

Oryza sativa

DESCRIPTION

Medicinal Parts: The medicinal parts of the plant are the seeds.

Flower and Fruit: The panicle is up to 30 cm long. The husk is 7 to 9 mm long with 5 clearly protruding veins. They have 8 cm long, light or dark red awns, or no awns at all. The seed is tightly covered by the layers of the husk and is compressed from the side.

Leaves, Stem, and Root: Rice is an annual. The stem is hollow, leafy, and erect. The leaves are clasping and sheath-like at the base and grow up to 1 m in length. The leaf surface is up to 60 cm long and 1.5 cm wide. The leaves have bristly ciliate spikelets at the base.

Habitat: Rice is probably native to China and India. Today it is cultivated widely in wet areas in the tropics and sub-tropics.

Production: Rice is the seed of *Oryza sativa.*

Other Names: Nivara

ACTIONS AND PHARMACOLOGY

COMPOUNDS

Starch (70%)

Proteins: including prolamines, glutelins, globulins, albumins

Fatty oil (1.0-1.8% in the entire fruit, 7–12 % in the germ): chief fatty acid linoleic acid (45%)

Polysaccharides, soluble: galactoarabinoxylan

Monosaccharides, oligosaccharides: glucose, fructose, saccharose

Flavonoids: including tricine, tricine-7-O-glucoside, tricinine

Steroids: sterols, including beta-sitosterol, gamma-sitosterol, campesterol

Diterpenes: momilactone A, momilactone B

Trigonelline

Trypsin inhibitors

Lectins

Vitamins of the B-group

EFFECTS

Rice has been shown to be effective for pain relief and sedation of the digestive tract.

INDICATIONS AND USAGE

Unproven Uses: Rice is used during recovery from disorders of the gastrointestinal tract, illnesses of the gastrointestinal tract, and diarrhea.

Chinese Medicine: Among uses in Chinese medicine are diabetes, spontaneous perspiration, diarrhea, and debility.

Indian Medicine: Rice is used for pneumonia, diarrhea, and diseases of the colon.

PRECAUTIONS AND ADVERSE REACTIONS

No health hazards or side effects are known in conjunction with the proper administration of designated therapeutic dosages.

DOSAGE

Preparation: Rice seeds are boiled in water before ingestion.

LITERATURE

Hikino H, Murakami M, Oshima Y, Konno C. Isolation and Hypoglycemic Activity of Oryzarans A, B, C and D: Glycans of *Oryza sativa* Roots. *Planta Med.* 52; 490-492. 1986

Huesing JE, Murdock LL, Shade RE, Rice and stinging nettle lectins - insecticidal activity similar to wheat germ agglutinin. In: *PH* 30:3565. 1991.

Kern W, List PH, Hörhammer L (Hrsg.), Hagers Handbuch der Pharmazeutischen Praxis, 4. Aufl., Bde. 1-8, Springer Verlag Berlin, Heidelberg, New York, 1969.

Marles RJ, Farnsworth NR. Antidiabetic plants and their active constituents. *Phytomedicine* 2 (2); 137-189. 1995

Perez G et al. Antidiabetic effect of compounds isolated from plants. *Phytomedicine* 5 (1); 55-75. 1998

Swaminathan S, Rice, This member of the grass family is one of three on which the human species largely subsists. In: *Scientific American* 250(1):80. 1984.

Vignols F, Wigger M, Garcia-Garrido JM, Grellet F, Kader JC, Delseny M, Rice lipid transfer protein (LTP) genes belong to a complex multigene family and are differentially regulated. *Gene,* 195:177-86, Aug 22, 1997.

Ricinus communis

See Castor Oil Plant

Rooibos

Aspalathus linearis

DESCRIPTION

Medicinal Parts: Leaves and twigs.

Botanical Description: A. linearis is a shrub of half a meter to two meters in height, with bright green, simple, needle-shaped leaves which turn a rich reddish-brown color upon fermentation. The small, yellow, typically pea-shaped flowers are produced in spring and early summer. The fruit is a flat, obliquely falcate, glabrous, single-seeded pod.

Habitat: Western parts of the Western Cape Province of South Africa, mainly in the Citrusdal, Clanwilliam and Nieuwoudtville regions. The production area stretches from Darling and Piquetberg in the south to Gifberg and Nieuwoudtville in the north.

Production: The tea is mostly harvested with sickles and tied into bundles. It is then chopped into 3 mm long segments, moistened, bruised and left in heaps to ''sweat'' or ''ferment'' for several hours until a sweet smell develops. So-called ''fermentation'' is actually an oxidation process, during which the phenolic compounds in the plant are enzymatically oxidized (Joubert 1996). When the tea maker is satisfied with the color and aroma, the tea is spread out thinly to sun-dry. Large quantities are available for export, including organic product, so-called ''green'' (unfermented) tea, and also spray-dried extract (powder).

Other Names: rooibos tea (English); rooibos (Afrikaans); aspalathus (French); Rotbusch, Rooibos (German); aspalathus (Italian)

ACTIONS AND PHARMACOLOGY

COMPOUNDS

Aspalathus linearis contains several flavonoid glycosides including orientin, isoorientin, and quercetin, but the dihydrochalcones aspalathin and nothofagin are the main constituents.

EFFECTS

Recent studies have shown significant activity of rooibos against negative effects related to mutagenesis and oxidative damage. The antioxidant activity and antiradical properties have been investigated and are linked to aspalathin, which showed significant activity when compared with other teas and commercial antioxidants. A recent animal study suggests the prevention of age-related accumulation of lipid peroxidases in the brain. Effects on cell division and dermatological conditions suggest a rationale for the cosmetic use of rooibos tea extracts.

INDICATIONS AND USAGE

Unproven Uses: Rooibos tea has been widely used as a milk substitute for infants who are prone to colic. It is considered to have significant antispasmodic activity. Rooibos has become very popular as a health beverage, because it free from harmful stimulants and is devoid of caffeine. Rooibos tea is widely used as an ingredient in cosmetics and is believed to be beneficial in cases of eczema. The main traditional use is as a health drink.

CONTRAINDICATIONS

None are known.

PRECAUTIONS AND ADVERSE REACTIONS

Pregnancy: Scientific evidence for the safe use of rooibos during pregnancy is not available.

DRUG INTERACTIONS

No human drug interaction data is available.

DOSAGE

Rooibos is prepared and consumed in the same way as ordinary tea.

LITERATURE

Blommaert, K.L.J. & Steenkamp, J. 1978. Tannien- en moontlike kafeïeninhoud van Rooibostee, Aspalathus linearis. Agroplantae 10: 49.

Bramati L, Minoggio M, Gardana C, Simonetti P, Mauri P, Pietta P (2002) Quantitative characterization of flavonoid compounds in Rooibos tea (Aspalathus linearis) by LC-UV/DAD. Journal of Agricultural and Food Chemistry 50: 5513-9.

Bramati L, Aquilano F, Pietta P (2003) Unfermented rooibos tea: quantitative characterization of flavonoids by HPLC-UV and determination of the total antioxidant activity. Journal of Agricultural and Food Chemistry 51: 7472-4.

Burger A, Wachter H (eds) (1998) Hunnius Pharmazeutisches Wörterbuch. 8th edn. Walter de Gruyter, Berlin, p. 148.

Dahlgren, R. 1968. Revision of the genus Aspalathus II. The species with ericoid and pinoid leaflets. Subgenus Nortieria. With remarks on Rooibos Tea Cultivation. Bot. Notiser 121: 165-208.

Dahlgren, R. 1988. Crotalarieae (Aspalathus). In: Flora of Southern Africa 16,3(6): 1-430. Botanical Research Institute, Pretoria.

Inanami O, Asanuma T, Inukai N, Jin T, Shimokawa S, Kasai N, Nakano M, Sato F, Kuwabara M (1995) The suppression of age-related accumulation of lipid peroxides in the rat brain by administration of rooibostea (Aspalathus linearis), Neuroscience Letters 196: 85-88.

Joubert, E. 1996. HPLC quantification of the dihydrochalcones, aspalathin and nothofagin in rooibos tea (Aspalathus linearis) as affected by processing. Food Chemistry 55: 403-411.

Joubert E, Winterton P, Britz TJ, Ferreira D (2003) Superoxide anion and α, α-diphenyl-β-picrylhydrazyl radical scavanging capacity of rooibos (Aspalathus linearis) aqueous extracts, crude phenolic fractions, tannin and flavonoids. Food Research International 37: 133-138.

Koeppen BH, Roux DG (1965) Aspalathin: a novel C-glycosylflavonoid from Aspalathus linearis. Tetrahedron Letters 6: 3497-3503.

Lamoš ová D, Juráni M, Greksák M, Nakano M, Vaneková M (1997) Effect of rooibos tea (Aspalathus linearis) on chick skeletal muscle cell growth in culture. Comparative Biochemistry and Physiology Part C: Pharmacology, Toxicology, Endocrinology 116: 39-45.

Marnewick JL, Gelderblom WCA, Joubert E (2000) An investigation of antimutagenic properties of South African herbal teas, Mutation Research/Genetic Toxicology and Environmental Mutagenesis 471: 157-166.

Marnewick JL, Joubert E, Swart P, van der Westhuizen F, Gelderblom WC (2003a) Modulation of hepatic drug metabolizing enzymes and oxidative status by rooibos (Aspalathus linearis) and honeybush (Cyclopia intermedia), green and black (Camellia sinensis) teas in rats. Journal of Agricultural and Food Chemistry 51: 8113-8119.

Marnewick JL, Batenburg W, Swart P, Joubert E, Swanevelder S, Gelderblom WCA (2003b) Ex vivo modulation of chemical-induced mutagenesis by subcellular liver fractions of rats treated with rooibos (Aspalathus linearis), honeybush (Cyclopia intermedia) tea, as well as, black (Camellia sinensis) teas. Mutation Research/Genetic Toxicology and Environmental Mutagenesis 558: 145-154.

Marnewick JL, Joubert E, Joseph S, Swanevelder S, Swart P, Gelderblom WC (2005) Inhibition of tumour promotion in mouse skin by extracts of rooibos (Aspalathus linearis) and honeybush (Cyclopia intermedia), unique South African herbal teas. Cancer Letters (in press)

Neethling HS, Theron HE, Geerthsen JMP (1988) Die Mutagenisiteit van Rooibostee. South African Journal of Science 84: 278-279.

Rabe C, Steenkamp JA, Joubert E, Burger JFW, Ferreira D (1994). Phenolic metabolites from Rooibos Tea (Aspalathus linearis). Phytochemistry 35: 1559-1565.

Rooi Tea Control Board. 1973. Eighty Rooi Tea Wonders. Muller & Retief, Cape Town.

Shindo Y, Kato.K, Effect of Rooibos Tea on Some Dermatological Diseases - Division of Dermatology, Shinonoi General Hospital, Nagano, Japan - 1991.

Snyckers, F.O. & Salemi, G. 1974. Studies of South African medicinal plants. Part. 1. Quercetin as the major in vitro active component of rooibos tea. J. S. Afr. Chem. Inst. 27: 5-7.

Standley L, Winterton P, Marnewick JL, Gelderblom WCA, Joubert E, Britz TJ (2001) Influence of processing stages on antimutagenic and antioxidant potentials of rooibos tea. J. Agric. Food Chem. 49: 114-117.

Van der Bank, M. et al. 1995. Biochemical genetic variation in four wild populations of Aspalathus linearis (Rooibos Tea). Biochem. Syst. Ecol. 23(3): 257-262.

Van der Walt, A. & Machado, R. 1992. New Marketing Success Stories. Southern Book Publishers, Halfway House.

Van Heerden FR, Van Wyk B-E, Viljoen AM, Steenkamp PA (2003) Phenolic variation in wild populations of Aspalathus linearis (rooibos tea). Biochemical Systematics and Ecology 31: 885-895.

Van Wyk B-E, Gericke N (2000) People's Plants: a guide to useful plants of southern Africa. Briza Publications, Pretoria, pp. 100-101.

Van Wyk B-E, Van Oudtshoorn B, Gericke N (1997) Medicinal plants of South Africa. Briza Publications, Pretoria, 48-49.

Van Wyk B-E, Wink, C, Wink, M. (2004) Handbuch der Arzneipflanzen. Wissenschaftliche Verlagsgesellschaft, Stuttgart, p. 59.

Van Wyk B-E, Wink, M. (2004) Medicinal Plants of the World. Briza Publications, Pretoria, p. 59.

Von Gadow A, Joubert E, Hansmann CF (1997) Comparison of antioxidant activity of rooibos tea (Aspalathus linearis) with green, oolong and black tea. Food Chemistry 60: 73-77.

Watt JM, Breyer-Brandwijk MG (1962) The Medicinal and Poisonous Plants of Southern and Eastern Africa. 2nd edn. Livingstone, London

Rosa canina

See Dog Rose

Rosa gallica & Rosa centifolia

See Rose

Rose

Rosa gallica & Rosa centifolia

DESCRIPTION

Medicinal Parts: The medicinal parts are the petals and the oil extracted from them. Rose is also used in homeopathic medicine.

Flower and Fruit: The flowers are usually solitary, more rarely in twos and threes, on 2- to 3-cm long, thickly glandular pedicles. The calyx is round to pear-shaped and is usually thickly covered with stem glands and gland bristles. The velvety petals are pink to purple, 2 to 3 cm long and wide. The style and stigma form the ovary that is surrounded by carpels enclosed in the calyx, forming woolly capitula. The ripe, red-brown false fruit is 1 to 1.5 cm long.

Leaves, Stem, and Root: The plant, a descendant of *Rosa gallica* is a low shrub with extensive runners and above ground reedlike shoots, which are erect and branched. They usually grow to between 0.5 to 1 m and are covered with long, revolute, or erect thorns and stem glands of different length. The leaves, which are usually penfoliate, less frequently trifoliate, have long glanular, dark green above, lighter and bluer below, leaflets. They grow together at the leaf stem that terminate in free tips.

Habitat: Rose is probably indigenous to Iran and is cultivated worldwide.

Production: Rose flowers consist of the dried petals of *Rosa gallica* and *Rosa centifolia* that are gathered prior to fully unfolding. The petals are harvested by hand and dried in the shade.

Other Names: Cabbage Rose, Damask Rose, French Rose, Hundred-Leafed Rose

ACTIONS AND PHARMACOLOGY

COMPOUNDS

Tannins: oligomeric proanthocyanidins

Volatile oil (in the fresh blossoms): chief components (-)-citronellol, geraniol, nerol, phenyl ethanol, Including as well (-)-linalool, and citral

EFFECTS

The astringent effect attributed to the drug is due to the tannin content.

INDICATIONS AND USAGE

Approved by Commission E:

- Inflammation of the mouth and pharynx

Unproven Uses: Rose flowers are used in folk medicine internally for diarrhea, tuberculosis of the lungs, pulmonary catarrh and asthma, hemorrhage and leukorrhea. Externally, it is used for inflammations of the oral and pharyngeal mucosa, suppurating wounds, and lid inflammation.

Indian Medicine: In India, Rose is used for coughs, bronchitis, asthma, fever, and general debility. It is also used for wounds and hyperhydrosis.

PRECAUTIONS AND ADVERSE REACTIONS

No health hazards or side effects are known in conjunction with the proper administration of designated therapeutic dosages.

DOSAGE

Mode of Administration: Rose flowers are available as whole, crude and powdered drug forms for internal and external use.

Preparation:

Tea – 1 to 2 g drug added to 1 cup (200 mL) water.

Rose vinegar – 60 g petals added to 750 mL red wine vinegar.

Daily Dosage:

Tea infusion – up to 3 cups per day. It is also used for rinses and washes.

Powder – 5 to 10 g with honey or liquid.

The leaves can be applied directly to the eyes.

Storage: Should be tightly sealed and stored in dry and cool place.

LITERATURE

Kern W, List PH, Hörhammer L (Hrsg.), Hagers Handbuch der Pharmazeutischen Praxis, 4. Aufl., Bde. 1-8: Springer Verlag Berlin, Heidelberg, New York, 1969.

Leung AY, Encyclopedia of Common Natural Ingredients Used in Food Drugs, Cosmetics, John Wiley & Sons Inc., New York 1980.

Madaus G, Lehrbuch der Biologischen Arzneimittel, Bde 1-3, Nachdruck, Georg Olms Verlag Hildesheim 1979.

Rosemary

Rosmarinus officinalis

DESCRIPTION

Medicinal Parts: The medicinal parts are the oil extracted from the leaves and the leafy stems, the flowering, dried twig tips, the dried leaves, the fresh leaves, the fresh aerial parts collected during flowering, and the flowering branches.

Flower and Fruit: Labiate flowers grow on tometose inflorescences in the leaf axils of the upper part of the branches. The calyx is 3 to 4 mm, green or reddish, initially tomentose, later 5 to 7 mm, and glabrous. The venation is conspicuous. The corolla is 10 to 12 mm long, bluish, occasionally pink or white. The nutlet is brown.

Leaves, Stem, and Root: The plant is an evergreen, branched subshrub, 50 to 150 cm high with erect, climbing, or occasionally decumbent brown branches. The leaves are linear, coriaceous, entire-margined, light green, and somewhat rugose above. They are tomentose, 15 to 40 mm by 1.2 to 3.5 mm.

Characteristics: The plant has a very pungent aroma.

Habitat: The plant is indigenous to the Mediterranean region and Portugal and is cultivated there as well as on the Crimea, in the Transcaucasus, Central Asia, India, Southeast Asia, South Africa, Australia, and the U.S.

Production: Rosemary leaves consist of the fresh or dried leaves of *Rosmarinus officinalis* collected after flowering as well as their preparations. The leaves are harvested after flowering on sunny, warm days and dried.

Not to be Confused With: May be confused with *Ledum palustre, Andromeda polifolia, Teucrium montanum, Taxus baccata, Santolina rosmarinfolia,* and *S. chamaecyparissus.*

ACTIONS AND PHARMACOLOGY

COMPOUNDS

Caffeic acid derivatives: chief component rosmarinic acid

Diterpenes (bitter): including carnosolic acid (picrosalvin), isorosmanol, rosmadial, rosmaridiphenol, rosmariquinone

Flavonoids: including cirsimarin, diosmin, hesperidin, homoplantiginin, phegopolin

Triterpenes: chief components oleanolic acid, ursolic acid and their 3-acetyl esters

Volatile oil (1.0 to 2.5%): chief components 1,8-cineole (20 to 50%), alpha-pinene (15 to 25%), camphor (10 to 25%), including as well camphene, borneol, bornyl acetate, beta-caryophyllene, p-cymene, limonene, linalool, myrcene, alpha-terpineol, verbenone

EFFECTS

The drug is mildly antimicrobial and antiviral (probably because of the diterpenes).

Animal tests have demonstrated spasmolytic effects on the gallbladder ducts and on the upper intestine. The tests have confirmed choleretic, liver-protective, anticonvulsive, antimutagenic, and tumor-inhibiting effects. The metabolism of the drug is accelerated by the presence of 1,8 cineol. In humans, Rosemary oil improves circulation when applied externally because of a certain skin irritating effect.

INDICATIONS AND USAGE

Approved by Commission E:

- Blood pressure problems
- Dyspeptic complaints
- Loss of appetite
- Rheumatism

Rosemary is used internally for dyspeptic disorders and externally for hypotonic circulatory disorders and rheumatic conditions.

Unproven Uses: Rosemary is used in folk medicine for digestive symptoms, headaches and migraine, dysmenorrhea, amenorrhea, and oligomenorrhea, states of exhaustion, dizziness, and poor memory. It is used externally as a poultice for poorly healing wounds, for eczema, as an analgesic for injuries of the mouth and throat, topically for myalgias, intercostal neuralgia, and sciatica.

Homeopathic Uses: Rosmarinus officinalis is used for gastrointestinal disorders.

CONTRAINDICATIONS

Rosemary preparations should not be used during pregnancy.

PRECAUTIONS AND ADVERSE REACTIONS

General: No health hazards or side effects are known in conjunction with the proper administration of designated therapeutic dosages. Contact allergies have been observed on occasion.

Pregnancy: Not to be used during pregnancy.

OVERDOSAGE

Very large quantities of rosemary leaves misused for the purpose of abortion, can lead to deep coma, spasm, vomiting, gastroenteritis, uterine bleeding, kidney irritation, and to death in humans.

DOSAGE

Mode of Administration: Rosemary is available as whole, crude and powdered drug forms for internal and external use. It is also available in compounded preparations.

How Supplied:

Liquid – 1:1

Preparation:

Tea – pour boiling water over 2 g finely cut drug and strain after 15 minutes (1 teaspoon corresponds to approximately 2 g drug).

Rosemary wine – Add 20 g drug in 1 liter wine, let stand for 5 days, shake occasionally.

Tincture – 1:5 with 70% ethanol (V/V)

Liquid extract – 1:1 45% ethanol (V/V)

Daily Dosage: The daily dose is 4 to 6 g drug.

Tea – 1 cup several times a day

Tincture (1:5) – single dose: 20 to 40 drops

Liquid extract – single dose: 2 to 4 mL

Externally – semi-solid and liquid forms with 6 to 10% essential oil

Bath additive – 50 gm drug to 1 liter hot water added to full or hip-depth bath

Washes – use 1% infusion

Homeopathic Dosage: 5 drops, 1 tablet, or 10 globules every 30 to 60 minutes (acute) or 1 to 3 times daily (chronic); parenterally: 1 to 2 ml sc acute: 3 times daily; chronic: once a day (HAB1)

Storage: Rosemary should be protected from light and moisture.

LITERATURE

Anonym, Phytotherapie:Pflanzliche Antirheumatika - was bringen sie? In: DAZ 136(45):4012-4015. 1996.

Aruoma OI, Halliwell B, Aeschbach R, Löligers J. Antioxidant and pro-oxidant properties of active rosemary constituents: carnosol and carnosic acid. *Xenobiotica* 22; 257-268. 1992

Chantraine JM, Laurent D, Ballivian C, Saavedra G, Ibanez R, Vilaseca LA. Insecticidal Activity of Essential Oils on Aedes aegypti Larvae. *Phytother Res.* 12 (5); 350-354. 1998

Czygan I, Czygan FC, Rosmarin - *Rosmarinus officinalis L.* In: ZPZ 18(3):182-186. 1997

Erenmemisoglu A, Sarymen R, Ustun H. Effect of a *Rosmarinus officinalis* leave extract on plasma glucose levels in normoglycaemic and diebetic mice. *Pharmazie* 52 (8); 645-646. 1997

Frankel EN, Huang SW, Aeschbach R, Prior E. Antioxidant Activity of a Rosemary Extract and Its Constituents, Carnosic Acid, Carnosol, and Rosmarinic Acid, in Bulk Oil and Oil-in-Water Emulsion. *J Agric Food Chem.* 44 (1); 131-135. 1996

Ganeva Y, Tsankova E, Simova S, Apostolova B, Zaharieva E. Rofficerone: A New Triterpenoid from *Rosmarinus officinalis. Planta Med.* 59; 276-277. 1993

Giachetti D, Taddei E, Taddei I. Pharmacological Activity of *Mentha piperita, Salvia officinalis* and *Rosmarinus officinalis* Essences on Oddi's sphincter. *Planta Med.* 52; 543-544. 1986

Haraguchi H et al., Inhibition of lipid peroxidation and superoxide generation by diterpenoids from *Rosmarinus officinalis.* In: *PM* 61(4):333-336. 1995.

Hiusman M, Lindberg Madsen H, Skibstedt LH, Bertelsen G. The combined effect of rosemary (*Rosmarinus officinalis L.*) and modified atmosphere packaging as protection against warmed over flavour in cooked minced pork meat. *Z Lebensm Unters Forsch.* 198; 57-59. 1994

Hjorther AB, Christophersen C, Hausen BM, Menne T. Occupational allergic contact dermatitis from carnosol, a naturally-occuring compound present in rosemary. *Contact Dermatitis* 37; 99-100. 1997

Houlihan CM et al., *J Am Oil Chem Soc* 62(1):96. 1985

Kreis P, Dietrich A, Mosandl A. Chiral compounds of essential oils. / Part 18: On the authenticity assessment of the essential oil of *Rosmarinus officinalis L. Pharmazie* 49; 761-765. 1994

Mastelic J, Kustrac D. Essential Oil and glycosidally bound volatiles in aromatic plants. II. Rosemary (*Rosmarinus officinalis L. Laminaceae*). *Acta Pharm.* 47; 139-142. 1997

Schwarz K, Ternes W. Antioxidative constituents of *Rosmarinus officinalis* and *Salvia officinalis* / I. Determination of phenolic diterpenes with antioxidative activity amongst tocochromanols using HPLC. *Z Lebensm Unters Forsch.* 195; 95-98. 1992

Rosinweed

Silphium laciniatum

DESCRIPTION

Medicinal Parts: The medicinal part is the root.

Leaves, Stem and Root: The plant is a stately 1- to 4-m high herbaceous perennial, with an almost leafless, round shaft. The leaves are 30 to 60 cm long. They are long-petioled, simple, or double-pinnate leaves. The leaves are alternate, with their edges turned upward and downward and their surfaces facing north and south.

Characteristics: The taste of the root is bitter and then acrid. The roots are odorless.

Habitat: The plant grows in the midwestern U.S., especially Ohio.

Other Names: Compass Weed, Polar Plant, Pilot Weed

ACTIONS AND PHARMACOLOGY

COMPOUNDS

Resins (smelling terpene-like, mastic-like)

Volatile oil

Inulin (in the root)

EFFECTS

The active agents are resin, with 19% terpene and 37% of a resin acid, and inulin in the root. The drug has antispasmodic, diuretic, and diaphoretic effects.

INDICATIONS AND USAGE

Homeopathic Uses: In homeopathy, the drug is used for the treatment of digestive disorders.

PRECAUTIONS AND ADVERSE REACTIONS

No health hazards or side effects are known in conjunction with the proper administration of designated therapeutic dosages.

DOSAGE

Mode of Administration: Rosinweed is available as a tincture or liquid extract.

LITERATURE

Kern W, List PH, Hörhammer L (Hrsg.), Hagers Handbuch der Pharmazeutischen Praxis, 4. Aufl., Bde. 1-8: Springer Verlag Berlin, Heidelberg, New York, 1969.

Madaus G, Lehrbuch der Biologischen Arzneimittel, Bde 1-3, Nachdruck, Georg Olms Verlag Hildesheim 1979.

Rosmarinus officinalis

See Rosemary

Round-Leafed Wintergreen

Pyrola rotundifolia

DESCRIPTION

Medicinal Parts: The medicinal parts are the leaves.

Flower and Fruit: The white, sometimes reddish flowers are in many-blossomed, nodding racemes turning to all sides. The calyx is divided in 5 almost to the base and has lanceolate, revolute, splayed tips. The corolla has 5 petals and is flatly campanulate. The 10 stamens are curved upward. The ovary is superior with 5 sections and a downward curving style. The fruit is a 5-sectioned capsule.

Leaves, Stem, and Root: The plant grows from 15 to 30 cm high. The stem is erect, obtusely angular, and glabrous; it has 2 sheathlike bracts. The leaves in the basal rosette are petiolate, orbicular, and glabrous. They are grass-green, glossy, somewhat cordate at the base, shallowly crenate, coriaceous, and evergreen.

Characteristics: The flowers have a slight, pleasant fragrance, and the leaves are astringent.

Habitat: The plant originated in the South Seas but is now naturalized in other climates.

Production: Wintergreen leaves are the leaves of *Pyrola rotundifolia*.

Other Names: Large Wintergreen

ACTIONS AND PHARMACOLOGY

COMPOUNDS

Hydroquinone derivatives (4-8%): chief components isohomoarbutin, additionally homoarbutin (arbutin)

Naphthacene derivatives (naphthoquinone): chimaphilin (2,7-dimethyl-1,4-naphthoquinone)

Tannins (up to 18%)

EFFECTS

No information is available.

INDICATIONS AND USAGE

Unproven Uses: Wintergreen is used for bladder inflammation and urinary tract diseases, diseases of the prostate, and kidney disorders.

PRECAUTIONS AND ADVERSE REACTIONS

No health hazards or side effects are known in conjunction with the proper administration of designated therapeutic dosages. The drug possesses a weak sensitizing effect due to its chimaphilin content. The drug is not suitable for long-term use because of its hydroquinone glycoside content.

DOSAGE

Mode of Administration: The drug is administered ground and as an extract.

LITERATURE

Hegnauer R, Chemotaxonomie der Pflanzen, Bde 1-11, Birkhäuser Verlag Basel, Boston, Berlin 1962-1997.

Kern W, List PH, Hörhammer L (Hrsg.), Hagers Handbuch der Pharmazeutischen Praxis, 4. Aufl., Bde. 1-8, Springer Verlag Berlin, Heidelberg, New York, 1969 (unter Pirola rotundifolia).

Madaus G, Lehrbuch der Biologischen Arzneimittel, Bde 1-3, Nachdruck, Georg Olms Verlag Hildesheim 1979 (unter Pirola rotundifolia).

Rubia tinctorum

See Madder

Rubus fruticosus

See Blackberry

Rubus idaeus

See Raspberry

Rue

Ruta graveolens

DESCRIPTION

Medicinal Parts: The medicinal parts are oil extracted from the herb, the herbal parts of the plant harvested after flowering, the fresh aerial parts of the plant collected at the beginning of the flowering season, and the whole plant.

Flower and Fruit: The yellow flowers are in cymes, which are on twining branches with entire or triple-lobed bracts. The calyx has 4 or 5 segments. The 4 to 5 petals are spoonlike, ovate, and end suddenly in the stem. The 8 to 10 stamens are in 2 circles. The single short, broadly ovate ovary has 4 to 5 grooves and is covered with hemispherical glands. The fruit is a globular, 4- to 5-valvular, many-seeded capsule. The seeds are angular and have a bumpy brown skin.

Leaves, Stem, and Root: The plant is a sturdy shrub 30 to 80 cm high with a woody root and a crooked, branched rhizome. The shoots are glabrous, pale green, and somewhat covered in oil glands. The stems are erect, rigid, round, lightly branched, and woody from below. The leaves are 4 to 11 cm long and 3 to 7 cm wide, odd-pinate, with 1 to 3 pinnatesect pinna. The terminal segments are spatulate to lanceolate. The front leaves are very finely crenate or serrate, somewhat fleshy, pale yellowish or bluish green.

Characteristics: The odor is tangy and the taste is hot, somewhat bitter and can cause skin irritation.

Habitat: The plant grows in the Balkans as far as Siebengebirge, upper Italy, and central Italy and is cultivated elsewhere. Rue is completely naturalized in the southern Alps, southern France, and Spain.

Production: Rue leaves consist of the dried leaves of *Ruta graveolens.* Rue herb consists of the dried above-ground parts of *Ruta graveolens.* Both are dried in the shade at a maximum of 35° C.

Not to be Confused With: Confusion can arise with other Ruta species.

Other Names: Bitter Herb, Common Rue, Countryman's Treacle, Garden Rue, Herb-of-Grace, Herbygrass

ACTIONS AND PHARMACOLOGY

COMPOUNDS

Alkaloids (0.4-0.4%): furoquinoline alkaloids including among others, skimmianin, gamma-fagarine, dictamnin, kokusaginine, ptelein

Acridine alkaloids: including arborinine- 2-arylquinoline

Quinazoline alkaloids: including among others, arborine

Quinoline alkaloids: including graveoline, graveolineine

Volatile oil (0.2-0.4%): chief components are nonan-2-one (50%), nonan-2-ylacetate, undecan-2-one, undec-2-ylacetate further including, among others, linalyl acetate, 1,8-cineole, menthol

Flavonoids: chief component is rutin (2-5%)

Hydroxycoumarins: umbelliferone, herniarin, gravelliferon, rutacultin

Furocoumarins: bergapten, psoralen, xanthotoxin, chalepensin, isopimpinellin, isoimperatorin, rutarin, rutaretine

Pyranocoumarins: including among others, xanthyletine

Lignans: savinin, helioxanthine

EFFECTS

The alkaloids in the drug are anti-exudative. Chalepensin inhibits fertility, and the coumarin derivatives and alkaloids are spasmolytic. In addition, the drug is antimicrobial, abortifacient, and photosensitizing.

INDICATIONS AND USAGE

Unproven Uses: Preparations of rue herb and/or leaves are used for menstrual disorders, as an effective uterine remedy and as an abortive agent. In folk medicine, Rue is used for menstrual complaints, as a contraceptive and as an abortive agent. The herb is also used for inflammation of the skin, oral and pharyngeal cavities, earache, toothache, for feverish infectious diseases, for cramps, as an obstetric remedy, dyspepsia, diarrhea, and intestinal worm infestations.

Homeopathic Uses: Among uses in homeopathy are contusions, sprains, bruising, varicose veins, and rheumatism (especially of the spine).

CONTRAINDICATIONS

Rue is not to be used during pregnancy.

PRECAUTIONS AND ADVERSE REACTIONS

General: No health hazards are known in conjunction with the proper administration of designated therapeutic dosages. The drug can lead to photosensitization, due to its furocoumarine and furoquinoline content; photodermatoses have been observed following skin contact with the fresh leaves. Sensitization is possible following skin contact.

Pregnancy: Vomiting, epigastric pain, liver damage, kidney damage, depression, sleep disorders, feelings of vertigo, delirium, fainting, tremor, and spasm, occasionally with fatal outcome, have occurred after misuse of extracts of the plant as an abortive agent.

OVERDOSAGE

Vomiting, epigastric pain, liver damage, kidney damage, depression, sleep disorders, feelings of vertigo, delirium, fainting, tremor, and spasm, occasionally with fatal outcome, have occurred in cases of overdose.

DOSAGE

Mode of Administration: Preparations of the leaves and root are used internally as a tea and also externally.

Preparation: Tea or a cold decoction is prepared by adding 1 heaping teaspoonful to 1/4 liter of water. (1 teaspoonful is roughly equivalent to 2.8 g drug).

Daily Dosage: 0.5 g of the drug is considered a medium single dose; 1.0 g the maximum daily dose. The tea may be taken several times a day.

Delayed menstruation— 2 cups per day of the infusion

For topical use, leaves are used to fill hollow teeth for toothache and juice from the leaves is used as an ear drop for earaches.

Homeopathic Dosage: 5 to 10 drops, 1 tablet, or 5 to 10 globules 1 to 3 times a day or 1 mL injection solution sc twice a week (HAB1)

LITERATURE

Baumert A, Gröger D, Schmidt J, Mügge C. Minor Alkaloids from Ruta graveolens Tissues. *Pharmazie* 42; 67-68. 1987

Baumert A, Maier W, Gröger D. Charakterization of Acridone-Specific Enzymes and Elictor-Stimulation of Acridone Formation in Cell Cultures of *Ruta graveolens. Planta Med.* 56; 494. 1990

Becela-Deller C, *Ruta graveolens L.* - Weinraute. In: *ZPT* 16(5):275-281. 1995.

Grundon, MF, In ''The Alkaloids Vol. 11'', Pub. *Royal Soc Chem.* 1981

Kong YC et al. Antifertility Principle of *Ruta graveolens. Planta Med.* 55; 176-178. 1989

Mascolo N et al., *Phytother Res* 1(1):28. 1987

Meckes M, Villarreal ML, Tortoriello J, Berlin B, Berlin A. A Microbiological Evaluation of Medicinal Plants used by the Maya People of Southern Mexico. *Phytother Res.* 9 (4); 244-250. 1995

Montagu M et al. Synchronous fluorescence spectrometry and identification of dihydrofuro(2,3-b)quinolinium alkaloids biosynthesized by *Ruta graveolens* cultures in vitro. *Pharmazie* 44; 342-344. 1989

Paulini H, Popp R, Schimmer O, Ratka O, Röder E. Isogravacridonchlorine: A Potent and Direct Acting Frameshift Mutagen from the Roots of *Ruta graveolens. Planta Med.* 57; 59-61. 1991

Paulini H, Eilert U, Schimmer O. Mutagenic compounds in an extract from Rutae Herba (*Ruta graveolens L.*). I. Mutagenicity is partiallc caused by furoquinoline alkaloids. *Mutagenesis* 2; 271-273. 1987.

Van Duuren BL et al., *J Natl Cancer Inst* 46:1039. 1971

Rumex acetosa

See Sorrel

Rumex aquaticus

See Water Dock

Rumex crispus

See Yellow Dock

Rupturewort

Herniaria glabra

DESCRIPTION

Medicinal Parts: The medicinal part is the fresh flowering plant.

Flower and Fruit: The flowers are in flat clusters of 7 to 10 in the leaf axils or opposite the leaves along the stem. They are yellow-white and very small. The fruit is a membranous capsule covered by the calyx and contains 1 seed.

Leaves, Stem, and Root: The plant is an annual small shrub of about 15 cm. The stem tends to be decumbent. It is round and branched. The leaves are sessile, entire-margined, elliptical, and opposite. The leaves are alternate.

Characteristics: The plant is yellow-green and glabrous; it creates suds when rubbed under water.

Habitat: The plant is found in the temperate and southern regions of Europe and in Asian Russia.

Production: Rupturewort is the complete aerial part of *Herniaria glabra* or *Herniaria hirsuta.*

Other Names: Flax Weed, Herniary

ACTIONS AND PHARMACOLOGY

COMPOUNDS

Triterpene saponins: herniaria saponins I-VII (aglycones medicagen, gypsogen, 16-hydroxy-medicagen)

Flavonoids: including hyperoside

Hydroxycoumarins: umbelliferone, herniarin

EFFECTS

The main active principles (saponins, flavonoids, coumarins, and small amounts of tannins) are reported to have mild spasmolytic and diuretic effects, which have not been scientifically proved.

INDICATIONS AND USAGE

Unproven Uses: Herniaria glabra is used for disorders of the efferent urinary tract, inflammatory disorders of the kidneys and bladder, respiratory disorders, nerve inflammation, gout, and rheumatism, and as a blood purifier.

PRECAUTIONS AND ADVERSE REACTIONS

Health risks or side effects following the proper administration of designated therapeutic dosages are not recorded.

DOSAGE

Mode of Administration: The drug is administered as an infusion and in tea mixtures, as an extract in drops and in urological pharmaceutical preparations.

Preparation: Put 1.5 g comminuted drug (1 teaspoonful is equal to 1.4 g) in cold water and bring briefly to a boil. Strain after 5 minutes.

Daily Dosage: Drink 1 cup 2 to 3 times daily as a diuretic.

LITERATURE

Cart J, Reznicek G, Korhammer S, Haslinger E, Jurenitsch J, Kubelka W, The first spectroscopically confirmed saponin from *Herniaria glabra.* In: *PM* 58(7):A709. 1992.

Cart J et al. A Further new Triterpenesaponine from *Herniaria glabra. Sci Pharm.* 60; 161. 1992

Freiler M et al., A new triterpenesaponin from *Herniaria glabra.* In: *PM* 61(Abstracts of 43rd Ann Congr):66. 1995.

Zoz et al., (1976) Rastit Resur 12(3):411 (via CA 85:174257). f Kern W, List PH, Hörhammer L (Hrsg.), Hagers Handbuch der Pharmazeutischen Praxis, 4. Aufl., Bde. 1-8, Springer Verlag Berlin, Heidelberg, New York, 1969.

Madaus G, Lehrbuch der Biologischen Arzneimittel, Bde 1-3, Nachdruck, Georg Olms Verlag Hildesheim 1979.

Steinegger E, Hänsel R, Pharmakognosie, 5. Aufl., Springer Verlag Heidelberg 1992.

Teuscher E, Biogene Arzneimittel, 5. Aufl., Wiss. Verlagsges. mbH Stuttgart 1997.

Wichtl M (Hrsg.), Teedrogen, 4. Aufl., Wiss. Verlagsges. Stuttgart 1997.

Ruscus aculeatus

See Butcher's Broom

Rust-Red Rhododendron

Rhododendron ferrugineum

DESCRIPTION

Medicinal Parts: The medicinal parts are the dried foliage leaves, the dried leafy branches, and the fresh leafy branches.

Flower and Fruit: The pink flowers are in umbel-like racemes. The calyx has 5 short ovate tips. The corolla is fused and funnel-shaped with an edge divided into 5 segments. It is covered on the outside with white or golden-yellow resin spots. There are 10 stamens and 1 superior ovary. The fruit is a 5-valved capsule. The seeds are fusiform, about 1 mm long and light brown.

Leaves, Stem, and Root: The plant is an evergreen shrub up to 1 m high and is richly branched from the base upward. The branches are sturdy and elastic with gray-brown bark. The leaves are oblong-lanceolate, tough, and glabrous. The margin is entire and involuted. The leaves are dark green above, densely scaled underneath, and sometimes rust-colored.

Characteristics: The leaves are not ciliate at the edge.

Habitat: The plant grows in the Alpine chain from the Pyrenees to the southern Croatian mountains, but not in the Carpathians.

Production: Rust-Red Rhododendron consists of the dried leaves of *Rhododendron ferrugineum.*

Not to be Confused With: The leaves of R. hirsutum. The plant product may be altered through the addition of cranberry leaves.

Other Names: Rosebay, Snow Rose, Yellow Rhodedendron

ACTIONS AND PHARMACOLOGY

COMPOUNDS: RHODODENDRON AUREUM

Diterpenes of the andromedan type (presence questionable)

Hydroquinone glycosides: arbutin (ericolin)

Flavonoids: including polystachoside, avicularin, myricetin, gossypetin, azaleatin

Phenol glycosides (bitter substances): rhododendrine (betuloside, 4-(3′-glucosyloxybutyl)-phenol)

COMPOUNDS: RHODODENDRON FERRUGINEUM

Diterpenes of the andromedan type (presence questionable, but probable)

Flavonoids: including myricetin, gossypetin, azaleatin

Phenol glycosides (bitter substances): rhododendrine (betuloside, 4-(3′-glucosyloxybutyl)-phenol)

COMPOUNDS: RHODODENDRON PONTICUM

Diterpenes of the andromedan type: grayanotoxin I (andromedotoxin, acetyl andromedol, asebotoxin, rhodotoxin), grayanotoxin II (andromedol), grayanotoxin III (andromedenol).

Flavonoids: including myricetin, gossypetin, azaleatin

Phenol glycosides (bitter substances): rhododendrine (betuloside, 4-(3′-glucosyloxybutyl)-phenol)

EFFECTS

No information is available.

INDICATIONS AND USAGE

Because the drug's composition is not fully known, its use cannot be recommended.

Unproven Uses: Rust-Red Rhododendron is used to treat rheumatic symptoms, kidney stones, geriatric complaints, gout, high blood pressure, meteorism, migraine, muscular pain, and neuralgia.

Homeopathic Uses: The drug is used for neuralgia, rheumatism, and inflammation of the testicles.

PRECAUTIONS AND ADVERSE REACTIONS

The Rhododendron species mentioned are considered poisonous. The grayanotoxins prevent the closure of the sodium channels and thus paralyze conduction.

OVERDOSAGE

Signs of poisoning could include cardiac arrhythmias, coordination disorders, diarrhea, hypotension, cold sweats, paresthesia, salivation, severe stupor, spasm bradycardia, vomiting, and eventually death through cardiac failure or apnea. Unambiguous proof of toxicity is available only for the foliage, blossoms, and sap of Rhododendron ponticum.

Following gastrointestinal emptying (inducement of vomiting, gastric lavage with burgundy-colored potassium permanganate solution, sodium sulphate), administration of activated charcoal and shock prophylaxis (quiet, warmth), therapy for poisonings consists of treating spasms with diazepam (IV), bradycardia with atropine, electrolyte substitution and treating possible cases of acidosis with sodium bicarbonate infusions. In case of shock, plasma volume expanders should be infused. Opiates should not be given. Monitoring of kidney function is essential. Intubation and oxygen respiration may also be necessary.

DOSAGE

Daily Dosage: The daily dosage is 5 to 6 gm of drug as an infusion.

LITERATURE

Bewuβtlos nach Verzehr eines Honigbrötchens. In: DAZ 132(27):1440. 1992.

Frohne D, Pfänder HJ, Giftpflanzen - Ein Handbuch für Apotheker, Toxikologen und Biologen, 4. Aufl., Wiss. Verlags-Ges. Stuttgart 1997.

Hänsel R, Keller K, Rimpler H, Schneider G (Hrsg.), Hagers Handbuch der Pharmazeutischen Praxis, 5. Aufl., Bde 4-6 (Drogen): Springer Verlag Berlin, Heidelberg, New York, 1992-1994.

Lewin L, Gifte und Vergiftungen, 6. Aufl., Nachdruck, Haug Verlag, Heidelberg 1992.

Madaus G, Lehrbuch der Biologischen Arzneimittel, Bde 1-3, Nachdruck, Georg Olms Verlag Hildesheim 1979.

Roth L, Daunderer M, Kormann K: Giftpflanzen, Pflanzengifte, 4. Aufl., Ecomed Fachverlag Landsberg Lech 1993.

Sasseville D, Nguyen KH. Allergic contact dermatitis from *Rhus toxicodendron* in a phytotherapeutic preparation. *Contact Dermatitis* 32; 182-183. 1995

Schulz R, Hänsel R, Rationale Phytotherapie, Springer Verlag Heidelberg 1996.

Tang W, Eisenbrand G, Chinese Drugs of Plant Origin, Springer Verlag Heidelberg 1992.

Teuscher E, Lindequist U, Biogene Gifte - Biologie, Chemie, Pharmakologie, 2. Aufl., Fischer Verlag Stuttgart 1994.

Wagner H, Wiesenauer M, Phytotherapie. Phytopharmaka und pflanzliche Homöopathika, Fischer-Verlag, Stuttgart, Jena, New York 1995.

Wichtl M (Hrsg.), Teedrogen, 4. Aufl., Wiss. Verlagsges. Stuttgart 1997.

Ruta graveolens

See Rue

Saccharomyces cerevisiae

See Brewer's Yeast

Safflower

Carthamus tinctorius

DESCRIPTION

Medicinal Parts: The medicinal parts are the flowers, seeds and the oil extracted from its embryos.

Flower and Fruit: Axillary flowers grow in the leaf axils. They are initially red-yellow, later bright orange. The heads are up to 4 by 3 cm and are encircled by upper leaves. The bracts are light green and have thorny tips with a thorny appendage. The fruit is 6 to 8 cm long, obovate or pear-shaped, and bluntly wedge-shaped at the base with protruding long ribs. The pappus consists of scales.

Leaves, Stem, and Root: Carthamus tinctorius is an annual plant that grows up to 90 cm high. It has a thin fusiform root. The stem is erect, simple, or branched at the top into stiff, glabrous, whitish-yellow, and glossy branches. The leaves are long, fairly soft, and glabrous with a thorny-serrate margin and tip.

Habitat: The plant is said to be indigenous to Iran, northwest India and possibly parts of Africa. It is also found in the Far East and North America, and can be cultivated.

Production: Safflower blooms are the dried flowers of *Carthamus tinctorius*. The flowers are gathered as they begin to wilt, the calyx and inferior ovary are removed, the remainder is put in the shade where it is mildly warm and left to dry. Direct sunlight destroys the coloring pigment. Safflower or thistle oil is the oil extracted from the embryos of the fruits of *Carthamus tinctorius*.

Other Names: American Saffron, Bastard Saffron, Dyer's Saffron, Fake Saffron, Zaffer

ACTIONS AND PHARMACOLOGY

COMPOUNDS: SAFFLOWER FLOWERS

Chalcones and their p-quinones: carthamin (yellow), carthamone (red-orange)

Flavonoids

EFFECTS: SAFFLOWER FLOWERS

No information is available.

COMPOUNDS: SAFFLOWER OIL

Fatty oil: chief fatty acids linoleic acid (55-88%), linolenic acid

Carotinoids

EFFECTS: SAFFLOWER OIL

Safflower oil lowers the serum cholesterol levels.

INDICATIONS AND USAGE

SAFFLOWER FLOWERS

Unproven Uses: In folk medicine, it is mainly used as a stimulant, purgative, antihydrotic, emmenagogue, abortifacient, expectorant, pneumonic, and for tumors. It is also added to teas for soothing coughs and bronchial conditions.

Chinese Medicine: In China, Safflower flowers treat amenorrhea and stomach tumors, as well as for external and internal wounds.

Indian Medicine: The flowers are used for scabies, arthritis, and chest pains.

SAFFLOWER OIL

Unproven Uses: Safflower oil is used for the prophylaxis of arteriosclerosis.

PRECAUTIONS AND ADVERSE REACTIONS

SAFFLOWER FLOWERS AND OIL

General: No health hazards or side effects are known in conjunction with the proper administration of designated therapeutic dosages.

SAFFLOWER FLOWERS

Pregnancy: Not to be used during pregnancy.

DOSAGE

SAFFLOWER FLOWERS

Daily Dosage: The average daily dose is 3 g of decoction; single dose is 1 g.

LITERATURE

SAFFLOWER FLOWER AND OIL

Akihisa T, Yasukawa K, Oinuma H, Kasahara Y, Yamanouchi S, Takido M, Kumaki K, Tamura T, Triterpene alcohols from the flowers of compositae and their anti-inflammatory effects. *Phytochemistry*, 12:1255-60, Dec. 1996

Chan, EH et al., (Eds.), Advances in Chinese Medicinal Materials Research, World Scientific Pub. Co. Singapore 1985.

Kern W, List PH, Hörhammer L (Hrsg.), Hagers Handbuch der Pharmazeutischen Praxis, 4. Aufl., Bde. 1-8, Springer Verlag Berlin, Heidelberg, New York, 1969.

Liu F, Wei Y, Yang XZ, Li FG, Hu J, Cheng RF, Hypotensive effects of safflower yellow in spontaneously hypertensive rats and influence on plasma renin activity and angiotensin II level. *Yao Hsueh Hsueh Pao*, 27:785-7, 1992.

Lu ZW, Liu F, Hu J, Bian D, Li FG, Suppressive effects of safflower yellow on immune functions. *Chung Kuo Yao Li Hsueh Pao*, 12:537-42, Nov. 1991

Martinez Flores H, Cruz Mondragon C, Larios Saldana A Reduction of crude fiber content in safflower meal (*Carthamus tinctorius L*) and its potential use in human food. *Arch Latinoam Nutr,* 284:295-8, Dec. 1996

Nose M, FuJimoto T, Takeda T, Nishibe S, Ogihara Y, Structural transformation of lignan compounds in rat gastrointestinal tract. *Planta Med*, 53:520-3, Dec. 1992

Shi M, Chang L, He G, Stimulating action of *Carthamus tinctorius L. Angelica sinensis (Oliv.) Diels and Leonurus sibiricus L.* on the uterus. *Chung Kuo Chung Yao Tsa Chih,* 20:173-5 192, Mar. 1995

Steinegger E, Hänsel R, Pharmakognosie, 5. Aufl., Springer Verlag Heidelberg 1992.

Teuscher E, Biogene Arzneimittel, 5. Aufl., Wiss. Verlagsges. mbH Stuttgart 1997.

Thomson RH, Naturally Occurring Quinones, 2nd Ed., Academic Press New York 1971.

Yasukawa K et al., Inhibitory effect of alkane-68-diols the components of safflower on tumor promotion by 12-O-tetradecanoylphorbol-13-acetate in two-stage carcinogenesis in mouse skin. *Oncology*, 53:133-6, Mar-Apr. 1996

Zhang HL, Nagatsu A, Watanabe T, Sakakibara J, Okuyama H, Antioxidative compounds isolated from safflower (*Carthamus tinctorius L.*) oil cake. *Chem Pharm Bull* (Tokyo), 45:1910-4, Dec. 1997

Zhang HL, Nagatsu A, Watanabe T, Sakakibara J, Okuyama H, Tinctormine a novel Ca2+ antagonist N-containing quinochalcone C-glycoside from *Carthamus tinctorius L. Chem Pharm Bull* (Tokyo), 45:3355-7, Dec. 1992

Saffron

Crocus sativus

DESCRIPTION

Medicinal Parts: The medicinal parts are the stigma and style.

Flower and Fruit: The lily-like flowers have two 2 bracts at the base. There is a pale violet-veined calyx, yellow anthers, and a white filament. The threadlike style is 10 mm long. The stigma is bright orange. The plant does not bear fruit.

Leaves, Stem, and Root: The grasslike plant is a perennial that grows 8 to 30 cm high. There is a large squat tuber, surrounded by reticulate and fibrous sheaths. The leaves are erect or splayed, narrow, and have a ciliate margin and keel.

Habitat: The plant is indigenous to India, the Balkans and the eastern Mediterranean region. It is cultivated in India, Spain, France, Italy, and the Middle East.

Production: Saffron is produced by drying the brown-red stigma over fire.

Not to be Confused With: The powdered drug is more or less always adulterated; *Calsendula officinalis, Carthamus tinctorius* are usually used.

Other Names: Spanish Saffron

ACTIONS AND PHARMACOLOGY

COMPOUNDS

Apocarotinoid glycosides: in particular crocin (crocetin-beta-digentiobioside), colored intensive yellow orange

Picrocrocin (glycosidic bitter principle, up to 4%): the apocarotinoids and picrocrocin are presumably breakdown products of a carotinoid-digentiobioside-diglucoside (protocrocin)

Volatile oil (0.4 to 1.3%): components 4,5-dehydro-beta-cyclocitral (safranal), 4-hydroxy-beta-cyclocitral (breakdown products of the picrocrocin)

Carotinoids: lycopene, alpha-, beta-, gamma-carotene

Fatty oil

Starch

EFFECTS

Small doses of Saffron stimulate the secretion of the gastric juices. Large doses stimulate the smooth muscle of the uterus.

INDICATIONS AND USAGE

Unproven Uses: Saffron is no longer of interest medicinally. It is sometimes used in folk medicine to stimulate digestion.

Chinese Medicine: Chinese uses include menorrhagia, amenorrhea, high-risk deliveries, and postpartum lochiostasis.

Indian Medicine: In India, Saffron is used for bronchitis, sore throat, headache, vomiting, and fever.

PRECAUTIONS AND ADVERSE REACTIONS

General: Health risks or side effects following the proper administration of designated therapeutic dosages are not recorded.

Pregnancy: The herb is not to be used during pregnancy.

OVERDOSAGE

Lethal poisonings can occur with overdoses or through the abuse of larger doses as an abortient (abortive dosage approximately 10 g, lethal dosage approximately 12 to 20 g). Symptoms of poisoning include vomiting, uterine bleeding, intestinal colic, bloody diarrhea, hematuria, severe schwere purpuras, hemorrhaging of skin of the nose, lips and eyelids, attacks of dizziness, stupor, yellowing of the skin and the mucous membranes (through inclusion of the apocarotinodermas), and central paralysis.

The treatment consists of stomach and intestinal emptying (gastric lavage, sodium sulfate) and the administration of activated charcoal; convulsions to be treated with diazepam, colics with atropine, and any eventual acidosis with sodium bicarbonate infusions. Intubation and oxygen respiration may also be necessary.

DOSAGE

Storage: It is stored in airtight, nonsynthetic containers and protected from light.

LITERATURE

Abdullaev FI. Inhibitory effect of crocetin on intracellular nucleic acid and protein synthesis in malignant cells. *Toxicol Lett.* 70; 243-251. 1994

Alonso GL, Salinas MR, Esteban-Infantes FJ, Sanchez-Fernandez MA. Determination of Safranal from Saffron (*Crocus sativus L.*) by Thermal Desorption-Gas Chromatography. *J Agric Food Chem.* 44 (1); 185-188. 1996

Corti P et al. High Performance Thin Layer Chromatographic Quatitative Analysis of Picrocrocin and Crocetin, Active Principles of Saffron (*Crocus sativus L.-Iridaceae*): A New Method. *Phytochem Anal.* 7; 201-203. 1996

Dufresne C, Cormier F, Dorion S, In vitro formation of crocetin glucosyl esters by *Crocus sativus* callus extract. *Planta Med,* 16:150-3, Apr. 1997

Escribano J, Alonso GL, Coca-Prados M, Fernandez JA, Crocin safranal and picrocrocin from saffron (*Crocus sativus L.*) inhibit the growth of human cancer cells in vitro. *Cancer Lett,* 100:23-30, Feb 27. 1996

Fenaroli's Handbook of Flavor Ingredients, Vol. 1, 2nd Ed., CRC Press 1975.

Frohne D, Pfänder HJ: Giftpflanzen - Ein Handbuch für Apotheker, Toxikologen und Biologen, 4. Aufl., Wiss. Verlagsges. mbH Stuttgart 1997.

Kern W, List PH, Hörhammer L (Hrsg.), Hagers Handbuch der Pharmazeutischen Praxis, 4. Aufl., Bde 1-8, Springer Verlag Berlin, Heidelberg, New York, 1969.

Leung AY, Encyclopedia of Common Natural Ingredients Used in Food Drugs and Cosmetics, John Wiley & Sons Inc., New York 1980.

Lewin L, Gifte und Vergiftungen, 6. Aufl., Nachdruck, Haug Verlag, Heidelberg 1992.

Liakopoulou-Kyriakides M, Skubas AI, Characterization of the platelet aggregation inducer and inhibitor isolated from Crocus sativus. Biochem Int, 22:103-10, 1990 Oct.

Morimoto S et al., Post-harvest degradation of carotenoid glucose esters in saffron. In: *PM* 60(5):438. 1994.

Nair SC, Kurumboor SK, Hasegawa JH, Saffron chemoprevention in biology and medicine: a review. *Cancer Biother*, 5:257-64, Winter. 1995

Nair SC, Pannikar B, Panikkar KR, Antitumor activity of saffron (*Crocus sativus*). *Cancer Lett,* 57:109-14, May 1, 1991

Nair SC, Salomi MJ, Panikkar B, Panikkar KR, Modulatory effects of *Crocus sativus* and *Nigella sativa* extracts on cisplatin-induced toxicity in mice. *J Ethnopharmacol,* 16:75-83, Jan. 1991

Roth L, Daunderer M, Kormann K, Giftpflanzen, Pflanzengifte, 4. Aufl., Ecomed Fachverlag Landsberg Lech 1993.

Salomi MJ, Nair SC, Panikkar KR, Inhibitory effects of *Nigella sativa* and saffron (*Crocus sativus*) on chemical carcinogenesis in mice. *Nutr Cancer,* 16:67-72, 1991.

Steinegger E, Hänsel R, Pharmakognosie, 5. Aufl., Springer Verlag Heidelberg 1992.

Tang W, Eisenbrand G, Chinese Drugs of Plant Origin, Springer Verlag Heidelberg 1992.

Teuscher E, Lindequist U, Biogene Gifte - Biologie, Chemie, Pharmakologie, 2. Aufl., Fischer Verlag Stuttgart 1994.

Teuscher E, Biogene Arzneimittel, 5. Aufl., Wiss. Verlagsges. mbH Stuttgart 1997.

Wichtl M (Hrsg.), Teedrogen, 4. Aufl., Wiss. Verlagsges. Stuttgart 1997.

Sage

Salvia officinalis

DESCRIPTION

Medicinal Parts: The medicinal parts are the fresh leaves and the fresh flowering aerial parts, the dried leaves, and the oils extracted from the flowers and stems.

Flower and Fruit: The medium-sized, pale violet, white or pink labiate flowers are in 6- to 12- blossomed false whorls, which are arranged above each other in 4 to 8 rows. The surrounding leaves fall early. The calyx is 10 to 14 mm long, funnel-shaped, downy, glandular punctate, and bilabiate. The upper lip has 3 throrny-awned teeth; the lower lip has 2. The corolla tube has a ring of hair inside. The upper lip is almost straight and the lower lip has 3 segments. There are 2 stamens with almost semicircular bent filaments.

Leaves, Stem, and Root: Sage grows as a bush up to 60 cm high. The stem is erect and woody at the base with leafy, quadrangular, white-gray tomentose branches. The leaves are simple, oblong or oblong-lanceolate, and narrowed at the base. They are petiolate, densely and finely crenate, ribbed-wrinkled, and white-gray tomentose initially, tough, and evergreen.

Characteristics: The leaves are aromatic, tangy, and bitterly astringent.

Habitat: The plant is indigenous to the Mediterranean region and has naturalized in all of Europe. It is cultivated in North America.

Production: Sage leaf consists of the fresh or dried leaf of *Salvia officinalis.* In the wild, sage is collected from the former Yugoslavia, the Adriatic coast and those areas that are farther from the coast but are still under Mediterranean influence. The harvest lasts from mid-July until December, depending on the area. October is recommended as the most favorable time to harvest Dalmatian sage.

When Sage is cultivated, it is recommended that the harvest take place beginning in the second vegetation year at the beginning of the flowering period and in the afternoon. Sage can be dried in direct sunlight, but up to 25% of the oil can be lost. Drying in shade reduces oil loss to 2 to 10%. Optimum drying conditions for preventing oil loss use a drying chamber with vertical incoming air currents at 50° C with 0.9% absolute humidity.

Not to be Confused With: Confusion can arise with the leaves of *Salvia triloba* and also with Salvia or Phlomis species.

Other Names: Dalmatian Sage, Garden Sage, Greek Sage, Red Sage, Shop Sage

ACTIONS AND PHARMACOLOGY

COMPOUNDS

Volatile oil (1.5-3.5%): chief constituents alpha-thujone and beta-thujone(20-60%), 1,8-cineole (6-16%), camphor (14-37%), borneol, isobutyl acetate, camphene, linalool, alpha- and beta-pinene, viridiflorol, alpha- and beta-caryophyllene (humulene)

Caffeic acid derivatives (3-6%): rosmarinic acid, chlorogenic acid

Diterpenes: chief components carnosolic acid (picrosalvin, 0.2-0.4%), rosmanol, safficinolide

Flavonoids: including, among others, apigenin- and luteolin-7-glucosides, numerous methoxylated aglycones, including among others, genkwanin, genkwanin-6-methylether

Triterpenes: chief components ursolic acid (5%)

EFFECTS

Sage has antibacterial, fungistatic, virostatic, astringent, secretolytic, and perspiration-inhibiting effects. In animal experiments, the herb was found to be antihypertensive and choleretic. It acts on the CNS and is a spasmolytic agent. Proof of an antidiabetic effect found in one study has not yet been confirmed. The essential oil has bactericidal, fungistatic, and virostatic.

INDICATIONS AND USAGE

Approved by Commission E:

- Loss of appetite
- Inflammation of the mouth and pharynx
- Excessive perspiration

Sage is used externally for inflammation of the mucous membranes of the nose and throat and internally for dyspeptic symptoms, and as a diaphoretic.

Unproven Uses: In folk medicine, the drug is used internally for gastric disorders such as bloating, flatulence, diarrhea, and enteritis. Externally, Sage is used as a rinse and gargle for light injuries and skin inflammation, bleeding gums, stomatitis, laryngitis, pharyngitis, and for firming the gums.

Homeopathic Uses: The most common application in homeopathy is for excessive perspiration.

CONTRAINDICATIONS

Sage preparations are contraindicated during pregnancy.

PRECAUTIONS AND ADVERSE REACTIONS

General: No health hazards or side effects are known in conjunction with the proper administration of designated therapeutic dosages.

Pregnancy: Sage preparations should not be taken during pregnancy.

OVERDOSAGE

A sense of heat, tachycardia, feelings of vertigo and epileptiform convulsions can occur following extended intake of ethanolic extracts of the drug or volatile oil, or through overdosage (corresponding to more than 15 g of the sage leaves).

DOSAGE

Mode of Administration: Cut herb for infusions, alcoholic extracts, and distillates for gargles, rinses, and other topical applications such as compresses or poultices. The pressed juice of fresh plants is also used. In folk medicine, Sage is used internally as an antihidrotic infusion and ''medicinal cigarettes'' are used for asthma.

How Supplied: Sage is available as an alcohol-free 1:1 liquid.

Preparation:

Tincture — prepared 1:10 with 70% ethanol.

Liquid extract — 1:1 with 45% ethanol.

The formulas for several ''generic'' folk medicine decoctions and infusions follows.

Decoction No. 1 — One spoonful of powdered drug scalded with 1 cup of water, quickly strained, and sweetened.

Decoction No. 2 — 15 g of the fresh leaves with 200 mL of water heated for 3 minutes.

Infusion No.1 — Scald 20 g dried leaves with 1 liter water, steep for 15 minutes, strain, press, and sweeten if required.

Infusion No. 2 — Pour 1 liter boiling water over 50 g drug, strain after 15 minutes and sweeten with honey.

Antihidrotic infusion — Scald 20 g of the dried leaves with 1 liter water, steep 15 minutes, strain, compress and sweeten if required.

Cardiac insufficiency — A tonic infusion is prepared by pouring 1 liter boiling water over 50 g of the drug, strain after 15 minutes, sweeten with sugar or honey.

Diabetes — Prepare a fortified wine made by boiling 100 g of the leaves with one liter wine for 2 minutes.

Inflammation of the bronchial mucous membranes — An expectorant honey is made by mixing 50 g of the powdered drug with 80 g of honey.

Nervous exhaustion — A fortified wine is manufactured using an 8-day maceration of 100 g of the leaves with one liter of wine.

Tumors — The drug is worked into an ointment base or pounded into a paste together with salt and vinegar to make an adhesive paste.

Wounds — The drug is prepared as a cleanser or rinse to heal wounds using a wine made by heating 100 g of the leaves with 0.5 liter white wine for 1 minute.

Daily Dosage: The average daily internal dose is 4 to 6 g of the drug; 0.1 to 0.3 g of the essential oil; 2.5 to 7.5 g of the tincture; 1.5 to 3 g of the liquid extract.

Antihidrotic — 0.25 g of the powdered drug (spoonful or capsules) taken before meals for excessive perspiration and nervous complaints.

Cardiac insufficiency — 1 glass of the tonic infusion can be taken 4 times daily. The decoction dosage (using No. 1 or No. 2) is 1 glass at hourly intervals.

Diabetes — 1 glass of the wine preparation after meals.

Halitosis — The leaves may be chewed occasionally.

Inflammation of the bronchial mucous membranes — 1 spoonful of the expectorant in the morning and at bedtime.

Nervous complaints — 0.25 g of the powdered drug (spoonful or capsules) before meals.

Externally, the following dosages/applications are often used:

Antihidrotic infusion — 200 mL of infusion 1 to three times daily.

Gargles and rinses — 2.5 g of the drug or 2 to 3 drops of essential oil in 100 mL of water as infusion or 5 g of the alcoholic extract in 1 glass of water.

Inflamed mucous membranes — Undiluted alcohol extract is applied repeatedly.

Homeopathic Dosage: 5 drops, 1 tablet, or 10 globules every 30 to 60 minutes (acute) or 1 to 3 times daily (chronic); parenterally: 1 to 2 ml sc acute: 3 times daily; chronic: once a day (HAB1), Special doses must be prepared for children.

Storage: Sage leaves are to be protected from light and humidity in sealed containers. Storage duration of coarsely cut drug is 18 months; powder, maximum 24 hours. The tincture is stored in tightly sealed containers away from light. The liquid extract may be kept for up to 2 years.

LITERATURE

Baricevic D et al. Topical anti-inflammatory activity of *Salvia officinalis L.* leaves: the relevance of ursolic acid. *J Ethnopharmacol* 75(2-3); 125-132. 2001

Darmati Z et al. 12-Deoxo-carnosol isolated from the wild type of sage from Dalmatia. *J Serb Chem Soc.* 59; 291-299. 1994

Darmati Z, Jankov RM, Djordjevic A, Ribar B, Lazar D, EngelP. Carnosic Acid 12-Methyl-Ether-gamma-Lactone, a Ferrugineol-Type Diterpene from *Salvia officinalis. Phytochemistry* 31; 1307-1309. 1992

Ivanic R, Savin K. A Comparative Analysis of Essential Oils from Several Wild Species of Salvia. *Planta Med.* 30; 25-31. 1976

Länger R, Mechtler C, Jurenitsch J. Composition of the Essential Oils of Commercial Samples of *Salvia officinalis L.* and *S. fruticosa Miller*: A Comparison of Oils Obtained by Extraction and Steam Distillation. Phytochem Anal. 7; 289-293. 1996

Länger R, Mechtler C, Tanzler HO, Jurenitsch J, Differences of the composition of the essential oil within an individium of *Salva officinalis.* In: PM 59(7):A635. 1993.

Males Z, Medic-Saric M. Optimisation of thin-layer chromatographic analysis of flavonoids and phenolic acids of *Salviae folium. Acta Pharm.* 48; 85-92. 1998

Paris A, Strukelj B, Renko M, Turk V, Puki M, Umek A, Korant BD, Inhibitory effect of carnosolic acid on HIV-1 protease in cell free assays. In: *JNP* 56(8):1426-1430. 1993.

Tada M et al., Antiviral diterpenes from *Salvia officinalis.* In: *PH* 35(2):539. 1994.

Vaverkova S, Holla M, Tekel J. The effect of herbocides on the qualitative properties of healing plants / Part 2: Content and composition of the essential oil from *Salvia officinalis L.* after application of Aflon(R) 50 WP. *Pharmazie* 50; 143-144. 1995

Salep

Orchis species

DESCRIPTION

Medicinal Parts: The medicinal parts of the plant are the tubers.

Flower and Fruit: The flowers form erect spikes. The surrounding leaves are sometimes large and longer than the flowers; they are often colored. The pollen mass is enclosed in 1 to 2 sectioned anthers. The ovary is almost always twisted. The seed skins can be with or without a reticulate thickening.

Leaves, Stem, and Root: The species are perennial, medium-sized, glabrous plants with a round, ovate or variously palmate tuber. The leaves are green, sheathlike, and tapering.

Habitat: The plant comes from central and southern Europe.

Production: Salep tubers are the subterranean parts of *Orchis morio* and other varieties of Orchis. They are gathered during flowering season, dried and processed into Salep powder.

Other Names: Cuckoo Flower, Levant Salep, Orchid, Sahlep, Saloop, Satyrion

ACTIONS AND PHARMACOLOGY

COMPOUNDS

Mucilage (Salep mannan, up to 50%): glucans, glucomannans (partially acetylized)

Starch (25%)

Proteins (5-15%)

EFFECTS

The mucilage is rich in mucine and polysaccharides, which act as a demulcent and have protective and sequestering effects on mucous membranes. In animal tests, a lowering of the plasma cholesterol effect was proved. In addition, the drug is said to be analgesic, cholagogic, and hypoglycemic, but no further details are available.

INDICATIONS AND USAGE

Unproven Uses: The drug is used for unspecified diarrhea, particularly in children, and for heartburn, flatulence, and indigestion.

Indian Medicine: Uses in Indian medicine include diabetes, hemiplegia, chronic diarrhea, neurasthenia, and general debility.

PRECAUTIONS AND ADVERSE REACTIONS

No health hazards or side effects are known in conjunction with the proper administration of designated therapeutic dosages.

DOSAGE

Mode of Administration: As a powdered formulation in medicinal preparations.

Daily Dosage: Dosage for commercial pharmaceutical preparations for heartburn, flatulence and indigestion is often 1 teaspoon of powder stirred into a glass of warm water and drunk before or after meals.

LITERATURE

Kern W, List PH, Hörhammer L (Hrsg.), Hagers Handbuch der Pharmazeutischen Praxis, 4. Aufl., Bde 1-8: Springer Verlag Berlin, Heidelberg, New York, 1969.

Steinegger E, Hänsel R, Pharmakognosie, 5. Aufl., Springer Verlag Heidelberg 1992.

Salix species

See White Willow

Salvia miltiorrhiza

See Red-Rooted Sage (Dan-Shen)

Salvia officinalis

See Sage

Salvia triloba

See Greek Sage

Sambucus ebulus

See Dwarf Elder

Sambucus nigra

See European Elder

Samphire

Crithmum maritimum

DESCRIPTION

Medicinal Parts: The aerial parts of the plant are the medicinal parts.

Flower and Fruit: The 10 to 20 radiating umbels are medium-sized, sturdy, and domed. The 1-mm long petals are yellow or greenish-white. The style is very short and barely visible. The fruit is ovate-oblong. The fruit wall is thick and filled with a spongy, air-retaining tissue.

Leaves, Stem, and Root: The plant is a perennial, glabrous shrub with woody base. The root is long, cylindrical, thick, hard, knotty, ringed, gray, branching upward, and polycephalous. The stem is erect, 20 to 50 cm high, round, tender, grooved, hollowed, woody, and has fewer branches higher up. The leaves are sea green, fleshy, and glossy.

Habitat: The plant grows on the Atlantic, Mediterranean, and Baltic coasts.

Production: Samphire herb is the above-ground part of *Crithmum maritimum.*

Other Names: Crest Marine, Peter's Cress, Pierce-Stone, Sampier, Sea Fennel

ACTIONS AND PHARMACOLOGY

COMPOUNDS

Volatile oil

Polyynes: including falcarindiol

Furanocoumarins

Ascorbic acid (high content)

EFFECTS

Samphire is a diuretic and also a source of vitamin C.

INDICATIONS AND USAGE

Unproven Uses: The herb is used for scurvy and states of general immune resistance.

PRECAUTIONS AND ADVERSE REACTIONS

Health risks or side effects following the proper administration of designated therapeutic dosages are not recorded.

DOSAGE

Mode of Administration: Samphire is used internally and is available as an extract and a food additive.

LITERATURE

Coiffard L, Piron-Frenet M, Amicel L. Geographical variations of the constituents of the essential oil of *Crithmum maritimum L., Apiaceae. Int J Cosmet Sci.* 15; 15-21. 1993

Guil JL, Torija ME, Gimenez JJ, Rodriguez-Garcia I, Gimenez A. Oxalic Acid and Calcium Determination in Wild Edible Plants. *J Agric Food Chem.* 44 (7); 1821-1823. 1996

Hegnauer R, Chemotaxonomie der Pflanzen, Bde 1-11, Birkhäuser Verlag Basel, Boston, Berlin 1962-1997.

Sandalwood

Santalum album

DESCRIPTION

Medicinal Parts: The medicinal parts are the oil extracted from the trunk wood, the heartwood freed from the sapwood and the bark, and the dried wood.

Flower and Fruit: The flowers are in numerous, small, short pedicled, odorless, erect paniculate inflorescences. There is no calyx. The perianth is 4 to 5 mm long, campanulate, and changes from yellow to deep red. There are 4 stamens at the mouth of the tube, which have simple hairs at their base. The semi-inferior ovary with 3 ovules is free in the bud and later enclosed in the disc. The fruit is a round, black, pea-sized drupe with a crown comprised of the perianth remains.

Leaves, Stem, and Root: The plant is a small evergreen tree up to 10 m high that flowers the whole year round. It has smooth bark and pendulous branches. The leaves are opposite, 4 to 6 cm long and 2 cm wide, lanceolate, entire-margined, and matte underneath. The petiole is approximately 1 cm long.

Characteristics: The wood has a characteristic odor.

Habitat: The tree grows wild in India and also is cultivated there and on Timor and the Sunda Islands.

Production: Sandalwood consists of the heartwood, the trunk and branches of *Santalum album* or *Pterocarpus santalinius*, which has been freed from the bark and sapwood.

Not to be Confused With: Confusion can arise with other sandalwoods, i.e. the heartwood of *Pterocarpus santalinus*. The white sapwood, which contains almost no essential oil, is occasionally marketed as Lignum santali albi. The brownish-yellow to brown-red root wood is, in contrast, rich in essential oil, but is disallowed as a drug in EB6.

Other Names: Sanderswood, White Saunders, Yellow Saunders

ACTIONS AND PHARMACOLOGY

COMPOUNDS

Volatile oil (3-5%): chief components santalols (50% cis-alpha-santalol, 20% cis-beta-santalol, 4% epi-beta-santalol), further including among others, alpha-bergamotol, alpha-bergamotal

Tannins

Resins

EFFECTS

The essential oil of Sandalwood has disinfecting effect on the urinary tract. However, if used in high doses and for long periods, it can be toxic to the kidneys.

INDICATIONS AND USAGE

Approved by Commission E:

■ Infections of the urinary tract

Sandalwood is used for inflammatory conditions of the efferent urinary tract. It is generally used in combination with other diuretic or urinary disinfecting drugs.

Chinese Medicine: The Chinese use Sandalwood primarily for epigastric pain, chest pain, and vomiting.

Indian Medicine: Internal uses include heat stroke, sunstroke, and resulting fever. It is used as an infusion mixed with honey (in Kerala); with water cooked in rice (in Nepal); in the treatment of gonorrhea and as an anti-aphrodisiac in ayurvedic medicine.

Homeopathic Uses: Uses of the drug in homeopathy include urethral inflammation. It is advisable to use Sandalwood in combination with other diuretic or urinary disinfecting drugs.

CONTRAINDICATIONS

Sandalwood is contraindicated in diseases of the kidney.

PRECAUTIONS AND ADVERSE REACTIONS

No health hazards are known in conjunction with the proper administration of designated therapeutic dosages. Intake can occasionally lead to skin itching, queasiness, gastrointestinal complaints, and hematuria. The drug possesses minimal potential for sensitization.

DOSAGE

Mode of Administration: Sandalwood is used internally in preparations derived from comminuted drug.

Preparation: Sandalwood oil should only be taken in an enteric-coated form.

Daily Dosage: The average daily dose is 10 g of the drug; 1 to 1.5 g of the essential oil.

Homeopathic Dosage: 5 drops, 1 tablet, or 10 globules every 30 to 60 minutes (acute) or 1 to 3 times daily (chronic); parenterally: 1 to 2 mL sc acute: 3 times daily; chronic: once a day (HAB34).

LITERATURE

Adams DR et al., *Phytochemistry* 14:1459 1975.

Demole DR et al., *Helv Chim Acta* 59:737. 1976

Hänsel R, Keller K, Rimpler H, Schneider G (Hrsg.), Hagers Handbuch der Pharmazeutischen Praxis, 5. Aufl., Bde 4-6 (Drogen), Springer Verlag Berlin, Heidelberg, New York, 1992-1994.

Lewin L, Gifte und Vergiftungen, 6. Aufl., Nachdruck, Haug Verlag, Heidelberg 1992.

Madaus G, Lehrbuch der Biologischen Arzneimittel, Bde 1-3, Nachdruck, Georg Olms Verlag Hildesheim 1979.

Patnikar SK, Naik CG, *Tetrahedron Letters* 15:1293. 1975

Roth L, Daunderer M, Kormann K, Giftpflanzen, Pflanzengifte, 4. Aufl., Ecomed Fachverlag Landsberg Lech 1993.

Steinegger E, Hänsel R, Pharmakognosie, 5. Aufl., Springer Verlag Heidelberg 1992.

Wagner H, Wiesenauer M, Phytotherapie. Phytopharmaka und pflanzliche Homöopathika, Fischer-Verlag, Stuttgart, Jena, New York 1995.

Sandarac

Tetraclinis articulata

DESCRIPTION

Medicinal Parts: The medicinal parts of the plant are the naturally flowing resin and the bark.

Flowers and Fruit: The inflorescences are apical on the lateral branches and conical. The male flowers are 4 to 5 mm wide. There are 4 stamens with very short filaments and scalelike anthers. The female flowers are very small, with 4 scales in 2 pairs arranged like whorls. The upper surface of the flower is fleshy, with a swelling at the base almost completely covering the ovules, which are on woody, dark-brown, 12-mm long cone scales. The seeds are narrow ovoid with large, membranous wings on both sides.

Leaves, Stem, and Root: Tetraclinis articulata grows as a monoclinous, monoecious evergreen shrub or tree, reaching a height of up to 12 m. The leaves are opposite, scaly, long, and down-turned. They grow close together in groups of 2 pairs on young branches in whorls. The branches are jointed and somewhat pressed together.

Habitat: North Africa, particularly Morocco and Algeria

Production: Sandarac gum is the resin that flows naturally from the branches and bark of *Tetraclines articulata.*

Other Names: Arartree, Alerce, Gharghar, Sandarac Gum Tree

ACTIONS AND PHARMACOLOGY

COMPOUNDS

Diterpenes (95%): diterpene acids: including pimaric acid, callitrolic acid, sandaracinic acid, sandaracinolic acid, sandaracolic acid, callitrisinic acid

Bitter substances

Volatile oil (1.3%): including alpha- and beta-pinene, limonene, thymoquinone

EFFECTS

The resin is said to be antibacterial and bacteriostatic in effect. Experimental data supporting these effects are not available.

INDICATIONS AND USAGE

Unproven Uses: Folk medicine uses include fever and diarrhea.

PRECAUTIONS AND ADVERSE REACTIONS

No health hazards are known in conjunction with the proper administration of designated therapeutic dosages.

DOSAGE

Mode of Administration: Whole and cut drug is either inhaled or used in the form of compresses.

LITERATURE

Ait Igri M, Holeman M, Ilidrissi A, Berrada M. Contribution a l'Etude chimique des Huiles essentielles des Rameaux et du Bois de Tetraclinis articulata (Vahl) Masters. *Plant med et phyt.* 24; 36-43. 1990

Blaschek W, Hänsel R, Keller K, Reichling J, Rimpler G, Schneider G (Eds), Hagers Handbuch der Pharmazeutischen Praxis. Folgebände 1 und 2. Drogen A-Z. Springer. Berlin, Heidelberg 1998.

Sanguinaria canadensis

See Bloodroot

Sanguisorba officinalis

See Great Burnet

Sanicula europaea

See European Sanicle

Santalum album

See Sandalwood

Santolina chamaecyparissias

See Lavender Cotton

Saponaria officinalis

See Soapwort

Sarracenia purpurea

See Pitcher Plant

Sarsaparilla

Smilax species

DESCRIPTION

Medicinal Parts: The medicinal parts are the dried roots, the entire underground part, and the tuberous swellings produced by the runners.

Flower and Fruit: The flowers are white to pale green, yellow, or brown. They are dioecious, usually in axillary cymes or racemes, and contain 6 petals in 2 circles. The ovate to lanceolate tepals are curved outward. The male flowers have 6 stamens with thick filaments and anthers, which are fused at the base of the petals. The female flowers have 6 (sometimes only 3) staminoids. The ovate ovary has 3 carpels, each with 1 to 2 atropic ovules and with an almost sessile, bent-back, triple-lobed stigma. The fruit is a globular, red, blue, or black berry with 1 to 6 seeds.

Leaves, Stem, and Root: The species are evergreen shrubs or semishrubs with climbing branches and stipular tendrils. They have a short, gnarled, perennial, creeping or ascending rhizome with numerous long roots stretching over many meters. The branched, thorny, nodular stem has the thickness of an arm and is yellowish-green. The leaves are in 2 rows. They are alternate, simple, and often hardy, with 3 to 5 reticulately joined main ribs. The leaf sheaths are ovate and cordate, sagittate and petiolate, or often stipulelike. They turn into climbing tendrils above and break off at this point when they die.

Habitat: The species is indigenous to tropical and subtropical regions of America, eastern Asia and India. In Europe, only the variety *S aspera* is found in the Mediterranean region.

Production: Sarsaparilla consists of the dried root of Smilax species, such as *Smilax aristolochiaefolii*, *Smilax regelii* and *Smilax febrifuga*. The plant is collected in the wild from January to May. The roots are cut up and air-dried.

Not to be Confused With: Adulterations and mistaken identity often occurs among the Smilax species.

ACTIONS AND PHARMACOLOGY

COMPOUNDS

Steroid saponins (0.5-3%): chief components are sarsaparilloside, along with parillin, as a breakdown product; also including desglucoparillin, desglucorhamnoparillin, and aglycones sarsapogenin

EFFECTS

The steroid saponins in the drug are responsible for its irritating effect on the skin and the strong diuretic and diaphoretic effect in high doses, as well as its effect as an emulsifier and foam stabilizer.

INDICATIONS AND USAGE

Unproven Uses: Preparations of Sarsaparilla root are used for skin diseases, psoriasis, rheumatic complaints, kidney diseases, and as a diuretic and diaphoretic.

Homeopathic Uses: In homeopathy Smilax is used for itching skin rashes, rheumatism, and inflammation of the urinary organs.

PRECAUTIONS AND ADVERSE REACTIONS

No health hazards are known in conjunction with the proper administration of designated therapeutic dosages. Stomach complaints and queasiness may occur in rare cases, as could kidney irritation.

DOSAGE

How Supplied:

Capsules: 425 mg

Tincture

Daily Dosage: Powder: 0.3 to 1.5 g drug; tea: 3 cups daily with meals; cold water extract: 500 mL mornings and evenings; decoction: 1 to 5 g 3 times daily; tincture: 5 to 15 g per day; liquid extract: 8 to 15 mL

Homeopathic Dosage: 5 drops, 1 tablet, or 10 globules every 30 to 60 minutes (acute) or 1 to 3 times daily (chronic); parenterally: 1 to 2 mL sc, acute: 3 times daily; chronic: once a day (HAB34)

LITERATURE

Bernardo RR, Pinto AV, Parente JP. Steroidal saponins from *Smilax officinalis. Phyto chemistry*, 43:465-9, Sep 1996

Chen G, Shen L, Jiang P. Flavanonol glucosides of *Smilax glabra* Roxb. *Chung Kuo Chung Yao Tsa Chih*, 21:355-7 383, Jun 1996

Fukunaga T, Miura T, Furuta K, Kato A. Hypoglycemic effect of the rhizomes of *Smilax glabra* in normal and diabetic mice. *Biol Pharm Bull*, 20:44-6, Jan 1997

Thurmon FM, *N Engl J Med* 227(4):128. 1942

Tschesche R, In: Pharmacognosy, Phytochemistry, Ed. H Wagner, L Hörhammer, Pub. Springer-Verlag. 1971

Sassafras

Sassafras albidum

DESCRIPTION

Medicinal Parts: The medicinal parts are the essential oil of the root wood, the peeled and dried root bark, and the root wood.

Flower and Fruit: The flowers appear before the leaves. They are dioecious, small and yellowish, and form loose cymes. The perigone has 6 tepals. The male flower has 6 filaments and the female has 1 ovate ovary and 6 bent stamens. The fruit is a pea-sized, oval drupe that is dark blue when ripe and appears in the beaker-shaped receptacle.

Leaves, Stem, and Root: Sassafras albidum is a deciduous tree up to 30 m tall with numerous branches. The bark of the trunk and of the thicker branches is rough, deeply grooved, and grayish. The bark of the outer branches is green. The alternate leaves are petiolate and 7 to 12 cm long. Some are simple ovate, others deeply 2- or 3-lobed. The root bark is a bright, rusty-brown, and its irregular pieces are soft, brittle, and corky. They grow in distinct layers and show numerous oil glands. The root itself is brownish-white with clear concentric rings traversed by narrow medullary rays.

Characteristics: The taste is sweet and slightly astringent and the odor is pleasantly aromatic. Sassafras's carcinogenic effect, however, has made its use inadvisable.

Habitat: The plant is common to eastern North America, Mexico, and Taiwan.

Production: Sassafras wood is the root wood of *Sassafras albidium*. The woody roots (up to 20 cm thick) are dug up in autumn, then shredded or cut into cubes. The wood must not be moistened when being cut because moisture will cause a deterioration of smell and taste in the later drying process.

Not to be Confused With: Sassafras root wood is sometimes confused with the wood of the tree's trunk, which has distinctive annual ring growth and marrow, or with the bark, which has calculus and primary fibers. Another difference is that the trunk wood and bark have little smell or taste.

Other Names: Ague Tree, Cinnamon Wood, Saloop, Sassafrax, Saxifrax

ACTIONS AND PHARMACOLOGY

COMPOUNDS

Volatile oil (6-9%): chief components safrole (up to 90%), 5-methoxyeugenol (up to 30%), asarone (up to 18%), camphor (up to 5%)

Isoquinoline alkaloids: representatives of the aporphine and reticuline type (less than 0.1%)

EFFECTS

The drug is said to have a mild diuretic effect, which is undocumented. The toxic characteristics are determined by the essential oil, which contains safrole (sassafras aetheroleum that is hepatatoxic and carcinogenic).

INDICATIONS AND USAGE

Unproven Uses: Sassafras is considered obsolete, but previously was used for disorders of the urinary tract. The drug, which was formerly an ingredient of "blood-cleaning tea," has also been used for skin disorders, inflammation of the mucous membranes, rheumatism, and syphilis.

PRECAUTIONS AND ADVERSE REACTIONS

Because of the carcinogenic effect of the safrole, neither the drug nor its volatile oil should be administered.

DOSAGE

Mode of Administration: The drug is a constituent of tea mixtures.

Storage: Keep Sassafras in a tightly sealed tin container.

LITERATURE

Albert K, Sassafrasöl zum Abtanzen? In: *PZ* 142(11):878. 1997.

Brophy JJ, Goldsack RJ, House APN, Lassak EV, *J Ess Oil Res* 5:117-122. 1993.

Chowdhury BK et al., *Phytochemistry* 15:1803. 1976

Kamdem DP et al., Chemical composition of essential oil from the root bark of *Sassafras albidum*. In: *PM* 61(6):574-575. 1995.

Kampen KR van, Sudan grass and sorghum poisoning of horse: a possible lathyrogenic disease. In: *J Am Vet Medic Assoc* 156, 629-630. 1970.

Miller EC et al., *Cancer Res* 43:1124 1983.

Segelman AB et al., *JAMA*. 236:477. 1976

Sassafras albidum

See Sassafras

Satureja hortensis

See Summer Savory

Saussurea costus

See Costus

Savin Tops

Juniperus sabina

DESCRIPTION

Medicinal Parts: The medicinal parts are the essential oil of the leaves and branch tips; the dried leafy branch tips; the fresh, youngest nonwoody branch tips with leaves; and the branches and leaves.

Flower and Fruit: The male and female flowers are at the end of the twigs, which are covered in leaf-scales. The male flowers are up to 2 mm wide and oblong to ovate. The female flowering branch bears the flowers erect when in bloom, later curved inward. The flowers have 4 carpels, which develop into pea-sized berry-cones with 4 ovate seeds. The seeds are ovate and striped with numerous edges.

Leaves, Stem, and Root: It is generally a 4.5-m high, dioecious, evergreen shrub with either an erect trunk, an irregular crown, or numerous low-lying branches with erect tips. The bark of the young branches are light brown, more mature branches are red-brown and peeling. The young plants up to 10 years have only needlelike 4-mm long, blue-green leaves whose tips stand out. Mature plants have triangular, scalelike, imbricate leaves.

Habitat: Found in southern and central Europe, the Caucasus and the southern mountains of Asian Russia, as well as in the northern U.S.

Production: Savin Tops is the young shoots and twig tips of *Juniperus sabina*.

Other Names: Savin, Savine

ACTIONS AND PHARMACOLOGY

COMPOUNDS

Volatile oil (3-5%): chief components sabinyl acetate, sabinene, further including among others beta-myrcene, terpin-4-ol, gamma-terpinene, alpha-pinene, limonene

Lignans: including among others deoxypodorhizone, deoxypodophyllotoxin, junaphtoinsäure, deoxypicropodophyllotoxin, and dehydropodophyllotoxin

Hydroxycoumarins: including among others cumarsabine, 8-methoxycumarsabine, siderin, 4-methoxy-5-methylcoumarin-propiophenone

Propiophenone derivatives: including among others 2-hydroxy-3,4-dimethoxy-6-methyl-propiophenone

EFFECTS

The drug is hyperemic both internally and externally, and is a strong irritant to the skin and mucous membranes. Lignans are also said to have antineoplastic and antiviral properties: The main substance is 3 to 5% essential oil with thujon acting as the principal ingredient, along with containing podophyllotoxin and other lignans.

A diuretic effect has been described for the essential oil and the drug is also said to be emmenagogic and hemostyptic.

The use of the drug on viral warts seems justified because of the podophyllotoxin content.

INDICATIONS AND USAGE

Unproven Uses: For external use only, in the treatment of venereal warts.

Homeopathic Uses: Juniperus sabina is used for metrorrhagia, gout, inflammation of the urogenital tract, rheumatism, and warts.

PRECAUTIONS AND ADVERSE REACTIONS

The drug is severely toxic. External administration, in particular of the volatile oil, can lead to severe skin irritation, blister formation, necroses, and resorbent poisonings.

OVERDOSAGE

One is cautioned against internal administration of the drug and of the volatile oil. Fatal poisonings have occurred repeatedly following administration of the drug in either powder form or infusion as an abortifacient. Symptoms include, among others, queasiness, cardiac rhythm disorders, spasm, kidney damage, and hematuria. Central paralysis, coma, and death ensue. The internal administration of 6 drops of the volatile oil is life-threatening for humans.

Following gastrointestinal emptying, (inducement of vomiting, gastric lavage, sodium sulfate) and instillation of activated charcoal, the therapy for poisonings consists of treating spasms with diazepam (IV), colic with atropine, electrolyte substitution and treating possible cases of acidosis with sodium bicarbonate infusions. Monitoring of kidney function, blood coagulation and liver values is essential. Intubation and oxygen respiration may also be necessary. The level of danger depends upon the age of the drug of the volatile oil, as the toxicity probably develops chiefly through the formation of terpene peroxides during storage. The fresh tips of the branches contain presumably very little toxicity.

DOSAGE

Mode of Administration: For external use, as a powdered drug. Internal application is obsolete because of the danger of intoxication.

Daily Dosage: maximum 1 g externally.

Savin Tops powder - Powder twice daily, put bandages into the folds of skin.

Skin ointment - Average content: 50% drug.

Homeopathic Dosage: 5 drops, 1 tablet, or 10 globules every 30 to 60 minutes (acute) or 1 to 3 times daily (chronic); parenterally: 1 to 2 mL sc acute, 3 times daily; chronic: once a day (HAB1).

LITERATURE

Banthorpe DV, Davies HF, Gatford C, Williams SR. Monoterpene pattern in *Juniperus* and *Thuja* species. *Planta Med.* 23; 64-69. 1973

Feliciano AS, Del Corral JMM, Gordaliza M, Castro A, Acid and phenolic lignans from *Juniperus sabina*. In: *PH* 30: 3483-3485. 1991.

Fournier G et al., Contribution to the Study of the Essential Oil of Various Cultivars of *Juniperus sabina. Planta Med.* 57;392-393 1991.

Frohne D, Pfänder HJ, Giftpflanzen - Ein Handbuch für Apotheker, Toxikologen und Biologen, 4. Aufl., Wiss. Verlags-Ges. Stuttgart 1997.

Hänsel R, Keller K, Rimpler H, Schneider G (Hrsg.), Hagers Handbuch der Pharmazeutischen Praxis, 5. Aufl., Bde 4-6 (Drogen): Springer Verlag Berlin, Heidelberg, New York, 1992-1994.

Lewin L, Gifte und Vergiftungen, 6. Aufl., Nachdruck, Haug Verlag, Heidelberg 1992.

Madaus G, Lehrbuch der Biologischen Arzneimittel, Bde 1-3, Nachdruck, Georg Olms Verlag Hildesheim 1979.

Roth L, Daunderer M, Kormann K, Giftpflanzen, Pflanzengifte, 4. Aufl., Ecomed Fachverlag Landsberg Lech 1993.

Steinegger E, Hänsel R, Pharmakognosie, 5. Aufl., Springer Verlag Heidelberg 1992.

Teuscher E, Lindequist U, Biogene Gifte - Biologie, Chemie, Pharmakologie, 2. Aufl., Fischer Verlag Stuttgart 1994.

Saw Palmetto

Serenoa repens

DESCRIPTION

Medicinal Parts: The medicinal parts are the partially dried ripe fruit, the ripe fresh fruit, and the ripe dried fruit.

Flower and Fruit: The inconspicuous cream flowers are in short, densely pubescent, paniculately branched inflorescences. The fruit is deep purple to almost black. It is an ovate, 3 cm long, 1-seeded berry. It has a hard but fragile pericarp that covers a pale brown, spongy pulp. The endocarp is thin and papery. The fruit is slightly wrinkled, 1.25 to 2.5 cm long and 1.25 cm in diameter. The hard seed is pale brown, oval or globular, and has a hilum near the base. The whole panicle can weigh up to 4 kg.

Leaves, Stem and Root: The plant is a bushy palm with a maximum height of 6 m. The large, yellow-green leaves have up to 20 segments and form a crown.

Characteristics: The taste of the seeds is soapy and unpleasant.

Habitat: The plant is indigenous to the coastal regions of the southern states of the U.S., from South Carolina to Florida and southern California.

Other Names: Sabal, Shrub Palmetto

ACTIONS AND PHARMACOLOGY

COMPOUNDS

Steroids: Sterols, including beta-sitosterol, beta-sitosterol-3-O-glucosides, beta-sitosterol-3-O-diglucoside, beta-sitosterol-fatty acid esters and their glucosides, for example beta-sitosterol-3-O-myristate, beta-sitosterol-3-O-(6-O-myristyl-beta-glucosides)

Flavonoids: including isoquercitrin, kaempferol-3-O-glucosides, rhoifolin

Water-soluble polysaccharides (galactoarabane with uronic acid)

Fatty oil: free fatty acids

The lipophilic components (fatty oil with phytosterines) can be found in ethanolic and hexane extracts. The anti-exudative components (polysaccharides) are found in aqueous extracts. Ethanolic extracts contain both component groups.

EFFECTS

In human studies, Saw Plametto's mechanism of action in the treatment of benign prostate hyperplasia (BPH) may have multiple sites of action and involves antiandrogenic, antiestrogenic, and estrogenic properties. Saw Plametto has been historically used as a treatment for prostate enlargement and chronic cystitis as well as a mild diuretic.

Antiandrogenic Effects

The lipophilic extract of the herb inhibits binding of dihydrotestosterone (DHT) to the cytosolic androgenic receptor and alpha1-adrenoceptor in the prostate, thus preventing accumulation of the steroid, which may lead to prostate hyperplasia (Carilla, 1984; Goepel, 1999). Antiandrogenic effects of the lipophilic extract also consist of 5-alpha-reductase and 3-ketosteroid reductase inhibition. These enzymes are responsible for the conversion of testosterone to DHT and for conversion of DHT to an androgen compound, respectively (Sultan, 1984).

Antiestrogenic Effects

The herb lowers cytosol and nuclear receptor values for estrogen, which result in an antiestrogen effect since progesterone receptor content is linked to estrogenic activity. Antiestrogenic agents inhibit stromatic prostate mass growth in patients with benign prostate hypertrophy (DiSilverio, 1992). There is also some evidence with inhibition of several steps involved in prolactin receptor signal transduction in ovary cells (Vacher, 1995).

Anti-Inflammatory Effects

The hexane extracts of the herb have demonstrated anti-inflammatory activity (Champault, 1984). Inhibition of the synthesis of arachidonic acid inflammatory metabolites, through a double blocking of cyclooxygenase and 5-lipoxygenase pathways, results in anti-inflammatory properties. (Breu, 1992). The drug also contains antispasmodic properties by inhibiting calcium influx and activation of the sodium/calcium ion exchanger. Induction of protein synthesis plays a role in the antispasmotic effect with cyclic AMP as a possible mediator. Extracts of the drug may also antagonize the contracting effect of acetylcholine on urinary bladders (Gutierrez, 1996).

CLINICAL TRIALS

Benign Prostatic Hyperplasia

No benefit of Saw Palmetto extract over placebo for benign prostatic hyperplasia (BPH) was found in a 12-month, randomized, and double-blind trial. The Saw Palmetto failed to improve symptoms or objective measures of BPH in the trial, in which 225 men (all over age 49) with moderate-to-severe BPH symptoms where randomly assigned to placebo or Saw Palmetto extract (160 mg twice daily). During the study, no significant difference between the herb and placebo was identified in change of scores on the American Urological Association Symptom Index, which is a validated, seven-item, self-administered questionnaire that measures symptoms relating to urinary obstruction. Significant differences were also not identified between the two groups in terms of maximal urinary flow rate, residual volume after voiding, prostate size, or serum prostate-specific antigen (PSA) levels. Quality of life, side effects, and laboratory values remained similar. While the extract of Saw Palmetto used in the study was similar to that of products commonly purchased by the more than 2 million men in the United States who use the herb for BPH, the authors note the possibility that the level of active ingredient in the herb may have been too low to produce a measurable effect (Bent, 2006).

A similar view was articulated in an accompanying editorial, "Proven and Unproven Therapy for Benign Prostatic Hyperplasia," which pointed out that different dosages or preparations may account for the negative results, and that more of such rigorous, placebo-controlled studies are needed before conclusive statements can be made regarding Saw Palmetto's potential for alleviating BPH symptoms. Long-term effectiveness and safety data also must be explored, the authors note (DiPaola, 2006).

A large review of evidence, also published in 2006, concludes that while recent well-designed trials don't illustrate significant benefits of Saw Palmetto for BPH, the weight of data nevertheless points to efficacy of this herb for this indication. Findings of most published trials are limited; most have been brief (just one to six months), involved a small number of participants, and failed to employ standardized outcome measurements (Ulbricht, 2006).

In one study involved 685 patients with severe BPH, the efficacy of Permixon®, a Saw Palmetto extract, was compared to that of tamsulosin. In the 12-month, double-blind, randomized study, subjects were assigned to receive Permixon (320 mg/day) or tamsulosin (0.4 mg/day). Permixon was found to be slightly superior to tamsulosin in reducing low urinary tract symptoms (Debruyne et al, 2004).

A prospective, single-blind, randomized, and parallel 12-month trial in 64 men (mean age 43.2) comparing the effectiveness of Saw Palmetto (325 mg daily) with Finasteride 5 mg daily in the treatment of category 111 prostatitis and chronic pelvic pain syndrome found no appreciable long-term improvement in those taking the herb (n=32). The Finasteride group (n=32), in contrast, experienced significant and ongoing relief for all measurements except urination. A placebo-controlled trial of Saw Palmetto for these indications is merited, the authors conclude (Kaplan, 2004).

In an earlier review, published in 2000, a systematic analysis of 18 randomized clinical trials comprising approximately 3,000 subjects conducted between 1983 and 1997 concluded that Saw Palmetto herbal combination products provided some benefit in controlling lower urinary tract symptoms and flow measures in men with BPH (Wilt et al, 2000).

In another, earlier study comparing Permixon® with tamsulosin, the lipido-sterolic extract of *Serenoa repens* (Permixon®) exhibited similar efficacy to alpha-blocker tamsulosin in the treatment of BPH in a 12-month, randomized, double-blind, multicenter, international trial (n=704, mean age 65.5 years). Following a 4-week placebo lead-in period, subjects were randomly assigned to oral therapy with 320 mg *Serenoa repens* daily or 0.4 mg tamsulosin daily for 12 months. Reductions of 4.4 in the International Prostate Symptom Score (IPSS) compared to baseline (mean IPSS=15.3 at baseline) were observed after treatment for 1 year in both groups (differences between groups were not significant). Significant differences between groups were not observed in IPS score for irritative or obstructive symptoms. Peak urinary flow was increased by 1.79 mL in subjects treated with *Serenoa repens* compared to a slight increase (0.22 mL) in subjects treated with tamsulosin, although this difference was not significant (Debruyne et al, 2002).

A lipido-serolic extract of *Serenoa repens* was effective in improving subjective and objective parameters of BPH in subjects with mild to moderate disease in an open-label study (n=75; 52 to 78 years) (Al-Shukri et al, 2000).

A combination product containing Saw Palmetto, cernitin, β-Sitosterol, and vitamin E improved subjective but not objective symptoms of BPH compared to placebo in a randomized clinical trial (n=144). Subjects were randomly assigned to receive 2 tablets of a combination product containing 286 mg of Saw Palmetto/phytosterol (Saw Palmetto standardized to 40% to 50% free fatty acids/β-sitosterol standardized to 43%), 378 mg cernitin, and 100 international units of vitamin E daily or placebo for 3 months. Improvement of 242% in daytime urinary frequency and 258% in nocturia were also observed compared to placebo over the 3-month treatment period (p=0.031 and p less than 0.001, respectively) (Pruess et al, 2001).

A fixed combination of extracts of Saw Palmetto fruit (*Serenoa repens*) and nettle root (Urtica dioica) (PRO 160/120) produced the same effect as the 5-alpha-reductase inhibitor finasteride in men with BPH, regardless of the baseline prostate volume. The study assessed a subgroup of men (n=431), 50 to 88 years, who participated in a 48-week randomized multicenter double-blind clinical trial (Sokeland, 2000).

INDICATIONS AND USAGE

Approved by Commission E:

- Irritable bladder
- Prostate complaints

This medication relieves only the difficulties associated with an enlarged prostate without reducing the enlargement.

Unproven Uses: In folk medicine, Saw Palmetto is used for inflammation of the urinary tract, bladder, testicles, and mammary glands. It has been used for nocturnal enuresis, persistent cough, eczema, and improvement of libido.

Homeopathic Uses: The herb is used for micturation problems and inflammation of the urinary tract.

PRECAUTIONS AND ADVERSE REACTIONS

Stomach complaints following intake have been observed in rare cases. Patients with hormone-dependent cancers should observe caution and speak to a physician regarding the use of Saw Palmetto because of its antiestrogenic, estrogenic, and antiandrogenic effects.

Pregnancy: The use of Saw Palmetto during pregnancy is not recommended due to its potential hormonal effects.

Breastfeeding: The use of Saw Palmetto during breastfeeding is not recommended due to its potential hormonal effects.

DRUG INTERACTIONS

MAJOR RISK

Warfarin: Concurrent use may result in increased risk of bleeding. *Clinical Management:* Caution is advised if Saw Palmetto is taken with warfarin. Monitor the INR and signs and symptoms of excessive bleeding.

POTENTIAL RISKS

Hormones, Hormone-Like Drugs, or Adrenergic Drugs: Concomitant use may interfere with therapy due to the possible estrogenic, androgenic, and alpha-adrenergic blocking effects of Saw Palmetto. *Clinical Management:* If concomitant use cannot be avoided, monitor patient for effects and adjust dose accordingly.

Iron: The tannin content of Saw Palmetto may complex with concomitantly administered iron, resulting in nonabsorbable, insoluble complexes that may lead to adverse sequelae on blood components. *Clinical Management:* Until more is known, patients who need iron supplementation should be advised to separate administration times of these 2 compounds by 1 to 2 hours.

DOSAGE

Mode of Administration: Comminuted herb and other galenic preparations for oral use.

How Supplied:

Capsule-80 mg, 125 mg, 160 mg, 227 mg, 250 mg, 320 mg 450 mg, 500 mg, 565 mg, 570 mg, 585 mg, 600 mg, 1000 mg

Liquid-1:1

Daily Dosage: The average daily dose is 1 to 2 g of the drug or 320 mg of the lipophilic extract (hexane or ethanol 90% v/v). Dosages used in studies demonstrated efficacy at 160 mg given twice daily or 320 mg given once daily (Carraro, 1996; Gerber, 1998; Grasso, 1995).

LITERATURE

Al-Shukri SH, Deschaseaux P. Kuzmin IV et al: Early urodynamic effects of the lipido-sterolic extract of *Serenoa repens* (Permixon® in patients with urinary tract symptoms due to benign prostatic hyperplasia. *Prostate Cancer Prostatic Dis*; 3(3):195-199. 2000.

Anonym: Welche Bedeutung haben pflanzliche Prostatamittel. In: *DAZ* 133(9):720. 1993.

Aso Y, Boccon-Gibob L, Brendler CB et al., Clinical research criteria. In: Cockett AT, Aso Y, Chatelain C, Denis L, Griffith K, Murphy G (eds.), Proceedings of the second international consultation on benign prostatic hyperplasia (BPH). Paris, *SCI S.* 345-355. 1993

Bach D, Medikamentöse Langheitbehandlung der BPH Ergebnisse einer prospektiven 3-Jahres-Studie mit dem Sabalextrakt IDS 89. *Urologe* [B]35:178-183. 1995

Bach D, Behandlung der benignen Prostatahypertrophie. In *ZPT* 17(4):209-218. 1996.

Bach D, Ebeling L, Long-term drug treatment of benign prostatic hyperplasia - Results of a prospective 3-year multicenter study using Sabal extract IDS 89. In: *Phytomedicine* 3(2):105-111. 1996.

Banz (Federal german Gazette) No.43; published 2 March 1989; revised 1 Feb 1990.

Bauer R, Neues von ''immunmodulierenden Drogen'' und ''Drogen mit antiallergischer und antiinflammatorischer Wirkung.'' In: *ZPT* 14(1):23-24. 1993.

Bazan NG, Authie D, Braquet P, Effect of *Serenoa repens* extract (Permixon®) on estradiol/testosterone-induced experimental prostate enlargement in the rat. In: *Pharmacol Res* 34(3/4):171-179. 1996.

Becker H, Ebeling L, Konservative Therapie der benignen Prostata-Hyperplasie (BPH) mit Cernilton (N) - Ergebnisse einer placebokontrollierten Doppelblindstudie. *Urologe* [B]28:301. 1988

Becker H, Ebeling L, Phytotherapie der BPH mit Cernilton(N) - Ergebnisse einer kontrollierten Verlaufsstudie. *Urologe* [B]31:113. 1991

Bent S, Shinohara C, Neuhaus K, et al. Saw palmetto for benign prostatic hyperplasia. *N Eng J Med*; 354 (6): 557-566. 2006.

Berges RR, Windeler J, Trampisch HJ, Senge TH, Randomised, placebo-controlled, double-blind clinical trial of β-sitosterol in patients with benign prostatic hyperplasia. *Lancet* 345:1529-1532. 1995

Breu W, Hagenlocher M, Redl K et al., Antiphlogistische Wirkung eines mit hyperkritischem Kohlendioxid gewonnenen Sabalfrucht-Extraktes. In vitro Hemmung des Cyclooxygenase-und 5-Lipoxygenase-Metabolismus. *Arzneimittelforschung*; 42:547. 1992

Breu W, Stadler F, Hagenlocher M et al., Der Sabalfrucht-Extrakt SG 291. Ein Phytotherapeutikum zur Behandlung der benignen Prostatahyperplasie. *Z Phytother*; 13:107-115. 1992.

Carraro JC et al., Comparision of phytotherapy (Permixon®) with finasteride in the treatment of benign prostate hyperplasia: a randomized international study of 1,098 patients. In: *Prostate* 29(4):231-240. 1996.

Carilla E, Briley M, Fauran F et al., Binding of Permixon®, a new treatment for prostatic benign hyperplasia, to the cytosolic androgen receptor in rat prostate. *J Steroid Biochem*; 20:521-523. 1984

Carraro J, Raynaud J, Koch G et al., Comparison of phytotherapy (Permixon®) with finasteride in the treatment of benign prostate hyperplasia: a randomized international study of 1,098 patients. *Prostate* Oct; 29(4):231-40. 1996.

Casarosa C, Cosci M, o di Coscio, Fratta M, (1988) Lack of effects of a lyposterolic extract of *Serenoa repens* on plasma levels of testosterone, follicle-stimulating hormone, luteinizing hormone. *Clin Ther* 10:5. 1988.

Cheema P, El-Mety O & Jazieh AR, Inoperative haemorrhage associated with the use of extract of Saw Palmetto herb: a case report and review of literature. In: *J Intern Med*; 250(2):167-169. 2001.

Debruyne F, Boyle P, Calais da Silva F, et al: Evaluation of the clinical benefit of Permixon® and tamsulosin in severe BPH patients. *Prog Urol*; 14(3):326-331. 2004.

Debruyne F, Koch G, Boyle P et al: Comparison of a phyotherapeutic agent (Permixon®) with an alpha-blocker (tamsulosin) in the treatment of benign prostatic hyperplasia: a 1-year randomized international study. *Eur Urol*; 41:497-507. 2002.

DiPaoloa RS, Morton RA. Proven and unproven therapy for benign prostatic hyperplasia. *N Eng J Med*; 354 (6): 632-634. 2006.

DiSilverio F, D'Eramo GD, Lubrano C et al., Evidence that Serenoa repens extract displays an anti-estrogenic activity in prostatic tissue of benign prostatic hypertrophy patients. *Eur Urol:* 21:309. 1992.

DiSilverio F, D'Eramo G, Flammia GP et al., Pharmacological combinations in the treatment of benign prostatic hypertrophy. *J Urol* (Paris); 99:316-320. 1993a.

Engelmann U, Phytopharmaka und Synthetika bei der Behandlung der benignen Prostatahypertrophie. In: *ZPT*; 18(1):13-19. 1997.

Gerber GS, Zagaja GP, Bales GT, et al., Saw Palmetto (*Seronoa repens*) in men with lower urinary tract symptoms: effects on urodynamic parameters and voiding symptoms. *Urology*; 51(6):1003-7. Jun 1998.

Goepel M, Hecker U, Krege S et al., Saw Palmetto extracts potently and noncompetitively inhibit human alpha1-adrenoceptors in vitro. In: *Prostate*; 15;38(3):208-15. Feb 15, 1999.

Grasso M, Montesano A, Buonaguidi A et al., Comparative effects of alfuzosin versus Serenoa repens in the treatment of symptomatic benign prostatic hyperplasia. *Arch Esp Urol*;48(1):97-103. Jan-Feb 1995.

Gutierrez M, Garcia De Boto MJ, Cantabrana B et al., Mechanisms involved in the spasmolytic effect of extracts from Sabal serrulata fruit on smooth muscle. In: *Gen Pharmacol*; 27:171-176. 1996.

Gutierrez M, Hidalgo A & Cantabrana B, Spasmolytic activity of a lipidic extract from Sabal serrulata fruits further study of the mechanism underlying this activity. *Planta Med*; 62:507-511. 1996.

Harnischfeger G, Stolze H, *Serenoa repens* - Die Sägezahnpalme. *Z Phytother* 10:71-76. 1989.

Kaplan SA, Volpe MA, Te AE. A prospective, 1-year trail using saw palmetto versus finasteride in the treatment of category 111 prostatitis/chronic pelvic pain syndrome. *J Urol*; 171: 284-288. 2004.

Koch E, Pharmakologie und Wirkmechanismen von Extrakten aus Sabalfrüchten (Sabal fructus): Brennesselwurzeln (Urticae radix) und Kürbissamen (Cucurbitae peponis semen) bei der Behandlung der benignen Prostatahyperplasie. In: Loew D, Rietbrock N (Hrsg) *Phytopharmaka in Forschung und klinischer Anwendung.* Steinkopff Verlag, Darmstadt, S 57-79. 1995.

Mattei FM, Capone M, Acconia A, Medikamentöse Therapie der benignen Prostatahyperplasie mit einem Exktrakt der Sägepalme. In: *Therapiewoche Urologie, Nephrologie* 2:346-350. 1990.

Miersch WDE, Benigne Prostatahyperplasie. In: *DAZ* 133(29):2653. 1993.

Nahrstedt A, Pflanzliche Urologica - eine kritische Übersicht. *Pharm Z* 138:1439-1450. 1993.

Niederprüm HJ, Schweikert HU, Zänker KS, Testosteron 5D-reductase inhibition by free fatty acids from Sabal serrulata fruits. *Phytomedicine* 1:127-133. 1994

Plosker GL, Brogden RN, Serenoa repens (Permixon®): A review of its pharmacological and therapeutic efficacy in benign prostatic hyperplasia. In: *Drugs & Aging* 9(5):379-395. 1996.

Preuss HG, Marcusen C, Regan J et al: Randomized trial of a combination of natural products (cernitin, Saw Plametto, β-sitosterol, vitamin E) on symptoms of benign prostatic hyperplasia (BPH). In: *Urol Nephrol*; 33(2):217-225. 2001.

Ravenna L et al., Effects of the lipidosterolic extract of Serenoa repens (Permixon®) on human prostatic cell lines. In: *Prostate* 29(4):219-230. 1996.

Rhodes L, Primka RL, Berman CH, Vergult F, Gabriel M, Pierre-Malice M, Gibelin B, Comparision of Finasteride (Proscar®), a 5alpha-reductase inhibitor, and various commercial plant extracts in in vitro and in vivo 5alpha reductase inhibition. In: *Prostate*; 22(1):43-51, 1993.

Schilcher H, Möglichkeiten und Grenzen der Phytotherapie am Beispiel pflanzlicher Urologika. *Urologe* [B] 27:316-319. 1987

Schilcher H, Pflanzliche Diuretika. *Urologe* [B]27:215-222. 1987.

Schilcher B, In: Schilcher H: *Phytotherapie in der Urologie*. Hippokrates Verlag Stuttgart. 1992.

Shimada H et al., Biological active acylglycerides from the berries of Saw Palmetto (*Serenoa repens*). In: *JNP* 60(4):417-418. 1997.

Sokeland J: combined sabal and Urtica extract compared with finasteride in men with benign prostate volume and therapeutic outcome. *BJU Int*; 86:439-432. 2000.

Sultan C, Terraza A, Devillier C et al., Inhibition of androgen metabolism and binding by a liposterolic extract of ''*Serenoa repens* B'' in human foreskin fibroblasts. *J Steroid Biochem*; 20:515-519. 1984.

Tyler VE, Brady LR, Robbers JE: *Pharmacognosy*, 8th edition. Lea and Febiger, Philadelphis, PA: 168. 1981.

Ulbricht C, Basch E, Bent E, et al. Evidence-based systematic review of saw palmetto by the Natural Standard Research Collaboration. *J Soc Integ Onc*; 4(4):170-186. 2006.

Vacher P, Prevarskaya N, Skryma R et al, The lipidosterolic extract from *Serenoa repens* interferes with prolactin receptor signal transduction. *J Biomed Sci;* 2:357-365. 1995.

Wagner H, Flachsbarth H, *Planta Med* 41:244. 1981.

Wichtl M, Pflanzliche Geriatrika. In: *DAZ* 132(30):1576. 1992.

Wilt TJ, Ishani A, Rutks I et al: Phytotherapy for benign prostatic hyperplasia. *Public Health Nutr*; 2(4a):459-472. 2000.

Yue QY, Jansson K: Herbal drug curbicin and anticoagulant effect with and without warfarin: possibly related to the vitamin E component. In: *J Am Geriatr Soc*; 49(6):838. 2001.

Scabiosa succisa

See Premorse

Scarlet Pimpernel

Anagallis arvensis

DESCRIPTION

Medicinal Parts: The medicinal part of the plant is the dried flowering herb, usually with the roots removed.

Flower and Fruit: The plant has 6 to 10 brick-red flowers in the leaf axils, which are up to 2.5 times as long as the bracts. The symmetrically radiating flower has a double perianth. It has 5 sepals that are 4 to 5 mm long, entire-margined, narrow-lanceolate, and acute. The wheel-shaped corolla is usually vermilion, but occasionally bluish, lilac, or white. The tip of the corolla is obovate to oval, about 7 mm long by 6 mm wide, overlapping at the base, entire-margined or slightly crenate with 50 to 70 glandular hairs. Its 5 stamens have a distinct awn and are fused to a funnel at the tube. The anthers are short, ellipsoid, and cordate at the base. The superior ovary is globose and one-valved with an oblong style and headlike stigma. The fruit is a globose pyxidum that is 4 to 5 mm in diameter and contains 20 to 22 rough, wartlike, brown seeds 1.3 mm long by 1 mm wide.

Leaves, Stem, and Root: Anagallis arvensis is an annual herb with prostrate, creeping, square stems up to 30 cm long. Its thinner, branched, ascending stems grow to a length of 6 to 30 cm. The square shoots, like the leaves, are thickly covered with short hairs when young; they later become glabrous. The leaves are opposite, occasionally in whorls of 3, ovate to lanceolate, up to 20 mm long by 10 mm wide, sessile, entire-margined, acute, and spotted black on the underside.

Characteristics: The flowers, which are poisonous, close at night and open at about 9:00 each morning. They also close at the first sign of rain.

Habitat: The plant is widely distributed throughout Europe, Asia, the U.S., and nontropical South America.

Production: Scarlet Pimpernel herb is the dried herb in flower of *Anagallis arvensis*, generally without the root but occasionally including the whole plant. It is collected in the wild and also cultivated.

Not to be Confused With: The blue flowering form of Scarlet Pimpernel is often confused with *Anagallis foemina*, and occasionally with *Stellaria media*.

Other Names: Adder's Eyes, Poor Man's Weatherglass, Red Chickweed, Red Pimpernel, Shepherd's Barometer

ACTIONS AND PHARMACOLOGY

COMPOUNDS

Triterpene saponins: including anagalline, chief sapogenine 13, 28-epoxy-16- oxooleanan

Cucurbitacins: including cucurbitacins E, B, D, I and L

Flavonoids

Caffeic acid derivatives

EFFECTS

In vitro and animal tests showed the drug (main constituents saponins and amaroids of the cucurbitacin group) to have fungitoxic, antiviral, taecidal, spermicidal, estrogenic, oxytocic, and hemolytic effects. The aqueous extract of the dried leaves is fungitoxic. Triterpenglycoside, anagalloside, and aglycon anagalligenones, when isolated from the drug, displayed inhibitory results against numerous microorganisms. Aqueous extracts showed uterine contracting activity in rats, guinea pigs, rabbits, and on strips of human uterine material. The triterpene saponins isolated from the drug demonstrated action against human sperm. The methanol extract of the drug demonstrated estrogen activity in the Allen-Doisy test. The saponins isolated from the powder drug with ethanol demonstrated hemolytic activity in human blood. The methanol extract of the dried powdered drug is antiviral against *Herpes simplex Type I, Adenovirus Type II,* and *Polio Type II*, among others. The saponins are the active constituents. The acetylsaponin isolated from the drug acts as a teniacide.

INDICATIONS AND USAGE

Unproven Uses: The drug is used to treat depression, disorders of the mucous membranes, hemorrhoids, herpes simplex, painful kidney and liver disorders (in particular, to increase urination), poorly healing wounds, and pruritus. The herb is used as a supporting treatment in various carcinomas. It is used both internally and externally (as a poultice) to treat pains in the joints.

Chinese Medicine: The herb is used for snake bites, dog bites, fish poisoning, joint ailments, and edema.

Indian Medicine: Employed as a treatment for menstruation disorders.

Homeopathic Uses: Used in the treatment of skin rashes, warts, and urinary tract infections.

Efficacy has not been proven.

PRECAUTIONS AND ADVERSE REACTIONS

No health hazards or side effects are known in conjunction with the proper administration of designated therapeutic dosages. Large doses or long-term administration could lead to gastroenteritis and nephritis, due to the cucurbitacins content of the drug.

OVERDOSAGE

Higher dosages (no amounts specified) are said to have a strong diuretic, diarrheic, and mildly narcotic effect.

DOSAGE

Mode of Administration: Scarlet Pimpernel topically as a poultice and internally as an infusion.

Preparation: For the treatment of liver and kidney disorders as well as dropsy, add one teaspoonful of the drug to a glass of hot water and let it steep for 10 minutes. Drink throughout the day.

Daily Dosage: The usual dosage is 1.8 g of the powder 4 times a day.

Homeopathic Dosage: The oral dosage is 5 to 10 drops, 1 tablet, or 10 globules daily. The parenteral dosage is 1 ml twice a week sc. Topically, ointment can be applied 1 to 2 times daily.

LITERATURE

Alimbaeva PK, Mukhamedziev MM, *Rast Resur* 5:380-385. 1996.

Aliotta G, De Napoli L, Giordano F, Piccialli G, Piccialli V, Santacroce C, An oleanen triterpene from *Anagallis arvensis.* In: *PH* 31(3):929-933. 1992.

Amoros M et al. Experimental Herpes Simplex Keratitis in Rabbits. *Planta Med.* 54; 128-131. 1988.

Amoros M, Fauconnier B, Girre RL, In vitro antiviral activity of a saponin from *Anagallis arvensis*, Primulaceae, against herpes simplex virus and poliovirus. In: *Antiviral Res* 8:13-25. 1987.

Büechi S, Antivirale Saponine, pharmakologische und klinische Untersuchungen. In: *DAZ* 136(2):89-98. 1996.

Lacaille-Dubois MA, Wagner H. A review of the biological and pharmacological activities of saponins. *Phytomedicine* 2 (4); 363-386. 1996

Mahato SB, Sahu NP, Roy SK, Sen S. Structure Elucidation of Four new Triterpenoid Oligoglycosides from *Anagallis arvensis. Tetrahedron* 47; 5215-5230 1991

Shoji N, Umeyama A, Yoshikawa K, Arihara S. Structures of Anagallosaponins I - V and Their Companion Substances from *Anagallis arvensis L. Chem Pharm Bull.* 42 (9); 1750-1755. 1994

Schinus molle

See California Peppertree

Schinus terebinthifolius

See Brazilian Pepper Tree

Schisandra (Wu-Wei-Zi)

Schisandra chinensis

DESCRIPTION

Medicinal Parts: The medicinal part of the plant is the fruit.

Flower and Fruit: The flowers are in clusters with a few blossoms in the axils of the bracts. There are 6 to 8 tepals. The perigone of the male flowers has 6 to 8 tepals that are 6 to 11 mm long and 5 mm wide, and 5 to 15 stamens. The female flowers have a similar perigone and 17 to 40 elongated, elliptical ovaries. The round, fleshy, berry-like fruit grows as a slim, hanging aggregate or as bloomed individual fruits. The fruit is deep red to black-brown and appears partly white-powdered. The fruit has a diameter of 5 to 8 mm and contains 1 to 2 reniform seeds.

Leaves, Stem and Root: This liana plant can be monoecious or dioecious. The leaves are alternate. They are arranged like whorls on short shoots. The petiole is 1 to 4 cm long. The lamina is 5 to 11 cm long, 3 to 9 cm wide, elongate to ovate-elliptical, serrate to dentate with up to 3 teeth per cm. The upper surface is green or brown. The lower surface is partly pubescent. The young branches are brown to purple.

Characteristics: The crushed seeds taste hot and are aromatic.

Habitat: The plant is indigenous to northeastern China and Korea.

Production: Northern schisandra fruit is the dried, ripe fruit of Schisandra chinensis. The fruit is harvested in autumn, then steamed before being dried in the sun.

Other Names: Chinese Mock-Barberry, Lemonwood

ACTIONS AND PHARMACOLOGY

COMPOUNDS

Volatile oil: containing among others, alpha- and beta-chamigrene, chamigrenal, sesquicarene, (+)-ylangene

Ascorbic acid (vitamin C)

Lignans (in the seeds 5 to 20%): dibenzo[a,c]cyclooctene derivatives, including schizandrine A to C, schizandrol A and B, schizantherine A and B, gomisins D to J, K1 to K3, L1 and L2, M1 and M2, N and O, P to T, the gomisins present to some extent as esters, among them those of angelic acid, benzoic acid and acetic acid; additional lignans with other parent substances, including pregomisin.

Fatty oil (in the seeds): chief fatty acids oleic acid and linoleic acid

EFFECTS

General: Schisandra chinensis has been used for thousands of years within the Chinese medical paradigm, which considers it a warming herb that strengthens the Qi, tonifies the lungs and kidneys, quiets the heart and spirit, and protects the liver. Historically used for chronic cough and wheezing, schisandra has also been used for diabetes, insomnia, and palpitations in Chinese medicine. Classified as an adaptogen or astringent, schisandra is said to increase the body's resistance and improve physiological processes by increasing energy and strength. Its more modern uses are as a liver protector and some research indicates that it may be useful in treating HIV-1 infections.

The lignans isolated from the drug (schizandrin, schizandrol) are liver-protective in effect, acting as radical scavengers and promoting liver regeneration. Anti-inflammatory and tumor-inhibiting characteristics have also been demonstrated. Schizandrol A is said to be neuroleptic, anticonvulsive and sedative in effect. Schisandra fruits and seeds are believed to bring about a non-specific increase in physical performance ability and to be antithelminthic in effect.

Liver protection

Various schizandrins from schisandra were tested for their ability to scavenge hydroxyl radicals and superoxide anions. Their ability to scavenge free radicals was stronger than that of vitamin C or vitamin E. The schizandrin Sin C was stronger than Sin B and the stereoisomers S(-) were stronger than R(+) forms. The ability to scavenge free radicals may partially explain the detoxification and protective ability of schisandra against liver injury. The authors also offer that in traditional Chinese medicine, mixtures of medicine are more effective than isolated components (Li et al, 1990).

It lowers elevated serum glutamic-pyruvic transaminase (SGPT) levels, increases liver protein and glycogen synthesis, is an anti-oxidant, and may induce P-450 enzymes. Schisandra has been used in China for the treatment of viral and chemical hepatitis. Liver protecting effects are associated with schisandra sinensis, and schisandra sphenanthera as well as other members of the Schisandraceae family (Li, 1991).

Anti-inflammatory

Gomisin C, isolated from the dried fruit of schisandra, inhibited the respiratory burst of rat neutrophils, but did not scavenge superoxide anion. The inhibitory effect of gomisin on the respiratory burst may be due to an inhibitory effect on NADPH oxidase as well as a reduction in the release of intracellular calcium ion. Stimulation of neutrophils is part of the inflammatory response (Wang et al, 1994).

CLINICAL TRIALS

While large, human clinical trials are lacking for *schisandra chinensis*, animal and in vitro studies support the use of Schisandra in liver protection and show potential benefit in treating intestinal flukes and HIV.

Short-term (3 weeks) oral administration of gomisin A, a lignan component of schisandra chinensis, inhibited both the level of glutathione-S-transferase placental form (GST-P), and the number and size of GST-P positive foci in rat livers after treatment with 3'-methyl-4-dimethylamino-azobenezine as compared with phenobarbital. Gomisin A also returned increased diploid nuclei and tetraploid nuclei to near the normal ploidy pattern. Results suggest gomisin A has an inhibitory effect on hepatocarcinogenesis as compared to phenobarbital and may be a candidate for a chemopreventive drug (Nomura, 1994).

Cardiomyopathy

Schisandra chinensis has also been investigated in human models regarding its use to improve cardiac function as well as exercise performance. In a single-blinded randomized clinical trial schisandra was used with digoxin as a treatment for cardiomyopathy. Preliminary results showed the group receiving schisandra to have improved cardiac function (Zeng, 1987). In another study, a single-blinded, randomized clinical trial showed that Sheng Mei, a Chinese herb preparation (Sheng Mei) containing schisandra, when used in combination with digoxin, significantly improved cardiac function (p less than 0.001) in patients with cardiomyopathy. Seven of 20 patients who received Sheng Mei plus digoxin improved in cardiac function (p less than 0.001) versus none in the control group receiving digoxin with inosine. All patients in the Sheng Mei group had a decrease in symptoms. No serious side effects were seen. Although these results were preliminary and published in abstract form, the authors suggest that Sheng Mei may be of value for long-term treatment of cardiomyopathy (Zeng, 1987).

Exercise Performance

Studying the content of nitric oxide (NO) and cortisol in blood and saliva during heavy physical exercise, standardized extracts of schisandra chinensis and Bryonia alba were used in a double-blind, placebo-controlled study. Results correlate with an increased physical performance in athletes taking schisandra and Bryonia versus placebo (Panossian, 1999).

INDICATIONS AND USAGE

In Chinese medicine, schisandra is an adaptogen and an astringent used mainly for conditions of the digestive tract such as intestinal inflammation, and also for insomnia, enuresis, urinary frequency, nightly ejaculation, coughs, chronic diarrhea, dyspnea, insomnia, spontaneous outbreaks of sweating, hepatitis, neurasthenia and anxiety states. Efficacy for these indications has not yet been proven. Miscellaneous reports of further uses of schisandra chinensis include the treatment of age-related memory deficits (Nishiyama, 1996) and the treatment of Clonorchis sinensis, the Chinese liver fluke (Rhee, 1982).

CONTRAINDICATIONS

Schisandra should not be used by people with epilepsy, severe hypertension, intercranial pressure or ''high acidity,'' in the terminology of Chinese medicine (Weiner & Weiner, 1994).

PRECAUTIONS AND ADVERSE REACTIONS

General: No health hazards are known in conjunction with the proper administration of designated therapeutic dosages. Rare side effects may include appetite suppression, stomach upset, and hives.

Interactions: No human interaction data available.

DOSAGE

Mode of Administration: Whole and powdered drug and their preparations for internal use.

Preparation: To prepare Cuwuweizi powder, the drug is evaporated in the ratio of 1:5 with vinegar in closed containers until the surface turns black. This substance is then ground to a powder.

Daily Dosage: Powder/tincture/extract: 1.5 to 6 g daily

Storage: Store in dry area with good air circulation to avoid fungal formation.

LITERATURE

Chang P & But P, Pharmacology and Applications of Chinese Materia Medica. Chinese University of Hong Kong: Singapore, 1987.

Hänsel R, Keller K, Rimpler H, Schneider G (Ed), Hagers Handbuch der Pharmazeutischen Praxis, 5. Aufl., Bde 4 - 6 (Drogen), Springer Verlag Berlin, Heidelberg, New York, 1992-1994.

Ip SP, Mak DH, Li PC, Poon MK, Ko KM, Determination and study of lignan distribution in the fruits of Schisandra chinensis (Turcz.). In: Baill Farmatsiia, 78:34-7, May-Jun 1972.

Ip SP, Mak DH, Li PC, Poon MK, Ko KM, Determination of lignans in the fruits of Schisandra chinensis (Trucz.) Baill. and S. Sphenanthern Rehd. et Wils. using HPLC and their chromatograms. In: Chung Kuo Chung Yao Tsa Chih, 78:611-4, 639-40, Oct 1989.

Ip SP, Mak DH, Li PC, Poon MK, Ko KM, Determination of the active ingredients in Chinese drug wuweizi (Schisandra chinensis) by TLC-densitometry. In: Yao Hsueh Hsueh Pao, 78:49-53, 1990.

Ip SP, Mak DH, Li PC, Poon MK, Ko KM, Ecological investigation on Schisandra chinensis (Turcz.) Baill. of the Changbai Mountain. In: Chung Kuo Chung Yao Tsa Chih, 78:204-5, 255, Apr 1992.

Ip SP, Mak DH, Li PC, Poon MK, Ko KM, Effect of a lignan-enriched extract of Schisandra chinensis on aflatoxin B1 and cadmium chloride-induced hepatotoxicity in rats. In: Pharmacol Toxicol, 78:413-6, Jun 1996.

Ip SP, Mak DH, Li PC, Poon MK, Ko KM, Pharmacological studies on an oil emulsion of Schisandra chinensis. In: Chung Yao Tung Pao, 78:185-6, Jul 1984.

Ip SP, Mak DH, Li PC, Poon MK, Ko KM, Preliminary studies on the processing of Schisandra chinensis. In: Chung Yao Tung Pao, 78:26-7, Mar1986.

Ip SP, Mak DH, Li PC, Poon MK, Ko KM, Schisandra chinensis-dependent myocardial protective action of sheng-mai-san in rats. In: Am J Chin Med, 78:255-62, 1996.

Ip SP, Mak DH, Li PC, Poon MK, Ko KM, The occurrence of some important lignans in Wu Wei Zi (Schisandra chinensis) and its allied species. In: Yao Hsueh Hsueh Pao, 78:138-43, Feb 1983.

Ip SP, Poon MK, Che CT, Ng KH, Kong YC, Ko KM, Anti-oxidant activity of dibenzocyclooctene lignans isolated from Schisandraceae. In: Planta Med, 21:311-3, Aug 1992.

Ip SP, Poon MK, Che CT, Ng KH, Kong YC, Ko KM, Schisandrin B protects against carbon tetrachloride toxicity by enhancing the mitochondrial glutathione redox status in mouse liver. In: Free Radic Biol Med, 21:709-12, 1996.

Jiaxiang N, Fujii K, Sato N et al, Inhibitory effect on reductive metabolism of halothane. In: J Appl Toxicol;13(6):385-388, Nov-Dec 1993.

Ko KM, Ip SP, Poon MK, Wu SS, Che CT, Ng KH, Kong YC, Effect of a lignan-enriched fructus schisandrae extract on hepatic glutathione status in rats: protection against carbon tetrachloride toxicity. In: Planta Med, 21:134-7, Apr 1995.

Li XJ, Zhao BL, Liu GT, Xin WJ. Scavenging effects on active oxygen radicals by schizandrins with different structures and configurations. In: Free Radic Biol Med; 9:99-104, 1990.

Li X-Y: Bioactivity of neolignans from Fructus Schizandrae. Mem Inst Oswaldo Cruz; 86sII:31-37, 1991.

Lin TJ: Antioxidation mechanism of schizandrim and tanshinonatic acid A and their effects on the protection of cardiotoxic action of adriamycin. In: Sheng Li Ko Hsueh Chin Chan; 22(4):342-345, 1991.

Liu CS, Fang SD, Huang MF, Kao YL, Hsu JS, Studies on the active principles of Schisandra sphenanthera Rehd. et Wils. The structures of schisantherin A, B, C, D, E and the related compounds. In: Sci Sin, 21:483-502, Jul-Aug 1978.

Liu G-T, Pharmacological actions and clinical use of Fructus Schizandrae. In: Chinese Med J; 102:740-749, 1989.

Nishiyama N, Chu P-J & Saito H, An herbal prescription, S-113m, consisting of biota, ginseng and Schizandra, improves learning performance in senescence accelerated mouse. In: Biol. Pharm Bull; 19:388-393, 1996.

Nishiyama N, Wang YL, Saito H, Beneficial effects of S-113m, a novel herbal prescription, on learning impairment model in mice. In: Biol Pharm Bull, 21:1498-503, Nov 1995.

Nomura M & Nakachiyama M, Gomisin A, a lignan component of schizandra fruits, inhibits development of preneoplactic lesions in rat liver by 3?-methyl-4- dimethylamino-azobenezene. In: Cancer Lett; 76(1):11-18, 1994.

Nomura M, Ohtaki Y, Hida T et al., Inhibition of early 3-methyl-4- dimethylaminoazobenzene-induced hepatocarcinogenesis by gomisin A in rats. In: Anticancer Res; 14(5A):1967-1971, 1994.

Ohtaki Y, Nomura M, Hida T et al., Inhibition of gomisin A, a lignan compound, of hepatocarcinogenesis by 3?-methyl-4-dimethylaminoazobenzene in rats. In: Biol Pharm Bull (6):808, Jun17, 1994.

Panossian AG, Oganessian AS, Ambartsumian M et al: Effects of heavy physical exercise and adaptogens on nitric oxide content in human saliva. In: Phytomedicine; 6(1):17-26, 1999.

Rhee JK, Woo KJ, Baek BK, et al: Screening of the wormicidal Chinese raw drugs on Clonorchis sinensis. In: Am J Chin Med; 9:277-284, 1982.

Tong Q, Deuteration of dimethyl 4,4'-dimethoxy-5,6,5',6'-dimethylenedioxybiphenyl-2,2'-dicarboxylate (BDD): a remedy for chronic hepatitis. In: Chung Kuo I Hsueh Ko Hsueh Yuan Hsueh Pao, 21:42-5, Feb1990.

Wang JP, Raung, SL, Hsu MF, et al, Inhibition by gomisin C (a lignan from Schizandra chinesis) of the respiratory burst of rat neutrophils. In: Br J Pharmacol; 113:945-953, 1994.

Weiner MA & Weiner JA: Herbs that Heal, Quantum Books, Mill Valley, CA; 1994.

Yasukawa K, Ikeya Y, Mitsuhashi H, Iwasaki M, Aburada M, Nakagawa S, Takeuchi M, Takido M, Gomisin A inhibits tumor promotion by 12-O-tetradecanoylphorbol-13-acetate in two-stage carcinogenesis in mouse skin. In: Oncology, 21:68-71, 1992.

Zeng X: Clinical observations of the effect of ''Sheng Mei'' in cardiomyopathy. Circulation; 76:153(abstract), 1987.

Schisandra chinensis

See Schisandra (Wu-Wei-Zi)

Schisandra sphenanthera

See Lemon-Wood

Scolopendrium vulgare

See Hartstongue

Scopolia

Scopolia carniolica

DESCRIPTION

Medicinal Parts: The medicinal part is the dried rhizome.

Flower and Fruit: The nodding flowers are solitary and axillary on long, bending pedicles. The calyx is campanulate with obtuse tips. The corolla is tubular-campanulate, glossy brown outside, and matte olive-green inside. The anthers are large and yellowish. The fruit is a bivalved pixidium. The seeds are 3 to 4 mm long, brownish-yellow, and bumpy.

Leaves, Stem, and Root: The erect perennial plant grows from 30 to 60 cm high. The rhizome is horizontal, slightly bent, and almost cylindrical. The rhizome grows up to 12 cm long and 5 cm thick, and is covered in tough, loose-skinned fibers. The color varies between yellowish-brown to dark brownish-gray. The stems bear scalelike stipules at the base that are bifurcated, fleshy, and glabrous or with scattered hairs. The 12 cm by 4 to 9 cm foliage leaves are petiolate, obovate, entire-margined or lightly sinuate, and dull green.

Characteristics: Scopolia is considered to be a narcotic. The taste is initially somewhat sweet, then bitter and biting. The plant is odorless.

Habitat: The plant is indigenous to southern Germany, Austria, Hungary, and southwest Russia.

Production: Scopolia root consists of the dried rhizome of *Scopolia carniolica.*

Other Names: Belladonna Scopola, Japanese Belladonna, Russian Belladonna, Scopola

ACTIONS AND PHARMACOLOGY

COMPOUNDS

Tropane alkaloids (0.2-0.5%): chief alkaloid (-)-hyoscyamine, which changes (to some extent) under drying conditions into atropine; also including scopolamine

Hydroxycoumarins: including among others, scopoletins, scopoline

Caffeic acid derivatives: chlorogenic acids

EFFECTS

The drug acts as a parasympatholytic/anticholinergic via competitive antagonism of the neuromuscular transmitter acetylcholine. Because of its parasympatholytic properties, Scopolia root relaxes the smooth muscle organs and eliminates spastic conditions, especially of the gastrointestinal tract and the bile ducts.

Conditions of muscular tremors and muscular rigidity caused by central nervous impulses, are alleviated. The action on the heart is positively chronotropic and positively dromotropic.

INDICATIONS AND USAGE

Approved by Commission E:

■ Liver and gallbladder complaints

The drug is used for spasms and coliclike pain of the gastrointestinal tract, bile ducts, and urinary tract for adults and for children over 6 years of age.

CONTRAINDICATIONS

The drug is contraindicated in narrow-angle glaucoma, prostatic adenoma with residual urine, tachycardia, mechanical stenosis in the area of the gastrointestinal tract, and megacolon.

PRECAUTIONS AND ADVERSE REACTIONS

General: No health hazards are known in conjunction with the proper administration of designated therapeutic dosages. However, accommodation disorders, heat buildup due to a decline in sweat secretion, micturition disorders, and obstipation can occur as side effects, particularly with overdosages. Scopolia should be used only under the supervision of an expert qualified in its appropriate use.

DRUG INTERACTIONS

POTENTIAL INTERACTIONS

Scopolia may increase the effectiveness of simultaneously administered tricyclic antidepressants, amantadine, and quinidine.

OVERDOSAGE

The four early warning symptoms of atropine poisoning are skin reddening, dryness of the mouth, and tachycardiac arrhythmias and mydriasis. In addition, other side effects, particularly with overdosages, can include accommodation disorders, heat buildup through decline in sweat secretion, micturition disorders, and obstipation. The intake of very high dosages leads to central excitation (restlessness, compulsive speech, hallucinations, delirium, manic episodes, followed by exhaustion and sleep). Potentially lethal dosages for adults start at 100 mg of atropine, depending upon alkaloid content, and may result from use of between 20 to 50 g of the drug; considerably less can prove lethal for children.

The treatment for poisonings includes gastric lavage; temperature-lowering measures with wet cloths (no antipyretics); oxygen respiration for respiratory distress; intubation; parenteral physostigmine salts as antidote; diazepam for spasms, and chlorpromazine for severe excitation.

DOSAGE

Mode of Administration: Comminuted root, powder and other galenic preparations for oral application.

Daily Dosage: The average daily dose is equivalent to 0.25 mg of total alkaloids, calculated as hyoscyamine. The maximum daily dose should not exceed the equivalent of 3.0 mg of total alkaloids, calculated as hyoscyamine. The maximum recommended single dose is equivalent to 1.0 mg of total alkaloids, calculated as hyoscyamine.

LITERATURE

Dräger B, Almsick Av, Mrachatz G. Distribution of Calystegines in Several Solanaceae. *Planta Med.* 61 (6); 577-579. 1995)

Frohne D, Pfänder HJ, Giftpflanzen - Ein Handbuch für Apotheker, Toxikologen und Biologen, 4. Aufl., Wiss. Verlags-Ges. Stuttgart 1997.

Kern W, List PH, Hörhammer L (Hrsg.), Hagers Handbuch der Pharmazeutischen Praxis, 4. Aufl., Bde. 1-8: Springer Verlag Berlin, Heidelberg, New York, 1969.

Lewin L, Gifte und Vergiftungen, 6. Aufl., Nachdruck, Haug Verlag, Heidelberg 1992.

Roth L, Daunderer M, Kormann K, Giftpflanzen, Pflanzengifte, 4. Aufl., Ecomed Fachverlag Landsberg Lech 1993.

Smart RG et al., *J Forens Sci* 32:303. 1987.

Teuscher E, Lindequist U, Biogene Gifte - Biologie, Chemie, Pharmakologie, 2. Aufl., Fischer Verlag Stuttgart 1994.

Scopolia carniolica

See Scopolia

Scotch Broom

Cytisus scoparius

DESCRIPTION

Medicinal Parts: The medicinal parts are the dried and stripped broom flowers, the dried aerial parts (broom herb), and freshly picked flowers.

Flower and Fruit: The bilabiate flowers are bright yellow, 20 to 25 mm long, large, solitary or in pairs. The flowers are on 2 or 3 obovate bracts on short stems, or singly in the leaf axils. They seem to form long racemes. The corolla is bright yellow, sometimes white. The standard is revolute, the wings obtuse. The ovary is short-stemmed and villous with a glabrous, strongly hooked style. The pod is oblong, compressed, glabrous on the surfaces, villous on the seams, and is matte black. There are numerous brown-black seeds.

Leaves, Stem, and Root: Scotch Broom is a shrub that grows from 0.5 to 2 m high. The taproot is very sturdy and woody. The bark of the root is brown. The branches are thick, usually crooked, and the bark is also brown. Young shoots are glabrous, later pubescent. The branchlets are canelike, erect, and pentangular. The leaves are small, short-petioled, with 3 obovate to lanceolate, pointed leaflets that are 1 to 2 cm long and 1.5 to 9 mm wide. The leaflets, particularly on the undersurface, are silky pubescent. After flowering, sessile and entire leaves form on the upper shoot.

Habitat: The herb is found in Europe, northern Africa, Canary Islands, North America, Chile, South Africa, and Japan.

Production: Scotch Broom herb consists of the aerial parts of *Cytisus scoparius*. Broom flowers consist of the flowers of *Cytisus scoparius*.

Not to be Confused With: The herb should not be confused with other Cytisus or Genista varieties. The flowers should not be confused with Spanish Broom.

Other Names: Basam, Besom, Bizzom, Breeam, Broom, Broomtops, Browme, Brum, Irish Tops, Scoparium

ACTIONS AND PHARMACOLOGY

COMPOUNDS: SCOTCH BROOM HERB

Quinolizidine alkaloids (0.5 to 1.6%): main alkaloid (-)-sparteine, including among others 11, 12-dehydrosparteine, 17-oxosparteine, lupanine, alpha-isosparteine

Biogenic amines: including tyramine, epinine, dopamine

Flavonoids: including spirasoside, isoquercitrin, scoparin

Isoflavonoids: including genistein, sarothamnoside

EFFECTS: SCOTCH BROOM HERB

No specific studies are available. Tyramine acts indirectly on the sympathetic nervous system as a vasoconstrictor and hypertensive.

COMPOUNDS: SCOTCH BROOM FLOWERS

Quinolizidine alkaloids (0.004%) (very small quantities): main alkaloid (-)-sparteine

Biogenic amines: including tyramine (0.13 to 2%)

Flavonoids: including scoparin (C-glycosylflavone)

EFFECTS: SCOTCH BROOM FLOWERS

The drug can contain over 2% tyramine. It contains small amounts of alkaloids. The main alkaloid is sparteine. Tyramine acts as an indirect sympathicomimetic, vasoconstrictoral and hypotensive. Sparteine acts negatively inotropic and negatively chronotropic; because of the very minimal amounts of sparteine, no intense effect can be expected.

INDICATIONS AND USAGE

SCOTCH BROOM HERB

Approved by Commission E:

- Circulatory disorders
- Hypertension

The herb is used for functional heart and circulatory disorders.

Unproven Uses: Folk medicine uses include as an adjunct in the stabilization of circulation and to raise blood pressure, pathological edema, cardiac arrhythmia, nervous cardiac complaints, low blood pressure, heavy menstruation, hemorrhaging after birth, as a contraction stimulant, for bleeding gums, hemophilia, gout, rheumatism, sciatica, gall and kidney stones, enlarged spleen, jaundice, bronchial conditions, and snake bites.

SCOTCH BROOM FLOWERS

Unproven Uses: The use of the pure drug cannot be recommended except as an inactive ingredient in teas. In folk medicine, the flowers are used for edema, rheumatism, gout, kidney stones, jaundice, liver disorders, enlarged spleen, and as a blood purifier.

CONTRAINDICATIONS

SCOTCH BROOM HERB AND FLOWERS

The drug is contraindicated in high blood pressure, A-V block, pregnancy, and with MAO inhibitor drugs.

PRECAUTIONS AND ADVERSE REACTIONS

SCOTCH BROOM HERB

General: Health risks or side effects following the proper administration of designated therapeutic dosages are not recorded. Scotch Broom preparations should not be used in cases of high blood pressure or with A-V block.

Pregnancy: The herb should not be used during pregnancy (abortive effect).

SCOTCH BROOM FLOWERS

Health risks or side effects following the proper administration of designated therapeutic dosages are not recorded. The drug should not be used in cases of high blood pressure or when the patient is being treated with monoamine oxidase inhibitors (amine content).

DRUG INTERACTIONS

POTENTIAL INTERACTIONS

Use of Scotch Broom herb with monoamine oxidase inhibitors (amine content) may cause a hypertensive crisis.

OVERDOSAGE

SCOTCH BROOM HERB

Doses corresponding to more than 300 mg sparteine (approximately 30 g of the drug), lead to dizziness, headache, palpitations, prickling in the extremities, feeling of weakness in the legs, outbreaks of sweat, sleepiness, pupil dilation, and ocular palsy. If no vomiting has occurred, poisonings are treated with gastric lavage and administration of activated charcoal. Spasms are to be treated with chlorpromazine or diazepam. In cases of asphyxiation, intubation and oxygen respiration are to be carried out. No deaths through poisonings with this drug have been proven beyond a doubt (though they certainly have been with sparteine).

DOSAGE

SCOTCH BROOM HERB

Mode of Administration: The herb is available in aqueous essential oil extracts for internal administration.

Preparation: Tea: Pour 150 ml boiling water over 1 to 2 gm drug and strain after 10 minutes

Decoction — from 1 to 2 g drug.

Liquid extract — 1:1 25% ethanol (V/V) (BHP83).

Tincture — 1:5 45% ethanol (V/V) (BHP83).

Daily Dosage: The daily dose of the infusion is 1 cup of fresh infusion 3 times daily. The liquid extract dosage is 1 to 2 mL daily. The tincture internal use dosage is 0.5 to 2 mL. Aqueous-ethanol extracts corresponding to 1:1.5 drug are also used.

Storage: Carefully protect from light and moisture.

SCOTCH BROOM FLOWERS

Mode of Administration: Since the efficacy for the claimed uses has not been documented, and considering the risks, a therapeutic application cannot be justified. To be used only under the supervision of an expert qualified in the appropriate use of this substance.

Preparation: To prepare an infusion, Pour 150 mL boiling water over 1 teaspoon of flowers and strain after 10 minutes.

Daily Dosage: Infusion dosage is 1 cup daily. For pathological edema, 1 liter infusion per day is administered in 4 portions during meals for 1 month.

LITERATURE

SCOTCH BROOM HERB AND FLOWERS

Brum-Bousquet M, Delaveau P, Plant Med Phytother 15(4):201. 1981

Gresser G, Der Besenginster - Cytisus scoparius (L.) LINK. Z Phytother 17 320-330. 1996

Konami Y, Yamamoto K, Osawa T, Irimura T, The primary structure of the *Cytisus scoparius* seed lectin and a carbohydrate-binding peptide. *J Biochem* (Tokyo), 112:366-75, Sep. 1992

Murakoshi I et al., *Phytochemistry* 25(2):521. 1986

Seeger R, Neumann HG, Spartein. In: *DAZ* 132(30):1577. 1992.

Vixcardi P et al., *Pharmazie* 39(11):781. 1984

Wink M, Heinen HJ, Vogt H, Schiebel HM, *Plant Cell Rep* 3:230-233. 1984.

Scotch Pine

Pinus species

DESCRIPTION

Medicinal Parts: The medicinal parts are the tar extracted from the trunks, branches, and roots. The oil extracted from the fresh needles, branch tips or fresh twigs is also used medicinally, as are the pine tips from fresh and dried shoots. The purified oil from the resin balsam, the tar extracted from the wood, the young shoots and the flowering branches of male and female flowers with pollen are also used.

Flower and Fruit: The male flowers are sulfur-yellow in the form of ovate catkins. The female flowers are purple and long-pedicled in erect, 5- to 6-mm long cones that hang down after flowering. The ripe cones are ovate-clavate, matte brown, and have rhomboid scales. The hilum is small, smooth, and light brown. The seeds are 3 to 4 mm long, oblong with wings, which are 3 times as long as the seed.

Leaves, Stem, and Root: The tree is 10 to 30 m high with a straight, slim, cylindrical trunk or a gnarled twisted one. It has a girth of 1.8 to 3.6 m. The crown is umbrella-shaped. The bark of the older trees is gray-brown on the outside and rust red on the inside. Bark of older trees is deeply fissured below and peeling. The bark of the young trees is red and thinly peeling. The buds are reddish, 6 to 12 mm long, oblong-oval, and somewhat resinous. The needles are in pairs and remain on the trees for 3 years. They are various lengths, rigid, twisted, bluish-green with interrupted rows on the outside and minimally dentate.

Habitat: Pinus sylvestris is found in Europe, Siberia, the Crimea, the Caucasus, and Iran.

Production: Pine shoots (*Pini turiones*) consist of the fresh or dried, 3- to 5-cm long shoots *of Pinus sylvestris.* Pine shoots are collected at the beginning of spring. The essential oil (*Pini aetheroleum*) is obtained from fresh needles, tips of the branches or fresh branches with needles and tips *of Pinus sylvestris, Pinus mugo ssp. pumilio, Pinus nigra* or *Pinus pinaster*. The oil is recovered form the fresh needles and branch tips using steam distillation with a successful yield of 0.15-0.6%. Purified turpentine oil (Terebinthinae aetheroleum rectificatum) is the essential oil obtained from the turpentine of *Pinus* species, especially *Pinus palustries* (syn. *Pinus australis*), and Pinus pinaster.

Not to be Confused With: Pine shoots should not be confused with the shoots of *Picea abies* and *Abies alba*. Pine oil should not be confused with ''pine oils'' that are synthetically produced.

Other Names: Dwarf-Pine, Pine Oils, Pix Liquida, Pumilio Pine, Scotch Fir, Stockholm Tar, Swiss Mountain Pine

ACTIONS AND PHARMACOLOGY

COMPOUNDS: PINE SHOOTS

Volatile oil (0.2-0.5%): including among others bornyl acetate, cadinene, Delta3 -carene, limonene, phellandrene, alpha-pinene

Resins

Bitter principles: pinicrin

Ascorbic acid (vitamin C)

EFFECTS: PINE SHOOTS

Pine shoots have secretolytic and mildly antiseptic effects and stimulate the peripheral circulation.

COMPOUNDS: PINE NEEDLE OIL

From Pinus mugo: chief components include Delta3-carene (up to 35%), alpha- and beta-pinene (20%), beta-phellandrene (15%)

From Pinus nigra: chief components include alpha-pinene (48-65%), beta-pinene (up to 32%), germacren D (up to 19%)

From Pinus palustris: chief components include alpha-and beta-pinene (95%)

From Pinus silvestris: chief components include alpha-pinene (10-50%), Delta3-carene (up to 20%), camphene (up to 12%), beta-pinene (10-25%), limonene (up to 10%), additionally including among others myrcene, terpinolene, bornyl acetate

EFFECTS: PINE NEEDLE OIL

The essential oil is secretolytic, hyperemic, and weakly antiseptic.

COMPOUNDS: TURPENTINE OIL, PURIFIED

Chief components of the raw turpentine oil yielded from turpentine from Pinus silvestris include: (-)-alpha-pinene (ca. 39-87%), Delta3-carene (ca. 14-33%), (-)-beta-pinene (share up to 27%), limonene (6%), camphene (ca. 5%), from out of which comes the volatile oils of other pine species' purified turpentine oil. Therebinthinae aetheroleum recticifactum is realized through fractional distillation. It must contain at least 90% pinenes, but no more than 0.5 % Delta3-carene.

EFFECTS: TURPENTINE OIL, PURIFIED

The essential oil is hyperemic, antiseptic, and increases bronchial secretion in animal tests.

INDICATIONS AND USAGE

PINE SHOOTS

Approved by Commission E:

- Blood pressure problems
- Common cold
- Cough/bronchitis
- Fevers and colds
- Inflammation of the mouth and pharynx
- Neuralgias
- Tendency to infection

Pine shoots are used internally for catarrhal conditions of the upper and lower respiratory tract. Externally, it is used for mild muscular pain and neuralgia, coughs, and acute bronchial diseases and topically for nasal congestion and hoarseness.

Homeopathic Uses: Homeopathic uses include weak ligaments of the upper ankle joint, inflammation of the respiratory tract, chronic rheumatism, eczema, and urticaria.

PINE NEEDLE OIL

Approved by Commission E:

- Common cold
- Cough/bronchitis
- Fevers and colds
- Inflammation of the mouth and pharynx
- Neuralgias
- Rheumatism
- Tendency to infection

The essential oil is used internally and externally for congestive diseases of the upper and lower respiratory tract. Externally, it is used for rheumatic and neuralgic ailments.

TURPENTINE OIL, PURIFIED

Approved by Commission E:

- Cough/bronchitis
- Inflammation of the mouth and pharynx
- Rheumatism

Purified turpentine oil is used internally and externally for chronic diseases of the bronchi with profuse secretion. It is used externally for rheumatic and neuralgic ailments.

Unproven Uses: Folk medicine uses include bladder catarrh, gallstones, and phosphorous poisoning. Externally, the oil is used for scabies, burns, frostbite, and skin injuries.

CONTRAINDICATIONS

PINE SHOOTS AND PINE NEEDLE OIL

Contraindications include bronchial asthma and whooping cough.

PRECAUTIONS AND ADVERSE REACTIONS

PINE SHOOTS

No health hazards or side effects are known in conjunction with the proper administration of designated therapeutic dosages. Patients with extensive skin injuries, acute skin diseases, feverish or infectious diseases, cardiac insufficiency or hypertonia should not use the drug as a bath additive.

PINE NEEDLE OIL

No health hazards are known in conjunction with the proper administration of designated therapeutic dosages. Signs of irritation could appear on skin and mucous membranes. Bronchial spasms could worsen. Patients with extensive skin injuries, acute skin diseases, feverish or infectious diseases, cardiac insufficiency, or hypertonia should not use the drug as a bath additive.

TURPENTINE OIL, PURIFIED

No health hazards or side effects are known in conjunction with the proper external administration of designated therapeutic dosages. However, resorptive poisonings, such as kidney and central nervous system damage, are possible with large-area administration. Where large skin injuries, severe feverish or infectious diseases, cardiac insufficiency, or hypertonia are present, entire-body baths with the volatile oil added should be carried out only following consultation with a physician.

Kidney damage is conceivable with internal administration of therapeutic dosages. Inhalation should be avoided with acute inflammation of the breathing passages.

Pediatric Use: Cases of death, in particular among children, following intake of the oil have been reported in the scientific literature.

DRUG INTERACTIONS

No drug interaction warnings were found.

OVERDOSAGE

TURPENTINE OIL, PURIFIED

Severe poisonings are possible with the intake of large dosages. Symptoms include albuminuria, diarrhea, dyspnea, dysuria, feelings of vertigo, hematuria, intestinal colic, queasiness, reddening of the face, salivation, skin efflorescences, sore throat, staggering walk, strangury, thirst, twitching, and vomiting. Poisonings can also occur through inhalation of the vapors or through skin contact. Fifty grams is the approximate lethal dosage for an adult. Cases of death, in particular among children, following intake of the oil are known from the scientific literature. Gastric lavage with bicarbonate of soda solution, intestinal emptying through administration of sodium sulphate, the administration of paraffin oil, activated charcoal and shock prophylaxis (suitable body position, quiet, warmth) should be instituted. Thereafter, therapy for poisonings consists of treating spasms with diazepam (IV), electrolyte substitution, and treating possible cases of acidosis with sodium bicarbonate infusions. In case of shock, plasma volume expanders should be infused. Monitoring of kidney function is essential. Intubation and oxygen respiration may also be necessary.

DOSAGE

PINE SHOOTS

Mode of Administration: Pine shoot is available as a comminuted herb for internal use in teas, syrups and tinctures. Alcoholic solutions, oils or ointments are used externally.

Daily Dosage:

Internal — daily dose: 2 to 3 g drug several times a day.

External — as a bath additive: 100 g alcoholic extract in a full bath.

Semi-solid preparations — 20 to 50% ointment to be rubbed in several times a day.

Homeopathic Dosage: 5 drops, 1 tablet or 10 globules every 30 to 60 minutes (acute) or 1 to 3 times daily (chronic); parenterally: 1 to 2 ml sc, acute: 3 times daily; chronic: once a day (HAB1). The dose is different for children.

PINE NEEDLE OIL

Mode of Administration: The essential oil is administered in alcoholic solutions, ointments, gels, emulsions, oils or as an inhalant. It is used externally as bubble baths and bath salts.

Daily Dosage: For internal use, the daily dose is 5 g drug. For inhalation therapy, add 2 g oil to 2 cups hot water and breathe in the vapors several times daily. When used externally, several drops of a liquid or semi-solid preparation containing 10 to 50% drug may be rubbed onto the affected area. To use as a bath additive, use 0.025 g drug per liter water and bathe for 10 to 20 minutes at a temperature 35 to 38° C.

Storage: Keep protected from light in tightly sealed containers.

TURPENTINE OIL, PURIFIED

Mode of Administration: Purified turpentine oil is administered externally in the form of ointments, gels, emulsions, oils, as a plaster and as an inhalant.

Daily Dosage:

External Dose — Varies according to the type and severity of the condition as well as the instructions of manufacturer.

As a bath additive and plaster — Use as directed by manufacturer.

Ointment/gel — 20% ointment/gel to be applied to the affected area several times a day.

Inhalation — 5 drops oil in hot water 3 times a day, inhale.

LITERATURE

PINE SHOOTS, OIL, AND TURPENTINE PURIFIED OIL

Glasl H et al., Gaschromatographische Untersuchung von Arzneibuchdrogen 7. Mitt.: GC-Untersuchung von Pinaceen-Ölen des Handels und Versuche zu ihrer Standardisierung. In: *DAZ* 120(2):64-67. 1980.

Ikeda RM, *J Food Sci* 27:455. 1962

Roschin VI et al., Khim Prir Soedin 1:122. 1985

Zinkel DF, *Chemtech* 5(4):235. 1975

Scotch Thistle

Onopordum acanthium

DESCRIPTION

Medicinal Parts: The medicinal parts are the herb and the root.

Flower and Fruit: The large, light-red composite flowers are terminal on the branches. The bracts are linear-lanceolate, thorny-tipped, splayed at the bottom, resembling cobwebs. The plant has only tubular androgynous flowers. The bristles of the hair calyx are reddish, short pinnate, and almost twice as long as the fruit. The flower heads fall after the fruit ripens and the seeds fall out.

Leaves, Stem, and Root: The plant is biennial and grows from 30 to 150 cm. The stem is erect and branched. It appears to be winged because of the downward leaves, which are broader than the stem. The leaves are rough, irregularly thorny, and dentate to pinnatisect. When young they appear almost white.

Habitat: The plant is indigenous to almost all of Europe, with the exception of the far north; it was introduced to North America.

Production: Scotch Thistle is the aerial part of *Onopordum acanthium.*

Other Names: Woolly Thistle

ACTIONS AND PHARMACOLOGY

COMPOUNDS

Sesquiterpene lactones (bitter principles): including, among others onopordopicrin

Flavonoids: including luteolin-7-O-glucoside

Hydroxycoumarins: esculin

Caffeic acid derivatives

Betaine: stachydrine

Polyynes

EFFECTS

A cardiotonic effect is questionable.

INDICATIONS AND USAGE

Unproven Uses: The drug is considered obsolete. In the religious system of anthroposophy, Scotch Thistle is used as a cardiac stimulant.

PRECAUTIONS AND ADVERSE REACTIONS

No health hazards or side effects are known in conjunction with the proper administration of designated therapeutic dosages.

DOSAGE

Mode of Administration: Scotch Thistle is available in the form of drops, ampules, and tablets. In anthroposophic medicine, a preparation of the fresh leaves is used internally.

LITERATURE

Kern W, List PH, Hörhammer L (Hrsg.), Hagers Handbuch der Pharmazeutischen Praxis, 4. Aufl., Bde 1-8, Springer Verlag Berlin, Heidelberg, New York, 1969.

Madaus G, Lehrbuch der Biologischen Arzneimittel, Bde 1-3, Nachdruck, Georg Olms Verlag Hildesheim 1979.

Scrophularia nodosa

See Figwort

Scullcap

Scutellaria lateriflora

DESCRIPTION

Medicinal Parts: The medicinal part of the plant is the herb.

Flower and Fruit: The pink or blue flowers are in short, chiefly lateral false spikes. The calyx is fluffy, dorsiventral and flattened, with 2 rounded, entire-margined lips. The lower lip has a helmet-shaped, concave appendage. The 4 ascending stamens have pairs of ciliated anthers. The fruit is a globular to flattened-ovoid warty nutlet.

Leaves, Stem, and Root: The perennial herb grows to 60 cm in height and is thickly covered with simple and glandular hairs. The stem is erect and heavily branched. The foliage leaves are usually ovate to lanceolate or linear, petioled, entire-margined, or crenate.

Characteristics: The herb has a bitter, slightly astringent taste.

Habitat: The plant is indigenous to North America and is cultivated in Europe.

Production: Scullcap is the aerial part of 3- to 4-year-old *Scutellaria lateriflora* and related species, which is harvested in June and then pulverized.

Other Names: Blue Pimpernel, Helmet Flower, Hoodwort, Mad-Dog Weed, Madweed, Quaker Bonnet, Side-Flowering Scullcap, Virginian Scullcap

ACTIONS AND PHARMACOLOGY

COMPOUNDS

Iridoids

Flavonoids: including among others, scutellarin

Volatile oil

Tannins

EFFECTS

Scullcap has sedative, antispasmodic (little research), anti-inflammatory, and also lipid peroxidation inhibitor effects.

INDICATIONS AND USAGE

Unproven Uses: The drug was formerly used for hysteria and nervous tension, epilepsy, chorea, and other nervous disorders. It has also been used as a bitter tonic and febrifuge.

PRECAUTIONS AND ADVERSE REACTIONS

No health hazards or side effects are known in conjunction with the proper administration of designated therapeutic dosages.

DOSAGE

Mode of Administration: The herb is available as a powder and liquid extract for internal use.

How Supplied:

Capsules – 425 mg, 429 mg, 430 mg

LITERATURE

Barberan FAT, *Fitoterapia* 57(2):67. 1986

Kimura Y et al., *Planta Med* 50:290. 1984

Kimura Y et al., *Planta Med* 51:132. 1985

Kimura Y et al., (1987) Phytother Res 1(1):48.

Kubo M et al., (1984) Chem Pharm Bull 32(7):2724.

Scurvy Grass

Cochlearia officinalis

DESCRIPTION

Medicinal Parts: The medicinal parts of the plant are the harvested and dried basal leaves of the first or second year; the aerial parts harvested shortly before or during flowering in the second year; or the fresh aerial parts of the plant collected at the onset of flowering.

Flower and Fruit: The flowers are arranged in racemes that are initially tight and somewhat hanging, which then grow longer. The flower is large, white, and fragrant. The sepals are about 1.5 to 2 mm long, narrowly elliptoid, with a white membranous edge. The petals are about 4 to 5 mm long and oblong-obovate. The stamens are yellow. The fruit is a 4- to -mm long, globular or ovate pod, crowned by the short style. The 2 to 4 seeds in each loculus are roundish-elliptoid, slightly compressed, and 1 to 3 mm long. The seed shell is usually red-brown and finely warty.

Leaves, Stem, and Root: The glabrous biennial or perennial plant is a 15 to 35 cm high evergreen. It has a fusiform, fibrous rhizome from which grows one or more stemmed shoots that are sterile or fertile. The leafy stems are ascending or almost erect, simple or branched, angular and grooved. The long-petioled basal leaves are in loose whorls. The fleshy, juicy cauline leaves are petiolate, ovate, angular-dentate, and the upper ones are stem-clasping.

Characteristics: The flowers have a strong taste and, when rubbed, a strong fragrance.

Habitat: The plant is found in central and northern Europe, Asia and North America.

Production: True Scurvy Grass consists of the dried basal leaves of *Cochlearia officinalis* harvested in the first year, or the aerial parts harvested during the flowering season in the second year. The cultivated plant is dried rapidly with artificial heat at temperatures below 35°C.

Not to be Confused With: Scurvy Grass is occasionally confused with *Ranunculus ficaria*.

Other Names: Scourbute-Grass, Scrubby Grass, Spoonwort

ACTIONS AND PHARMACOLOGY

COMPOUNDS

Glucosinolates: chief components in the freshly harvested, unbruised plant include glucocochlearin; with the destruction of the cells, the plants yield secretions of butyl mustard oil, and among others, glucotropaeolin (yielding butyl mustard oil) and sinigrin (yielding allyl mustard oil).

Flavonoids

Tropane alkaloids: tropine, m-hydroxybenzoyl-tropine (cochlearin)

Vitamin C

EFFECTS

The mustard oil glycosides in the drug, in ethereal oil and in an ethanol solution are strong external skin and mucous membrane irritants.

INDICATIONS AND USAGE

Unproven Uses: Scurvy Grass is used internally for vitamin C deficiency, and was used in folk medicine primarily as an agent for scurvy and scrofula. However, it was also valued for nosebleeds, rheumatism, gonorrhea, "blood-cleansing or purification" cures, gout, rheumatism, stomachache, and as a diuretic. External applications include use as a mouthwash for gum disease and as a poultice for ulcers.

Homeopathic Uses: Among uses in homeopathy are eye inflammation and stomach disorders.

Efficacy has not been proved.

PRECAUTIONS AND ADVERSE REACTIONS

Health risks or side effects following the proper administration of designated therapeutic dosages are not recorded. The administration of higher dosages can lead to irritation of the mucous membrane of the gastrointestinal tract.

DOSAGE

Mode of Administration: Alcoholic extracts of Scurvy Grass are used topically. Freshly pressed juice is for internal use.

Homeopathic Dosage: 5 to 10 drops, 1 tablet, 5 to 10 globules 1 to 3 times a day; or 1 mL injection solution sc twice weekly; as an eye drop: 1 drop 1 to 3 times daily (HAB1)

LITERATURE

Hänsel R, Keller K, Rimpler H, Schneider G (Hrsg.), Hagers Handbuch der Pharmazeutischen Praxis, 5. Aufl., Bde 4-6 (Drogen): Springer Verlag Berlin, Heidelberg, New York, 1992-1994.

Madaus G, Lehrbuch der Biologischen Arzneimittel, Bde 1-3, Nachdruck, Georg Olms Verlag Hildesheim 1979.

Scutellaria lateriflora

See Scullcap

Sea Buckthorn

Hippophaë rhamnoides

DESCRIPTION

Medicinal Parts: The medicinal parts are the ripe, yellow-red berries.

Flower and Fruit: The plant is dioecious and has greenish-yellow, insignificant flowers in numerous, sturdy clusters in the axils of scales. There are 2 bracts and a simple calyx. The male calyx is divided in half down to the base, with brown-spotted ovate sepals; it has 4 stamens attached to the base. The female calyx is a tight tube clasping the ovary with erect, inward-inclined tips. The fruit is a bright orange, globular, ellipsoid, false berry.

Leaves, Stem, and Root: The plant is an angular, thorny, 1.5- to 4.- m high shrub with numerous thorn-tipped and thorny branches. The leaves are 5 to 8 cm long, linear-lanceolate, short petioled, glabrous above, tomentose beneath. The plant spreads by underground runners.

Habitat: Hippophaë rhamnoides is indigenous to Europe and some northern regions of Asia.

Production: Sea Buckthorn berries are the false fruit of *Hippophaë rhamnoides*. The fatty oil is extracted from both the seeds and the fruit flesh. The harvest is from August to December, until the first snow. As soon as the fruit has been picked, it is immediately processed. The juice is produced without any contact with metal substances.

Other Names: Sallow Thorn

ACTIONS AND PHARMACOLOGY

COMPOUNDS

Fruit acids: chiefly malic acid, additionally acetic acid, quinic acid

Ascorbic acid (Vitamin C): 0.2-1.4%

Flavonoids: in particular kaempferol, isorhamnetin-as well as quercetin tri- and tetra-glycosides

Carotinoids: beta-carotine, gamma-carotine, lycopene

Fatty oil (in the seeds 12%): chief fatty acids oleic acid, isolinol acid, linolenic acid, stearic acid

Sugar alcohols: mannitol, quebrachit

EFFECTS

The drug is used as a vitamin C supplement. The vitamin C constituent encourages the healing of wounds and epithelization. The oil has a liver-protective, ulcer-protective, tumor-protective, antioxidative and wound-healing effect. The oil is said to be anticoagulative. The flavones are said to improve the contractility and pumping ability of cardiac muscle, reduce peripheral resistance, and promote vascular elasticity.

INDICATIONS AND USAGE

Unproven Uses: The drug is used as an infection prophylaxis, in particular during the time just before spring and during periods of convalescence. It is used externally as a treatment for radiation damage, such as x-ray damage and sunburn, and as fatty oil for the treatment of wounds.

PRECAUTIONS AND ADVERSE REACTIONS

No health hazards or side effects are known in conjunction with the proper administration of designated therapeutic dosages.

DOSAGE

Mode of Administration: Buckthorn is an extract constituent in various vitamin C concentrates and juices.

Daily Dosage: The recommended daily dose is 5 to 10 g of one of the Buckthorn products.

LITERATURE

Kern W, List PH, Hörhammer L (Hrsg.), Hagers Handbuch der Pharmazeutischen Praxis, 4. Aufl., Bde. 1-8, Springer Verlag Berlin, Heidelberg, New York, 1969.

Sedum acre

See Common Stonecrop

Selenicereus grandiflorus

See Night-Blooming Cereus

Self-Heal

Prunella vulgaris

DESCRIPTION

Medicinal Parts: The medicinal part is the whole flowering plant.

Flower and Fruit: The blue-violet or brownish-blue labiate flowers are clustered in semi-whorls at the end of stems and lateral branches. The accompanying leaves are red-brown. The upper lip of the calyx has 3 tips and the lower lip has 2 tips. The corolla is about 1 cm longer than the domed upper lip. The lower lip has 3 lobes. There are 4 stamens, the longer ones have a straight awl-shaped tip. The style is divided into two. The small fruit is flung out of the calyx.

Leaves, Stem, and Root: The plant grows from 10 to 30 cm high. The stems are usually ascendant, sometimes creeping. The leaves are petiolate, ovate to lanceolate, dentate or entire-margined, and crossed opposite.

Habitat: Prunella vulgaris is indigenous to Europe and Asia and practically all temperate regions of the world.

Production: Self-Heal is the complete plant in flower of *Prunella vulgaris.*

Other Names: All-Heal, Blue Curls, Brownwort, Brunella, Carpenter's Herb, Carpenter's Weed, Heal-All, Heart of the Earth, Hook-Heal, Prunella, Sicklewort, Slough-Heal, Woundwort

ACTIONS AND PHARMACOLOGY

COMPOUNDS

Bitter principles

Flavonoids: including rutin, hyperoside.

Tannins

Triterpene saponins

Triterpenes, ursolic acid, oleanolic acid

EFFECTS

There is no information available.

INDICATIONS AND USAGE

Unproven Uses: Self-Heal is used for inflammatory diseases and ulcers in the mouth and throat, gastrointestinal catarrh, as a remedy for diarrhea, hemorrhage, and gynecological disorders.

PRECAUTIONS AND ADVERSE REACTIONS

No health hazards or side effects are known in conjunction with the proper administration of designated therapeutic dosages.

DOSAGE

Mode of Administration: Self-Heal is available as crude drug, as an extract and as a gargle solution.

Preparation: To prepare a tea, use 1 dessertspoon of the drug per cup of water.

LITERATURE

Hegnauer R, Chemotaxonomie der Pflanzen, Bde 1-11, Birkhäuser Verlag Basel, Boston, Berlin 1962-1997.

Kern W, List PH, Hörhammer L (Hrsg.), Hagers Handbuch der Pharmazeutischen Praxis, 4. Aufl., Bde. 1-8, Springer Verlag Berlin, Heidelberg, New York, 1969.

Kojima H. et al., *Phytochemistry* 26(4):1107. 1987

Meckes M, Villarreal ML, Tortoriello J, Berlin B, Berlin A. A Microbiological Evaluation of Medicinal Plants used by the Maya People of Southern Mexico. Phytother Res. 9 (4); 244-250. 1995

Tabba HD, Chang RSh, Smith KM, Isolation, purification and partial characterization of prunellin, an anti-HIV component from aqueous extracts of *Prunella vulgaris*. In: *Antiviral Res* 11:263-274. 1989.

Sempervivum tectorum

See Houseleek

Senburi

Swertia japonica

DESCRIPTION

Medicinal Parts: The medicinal parts of the plant are the leaves and stems, which are used as an amaroid and tonic.

Flower and Fruit: The flowers are in dense apical panicles. The flowers are radial and fused, and appear in groups of five. The 5 calyx tips are up to 5 mm long and linear-to-lanceolate. The petals are 12 to 17 mm long, fused to a tube, with 5 broadened, elongate elliptical tips. The petals are white with reddish veins at the margin. Pairs of villous glandular scales are ciliate and twisted in the bud. There are 5 stamens and a superior, single-chambered ovary. The style is very short and the stigma double-lobed. The fruit is a capsule; the seeds are ovate to clavate.

Leaves, Stem, and Root: The herbaceous plant grows to approximately 20 cm high. The leaves are opposite and simple. The lower leaves are small and lanceolate. The cauline leaves are 1.5 to 3.5 cm long and 1 to 3 mm wide, linear to elongate-lanceolate, and acuminate with an involute margin. The stem is square in cross-section, 2 mm thick, dark green to dark red. The root is woody.

Characteristics: All parts of the plant taste very bitter.

Habitat: Swertia japonica is found in Korea, China, and Japan.

Production: Japanese chirata is the dried herb of *Swertia japonica* harvested during its flowering season.

ACTIONS AND PHARMACOLOGY

COMPOUNDS

Iridoids (bitter substances): secoiridoid glycosides, including amarogentin (0.01 to 0.05%) and amaroswerin (0.05 to 0.3%), the representatives that are chiefly responsible for the bitter taste, as well as the less bitter representatives swertiamarin (1.0 to 2.5%), gentiopicroside (0.5%) and sweroside (0.2%)

Flavonoids: including swertisin, isoswertisin, swertiajaponin, isovitexin

Xanthone derivatives (yellow): including swertianin, norswertianin, methyl swertianin, swertianol (bellidifolin)

Monoterpene alkaloids

EFFECTS

The use of the drug as an amarum is traceable to the bitter substances it contains (secoiridoid glucoside). The allergenic effect connected with topical application should be taken into consideration.

INDICATIONS AND USAGE

Unproven Uses: Uses in folk medicine include poor digestion and loss of appetite.

Chinese Medicine: Insomnia and poor digestion are considered indications for use in Chinese medicine. Efficacy for these indications has not yet been proved.

PRECAUTIONS AND ADVERSE REACTIONS

No health hazards are known in conjunction with the proper administration of designated therapeutic dosages.

DOSAGE

Mode of Administration: Whole, cut, and powdered drug.

How Supplied: Forms of: Drops (commercial pharmaceutical preparations).

Daily Dosage: 30 to 50 mg of the powder.

LITERATURE

Basnet P, Kadota S, Shimizu M, Takata Y, Kobayashi M, Namba T, Bellidifolin stimulates glucose uptake in rat 1 fibroblasts and ameliorates hyperglycemia in streptozotocin (STZ)-induced diabetic rats. *Planta Med,* 61:402-5, 1995 Oct.

Blaschek W, Hänsel R, Keller K, Reichling J, Rimpler G, Schneider G, (Eds) Hagers Handbuch der Pharmazeutischen Praxis. Folgebände 1 und 2. Drogen A-Z. Springer. Berlin, Heidelberg 1998.

el-Sedawy AI, Shu YZ, Hattori M, Kobashi K, Namba T, Metabolism of swertiamarin from *Swertia japonica* by human intestinal bacteria. *Planta Med,* 33:147-50, Apr. 1989

Hase K, Li J, Basnet P, Xiong Q, Takamura S, Namba T, Kadota S, Biologically active principles of crude drugs: pharmacological actions of *Swertia japonica* extracts, swertiamarin and gentianine (author's transl.). *Yakugaku Zasshi,* 45:1446-51, Nov. 1978

Hase K, Li J, Basnet P, Xiong Q, Takamura S, Namba T, Kadota S, Biosynthesis of C-glucosylflavones in *Swertia japonica* (author's transl.). *Yakugaku Zasshi,* 45:165-71, Feb. 1979

Hase K, Li J, Basnet P, Xiong Q, Takamura S, Namba T, Kadota S, Hepatoprotective principles of *Swertia japonica* Makino on D-galactosamine/lipopolysaccharide-induced liver injury in mice. *Chem Pharm Bull* (Tokyo), 45:1823-7, Nov. 1997

Yamahara J, Kobayashi M, Matsuda H, Aoki S, Anticholinergic action of *Swertia japonica* and an active constituent. *J Ethnopharmacol,* 33:31-5, May-Jun. 1991

Seneca Snakeroot

Polygala senega

DESCRIPTION

Medicinal Parts: The medicinal part is the dried root.

Flower and Fruit: The raceme is 8 cm long and is smaller than the bracts. The petals are pale red, the wings are yellowish-white with green veins.

Leaves, Stem, and Root: The plant is a perennial herb with up to 40 cm high stems, which sprout in the axils of the scalelike bracts of the previous year's growth. The leaves are 8 cm long and 3 cm wide, alternate, ovate-lanceolate to lanceolate, acuminate, and denticulate. The upper surface is rich green; the under surface somewhat paler. The root varies in color from pale yellowish-gray to brownish-gray. It is usually twisted or almost spiral and has a thick, irregular, gnarled crown.

Habitat: Polygala senega is indigenous to the central and western U.S.

Production: Seneca Snakeroot consists of the dried root with remains of aerial stems of *Polygala senega* and/or other closely related species or a mixture of Polygala species.

Not to be Confused With: The roots of other Polygala species.

Other Names: Milkwort, Mountain Flax, Rattlesnake Root, Seneca, Senega Snake Root, Senega, Seneka, Snake Root

ACTIONS AND PHARMACOLOGY

COMPOUNDS: SNAKEROOT (SENEGA SPECIES)

Triterpene saponins (6-12%): chief components senegins II to IV, chief aglycone presenegin

Oligosaccharide esters: senegosene A-I

Xanthone derivatives

Methyl salicylate (traces) and its glucoside

COMPOUNDS: SNAKEROOT (TENUIFOLIA SPECIES)

Triterpene saponins (6-12%): chief components onjisaponine aglycone presenegenin

Oligosaccharide esters: tenuifolosen A-P

Polygalite (acerite, 1.5-anhydrosorbite) and its glycosides, for example polygalite-2-alpha-galactoside

EFFECTS

The rhizome is secretolytic and works as an expectorant.

INDICATIONS AND USAGE

Approved by Commission E:

- Cough/bronchitis

The drug is used for congestion of the respiratory tract, as an expectorant in cases of bronchitis with minor sputum output

Unproven uses: The drug is also used for tracheitis.

PRECAUTIONS AND ADVERSE REACTIONS

General: No health hazards or side effects are known in conjunction with the proper administration of designated therapeutic dosages. With prolonged use, gastrointestinal irritation can occur.

Pregnancy: Not to be used during pregnancy.

OVERDOSAGE

Overdosage leads to nausea, diarrhea, gastric complaints and queasiness.

DOSAGE

Mode of Administration: As a comminuted root for decoctions and other galenic preparations for internal use or as an extract. It is a component of various standardized antitussive preparations.

Preparation: To make an infusion, place 0.5 g comminuted drug in cold water, heat to a simmer and strain after 10 minutes (1 teaspoonful = 2.5 g drug).

Daily Dosage: The daily dosage is 1.5 to 3.0 g root or liquid extract (1:2) or 2.5 to 7.5 g tincture (1:10). To use the infusion as an expectorant, drink 1 cup of tea 2 to 3 times daily. In serious cases, the tea can be taken every two hours if the patient is observed for side effects.

LITERATURE

Favel A et al. In Vitro Antifungal Activity of Triterpenoid Saponins. *Planta Med.* 60; 50-53. 1994

Kako M et al., Hypoglycemic effect of the rhizomes of *Polygala senega* in normal and diabetic mice and its main component, the triterpenoid glycoside senegin-II. In: *PM* 62(5)440-443. 1996.

Karl J. Bronchitis und Phytotherapie. *Naturheilpraxis* 46; 167-173. 1993

Saitoh H, Miyase T, Ueno A. Senegoses F-I, Oligosaccharide Multi-Esters from the Roots of *Polygala senega var. latifolia Torr. et Gray. Chem Pharm Bull.* 41; 2125-2128. 1993

Saitoh H et al. Senegoses J - O, Oligosaccharide Multi-Esters from Roots of *Polygala senega L. Chem Pharm Bull.* 42; 641-645. 1994

Shibata S, In: Progress in Phytochemistry, Vol. 6, Ed. Reinhold et al., Pergamon Press 1980.

Yoshikawa M, Murakami T, Ueno T, Kadoya M, Matsuda H, Yamahara J, Murakami N. E-Senegasaponins A and B, Z-Senegasaponins A and B, Z-Senegins II and III, New Type Inhibitors of Ethanol absortpion in Rats from Senegae radix, The Roots of *Polygala senega L. var. latifolia Torr. et Gray. Chem Pharm Bull.* 43 (2); 350-352 1995

Senecio aureus

See Golden Ragwort

Senecio bicolor

See Dusty Miller

Senecio jacoboea

See Ragwort

Senecio nemorensis

See Alpine Ragwort

Senecio vulgaris

See Groundsel

Senna

Cassia species

DESCRIPTION

Medicinal Parts: The medicinal parts are the leaves, fruit, and flowers.

Flower and Fruit: The flowers are yellow, occasionally white or pink. They are located in axillary or terminal positions on erect racemes. The calyx is deeply divided with a short tube and 5 regular, imbricate sepals. There are 5 layered petals. The 4 to 10 stamens are often irregular and partially sterile. The ovary is sessile or short-stemmed with a short or oblong style. The pod can be cylindrical or flat, angular or winged, and often with horizontal walls between the seeds. The seeds are numerous and either horizontally or vertically compressed.

Leaves, Stem, and Root: The genus Cassia comprises shrubs, subshrubs, and herbaceous perennials with paired-pinnate leaves. There are axes with stem glands either between the leaflets or on the petiole. The stipules have varying shapes.

Habitat: Cassia species is found in the tropical and subtropical regions of all continents except Europe. Most varieties are indigenous to North, Central, and South America.

Other Names: Alexandrian Senna, India Senna, Khartoum Senna, Tinnevelly Senna

ACTIONS AND PHARMACOLOGY

COMPOUNDS

Anthracene derivatives (2.5-3.5%): chief components sennosides A, A1 and B, as well as sennosides C and D

Naphthacene derivatives: including 6-hydroxymusizin glucoside (0.85% in Cassia senna), tinnevellin-6-glucosides (0.3% in Cassia angustifolia)

EFFECTS

Laxative Effects

Senna is an anthranoid-type stimulating laxative. The laxative effect is due to the action of sennosides and their active metabolite, rhein anthrone, in the colon. The laxative effect is realized by inhibition of water and electrolyte absorption from the large intestine, which increases the volume and pressure of the intestinal contents. This will stimulate colon motility resulting in propulsive contractions.

In addition, stimulation of active chloride secretion increases water and electrolyte content of the intestine. These changes in active electrolyte transport are dependent on calcium in the serosal surface (Donowitz, 1984; Yamauchi, 1993). The laxative action of Senna is partially via stimulation of colonic fluid and electrolyte secretion, and this secretion is mediated by stimulation of endogenous prostaglandin E2 formation (Beubler, 1988; Yamauchi, 1993).

CLINICAL TRIALS

Laxative Use

A Cochrane Collaboration review of randomized clinical trials comparing laxatives for constipation in palliative care patients failed to produce sufficient data to determine relative treatment efficacy. Senna was among the laxatives used in the four trials included in the review, which involved a total of 280 people and, among other items, assessed number and frequency of bowel movements and relative ease of defecation. Senna and other laxatives in the comparison—danthron combined with poloxamer, magnesium hydroxide combined with liquid paraffin, and Misrakasneham—demonstrated a limited level of effectiveness. Only significantly different results were identified in the trial in which lactulose plus Senna proved more effective than danthron combined with poloxamer—although patients did not prefer one over the other. The authors conclude that the treatment of constipation in palliative care is based on inadequate experimental evidence (Miles, 2007).

A comparative study was performed to compare the efficacy of Senna tablets and sodium phosphate solution for bowel preparation before colonoscopy. A total of 134 patients were randomly allocated to take 180 mg senna tablet or 95 mL sodium phosphate solution one day before colonoscopy. To assess the efficacies of both laxatives, the comparison of mean differences of colon-cleanliness score of the rectum, sigmoid segments, descending solon, transverse colon, and cecum was used. The scores were rated by two observers, who were blinded to the laxatives administered. Intention-to-treat analysis revealed that the mean cleanliness scores in the four segments of colon except the cecum were higher in the sodium phosphate group than those in the senna group. The 95% confidence intervals (95% CI) of mean difference in each segment of colon were not found to lie within 1 point, which indicated that their efficacies were not equivalent. Administration of senna led to fewer side effects than sodium phosphate solution (Kosichaiwat et al, 2006).

A randomized clinical trial showed that a high oral dose of Senna was a valid alternative to conventional polyethylene glycol-electrolyte solution (PEG-ES) for outpatient colonoscopy preparation, resulting in better quality of colon cleansing, overall tolerance of the preparation, and compliance. A total of 191 participants were assigned to receive 24 tablets of 12 mg Senna (divided into 2 doses), and 92 were assigned to receive the standard PEG-ES solution. Investigators (endoscopists), who were blinded to the group assignments, rated the quality of the overall cleansing as "excellent or good" in 90.6% of the Senna group, and in 79.7% of the PEG-ES group (p=000.3). The incidence of adverse events was similar for both groups (Radaelli, 2005).

An earlier, randomized, single-blind study evaluated the efficacy of Senna compared to polyethylene glycol (PEG) for mechanical preparation for elective colorectal resection. Five hundred twenty-three patients included in the study were undergoing resection, followed by anastomosis. All patients received 5% providone iodine antiseptic enema before surgery, and ceftriaxone sodium and metronidazole were given at anesthesia induction. Senna was significantly better than PEG with regard to colonic cleanliness and less fecal matter in the colonic lumen. The risk for moderate or large intraoperative fecal soiling was lower with Senna and overall clinical tolerance did not differ significantly between the treatment groups. Senna was better tolerated in patients with stenosis. There was no statistical difference between the treatment groups with postoperative infective complications or anastomotic leakage (Valverde, 1999).

A prospective randomized trial evaluated the efficacy of the addition of Senna to a polethylene glycol electrolyte lavage solution (PEG-ELS). One hundred and twenty patients received either a Senna extract with PEG-ELS or placebo with PEG-ELS before a total colonoscopy. Superiority by physician assessment was seen in the group with Senna. The colon was free of solid debris in 66.7% of patients after PEG-ELS and in 90% after Senna/PEG-ELS administration, which was a significant difference. Patient tolerance was similar in both groups, and significantly less lavage fluid was needed in the Senna/PEG-ELS treatment group (Ziegenhagen, 1991).

A randomized, open, parallel group study was conducted to determine the efficacy of Senna compared to lactulose in terminal cancer patients treated with opioids. Ninety-one terminal cancer patients were treated with either Senna (starting with 0.4 mL daily) or lactulose (starting with 15 mL daily) for a 27-day period. The main outcome measures were defecation-free intervals of 72 hr, days with defecation, general health status, and treatment cost. Both treatment groups had similar scores for defecation-free intervals and in days with defecation. The final scores for general health status were similar in both groups (Agra, 1998).

INDICATIONS AND USAGE

Commission E Approved:

- Constipation

Senna is used for constipation and for evacuation of the bowel prior to diagnostic tests of the gastrointestinal and colorectal area.

Indian Medicine: The herb is used for constipation, liver disease, jaundice, splenomegaly, anemia, and typhoid fever.

Note: Stimulating laxatives must not be used over a period of more than 1 to 2 weeks without medical advice.

CONTRAINDICATIONS

The herb is not to be administered in the presence of intestinal obstruction, acute inflammatory intestinal diseases or appendicitis.

PRECAUTIONS AND ADVERSE REACTIONS

General: Spasmodic gastrointestinal complaints can occur as a side effect to the drug's purgative effect or from overdosage. In rare cases, prolonged use may lead to cardiac arrhythmias, nephropathies, edema, and accelerated bone deterioration. Senna abuse has also resulted in tetany, aspartylglucosamine excretion, and hypogammaglobulinemia (Levine, 1981; Malmquist, 1980; Prior, 1978).

Electrolyte Abnormalities: Long-term use leads to loss of electrolytes, in particular potassium ions. As a result of hypokalemia, hyperaldosteronism, albuminuria, hematuria, inhibition of intestinal motility, and muscle weakness may occur. Enhancement of cardioactive glycosides and antiarrythics may also occur with hypokalemia.

Finger Clubbing: Senna abuse has resulted in finger clubbing, which was reversible upon discontinuation of the drug (Levine, 1981; Malmquist, 1980; Prior, 1978; Currie 2006).

Cathartic Colon: Anatomic alteration of the colon is seen secondary to chronic use with Senna (more than three times weekly for 1 year or longer). The result is a loss of haustral folds, a finding that suggests neuronal injury or damage to colonic longitudinal musculature (Joo, 1998).

Carcinogenesis: Carcinogenic activity in the colon following long-term administration of anthracene drugs has not yet been fully clarified. Study findings are controversial regarding the correlation between the administration of anthracene drugs and the frequency of carcinomas in the colon (al-Dakan, 1995; Mereto, 1996).

Melanosis Coli: Prolonged use of Senna may lead to melanosis coli. Precursors of the melanic substance in melanosis coli may be derived from anthranoid laxatives (Benavides, 1997).

Occupational Sensitization: IgE-mediated allergy, asthma, and rhinoconjunctivitis have been reported after occupational exposure to Senna products (Helin, 1996, Marks, 1991).

Tissue Damage: Chronic treatment with anthranoids in high doses reduces vasoactive intestinal polypeptide and somatostatin levels in the colon, which may represent damage to the enteric nervous tissue (Tzavella, 1985).

Pregnancy: The drug should not be used during pregnancy or while nursing.

Pediatric Use: Not to be used by children under 2 years of age.

Elderly: Elderly patients should initially take half of the normal prescribing dose.

DRUG INTERACTIONS

MAJOR RISK

Licorice: Concurrent use may result in increased risk of hypokalemia. *Clinical management:* Avoid concomitant use of licorice and laxatives.

MODERATE RISK

Digoxin: Concurrent use may result in increased risk of digoxin toxicity. *Clinical management:* Patients who are taking digoxin should be advised to avoid concomitant use with Senna. If digoxin toxicity occurs, potassium should be monitored and supplemented if necessary while discontinuing Senna.

DOSAGE

Mode of Administration: Comminuted herb, powder or dried extracts for teas, decoctions, cold macerates, or elixirs. Liquid or solid forms of medication exclusively for oral use.

How Supplied:

Capsule — 25 mg, 450 mg

Chewable tablet — 15 mg sennosides

Granules — 15 mg sennosides per teaspoon

Liquid — 2.5 oz. (alcohol 7% by volume), 8.8 mg sennosides per teaspoon

Tablet — 8.6 mg sennosides, 15 mg sennosides, 17 mg sennosides, 25 mg sennosides

Preparation: To prepare an infusion, pour hot water (not boiling) over 0.5 to 2 g of comminuted drug, steep for 10 minutes, then strain; or steep in cold water for 10 to 12 hours, then strain. The cold water method, according to various authors, should result in a solution containing less resin, which is responsible for abdominal pain. The drug takes effect after a latency period of 10 to 12 hours.

Daily Dosage:

Constipation — The average dose is 20 to 40 mg sennosides.

Chewable Tab — Adults and children 12 years of age and over, chew 2 tabs once or twice daily. Children 6 to under 12 years of age, chew 1 tab once or twice daily (Prod Info Ex-Lax®, 1998).

Granules (15 mg sennosides per teaspoon) — Adults and children 12 years of age, administer 1 teaspoon once daily with a maximum of 2 teaspoons twice daily. Children 6 to 12 years of age, administer 1/2 teaspoon once daily with a maximum of 1 teaspoon twice a day. Children 2 to 6 years of age, administer 1/4 teaspoon daily with a maximum of 1/2 teaspoon twice daily (Prod Info Senokot®, 1993).

Liquid (8.8 mg sennoside per teaspoon) — Children 6 to 12 years of age, administer 1 to 1 1/2 teaspoon once daily with a maximum of 1 1/2 teaspoon twice daily. Children 2 to 6 years of age, administer 1/2 to 3/4 teaspoon once daily with a maximum of 3/4 teaspoon twice daily (Prod Info Senokot®, 1991).

Pills — Adults and children 12 years of age and over should take 2 pills once or twice daily with a glass of water. Children 6 to under 12 years of age: take 1 pill once or twice daily with a glass of water. Children under 6 years of age: consult a doctor (Prod Info Ex-Lax®, 1998).

Tablets (8.6 mg sennosides) — Adults and children 12 years of age, administer 2 tablets once daily with a maximum of 4 tablets twice daily. Children 6 to 12 years of age, administer 1 tablet once daily, with a maximum of 2 tablets twice daily. Children 2 to 6 years of age, adminster 1/2 tablet once daily with a maximum of 1 tablet twice daily (Prod Info Senokot®, 1993).

Tablets (17 mg sennosides) — Adults and children 12 years of age, administer 1 tablet once daily with a maximum of 2 tablets twice daily. Children 6 to 12 years of age, administer 1/2 tablet once daily with a maximum of 1 tablet twice daily (Prod Info SenokotXTRA®, 1993).

Bowel Evacuation:

Liquid (alcohol 7% by volume) — Adults and children 12 years of age and older should take one bottle between 2 and 4 p.m. on day prior to x-ray or other diagnostic procedures. Drink entire contents of bottle. A strong bowel action can be expected approximately 6 hours after drinking the preparation (Prod Info X-Prep®,1998).

Storage: Senna should be protected from light stored for a maximum of 3 years.

LITERATURE

Agra Y; Sacristan A; Gonzalez M et al. Efficacy of senna versus lactulose in terminal cancer patients treated with opioids. *J Pain Symptom Manage* Jan;15(1):1-7. 1998

al-Dakan AA; al-Tuffail M; Hannan MA. *Cassia senna* inhibits mutagenic activities of benzo[a]-pyrene, aflatoxin B1, shamma and methyl methanesulfonate. *Pharmacol Toxicol* Oct;77(4):288-92. 1995

Benavides SH; Morgante PE; Monserrat AJ et al. The pigment of melanosis coli: a lectin histochemical study. *Gastrointest Endosc* Aug;46(2):131-8. 1997

Beubler E, Kollar G. Stimulation of PGE2 synthesis and water and electrolyte secretion by senna anthraquinones is inhibited by indomethacin. *J Pharm Pharmacol* Apr;37(4):248-51. 1985

Beubler E; Kollar G. Prostaglandin-mediated action of sennosides. *Pharmacology*;36 Suppl 1:85-91. 1988

Choi JS et al., In vitro antimutagenic effects of anthraquinone aglycones and naphthoquinones. In: *PM* 63(1):11-14. 1997.

Dufour P, Gendre P, Long-Termin mucosal alterations by sennosides, related compounds. *Pharmacology* 36(Suppl 1):194-202. 1988

Helin T; Makinen-Kiljunen. Occupational asthma and rhinoconjunctivitis caused by senna. *Allergy* Mar;51(3):181-4. 1996

Jahn K et al., Toxicology of Cassia fikifiki Aubréville 6 Pellegrin in relation to other species of the genus Cassia (s.l.). In: PM 62, Abstracts of the 44th Ann Congress of GA, 57. 1996.

Jeko ZB, Mate M, Krausz E, Bene M. Development and scale up of a new film coated tablet containing dry herba extract. *Pharmazie* 54 (2); 148-150. 1999

Joo JS; Ehrenpreis ED; Gonzalez L et al. Alterations in colonic anatomy induced by chronic stimulant laxatives: the cathartic colon revisited. *J Clin Gastroenterol* Jun;26(4):283-6. 1998

Kositchaiwat S, Suwanthanmma W, Suvikapakornkul R, Tiewthanom V, Rerkpatanakit P, Tinkornrusmee C. Comparative study of two bowel preparation regimens for colonoscopy: senna tablets vs sodium phosphate solution. *World J Gastroenterol*; 12(34): 5536-5539. 2006.

Levine D; Goode AW; Wingate DL. Purgative abuse associated with reversible cachexia, hypogammaglobulinaemia, and finger clubbing. *Lancet* Apr 25;1(8226):919-20. 1981

Lewis SJ, Oakey RE, Heaton KW. Intestinal absorption of estrogen: the effect of altering transit-time. *Eur J Gastroenterol Hepatol* Jan;10(1):33-9. 1998

Malmquist J; Ericsson B; Hulten-Nosslin MB et al. Finger clubbing and aspartylglucosamine excretion in a laxative-abusing patient. *Postgrad Med J* Dec;56(662):862-4. 1980

Marks GB; Salome CM; Woolcock AJ. Asthma and allergy associated with occupational exposure to ispaghula and senna products in a pharmaceutical work force. *Am Rev Respir Dis* Nov;144(5):1065-9. 1991

Mengs U. Toxic Effect of Sennosides in Laboratory Animals and in vitro. *Pharmacology* 36; Suppl.1; 180-187. 1988

Mereto E; Ghia M; Brambilla G. Evaluation of the potential carcinogenic activity of Senna and Cascara glycosides for the rat colon. *Cancer Lett* Mar 19;101(1):79-83. 1996

Prior J, White I. Tetany and clubbing in patient who ingested large quantities of senna. *Lancet*. Oct 28:2(8096):947. 1978

Product Information: Ex-Lax®, chocolated laxative pieces. Novartis, Summit, NJ, USA, 1998.

Product Information: Ex-Lax®, regular and maximum strength laxative pills. Novartis, Summit, NJ, USA, 1998.

Product Information: SenokotXTRA®, standardized senna concentrate. Purdue Frederick, Norwalk, CT, USA, 1993.

Product Information: Senokot®, extract of standardized senna. Purdue Frederick, Norwalk, CT, USA, 1991.

Product Information: Senokot®, standardized senna concentrate. Purdue Frederick, Norwalk, CT, USA, 1993.

Product Information X-Prep®, extract of standardized senna. Gray Pharmaceuticals, Norwalk, CT, USA, 1998.

Schultze W, Jahn K, Richter R, Volatile constituents of the dried leaves of *Cassia angustifolia* and *C. acutifolia* (Sennae folium). In: *PM* 61(6):540-543. 1996.

Sydiskis RJ, Owen DG, Lohr JL, Rosler KHA, Blosmster RN, Inactivation of enveloped viruses by anthraquinones extracted from plants. In: *Antimicrob Agents Chemother* 35:2463-2466. 1991.

Tzavella K; Schenkirsch G; Riepl RL et al. Effects of long-term treatment with anthranoids and sodium picosulphate on the contents of vasoactive intestinal polypeptide, somatostatin and substance P in the rat colon. *Eur J Gastroenterol Hepatol* Jan;7(1):13-20. 1995

Valverde A; Hay JM; Fingerhut A et al. Senna vs polyethylene glycol for mechanical preparation the evening before elective colonic or rectal resection: a multicenter controlled trial. French Association for Surgical Research. Arch Surg May;134(5):514-9. 1999

Yamauchi K; Yagi T; Kuwano S. Suppression of the purgative action of rhein anthrone, the active metabolite of sennosides A and B, by calcium channel blockers, calmodulin antagonists and indomethacin. *Pharmacology* Oct;47 Suppl 1:22-31. 1993

Ziegenhagen DJ; Zehnter E; Tacke W et al. Addition of senna improves colonoscopy preparation with lavage: a prospective randomized trial. *Gastrointest Endosc* Sep-Oct;37(5):547-9. 1991

Serenoa repens

See Saw Palmetto

Sesame

Sesamum orientale

DESCRIPTION

Medicinal Parts: The medicinal part of the plant is the seed.

Flower and Fruit: The flowers are short-pedicled, single or in groups of 2 or 3 in the leaf axils. The flowers are zygomorphic; the calyx 5-tipped, 2 to 5 mm long, pubescent and does not drop. The corolla is campanulate, 5-lobed, and distinctly bilabiate. It is 1.5 to 3.5 cm long, white or reddish. The lower lobes are the longest. There are 4 stamens. The ovary is usually double-chambered (but can have up to 10 chambers) with a false septum, 1 to 1.5 mm long, and pubescent. The fruit is a square, brownish, 2 to 3 cm long, and up to 1 cm wide, multiseeded capsule. The seeds are yellowish-white, brownish, reddish or black, 1.5 to 4 mm long, 1 to 2 mm wide, 0.5 to 1 mm thick, and smooth or finely ribbed.

Leaves, Stem, and Root: The herb grows upright to a height of 1.2 m. The lower leaves are opposite and the petiole is 3 to 11 cm long. The lamina 4 to 20 cm long and 2 to 10 cm wide. It is elongate-ovate, entire or 3-lobed, then dentate. The upper leaves are opposite or alternate. The petiole is up to 3 cm long. The lamina is 0.5 to 2.5 cm wide, lanceolate, and usually entire. Young leaves are pubescent and sticky. The stem is square to hexagonal, either completely pubescent or only on the upper section. The taproot grows down to a depth of almost 1 m. The stem is branched or unbranched.

Characteristics: The plant's oily seeds are odorless with a sweet taste.

Habitat: Sesame orientale is cultivated worldwide in tropical and subtropical temperate zones, but the main sesame oil-producing countries are India, Sudan, Myanmar, and China.

Production: Sesame oil is the oil of *Sesamum orientale*, which is pressed or extracted from the ripe seeds and refined.

Other Names: Beniseed, Gingelly, Oriental Sesame

ACTIONS AND PHARMACOLOGY

COMPOUNDS

Fatty oil (97 to 98%): chief fatty acids are oleic acid (35 to 50%), linoleic acid (35 to 50%), palmitic acid (7 to 12%), stearic acid (3 to 6%)

Lignans (0.8 to 1.7%): including sesamine sesamolin

Steroids: sterols, including beta-sitosterol (0.4%), campesterol

EFFECTS

The lignan sesamine contained in the drug is immunosuppressive in vitro. In view of its oily nature, use as a clysma for softening the stool and topically on dry skin diseases is plausible. Its effect as a purgative seems logical but has not been clinically proved. Sesame oil treated with lipase is cytotoxic in vitro. Because of its high levels of linoleic acid, sesame oil is a valuable dietetic.

INDICATIONS AND USAGE

Unproven Uses: Folk medicine internal uses include treating constipation, especially dyschezia; external uses include removal of scabs and crust formations, for swellings, rheumatism and as a massage oil. Its use as a laxative is considered obsolete.

PRECAUTIONS AND ADVERSE REACTIONS

No health hazards are known in conjunction with the proper administration of designated therapeutic dosages. The drug possesses a limited potential for sensitization.

DOSAGE

Mode of Administration: Preparations are available for internal and external use.

Preparation: Sesame oil for parenteral application is produced from *Sesamum orientale* by heating in a drying chamber to 140°C or by means of germ filtration with the addition of 5% benzyl alcohol followed by heating at 120° C for 1 hour in the drying chamber.

Daily Dosage 30 to 60 g of drug for constipation.

Storage: Store in tightly sealed containers and protect from light.

LITERATURE

Aregheore EM, A review of implications of antiquality and toxic components in unconventional feedstuffs advocated for use in intensive animal production in Nigeria. *Vet Hum Toxicol*, 40:35-9, Feb. 1998

Badifu GI, Akpagher EM, Effects of debittering methods on the proximate composition, organoleptic and functional properties of sesame (*Sesamum indicum L.*) seed flour. *Plant Foods Hum Nutr,* 51:119-26, Feb. 1996

Bhatnagar A, Gupta A, Chlorpyriphos, quinalphos and lindane residues in sesame seed and oil (*Sesamum indicum L.*). *J Sci Food Agric,* 60:596-600, Apr. 1998

Bhatnagar A, Gupta A, Dissociation and denaturation behaviour of sesame alpha-globulin in sodium dodecyl sulphate solution. *Int J Pept Protein Res,* 60:385-92, Apr. 1998

Chambers SJ, Carr HJ, Lambert N, An investigation of the dissociation and denaturation of legumin by salts using laser light scattering and circular dichroism spectroscopy. *Biochim Biophys Acta,* 1037:66-72, Jan 19, 1990

Egbekun MK, Ehieze MU, Proximate composition and functional properties of fullfat and defatted beniseed (*Sesamum indicum L.*) flour. *Plant Foods Hum Nutr*, 51:35-41, 1997.

Guerra MJ, Jaffe WG, Sangronis E, Obtaining protein fractions from commercial sesame cakes (*Sesamum indicum*). *Arch Latinoam Nutr*, 34:477-87, Sep. 1984

Guerra MJ, Jaffe WG, Sangronis E, Os sesamum genus proximale tibiale. *Cesk Radiol,* 34:477-87, Sep. 1984

Hansel R, Keller K, Rimpler H, Schneider G (Ed), Hagers Handbuch der Pharmazeutischen Praxis, 5. Aufl., Bde 4 - 6 (Drogen), Springer Verlag Berlin, Heidelberg, New York, 1992-1994.

Lakshmi TS, Nandi PK, Prakash V, Interactions of sugars with alpha-globulin from *Sesamum indicum L. Indian J Biochem Biophys,* 51:135-41, Jun. 1985

Marston A, Potterat O, Hostettmann K, Isolation of biologically active plant constituents by liquid chromatography. *J Chromatogr,* 60:3-11, Oct 19, 1988

Otaiza ER, Valeri H, Cumare V, Selenium content in the blood of cattle from Venezuela. I. Central and Portuguese zones. *Arch Latinoam Nutr*, 60:233-46, Jun. 1977

Perez C, Saad R, Enzymatic modification of proteins of commercial sesame meals (*Sesamum indicum, L.*). *Arch Latinoam Nutr,* 34:735-48, Dec. 1984

Plietz P, Damaschun G, Zirwer D, Gast K, Schwenke KD, Prakash V, Shape and quaternary structure of alpha-globulin from sesame (*Sesamum indicum L.*) seed as revealed by small angle x-ray scattering and quasi-elastic light scattering. *J Biol Chem,* Sep 25; 261(27):12686-91. 1986

Prakash V, Nandi PK, Association-dissociation behavior of sesame alpha-globulin in electrolyte solutions. *J Biol Chem,* 60:240-3, Jan 10. 1977

Prakash V, Nandi PK, Dissociation, aggregation and denaturation of sesame alpha-globulin in urea and guanidine hydrochloride solutions. *Int J Pept Protein Res,* 60:97-106, 1977.

Prakash V, Nandi PK, Jirgensons B, Effect of sodium dodecyl sulfate, acid, alkali, urea and guanidine hydrochloride on the circular dichroism of alpha-globulin of *Sesamum indicum L. Int J Pept Protein Res,* 51:305-13, Apr. 1980

Rajamohan T, Kurup PA, Lysine: arginine ratio of a protein influences cholesterol metabolism. Part 1 - Studies on sesame protein having low lysine: arginine ratio. *Indian J Exp Biol,* 35:1218-23, Nov. 1997

Saad R, Perez C, Functional and nutritional properties of modified proteins of sesame (*Sesamum indicum, L.*). *Arch Latinoam Nutr,* 34:749-62, Dec. 1984

Saad R, Perez C, Persistance of antibiotics in leaves of sesamum (*Sesamum indicum L.*). *Hindustan Antibiot Bull,* 34:107-8, Aug-Nov. 1984

Salgado JM, Goncalves CM, Sesame seed (*Sesamum indicum, L.*). I. Methods for preparing an edible white flour. *Arch Latinoam Nutr,* 38:306-11, Jun. 1988

Sheela P, Amuthan G, Mahadevan A, Cloning of extracellular lipase gene from *Xanthomonas campestris pathovar sesami* on to *Escherichia coli. Indian J Exp Biol*, 60:27-31, Jan. 1996

Tasneem R, Prakash V, Aggregation, dissociation and denaturation of sesame (*Sesamum indicum L.*) alpha-globulin in cetyl trimethyl ammonium bromide solution. *Int J Pept Protein Res,* 8:120-8, 1977.

Tasneem R, Prakash V, Association-dissociation and denaturation behaviour of an oligomeric seed protein alpha-globulin of *Sesamum indicum L.* in acid and alkaline solutions. *Int J Pept Protein Res,* 8:319-28, 1977.

Tasneem R, Prakash V, Resistance of alpha-globulin from *Sesamum indicum L.* to proteases in relationship to its structure. *J Protein Chem,* 8:251-61, Apr. 1989

Tasneem R, Prakash V, The nature of the unhydrolysed fraction of alpha-globulin, the major protein component of *Sesamum indicum L.* hydrolysed by alpha-chymotrypsin. *Indian J Biochem Biophys,* 29:160-7, Apr. 1992

Thompson EW, Richardson M, Boulter D, The amino acid sequence of sesame (*Sesamum indicum L.*) and castor (Ricinus communis L.) cytochrome c. *Biochem J,* 51:439-46, Feb. 1971

Wankhede DB, Tharanathan RN, Sesame (*Sesamum indicum*) carbohydrates. *J Agric Food Chem,* 51:655-9, May-Jun. 1976

Yukawa Y, Takaiwa F, Shoji K, Masuda K, Yamada K, Structure and expression of two seed-specific cDNA clones encoding stearoyl-acyl carrier protein desaturase from sesame, *Sesamum indicum L. Plant Cell Physiol,* 37:201-5, Mar. 1996

Yun TK, Kim SH, Lee YS, Trial of a new medium-term model using benzo(a)pyrene induced lung tumor in newborn mice. *Anticancer Res,* 15:839-45, May-Jun. 1995

Sesamum orientale

See Sesame

Shepherd's Purse

Capsella bursa-pastoris

DESCRIPTION

Medicinal Parts: The medicinal part is the aerial portion of the plant.

Flower and Fruit: The plant stays in bloom for almost the whole year. The flowers are white and about 4 to 6 mm long. The 4 sepals are 1 to 2 mm long and the 4 petals are 2 to 3 mm long. There are 6 stamens. The inflorescence is extended after flowering. The many-seeded pod is 4 to 9 mm long and almost as wide. It is glabrous, flattened, long-stemmed, triangular, and obcordate. The seeds are 0.8 to 1 mm long and red-brown with a short style.

Leaves, Stem, and Root: Shepard's purse is a 2 to 40 cm high plant with a simple fusiform root and a simple upright stem. The stem is glabrous or has scattered hairs on the lower section. The basal leaves form a rosette and are petioled, entire-margined, or pinnatifid. The few cauline leaves are alternate, smaller, sessile, entire, very wrinkled, and involute.

Habitat: Worldwide, except tropical regions.

Production: Shepherd's Purse herb consists of the fresh or dried aboveground parts of *Capsella bursa*, collected in the wild during the summer and dried rapidly.

Other Names: Blindweed, Case-Weed, Cocowort, Lady's Purse, Mother's Heart, Pepper-and-Salt, Pick-Pocket, Poor Man's Parmacettie, Rattle Pouches, Sanguinary, Shepherd's Scrip, Shepherd's Heart, Shepherd's Sprout, St. James' Weed, Toywort, Witches' Pouches,

ACTIONS AND PHARMACOLOGY

COMPOUNDS

Cardioactive steroids: presumably only in the seeds

Glucosinolates, sinigrin: 9-methyl sulfinyl nonyl glucosinolate, 9-methyl sulfinyl decyl glucosinolate

Flavonoids: including rutin, luteolin-7-rutinoside

Caffeic acid derivatives: including chlorogenic acid.

The plant very often acts as a host to endophytic fungi (*Albugo candida, Peronospora parasitica*), so the presence of mytotoxins is a possibility.

EFFECTS

A number of different studies have shown both a lowering and elevation of blood pressure, positive inotropic and chronotropic cardiac effects, and increased uterine contraction. An antibacterial effect against gram-negative pathogens has been shown with formulations of the root constituents (Park 2000). Despite numerous studies a clear therapeutic use could not be identified.

INDICATIONS AND USAGE

Approved by Commission E:

- Nosebleeds
- Premenstrual syndrome (PMS)
- Wounds and burns

Unproven Uses: Internally, the plant is used for mild menstrual irregularities such as menorrhagia and metrorrhagia. Externally, it is used for nosebleeds and superficially bleeding skin injuries. Shepherd's Purse is seldom used in folk medicine today. In America it is used for headaches. In Spain a decoction of the fresh plant is used for bladder inflammation.

Homeopathic Uses: Capsella bursa-pastoris is used for uterine and mucous membrane bleeding as well as for calculosis.

PRECAUTIONS AND ADVERSE REACTIONS

General: No health hazards or side effects are known in conjunction with the proper administration of designated therapeutic dosages.

Pregnancy: Not to be used during pregnancy.

DOSAGE

Mode of Administration: Comminuted drug for tea and other galenic preparations for internal use and external administration.

Daily Dosage: Internally, the average daily dose is 10 to 15 g of drug. The liquid extract daily dose is 5 to 8 g drug. The infusion may be drunk throughout the day. Externally an infusion is prepared by adding 3 to 5 g drug to 150 mL water.

Homeopathic Dosage: 5 drops or 1 tablet, or 10 globules every 30 to 60 minutes (acute) or 1 to 3 times a day (chronic); parenterally: 1 to 2 mL 3 times a day sc (HAB1)

Storage: Shepard's Purse should be protected from light and moisture.

LITERATURE

Hill RK, in ''The Alkaloids Vol. 2'', Ed. SW Pelletier, John Wiley 1984.

Kuroda K, Tagaki K, *Nature* 220:707. 1968

Kuroda K et al., *Cancer Res* 36:1900. 1976

Park CJ et al. Characterization and cDNA cloning of two glycine- and histidine-rich antimicrobial peptides from the roots of sheperd's purse, *Capsella bursa-pastoris. Plant Mol Biol* (2000), 44: 187-197

Vermathen M, Glasl H, Effect of the herb extract of *Capsella bursa pastoris* on blood coagulation. In: *PM* 59(7):A670. 1993.

Short Buchu

Barosma species

DESCRIPTION

Medicinal Parts: The medicinal parts are the leaves of *Barosma betulina, Barosma crenulata,* and *Barosma serratifolia* gathered during the flowering season, as well as the ethereal oil extracted from the dried leaves of *Barosma betulina.*

Flower and Fruit: The pentamerous flowers of *Barosma betulina* form a white or pink corolla 12 mm in diameter with lanceolate petals. The fruit is a 7 mm long capsule with 5 chambers and one seed per chamber. The upper surface is greenish-brown and rough. The fruit springs open at the 5 valves. The seeds are ovoid, oblong, about 5 mm long and 2 mm wide, glossy black and hard with no endosperm. The flowers of *Barosma crenulata* are pink or white and attached to short leafy side branches.

Leaves, Stem, and Root: Barosma betulina is a small shrub with light green to yellowish leaves. The leaves are 12 to 20 mm in length, opposite, rigid, and coriaceous. They are rhomboid or obovate, short-petioled, and slightly pubescent, blunt and revolute at the apex. Each indentation has an oil gland. The oil glands form small raised structures on the leaf surface. The stem is about 2 to 3 mm in diameter, reddish-brown, and rough (due to the oil glands) with 4 long grooves. The internodes are 8 to 20 mm long.

Barosma crenulata is a slender glabrous bush 2 to 3 m high. It is branched somewhat angularly. The bark is violet-brown. The leaves of *Barosma crenulata* vary in form, and are opposite and pubescent on both surfaces. They reach up to 3 cm in length with an obtuse, but not a revolute, tip.

The *Barosma serratifolia* bush is very similar to *Barosma crenulata*, although the leaves are longer, obtuse at the tip, and narrowed on both edges. The leaves are lanceolate, have a long, serrated, saw-shaped margin, and a blunt apex. They are yellowish green and up to 4 cm long with an oil gland at the apex and indentations on the margin. There are smaller oil glands spread over the leaf blade.

Characteristics: The leaves have a peppermint odor.

Habitat: The plant is indigenous to the Cape region of South Africa.

Production: Short Buchu leaf consists of the dried leaves of *Barosma betulina* harvested when in flower and in fruit. In South Africa, collection of the leaves is strictly controlled by the government to prevent destruction of the plant in the wild.

Not to be Confused With: Other Barosma and Diosma species.

Other Names: Buchu, Bucku, Long Buchu, Ovate Buchu, Round Buchu

ACTIONS AND PHARMACOLOGY

COMPOUNDS

Volatile oil: chief components diosphenol and psi-diosphenol (as a mixture known as buccocamphor), limonene, (+)-menthone, 8-9-isomenthone, pulegone, furthermore (-)- cis- and (+)-trans-8-mercapto-p-menth-3-one (odor-determining, so-called cassis aroma)

Flavonoids: including rutin and diosmetin

EFFECTS

No studies of the drug are currently available.

INDICATIONS AND USAGE

Unproven Uses: Short Buchu leaf is used for inflammation and infection of the kidneys and urinary tract, for bladder irritation, as a disinfectant of the urinary tract, and as a diuretic. In Europe the drug has been in use since the 16th century for the treatment of gout, various bladder disorders and rheumatism, and for the prostate gland. In South Africa it is still widely used, typically as a brandy made from the plant and used to treat stomach complaints.

CONTRAINDICATIONS

Short Buchu is not to be used during pregnancy.

PRECAUTIONS AND ADVERSE REACTIONS

No health hazards or side effects are known in conjunction with the proper administration of designated therapeutic dosages, but it is noted that the volatile oil could lead to signs of irritation.

DOSAGE

Mode of Administration: Since the claimed efficacy has not been documented, the application of Buchu leaf cannot be recommended. Buchu is used in various preparations and combinations.

How Supplied: Short Buchu is available as an extract, tincture and infusion.

Preparation: A fluid extract is prepared using 1,000 parts powdered Buchu leaves plus 400 parts 90% ethanol (V/V) 7:3 water produce 1,000 parts fluid extract (EB6).

Infusion — fluid extract 1:1 90% ethanol (V/V) (BHP83).

Buchu leaf tincture — 1:5 60% ethanol (V/V) (BHP83).

Daily Dose: The daily dose of the drug is 1 g to 2 g. Fluid extracts of 0.3 to 1.2 mL are taken 3 times daily. Dosage for the tincture is 2 to 4 mL up to 3 times daily. Infusion usage is typically 1 g per cup.

Homeopathic Dosage: 5 drops, 1 tablet, 10 globules every 30 to 60 minutes (acute) or 1 to 3 times daily (chronic); parenterally: 1 to 2 mlL3 times daily sc (HAB34).

Storage: The drug must be kept cool, dry, and away from the light in sealed containers.

LITERATURE

Didry N, Pinkas M, *Plant Med Phytother* 16 (4): 249. 1982

Hänsel R, Keller K, Rimpler H, Schneider G (Hrsg.), Hagers Handbuch der Pharmazeutischen Praxis, 5. Aufl., Bde 4-6 (Drogen), Springer Verlag Berlin, Heidelberg, New York, 1992-1994.

Kaiser R et al., *J Agric Food Chem* 23: 943-950. 1975

Leung AY, Encyclopedia of Common Natural Ingredients Used in Food Drugs and Cosmetics, John Wiley & Sons Inc., New York 1980.

Madaus G, Lehrbuch der Biologischen Arzneimittel, Bde 1-3, Nachdruck, Georg Olms Verlag Hildesheim 1979.

Steinegger E, Hänsel R, Pharmakognosie, 5. Aufl., Springer Verlag Heidelberg 1992.

Wichtl M (Hrsg.), Teedrogen, 4. Aufl., Wiss. Verlagsges. Stuttgart 1997.

Siam Benzoin

Styrax tonkinensis

DESCRIPTION

Medicinal Parts: The medicinal part of the plant is the resin obtained from the trunk.

Flower and Fruit: Styrax tonkinensis is a tree that grows up to 20 m high. It is very similar to *Styrax benzoin,* but the flowers are smaller, the calyx is 3 to 4 mm long, the corolla is white and up to 9 mm long. The fruit is up to 12 mm long.

Leaves, Stem, and Root: The leaves are oval, 4.5 to 10 cm long and 2 to 6 cm wide.

Habitat: Laos

Production: Siam Benzoin is the balsam of *Styrax tonkinensis*, or other related species, obtained by making cuts in the trunk. The optimal age of tree to be harvested is 7 years. The tree is cut, which stimulates it to exude resin to heal the cuts. The resin is then collected in a vessel, and left to melt to a homogenous mass in the sun.

Other Names: Gum Benjamin Siam

ACTIONS AND PHARMACOLOGY

COMPOUNDS

Ester mixture (90%): bestehend aus coniferyl benzoate (60 to 70%), p-cumaryl benzoate (10 to 15%), as well as cinnamyl benzoate, cinnamyl cinnamate

Benzoic acid (10 to 20%)

Vanillin (0.5%)

Triterpenes: alpha-siaresinolic acid (5%)

EFFECTS

The expectorant effect with which the drug is credited could not be proved experimentally (it possibly originated in connection with an ''aroma therapy,'' due to its vanilla content).

INDICATIONS AND USAGE

Unproven Uses: Siam Benzoin is used for respiratory catarrh.

Chinese Medicine: In China, preparations are used for stroke, syncope, post partal syncope due to heavy loss of blood, and chest and stomach pain.

PRECAUTIONS AND ADVERSE REACTIONS

No health hazards are known in conjunction with the proper administration of designated therapeutic dosages.

DOSAGE

Mode of Administration: Whole herb, powdered drug and other galenic preparations for internal use.

Preparation: To prepare a tincture, use powder in 90% ethanol (V/V) 1:5 macerate (DAB9).

Daily Dosage: 0.5 g; single dose: 0.05 g

Storage: Should be tightly sealed, and protected from light.

LITERATURE

Hänsel R, Keller K, Rimpler H, Schneider G (Ed), Hagers Handbuch der Pharmazeutischen Praxis, 5. Aufl., Bde 4 - 6 (Drogen), Springer Verlag Berlin, Heidelberg, New York, 1992-1994.

Hausen BM, Simatupang T, Bruhn G, Evers P, Koenig WA. Identification of New Allergenic Constituents and Proof of Evidence for Coniferyl Benzoate in Balsam of Peru. *Am J Contact Dermatitis* 6 (4); 199-208. 1995

James WD, White SW, Yanklowitz B, Allergic contact dermatitis to compound tincture of benzoin. *J Am Acad Dermatol*, 11:847-50, Nov. 1984

Siberian Ginseng

Eleutherococcus senticosus

DESCRIPTION

Medicinal Parts: The medicinal parts are the pulverized root rind, the pulverized root and an alcoholic fluid extract of the rhizome and the roots.

Flower and Fruit: The flowers are in umbels. The central umbel is on a long, thick peduncle. The style is fused into a column to the tip and has 5 small stigma lobes.

Leaves, Stem and Root: Siberian Ginseng is a 1 to 3 m high shrub whose branches are thickly covered with pale, thorny bristles pointing downward at an angle. The leaves are in groups of 5 and are thorny-serrate. The petiole is covered in fine bristles.

Habitat: Siberian Ginseng grows in Siberia, northern China, Korea, and Japan.

Production: Siberian Ginseng consists of the dried roots and/or rhizome of *Eleutherococcus senticosus* as well as their preparations in effective dosage.

ACTIONS AND PHARMACOLOGY

COMPOUNDS

Caffeic acid derivatives: including chlorogenic acid

Hydroxycoumarins: isofraxidin

Lignans: sesamine, eleutheroside D (epimeric diglucosides of syringaresinols)

Steroids: including beta-sitosterol-3-O-beta-D-glucoside (daucosterol, eleutheroside A, 0.1%)

Phenylacrylic acid derivatives: eleutheroside B (syringin)

Polysaccharides: immunostimulatingly effective polysaccharides (eleutherane A-G)

Steroid glycosides: eleutheroside A (daucosterol, beta-stigmasterol-3-O-beta-D-glucoside)

Triterpene saponins: eleutheroside I, eleutheroside K (beta-hederin), eleutheroside L, eleutheroside M (hederasaponin B), for all of these aglycone oleanolic acid

EFFECTS

The liquid extract of the drug has an immune-stimulating/immune-modulating and antiviral effect. In various stress models, e.g., immobilization test and coldness test, the endurance of rodents was enhanced. Learning and memory capability in rats was also shown. Inhibition of histamine, enhanced cytokine synthesis, and inducement of interleukin-1 and interleukin-2 production in vitro has been demonstrated. With healthy volunteers, the lymphocyte count, especially that of T-lymphocytes, increased following intake of liquid extracts.

Hypoglycemic effects have also been demonstrated with the herb along with enhancement of platelet aggregation-inhibiting effects (Hikino, 1986; Yun-Coi, 1987).

CLINICAL TRIALS

Adaptogenic qualities

Siberian ginseng's adaptogenic powers were tested for measures of improvements in quality of life in a group of Italian adults, age 65 and older. In this double-blind study, 20 healthy, elderly adults with hypertension (and taking antihypertensive medicines and digitalis) were randomized to either Siberian ginseng daily (dry extract 300 mg) or placebo for eight weeks. The participants completed surveys to assess their quality of life at the start of the study, at four weeks, and then at eight weeks. At four weeks, but not eight weeks, those assigned to Siberian ginseng had significantly better mental health and social functioning ($p = 0.02$). The herb was well-tolerated and safe, with no influence noted in terms of blood levels of digoxin (Cicero, 2004).

Fatigue

A blinded and controlled trial looked at 96 adults (76 completed the study), recruited both from advertisements and from chronic fatigue support groups, who reported substantial fatigue of unknown cause for six months or more. While fatigue appreciably lessened over the course of the two-month study in subjects randomized to take Siberian Ginseng capsules (powdered extract; four 500 mg capsules standardized to a total intake of 2.24 mg of the active ingredient, eleutherosides), differences between the treatment and placebo groups were not statistically significant. For the 45 individuals with less severe fatigue ($p=0.04$) at study start and the 41 participants with long-standing fatigue (5 years or more; $p=0.09$), Siberian Ginseng led to improvement at two months. While overall efficacy for Siberian Ginseng was not shown, the authors note that fatigue is subjective and hard to measure, and that the causes of fatigue in this study were diverse and multifactorial (Hartz, 2004).

INDICATIONS AND USAGE

Approved By Commission E:

- Lack of stamina
- Tendency to infection

Unproven Uses: Siberian Ginseng is used as a tonic for invigoration and fortification in times of fatigue and debility or declining capacity for work and concentration, and during convalescence.

Chinese Medicine: Siberian Ginseng is used for kidney pain, retention of urine, impotence, sleep disturbance, loss of appetite, pain and weakness in the hip and knee joints, rheumatoid arthritis, and as a stimulant for the immune system.

CONTRAINDICATIONS

The drug should not be administered to patients with hypertension.

PRECAUTIONS AND ADVERSE REACTIONS

Health risks or side effects following the proper administration of designated therapeutic dosages are not recorded.

DRUG INTERACTIONS

POTENTIAL INTERACTIONS

Antidiabetic Agents/Insulin – may potentiate effects (Hikino, 1986)

Anticoagulants/Antiplatelets/Antithrombotics – may enhance effects (Yun-Choi, 1987)

DRUG-LAB MODIFICATIONS

Digoxin Assay: Concurrent use of digoxin and eleuthrococcus may result in false reading sin digoxin concentrations. Eleutherococcus falsely increased serum digoxin levels using the fluorescence polarization immunoassay and falsely decreased levels using the microparticle enzyme immunoassay ex vivo (Dasgupta et al, 2003). A case report described elevation of Digoxin levels following concomitant use of a product purported to be eleutherococcus (McRae, 1996). Glycosides in eleutherococcus have structural similarity to digoxin (Dasgupta et al, 2003). *Clinical Management:* Patients should be asked about eleutherococcus use when unanticipated serum digoxin concentrations are obtained.

DOSAGE

Mode of Administration: Powdered or cut root for teas, as well as aqueous-alcoholic extracts for internal use.

Preparation:

Extract (Siberian Ginseng) — root powder 1:7 75% ethanol extracted with back flow to which is added a 10% alpha-naphthol solution until there is no reaction. It is then evaporated to a paste (ChinP IX).

Liquid extract — medium fine root powder can be produced using a through flow procedure with 40% ethanol (V/V) (1000 gm drug to 1 Liter extract), (Ross XI).

Daily Dosage: 9 to 15 g root bark; 9 to 27 g root; 0.3 to 0.5 g drug extract 3 times daily. The average daily dosage is 2 to 3 g of root.

Storage: Should be stored in well-aired, dry place, protected from light

LITERATURE

Bohn B, Nebe Cr, Birr C, Flow-cytometric studies with Eleutherococcus senticosus extract as an immunomodulatory agent. *Arzneim Forsch* (Drug Res) 37:1193-1196. 1987

Cicero AF, Derosa G, Brillante R, et al. Effects of Siberian ginseng (Eleutherococcus senticosus maxim.) on elderly quality of life: a randomized clinical trial. *Arch Gerontol Geriatr Suppl*; (9):69-73. 2004.

Hikino H, Takahashi M, Otake K, Konno C, Isolation and hypoglycemic activity of A, B, C, D, E, F, and G: glycans of *Eleutherococcus senticosus* roots. *J Nat Prod* Mar-Apr; 49(2):293-7. 1986

Hartz AJ, Bentler S, Noyes R, et al. Randomized controlled trial of Siberian ginseng for chronic fatigue. *Psychol Med*; 34:51—61. 2004.

Koch HP, Eidler S, *Eleutherococcus Senticosus*. Sibirischer Ginseng. Wissenschaftlicher Bericht. Kooperation Phytopharmaka, Köln Bonn Frankfurt Bad Homburg. 1988

McRae S, Elevated serum digoxin levels in a patient taking digoxin and Siberian ginseng. *CMAJ* Aug 1;155(3):293-5. 1996

Wagner H, Nörr H, Winterhoff H, Drogen mit ''Adaptogenwirkung'' zur Stärkung der Widerstandskräfte. In: ZPT 13(2):42. 1992.

Yun-Choi HS, Kim JH, Lee, Potential inhibitors of platelet aggregation from plant sources, III. *J Nat Prod* Nov-Dec;50(6):1059 1987

Zorikov PS, Lyapustina TA, (1974) Change in a concentration of protein and nitrogen in the reproductive organs of hens under the effect of *Eleutherococcus* extract. Deposited DOC VIN1:732-774, 58-63: ref *Chem Abstracts* 86 (1977).

Silphium laciniatum

See Rosinweed

Silphium perfoliatum

See Cup Plant

Silybum marianum

See Milk Thistle

Simaruba

Simaruba amara

DESCRIPTION

Medicinal Parts: The medicinal part is the dried root bark.

Flower and Fruit: The flowers grow in small racemes with dense matte-white petals.

Leaves, Stem, and Root: Simaruba amara is a tree that grows over 18 m high. The roots are long and spread horizontally. The leaves are 22 to 27 cm long. The tree has numerous long, bent branches covered in smooth, grayish bark. The bark that is used commercially is thin and flat with a yellowish or grayish-yellow color. The bark is tough, fibrous, and almost impossible to break.

Characteristics: The taste is very bitter and odorless.

Habitat: The plant grows on the Caribbean islands and the northern parts of South America.

Other Names: Bitter Damson, Dysentery Bark, Mountain Damson, Slave Wood, Stave Wood, Sumaruba

ACTIONS AND PHARMACOLOGY

COMPOUNDS

Bitter substances: quassinoids (breakdown products of triterpenes), including among others simarubin (1%), simarubidin, simarolide, 13,18-dehydro-glaucarubinone

Tannins (20-27%)

Volatile oil (0.1-0.2%)

5-hydroxy-canthin-6-one

Alkaloids

EFFECTS

The active agents are tannin, simarubin, essential oil and fat. The drug has a sedative effect on the smooth muscle of the intestine. It constricts the vessels of the intestinal tract. Simaruba is a tonic and febrifuge.

INDICATIONS AND USAGE

Unproven Uses: Simaruba was formerly used in the treatment of febrile illnesses and dysentery. Recent research indicates that it may be effective in treating malaria. The drug is used for unspecified enteritis, diarrhea, and as a bitter. It may cause vomiting, and is also used as an abortifacient.

PRECAUTIONS AND ADVERSE REACTIONS

No health hazards or side effects are known in conjunction with the proper administration of designated therapeutic dosages. The drug triggers vomiting in high dosages.

DOSAGE

Mode of Administration: The drug is available as a liquid extract for internal use.

Daily Dosage: The average dose is 1 g of the drug to be taken internally.

Storage: Protect against dampness.

LITERATURE

Dou J, Khan IA, McChesny JD, Burandt jr, CL. Qualitative and Quantitative High Performance Liquid Chromatographic Analysis of Quassinoids in Simaroubaceae Plants. *Phytochem Anal.* 7; 192-200. 1996

Hegnauer R, Chemotaxonomie der Pflanzen, Bde 1-11: Birkhäuser Verlag Basel, Boston, Berlin 1962-1997.

Kern W, List PH, Hörhammer L (Hrsg.), Hagers Handbuch der Pharmazeutischen Praxis, 4. Aufl., Bde 1-8: Springer Verlag Berlin, Heidelberg, New York, 1969.

Simaruba amara

See Simaruba

Simmondsia chinesis

See Jojoba

Sinapis alba

See White Mustard

Sisymbrium officinale

See Hedge Mustard

Sium sisarum

See Skirret

Skirret

Sium sisarum

DESCRIPTION

Medicinal Parts: The medicinal part is the root.

Flower and Fruit: The inflorescence has 10- to 30-rayed umbels with 1 to 5 lanceolate-narrow involucral bracts. The petals are white, about 1 mm long, and broad orbicular-elliptical. The fruit is broad-ovate, about 3.5 by 2 to 2.5 mm in diameter, and brownish with light ribs. The fruit segments in cross-section are obtuse pentagons with thin walls.

Leaves, Stem, and Root: Sium sisarum is a perennial glabrous plant on a stubby rhizome with clustered, often tuberous roots. The stem is about 30 to 80 cm high, round, and branched. The lower leaves are simple pinnate, oblong, and serrate. The upper leaves are narrower and more acuminate, and are usually lanceolate.

Habitat: The plant is indigenous to China; it is cultivated in Europe.

Production: Skirret root is the root of *Sium sisarum.*

ACTIONS AND PHARMACOLOGY

COMPOUNDS

Oligosaccharides: saccharose (4-8%)

Starch (4-18%)

Mucilage

EFFECTS

No information is available.

INDICATIONS AND USAGE

Unproven Uses: The drug is used for digestive disorders and loss of appetite.

PRECAUTIONS AND ADVERSE REACTIONS

No health hazards or side effects are known in conjunction with the proper administration of designated therapeutic dosages.

DOSAGE

Mode of Administration: Skirret root is available as cut drug for internal use.

LITERATURE

Kern W, List PH, Hörhammer L (Hrsg.), Hagers Handbuch der Pharmazeutischen Praxis, 4. Aufl., Bde. 1-8: Springer Verlag Berlin, Heidelberg, New York, 1969.

Skunk Cabbage

Symplocarpus foetidus

DESCRIPTION

Medicinal Parts: The medicinal parts are the seeds, the rhizome, and the roots.

Flower and Fruit: The plant has numerous small purple flowers in a red-brown, oval, high, spadixlike inflorescence.

Leaves, Stem, and Root: The plant is a perennial and grows up to 75 cm high. It has a thick tuberous rhizome, which is truncate at both ends, dark brown and up to 4 cm in diameter. The rhizome is gnarled and woody and bears numerous roots and root scars. The roots are up to 8 cm long, 0.5 cm in diameter, and transversely wrinkled. The leaves are similar to cabbage leaves and they surround the inflorescence.

Characteristics: The taste is hot and the odor is unpleasant.

Habitat: The plant is indigenous to the northern U.S.

Production: Skunk Cabbage root and rootstock are the rhizome and roots of *Symplocarpus foetidus.*

Other Names: Dracontium, Meadow Cabbage, Polecatweed, Skunkweed

ACTIONS AND PHARMACOLOGY

COMPOUNDS

Volatile oil (bad-smelling)

Resins

The constituents of the drug have not been fully investigated.

EFFECTS

Skunk Cabbage is an antispasmodic, a diaphoretic, an expectorant, and a sedative.

INDICATIONS AND USAGE

Unproven Uses: The plant is used for bronchitis and asthma.

PRECAUTIONS AND ADVERSE REACTIONS

No health hazards or side effects are known in conjunction with the proper administration of designated therapeutic dosages.

OVERDOSAGE

Overdosage results in queasiness and vomiting.

DOSAGE

Mode of Administration: Skunk Cabbage is administered as a liquid extract in various medicinal preparations.

LITERATURE

Adolf A, Hecker E. *Tetrahedron Letters* 21:2887 1980

Hegnauer R, Chemotaxonomie der Pflanzen, Bde 1-11: Birkhäuser Verlag Basel, Boston, Berlin 1962-1997.

Kern W, List PH, Hörhammer L (Hrsg.), Hagers Handbuch der Pharmazeutischen Praxis, 4. Aufl., Bde 1-8: Springer Verlag Berlin, Heidelberg, New York, 1969.

Slippery Elm

Ulmus rubra

DESCRIPTION

Medicinal Parts: The medicinal part is the dried inner rind separated from the outer bark.

Flower and Fruit: The flowers are in dense, almost sessile clusters. There are 5 to 9 tepals and the same number of stamens. The stigmas are bright red. The fruit is almost top-shaped to broad-elliptical, 1 to 2 cm long, wide and glabrous, except for the rust-red downy center. The seeds are inserted in the center.

Leaves, Stem, and Root: The tree is medium-sized and grows up to 20 m tall with spread branches forming an open crown. The younger branches are red-brown or orange and more or less downy. The bark is deeply fissured. The buds are large, rust-red, and downy. The leaves are obovate to oblong, 10 to 20 cm long, and have a double-serrate margin. The lamina is long acuminate and sharply asymmetrical at the base. The leaves are dark green above and very rough, densely downy beneath. They darken in autumn.

Characteristics: The texture is mucilaginous and the odor slight but characteristic. The powdered inner bark is used for its mucilaginous quality. Taken as a drink, it relieves irritation of the mucous membrane. The same water-retaining properties allow the powder to be used as an emollient poultice.

Habitat: The plant is indigenous to North America.

Production: Slippery Elm bark is the inner bark and wood of *Ulmus fulva*.

Other Names: Red Elm, Sweet Elm

ACTIONS AND PHARMACOLOGY

COMPOUNDS

Steroids: sterols, including cholesterol, campesterol, beta-sitosterol

Sesquiterpenes: including 5-isopropyl-3,8-dimethyl-2-naphthol, 2-hydroxy-5-isopropyl-8-methyl-5,6,7,8-tetrahydro-3-naphthyl aldehyde

Tannins (very little)

EFFECTS

Slippery elm contains large amounts of mucilage, which will coat the surface of the mucous membranes or surface of wounds and sores when it comes in contact with water (Gallagher, 1997). Slippery elm has been successfully used as a demulcent and emollient. The primary indication for slippery elm is in the treatment of irritated and inflamed mucous membranes such as the lining of the throat and digestive tract. This functional herb is utilized for its mucilagenous comforting properties. Used externally as a poultice, slippery elm is used to expedite healing of wounds, draw out impurities, and soothe inflammation.

Most data on the antitussive actions of slippery elm are anecdotal rather than clinically proven. Slippery elm is included in the herbal antineoplastic compound essiac, but its role in the mixture is uncertain. In a 1977 study approved by the Canadian Health Protection Branch, a study of the effectiveness of essiac showed that it did not stop the progression of cancer, did not cure cancer, and was not palliative (Locock, 1997).

Demulcent Effects: The mucilage in slippery elm bark works as a demulcent by soothing and decreasing irritation of the intestinal tract, throat, esophagus, and other mucous membranes. It is often included in antitussive remedies such as lozenges. A sore throat can be treated by taking 200 mg slippery elm 3 times daily as a tea. It is thought that slippery elm causes a reflex in the gastrointestinal and urinary tracts that causes mucous secretion. Tannins found in slippery elm preparations may provide an astringent effect (Chevallier, 1996).

Nutritive Effects: The starch and other constituents in slippery elm are nutritive and have been given to babies and to convalescent or debilitated patients (Chavallier, 1996).

Wound-Healing Effects: A poultice containing the mucilage of slippery elm bark is applied to wounds and sores to protect the area and allow healing (Anon, 1999). It is also thought to draw out toxins or irritants but no studies could be found to confirm this effect. When applied to the skin it acts as an emollient, softening the skin (Chavallier, 1996). Mix the powdered bark with boiling water to create a paste and apply liberally to the affected area.

CLINICAL TRIALS

Cancer

Slippery elm is part of the herbal antineoplastic remedy called Essiac. This remedy also contains sheep sorrel (*Rumex acetosella*), burdock root (*Arctium lappa*), and turkey rhubarb (*Rheum palmatum*). Of 360 cancer patients surveyed, 16.3% had taken the herb and 20% had heard of it. Patients were more likely to be taking the herb if undergoing treatment and gastrointestinal cancer patients were the most likely group to be using Essiac. Of those taking Essiac, 30% thought the herb had helped them. About 54% of these thought the benefit was psychological and 29% thought it was physical. Seventeen percent described other benefits (Karn & Moore, 1997). The role that slippery elm plays in this mixture is uncertain. There were no objective measurements.

INDICATIONS AND USAGE

Unproven Uses: Internally, the drug is used in the treatment of gastritis and gastric or duodenal ulcers. Externally, it is used in the treatment of wounds, burns, skin conditions, swollen glands, gout, and rheumatism.

CONTRAINDICATIONS

There are no known contraindications to the use of slippery elm bark.

PRECAUTIONS AND ADVERSE REACTIONS

General: No health hazards or side effects are known in conjunction with the proper administration of designated therapeutic dosages.

Dermatologic Effects: Contact dermatitis has been reported after exposure to an oleoresin contained in the bark (Lewis & Elvin Lewis, 1977).

Pregnancy: Slippery elm should not be used during pregnancy. Spontaneous abortions have occurred from the use of whole bark preparations and the agent has been used as an abortifacient (Fetrow & Avila, 1999; Hutchens, 1973).

Breast Milk: Scientific evidence for the safe use of slippery elm during lactation is not available.

DRUG INTERACTIONS

POTENTIAL INTERACTIONS

Iron: Taking iron and slippery elm together may affect iron absorption. This interaction has been reported when herbal teas containing tannins (such as slippery elm) and iron were taken together. This interaction has been reported in people (Koren 1982; Pizarro 1994). Until more is known, patients who need iron supplementation should be advised to separate administration times of these two compounds by one to two hours.

DOSAGE

Mode of Administration: Whole and cut drug is available in the form of a decoction for internal use and poultices for external use.

How Supplied: Capsules — 370 mg

Preparation: A decoction is made in a ratio of 1:8 with ethanol.

Daily Dosage: The dose for the decoction is 4 to 16 mL per day. Externally, the coarsely ground drug is used as a poultice.

LITERATURE

Anon. British Herbal Pharmacopoeia. Diddles Ltd, Guildford and King's Lynn, Exeter, England. 1996.

Chevallier A. The Encyclopedia of Medicinal Plants. DK Publishing Company, New York, NY. 1996.

DerMarderosian A (ed). The Review of Natural Products. Facts and Comparisons Inc, St Louis, MO. 1999.

Fetrow CW, Avila JR. Professional's Handbook of Complementary and Alternative Medicines. Springhouse Corp, Springhouse, PA. 1999.

Gallagher R. Use of herbal preparations for intractable cough. *J Pain Symptom Manage* 14(1):1-2. 1997.

Karn H, Moore MJ. The use of the herbal remedy ESSIAC in an outpatient cancer population. *Proceed ASCO* 16:71a. 1997.

Kim JP, Kim WG, Koshino H, et al. Sesquiterpene O-naphthoquinones from the root bark of Ulmus davidiana. *Phytochemistry* 43:425-430. 1996.

Koren G, Boichis H, Keren G. Effects of tea on the absorption of pharmacological doses of an oral iron preparation. *Sci Meet Israel* 18:547. 1982.

Locock RA Essiac. *Can Pharm J* 130:18-20. 1997.

Pizarro F, Olivares M, Hertrampf E, Walter T. Factors which modify the nutritional state of iron: tannin content of herbal teas. *Arch Latinoam Nutr* 44:277-80. 1994.

Sloe

Prunus spinosa

DESCRIPTION

Medicinal Parts: The medicinal parts are the flowers.

Flower and Fruit: The white, pedicled flowers are solitary but appear close to each other on the branches. The bush finishes flowering before the leaves unfold. The calyx is campanulate with long tips, which are twice as long as the tips of the 5 petals. The fruit is dark blue, frosted, globular, diameter approximately 10 mm.

Leaves, Stem, and Root: Sloe is a bulky bush about 3 m high. The branches are velvet-haired when young. The numerous lateral branches are almost horizontal and end in sharp thorns. The bark is black-brown.

Characteristics: The fruit tastes exceptionally sour and is only edible after several frosts.

Habitat: The plant grows in Europe and parts of Asia.

Production: Sloe fruit consists of the fresh or dried ripe fruit of *Prunus spinosa* as well as its preparations. Sloe flower consists of the dried flowers of *Prunus spinosa* as well as its preparations.

Not to be Confused With: May be confused with the flowers of *Prunus padus* syn. *Padus avium.*

Other Names: Blackthorn, Wild Plum

ACTIONS AND PHARMACOLOGY

COMPOUNDS: SLOE FRUIT

Cyanogenic glycosides: amygdalin, only in the seeds

Fruit acids

Monosaccharides/oligosaccharides

Tannins

EFFECTS: SLOE FRUIT
Sloe fruit has an astringent effect.

COMPOUNDS: SLOE FLOWER
Cyanogenic glycosides: amygdalin (traces, likely only in the fresh blossoms)

Flavonoids: including quercitrin, rutin, and hyperoside

EFFECTS: SLOE FLOWER
There is no reliable information available.

INDICATIONS AND USAGE

SLOE FRUIT
Approved by Commission E:

■ Inflammation of the mouth and pharynx

Sloe fruit is used externally for inflammation of the oral and pharyngeal mucosa (as a gargle).

Unproven Uses: In folk medicine the fruit juice is used as a gargle for mouth, throat, and gum inflammation. Syrup and wine are employed as a purgative or diuretic and as jam for a weak stomach.

SLOE FLOWER
Unproven Uses: Preparations of Sloe flower are used for common colds, diseases and ailments of the respiratory tract, as a laxative, for diarrhea, for prophylaxis and treatment of gastric spasms, flatulence, intestinal diseases, and gastric insufficiency.

Homeopathic Uses: Prunus spinosa is used for cardiac insufficiency and ''nervous headaches''.

PRECAUTIONS AND ADVERSE REACTIONS

SLOE FRUIT AND FLOWER
No health hazards or side effects are known in conjunction with the proper administration of designated therapeutic dosages.

DOSAGE

SLOE FRUIT
Mode of Administration: Sloe fruit is available as crude drug for infusions and other galenic preparations for mouth rinses.

Daily Dosage: External use — 2 to 4 g drug

SLOE FLOWER
Mode of Administration: Sloe flower preparations are available in various commercial compounded preparations.

Preparation: Tea: pour boiling water over 1 to 2 heaped teaspoons, stir occasionally for 5 to 10 minutes and strain.

Daily Dosage: Drink 1 to 2 cups during the day or 2 cups in the evening. (1 teaspoon corresponds approximately to 1 gm drug)

Storage: Should be protected from light and moisture, at best not longer than 1 year.

LITERATURE

SLOE FLOWER AND FRUIT
Hartisch C, Kolodziej H, Bruchhausen Fvon. Dual Inhibitory Activities of Tannins from Hamamelis virginiana and Related Polyphenols on 5-Lipoxygenase ans Lyso-PAF: Acetyl-CoA Acetyltransferase. *Planta Med.* 63 (2); 106-110. 1997

Irizar AC, Fernandez MF, Constituents of *Prunus spinosa.* In: *JNP* 55:450-454. 1992.

Kern W, List PH, Hörhammer L (Hrsg.), Hagers Handbuch der Pharmazeutischen Praxis, 4. Aufl., Bde. 1-8, Springer Verlag Berlin, Heidelberg, New York, 1969.

Madaus G, Lehrbuch der Biologischen Arzneimittel, Bde 1-3, Nachdruck, Georg Olms Verlag Hildesheim 1979.

Steinegger E, Hänsel R, Pharmakognosie, 5. Aufl., Springer Verlag Heidelberg 1992.

Teuscher E, Biogene Arzneimittel, 5. Aufl., Wiss. Verlagsges. Stuttgart 1997.

Wichtl M (Hrsg.), Teedrogen, 4. Aufl., Wiss. Verlagsges. Stuttgart 1997.

Smartweed

Persicaria hydropiper

DESCRIPTION

Medicinal Parts: The medicinal parts are the leaves and the whole plant harvested during the flowering season.

Flower and Fruit: The greenish pink flowers are in sparse, thin, hanging false ears. The 4-bract involucre is inconspicuous with a reddish tip and is glandular-punctate. The flowers are androgynous. There are 6 to 8 stamens, 2 of which have no function. The fruit has a flat and a domed side. It is black, punctate, nutlike, roughly bumpy, and surrounded by a remaining epicalyx.

Leaves, Stem, and Root: The plant grows from 30 to 50 cm high. The branched stems, which are from 60 to 90 cm long, are first creeping and later semi-erect and often tinged red. The leaves are oblong-lanceolate, short petioled, narrowed at both ends and alternate; they are glandular and ciliate on the under surface. The leaf sheaths at the base of the leaves are loose, glabrous, and ciliated at the margin.

Characteristics: Smartweed has an extraordinarily hot, pepperlike taste and is often used as a pepper substitute. The plant has characteristic long, thinly curved, hanging, flowering branches.

Habitat: The plant is indigenous to large parts of Europe, Asian Russia, and Arctic regions.

Production: Smartweed is the fresh plant, in flower, of *Polygonum hydropiper*. The flowering herb is cut and washed, the roots are removed and discarded and the herb is dried in the shade.

Not to be Confused With: Polygonum hydropiper is sometimes adultered with polygonum persicaria, *P. mite* and *P. minus.*

Other Names: Arsesmart, Water Pepper

ACTIONS AND PHARMACOLOGY

COMPOUNDS

Flavonoids: including rhamnazin, rhamnazin bisulfate, persicarin (isorhamnetine sulfate) quercitrin, and hyperoside

P-cumaroyl glycosides: hydropiperoside

Sesquiterpenes: sesquiterpene aldehydes (pungent substances), polygoidal (tadeonal), and warburganal

Tannins

EFFECTS

Smartweed is a hemostyptic.

INDICATIONS

Unproven Uses: In folk medicine Smartweed is used internally for uterine bleeding, menstrual bleeding, bleeding of hemorrhoids (piles), gastrointestinal bleeding, rheumatic pain, as a diuretic, for bladder and kidney disease and gout; and used externally for poorly healing wounds, sprains, contusions, rheumatism, and gout.

Chinese Medicine: Smartweed is used for severe digestive problems, vomiting, diarrhea, dysentery, scabies, and external wounds.

Homeopathic Uses: Polygonum hydropiper is used to treat varicose veins.

PRECAUTIONS

No health hazards or side effects are known in conjunction with the proper administration of designated therapeutic dosages. The consumption of larger quantities of the fresh kraut can lead to gastroenteritis. External use is not advisable because of the drug's irritant effect on the skin.

DOSAGE

Mode of Administration: Smartweed is available in crude powder form for oral intake and in parenteral form for homeopathic use.

Preparation: Tea — Pour 1/4 Liter hot water over 1 heaped teaspoon drug and strain after 10 minutes.

Daily Dosage: Tea — 3 times a day.

Homeopathic Dosage: 5 drops, 1 tablet, or 10 globules every 30 to 60 minutes (acute) or 1 to 3 times daily (chronic); parenterally: 1 to 2 mL sc acute: 3 times daily; chronic: once a day (HAB34)

LITERATURE

Furuta, T. et al., *Phytochemistry* 25(2):517. 1986

Fukujama Y et al., Hydropiperoside, a novel coumaroly glycoside from the root of *Polygonum hydropiper*. In: *PH* 22:549-552. 1983.

Smilax species

See Sarsaparilla

Sneezewort

Achillea ptarmica

DESCRIPTION

Medicinal Parts: The medicinal part is the dried root.

Flower and Fruit: The flowers are white, composite and in cymes at the tip of the stem. The bracts are lanceolate and short-haired. The ray florets are linguiform and female. The disc florets are tubular and androgynous. The chaff scales are lanceolate and hairy-tipped. The fruit is hairless.

Leaves, Stem, and Root: The plant grows from 30 to 80 cm high. The rhizome is creeping, and the stem is upright and glabrous. The leaves are glabrous, alternate, simple, lanceolate, acute, sessile, and finely serrated. They are slightly glossy and dark green.

Habitat: The plant is indigenous to northern and central Europe.

Production: The rhizome is dug up in the autumn of its second year of bearing fruit, washed, freed of any green areas and dried in the shade at a temperature of 35° C.

ACTIONS AND PHARMACOLOGY

COMPOUNDS

Volatile oil

Polyynes: including pontica expoxide, tridecatrien-(1,3,5)-triin-(7,9,11)-cis-dehydromatricaria ester

Alkamides: including trans-dehydromatricaria acid isobutylamide

EFFECTS

No information is available.

INDICATIONS AND USAGE

Unproven Uses: In the past, Sneezewort was used as a remedy for tiredness, loss of appetite, urinary tract complaints, nausea, vomiting, diarrhea, rheumatism, and other painful disorders. Today it is considered a remedy for toothache, flatulence, and problems with elimination; the herb also helps to regulate bowel movements.

PRECAUTIONS AND ADVERSE REACTIONS

No health hazards or side effects are known in conjunction with the proper administration of designated therapeutic dosages, although persons with compound allergies should avoid salves prepared from the drug.

DOSAGE

Mode of Administration: Sneezewort is available as a topical preparation and in alcoholic extracts.

Preparation: To prepare an infusion, use 2 teaspoonfuls of the comminuted drug to 2 cups of water.

Daily Dosage: A daily infusion can be drunk, or the fresh root can be chewed.

LITERATURE

Kuropka G, Neugebauer M, Glombitza KW, Essential oils of *Achillea ptarmica*. In: *PM* 57:492. 1991.

Rücker G et al., trans-Pinocarveylhydroxid aus *Achillea ptarmica*. In: *PM* 60(2):194. 1994.

Valant-Vetschera KM. Review: Therapeutic Significance of C-Glycosylflavone Accumulation in Achillea (Compositae - Anthemideae). *Sci Pharm*. 62; 323-330. 1994

Snowdrop

Galanthus nivalis

DESCRIPTION

Medicinal Parts: Although disputed, some attribute medicinal properties to the bulb.

Flower and Fruit: The flowers are single on approximately 10 cm long peduncles, are campanulate, drooping, and shorter than the hoodlike bract. The perigone has 6 tepals, the outer 3 oval, white, 14 to 18 mm long, and free. The inner 3 tepals are shorter, with an indentate tip, a green longitudinal stripe on the inside, and a green halfmoon-shaped spot on the outside. The 6 stamens are short and inclined toward each other. The ovary is barrel-shaped and has 1 style. The fruit is a yellowish-green, 3-chambered capsule with up to 12 seeds in each chamber. It is initially fleshy, and later springs open in folds. The seeds are elliptical, 3 to 4 mm long, with a thin membranous skin and a small and narrow hornlike appendage.

Leaves, Stem, and Root: This bulb plant is hardy and grows to 10 to 25 cm high. There are only 2 basal leaves, up to 0.8 cm wide and up to 10 cm long, with a blue-green bloom. They are linear and slightly keeled on the underside. The outer leaf has an open sheath, the inner leaf a closed sheath. The bulb is globose to ovoid and approximately 1.5 cm wide.

Habitat: The plant is native to Switzerland and Austria as well as other sections of southern Europe, but also has spread to other parts of Europe including Bulgaria and the Commonwealth of Independent States.

Production: The Snowdrop bulb is the fresh bulb of *Galanthus nivalis*, which is harvested in the flowering season.

ACTION AND PHARMACOLOGY

COMPOUNDS

Amaryllidaceae alkaloids (0.2 to 1.6%): including galanthamine, hemanthamin, narwedine, nivalidine, hippeastrine, lycorine, nivaline, narciclasine, pretazettine. The alkaloid spectrum depends greatly upon the variety.

Lectins

EFFECTS

The drug is considered toxic. Previous use was based on the effect of the alkaloid galanthamine contained in the drug as a competitive inhibitor of true cholinesterase. The administration of this isolated alkaloid for decurarization in connection with anesthetics thus appeared plausible, as did use for postoperative atonia of the gastrointestinal tract and of the bladder, myasthenia, and other conditions. The effects of other alkaloids contained in the drug are virostatic, tumor-inhibiting, positively inotropic, and negatively chronotropic, as well as being respiratory analeptics.

INDICATIONS AND USAGE

Unproven Uses: The drug is no longer in use. Snowdrop was used in the past for myasthenia, myopathy, symptoms resulting from polyneuropathy, neuritis, myelitis, and injuries to the spine, as well as postoperative intestinal, gastric, and bladder atonia. It has also been used in anesthetics, for thrombosis and thromboembolism, glaucoma (rare), and Alzheimer's disease.

DOSAGE

The drug is no longer used therapeutically. The literature includes mention of previous use of an aqueous solution of Galanthamine hydrobromide 0.15 to 0.35 mg per kg of body weight IV, IM, sc.

PRECAUTIONS AND ADVERSE REACTIONS

The drug is toxic. Oral ingestion leads to symptoms resembling those of physostigmine poisoning: diarrhea, colic and vomiting (acetylcholine esterase inhibition through galanthamine). Fatal poisonings have not been recorded.

LITERATURE

Amin K, Beillevaire D, Mahmoud E, Hammar L, Mardh PA, Frman G, Binding of *Galanthus nivalis* lectin to Chlamydia trachomatis and inhibition of in vitro infection. *APMIS*, 103:714-20, Oct. 1995

Hänsel R, Keller K, Rimpler H, Schneider G (Ed.), Hagers Handbuch der Pharmazeutischen Praxis, 5. Aufl., Bde 4 - 6 (Drogen), Springer Verlag Berlin, Heidelberg, New York, 1992-1994.

Kalashnikov ID, Isolation of alkaloids from *Galanthus nivalis L Farm Zh*, 103:40-4, 1970

Plaitakis A, Duvoisin RC, Homer's moly identified as *Galanthus nivalis L.*: physiologic antidote to stramonium poisoning. *Clin Neuropharmacol*, 6:1-5, Mar. 1983

Venturi VM, Piccinin GL, Taddei I, Pharmacognostic study of self-sown *Galanthus nivalis* (var. gracilis) in Italy Boll *Soc Ital Biol Sper*, 103:593-7, Jun 15. 1965

Soapwort

Saponaria officinalis

DESCRIPTION

Medicinal Parts: The medicinal parts are the fresh or dried roots, and the leaves harvested in summer before or during the flowering season of the first and second year of growth.

Flower and Fruit: The flowers generally are flesh-colored, sometimes white, grow in racemes, and have a 5-tipped fused calyx. The petals have long stems. The ovary is superior and has 1 style. The fruit is a capsule with 4 teeth at the tip and bursts open when ripe. The seeds are reniform-globular and black-brown.

Leaves, Stem, and Root: The perennial plant is leafy and grows about 100 cm high. The stems are round, erect, and are covered with fine down. The leaves are crossed opposite, oblong to lanceolate, acute, entire-margined, triple-veined, and taper to a short petiole.

Characteristics: The plant has a weak fragrance. The leaves and root contain bitter tasting saponine and produce suds when rubbed under water.

Habitat: The plant is indigenous to the temperate regions of North America, Asia, and Europe.

Production: Soapwort herb consists of the dried, above ground parts of *Saponaria officinalis*. The herb is harvested in the summer before flowering in the first and second years of the plant's growth. Soapwort root consists of the dried roots, rhizomes and runners of *Saponaria officinalis*. The roots are plowed up in autumn, after the herb has been mown. The root is cleaned and then dried artificially at 50° C.

White Soapwort root consists of the dried, underground parts of *Gypsophila* species, particularly *Gypsophila paniculata.* The roots of *Gypsophilae radix* are dried quickly under high temperatures or in direct sunlight. The roots are cut into 5 mm thick slices to avoid a separation of the sugars from the saponines.

Not to be Confused With: Saponaria officinalis should not be confused with *Gypsophilae* species and *Solanum dulcamara.*

Other Names: Bouncing Bet, Bruisewort, Crow Soap, Dog Cloves, Fuller's Herb, Latherwort, Old Maids' Pink, Soapwood, Soap Root, Sweet Betty, Wild Sweet William

ACTIONS AND PHARMACOLOGY

COMPOUNDS: SOAPWORT HERB

Triterpene saponins: chiefly aglycone quillaic acid

Flavonoids: including among others, saponarine (C-glycosylflavone)

Ribosome-inactivating proteins (in the seeds)

EFFECTS: SOAPWORT HERB

Because of the high saponin content, the drug is antibiotic, expectorant, antiphlogistic, cholesterol-lowering and spermicidal. In high doses, it becomes irritating to the mucous membrane, cytotoxic, and emetic.

COMPOUNDS: SOAPWORT ROOT

Triterpene saponins (2 to 8%): aglycones quillaic acid, gypsogenic acid

EFFECTS: SOAPWORT ROOT

Because of the high saponin content, the Soapwort root is antibiotic, expectorant, antiphlogistic, cholesterol-lowering, and spermicidal. The drug is expectorant because of its effect on the gastric mucosa. In high concentrations, it has been shown to be irritating to the mucous membranes, cytotoxic, and emetic.

INDICATIONS AND USAGE

SOAPWORT HERB

Unproven Uses: In addition to uses as an expectorant for cough and other diseases of the respiratory tract, folk medicine internal uses also encompass constipation, gastrointestinal disorders, liver and kidney disorders, rheumatic gout, neurasthenia, and oxyuriasis (pinworms). External folk medicine indications include skin rashes, eczema, and as a gargle for tonsillitis.

SOAPWORT ROOT

Approved by Commission E:

■ Cough/bronchitis

The drug is used for inflammation of the mucous membranes of the upper respiratory tract.

Unproven Uses: In addition to respiratory applications, internal folk medicine uses occasionally include diseases of the liver, gallbladder and kidney, constipation, gout, and as an emmenagogue. Among external uses are skin disorders, lingual mycoses, and rheumatic complaints.

PRECAUTIONS AND ADVERSE REACTIONS

SOAPWORT HERB AND ROOT

No health hazards are known in conjunction with the proper administration of designated therapeutic dosages. Localized skin and mucus membrane irritations are possible with the administration of larger dosages.

DOSAGE

SOAPWORT HERB

Daily Dosage: As an aqueous extract, take 1 to 2 g daily.

Constipation – 2 glasses daily of a decoction, (Preparation instructions are not given.)

Storage: The herb should be stored in a container that protects it from light and moisture.

SOAPWORT ROOT

Mode of Administration: Comminuted herb for teas and other galenic preparations for internal use. Drug extracts are contained in a few standardized preparations of antitussives.

Preparation: To prepare tea, use 0.4 g of medium fine cut (1 teaspoonful is approximately equal to 2.6 g of the drug).

Decoction – 10 g/180 g drug with the addition of 1 g sodium carbonate and simple syrup to 200 g.

Daily Dosage: The average daily dose is 30 to 150 mg of the drug corresponding to 3 to 15 mg of gypsophilia saponin. As an expectorant, 1 dessertspoonful of the decoction is taken every 2 hours.

Storage: The root should be stored tightly sealed and protected from light.

LITERATURE

SOAPWORT HERB AND ROOT

Henry M, Chantalat-Dublanche I. Isolation of Spinasterol and its Glucoside from Cell Suspension Cultures of Saponaria officinalis:

13C-NMR Spectral Data and Batch Culture Production. *Planta Med.* 51; 322-325. 1985

Kern W, List PH, Hörhammer L (Hrsg.), Hagers Handbuch der Pharmazeutischen Praxis, 4. Aufl., Bde. 1-8: Springer Verlag Berlin, Heidelberg, New York, 1969.

Lewin L, Gifte und Vergiftungen, 6. Aufl., Nachdruck, Haug Verlag, Heidelberg 1992.

Madaus G, Lehrbuch der Biologischen Arzneimittel, Bde 1-3, Nachdruck, Georg Olms Verlag Hildesheim 1979.

Roth L, Daunderer M, Kormann K: Giftpflanzen, Pflanzengifte, 4. Aufl., Ecomed Fachverlag Landsberg Lech 1993.

Teuscher E, Biogene Arzneimittel, 5. Aufl., Wiss. Verlagsges. Stuttgart 1997.

Wichtl M (Hrsg.), Teedrogen, 4. Aufl., Wiss. Verlagsges. Stuttgart 1997.

Solanum dulcamara

See Bittersweet Nightshade

Solanum nigrum

See Black Nightshade

Solidago canadensis

See Canadian Golden Rod

Solidago virgaurea

See European Golden Rod

Solomon's Seal

Polygonatum multiflorum

DESCRIPTION

Medicinal Parts: The medicinal parts of the plant are the dried rhizome and roots.

Flower and Fruit: The odorless, greenish-white campanulate flowers are in 2 to 6 blossomed racemes, usually without an accompanying leaf. The perigone tube is tightly cylindrical, 9 to 20 mm long, and 2 to 4 mm wide. It is drawn together over the ovary and opens out like a funnel at the top. The tepals at the tip are pubescent on the inside, and the filaments are softly pubescent. The fruit is a blue-black, frosted berry, 8 to 9 mm in diameter with a disgusting, sweet taste.

Leaves, Stem, and Root: The plant is a perennial 30 to 80 cm high herb. The stems are sturdy, round, and glabrous. The leaves are ovate to elliptical, 5 to 15 cm long, and 3 to 7.5 cm wide, narrowing suddenly at the base. They are glabrous, dark green above, and gray-green frosted beneath.

Habitat: The plant is indigenous to Europe, the Near East, eastern Asia, the Himalayas, Siberia, and North America.

Production: Solomon's Seal rhizome is the rhizome of *Polygonatum multiflorum*. The rootstocks should be dug up during the dormant seasons–autumn and spring. Earth and roots are removed and the rhizomes cut into pieces of a few centimeters in length.

Other Names: Dropberry, Lady's Seals, Sealroot, Sealwort, St. Mary's Seal

ACTIONS AND PHARMACOLOGY

COMPOUNDS

Steroid saponins (2.5%): 2 unnamed saponins, aglycones diosgenin, or else (25R)-furost-5-en-3beta,22alpha,26-triole

Mucilages

Acetidin-2-carboxylic acid

EFFECTS

The steroid saponins may be responsible for the anti-inflammatory effect of the drug. It works as a tonic, and relieves and soothes upset stomach.

INDICATIONS AND USAGE

Unproven Uses: Obsolete today as a drug, the plant was formerly used in the treatment of respiratory and lung disorders. It was used externally in the treatment of bruises, ulcers or boils on the fingers, hemorrhoids, redness of the skin, and for hematomas.

PRECAUTIONS AND ADVERSE REACTIONS

No health hazards or side effects are known in conjunction with the proper administration of designated therapeutic dosages. Extended administration of the drug in therapeutic dosages can lead to gastrointestinal irritation.

OVERDOSAGE

Overdosage leads to nausea, diarrhea, gastric complaints, and queasiness.

DOSAGE

Mode of Administration: The drug has been used internally as an infusion and externally as a poultice, but is now obsolete.

Storage: Store in paper and cloth sacks.

LITERATURE

Janeczko Z, The structure of the sugar moiety of steroidal saponosides isolated from the roots of *Polygonatum multiflorum L. Planta Med.* 36; 266. 1979

Kato A, Miura T, Hypoglycemic action of the rhizomes of *Polygonatum officinale* in normal and diabetic mice. In: *PM* 60(3):201. 1994.

Miura T, Kato A. Medicinal Polygonatum in northwest China. *Chung Kuo Chung Yao Tsa Chih*, 31:202-4 253, Apr 1991

Miura T, Kato A. The difference in hypoglycemic action between polygonati rhizoma and polygonati officinalis rhizoma. Biol Pharm Bull, 31:1605-6, Nov 1995

Sugiyama M et al., *Chem Pharm Bull* 32:1365-1372. 1984.

Sophora japonica

See Pagoda Tree

Sorb Apple

Sorbus domestica

DESCRIPTION

Medicinal Parts: The medicinal part is the ripe fruit.

Flower and Fruit: The inflorescence is umbelliferous-racemous and tomentose. The sepals and petals are also tomentose. The petals are white to light red, and the carpels are pubescent. The dividing membranes are not split. There are 2 ovules in each ovary chamber. The fruit is false pear-shaped/ globular, yellow, and speckled red on the sun side. The seed is flat, brown, and sharp-edged.

Leaves, Stem, and Root: Sorbus domestica is a bush or tree up to 13 m high, with branches that are initially gray-tomentose, later glabrous. The winter buds are glabrous or have hairy tips, and are sticky. The leaves are pinnatifid with 13 to 21 sessile, serrate, and acuminate leaflets. The serrate teeth are long and finely acuminate. The lower surface is bluish-green and initially villous-cobweb pubescent, later glabrous.

Habitat: The plant is cultivated in Europe and elsewhere.

Production: Sorb Apple berries are the fruit of *Sorbus domestica.*

Other Names: Ash, Cheque Tree, Sorvice Tree,

ACTIONS AND PHARMACOLOGY

COMPOUNDS

Sugar alcohols: sorbitol

The fruits do not contain parasorboside, in contrast to those of *Sorbus aucuparia.*

The drug has not been fully researched.

EFFECTS

The active agents are pectin, tannin, organic acids (sorbic acid) and sorbitol. The fruit has astringent, anti-inflammatory, and pain-relieving properties.

INDICATIONS AND USAGE

Unproven Uses: Internally, the berries act as an astringent for the intestinal tract. Externally, preparations are used for skin cleansing.

PRECAUTIONS AND ADVERSE REACTIONS

No health hazards or side effects are known in conjunction with the proper administration of designated therapeutic dosages.

DOSAGE

Mode of Administration: Fresh juice from the berries and a decoction made from the dried fruit are used internally. The decoction is also applied externally as a wash to the affected areas. See also Mountain Ash Berry (Sorbus aucuparia).

Daily Dosage: Fresh juice: 50 to 80 g; decoction: add 5 g of drug to 100 mL of water and drink 1 to 2 cups.

LITERATURE

No literature is available.

Sorbus aucuparia

See Mountain Ash Berry

Sorbus domestica

See Sorb Apple

Sorbus torminalis

See Wild Service Tree

Sorghum vulgare

See Broomcorn

Sorrel

Rumex acetosa

DESCRIPTION

Medicinal Parts: The medicinal parts are the fresh leaves and the whole herb.

Flower and Fruit: The plant has small greenish unisexual, dioecious flowers growing in narrow, loose panicles. There are 6 tepals. The 3 inner ones are longer, closer together, and turn red when the fruit ripens. When mature they are often red-tinged, membranous, entire-margined, and have a scale-like downwardly curved welt at the base. The 3 outermost tips are revolute. There are 6 stamens and 3 styles with a stigma that resembles a paintbrush. The fruit is a triangular, brown-black nut enclosed in the winglike enlarged inner tepal.

Leaves, Stem, and Root: The plant can grow up to 100 cm high. The leaves alternate on the erect, grooved stems, which are unbranched up to the panicles. The leaves are fleshy, grass green, hastate, or spit-shaped. The lower leaves are long-petioled; the upper ones are short-petioled, sessile, and clasping. There is a membranous, dentate, or fringed cone at the base of the leaves.

Characteristics: The stem is red-tinged, and the herb has a sour taste. It gets its acidity from the same salt that is present in Rhubarb.

Habitat: The plant is common in Europe.

Production: Sorrel is the aerial part of *Rumex acetosa.*

ACTIONS AND PHARMACOLOGY

COMPOUNDS

Oxalates: oxalic acid, calcium oxalate

Tannins (7-10%)

Flavonoids

Anthracene derivatives: anthranoids, aglycones, physcion, chryosphanol, emodin, aloe-emodin, rhein, and their glucosides, as well as aloe-emodin acetate

EFFECTS
Sorrel acts as a diuretic. It stimulates secretion, and improves resistance to infections (antibacterial), although some of these effects are questionable.

INDICATIONS AND USAGE
Unproven Uses: The herb is used for acute and chronic inflammation of the nasal passages and respiratory tract. It is also used as an adjuvant in antibacterial therapy.

PRECAUTIONS AND ADVERSE REACTIONS
No health hazards or side effects are known in conjunction with the proper administration of designated therapeutic dosages.

OVERDOSAGE
Oxalate poisonings are conceivable only with the consumption of very large quantities of the leaves as a salad.

DOSAGE
Mode of Administration: The drug is described as obsolete.

How Supplied:

Tablets

Liquid – 1:4

Daily Dosage: The dosage for adults is 2 coated tablets or 50 drops (drops with 19% Ethanol) taken 3 times daily.

LITERATURE

Ernst E, März R, Sieder C. A controlled multi-centre study of herbal versus synthetic secretolytic drugs for acute bronchitis. *Phytomedicine* 4 (4); 287-293. 1997

Ito H. Effects of the antitumor agents from various natural sources on drug-metabolizing system, phagocytic activity and complement system in sarcoma 180-bearing mice. *Jpn J Pharmacol*, 40:435-43, Mar 1986.

Southern Bayberry

Myrica cerifera

DESCRIPTION
Medicinal Parts: The medicinal parts are the dried root bark and the wax extracted from the berries.

Flower and Fruit: The flowers are unisexual and have no calyx or corolla. They are small and yellowish in scaly catkins. The fruit is small groups of round, gray-white berries containing numerous black seeds, which have a crust of usable greenish-white wax. The wax helps keep the berries in a suitable state for germination for a period of 2 to 3 years.

Leaves, Stem, and Root: Southern Bayberry is an evergreen shrub or small tree that grows up to 10 m high. The bark has a white, peeling outer layer, which covers a red-brown inner layer. The leaves are lanceolate to oblong-lanceolate, glossy or resinous, and punctate on both sides.

Characteristics: The taste is astringent and bitter. The leaves have an aromatic odor.

Habitat: The plant is found in the eastern and southern regions of the U.S. and around Lake Erie.

Production: Bayberry bark is the bark from the trunk and branches of *Myrica cerifera.*

Other Names: Bayberry, Candleberry, Myrica, Tallow Shrub, Vegetable Tallow, Waxberry, Wax Myrtle,

ACTIONS AND PHARMACOLOGY
COMPOUNDS
Volatile oil (traces)

Tannins

Resins

The constituents of the drug have not been extensively investigated.

EFFECTS
The active compounds have diaphoretic, stimulant and astringent effects.

INDICATIONS AND USAGE
Unproven Uses: The drug is used internally for coughs and colds, and externally for skin diseases and ulcers.

PRECAUTIONS AND ADVERSE REACTIONS
No health hazards or side effects are known in conjunction with the proper administration of designated therapeutic dosages. Higher dosages of the drug are said to trigger vomiting, and are used as an emetic.

DOSAGE
Mode of Administration: The drug is available as a liquid extract for internal use, and in powder form.

How Supplied:

Capsules — 450 mg, 475 mg

Liquid Extract — 1:1

LITERATURE

Sakurawi K et al. Endothelin Receptor Antagonist Triterpenoid, Myriceric Acid A. Isolated from *Myricera cerifera*, and Structure Activity Relationships of Its Derivatives. *Chem Pharm Bull.* 44 (2); 343-351. 1996

Tortoriello J, Meckes-Fischer M, Villarreal ML, Berlin B, Berlin E. Spasmolytic Activity of Medicinal Plants Used to Treat Gastrointestinal and Respiratory Diseases in the Highland of Chiapas. *Phytomedicine* 2 (1); 57-66. 1995

Southern Tsangshu (Cang-Zhu)

Atractylodes lancea

DESCRIPTION
Medicinal Parts: The medicinal parts of the plant are the whole plant and roots.

Flower and Fruit: The composite flowers are surrounded by bracts. The capitulas are apical and upright, with a diameter of

1.5 to 2 cm. The calyx is double-rowed and double-pinnate. The lingual florets are in 7 or 8 rows, whitish and 1 to 1.2 cm long. The fruit is an achaene. The pappus is brownish and 8 to 9 mm long.

Leaves, Stem, and Root: Southern Tsangshu is an upright, herbaceous perennial with a rhizome that extends up to 1 m high. The basal leaves wilt rapidly, the upper cauline leaves are alternate, small, usually simple and sessile. The lower leaves are long-petiolate and 8 to 10 cm long. The lamina is pergamentlike, single pinnate with 3 to 5 elongate-elliptical leaflets. The apical leaflet is larger with short thorns on the margin. The rhizome is elongate, gnarled, 2 to 3 cm thick, and up to 8 cm long.

Habitat: Cang-Zhu is indigenous to Japan and China.

Production: Southern Tsangshu rhizome is the dried rhizome of *Atractylodes lancea.* The rhizome is dug up in spring or autumn and dried. In order to obtain the cut drug, the rhizome is soaked after being cleaned and cut into slices.

ACTIONS AND PHARMACOLOGY

COMPOUNDS

Volatile oil (1.5%): components including p-cymol, beta-selinene, alpha curcumene, elemol, hinesol, beta-eudesmol

Sesquiterpenes: 3 beta-hydroxyatractylon, 3beta-acetoxy-atractylon

Polyynes: including atractylodin, atractylodinol, acetylatratylodinol

EFFECTS

The sesquiterpenes and furanosesquiterpenes contained in the essential oil of the drug have hepatoprotective, immunostimulating, and intestinal motility-enhancing effects, while also inhibiting the secretion of gastric juices. The smoke of the drug is said to have antiseptic characteristics, while the essential oil is additionally credited with a sedative effect, derived from its beta-eudesmol and hinesol content.

INDICATIONS AND USAGE

Unproven Uses: Southern Tsangshu is used for diarrhea, feelings of fullness in the lower abdomen, lack of strength including atrophy, rheumatic pain, colds, and night blindness.

Chinese Medicine: The herb is used for gastroenteritis, edema, disturbances of renal function, and generalized pain.

PRECAUTIONS AND ADVERSE REACTIONS

No health hazards are known in conjunction with the proper administration of designated therapeutic dosages.

DOSAGE

Mode of Administration: Whole herb, cut and powdered drug for internal use.

Preparation: The powder is prepared in accordance with Jap XI or ChinP IX. It is roasted using the Fuchao method.

Dosage: 3 to 9 of g of drug

Storage: Should be stored in a dry and cool place and in tightly sealed containers.

LITERATURE

Blaschek W, Hänsel R, Keller K, Reichling J, Rimpler G, Schneider G (Eds), Hagers Handbuch der Pharmazeutischen Praxis. Folgebände 1 und 2. Drogen A-Z. Springer. Berlin, Heidelberg 1998.

Gong QM, Wang SL, Gan C, A clinical study on the treatment of acute upper digestive tract hemorrhage with wen-she decoction. *Chung Hsi I Chieh Ho Tsa Chih*, 29:272-3, 260, May. 1989

Hiraoka N, *Atractylodes lancea* autotetraploids induced by colchicine treatment of shoot cultures. *Biol Pharm Bull*, 16:479-83, May. 1998

Hwang JM, Tseng TH, Hsieh YS, Chou FP, Wang CJ, Chu CY, Inhibitory effect of atractylon on tert-butyl hydroperoxide induced DNA damage and hepatic toxicity in rat hepatocytes. *Arch Toxicol*, 70:640-4, 1996.

Kimura M, Diwan PV, Yanagi S, Kon-no Y, Nojima H, Kimura I, Potentiating effects of beta-eudesmol-related cyclohexylidene derivatives on succinylcholine-induced neuromuscular block in isolated phrenic nerve-diaphragm muscles of normal and alloxan-diabetic mice. *Biol Pharm Bull,* 18:407-10, Mar. 1995

Kimura M, Nojima H, Muroi M, Kimura I, Mechanism of the blocking action of beta-eudesmol on the nicotinic acetylcholine receptor channel in mouse skeletal muscles. *Neuropharmacology*, 30:835-41, Aug. 1991

Kiso Y, Tohkin M, Hikino H, Antihepatotoxic principles of Atractylodes rhizomes. *J Nat Prod,* 46:651-4, Sep-Oct. 1983

Muroi M, Tanaka K, Kimura I, Kimura M, Anti-inflammatory principles of Atractylodes rhizomes. *Chem Pharm Bull* (Tokyo), 50:2954-8, Dec. 1979

Muroi M, Tanaka K, Kimura I, Kimura M, Beta-eudesmol (a main component of *Atractylodes lancea*)-induced potentiation of depolarizing neuromuscular blockade in diaphragm muscles of normal and diabetic mice. *Jpn J Pharmacol,* 50:69-71, May. 1989

Nojima H, Kimura I, Kimura M Blocking action of succinylcholine with beta-eudesmol on acetylcholine-activated channel activity at endplates of single muscle cells of adult mice. *Brain Res*, 575:337-40, Mar 20. 1992

Resch M, Steigel A, Chen ZL, Bauer R 5-Lipoxygenase and cyclooxygenase-1 inhibitory active compounds from *Atractylodes lancea. J Nat Prod*, 61:347-50, Mar. 1998

Sakamoto S, Kudo H, Suzuki S, Sassa S, Yoshimura S, Nakayama T, Maemura M, Mitamura T, Qi Z, Liu XD, Yagishita Y, Asai A Pharmacotherapeutic effects of toki-shakuyaku-san on leukorrhagia in young women. *Am J Chin Med,* 24:165-8, 1996.

Satoh K, Nagai F, Ushiyama K, Kano I Specific inhibition of Na+,K(+)-ATPase activity by atractylon, a major component of byaku-jutsu, by interaction with enzyme in the E2 state. *Biochem Pharmacol*, 51:339-43, Feb 9. 1996

Usuki S Blended effects of herbal components of tokishakuyakusan on rat corpus luteum function in vivo. *Am J Chin Med,* 16:107-16, 1988.

Wang GT Antianoxic action and active constituents of atractylodis lanceae rhizoma. *Chem Pharm Bull* (Tokyo), 10:2033-4, Jul. 1990

Yamahara J, Matsuda H, Huang Q, Li Y, Fujimura H Intestinal motility enhancing effect of *Atractylodes lancea* rhizome. *J Ethnopharmacol*, 29:341-4, Jul. 1990

Soybean

Glycine soja

DESCRIPTION

Medicinal Parts: The medicinal parts are the Soya lecithin extracted from the Soya bean, the Soya oil, and the Soya seed.

Flower and Fruit: The flowers are small, inconspicuous, short pedicled, upright, axillary, and appear in 3 to 8 blossomed clusters. The sepals are campanulate or tubular-campanulate and somewhat bilabiate. The corolla is usually purple, exceeding the calyx only slightly or not at all. The stamens are diadelphous or monodelphous. The style is glabrous. The pod is linear or oblong and constricted between the seeds. The pod is septate and dehiscent. There are 2 to 4 seeds, which are oblong-ovate, white, yellow or black-brown.

Leaves, Stem, and Root: The Soya plant is an erect or twining annual bushy plant. The stem and leaves are thickly villous. The leaves are trifoliate, the leaflets are large, ovate, entire-margined and, particularly on the margins and on the ribs of the lower surface, pubescent.

Habitat: The Soya plant is indigenous to east Asia but has never been found in the wild. *Glycine soja* is found in the Amur-Ussuri area, northern China, Taiwan, Korea, and Japan.

Production: Lecithin consists of the phospholipid mixture from *Glycine soja* seeds and its preparations. Virgin Soybean oil is mixed with 2% water at 60° to 80° C. After the swelling times it is separated by centrifugation and the lecithin paste is evaporated at 100° C in a vacuum until the remaining water content is 0.2 to 0.8%.

ACTIONS AND PHARMACOLOGY

COMPOUNDS

Phospholipids (45-60%): in particular phosphatidylcholine, phosphatidylethanolamine, phosphatidylinositol

Fatty oil (30-35%)

Steroids: Phytosterols (2-5%)

EFFECTS

Soy contains high amounts of protein, phytochemicals, and isoflavones, such as genistein and diadzein. In certain hormone-related cancers, the isoflavones in Soy act as antiestrogens and block the uptake of estrogen into tissues such as that of the breast. Soy reduces the effects of androgens on the prostate gland. However, whether Soy is beneficial for breast and prostate cancer remains questionable. Epidemiological studies report a link between Soy consumption and reduction of breast and prostate cancer, but clinical studies are lacking. Soy has a potential use as a protein source to reduce weight loss and diarrhea during chemotherapy based on animal studies.

The FDA has approved health claims that Soy products can lower coronary heart disease by lowering blood cholesterol levels. Germany's Commission E approves of its use for elevated cholesterol as well. Soy may have a beneficial effect on cognitive function, but its role in this capacity needs much more elucidation. Soy protein may improve insulin resistance and glycemic control and may have a use as part of a diabetic regime. Soy is mostly beneficial for use in menopause, but not all clinical trials demonstrate positive results. More studies are needed to further define its role. Soy failed to reduce hot flushes in breast cancer patients. Mild to moderate hypertensive patients supplemented with Soy milk experienced a modest reduction in blood pressure. Soy's role in infant diarrhea is not fully clear. A combination product containing Soy, Dong Quai, and black cohosh improved menstrual migraines dramatically; more study is needed to support this data. Soy has demonstrated small, but significant, effects on bone mineral density in postmenopausal women. Soy protein diets may have advantages over animal protein in renal disease. Several in vitro and in vivo studies reported potential benefits of genistein in the treatment of cystic fibrosis and HIV-1 (Gozlan et al, 1998; Hwang et al, 1997; Illek et al, 1997).

Antineoplastic Effects: The chemopreventive effects of the isoflavone genistein may be due to its action as an estrogen agonist or antagonist. However, a variety of nonestrogenic mechanisms, including inhibition of protein tyrosine phosphorylation, induction of differentiation, inhibition of DNA topoisomerases, inhibition of specific cell cycle events, induction of apoptosis, inhibition of angiogenesis, and antioxidant activity have been proposed (Tham et al, 1998). In terms of breast cancer, Soy isoflavones are converted in the bowel to antineoplastic agents, which demonstrated cytostatic actions on estrogen receptor-positive and negative human mammary cancer cell lines. The chemopreventive potential of genistein in breast cancer has been demonstrated in numerous in vitro and in vivo studies but few clinical studies are available. Epidemiologic studies have shown an inverse association between hormone-dependent breast cancer incidence and mortality and a Soy-rich Asian diet (Stoll, 1997). In one human study, increased proliferation of breast epithelium was demonstrated. (McMichael-Phillips et al, 1998). High tyrosine kinase activity is associated with tumor tissue. Tyrosine kinase inhibitors (such as genistein) can block the action of growth factors on cells (Wardle, 1998; Helms & Gallaher, 1995).

Genistein was an effective in vitro suppresser of bladder tumor growth and motility, irrespective of epidermal growth factor receptor expression levels. The inhibition of motility was dependent on epidermal growth factor receptor but not p21ras gene expression (Theodurescu et al, 1998; Theodorescu et al, 1998a). The mechanism of the cytotoxic effect of genistein on human prostate cancer cell lines LNCaP, PC3, and DU145 was examined in vitro with non- toxic genistein concentrations ranging between 1.85 to 93 micromoles. An involvement of p53 in growth inhibition of LNCaP, but not PC3 or DU145, by genistein, has been observed (Davies et al, 1998). Genistein induced an antiproliferative effect with a partial G2-M block and apoptosis in human uterine adenocarcinoma cell lines HEC 1A, HEC-1B, AN3Ca, and RL95-2. The antiproliferative effect of genistein was independent of its estrogenic activity but interactions with tyrosine kinase and topoisomerase II were relevant (Muratori et al, 1997).

Cholesterol-Lowering Effects: Soy protein can lower cholesterol in hypercholesterolemic subjects (Morelli et al, 2000). The FDA approved the ''health claim'' that Soy products (which contain at least 6.25 g of Soy/serving and are low in fat, saturated fat, and cholesterol) can reduce the risk of coronary heart disease by lowering cholesterol. The mechanism by which Soy lowers cholesterol is unknown. The effects are modest (6% to 7%) and 25 g of Soy protein must be consumed a day in order to derive benefit. Examples of estimated Soy protein content are 3 to 10 g/cup of Soy milk and 5 to 13 g of Soy protein/4 ounces of tofu (FDA, 2003; Stone, 2002).

Effects on Cognitive Function: Memory improved, but not other measures of cognitive function, in postmenopausal women supplemented with Soy isoflavones; larger trials are needed (Kritz- Silverstein et al, 2003). In young healthy adults supplemented with Soy isoflavones, there were improvements in memory and mental flexibility, but not attention and category generation task (File et al, 2001)

Estrogenic Effects: Soy contains several isoflavones that degrade to genistein, glycitein, and daidzein. These molecules are structurally related to estradiol (Grauds, 1999). In one study, isoflavones altered estrogen metabolism. Eighteen post menopausal women were given three diets for 93 days each, separated by a 25-day washout period between the diets. The three diets contained Soy protein isolate in concentrations of 0.1 mg/kg/d, 1 mg/kg/d, or 2 mg/kg/d (Xu et al, 2000). Premenopausal women fed a diet containing 60 g of Soy protein/day (equivalent to about 45 mg of isoflavones) had reduced luteinizing and follicle-stimulating hormone levels during their midcycles (Wardle, 1998).

Renal Effects: Soy protein contains, in small amounts, several agents that may contribute to its beneficial actions in renal disease. Nicotinamide-N, N-(3-amino-3-carboxypropyl) azetidine-2-carboxylic acid is an angiotensin-converting enzyme inhibitor; phytic acid controls serum phosphate for chronic renal patients and proteinase inhibitors help control inflammatory reactions (Wardle, 1998).

CLINICAL TRIALS

Body Composition/Weight Loss/Lipid profile

Soy protein supplementation was found to have no influence on indicators of body composition but did favorably affect lipid levels. Forty-six postmenopausal women were enrolled in a randomized, placebo-controlled study and assigned to one of four groups: 25 g soy protein (SP); 25 g of soy protein plus resistance exercise (SPE); 25 g of maltodextrine (placebo), or placebo plus resistance exercise (PLE). At baseline and after 16 weeks, body mass index, waist circumference, body fat, muscle mass, and serum lipid levels were measured. To confirm isoflavone absorption, urinary concentrations were determined. After 16 weeks of intervention, both SPE and PLE groups showed a significant increase of 1.3 kg in muscle mass and reduction of waist circumference of -1.4 and -2.1 cm, respectively ($p<0.05$). Significant decreases in the mean values of total cholesterol and LDL were observed in the users of soy protein alone, indicating the favorable effects of soy protein on lipid profile in postmenopausal women (Maesta et al, 2007).

Forty-three women with body mass index values between 30 and 40 kg/m^2 were randomized in intensive dietary interventions using either casein (placebo) or soy shakes. The subjects were instructed to consume three shakes, one prepacked entrée, and five servings of fruit and vegetables daily to achieve an energy intake of 4.5 to 5.0 MJ/d. Weight, body fat, lipid, and glucose measurements were obtained at baseline and at eight and 16 weeks. For both groups combined, subjects lost 8.1% of initial body weight (7.7 kg) at eight weeks and 13.4% (12.7 kg) at 16 weeks. Differences in weight loss and body composition changes between casein and soy treatments were not significant (Anderson et al, 2007).

In another study by the same author and colleagues, a Soy meal replacement (MR) was associated with significant reductions in serum triglycerides at six and 12 weeks. Researchers looked at the effects of a soy-based meal replacement MR on body weight and fat distribution in 90 overweight or obese adults. Participants were randomly assigned to LED (low-energy-diet) providing 1200 kcal/day, with consumption of five soy-based MR or two milk-based MR for the 12-week study. Serum lipoprotein measurements were obtained at baseline, six and 12 weeks. After the end of treatment, participants who used soy MR lost 9.0% of initial body weight, while participants taking milk lost 7.9% of initial body weight. Reductions of serum cholesterol and LDL cholesterol were significantly greater ($p<0.015$) with soy MR (15% and 17.4%) than with milk MR (7.9 and 7.7%) (Anderson & Hoie, 2005).

Bone Mineral Density

The effects of soy isoflavone supplementation on bone mineral density was investigated in a controlled, parallel-arm, double-blind, trial of 145 adults between the ages of 50 and 80. After 12 months of treatment, soy protein containing isoflavones resulted in a modest benefit in preserving bone mineral density in the spine, but not the hip, in older women (Newton et al, 2006).

Breast Cancer

Seventy-two patients with a histologically confirmed preexisting diagnosis of breast cancer were randomized to either soy capsules or placebo during a 12-week period. Quality of life and menopausal symptom scores were assessed at baseline, four, eight, and 12 weeks. Results showed no statistical difference in menopausal symptom scores or quality of life between the two arms of the study (MacGregor et al, 2005).

Dietary intervention with Soy led to significant changes in the regulation of the menstrual cycle of six premenopausal women (21 to 29 years) with regular ovulatory cycles in this controlled study. During the first month of the study, each subject consumed a constant daily diet of non-Soy-containing foods and the first complete menstrual cycle served as a control period. Daily supplementation of 60 g of Soy, containing 45 mg of isoflavones, during the following month, caused a significant increase of follicular phase length ($p<0.01$), plasma estradiol concentrations during the follicular phase and cholesterol concentrations (9.6%), a significant suppression of midcycle surges of luteinizing and follicle stimulating hormone, and delayed menstruation. These effects may be due to nonsteroidal estrogens of the isoflavone class, which may possess partial estrogen agonistic and antagonistic effects. The authors suggested that a diet rich in dietary estrogens may be protective against breast cancer (Cassidy et al, 1994).

A case control study of 18 post menopausal women with breast cancer and 20 healthy women showed that breast cancer subjects had lower urinary Soy isoflavones in a 24-hour urine collection. Significant differences in urinary daidzein levels existed between the two treatment groups. Breast cancer subjects excreted 31 nanomoles/day (nmol/d) and controls excreted 427 nmol/d. Breast cancer patients also showed lower urinary genistein levels (25 nmol/d) compared to control patients (155 nmol/d). Serum testosterone levels were elevated in breast cancer subjects although the difference did not reach statistical significance. Dietary analysis was performed and showed no significant differences in carbohydrate, fat, protein, or fiber consumption between the two groups (Murkies et al, 2000).

Dietary Soy supplementation significantly increased the proliferation rate of breast lobular epithelium and progesterone receptor expression in a randomized, controlled study of 48 women with benign or malignant breast disease. The patients were assigned to continue their normal diet or receive additional 60 g of Soy supplement containing 45 mg of isoflavones. After 14 days, serum concentrations of the phytoestrogens genistein and daidzein increased significantly ($p<0.05$) in the Soy group. Short-term Soy treatment of premenopausal human breast tissue caused an up-regulation in progesterone receptor expression and an elevation in the number of proliferating epithelial cells. A trend toward increased expression of the proliferation antigen Ki67LI was observed. Radiographic, echographic, cytologic, and histologic examinations were performed for diagnosis. No estrogen antagonistic effects were found (McMichael-Phillips et al, 1998).

Cognitive Function/Mood in Postmenopausal Women

A randomized, double-blind, placebo-controlled crossover study was performed to investigate the effects of Soy isoflavones on mood and cognitive function in 78 postmenopausal women. Investigators administered 60 mg/day isoflavones or placebo for six months. After a wash-out period of one month, the patients who had been treated with phytoestrogens received placebo and vice versa. At the end of each treatment a battery of tests was carried out. The results revealed that of the 17 scores on cognitive performance test and the six for mood assessments, six showed an advantage for the treatment with isoflavones. Of the eight visual analog scales used to indicate mood, seven improved significantly after the treatment with phytoestrogens. This study suggests that isoflavones may have a positive effect on postmenopausal women improving cognitive performance and mood (Casini et al, 2006).

A relatively long-term (12-month), large, double-blind and placebo-controlled trial in which 202 healthy postmenopausal women age 60 to 75 were randomly assigned to a placebo or 25.6 g of soy protein daily (containing 99 mg of isoflavones [52 mg genistein, 41 mg daidzein, and 6 mg glycerin) or total milk protein (as a powder) daily did not find evidence that the Soy protein improved cognitive function, bone mineral density, or plasma lipids when started at age 60 or later. While isoflavones from Soy appear to cause fewer adverse effects than postmenopausal estrogen therapy may, these findings indicate that they don't confer clear positive effects. Cognitive testing results at the final visit were essentially the same as they were at baseline, with assessments for verbal skills, concentration, and visual attention showing no significant inter-group differences or improvements at the final visit. The same was true when women with depression were excluded from the analysis, as this can affect cognition test results). Adherence to the regimen was good. Ultimately, no significant difference was found between the soy protein supplement and placebo groups after a full year (Kreijkamp-Kasper, 2004).

In contrast, postmenopausal women supplemented with Soy isoflavones demonstrated improved verbal memory, but not in other measurements of cognitive function, in a double-blind, randomized, placebo-controlled trial. Postmenopausal women, not on estrogen replacement and in good health, were supplemented with 110 mg of Soy-extracted isoflavones/day ($n=27$) or an identical placebo ($n=26$) for 6 months. A trend toward improved cognitive function (visuomotor tracking and attention) was noted in the treatment group as it related to baseline values and between placebo and treatment groups. Significant improvements in category fluency (verbal memory) was noted between treatment and placebo groups ($p=0.02$) (Kritz- Silverstein et al, 2003).

A short-term supplementation of Soy to young men and women demonstrated significant improvements in memory and mental flexibility in a randomized controlled trial. Student volunteers (15 men, 12 women) were randomized to either receive high-Soy (100 mg total isoflavones/day) or low-Soy diet (0.5 mg total isoflavones/day) for 10 weeks. Significant improvements in short term and long term memory as well as mental flexibility were noted in both men and women who were on the high-Soy diet ($p<0.05$). Females in the high-Soy diet also significantly improved in letter fluency and planning test. Tests of attention and category generation task did not improve with Soy supplementation (File et al, 2001).

Tofu (a Soy-based product) was associated with reduced cognitive function and organic brain changes in a longitudinal study. Japanese-American men, originally enrolled in the Honolulu Heart Program (HHP) and the Honolulu-Asia Aging Study (HAAS), were assessed for cognitive changes (n=3734) and brain atrophy (neuro-image: n=574; autopsy: n=290) after a review of their dietary habits from 1965 to 1967 and 1971 to 1974. Men with the highest tofu consumption (2 or more servings a week) were more likely to develop cognitive impairment than those with low or no tofu consumption ($p<0.05$). Low brain weight and enlargement of ventricles were also associated with higher tofu consumption. The authors determined an odds ratio of 1.6 to 2 for having poor cognitive test scores, low brain weight, or ventricular enlargement later in life (White et al, 2000).

Diabetes

Soy protein significantly improved insulin resistance, glycemic control, and serum lipoproteins in women with type 2 diabetes in a randomized, double-blind, placebo-controlled, crossover trial. Postmenopausal women (n=32) with type 2 diabetes were randomized to 30 g of isolated Soy protein (containing 132 mg of isoflavones) or placebo (cellulose) daily for 12 weeks and then crossed over to the opposite treatment for an additional 12 weeks. Isoflavones consisted of genistein (53%), daidzein (37%), and glycitein (10%). Modest yet significant improvements were noted during Soy supplementation for fasting insulin, insulin resistance, glycosylated hemoglobin, total cholesterol, LDL cholesterol, cholesterol/HDL ratio and free thyroxine ($p<0.05$). No significant changes were noted in HDL cholesterol, triglycerides, weight, blood pressure, creatinine, dehydroepiandrosterone sulfate, androstenedione, or the hypothalamic-pituitary-ovarian axis hormones (Jayagopal et al, 2002).

Diarrhea, Infant

Infants over 6 months of age had a significantly shorter duration of diarrhea (9.7 hours) while taking a Soy with fiber product than with a Soy-alone product (23.1 hours) ($p<0.05$). These differences were not statistically significant with the children under 6 months of age. Patients with acute infant diarrhea were given either a Soy or a Soy and Soy fiber diet for 10 days in the rehydration phase of their illness. Acute infant diarrhea was defined as less than 24 months old with acute diarrhea under 3 days of duration and more than 3 watery stools in 24 hours. Three times the usual number of stools/24 hours also qualified. A child was disqualified if there was a pre-existing gastrointestinal illness. The two products used were similar in fat, protein, and carbohydrate composition but Soy fiber (6 g/L) was added to the second formula (Vanderhoof et al, 1997).

Soy-based formula decreased the duration of infant diarrhea when compared to a cow's milk product in this randomized, controlled, double-blind study of infants 2 to 12 months old with diarrhea of less than 1 week. The infants had mild to moderate dehydration from the diarrhea. Seventy-three children were included in the study; 39 of these received a Soy-based formula and 34 received a cow's milk formula after rehydration with an oral or intravenous glucose-electrolyte solution. The duration of diarrhea was shorter in the Soy-based product (4.5 days) than in the cow's milk product (6.6 days) ($p=0.03$). The number of treatment failures did not differ significantly. The amount of formula eaten and weight gain at 14 days did not differ significantly (Allen et al, 1994).

Hot Flushes, Breast Cancer

No improvement of hot flushes was noted in women with breast cancer supplemented with Soy in a double-blind, placebo-controlled trial. Post menopausal women (mean age approximately 55 years) not on hormone replacement and with a history of breast cancer who were reporting moderate hot flushes were randomized to receive either a Soy beverage (90 mg of isoflavones; n=59) or placebo (rice beverage; n=64) daily for 12 weeks. While both groups reported a reduction in hot flushes and hot flash score, the use of the Soy supplement did not reach significance compared to the placebo group (Van Patten et al, 2002).

A double-blind, placebo-controlled, crossover study of 177 breast cancer survivors 18 years and older found that Soy was no more effective than placebo in the treatment of substantial hot flushes. At baseline, patients averaged 7 hot flushes/day. Seventy percent of patients were on tamoxifen or raloxifene. The women were split into 2 groups; group 1 (n=87) received Soy 600 mg (with 50 mg Soy isoflavones including 40% to 45% genistein, 40% to 45% diadzein, and 10% to 20% glycitein) 3 times daily for 4 weeks and then placebo for 4 weeks. Group 2 (n=88) received placebo for 4 weeks and then Soy for 4 weeks. Response criteria were based on a hot flush patient questionnaire from baseline to 9 weeks. Similar results were demonstrated in hot flush frequency and severity scores in both groups, with a trend toward better results with placebo (Quella et al, 2002).

Hyperlipidemia, Adult

Replacing high-fat animal protein with soy protein may help improve atherogenic profiles in postmenopausal women. In a randomized, double-blind, placebo-controlled study, 216 postmenopausal women first consumed casein protein-based supplements for four weeks. After a four-week run-in period, participants were randomly assigned to continue the casein placebo or receive soy protein-containing isoflavones for 12 weeks. Results showed total cholesterol, LDL cholesterol, and low-density lipoprotein particle number decreased significantly as compared to placebo at six weeks. Although this decrease continued at 12 weeks in the soy group, the difference from placebo group was attenuated for total cholesterol and low-density lipoprotein particle number (Allen et al, 2007).

To examine the effects on LDL cholesterol and arterial function as the result of dietary supplementation, a randomized, double-blind, placebo-controlled study was performed on 100 hypercholesterolemic but otherwise healthy subjects who were assigned to 24 weeks of daily intake of either Soy supplement, Abalon (30 g Soy protein, 9 g cotyledon fibre and 100 mg isoflavones), or placebo (30 g of casein). No difference in fasting plasma lipid levels or insulin sensitivity was found between treatment groups. Investigators did observe a significant postprandial increase in GIP (glucose-dependent insulinotropic peptide) in the Soy group ($p<0.05$). They concluded that markers of arterial function were not influenced by soy (Hermansen et al, 2005).

Water-washed Soy protein concentrate had no significant effect on blood lipids in moderately hypercholesterolemic adults compared to a milk-protein based control. This was observed in a randomized, double-blind, controlled clinical trial involving 159 subjects over a period of five weeks (Ma et al, 2005).

Somewhat different results were generated in another 2005 study, in which Soy protein (25 g daily) was determined to be twice as effective as 15 g daily in reducing serum cholesterol levels in 117 men and women with hypercholesterolemia as part of an eight-week, randomized and placebo-controlled trial. Not only did low-density lipoprotein cholesterol levels drop significantly by 5.9% and 1.1%, respectively, but total serum cholesterol and apolipoprotein B levels changed similarly as well. Compared with baseline, levels of high-density lipoprotein cholesterol, homocysteine, triglycerides, folic acid, and vitamin B12 did not alter significantly with either Soy or placebo groups. No serious adverse effects were recorded. The findings suggest that soy protein supplements may offer an uncomplicated method for lowering cardiovascular disease risk (Hoie, 2005).

An earlier, randomized, crossover study found that plasma and urinary isoflavone levels markedly increased with regular consumption of whole Soybean extracts in adults (23 men and 10 post-menopausal women). However, no overall differences in plasma lipids, blood pressure, or arterial compliance were identified as compared to the group consuming a control (dairy) diet. The whole Soybean contained not only Soy protein with isoflavones but polyunsaturated fat and soluble fiber that might further enhance cardiovascular benefits. The soy intervention component involved consumption of four servings daily (250 ml per serving) of either or both Soy milk or yogurt as part of the normal diet. After five weeks, the group switched to a dairy diet (or vice versa) that included four servings daily (250 ml per serving) of either or both low-fat dairy milk or yogurt. The 23 volunteers who completed the crossover trial were mildly hypercholesterolemic (total plasma cholesterol >5.5 mmol/l and (or) mildly hypertensive (blood pressure >140/90 mm Hg) but not taking medication for either at study start. The authors assert that this may have been the first assessment of the power of whole Soybean to affect vessel function. All participants appeared to comply with the diet instructions. Of note is that a later analysis of the data indicated that participants who were equol-positive had significant improvements in plasma lipids; equol is a metabolite of daidzein produced by digestion of bacteria in the gut, and the ability to produce it may be linked to certain health benefits. More research on the potential role of equol in lowering lipid levels are merited (Meyer, 2004).

Soy isoflavones decreased lipid levels in a randomized, double-blind, placebo-controlled study of 80 healthy women aged 45 to 55 years. Subjects received isoflavones 100 mg (including genistein 69.9 mg, daidzein 18.6 mg, and glycitein 11.4 mg) (n=40) or placebo (n=40) daily for 5 months. Total cholesterol (TC) and LDL cholesterol decreased significantly in the isoflavone group (TC=199; LDL=120) compared to placebo (TC=227; LDL=139) and baseline (TC=226; LDL=134) ($p<0.001$). No side effects were observed (Han et al, 2002).

Total cholesterol did not change but HDL (''good'') cholesterol increased and non-HDL cholesterol decreased in this study of 66 hypercholesterolemic, post-menopausal women who were studied in a 6-month, double-blind study. All subjects had a normalization period for 2 weeks, then received National Cholesterol Education Program (NCEP) Step 1 diet with either protein from casein and nonfat dry milk (control group), protein from Soy containing moderate 1.39 mg/g of protein) amounts of isoflavones (MI group), or a Soy protein group with high (2.25 mg/g) amounts of isoflavones (HI) group. Non-HDL cholesteral was reduced in both groups compared to the controls ($p<0.05$) but total cholesterol was not changed. HDL cholesterol increased in both Soy groups (p less than 0.05). The total cholesterol to HDL cholesterol ratio was also decreased compared to the control ($p<0.05$) (Baum et al, 1998).

A Soy protein diet reduced LDL cholesterol, and the LDL to HDL ratio in one study of 26 men. The reductions were independent of age, weight, and pretreatment lipid concentrations. Thirteen men with hypercholesterolemia and 13 normocholesterolemic patients (20 to 50 years) were randomly given either an NCEP Step 1 diet with animal protein or the NCEP diet with Soy protein for 5 weeks. Either animal or Soy protein represented 75% or more of the total protein in the diet. After a 10 to 15 week washout period, subjects were crossed over to the other study diet (Wong et al, 1998).

Twice-weekly topical administration of a purified Soy phosphatidylcholine in ethanol solution with butylated hydroxytoluene 0.01% to 20 men and 20 women with serum cholesterol greater than 250 mg/dL produced a 25% reduction in serum cholesterol ($p<0.01$) and a 23% reduction LDL cholesterol ($p<0.01$). The trial was 8 weeks long (Hsia et al, 1995).

Dietary isoflavonoid phytoestrogen supplementation did not alter serum lipid and lipoprotein (a) concentrations in a randomized, double-blind, placebo-controlled study of 59 healthy volunteers with average serum cholesterol concentrations (Hodgson et al, 1998).

Oral daily administration of 60 g of a Soy protein isolate beverage powder for 28 days had no beneficial effects on plasma cholesterol and platelet aggregation in a randomized, controlled study of 20 healthy male subjects. Although genistein (907 nmol/L) and daidzein (498 nmol/L) plasma levels in the Soy group were higher than plasma levels obtained with traditional Japanese diets, no significant differences in collagen or 9,11-dideoxy-11-alpha,9-alpha-epoxy-methanoprostaglandin F2- alpha (U46619)-induced platelet aggregation were observed in both groups. Plasma total cholesterol and HDL-cholesterol concentrations and plasma phospholipid polyunsaturated fatty acid composition showed no differences between Soy protein and casein supplementation (Gooderham et al, 1996).

Hyperlipidemia, Pediatric

An average drop in total cholesterol of 21.8% was found in 16 children with familial hypercholesterolemia who were given a Soy diet for 8 weeks. The children were first stabilized on a control, low lipid and cholesterol diet, then given the Soy protein diet with similar low lipids. Slight changes were noted in triglyceridemia and in HDL cholesterol concentration (Gaddi et al, 1987).

Soy formula diets fed to infants through the first 6 months of life resulted in lower total serum cholesterol and serum triglycerides ($p<0.05$) than in whey-based diets. Infants were divided into 5 groups: human milk (HM)(n=29), Soy formula (SF)(n=25), whey-based low-degree hydrolysate (Why)(n=15), casein-based high-degree hydrolysate (Chy)(n=13), and Soy plus collagen-based high-degree hydrolysate (SHy) (n=10). The mean total cholesterol level was lowest in the SHy group (3.0 mmol/L), followed by the SF and HM groups (3.3 mmol/L), the Chy group (3.4 mmol/L), and then the Why group (3.8 mmol/L). The similar order for triglycerides was 0.9 mmol/L for Soy, 1.2 mmol/L for HM and Why, and 1.6 for the Chy and Shy groups (Giovannini et al, 1994).

Hypertension

To examine the effects of dietary Soy/isoflavones on 24-hour blood pressure profiles and arterial function, a six-month, double-blind, placebo-controlled, crossover trial was performed. Forty-one hypertensive subjects received either Soy cereal (40 g Soy protein, 118 isoflavones) or gluten placebo cereal for three months. Soy dietary supplementation had no effect on arterial function, ambulatory blood pressure parameters, or central blood pressure (Teede et al, 2006).

By contrast, a cookie containing 40 g of Soybean protein resulted in a reduction in blood pressure in a randomized, double-blind controlled trial in three communities in China. The study involved 302 adults (35 to 64 years old) with high-normal or mildly elevated untreated systolic blood pressure of 130 to 159 mm Hg and diastolic pressure of 80 to 99 mm Hg or both. The participants were randomized to consume the Soybean protein cookies or a control cookie (a complex carbohydrate) daily for 12 weeks. Blood pressure was measured at baseline, six weeks, and 12 weeks. At this final reading, the time in which the Soybean cookies was consumed were linked to reduced diastolic and systolic blood pressure values by approximately 3 to 4 mm Hg more than the time that the carbohydrate cookies were consumed. Most participants ate the cookies in place of their usual breakfasts (He, 2005).

In a similar finding, supplemental Soy milk demonstrated a modest but significant reduction in blood pressure in a placebo-controlled, randomized trial. Patients with mild to moderate essential hypertension (n=40; 25 male, 15 female) were randomly assigned to receive 500 mL of Soy milk (containing 63 mg daidzein, 80 mg genistein), or 500 mL cow's milk twice daily for 3 months, following a 4-week washout period (without any medications, including antihypertensives). The Soy group significantly ($p<0.001$) reduced systolic blood pressure by 18.4 mm/Hg (± 10.7), diastolic blood pressure by 15.9 mm/Hg (± 9.8), and mean blood pressure by 16.7 mm/Hg (± 9.0) compared to 1.4 mm/Hg (± 7.2), 3.7 mm/Hg (± 5.0), 3.0 mm/Hg (± 4.6), respectively, for cow's milk. Reductions in blood pressure were associated with urinary genistein excretion but not daidzein (Rivas et al, 2002).

Menopausal Symptoms/Hot Flushes

A systematic review and meta-analysis of nonhormonal therapies for menopausal hot flushes found mixed results for the ability of Soy isoflavone extracts to lessen this common symptom. In fact, results for Soy isoflavone extracts were contradictory overall—even among the largest and highest quality trials, the authors concluded. The weak estrogenic and anti-estrogenic activities and ability to bind to estrogen receptors of isoflavones from Soy (and red clover) could potentially mediate hot flushes triggered by estrogen deficiency in menopause, but this action also could cause adverse effects. Evidence as a whole, the authors conclude, does not support recommending Soy in any form (flour, powder, in foods) for relieving hot flushes and is not an optimal choice for most women (Nelson 2006).

A systematic review of 10 clinical trials involving monotherapy of Soy or Soy isoflavones for perimenopausal symptoms, with focus on hot flushes, demonstrated equivocal results. Four of the randomized trials had beneficial effects, while six did not. Authors reported a dosing range of the studies of 34 to 134.5 mg a day of Soy isoflavones. Of the 6 that did not demonstrate beneficial effects, one of them demonstrated a positive trend that did not reach significance. Adverse events were insignificant, with no serious side effects other than mild gastrointestinal complaints (Huntley and Ernst, 2004).

Soy isoflavones decreased menopausal symptoms in a randomized, double-blind, placebo-controlled study of 80 healthy women 45 to 55 years. Subjects received isoflavones 100 mg (including genistein 69.9 mg, daidzein 18.6 mg, glycitein 11.4 mg) (n=40), or placebo (n=40) daily for five months. Subjects taking isoflavones experienced a significant decrease in menopausal symptoms measured using the Kupperman index compared with placebo and baseline (24.9 with isoflavones, 41.6 with placebo, and 44.6 at baseline) (p<0.01). The Kupperman index rates hot flushes, paresthesia, insomnia, nervousness, melancholia, vertigo, weakness, arthralgia or myalgia, headache, palpitations, and formication. No side effects were observed (Han et al, 2002).

Soy isoflavone extract reduced the frequency of hot flushes in postmenopausal women in a double-blind, placebo-controlled trial. Postmenopausal women, who not on hormone replacement therapy who requested treatment for hot flushes and with no menstrual period for at least 6 months, were randomized to receive four, 325 mg PhytoSoya® (for a total of 70 mg isoflavones/day; n=38) or placebo (cellulose; n=34) for 16 weeks. The authors claimed a mean reduction in hot flush frequency using last observation carried forward for the intention to treat analysis (p=0.0103; -3.6 (95% confidence interval - 6.2; -.9), but significance was not reached using 16-week observed data (Drapier-Faure, et al, 2002).

Soy had no effect on menopausal symptoms in a double-blind, placebo-controlled, trial. Women (42 to 62 years), not on hormone replacement, were randomized to receive either isoflavone-rich Soy protein (80.4 milligrams a day of aglycone components; n=24), isoflavone-poor Soy protein (4.4 milligrams a day of aglycone components; n=24) or whey protein control (n=21) for 24 weeks. No significant changes were noted for those women taking Soy for reductions in hot flushes or night sweat frequency, duration, or severity. All symptoms in all groups improved with time, suggesting a placebo effect or time as a factor in improvement (Germain et al, 2001).

Hot flushes were reduced in frequency and severity in postmenopausal women treated with a Soy isoflavone extract containing 50 mg of genistein and daidzein/day in a double-blind, randomized, placebo-controlled study. Subjects were randomized to receive the Soy extract treatment (n=89) or placebo (n=86) daily for 12 weeks. The Soy group experienced a significant decrease in hot flash severity (p=0.01) in comparison to the placebo group (Upmalis et al, 2000). An earlier double-blind, placebo-controlled, parallel, multicenter, randomized study of post menopausal women also showed a reduction in hot flushes (Albertazzi et al, 1998).

Migraine, Menstrual

A combination Soy, Donq quai, and Black Cohosh supplement successfully reduced migraine frequency in a double-blind, randomized, placebo-controlled trial. Following a 4-week placebo run-in period, patients were randomized to receive either a phytoestrogen supplement (n =20) containing: 75 mg Soy extract (40% isoflavones), 50 mg Dong Quai extract (standardized to 1% ligustilide), and 25 mg Black Cohosh (standardized to 8% triterpenes) or an identical looking placebo (n=18) twice daily for 24 weeks. Significant reductions in the primary outcome measure of mean number of menstrual migraine attacks (weeks 9 to 24) was observed in the supplemented group compared to placebo (4.7 (95% confidence interval 1.59 to 7.81) vs 10.3 (6.12 to 14.48); p<0.01). Secondary outcomes including frequency of any migraine attack (weeks 20 to 24), mean headache severity score (weeks 20 to 24), self-medicated triptans doses (weeks 20 to 24), and doses of analgesics (weeks 20 to 24) were all significantly reduced compared to placebo (p less than 0.01) (Burke et al, 2002).

Osteoporosis Prevention

Soy had a mildly beneficial effect on bone mineral content in women in a randomized, double-blind, placebo-controlled trial. Post menopausal Chinese women (48 to 62 years) were randomly assigned to receive either a 0.5 g Soy extract (40 mg isoflavones) (n=68), a 1 g Soy extract (80 mg isoflavones) (n=68), or placebo (n=67) daily for 1 year. Isoflavones consisted of daidzein (46.4%), glycetein (38.8%), and genistein (14.7%). All women also took calcium 500 mg/day and vitamin D 125 international units/day for a year. No statistically significant difference in bone mineral density (BMD) was noted. Positive changes to bone mineral content (BMC) were noted at the trochanter in subjects in the high-dose group compared to placebo and mid-dose groups (p<0.05) (Chen et al, 2003).

Soy protein exerted a beneficial effect on serum and urinary biomarkers of bone metabolism in women in a double-blind, parallel design study. Forty-two postmenopausal women (mean age 62.4 years) were randomly assigned to receive either 40 g Soy protein (n=20) or 40 g milk-based protein (n = 22) daily for 3 months. Soy protein had the greatest effects on women who were not on hormone replacement therapy. In this sub-roup, a significant decrease in urinary deoxypyridinoline (Dpd) excretion (p =0.0041) and a substantial increase in serum IGF-I (p= 0.0001) were noted compared to baseline, while corresponding changes were not noted in those on milk-based protein (Arjmandi et al, 2003).

A randomized trial of 187 healthy postmenopausal women demonstrated that a diet rich in Soy is not as effective as hormone replacement therapy (HRT) on the main biomarkers of bone turnover, but the Soy diet did stimulate osteoblastic activity. The women were divided into 3 groups and were followed for 6 months; diet intervention group (average 47 mg/day of isoflavones) (n=53), HRT group (n=53, type and dose not specified), and control group (n=58). The biomarkers of bone turnover measured were osteocalcin, N-telopeptide-C, hydroxyproline, and cortical and trabecular bone mineral density. A significant decrease in bone turnover was demonstrated only in the HRT group (p<0.05). Osteocalcin levels significantly increased in the Soy diet group (5.45; CI=0.36 to

10.5; p<0.05). Bone mineral density decreased significantly only in the control group (-.03; CI=-.06 to .001, p<0.05). Fifty-five percent of subjects in the Soy-rich diet group did not complete the study due to dislike of Soy and difficulty finding and cooking Soy foods (Chiechi et al, 2002).

Treatment with Soy protein decreased bone loss from the lumbar spine in postmenopausal women in a randomized, double-blind trial (Alekel et al, 2000). Limited increases in bone density and mineralization occurred in 66 hypercholesterolemic, postmenopausal women who were given 40 g/day of moderate to high isoflavone containing Soy protein in a 6-month, double-blind, parallel-group study (Potter et al, 1998).

Six months of treatment with 40 g of Soy protein/day (containing 90 mg of isoflavone) produced increased lumbar spine mineral content and density. A dose with 56 mg of isoflavones did not have this effect (Finkel, 1998).

Prostate Cancer

The incidence of prostate cancer is much lower in Asian than Western men, suggesting a possible link to environmental factors such as diet. This population-based prospective examination in 43,509 men from Japan aged 45 to 74 years old looked at the intake of Soy isoflavones in the diet and the incidence of prostate cancer over time. The participants filled out a validated questionnaire that included questions about 147 food items at various times from 1995 through 2004. While consumption of Soy food, miso soup, genistein and and daidzein were not associated with the incidence of total prostate cancer, consumption did decrease the risk of localized prostate cancer. Notably, in men over age 60, consumption of isoflavones and Soy foods were linked to a dose-dependent decrease in the risk of localized cancer. Also, men with the highest intake of isoflavones (specifically, as genistin equal to or greater than 32.8 mg/d) had a decreased risk of prostate cancer compared with those with the lowest intake (as genistein less than 13.2 mg/d). This inverse association between isoflavone and localized prostate cancer in Japan may be the first prospective study to show this association, Notably, however, the isoflavone intake did also tend to be associated with an increased risk of advanced prostate cancer. More research in the form of clinical trials is needed to clarify these effects (Kurahashi, 2007).

In earlier research, Soy had no effect of serum prostate specific antigen (PSA) in a series of randomized, crossover trials. Healthy men (n=46) with various baseline PSA levels were recruited for studies on the effects of Soy on blood lipids. Pooled analysis from four studies showed treatment phases that lasted from 3 to 4 weeks, with average Soy protein consumption of 44 g (116 mg isoflavones) daily. Although Soy consumption was significant enough to reduce serum cholesterol and oxidized low-density lipoprotein concentration, no effect on PSA values were seen (Jenkins et al, 2003).

Treatment with isolated Soy protein (ISP) beverages in 34 elderly men (>55 years) with elevated PSA (> 4 nanogram/milliliter) had no effect on either PSA or p105 (pro-oncogene) in a randomized, double-blind, crossover study (Urban et al, 2001).

Quality of Life, Postmenopausal

No particular or marked overall benefit of one-year supplementation with Soy protein containing isoflavones on quality of life was observed in 202 postmenopausal women (age 60 to 75) in this double-blind, randomized and placebo-controlled trial. The daily Soy protein supplement was a powder that contained 25.6 g Soy protein with 52 mg genistein, 41 mg daidzein, and 6 mg glycein. The placebo was milk protein. A questionnaire was used to assess changes in quality of life such as health status, depression, and life satisfaction (Kok. 2005).

Renal Failure

A Soy-based, low-protein, vegetarian diet was well tolerated, maintained renal function, and improved some nutritional aspects in patients with chronic renal failure. Patients were more compliant with recommended caloric, protein, and phosphate intakes on the Soy diet versus the animal protein diet (p<0.05). These results translate to higher caloric diets, which were lower in protein and phosphate that are essential for patients with chronic renal failure. Nine patients with chronic renal failure (glomerular filtration rate (GFR) of 15 to 50 mL/minute/1.73 m2) completed testing in a randomized, crossover trial of 2 different diets. Both diets were low protein; one contained Soy and the other contained animal-based protein. The GFR was the same at 6 months and remained the same throughout the study in both groups. Nutritional status (body mass, midarm circumference, lean body mass, percent body fat) remained the same over the one year of the study. The Soy group had a higher calorie intake, a lower protein intake, and a lower protein intake/kg than either prediet baseline or the animal protein diet (p<0.05). The Soy diet also lowered blood urea nitrogen, urine urea nitrogen, protein catabolic rate, 24-hour urine creatinine, and phosphate more than the animal protein diet (Soroka et al, 1998).

INDICATIONS AND USAGE

Approved by Commission E:

- Raised levels of cholesterol

Unproven Uses: Soybean is used for less severe forms of hypercholesterolemia when dietary measures are required. Soybean is also used for liver and gallbladder complaints, anemia, poor concentration, cerebral and nerve conditions, and general debility.

Chinese Medicine: Soybean is used for hyperhidrosis, night sweats, confusion, and joint pain.

CONTRAINDICATIONS

There are no known contraindications to the use of Soy.

PRECAUTIONS AND ADVERSE REACTIONS

Minor side effects may include occasional gastrointestinal effects, such as stomach pain, loose stool and diarrhea.

Lower circulating estrogen levels and longer menstrual cycles have been reported with Soy-rich diets. Vomiting has been reported, as has contact dermatitis. Gastrointestinal symptoms and atopic dermatitis may occur with the use of Soy formulas but anaphylaxis is extremely rare. A meta analysis of 17 studies on allergy to Soy formulas was represented by 27% history- based studies, 4% challenged test based studies, and about 3% skin prick tests (Cantani & Lucenti, 1997).

Carcinogenicity: A meta analysis of 14 trials determined that there is a link between the consumption of fermented Soy foods and risk of stomach cancer in Asian populations. The inverse relationship between stomach cancer and non-fermented Soy foods was also present. The authors of the analysis state that none of the studies have taken into account such confounders as salt, N-nitroso compounds, and additional plant foods that might be eaten in conjunction with non-fermented Soy foods and, therefore, makes these conclusions suspect (Wu et al, 2000).

Central Nervous System Effects: A prospective cohort study of 3,734 Japanese-American men found that those who consumed higher amounts of tofu in middle life were significantly more likely to demonstrate poor cognitive test performance, enlargement of ventricles, and low brain weight. The investigators hypothesized that the result may be due to the ability of some Soy isoflavones to inhibit tyrosine kinase, an enzyme that is involved with neuronal plasticity (White et al, 2000).

Endocrine Effects: Lower estrogen levels and longer menstrual cycles have been reported with Soy-rich diets (Cassidy et al, 1994).

Kidney/Genitourinary Effects: Dietary Soy consumption was associated with greater than a twofold increased risk of bladder cancer in the Singapore Chinese Health Study of 63,257 Chinese men and women (Sun et al, 2002).

Thyroid Effects: An epidemiologic study suggests that early Soy formula feeding may be associated with autoimmune thyroid disorders later in life (Fort et al, 1990). In a review article, this hypothesis was supported by animal and in vitro studies that suggested genistein may stimulate immune function by antigen formation through covalent binding of genistein to thyroid peroxidase (TPO) (Doerge & Chang, 2002; Doerge & Sheehan, 2002). Soy-containing formulas were associated with goiter and hypothyroidism in infants in the 1960s until the addition of iodine to formulas. The relationship between Soy and goiter is well known in animals and appears to be related to iodine deficiency (Doerge & Sheehan, 2002).

DRUG INTERACTIONS

MODERATE RISK

Levothyroxine: Concurrent use of soy and levothyroxine may result in decreased effectiveness of levothyroxine. *Clinical Management:* Soy administered either as a supplement or as a dietary component may impair absorption of levothyroxine. It is thought that this effect would be minimized if administration times were separated by two hours or more, but no data exists to verify this assumption. Patients should be advised to avoid the combination. Thyroid function tests should be monitored in patients who elect to use soy with levothyroxine. Levothyroxine dose requirements may increase. Serum thyroxine and thyrotropin levels should be obtained within 6 weeks of soy discontinuation to determine if levothyroxine dose requirements have decreased.

Warfarin: Concurrent use of soy and warfarin may result in reduced warfarin effectiveness. *Clinical Management:* Monitor the INR closely whenever initiating or discontinuing soy milk or other soy foods or supplements in a patient taking warfarin. One case report described a decreased INR in a patient taking warfarin after starting Soy milk (Cambria-Kiely, 2002).

MINOR RISK

Iron: Concurrent use of soy and iron may result in reduced iron absorption. *Clinical Management:* Soy administered either as a supplement or as a dietary component may impair absorption of iron. It is thought that this effect would be minimized if administration times were separated by two hours or more, but no data exists to verify this assumption. Patients should be advised to avoid the combination.

OTHER POSSIBLE RISKS

Tamoxifen: Concurrent use of soy and tamoxifen may result in decreased tamoxifen effectiveness. Clinical Management: Avoid concomitant use of soy and tamoxifen.

DOSAGE

Mode of Administration: Preparations for oral administration.

Daily Dosage: The average dose is 3.5 g of phospholipids (phosphatidylcholine).

Storage: Soybean preparations must be protected from light and tightly sealed.

LITERATURE

Alarcon P, Montoya R, Perez F, et al: Clinical trial of home available, mixed diets versus a lactose-free, Soy protein formula for the dietary management of acute childhood diarrhea. *J Pediatr Gastroenterol* Nutr 12(2):224-232. 1991.

Albertazzi P, Pansini F, Bonaccorsi G, et al: The effect of dietary Soy supplementation on hot flashes. *Obstet Gynecol* 91(1):6-11. 1998.

Alekel DL, St Germain A, Peterson CT, et al: Isoflavone-rich Soy protein isolate attenuates bone loss in the lumbar spine of perimenopausal women. *Am J Clin Nutr* 72(3):844-852. 2000.

Alhasan S, Alonso MD, Ensley J, et al: Genistein induced growth inhibition and apoptosis in squamous cell carcinoma cell line of the head and neck. *Proc Am Assoc Cancer Res* 39:585. 1998.

Allen JK, Becker DM, Kwiterovich PO, et al. Effect of soy protein-containing isoflavones on lipoproteins in postmenopausal women. *Menopause*; 14(1): 106-114. 2007.

Allen UD, McLeod K, Wang EL. Cow's milk versus Soy-based formula in mild and moderate diarrhea: a randomized, controlled trial. *Acta Paediatr* 83(2):183-187.1994.

Anderson J, Ambrose W, Garner SC. Biphasic effects of genistein on bone tissue in the ovariectomized, lactating rat model. *PSEBM* 1998; 217(3):345-350.

Anderson J, Garner SC. The effects of phytoestrogens on bone. *Nutr Res* 17:1617-1632. 1997.

Anderson J, Blake JE, Turner J, et al: Effects of Soy protein on renal function and proteinuria in patients with type 2 diabetes. *Am J Clin Nutr* 68(6 suppl):1347S-1353S. 1998.

Anderson J, Johnstone BM, Cook-Newell ME. Meta-analysis of the effects of Soy protein intake on serum lipids. *N Engl J Med* 333(5):276-282. 1995.

Anderson J, Smith BM, Washnock CS: Cardiovascular and renal benefits of dry bean and Soybean intake. *Am J Clin Nutr* 70(3 suppl):464S-474S. 1999.

Anderson JW, Fuller J, Patterson K, et al. Soy compared to casein meal replacement shakes with energy-restricted diets for obese women: randomized controlled trial. *Metabolism*; 56(2): 280-288. 2007.

Anderson JW, Hoie LH. Weight loss and lipid changes with low-energy diets: comparator study of milk-based versus soy-based liquid meal replacement interventions. *J Am Coll Nutr*; 24(3): 210-216. 2005.

Anon: Clinical Develpment Plan - National Cancer Institute: Genistein. *J Cell Biochem Suppl* 26:114-126. 1996.

Arjmandi BH, Khalil DA, Smith BJ, et al: Soy protein has a greater effect on bone in postmenopausal women not on hormone replacement therapy, as evidenced by reducing bone resorption and urinary calcium excretion. J Clin Endocrinol Metab 88(3):1048-1054. 2003.

Baird DD, Umbach DM, Lansdell L, et al: Dietary intervention study to assess estrogenicity of dietary Soy amoung postmenopausal women. *J Clin Endocrinol Metab* 80(5):1685-1690. 1995.

Bakhit R, Potter SM. In vitro inhibition of LDL oxidation by means of SOY isoflavones genistein and genistin. *FASEB J* 11:A271.1997.

Barnes S, Petersen G, Coward L. Rationale for the use of genistein-containing SOY matrices in chemoprevention trials for breast and prostate cancer. *J Cell Biochem Suppl* 22:181-187. 1995.

Baum JA, Teng H, Erdman JW Jr., et al: Long-term intake of Soy protein improves blood lipid profiles and increases mononuclear cell low-densitiy-lipoprotein receptor messenger RNA in hypercholesterolemic, postmenopausal women. *Am J Clin Nutr* 68(3):545-551. 1998.

Bhutta ZA, Molla AM, Issani Z, et al: Nutrient absorption and weight gain in persistent diarrhea: comparison of a traditional rice-lentil/yogert/milk diet with Soy formula. *J Pediatr Gastroenterol Nutr* 18(1):45-52. 1994.

Bingham SA, Atkinson C, Liggins J, et al: Phyto-oestrogens: where are we now? *Br J Nutr* 79(5):393-406. 1998.

Bosland MC, Davies JA, Voermans C. Inhibition of human prostate cancer cell proliferation by genistein. *Proc Am Assoc Cancer Res* 38:1997. 1998.

Brown A, Jolly P, Wie H. Genistein modulates neuroblastoma cell proliferation and differentiation through induction of apoptosis and regulation of tyrosine kinase activity and N-myc expression. *Carcinogenesis* 19(6):991-997. 1998.

Brzezinski A, Adlercreutz H, Shaoul R, et al: Short-term effects of phytoestrogen-rich diet on postmenopausal women. *Menopause* 4(2):89-94. 1997.

Burke BE, Olson RD, Cusack M. Randomized, controlled trial of phytoestrogen in the prophylactic treatment of menstrual migraine. *Biomed Pharmacother* 56(6):283-288. 2002.

Burks AW, Casteel HB, Fiedorek SC, et al: Prospective oral food challenge study of two Soybean protein isolates in patients with possible milk or Soy protein enterocolitis. *Pediatr Allergy Immunol* 5(1):40-45. 1994.

Cambria-Kiely JA, Effect of Soy milk on warfarin efficacy. *Ann Pharmacother* 36(12):1893-1896. 2002.

Cantani A, Lucenti P. Natural history of Soy allergy and/or intolerance in children, and clinical use of Soy-protein formulas. *Pediatr Allergy Immunol* 8(2):59-74. 1997.

Casini ML, Marelli G, Papaleo E, et al. Psychological assessment of the effects of treatment with phytoestrogens on postmenopausal women: a randomized, double-blind, crossover, placebo-controlled study. *Fertil Steril*; 85(4): 972-978. 2006.

Cassidy A, Bingham S, Setchell KR. Biological effects of a diet of Soy protein rich in isoflavones on the menstrual cycle of premenopausal women. *Am J Clin Nutr* 60(3):333-340. 1994.

Chen YM, Ho SC, Lam SSH et al: Soy isoflavones have a favorable effect on bone loss in Chinese postmenopausal women with lower bone mass: a double-blind, randomized, controlled trial. *J Clin Endocrinol Metab* 88(10):4740-4747. 2003.

Chiechi Lm, Secreto G, D'Amore et al: Efficacy of a Soy rich diet in preventing postmenopausal osteoporosis: the Menfis randomized trial. *Maturitas* 42(4):295-300. 2002.

Choi YH, Zhang L, Lee WH, et al: Genistein-induced G2/M arrest is associated with the inhibition of cyclin B1 and the induction of p21 in human breast carcinoma cells. *Int J Oncol* 13(2):391-396. 1998.

Clarkson TB, Anthony MS, Williams JK, et al: The potential of Soybean phytoestrogens for postmenopausal hormone replacement therapy (44246). *PSEBM* 7(3):365-368. 1998.

Clifford HG, Shand N, Fitzpatrick MG, et al: Daily intake and urinary excretion of genistein and daidzein by infants fed Soy- or dairy-based infant formulas. *Am J Clin Nutr* 68(6 suppl):1462S-1465S. 1998.

Constantinou AI, Kamath N, Murley JS. Genistein inactivates bcl-2, delays the G2-M phase of the cell cycle, and induces apoptosis of human breast adenocarcinoma MCF-7 cells. *Eur J Cancer* 34(12):1927-1934. 1998.

Constantinou AI, Krygier AE, Mehta RR. Genistein induces maturation of cultured human breast cancer cells and prevents tumor growth in nude mice. *Am J Clin Nutr* 68(6 suppl):1426S-1430S. 1998.

Costa RL, Summa MA: Soy protein in the management of hyperlipidemia. Ann Pharmacother 34(7-8):931-935. 2000.

Craig WJ: Phytochemicals: guardians of our health. *J Am Diet Assoc* 97(10 suppl 2):S199-S204. 1997.

Dalu A, Haskell JF, Lamartiere CA. Soy and cancer. *Am J Clin Nutr* 68(6 suppl):1524S-1530S. 1998.

D'Amico G, Gentile MG. Effect of dietary manipulation on the lipid abnormalities and urinary protein loss in nephrotic patients. *Miner Electrolyte Metab* 18(2-5):203-206. 1992.

Davies JA, Walden P, Bosland MC. Role of BTG2 and possibly p53 in growth inhibition by genistein in LNCaP, PC3 and DU145 human prostate cancer cells. *Proc Am Assoc Cancer Res* 39:389. 1998.

Dees C, Foster JS, Ahamed S, et al: Dietary estrogens stimulate human breast cells to enter the cell cycle. *Environ Health Perspect* 105(suppl 3):633-636. 1997.

Dewell A, Hollenbeck CB, Bruce B. The effects of Soy-derived phytoestrogens on serum lipids and lipoproteins in moderately hypercholesterolemic postmenopausal women. *J Clin Endocrinol Metab* 87(1):118-121. 2002.

Divi RL, Chang HC, Doerge DR. Anti-thyroid isoflavones from Soybean. *Biochem Pharmacol* 54(10):1087-1096. 1997.

Doerge D, Chang H. Inactivation of thyroid peroxidase by Soy isoflavones, in vitro and in vivo. *J Chromatog* 777(1-2):269-279. 2002.

Donovan GK, Torres-Pinedo R. Chronic diarrhea and Soy formulas. *Am J Dis Child* 141(10):1069-1071. 1987.

Engel PA. New onset migraine associated with use of Soy isoflavone supplements. *Neurology* 59(8):1289-1290. 2002.

Erdman JW. Control of serum lipids with Soy protein. *N Engl J Med* 333(5):313-315. 1995.

Erdman JW. Soy protein and cardiovascular disease, a statement for healthcare professionals from the nutrition committee of the AHA. *Circulation* 102(20):2555-2559. 2000.

Fair WR, Fleshner NE, Heston W. Cancer of the prostate: a nutritional disease? *Urology* 50(6):840-848. 1997.

Faure ED, Chantre P, Mares P. Effects of a standardized Soy extract on hot flushes: a multicenter, double-blind, randomized, placebo-controlled study. Menopause 9(5):329-334. 2002.

FDA: FDA Talk Paper FDA: approves new health claim for Soy protein and coronary heart disease. October 20, 1999 accessed at http://www.fda.gov/bbs/topics/answers/ans00980.html (cited 2/28/2003).

File S, Jarrett N, Fluck E. Eating Soya improves human memory. *Psychopharmacology* 157(4):430-436. 2001.

Finkel E. Phyto-oestrogens: the way to postmenopausal health? *Lancet* 352(9142):1762. 1998.

Gaddi A, Descovich GC, Noseda G, et al: Hypercholesterolaemia treated by Soybean protein diet. *Arch Dis Child* 62(3):274-278. 1987.

Geller J, Sionit L, Partido C, et al: Genistein inhibits the growth of human-patient BPH and prostate cancer histoculture. *Prostate* 34(2):75-79. 1998.

Gentile MG, Fellin G, Cofano F, et al: Treatment of proteiuric patients with a vegetarian Soy diet and fish oil. *Clin Nephrol* 40(6):315-320. 1993.

Gescher A, Pastorino U, Plummer S, et al: Suppression of tumor development by substances derived from the diet - mechanisms and clinical implications. *Br J Clin Pharmacol* 45(1):1-12. 1998.

Giovannini M, Agostoni C, Fiocchi A, et al: Antigen-reduced infant formulas versus human milk: growth and metabolic parameters in the first 6 months of life. *J Am Coll Nutr* 13(4):357-363. 1994.

Gooderham MJ, Adlercreutz H, Ojala ST et al: A Soy protein isolate rich in genistein and daidzein and its effects on plasma isoflavone concentrations, platelet aggregation, blood lipids and fatty acid composition of plasma phospholipid in normal men. *J Nutr* 126(18):2000-2006. 1996.

Gozlan J, Lathey JL, Spector SA. Human immunodeficiency virus type 1 induction mediated by genistein is linked to cell cycle arrest in G2. *J Virol* 72(10):8174-8180. 1998.

Grauds C. Soy monograph. *Pharm Times* 10:59-60. 1999.

Haffejee IE. Cow's milk-based formula, human milk, and Soya feeds in acute infantile diarrhea: a therapeutic trial. *J Pediatr Gastroenterol Nutr* 10(2):193-198. 1990.

Han KK, Soares JM, Haidar MA, et al: Benefits of Soy isoflavone therapeutic regimen on menopausal symptoms. *Obstet Gynecol* 99(3):389-394. 2002.

He J, Gu D, Wu X, et al. Effect of soybean protein on blood pressure: a randomized controlled trial. *Ann Intern Med*; 143: 1-9. 2005.

Hebert JR, Hurley TG, Olendzi BC, et al: Nutritional and socioeconomic factors in relation to prostate cancer mortality: a cross-national study. *J Natl Cancer Inst* 90(24):1637-1647. 1998.

Hermansen K, Hansen B, Jabobsen, R, et al. Effects of soy supplementation on blood lipids and arterial function in hypercholesterolaemic subjects. *Eur J Clin Nutr*; 59(7): 843-850. 2005.

Hilakivi-Clarke L, Cho E & Clarke R: Maternal genistein exposure mimics the effects of estrogen on mammary gland development in female mouse offspring. *Oncol Rep* 5(3):609-616. 1998.

Hodgson JM, Puddey IB, Beilin LJ, et al: Supplementation with isoflavonoid phytoestrogens does alter serum lipid concentrations: a randomized controlled trial in humans. *J Nutr* 128:728-732. 1998.

Ho SC, Woo JF, Leung SF, et al: Intake of Soy products is associated with better plasma lipid profiles in the Hong Kong Chinese population. *J Nutr* 130(10):2590-2593. 2000.

Hoie L, Graubman H, Wernecke K. Lipid-lowering effect of 2 dosages of a Soy protein supplement in hypercholesterolemia. Adv Nat Ther; 22(2):175-186. 2005.

Hsia SL, He J-L, Xu X, et al: Topical treatment for hypercholesterolemia with Soy lecithin. *J Nutr* 125:801-802. 1995.

Huntley A, Ernst E. Soy for the treatment of perimenopausal symptoms-a systematic review. *Maturitas* 47(1):1-9. 2003.

Hurrell RF, Davidsson L, Reddy M, et al: A comparison of iron absorption in adults and infants consuming identical infant formulas. *Br J Nutr* 79(1):31-36. 1998.

Hurrell RF, Juillerat MA, Reddy MB, et al: Soy protein, phytate, and iron absorption in humans. *Am J Clin Nutr* 56(3):573-578. 1992.

Hwang TC, Wang F, Yang IC et al: Genistein potentiates wild-type and delta F508-CFTR channel activity. *Am J Physiol*; 273(3 pt 1):C988-998. 1997

Illek B, Yankaskas JR, Machen TE: cAMP and genistein stimulate HCO3-conductance through CFTR in human airway epithelia. *Am J Physiol*; 272(4 pt 1):L752-L761. 1997

Jabbar MA, Larrea J, Shaw RA. Abnormal thyroid function tests in infants with congenital hypothyroidism: the influence of Soy-based formula. *J Am Coll Nutr* 16:280-282. 1997.

Jayagopal V, Albertazzi P, Kilpatrick ES, et al: Beneficial effects of Soy phytoestrogen intake in postmenopausal women with type 2 diabetes. *Diabetes Care* 25(10):1709-1714. 2002.

Jenkins D, Kendall C, D'Costa M, et al: Soy consumption and phytoestrogens: effect on serum prostate specific antigen when blood lipids and oxidized low-density lipoprotein are reduced in hyperlipidemic men. *Journal of Urology* 169(2):507-511. 2003.

Ju YH, Doerge DR, Allred KF, et al: Dietary genestein negates the inhibitory effect of tamoxifen on growth of estrogen-dependent human breast cancer (MCF-7) cells implanted in athymic mice. *Cancer Res* 62(9):2474-2477. 2002.

Kapiotis S, Hermann M, Held I, et al: Genistein, the dietary-derived angiogenesis inhibitor, prevents LDL oxidation and protects endothelial cells from damage by atherogenic LDL. *Arterioscler Thromb Vasc Biol* 17(11):2868-2874. 1997.

Karr SC, Lampe JW, Hutchins AM, et al: Urinary isoflavonoid excretion in humans is dose-dependent at low to moderate levels of Soy protein. *Am J Clin Nutr* 66(1):46-51. 1997.

Kennedy AR. The evidence for Soybean products as cancer preventive agents. *J Nutr* 125(suppl):733S-743S. 1995.

King RA, Bursill DB: Plasma and urinary kinetics of the isoflavones daidzein and genistein after single Soy meal in humans. *Am J Clin Nutr* 67(5):867-872. 1998.

Knight DC, Eden JA. A review of the clinical effects of phytoestrogens. *Obstet Gynecol* 87(5 pt 2):897-904. 1996.

Kok L, Kreijkamp-Kaspers S, Grobbee DE, et al. A randomized, placebo-controlled trial on the effects of soy protein containing isoflavones on quality of life in postmenopausal women. *J North Amer Menopause Soc*; 12 (1): 56-62. 2005.

Kotsopoulos D, Dalais FS, Liang YL, et al: The effects of Soy protein containing phytoestrogens on menopausal symptoms in postmenopausal women. *Climacteric* 3(3):161-167. 2003.

Kreijkamp-Kaspers S, Kok L, Grobbee DE, et al. Effect of Soy protein containing isoflavones on cognitive function, bone mineral density, and plasma lipids in postmenopausal women. A randomized controlled trial. *JAMA*; 292(1): 65-74. 2004.

Kritz-Silverstein D, Von Muhlen D, Barrett-Connor E, et al: Isoflavones and cognitive function in older women: the Soy and Postmenopausal Health in Aging (SOPHIA) Study. *Menopause* 10(3):196-202. 2003.

Kurahashi N, Iwasaki M, Sasazuki S, et al. Soy product and isoflavone consumption in relation to prostate cancer in Japanese men. *Cancer Epidemiol Biomarers Prev*; 16(3):538-545. 2007.

Kurowska EM, Jordan J, Spence JD, et al: Effects of substituting dietary Soybean protein and oil for milk protein and fat in subjects with hypercholesterolemia. *Clin Invest Med* 20(3):162-170. 1997.

Kwiterovich PO Jr., Motevalli M. Differential effect of genistein on the stimulation of cholesterol production by basic protein II in normal and hyperapoB fibroblasts. *Arterioscler Thromb Vasc Biol* 18(1):57-64. 1998.

Lamartiniere CA, Murrill WB, Manzolillo PA, et al: Genistein alters the ontogeny of mammary gland development and protects against chemically-induced mammary cancer in rats. *PSEBM* 217(3):358-364. 1998.

LeCoz CJ, Lefebvre C: Contact dermatitis from maleated Soybean oil: last gasps of an expiring cosmetic allergen. *Contact Dermatitis* 43(2):118-119. 2000.

Lenn J, Uhl T, Mattacola C, et al: The effects of fish oil and isoflavones on delayed onset muscle soreness. *Med Sci Sports Exerc* 34(10):1605-1613. 2002.

Li W, Weber G. Synergistic action of tiazufurin and genistein in human ovarian carcinoma cells. *Oncol Res* 10(3):117-122. 1998.

Li W, Weber G: Synergistic action of tiazufurin and genistein on growth inhibition and differentiation of K-562 human leukemic cells. *Life Sci* 63(22):1975-1981. 1998.

Macfarlane BJ, van der Riet WB, Bothwell TH, et al: Effect of traditional oriental Soy products on iron absorption. Am J Clin Nutr 51(5):873-880. 1990.

Ma Y, Chiriboga D, Olendzki BC, et al. Effect of soy protein containing isoflavones on blood lipids in moderately hypercholesterolemic adults: a randomized controlled trial. J Am Coll Nutr: 24(4): 275-285. 2005.

MacGregor CA, Canney PA, Patterson G, McDonald R, Paul J. A randomized double-blind controlled trial of oral soy supplements versus placebo for treatment of menopausal symptoms in patients with early breast cancer. *Eur J Cancer*; 41(5): 708-714. 2005.

Maesta N, Nahas EA, Nahas-Neto J, et al. Effects of soy protein and resistance exercise on body composition and blood lipids in postmenopausal women. *Maturitas*; 56(4): 350-358. 2007.

Magnolfi CF, Zani G, Lacava L, et al: Soy allergy in atopic children. *Ann Allergy Asthma Immunol* 77(3):197-201. 1996.

Maskarinec G, Williams AE, Inouye JS. A randomized isoflavone intervention among premenopausal women. *Cancer Epidemiol Biomarkers Prev* 11(2):195-201. 2002.

Maulen-Radovan I, Brown KH, Acosta MA, et al: Comparison of a rice-based, mixed diet versus a lactose-free, Soy-protein isolate formula for young children with acute diarrhea. *J Pediatr* 125(5 pt 1):699-706. 1994.

McMichael-Phillips DF, Harding C, Morton M, et al: Effects of Soy-protein supplementation on epithelial proliferation in the histologically normal human breast. *Am J Clin Nutr* 68(6 suppl):1431S-1436S. 1998.

Messina M, Barnes S. The roles of Soy products in reducing risk of cancer. J Natl Cancer Inst 83(8):541-546. 1991.

Messina M, Messina V. Soyfoods, Soybean isoflavones, and bone health: a brief overview. *J Ren Nutr* 10(2):63-68. 2000.

Meyer BJ, Larkin T, Owen AJ, et al. Limited lipid-lowering effects of regular consumption of whole soybean foods. *Ann Nutr Metab*; 48:67-78. 2004.

Morelli V, Zoorob RJ. Alternative therapies: Part II. Congestive heart failure and hypercholesterolemia. Am Fam Physician 15;62(6):1325-1330. 2000.

Murkies A, Dalais FS, Briganti EM, et al: Phytoestrogens and breast cancer in postmenopausal women, a case control study. *Menopause* 7(5):289-296. 2000.

Murkies AL, Lombard C, Strauss BJ, et al: Dietary flour supplementation decreases post-menopausal hot flushes: effect of Soy and wheat. Maturitas 21(3):189-195. 1995.

Nagata C. Ecological study of the association between Soy product intake and mortality from cancer and heart disease in Japan. *Int J Epidemiol* 29(5):832-836. 2000.

Nelson HD, Vesco KK, Haney E, et al. Nonhormonal therapies for menopausal hot flashes. Systematic review and meta-analysis. *JAMA*; 295 (17): 2057-2071. 2006.

Nestel PJ, Yamashita T, Sasahara T, et al: Soy isoflavones improve systemic arterial compliance but not plasma lipids in menopausal and perimenopausal women. *Arterioscler Thromb Vasc Biol* 17(12):3392-3398. 1997.

Newton KM, LaCroix AZ, Levy L, et al. Soy protein and bone mineral density in older men and women: a randomized trial. *Maturitas*; 55(3): 270-277. 2006.

Nizami SQ, Bhutta AZ, Molla AM: Efficacy of traditional rice-lentil-yogurt diet, lactose free milk protein-based formula and Soy protein formula in management of secondary lactose intolerance with acute childhood diarrhoea. *J Trop Pediatr* 42(3):133-137. 1996.

Peterson TG, Ji GP, Kirk M, et al: Metabolism of the isoflavones genistein and bioachnin A in human breast cancer cell lines. *Am J Clin Nutr* 68(6 suppl):1505S-1511S. 1998.

Porch MC, Shahane AD, Leiva LE, et al: Influence of breast milk, Soy or two hydrolyzed formulas on the development of allergic manifestations in infants at risk. *Nutr Res* 18(8):1413-1424. 1998.

Potter SM, Baum JA, Teng H, et al: Soy protein and isoflavones: their effects on blood lipids and bone density in postmenopausal women. *Am J Clin Nutr* 68(6 suppl):1375S-1379S. 1998.

Quak SH, Low PS, Quah TC, et al: Oral refeeding following acute gastro-enteritis: a clinical trial using four refeeding regimes. *Ann Trop Paediatr* 9(3):152-155. 1989.

Quella SK, Loprinizi CL, Barton DL, et al: Evaluation of Soy phytoestrogens for the treatment of hot flashes in breast cancer survivors: a north central cancer treatment group trial. *J Clin Oncol* 18:1068-1074. 2000.

Rauth S, Kichina J, Green A. Inhibition of growth and induction of differentiation of metastatic melanoma cells in vitro by genistein: chemosensitivity is regulated by cellular p53. *Br J Cancer* 75(11):1559-1566. 1997.

Rivas M, Garay R, Escanero J, et al: Soy milk lowers blood pressure in men and women with mild to moderate essential hypertension. *J Nutr* 132(7):1900-1902. 2002.

Rygwelski JM, Smith MA. Dietary Soy and hot flushes. *J Fam Pract* 46(4):276-277. 1998.

Santell RC, Kieu N, Helferich WG. The effect of genistein upon estrogen receptor negative human breast cancer cell growth in vitro and in vivo. *Physiol Pharmacol Effects Food Components* 12:3807. 1998.

Santosham M, Goepp J, Burns B, et al: Role of a Soy-based lactose free formula in the outpatient management of diarrhea. *Pediatrics* 87(5):629-622. 1991.

Santti R, Makela S, Strauss L et al: Phytoestrogens: potential endocrine disruptors in males. *Toxicol Ind Health* 14(1-2):223-237. 1998.

Sarkar FH, Odenwaller R, Singh B, et al: Up-regulation of p21(waf) by isoflavone genistein in prostate cancer (Pca) cells. *J Urol* 4:21. 1997.

Schricker BR, Miller DD, Van Campen D. Effects of iron status and Soy protein on iron absorption by rats. *J Nutr* 113(5):996-1001. 1983.

Seidl MM, Stewart DE: Alternative treatments for menopausal symptoms. *Can Fam Physician* 44:1299-1308. 1998.

Setchell KR, Zimmer-Nechemias L, Cai J, et al: Exposure of infants to phyto-estrogens from Soy-based infant formula. *Lancet* 350(9070):23-27. 1997.

Shao ZM, Alpaugh ML, Fontana JA, et al: Genistein inhibits proliferation similarly in estrogen receptor-positive and negative human breast carcinoma cell lines characterized by P21(WAF/CIP1) induction, G2)/M arrest, and apoptosis. *J Cell Biochem* 69(1):44-54. 1998.

Shen F, Weber G. Synergistic action of quercitin and genistein in human ovarian carcinoma cells. *Oncol Res* 9(11-12):597-602. 1997.

Shige H, Ishikawa T, Higashi K, et al: Effects of Soy protein isolate (SPI) and casein on the postprandial lipemia in normlipidemic men. *J Nutr Sci Vitaminol* (Tokyo) 44(1):113-127. 1998.

Singletary K, Li J, Faller J. Inhibition of human mammary epithelial cell proliferation by genistein. *Physiol Pharmacol Effects Food Components* 12:3809. 1998.

Sirtori CR, Agradi E, Conti F, et al: Soybean-protein diet in the treatment of type-II hyperlipoprotenaemia. *Lancet* 8006):275-277. 1977.

St. Germain A, Peterson C, Robinson JG, et al: Isoflavone-rich or isoflavone-poor Soy protein does not reduce menopausal symptoms during 24 weeks of treatment. *Menopause* 8(1):17-26. 2001.

Stoll BA. Eating to beat breast cancer: potential role of Soy supplements. *Ann Oncol* 8(3):223-225. 1997.

Stone NJ. Approach to the Patient with Hyperlipidemia, in Gotto A (ed.): DiseaseDex™ - General Medicine, May 23, 2002. MicroMedex, Greenwood Village, Colorado. 2002.

Strom B, Schinnar R, Ziegler E, et al: Exposure to Soy-based formula in infancy and endocrinological and reproductive outcomes in young adulthood. *JAMA* 286(7):807-814. 2001.

Sun CL, Yan JM, Arakawa K, et al: Dietary Soy and increased risk of bladder cancer: the Singapore Chinese Health Study. *Cancer Epidemiol Biomarkers Prev* 11:1674-1677. 2002.

Taramarcaz P, Hauser C & Eigenmann PA. Soy anaphylaxis. *Allergy* 56(8):792. 2001.

Taubman B. Parental counseling compared with elimination of cow's milk or Soy milk protein for the treatment of infant colic syndrome: a randomized trial. *Pediatrics* 81(6):756-761. 1988.

Teede HJ, Giannopoulos D, Dalais FS, Hodgson J, McGrath BP. Randomised, controlled, cross-over trial of soy protein with isoflavones on blood pressure and arterial function in hypertensive subjects. *J Am Coll Nutr*; 25(6): 533-540. 2006.

Tham DM, Gardner CD & Haskell WL. Potential health benefits of dietary phytoestrogens: a review of the clinical, epidemiological, and mechanistic evidence. *J Clin Endocrinol Metab* 83(7):2223-2235. 1998.

Theodorescu D, Gulding KM. Genistein inhibits the growth and motility of human bladder cancer cells irrespective of EGF receptor expression. *J Urol* 159:287. 1998.

Theodorescu D, Laderoute KR, Calaoagan JM, et al: Inhibition of human bladder cell motility by genistein is dependent on epidermal growth factor but not p21ras gene expression. Int J Cancer 78(6):775-782. 1998.

Tolia V, Ventimiglia J, Kuhns L. Gastrointestinal tolerance of a pediatric fiber formula in developmentally disabled children. *J Am Coll Nutr* 16(3):224-228. 1997.

Umland EM, Cauffield JS, Kirk JK, et al: Phytoestrogens as therapeutic alternatives to traditional hormone replacement in postmenopausal women. *Pharmacotherapy* 20(8):981-990. 2000.

Upmalis DH, Lobo R, Bradley L, et al: Vasomotor symptom relief by Soy isoflavone extract tablets in postmenopausal women: a multicenter, double-blind, randomized, placebo- controlled study. *Menopause* 7(4):236-242. 2000.

Urban D, Irwin W, Kirk M, et al: The effect of isolated Soy protein on plasma biomarkders in elderly men with elevated serum prostate specific antigen. *J Urol* 2001; 165(1):294-300. 2001.

Vanderhoof JA, Murray ND, Paule CL, et al: Use of Soy fiber in acute diarrhea in infants and toddlers. *Clin Pediatr* (Phila) 36(3):135-139. 1997.

Van Patten C, Olivotto IA, Chambers GK, et al: Effect of Soy phytoestrogens on hot flashes in postmenopausal women with breast cancer: a randomized, controlled clinical trial. *J Clin Oncol* 20(6):1449-1455. 2002.

Viall C, Porcelli K, Teran JC, et al: A double-blind clinical trial comparing the gastrointestinal side effects of two enteral feeding formulas. *J Parenter Enteral Nutr* 14(3):265-269. 1990.

Wagner JD, Zhang L, Greaves KA, et al: Soy protein reduces the arterial low-density lipoprotein (LDL) concentration and delivery of LDL cholesterol to the arteries of diabetic and nondiabetic male cynomolgus monkeys. *Metabolism* 49(9):1188-1196. 2000.

Wangen KE, Duncan AM, Merz-Demlow BE, et al: Effects of Soy isoflavones on markers of bone turnover in premenopausal and postmenopausal women. *J Clin Endocrinol Metab* 85(9):3043-3048. 2000.

Wardle EN. Soyprotein diet therapy in renal disease. *Nephron* 78(3):328-331. 1998.

Wei H: American Academy of Dermatology 1998 Awards for Young Investigators in Dermatology. Photoprotective action of isoflavone genistein: models, mechanisms, and relevance to clinical dermatology. *J Am Acad Dermatol* 39(2 pt 1):271-272. 1998.

White LR, Petrovitch H, Ross GW et al: Brain aging and midlife tofu consumption. *J Am Coll Nutr* 19(2):242-255. 2000.

White LR, Petrovitch H, Ross GW et al: Brain aging and midlife tofu consumption. *J American College* Nutr 19(2):242-255. 2000.

Whitington PF, Gibson R. Soy protein intolerance; four patients with concomitant cow's milk intolerance. *Pediatrics* 59(5):730-732. 1977.

Wilcox G, Wahlqvist ML, Burger HG, et al: Oestrogenic effects of plant foods in postmenopausal women. *BMJ* 301(6757):905-906. 1990.

Wong WW, Smith EB, Stuff JE, et al: Cholesterol-lowering effect of Soy protein in normocholesterolemic and hypercholesterolemic men. *Am J Clin Nutr* 68(6 suppl):1385S-1389S. 1998.

Wu AH, Yang D, Pike MC: A meta-analysis of Soyfoods and risk of stomach cancer: the problem of potential confounders. *Cancer Epidemiol Biomarkers Prev* 9(10):1051-1058. 2000.

Xu X, Duncan AM, Wangen KE, et al: Soy consumption alters endogenous estrogen metabolism in postmenopausal women. *Cancer Epidemiol Biomarkers Prev* 9:781-786. 2000.

Xu X, Wang H-J, Murphy PA et al: Daidzein is a more bioavailable Soymilk isoflavone than is genistein in adult women. *J Nutr* 1994; 124(6):825-832.

Yamamoto S, Sobue T, Kobayashi M, et al: Soy, isoflavones, and breast cancer risk in Japan. *J Natl Cancer Institute* 95(12):906-913. 2003.

Yamori Y, Moriguchi EH, Teramoto T, et al: Soybean isoflavones reduce postmenopausal bone resorption in female Japanese immigrans in Brazil: a ten-week study. *J Am Coll Nutr* 21(6):560-563. 2002.

Zava DT, Dollbaum CM, Blen M. Estrogen and progestin bioactivity of foods, herbs, and spices. *Proc Soc Exp Biol Med* 217(3):369-378. 1998.

Zhou Y, Lee AS: Mechanism for the suppression of the mammalian stress response by genistein, an anticancer phytoestrogen from Soy. *J Natl Cancer Inst* 90(5):381-388. 1998.

Spanish Chestnut

Castanea sativa

DESCRIPTION

Medicinal Parts: The medicinal parts are the leaves collected and dried in autumn, and preparations of the fresh leaves.

Flower and Fruit: The male, monoecious, yellowish-white flowers are in 12 to 20 cm long, erect catkins consisting of numerous, 7-flowered clusters. These are located in the leaf axils of the upper branches. There are 3 to 6 female flowers at the base of unopened male catkins. When the fruit ripens in October, the outer soft thorny husk bursts into 4 lobes, revealing a brown-skinned sweet chestnut that needs ''wine weather'' to ripen.

Leaves, Stem, and Root: The tree grows from 15 to 30 m high. The bark is smooth at first, olive green, later dark brown and vertically reticulate. The leaves are 8 to 25 cm long, coriaceous, oblong-lanceolate with long, pointed, serrated teeth.

Habitat: Northern temperate hemispheres; prefers maritime climate.

Production: Spanish Chestnut leaves consist of the leaves of *Castanea sativa* collected from September to October. The leaves are collected and air-dried.

Other Names: Chestnut, Husked Nut, Jupiter's Nut, Sardian Nut, Sweet Chestnut

ACTIONS AND PHARMACOLOGY

COMPOUNDS

Tannins (6 to 8%): ellagitannins, including pedunculagin, tellimagrandin I and II, casuarictin, potentillin, castalagin, vescalagin

Flavonoids: including rutin, quercitrin, myricetin

EFFECTS

No information is available.

INDICATIONS AND USAGE

Unproven Uses: Spanish Chestnut leaves are used for complaints affecting the respiratory tract such as bronchitis and whooping cough, leg pain, circulation disorders, and diarrhea, and as a gargle for sore throats.

PRECAUTIONS AND ADVERSE REACTIONS

No health hazards or side effects are known in conjunction with the proper administration of designated therapeutic dosages.

DOSAGE

Preparation: An infusion is prepared by pouring boiling water over 5 gm of comminuted drug and then straining it.

Daily Dosage: The average single dose is 5 g of drug or 5 g of liquid extract.

LITERATURE

Beier C, Disch R. Latex-Kontakturtikaria mit gleichzeitig vorliegender Typ-I-Sensibilisierung gegenüber Bananen, Avocado und Maronen / Der interessante Fall. *Allergologie* 17; 268-270. 1994

Hänsel R, Keller K, Rimpler H, Schneider G (Hrsg.), Hagers Handbuch der Pharmazeutischen Praxis, 5. Aufl., Bde 4-6 (Drogen), Springer Verlag Berlin, Heidelberg, New York, 1992-1994.

Leung AY, Encyclopedia of Common Natural Ingredients Used in Food Drugs and Cosmetics, John Wiley & Sons Inc., New York 1980.

Madaus G, Lehrbuch der Biologischen Arzneimittel, Bde 1-3, Nachdruck, Georg Olms Verlag Hildesheim 1979.

Marsili A, Morelli I. Some Constituents of the Leaves of *Castanea sativa. Phytochemistry* 11; 2633-2634. 1972

Wichtl M (Hrsg.), Teedrogen, 4. Aufl., Wiss. Verlagsges. Stuttgart 1997.

Spearmint

Mentha spicata

DESCRIPTION

Medicinal Parts: The medicinal parts are the steamed distillation of the fresh, flowering, aerial parts, and the leaves collected during the flowering season and dried.

Flower and Fruit: The spikelike inflorescence consists of false whorls in the axils of the bracts. The 5-tipped calyx is campanulate, glabrous, or pubescent and is surrounded by a 5-tipped, pale lilac, pink, or white corolla, which is almost half as long again as the calyx. The nutlet is reticulate in pubescent plants and smooth in glabrous plants.

Leaves, Stem, and Root: The plant is 30 to 60 cm during the flowering season. Runners grow from the buds at the base of the stem. The quadrangular stem is ascendent or erect and usually thickly pubescent. The leaves are oblong-ovate or lanceolate, decussate, smooth or wrinkled, regularly serrate, and glabrous to thickly pubescent. The upper leaves are sessile, the lower ones short petiolate.

Habitat: The plant probably originates from the Mediterranean region and is now naturalized in large parts of Europe and North America.

Production: Spearmint is the aerial part of *Mentha spicata*. Spearmint oil is the essential oil extracted from the plant.

Other Names: Curled Mint, Fish Mint, Garden Mint, Green Mint, Lamb Mint, Mackerel Mint, Our Lady's Mint, Sage of Bethlehem, Spire Mint,

ACTIONS AND PHARMACOLOGY

COMPOUNDS: IN THE FOLIAGE

Volatile oil (0.8-2.5%)

Flavonoids: thymonin

Caffeic acid derivatives: including among others rosmaric acid in the volatile oil

Chief components: L-carvone (40-80%, aroma-carrier), (-)-limonene (5-15%), additionally including among others beta-bourbonene, cis- and transcarvylacetate, caryophyllene, 1,8-cineole, dihydrocarveol, trans-sabinene hydrate

EFFECTS

The oil produced contains a high proportion of carvon, which produces the spearmint smell. It has antispasmodic, carminative, and stimulant effects.

In vitro, an antimicrobial effect was observed. The drug is insecticidal and shows a neurodepressive effect in animal experiments (increased duration of sleep).

INDICATIONS AND USAGE

Unproven Uses: Spearmint is used for digestive disorders and as a remedy for flatulence. The essential oil is used as an aromatic preparation. Spearmint leaves are used as carminative.

PRECAUTIONS AND ADVERSE REACTIONS

No health hazards or side effects are known in conjunction with the proper administration of designated therapeutic dosages. The volatile oil possesses a weak potential for sensitization due to its menthol and L-carvone content.

DOSAGE

Mode of Administration: Spearmint is mainly used internally in the form of an oil or concentrate.

LITERATURE

Amelunxen F, Intert F. The Filament Bundle of *Mentha piperita*. *Planta Med.* 59; 86-89. 1993

Avato P, Sgarra G, Casadoro G. Chemical composition of the essential oils of *Mentha* species cultivated in Italy. *Sci Pharm.* 63; 223-230. 1995

Caceres A, Cano O, Samayoa B, Aguilar L. Plants used in Guatemala for the Treatment of Gastrointestinal Disorders. 1.Screening of 84 Plants against Enterobacteria. *J Ethnopharmacol.* 30; 55-73. 1990

Ciobanu V, Pisov M, Peleah E. New advanced hybrids of mentha plants for medicine. *Pharm Pharmacol Lett.* 7 (2/3); 109-110. 1997

Speedwell

Veronica officinalis

DESCRIPTION

Medicinal Parts: The medicinal parts are the dried herb collected during the flowering season, the fresh aerial parts of the flowering plant, and the dried aerial parts collected during the flowering season.

Flower and Fruit: The erect bright blue or lilac flowers are in axillary, peduncled, spikelike racemes. The flowers are small, pedicled and have 4 slightly fused sepals. The corolla has a very short tube, is flatly splayed, and has 4 uneven tips. There are 2 stamens and 1 superior ovary. The fruit is a triangular capsule narrowed at the base. The fruit chambers each have 5 to 10 seeds. The seeds are about 1 mm long, oval and flat; the back of the seed is smooth.

Leaves, Stem, and Root: The plant is a 10 to 20 cm high herbaceous perennial with runners that tend to form grass. The root system consists mainly of shoot-producing roots. The stem is creeping, and the flower-bearing branches are erect. The whole plant is roughly pubescent. The leaves are obovate-ovate, elliptical or oblong, short-petioled and serrate.

Habitat: The plant is indigenous to almost all of Europe, parts of Asia and North America. The sources of the drug are Bulgaria, the former Yugoslavia and Hungary.

Production: Speedwell consists of the above-ground parts of *Veronica officinalis* imported from Bulgaria, the former Yugoslavia, and Hungary. Only the flowering herb is harvested (without roots or lower parts) and subsequently dried fully in the shade before it is cut.

Not to be Confused With: Veronica chamaedrys or *Veronica allionii.*

ACTIONS AND PHARMACOLOGY

COMPOUNDS

Iridoide monoterpenes (0.5-1.0%): including among others aucubin, catalpol, catalpol esters (including among others minecoside, verminoside, veronicoside), mussaenoside, ladroside

Flavonoids (0.7%): including among others luteolin-7-O-glucosides (cinaroside), 6-hydroxyluteolin-7-monoglucoside

Triterpene saponins (10%)

Caffeic acid derivatives: chlorogenic acid (0.5%)

EFFECTS

Speedwell exhibits a protective effect against ulcers and accelerates ulcer healing. Its use as an astringent in the treatment of wounds and as a gargle for inflammations of the mouth and throat is plausible because of the amaroidlike properties of the drug.

INDICATIONS AND USAGE

Unproven Uses: Speedwell preparations are used for diseases and discomfort of the respiratory, gastrointestinal, and lower urinary tracts. It is also used for the liver and kidneys, and to treat gout and rheumatic complaints.

In addition, Speedwell is used internally to improve metabolism (''blood-purifying'') and for nervous agitation. Externally, the herb is used as a gargle for inflammation of the oral and pharyngeal mucosa, promotion of wound healing, chronic skin complaints, itching, and sweating of the feet.

PRECAUTIONS AND ADVERSE REACTIONS

No health hazards or side effects are known in conjunction with the proper administration of designated therapeutic dosages.

DOSAGE

Mode of Administration: The herb is available as a whole, cut and powdered drug for internal and external use in compound preparations.

Preparation: To prepare a tea, pour 1 cup of boiling water over 1.5 g of drug (1 gm is approximately 1 teaspoonful). For the preparation of external lavages and compresses for ulcers, wounds and eczema, add 1 handful of drug to1 liter of water and boil for 10 minutes.

Daily Dosage: The average single dose is 1.5 g of drug. The dose of the tea (used as an expectorant) is 1 cup taken 2 to 3 times daily.

Storage: Speedwell must be protected from light sources.

LITERATURE

Afifi-Yazar F, Sticher O, *Helv Chim Acta* 63:1905. 1980

Afifi-Yazar FÜ et al., *Helv Chim Acta* 64:16. 1981.

Brantner A, Grein E. Antibacterial activity of plant extracts used externally in traditional medicine. *J Ethnopharmacol.* 44; 35-40. 1994

Sticher O et al., (1982) Planta Med 45:159.

Spergularia rubra

See Arenaria Rubra

Spigelia anthelmia

See Wormwood Grass

Spigelia marilandica

See Pink Root

Spikenard

Aralia racemosa

DESCRIPTION

Medicinal Parts: The medicinal parts are the fresh and dried rhizome and roots.

Flower and Fruit: The inflorescence is a large panicle, each branch of which carries a simple, round, 10 to 15 flower umbel. The flowers are small and have greenish-white petals. The drupes are dark red to crimson, roundish, and have 5 ribs. The seeds are compressed and have a similarly formed endosperm.

Leaves, Stem, and Root: Aralia racemosa is a herbaceous, bushy, stiffly branched perennial with a woody base. The stem extends up to 2 m high and is glabrous and grooved. The leaflets are thin and oval. The leaflets can grow up to 20 cm long and 16 cm wide, but are usually much smaller and cordate at the base. The rhizome is up to 15 cm long and has a diameter of roughly 2.5 cm with prominent concave scars. The roots are about 2 cm thick at the base, pale brown, and wrinkled. The root fracture is short and whitish.

Characteristics: Spikenard has an aromatic odor and taste.

Habitat: The plant grows in North America from central Canada southward to Virginia.

Production: The root and rhizome of *Aralia racemosa* are gathered from the wild in summer and autumn and chopped while fresh. The freshly chopped roots and rhizomes are either dried or processed immediately to form a thick paste.

Not to be Confused With: It is possible to confuse Spikenard with the *Aralia nudicaulis* root. However, Spikenard can be distinguished by its lack of spotted hypodermis cells, which are a feature of the *Aralia nudicaulis* root.

Other Names: Indian Root, Life of Man, Old Man's Root, Petty Morell, Spignet

ACTIONS AND PHARMACOLOGY

COMPOUNDS

Polyynes: including falcarinole, falcarindiole

Triterpene saponins

Volatile oil (very little)

EFFECTS

Due to its saponin content, the drug's effectiveness as a reflex expectorant for colds seems plausible. It is also diaphoretic and stimulates tissue renewal. Its efficacy has not been proved.

INDICATIONS AND USAGE

Unproven Uses: Preparations are used internally for colds, chronic coughs, and asthma. It is used as an alternative to sarsaparilla in the treatment of skin diseases and for rheumatic conditions. North American Indians use Spikenard internally to treat backache and externally for bruises, wounds, swellings, and inflammations.

Homeopathic Uses: Spikenard is used for colds, hay fever and asthma. Efficacy for colds appears plausible; efficacy for other uses has not been documented.

PRECAUTIONS AND ADVERSE REACTIONS

General: No health hazards or side effects are known in conjunction with the proper administration of designated therapeutic dosages. Because of the polyyne spectrum, sensitization and dermatoses connected with the plant are also possible through skin contact.

Pregnancy: The drug is not to be used during pregnancy.

DOSAGE

Mode of Administration: The drug is administered internally as a fluid extract.

Preparation: It is prepared as a liquid extract (1:1); information on the ethanol content is unavailable.

Daily Dosage: When the drug is prepared as an infusion, the recommended daily dosage is approximately 15 g per 500 mL, to be drunk one cup at a time during the course of the day. The recommended dosage of the liquid extract is 0.9 g to 1.8 g.

Homeopathic Dosage: 5 to 10 drops, 1 tablet, 5 to 10 globules, 1 to 3 times daily or 1 ml injection solution twice a week sc (HAB1).

LITERATURE

Ahn Y-J, Kim M-J, Yamamoto T, Fujiwawa T, Mitsouka T, Selective growth responses of human intestinal bacteria to Araliaceae extracts. *Microbial Ecol Health Disease* 3:223-229. 1990

Spinach

Spinacia oleracea

DESCRIPTION

Medicinal Parts: The medicinal parts are the leaves.

Leaves, Stem and Root: Spinach is an annual plant that can be planted at various times during the vegetation period to guarantee a year-round supply. The stems may grow up to 1 m or more and are erect. The leaves are ovate to deltoid-hastate, entire, or dentate. When the plant ripens, the bracteoles are almost orbicular-obovate, usually wider than long. They often have a divergent spine at the apex.

Habitat: The plant probably originated in Iran and is cultivated worldwide today.

Production: Spinach consists of the fresh or dried leaf of *Spinacia oleracea*.

ACTIONS AND PHARMACOLOGY

COMPOUNDS

Triterpene saponins: including among others spinach saponins A and B

Oxalic acid (in young leaves 6-8%, in older leaves up to 16%)

Histamine (up to 140 mg/100 g fresh weight)

Flavonoids: including among others patuletin, spinacetin, spinatoside

Chlorophyll (0.3-1.0%)

Vitamins: including among others ascorbic acid (vitamin C, 40-155 mg/100 g)

Nitrates (depending on the fertilizer, 0.3-0.6%)

EFFECTS
No information is available.

INDICATIONS AND USAGE
Unproven Uses: Spinach preparations are used for ailments and complaints of the gastrointestinal tract, to stimulate growth in children, as an appetite stimulant, for fatigue and for supporting convalescence.

PRECAUTIONS AND ADVERSE REACTIONS
General: No health hazards or side effects are known in conjunction with the proper administration of designated therapeutic dosages. The relatively high nitrate content makes it advisable to forgo consuming spinach as a foodstuff too often. Circumstances that lead to reduction (e.g., leaving spinach standing at room temperature) should also be avoided to prevent nitrite formation. In addition, the oxalate content of spinach could reduce calcium resorption.

Pediatric Use: Infants should not receive spinach as a foodstuff until after their fourth month (danger of methemoglobin formation through nitrites).

DOSAGE
No information is available.

LITERATURE

Hegnauer R, Chemotaxonomie der Pflanzen, Bde 1-11: Birkhäuser Verlag Basel, Boston, Berlin 1962-1997.

Kern W, List PH, Hörhammer L (Hrsg.), Hagers Handbuch der Pharmazeutischen Praxis, 4. Aufl., Bde. 1-8: Springer Verlag Berlin, Heidelberg, New York, 1969.

Teuscher E, Lindequist U, Biogene Gifte - Biologie, Chemie, Pharmakologie, 2. Aufl., Fischer Verlag Stuttgart 1994.

Spinacia oleracea

See Spinach

Spiny Rest Harrow

Ononis spinosa

DESCRIPTION
Medicinal Parts: The medicinal parts are the roots and flowering branches.

Flower and Fruit: The pink flowers are solitary or in pairs in the leaf axils. The calyx is campanulate with 5 segments. The standard is large and has dark stripes. The ovoid, erect fruit is a pod as long as or longer than the calyx.

Leaves, Stem, and Root: The plant is a low subshrub of about 30 to 60 cm with a long taproot. The branches are erect, spreading, villous, and densely covered in short shoots, which terminate in straight thorns. The leaves are trifoliate with 3 small, dentate, oblong leaflets. The upper leaves are entire.

Characteristics: The plant has an unpleasant smell.

Habitat: Spiny Rest Harrow is common in almost all of Europe, as well as in North Africa and western Asia.

Production: Spiny Rest Harrow root consists of the dried roots and rhizomes of *Ononis spinosa*. The plant is harvested in autumn.

Other Names: Cammock, Ground Furze, Land Whin, Petty Whin, Rest-Harrow, Stayplough, Stinking Tommy, Wild Liquorice

ACTIONS AND PHARMACOLOGY
COMPOUNDS
Isoflavonoids: glycosides, including among others, trifolirhizin (maackiain-7-0-glucoside), ononin (formononetin-7-0-glucoside), ononin-6-malonylester, homopterocarpin-7-0-glucoside

Free isoflavonoids: including among others, formononetin, genistein, biochanin

Volatile oil (0.02-0.2%): chief components anethole, carvone, menthol

Triterpenes: including among others, alpha-onocerin (alpha-onoceradiendiol)

Lectins

EFFECTS
In combination with sufficient liquid intake, the drug is said to be diuretic. The diuretic effect is disputed because it is not sufficiently documented and can be attributed neither to the essential oil nor to the flavonoids. In animal tests, an anti-edemic effect was proved. The genistein is mildly estrogenic.

INDICATIONS AND USAGE
Approved by Commission E:

- Infections of the urinary tract
- Kidney and bladder stones

Preparations of the drug are used for irrigation therapy for inflammatory diseases of the lower urinary tract and also for prevention and treatment of kidney gravel.

Unproven Uses: Spiny Rest Harrow is popularly used for gout, rheumatic complaints, as a irrigation therapy for inflammatory diseases of the lower urinary tract, and for prevention and treatment of kidney gravel.

CONTRAINDICATIONS
The drug should not be used in the presence of edema resulting from reduced cardiac or renal activity.

PRECAUTIONS AND ADVERSE REACTIONS
No health hazards or side effects are known in conjunction with the proper administration of designated therapeutic dosages.

DOSAGE

Mode of Administration: The drug is ground for teas and other galenic preparations for internal use. Ample liquid intake (at least 2 liters per day) should accompany use of the drug.

Preparation: To prepare an infusion (tea), pour boiling water over 2 to 2.5 g finely cut or coarsely powdered drug and strain after 20 to 30 minutes (1 teaspoonful equals approximately 3 g).

Daily Dosage: 6 to 12 g of drug.

LITERATURE

Dannhardt G, Schneider G, Schwell B. Identification and 5-lipoxygenase inhibiting potency of medicarpin isolated from roots of *Ononis spinosa L. Pharm Pharmacol Lett.* 2; 161-162. 1992

Haznagy A, Thot G, Tamas J, Constituents of the aqueous extracts from *Ononis spinosa L.* In: *Arch Pharm* 311(4):318-323. 1978.

Kartnig T, Gruber A, Preuss M. Flavonoid-O-Glykoside in *Ononis spinosa L.* (Fabaceae). *Pharm Acta Helv.* 60; 253-255. 1985

Kirmizigül S et al., Spinonin, a novel glycoside from *Ononis spinosa subsp. leiosperma.* In: *JNP* 60(4):378-381. 1997.

Spruce

Picea species

DESCRIPTION

Medicinal Parts: The medicinal parts are the oil extracted from the needles, branch tips or branches, and the fresh Spruce shoots.

Flower and Fruit: The male flowers are strawberry colored, the female are crimson or green. The male flowers are in short-stemmed, cylindrical catkins scattered over the crown. The female flowers are in elliptical-cylindrical cones at the top of the crown. The ripe cones are sessile, hanging, globular-clavate, and covered in rhomboid scales, which are thin, undulating at the tip, and dentate. The wings of the small seeds are 3 times as long as the seeds themselves.

Leaves, Stem, and Root: Picea excelsa is a tree that grows from 30 to 60 m high and has a columnlike trunk with brown-red bark and a girth of about 2 m. The trunk is usually branched. The branches are horizontal and flat. The young shoots are reddish-brown or orange-red. The crossed-opposite leaves are scaly and imbricate. The needles remain on the tree for a number of years. On the upper surface of the shoots they are pointed forward, on the lower surface they are pointed toward the sides. They are 1.3 to 2.5 cm long, rigid or curved, rich green, and have a blunt hornlike tip.

Habitat: The tree is found in northern and central Europe.

Production: The essential oil is obtained from the fresh needles and twig tops or branches of *Picea abies* (syn: *Picea excelsa*), *Abies alba, Abies sachalinensis* or *Abies sibirica.* The essential oil is recovered from the needles by a 5 to 6 hour continuous process of aqueous steam distillation on a sieve base of layered and crushed fresh twigs. Preparations from the fresh 10 to 15 cm long shoots of *Picea abies* and/or *Abies alba* (syn.: *Abies pectinata*) are collected in the spring.

Other Names: Balm of Gilead Fir, Balsam Fir, Canada Balsam, Fir Tree, Hemlock Spruce, Norway Pine, Norway Spruce, Spruce Fir

ACTIONS AND PHARMACOLOGY

COMPOUNDS: SPRUCE NEEDLE OIL

From Picea abies:

Bornyl acetate (5-25%)

Limonene (10-30%)

Camphene (10-25%)

Alpha-pinene (10-25%): additionally, including among others santene, beta-pinene, Delta3-carene, myrcene

From Picea mariana:

Bornyl acetate (37-49%)

Camphene (10-17%)

Alpha-pinene (10%): additionally, including among others beta-pinene, limonene, Delta3-carene, myrcene, santene

From Abies alba:

Bornyl acetate (2-10%)

Limonene (25-55%)

Camphene (9-20%)

Alpha-pinene (6-35%): additionally, including among others beta-pinene, beta-phellandrene, Delta-carene, myrcene, santene

EFFECTS: SPRUCE NEEDLE OIL

The plants are secretolytic, antibacterial and hyperemic.

COMPOUNDS: SPRUCE SHOOTS (FRESH)

Volatile oil (0.2-0.5%): chief components limonene, alpha-pinene, borneol, bornyl acetate

Ascorbic acid (vitamin C)

EFFECTS: SPRUCE SHOOTS (FRESH)

The essential oil has a secretory, mild antiseptic and hyperemic effect.

INDICATIONS AND USAGE

SPRUCE NEEDLE OIL

Approved by Commission E:

- Common cold
- Cough/bronchitis
- Fevers and colds
- Inflammation of the mouth and pharynx
- Neuralgias
- Rheumatism
- Tendency to infection

The essential oil is used internally for catarrhal conditions of the respiratory tract. Externally, it is used for catarrhal conditions of the respiratory tract, rheumatic and neuralgic pain.

Unproven Uses: For tension states.

SPRUCE SHOOTS (FRESH)
Approved by Commission E:

- Common cold
- Cough/bronchitis
- Fevers and colds
- Inflammation of the mouth and pharynx
- Muscular and nerve pains
- Tendency to infection

The drug is used internally as a respiratory tract catarrh and externally for muscle pains and neuralgia.

Unproven Uses: In folk medicine, it is used internally for tuberculosis and externally as a bath additive for patients with neurological illnesses.

CONTRAINDICATIONS

Contraindications include bronchial asthma and whooping cough. Patients with extensive skin injuries, acute skin diseases, feverish or infectious diseases, cardiac insufficiency, or hypertonia should not use the drug as a bath additive.

PRECAUTIONS AND ADVERSE REACTIONS

No health hazards or side effects are known in conjunction with the proper administration of designated therapeutic dosages, although bronchial spasms could be worsened.

DOSAGE

SPRUCE NEEDLE OIL
Mode of Administration: Embrocations of alcohol solutions, ointments, gels, emulsions and oils are available, as well as bath additives and inhalants.

Daily Dosage:

Infusion — Place 4 drops of oil on a lump of sugar or in a little water and take 3 times a day.

External application — A 20 to 30% ointment is rubbed onto the affected area several times a day.

Inhalation — Add 2 g of oil to hot water and inhale several times a day.

Bath additive — Add 5 g oil to a full bath at a temperature of 35 to 38° C.

Storage: Store in a cool place, in a tightly sealed container, protected from light.

SPRUCE SHOOTS (FRESH)
Mode of Administration: In galenic preparations for internal and external application.

Preparation: For inhalation therapy, place 2 g of oil in hot water and inhale the vapors. To make a bath additive, boil 200 to 300 g drug in 1 liter water and strain after 5 minutes; add to a full bath. Make sure it is possible to relax after the bath.

Daily Dosage: For internal use: 5 to 6 g of drug is administered per day.

Four drops of the essential oil may be placed in a little water or on a lump of sugar and taken 3 times a day.

The inhalation therapy mentioned in the *Preparation* section can be used several times a day.

LITERATURE

SPRUCE NEEDLE OIL AND SHOOTS (FRESH)
Glasl H, Wagner H, *DAZ* 120:64-67. 1980.

Hänsel R, Keller K, Rimpler H, Schneider G (Eds.), Hagers Handbuch der Pharmazeutischen Praxis, 5. Aufl., Bde 4-6 (Drogen), Springer Verlag Berlin, Heidelberg, New York, 1992-1994.

Kubeczka KH, Schultze W, *Flavour Fragrance J*:2.137-148. 1987.

Madaus G, Lehrbuch der Biologischen Arzneimittel, Bde 1-3, Nachdruck, Georg Olms Verlag Hildesheim 1979.

Steinegger E, Hänsel R, Pharmakognosie, 5. Aufl., Springer Verlag Heidelberg 1992.

Teuscher E, Biogene Arzneimittel, 5. Aufl., Wiss. Verlagsges. Stuttgart 1997.

Wagner H, Wiesenauer M, Phytotherapie. Phytopharmaka und pflanzliche Homöopathika, Fischer-Verlag, Stuttgart, Jena, New York 1995.

Spurge

Euphorbia resinifera

DESCRIPTION

Medicinal Parts: The medicinal part of the plant is the milky resin that is exuded when the plant is cut.

Flower and Fruit: The inflorescence is arranged in a dichasium above the thorn-bearing scales. They are typical cyathia of the Euphorbia species, which have one female and a number of male flowers surrounded by 5 greenish-yellowish, tubularly fused bracts. The female flower has a 3-carpeled ovary with 3 styles; the male flower consists of only 1 stamen. The fruit separates into 3 mericarps.

Leaves, Stem, and Root: This diclinous, monoecious leafless shrub has the appearance of cactus and grows to a height of up to 2.5 m. The trunk is thick at the base, and only slightly branched higher up. The fleshy branches are 2 cm in diameter and have 3 or 4 edges. There are scales at intervals of 1 cm at the edges, each with 2 short thorns, which are splayed and approximately 5 mm long.

Characteristics: The plant produces a milky latex when the surface is scored.

Habitat: The shrub grows in the folds of the Great Atlas Mountains in Morocco and also in North America and the Canary Islands.

Production: Spurge is the air-dried latex of *Euphorbia resinifera*. The plant is cut in late summer to produce the latex.

Other Names: Gum Euphorbium

ACTIONS AND PHARMACOLOGY

COMPOUNDS

Diterpenes: diterpene esters of the ingenan-, tiglic- and daphnan-types (0.1 to 2%): resinifera factors RL 1 to RL 23, among them resiniferatoxin, 12-desoxyphorbol-13-isobutyrate-20-acetate, 12-Desoxyphorbol-13-phenylacetate-20-acetate

Triterpenes: particularly alpha- and beta-euphorbol, beta-amyrin, resiniferol

Fruit acids: including malic acid, succinic acid, citric acid

Resins (40%)

Polyterpenes

EFFECTS

The diterpene esters contained in the drug have laxative and nonspecific immunostimulating effects. Severe skin and mucous membrane irritation arises in conjunction with topical administration.

INDICATIONS AND USAGE

Use of the medication has been discontinued because of the related dangers. Because of its harsh effects, the plant's resin is no longer administered internally despite its properties as a strong emetic and laxative.

Unproven Uses: External uses in folk medicine have included application to remove proliferating flesh, warts, and malignant ulcers, as well as for chronic inflammatory conditions. It was also used as a plaster for gout. Internal uses included the treatment of dropsy, chronic headaches, and ear or eye complaints.

Homeopathic Uses: The drug is used homeopathically for acute inflammation of the respiratory tract and skin.

Indian Medicine: Uses include constipation and menstrual complaints and also as an abortifacient. Because of the danger of rapid intoxication, the drug's use is not advised. Efficacy for these indications has not been proved.

PRECAUTIONS AND ADVERSE REACTIONS

The drug is severely irritating to mucous membranes and skin. Ingestion leads to salivation, burning pains in the stomach, colic, diarrhea, and nephritis. One case of death has been reported. Chronic application of the drug promotes tumor formation, so its administration in human medicine is no longer advised.

DOSAGE

Mode of Administration: Administration of preparations of Spurge are no longer recommended.

How Supplied: Skin stimulating ointment: 5% drug content

Homeopathic Dosage: 5 drops, 1 tablet, 10 globules every 30 to 60 minutes (acute from D4) and 1 to 3 times daily (chronic); parenterally: 1 to 2 mL sc; IV; IM acute: 3 times daily; chronic once a day (HAB1); children are given special doses.

Storage: Due to the plant's poisonous nature, store securely.

LITERATURE

Blaschek W, Hänsel R, Keller K, Reichling J, Rimpler G, Schneider G (Eds), Hagers Handbuch der Pharmazeutischen Praxis. Folgebände 1 und 2. Drogen A-Z. Springer. Berlin, Heidelberg 1998.

Galeffi C. The Contribution of American Plants to pharmaceutical Sciences / Review Article. *Il Farmaco* 48; 1175-1195. 1993

Hergenhahn M, Kusumoto S, Hecker E, New constituents of *Euphorbia resinifera* Berg. *Acta Chem Scand,* 108:3609, 1984.

Hergenhahn M, Kusumoto S, Hecker E, On the active principles of the spurge family (Euphorbiaceae). V. Extremely skin-irritant and moderately tumor-promoting diterpene esters from *Euphorbia resinifera* Berg. *J Cancer Res Clin Oncol,* 108:98-109, 1984.

Squill

Urginea maritima

DESCRIPTION

Medicinal Parts: The medicinal parts come from the bulbs of the white latex variety collected after flowering and the fresh, fleshy bulb scales of the white variety and of the red variety.

Flower and Fruit: The flowering stem is erect and 50 to 150 cm high. It is often a washed purple color and glabrous. The flowers, which often number 100, are arranged in richly flowered, dense racemes up to 60 cm long. The bracts are membranous and pointed. They are shorter than the pedicles and drop early. The pedicles are up to 3 cm long, thin, and smooth. The flowers are white, radial, and star-shaped. The ovary is ovate to oblong triangular. The capsule is ovate to oblong, 3-valved, obtuse, or almost pointed. Each chamber has 1 to 4 seeds, which are elongate, flattened, smooth, glossy, and winged.

Leaves, Stem, and Root: The plant is a perennial bulb plant. The bulbs are pear-shaped, about 15 to 30 cm in diameter. They are rarely sold whole commercially, as they tend to start growing. The fracture is short, tough and flexible.

Characteristics: The taste is bitter and acrid.

Habitat: Indigenous to the Mediterranean and is cultivated there too.

Production: Squill consists of the sliced, dried, fleshy middle scales of the onion of the white variety of *Urginea maritima,* harvested during the flowering season. It is collected mostly from uncultivated regions.

Other Names: Indian Squill, Maritime Squill, Sea Onion, Red Squill, Scilla, White Squill

ACTIONS AND PHARMACOLOGY

COMPOUNDS

Cardioactive steroid glycosides (bufadienolides, 1-3%): chief components glucoscillarene A, proscillaridin A, scillarene A; including among others, scillicyanoside, scilliglaucoside

Mucilage

EFFECTS

The drug is inotropic on myocardial work capacity and negatively chronotropic. The overall effect is economy of heart action. There is a lowering of increased, left ventricular diastolic pressure and pathologically elevated venous pressure.

INDICATIONS AND USAGE

Approved by Commission E:

- Cardiac insufficiency NYHA I and II
- Arrhythmia
- Nervous heart complaints

Unproven Uses: Squill is used for reduced kidney capacity. In folk medicine it is used for catarrhal conditions of the upper respiratory tract, bronchitis, asthma, and whooping cough, also for wounds and fractures, back pain, and hemorrhoids, and for the disinfection of septic wounds.

CONTRAINDICATIONS

The drug and pure glycosides, among others, should not be administered in the presence of second or third degree atrioventricular block, hypercalcemia, hypokalemia, hypertrophic cardiomyopathy, carotid sinus syndrome, ventricular tachycardia, thoracic aortic aneurysm, or WPW-syndrome.

PRECAUTIONS AND ADVERSE REACTIONS

General: No health hazards are known in conjunction with the proper administration of designated therapeutic dosages. Because of the narrow therapeutic range of cardioactive steroid glycosides, side effects could appear even with therapeutic dosages. Side effects include tonus elevation of the gastrointestinal area, loss of appetite, vomiting, diarrhea, headache, and irregular pulse.

Contact with the juice of the fresh bulb can lead to skin inflammation (squill dermatitis). The administration of pure glycoside is preferable due to the difficulties of standardizing the drug (proscillaridin A).

DRUG INTERACTIONS

MAJOR RISK

Digoxin: Concurrent use may result in increased risk of digoxin toxicity (nausea, vomiting, abnormal vision, cardiac arrhythmias, unexplained hyperkalemia). *Clinical Management:* A digoxin level may confim the diagnosis, but may not quantify the severity. Treatment with digoxin-specific Fab (dsFab) antibody fragments has been successful in toxic ingestion of other cardiac glycoside-containing plants.

POTENTIAL INTERACTIONS

Quinidine, Calcium, Saluretics, Laxatives, and Extended Therapy with Glucocorticoids: Concurrent use may result in increased effectiveness and side effects of these substances.

Arrhythmogenic Substances (sympathomimetics, methylxanthines, phosphodiesterase inhibitors, and quinidine): Concurrent use may result in an increased risk of cardiac arrhythmias.

OVERDOSAGE

Besides the above-mentioned symptoms, overdosage can lead to cardiac rhythm disorders, life-threatening ventricular tachycardia, atrial tachycardia with atrioventricular block, stupor, vision disorders, depression, confused states, hallucinations, and psychosis. Fatal dosages lead to cardiac arrest or asphyxiation.

Treatment of poisoning includes gastric lavage and instillation of activated charcoal. All other measures are to be carried out according to the symptoms. In case of potassium loss, replenish carefully; for ectopic impulse formation in the ventricle, administer phenytoin as an antiarrhythmic drug; use lidocaine for ventricular extrasystole; for pronounced bradycardia, use atropine or orciprenaline. The prophylactic use of a pacemaker is recommended. Hemoperfusion for eliminating the glycosides or the administration of cholestyramine for interrupting the enterohepatic circulation are possible.

DOSAGE

Mode of Administration: Comminuted drug and other galenic preparations for internal use.

Preparation: Stabilized powder is standardized according to content, there are no more exact specifications in the literature, standardization according to DAB10.

Squill Extract — Evaporated extract 1:4; drug: diluted spirit of wine (EB6)

Acetum Scillae — drug: spirit of wine 1:1 (EB6)

Oxymel Scillae — 5 parts Acetum Scillae: 10 parts purified honey evaporated in a water bath to 10 parts

Daily Dosage: Single dose: 60 to 200 mg; Daily dose: 180 to 200 mg; Average daily dosage: 0.1 to 0.5 g of standardized sea onion powder.

Squill Extract: 1.0 g; Liquid extract: 0.03 to 2.0 mL; Tincture: 0.3 to 2.0 mL; Acetum Scillae: 1.0 g; Acetic acid maceration: 0.6 to 2.0 mL

Oxymel Scillae: 2.5 g

Storage: Squill should be protected from light and moisture at temperatures below 25°C.

LITERATURE

Garcia-Casado P et al., Proscillaridin A Yield from Squill Bulbs. *Pharm Acta Helv.* 52; 218-221. 1977

Hakim FS, Evans FJ, The potency and phytochemistry of Indian squill soft extract. *Pharm Acta Helv.* 51; 117-118 1976

Joubert JP, Schultz RA. Detection of scilliroside in the preparation of maritime Scille. (*Urginea maritima* Baker) *Ann Pharm Fr,* 42:17-21, Jan 1967

Kamano Y, Satoh N, Nakayoshi H, Pettit GR, Smith CR, Rhinovirus inhibition by bufadienolides. In: *Chem Pharm Bull* 36:326-332. 1988.

Kopp B et al Bufadienolides from *Urginea maritima* from Egypt. *Phytochemistry* 42 (2); 513-522. 1996

Krenn L, Ferth R, Robien W, Kopp B, Bufadienolide aus Urginea-maritima-sensu-strictu. In: *PM* 57:560. 1991.

Krenn L, Kopp B, 9-Hydroxyscilliphaeosid, a new bufadienolide from Urginea maritima. In: *JNP* 59(6):612-613. 1996.

Majinda RRT et al., Bufadienolides and other constituents of *Urginea sanguinea.* In: *PM* 63(2):188-190. 1997.

Sato, Muro T, Antiviral activity of scillarenin, a plant bufadienolide. In: *Jap J Microbiol* 18:441-448. 1974.

Spies T, Praznik W, Hofinger A, Altmann F, Nitsch E, Wutka R. The structure of the fructan sinistrin from *Urginea maritima. Carbohydr Res,* 235:221-30, Nov 4, 1992

Spies T, Praznik W, Hofinger A, Altmann F, Nitsch E, Wutka R A new bufadienolide from Urginea pancration. *Planta Med,* 235:284-5, Jun, 1992.

Tuncok Y, Kozan O, Cavdar C, Guven H, Fowler J. *Urginea maritima* (squill) toxicity. *J Toxicol Clin Toxicol,* 33:83-6, 1995

Wälli F, Grob PJ, Müller-Schoop J Antineoplastic constituents of some Southern African plants. *J Ethnopharmacol,* 111:323-35, Dec, 1980.

Wälli F, Grob PJ, Müller-Schoop J Pseudo-(venocuran-)lupus - a minor episode in the history of medicine. *Schweiz Med Wochenschr,* 111:1398-405, Sep 19, 1981.

Wälli F, Grob PJ, Müller-Schoop J Traditional medicine in health care. *J Ethnopharmacol,* 111:19-22, Mar, 1980.

Wawrosch C, Kolar M, Kopp B, Kubelka W. Micropropagation of Urginea aphylla (Forskal) Speta and Protoplast Isolation. *Sci Pharm.* 60; 169. 1992

Stachys palustris

See Woundwort

Star Anise

Illicium verum

DESCRIPTION

Medicinal Parts: The medicinal parts are the oil extracted from the ripe fruit, the whole dried fruit and the seeds.

Flower and Fruit: The flowers are yellowish or reddish-white. The follicles have a diameter of about 2 cm. They are star-like and formed from eight cybiform carpels. The follicles open when ripe, each containing one smooth, polished, brown seed. The pericarp of the seed is brown and wrinkled below.

Leaves, Stem and Root: The plant is an evergreen tree up to 10 m tall with white, birch-like bark. The leaves are 7.5 cm long, entire-margined, glossy, elliptic-lanceolate and acuminate.

Habitat: The plant is only known in its cultivated form. It is cultivated in China and Vietnam.

Production: Star anise consists of the ripe syncarp of Illicium verum, as well as its preparations in effective dosage. The fruit is harvested shortly before it is fully ripe (August to October).

Not to be Confused With: Should not be confused with the smaller Japanese star anise (I. lanceolatum or I. religiosum), which is poisonous.

Other Names: Aniseed Stars, Badiana

ACTIONS AND PHARMACOLOGY

COMPOUNDS

Volatile oil: chief constituent trans-anethol, chavicol methyl ether (estragole), d-limonene, l-limonene, d-fenchone, d-pinene, dl-limonene, anisaldehyde

Fatty oil

Flavonoids: including rutin, kaempferol-3-O-rutinoside

Tannins

EFFECTS

Star Anise is a bronchial expectorant and antispasmodic for the gastrointestinal tract. The essential oils (star anise oil) and flavonoids act on the smooth muscle of the gastrointestinal tract and the mucous membrane of the respiratory tract.

INDICATIONS AND USAGE

Approved by Commission E:

- Loss of appetite
- Cough/bronchitis

Unproven Uses: Star Anise is used for catarrh of the respiratory tract and peptic discomfort.

Indian Medicine: Star Anise is used for dyspeptic complaints, flatulence, spasmodic colon pain, dysentery, facial paralysis, hemiparesis and rheumatoid arthritis.

PRECAUTIONS AND ADVERSE REACTIONS

No health hazards or side effects are known in conjunction with the proper administration of designated therapeutic dosages. Sensitization has occurred very rarely in cases of repeated administration. Berries of Illicium anisatum are similar, but contain spasmogenic sesquiterpene lactones; confusions with Star Anise have been observed.

DOSAGE

Mode of Administration: Herb, ground fresh just prior to use, and other galenic preparations for internal use.

Daily Dosage: 3 gm of drug or 0.3 gm of essential oil. Single dose: 0.5 to 1 gm prepared as tea.

Storage: Keep Star Anise protected from light.

LITERATURE

Czygan FC. Anis (Anisi fructus DAB 10) - Pimpinella anisum L. Z Phytother. 13; 101-106 (1992)

Frohne D, Pfänder HJ, Giftpflanzen - Ein Handbuch für Apotheker, Toxikologen und Biologen, 4. Aufl., Wiss. Verlags-Ges Stuttgart 1997.

Hänsel R, Keller K, Rimpler H, Schneider G (Hrsg.), Hagers Handbuch der Pharmazeutischen Praxis, 5. Aufl., Bde 4-6 (Drogen), Springer Verlag Berlin, Heidelberg, New York, 1992-1994.

Leung AY, Encyclopedia of Common Natural Ingredients Used in Food Drugs and Cosmetics, John Wiley & Sons Inc., New York 1980.

Okuyama E, Nakamura T, Yamazaki M. Convulsants from Star Anise (Illicium verum HOOK.F.). *Chem Pharm Bull.* 41; 1670-1671. 1993

Schulz R, Hänsel R, Rationale Phytotherapie, Springer Verlag Heidelberg 1996.

Steinegger E, Hänsel R, Pharmakognosie, 5. Aufl., Springer Verlag Heidelberg 1992.

Teuscher E, Lindequist U, Biogene Gifte - Biologie, Chemie, Pharmakologie, 2. Aufl., Fischer Verlag Stuttgart 1994.

Teuscher E, Biogene Arzneimittel, 5. Aufl., Wiss. Verlagsges. Stuttgart 1997.

Wichtl M (Hrsg.), Teedrogen, 4. Aufl., Wiss. Verlagsges. Stuttgart 1997.

Zänglein A, Schultze W, Illicium verum - Sternanis. In: ZPT 10(6):191. 1989.

Stavesacre

Delphinium staphisagria

DESCRIPTION

Medicinal Parts: The medicinal parts are the ripe, dried seeds.

Flower and Fruit: The flowers are deep blue. The sections of the involucres are 13 to 20 mm long. The limb of the lateral honey-leaves gradually narrows to a claw. The follicles are 8 to 11 mm wide and swollen. The seeds are grayish-black, wrinkled, and pitted. They are triangular or square and convex at the back. The seeds are about 2 cm long.

Leaves, Stem, and Root: The plant is annual and has a 30 to 100 cm high stem that is stout and sparsely pubescent. The leaves are are palmatiform digitate with 5 to 7 lobes, pubescent on both surfaces with a mixture of very short and longer hairs. The segments are entire-margined or are made up of ovate-lanceolate or oblong, sharp-edged lobes.

Characteristics: The seeds are poisonous. They taste bitter and tingling, and are odorless.

Habitat: The plant is found in Asia Minor and Europe, and is cultivated in Italy and France.

Production: Stavesacre seeds are the seeds of *Delphinium staphisagria.*

Other Names: Lousewort

ACTIONS AND PHARMACOLOGY

COMPOUNDS

Diterpene alkaloids: main alkaloid delphinine, including among others the bi-diterpene alkaloids staphisine, staphisagroine

EFFECTS

Stavesacre is arrythmogenic and has an effect similar to aconitine.

INDICATIONS AND USAGE

Unproven Uses: The herb is used for neuralgia.

Homeopathic Uses: Stavesacre is used for the treatment of anxiety, urinary tract diseases, acute or acutely recurring hordeolum or chalazion, seborrheal skin with a tendency to inflammation, odorous perspiration, nervous exhaustion, neurasthenia with poor memory and hypochondria, sexual neurasthenia, gonorrhea, melancholia, hysteria, leukorrhea, headaches, general debility and delicate health, weak bladder, scrofulous and swollen glands, hair loss, rheumatism, nervous diarrhea, habitual obstipation, gastric ulcer, gastritis, trigeminal neuralgia, and conditions of the eyelids.

PRECAUTIONS AND ADVERSE REACTIONS

External administration of extracts of the drug leads to reddening, inflammation and eczema. Internal administration could lead to inflammation of the throat, salivation, nausea, ructus, skin itching, and urinary, and stool urgency.

OVERDOSAGE

The intake of 2 teaspoonfuls of seeds leads to weakened pulse, stomach pain, labored breathing, and collapse.

Treatment of poisoning consists of stomach and intestinal emptying (gastric lavage, sodium sulphate), and the administration of activated charcoal. Further treatment should proceed symptomatically (i.e., diazepam for spasms, sodium bicarbonate for acidoses, intubation, and oxygen respiration may also be required).

DOSAGE

Mode of Administration: An extract from the seeds is used in homeopathic dilutions.

Storage: The drug should be stored cautiously, as it is poisonous.

LITERATURE

Kern W, List PH, Hörhammer L (Hrsg.), Hagers Handbuch der Pharmazeutischen Praxis, 4. Aufl., Bde. 1-8, Springer Verlag Berlin, Heidelberg, New York, 1969.

Lewin L, Gifte und Vergiftungen, 6. Aufl., Nachdruck, Haug Verlag, Heidelberg 1992.

Madaus G, Lehrbuch der Biologischen Arzneimittel, Bde 1-3, Nachdruck, Georg Olms Verlag Hildesheim 1979.

Micovic IV, *J Serb Chem Soc* 51:355. 1986.

Roth L, Daunderer M, Kormann K, Giftpflanzen, Pflanzengifte, 4. Aufl., Ecomed Fachverlag Landsberg Lech 1993.

Teuscher E, Lindequist U, Biogene Gifte - Biologie, Chemie, Pharmakologie, 2. Aufl., Fischer Verlag Stuttgart 1994.

Wagner H, Wiesenauer M, Phytotherapie. Phytopharmaka und pflanzliche Homöopathika, Fischer-Verlag, Stuttgart, Jena, New York 1995.

Stellaria media

See Chickweed

Stevia

Stevia rebaudiana

DESCRIPTION

Medicinal Parts: The medicinal part of the plant is the dried leaves.

Flower and Fruit: The composite flowers are surrounded by an involucre. The capitula are in loose, irregular, sympodial cymes. There are 5 overlapping epicalyx sepals, with 5 tubular florets per composite flower. The flowers have light purple rhacis, white tips, and 5 stamens. The fruit is a 5-ribbed, spindle-shaped achene with 15 to 17 awns.

Leaves, Stem, and Root: Stevia rebaudiana is a semishrub that grows up to 30 cm high. The leaves are sessile, 3 to 4 cm long with an elongate-lanceolate or spatulate, blunt-tipped lamina. The leaves are serrate from the middle to the tip and entire below. The upper surface of the leaf is slightly glandular pubescent. The stem is weakly downy-pubescent at the bottom and woody. The tough rhizome has slightly branching roots.

Characteristics: All plant parts taste intensively sweet.

Habitat: The plant is indigenous to Paraguay.

Production: Stevia leaves are the dried leaves of *Stevia rebaudiana.*

Other Names: Sweet Herb, Sweetleaf

ACTIONS AND PHARMACOLOGY

COMPOUNDS

Diterpenes: diterpene glycosides, particularly stevioside (5 to 10%), rebaudoside A (2 to 4%), including as well rebaudoside C and dulcoside A

Volatile oil (0.1%): chief components nerolidol and caryophyllene oxide

Flavonoids: including apigenin-4'-O-glucoside, luteolin-7-O-glucoside

EFFECTS

Stevia rebaudiana Bert. is a strong sweetening agent. The glycosides stevioside and steviol affect several mitochondrial functions. The questionable hypoglycemic effect may be due to inhibition of glucogenesis leading to hypoglycemia (Curi et al, 1986). Stevia's effect on blood glucose is inconclusive in human studies. Stevia may have antihypertensive effects. Animal studies suggest effectiveness in fertility reduction and diuresis, but few human studies are available. Stevia has also been tested as a spasmolytic, antibiotic, and as an adjunct in vein surgery.

Antidiabetic and Sweetening Effects: The use of the drug as a noncaloric sweetener is based upon the glycosidal diterpenes present: stevioside and rebaudioside A. Rebaudioside A is even sweeter than stevioside (Tanaka, 1997; Ishikawa et al, 1991; Yamamato et al, 1985; Planas & Kuc, 1968). Stevioside is composed of three glucose molecules and a diterpenic carboxylic alcohol (aglycone). Slight modification to these glycosides may produce a bitter taste (Tanaka, 1997; Kinghorn et al, 1997).

Stevioside is 300 times as sweet as a 0.4% sucrose solution, 150 times as sweet as a 4% sucrose solution, and 100 times as sweet as a 10% sucrose solution (Lung & Foster, 1996). Compared to other sweet plant extracts *Stevia rabaudiana* is sweeter than *Thaladiantha grosvenorii* and *Abrus precatorius* (Jakinovich & Moon, 1990).

Hypotensive Effects: Pure stevioside has caused bradycardia and hypotension in humans and rats (Melis, 1996). Stevioside's action on mean arterial pressure and renal function is similar to that of a calcium antagonist such as verapamil (Melis, 1996; Melis & Sainati, 1991). In animal experiments, stevioside significantly elevated the glucose clearance while at the same time increasing both salt excretion and urine flow (measured in percentage of glomerular filtration rate), which led to a significant lowering of blood pressure.

Fertility Reducing Effects: Stevia leaves (a 5% decoction) reduced fertility in female rats by as much as 65%, but purified stevoside had no effect on pregnancy or rat fetus development (Suttajit et al, 1993). In a controversial study, fertility in rats was decreased by 57% to 79% after administration of a Stevia decoction when compared to rats given water. This decrease occurred across 3 differently treated experimental groups. The reduction in fertility was still evident 50 to 60 days after discontinuation of Stevia (Planas & Kuc, 1968). In a separate study, an infusion of Stevia was tested in a cell cycle test model (Allium cepa meristems) to determine if the mechanism of action involved c-mitotic effects. No adverse effect on the cell cycle was observed with the administration of Stevia suggesting that the contraceptive effects may not be due to changes in the chromosome cycle (Schvartzman et al, 1977).

CLINICAL TRIALS

Diabetes

Investigators studied the acute effects of stevioside in 12 patients with type 2 diabetes, hypothesizing that supplementation with stevioside could cause a reduction in postprandial blood glucose. In the acute, paired, crossover study, patients consumed a test meal supplemented with either 1 g of stevioside of 1 g of maize starch (control). Blood samples were drawn at 30 minutes before and for 240 minutes after ingestion of the meal. Compared to control, stevioside reduced the incremental area under the glucose response curve by 18% (P=.013). The insulinogenic index (AUC[i,insulin]/AUC[I, glucose] was increased by approximately 40% by stevioside, compared to control (P<.001).

Stevioside tended to decrease glucagon levels, while it did not significantly alter the area under the insulin, glucagon-like peptide 1, and glucose-dependent insulinotropic polypeptide curves. The researchers concluded that the herb reduces postprandial blood glucose levels in patients with type 2 diabetes, indicating beneficial effects on glucose metabolism (Gregersen et al, 2004).

Stevia extract induced significant changes in glucose, insulin, and electrolytes in a double-blind study of 60 healthy volunteers. Patients were tested in both an anabolic phase (after meals) and catabolic (fasting overnight) phase. The changes observed were still within physiological limits. One group received a minimum of 50 mg of Stevia extract 4 times daily (27.7 mg of stevioside), another group received 200 mg of Stevia extract 4 times daily (110.8 mg of stevioside), and the final group served as control. Compared to the placebo group, a dose corresponding to 110.8 mg of stevioside induced only a slight reduction in plasma glucose and insulin during the catabolic phase and plasma free fatty acids were increased in the anabolic phase. Plasma potassium and sodium levels were slightly increased. Significant reductions in blood glucose were found in both the anabolic and catabolic phases with the 200-mg mg dose (68.3 mg/100 mL) and 67.8 mg/mL, respectively) but not the 50-mg dose (75.1 mg/mL and 73.1 mg/mL, respectively) (Boeckh-Haebisch, 1992).

Hypertension

The antihypertensive effect of crude stevioside obtained from leaves of Stevia rebaudiana on patients with untreated mild hypertension was investigated. Patients were submitted to a placebo phase for 4 weeks. Participants selected in this phase were randomly assigned to receive either capsules containing placebo during 24 weeks or crude stevioside 3.75 mg/kg/day (7 weeks), 7.5 mg/kg/day (11 weeks), and 15.0 mg/kg/day (6 weeks). Systolic and diastolic BP decreased (P<0.05) during the treatment with crude stevioside, but a similar effect was observed in the placebo group. Therefore, crude stevioside up to 15.0 mg/kg/day did not show an antihypertensive effect, but can be regarded as safe and tolerable during long term use as a sweetener (Ferri et al, 2006).

Stevia significantly decreased the systolic and diastolic blood pressure in hypertensive subjects in a multicenter, randomized, double-blind, placebo-controlled study. One hundred and six (106) subjects (28 to 75 years) with mild to moderate essential hypertension were enrolled in the study. They entered a 4-week, single-blind, placebo wash-out period. Subjects with a sitting diastolic blood pressure between 95 and 115 mmHg at the last two visits of the placebo period were randomized to receive stevioside capsules 250 mg (n=60) or placebo (n=46) 3 times a day and were followed monthly for 1 year. In the active treatment group, systolic and diastolic blood pressure decreased significantly after 3 months (systolic: 166 mm Hg [± 9.4] to 152.6 mm Hg [± 6.8]; diastolic: 104.7 mm Hg [± 5.2] to 90.3 mm Hg [± 3.6], p<0.05). This effect continued throughout the trial period (Chan et al, 2000).

INDICATIONS AND USAGE

Unproven Uses: Folk medicine uses include hypertension, diabetes, and as a contraceptive.

PRECAUTIONS AND ADVERSE REACTIONS

Adverse cardiovascular and kidney/genitourinary effects have been documented with Stevia.

Cardiovascular: A slight decrease in mean arterial pressure (approximately 9.5%) and bradycardia was reported in healthy subjects (age 24 to 40 years) after ingestion of a tea made from Stevia leaves for 30 days (Kinghorn, 1985).

Kidney/Genitourinary Effects: Intravenous administration of stevioside to rats has resulted in natriuresis. This effect is partially dependent on prostaglandins (Melis & Saninati, 1991a). Kaliuresis has also been reported in animal studies (Mauri, 1996).

DRUG INTERACTIONS

No information is available.

DOSAGE

Mode of Administration: Stevia is available as cut drug for oral administration.

LITERATURE

Bailey CJ, Day C. Traditional plant medicines as treatments for diabetes. *Diabetes Care* 12(8):553-564. 1989.

Boeckh-Haebisch EMA. Pharmacological trial of concentrated crude extract of *Stevia rebaudiana* (Bert.) Bertoni in healthy volunteers. *Arg Biol Tecnol* 35(2):299-314. 1992.

Brandle JE, Starratt AN, Gijzen M. *Stevia rebaudiana*: its biological, chemical and agricultural properties. *Can J Plant Sci* 78:527-536. 1998.

Chan P, Tomlinson B, Chen YJ, et al: A double-blind placebo-controlled study of the effectiveness and tolerability of oral stevioside in human hypertension. Br J Clin Pharmacol 50(3):215-220. 2000.

Constantin J, Ishii-Iwamoto EL, Ferraresi-Filho O, et al: Sensitivity of ketogenesis and citric acid cycle to stevioside inhibition of palmitate transport across the cell membrane. *Braz J Med Biol Res* 11:767-771. 1991.

Curi R, Alvarez M, Bazotte RB, et al: Effect of *Stevia rebaundiana* on glucose tolerance in normal adult humans. *Braz J Med Biol Res* 19:771-774. 1986.

Das S, Das AK, Murphy RA, et al: Evaluation of the cariogenic potential of the intense natural sweeteners stevioside and rebaudioside A. *Caries Res* 26:363-366. 1992.

Ferri LA, Alves-Do-Prado W, Yamada SS, et al. Investigation of the antihypertensive effect of oral crude stevioside in patients with mild essential hypertension. *Phytother Res*. Sep;20(9):732-6. 2006.

Gregersen S, Jeppesen PB, Holst JJ, Hermansen K. Antihyperglycemic effects of stevioside in type 2 diabetic subjects. Metabolism; 53(1): 73-76. 2004.

Ishii EL, Bracht A. Stevioside, the sweet glycoside of Stevia rebaudiana, inhibits the action of atractyloside in the isolated perfused rat liver. Res Commun Chem Pathol Pharmacol, 34:79-91. 1986.

Ishii-Iwamoto EL, Bracht A. Stevioside is not metabolized in the isolated perfused rat liver. *Res Commun Mol Pathol Pharmaco l* 82:167-175. 1995.

Ishikawa H, Kitahata S, Ohtani K, et al: Transfructosylation of rebaudioside A (a sweet glycoside of Stevia leaves) with Microbacterium beta-fructofuranosidase. *Chem Pharm Bull* (Tokyo), 6:2043-2045. 1991.

Jakinovich W Jr, Moon C, Choi YH, et al: Evaluation of plant extracts for sweetness using the Mongolian gerbil. *J Nat Prod* 82:190-195. 1990.

Kawano T, Simoes LC. Effect of *Stevia rebaudiana* in Biomphalaria glabrata. Rev Bras Biol 34:555-562. 1986.

Kelmer Bracht A, Alvarez M, Bracht A. Effect of Stevia rebaudiana on glucose tolerance in normal adult humans. *Braz J Med Biol Res* 34:771-774. 1986.

Kelmer Bracht A, Alvarez M, Bracht A. Effects of Stevia rebaudiana natural products on rat liver mitochondria. *Biochem Pharmacol* 34:873-882. 1985.

Kelmer Bracht A, Alvarez M, Bracht A. Sterols in Stevia rebaudiana Bertoni. *Boll Soc Ital Biol Sper* 34:2237-2240. 1984.

Kim KK, Sawa Y, Shibata H. Hydroxylation of ent-kaurenoic acid to steviol in Stevia rebaudiana Bertoni - purification and partial characterization of the enzyme. *Arch Biochem Biophys* 34:223-230. 1996.

Kinghorn AD, Nanayakara NPD, Soejarto DD, et al: Potential sweetening agents of plant origin. I. Purification of Stevia rebaudiana sweet constituents by droplet counter-current chromatography. *J Chromatogr* 237:478-483. 1982.

Klongpanichpak S, Temcharoen P, Toskulkao C, et al: Lack of mutagenicity of stevioside and steviol in Salmonella typhimurium TA 98 and TA 100. *J Med Assoc Thai*, 82:S121-8128. 1997.

Matsui M, Matsui K, Kawasaki Y, et al: Evaluation of the genotoxicity of stevioside and steviol using six in vitro and one in vivo mutagenicity assays. *Mutagenesis* 11:573-579. 1996.

Mauri P, Catalano G, Gardana C, et al: Analysis of Stevia glycosides by capillary electrophoresis. *Electrophoresis* 17:367-371. 1996.

Melis MS. A crude extract of Stevia rebaudiana increases the renal plasma flow of normal and hypertensive rats. *Braz J Med Biol Res*. 29:669-675. 1996.

Melis MS. Chronic administration of aqueous extract of Stevia rebaudiana in rats: renal effects. *J Ethnopharmacol* 47:129-134. 1995.

Melis MS. Renal excretion of stevioside in rats. *J Nat Prod* 26:688-690. 1992.

Melis MS. Stevioside effect on renal function of normal and hypertensive rats. J Ethnopharmacol 26:213-217. 1992.

Melis MS, Sainati AR. Effect of calcium and verapamil on renal function of rats during treatment with stevioside. *J Ethnopharmacol.* 11:257-262. 1991.

Oliveira-Filho RM, Uehara OA, Minetti CA, et al: Chronic administration of aqueous extract of Stevia rebaudiana (Bert.) Bertoni in rats: endocrine effects. *Gen Pharmacol* 34:187-191. 1989.

Pezzuto JM, Compadre CM, Swanson SM, et al: Metabolically activated steviol, the aglycone of stevioside, is mutagenic. *Proc Natl Acad Sci* U S A 82:2478-2482. 1985.

Pezzuto JM, Nanayakkara NP, Compadre et al: Characterization of bacterial mutagenicity mediated by 13-hydroxy-ent-kaurenoic acid (steviol) and several structurally related derivatives and evaluation of potential to induce glutathione S-transferase in mice. *Mutat Res* 169:93-103. 1986.

Planas GM, Kuc J. Contraceptive properties of *Stevia rebaudiana. Science* 162(857):1007. 1968.

Procinska E, Bridges BA, Hanson JR: Interpretation of results with the 8-azaguanine resistance system in Salmonella typhimurium: no evidence for direct acting mutagenesis by 15-oxosteviol, a possible metabolite of steviol. *Mutagenesis* 6(2):165-167. 1991.

Sakaguchi M, Kan T. Japanese research on *Stevia rebaudiana* (Bert.) Bertoni and the stevioside. *Cienc Cult* 34:235-248. 1982.

Schvartzman JB, Krimer DB, Azorero RM. Cytological effects of some medicinal plants used in the control of fertility. *Experientia* 33(5):663-665. 1977.

Shibata H, Sawa Y, Oka T, et al: Steviol and steviol-glycoside: glucosyltransferase activities in Stevia rebaudiana Bertoni - purification and partial characterization. *Arch Biochem Biophys* 34:390-396. 1995.

Smoliar VI, Karpilovskaia ED, Sali NS, et al:, Effect of a new sweetening agent from Stevia rebaudiana on animals. *Planta Med* 32:60-63. 1992.

Suttajit M, Vinitketkaumnuen U, Meevatee U, et al: Mutagenicity and human chromosomal effect of stevioside, a sweetener from Stevia rebaudiana Bertoni. Environ Health Perspect 101(suppl 3):53-56. 1993.

Tanaka O. Improvement of taste of natural sweeteners. *Pure Appl Chem* 69(4):675-683. 1997.

Tomita T, Sato N, Arai T, et al: Bactericidal activity of a fermented hot-water extract from Stevia rebaudiana Bertoni towards enterohemorrhagic Escherichia coli O157:H7 and other food-borne pathogenic bacteria. *Microbiol Immunol* 34:1005-1009. 1997.

Toskulkao C, Deechakawan W, Leardkamolkarn V, et al: The low calorie natural sweetener stevioside: nephrotoxicity and its relationship to urinary enzyme excretion in the rat. *Phytother Res* 8:281-286. 1994.

White Jr, Kramer J, Campbell RK, et al: Oral use of a topical preparation containing an extract of Stevia rebaudiana and the chrysanthemum flower in the management of hyperglycemia. *Diabetes Care* 17(8):940. 1994.

Xili L, Chengjiany B, Eryi X, et al: Chronic oral toxicity and carcinogenicity study of stevioside in rats. *Ed Chem Toxic* 30(11):957-965. 1992.

Yamamoto NS, Kelmer-Bracht AM, Ishii EL, et al: Effect of steviol and its structural analogs on glucose production and oxygen uptake in rat renal tubules. *Experientia* 41:55-57. 1985.

Yodyingyuad V, Bunyawong S. Analysis of Stevia glycosides by capillary electrophoresis. *Electrophoresis* 6:367-371. 1996

Yodyingyuad V, Bunyawong S. Effect of stevioside on growth and reproduction. *Hum Reprod* 6:158-165. 1991.

Yodyingyuad V, Bunyawong S. Potential sweetening agents of plant origin. III. Organoleptic evaluation of Stevia leaf herbarium samples for sweetness. *J Nat Prod* 6:590-599. 1982.

Stevia rebaudiana

See Stevia

Stillingia

Stillingia sylvatica

DESCRIPTION

Medicinal Parts: The medicinal part is the fresh or dried root.

Flower and Fruit: The yellow flowers are in terminal spikes and are apetalous. The fruit is a 3-seeded capsule.

Leaves, Stem, and Root: The plant is a perennial herb up to 100 cm high. It has an angular, smooth stem, which contains a milky latex. The leaves are sessile, coriaceous, and narrow at the base. They are variable in form and color and are 3 to 11 cm long. The root is usually reddish-white on the outside and has numerous resin glands.

Characteristics: The taste is bitter and acrid; the smell is characteristic and unpleasant.

Habitat: The plant is indigenous to the southern U.S.

Production: Stillingia root is the root of *Stillingia sylvatica.*

Other Names: Cockup Hat, Marcory, Silver Leaf, Queen's Delight, Yaw Root

ACTIONS AND PHARMACOLOGY

COMPOUNDS

Diterpenes: diterpene esters of the tiglic or daphnan type, including diesters of 12-deoxyphorbol, of 12-deoxy-5β-hydroxyphorbol, of 5β, 12β-dihydroxyresiniferonol-6α,7α-oxide, referred to as stillingia factors S1 to S9 (S6 = gniditilactin, yuanhuacin, S7 = prostratin)

Volatile oil

Tannins (10 to 12%)

EFFECTS

The juice of the green root causes inflammation of the skin and swelling. The drug has laxative, tonic, and diuretic properties.

INDICATIONS AND USAGE

Unproven Uses: The herb is used as a "blood purifier," for digestive disorders, and for the treatment of liver, billiary, and skin diseases.

Homeopathic Uses: Stillingia sylvatica is used for secondary and tertiary syphilis.

PRECAUTIONS AND ADVERSE REACTIONS

General: The drug is strongly irritating to skin and mucous membranes. Taken internally, it triggers vomiting (it is used as an emetic) and diarrhea (it is used as a laxative). Skin contact leads to inflammation and swelling. The diterpenes cause inflammation and are likely to be carcinogenic and virus-activating.

Breastfeeding: Stillingia should not be administered to nursing mothers.

DOSAGE

Mode of Administration: As a liquid extract or tincture.

Storage: The drug should not be kept longer than 2 years.

LITERATURE

Adolf A, Hecker E, *Tetrahedron Letters* 21:2887. 1980

British Herbal Pharmacopoeia, British Herbal Medicine Association, UK 1983.

Hegnauer R, Chemotaxonomie der Pflanzen, Bde 1-11: Birkhäuser Verlag Basel, Boston, Berlin 1962-1997.

Kern W, List PH, Hörhammer L (Hrsg.), Hagers Handbuch der Pharmazeutischen Praxis, 4. Aufl., Bde. 1-8: Springer Verlag Berlin, Heidelberg, New York, 1969.

Lewin L, Gifte und Vergiftungen, 6. Aufl., Nachdruck, Haug Verlag, Heidelberg 1992.

Madaus G, Lehrbuch der Biologischen Arzneimittel, Bde 1-3, Nachdruck, Georg Olms Verlag Hildesheim 1979.

Teuscher E, Lindequist U, Biogene Gifte - Biologie, Chemie, Pharmakologie, 2. Aufl., Fischer Verlag Stuttgart 1994.

Zahn P et al., Investigations of homeopathic drugs derived from *Hippomane mancinella* and *Stillingia sylvatica*: A potential iatrogenic risk of cancer? In: *PM* 59(7):A684. 1993.

Stillingia sylvatica

See Stillingia

Stinging Nettle

Urtica dioica

DESCRIPTION

Medicinal Parts: The medicinal parts are the fresh and dried flowering plant and the roots.

Flower and Fruit: The flowers are greenish-white in axillary, clustered, hanging panicles. The perigone has 4 tepals. There are 4 stamens and 1 ovary with a brushlike stigma. The flowers are dioecious. The male flowers have only stamens and the female flowers have only a style or a seed-producing organ. The male flower consists of a perianth of 4 segments, which enclose an even number of stamens. The stamens curve inward in the bud stage and spring back at the end of flowering for the anthers to fling out the pollen. The fruit is a small single-seeded nutlet.

Leaves, Stem, and Root: The plant grows from 60 to 150 cm high and has a hard rhizome. The leaves are opposite, oblong-cordate, and roughly serrate. The whole plant is covered in stinging hairs.

Habitat: The plant is common in most temperate regions of the world.

Production: Stinging Nettle herb consists of the fresh or dried above-ground parts of *Urtica dioica, Urtica urens,* and/or hybrids of these species, collected during flowering season. Stinging Nettle leaf consists of fresh or dried leaves of *Urtica dioica, Urtica urens,* and/or hybrids of these species, gathered during flowering season.

Not to be Confused With: The leaves of *Laminum album.*

Other Names: Nettle

ACTIONS AND PHARMACOLOGY

COMPOUNDS: STINGING NETTLE FLOWERING PLANT

In the stings of the fresh plant: histamine, serotonin, acetylcholine, formic acid, leukotriens (LTB4, LTC4, LTD4)

Flavonoids (0.7-1.8%): including rutin, isoquercitrin (0.02%), astragalin, kaempferol-3-O-rutinoside

Silicic acid (1-4%): partially water-soluble

Volatile oil: chief components are ketones, including, among others, 2-methylhept-2-en-6-on

Potassium-ions (0.6% in the fresh foliage)

Nitrates (1.5 to 3%)

COMPOUNDS: STINGING NETTLE ROOT

Steroids: sterols, including beta-sitosterol (0.03 to 0.06%), beta-sitosterol-3-O-beta-glucoside (0.03 to 0.5%), (6'-Palmitoyl)-sitosterol-3-O-beta-D-glucoside (0.003%), 7alpha-hydroxysitosterol (0.001%), 7eta-Hydroxysitosterol (0.001%), stigmasterol, campesterol, stigmast-4-en-3-one

Lectins (0.1%): UDA (Urtica dioica Agglutinin, isolectine mixture)

Polysaccharides: glucans, glucogalacturonans, acidic arabinogalactans water-soluble with immunostimulating effect)

Hydroxycoumarins: scopoletin

Lignans: including secoisolariciresinol-9-O-glucoside (0.004%), neo-olivil (0.003%), neo-olivil-4-O-glucoside (0.004%)

Ceramides

EFFECTS: STINGING NETTLE FLOWERING PLANT

The fresh leaves contain acetylcholine, serotin, and histamine. The pressed juice (main active principles scopoletine, beta-sitosterol, and caffeoyl malic acid) is diuretic in combination with sufficient fluid intake. The fresh leaf may cause painful stings, but these may have anti-inflammatory and analgesic effects. Caffeoyl acid in vitro, inhibits 5-lipoxygenase-dependent leukotriene synthesis In animal experiments, a local anaesthetic and analgesic effect has been observed. Topical use of fresh nettle leaves as a counterirritant has been reported but not investigated systematically.

In various studies, an antirheumatic and anti-arthritic effect was demonstrated. Preliminary studies suggest possible benefit in osteoarthritis and rheumatoid arthritis.

Anti-inflammatory Effects: In one study, an extract from Stinging Nettle leaves (IDS 23) and its main phenolic component, caffeic malic acid, were tested for their ability to inhibit the biosynthesis of arachidonic acid metabolites in vitro. IDS 23 showed a strong concentration dependent inhibition of cyclooxygenase derived reactions. A phenolic acid isolate from the extract inhibited the synthesis of leukotriene B4 in a concentration dependent manner. This study demonstrates that the antiphlogistic properties of *Urtica dioica* are due to enzymatic action on more than one pathway. There may have been other active components aside from the caffeic malic acid in the plant extract (Obertreis, 1996).

EFFECTS: STINGING NETTLE ROOT

The aqueous extract of nettle yields 5 immunologically active polysaccharides and a mixture of lectins. Nettle agglutinin (UDA) was isolated from fresh and dried roots by affinity chromatography on crude chitin. Ion-exchange chromatography further separated 2 lectins that have different hemagglutination activities and stimulate human lymphocytes lectins (Willer & Wagner, 1990). A (N-acetylglucosamine)(n)-specific lectin inhibited the cytopathicity of human immunodeficiency viruses in vitro. Lectins are thought to interfere with fusion between virion and target cell membrane (Balzarini et al, 1992). The polysaccharide fraction shows anti-inflammatory and immunostimulating abilities (Lichius & Muth, 1997). Scopoletin has known anti-inflammatory activity.

Nettle administration seems to effectively alleviate the symptoms of benign prostatic hyperplasia (BPH) whether used alone or in conjunction with other herbals (Sokeland & Albrecht, 1997; Schneider et al, 1995).

Antifungal Effects: The lectin nettle agglutinin (UDA) has shown antifungal activity as well as the ability to bind chitin (Bombardelli & Morazzoni, 1997).

Effects on Prostate Tissue: The root has been show to cause an increase in the volume of urine, increase of maximum urinary flow and reduction of residual urine. One study found that an aqueous extract of the root was the most effective in treating BPH. The extract inhibited the binding of sex hormone-binding globulin (SHBG) to its receptor on human prostatic membranes in a dose-related manner. Inhibition was noted at 0.6 mg/mL and complete inhibition was achieved at 10 mg/mL (Hryb et al, 1995.) In a second study, most ligans that were tested were found to have an affinity for SHBG. The affinity of (-)-3,4-divanillyltetrahydrofuran was found to be extremely high (Schottner, 1997.) Other steroids (stigmasterol, campesterol, and hecogenin) found in Stinging Nettle roots also showed inhibitory properties, although not as potently (Hirano et al, 1994). Additionally, the isolectin mixture *Urtica dioica* agglutinin (UDA), present in substantial amounts in the root, may contribute to anti-inflammatory and antiprostatic activities. UDA has been found to suppress lymphocyte proliferation in a concentration of 30 mcg/mL and to stimulate proliferation at a concentration of 10 mcg/mL if treated with hydrochloric acid first (Wagner et al, 1994).

Various constituents of the methanolic extract of the root show weak to moderate inhibitory activity on aromatase, a critical enzyme in steroid-hormone metabolism (Bombardelli & Morazzoni, 1997). Nettle root extract WS 1031 more strongly inhibited the activity of aromatase in vitro than Serenoa repens extract WS 1473 (Koch & Biber, 1994). Aromatase converts androgens to estrogens and thus may contribute to the pathogenesis of BPH.

Viral Inhibiting Effects: The (N-acetylglucosamine) n-specific lectin from Stinging Nettle was found to be inhibitory to HIV-1, HIV-2, CMV, RSV, and influenza A virus in vitro at an EC-50 (50% inhibitory concentration) ranging from 0.3 to 0.9 mcg/mL (Balzarini, 1992.). Nettle agglutinin is a lectin with immunostimulating activity and ability to bind to the epidermal growth factor receptor (Lichius & Muth, 1997).

Effects on Systemic Lupus Erythematosus-like Pathology: Urtica dioica agglutinin (UDA)-treated MRL lpr/lpr mice were shown to be protected from developing clinical signs of lupus and nephritis (Musette, 1996.)

CLINICAL TRIALS

Arthritis

Nettle leaf extract had a synergistic action with diclofenac in one open study. Patients were randomly assigned in a nonblind fashion to take 200 mg diclofenac with misoprostol for gastroprotection or 50 mg diclofenac with 50 g freeze-dried, aqueous extract of Nettle leaf. A total of 40 patients with acute joint pain related to osteoarthritis, rheumatoid arthritis, or gout volunteered for this 2-week study. Both treatment groups improved under treatment compared to baseline based on C-reactive protein (CRP) levels and symptom scores. There was no significant difference between the groups on CRP levels (p=0.34) or various symptom scores p=0.38 to 0.71) (Chrubasik et al, 1997).

In an open, 3-week study of 1,528 patients with arthrosis (majority of patients) or rheumatoid arthritis, the use of Nettle leaf extract led to significant improvement of symptoms in patients on monotherapy as well as those on combination therapy with other nonsteroidal anti-inflammatory drugs (NSAIDS). Pain while resting, pain during movement, and movement limitations were parameters used to evaluate the efficacy of treatment. After 3 weeks of twice -aily administration of 770 mg Nettle extract IDS 23 (Rheumahek®), a 50% reduction in NSAID use by the combination therapy group was recorded; 29% of patients in this group were not able to lower their concurrent NSAID dose. Symptom scores were reduced by an average of 45% in the monotherapy group and 42% in the combination therapy group. No significant difference in efficacy was noted between the two treatment groups. Overall, resting pain decreased by 52%, pain during movement by 44%, and movement limitations were improved in 37% of patients. Seventy-five percent of physicians and patients reported very good and/or good results with Nettle treatment. Five patients in the monotherapy and 5 in the combination therapy group reported gastrointestinal discomfort. Six patients experienced allergic reactions (primarily dermatologic in nature) and 3 patients reported increased diuresis (Ramm & Hansen, 1996).

Benign Prostatic Hyperplasia (BPH)

A prospective, randomized and double-blind, crossover trial compared the effectiveness of *Urtica dioica* with placebo for symptomatic relief of lower urinary tract symptoms (LUTS) secondary to BPH of a minimum of 1-3 years duration. Of the 558 patients (mean age 63 years) who completed the study, 232 (81%) of 287 patients in the *Urtica dioica* group reported improved LUTS compared with 43 (16%) of the 271 patients in the placebo group (P<0.001). Participants in the treatment group continued to have favorable outcomes over the long term, although there was no added effect from extended (18 months) treatment. No side effects were reported in either group. The authors recommend that future trials be conducted to confirm this apparent positive effect of *Urtica dioica* on BPH-related lower urinary tract symptoms. (Safarinejad, 2005).

Another randomized, double-blind, placebo-controlled multicenter study demonstrated that Bazaton Uno, a Stinging Nettle root extract, is effective in the reduction of irritative symptoms and BPH-associated complications due to the antiphlogistic and antiproliferative effects of *Urtica dioica*. After the treatment of 246 patients with Bazaton Uno (459 mg dry extract of Stinging Nettle roots), International Prostrate Symptom Score (IPSS) decreased on average from 18.7±0.3 to 13.0±0.5 with a statistically significant difference compared to placebo (18.5±0.3 to 13.8±0.5; p=0.0233). Increase of median Qmax and median volume of residual urine was not statistically significant between both treatment groups. The number of adverse events (29/38) as well as urinary infections etc (3/10 events) was smaller under Bazaton Uno therapy compared with placebo. Bazoton Uno can therefore be considered a safe therapeutic option for BPH (Schneider & Rubben, 2004).

One randomized, reference-controlled, multicenter, double-blind clinical trial compared therapeutic efficacy of a Sabal and Urtica extract (PRO 160/120) with finasteride in BPH (Aiken stages I to II). The study involved 543 patients that were treated for 48 weeks with either the PRO 160/120 extract or finasteride in a double-blind design. The primary marker was the change of maximum urinary flow after 24 weeks of therapy. Secondary markers included average urinary flow, miction volume, and miction time. Urinary symptoms were recorded by the International-Prostate-Symptom-Score (I-PSS). There was also a quality-of-life (QOL) questionnaire that was developed by the American Urological Association Measurement Committee (1991). Results were similar for both groups. There was an increase in urinary flow rate (1.9 mL with PRO 160/120; 2.4 mL with finasteride). Urinary flow increase and miction time decreases were comparable for both groups. The I-PSS decreased from 11.3 at the start to 8.2 at 24 weeks and 6.5 by week 48 for the PRO 16/120 group, and went from 11.8 to 8.0 and 6.2 respectively for the finasteride group. The QOL scores went from 7.5 at the start of treatment, to 4.2 in the PRO 160/120 group, and from 7.7 to 4.1 in the finasteride group. The most notable differences between the groups were in the lower adverse events categories where the PRO 160/120 group reported less events, in particular in the areas of diminished ejaculation volume, erectile dysfunction and headache (Sokeland & Albrecht, 1997.)

In an open, prospective, multicenter, observational study of 2,080 patients with Alken's stage I or II BPH, a combination product of Nettle and Saw Palmetto extracts improved QOL and uroflow, and reduced nocturia. Treatment continued for 12 weeks with one capsule Prostagutt® forte (120 mg Nettle extract plus 160 mg Saw Palmetto extract) twice daily in 5% of patients (4% other dose, 1% no dose reported). Mean uroflow values increased 47%, residual urine decreased in 66%, and nocturia episodes in 49%. A total of 85% of participants reported symptomatic improvement and 80% reported an improvement in QOL. Fifty percent of patients echographically revealed a decrease in the size of the prostate. Fifteen cases of adverse effects were reported, primarily gastrointestinal in nature (6 of 12 patients discontinued treatment as a result), and one case of allergic urticaria due to a confirmed nettle allergy. Other adverse effects reported could not conclusively be linked to the extract (Schneider et al, 1995).

INDICATIONS AND USAGE

STINGING NETTLE FLOWERING PLANT

- Infections of the urinary tract
- Kidney and bladder stones
- Rheumatism

The drug is used internally and externally as supportive therapy for rheumatic ailments. It is used internally as irrigation therapy for inflammatory diseases of the lower urinary tract. Also used as irrigation therapy for prevention and treatment of kidney stones.

Unproven Uses: In folk medicine, the plant is used internally as a hematogenic remedy, diuretic for arthritis, rheumatism of the joints and muscles, and as a component of diabetic teas (this indication is not recommended). Externally, the drug is used as a hair and scalp remedy against oily hair and dandruff.

STINGING NETTLE ROOT

Approved by Commission E:

- Prostate complaints, irritable bladder

Preparations of the root are used for micturition disorders in prostate adenoma stages I to II. This drug only relieves the symptoms of an enlarged prostate without eliminating the enlargement itself. Specifically, according to Commission E, it it reduces residual urine and increases urinary flow.

Unproven Uses: In folk medicine, the root is used for edema, rheumatism, gout, and prostatitis.

CONTRAINDICATIONS

STINGING NETTLE FLOWERING PLANT

The drug is contraindicated when there is fluid retention resulting from reduced cardiac or renal function.

Pregnancy: Not to be used during pregnancy.

STINGING NETTLE ROOT

Pregnancy: Not to be used during pregnancy.

PRECAUTIONS AND ADVERSE REACTIONS

STINGING NETTLE FLOWERING PLANT

Gastric irritation is the most commonly reported adverse effect. Possible allergic reactions (skin afflictions, edema) have been observed in rare cases following intake of the drug. Topical irritation and allergic contact reaction from drinking tea has been reported. Contact urticaria frequently occurs when skin is exposed to the plant. The urticaria may be treated with gentle washing in mild soapy water; systemic antihistamines and topical steroids may be useful but are rarely necessary.)

Gingival Effects: A diffuse edematous gingivostomatitis developed in an 82-year-old man who regularly drank a tea made from Stinging Nettle. The authors consider the patient's reaction to be an allergic contact reaction, rather than an irritant, because of negative patch tests in 2 control subjects (Bossuyt & Dooms-Goossens, 1994).

Kidney/Genitourinary Effects: Increased diuresis and a strong diuretic effect have been reported in patients with arthritic conditions and those with myocardial or chronic venous insufficiency, respectively (Ramm & Hansen, 1996).

DRUG INTERACTIONS

POTENTIAL INTERACTIONS

Iron: Nettle contains an unspecified amount of tannins. Its tannin content may complex with concomitantly administered iron, resulting in nonabsorbable insoluble complexes and may result in adverse sequelae on blood components. It is unknown to what extent the amount of tannin in nettle may affect iron absorption clinically. *Clinical Management:* Until more is known, patients who need iron supplementation should be advised to separate administration times of these compounds by 1 to 2 hours.

STINGING NETTLE ROOT

No health hazards are known in conjunction with the proper administration of designated therapeutic dosages. Occasional, mild gastrointestinal complaints may occur as side effects of drug intake. Diminished urine formation has been reported infrequently, and edema rarely (Anon, 1997).

Gastrointestinal Effects: In an open, 12-week prospective, multicenter observational study of 2,080 patients with Alken's stage I or II BPH, a combination product of Nettle and Saw Palmetto extracts was taken; 15 cases of adverse effects were reported, primarily gastrointestinal in nature (Schneider et al, 1995).

Pregnancy: Not to be used during pregnancy.

DRUG INTERACTIONS

POTENTIAL INTERACTIONS

Iron: See Drug Interactions for Stinging Nettle Flowering Plant, above.

DOSAGE

STINGING NETTLE FLOWERING PLANT

Mode of Administration: Comminuted herb for infusions and other galenic preparations for internal use; as Stinging Nettle spirit for external application. Drug extracts are contained in diuretic tea mixtures and in blood-purifying teas.

Preparation: To prepare an infusion, use 1.5 g finely cut herb in cold water, briefly bring to a boil and steep for 10 minutes, then strain.

Daily Dose: The average daily dose is 8 to 12 g of drug. Observe ample intake of liquid (minimum 2 liters/day). One cup several times daily as a diuretic (1 teaspoonful = 0.8 g drug). For external application, a tincture/spiritus (1:10) may be administered.

STINGING NETTLE ROOT

Mode of Administration: Comminuted drug from the root for infusions as well as other galenic preparations for oral use.

Preparation: To prepare an infusion, use 1.5 g of coarse powdered drug in cold water, heat to boiling point for 1 minute, then steep, covered, for 10 minutes, and strain. (1 teaspoonful = 1.3 g of drug)

Daily Dose: 4 to 6 g.

Tea - 1.5 g of coarse powdered drug added to boiling water.

Dry Extract - 120 mg twice daily.

LITERATURE

Anon. Nettles. *The Review of Natural Products.* Facts and Comparisons, St. Louis, MO. 1997.

Anon. *Vet Hum Toxicol* 24:247. 1982.

Anon. Extrakt aus Brennesselwurzel wirksam bei benigner Prostatahyperplasie. *ZPT* 12(5):8. 1991.

Anon. Phytotherapie: Pflanzliche Antirheumatika - was bringen sie? *DAZ* 136(45):4012-4015. 1996.

Anon. Welche Bedeutung haben pflanzliche Prostatamittel. *DAZ*; 133(9):720. 1993.

Balzarini J, Neyts J, Schols D, et al: The mannose-specific plant lectins from Cymbidium hybrid and Epipactishelleborine and the (N-acetylglucosamine)(n)-specific plant lectin from *Urtica dioica* are potent and selective inhibitors of human immunodeficiency virus and cytomegalovirus replication in vitro. *Antivir Res* 18(12):191-207. 1992.

Belaiche P, Lievoux O. Clinical studies on the palliative treatment of prostatic adenoma with extract of Urtica root. *Phytother Res* 5:267-269. 1991.

Bombardelli E, Morazzoni P: *Urtica dioica L. Fitoterapia* 68(5):387-402. 1997.

Bossuyt L, Dooms-Goossens A. Contact sensitivity to nettles and camomile in ''alternative'' remedies. *Contact Dermatitis* 31:131-132. 1994.

Chaurasia N, Wichtl M. *PM* 53:432. 1987.

Chrubasik S, Enderlein W, Bauer R, et al: Evidence for the antirheumatic effectiveness of herba *Urticae dioicae* in acute arthritis: A pilot study. *Phytomedicine* 4:105-108. 1997.

Dathe G, Schmid H. Phytotherapie der benignen Prostatahyperplasie (BPH). Doppelblindstudie mit Extraktum Radicis Uricae (ERU). *Urologe* [B]27:223-226. 1987.

Fessler B. Brennesselwurzel bei Prostataadenom. *Med Mo Pharm* 16(9):287. 1993.

Gan ber D, Spiteller G. Aromatase inhibitors from *Urtica dioica. PM* 61(2):138-140. 1995.

Goetz P. Die Behandlung der benignen Prostatahyperplasie mit Brennesselwurzeln. *ZPT* 10(6):175. 1990.

Hirano T, et al: Effect of Stinging Nettle root extract and their steroidal components on the Na+,K+-ATPase of the benign prostic hyperplasia. *PM* 60:30. 1994.

Hryb DJ, Khan MS, Romas NA, et al: The Effect of Extracts of the Roots of the Stinging Nettle (*Urtica dioica*) on the Interaction of SHBG with 1st Receptor on Human Prostatic Membranes. *Planta Med* 61:31-32. 1995.

Huesing JE, Murdock LL, Shade RE. Rice and Stinging Nettle lectins - insecticidal activity similar to wheat germ agglutinin. *PH* 30:3565. 1991.

Hughes RE, et al. *J Sci Food Agric* 31:1279. 1980.

Koch E. Pharmakologie und Wirkmechanismen von Extrakten aus Sabalfrüchten (Sabal fructus): Brennesselwurzeln (Urticae radix) und Kürbissamen (Cucurbitae peponis semen) bei der Behandlung der benignen Prostatahyperplasie. In: Loew D, Rietbrock N (Hrsg.) Phytopharmaka in Forschung und klinischer Anwendung. Steinkopff Verlag, Darmstadt, S 57-79. 1995.

Koch E, Biber A. Pharmacological effects of Sabal and Urtica extracts as a basis for rational medication of benign prostatic hyperplasia. *Urologe* 34:90-95. 1994.

Krzeski T, Kazon M, Borkowski A, et al: Combined extracts of *Urtica dioica* and *Pygeum africanum* in the treatment of benign prostatic hyperplasia: Double-blind comparison of two doses. *Clin Ther* 15:1011-1020. 1993.

Lepik K. Safety of herbal medications in pregnancy. *Can Pharm* J 130(3):29-33. 1997.

Lauel H. Extrakt aus Radix Urticae normalisiert Hormonhaushalt. *DAZ* 130(51/52):2789. 1990.

Lichius JJ, et al: Inhibition of experimentally induced mouse prostatic hyperplasia by methanolic extracts of *Urtica dioica* roots. *PM* 61(Abstracts of 43rd Ann Congr):89. 1995.

Lichius JJ, Muth C. The inhibiting effects of *Urtica dioica* root extracts on experimentally induced prostatic hyperplasia in the mouse. *Planta Med* 63(4):307-310. 1997.

Lichius JJ, Muth C. A new biological evaluation of Urtica dioica root-extracts. In: PM 62, Abstracts of the 44th Ann Congress of GA, 20. 1996.

Miersch WE. Benigne Prostatahyperplasie. *DAZ* 133(29):2653. 1993.

Mittman P. Randomized, double-blind study of freeze-dried *Urtica dioica* in the treatment of allergic rhinitis. *Planta Med* 56(1):44-47. 1990.

Musette P, Galelli A, Chabre H, et al: Urtica dioica agglutinin, a V beta 8.3-specific superantigen, prevents the development of the systemic lupus erythematosus-like pathology of MRL lpr/lpr mice. *Eur J Immunol* 26:1707-1711. 1996.

Nahrstedt A. Pflanzliche Urologica - eine kritische Übersicht. *Pharm Z* 138: 1439-1450. 1993.

Nöske HD. Die Effektivität pflanzlicher Prostatamittel am Beispiel von Brennesselwurzelextrakt. ÄrzteZ Naturheilverfahren 35 (1):18-27. 1994.

Obertreis B, Giller K, et al: Anti-inflammatory effect of *Urtica dioica* folia extract in comparison to caffeic malic acid. *Arzneimitte-Forsch*; 46(1):52-56.1996.

Oliver F, Amon EU, Breathnach A, et al: Contact urticaria due to the common Stinging Nettle (*Urtica dioica*)–histological, ultrastructural and pharmacological studies. *Clin Exp Dermatol*; 16:1-7. 1991.

Ramm S, Hansen C. Stinging Nettle leaf extract for arthritis and rheumatic arthritis. *Therapiewoche* 28:3-6. 1996.

Sabo A, et al: Radix Urticae (Urtica dioica): Influence on erythrocyte deformability and enzymes. *PM* 62, Abstracts of the 44th Ann Congress of GA, 60. 1996.

Safarinejad MR. Urtica dioica for treatment of benign prostatic hyperplasia: a prospective, randomized, double-blind, placebo-controlled, crossover study. *J Herb Pharmacother 5:1*-11. 2005.

Schiebel-Schlosser G. Die Brennessel. *PTA* 8(1):53. 1994.

Schilcher H. Pflanzliche Diuretika. *Urologe* [B]27:215-222.

Schlicher H. Möglichkeiten und Grenzen der Phytotherapie am Beispiel pflanzlicher Urologika. *Urologe* [B]27:316-319. 1987.

Schilcher H, Boesel R, Effenberger ST, et al: Neuere Untersuchungsergebnisse mit aquaretisch, antibakteriell und prostatotrop wirksamen Arzneipflanzen. *ZPT* 10(3):77. 1989.

Schilcher H. Urtica-Arten - Die Brennessel. *ZPT* 9(5):160. 1988.

Schmidt K. Die Wirkung eines Radix Urticae-Extrakts und einzelner Nebenextrakte auf das SHBG des Blutplasmas bei der benignen Prostatahyperplasie. *Fortschr Med* 101:713-716. 1983.

Schneider T, Rubben H. Stinging nettle root extract (Bazoton Uno) in long term treatment of benign prostatic syndrome (BPS). Results of a randomized, double-blind, placebo controlled multicenter study after 12 months. *Urologe A*; 43(3): 302-306. 2004.

Schomakers J, Bollbach FD Hagels H. Brennesselkraut - Phytochemische und anatomische Unterscheidung der Herba-Drogen von Urtica dioica und U. urens. *DAZ* 135(7):578-584. 1995.

Schneider HJ, Honold E, Masuhr T. Treatment of benign prostatic hyperplasia: Results of a surveillance study in the practices of urological specialists using a combined plant-based preparation (Sabal extract WS 1473 and Urtica extract WS 1031). *Fortschr Med* 113:37-40. 1995.

Schoettner M, Gansser D, Spiteller G. Lignans from the roots of Urtica dioica and their metabolites bind to human sex hormone binding globlin (SHBG). *Planta Med* 63:529-532. 1997.

Sokeland J, Albrecht J. Combination of Sabal and Urtica extract vs. finasteride in benign prostatic hyperplasia (Aiken stages I to II). Comparison of therapeutic effectiveness in a one year double-blind study. *Urologe A* 36(4):327-333. 1997.

Sonnenschein R. Untersuchung der Wirksamkeit eines prostatotropen Phytotherapeutikums (Urtica plus) bei benigner Prostatahyperplasie und Prostatitis - eine prospektive multizentrische Studie. *Urologe* [B]27:232-237. 1987.

Wagner H, et al: Studies on the binding of Urtica dioica agglutinin (UDA) and other lectins in an in vitro epidermal growth factor receptor test. *Phytomedicine* 1:287-290. 1994.

Wagner H, Willer F, Samtleben R, et al: (Search for the antiprostatic principle of Stinging Nettle (*Urtica dioica*) roots. *Phytomedicine* 1:213-224. 1994.

Willer F, Wagner H, Schecklies E, et al: Urtica-Wurzelextrakte. *DAZ* 131(24):1217. 1991.

Willer F, Wagner H. Immunologically active polysaccharides and lectins from the aqueous extract of *Urtica dioica*. *Planta Med* 56(6):669. 1990.

St. John's Wort

Hypericum perforatum

DESCRIPTION

Medicinal Parts: The medicinal parts include the fresh buds and flowers separated from the inflorescences, the aerial parts collected during the flowering season and dried, and the entire fresh flowering plant.

Flower and Fruit: The golden yellow flowers are in sparsely blossomed terminal cymes. The 5 sepals are ovate-lanceolate to lanceolate and very pointed. The sepals are also smooth, serrate at the tip, and marked by many light and dark glands. The 5 petals and numerous stamens are fused into 3 bundles. The ovary has a broad or narrow oval shape. The fruit is a 3-valvular capsule, which is triangular and oval. The seeds are cylindrical and shortly pointed at both ends. The seeds are 1 to 3 mm long, either black or dark brown, and covered in small warts.

Leaves, Stem, and Root: The perennial plant is 30 to 60 cm and contains a long-living branched root and rhizome, which tapers toward each end. The reddish stem is erect, has 2 raised edges, and can reach 100 cm in height. The oval-shaped, translucent, punctate leaves are attached directly at the base and often covered in black glands.

Characteristics: The flowers release an odorless red juice when squeezed, which tastes weakly bitter and irritating.

Habitat: The plant is indigenous to all of Europe, western Asia and northern Africa. It has been introduced to eastern Asia, Australia and New Zealand, and it is cultivated in Poland and Siberia.

Production: St. John's Wort consists of the dried above-ground parts of *Hypericum perforatum* gathered during flowering season. The herb is cut at the start of the flowering season and dried quickly in bunches in order to preserve the oil and secreted contents.

Not to be Confused With: The plant may be mistaken for other Hypericum species, such as *Hypericum barbatum, Hypericum hirsutum, Hypericum maculatum, Hypericum montanum*, and *Hypericum tetrapterum.*

Other Names: Amber, Hardhay, Goatweed, Klamath Weed, Saint John's Word, St. Johnswort, Tipton Weed

ACTIONS AND PHARMACOLOGY

COMPOUNDS

Anthracene derivatives (0.1-0.15%): favoring naphthodianthrones, especially hypericin, pseudohypericin

Flavonoids (2-4%): in particular, hyperoside, quercitrin, rutin, isoquercitrin, and also biflavonolids, including amentoflavone

Xanthones (0.15-0.72%): 1,3,6,7-tetrahydroxy-xanthone

Acylphloroglucinols: hyperforin with small quantities of adhhyperforin

Volatile oil: chief components are aliphatic hydrocarbons, including, among others, 2-methyloctane, undecane; also dodecanol, mono- and sesquiterpenes, including, among others, alpha-pinene, caryophyllene; also 2-methyl-3-but-3-en-2-ol

Oligomers

Procyanidines and other catechin tannins (6.5-15%)

Caffeic acid derivatives: including chlorogenic acid

EFFECTS

St. John's Wort extracts were more effective than placebo in the treatment of mild to moderate depression in multiple controlled clinical trials. St. John's Wort demonstrated similar efficacy to amitriptyline, imipramine, maprotiline, and fluoxetine as well as to diazepam and desipramine when combined with valerian. Antimicrobial and antifungal effects have been studied in vitro. St. John's Wort was effective against cancer in vitro. The herb has shown anti-inflammatory, antioxidant, and cardiac effects as well.

Serotonin reuptake inhibition and monoamine oxidase inhibition have been reported. The antidepressant effect of St. John's Wort may also be mediated via reduction of corticotropin releasing hormone (CRH) secretion through suppression of interleukin-6 release. Anti-inflammatory activity may be related to inhibited release of arachidonic acid from membrane phospholipids, inhibition of nuclear factor-kappa B and protein kinase C. The cardiac effect may be due to inhibition of cellular phosphodiesterase, with positive inotropic effects at low concentrations and negative inotropic effects at high concentrations. A 2006 systematic review of prospective clinical trials found reasonable evidence to suggest that high-dose hyperforin extracts induce CYP3A (Whitten, 2006). St. John's Wort may induce cytochrome P450 3A4 and other isoenzymes in humans through the induction of the pregnane X receptor, which regulates CYP3A4 transcription. St. John's Wort also may induce CYP1A2, 2E1, and 2D6. St. John's Wort has demonstrated ability to induce P-glycoprotein. Antimicrobial action of St. John's Wort may be due to hyperforin, a phloroglucin derivative.

Antianxiety Effects: The anxiolytic effect of St. John's Wort may be due to benzodiazepine receptor activation. The antidepressant mechanism of action may be due to effects on many neurotransmitters including serotonin, norepinephrine, dopamine, L-glutamate, and GABA. *Hypericum perforatum* extract increased rearing in open field tests with rats and latency time was significantly enhanced in the light-dark model of anxiety. Individual components of this extract did not demonstrate the same effect. Administration of the benzodiazepine antagonist flumazenil, with *Hypericum perforatum,* completely negated the anxiolytic activity. Investigators concluded that benzodiazepine receptor activation is the basis for the use of St. John's Wort in the treatment of anxiety (Zanoli et al, 1998).

Antidepressant Effects: The mechanism of the antidepressant effect of St. John's Wort has not been fully determined. It is likely a result of synergistic and/or additive effects of several different constituents of St. John's Wort. In vitro, hyperforin inhibited the uptake of norepinephrine, dopamine, L-glutamate, and GABA (Wonnemann et al, 2000). Hyperforin inhibited dopamine receptors D1 and D5 and selectively inhibited the norepinephrine transporter in vitro. Hypericin inhibited dopamine receptors D3 and D4 and the flavonoid rutin inhibited D2. The bioflavonoid amentoflavone was the only substance studied that demonstrated significant inhibition at serotonin receptors, specifically 5-HT(1D) and 5-HT(2C). Amentoflavone also inhibited the benzodiazepine receptor and opioid receptor subtype h-delta (Butterweck et al, 2002). Rutin was necessary for the antidepressant activity of a methanolic St. John's Wort extract in rats, but was not effective alone. Rutin may increase the bioavailability of other essential constituents in St. John's Wort through effects on transport through biological membranes, P-glycoprotein, or the cytochrome P450 system (Noldner & Schotz, 2002).

An elevated level of corticotropin releasing hormone (CRH) has been implicated in the pathogenesis of depression. When human blood cells from patients with depression and healthy subjects were stimulated with phytohemagglutinin or lipopolysaccharides and treated with hypericum extract, interleukin-6 (IL-6), and, to a lesser extent, interleukin 1 beta (IL-1b) and tumor necrosis factor alpha (TNF-alpha) were suppressed. IL-6 production was suppressed in all blood samples (from patients with depression and healthy subjects) treated with hypericum extract. IL-1b production was suppressed in the blood of 2 of 4 patients with depression while no change was observed in healthy subjects (n=5). TNF-alpha release was suppressed in all but one blood sample (from a healthy patient) treated with hypericum extract. If hypericum extract reduces IL-6 production in vivo, the antidepressant effects of St. John's Wort may be mediated via reduction of CRH secretion, as IL-6 induces the release of CRH (Thiele et al, 1994).

It has been demonstrated in rats that the antidepressant activity of St. John's Wort depends on its hyperforin content, possibly due to its effects on serotonergic transmission. Other central nervous system activity is mediated by other components of St. John's Wort. Hyperforin is not involved in the dopaminergic activity of alcoholic extracts (Bhattacharya et al, 1998). Dopamine-mediated CNS activity of *Hypericum perforatum* extract LI160 was again demonstrated in mouse bioassays with the help of dopamine receptor antagonists (Butterweck et al, 1997).

Anti-inflammatory Effects: Amentoflavone, found in St. John's Wort, has anti-inflammatory and anti-ulcerogenic properties (Berghofer & Holzl, 1989). A St. John's Wort extract suppressed leukocyte infiltration in mice treated with carageenan and prostaglandin E1 (Shipochliev et al, 1981). Hypericin dose-dependently inhibited the release of arachidonic acid from membrane phospholipids in calcium ionophore-stimulated human granulocytes. The calcium ionophore was not the only inducer. Inhibitory activities were noted in concentrations of hypericum under 0.4 micromoles. This inhibition resulted in the suppression of leukotriene B and interleukin production but did not affect prostaglandin E2. The end result is an immunosuppressive effect (Panossian et al, 1996). Anti-inflammatory effects of hypericin may be partly due to nuclear factor-kappa B (NF-kB) inhibition. Hypericum may inhibit protein kinase C (PKC), suggesting an inhibitory effect on PKC-regulated transcription factors. Hypericin was not confirmed as an antioxidant since it did not affect hydrogen peroxide-induced NF-kB activation (Bork et al, 1999).

Antimicrobial Effects: Hyperforin, an extract isolated from St. John's Wort, has demonstrated significant antimicrobial activity against strains of *Staphylococcus aureus.* A butanol fraction of St. John's Wort inhibited the growth of *Helicobacter pylori.* Antibacterial effects of St. John's Wort may be related to the simultaneous effects of radiation from the sun (Reichling et al, 2001). In vitro antibacterial activity of hyperforin against methicillin-resistant *Staphylococcus aureus* (MRSA) has been documented at a minimum inhibitory concentration of 1 mcg/mL. Standard therapeutic dosing of 300 mg 3 times daily resulted in a steady-state plasma concentration of 100 ng/mL, lower than that necessary for therapeutic antibacterial activity (Reichling et al, 2001; Voss & Verweij, 1999).

Antineoplastic Effects: In vitro studies demonstrated cytoxicity against human colon carcinoma. Hypericin was studied for antitumor effects in A431 human cancer cells. Hypericin inhibited leukemia cells and gastrointestinal tumor cells. Hypericin also inhibited autophosphorylation of the epidermal growth factor (EGF) receptor as well as the tyrosine phosphorylation of peptides catalyzed by the EGF receptor. The T cell, PTK, P56, was also dose-dependently inhibited by hypericin. The study concluded hypericin has direct inhibitory effects on tumor cells (Kil et al, 1996).

Antioxidant Effects: Dilutions of Hypericum extract, standardized to either hypericin or hyperforin, demonstrated significant antioxidant effects in both cell-free and human vascular tissue (Hunt et al, 2001). *Cytochrome P450 Induction Effects:* St. John's Wort significantly induced cytochrome P450 1A2, 3A4, 2E1, and 2D6 in a randomized, open-label trial of 12 healthy subjects (Durr et al, 2000).

Neuroendocrine Effects: Oral administration of 600 mg of a St. John's Wort extract containing hyperforin (WS 5570) stimulated cortisol secretion 30 to 90 minutes following intake. No cortisol stimulation was observed following oral intake of 300 mg WS 5570. The results of this study suggested that hyperforin (not hypericin) is the active component in St. John's Wort extracts which influence certain neurotransmitters in the central nervous system (Schule et al, 2001). *Norepinephrine Reuptake Inhibition Effects:* Alteration of biogenic amine synthesis was proposed as a possible mechanism of action. Hypericum extract (0.01% to 0.1%) demonstrated 50% synaptosomal norepinephrine reuptake inhibition and some beta-adrenergic and muscarinic receptor inhibition at higher concentrations (Mueller & Schaefer, 1996).

P-Glycoprotein Induction Effects: A single dose of St. John's Wort (900 mg) significantly inhibited p-glycoprotein while long term use of St. John's Wort nonsignificantly induced p-glycoprotein in an open-label study of 12 healthy subjects. Fexofenadine (60 mg) was studied as a marker p-glycoprotein substrate. Fexofenadine Cmax increased 45% and oral clearance decreased 20% (both $p<0.05$ compared to pretreatment) (Wang et al, 2002).

St. John's Wort significantly increased P-glycoprotein expression and associated drug efflux in a randomized, single-blinded, placebo-controlled trial of 22 healthy subjects (13 female, 9 male). Subjects received St. John's Wort (Good n' Natural, standardized to 0.15% hypericin) 600 mg (n=15) or placebo (n=7) three times daily for 16 days. P-glycoprotein expression in peripheral blood mononuclear cells increased 4.2-fold with St. John's Wort after 16 days (29.5 ± 14.3 median fluorescence intensity (MFI, a measure of P-glycoprotein expression) versus 7 ± 1.9 MFI, $p<0.05$, 95% confidence interval (CI): 13.5, 31.6) (Hennessy et al, 2002). In 8 healthy male volunteers, St. John's Wort significantly induced intestinal P-glycoprotein/MDR1 and hepatic cytochrome P450 3A4. Subjects were nonsmokers, ages 23 to 35 years, and abstained from caffeine, alcohol, citrus fruits, and medications for 5 days prior to and during the study (Durr et al, 2000).

Wound-Healing Effects: In a comparative study in rats, oral St. John's Wort was more effective for wound healing than a topical tincture of calendula (marigold). Primary endpoints of the study were rates of wound contraction, epithelization time, and wound breaking strength; incision, excision, and dead space wounds were investigated. Both treatments demonstrated greater wound healing compared with placebo (Rao et al, 1991).

CLINICAL TRIALS

Anxiety

Three cases have been reported of patients with generalized anxiety disorder experiencing relief of symptoms with St.

John's Wort at doses of 900 mg twice daily. Two patients had taken kava previously without effectiveness. The 900-mg dose improved sleep, ability to relax, and ability to cope with daily stress, and reduced worry within 4 weeks in a 45-year-old female with chronic anxiety for 8 years. At 12 months of therapy with St. John's Wort, the patient continued to report effectiveness without side effects or relapse. St. John's Wort 900 mg twice daily reduced anxiety symptoms on the Symptoms Checklist 90 from 74 to 25 by week 9 in a 43-year-old female. Prior to treatment, she had persistent tension, worry, irritability, muscle tightness, bruxism, and insomnia. After 9 weeks of treatment, she slept better and had increased ability to cope (Davidson & Connor, 2001).

Cognitive Function

Hypericum extract containing 5% hyperforin increased quantitative pharmaco electroencephalogram (qEEG) power performances to a greater extent than the 0.5% extract but overall differences only reached statistical significance compared to placebo. In a double-blinded, placebo-controlled, parallel group comparison, the effect of hyperforin content on the pharmacological effects of St. John's Wort was measured via the qEEG. Fifty-five volunteers received 900 mg hypericum extract containing 0.5% or 5% hyperforin as a single dose for 1 week. qEEG data represented the mean power values of the absolute electrical power of 17 electrodes during 10-minute intervals of "eyes open" and "eyes shut" conditions. Increases in power were recorded in delta, theta, and alpha-1 frequencies with the most significant effect occurring in the theta frequency band during "eyes closed" conditions. The most significant power increases occurred 6 hours after extract administration. Alpha-2 frequency power values for the extracts were not appreciably different from placebo. Both extracts were well tolerated and no relevant adverse effects were reported (Schellenberg et al, 1998).

St. John's Wort extract demonstrated a trend toward greater cognitive ability in a placebo-controlled, double-blinded, multicenter 4-week trial of 50 patients with neurotic depression. St. John's Wort not only prevented a further reduction in cognitive ability but also improved it. It was also noted that this patient group, which included treatment-resistant cases, were selected from general practice, not from neurological practice, where a higher response rate is usually seen due to better patient selection (Lehrl et al, 1993).

Depression

The evidence from quality clinical trials to date is inconsistent and confusing as to whether St. John's Wort extracts are better than placebo or standard antidepressants in alleviating depression in adults, the authors of a 2005 Cochrane Database review of current publications conclude. Several specific extracts of the herb may help with mild to moderate depression, they found; the studies overall seem to show that they are more effective than placebo and similarly effective as prescription antidepressants for depression that is mild to moderate in severity. But benefits for treating major depression are likely minimal. Trials were included in the analysis if they were randomized, double-blind, included people with depression and outcomes such as symptoms, and compared the herb to a placebo or standard antidepressant. A total of 37 trials were identified. The 12 trials that compared the extract to placebo in people with major depression found the herb to be more effective than placebo, but the bigger and more precise trials indicated only a small benefit [rate ratio 1.15]. But trials that included not only people with major depression but those with mild and moderate symptoms as well indicated notable benefits for St. John's Wort. While side effects from the herb are uncommon and usually mild, there is a substantial risk of unwanted and risky interactions with a number of other medicines, so consultation with a physician before starting to take the herb is crucial. Also, effectiveness and safety indicated in this review hinge on the use of certain marketed preparations, which may vary notably from those sold in most venues (Linde, 2005).

The authors of a 2006 review of evidence from the above Cochrane database review and other (primarily) English-language literature—25 systematic reviews, 10 meta-analyses, one qualitative research study—for St. John's wort in treating depression conclude that intensive and regular publications of this kind have been published over the past decade. Overall, most report positive findings for the extract when compared with placebo for mild to moderate depression. Recently, however, the focus of studies has shifted from questions of effectiveness to potential interactions and safety of St. John's Wort. The authors of a 2004 review of adverse effects (from case reports) conclude that the most relevant risks involve interactions with other medicines, such as with cyclosporine in people with organ transplants. St. John's Wort increases metabolism and consequently reduced plasma concentrations of drugs that are metabolized by the cytochrome P450 enzyme system. Of all the research published on St. John's Wort for depression, only one was identified that focused on the patient's motivation in considering the herb over standard medications. The authors note that this area of examination warrants more attention (Pilkington, 2006).

A systematic large-scale observational study of St. John's Wort extract a year earlier found the herb extracts to be well tolerated and apparently effective in routine treatment of mild to moderate depression. The review was based on 16 observational (nonrandomized) and phase IV studies in primary care settings that included a minimum of 100 patients with primarily depressive illnesses and treated with a St. John's Wort extract. Altogether, 34,804 patient experiences with the extract were included in the pooled analysis. The daily extract dosage used varied from 360 to 1200 mg, and most studies were 4 to 6 weeks long. No serious side effects or interactions were reported; the most common side effect reported was gastrointestinal upset, and the second most common was increased sensitivity to light and skin reactions (Linde & Knuppel, 2005).

The same author of an earlier systematic review, in 2002, found thtat St. John's Wort was significantly more effective than placebo (17 trials; n = 1168) and similarly effective as tricyclic antidepressants and benzodiazepines, with fewer adverse effects, in 8 trials including 1,132 patients with mild-to-moderate depression. St. John's Wort preparations were tested at doses ranging from 350 milligrams (mg) to 1800 mg daily. Limitations of the trials reviewed included heterogeneity of the patient population and St. John's Wort extracts and doses used, low doses of comparison antidepressants, and short observation periods of 4 to 6 weeks (Linde & Mulrow, 2002).

A meta-analysis concluded that St. John's Wort was more effective than placebo and similarly effective as tricyclic antidepressants in moderate depression. Two German trials comparing St. John's Wort and placebo and 4 trials (3 German) comparing St. John's Wort to amitriptyline, maprotiline, and imipramine were included. The usual St. John's Wort dose used was 300 mg 3 times daily (total daily dose ranged from 200 mg to 900 mg). To be included in the analysis, the studies had to be blinded and controlled with placebo or standard antidepressants; patients (n=651 combined) had to have depressive disorders diagnosed using ICD-10, DSM-IIIR, or DSM-IV criteria; patients had to have similar sociodemographic backgrounds; and the clinical outcome had to be measured using the Hamilton Depression Scale (HAMD). Baseline HAMD scores ranged from 15 to 24. When compared with placebo, St. John's Wort demonstrated a significantly higher response rate (73.2% versus 37.9%) and had a lower dropout rate (12.2% versus 19.5%). St. John's Wort demonstrated a similar response rate when compared to tricyclic antidepressants (64% versus 66.4%) and a lower dropout rate due to side effects or inadequate efficacy (12.6% versus 16.2%) (Kim et al, 1999). The studies included in this meta-analysis are also included in the systematic review by Linde & Mulrow, 2000; however, this meta-analysis reflects a less heterogenous patient population due to more stringent inclusion criteria.

St. John's Wort significantly reduced symptoms of depression in a randomized, double-blinded, placebo-controlled trial of 375 patients with mild-to-moderate depression. Patients had a single-blind, placebo run-in phase for 3 to 7 days. Responders to the placebo phase, defined as 25% or greater reduction in the Hamilton depression scale, were excluded from continuing the trial. Remaining patients were randomized to receive St. John's Wort extract WS 5570 300 mg 3 times daily for 6 weeks. WS 5570 is a hydroalcoholic extract standardized to contain 3% to 6% hyperforin and 0.12% to 0.28% hypericin. Previous studies have generally used extracts standardized to 0.3% hypericin and/or 3% hyperforin. The mean Hamilton depression scale (HAMD) score for all patients decreased from baseline 21.9 ± 1.7 by a mean of 9.9 ± 6.8 with WS 5570 and 8.1 ± 7.1 with placebo (p=0.03 versus placebo). In patients with a baseline HAMD score of at least 22, the HAMD decreased by 10.5 ± 7.0 with WS 5570 and 8.5 ± 7.7 with placebo (p = 0.04). In patients with baseline HAMD score <22, no significant difference was noted between WS 5570 and placebo. In the intention-to-treat analysis, 52.7% of patients were responders (defined as a decrease of at least 50% in HAMD score from baseline) to WS 5570 versus 42.3% with placebo (p less than 0.05 versus placebo). Patients withdrawing from the trial included 18 (9.7%) WS 5570 patients and 25 (13.2%) placebo patients. Adverse events were reported by 30.6% of WS 5570 patients compared with 37% of placebo patients. Two patients taking WS 5570 were withdrawn and hospitalized due to worsening symptoms (Lecrubier et al, 2002).

St. John's Wort in 3 different daily doses reduced the symptoms of mild-to-moderate depression in a randomized, double-blinded, multicenter, parallel-group study (Lenoir et al, 1999).

Depressive symptoms continued to be controlled with open-label St. John's Wort therapy given for an additional 6 months following a 7-week double-blinded trial comparing St. John's Wort with sertraline in 18 patients with mild-to-moderate depression (Brenner et al, 2002).

Other trials have shown similar results in the treatment of mild-to-moderate depression (Schrader et al, 1998; Laakmann et al, 1998; Harrer, 1999, 1994; Vorbach, 1997, 1994; Steger, 1985; Behnke et al, 2002; Philipp et al, 1999) No significant difference was demonstrated between St. John's Wort and imipramine in the treatment of depression in a randomized, double-blind, parallel-group, multicenter trial of 324 patients. Patients received Hypericum extract (ZE 117, standardized to 0.2% hypericin) 250 mg or imipramine 75 mg twice daily for 6 weeks.

No significant differences were found between groups using the Hamilton Depression Scale, Clinical Global Impression scale, and the patient's global impression scale. Adverse effects were reported by 39% (62/157) of patients taking St. John's Wort and 63% (105/167) of patients taking imipramine (Woelk, 2000).

Depression, Major

A multicenter, randomized, double-blind phase III study was conducted to test and compare the efficacy and safety of Hypericum extract WS 5570 to paroxetine in patients suffering from moderate or severe depression according to DSM-IV criteria. One hundred thirty patients were included. The results showed that WS 5570 and paroxetine were similar in preventing relapse in a continuation treatment after recovery from an episode of moderate to severe depression (Anghelescu et al, 2006).

The objective of a double-blind, randomized, placebo-controlled trial was to study the antidepressant efficacy and safety of *Hypericum perforatum* extract WS 5570 at doses of 600 mg/day (once daily) and 1200 mg/day (600 mg twice daily). Patients (n=332) with an episode of mild or moderate major depressive episode were randomized to take either WS 5570

600 mg/day, WS 5570 1200 mg/day, or placebo over a period of six weeks. The primary outcome measure was the change in total score on the Hamilton Rating Scale for Depression (HAM-D, 17 item version). Significantly more patients in the WS 5570 groups showed treatment response and remission. St. John's wort was consistently more effective than placebo in patients with either less severe or more severe baseline impairment. Patients in the WS 5570 1200 mg/day group experienced higher remission than in the group receiving WS 5570 600 mg/day. Incidence of adverse events was low in all groups (Kasper et al, 2006).

In a postmarketing surveillance study, single-dose-administration of highly dosed St. John's wort was studied in 4,337 patients with depressive symptoms over a 12-week period. States of mental and physical health were documented using the SF-12-sumscore as a measure for quality of life. Physicians and patients rated efficacy and tolerability. Results showed that SF-12-sumscore improved significantly. About 80% of the physicians and patients judged the efficacy and safety of the drug as "good" or "very good". Tolerability was assessed as "good" or "very good" in more than 95% (Rudolf & Zeller, 2004).

The antidepressant efficacy of *Hypericum perforatum* was investigated in an 8-week, double-blind, placebo-controlled study and compared to the antidepressant, fluoxetine. Seventy-two outpatients were randomly assigned to receive *Hypericum perforatum* 900 mg/day, fluoxetine 20 mg/day, or placebo. Efficacy measures included the HAM-D21 scale, the Montgomery-Asberg Rating Scale, and the Clinical Global Impression. Safety was assessed with the UKU Side Effect Rating Scale. In the intention-to-treat analysis, no differences between the mean scores of the three treatment groups were found. In the analysis of observed cases, patients receiving Hypericum had the lowest remission rates (12%, p=0.016) compared to fluoxetine (34.6%) and placebo (45%). In conclusion, *Hypericum perforatum* was less efficacious than both fluoxetine and placebo (Moreno et al; 2006). A previous well-designed trial by Bjerkenstedt et al revealed different results. One-hundred sixty outpatients received the same doses as above over four weeks. Treatment with hypericum was still not more effective in short-term treatment in mild to moderate depression than placebo, but remission rates were higher with 24% compared to fluoxetine (28%) and placebo (7%). In this trial, hypericum was furthermore significantly better tolerated than fluoxetine (Bjerkenstedt et al, 2005).

In contrast, St. John's wort was assessed to be more effective than fluoxetine in a study by Fava et al. In a double-blind, placebo-controlled study, patients with major depressive disorders were randomized to 12 weeks of double-treatment with LI 160 St. John's wort extract (900 mg/day), fluoxetine (20 mg/day), or placebo. Remission rates of 38% for hypericum, 30% for fluoxetine and 21 % for placebo were found (Fava et al, 2005).

A 2005 randomized and double-blind trial concluded that a specific extract of St. John's wort—WS 5570—is at least as effective as paroxetine, a selective serotonin reuptake inhibitor (SSRI), and also is better tolerated than this drug, when taken over the course of six weeks in people with moderate or severe depression. In all, 251 adults with acute major depression at 21 psychiatric primary care practices in Germany were randomized to St. John's wort [900 mg three times daily) or paroxetine (20 mg once daily). Those who did not respond sufficiently to the initial dose after two weeks got benefit from an increased dose. By the end of six weeks, 71% of those randomized to take St. John's Wort compared to 60% of those rancomized to take paroxetine had a 50% or greater reduction in depression symptoms (Szegedi, 2005).

A comparison with sertraline found favorable effects of a hypericum extract (STW3) found. A once-daily dose of 612 mg of hypericum was not inferior to sertraline in 241 patients with moderate depressive disorders in a long-term treatment (Gastpar et al, 2005).

Safety and efficacy of hypericum extract STW-VI in comparison to the SSRI citalopram was assessed using a double-blind, randomized, multicenter, placebo-controlled study design. Outpatients (n=388) suffering from moderate depression received hypericum extract (900mg/day), citalopram (20 mg/daily), or placebo. The statistical significant therapeutic equivalence of hypericum extract STW3-VI to citalopram (p<0.0001) and the superiority of this hypericum extract over placebo (p<0.0001) was demonstrated. At the end of the treatment, 54.2% (hypericum extract), 55.9% (citalopram), and 39.2% (placebo) of the patients were assessed as therapy responders. In most cases, the investigators judged the tolerability of hypericum extract, citalopram, and placebo as "good" or "very good." Thus, hypericum extract STW3-VI is a good alternative to chemically defined antidepressants in the treatment of outpatients with moderate depression (Gastpar et al, 2006). These findings support the results of a previous study carried out by Uebelhack et al (Uebelhack et al, 2004).

By contrast, St. John's Wort was no more effective than placebo or sertraline for major depression in a randomized, double-blinded, placebo-controlled, multicenter trial. After a one-week, single-blind, placebo run-in phase including 428 patients, nonresponding patients (n=340) were randomized to receive either hypericum extract (LI 160, Lichtwer Pharma, Berlin, Germany) 900 mg daily divided into 3 doses (n=113), sertraline 50 mg daily (with two placebo doses; n=109), or placebo 3 times daily for 8 weeks (n=116). After weeks 3 or 4, daily hypericum doses could be increased to 1200 mg and sertraline doses to 75 mg. The average hypericum and sertraline doses received between week 3 and 8 were 1299 mg and 75 mg, respectively. During the continuation phase, the hypericum and sertraline doses could be increased to 1800 mg and 150 mg daily (Hypericum Depression Trial Study Group, 2002).

St. John's Wort was not more effective than placebo for the treatment of major depression in a randomized, double-blinded, placebo-controlled trial of 200 patients (Shelton et al, 2001).

Depression, Pediatric

A notable improvement in symptoms of depression and psychovegetative disorders in children was noted during a 6-week treatment with St. John's Wort extract (LI 160 Lichtwer Pharma). Seventy-four children ages 1 to 12 years (median age 9) with symptoms of depression, psychovegetative disturbance, anxiety, and/or restlessness were administered St. John's Wort extract at doses ranging from 300 mg daily to 900 mg daily, at the discretion of their physician, for an intended 4-week study period that was extended to 6 weeks. Efficacy and tolerance of treatment were evaluated based on the terms ''worsened,'' ''unchanged,'' ''good,'' and ''excellent,'' as assessed by both physicians and parents. In addition to the four general symptoms assessed, 8 specific symptoms, including listlessness, exhaustion, irritability, sleep disturbance, nervousness, concentration disturbance, dejection, and lack of drive were evaluated. Physicians rated overall efficacy either good or excellent in 72% of children by week 2, 97% after 4 weeks of treatment, and 100% after 6 weeks. Parents' ratings were similar at 65% improvement after 2 weeks, 93% after 4 weeks, and 98% after 6 weeks. Treatment was well tolerated and no adverse effects were reported. One case of worsening of nervousness presented when symptoms changed from ''not present'' at baseline to ''mild'' at 2 weeks. This was self-limiting (Hubner & Kirste, 2001).

Dermatitis

A significant improvement in symptoms of subacute atopic dermatitis was noted in patients following a 4-week treatment with a cream containing Hypericum extract standardized to 1.5% hyperforin (verum). Twenty-one patients with mild-to-moderate atopic dermatitis randomly applied verum or placebo twice daily to the left or right side of the body, respectively. Eighteen patients completed the double-blind trial. Intensity of eczematous lesions was compared and evaluated at days 7, 14, and 28. At each clinic visit, the hypericum cream was significantly superior to placebo ($p<0.05$), with a lack of anti-*Staphylococcal aureus* activity ($p=0.064$). Tolerance of the hypericum cream as well as placebo was good or excellent (Schempp et al, 2003).

Fatigue

Hypericum significantly reduced fatigue, anxiety, and depression in an open, uncontrolled study. Patients ($n=20$) with self-reported complaints of fatigue, tiredness, and exhaustion of at least 2 weeks duration (but no self-reported depression) received Hypericum (135 to 225 mg dried extract) 3 times daily for 6 weeks. The study concluded with a reduction of fatigue, depression, and anxiety. Without a control group, it was difficult to determine which results were from Hypericum or from a placebo effect. Further controlled studies were recommended (Stevinson et al, 1998).

Menopausal Symptoms

The efficacy of a fixed combination of black cohosh (Cimicifuga racemosa) and St. John's wort (*Hypericum perforatum*) extracts in women with climacteric complaints with a pronounced psychological component was investigated in a double-blind, randomized, placebo study involving 301 women. The treatment was superior to placebo ($P<0.001$) in alleviating climacteric complaints (Uebelhack et al, 2006).

Marked improvement of subjective and physical symptoms of menopause was observed in pre- and postmenopausal women following a 12-week treatment with Kira®, a St. John's Wort extract standardized to a total hypericin content of 300 mcg/tablet. One hundred and six women, 43 to 65 years old, were supplemented with 1 tablet St. John's Wort extract orally 3 times daily for a total of 12 weeks. Patients were excluded from the study if they were using hormone replacement therapy with estrogens or estrogen-progestogen combinations. The Menopause Rating Scale (MRS) (including changes in libido, dryness of the vagina, and urinary complaints) ranked symptoms from ''not present'' to ''very marked.'' The average total MRS score fell from marked intensity of symptoms to slight intensity after 12 weeks of St. John's Wort treatment ($p<0.001$) (Grube et al, 1999).

Otalgia, Pediatric

A reduction in ear pain in children was noted following the use of naturopathic herbal extract eardrops (NHED) containing St. John's Wort extract. One hundred and seventy-one children ages 5 to 18 years with otalgia related to acute otitis media (AOM) were randomly divided into 4 groups and treated with NHED (containing *allium sativum* (0.05%), *verbascum thapsus* (25%), *calendula flores* (28%), *hypericum perforatum* (30%), lavender (5%), and vitamin E (2%) in olive oil) 5 drops 3 times daily, alone; topical anesthetic (amethocaine and phenazone in glycerin) 5 drops 3 times daily, alone; NHED with oral amoxicillin 80 mg/kg/day; or topical anesthetic with oral amoxicillin 80 mg/kg/day. All treatments were for 3 days. The study was double-blinded and randomized. A 93.4% reduction in ear pain in the NHED group compared to an 80.9% reduction in the anesthetic group was observed. Visual analog scale was used to assess pain. Treatment was considered successful when the subjects or parents reported a reduction in ear pain after 48 hours. On both days 2 and 3, the NHED group reported less pain than the anesthetic group. Both groups who received drops alone reported significantly greater pain relief on both days 2 and 3 than the patients who were given eardrops plus oral antibiotics. No adverse effects were documented in any of the groups. The results of the NHED group cannot be directly correlated to the activity of St. John's Wort since the drops contained multiple herbal extracts. Another consideration the authors had taken into account was that AOM is usually a self-limiting condition that abates within 2 to 3 days on its own, suggesting that time alone may account for much of the reduction in pain (Sarrell et al, 2003).

A 3-day course of herbal ear drops that contained extract of *Hypericum perforatum* was as effective as a topical anesthetic in reducing ear pain in children. One hundred and three children 6 to 18 years completed this randomized trial. Sixty-one children received the combination herbal ear drops (Otikon Otic Solution), which contained *Allium sativum, Verbascum thapsus, Calendula flores,* and *Hypericum perforatum* in olive oil. Forty-two children received anesthetic eardrops containing amethocaine and phenazone in glycerin. The dose for both groups was 5 drops of Otikon or anesthetic applied to the affected ear canal three times daily. A significant reduction in ear pain for both groups ($p<0.007$) was observed. There was not a significant difference between the 2 groups although there was less pain 30 minutes following instillation with Otikon ($p=0.007$). No adverse effects were reported (Sarrell et al, 2001).

Premenstrual Syndrome

St. John's Wort significantly reduced symptoms of premenstrual syndrome in an observational study of 19 women. Subjects were given one 300 mg tablet of St. John's Wort daily, standardized to 900 mcg hypericin. Daily symptom ratings recorded by the subjects were significantly reduced ($p<0.01$) from a baseline of 128.42 to 70.11 after one menstrual cycle. Significant improvements were also demonstrated by scores on the Hospital Anxiety and Depression scale ($p<0.01$) and the modified Social Adjustment Scale ($p<0.05$). Improvements were greatest after one cycle of treatment (Stevinson & Ernst, 2000).

Sleep Quality

Hypericum extract increased slow-wave sleep but had no effect on REM sleep in a double-blinded, placebo-controlled, randomized, crossover study of 12 healthy female volunteers (mean age 59.8 years). Subjects received Hypericum extract LI 160 (Jarsin®) 300 mg 3 times daily for 4 weeks. Sleep onset and total sleep time did not change following supplementation. There was a slight drop in the total sleep amount and a corresponding increase in waking period occurred. Slow-wave sleep (sleep stages 3 and 4) increased from 1.5% to 6.0%. This increase in slow-wave sleep has been postulated by several investigators to be a significant contributor to the antidepressant effect of St. John's Wort (Schulz & Jobert, 1994).

Somatoform Disorders

A prospective, randomized, double-blind and placebo-controlled trial concluded that 600 mg of St. John's Wort extract LI 160 daily is both effective and safe in treating acute mild to moderately severe somatoform disorders. Statistically significant medium to large-sized superiority of St. John's wort treatment over placebo was shown ($p<.0001$) for each of the six primary efficacy measures as well as for the combined test in the intention-to-treat populations ($n=173$). All were adults being treated as outpatients. The findings confirm the results of a 2002 study in the journal *Phamacology* (by Volz HP, et al) In the current study, St. John's Wort was as safe and well-tolerated as the placebo (Muller, 2004).

Weight Loss

In a randomized, double-blinded, placebo-controlled trial, subjects taking a combination supplement containing St. John's Wort lost a statistically significant amount of body weight (1.4 kg; $p<0.05$) and body fat (2.9% change; $p>0.05$). Twenty-three subjects were assigned to 1 of 3 groups. Group A, the treatment group, received *Citrus aurantium* extract 975 mg, caffeine 528 mg, and St. John's Wort 900 mg daily. Group B received a placebo while group C served as the control and received nothing. All subjects participated in a circuit training exercise program 3 times a week for 45 minutes. Subjects also received instructions to follow the 1,800 kilocalorie/day American Heart Association Step One diet. The treatment group experienced an insignificant decrease in both plasma cholesterol and triglycerides. Neither the placebo nor control group lost a significant amount of body weight or body fat (Colker et al, 1999).

INDICATIONS AND USAGE

Approved by Commission E:

- Anxiety
- Depressive moods
- Inflammation of the skin
- Blunt injuries
- Wounds and burns

Internally, the drug is used for psychovegetative disturbances, depressive moods, anxiety and nervous unrest. Externally, the oily Hypericum preparations are used for treatment and post-therapy of acute and contused injuries and for first-degree burns.

Unproven uses: The herb has been used for worm infestation, bronchitis and asthma, gallbladder disease, gastritis (also diarrhea), nocturnal enuresis, gout, and rheumatism. Oily Hypericum preparations are used internally for dyspeptic complaints, and externally for the treatment of myalgia.

Chinese Medicine: In a gargle solution, the herb is used externally for tonsillitis. The herb is also administered externally as a lotion for dermatoses.

Homeopathic Uses: The herb has been used for treatment of peripheral and central nervous system injuries, depressive moods, asthma and cerebral-vascular calcification.

CONTRAINDICATIONS

Contraindications to use include a history of photosensitivity or a hypersensitivity to St. John's Wort.

PRECAUTIONS AND ADVERSE REACTIONS

The potential risk for adverse interactions with other medicines (antidepressants, anticoagulants, cyclosporine, others) has emerged as an important risk and precaution in the use of St. Johns Wort (Schulz 2006; Pilkington 2006, Whitten 2006, Linde 2005).

The tannin content of the drug can lead to digestive complaints, such as feeling of fullness or constipation. Photosensitization has been demonstrated in a controlled clinical trial using metered doses of hypericin and subsequent exposure to UVA/UVB radiation (Roots, 1996). Patients with a previous history of photosensitization to various chemicals should be cautious of direct sun exposure (Wheatley, 1998). Also, concomitant use of St. John's Wort and drugs metabolized by cytochrome P450 3A4, 1A2, or 2E1 may result in decreased drug concentrations and subsequent loss of drug effectiveness (Gurley et al, 2002).

Cardiac Effects: Swelling (edema) was reported by 21 of 113 patients taking St. John's Wort versus 9 of 116 patients taking placebo (p=0.02) for major depression in a randomized, double-blinded, placebo-controlled, multicenter trial (Hypericum Depression Trial Study Group, 2002). A case of hypertensive crisis possibly related to the consumption of wine and aged cheese with St. John's Wort therapy has been reported (Patel et al, 2002). The significance of any monoamine oxidase inhibition by St. John's Wort is controversial, though constituents of St. John's Wort have demonstrated mild monoamine oxidase inhibitory effects (Thiede & Walper, 1994; Demisch et al, 1989; Suzuki et al, 1984). Although St. John's Wort was initially characterized as a monoamine oxidase inhibitor (MAOI), it is believed that insufficient MAO inhibition occurs to explain the clinical activity of St. John's Wort as an antidepressant (DeSmet & Nolen, 1996; Bladt & Wagner, 1994). It remains possible that the mild MAOI property of St. John's Wort may lead to hypertensive crisis when combined with tyramine-containing foods (Demisch et al, 1989). Advise patients to use caution if they consume tyramine-containing foods while taking St. John's Wort and to immediately report any unusual symptoms to their healthcare provider.

Central Nervous System Effects: Restlessness (0.3%) and fatigue (0.4%) occurred in 3,250 patients in one study of depressed patients (Woelk, 1994). In another study, fatigue/tiredness was reported in 5% of subjects, and restlessness in 6% (Vorbach, 1997). Symptoms are difficult to evaluate since the herb is being used to treat depression, which may have similar symptoms. Headache was noted in 7% of studies reviewed (Wheatley, 1998).

Dermatologic Effects: Multiple studies have reported photosensitivity (Jacobson, 2001; Brockmoller et al, 1997; Roots et al, 1996) while other studies demonstrated a lack of photosensitivity with St. John's Wort (Schempp et al, 2001; Schempp et al, 2000; Kerb et al, 1996). Hypericin is an active, photodynamic pigment and is considered the phototoxic constituent of St. John's Wort (Siegers, 1993). No significant phototoxic effects occurred from ingestion of a hypericum extract in both a single-dose and multiple-dose study (Schempp et al, 2001).

Genitourinary Effects: Frequent urination was reported by 30 of 113 patients taking St. John's Wort versus 13 of 116 patients taking placebo (p=0.003) for major depression in a randomized, double-blinded, placebo-controlled, multicenter trial (Hypericum Depression Trial Study Group, 2002). Anorgasmia was reported by 28 of 113 patients taking St. John's Wort versus 16 of 116 patients taking placebo (p=0.04) for major depression in a randomized, double-blinded, placebo-controlled, multicenter trial (Hypericum Depression Trial Study Group, 2002).

Neurological Effects: Headache was noted in 7% of studies reviewed (Wheatley, 1998). Nerve hypersensitivity reactions were reported in 6% (4/70) of patients treated with high dose hypericum by one practitioner. These reactions only occurred in patients who ingested liquid hypericum preparations with sediment. The practitioner linked this adverse effect to substances contained in the sediment. This reaction involved hypersensitivity of the hands and feet to cold, heat, and touch, to the point of being painful (Baillie, 1998).

Coordination, concentration, and attentiveness (necessary for the safe operation of motor vehicles) were *not* impaired in 32 depressed patients receiving 900 mg hypericum extract daily (1080 micrograms hypericin content) for 4 weeks in a double-blinded, placebo-controlled study (Schmidt, 1991). A case was reported of acute neuropathy following concomitant use of St. John's Wort and sun exposure. A 35-year-old woman took 500 milligrams/day of St. John's Wort for 4 weeks. She developed stinging pain on her face and hands, areas exposed to sun. During an examination, she had painful reactions to light brushing, air gusts at room temperature, and exposure to cold (5 to 10 degrees Celsius). Three weeks after discontinuing St. John's Wort, her symptoms improved and completely disappeared in 2 months (Bove, 1998).

Psychiatric Effects: Numerous cases of mania, hypomania, anxiety, and schizophrenia relapse have been reported (van Gurp et al, 2002; Brown, 2000; Lal & Iskandar, 2000; Anon, 1999; O'Bresail & Argouarch, 1998).

Thyroid Hormone Effects: St. John's Wort was weakly associated with increased thyroid stimulating hormone (TSH) levels in two cases in a retrospective case control study involving 37 patients with elevated TSH levels and 37 control patients matched for gender and age (Ferko & Levine, 2001). The design and conclusions of the study by Ferko and Levine were criticized in a commentary article (Hauben, 2002).

Pregnancy: St. John's Wort is contraindicated during pregnancy. High concentrations of St. John's Wort in vitro were mutagenic to sperm cells and adversely effected oocytes. The data suggest that St. John's Wort given at high concentrations damages reproductive cells (Ondrizek, 1999).

DRUG INTERACTIONS

CONTRAINDICATED

Irinotecan: Concurrent use may result in reduced irinotecan effectiveness and treatment failure. *Clinical Management*: Avoid concomitant use of St. John's Wort with irinotecan. The effect of St. John's Wort on metabolizing enzymes of irinotecan may last several weeks after St. John's Wort is discontinued. If a patient is to receive a course of therapy with irinotecan and is found to be taking St. John's Wort, discontinue St. John's Wort and if possible, delay the course of irinotecan for at least 2 weeks. An appropriate dose increase has not been determined in the case that the irinotecan course cannot be delayed.

Non-Nucleoside Reverse Transcriptase Inhibitors: Concurrent use may result in decreased non-nucleoside reverse transcriptase inhibitor concentrations and an increased risk of antiretroviral resistance and treatment failure. *Clinical Management*: Patients receiving therapy with non-nucleoside reverse transcriptase inhibitors should be advised to avoid the use of St. John's Wort. Coadministration of non-nucleoside reverse transcriptase inhibitors with St. John's Wort is expected to decrease non-nucleoside reverse transcriptase inhibitor concentrations leading to suboptimal serum concentrations of non-nucleoside reverse transcriptase inhibitors and an increased risk of antiretroviral resistance and treatment failure.

Protease Inhibitors: Concurrent use may result in decreased protease inhibitor concentrations and an increased risk of antiretroviral resistance and treatment failure. *Clinical Management*: Avoid concomitant use of St. John's Wort and protease inhibitors.

Rasagiline: Concurrent use may result in an increased risk of serotonin syndrome (hypertension, hyperthermia, myoclonus, mental status changes) and/or an increased risk of hypertensive crisis. *Clinical Management*: The concurrent administration of rasagiline and St John's Wort is contraindicated. Allow at least a 14-day washout period after stopping rasagiline before starting St John's Wort. Given the terminal half-life of St John's Wort of 41.7 hours, wait at least 5 half-lives (9 days) after stopping St John's Wort before initiating rasagiline.

Selegiline: Concurrent use may result in an increased risk of serotonin syndrome (hypertension, hyperthermia, myoclonus, mental status changes) and/or an increased risk of hypertensive crisis. *Clinical Management:* The concurrent administration of selegiline and St John's Wort is contraindicated. Allow at least a 14-day washout period after stopping selegiline before starting St John's Wort. Given the terminal half-life of St John's Wort of 41.7 hours, wait at least 5 half-lives (9 days) after stopping St John's Wort before initiating selegiline.

MAJOR RISK

Amiodarone: Concurrent use may result in reduced amiodarone levels. *Clinical Management*: Concurrent use of amiodarone and St. John's Wort is not recommended. Given the extended half-life of amiodarone, potential for drug interaction may exist even after discontinuation of amiodarone.

Amsacrine: Concurrent use may result in reduced effectiveness of amsacrine. *Clinical Management*: Avoid concomitant use of St. John's Wort and amsacrine.

Anesthetics: Concurrent may result in an increased risk of cardiovascular collapse and/or delayed emergence from anesthesia. *Clinical Management*: Discontinue St. John's Wort at least 5 days before surgery using anesthetics.

Anticoagulants: Concurrent use may result in decreased warfarin plasma concentrations leading to reduced anticoagulant effectiveness. *Clinical Management*: Concomitant use of anticoagulants with St. John's Wort is not recommended. If patients elect to remain on St. John's Wort, symptoms of decreased anticoagulant efficacy and prothrombin times should be closely monitored. Upward dose titration of the anticoagulant should be undertaken only if the patient takes a consistent daily dose of St. John's Wort with a reputable product containing a consistent amount of active ingredients of St. John's Wort. Patients should be advised that if they discontinue use of St. John's Wort, they may have an increased risk of bleeding complications. Patients should not discontinue St. John's Wort without notifying their health care provider.

Cyclophosphamide: Concurrent use may result in reduced cyclophosphamide effectiveness. *Clinical Management*: Avoid concomitant use of St. John's Wort and cyclophosphamide.

Cyclosporine: Concurrent use may result in decreased cyclosporine levels, acute transplant rejection, and graft loss. *Clinical Management*: Extreme caution is advised when cyclosporine to patients who are taking St. John's Wort as concomitant use has resulted in significantly decreased cyclosporine levels, organ transplant rejection, and graft loss. If concurrent use is warranted, monitor cyclosporine blood levels and adjust cyclosporine dose as necessary (Prod Info NEORAL® soft gelatin oral capsules, oral solution, 2006; Prod Info SANDIMMUNE® oral capsules, oral solution, IV injection, 2006).

Darunavir: Concurrent use may result in decreased darunavir plasma concentrations and potential loss of darunavir efficacy. *Clinical Management*: Coadministration of darunavir/ritonavir and St. John's Wort (*Hypericum perforatum*) may result in significantly decreased darunavir plasma concentrations due to induction of CYP3A-mediated darunavir metabolism by St. John's Wort. As this may lead to loss of darunavir efficacy, darunavir/ritonavir and St. John's Wort should not be used concurrently.

Digoxin: Concurrent use may result in reduced digoxin efficacy. *Clinical Management*: Avoid concomitant use of St. John's Wort and digoxin. If patients elect to combine products despite this advice, digoxin levels should be monitored closely, noting that by day 10, trough digoxin concentrations may be decreased by 33% with further reductions possible. Upward dosage titration of digoxin should be undertaken only if the patient engages in consistent daily intake of St. John's Wort with a reputable product containing a constant amount of active ingredients of St. John's Wort. Under these circumstances, patients should be advised that if they discontinue use of St. John's Wort, that digoxin blood levels may escalate to toxic levels. Patients should not discontinue St. John's Wort without notifying their physician.

Erlotinib: Concurrent use may result in increased erlotinib clearance and reduced serum concentrations. *Clinical Management*: Avoid concomitant use of erlotinib and St. John's Wort. If concomitant erlotinib and St. John's Wort is not avoidable, doses of erlotinib greater than 150 mg may be required.

Etoposide: Concurrent may result in reduced effectiveness of etoposide. *Clinical Management*: Avoid concomitant use of St. John's Wort with etoposide.

Imatinib: Concurrent use may result in increased imatinib clearance. *Clinical Management*: Coadministration of imatinib and St. John's Wort, a CYP3A4 inducer, may result in a significant reduction in exposure to imatinib. Caution is advised when these two agents are coadministered. Consider using alternatives to St. John's Wort with less enzyme induction potential. However, if imatinib is used concurrently with St. John's Wort, consider an increase in imatinib dose by at least 50% to maintain therapeutic efficacy and monitor clinical response closely.

Lapatinib: Concurrent use may result in decreased lapatinib exposure or plasma concentrations. *Clinical Management*: Coadministration of lapatinib with St. John's Wort, a CYP3A4-inducer, may result in significantly decreased lapatinib AUC and should be avoided. However, if concurrent use is warranted, then consider titrating the dose of lapatinib gradually from 1250 mg/day up to 4500 mg/day, depending on tolerability. Once St. John's Wort is discontinued, reduce the increased lapatinib dose to the indicated dose (Prod Info TYKERB® oral tablets, 2007).

Linezolid: Concurrent use may result in CNS toxicity or serotonin syndrome (hypertension, hyperthermia, myoclonus, mental status changes). *Clinical Management*: Concurrent use of linezolid and St John's Wort may result in serotonin syndrome. Monitor for serotonin syndrome effects including confusion, delirium, restlessness, tremors, blushing, diaphoresis, and hyperpyrexia. Consider a waiting period of 14 days between administration of these drugs.

Monoamine Oxidase Inhibitors: Concurrent use may result in an increased risk of serotonin syndrome (hypertension, hyperthermia, myoclonus, mental status changes) and/or an increased risk of hypertensive crisis. *Clinical Management*: Avoid concomitant use of St. John's Wort and monoamine oxidase inhibitors (MAOIs). Allow at least a 14-day washout period after stopping the MAOI before starting St. John's Wort. Given the terminal half-life of St. John's Wort of 41.7 hours, if an MAOI is to replace St. John's Wort, wait at least 5 half-lives (9 days) after stopping St. John's Wort.

Paclitaxel: Concurrent use may result in reduced paclitaxel effectiveness. *Clinical Management*: Avoid concomitant use of St. John's Wort and paclitaxel.

Phenytoin: Concurrent use may result in reduced phenytoin effectiveness. *Clinical Management*: Avoid concomitant use of St. John's Wort and phenytoin. If patients elect to continue St. John's Wort while taking phenytoin, they must take a consistent dose of St. John's Wort with a reputable product containing a constant about of active ingredients of St. John's Wort. Phenytoin levels should be monitored and stabilized, and symptoms of reduced effectiveness (e.g. increased seizure activity) should be carefully monitored. If patients discontinue St. John's Wort, dosage of phenytoin may need to be decreased, and symptoms of phenytoin toxicity (e.g. nystagmus, ataxia, dysarthria, hyperreflexia, CNS depression, mental status changes, and hallucinations) should be monitored.

Selective Serotonin Reuptake Inhibitors: Concurrent use may result in an increased risk of serotonin syndrome (hypertension, hyperthermia, myoclonus, mental status changes). *Clinical Management*: Patients should be advised to wait two weeks after stopping St. John's Wort before restarting selective serotonin reuptake inhibitor therapy. If a patient plans to replace selective serotonin reuptake inhibitor (SSRI) therapy with St. John's Wort, the half-life of the specific SSRI should be taken into consideration, waiting at least 5 half-lives for the SSRI to be metabolized out of the body.

Sirolimus: Concurrent use may result in subtherapeutic sirolimus levels resulting in possible transplant rejection. *Clinical Management*: Patients should be advised not to take St. John's Wort concurrently with sirolimus. If patients are found to be taking St. John's Wort and sirolimus, discontinue St. John's Wort and monitor sirolimus blood levels as sirolimus dosage may need to be reduced.

Sunitinib: Concurrent use may result in decreased sunitinib plasma concentrations. *Clinical Management*: The concomitant administration of sunitinib and St. John's Wort may result in an unpredictable decrease in sunitinib concentrations and is not recommended.

Tacrolimus: Concurrent use may result in subtherapeutic tacrolimus levels resulting in possible transplant rejection. *Clinical Management*: Advise patients not to take St. John's Wort concurrently with tacrolimus. If patients are found to be taking St. John's Wort and tacrolimus, discontinue St. John's Wort and monitor tacrolimus blood levels as tacrolimus dosage may need to be reduced.

Tamoxifen: Concurrent use may result in reduced tamoxifen effectiveness. *Clinical Management*: Avoid concomitant use of St. John's Wort and tamoxifen.

Trazodone: Concurrent use may result in an increased risk of serotonin syndrome (hypertension, hyerthermia, myoclonus, mental status changes). *Clinical Management:* Avoid concomitant use of St. John's Wort and trazodone. Given the half-life of trazodone of up to 15 hours, St. John's Wort should be avoided for at least 5 half-lives (3 days) following trazodone discontinuation.

MODERATE RISK

Aminoleuvulinic acid: Concurrent use may result in increased risk of phototoxic reaction. *Clinical Management*: Avoid concomitant use of St. John's Wort and aminolevulinic acid.

Amitryptyline: Concurrent use may result in decreased effectiveness of amitriptyline and possible increased risk of serotonin syndrome (hypertension, hyperthermia, myoclonus, mental status changes). *Clinical Management*: Avoid concomitant use of St. John's Wort with amitriptyline.

Antidiabetic agents: Concurrent use may result in hypoglycemia. *Clinical Management*: Caution is advised if patients take St. John's Wort with antidiabetic agents. Monitor closely for signs and symptoms of hypoglycemia.

Atorvastatin: Concurrent use of may result in reduced effectiveness of atorvastatin. *Clinical Management*: Advise patients taking atorvastatin not to start therapy with St. John's Wort without consulting their health care provider. Patients taking St. John's Wort with atorvastatin may require a higher dose of atorvastatin to retain effectiveness. If a patient has been taking atorvastatin and St. John's Wort, advise the patient not to stop St. John's Wort without consulting their health care provider, as atorvastatin levels may increase, leading to adverse effects.

Benzodiazepines: Concurrent use may result in reduced benzodiazepine effectiveness. *Clinical Management*: If patients take St. John's Wort with a benzodiazepine, monitor for alterations in the therapeutic and adverse effects of the benzodiazepine. If a patient is found to be taking St. John's Wort at the time of surgery during which midazolam or any other benzodiazepine is to be used for sedation, monitor the patient closely for signs of reduced benzodiazepine effectiveness and adjust the benzodiazepine dose if necessary.

Beta-Adrenergic Blockers: Concurrent use may result in decreased effectiveness of beta-adrenergic blockers. *Clinical Management*: Concomitant use of St. John's Wort and beta-adrenergic blockers is not recommended. If patients elect to take St. John's Wort and a beta-adrenergic blocker, increased dosage of the beta-adrenergic blocker may be necessary to achieve therapeutic goals. Patients should not discontinue St. John's Wort without consulting their physician as downward dose adjustment of the beta-adrenergic blocker may be required.

Buspirone: Concurrent use may result in an increased risk of serotonin syndrome (hypertension, hyperthermia, myoclonus, mental status changes) or hypomania. *Clinical Management*: Caution patients taking buspirone to discuss the use of nonprescription medicines, herbs, and dietary supplements with their doctor or pharmacist. If a patient presents with hypomanic or serotonergic symptoms when taking buspirone, inquire about the use of nonprescription medicines, herbs, and dietary supplements. It is recommended to avoid St. John's Wort in patients taking buspirone, especially in combination with other psychotropic medicines.

Calcium Channel Blockers: Concurrent use may result in reduced bioavailability of calcium channel blockers. *Clinical Management*: Caution is advised if St. John's wort and calcium channel blockers are taken together. Monitor for continued effectiveness of the calcium channel blocker.

Carbamazepine: Concurrent use may result in altered carbamazepine blood concentrations. *Clinical Management*: Caution is advised if St. John's Wort and carbamazepine are taken concomitantly. Patients must take a consistent dose of St. John's Wort with a reputable product containing a consistent amount of active ingredients of St. John's Wort. Carbamazepine concentrations should be monitored if patients report the loss of seizure control or new side effects while taking St. John's Wort concomitantly. When patients discontinue St. John's Wort, carbamazepine levels and symptoms of carbamazepine toxicity (e.g. drowsiness, ataxia, slurred speech, nystagmus, dystonic reactions, hallucinations and vomiting) should be monitored.

Cerivastatin: Concurrent use may result in reduced effectiveness of cerivastatin. *Clinical Management*: Cerivastatin is no longer available in the United States; however, there may be a few patients who remain taking cerivastatin. Advise patients taking cerivastatin not to start therapy with St. John's Wort without consulting their health care provider. Patients taking St. John's Wort with cerivastatin may require a higher dose of cerivastatin to retain effectiveness. If a patient has been taking cerivastatin and St. John's Wort, advise the patient not to stop St. John's Wort without consulting their health care provider, as cerivastatin levels may increase, leading to adverse effects.

Clozapine: Concurrent use may result in reduced clozapine efficacy. *Clinical Management*: Avoid concomitant use of clozapine with St. John's Wort. If patients elect to remain on St. John's Wort, they should maintain consistent dosing. Clozapine dosage may need to be increased. Patients should not discontinue St. John's Wort without first consulting their clinician as downward adjustments in clozapine dose may be necessary as well as monitoring for increased side effects of clozapine (e.g. decreased white blood cell count, increased salivation, orthostatic hypotension, tachycardia, sedation, seizures).

Contraceptives, Combination: Concurrent use may result in decrease in plasma concentrations of estrogens and in contraceptive effectiveness. *Clinical Management*: Avoid concomitant use of St. John's Wort and hormonal contraceptives. Advise patient to use an alternate nonhormonal contraceptive method of birth control. Monitor patient closely for signs of breakthrough bleeding and/or pregnancy.

Estrogens: Concurrent use may result in decrease in plasma concentrations of estrogens and in estrogen effectiveness. *Clinical Management*: Caution is advised if St. John's Wort is taken with estrogen. Monitor the patient for a decreased response to estrogen replacement therapy (i.e. increase in vasomotor symptoms).

Fenfluramine: Concurrent use may result in an increased risk of serotonin syndrome (hypertension, hyperthermia, myoclonus, mental status changes). *Clinical Management*: Avoid concomitant use. Given the half-life of fenfluramine of 20 hours (Prod Info Pondimin®, 1997), St. John's Wort should be avoided for at least 5 half-lives (4 to 5 days) following fenfluramine discontinuation. Given the terminal half-life of St. John's Wort of 41.7 hours (Wheatley, 1998), St. John's Wort should be avoided for at least 5 half-lives (9 days) before starting fenfluramine.

Fluvastatin: Concurrent use may result in reduced effectiveness of fluvastatin. *Clinical Management*: St. John's Wort may not affect the metabolism of fluvastatin. However, patients taking St. John's Wort with fluvastatin should be monitored for continued lipid-lowering effectiveness. If a patient has been taking fluvastatin and St. John's Wort, advise the patient not to stop St. John's Wort without consulting their health care provider, as fluvastatin levels may increase, leading to adverse effects.

Ginkgo: Concurrent use may result in changes in mental status. *Clinical Management*: If a patient presents with hypomanic symptoms, inquire about the use of nonprescription medicines, herbs, and dietary supplements.

Loperamide: Concurrent use may result in delirium with symptoms of confusion, agitation, and disorientation. *Clinical Management:* Caution is advised if St. John's Wort and loperamide are taken together. Monitor the patient closely for signs of altered mental status.

Lovastatin: Concurrent use may result in reduced effectiveness of lovastatin. *Clinical Management*: Advise patients taking lovastatin not to start therapy with St. John's Wort without consulting their health care provider. Patients taking St. John's Wort with lovastatin may require a higher dose of lovastatin to retain effectiveness. If a patient has been taking lovastatin and St. John's Wort, advise the patient not to stop St. John's Wort without consulting their health care provider, as lovastatin levels may increase, leading to adverse effects.

Methadone: Concurrent use may result in reduced methadone levels and increased risk of withdrawal symptoms. *Clinical Management*: Advise patients taking methadone to avoid concomitant St. John's Wort use. In patients presenting with symptoms of methadone withdrawal or requesting increased methadone doses, inquire about the use of St. John's Wort. If St. John's Wort and methadone are used concomitantly, advise the patient to take a consistent daily dose of St. John's Wort with a reputable product containing a standardized amount of active ingredients of St. John's Wort.

Nefazodone: Concurrent use may result in an increased risk of serotonin syndrome (hypertension, hyperthermia, myoclonus, mental status changes). *Clinical Management*: Avoid concomitant use. Given the half-life of nefazodone and its active metabolites of up to 33 hours, St. John's Wort should be avoided for at least 5 half-lives (6 to 7 days) following nefazodone discontinuation. A two-week washout period is suggested after discontinuing St. John's Wort before starting an SSRI, and may be applied to nefazodone as well.

Nortriptyline: Concurrent use may result in decreased effectiveness of nortriptyline and possible increased risk of serotonin syndrome (hypertension, hyperthermia, myoclonus, mental status changes). *Clinical Management*: Avoid concomitant use of St. John's Wort with nortriptyline.

Olanzapine: Concurrent use may result in reduced olanzapine efficacy. *Clinical Management*: Avoid concomitant use of olanzapine with St. John's Wort. If patients elect to remain on St. John's Wort, they should maintain consistent dosing. Olanzapine dosage may need to be increased. Patients should not discontinue St. John's Wort without first consulting their clinician, as downward adjustments in olanzapine dose may be necessary as well as monitoring for increased side effects of olanzapine (e.g. somnolence, nausea, constipation, dry mouth, asthenia).

Omeprazole: Concurrent use may result in decreased serum concentration of omeprazole. *Clinical Management*: Advise patients taking omeprazole to not start therapy with St. John's wort without consulting their health care provider. Patients taking omeprazole with St. John's wort may require a higher dose of omeprazole to retain effectiveness.

Opioid Analgesics. Concurrent use may result in increased sedation. *Clinical Management*: Caution is advised if St. John's Wort is taken with opioid analgesics. Monitor the patient closely for signs of excessive central nervous system sedation.

Pravastatin: Concurrent use may result in reduced effectiveness of pravastatin. *Clinical Management*: St. John's Wort did not affect the metabolism of pravastatin in one study. However, patients taking St. John's Wort with pravastatin should be monitored for continued lipid-lowering effectiveness. If a patient has been taking pravastatin and St. John's Wort, advise the patient not to stop St. John's Wort without consulting their health care provider, as pravastatin levels may increase, leading to adverse effects.

Reserpine: Concurrent use may result in reduced reserpine effectiveness. *Clinical Management*: Caution is advised if reserpine and St. John's wort are used concomitantly. Monitor for continued effectiveness of reserpine.

Rosuvastatin: Concurrent use may result in reduced effectiveness of rosuvastatin. *Clinical Management*: St. John's Wort may not affect the metabolism of rosuvastatin. However, patients taking St. John's Wort with rosuvastatin should be monitored for continued lipid-lowering effectiveness. If a patient has been taking rosuvastatin and St. John's Wort, advise the patient not to stop St. John's Wort without consulting their health care provider, as rosuvastatin levels may increase, leading to adverse effects.

Serotonin Agonists: Concurrent use may result in additive serotonergic effects and risk of cerebral vasoconstriction disorders. *Clinical Management*: It is recommended to avoid concomitant use of St. John's Wort and serotonin receptor agonists. If both agents are necessary, monitor closely for symptoms of serotonin syndrome and cerebral vasoconstriction.

Simvastatin: Concurrent use may result in reduced effectiveness of simvastatin. *Clinical Management*: Advise patients taking simvastatin not to start therapy with St. John's Wort without consulting their health care provider. Patients taking St. John's Wort with simvastatin may require a higher dose of simvastatin to retain effectiveness. If a patient has been taking simvastatin and St. John's Wort, advise the patient not to stop St. John's Wort without consulting their health care provider, as simvastatin levels may increase, leading to adverse effects.

Sorafenib: Concurrent use of may result in decreased sorafenib concentrations. *Clinical Management*: Coadministration of St. John's wort and sorafenib may result in decreased sorafenib concentrations due to induction of cytochrome P450-mediated sorafenib metabolism by St. John's wort. Use caution if St. John's wort and sorafenib are administered concurrently. Monitor patients for clinical response to sorafenib.

Theophylline: Concurrent use may result in reduced theophylline efficacy. *Clinical Management*: Concomitant use of theophylline with St. John's Wort is not recommended. If patients elect to remain on St. John's Wort, symptoms of decreased theophylline efficacy and theophylline levels should be closely monitored. A stable dose of St. John's Wort is recommended and patients should be advised not to abruptly discontinue St. John's Wort without consulting with their physician. Patients who experience decreased theophylline levels without apparent reason should be questioned about taking St. John's Wort. Theophylline doses may need to be increased to maintain a therapeutic level.

Tramadol: Concurrent may result in decreased tramadol exposure. *Clinical Management*: Monitor patients for tramadol efficacy.

Trycyclic Antidepressants: Concurrent use may result in an increased risk of serotonin syndrome (hypertension, hyperthermia, myoclonus, mental status changes). *Clinical Management*: Avoid concomitant use of St. John's Wort with tricyclic antidepressants.

Venlafaxine: Concurrent use may result in an increased risk of serotonin syndrome (hypertension, hyperthermia, myoclonus, mental status changes). *Clinical Management*: Avoid concomitant use. Given the half-life of venlafaxine of up to 11 hours, St. John's Wort should be avoided for at least 5 half-lives (one to two days) following venlafaxine discontinuation. A two-week washout period is suggested after discontinuing St. John's Wort before starting a SSRI, and may be applied to venlafaxine as well.

Verapamil: Concurrent use may result in reduced bioavailability of verapamil. *Clinical Management*: Caution is advised if St. John's wort and verapamil or similar calcium channel blockers are taken together. Monitor for continued effectiveness of the calcium channel blocker.

MINOR RISK

Barbiturates: Concurrent use may result in decreased central nervous system depressive effect of barbiturates. *Clinical Management*: If patients take St. John's Wort with a barbiturate, monitor for alterations in the therapeutic and adverse effects of the barbiturate.

Chlorzoxazone: Concurrent use may result in reduced chlorzoxazone effectiveness. *Clinical Management*: Monitor patients for continued effectiveness of chlorzoxazone.

POTENTIAL INTERACTIONS

Acitretin: Concurrent use of St. John's Wort and acitretin may result in unplanned pregnancy and birth defects. *Clinical Management:* Avoid concomitant use of St. John's Wort and acitretin in female patients. Advise female patients starting acitretin therapy not to self-medicate with St. John's Wort.

Debrisoquin: Concurrent use of St. John's Wort and debrisoquin may result in reduced debrisoquin effectiveness. *Clinical Management:* Monitor patients taking St. John's Wort with debrisoquin for continued effectiveness of debrisoquin.

Fexofenadine: Investigators concluded that the modest changes in fexofenadine disposition with long term St. John's Wort use would not likely result in a clinically significant drug interaction. Long term administration of St. John's Wort (300 milligrams three times daily for 14 days) did not significantly alter bioavailability of fexofenadine, a selective P-glycoprotein substrate, compared to pretreatment (Wang et al, 2002).

Iron: The tannin content of St. John's Wort may complex with concomitantly administered iron, resulting in nonabsorbable insoluble complexes and may result in adverse sequelae on blood components. *Clinical Management:* It is unknown to what extent the amount of tannin in St. John's Wort may affect iron absorption clinically. Until more is known, patients who need iron supplementation should be advised to separate administration times of these two compounds by one to two hours.

DRUG-FOOD INTERACTIONS

MINOR RISK

Caffeine: Concurrent use of St. John's Wort and caffeine may result in increased caffeine metabolism. St. John's Wort significantly increased metabolism of caffeine, studied as a marker substance for metabolism through cytochrome P450 1A2, after 4 weeks in a randomized, open-label study of 12 healthy subjects (Gurley et al, 2002). In contrast, St. John's Wort did not affect pharmacokinetic parameters of caffeine after 2 weeks in an open-label study of 12 healthy volunteers (Wang et al, 2001).

Tyramine foods: Concurrent use may result in increased risk of hypertensive crisis. *Clinical Management*: The significance of the single case report of hypertensive crisis associated with consumption of St. John's Wort with tyramine containing foods (wine, aged cheese, others) is unknown. Advise patients to use caution if they consume tyramine containing foods while taking St. John's Wort, and to immediately report any unusual symptoms to their health care provider.

DOSAGE

Mode of Administration: Comminuted drug, herb powder, liquid and solid preparations for internal use; liquid and semi-solid preparations for external use; preparations made with fatty oils for external and internal use.

How Supplied:

Capsules - (standardized at 0.3% hypericin) 125mg, 150mg, 250mg, 300mg, 350mg, 370mg, 375mg, 400mg, 424mg, 434mg, 450mg, 500mg, 510mg

Capsules, Extended Release - (standardized at 0.3% hypericin) 450mg, 900mg, 1000mg

Dried Herb

Extract - 1:1

Injection - 1%

Liquid - 300 mg/5ml, 250 mg/ml

Liquid Dilutions - 3x, 6x, 30x, 12c, 30c

Pellets - 3x, 6x, 12x, 12c, 30c

Tablets - (standardized at 0.3% hypericin) 100mg, 150mg, 300mg, 450mg

Tincture - 1:10

Transdermal - 900 mg/24 hr

Preparation: To prepare an infusion, use 2 teaspoonfuls of drug in 150 mL boiling water and steep for 10 minutes.

Daily Dosage: In general, a range of 200 to 1,000 mcg/day of hypericin is recommended for treatment of depression (Anon, 1996). Total hypericin concentrations of Hypericum extracts may vary widely; therefore caution should be taken in determining dosage (Fachinfo Helarium Hypericum, 1996; Fachinfo Remotiv, 1996; Hansgen, 1993; Schmidt & Sommer, 1993; Vorbach, 1994; Woelk, 1994).

For depressive moods, it is recommended the herb be administered for the duration of 4 to 6 weeks; if no improvement is apparent, a different therapy should be initiated.

Depression:

Capsules/tablets - 300 mg of the standardized extract should be administered 3 times daily (Clausson & Muller, 1997; Fachinfo Helarium Hypericum, 1996).

Dried herb - 2 to 4 g taken 3 times daily (Fachinfo Helarium Hypericum, 1996; Fachinfo Remotiv, 1996; Hansgen, 1993; Schmidt & Sommer, 1993; Vorbach, 1994; Woelk, 1994).

Tea - St. John's Wort as a tea is the traditional method of administration, with a single dose of 2 to 3 g dried herb placed in boiling water. If dried herb of 2 g is used, and the dried herb to extract ratio is 6, a usual dose of the extract would be 300 mg (Schultz, 1997).

Liquid extract 1:1 in 25% ethanol - 2 to 4 mL taken 3 times daily (Fachinfo Helarium Hypericum, 1996; Fachinfo Remotiv, 1996; Haensgen, 1993; Schmidt & Sommer, 1993; Vorbach, 1994; Woelk, 1994).

Tincture: (1:10) in 45% ethanol - 2 to 4 mL, 3 times a day (Fachinfo Helarium Hypericum, 1996; Fachinfo Remotiv, 1996; Hansgen, 1993; Schmidt & Sommer, 1993; Vorbach, 1994; Woelk, 1994).

Wounds, bruising, and swelling:

The herb is applied topically and locally for treatment. The activity of the topical preparations is based on the hyperforin content, which is highly variable depending on the method of oil preparation. The preparation may be stable for a few weeks up to 6 months. (Maisenbacher & Kovar, 1992)

Homeopathic Dosage: The daily dosage for homeopathic indications is 5 drops, 1 tablet or 10 globules every 30 to 60 minutes for acute therapy, and 1 to 3 times daily for chronic use. Parenterally, 1 to 2 mL subcutaneously administered 3 times daily for acute therapy and once daily for chronic therapy. The ointment is applied 1 to 2 times daily for acute and chronic use (HAB1).

Storage: Store at room temperature, away from heat, moisture and direct light. *Hyperici oleum* has a limited shelf life. One study showed that a sample containing 62 mg of hyperforin (the active ingredient in the oil) contained no hypericin in 14 days. If sunlight is not used to prepare the oil, then the breakdown is slower, but still less than 30 days. Various oil preparation methods have been described, including one with eutanol G, which showed stability for 6 months. Researchers evaluated 6 commercial samples of oil of Hypericum containing 2.2 to 20.8 milligrams/deciliter. All hyperforin was gone by the end of five weeks (Maisenbacher, 1992).

LITERATURE

Agostinis P, Vandenbogaerde A, Donella-Deana A, et al: Photosensitized inhibition of growth factor-regulated protein kinases by hypericin. *Biochem Pharmacol* 49(11):1615-1622. 1995.

Alscher DM, Klotz U: Drug interaction of herbal tea containing St. John's wort with cyclosporine. *Transpl Int* 16(7):543-544. 2003.

Andreas J, J. Brockmoller, et al: Pharmacokientic interaction of digoxin with an herbal extract from St. John's wort. *Clin Pharm Ther* 66:338-345. 1999.

Anghelescu IG, Kohnen R, Szegedi A, et al. Comparison of Hypericum extract WS 5570 and paroxetine in ongoing treatment after recovery from an episode of moderate to severe depression: results from a randomized multicenter study. Pharmacopsychiatry; 39(6): 213-219. 2006.

Anon: ABDA-Datenbank; WuV, Eschborn and Micromedex, Inc. 1996.

Anon: Another adverse effect with St. John's Wort. *Adverse Drug Reaction Reports* 34:694-696. 1999.

Anon: *Drug Facts & Comparisons.* Facts & Comparisons Inc, St. Louis, MO 264d. 1999.

Anon: Risk of drug interactions with St. John's Wort. *JAMA* 283(13):1679. 2000.

Anon: St. John's Wort: drug interactions and safety. *Alt Med Alert* 3(6):71-72. 2000.

Anon: St. John's wort extract found not helpful for hepatitis C. *Tr Upd* 12(11):4-5. 2001.

Anon: St. John's Wort may influence other medication. Medical Products Agency, Sweden. Feb 6, 2002. Accessed at: http://www3.mpa.se/ieengindex.html (cited 2/14/2002).

Anon: *The Lawrence Review of Natural Products.* Facts and Comparisons, St. Louis, MO. 1995.

Araya OS, Ford EH: An investigation of the type of photosensitization caused by the ingestion of St. John's Wort (hypericum perforatum) by calves. *J Comp Pathol* 91:135-141. 1981.

Baillie N: Hypericum - Four hypersensitivity reactions. *Modern Phytotherapist* 25:1-3. 1998.

Barbagallo C, Chisari G: Antimicrobial activity of three hypericum species. *Fitoterapia* 58(3):175-177. 1987.

Barbanel DM, Yusufi B, O'Shea D, et al: Mania in a patient receiving testosterone replacement post-orchidectomy taking St. John's Wort and sertraline. *J Psychopharmacol* 14:84-86. 2000.

Barone GW, Gurley BJ, Ketel BL, et al: Drug interaction between St. John's Wort and cyclosporine. *Ann Pharmacother* 34(9):1013-1016. 2000.

Bauer S, Stormer E, Johne A, et al: Alterations in cyclosporin A pharmacokinetics and metabolism during treatment with St. John's wort in renal transplant patients. *Br J Clin Pharmacol* 55(2):203-211. 2003.

Beaubrun G, Gray GE. A review of herbal medicines for psychiatric disorders. *Psychiatr Serv* 51(9):1130-1134. 2000.

Beckman SE, Sommi RW, Switzer J. Consumer use of St. John's Wort: A survey on effectiveness, safety, and tolerability. *Pharmacotherapy* 20(5):568-574. 2000.

Beer AM, Ostermann T. Cyclosporine interaction with St. John's Wort (Hypericum perforatum) increases the risk of graft rejection and causes a raise of the daily medication costs. *Med Klinik* 96(8):480-484. 2001.

Behnke K, Jensen GS, Graubaum HJ, et al: Hypericum perforatum versus fluoxetine in the treatment of mild to moderate depression. Adv Ther 19(1):43-52. *Adv Ther* 19(1):43-52. 2002.

Berghofer R, Holzl J. Bioflavonoids in Hypericum perforatum. Part 1. Isolation of 13,II8-biapigenin. *Planta Med* 53: 216-217. 1987.

Berghofer R, Holzl J. Isolation of 13',II8-biapigenin (amentoflavone) from *Hypericum perforatum. Planta Med* 55:91. 1989.

Bergmann R, Nubner JC, Demling J. Behandlung leichter bis mittelschwerer depressionen. *Therapiewoche Neurologie-Psychiatrie* 7:235-240. 1993.

Bhattacharya S, Chakrabart A, Chatterjee S. Activity profiles of two hyperforin-containing hypericum extracts in behavioral models. *Pharmacopsychiatry* 31(supp):22-29. 1998.

Biber A, Fischer H, Romer A, et al: Oral boavailability of hyperforin from hypericum extracts in rats and human volunteers. *Pharmacopsychiatry* 31(supp):36-43. 1998.

Biffignandi PM, Bilia AR: The growing knowledge of St. John's Wort (*Hypericum perforatum L.*) drug interactions and their clinical significance. *Curr Ther Res* 61(7):389-394. 2000.

Bisset NG: *Herbal Drugs and Phytopharmaceuticals: A Handbook for Practice on a Scientific Basis.* Medpharm Scientific Publishers, CRC Press, Stuttgart, Germany, 1994.

Bjerkenstedt L, Edman GV, Alken RG, Mannel M. Hypericum extract LI 160 and fluoxetine in mild to moderate depression: a randomized, placebo-controlled multicenter study in outpatients. *Eur Arch Psychiatry Clin Neurosci*; 255(1): 40-47. 2005.

Bladt S, Wagner H: Inhibition of MAO by fractions and constituents of hypericum extract. *J Geriat Psych Neurol* 7(1):57-59. 1994.

Blumenthal M, Busse WR, Goldberg A, et al: *The Complete German Commission E Monographs.* American Botanical Council, Austin, TX 214-215. 1998.

Blumenthal M, Goldberg A, Brinckmann J (eds): *Herbal Medicine, Expanded Commission E monographs*, 1st ed. Integrative Medicine Communications, Newton, MA; 2000.

Bolley R, Zulke C, Kammerl M, et al: Tacrolimus-induced nephrotoxicity unmasked by induction of the CYP3A4 system with St. John's Wort. *Transplantation* 73(6):1009. 2002.

Bombardelli E, Morazzoni P: Hypericum perforatum. *Fitoterapia* 66(1):43-68. 1995.

Bork P, Bacher S, Schmitz M, et al: Hypericin as a non-oxidant inhibitor of NF-kB. *Planta Med* 65:297-300. 1999.

Bourke CA: Sunlight associated hyperthermia as a consistent and rapidly developing clinical sign in sheep intoxicated by St. John's Wort (hypericum perforatum). *Aust Vet J* 78(7):483-488. 2000.

Bove G. Acute neuropathy after exposure to sun in a patient treated with St John's Wort. *Lancet* 352(9134):1121-1122. 1998.

Brantner A, Kartnig T, Quehenberger F. Vergleichende phytochemische Untersuchungen an *Hypericum perforatum* L., und *Hypericum maculatum* (Crantz). *Sci Pharm* 62:261-276. 1994.

Breidenbach T, Hoffmann MW, Becker T, et al: Drug interaction of St. John's Wort with cyclosporine (letter). *Lancet* 355(9218):1912. 2000.

Breidenbach T, Kliem V, Burg M, et al: Profound drop of cyclosporin A whole blood trough levels caused by St. John's Wort (Hypericum perforatum). *Transplantation* 69(10):2229-2230. 2001.

Brenner R, Azbel V, Madhusoodanan S, et al: Comparison of an extract of hypericum (LI 160) and sertraline in the treatment of depression: a double-blind, randomized pilot study. *Clin Ther* 22(4):411-419. 2000.

Brenner R, Madhusoodanan S, Pawlowska M. Efficacy of continuation treatment with hypericum perforatum in depression. *J Clin Psychiatry* 63(5):455. 2002.

Briggs GG, Freeman RK, Yaffe SJ. St. John's Wort. In: *Drugs in Pregnancy and Lactation Update* 12(3):17-19. 1999.

Brinker F. *Herb Contraindications and Drug Interactions*, 2nd ed. Eclectic Medical Publications, Sandy, OR. 1998.

Brinker F. *The Toxicology of Botanical Medicines*, 2nd ed. Eclectic Medical Publications, Sandy, OR. 1983.

Brockmoller J, Reum T, Bauer S, et al: Hypericin and pseudohypericin: pharmacokinetics and effects on photosensitivity in humans. *Pharmacopsychiat* 30 (Suppl):94-101. 1997.

Brolis M, Gabetta B, Fuzzati N, et al: HPLC-DAD-MS identification and HPLC-UV quantification of the major constituents of Hypericum perforatum. *Fitoterapia* 69(5):27-28. 1998.

Brondz I. n-Alkanes of Hypericum perforatum: revision. *Phytochemistry* 22: 295-296. 1983.

Brown D. St. John's Wort extract continues to compare favorably to SSRIs. *Healthnotes* 7(3):192-193. 2000.

Brown TM. Acute St. John's Wort toxicity (letter). *Am J Emer Med* 18(2):231-232. 2000a.

Budzinski JW, Foster BC, Vandenhoek S, et al: An in vitro evaluation of human cytochrome P450 3A4 inhibition by selected commercial herbal extracts and tinctures. *Phytomedicine* 7(4):273-282. 2000.

Burstein AH, Horton RL, Dunn T, et al: Lack of effect of St. John's Wort on carbamazepine pharmacokinetics in healthy volunteers. *Clin Pharmacol Ther* 68(6):605-612. 2000.

Butterweck V, Nahrstedt A, Evans J, et al: In vitro receptor screening of pure constituents of St. John's Wort reveals novel interactions with a number of GPCRs. *Psychopharmacology* (Berl) 162(2): 193-202. 2002.

Butterweck V, Wall A, Lieflaender-Wulf U, et al: Effects of the total extract and fractions of *Hypericum perforatum* in animal assays for antidepressant activity. *Pharmacopsychiatry* 30:117-124. 1997.

Calapai G, Crupi A, Firenzuoli F, et al: Effects of *Hypericum perforatum* on levels of 5-hydroxytryptamine, noradrenaline and dopamine in the cortex, diencephalon and brainstem of the rat. *J Pharm Pharmacol* 51:723-728. 1999.

Carpenter S, Kraus G: Photosensitization is required for inactivation of equine infectious anemia virus by hypericin. *Photochem Photobiol* 53(2):169-174. 1991.

Chatterjee S, Noldner M, Koch E, et al: Antidepressant activity of hypericum perforatum and hyperforin: the neglected possibility. *Pharmacopsychiatry* 31(supp):7-15. 1998.

Chatterjee SS, Bhattacharya SK, Singer A, et al: Hyperforin inhibits synaptosomal uptake of neurotransmitter in vitro and shows antidepressant activity in vivo. *Pharmazie* 53 (suppl. 1): 9. 1998.

Chatterjee SS, Bhattacharya SK, Wonnemann M et al: Hyperforin as a possible antidepressant component of hypericum extracts. *Life Sci* 63(6):499-510. 1998.

Colker CM, Kalman DS, Torina GC, et al: Effects of Citrus aurantium extract, caffeine, and St. John's Wort on body fat loss, lipid levels, and mood states in overweight healthy adults. *Curr Ther Res* 60(3):145-153. 1999.

Constantine GH, Karechesy J. Variations in hypericin concentrations in *Hypericum perforatum L.* and commercial products. *Pharmaceutical Biol* 36(5):365-367. 1998.

Cooper WC, James J. An observational study of the safety and efficacy of hypericin in HIV+ subjects. *Int Conf AIDS* 6(2):369 (abstract 2063). 1990.

Cott JM. In vitro receptor binding and enzyme inhibition by *Hypericum perforatum* extract. *Pharmacopsychiatry* 30(suppl):108-112. 1997.

Cott J. Natural products formulations available in Europe for psychotropic indications. *Psychopharmacology* Bull 31(4):745-751. 1995.

Crowe S, McKeating K. Delayed emergence and St. John's Wort. *Anesthesiology* 96(4):1025-1027. 2002.

Czekalla J, Gaastpar M, Hubner WD, et al: The effect of hypericum extract on cardiac conduction as seen in the electrocardiogram compared to that of imipramine. *Pharmacopsychiatria* 20(S):86-88. 1997.

Dannawi M. Possible serotonin syndrome after combination of buspirone and St. John's Wort. *J Psychopharmacol* 16(4):401. 2002.

Davidson JT, Connor KM. St. John's Wort in generalized anxiety disorder: three case reports (letter). *J Clin Psychopharmacol* 21(6): 635-636. 2001.

Decosterd LA, et al: Isolation of new cytotoxic constituents from Hypericum revolutum and Hypericum calycinum by liquid-liquid chromatography. *Planta Med* 54: 560. 1988.

De Maat MR, Hoetelmans RW, Mathot RA, et al: Drug interaction between St. John's Wort and nevirapine. *AIDS* 15(3):420-421. 2001.

Demisch L, Holzl J, Gollnik B, et al: Identification of selective MAO-type A inhibitors in *Hypericum perforatum L.* (Hyperforat®). *Pharmacopsychiatry* 22:194. 1989.

DeMott K. St John's Wort tied to serotonin syndrome. *Clin Psychiatry* 26:28. 1998.

Denke A, Schempp H, Weiser D, et al: Biochemical activities of extracts from hypericum perforatum L. 5th communication: dopamine- beta-hydroxylase product quantification by HPLC and inhibition by hypericins and flavonoids. *Arzneim-Forsch Drug Res* 50(5):415-419. 2000.

DeSmet PM, Touw DJ. Safety of St. John's Wort (*Hypericum perforatum*) (letter). *Lancet* 355(9203):575-576. 2000.

DeSmet PA, Nolen W. St. John's Wort as an antidepressant. *BMJ* 313:241-242. 1996.

Dimpfel W, Schober F, Mannel M. Effects of a methanolic extract and a hyperforin-enriched CO2 extract of St. John's wort (Hypericum perforatum) on intracerebral field potentials in the freely moving rat (tele-stereo-EEG). *Pharmacopsychiatry* 31(supp):30-35. 1998.

Dittmer T. Die Behandlung von psychovegetativen Stoerungen mit Johanniskraut-Oel (Jukunda-Rot-Oel-Kapseln). *Naturheilpraxis* 2:118-122. 1991.

Duran N, Song P-S. Hypericin and its photodynamic action. *Photochem Photobiol* 43(6): 677-680. 1986.

Durr D, Stiger B, Kullak-Ublick GA, et al: St. John's Wort induces intestinal P-glycoprotein/MDR1 and intestinal and hepatic CYP3A4. *Clin Pharmacol Ther* 68(6):598-604. 2000.

Eich-Hochli D, Oppliger R, Golay KP, et al: Methadone maintenance treatment and St. John's Wort. *Pharmacopsychiatry* 36(1):35-37. 2003.

Erdelmeier C: Hyperforin, possibly the major non-nitrogenous secondary metabolite of *Hypericum perforatum L. Pharmacopsychiatry* 31(supp):2-6. 1998.

Ernst E. Second thoughts about safety of St. John's Wort. *Lancet* 354(9195):2014-2015. 1999.

Ernst E. St. John's Wort, an antidepressant? A systemic, criteria based review. *Phytomedicine* 2(1):67-71. 1995.

Fachinformation. Cesradyston® 200, hypericum extract. Cesara-Arzneimittelfabrik GmbH & Co, Baden-Baden. 1997.

Fachinformation. Esbericum® forte, hypericum extract. Schaper & Bruemmer GmbH & Co, KG, Salzgitter. 1997.

Fachinformation. Helarium® Hypericum, hypericum extract. Bionorica GmbH, Neumarkt. 1996.

Fachinformation. Hyperimerck® 260 mg, hypericum extract. Merck Generika GmbH, Darmstadt. 1997.

Fachinformation. Remotiv®, hypericum extract. Bayer AG, Pharma Deutschland, Leverkusen. 1996.

Fava M, Alpert J, Nierenberg AA, et al. A double-blind, randomized trial of St. John's wort, fluoxetine, and placebo in major depressive disorder. J Clin Psychopharmacol; 25(5): 441-447. 2005.

Ferko N, Levine MA. Evaluation of the Association between St. John's Wort and elevated thyroid-stimulating hormone. *Pharmacotherapy* 21(12):1574-1578. 2001.

Gaster B, Holroyd J. St. John's Wort for depression: a systematic review. *Arch Intern Med* 160(2):152-156. 2000.

Gastpar M, Singer A, Zeller K. Efficacy and tolerability of hypericum extract STW3 in long-term treatment with a once-daily dosage in comparison with sertraline. *Pharmacopsychiatry*: 38(2): 78-86. 2005.

Gastpar M, Singer A, Zeller K. Comparative efficacy and safety of a once-daily dosage of hypericum extract STW3-VI and citalopram in patients with moderate depression: a double-blind, randomized, multicentre, placebo-controlled study. *Pharmacopsychiatry*; 39(2): 66-75. 2006.

Giese AC. Hypericism. *Photochem Photobiol Rev* 5(6):229-255. 1980.

Gill M, LoVecchio F, Selden B. Serotonin syndrome in a child after a single dose of fluvoxamine. *Ann Emerg Med* 33:457-459. 1999.

Gordon J. SSRIs and St. John's Wort: possible toxicity? *Am Fam Physician* 57(5):950-953. 1998.

Gorski J, Hamman M, Wang Z, et al: The effect of St. John's Wort on the efficacy of oral contraception (abstract MPI-80). *Clin Pharmacol Ther* 71(2):P25. 2002.

Graber MA, Hoehns TB, Perry PJ: Sertraline-phenelzine drug interaction: a serotonin syndrome reaction. *Ann Pharmacother* 28:732-735. 1994.

Grube B, Walper A, Wheatley D. St. John's wort extract: efficacy for menopausal symptoms of psychological origin. *Adv Ther* 16(4):177-186. 1999.

Grush LR, Nierenberg A, Keefe B, et al: St. John's Wort during pregnancy. *JAMA* 280(18):1566. 1998.

Gulick R, McAuliffe V, Holden-Wiltse J, et al: Phase 1 studies of hypericin, the active compound in St. Johns Wort, as an antiretroviral agent in HIV-infected adults. *Ann Intern Med* 130(6):510-514. 1999.

Gurley BJ, Gardner SF, Hubbard MA, et al: Cytochrome P450 phenotypic ratios for predicting herb-drug interactions in humans. *Clin Pharmacol Ther* 72(3):276-287. 2002.

Hainsgen KD, Vesper J, Ploch M. Multicenter double-blind study examining the antidepressant effectiveness of the hypericum extract LI 160. *Nervenheilkunde* 12(6A):285-289. 1993.

Halama P. Wirksamkeit des Johanniskrautextraktes LI 160 bei depressiver Verstimmung. Plazebokontrollierte Doppelblindstudie mit 50 Patienten. *Nervenheilkunde* 10:250-253. 1991.

Hansgen KD, Vesper J. Antidepressive Wirksamkeit eines hochdosierten Hypericum-Extraktes. *Munch Med Wschr* 138(3):29-33. 1996.

Harrar G, Huebner WD, Podzuweit H. Effectiveness and tolerance of the hypericum extract LI 160 compared to maprotiline: a multicenter double-blind study. *J Geriatr Psychiatry Neurol 7* (suppl 1): S24-S28. 1994.

Harrar G, Schmidt U, Kuhn U, et al: Alternative Depressionsbehnadlung mit einem HypericumExtrakt. TW *Neurologie Psychiatrie* 5:710-716. 1991.

Harrer G, Schmidt U, Kuhn U, et al: Comparison of equivalence between the St. Johns Wort extract LoHyp-57 and fluoxetine. *Arzneimittelforschung* 49(4):289-296. 1999.

Harrer G, Sommer H: Treatment of mild/moderate depressions with Hypericum. *Phytomed* 1:3-8. 1994.

Hauben M. The association of St. John's wort with elevated thyroid-stimulating hormone. *Pharmacotherapy* 22(5):673-675. May 2002. (Summation available at http://www.medscape.com/viewarticle/434468.)

Hebert MF, Park JM, Chen YL, et al: Effects of St. John's Wort (*Hypericum perforatum*) on tacrolimus pharmacokinetics in healthy volunteers. *J Clin Pharmacol* 44:89-94. 2004.

Hennessy M, Kelleher D, Spiers JP, et al: St. John's Wort increases expression of P-glycoprotein: implications for drug interactions. *Br J Clin Pharmacol* 53(1):75-82. 2002.

Hiller K, Rahlfs V. Therapeutische Aequivalenz eines hochdosierten Phytopharmakons mit Amitriptylin bei aengstlich-depressiven Verstimmungen - Reanalyse einer randomisierten Studie unter besonderer Beachtung biometrischer und klinischer Aspekte. *Forsch Komplementaermed* 2:123-132. 1995.

Hobbs C. St. John's wort. Hypericum perforatum L. *HerbalGram* 18/19:24-33. 1988.

Hoelzl J, Demisch L, Gottnik B: Investigations about antidepressive and mood changing effects of *Hypericum perforatum. Planta Med* 55:643. 1989.

Hoelzl J, Ostrowski E: Analysis of the essential compounds of *Hypericum perforatum. Planta Med* 6:531. 1986.

Holme SA, Roberts DL. Erythroderma associated with St. John's wort. *Br J Dermatol* 143(5):1127-1128. 2000.

Holzl J, Demisch L, Stock S. Comparison of the hypericin and peroxide concentration of commercial and self-produced oleum hyperici and its effect on serotonin uptake. *Planta Med* 55:601-602. 1989.

Hubner WD, Kirste T. Experience with St. John's wort (*Hypericum perforatum*) in children under 12 years with symptoms of depression and psychovegetative disturbances. *Phytother Res* 15(4):367-370. 2001.

Hudson J, Graham E, Towers G. Antiviral assays on phytochemicals: The influence of reaction parameters. *Planta Med* 60:329-332. 1994.

Huebner WD, Lande S, Podzuweit H. Hypericum treatment of mild depressions with somatic symptoms. *J Geriatric Psychiatry Neurol* 7(suppl 1):S12-S24. 1994.

Hunt EJ, Lester CE, Lester EA, et al: Effect of St. John's wort on free radical production. *Life Sci* 69(2):181-190. 2001.

Hussain MD. Saint John's Wort and analgesia: effect of St. John's Wort on morphine induced analgesia. *AAPS* Pharm Sci 2(2):Abstract 1810. 2000.

Hypericum Depression Trial Study Group. Effect of *hypericum perforatum* (St. John's Wort) in major depressive disorder. *JAMA* 287(14):1807-1814. 2002.

Irefin S, Sprung J. A possible cause of cardiovascular collapse during anesthesia: Long-term use of St. John's Wort. *J Clin Anesth* 12:498-499. 2000.

Ishiguro K, Yamaki M, Kashihara M, et al: A chromene from Hypericum japonicum. *Phytochemistry* 29:1010-1011. 1990.

Ishiguro K, Yamaki M, Kashihara M, et al: Saroaspidin A, B, and C - additional antibiotic compounds from *Hypericum japonicum. Planta Med* 53(5):415-417. 1987.

Ishiguro K, Yamaki M, Kashihara M, et al: Sarothalin G - a new antimicrobial compound from *Hypericum japonicum. Planta Med* 56(3):274-276. 1990a.

Ishiguro K, Yamaki M, Kashihara M, et al: Sarothralen A & B, new antibiotic compounds from *Hypericum japonicum. Planta Med* 52:288-290. 1986.

Jacobson JM, Feinman L, Liebes L, et al: Pharmacokinetics, safety, and antiviral effects of hypericin, a derivative of St. John's wort plant, in patients with chronic hepatitis C virus infection. *Antimicrob Agents Chemother* 45(2):517-524. 2001.

Jayasuriya H, McChesney JD, Swanson SM, et al: Antimicrobial and cytotoxic activity of rotterin-type compounds from *Hypericum drummondii. J Nat Prod* 52(2):325-331. 1989.

Johne A, Brockmoller J, Bauer S, et al: Pharmacokinetic interaction of digoxin with an herbal extract from St. John's Wort (*hypericum perforatum*). *Clin Pharmacol Ther* 66(4):338-345. 1999.

Johnson D, Ksciuk H, Woelk H, et al: Effects of Hypericum extract LI 160 compared with maprotiline on resting EEG and evoked potentials in 24 volunteers. *J Geriat Psych Neurol* 7(1):44-46. 1994.

Johnson D, Siebenhuner G, Hofer E, et al: Einfluss von Johanniskraut auf die ZNS-Aktivitaet. Ergebnisse einer Studie mit dem Johanniskraut-Extrakt LI 160. *Neurol Psychiat* 6:436-444. 1992.

Jokovljevic V, Popovic M, Mimica-Dukic N, et al: Pharmacodynamic study of Hypericum perforatum L. *Phytomedicine* 7(6):449-453. 2000.

Josey ES, Tackett RL. St. John's Wort: a new alternative for depression? *Int J Clin Pharmacol Ther* 37(3):111-119. 1999.

Kasper S, Anghelescu IG, Szegedi A, et al. Superior efficacy of St. John's wort extract WS 5570 compared to placebo in patients with major depression: a randomized, double-blind, placebo-controlled, mutli-center trial. *BMC Med*; 4: 14. 2006.

Karliova M, Treichel U, Malago M, et al: Interaction of *hypericum perforatum* (St. John's Wort) with cyclosporin A metabolism in a patient after liver transplantation. *J Hepatol* 33(5):853-855. 2000.

Kerb R, Bauer J, Brockmoller J, et al: Urinary 6 beta-hydroxycortisol excretion rate is affected by treatment with hypericum extract (Abstract). *Eur J Clin Pharmacol* 52:A186. 1992.

Kerb R, Brockmoller J, Staffeldt B, et al: Single-dose and steady-state pharmakokinetics of hypericin and pseudohypericin. *Antimicrob Agents and Chemother* 40(9):2087-2093. 1996.

Khawaja IS, Marotta RF, Lippmann S. Herbal medicines as a factor in delirium (letter). *Psychiatr Serv* 50(7):969-970. 1999.

Khosa RL, Bhatia N. Antifungal effects of *Hypericum perforatum Linn. J Sci Res Plant & Med* 3(2-3):49-50. 1982.

Kil KS, Yum YN, Seo SH, et al: Antitumor activities of hypericin as a protein tyrosine kinase blocker. *Arch Pharm* Res 19(6):490-496. 1996.

Kim HL, Streltzer J, Goebert D. St. John's Wort for depression: a meta-analysis of well-defined clinical trials. *J Nerv Ment Dis* 187(9):532-539. 1999.

Klier CM, Schafer MR, Schmid-Siegel B, et al: St. John's Wort (*Hypericum perforatum*)-is it safe during breastfeeding? *Pharmacopsychiatry* 35(1):29-30. 2002.

Kniebel R, Burchard J. Zur Therapie depressiver Verstimmungen in der Praxis. Multizentrischer Doppelblindvergleich des Baldrian-Johanniskraut-Konzentrats mit dem Standard- Antidepressivum Amitriptylin. Z *Allg Med* 64:689-696. 1988.

Kolesnikova AG. Bacterial and immunocorrective properties of plant extracts. *Zh Mikrobiol Epidemiol Immunobiol* 3:75-78. 1986.

Konopa J, Jereczek E, Matuszkiewicz A, et al: Screening of antitumor substances from plants. *Arch Immunol Ther Exp* 15:129-132. 1967.

Laakmann G, Schule C, Baghai T, et al: St. John's Wort in mild to moderate depression: the relevance of hyperforin for the clinical efficacy. *Pharmacopsychiatry* 31(suppl):54-59. 1998.

Ladner DP, Klein SD, Steiner RA, et al: Synergistic toxicity of delta-aminolaevulinic acid-induced protoporphyrin IX used for photodiagnosis and hypericum extract, a herbal antidepressant. *Br J Dermatol* 144(4):916-918. 2001

Lal S, Iskandar H. St. John's Wort and schizophrenia. *Can Med Assn J* 163(3):262-263. 2000.

Lantz M, Buchalter E, Giambanco V. St. John's Wort and antidepressant drug interactions in the elderly. *J Geriatr Psychiatry Neurol* 12(1):7-10. 1999.

Lecrubier Y, Clerc G, Didi R, et al: Efficacy of St. John's Wort extract WS 5570 in major depression: a double-blind, placebo-controlled trial. *Am J Psychiatry* 159(8):1361-1366. 2002.

Lehrl S, Willemsen A, Papp R et al: Results from measurements of the cognitive capacity in patients during treatment with hypericum extract. *Nervenheilkunde* 12:281-284. 1993.

Lenoir S, Degenring F, Saller R. A double-blind randomised trial to investigate three different concentrations of a standardized fresh plant extract obtained from the shoot tips of *Hypericum perforatum L. Phytomed* 6(3):141-146. 1999.

Leuschner G. Preclinical toxicology profile of Hypericum extract LI 160 (abstract). *Phytomedicine Int J Phytother Phytopharmacol* 3(suppl 1):104. 1996/1997.

Levine M, Ferko N. The association of St. John's Wort with elevated thyroid-stimulating hormone (reply). *Pharmacotherapy* 22(5):675. 2002.

Lieberman S. Nutriceutical review of St. John's Wort (*Hypericum perforatum*) for the treatment of depression. *J Women's Health* 7(2):177-181. 1998.

Linde K, Mulrow CD. St. John's Wort for depression (Cochrane Review). In: The Cochrane Library, Issue 3, 2000. Oxford: Update Software. 2000.

Linde K, Mulrow CD, Berner M, et al. St John's Wort for depression (Review). Cochrane Database of Systematic Reviews 2. CD000448: 2005.

Linde K, Knuppel L. Large-scale observational studies of hypericum extracts in patients with depressive disorders—a systematic review. *Phytomed*; 12: 148-157. 2005.

Linde K, Ramirez G, Mulrow CD, et al: St. John's Wort for depression - an overview and meta-analysis of randomized clinical trials. *BMJ* 313(7052):253-258. 1996.

Lopez-Bazzocchi I, Hudson JB, Towers GN. Antiviral activity of the photoactive plant pigment hypericin. *Photochem Photobiol* 54(1):95-98. 1991.

Lumpkin M. Public Health Advisory: Risk of drug interactions with St. John's Wort and indinavir and other drugs. Feb 10, 2000. Accessed at: http://www.fda.gov/cder/drug/advisory/sjwort.htm. (cited 2/10/2000).

Mai I, Kruger H, Budde K, et al: Hazardous pharmacokinetic interaction of Saint John's Wort (*Hypericum perforatum*) with the immunosuppressant cyclosporin. *Int J Clin Pharm Thera* 38(10):500-502. 2000.

Mai I, Stormer E, Bauer S, et al: Impact of St. John's Wort treatment on the pharmacokinetics of tacrolimus and mycophnolic acid in renal transplant patients. *Nephrol Dial Transplant* 18:819-822. 2003.

Maisenbacher HJ, Kuhn U. Therapie von Depressionen in der Praxis. Ergebnisse einer Anwendungsbeobachtung mit Herba Hyperici. *Natura Med* 7(5):394-399. 1992.

Maisenbacher P, Kovar KA. Analysis and stability of *Hyperici Oleum. Planta Med* 58(4):351-354. 1992.

Mandelbaum A, Pertzborn F, Martin-Facklam M, et al: Unexplained decrease of cyclosporin trough levels in a compliant renal transplant patient. *Nephrol Dial Transplant* 15(9):1473-1474. 2000.

Markowitz JS, Devane CL, Boulton DW, et al: Effect of St. John's Wort (*Hypericum perforatum*) on cytochrome P450 2D6 and 3A4 activity in healthy volunteers. *Life Sci* 66(9):133-139. 2000.

Markowitz JS, Donovan JL, DeVane CL, et al: Effect of St. John's Wort on drug metabolism by induction of cytochrome P450 3A4 enzyme. *JAMA* 290(11):1500-1504. 2003.

Martinez B, Kasper S, Ruhrmann S, et al: Hypericum in the treatment of seasonal affective disorders. J *Geriat Psych Neurol* 7(1):29-33. 1994.

Mathew NT, Tietjen GE, Lucker C. Serotonin syndrome complicating migraine pharmacotherapy. *Cephalalgia* 16:323-332. 1996.

Mathijssen RHJ, Verweij J, DeBruijn P, et al: Effects of St. John's Wort on irinotecan metabolism. *J Natl Cancer Inst* 94(16):1247-1249. 2002.

Maurer A, Johne A, Bauer S, et al: Interaction of St. John's wort extract with phenprocoumon (abstract). *Eur J Clin Pharmacol* 55:A22. 1999.

McGuffin M, Hobbs C, Upton R et al (eds): *The American Herbal Products Association's Botanical Safety Handbook: Guidelines for the Safe Use and Labeling for Herbs in Commerce*. CRC Press, Boca Raton, FL. 1997.

McTaggart F, Buckett L, Davidson R, et al: Preclinical and clinical pharmacology of rosuvastatin, a new 3-hydroxy-3-methylglutaryl coenzyme A reductase inhibitor. *Am J Cardiol* 87(suppl):28B-32B. 2001.

Melzer R, Fricke U, Holzl J et al: Proanthrocyanidins from *Hypericum perforatum* - effects on isolated pig coronary arteries. *Planta Med* 55:572-573. 1988.

Melzer R, Fricke U, Holzl J, et al: Procyanidins from *Hypericum perforatum*: Effects on isolated guinea pig hearts. *Planta Med* 55:655-656. 1989.

Melzer R, Fricke U, Holzl J, et al: Vasoactive properties of procyanidins from *Hypericum perforatum L.* in isolated porcine coronary arteries. *Arzneimittelforschung* 41(5 pt 1):481-483. 1991.

Meruelo D, Lavie D, Lavie E. Therapeutic agents with dramatic antiretroviral activity and little toxicity at effective doses. Aromatic polycyclic diones hypericin and pseudohypericin. *Proc Natl Acad Sci* USA 85:5230-5234. 1989.

Miller ER. The volatile oil of *Hypericum perforatum. J Am Pharm Assoc* 16(9):824-828. 1924.

Mishenkova EL. Antiviral properties of St. John's wort and preparations produced from it. *Tr S'ezda Mikrobiol Ukr* 222-223. 1975.

Moore LB, Goodwin B, Jones SA, et al: St. John's Wort induces hepatic drug metabolism through activation of the pregnane X receptor. *Proc Nat Acad Sci* 97(13):7500-7502. 2000.

Moschella C. Jaber BL. Interaction between cyclosporine and *Hypericum perforatum* (St. John's Wort) after organ transplantation. Am J Kidney Dis 38(5):1105-1107. 2001.

Mueller WE, Schaefer C: Johanniskraut. In vitro Studie ueber Hypericum- Extrakt, Hypericin, und Kaempferol als Antidepressiva. *Dtsch Apoth Z* 136:1015-1022. 1996.

Muldner VH, Zoller M. Antidepressive Wirkung eines auf den Wirkstoffkomplex Hypericin standardisierten Hypericum-Extraktes. Biochemische und lkinische Untersuchungen. *Arzneimittelforschung* 34(8): 918-920. 1984.

Muller T, Mannel M, Murck H, et al. Treatment of somatoform disorders with St. John's Wort: a randomized, boudl-blind, and placebo-controlled trial. *Psychosomat Med*; 66: 538-547. 2004.

Muller JL, Clauson KA. Pharmaceutical considerations of common herbal medicine. *Am J Man Care* 3(11):1753. 1997.

Muller WE, Rolli M, Schafer C, et al: Effects of Hypericum extract (LI 160) in biochemical models of antidepressant activity. *Pharmacopsychiatry* 30(Suppl):102-107. 1997.

Muller W, Rossol R: Effects of hypericum extract on the expression of serotonin receptors. J *Geriat Psych Neurol* 7(1):63-64. 1994.

Muller W, Singer A, Wannemann M, et al: Hyperforin represents the neurotransmitter reuptake-inhibiting constituent of hypericum extract. *Pharmacopsychiatry* 31:16-21. 1998.

Murch S, Simmons C, Saxena P: Melatonin in feverfew and other medicinal plants. *Lancet* 350(9091):1598-1599. 1997.

Murphy PA. St. John's Wort and oral contraceptives: reasons for concern? *J Midwifery Womens Health* 47(6):447-450. 2002.

Nebel A, Schneider BJ, Baker RK, et al: Potential metabolic interaction between St. John's Wort and theophylline. *Ann Pharmacother* 33(4):502. 1999.

Negrash AK. Comparative study of chemotherapeutic and pharmacological properties of antimicrobial preparation from common St. John's wort. *Fitontsidy Mater Soveshch* 198-200. 1969.

Newall CA, Anderson LA, Phillipson JD. Herbal Medicines. A Guide for Health-care Professionals. Pharmaceutical Press, London, UK; 1996.

Niesel S, Schilcher H. Johanniskraut. Vergleich der Freisetzung von Hypericin und Psuedohypericin in Abhaengigkeit verschiedener Extraktbedingungen. *Arch Pharm* 323(9):755. 1990.

Noldner M, Schotz K. Rutin is essential for the antidepressant activity of Hypericum extracts in the forced swimming test. *Planta Med.* 68(7):577-580. 2002.

Obach RS. Inhibition of human cytochrome P450 enzymes by constituents of St. John's Wort, an herbal preparation used in the treatment of depression. *J Pharmacol Exp Ther* 294(1):88-95. 2000.

O'Breasail AM, Argouarch S. Hypomania and St. John's Wort (letter). *Can J Psychiatry* 43(7):746-747. 1998.

Okpanyi SN, Lidzba H, Scholl BC, et al: Genotoxizitaet eines standardisierten Hypericum-Extraktes. *Arzneimittelforschung* 40(8 pt 2):851-855. 1990.

Okpanyi VN, Weischer ML. Tierexperimentelle Untersuchungen zur psychotropen Wirksamkeit eines Hypericum-Extraktes. *Arzneimittel-Forsch* 37(1):10-13. 1987.

Ondrizek R, Chan P, Patton W. An alternative medicine study of herbal effects on the penetration of zona-free hamster oocytes and the integrity of sperm deoxyribonucleic acid. *Fertil Steril* 71(3):517-522. 1999.

Osterheider M, Schmidtke A, Beckmann H. Behandlung depressiver Syndrome mit Hypericum (Johanniskraut - Eine placebokontrollierte Doppelblindstudie. *Fortschr Neurol Psychiat* 60(2):210-211. 1992.

Ozturk Y, Aydin S, Baser KC, et al: Hepatoprotective activity of *Hypericum perforatum L.* alcoholic extract in rodents. *Phytother Res* 6:44-46. 1992.

Ozturk Y, Aydin S, Beis R, et al: Effects of Hypericum perforatum L. and Hypericum calycinum L. extracts on the central nervous system in mice. *Phytomedicine* 3(2):139-146. 1996.

Panijel M. Die Behandlung mittelschwerer Angstzustaende. Randomisierte Doppelblindstudie zum klinischen Wirksamskeitvergleich eines Phytotherapeutikums mit Diazepam. *Therapiewoche* 41:4659-4668. 1985.

Panossian AG, Gabrielian E, Manvelian V, et al: Immunosuppressive effects of hypericin on stimulated human leukocytes: inhibition of the arachidonic acid release, leukotriene B4 and interleukin-1 alpha production, and activation of nitric oxide formation. *Phytomedicine* 3(1):19-28. 1996.

Patel S, Robinson R, Burk M: Hypertensive crisis associated with St. John's Wort. *Am J Med* 112(6):507-508. 2002.

Peebles KA, Baker RK, Kurz Eu, et al: Catalytic inhibition of human DNA topoisomerase IIalpha by hypericin, a naphthodianthrone from St. John's Wort. *Biochem Pharmacol* 62(8):1059-1070. 2001.

Perovic S, Muller WG. Pharmacological profile of Hypericum extract. Effect on serotonin uptake by postsynaptic receptors. *Arzneimittelforschung* 45(11):1145-1148. 1995.

Philipp M, Kohnen R, Hiller KO. Hypericum extract versus imipramine or placebo in patients with moderate depression: randomized multicentre study of treatment for eight weeks. *BMJ* 319(7224):1534-1538. 1999.

Pieschel D, Angersbach P, Toman M. Zur Behandlung von Depressionen. Verbundstudie mit einem pflanzlichen Extrakt aus Johanniskraut. *Therapiewoche* 39:2567-2571. 1989.

Pilkington K, Boshnakova A, Richardson J. St John's wort for depression: Time for a different perspective? *Comp Ther Med*; 14: 268-281. 2006.

Piscitelli S, Burstein A, Chaitt D, et al: Indinavir concentrations and St. John's Wort. *Lancet* 355(9203):547-548. 2000.

Poginsky B, Westendorf, J, Prosenc N, et al: Johanniskraut (Hypericum perforatum L.) Genotoxizitaet bedingt durch den Quercetingehalt. *Dtsch Apoth Ztg* 128:(126) 1364-1366. 1988.

Product Information: Amerge (naratriptan hydrochloride). Glaxo Wellcome Inc, Research Triangle Park, NC. 1999.

Product Information: Cordarone (amiodarone). Wyeth-Ayerst, Philadelphia, PA; (PI revised 08/2001) reviewed 12/2003.

Product Information: Femring (estradiol acetate). Warner Chilcott Inc, Rockaway, NJ; revised 4/2002.

Product Information: Gleevec (imatinib mesylate). Novartis Pharmaceuticals, East Hanover, NJ; 2003.

Product Information: Imitrex (sumatriptan tablets). Glaxo Wellcome Inc, Research Triangle Park, NC; 1999.

Product Information: Maxalt-MLT (rizatriptan benzoate orally disintegrating tablets). Merck & Co, West Point, PA; 1998.

Product Information: Ortho Evra (norelgestromin/ethinyl estradiol). Ortho-McNeil Pharmaceutical, Inc, Raritan, NJ; (PI revised 11/2001) reviewed 3/2002.

Product Information: Prograf (tacrolimus). Fujisawa Healthcare, Inc, Deerfield, IL; (PI revised 10/2001) reviewed 11/2001.

Product Information: Reyataz (atazanavir). Bristol-Myers Squibb Company, Princeton, NJ (PI issued 6/2003) reviewed 7/2003.

Product Information: Soriatane (acitretin). Roche Laboratores, Inc, Nutley, NJ; 4/2003.

Product Information: Zomig (zolmitriptan tablets). Zeneca Pharmaceuticals, Wilmington, DE; 1999.

Prost N, Tichadou L, Rodor F, et al: Interaction millepertuis-venlafaxine (Article in French). *Presse Med* 29:1285-1286. 2000.

Quandt J, Schmidt U, Schenk N. Ambulante Behandlung leichter und mittelschwerer depressiver Verstimmungen. *Allgemeinarzt* 2:97-102. 1993.

Raffa RB. Screen of receptor and uptake-site activity of hypericin component of St. John's Wort reveals sigma receptor binding. *Life Sci* 62(16):PL265-PL270. 1998.

Rao SG, Laxminarayana AU, Saraswathi LU, et al: Calendula and Hypericum: two homeopathic drugs promoting wound healing in rats. *Fitoterapia* 6:508-510. 1991.

Rayburn WF, Christensen HD, Gonzalez CL. Effect of antenatal exposure to Saint John's Wort (hypericum) on neurobehavior of developing mice. *Am J Obstet Gynecol* 183(5):1225-1231. 2000.

Reh C, Laux P, Schenk N. Hypericum-Extrakt bei Depressionen - eine wirksame Alternative. *Therapiewoche* 42(25):1576-1581. 1992.

Reichling J, Weseler A, Saller R. A current review of the antimicrobial activity of *Hypericum perforatum L. Pharmacopsychiatry* 34(supp 1):116-118. 2001.

Roby CA, Anderson GD, Kantor E, et al: St. John's Wort: effect on CYP3A4 activity. *Clin Pharmacol Ther* 67(5):451-457. 2000.

Roots I, Johne A, Schmider J, et al: Interaction of a herbal extract from St. John's Wort with amitriptyline and its metabolites (abstract). *Clin Pharmacol Ther* 67(2):159. 2000.

Roots T. Evaluation of photosensitization of the skin and multiple dose intake of Hypericum extract. Second International Congress on Phytomedicine. Munich, Germany. 1996.

Ruschitzka F, Meier P, Turina M, et al: Acute heart transplant rejection due to St. John's wort. *Lancet* 355:548-549. 2000.

Sakar MK, et al: Antimicrobial activities of some Hypericum species growing in Turkey. *Fitoterapia* 59:49-52. 1988.

Sarrell EM, Cohen HA, Kahan E. Naturopathic treatment for ear pain in children. *Pediatrics* 111(5):e574-e579. 2003.

Sarrell EM, Mandelberg A, Cohen HA. Efficacy of naturopathic extracts in the management of ear pain associated with acute otitis media. *Arch Pediatr Adolesc Med* 155(7):796-799. 2001.

Schellenberg R, Sauer S, Dimpfel W. Pharmacodynamic effects of two different hypericum extracts in healthy volunteers measured by quantitative EEG. *Pharmacopsychiatry* 31:44-53. 1998.

Schempp CM, Ludtke R, Winghofer B, et al: Effect of topical application of hypericum perforatum extract (St. John's Wort) on skin sensitivity to solar stimulated radiation. *Photodermatol Photoimmunol Photomed* 16(3):125-128. 2000.

Schempp CM, Muller K, Windhofer B, et al: Single-dose and steady-state administration of hypericum perforatum extract (St. John's Wort) does not influence skin sensitivity to UV radiation, visible light, and solar- stimulated radiation. *Arch Dermatol* 137(4):512-513. 2001.

Schempp M, Hezel S, Simon C. Topical treatment of atopic dermatitis with Hypericum cream: a randomized, placebo-controlled, double-blind half-side comparison study. *Hautarzt* 54(3):248-253. 2003.

Schmidt U, Harrer G, Kuhn U, et al: Interaction of hypericum extract with alcohol. Placebo controlled study with 32 volunteers. *Nervenheilkunde* 12:314-319. 1993.

Schmidt U. Konstantes Reaktionsvermoegen unter antidepressiver Therapie mit Hypericum Praeparat LI 160. Nervenheilkunde 10:311-312. 1991.

Schmidt U, Sommer H. Johanniskraut-Extract zur ambulanten Therapie der Depression. *Fortschr Med* 111(19):339-342. 1993.

Schrader E, Meier B, Brattstrom A. Hypericum treatment of mild-moderate depression in a placebo-controlled study. A prospective, double-blind, randomized, placebo-controlled, mulitcentre study. *Hum Psychopharmacol Clin Exp* 13:163-169. 1998.

Schule C, Baghai A, Ferrera A, et al: Neuroendocrine effects of hypericum extract WS 5570 in 12 healthy male volunteers. *Pharmacopsychiatry* 34(supp 1):127-133. 2001.

Schulz V. Safety of St. John's Wort extract compared to synthetic antidepressants. *Phtyomed;* 13:199-204. 2006.

Schulz H, Jobert M. Effects of hypericum extract on the sleep EEG in older volunteers. *J Geriat Psych Neurol* 7(1):39-43. 1994.

Schulz V, Huebner WD, Ploch M. Clinical trials with phytopsychopharmacological agents. *Phytomedicine* 4(4):379-387. 1997.

Schwarz UI, Buschel B, Kirch W: Unwanted pregnancy on self-medication with St. John's wort despite hormonal contraception (letter). *Br J Clin Pharmacol* 55(1):112-113. 2003.

Serkedjieva J, Manolova N, Nowosielska IZ, et al: Antiviral activity of the infusion (SHS-174) from flowers of Sambucus nigra L, aerial parts of Hypericum perforatum, and roots of Saponaria officinalis L. against influenza and Herpes simplex viruses. *Phytother Res* 4:97-101. 1990.

Shelton RC, Keller MB, Gelenberg A, et al: Effectiveness of St. John's Wort in major depression, a randomized controlled trial. *JAMA* 285(15):1978-1986. 2001.

Shiplochliev T, Dimitrov V, Aleksandrova E. Anti-inflammatory action of a group of plant extracts. *Vet Med Nauki* 18(6): 87-94. 1981.

Shiplochliev T. Extracts from a group of medicinal plants enhancing the uterine tonus. *Vet Med Nauki* 18(8): 94-98. 1981a.

Siegers CP, Biel S, Wilhelm KP. Phototoxicity caused by hypericum. *Nervenheilkunde* 12:320-322. 1993.

Siepman M, Krause S, Joraschky P, et al: The effects of St. John's wort extract on heart rate variability, cognitive function and quantitative EEG: a comparison with amitriptyline and placebo in healthy men. *Br J Clin Pharmacol* 54(3):277-282. 2002.

Singer A, Wonnemann M, Muller WE. Hyperforin, a major antidepressant constituent of St. John's wort, inhibits serotonin uptake by elevating free intracellular Na+. *J Pharmacol Exp Ther* 290(3):1361-1368. 1999.

Singhal AB, Caviness VS, Begleiter AF, et al: Cerebral vasoconstriction and stroke after use of serotonergic drugs. *Neurology* 58(1):130-133. 2002.

Smith M, Lin KM, Zheng YP. An open trial of nifedipine-herb interactions: nifedipine with St. John's Wort, ginseng, or Ginkgo biloba (abstract). *Clin Pharmacol Ther* 69(2):P86. 2001.

Sommer H, Harrer G: Placebo-controlled double-blind study examining the effectiveness of an Hypericum preparation in 105 mildly depressed patients. *J Geriatr Psychiatry Neurol* 7 (suppl 1):S9-S11. 1994.

Southwell IA, Campbell MH: Hypericin content variation in *Hypericum perforatum* in Australia. *Phytochemistry* 30(2):475-478. 1991.

Spinella M, Eaton LA. Hypomania induced by herbal and pharmaceutical psychotropic medicines following mild traumatic brain injury. i 16(4):359-367. 2002.

Staffeldt B, Kerb R, Brockmoller J, et al: Pharmacokinetics of hypericin and pseudohypericin after oral intake of the hypericum perforatum extract LI 160 in healthy volunteers. *J Geriat Psych Neurol* 7(1):47-53. 1994.

Steger W. Depressive Verstimmungen. Randomisierte Doppelblindstudie zum Wirksamskeitvergleich einer pflanzlichen Wirkstoffkombination und eines synthetischen Antidepressivums. *Z Allg Med* 61:914-918. 1985.

Sternbach H. Danger of MAOI therapy after fluoxetine withdrawal (letter). *Lancet* 2:850-851. 1988.

Sternbach H. The serotonin syndrome. i 148:705-713. 1991.

Stevinson C, Dixon M, Ernst E. Hypericum for fatigue - a pilot study. *Phytomedicine* 5(6):443-447. 1998.

Stevinson C, Ernst E. A pilot study of Hypericum perforatum for the treatment of premenstrual syndrome. *Br J Obstet Gynaecol* 107(7):870-876. 2000.

Stock S, Holzl J. Pharmacokinetic test of (14 C)-labeled hypericin and pseudohypericin from Hypericum perforatum and serum kinetics of hypericin in man. *Planta Med* 57 (suppl 2): A61-A62. 1991.

Sugimoto K, Ohmori M, Tsuruoka S, et al: Different effects of St. John's Wort on the pharmacokinetics of simvastatin and pravastatin. *Clin Pharmacol Ther* 70(6):518-524. 2001.

Suzuki O, Katsumata Y, Oya M, et al: Inhibition of monoamine oxidase by hypericin. *Planta Med* 50(3): 272-274. 1984.

Szegedi A, Kohnen R, Dienel A, et al. Acute treatment of moderate to severe depression with hypericum extract WS 5570 (St John's wort): randomized controlled double blind non-inferiority trial versus paroxetine. BMJ; 330(7490): 503. 2005.

Thiede HM, Walper A. Inhibition of MAO and COMT by hypericum and hypericum extracts. *J Geriatr Psychiatry Neurol* 7 (suppl 1):S54-S56. 1994.

Thiele B, Brink I, Ploch M. Modulation of cytokine expression by hypericum extract. *J Geriatr Psychiatry Neurol* 7(suppl 1):S60-S62. 1994.

Uebelhack R, Blohmer JU, Graubaum HJ, et al. Black cohosh and St. John's wort for climacteric complaints: a randomized trial. Obstet Gynecol; 107(2 Pt)1): 247-255. 2006.

Uebelhack R, Gruenwald J, Graubaum HJ, Busch R. Efficacy and tolerability of Hypericum extract STW 3-VI in patients with moderate depression: a double-blind, randomized, placebo-controlled clinical trial. Adv Ther; 21(4): 265-275. 2004.

Uehleke B, Mueller SC, Uehleke B, et al: Interaction of St. John's Wort with digoxin, the relation to dosage and formulation (abstract). *Phytomedicine* 7(SII):20. 2000.

Upton R (ed): St. John's Wort, Hypericum perforatum: quality control, analytical and therapeutic monograph. Am Herbal Pharmacopoeia, Santa Cruz, CA. 1-32. 1997.

van Gurp G, Meterissian GB, Haiek LN, et al: St John's wort or sertraline? *Can Fam Physician* 48:905-912. 2002.

Vasilchenko EA. Analgesic action of flavonoids of Rhododendron luteum Sweet, *Hypericum perforatum L.,* Lespedeza bicolor Turcz. and L. hedysaroides (Pall.) Kitag. *Rastit Resur* 1986; 22:12-21. 1986.

Verotta L, Appendino G, Belloro E, et al: Furohyperforin, a prenylated phloroglucinol from St. John's wort (*Hypericum perforatum*). *J Nat Prod* 62:770-772. 1999.

Vitiello B. *Hypericum perforatum* extracts as potential antidepressants. J Pharm Pharmacol 51(5):513-517. 1999.

Volz HP. Controlled clinical trials of hypericum extracts in depressed patients - an overview. *Pharmacopsychiatry* 30 (suppl):72-76. 1997.

Vorbach EU, Arnold KH, Hubner WD. Efficacy and tolerability of St. John's Wort extract hypericum extract LI 160 in patients with severe depressive incidents according to ICD-10. *Pharmacopsychiatry* 30 (suppl 1):S81-S85. 1997.

Vorbach EU, Huebner WD, Arnoldt KH. Effectiveness and tolerance of the hypericum extract LI 160 in comparison with imipramine: randomized double- blind double-blind study to 135 outpatients. *J Geriatr Psychiatry Neurol* 7(suppl 1): S19-S23. 1994.

Voss A, Verweij P. Antibacterial activity of hyperforin from St. John's wort. *Lancet* 354:777. 1999.

Wagner H, Bladt S. Pharmaceutical quality of hypericum extracts. *J Geriatr Psychiatry Neurol* 7 (suppl 1):S65-S68. 1994.

Waksman JC, Heard K, Jolliff H, et al: Serotonin syndrome associated with the use of St. John's Wort (*Hypericum perforatum*) and paroxetine (abstract). *Clin Toxicol* 38(5):521. 2000.

Wang Z, Gorski JC, Hamman MA, et al: The effects of St. John's Wort (Hypericum perforatum) on human cytochrome P450 activity. *Clin Pharmacol Ther* 70(4):317-326. 2001.

Wang Z, Hamman MA, Huang SM, et al: Effect of St. John's wort of the pharmacokinetics of fexofenadine. *Clin Pharmacol Ther* 71(6): 414-420. 2002.

Warnecke G. Beeinflussung klimakterischer Depressionen. Therapieergebnisse mit Hypericin (Johanniskraut-Extract). *Z Allg Med* 62:1111-1113. 1986.

Wentworth JM, Agostini M, Love J, et al: St. John's Wort, a herbal antidepressant, activates the steroid X receptor. *J Endocrinol* 166(3):R11-R16. 2000.

Werth W. Psychotonin(R) versus Imipramin in der Chirurgie. *Der Kassenarzt* 15(64):64-68. 1989.

Wheatley D. Hypericum extract: potential in the treatment of depression. *CNS Drugs* 9(6):431-440. 1998.

Wheatley D. Hypericum in seasonal affective disorder (SAD). *Curr Med Res Opin* 15(1):33-37. 1999.

Wheatley D. LI 160, an extract of St. John's Wort, versus amitriptyline in mildly to moderately depressed outpatients - a controlled 6-week clinical trial. *Pharmacopsychiatry* 30(suppl II):S77-S80. 1997.

Whitten DL, Myers SP, Hawrelak JA, et al. The effect of St. John's wort extract on CYP3A: a systematic review of prospective clinical trials. Br J Clin Pharmacol; 62: 5: 1365-2125. 2006.

Winterhoff H, Hambrugge M, Vahlensieck U. Pharmacological screening of *Hypericum perforatum L.* in animals. *Nervenheilkunde* 12:341-345. 1993.

Woelk H, Burkard G, Gruenwald J. Benefits and risks of the Hypericum extract LI 160: drug monitoring with 3250 patients. *J Geriatr Psychiatry Neurol* 7(suppl 1):534-538. 1994.

Woelk H. Comparison of St. John's Wort and imipramine for treating depression: randomised controlled trial. *BMJ* 321:536-539. 2000.

Wonnemann M, Singer A, Muller WE. Inhibition of synaptosomal uptake of H-L-glutamate and H- GABA by hyperforin, a major constituent of St. John's Wort: the role of amiloride sensitive sodium conductive pathways. *Neuropsychopharmacology* 23(2):188-197. 2000.

Wood S, Huffman J, Weber N, et al: Antiviral activity of naturally occurring anthraquinones and anthraquinone derivatives. *Planta Med* 56:651-652. 1990.

Yu DK. The contribution of P-glycoprotein to pharmacokinetic drug-drug interactions. *J Clin Pharmacol* 39:1203-1211. 1999.

Yue QY, Bergquist C, Gerden B. Safety of St. John's Wort (Hypericum perforatum) (letter). *Lancet* 355(9203):576-577. 2000.

Zanoli P, Truzzi C, Cannazza G, et al: Evidence that hypericum perforatum extracts exert anxiolytic effects in rats. *Fitoterapia* 69(5):30. 1998.

Zhang W, Lawa R, Hintona D, et al: Growth inhibition and apoptosis in human neuroblasoma SK-N-SH cells induced by hypericin, a potent inhibitor of protein kinase C. *Cancer Lett* 96:31-35. 1995.

Stone Root

Collinsonia canadensis

DESCRIPTION

Medicinal Parts: The medicinal parts of the plant are the fresh or dried roots and rhizomes.

Flower and Fruit: The flowers are dirty yellow, labiate, with red venation on the inside in richly blossomed panicles. The upper lip has an obtuse tip. The side tips of the lower lip are small and rounded; the middle tips are larger and fringed. The calyx is acuminate and has 2 stamens. The fruit is a small globose nutlet.

Leaves, Stem, and Root: The plant is a perennial that grows 90 to 120 cm high. The rhizome is grayish-brown, very hard, fibrous, and up to 8 cm long. The shoots are glabrous, often tinged red, with few side shoots. The bark is very thin. The leaves are light green above and pale green, glabrous, broad, cordate, or ovate below, becoming narrower and shorter above.

Characteristics: The smell is strongly aromatic and unpleasant. The taste is unpleasantly bitter.

Habitat: The plant is indigenous to North America from Canada to the Carolinas in the U.S. It is also found in central Europe.

Production: Stone Root, the rhizome and root of *Collinsonia canadensis*, is gathered and dried in autumn.

Other Names: Archangel, Canadian Horsemint, Hardback, Hardhack, Horseweed, Heal-All, Knob Grass, Knob Root, Knobweed, Richweed, Richleaf, Rock-Weed

ACTIONS AND PHARMACOLOGY

COMPOUNDS

Volatile oil: chief components are caryophyllene, germacrene D, limonene, alpha- and beta-pinenes

Caffeic acid derivatives: including rosmaric acid

EFFECTS

Stone Root has stomachic, tonic, and diuretic effects, probably due to the presence of the essential oil and rosmaric acid.

INDICATIONS AND USAGE

Unproven Uses: Stone Root is used for gastrointestinal disorders, kidney stones, and bladder inflammation.

Homeopathic Uses: Preparations of *Collinsonia canadensis* are used for hemorrhoids and constipation.

DOSAGE

Mode of Administration: The drug is used internally as an extract, infusion, or tincture.

Preparation: Liquid extract (1:1) 1 mL to 4 mL; tincture (1:5) 2 mL to 8 mL.

Daily Dosage: The drug is generally used as a single dose, 1 to 4 g, internally as an infusion.

Homeopathic Dosage: 5 to 10 drops, 1 tablet, or 5 to 10 globules 1 to 3 times daily; or 1 mL injection solution sc twice weekly (HAB1).

LITERATURE

Joshi BS, Moore KM, Pelletier SW, Saponins from *Collinsonia canadensis*. In: *JNP* 55(10):1468-1476. 1992.

Lamaison JL, Petitjean-Freytet C, Duke JA, Walker J. Hydroxycinnamic Derivative Levels and antioxidant Activity in North American Laminaceae. *Plant med et phyt.* 26; 143-148. 1993

Hänsel R, Keller K, Rimpler H, Schneider G (Hrsg.), Hagers Handbuch der Pharmazeutischen Praxis, 5. Aufl., Bde 4-6 (Drogen), Springer Verlag Berlin, Heidelberg, New York, 1992-1994.

Madaus G, Lehrbuch der Biologischen Arzneimittel, Bde 1-3, Nachdruck, Georg Olms Verlag Hildesheim 1979.

Wolters B, Zierpflanzen aus Nordamerika. In: DAZ 137(26):2253-2261. 1997.

Storax

Liquidambar orientalis

DESCRIPTION

Medicinal Parts: The medicinal part is the balsam from the trunk and the inner bark.

Flower and Fruit: The flowers and inflorescences are unisexual, monoecious, and arranged in small, round, solitary capitula. The flowers are yellow. The male flowers show no signs of a calyx or corolla. The female flowers have tiny scaly sepals, and the floret tubes are fused. There are numerous stamens, and the ovary is semi-inferior. The fruit is a hard, globular schizocarp.

Leaves, Stem, and Root: Liquidambar orientalis is a deciduous tree about 12 m tall with many branches and a thick reddish-gray bark. It has alternate, usually 5-lobed leaves. The leaf blades are roughly toothed.

Characteristics: Raw Storax is a thick, viscous, sticky, aromatic, and somewhat bitter-tasting gray-brown substance. When stored, the drug becomes more clear, an effect caused by a reduction in the water content.

Habitat: The tree is indigenous from Asia Minor to Syria.

Production: Storax (amber tree balm) is extracted from *Liquidambar orientalis*. To extract the balsam, the trunk is beaten, causing the bark to soak up the exuding resin. The bark is then boiled and the resulting decoction further refined.

Not to be Confused With: Fir resin, turpentine, colophony, or olive oil

Other Names: Balsam Styracis, Sweet Gum, Copalm, Gum Tree, Levant Storax, Liquid Amber, Opossum Tree, Red Gum, White Gum

ACTIONS AND PHARMACOLOGY

COMPOUNDS

Aromatic alcohols: phenylpropyl-, cinnamic-, benzyl alcohol

Cinnamic acid (up to 30%): cinnamic acid esters, including among others cinnamylcinnamate (styracine), cinnamic acid ethyl esters

Styrene

Triterpenes: oleanolic acid, 3-epioleanolic acid (resin fraction)

Vanillin (up to 2%)

Volatile oil (depending upon source, 1 to 20%): with styrol, benzyl alcohol, cinnamic alcohol

EFFECTS

Storax has anti-inflammatory, diaphoretic, and stimulant effects.

INDICATIONS AND USAGE

Unproven Uses: Storax is used for coughs and bronchitis as an inhalation, externally for wounds and ulcers.

Chinese Medicine: In China, Storax is used in the treatment of syncope, epilepsy, and lactose intolerance in young children.

Indian Medicine: In India, Storax is used for itching, suppurating wounds, leprosy, chronic coughs, and fever.

PRECAUTIONS AND ADVERSE REACTIONS

No health hazards are known in conjunction with the proper administration of designated therapeutic dosages. Internal administration of the drug occasionally leads to diarrhea. Storax can also trigger contact allergies.

OVERDOSAGE

External administration over large areas can lead to absorptive poisonings that are characterized by kidney damage (albuminuria, hemorrhagic nephritis).

DOSAGE

Mode of Administration: Storax is used in combination preparations for coughs and bronchitis as an inhalation, externally for wounds and ulcers.

LITERATURE

Hänsel R, Keller K, Rimpler H, Schneider G (Hrsg.), Hagers Handbuch der Pharmazeutischen Praxis, 5. Aufl., Bde 4-6 (Drogen), Springer Verlag Berlin, Heidelberg, New York, 1992-1994.

Leung AY, Encyclopedia of Common Natural Ingredients Used in Food Drugs and Cosmetics, John Wiley & Sons Inc., New York 1980.

Lewin L, Gifte und Vergiftungen, 6. Aufl., Nachdruck, Haug Verlag, Heidelberg 1992.

Mitscher LA, Telikepalli H, McGhee E, Shankel DM. Natural antimutagenic agents. *Mutation Res.* 350; 143-152. 1996

Strawberry

Fragaria vesca

DESCRIPTION

Medicinal Parts: The medicinal parts are dried leaves collected during the flowering season, the dried rhizome, and ripe fruit.

Flower and Fruit: The small white flowers are arranged on a repeatedly bifurcated pedicle. They are usually androgynous. There are 5 sepals and 5 petals. The sepals are triangular, pointed, or appressed pubescent. The petals are oribicular or ovate, glabrous, and pure white. There are 20 stamens and numerous ovate, glabrous carpels and a style at the side. After flowering the receptacle turns into a fleshy false fruit. The receptacle is 2 cm long, ovate, globular or clavate, and red when ripe. The nutlets are ovate, 0.8 to 1.5 mm long, brown and matte.

Leaves, Stem, and Root: The perennial, herbaceous plant grows from 20 to 30 cm high. The rhizome is cylindrical, horizontal, or crooked and thickly covered with the residual dead leaves and stipules. Long runners grow from the axils of the basal leaves. The stem is erect and is slightly longer than the basal leaves. The cauline leaves are trifoliate and roughly serrate from the first quarter upward. The petioles are very long and, like the stem, have patent hairs. The stipules are lanceolate, long-acuminate, entire-margined, reddish brown, glabrous above and hairy beneath.

Habitat: Found in almost all of the temperate zones of Europe and Asia.

Production: Strawberry leaf consists of the dried leaf of *Fragaria* species, mainly *Fragaria vesca*. The leaves are collected in the wild and air-dried in a shady place.

Not to be Confused With: Other *Fragaria* species, although they have the same value.

Other Names: Alpine Strawberry, Mountain Strawberry, Wild Strawberry, Wood Strawberry

ACTIONS AND PHARMACOLOGY

COMPOUNDS

Caffeic acid derivatives: including chlorogenic acid

Flavonoids: including rutin, quercetin

Tannins: ellagic acid tannins, oligomeric proanthocyanidins

EFFECTS

Strawberry leaf has astringent and diuretic properties; but no studies are available.

INDICATIONS AND USAGE

Unproven Uses: Preparations of strawberry leaf are used externally as compresses for rashes, and internally for catarrh of the gastrointestinal tract, diarrhea, intestinal sluggishness, liver disease, jaundice, catarrh of the respiratory tract, gout, rheumatoid arthritis, nervous tension, kidney ailments involving gravel and stones, and as a diuretic. Because of the tannin content, its efficacy in treating mouth and throat inflammation and diarrhea is plausible.

PRECAUTIONS AND ADVERSE REACTIONS

Health risks or side effects following the proper administration of designated therapeutic dosages are not recorded. The drug should not be taken in presence of strawberry allergy.

DOSAGE

Mode of Administration: Strawberry leaves are only used occasionally in folk medicine; the berries are used more commonly.

Preparation: Pour boiling water over 1 g of comminuted drug and strain after 5 to 10 minutes.

Decoction — boil 375 g green leaves with 1.15 liter water until only 550 mL remains.

Infusion — add 4 g drug to 150 mL boiling water.

Extract — boil 20 g drug with 500 mL water until only half remains.

Daily Dosage: Tea: As an antidiarrheal agent, several cups per day.

Decoction — for diarrhea, 1 teaspoon every 3 to 4 hours.

Extract — for diarrhea, a spoonful before bed and on rising.

Infusion — one dose only for children with diarrhea. The decoction is used as a gargle.

LITERATURE

Hänsel R, Keller K, Rimpler H, Schneider G (Hrsg.), Hagers Handbuch der Pharmazeutischen Praxis, 5. Aufl., Bde 4-6 (Drogen), Springer Verlag Berlin, Heidelberg, New York, 1992-1994.

Lund K, Dissertation Universität Freiburg i. Br. 1986.

Teuscher E, Biogene Arzneimittel, 5. Aufl., Wiss. Verlagsges. mbH Stuttgart 1997.

Vennat B, Pourrat A, Pourrat H, Gross D, Bastide P, Bastide J. Procyanidins from the Roots of Fragaria vesca: Characterization and Pharmacological Approach. *Chem Pharm Bull.* 36 (2); 828-833. 1988

Wichtl M (Hrsg.), Teedrogen, 4. Aufl., Wiss. Verlagsges. Stuttgart 1997.

Strophanthus

Strophanthus species

DESCRIPTION

Medicinal Parts: The medicinal parts are the ripe seeds that have been removed from their appendages and dried. Most of the species are poisonous.

Flower and Fruit: The flowers are in terminal or lateral panicles with few flowers or in richly blossomed, umbelliferous panicles. They appear in groups of fine and are white or yellowish, radially symmetrical, and sometimes fragrant. The calyx has 5 elliptical/lanceolate to obovate sepals and a short tube with a campanulately splayed upper part, which has 10 scales on the margin. The anthers are acute with a partly tailed middle section. The ovary is bivalved, semi-inferior, and has numerous ovules. The fruit has 1 to 2 follicles, which are oblong, 8 to 58 cm long, splayed or horizontal on one level. The greenish-brown seeds are 8 to 25 mm long, fusiform, and often flattened. The seeds have an awnlike appendage and a long tuft of hair at the base, which eventually drops off.

Leaves, Stem and Root: The plants are climbing lianes, occasionally erect shrubs, subshrubs, or trees. They contain milky latex. The leaves are opposite, ovate to elliptical, short-petioled, simple, entire-margined,and usually coriaceous.

Habitat: Strophanthus is indigenous to tropical Africa.

Production: Strophanthus seeds are the seeds of *Strophanthus gratus*. Kombe-Strophanthus seeds are the seeds of *Strophanthus kombé*. The plant is harvested mostly by African tribes in the wilderness or in protected areas in the vicinity of African settlements.

Not to be Confused With: Strophanthi semen should not be confused with African Strophantus species.

Other Names: Kombé

ACTIONS AND PHARMACOLOGY

COMPOUNDS: STROPHANTHUS GRATUS SEEDS

Cardioactive steroid glycosides (cardenolides, 3-8%): chief glycoside strophanthin-G (ouabain, over 80%), further including acolongifloroside K, strogoside, among others

Saponins (0.2%)

Fatty oil (35%)

EFFECTS: STROPHANTHUS GRATUS SEEDS

The active agent, Strophanthin-G, is a cardioactive glycoside that has actions similar to digitalis, but is milder. No clinical test results are available. The drug is poorly absorbed by the gastrointestinal tract.

COMPOUNDS: STROPHANTHUS KOMBE SEEDS

Cardioactive steroid glycosides: (cardenolides, 4.0-4.5%, the mixture known as Strophanthin-K) chief glycoside K-strophanthoside (60-80%), erysimoside (15-25%), strophoside, (10-15%)

Saponins (0.2%)

Fatty oil (35%)

EFFECTS: STROPHANTHUS KOMBE SEEDS

The effects are similar to *Strophanthus gratus,* but milder.

INDICATIONS AND USAGE

STROPHANTHUS GRATUS SEEDS

Unproven Uses: Strophanthus is used for arteriosclerosis, cardiac insufficiency, gastrocardial symptoms, hypertension, and neurodystonia.

Homeopathic Uses: Strophanthus gratus is used for cardiac insufficiency and anxiety.

PRECAUTIONS AND ADVERSE REACTIONS

General: No health hazards are known in conjunction with the proper administration of designated therapeutic dosages. Queasiness, vomiting, headache, stupor, disturbance of color vision, and cardiac arrhythmias could occur as side effects, in particular through overdosages connected with parenteral administration of strophanthin-G or glycoside mixtures.

DRUG INTERACTIONS

POTENTIAL INTERACTIONS

Simultaneous administration of quinidine, calcium salts, saluretics, laxatives, and glucocorticoids may enhance both effects and side effects.

OVERDOSAGE

Queasiness, vomiting, headache, stupor, disturbance of color vision and cardiac arrhythmias are the most likely consequences of overdosage, which is more likely to occur with parenteral administration of strophanthin-G or glycoside mixtures.

For a review of symptoms of an acute poisoning and therapy, see *Digitalis folium.* The danger of poisoning after oral administration is relatively low, due to the poor absorption of the glycosides.

DOSAGE

STROPHANTHUS GRATUS SEEDS

Mode of Administration: The drug is available as injection solutions and capsules and in combination preparations.

Preparation: A tincture is prepared by using 1 part coarsely ground powder (previously specially treated) stabilized for content with 10 parts 70% ethanol (V/V) (DAB6)

Daily Dosage: Tincture daily dose is 1.5 g. The single dose is 0.5 g.

Homeopathic Dosage: From D4: 5 drops, 1 tablet, or 10 globules (from D2); Tincture: single dose: 0.5 g and daily dose: 1.5 g.

STROPHANTHUS KOMBE SEEDS

Mode of Administration: The drug is available in monopreparations, and is rarely used in combinations.

Homeopathic Dosage: From D4: 5 drops, 1 tablet, or 10 globules (from D2) every 30 to 60 minutes (acute) or 1 to 3 times daily (chronic); parenterally: 1 to 2 mL sc, acute: 3 times daily; chronic: once a day (HAB1).

LITERATURE

STROPHANTHUS GRATUS SEEDS AND STROPHANTHUS KOMBE SEEDS

Brisse B, Anwendung pflanzlicher Wirkstoffe bei kardialen Erkrankungen. In: *ZPT* 10(4):107. 1989.

Norton SA. Useful plants of dermatology. III. Corticosteroids Strophanthus and Dioscorea. *J Am Acad Dermatol*, 38:256-9, Feb 1998

Strophanthus hispidus

See Kombe Seed

Strophanthus species

See Strophanthus

Strychnos ignatii

See Ignatius Beans

Strychnos nux vomica

See Nux Vomica

Styrax benzoin

See Benzoin

Styrax paralleloneurum

See Sumatra Benzoin

Styrax tonkinensis

See Siam Benzoin

Sumatra Benzoin

Styrax paralleloneurum

DESCRIPTION

Medicinal Parts: The medicinal part of the plant is the balsamic resin obtained from the damaged trunk.

Flower and Fruit: Styrax paralleloneurum is a tree that grows up to 35 m high. The flowers are small, the corolla is violet, and the calyx is 3 to 4.5 mm high. The fruit is 5 to 9 mm in diameter.

Leaves, Stem, and Root: The leaves are ovate or lanceolate and 6 to 16 cm long.

Habitat: Sumatra

Production: Sumatra Benzoin (Gum Benzoin) is the balsamic resin from the damaged trunk of *Styrax benzoin* and *Styrax paralleloneurum.* The optimal age of a tree to be harvested is 7 years. The tree is cut, which causes it to exude resin to heal the cuts. The resin is then collected in a vessel and left in the sun to melt to a homogenous mass.

ACTIONS AND PHARMACOLOGY

COMPOUNDS

Ester mixture (70 to 80%): composed of coniferyl benzoate and cinnamyl benzoate, as well as cinnamyl cinnamoate (styracine), propyl cinnamoate

Phenylacrylic acids: cinnamic acid (10 to 20%)

Vanillin (0.4 to 0.6%)

Triterpenes: including sumaresinolic acid

EFFECTS

Sumatra Benzoin has a mild expectorant effect possibly due to its vanilla content.

INDICATIONS AND USAGE

Unproven Uses: Preparations of the resin have been used for respiratory catarrh.

Chinese Medicine: Sumatra Benzoin preparations are used for stroke, syncope, postpartum syncope due to heavy loss of blood, and chest and stomach pain.

PRECAUTIONS AND ADVERSE REACTIONS

No health hazards are known in conjunction with the proper administration of designated therapeutic dosages.

DOSAGE

Mode of Administration: Whole herb preparations for internal use.

Storage: Should be tightly sealed and stored below 25° C.

LITERATURE

Bacchi EM, Sertié JA, Villa N, Katz H. delta7-stigmasteryl-3 betaD-glucoside from *Styrax officinalis*. Part II. *Planta Med*, 61:221-2, Nov 1976

Bacchi EM, Sertié JA, Villa N, Katz H. Preliminary investigations on the herba of *Styrax officinalis*. I. *Planta Med*, 61:290-3, Nov 1973

Hänsel R, Keller K, Rimpler H, Schneider G (Ed), Hagers Handbuch der Pharmazeutischen Praxis, 5. Aufl., Bde 4 - 6 (Drogen), Springer Verlag Berlin, Heidelberg, New York, 1992-1994.

James WD, White SW, Yanklowitz B, Allergic contact dermatitis to compound tincture of benzoin. *J Am Acad Dermatol*, 11:847-50, Nov. 1984

Pastorova I, Koster CG de, Boon JJ. Analytical Study of Free and Ester Bound Benzoic and Cinnamic Acids of Gum Benzoin Resins by GC-MS and HPLC-frit FAB-MS. *Phytochem Anal*. 8; 63-73. 1997

Sumbul

Ferula sumbul

DESCRIPTION

Medicinal Parts: The medicinal part is the rhizome with the roots.

Leaves, Stem and Root: The plant is a 2.5 m tall shrub. It has a solid, cylindrical, thin stem, which produces about 12 branches. The fernlike leaflets are blue-gray. The basal leaves are about 50 cm long and triangular while the cauline leaves reduce gradually in size until they are little more than sheath leaves. The roots are 2.5 to 7.5 cm thick. They are covered on the outside with a blackish-brown, paperlike, horizontally folded cork, which is sometimes fibrous. The fracture is spongy and roughly fibrous with white spots and resin drops.

Characteristics: The odor is strong and musklike; the taste is bitter and aromatic.

Habitat: The plant is found in some parts of Russia, Turkestan, and northern India.

Production: Sumbul or Musk root is the root of *Ferula moschata* (Reinsch, Kozo) or *Ferula sumbul*.

Other Names: Ferula, Musk Root

ACTIONS AND PHARMACOLOGY

COMPOUNDS

Volatile oil (0.3-0.5%)

Resins (17%)

Bitter substances

Hydroxycoumarins: including among others, umbelliferone

Short-chained acids: butyric acid, angelic acid, methylcrotonic acid, and valeric acid

EFFECTS

The active agents include essential oil, resin, angelic acid, and umbelliferon.

The effects are unclear; and sedative effect has not been proved.

INDICATIONS AND USAGE

Indian Medicine: Sumbul root is used for states of debility, asthma, bronchitis, pneumonia, dysmenorrhea, diarrhea, hypertension. and excessive excitability.

Homeopathic Uses: Ferula sumbul is used to treat nervous cardiac symptoms.

PRECAUTIONS AND ADVERSE REACTIONS

No health hazards or side effects are known in conjunction with the proper administration of designated therapeutic dosages.

DOSAGE

Mode of Administration: Sumbul is used as liquid extract or tincture.

LITERATURE

Kern W, List PH, Hörhammer L (Hrsg.), Hagers Handbuch der Pharmazeutischen Praxis, 4. Aufl., Bde. 1-8: Springer Verlag Berlin, Heidelberg, New York, 1969.

Madaus G, Lehrbuch der Biologischen Arzneimittel, Bde 1-3, Nachdruck, Georg Olms Verlag Hildesheim 1979.

Summer Savory

Satureja hortensis

DESCRIPTION

Medicinal Parts: The medicinal part is the fresh or dried plant harvested during the flowering stage.

Flower and Fruit: The lilac or whitish labiate flowers are in axillary, 5-blossomed, false whorls. The calyx is tubular-campanulate, regular, and has 5 tips. The corolla does not have a ring of hair. The upper lip is straight and margined. The lower lip has 3 divisions and is red-spotted at the mouth of the tube.

Leaves, Stem, and Root: The herb grows 30 to 45 cm in height with erect, heavily branched, and shortly pubescent stems. The leaves are crossed opposite, up to 3 cm long, short-petioled, lanceolate to linear-lanceolate, and entire-margined. They are rather thick with a ciliate margin and are glandular-punctate on both surfaces.

Characteristics: Summer Savory has a spicy scent and a taste that is spicy and peppery.

Habitat: The plant is indigenous to southern Europe and northern Africa, and is extensively cultivated elsewhere.

Production: Summer Savory is the aerial part of *Satureja hortensis*.

Other Names: Bean Herb, Garden Savory, Savory, Winter Savory

ACTIONS AND PHARMACOLOGY

COMPOUNDS

Volatile oil (0.2-3.0%): chief components carvacrol (30%), p-cymene (20-30%), alpha-thujene, alpha-pinene, beta-myrcene, alpha- and beta-terpinene, beta-caryophyllene, thymol

Caffeic acid derivatives: rosmarinic acid (0.2 to 1.3%), chlorogenic acid

EFFECTS

The tannin content of the drug provides astringent qualities. Summer Savory also has a mild antiseptic effect due to the presence of cymol and carvacrol in the essential oil. An aqueous extract of the herb has antiviral properties.

INDICATIONS AND USAGE

Unproven Uses: Savory is used for acute gastroenteritis.

PRECAUTIONS AND ADVERSE REACTIONS

No health hazards or side effects are known in conjunction with the proper administration of designated therapeutic dosages.

DOSAGE

Mode of Administration: The drug is used internally as an infusion that is prepared from ground plant.

Daily Dosage: Three teaspoonfuls of the drug can be taken daily in the form of a hot tea. To prepare the tea, do not boil but leave the drug to steep in scalding hot water.

LITERATURE

Deans SG, Svoboda KP, Kennedy AI. Biological Activity of Plant Volatile Oils and their Constituents. *Planta Med.* 55; 588. 1989

Kern W, List PH, Hörhammer L (Hrsg.), Hagers Handbuch der Pharmazeutischen Praxis, 4. Aufl., Bde 1-8: Springer Verlag Berlin, Heidelberg, New York, 1969.

Leung AY: Encyclopedia of Common Natural Ingredients Used in Food, Drugs, Cosmetics, John Wiley & Sons Inc., New York 1980.

Madaus G: Lehrbuch der Biologischen Arzneimittel, Bde 1-3, Nachdruck, Georg Olms Verlag Hildesheim 1979.

Opdyke DLJ. *Food Cosmet Toxicol*: 14. 1976

Sattar AA, Bankova V, Kujumgiev A, Galabov A, Ignatova A, Todorova C, Popov S. Chemical composition and biological activity of leaf exudates from some Lamiaceae plants. *Pharmazie* 50; 62-65. 1995

Zani F et al., Studies on the genotoxic properties of essential oils with Bacillus subtilis recassay and Salmonella/microsome reversion assay. *Planta Med*, 57:237-41, Jun 1991

Sundew

Drosera ramentacea

DESCRIPTION

Medicinal Parts: The medicinal part is the whole herb.

Flower and Fruit: Size: The plant is from 7 to 20 cm tall. The flowers are white and arranged in racemes turned to one side. There are 5 sepals, 5 petals, and 1 ovary with 3 to 5 styles. The fruit is capsular.

Leaves, Stem, and Root: The leaves are basal rosette, long-petioled, and thickly covered in red glandular hairs. The thickened ends have a drop of viscous juice to trap insects.

Characteristics: The herb has a sour, bitter, hot taste.

Habitat: Europe, India, China, and North and South America.

Production: Sundew consists of the dried, above- and underground parts of *Drosera ramentacea.*

Not to be Confused With: Asian varieties.

Other Names: Dew Plant, Lustwort, Red Rot, Youthwort

ACTIONS AND PHARMACOLOGY

COMPOUNDS

Naphthaquinone derivatives:

If the source is *Drosera rotundifolia*: plumbagin, ramentaceone

If the source is *Drosera ramentacea*: ramentone, ramentaceone, biramentaceone, plumbagin

If the source is *Drosera madagascariensis*: 7-methyl juglone, plumbagin

If the source is *Drosera peltata*: plumbagin, droserone, 8-hydroxydroserone

EFFECTS

The drug has secretolytic, broncho-spasmolytic, and antitussive effects. The pharmacological mode of action can be traced to 1, 4 naphtoquinone and plumbagin. Plumbagin showed an antiphlogistic effect in vitro through the inhibition of prostaglandin synthesis and an antimicrobial and cytostatic effect in animal experiments.

A possible immune-stimulating effect is the subject of recent studies, the results of which are not yet available.

INDICATIONS AND USAGE

Approved By Commission E:

- Cough/Bronchitis

Sundew is used for respiratory problems, particularly for coughing fits and dry coughs.

Unproven Uses: In folk medicine, Sundew is used for asthma and warts.

PRECAUTIONS AND ADVERSE REACTIONS

Health risks or side effects following the proper administration of designated therapeutic dosages are not recorded.

DOSAGE

Mode of Administration: Liquid and solid preparations are available for external and internal application. The plant is a protected species and is in danger of extinction.

Preparation: To prepare an infusion, pour boiling water over 2 to 10 g drug and strain after 10 minutes.

Daily Dosage: The average daily dose is 3 g drug. The dosage of the infusion when used as a broncholytic is 1 cup, 3 to 4 times daily.

LITERATURE

Bendz G, Lindberg G. Note on the Pigments of Some Drosera Species. *Acta Chem Scand*. 24; 1082-1083. 1970

Budzianowski J. Naphthohydroquinone glucosides of *Drosera rotundifolia* and *D. intermedia* from in vitro cultures. *Phytochemistry* 42 (4); 1145-1147. 1996

Budzianowski J. 2-Methylnaphthazarin 5-O-Glucoside from the Methanol Extracts of in vitro Cultures of *Drosera* Species. *Phytochemistry* 44 (1); 75-77. 1997

Budzianowski J et al., Ellagic acid derivatives and further naphthoquinones from *Dionea muscipula* and four species of the genus *Drosera* in vitro cultures. In: *PM* 59(7):A654. 1993.

Caniato R, Filippini R, Cappelletti EM. Naphthochinone Contents of Cultivated *Drosera* species *Drosera binata, D. binata var. dichotoma* and *D. capensis*. *Int J Crude Drug Res.* 27; 129-136. 1989

Croft S et al., *Ann Trop Med Parasitol* 79(6):651. 1985

Didry N, Dubreuil L, Trotin F, Pinkas M. Antimicrobial of aerial parts of *Drosera peltata Smith* on oral bacteria. *J Ethnopharmacol*; 60: 91-96. 1998

Leclerqu J, Angenot L. About *Drosera peltata* and the Standardization of the Sundew's Tincture (Tinctura Droserae). *Farm Tijdschr Belg*. 61; 357. 1984

Schilcher H, Elzer M, Drosera - der Sonnentau, ein bewährtes Antitussivum. In: ZPT 14(1):50. 1993.

Wunderer H, Zentral und peripher wirksame Antitussiva: eine kritische Übersicht. In: PZ 142(11):847-852. 1997.

Sunflower

Helianthus annuus

DESCRIPTION

Medicinal Parts: The medicinal parts of the plant are the ray florets, the leaves, the ripe fruit, the oil extracted from the seeds, and the mature flower heads.

Flower and Fruit: The very large, composite flowers are solitary or in small clusters, usually nodding, and 10 to 40 cm wide on the stems. The bracts appear in a number of rows and are leaflike, ovate, acute, and sparsely bristly. The 20 to 70 asexual, linguiform golden-yellow ray florets are 3 to 10 cm long and 1 to 3 cm wide. The numerous tubular disc florets are androgynous. They may be brown, purple, or yellow, with black or purple anthers. There are small 3-pointed paleas on the base of the capitula. The fruit is compressed at the sides, obovate to almost wedge-shaped; it is an achaene. It is densely appressed, downy and whitish, straw yellow or gray to black.

Leaves, Stem, and Root: The sunflower is a 1 to 3 m high annual plant with a long primary root and numerous lateral roots. The stem is erect, branchless, or branched higher up, densely covered in hairs, and filled with thin white pith. The leaves are alternate, cordate-triangular, long-petioled, irregularly serrated and covered with short bristles on both sides.

Habitat: Helianthus annuus is indigenous to central and eastern North America and is cultivated worldwide.

Production: Sunflower oil is the fatty oil of the achenes of *Helianthus annuus*, which is recovered from the fruits, excluding the shell, by cold pressing. The ray florets and leaves are collected at the beginning of the flowering season.

Other Names: Corona Solis, Helianthus, Marigold of Peru, Sun Rose

ACTIONS AND PHARMACOLOGY

COMPOUNDS: SUNFLOWER OIL

Triglycerides: chief fatty acids linoleic acid (35-62%), oleic acid (25-42%), palmitic acid (4-7%)

Steroids: Sterols including campesterol, cholesterol, beta-sitosterol

EFFECTS: SUNFLOWER OIL

Useful as a dietary supplement.

INDICATIONS AND USAGE

SUNFLOWER OIL

Sunflower oil is used internally to alleviate constipation (as a lubricant). It is used externally as massage oil, for poorly healing wounds (as an oil dressing), and in the treatment of skin lesions, psoriasis, and rheumatism. Sufficient information on the efficacy of the drug is not available.

PRECAUTIONS AND ADVERSE REACTIONS

SUNFLOWER OIL

Health risks or side effects following the proper administration of designated therapeutic dosages are not recorded.

DOSAGE

SUNFLOWER OIL

Mode of Administration: In folk medicine, the drug is mainly for external use. In other areas, it is used as an inactive ingredient in pharmaceutical preparations.

Storage: Keep protected from light, in tightly sealed containers. Oils from different deliveries should not be mixed.

LITERATURE

Akihisa T et al. Helianol [3,4-seco-19(10–>9)abeo-8à,9β,10à-eupha-4,24-dien-3-ol], a Novel Triterpene Alcohol from the Tabular Flowers of *Helianthus annus L. Chem Pharm Bull.* 44 (6); 1255-1257. 1996

Bader G, Streich S, Gründemann E, Flatau S, Hiller K, Enzymatic degradation of the triterpenoid saponin helianthoside 2. *Pharmazie*, 52:836-8, Nov. 1997

Bader G, Zieschang M, Wagner K, Gründemann E, Hiller K. Neue Triterpensaponine aus *Helianthus annuus* / New Triterpenoid Saponins from *Helianthus annuus. Planta Med.* 57; 471-474. 1991

Durán S et al. Contact urticaria from sunflower seeds. *Contact Dermatitis* 37; 184. 1997

Gomez E, Garçia R, Galindo PA, Feo F, Fernandez FJ. Occupational allergic contact dermatitis from sunflower. *Contact Dermatitis* 35; 189-190. 1996

Grotjohann N, Janning A, Eising R, In vitro photoinactivation of catalase isoforms from cotyledons of sunflower (*Helianthus annuus L.*). *Arch Biochem Biophys,* 346:208-18, Oct 15. 1997

Kato T, Takahasi W, Suzuki Y. Isolation and Synthesis of a New Antioxidants from Sunflower Seeds. *Nat Prod Lett.* 9; 161-165. 1997

Macias FA, Molinillo JMG, Torres A, Varela RM, Castellano D. Bioactive Flavonoids from *Helianthus annuus* cultivars. *Phytochemistry* 45 (4); 683-687. 1997

Macias FA, Varela RM, Torres A, Oliva RM, Molinillo MG. Bioactive Norsesquiterpenes from *Helianthus annuus* with potential allelopathic activity. *Phytochemistry* 48 (4); 631-636. 1998

Nandakishore T, Pasricha JS. Pattern of cross-sensitivity between 4 Compositae plants, *Parthenium hysterophorus, Xanthium strumarium, Helianthus annuus* and *Chrysanthemum coronarium,* in Indian patients. *Contact Dermatitis* 30; 162-167. 1994

Plohmann B, Bader G, Hiller K, Franz G, Immunomodulatory and antitumoral effects of triterpenoid saponins. *Pharmazie*, 52:953-7, Dec. 1997

Surinam Cherry

Eugenia uniflora

DESCRIPTION

Medicinal Parts: The medicinal parts are the bark of the plant's main stem, the leaves, and its fruit.

Flower and Fruit: The flowers are radial, in clusters of 1 to 8. The sepals are fused; the calyx has 4 or 5 points and a tube approximately 1.5 mm long. The sepals are ovate-elliptical, revolute, and up to 4 mm long. The 4 or 5 petals are white, elongate-ovate, and 8 to 12 mm long. There are numerous conspicuous stamens. The ovary is an inferior coenocarp. The fruit is a red, juicy berry with 8 vertical grooves and a diameter of 1 to 3 cm; it usually contains a single seed.

Leaves, Stem, and Root: The plant grows as a shrub or low evergreen tree, which reaches a height of 3 to 10 m. The leaves are opposite, 2.5 to 7 cm long and 1.5 to 4.5 cm wide, short-petiolate, elliptical-ovate, blunt-tipped, slightly cordate at the base, entire, and densely and translucently punctate. The trunk is slim (about the thickness of an arm); the bark is smooth and light brown.

Characteristics: The plant produces a shiny, red cherry-sized vitamin-rich fruit, whose strongly acidic taste is like that of a nectarine.

Habitat: The plant grows abundantly in the tropics, especially in Brazil, Uruguay, and Paraguay.

Production: Surinam Cherries are the fresh fruit of *Eugenia uniflora*, and Surinam Cherry leaves are the dried leaves of the same plant.

ACTIONS AND PHARMACOLOGY

COMPOUNDS: SURINAM CHERRY LEAVES

Volatile oil (0.2 to 1%): composition very dependent on the variety.

Components of an African variety include: furanodien (20%), selina-1,3,7(11)-trien-8-one (17%), oxidoselina-1,3,7(11)-trien-8-one (14%), in addition to caryophyllene, germacrene B, germacrene D, cis- and trans-ocimene, beta-selinene, spathulenol and viridiflorol

In a South American variety, the chief components include carvone, pulegone, nerolidol, limonene and verbenone, flavonoids: including quercitrin, myricitrin, and tannins.

EFFECTS: SURINAM CHERRY LEAVES

The flavonoids quercitrin and myricitrin contained in the drug have an inhibiting effect on the xanthine oxidase; the essential oil exhibits antimicrobial and antimycotic effect. A possible protective effect in relation to hyperlipidemia has been proposed. The drug may also exhibit astringent effects due to tannins and flavonoids, whose identities have not yet been determined.

COMPOUNDS: SURINAM CHERRY FRUIT

Volatile oil: components including isofuranodiene, germacrene B, selina-4(14),7(11)-diene

Monosaccharides/oligosaccharides (6%): L-fructose, D-glucose, saccharose

Carotinoids: including lycopine, gamma-carotine, beta-cryptoxanthine

Fatty oil (in the seeds and the pulp)

Fruit acids: citric acid (2%)

EFFECTS: SURINAM CHERRY FRUIT
The fruit contains vitamin C, tannins, and citric acid, which explain its use as a dietetic. The essential oil of the fruit is said to have an antimicrobial effect.

INDICATIONS AND USAGE

SURINAM CHERRY LEAVES
Unproven uses: Folk medicine practices include use of the bark as an astringent in the treatment of diarrhea, gout, fever, hypertension, gastrointestinal complaints, and edema.

SURINAM CHERRY FRUIT
Unproven Uses: Folk medicine includes use as a dietetic, but efficacy for that use has not yet been proved.

PRECAUTIONS AND ADVERSE REACTIONS

No health hazards are known in conjunction with the proper administration of designated therapeutic dosages of either drug.

DOSAGE

There is no information in the literature.

LITERATURE

Hänsel R, Keller K, Rimpler H, Schneider G (Ed.), Hagers Handbuch der Pharmazeutischen Praxis, 5. Aufl., Bde 4 - 6 (Drogen), Springer Verlag Berlin, Heidelberg, New York, 1992-1994.

Wazlawik E, Da Silva MA, Peters RR, Correia JF, Farias MR, Calixto JB, Ribeiro-Do-Valle RM, Analysis of the role of nitric oxide in the relaxant effect of the crude extract and fractions from *Eugenia uniflora* in the rat thoracic aorta. *J Pharm Pharmacol*, 49:433-7, Apr. 1997

Weyerstahl P, Marschall-Weyerstahl H, Christiansen C, Oguntimein BO, Adeoye AO. Volatile Constituents of *Eugenia uniflora* Leaf Oil. *Planta Med.* 54; 546-549. 1988

Swamp Milkweed

Asclepias incarnata

DESCRIPTION

Medicinal Parts: The medicinal parts are the rhizome with roots.

Flower and Fruit: The flowers are reddish-purple and are located on terminal umbels in clusters of 2 to 6 on a 5-cm long peduncle. The umbels consist of 10 to 20 small florets. The fruit is a long pod.

Leaves, Stem, and Root: The herbaceous plant grows up to 80 cm high. The stem is erect and smooth. The upper part of the stem is branched and very leafy. The leaves are opposite, petiolate, oblong, lanceolate, hairy, acute and cordate at the base. They are 10 to 18 cm long, 2.5 to 5 cm wide, and sharp-edged. The rhizome is about 2 to 3 cm in diameter, yellowish-brown, irregularly globular or oblong, hard and knotty. The rhizome is covered with a thin, tough bark and is surrounded by light brown rootlets that are about 10 cm long.

Characteristics: The taste is sweetish, acrid, and bitter. The plant's roots exude a latex that is typical of the genus (and giving rise to the name Milkweed,) which is slightly acrid and has a strong odor that decreases on drying.

Habitat: Swamp Milkweed is indigenous to America, Canada, and Asia.

Other Names: Rose-Colored Silkweed, Swamp Silkweed

ACTIONS AND PHARMACOLOGY

COMPOUNDS
Cardioactive steroids (cardenolids): including asclepiadin

EFFECTS
The root is said to contain asclepiadin (cardiac glycoside), which is positively inotropic and emetic.

INDICATIONS AND USAGE

Unproven Uses: Similar to other Asclepiadaceae, Swamp Milkweed is mainly used for digestive disorders.

Homeopathic Uses: The main importance of medicinal use of the American varieties is in homeopathy, but further details are not available.

PRECAUTIONS AND ADVERSE REACTIONS

No health hazards or side effects are known in conjunction with the proper administration of designated therapeutic dosages. The drug has an emetic effect in higher dosages, and digitalislike poisonings are possible due to the cardioactive steroid content. For possible symptoms and treatments for poisonings, see *Digitalis folium*.

LITERATURE

Kern W, List PH, Hörhammer L (Hrsg.), Hagers Handbuch der Pharmazeutischen Praxis, 4. Aufl., Bde. 1-8, Springer Verlag Berlin, Heidelberg, New York, 1969.

Sweet Cicely

Myrrhis odorata

DESCRIPTION

Medicinal Parts: The medicinal parts of the plant are the entire herb and the seeds.

Flower and Fruit: The white flowers appear in early summer. The complex umbels are flattened on top, many-rayed, and more cymelike at the end of the branches. The rays of the androgynous flowers are covered in thick down. The pedicles of the male flowers are hollow. In the flowering season, the umbels are erect and closed. The fruit is pyramid-shaped, 2 to 2.5 cm long, compressed at the sides and brown to glossy black.

Leaves, Stem, and Root: The plant is a perennial with a thick, gnarled, brown, branched, and polycephalous rhizome. The stem is erect, 50 to 120 cm high, canelike and, higher up, is glabrous or villous and branched. The nodes are covered in long, fine hairs. The 2- to 4-pinnatisect leaves are large, soft, triangular, and covered underneath with short, soft bristles.

Characteristics: The leaves smell like garden lovage and taste like anise.

Habitat: The herb is found in mountainous regions from the Pyrenees to the Caucasus and is cultivated elsewhere.

Production: Sweet Cicely root and herb are the whole plant of *Myrrhis odorata.*

Other Names: British Myrrh, Cow Chervil, Great Chervil, Sweet Chervil, Sweet Bracken, Sweet-Cus, Sweet-Fern, Sweet-Humlock, Sweets, Shepherd's Needle, The Roman Plant

ACTIONS AND PHARMACOLOGY

COMPOUNDS

Volatile oil: chief components are trans-anethole, additionally germacrene-D, anisaldehyde, limonene, chavicolmethyl ether, beta-caryophyllene, alpha-pinene, alpha-farnesene, myrcene. Also, in the roots, trans-isoosmorhizol.

Flavonoids: apigenine-7-O-glucoside, luteolin-7-O-glucoside

EFFECTS

The drug is said to be a carminative, a digestive, and an expectorant.

INDICATIONS AND USAGE

Unproven Uses: The herb is used as a blood purifier and an expectorant, as well as for asthma and other breathing difficulties. Balms and salves made from it are used to treat fresh wounds and sores and relieve the pains of gout. The roots are used to treat chest and throat complaints and also urinary complaints. The fresh herb is used externally for gout swelling and indurations. Previous folk medicine uses also included use of a decoction from the roots for snake and dog bites.

PRECAUTIONS AND ADVERSE REACTIONS

No health hazards or side effects are known in conjunction with the proper administration of designated therapeutic dosages.

DOSAGE

Mode of Administration: Ground root is used to make tonics and infusions for internal and external use. Salves are used externally.

LITERATURE

Hegnauer R, Chemotaxonomie der Pflanzen, Bde 1-11, Birkhäuser Verlag Basel, Boston, Berlin 1962-1997.

Kern W, List PH, Hörhammer L (Hrsg.), Hagers Handbuch der Pharmazeutischen Praxis, 4. Aufl., Bde. 1-8, Springer Verlag Berlin, Heidelberg, New York, 1969.

Sweet Clover

Melilotus officinalis

DESCRIPTION

Medicinal Parts: The medicinal part is the flowering herb.

Flower and Fruit: The small yellow flowers are in many-blossomed, long-peduncled racemes. The standard and wings are the same length, but longer than the carina. Of the 10 stamens, 9 are fused. The fruit is an obtuse, glabrous, light brown to black, thorny-tipped, and horizontally wrinkled pod that usually has 1 seed.

Leaves, Stem, and Root: The plant is perennial and 60 to 120 cm high. The smooth ascending or decumbent stems are heavily branched. The leaves are alternate, glabrous, trifoliate, and long petioled. The leaflets are obovate and dentate. The stipules are awl-like bristly.

Characteristics: The plant has a fragrance similar to woodruff or hay.

Habitat: The plant is found all over Europe, Australia, and North America, as well as in temperate regions of Asia.

Production: Sweet Clover consists of the dried or fresh leaf and flowering branches of *Melilotus officinalis*, and/or *Melilotus altissimus.*

Other Names: Common Melilot, Corn Melilot, Field Melilot, King's Clover, Hart's Tree, Hay Flowers, Ribbed Melilot, Sweet Lucerne, Wild Laburnum, Yellow Sweet Clover

ACTIONS AND PHARMACOLOGY

COMPOUNDS: IN THE FRESH PLANT

Coumarinic acids glycosides: including melilotoside

COMPOUNDS: IN THE DEHYDRATED DRUG

Free coumarin (0.4-0.9%): formed from the coumarinic acids during dehydration, furthermore 3,4-dihydrocoumarin, melilotol, melilotin

Hydroxycoumarins: including among others umbelliferone, scopoletin, herniarin, fraxidin

Flavonoids: including kampferol- and quercetin glycosides

Triterpene saponins: including azuki saponin-V-carboxylate, azuki saponin II, aglycones soya sapogenols B and E, melilotigenin

Volatile oil: traces of very complex composition

COMPOUNDS: IN THE SEEDS

Canavanin

Trigonelline

EFFECTS

The drug has an antiphlogistic, antiexudative, and antiedematous effect, which explain its use for inflammatory and congestive edema. It increases venous reflux and improves lymphatic kinetics.

Animal experiments showed an increase in healing wounds.

INDICATIONS AND USAGE

Approved by Commission E:

- Blunt injuries
- Hemorrhoids
- Venous conditions

The drug is used internally for problems arising from chronic venous insufficiency, such as pain and heaviness in legs, night cramps in the legs, itching and swelling; for the supportive treatment of thrombophlebitis, post-thrombotic syndromes, hemorrhoids, and lymphatic congestion. Externally, the drug is used for contusions, sprains, and superficial effusions of blood.

Unproven Uses: In folk medicine, Sweet Clover is used as a diuretic.

PRECAUTIONS AND ADVERSE REACTIONS

No health hazards or side effects are known in conjunction with the proper administration of designated therapeutic dosages. Administration of the drug in higher dosages can lead to headache and stupor. Transitory liver damage is possible for particularly susceptible patients. Elevated liver enzyme values usually disappear following discontinuance of the drug. (Monitoring liver enzyme values is recommended.)

DOSAGE

Mode of Administration: Comminuted drug for infusions and other galenic preparations for oral use; liquid forms of medication for parenteral application; ointments, liniments, cataplasms, and herbal sachets for external use; ointments and suppositories for rectal use.

Preparation: To prepare an infusion, pour boiling water over 1 to 2 teaspoonfuls of comminuted, cut drug, then strain after 5 to 10 minutes.

Daily Dosage: The average daily dose of the herb or preparation in amounts corresponding to 3 to 30 mg of coumarin; parenteral application corresponding to 1.0 to 7.5 mg of coumarin.

Infusion — As a therapy for varicose veins, 2 to 3 cups daily.

External — As a poultice for hemorrhoids.

Storage - The drug must be stored away from light in sealed containers to prevent loss of coumarin.

LITERATURE

Abou-Donia AHA. Ph. D. Thesis, Faculty of Pharmacy, University of Alexandria, Egypt. 1976

Borzeix MG, Angignard J, Dedieu F, Dupont JM, Miloradovich T, Leutenegger E. Effect of a Combination of Coumarin Derivatives and Rutoside on Venous and Lymphatic Circulations during Severe Constriction of the Caudal Vena Cava in Rabbits. *Arzneim Forsch.* 45 (3); 262-266. 1995

Bos R et al., Analysis of coumarin in *Melilotus officinalis*. In: *PM* 61(Abstracts of 43rd Ann Congr):68. 1995.

Brantner A, Lücke W. Influence of physical parameters on the germ-reducing effect of microwave irridation on medicinal plants. *Pharm Ind.* 50 (11); 762-765 1995

Hammouda FM, Rizk AM, Seif EL-Nazar MM, Abou-Youssef AA, Ghaleb HA, Madkour MK, Pholand AE, Wood G, Flavonoids and coumarins from elilotus. In: *Fitotherapia* 54(6):249-255. 1983.

Marshall M, Wüstenberg P, Klinik und Therapie der chronischen enösen Insuffizienz. In: Klinik und Therapie der chronischen venösen Insuffizienz, Braun Fachverlage, Karlsruhe 1994.

Sweet Gale

Myrica gale

DESCRIPTION

Medicinal Parts: The medicinal parts are the leaves and branches as well as the wax extracted from the catkins.

Flower and Fruit: Sweet Gale plants are either male or female. The male plants produce groups of stemless catkins on the leafless branches of the previous year's growth. The fruit catkins are about the same size but somewhat thicker and grow in closely packed resinous nutlets. They are dry and compressed.

Leaves, Stem, and Root: The plant is usually dioecious, but plants may change sex from year to year. Sweet Gale is a deciduous shrub up to 2.5 m high. The branches have scattered yellowish glands. The leaves are 2 to 6 cm long, almost lanceolate, cuneate at the base, and serrate near the apex. They are pubescent beneath with shiny yellow, fragrant glands on both surfaces.

Characteristics: The branches and leaves are fragrant when bruised.

Habitat: Sweet Gale is indigenous to the higher latitudes of the northern hemisphere.

Production: Sweet Gale is the aerial part of *Myrica gale*.

Other Names: Bog Myrtle, Dutch Myrtle, Bayberry

ACTIONS AND PHARMACOLOGY

COMPOUNDS

Volatile oil (0.4-0.7%): including among others alpha-pinene, delta-cadinene, gamma-cadinene, limonene, beta-myrcene, alpha-phellandrene, beta-phellandrene, 1,8-cineole, nerolidol, p-cymene, alpha-copaene, beta-caryophyllene

Flavonoids: including myricitrin

Triterpenes: including ursolic acid, oleanolic acid

EFFECTS

Sweet Gale has an astringent and aromatic effect.

INDICATIONS AND USAGE

Unproven Uses: Sweet Gale has been used in digestive disorders. A strong brew of dried bark is also used in Sweden for intestinal worms and to cure itching.

PRECAUTIONS AND ADVERSE REACTIONS

The volatile oil of the drug is considered toxic. Mixing plant extracts with beer, as practiced in the Middle Ages, is said to have led to manic episodes.

DOSAGE

Mode of Administration: The drug is ground. Information on preparations is not available.

LITERATURE

Hegnauer R, Chemotaxonomie der Pflanzen, Bde 1-11, Birkhäuser Verlag Basel, Boston, Berlin 1962-1997.

Kern W, List PH, Hörhammer L (Hrsg.), Hagers Handbuch der Pharmazeutischen Praxis, 4. Aufl., Bde. 1-8, Springer Verlag Berlin, Heidelberg, New York, 1969.

Lawrence BM, Weaver KM. Essential Oils and their Constituents; XII: A Comparative Chemical Composition of the Essential Oils of *Myrica gale* and *Comptonia peregrina*. *Planta Med.* 25; 385-388. 1974

Malterud KE. C-methylated dihydrochalcones from *Myrica gale* fruit exudate. *Acta Pharm Nord.* 4; 65-68. 1992

Mathisen L, Malterud KE, Sund RB. Antioxidant Activity of Fruit Exudate and C-Methylated Dihydrochalcones from *Myrica gale*. *Planta Med.* 61 (6); 515-518 1995

Morihara M, Sakurai N, Inoue T, Kawai KI, Nagai M. Two Novel Diarylheptanoid Glucosides from *Myria gale var. tomentosa* and Absolute Structure of Plane-Chiral Galeon. *Chem Pharm Bull.* 45 (5); 820-823. 1997

Roth L, Daunderer M, Kormann K, Giftpflanzen, Pflanzengifte, 4. Aufl., Ecomed Fachverlag Landsberg Lech 1993.

Sweet Marjoram

Origanum majorana

DESCRIPTION

Medicinal Parts: The medicinal parts of the plant are the leaves and flowers, the fresh aerial parts of the flowering plant, and the whole of the fresh, flowering plant.

Flower and Fruit: The inconspicuous, sessile flowers barely extend above the surrounding gray tomentose bracts. The calyx appears to have only 1 sepal because the 2 lower sepals are almost nonexistent and the upper 3 are completely fused. The calyx is 2.5 cm long and otherwise resembles the bracts. The corolla is white to pale lilac or pink, 4 mm long, with a few uneven, pointed tips. The 2 upper tips are fused together to form a lip. The stamens are enclosed in the corolla or extend above it. The fruit is a smooth, light brown nutlet, 0.75 to 1 mm long.

Leaves, Stem, and Root: The plant is biennial with a main shoot that is heavily branched. It grows 20 to 25 cm high. The downy-to-tomentose shoots are gray-green to whitish, and sometimes tinged with red. The leaves are spatulate, short-petioled, 0.5 to 2 cm long and 0.5 to 1 cm wide, entire-margined, and rounded. They are gray-tomentose on both surfaces, somewhat thick and usually without distinct ribs. The false whorls are mostly covered by the 3 to 4 wide, circular, gray-green bracts, which are fused to globular, racemous or panicled capitula.

Characteristics: The plant has a distinctive tangy odor and a bitter taste.

Habitat: The plant is indigenous to the southeastern Mediterranean region and is cultivated in Germany.

Production: Marjoram herb consists of the dried leaf and flower of *Origanum majorana* (syn. *Majorana hortensis*), gathered during the flowering season and stripped off the stems. Drying must happen fast to avoid blackening of the leaves. Marjoram oil consists of the essential oil of *Origanum majorana* obtained by aqueous steam distillation of the fresh or dried leaves and flowers stripped from the stems and harvested during flowering season. Depending on the area of cultivation, there may be two crops of the aerial plant parts per year.

ACTIONS AND PHARMACOLOGY

COMPOUNDS: MARJORAM HERB

Chief components in the volatile oil of the foliage: cis-sabinene hydrate (40 to 50%), cis-sabinene hydrate acetate (20 to 30%), sabinene (10%) and trans-sabinene hydrate (2%); cis-sabinene hydrate acetate transforms itself with steam distillation into (among others) terpinene-4-ol (in volatile oil yielded through steam distillation, 15 to 40%), gamma-terpinene (in volatile oil yielded through steam distillation, 2 to 12%), alpha-terpinene, limonene and terpinols, which leads toa change of aroma.

COMPOUNDS: MARJORAM OIL

Volatile oil (1 to 3%)

Flavonoids: including diosmetin, luteolin, apigenin and their C- and O-glycosides, including vitexin, orientin, thymonine

Hhydroquinone glycosides: including arbutin (0.15 to 0.45%), methyl arbutin

Caffeic acid derivatives: rosmarinic acid, chlorogenic acid

Water soluble polysaccharides (13%)

Triterpenes: including ursolic acid (0.5%), oleanolic acid (0.2%)

EFFECTS: MARJORAM HERB AND OIL

In vitro, Marjoram is antimicrobial, antiviral and insecticidal.

INDICATIONS AND USAGE

Unproven Uses: In folk medicine, Majoram herb and oil are used for cramps, depression, dizziness, gastrointestinal disorders, migraine, nervous headaches, neurasthenia, paralysis, paroxysmal coughs, colds, and as a diuretic.

Homeopathic Uses: Homeopathy sometimes uses Marjoram to increase sexual excitability.

PRECAUTIONS AND ADVERSE REACTIONS

General: No health hazards or side effects are known in conjunction with the proper administration of designated therapeutic dosages. The drug is not suitable for longer-term use because of its arbutin content.

Pediatric Use: Marjoram salve should not be administered to infants or small children.

DOSAGE

Mode of Administration: Marjoram herb is used as an infusion for teas, mouthwashes and poultices (5% infusion). The oil is used in ointments and a few compound preparations.

Preparation: To prepare a tea, pour 250 mL boiling water over 1 to 2 teaspoonfuls of Marjoram herb and strain after 5 minutes. An ointment is prepared by leaving 20 parts

Marjoram herb to stand with 1 part ammonia and 10 parts spirit of wine for a few hours. It is then heated with 100 parts petroleum jelly in a water bath until the spirit of wine and ammonia have evaporated. Then the ointment is filtered (EB6).

Daily Dosage: Sip 1 to 2 cups of tea throughout the day.

Homeopathic Dosage: 5 to 10 drops, 1 tablet, or 5 to 10 globules 1 to 3 times a day or 1 mL injection solution sc twice weekly (HAB1).

Storage: Dried Marjoram herb may be stored for up to 2 years in airtight containers.

LITERATURE

Assaf MH, Ali AA, Makboul MA, Beck JP, Anton R. Preliminary Study of Phenolic Glycosides from *Origanum majorana*; Quantitative Estimation of Arbutin; Cytotoxic Activity of Hydrochinone. *Planta Med.* 55; 343-345. 1987

Deans SG, Svoboda KP. The Antimicrobial Properties of Majoram (*Origanum majorana L.*) Volatile Oil. *Flav Fragr J.* 5; 187-190. 1990

Hänsel R, Keller K, Rimpler H, Schneider G (Hrsg.), Hagers Handbuch der Pharmazeutischen Praxis, 5. Aufl., Bde 4-6 (Drogen), Springer Verlag Berlin, Heidelberg, New York, 1992-1994 (unter Orignum majorana).

Leung AY, Encyclopedia of Common Natural Ingredients Used in Food Drugs and Cosmetics, John Wiley & Sons Inc., New York 1980.

Madaus G, Lehrbuch der Biologischen Arzneimittel, Bde 1-3, Nachdruck, Georg Olms Verlag Hildesheim 1979.

Steinegger E, Hänsel R, Pharmakognosie, 5. Aufl., Springer Verlag Heidelberg 1992.

Teuscher E, Biogene Arzneimittel, 5. Aufl., Wiss. Verlagsges. Stuttgart 1997.

Sweet Orange

Citrus sinensis

DESCRIPTION

Medicinal Parts: The medicinal parts are the fresh and dried peel as well as the oil extracted from the peel.

Flower and Fruit: The fragrant flowers are arranged singly or in short, limp racemes. The fruit is depressed-globose to shortly ovoid, 10- to 13-locular. The peel is thin to rather thick, nearly smooth, orange to orange-yellow when ripe. The pulp is sweet. The core remains solid when ripe.

Leaves, Stem, and Root: Citrus sinensis is an evergreen tree with rounded crown. The branches are angular when young, then become cylindrical, with a few slender, rather flexible axillary spines. The leaves are acute and rounded below; the petioles are narrowly winged.

Habitat: Like other Citrus varieties, the plant is indigenous to Asia and is cultivated in the Mediterranean and other subtropical regions in many parts of the world.

Production: Orange peel consists of the fresh or dried outer peel of ripe fruits of *Citrus sinensis*, separated from the white pith layer, as well as its preparations in effective dosage.

Other Names: China Orange, Citrus Dulcis, Orange

ACTIONS AND PHARMACOLOGY

COMPOUNDS

Volatile oil: chief components in the fresh pericarp include (+)-limonene, furthermore citral (as an odor-bearer), citronellal, nootkatone, sinesal, n-nonanal, n-decanal, n-dodecanal, linalyl acetate, geranyl acetat, citronellyl acetat, methyl anthranilate. Pressed oils also contain lipophilic flavonoids and furocoumarins.

Flavonoids

EFFECTS

Sweet Orange promotes gastric juice secretion.

INDICATIONS AND USAGE

- Dyspeptic complaints
- Loss of appetite

PRECAUTIONS AND ADVERSE REACTIONS

No health hazards or side effects are known in conjunction with the proper administration of designated therapeutic dosages. There is a low potential for sensitization through skin contact with the volatile oil.

DOSAGE

Mode of Administration: Comminuted herb for teas and other bitter-tasting galenic preparations for oral administration.

Daily Dosage: 10 to 15 g of drug.

LITERATURE

Fouche SD, Dubery IA. Chalcone Isomerase from *Citrus sinensis*: Purification and Characterization. *Phytochemistry* 37; 127-132. 1994

Ihrig M, Qualitätskontrolle von süβem Orangenschalenöl. In: *PZ* 140(26):2350-2353. 1995.

Hausen B, Allergiepflanzen, Pflanzenallergene, ecomed Verlagsgesellsch. mbH, Landsberg 1988.

Kern W, List PH, Hörhammer L (Hrsg.), Hagers Handbuch der Pharmazeutischen Praxis, 4. Aufl., Bde. 1-8, Springer Verlag Berlin, Heidelberg, New York, 1969.

Trovato A, Monforte MT, Barbera R, Rossitto A, Galati EM, Forestieri AM. Effects of fruit juices of *Citrus sinensis L.* and *Citrus limon L.* on experimental hypercholesterinaemia in the rat. *Phytomedicine* 2 (3); 221-227 (1996)

Sweet Sumach

Rhus aromatica

DESCRIPTION

Medicinal Parts: The medicinal parts are the dried and fresh root bark.

Flower and Fruit: The flowers are in 1- to 1.5-cm false spikes. They are yellow-green and often appear before the leaves are fully developed. The fruit is a globular, yellow-red, pubescent drupe.

Leaves, Stem, and Root: The plant is a fragrant 1- to 2.4-m shrub with glabrous red-brown annual growth and small to 10-cm trifoliate leaves. The leaflets are oval and the middle one is cuneate at the base. The leaflets are irregularly dentate and initially pubescent on both sides. Later the leaflets turn glabrous on the upper surface and eventually pubescent only on the ribs of the lower surface.

Habitat: The plant is indigenous to Atlantic North America.

Production: Sweet Sumach root-bark is the root-bark of *Rhus aromatica*.

Other Names: Polecat-Bush, Sumach, Sumac, Sweet Fragrant,

ACTIONS AND PHARMACOLOGY

COMPOUNDS

Phenol glycosides: orcin-O-beta-D-glucoside

Steroids: sterols, including beta-sitosterol, stigmast-7-en-3beta-ole

Tannins

Triterpenes: including oleanolic aldehyde

Volatile oil (0.01 to 0.07%); very complex in mixture, with constituents including delta-cadinene, camphene, delta3-carene, beta-elemene, farnesyl acetone, alpha- and beta-pinene, fatty acids

EFFECTS

The drug has an antimicrobial and antiviral effect due to the tannins (gallic acid). In animal experiments it increased contraction of the smooth muscles of ileum. Two older studies describe an improvement in the symptoms of urinary incontinence.

INDICATIONS AND USAGE

Unproven Uses: In folk medicine Sweet Sumach is used for irritable bladder, urinary incontinence, enuresis nocturna, and uterine bleeding.

Homeopathic Uses: Rhus aromatica is used for weak bladder conditions.

PRECAUTIONS AND ADVERSE REACTIONS

No health hazards or side effects are known in conjunction with the proper administration of designated therapeutic dosages.

DOSAGE

Mode of Administration: Sweet Sumach is available in crude powder form and in compounded preparations for oral use. It is also available in parenteral form for homeopathic use.

Daily Dosage: Single dose is 1 g.

Bed-wetting—5 to 20 drops depending on age, to be taken 2 to 3 times daily, over an extended period.

Homeopathic Dosage: 5 drops, 1 tablet, or 10 globules every 30 to 60 minutes (acute) or 1 to 3 times daily (chronic); parenterally: 1 to 2 mL sc acute: 3 times daily; chronic: once a day (HAB34)

Storage: Should be stored in dry place, protected from direct light.

LITERATURE

Baer H, In: Toxic Plants, Ed. AD Kinghorn, Columbia Press 1979.

Effenberger S, Schilcher H, Gewürzsumachrinde. In: *ZPT* 11(4):113. 1990.

Hänsel R, Keller K, Rimpler H, Schneider G (Hrsg.), Hagers Handbuch der Pharmazeutischen Praxis, 5. Aufl., Bde 4-6 (Drogen): Springer Verlag Berlin, Heidelberg, New York, 1992-1994.

Madaus G, Lehrbuch der Biologischen Arzneimittel, Bde 1-3, Nachdruck, Georg Olms Verlag Hildesheim 1979

Schilcher H, Boesel R, Effenberger ST Segebrecht S, Neuere Untersuchungsergebnisse mit aquaretisch, antibakteriell und prostatotrop wirksamen Arzneipflanzen. In: *ZPT* 10(3):77. 1989.

Sweet Vernal Grass

Anthoxanthum odoratum

DESCRIPTION

Medicinal Parts: The whole plant is considered to have medicinal properties.

Flower and Fruit: The green, solitary, flowered spikelet has 4 spelts, the lower half of which are as large as the upper and taller than the flowers. Both of the upper spelts are awned, with 2 stamens. The style is long, the stigma pinnate, and spikelets form an oblong false ear.

Leaves, Stem, and Root: The plant size ranges from 15 to 50 cm. The plant grows as thick grass. The leaves are ciliate at the base of the lamina. The leaf sheath is deeply grooved and hairy.

Characteristics: Sweet Vernal Grass has a scent of dried woodruff or new-mown hay and a tangy taste.

Habitat: The plant is indigenous to Britain, Europe, and temperate Asia.

Production: Sweet Vernal Grass is the whole *Anthoxanthum odoratum* plant in flower.

ACTIONS AND PHARMACOLOGY

COMPOUNDS

Hydroxy cinnamic acid glycosides: in the fresh plant

Melilotoside and coumarin: triggered by a beta-glucosidase during dehydration of the plant

Iridoids: asperuloside, monotropein, scandoside

EFFECTS

No information is available.

INDICATIONS AND USAGE

Unproven Uses: The drug is used for headache, nausea, sleeplessness, and conditions of the urinary tract.

PRECAUTIONS AND ADVERSE REACTIONS

The freshly harvested plant contains glycosidic precursors of coumarin, which release coumarin in the process of dehydration (the drug contains up to 1.5% coumarin). No health hazards or side effects are known in conjunction with the proper administration of designated therapeutic dosages.

OVERDOSAGE

The administration of higher levels of the drug can lead to headache and dizziness. Liver injuries are possible among susceptible patients during long-term treatment. The abnormal liver values disappear when the drug is discontinued, but ongoing observation of liver enzyme values is recommended.

DOSAGE

Mode of Administration: The drug is used externally as an extract.

LITERATURE

Fentem JH, Fry JR, Thomas NW, Species differences in the hepatotoxicity of coumarin-a comparision of rat and Mongolian gerbil. In: *Toxicology* 71(1-2):129. 1992.

Kern W, List PH, Hörhammer L (Hrsg.), Hagers Handbuch der Pharmazeutischen Praxis, 4. Aufl., Bde. 1-8, Springer Verlag Berlin, Heidelberg, New York, 1969.

Lewin L, Gifte und Vergiftungen, 6. Aufl., Nachdruck, Haug Verlag, Heidelberg 1992.

Poisonous Plants in Britain and their effects on Animals and Man, Ministry of Agriculture Fisheries and Food, Pub; HMSO (1984) UK.

Roth L, Daunderer M, Kormann K, Giftpflanzen, Pflanzengifte, 4. Aufl., Ecomed Fachverlag Landsberg Lech 1993.

Teuscher E, Lindequist U, Biogene Gifte - Biologie, Chemie, Pharmakologie, 2. Aufl., Fischer Verlag Stuttgart 1994.

Sweet Violet

Viola odorata

DESCRIPTION

Medicinal Parts: The medicinal parts are the essential oil from the leaves, the dried flowers, the air-dried leaves collected during the flowering season, the flowering herb, the dried rhizome, the fresh aerial parts collected during the flowering season, and the whole plant.

Flower and Fruit: The dark violet flowers are solitary on 3 to 7 cm long pedicles. The flowers are 1.5 to 2 cm long and fragrant. The 5 sepals are obtuse, glabrous, and have an appendage. There are 5 uneven petals that are unevenly spurred and which have a broad margin. The 5 stamens have an appendage at the tip. The flower has 3 fused ovaries. The fruit is a globular capsule, approximately 7.5 mm. It is 3- to 6-sided, clearly and densely short-pubescent, and often violet. It can be found pressed to the receptacle.

Leaves, Stem, and Root: Violet is 5 to 10 cm high, a rosette plant with a short, thick yet soft ground axis. The rooting runners are 10 to 20 cm long and 1.5 mm thick. They produce flowers in the second year. The shoots are a strong dark green with scattered appressed hairs or almost glabrous. The leaves are petiolate, broadly cordate, obtuse, or short-acuminate and crenate. The leaves, which appear first, are reniform-cordate and the younger ones are rolled up. There are lanceolate stipules at the base of the leaves.

Characteristics: The plant is strongly scented.

Habitat: The plant is indigenous to or naturalized in large parts of Europe and the Middle East as far as central Asia; it is also found in North America.

Production: Sweet Violet root consists of the dried root of *Viola odorata*. Sweet Violet herb is the dried plant section of *Viola odorata*. The rhizome is imported from the former Czechoslovakia and Romania. The rootstock is dug up, pounded to remove any soil residue, washed and air-dried.

Other Names: Garden Violet

ACTIONS AND PHARMACOLOGY

COMPOUNDS: SWEET VIOLET RHIZOME AND HERB

Volatile oil (0.04%): salicylic acid methyl ester (formed out of glycosidic precursors during plant drying), beta-nitropropionic acid

Saponins

Alkaloids

EFFECTS: SWEET VIOLET RHIZOME AND HERB

The drug acts as an expectorant due to its saponin content. The alkaloid violin has an emetinelike effect.

COMPOUNDS: SWEET VIOLET FLOWER

Volatile oil (0.003%): aroma-carrier trans-alpha-ionone (parmone), chief constituents (-)-zingiberene, (+)-curcumene, dihydro-beta-ionone, 2,6-nonadien-1-al, undecan-2-one, isoborneol

EFFECTS: SWEET VIOLET FLOWER

The drug has antimicrobial and broncho-secretolytic effects due to the saponin content.

INDICATIONS AND USAGE

SWEET VIOLET RHIZOME AND HERB

Unproven Uses: The rhizome is used for conditions of the respiratory organs, particularly for dry catarrh and rheumatism of the minor joints; it is also used for fever, skin diseases, inflammation of the oral mucosa, nervous complaints, headache, and insomnia. The herb is used internally for coughs, hoarseness, pneumonia, throat inflammations, bronchitis accompanied by fixed mucous, nervous strain, insomnia and hysteria. It is also used to induce sweating. Externally, the herb is used to treat various skin diseases.

SWEET VIOLET FLOWER

Unproven Uses: The flowers are used to prepare an infusion tea, which is used as an expectorant for bronchial catarrh; as an antitussive for chronic bronchitis; and for whooping cough, asthma, and migraine. Sweet Violet syrup is used as an expectorant and to lessen irritation for bronchial catarrh (children's remedy).

Homeopathic Uses: The flowers are used for inflammation of the respiratory tract and rheumatism of the wrist.

PRECAUTIONS AND ADVERSE REACTIONS

SWEET VIOLET RHIZOME, HERB, AND FLOWER

No health hazards or side effects are known in conjunction with the proper administration of designated therapeutic dosages.

DOSAGE

SWEET VIOLET RHIZOME AND HERB

Preparation: An herbal tea is prepared by adding 2 teaspoonfuls Sweet Violet herb with 1/4 liter water.

Daily Dosage: The average single dose of the rhizome is 1 g orally. The 5% rhizome decoction dosage is 20 g. The 5% rhizome infusion dosage is 1 dessertspoonful 5 to 6 times daily. The herbal tea dosage is 1 cup 2 to 3 times daily.

SWEET VIOLET FLOWER

Preparation: To prepare an infusion, decoction or tea, use 1 heaping teaspoonful of drug with 1 cup of water.

Daily Dosage: The dosage for the infusion, decoction or tea is 1 cup twice daily, or taken in sips 1 to 2 times per hour. The dosage of Sweet Violet syrup is 1 to 2 dessertspoonfuls every 2 hours.

Homeopathic Dosage: 5 drops, 1 tablet, or 10 globules every 30 to 60 minutes (acute) or 1 to 3 times daily (chronic); parenterally: 1 to 2 mL sc, acute: 3 times daily; chronic: once a day (HAB34).

LITERATURE

SWEET VIOLET RHIZOME, HERB AND FLOWER

Farnsworth NR, *Lloydia* 246. 1968

Hänsel R, Keller K, Rimpler H, Schneider G (Hrsg.), Hagers Handbuch der Pharmazeutischen Praxis, 5. Aufl., Bde 4-6 (Drogen): Springer Verlag Berlin, Heidelberg, New York, 1992-1994.

Madaus G, Lehrbuch der Biologischen Arzneimittel, Bde 1-3, Nachdruck, Georg Olms Verlag Hildesheim 1979.

Watt JM, Breyer-Brandwijk MG, The Medicinal, Poisonous Plants of Southern, Eastern Africa, 2nd Ed, Livingstone 1962.

Willaman JJ, Hui-Li L, *Lloydia* 33 (3A):1. 1970

Sweet Woodruff

Galium odoratum

DESCRIPTION

Medicinal Parts: The medicinal parts are the dried or fresh aerial parts collected during or shortly before the flowering season.

Flower and Fruit: The flowers are in loose terminal cymes. The petals are fused to a white, funnel-shaped, 1.5-mm tube. The border of the tube is divided in 4 and is 2 to 3.5 mm long. The 4 stamens are fused with the corolla. The involucre bracts are small, lanceolate, or almost bristlelike. The 2-seeded indehiscent fruit is globular, 2 to 3 mm long, and thickly covered with white barbed bristles.

Leaves, Stem, and Root: Sweet Woodruff is a 10 to 35 cm herbaceous perennial with a thin cylindrical circular rhizome. The stem is erect, quadrangular, and smooth. Apart from the bristly nodes, the stem is glabrous and glossy. The leaves are in false whorls of 6 to 9, the lower ones are obovate-oblong, the middle and upper ones are lanceolate to oblong-lanceolate. They are entire-margined, thorny tipped, glabrous, and rough-edged.

Characteristics: Sweet Woodruff is aromatic when dried; the taste is bitter and tangy.

Habitat: The plant grows in northern and central Europe, Siberia, and northern Africa.

Production: Sweet Woodruff herb is the fresh or dried aerial part of *Galium odoratum*. It is gathered during or shortly before flowering. The herb must be turned regularly while being dried.

Not to be Confused With: Gallium mollugo or *Gallium sylvaticum*

Other Names: Master of the Wood, Woodwrad, Woodruff

ACTIONS AND PHARMACOLOGY

COMPOUNDS: IN THE FRESH PLANT

O-hydroxycinnamic acid glucoside: melilotoside

COMPOUNDS: IN THE DRIED PLANT

Coumarin (0.4-1%)

Iridoids: asperuloside (0.05-0.3%), monotropein (0.04%), scandoside

EFFECTS

The coumarin content may impart antiphlogistic, antiedematic, spasmolytic, and lymphokinetic properties. However, due to the low level of coumarin, the therapeutic effect is doubtful.

INDICATIONS AND USAGE

Unproven Uses: Sweet Woodruff is used as a treatment for nervous agitation, sleeplessness, nervous menstrual disorders, congested liver, jaundice, hemorrhoids, circulation disorders, and venous conditions.

PRECAUTIONS AND ADVERSE REACTIONS

The freshly harvested plant contains melilotoside as a glycosidic precursor of coumarin. In the process of dehydration, coumarin is released (content up to 1% coumarin in freshly dried drug). Health risks or side effects following the proper administration of designated therapeutic dosages are not recorded. Headache and stupor can occur with the administration of higher dosages of the drug. Susceptible patients could experience liver damage following long-term administration. This effect is reversible following discontinuation of the drug. Liver enzyme values should be monitored.

DOSAGE

Mode of Administration: The herb is obsolete as a drug in many countries.

Preparation: To make a tea, place 2 teaspoonfuls (1.8 g drug) in one glass water. An infusion of 5% drug is used for insomnia, and a forehead poultice made of crushed herb is used for headache.

Daily Dosage: The average single dose is 1.0 g drug. The preparations can be taken during the day or shortly before going to bed.

Storage: The drug should be protected from light sources to avoid brown coloring.

LITERATURE

Berkowitz WF et al., *J Org Chem* 47:824. 1982

Casley-Smith JR, Casley-Smith JR, Effects of varying doses of 7-hydroxy-coumarin and coumarin in acute lymphoedema and other high-protein oedemas. In: Progress in Lymphology, X, Adelaide, 194-196. 1985.

Cox D, O'Kennedy R, Thornes RD, The rarity of liver toxicity in patients treated with coumarine (1,2-Benzopyrone). In: *Human Toxikol* 8:501-506. 1989.

Egan D, O'Kennedy R, Moran E, Cox D, Prosser E, Thornes RD, The pharmacology, metabolism, analysis, and applications of coumarin and coumarin-related compounds. In: *Drug Metabolism Reviews* 22(5):503-529. 1990.

Fentem JH, Fry JR, Thomas NW, Species differences in the hepatotoxicity of coumarin - a comparision of rat and Mongolian gerbil. In: *Toxicology* 71(1-2):129. 1992.

Hardt TJ, Ritschel WA, The effect of coumarin and 7-hydroxycoumarin on in vitro macrophage phagocytosis of latex particles. In: *Methods Find Exp Clin Pharmacol* 5(1):39-43. 1983.

Hausen BM, Schmieder M, The sensitizing capacity of coumarins. In: *Contact Dermatitis* 15(3):157-163. 1986.

Hazleton LW, Tusing TW, Zeitlin BR, Thiesen R, Murer HK, Toxicity of coumarin. In: *J Pharmacol Exp Ther* 116:348-358. 1956.

Rosskopf F, Kraus J, Franz G, Immunological and antitumor effects of coumarin and some derivatives. In: *PA* 47(2):139-142. 1992.

Wüstenberg, P, Baumann G, Verdacht der Toxizität von Cumarin nicht bestätigt. In: PZ 139(13):1058. 1994.

Swertia chirata

See Chiretta

Swertia japonica

See Senburi

Symphytum officinale

See Comfrey

Symplocarpus foetidus

See Skunk Cabbage

Syzygium aromaticum

See Clove

Syzygium cumini

See Jambol

Tamarind

Tamarindus indica

DESCRIPTION

Medicinal Parts: The medicinal parts are the fruit pulp and the dried seeds.

Flower and Fruit: The flowers form a terminal raceme and have 3 petals that are 1 cm in length, initially whitish, then yellowish with light-red stripes. They have a calyx with a narrow, top-shaped base, and 4 thickly covered segments. The stamens are fused in a sheath, which is open at the top. The fruit is a 20-cm long by 3-cm wide, matte-brown, slightly compressed, indehiscent, beanlike pod. The fruit has 3 to 12 seeds that are very hard and glossy brown. The seeds are 14 mm long and have an irregular, roundish-quadrangular shape. The mesocarp is odorless, mushy, and sweet.

Habitat: The plant is indigenous to tropical Africa and is naturalized in North and South America from Florida to Brazil. It is cultivated in subtropical China, India, Pakistan, Vietnam, the Phillippines, Java, and Spain.

Production: Tamarind paste is derived from the fruit of *Tamarindus indica.* The fruit is fermented for a long time in the sun. The initially red-brown fruit attains a black or black-brown hue and becomes more aromatic and sour. The paste is boiled to a glutinous mass, which is the finished product.

Other Names: Imlee

ACTIONS AND PHARMACOLOGY

COMPOUNDS

Fruit acids: tartaric acid (3-10%); including among others, malic acid, citric acid, lactic acid

Invert sugar (25-30%)

Pectin

Pyrazines and thiazols (aromatic substances)

EFFECTS

The drug, which contains organic acids and pectine, is said to be laxative; however, the mode of action has not been documented. Various extracts have shown inflammation-inhibiting effects in animals. Antimicrobial and immunomodulating effects have also been seen, as have wound-healing properties.

INDICATIONS AND USAGE

Unproven Uses: The drug is used for chronic or acute constipation and liver and gallbladder ailments.

Indian Medicine: The drug is used for bilious vomiting, alcohol intoxication, fever, pharyngitis, stomatitis, constipation, and hemorrhoids.

Homeopathic Uses: Tamarindus indica is used for stomachaches.

PRECAUTIONS AND ADVERSE REACTIONS

No health hazards or side effects are known in conjunction with the proper administration of designated therapeutic dosages.

DOSAGE

Mode of Administration: Tamarind is taken orally and is usually used in combination with other laxatives, such as figs.

Preparation: To make a clean paste, soften the raw tamarind paste in hot water, strain through a sieve, and steam to a soft consistency in a water bath; mix the paste with sugar.

Daily Dosage: 10 to 50 g of cleaned tamarind paste, pure or with other purgatives, is taken in fruit cubes.

Homeopathic Dosage: 5 drops, 1 tablet, or 10 globules, every 30 to 60 minutes (acute) or 1 to 3 times daily (chronic); parenterally: 1 to 2 mL sc, acute: 3 times daily; chronic: once a day (HAB34).

Storage: Store in a tightly sealed container.

LITERATURE

Burgalassi S, Raimondi L, Pirisino R, Banchelli G, Boldrini E, Saettone MF. Effect of xyloglucan (tamarind seed polysaccharide) on conjunctival cell adhesion to laminin and on corneal epithelium wound healing. *Eur J Ophthalmol*;10: 71-76. 2000

De M, Krishna Se A, Banerjee AB. Antimicrobial screening of some Indian spices. *Phytother Res.* 13: 616-618. 1999

Kobayashi A, Adenan MI, Kajiyama SI, Kanzaki H, Kawazu K. A Cytotoxic Principle of *Tamarindus indica*, Di-n-butyl Malate and the Structure-Activity Relationship of Its Analogues. Z Naturforsch. 51c; 233-242. 1996

Mustapha A, Yakasai IA, Aguye IA. Effect of *Tamarindus indica L.* on the bioavailability of aspirin in healthy human volunteers. *Eur J Drug Metab Pharmacokinet*; 21: 223-226. 1996

Sreelekha TT, Vijayakumar T, Ankanthil R, Vijayan KK, Nair MK. Immunomodulatory effects of a polysaccharide from *Tamarindus indica. Anti-Cancer Drug.*; 4: 209-212. 1993

Strickland FM, Darvill A, Albersheim P, Eberhard S, Pauly M, Pelley RP. Inhibition of UV-induced immune suppression and interleukin-10 production by plant oligosaccharides and polysaccharides. *Phytochem Phytobiol.* 1999; 69: 141-7

Tamarindus indica

See Tamarind

Tamus communis

See Black Bryony

Tanacetum parthenium

See Feverfew

Tanacetum vulgare

See Tansy

Tansy

Tanacetum vulgare

DESCRIPTION

Medicinal Parts: The medicinal part consists of the dried flowering herb.

Flower and Fruit: The inflorescences are flat, round, and buttonlike composite flowers in cymes. The bright golden yellow flowers consist only of tubular flowers. The fruit has 5 ribs without tufts of hair.

Leaves, Stem, and Root: The plants grow from 60 to 120 cm high. The stem is erect, glabrous, angular, red-tinged, and leafy. The leaves are alternate, simple or double pinnatifid, 15 cm long and 12 cm wide, and have a long emarginate tip.

Characteristics: The herb has a strong aromatic smell. The taste is bitter and camphor-like. The plant is poisonous.

Habitat: The plant is indigenous to Europe.

Production: Tansy flower consists of the inflorescence of *Chrysanthemum vulgare* (syn. *Tanacetum vulgare*). Tansy herb consists of the above-ground parts of *Chrysanthemum vulgare* (syn. *Tanacetum vulgare*). Tansy oil is the oil extracted from *Tanacetum vulgare.*

Other Names: Buttons, Daisy, Hindheal, Parsley Fern

ACTIONS AND PHARMACOLOGY

COMPOUNDS: TANSY FLOWER AND HERB

Volatile oil (0.5 to 0.9% in the foliage, 0.8 to 1.8% in the blossoms): constituents of the volatile oil vary greatly according to variety. The following could appear as main constituents: artemisia ketone, (-)-thujone, (+)-isothujone, 1,8-cineole, alpha-pinene, alpha-terpinyl acetate, borneol, bornyl acetate, davanone, germacrene D, L-camphor (+) umbellulone, camphor, lyratol (+) lyratol acetate, piperitone, sabinene, thuj-4-en-2-ylacetate (+) trans-Carveyl acetate, trans-chrysanthenol (+) trans-chrysanthenyl acetate, umbellulone, as well as (+)-vulgarol A (8%), vulgaron B (up to 12%). Hybrid varieties exist.

Sesquiterpenes: sesquiterpene lactones, including crispolid, deacetyl crispolid, tatridins A and B, tavulin, artemorin, parthenolide (in some varieties), reynosine, armefoline, dentatin A, santamarin, chrysanthemine

Flavonoids: including cosmosiin, apigenin-7-O-glycoside, cynaroside, luteolin-7-O-glucoside, quercimetrin, eupatilin, acacetin-7-glucobioside

Hydroxycoumarins: including scopoletin

Polyynes: including diterthiophene, triterthiophene (phototoxic)

EFFECTS: TANSY FLOWER AND HERB

The oil, which contains thujone, is an insect repellent. The sesquiterpenes in the leaves are antimicrobial. A leaf extract has displayed an antiedemic effect, and the polysaccharide fraction is said to have an ulcer-protective effect in rats.

COMPOUNDS: TANSY OIL

Constituents of the volatile oil vary greatly according to variety. The following could appear as chief constituents: artemisia ketone, (-)-thujone, (+)-isothujone, 1,8-cineole, alpha-pinene, alpha-terpinyl acetate, borneol, bornyl acetate, davanone, germacrene D, L-camphor (+) umbellulone, L-camphor, lyratol (+) lyratol acetate, piperitone, sabinene, thuj-4-en-2-ylacetate (+) trans-carvyl acetate, trans-chrysanthenol (+) trans-chrysanthenyl acetate, umbellulone, among others. Hybrid varieties exist.

EFFECTS: TANSY OIL

The thujone-type oil is antimicrobial, anthelmintic, and repellent to various insects.

INDICATIONS AND USAGE

TANSY FLOWER AND HERB

Unproven Uses: Tansy preparations are used as an anthelmintic, for migraine, neuralgia, rheumatism, meteroism, and loss of appetite.

TANSY OIL

Unproven Uses: Tansy oil is used internally for gout, rheumatic complaints, joint pains, stomach cramps, gastrointestinal infections, intermittent fever, dizziness, and dysmenorrhea. It is used externally for rheumatism, gout, contusions, sprains, and wounds.

CONTRAINDICATIONS

The drug should not be used during pregnancy.

PRECAUTIONS AND ADVERSE REACTIONS

TANSY FLOWER AND HERB

The administration of therapeutic dosages of drugs that have a high thujone content (see *Tanaceti aetheroleum*) can lead to poisoning. Beyond that, there is a medium potential for sensitization via skin contact with the drug. Internal administration of the drug in allopathic dosages is to be avoided.

TANSY OIL

Particularly toxic are volatile oils with high thujone content. Poisonings occur chiefly through the misuse of the drug as an abortifacient. Administration in allopathic dosages is to be avoided.

OVERDOSAGE

TANSY OIL

Symptoms of poisoning include vomiting, abdominal pain, gastroenteritis, severe reddening of the face, mydriasis, fixed pupil, tonic-clonic spasms, cardiac arrhythmias, uterine bleeding, kidney damage, and liver damage. Death occurs after 1 to 3.5 hours. The lethal dosage is approximately 15-30 g. The treatment for poisonings can only proceed symptomatically.

DOSAGE

TANSY FLOWER AND HERB

Daily Dosage: Administration in allopathic dosages is to be avoided.

TANSY OIL

Mode of Administration: The drug is found in extract form in a small number of combination preparations.

Daily Dosage: Administration in allopathic dosages is to be avoided. The documented single dose is 0.1 g.

LITERATURE

TANSY FLOWER, HERB AND OIL

Brown AMG et al., Tissue culture, biochemistry and pharmacology of *Tanacetum ssp.* In: *PM* 62, Abstracts of the 44th Ann Congress of GA, 33. 1996.

Ognyanov I, Tochorova M, *Planta Med* 48:181. 1983

Schearer WR, *J Nat Prod* 47(6):964. 1984

Taraxacum officinale

See Dandelion

Taumelloolch

Lolium temulentum

DESCRIPTION

Medicinal Parts: The medicinal parts are the ripe seeds.

Flower and Fruit: The green spikes are 30 cm long and uninterrupted; 5 to 7 spikelets form the ear. The glume is longer than the spikelet, which has 7 ribs and no awn. The husk is cartilaginous, with 5 ribs and a stiff, straight awn.

Leaves, Stem, and Root: The stalk is rigid and erect. The leaf sheaths are rough and weakly bulbous on the upper leaves.

Characteristics: The spikelets have their narrow sides turned toward the main axis (in contrast to the couch grass). A parasitic fungus, which is often present on the plant, forms an alkaloid, making the plant poisonous.

Habitat: The plant grows in Europe and Mediterranean regions.

Production: Taumelloolch seeds are the ripe seeds of *Lolium temulentum.*

Other Names: Bearded Darnel, Cheat, Drake, Ray-Grass, Tare

ACTIONS AND PHARMACOLOGY

COMPOUNDS

The active ingredients are not known. However, the toxicity of *Lolium rigidum* is caused by bacterial toxins, the so-called kidney toxins, which are unusual nucleosides with uracil as the base.

EFFECTS

The active agents are temulentin, temulentic acid, free fatty acids, tannin and glycosides. The fruit has been suspected of poisoning for some time; however, the toxic principle generally remains unexplained. The drug's ability to relieve gastroenteritis can possibly be attributed to the free fatty acids.

INDICATIONS AND USAGE

Unproven Uses: Taumelloolch is used for dizziness, nerve pain, nosebleeds, sleeplessness, stomach cramps, and urinary incontinence.

PRECAUTIONS AND ADVERSE REACTIONS

The drug can be toxic. In earlier times, poisonings were frequently caused by the presence of the plant's berries in grain. No cases of poisoning are known in recent times. The plant has now become extremely rare through intensive seed-corn purification.

OVERDOSAGE

Symptoms of poisoning include dizziness, headache, colic, confusion, staggering, vision and speech disorders, somnolence, and, in rare cases, death through respiratory failure. The treatment of poisoning consists of gastrointestinal emptying (inducement of vomiting, gastric lavage with burgundy-colored potassium permanganate solution, sodium sulphate), administration of activated charcoal and shock prophylaxis (quiet, warmth). Further management consists of treating spasms with careful administration of diazepam (IV) and icepacks for fever. Phenothiazines and analeptics should not be administered. Intubation and oxygen therapy may be required.

DOSAGE

Mode of Administration: The plant is administered ground and as a liquid extract.

LITERATURE

Dannhardt G, Lehr M, Mayer KK, Steindl L. Volatile alkaloids of the caryopses of *Lolium temulentum*: genuine compounds and artifacts. *Pharm Pharmacol Lett.* 1; 7-10. 1991

Frohne D, Pfänder HJ, Giftpflanzen - Ein Handbuch für Apotheker, Toxikologen und Biologen, 4. Aufl., Wiss. Verlags-Ges Stuttgart 1997.

Hammouda FM et al. Poisonous Plants Contaminating Edible Ones and Toxic Substances in Plant Foods IV. Phytochemistry and Toxicity of *Lolium temulentum. Int J Crude Drug Res.* 26; 240-245. 1988

Kern W, List PH, Hörhammer L, (Hrsg.), Hagers Handbuch der Pharmazeutischen Praxis, 4. Aufl., Bde 1-8, Springer Verlag Berlin, Heidelberg, New York, 1969.

Lewin L, Gifte und Vergiftungen, 6. Aufl., Nachdruck, Haug Verlag, Heidelberg 1992.

Madaus G, Lehrbuch der Biologischen Arzneimittel, Bde 1-3, Nachdruck, Georg Olms Verlag Hildesheim 1979.

Roth L, Daunderer M, Kormann K, Giftpflanzen, Pflanzengifte, 4. Aufl., Ecomed Fachverlag Landsberg Lech 1993.

Teuscher E, Lindequist U, Biogene Gifte - Biologie, Chemie, Pharmakologie, 2. Aufl., Fischer Verlag Stuttgart 1994.

Taxus baccata

See Yew

Tea Tree

Melaleuca alternifolia

DESCRIPTION

Medicinal Parts: The medicinal parts of the plant are the leaves and branch tips from which the oil is extracted by steam distillation.

Flower and Fruit: The inflorescence is a 3- to 5-cm long spike. The flowers are sessile with a campanulate epicalyx on which the sepals sit. The tips are 3 to 4 mm long. The petals are free, approximately twice as large as the calyx tips. There are numerous conspicuous stamens, in 5 bundles approximately 2 cm long. The ovary is inferior and partially fused with the hollow receptacle. It is in 3 parts with a thick pistil and a capitular stigma. The fruit is a woody, cylindrical capsule with a diameter of 3 to 4 mm.

Leaves, Stem, and Root: This tree reaches heights up to 7 m. The leaves are simple, coriaceous, 1 to 2.5 cm long, acute-lanceolate, and sometimes slightly sickle-shaped with oil glands. The young shoots are tomentose, the older branches glabrous. The trunk has a paperlike, whitish bark.

Habitat: Melaleuca alternifolia is indigenous to Australia.

Production: Tea Tree oil is the essential oil extracted from the leaves and branch tips of *Melaleuca alternifolia*, *Melaleuca dissitifolia*, and other Melaleuca species by aqueous steam distillation. Ideally, the leaves and shoots have first been stored for 6 weeks.

ACTIONS AND PHARMACOLOGY

COMPOUNDS

Terpinenes: Primarily terpinene-4-ol (45%), gamma-terpinene (18%), alpha-terpinene (8%), 1.8-cineole (6%), alpha-terpineol (5%), as well as alpha-pinene, limonene, p-cymol, terpinolene, viridiflorene

EFFECTS

The in vitro data regarding the antimicrobial activity of Tea Tree oil is extensive, documenting it to be active against a wide range of bacteria, fungi, and yeast causing superficial skin infections. Tea Tree oil causes autolysis of bacteria during both the exponential and stationary phase of bacterial cell growth. Its effectiveness on the skin may also be attributed to its lipophilic nature causing it to penetrate the skin surface. However, few clinical studies have been done to confirm effectiveness and skin tolerance. The minimum bactericidal concentrations are typically close to 0.25% and many skin care products contain a concentration ranging from 1% to 10%.

As an antifungal, Tea Tree oil is rarely used as a monotherapy but instead combined with other antifungal natural products. Three comparative blinded trials showed Tea Tree oil to be effective in relieving the symptoms of athlete's foot, and in treating toenail onychomycosis.

Tea Tree oil is frequently recommended in either suppository or douche form as part of a treatment protocol for women with vaginal candidiasis or trichomoniasis; however, there is little documentation of the efficacy of this approach. Another use is as a ''swish and spit'' for patients with oral candidiasis. This is used in immunocompetent and immunocompromised patients.

Tea Tree oil is effective for treating acne vulgaris, with slightly less efficacy than benzoylperoxide. The oil had fewer side effects than benzoylperoxide. In a separate study, Tea Tree oil was found to be effective against head lice (Veal, 1996).

Antimicrobial Effects: One study suggested that Tea Tree oil is similar in mechanism to the membrane-active disinfectants such as chlorhexidine and quaternary ammonium compounds by denaturing proteins and disrupting membrane structure. This is based on microscopic observation showing a loss of cell constituents and a breakdown of the cell wall after treatment of *E coli* cells with Tea Tree oil as well as the observation that cells were killed prior to autolysis. Tea Tree oil was also able to kill *E coli* cells in both the exponential phase and in the stationary phase of growth. Cells in the exponential phase of growth were killed after 30 minutes of Tea Tree oil treatment using the known minimum bactericidal concentration of 0.25% and in the stationary phase of growth in 45 minutes using twice the minimum bactericidal concentration (Gustafson et al, 1998).

Tea Tree oil inhibits cellular respiration and causes potassium leakage in *E coli* cells, further evidence that it is a membrane-active antibiotic. A concentration of 0.5% or 2x the minimum inhibitory concentration (MIC) caused exponentially growing cells to completely cease glucose-dependent oxygen consumption. In stationary phase cells, glucose-dependent oxygen consumption was decreased by 43% after increasing the concentration of Tea Tree oil to 1%, or 4x the MIC. This was accompanied by a leakage of potassium ions from the *E coli* cells that reached 75% using 0.25% Tea Tree oil on exponentially growing cells. Stationary phase cells are slightly resistant to Tea Tree oil, possibly due to alterations in the cell membrane that occur during this phase of growth (Cox et al, 1998).

Concentrations of Tea Tree oil greater than 300 mcg/mL had cytotoxic effects on fibroblasts and epithelial cells. Because this concentration also corresponded with the concentration that was cytotoxic to *Staphylococcus aureus*, the authors suggested that the mode of action for cytotoxicity is a membrane-associated event (Soderberg et al, 1996).

When eight components of Tea Tree oil were analyzed for antimicrobial activity, terpinen-4-ol inhibited all 12 of the test organisms, which were: *Bacillus subtilis, Bacteriodes fragilis, Candida albicans, Clostridium perfringens, Enterococcus faecalis, Escherichia coli, Lactobacillus acidophilus, Moraxella catarrhalis, Mycobacterium smegmatis, Pseudomonas aeruginosa, Serratia marcescens*, and *Staphylococcus aureus*. Linalool and alpha-terpineol were the next most effective, killing 11 of the 12 organisms. p-cymene was the least effective. The minimum cidal concentrations for linalool, terpinen-4-ol, and alpha terpineol were all 0.25% or less. Although it was previously stated that the antimicrobial activity of Tea Tree oil was due to terpinen-4-ol, this shows that linalool and alpha-terpineol are also very active, although there concentrations in Tea Tree oil are low (Carson & Riley, 1995).

Tea Tree oil was found to be active against a wide range of skin flora. These organisms include: *A baumannii, Corynebacterium spp, K pneumoniae, M luteus, M varians, Micrococcus spp, P aeurginosa, S marcescens, S aureus, S capitis, S epidermidis, S haemolyticus, S hominis, S saprophyticus, S warneri*, and *S xylosus*. The MIC ranged from 0.06% to 5% while the minimum bactericidal concentrations ranged from 0.25% to 8%. Generally, the gram-negative organisms were more susceptible to Tea Tree oil. The authors suggest that Tea Tree oil may be useful in hygienic hand disinfection by removing transient skin flora while maintaining protective resident flora. The technique used here was the broth microdilution method (Hammer et al, 1996).

Several species of Streptococcus were found to be susceptible to Tea Tree oil. *Streptococcus pyogenes,* a causative agent in impetigo, with an MIC of 0.12% Tea Tree oil and a minimum bactericidal concentration of 0.25% (Carson et al, 1996). Tea Tree oil was found to be effective against a number of oral bacterium, both anaerobic and capnophilic. The MIC for all 15 bacterial species tested was less <0.6% Tea Tree oil (Shapiro et al, 1994).

Antifungal/Antiyeast Effects: Tea Tree oil was found to be active against *Malassezia furfur,* the fungal agent implicated for pityriasis versicolor, folliculitis, and intertrigo, as well as seborrheic dermatitis and dandruff. Using an agar dilution assay, 52 isolates of *M furfur* gave an average MIC of Tea Tree oil of 0.25% after 72 hours. Using a broth macrodilution assay, 16 isolates were found to have an MIC of 0.12% and a minimum fungicidal concentration of 1.0% Tea Tree oil after 24 hours (Hammer et al, 1997).

Tea Tree oil was active against a variety of dermatophytes and yeasts. Clinical samples were collected from patients suffering dermatophytic disease and included 26 fungal specimens including *Trichophyton rubrum, Trichophyton mentagrophytes,* and *Microsporum canis;* 31 strains from the Candida genus and one Trichosporon and 31 different *Malassezia furfur* strains. The MIC ranged from 0.11% (1,112 mcg/mL) to 0.44% (4,450 mcg/mL) of Tea Tree oil. When compared to the antibiotic miconazole, minimum inhibitory values were lower, ranging from 0.1 to 0.78 mcg/mL (Nenoff et al, 1996).

Tea Tree oil was able to completely inhibit the growth of *Candida albicans* on agar. Tea Tree oil was diluted 1:5 in 90% ethanol and then 1:8 in agar plates. A dilution of 1:16 was the MIC. It was noted that Tea Tree oil from different sources gave variable results (McFadden, 1996).

Antipedicular Effects: Various essential oils were tested at 1% in 40% ethanol. Lice were dipped into the solution for 10 seconds, blotted dry, and then incubated for 17 hours. At this time the lice were washed, rinsed, and incubated for another 4 hours at which time live, dead, and morbid lice were counted. Similar procedures were done for lice eggs. A mixture of 50% Tea Tree oil and 50% Cinnamon Leaf oil killed 100% of the lice and 96% of the eggs. The dilution of Tea Tree oil alone killed 93% of the lice and 83% of the eggs. Although the results seem impressive, it is questionable as to whether appropriate controls were run or whether the procedure is relevant to how a product might be used in a clinical condition (Veal, 1996).

CLINICAL TRIALS

Acne

The efficacy of a 5% topical tea tree oil gel in mild to moderate acne vulgaris was investigated in a randomized, double-blind, placebo controlled study. Sixty patients were randomly divided into two groups and treated with tea tree oil gel (n=30) or placebo (n=30) over a period of 45 days. There was a statistically significant difference between tea tree oil and placebo in the improvement of the Total Acne Lesions Count (TLC) and Acne Severity Index (ASI). In terms of TLC and ASI, tea tree oil was 3.55 times and 5.75 times more effective than placebo respectively. Side-effects were similar in both groups (Enshaieh et al, 2007).

A 5% solution of Tea Tree oil was effective in treating acne vulgaris in a study of 124 patients who were randomized to receive either Tea Tree oil or 5% benzoylperoxide lotion for 3 months. It was not mentioned how often the treatment was used. Both groups showed improvement in the number of inflamed lesions, the number of noninflamed lesions, and skin oiliness (Bassett et al, 1990).

According to more recent interviews with 62 patients recruited from Australian general practice and dermatology offices, the use of tea tree oil and other complementary and alternative therapies for acne, psoriasis, and atopic eczema is far more common than physicians expected (Magin et al, 2006).

Clearance of Skin

Two topical MRSA eradication regimes were compared: a standard treatment including mupirocin 2% nasal ointment, chlorhexidine gluconate 4% soap, silver sulfadiazine 1% cream versus a tea tree oil regimen, which included tea tree 10% cream, tea tree 5% body wash, both given for five days. Mupirocin was significantly more effective at clearing nasal carriage (78%) than tea tree cream (47%, p=0.0001), but tea tree treatment was more effective than chlorhexidine or silver sulfadiazine at clearing superficial skin sites and skin lesions (Dryden et al, 2004).

Gingivitis

A double-blind, longitudinal study of 49 nonsmokers assessed the effect of a gel containing tea tree oil on plaque and chronic gingivitis. The volunteers were randomly assigned to 1 of 3 groups designated to apply (without supervision) 1 of 3 gel formulations: tea tree oil gel (2.5%); gel with chlorhexidine (CHX; 0.2%); or a placebo gel. Participants were instructed to apply the gel with a toothbrush twice daily to inflamed gums. Over the course of eight weeks, those using the tree tee oil gel experienced more of a reduction in gingival inflammation than did those in the other groups. However, there was no reduction in plaque level with tea tree oil, suggesting that its antibacterial effects *in vitro* do not translate to plaque inhibition *in vivo*. The authors hypothesize that anti-inflammatory properties of tea tree oil helped to reduce gingivitis. No adverse reactions to any of the gels were reported. (Soukoulis, 2004).

Toenail Fungus (Onychomycosis)

A 100% solution of Tea Tree oil was effective in treating onychomycosis. In this double-blind randomized trial, 117 patients with distal subungual onychomycosis, proved by culture, applied either 100% Tea Tree oil or 1% clotrimazole twice daily for 6 months. At the end of 6 months, 11% of the clotrimazole group had a negative culture and 18% of the Tea Tree oil group was negative. Nail appearance improved in 61% of clotrimazole patients and 60% of Tea Tree oil patients. A 3-month follow-up showed that a positive resolution was still present in 55% of the clotrimazole patients and 56% of the Tea Tree oil patients (Buck et al, 1994).

Skin Inflammation (Histamine-Induced)

Tea Tree oil significantly decreased histamine-induced skin inflammation in 21 subjects 20 minutes after histamine injection in an open trial. Twenty-seven subjects were injected intradermally with histamine diphosphate (5 mcg/50 mcL) on each forearm. Flare area and weal volume was calculated after measuring weal diameters and double skin thickness every 10 minutes for 1 hour. Twenty-one subjects had 25 mcL of 100% Tea Tree oil topically applied to one forearm at 20 minutes while 6 subjects had 25 mcL paraffin oil topically applied to a forearm. The percentage weal volume of Tea Tree oil-treated arms was statistically significantly lower than that of the control arms (p=0.0004, Mann-Whitney U-test) at 30 minutes and at 60 minutes (p=0.017) (Koh et al, 2002).

INDICATIONS AND USAGE

Unproven Uses: Tea Tree Oil is used for conditions of the respiratory tract and for skin conditions. It is also used as a disinfectant. Folk medicine internal uses have included tonsillitis, pharyngitis, colitis, and sinusitis. Externally, Tea Tree Oil is used for ulcers of the oral mucous membrane, gingivitis, root canal treatment, mycosis of the nail, skin infections, ulcers, burns, and insect bites.

CONTRAINDICATIONS

Tea Tree oil should definitely not be applied to eczematous skin as it can cause irritation. It is contraindicated for hypersensitivity or known allergy to turpentine (DeGroot, 1996). Although Tea Tree oil has been used orally for infections, this usage is not recommended due to its toxicity;

the essential oil should not be used internally other than in the form of an oral rinse that is not swallowed or as vaginal douche. (Lininger et al, 1998).

PRECAUTIONS AND ADVERSE REACTIONS

Allergic contact dermatitis is said to be a common side effect of Tea Tree oil seen by Australian dermatologists. If sufficient quantities are ingested, diarrhea, central nervous system toxicity, and coma may occur (Moss 1994).

Cytotoxicity experiments found that the most toxic component of Tea Tree oil is alpha-terpineol and the least toxic is 1,8-cineole. HeLa cells (epithelial) were least affected while Hep G2 (liver) cells were most affected. This may or may not represent toxicity to the corresponding organs. The findings also suggest that 1,8-cineole is incorrectly credited with toxicity (Hayes et al, 1997). Except for mild irritation, there is no toxicity from using even 50% solutions as a douche for most patients.

Central Nervous System Effects: In one case report, a patient swallowed approximately half a teacup of Tea Tree oil and was in a coma for 12 hours, followed by 36 hours in a semiconscious state. This was accompanied by hallucinations, abdominal pain, and diarrhea. No further information was given (Seawright, 1993). In a separate case, a 4-year-old boy became ataxic and unresponsive about 2 hours after erroneously being given approximately 2 teaspoons 100% pure Tea Tree oil with a glass of water. After intubation, he began to move all limbs, muscle tone was normal, and pupils were sluggishly reactive. He was admitted to the intensive care unit for further observation and within several hours was weaned from the ventilator. Forty-eight hours after admission, he was discharged after having a normal physical examination (Morris et al, 2003).

Dermatologic Effects: Although 1,8-cineole has been credited for skin irritation associated with Tea Tree oil, a study showed that 1,8-cineole was not an irritant in concentrations up to 28.1%. This study was conducted on 28 human subjects for 21 days. However, three subjects showed signs of allergic responses to Tea Tree oil, which were due to the sesquiterpene hydrocarbon fraction of the oil (Southwell, 1997).

A report treating acne with 5% Tea Tree oil reported skin dryness, pruritis, stinging, burning, and redness as side effects (Bassett et al, 1990). Allergic contact dermatitis occurred from inhaling Tea Tree oil vapors. The patient had inhaled Tea Tree oil for several minutes, several times a day for 2 days as a treatment for bronchitis. The patient was previously atopic, with hand eczema and a known allergy to turpentine. He was also found to be allergic to several other essential oils (DeGroot, 1996).

Hormonal Effects: Three case reports indicate that the common use of products containing Tea Tree oil, Lavender oil, or the two combined may result in prepubertal gynecomastia. The authors hypothesize that endocrine-disrupting activity of the topically applied oils led to an imbalance in estrogen and androgen pathway signaling in the case reports they describe—a hypothesis reinforced by the resolution of the gynecomastia within months of ceasing product use. *In vitro* data indicate that Tea Tree oil possesses weak estrogenic and antiandrogenic properties, as does lavender oil (Henley et al, 2007).

DRUG INTERACTIONS

No human interaction data available.

OVERDOSAGE

In several cases involving children, overdosage (10 mL for a child) led to coordination weakness and a state of confusion. A very high dosage (70 mL) led to coma.

DOSAGE

Mode of Administration: Preparations of the oil are used internally and externally.

Storage: Store tightly sealed and protected from light.

LITERATURE

Anon. Tea Tree Oil-Skin Reactions *SADRAC Bulletin* 66:4. 1996.

Bassett IB, Pannowitz DL, Barnetson RStC. A comparative study of tea-tree oil versus benzoylperoxide in the treatment of acne. *Med J Aust* 153:455-458. 1990.

Bhushan M, Beck MH. Allergic contact dermatitis from Tea Tree oil in a wart paint. *Contact Dermatitis* 36:117-118. 1997.

Blackwell AL. Tea Tree oil and anaerobic (bacterial) vaginosis. *Lancet* 337:300. 1991.

Buck DS, Nidorf DM, Addino JG. Comparison of two topical preparations for the treatment of onychomycosis: *melaleuca alternifolia* (Tea Tree) oil and clotrimazole. *J Fam Pract* 38:601-605. 1994.

Carson CF, Cookson BD, Farrelly HD, et al: Susceptibility of methicillin-resistant Staphylococcus aureus to the essential oil of *Melaleuca alternifolia. J Antimicrob Chemother* 35:421-424. 1995.

Carson CF, Hammer KA, Riley TV. In-vitro activity of the essential oil of *Melaleuca alternifolia* against Streptococcus spp. *J Antimicrob Chemother* 37:1177-1178. 1996.

Carson CF, Hammer KA, Riley TV. Broth micro-dilution method for determining the susceptibility of Escherichia coli and Staphylococcus aureus to the essential oil of *Melaleuca alternifolia* (Tea Tree oil). *Microbios*, 82:181-185, 1995.

Carson CF, Riley TV. Antimicrobial activity of the major components of the essential oil of *Melaleuca alternifolia. J Appl Bacteriol,* 78:264-269. 1995.

Carson CF, Riley TV. Toxicity of the essential oil of Melaleuca alternifolia or Tea Tree oil. letter; comment. *J Toxicol Clin Toxicol* 33:193-194. 1995.

Chan CH, Loudon KW. Activity of Tea Tree oil on methicillin-resistant *Staphylococcus aureus* (MRSA). *J Hosp Infect* 3:244-245. 1998.

Cox SD, Gustafson JE, Mann CM, et al: Tea Tree oil causes K+ leakage and inhibits respiration in *Escherichia coli. Lett Appl Microbiol* 1998; 26:355-358.

DeGroot AC. Airborne allergic contact dermatitis from Tea Tree oil. *Contact Dermatitis* 35:304-305. 1996.

Dryden MS, Dailly S, Crouch M. A randomized, controlled trial of tea tree topical preparations versus a standard topical regimen for the clearance of MRSA colonization. J Hosp Infect; 56(4): 283-286. 2004.

Elliott C. Tea Tree oil poisoning. *Med J Aust* 159:830-831. 1993.

Enshaieh S, Jooya A, Siadat AH, Iraji F. The efficacy of 5% topical tea tree oil gel in mild to moderate acne vulgaris: a randomized, double-blind placebo-controlled study. Indian J Dermatol Venereol Leprol; 73(1): 22-25. 2007.

Hammer KA, Carson CF, Riley TV. Susceptibility of transient and commensal skin flora to the essential oil of *Melaleuca alternifolia* (Tea Tree oil). *Am J Infect Control* 24:186-189. 1996.

Hayes AJ, Leach DN, Markham JL. In vitro cytotoxicity of Australian Tea Tree oil using human cell lines. *J Essent Oil Res* 9:575-582. 1997.

Henley DV, Lipson N, Korach KS, et al. Prepubertal gynecomastia linked to lavender and tea tree oils. *NEJM* 365;5. 2007.

Jandourek A, Vaishampayan JK, Vazquez JA. Efficacy of melaleuca oral solution for the treatment of fluconazole refractory oral candidiasis in AIDS patients. *AIDS* 12:1033-1037. 1998.

Knight TE, Hausen BM. Melaleuca oil (Tea Tree oil) dermatitis. *J Am Acad Dermatol* 30:423-427. 1994.

Koh KJ, Pearce AL, Marshman G, et al: Tea Tree oil reduces histamine-induced skin inflammation. *Br J Dermatol* 147:1212-1217. 2002.

Magin PJ, Adams J, Heading GS, et al. Complementary and Alternative Medicine Therapies in Acne, Psoriasis, and Atopic Eczema: Results of a Qualitative Study of Patients' Experiences and Perceptions. *J Alt Comp Med.* 12(5):451-457. 2006.

McFadden R: Comparison of the inhibitory effects of various plant extracts on the growth of *Candida albicans* - in vitro. *Eur J Herbal Med* 1:26-31. 1995.

Morris M, Donoghue A, Markowitz J, et al: Ingestion of Tea Tree oil (Melaleuca oil) by a 4-year-old boy. *Pediatr Emerg Care* 19(3):169-171. 2003.

Moss A. Tea Tree oil poisoning. *Med J Aust* 160:236. 1994.

Nenoff P, Haustein UF, Brandt W. Antifungal activity of the essential oil of *Melaleuca alternifolia* (Tea Tree oil) against pathogenic fungi in vitro. *Skin Pharmacol*, 9:388-394. 1996.

Osborne F, Chandler F. Australian Tea Tree oil. *Herbal Medicine.* March:42-46. 1998.

Pena EO. *Melaleuca alternifolia* oil: uses for trichomonal vaginitis and other vaginal infections. *Obstet Gynecol* 19:793-795. 1962.

Seawright A. Editorial comment. *Med J Aust* 159:831. 1993.

Selvaag E, Eriksen B, Thune P. Contact allergy due to Tea Tree oil and cross-sensitization to colophony. *Contact Dermatitis* 31:124-125. 1994.

Shapiro S, Meier A, Guggenheim B: The antimicrobial activity of essential oils and essential oil components towards oral bacteria. *Oral Microbiol Immunol* 9:202-208. 1994.

Soderberg TA, Johansson A, Gref R. Toxic effects of some conifer resin acids and Tea Tree oil on human epithelial and fibroblast cells. *Toxicology* 107:99-109. 1996.

Soukoulis S, Hirsch R. The effect of a tea tree-oil containing gel on plaque and chronic gingivitis. *Australian Dental J* 49(2):78-83. 2004.

Southwell IA. Skin irritancy of Tea Tree oil. *J Essent Oil Res* 9:47-52. 1997

Tong MM, Altman PM, Barnetson RStC. Tea Tree oil in the treatment of tinea pedis. *Australas J Dermatol* 33:145-149. 1992.

Veal L. The potential effectiveness of essential oils as a treatment for headlice, *Pediculus humanus capitis. Complement Ther Nursing Midwifery* 2:97-101. 1996.

Williams L, Home V. A comparative study of some essential oils for potential use in topical applications for the treatment of the yeast *Candida albicans. Aust J Med Herbalism* 7:57-62. 1995.

Teazle

Dipsacus silvestris

DESCRIPTION

Medicinal Parts: The medicinal part is the whole flowering plant with root.

Flower and Fruit: The flowers are lilac in color, with 8-cm cylindrical capitula. The thorny bracts are lanceolate/awl-shaped, curved upward, and longer than the capitula. The outer bracts with their straight, flexible, thorny tips are longer than the flowers. The calyx is basin-shaped, and the corolla is fused with 4 tips. There are 4 stamens and 1 inferior ovary. The fruit is a nutlet.

Leaves, Stem, and Root: The plant is a biennial that grows 80 to 150 cm high. The stem is erect, angular, and thorny. The basal leaves are rosettelike and crenate-serrate. The cauline leaves are oblong with a thorny midrib underneath.

Habitat: With the exception of northern Norway, Sweden, and Finland, wild Teazle grows throughout all of Europe, North Africa, and Asia Minor.

Production: Common Teazle root is the underground part of *Dipsacus silvestris.*

Other Names: Barber's Brush, Brushes and Combs, Card Thistle, Church Broom, Common Teazle, Fuller's Teazle, Venus' Basin

ACTIONS AND PHARMACOLOGY

COMPOUNDS

Iridoide monoterpenes: including cantleyoside, loganin, sweroside, sylvestroside III and IV

Caffeic acid derivatives: including chlorogenic acid

EFFECTS

No information is available.

INDICATIONS AND USAGE

Unproven Uses: Teazle is used externally for small wounds, fistulae, eczema, and as a rub in the treatment of rheumatism.

PRECAUTIONS AND ADVERSE REACTIONS

Health risks or side effects following the proper administration of designated therapeutic dosages are not recorded.

DOSAGE

Mode of Administration: Teazle is used externally in alcoholic extracts.

LITERATURE

Hegnauer R, Chemotaxonomie der Pflanzen, Bde 1-11, Birkhäuser Verlag Basel, Boston, Berlin 1962-1997.

Kern W, List PH, Hörhammer L (Hrsg.), Hagers Handbuch der Pharmazeutischen Praxis, 4. Aufl., Bde. 1-8, Springer Verlag Berlin, Heidelberg, New York, 1969.

Madaus G, Lehrbuch der Biologischen Arzneimittel, Bde 1-3, Nachdruck, Georg Olms Verlag Hildesheim, 1979.

Suh HW, Song DK, Son KH, Wie MB, Lee KH, Jung KY, Do JC, Kim YH, An iridoid glucoside from *Dipsacus asperoides*. *Phytochemistry*, 27:239-40, May 1996

Suh HW, Song DK, Son KH, Wie MB, Lee KH, Jung KY, Do JC, Kim YH, Studies on the chemical constituents of *Dipsacus asper* Wall. *Yao Hsueh Hsueh Pao*, 27:1167-72, Oct. 1996

Zhang Y, Kiyohara H, Matsumoto T, Yamada H, Fractionation and chemical properties of immunomodulating polysaccharides from roots of *Dipsacus asperoides*. *Planta Med*, 27:393-9, Oct. 1997

Terminalia arjuna

See Arjun Tree

Terminalia chebula

See Tropical Almond

Tetraclinis articulata

See Sandarac

Teucrium chamaedrys

See Germander

Teucrium polium

See Poley

Teucrium scordium

See Water Germander

Teucrium scorodonia

See Wood Sage

Theobroma cacao

See Cocoa

Thuja

Thuja occidentalis

DESCRIPTION

Medicinal Parts: The medicinal parts are the oil extracted from the leaves and branch tips, the young dried branches, the fresh, leafy annual branches, and the fresh, leafy branches collected in spring.

Flower and Fruit: The male flowers are dark brown and the female flowers are yellow-green; both are monoecious. The male flowers are arranged in small, terminal catkins and the female flowers are almost star-shaped. The ripe cones are brown-yellow, 6 to 8 mm long, ovate, and covered in coriaceous, obtuse scales. The lower ones are patent at the tips. The seeds are brown-yellow, 3 to 5 mm long, and approximately 1 mm wide. They are narrowly winged the whole way around.

Leaves, Stem, and Root: The plant is a narrowly clavate, 12- to 21-m high tree with short horizontally spread branches and red-brown, striped, peeling trunk. The trunk is usually branched from the base up. The leaves are scalelike, crossed opposite, imbricate, flattened on the branch side and folded at the margins. They are dark green above and matte-green beneath. The scales on the upper part of the branches have a globular glandular swelling.

Habitat: The plant originated from eastern North America and is found in Europe mainly as an ornamental plant and is partly naturalized.

Production: Thuja herb is the young branch tips and young shoots of *Thuja occidentalis*. The harvest should take place in spring when the content of the active agents is optimal. The herb should be dried in the shade and handled with care.

Not to be Confused With: Other forms of Thuja.

Other Names: Arborvitae, Eastern White Cedar, False White Cedar, Hackmatack, Northern White Cedar, Swamp Cedar, Tree of Life, White Cedar, Yellow Cedar

ACTIONS AND PHARMACOLOGY

COMPOUNDS

Water-soluble immunostimulating polysaccharides and glycoproteins

Water-soluble immunostimulating glycoproteins

Volatile oil (1.4-4%): chief components (-)-thujone (alpha-thujone, 59%), (+)-isothujone (beta-thujone, 7-10%), fenchone (10-15%)

Flavonoids: including among others, quercitrin, mearusitrin, the biflavonoids hinoki flavone, amentoflavone, bilobetin-procyanidins

Lignans

Tannins

EFFECTS

The antiviral effect of the drug is attributed to many things. The topical use for viral wart growth is plausible. Proliferation of T cells caused by polysaccharides (esp. CD4 and T-helper/inducer-cells) and an increase in the production of interleukin-2 has been demonstrated.

Because of its thujone content, the essential oil causes spasms and leads in high doses to clonic-tonic convulsions, severe metabolism disturbances through fatty degeneration of the liver, and damage of the renal parenchyma.

INDICATIONS AND USAGE

Unproven Uses: Thuja is used for respiratory tract infections and in conjunction with antibiotics in the treatment of bacterial skin infections and *herpes simplex*. Other possible uses include the treatment of rheumatism, trigeminal neuralgia, strep throat, gout, pruritus, blepharitis, conjunctivitis, otitis media, pertussis, tracheitis, kidney and bladder complaints, enuresis, psoriasis, amenorrhea, and cardiac insufficiency. The drug is used externally as an ointment for treating pains in the joints, arthritis, and muscle rheumatism, as well as infected wounds and burns.

Homeopathic Uses: Thuja occidentalis is used for rheumatism, depressive states, poor digestion, and skin and mucous membrane conditions.

CONTRAINDICATIONS

The drug should not be used during pregnancy.

PRECAUTIONS AND ADVERSE REACTIONS

General: The drug's toxic effect is due to the thujone content. The doses should be strictly followed because of the toxicity of the drug. Allopathic preparations do not contain any thujone.

The toxicological limit, up to which thujone can be administered orally without risk to health, has been established at 1.25 mg/kg body weight. Only poisonings connected with the consumption of the leaves and shoots of fresh plants have been recorded since 1980. In therapeutic dosages of medications, the thujone content is far below the toxicological limit.

Use in Pregnancy: The drug is misused as an abortifacient. Thuja should not be taken during pregnancy.

OVERDOSAGE

Symptoms of poisoning, often seen after misuse of the drug as an abortifacient, include queasiness, vomiting, painful diarrhea, and mucous membrane hemorrhaging. Instances of death have been reported.

Following gastrointestinal emptying (inducement of vomiting, gastric lavage with burgundy-colored potassium permanganate solution, sodium sulphate), administration of activated charcoal, and shock prophylaxis (appropriate body position, quiet, warmth), the treatment for poisoning consists of treating spasms with diazepam (IV), colic with atropine, administering electrolytes and treating possible cases of acidosis with sodium bicarbonate infusions. Monitoring of kidney function is essential. Intubation and oxygen respiration may also be necessary.

DOSAGE

Mode of Administration: Whole, cut, and powdered drug is found in compound preparations.

Preparation: To make an extract of 1:1, use 50% ethanol; for an extract of 1:10, use 60% ethanol. To make a tincture, mix 100 parts Thuja powder and 1,000 parts diluted spirit of wine (EB6).

Daily Dosage: The daily dose for the extract is 1 to 2 mL 3 times daily.

Homeopathic Dosage: 5 drops, 1 tablet, or 10 globules every 30 to 60 minutes (acute) or 1 to 3 times daily (chronic); parenterally: 1 to 2 mL sc, acute: 3 times daily; chronic: once a day (HAB1).

Storage: Mark the container as ''poisonous'' and protect from light and excessive heat.

LITERATURE

Baba T et al. Inhibitory effect of beta-thujaplicin on ultraviolet B-induced apoptosis in mouse keratinocytes. *J Invest Dermatol,* 110:24-8, Jan 1998

Beuscher N, Kopanski L, Purification and biological characterization of antiviral substances from *Thuja occidentalis*. In: *PM* 52:555-556. 1986.

Bodinet K, Freudenstein J. Effects of an orally applied aqueous-ethanolic extract of a mixture of *Thujae occidentalis herba, Baptisiae tinctoriae radix, Echinaceae purpureae radix* and *Echinaceae pallidae radix* on antibody response against sheep red blood cells in mice. *PM* 65. 1999

Cartier A, Chan H, Malo JL, Pineau L, Tse KS, Chan-Yeung M. Occupational asthma caused by eastern white cedar (*Thuja occidentalis*) with demonstration that plicatic acid is present in this wood dust and is the causal agent. *J Allergy Clin Immunol,* 77:639-45, Apr 1986

Gan OI, Drize NI, Gohla SH, Shrum S, Neth R. Effects of polysaccharide from *Thuja occidentale L.* on stromal precursor cells of hematopoietic microenvironment in mice *Bioll Eksp Biol Med,* 112:635-7, Dec 1991

Gohla SH, Haubeck HD, Neth RD. Mitogenic activity of high molecular polysaccharide fractions isolated from the *Cupressaceae Thuja occidentale L.* I. Macrophage-dependent induction of CD-4-positive T-helper (Th+) lymphocytes. *Leukemia*, 2:528-33, Aug 1988

Gohla SH, Haubeck HD, Schrum S, Soltau H, Neth RD. Activation of CD4-positive T cells by polysaccharide fractions isolated from the *Cupressaceae Thuja occidentalis L.* (Arborvitae). *Hamatol Bluttransfus,* 50:268-72, 1989

Hassan HT, Drize NJ, Sadovinkova EYu, Gan OI, Gohla S, Schrum S, Neth RD. TPSg, an anti-human immunodeficiency virus (HIV-1) agent, isolated from the *Cupressaceae Thuja occidentale L.* (Arborvitae) enhances in vivo hemopoietic progenitor cells recovery in sublethally irradiated mice. *Immunol Lett,* 50:119-22, Apr 1996

Khurana SMP, Effect of homoeopathic drugs on plant viruses. In: PM 20:142-146. 1971.

Schubert W, Die Inhaltsstoffe von *Thuja occidentalis*. In: Dissertation Technische Universität Braunschweig. 1987.

Tachibana Y et al., Mitogenic activities in African traditional herbal medicines. In: *PM* 59(4):354. 1993.

Thuja occidentalis

See Thuja

Thuja orientalis

See Oriental Arborvitae

Thyme

Thymus vulgaris

DESCRIPTION

Medicinal Parts: The medicinal parts are the oil extracted from the fresh, flowering herb, the dried leaves, the stripped and dried leaves, and the fresh aerial part of the flowering plant.

Flower and Fruit: The blue-violet to bright red labiate flowers are arranged in 3- to 6-blossomed axillary clusters. The calyx is bilabiate with a 3-tipped upper lip and a 2-tipped lower lip. The upper lip of the corolla is straight and the lower lip is divided in 3. The stamens are splayed from the base.

Leaves, Stem, and Root: The plant is a dwarf shrub that grows up to 50 cm high with an erect, woody, and many branched/bushy, downy stem that never roots. The leaves are short-petioled, linear, or oblong-round, acute, glandular-punctate with an involute margin and a tomentose undersurface.

Characteristics: The odor is aromatic and the taste tangy, somewhat bitter and camphorlike.

Habitat: The plant is indigenous to the Mediterranean region and neighboring countries, northern Africa, and parts of Asia. It is extensively cultivated.

Production: Thyme consists of the stripped and dried leaves and flowers of *Thymus vulgaris, Thymus zygis,* or both species.

Other Names: Common Thyme, Garden Thyme, Rubbed Thyme

ACTIONS AND PHARMACOLOGY

COMPOUNDS

Volatile oil (1.0-2.5%): chief components thymol (20-55%), p-cymene (14-45%), carvacrol (1-10%), gamma-terpinene (5-10%), borneol (up to 8%), linalool (up to 8%)

Caffeic acid derivatives: rosmarinic acid (0.15-1.35%)

Flavonoids: including among others, luteolin, apigenin, naringenin, eriodictyol, cirsilineol, salvigenin, cirsimaritin, thymonine, thymusine, partially present as glycosides

Triterpenes: including among others, ursolic acid (1.9%), oleanolic acid (0.6%)

EFFECTS

Thyme is a bronchial antispasmodic and an expectorant. It has shown antibacterial, antifungal, antiviral, antiprotozoan, and antioxidant properties. In animal experiments, a spasmolytic effect was demonstrated for the flavone fraction and an expectorant effect on ciliary activity for the terpenes.

INDICATIONS AND USAGE

Approved by Commission E:

- Cough
- Bronchitis

Unproven Uses: The herb is used internally for catarrh of the upper respiratory tract, dyspeptic complaints, asthma, laryngitis, chronic gastritis, and whooping cough. Externally, it is used as a mouthwash and gargle for inflammations of the mouth and throat, pruritus, and dermatoses. It is also used externally for tonsillitis and poorly healing wounds.

PRECAUTIONS AND ADVERSE REACTIONS

No health hazards or side effects are known in conjunction with the proper administration of designated therapeutic dosages. The drug possesses a low potential for sensitization. Avoid whole-body baths except with doctor's permission in cases involving large skin injuries, acute skin illnesses, severe feverish or infectious diseases, cardiac insufficiency, or hypertonia.

DOSAGE

Mode of Administration: Thyme is available as a comminuted drug, powder, liquid extract or dry extract for infusions and other galenic preparations. Liquid and solid medicinal forms for internal and external application are available. Combinations with other herbs, which have expectorant action, are also available. Extracts of the drug are components of standardized preparations of antitussive and cough remedy teas.

How Supplied:

Oil — 100%

Liquid — 1:1, 1:5

Preparation: To prepare a tea, use 1.5 to 2 g drug with boiling water, steep for 10 minutes, then strain. (1 teaspoonful is equivalent to 1.4 g drug.) To prepare an infusion, add 1 to 2 g drug to 150 mL of water. For a bath, add a minimum of 0.004 g thyme oil to 1 liter of water, filter, then add to bath water drawn at a temperature of 35-38° C. Alternatively, add 500 g of drug to 4 liters of boiling water, filter, then add to bath water.

Daily Dosage: The recommended daily dosage is 10 g drug with 0.03% phenol, calculated as thymol. When using a liquid extract, 1 to 2 g is taken 1 to 3 times daily. The single dose for the infusion is 1.5 g drug, or 1 to 2 g drug per cup of water taken several times a day. The dose for the powder is 1 to 4 g drug twice daily.

The tea can be taken several times a day as needed. A 5% infusion can be used for compresses. Baths should be taken for 10 to 20 minutes.

Storage: Keep the herb in a tightly sealed container, and protect from light and moisture.

LITERATURE

Broucke CO van den, Lemli JA. Pharmacological and Chemical Investigations of Thyme Liquid Extracts. *Planta Med.* 41; 129-135. 1981

Broucke CO van den, Lemli JA. Spasmolytic activity of the flavonoids from *Thymus vulgaris. Pharm Weekbl Sci Ed.* 5; 9-14. 1983

Broucke CO van den, Dommisse RA, Esmans EL, Lemli JA. Three Methylated Flavones from *Thymus vulgaris. Phytochemistry* 21; 2581-2583. 1982

Ernst E, März R, Sieder C. A controlled multi-centre study of herbal versus synthetic secretolytic drugs for acute bronchitis. *Phytomedicine* 4 (4); 287-293. 1997

Haraguchi H et al., Antiperoxidative components in *Thymus vulgaris*. In: *PM* 62(3):217-221. 1996.

Mossa JS, Al-Yahya MA, Hassan MM. Phytochemical Characteristics and Spectroscopy of the Volatile Oil of *Thymus vulgaris* Growing in Saudi Arabia. *Int J Crude Drug Res.* 25; 26-34. 1987

Thymus serpyllum

See Wild Thyme

Thymus vulgaris

See Thyme

Tiarella cordifolia

See Coolwort

Tilia species

See Linden

Tobacco

Nicotiana tabacum

DESCRIPTION

Medicinal Parts: The medicinal parts are the dried leaves.

Flower and Fruit: The numerous flowers are in many-branched panicles. The sepals are 12 to 25 mm long and tubular to tubular-campanulate. The tips are triangular, pointed and unequal. The corolla is 30 to 55 mm long, funnel-shaped, pale greenish-cream. The limb is 10 to 15 mm with pointed lobes, which are not always entire. The four stamens are unequal and sometimes slightly exerted. The capsule is 15 to 20 mm long, ellipsoid to globose.

Leaves, Stem, and Root: Tobacco is an annual or biennial plant, 1 to 3 m in height. The plant has a long fibrous root and an upright, round, pubescent and stick stem, which is heavily branched at the top. The leaves are up to 50 cm in length. They are ovate to elliptical or lanceolate, pointed, alternate, and sessile. They sometimes have a short, winged petiole.

Habitat: The plant originates from tropical America and is cultivated worldwide, in particular in the U.S., China, Turkey, Greece, Holland, France, Germany, and most subtropical countries.

Production: Tobacco leaves are the cultivated, unfermented leaves of *Nicotiana tabacum*.

ACTIONS AND PHARMACOLOGY

COMPOUNDS

Pyridine alkaloids (0.5-8.0%, among select cultivars 1.5%): chief alkaloid nicotine (30-60% share of the alkaloid mixture) including among others N-formyl nor-nicotine, cotinine, myosmine, nicotyrine, anabasine, nicotelline

EFFECTS

In small doses, Tobacco increases blood pressure and the activity of the gastric mucous membrane. In larger doses, it reduces blood pressure and lowers muscle tone of the gastrointestinal tract. Tobacco is a stimulant to the respiratory and central nervous system.

INDICATIONS AND USAGE

Unproven Uses: Nicotine is used to help break the smoking habit.

Apache Indians use the drug to treat toothache, mosquito bites, and bee stings. In Brazil and Guyana, Tobacco is used for worm infestation, skin parasites, and biliary flow disturbances. The drug's use in these conditions is not advised because of the risk of toxicity.

Indian Medicine: Tobacco is used for toothache, dental caries, earache, suppurating rhinitis, hernias, and painful swellings.

Homeopathic Uses: Tobacco is used for angina pectoris, low blood pressure and vomiting with diarrhea.

PRECAUTIONS AND ADVERSE REACTIONS

Tobacco leaves are severely poisonous. The chief toxin is nicotine, a liquid alkaloid, which can be resorbed through the skin.

OVERDOSAGE

The lethal dosage for nicotine for an adult is 40 to 100 mg, although this can be considerably elevated through habituation (with smoking Tobacco, 2 to 7 g of the drug; one cigarette contains 10 mg nicotine, of which 1 to 2 mg are inhaled during smoking). Symptoms of an acute poisoning include dizziness, salivation, vomiting, diarrhea, trembling of the hands and feelings of weakness in the legs; very high dosages can lead rapidly to spasms, unconsciousness, cardiac arrest and respiratory failure. Poisonings occur in particular through the ingestion of cigarettes by children, the handling of insecticides containing nicotine (through skin contact), and in connection with the harvesting of Tobacco (also through cutaneous resorption). Nicotine patches also represent a danger for children.

Following gastric lavage with burgundy-colored potassium permanganate solution, instillation of activated charcoal and sodium sulphate solution, the therapy for poisonings consists of treating spasms with diazepam (IV), chloral hydrate for children (rectal); cardiac massage; administration of orciprenaline; and atropine for severe sympathetic excitation. Intubation and oxygen respiration may also be necessary. No centrally effective analeptics are to be given.

DOSAGE

Mode of Administration: The nicotine alkaloid is used internally as a gum and externally as a transdermal patch.

Preparation: Nicorette (chewing gum); also as transdermal patches.

Daily Dosage: Nicotine as a pure alkaloid in smoker's remedies; nicotine (2 to 4 mg) bound by polacrilin (8 to 16 mg). Nicotine gum is an ion exchanger and therefore causes the slow release of nicotine, which is absorbed in the saliva over and over again. Eventually, the doses are reduced as the breaking of the habit progresses.

Homeopathic Dosage: 5 drops, 1 tablet, or 10 globules every 30 to 60 minutes (acute) or 1 to 3 times daily (chronic); parenterally: 1 to 2 mL sc, acute: 3 times daily; chronic: once a day (HAB1).

LITERATURE

Bakoula C et al., Objective passive smoking indicators and respiratory morbidity in young children. In: *DAZ* 135(46):4330-4331 et 4334. 1995.

Borisjuk NV, Davidjuk YM, Kostishin SS, Miroshnichenco GP, Velasco R, Hemleben V, Volkov RA, Structural analysis of rDNA in the genus Nicotiana. *Plant Mol Biol,* 35:655-60. Nov. 1997

Devarenne TP, Shin DH, Back K, Yin S, Chappell J, Characterization of cucumber mosaic virus. IV. Movement protein and coat protein are both essential for cell-to-cell movement of cucumber mosaic virus. Virology, 349:237-48. Oct 27. 1997

Klotz KL, Liu TT, Liu L, Lagrimini LM, Expression of the Tobacco anionic peroxidase gene is tissue-specific and developmentally regulated. *Plant Mol Biol,* 36:509-20. Mar. 1998

Lippiello, Buch. In: The Biology of Nicotine. Current Research Issue. Lippiello PM, Collins AC, Gray JA, Robinson JH (Eds.). Raven Press New York. 1992.

Matsushima S, Ohsumi T, Sugawara S, *Agric Biol Chem* (Tokyo) 47:507. 1983.

Olbrich A, Das Lungenemphysem - Neuere Apsekte zu Pathogenese und Therapie. In: *DAZ* 135(47):4393-4405. 1995.

Piotrowski M, Oecking C, Five new 14-3-3 isoforms from *Nicotiana tabacum L.*: implications for the phylogeny of plant 14-3-3 proteins. *Planta Med,* 204:127-30. Jan. 1998

Tolu Balsam

Myroxylon balsamum

DESCRIPTION

Medicinal Parts: The medicinal parts are the resin balsam from the trunks.

Flower and Fruit: The androgynous flowers grow on pedicles approximately 12 cm long on simple, richly blossomed racemes. The calyx is inferior, broadly tubular or oblong-campanulate, dark green with short, rough hairs. The 5 petals are white and stemmed. The standard is almost circular. The stamens are bright red and the 1-valve ovary is on a long stem. The fruit is a single-seeded, indehiscent, winged pod. The seeds are distinctly curved, red, and reniform.

Leaves, Stem, and Root: These balsam trees grow to 25 m tall with a round, spreading crown that only starts to branch at a height of 13 to 19 m. The bark is smooth, yellow-gray, or brown with numerous lenticles. The leaves are usually odd-pinnate and have 4 to 7 obovate, acuminate, coreacious, short-petioled leaflets. The upper surface is dark green and the lower surface pale green.

Characteristics: Before drying, the resin smells strongly of vanilla or benzoin.

Habitat: Myroxylon balsamum is indigenous to South and Central America, Sri Lanka, and Jamaica.

Production: Peruvian balsam consists of the balsam generated from scorched tree trunks of *Myroxylon balsamum.* The bark of 10-year-old trees is removed just above ground level and this area is scorched with a flame, after which the balsam is collected in cloths placed on the scorched area. Tolu Balsam consists of the balsam generated from the incised tree trunks of *Myroxylon balsamum.* The balsam is purified by melting, straining, and solidifying. A V-shaped incision is made in the tree trunk, and a vessel is secured under the incision to collect the resin, which is then cleaned.

Other Names: Balsam of Peru, Balsam Tree, Peruvian Balsam, Tolu

ACTIONS AND PHARMACOLOGY

COMPOUNDS: PERUVIAN BALSAM

Ester mixture, so-called cinnamein (50-70%): made up of benzyl benzoate and benzyl cinnamoate

Resins (20-30%): chief constituent cinnamic acid ester of the so-called peruresitannols (polymer)

Volatile oils: including some with nerolidol

EFFECTS: PERUVIAN BALSAM

The drug has an antibacterial/antiseptic effect, promotes the granulation process, and is antiparasitic (especially for scabies). The main active constituent is an ester mixture that mainly contains benzyl benzoate.

COMPOUNDS: TOLU BALSAM

Ester mixture (10-20%): made up of benzyl benzoate and benzyl cinnamoate

Free benzoic acid/free cinnamic acid (10 to 30%)

Resins (up to 80%)

Volatile oil

EFFECTS: TOLU BALSAM

The undiluted oil showed antibacterial and fungicidal effects in the diffusion test. The drug also acts as an expectorant. The effect on the respiratory tract appears to work in the field of aromatherapy.

INDICATIONS AND USAGE

PERUVIAN BALSAM

Approved by Commission E:

- Wounds and burns

■ Hemorrhoids

External Use: for infected and poorly healing wounds, for burns, decubitus ulcers, frostbite, leg ulcers, and bruises caused by prostheses and hemorrhoids.

Unproven Uses: Although no longer used internally, it was used previously for fevers, colds, coughs, bronchitis, inflammation of the mouth and pharynx, and a tendency to infection. External folk medicine uses are the treatment of eczema and itching. Outdated uses include treatment of scabies; as a liniment for headaches, toothache and rheumatic symptoms; and use of the resin for uterine and umbilical venous bleeding.

Homeopathic Uses: Indications in homeopathy include chronic mucous membrane inflammation of the respiratory and urinary organs.

TOLU BALSAM
Approved by Commission E:

■ Cough/Bronchitis

Tolu Balsam is used to treat inflammation of the mucous membranes of the respiratory tract.

Unproven Uses: Folk medicine external uses include the approved indications above, as well as the treatment of wounds.

PRECAUTIONS AND ADVERSE REACTIONS

PERUVIAN BALSAM
Peruvian balsam often causes contact allergies. Urticaria, recurring aphthoid oral ulcers, Quincke's disease, and diffuse purpura can all occur, among other ailments (possibly also following internal administration, for example, of foods containing Peruvian Balsam). Photodermatoses and phototoxic reactions are possible without ingestion. Kidney damage has been observed following internal as well as external use of large dosages (such as albuminuria, pyelitis, and necroses of the canaliculus epithelia).

TOLU BALSAM
No health hazards or side effects are known in conjunction with the proper administration of designated therapeutic dosages. However, just as is the case with Peruvian Balsam, allergic reactions are possible.

DOSAGE

PERUVIAN BALSAM
Mode of Administration: Galenic preparations for external use.

How Supplied: Commercial pharmaceutical preparations include ointments and suppositories.

Homeopathic Dosage: 5 drops, 1 tablet or 10 globules every 30 to 60 minutes (acute) or 1 to 3 times daily (chronic); parenterally: 1 to 2 mL sc acute, 3 times daily; chronic: once a day (HAB34).

Daily Dosage: Galenic preparations containing 5 to 20% Peruvian Balsam, for extensive surface application not more than 10% Peruvian Balsam. Duration of application should not exceed 1 week.

Storage: Store Peruvian Balsam in a container that seals tightly and prevents exposure to light.

TOLU BALSAM
Mode of Administration: Various preparations of Tolu Balsam are used internally.

Preparation: To prepare Tolu Balsam syrup, dissolve the drug in 96% alcohol in a water bath with reflux; add 85% glycerol and water, then warm the mixture. Let stand for a week before adding saccharose. Prepare a 1,000 mL tincture with 200 g Tolu Balsam and 92.3% ethanol.

Daily Dosage: Average daily dosage is 0.6 g of drug, depending on the preparation.

Storage: Store protected from light in tightly sealed containers with a suitable drying agent. Do not store Tolu Balsam in powder form.

LITERATURE

PERUVIAN BALSAM AND TOLU BALSAM
Galeffi C. The Contribution of American Plants to pharmaceutical Sciences / Review Article. *Il Farmaco* 48; 1175-1195. 1993

Harkiss KJ, Linley PA, *PM* 35:61-65. 1979.

Lund K, Rimpler H, *Dtsch Apoth Ztg* 125(3):105. 1985

Morton JF, An Atlas of Medicinal Plants of Middle America, Charles C. Thomas, USA 1981.

Rudski E, Grzywaz Z, *Dermatologia* 155(2):115. 1977

Tomato

Lycopersicon esculentum

DESCRIPTION

Medicinal Parts: The medicinal parts are the fresh leaves, the fresh herb collected during the flowering season, or the whole plant.

Flower and Fruit: The flowers are in lateral, cymelike coils. The tips of the calyx are linear-lanceolate. The corolla is yellow, as long as the calyx, and has a very short tube. It is divided into pointed, lanceolate lobes. The stamens are fused to the tube. The stigma is greenish and capitular. The fruit is a large, juicy, smooth, round to ovoid berry with a short, obtuse tip. It is scarlet, occasionally yellow or whitish with a diameter of 2 to 10 cm. The seeds are reniform, flattened, whitish-gray-yellow, and villous-tomentose.

Leaves, Stem, and Root: The Tomato plant is an annual with a fusiform, fibrous root. The stem grows to 120 cm, and is leafy and heavily branched, with glandular hairs. The leaves are broad-petiolate, odd-pinnate, petiolate, ovate-lanceolate, pinnatifid, dentate, and slightly involute leaflets. The leaves have a gray-green underside.

Habitat: The plant probably originated in southern or Central America; today it is only cultivated.

Production: Tomato tincture is the homeopathic mother tincture of the whole plant *Lycopersicon esculentum.*

Other Names: Love Apple

ACTIONS AND PHARMACOLOGY

COMPOUNDS

Steroid alkaloid glycosides: chief alkaloid alpha-tomatine

EFFECTS

Some studies are showing a relationship between high Tomato consumption and lower levels of cancer. While a number of epidemiological studies demonstrated some benefits for cancer treatment with lycopene, the carotenoid that is plentiful in Tomatoes and certain other fruits and vegetables, other studies showed no effect. The majority of evidence, however, supports the use of lycopene in cancer prevention. Lycopene levels have been shown to be inversely proportional to cancers of the prostate, cervix, pancreas, and stomach.

There is a fair amount of epidemiologic evidence to document a possible correlation between lycopene ingestion and protection from cardiovascular disease. Similarly, there is fair documentation to indicate a possible effectiveness of lycopene in reducing cholesterol in adults and animals. Lycopene may have anticholesterol effects due to inhibition of HMG CoA reductase activity and antineoplastic activity due to its inhibition of DNA synthesis, antioxidant effects, modulation of intercellular communication, and induction of cell differentiation. Lycopene has the highest singlet oxygen-quenching capacity in vitro (antioxidant).

The content of lycopene, a common carotenoid found in tomatoes as well as other fruits (apricot, cranberry, eggplant, grape, papaya, peach, guava, watermelon) varies by the color of the tomato. The very red varieties having as much as 50 mg/100 g, and the yellow varieties as little as 5 mg/100 g (Clinton, 1998).

Seventy-two to 92% of lycopene in the tomato is associated with the water insoluble fraction and the skin of the fruit. In one test, the tomato pulp had 42.3 mg/100 g of tomato, while the water-soluble portion contained only 4 mg/100 g. Five different strains were used. The concentrations of lycopene in the tomato pulp ranged from 6.46 to 10.19 mg/100 g. The concentration in the insoluble fraction ranged from 35.4 to 53.56 mg/100 g and in the soluble fraction from 0.0074 to 0.034 mg/100 g. When a commercial sample of pulp was tested the lycopene concentration was 12.46 mg/100 g (Sharma & LeMaguer, 1996).

Lycopene is susceptible to oxidation and elevated temperature, exposure to light, oxygen, pH extremes, and active surfaces will degrade it. Lycopene also undergoes cis-trans isomerization the cis form is less thermo-stable. Twenty percent to 57% of lycopene has been lost in processing tomato fruit pulp according to some studies, but others have shown lycopene to be relatively heat stable. Lycopene is more stable in the tomato or fruit than it is in isolated form (Nguyen & Schwartz, 1999). Store at room temperature, away from heat, moisture, and direct light.

Tomato's tomatin content has been shown to be antibacterial. In animal experiments, a lowering of blood pressure was observed after IV administration of tomatin hydrochloride. Lectin isolated from the fruit is said to have an effect on cell division and DANN synthesis in human leukocyte cultures.

Anticholesterol Effects: In one murine study, reduced atherosclerosis risk was estimated due to reduced lipid oxidation in animals treated with a Tomato supplement. Male ICR mice were fed a control diet for 4 months or an atherogenic diet for the same time period. Blood from the mice was drawn every 2 months and analyzed for lipid oxidation. The atherogenic diet produced a reduction in body weight for both groups 2 and 3 when compared to controls. The reduction was significant ($p<0.05$) after 2 months and continued until the end of the experiment. There were no growth differences between groups 2 and 3. Serum cholesterol increased significantly during the study in both groups 2 and 3. The increase in thiobarbituric acid-reactive substances (TBARS) (oxidation) in the Tomato group was only slightly greater than that of the control group (Suganuma & Inakuma, 1999).

When tested in the J-774A cell line, lycopene was shown to augment the activity of LDL receptors, similar to the anticholesterol drug fluvastatin. The mechanism was thought to be inhibition of macrophage 3-hydroxy-3-methyl glutaryl coenzyme A (HMG CoA) reductase. This enzyme is used in the rate-limiting step of cholesterol synthesis (Fuhrman et al, 1997).

The susceptibility of low-density lipoproteins to oxidation was not changed by increased lycopene plasma concentrations caused by supplementation with Tomato juice. Fifteen renal transplant patients were given either a synthetic orange drink or Tomato juice for 4 weeks in a crossover study. Plasma lycopene levels increased significantly ($p<0.015$). LDL oxidation was measured by fluorescent lipid oxidation products (FLOP) and by thiobarbituric acid reacting substances (TBARS) in the serum. The lag time to LDL oxidation was also measured. None of the measures showed decreased LDL oxidation (Sutherland et al, 1999).

Antineoplastic Effects: Tomato juice containing lycopene, but not an equal amount of lycopene alone, protected against development of induced colon cancer. Seven-week-old female F344/NSlc rats were given an intrarectal dose of 2 or 4 mg of N-methylnitrosourea (NMN) 3 times a week for 3 weeks to induce cancer. The animals were allowed to drink unlimited amounts of either water (controls), water containing 17 ppm lycopene (LY group), diluted Tomato juice containing the same 17 ppm lycopene (TJ), or 3.4 ppm lycopene as Tomato juice (LTJ). At 35 weeks after treatment with the 2 mg NMN dose there was a significantly lower incidence (compared to controls (54%)) in the TJ group (21%), but not in the LY group (33%). At the higher NMN dose, there was also a significant difference between the TJ group (40%) and the controls (84%) or the LTJ groups (72%). When the colon mucosa of the rats was examined, a significant amount of lycopene was found in TJ group but not the LTJ group (Narisawa et al, 1998). In another study, lycopene in combination with the drug piroxicam, but not lycopene alone, or lycopene with beta-carotene, produced a cancer preventative effect against induced urinary bladder cancers in rats (Okajima et al, 1997).

The serum level of lycopene was reduced when exposed to the oxidative stress of a meal or smoking. The lipid peroxidation expressed as thiobarbituric acid reactive substances (TBARS) was taken in 20 healthy human subjects before and after a meal. Serum lycopene levels between smokers and nonsmokers were not statistically different but after smoking three cigarettes, serum lycopene levels dropped 40%, and TBARS increased (increased lipid peroxidation) 40%. After a meal lycopene levels dropped 25% when compared to fasting levels. Eating a meal and smoking, both of which produce oxidative stress, reduced lycopene levels (Rao & Agarwal, 1998).

Antioxidant Effects: The antiproliferative effect of lycopene is secondary to its inhibition of DNA synthesis (Levy et al, 1995). Much of its activity is attributed to its antioxidant properties (Clinton, 1998). Modulation of intercellular communication, which has been demonstrated in cell cultures, may be another mechanism for the antiproliferative effect of lycopene (Stahl et al, 2000; Krutovskikh et al, 1997). Another postulated mechanism for its antiproliferative effect is that it can induce differentiation of cancer cells. This induction of differentiation has been observed in leukemic cell cultures exposed to a combination of both lycopene and 1,25 dihydroxyvitamin D3 (Amir et al, 1999).

When tested for antioxidant properties in a multilamellar liposome system, lycopene was found to have the greatest antioxidant activity of the carotenoids. The ranking (greatest to least) was lycopene, alpha-tocopherol, alpha carotene, beta-cryptoxanthin, zeaxanthin, beta-carotene, and lutein (Stahl et al, 1998).

Lycopene was not associated with a reduced risk of nuclear cataracts in the aged. Lycopene has been shown to have a protective antioxidant effect on cataracts in experimental animals. A nuclear opacity test was done using lens photographs taken in 1988 to 1990 and compared to photographs taken in 1993 to 1995. Nonfasting concentrations of various carotenoids and tocopherols were determined from serum obtained at baseline. A comparison was made between those that developed cataracts and those that did not. No statistically significant relationship was found with lycopene (Lyle et al, 1999).

Lymphocyte oxidative DNA damage was lessened in 10 healthy women who ate a lycopene-containing Tomato puree. The study had a crossover design, with one group receiving a diet containing 16.5 mg of lycopene while the other had a Tomato-free diet for 21 days. Plasma lycopene concentrations and primary resistance to oxidative stress was analyzed before and after each diet. Oxidative stress was determined by single-cell gel electrophoresis. Lycopene levels increased by 0.5 mcmol/liter during the supplementation trial while during the Tomato-free diet lycopene dropped 0.2 mcmol/L ($p<0.01$). Lymphocyte DNA damage after ex vivo treatment with hydrogen peroxide decreased by 33% and 42% in the two groups of subjects (Riso et al, 1999).

Lycopene may play a role in preventing oxidative damage in skin produced by exposure to ultraviolet light. The volar forearm of 16 healthy Caucasian women was exposed to 3x their minimal erythema dose (determined previously) of ultraviolet light. This produced a 31% to 46% reduction in skin concentrations of lycopene. This same dose of light did not appreciably affect the concentration of skin beta-carotene, another carotenoid. Three days after the ultraviolet exposure a 6-mm skin biopsy was obtained and levels of lycopene and beta-carotene determined (Ribaya-Mercado et al, 1995).

CLINICAL TRIALS

Breast Cancer

A cohort epidemiological study of 88 Finish patients evaluated the relative risk (RR) of developing breast cancer. The comparison was between those in the third tertile (highest) versus those in the first tertile of serum lycopene levels. The RR was approximately 1. The cases were adjusted for age, body mass, parity, occupation, smoking status, and region of the country (Jarvinen et al, 1997).

A case-control study of 46 American patients evaluated the relative risk (RR) of developing breast cancer. The comparison was between those with higher than the mean breast adipose tissue levels of lycopene versus those with lower than the mean. The RR was 0.32 with a 95% confidence interval of 0.11 to 0.94. The cases were adjusted for age, smoking status, and menopause status (Zhang et al, 1997).

A cohort epidemiological study of 105 American patients evaluated the relative risk (RR) of developing breast cancer. The comparison was between those with a serum lycopene level greater than 0.51 mcmol/liter and those with a serum level 22 mcmol/liter. The RR was 0.5 with a 95% confidence interval of 0.2 to 1.2 and a p value of 0.02. The cases were adjusted for age, serum cholesterol level, body mass, breast disease, and smoking status (Dorgan et al, 1998).

Cardiovascular Disease

An epidemiological study from 10 European countries showed a correlation between lycopene lipid levels and reduced risk of myocardial infarction. A multicenter, case-control study was performed evaluating the content of lycopene in buttock tissue taken after myocardial infarction. Analyses using conditional logistic regression models controlling for age, body mass index, socioeconomic status, smoking, hypertension, and maternal and paternal history of disease showed lycopene to be protective with an odds ratio of 0.52 for the contrast of the 10th and 90th percentiles (95%

confidence interval 0.33-0.82, p<0.005). The median lycopene adipose tissue concentration for controls was 0.27 mg/g of fatty acid. The effect of lycopene was strongest in nonsmokers. The protective effect of lycopene increased at each increasing level of polyunsaturated fat and was significant in individuals whose fat tissue contained more than 16.1% polyunsaturates. Levels of lycopene in the fatty tissue provide a better measure of long-term lycopene intake than does serum levels or dietary records (Kohlmeier et al, 1997).

Cervical Cancer

A trend toward decreased lycopene levels was found in a study of Latin American women with cervical cancer. Newly diagnosed cases of cervical cancer from Latin America were included in the study. Patients were under 70 years of age. Lycopene was determined in plasma using high performance liquid chromatography. Lycopene values trended toward lower values with more advanced disease. Early-stage cases had levels not very different from controls. There were 696 cervical cancer patients in the study and 1,217 controls. The age adjusted mean value of lycopene in controls was 10.9 mcg/dL in the cervical cancer patients it was 9.9 mcg/dL. When lycopene levels were determined for each stage of the cancer, plasma values were 12.5 mcg/dL for stage one, 10.4 mcg/dL for stage 2, 8.4 mcg/dL for stage 3, and 8.3 mcg/dL for stage 4 (Potischman et al, 1994).

Colorectal Cancer

A case-control epidemiological study of 629 Italian rectal cancer subjects and 955 colon cancer patients compared the RR of developing colorectal cancer between the fourth and first quartile of Tomato eaters. The RR for the colon cancer patients was 0.39 (95% confidence interval of 0.31 to 0.49) and for the rectal cancer patients was 0.42 (confidence interval of 0.32 to 0.55). The cases were adjusted for sex, study center where the case occurred, educational level, alcohol usage, smoking status, caloric intake, and age (Franceschi et al, 1997).

A case-control epidemiological study of 453 colon cancer and 365 rectal cancer patients compared the relative risk (RR) of developing colorectal cancer between the 2 groups. One group reported eating any amount of Tomatoes each week compared to those that ate none. The RR for the colon cancer group was 1.15 with a p for trend equal to 0.31. The RR for the rectal cancer patients groups was 1.03 with a p=0.84. The same cases were evaluated again using Tomato paste instead of Tomatoes as the criteria. The RR for the colon cancer group was 0.78 (p=0.12) and for the rectal cancer group the RR was 0.93 (p=0.93). The cases were adjusted for sex, region, and age (Tuyns et al, 1988).

Esophageal Cancer

A case-control epidemiological study of 217 male and 127 female patients evaluated the RR of developing esophageal cancer. The comparison was between those who ate one or more Tomatoes per day (minimum of 7/week) and those that ate one or less than 1 per month. The RR for the males was 0.61 with a 95% confidence interval of 0.43 to 0.86. The RR for the females was 1.08 with a 95% confidence interval of 0.69 to 1.67. The cases were adjusted for age and region of Iran (Cook-Mozaffari et al, 1989).

A case-control epidemiological study of 207 American male patients evaluated the RR of developing esophageal cancer. The comparison was between those who had ''high'' intake of Tomatoes versus those with ''low'' intake. The RR was 0.70 with a 95% confidence interval of 0.4 to 1.4. The cases were adjusted for age, alcohol intake, and smoking status (Brown et al, 1988).

Hypercholesterolemia

No significant change in lipids was noted when supplementation with 5 mg of lycopene daily was used by 22 female adults for 6 weeks. Lycopene supplementation did not affect lipid status. The antioxidant activity of the subject's plasma was not altered (Bohm & Bitsch, 1999).

A 14% reduction in plasma LDL cholesterol concentrations was noted when 6 males were given Tomato lycopene supplementation of 60 mg daily for 3 months (Fuhrman et al, 1997).

Oxidation of LDL cholesterol was significantly reduced by the administration of lycopene in the diet of 19 healthy subjects not taking other drugs. Administration of dietary lycopene increased serum lycopene by at least twofold. There was no change in the levels of LDL cholesterol, HDL cholesterol, or total cholesterol in these subjects. This was a crossover design study. Lycopene was administered in the diet as Tomato juice, spaghetti sauce, and Tomato oleoresin. The study was randomized and crossover in design. There were four test groups in the study. Group 1 received no lycopene, group 2 received 39.2 mg of lycopene as spaghetti sauce, group 3 received 50.4 mg of lycopene as Tomato juice, and group 4 received 75 mg of lycopene as a 6% lycopene Tomato oleoresin. Although the differences in serum lycopene levels were significant (p<0.05) between the placebo and each of the lycopene supplements, there was no significant difference between the various supplements, despite the varied amounts of lycopene administered. Oxidation of DNA and protein was measured using protein thiols and 8-oxodeoxyguanosine contents of lymphocyte DNA. A tendency toward lower oxidation in these groups was noted but the results were not statistically significant (Agarwal & Rao, 1998; Rao & Agarwal, 1998a).

Lung Cancer

A case-control, epidemiologic study of non-small cell lung carcinoma showed a relative risk of 0.37 (p=0.01) between a group that had plasma lycopene levels in the third tertile when compared to those in the first tertile. When the data was analyzed for African Americans, the relative risk was 0.12 (p=0.001). Ninety-three cases in the United States were reviewed. The cases were adjusted for age, sex, and race (Li et al, 1997).

A case-controlled epidemiological study of 103 cases from Spain compared the risk of developing lung or pleural cancer between the third (highest) and first (lowest) tertile of Tomato eaters. The RR was 0.45 with a p for trend of 0.026 and a 95% confidence interval of 0.22 to 0.91. Cases were adjusted for age, smoking, and the total number of pack years smoked (Agudo et al, 1997).

In another study measuring relative risk, when the fifth quintile of patients with high serum lycopene were compared to the first quintile (lowest serum levels), there was no noticeable benefit from lycopene. The RR for developing lung or pleural cancer for this group was 1.01 and the p value for the trend was 0.97. This was a cohort study of 258 Maryland patients matched for age, race, sex, date of blood donation, and smoking status (Comstock, 1997).

Mesothelioma

In a case-control epidemiological study of mesothelioma, Tomato or Tomato juice consumption of greater than 16 ''doses'' per month was compared to no doses. The RR for the Tomato group was 0.6 with a 95% confidence interval of 0.2 to 1.9. Ninety-four cases were examined and adjusted for age, religion, occupation, and educational level (Muscat & Huncharek, 1996).

Oral/Pharyngeal Cancer

A case-control epidemiological study of 266 male and 36 female Italian patients evaluated the RR of developing oral or pharyngeal cancer. The comparison was between the third and first tertile of Tomato eaters. The RR was 0.5 with a p for trend of less than 0.01. The cases were adjusted for sex, age, occupation, alcohol intake, smoking status, and other foods with significant effects (Franceschi et al, 1991).

A case-control epidemiological study of 404 Chinese patients evaluated the RR of developing oral cancer. The comparison was between those who ate one or more Tomatoes per day (minimum of 7/week) and those that ate less than 3 per week. The RR was 0.49 with a 95% confidence interval of 0.26 to 0.94. The cases were adjusted for sex, age, body mass, dentition, educational level, alcohol intake, smoking status, and energy (Zheng et al, 1993).

Ovarian Cancer

A cohort epidemiological study of 35 American patients evaluated the RR of developing ovarian cancer. The comparison was between those with a serum lycopene level greater than 35.2 mcg/dL and those with a serum level 21.9 mcg/dL. The RR was 1.36 with a 95% confidence interval of 0.4 to 4.3 (p=0.59). The cases were adjusted for age, menstrual status, and the time since the subjects had last eaten (Helzlsourer et al, 1996).

Pancreatic Cancer

A case-control epidemiological study of 164 European patients evaluated the RR of developing pancreatic cancer. The comparison was between those in the fifth quintile of those who ate Tomatoes versus those in the first quintile. The RR was 0.23 ($p<0.05$). The cases were adjusted for sex, age, smoking status, and energy (Bueno de Mesquita et al, 1989).

Prostate Cancer

Lycopene was the only carotenoid in the plasma that was associated with reduced risk of prostate cancer. Subjects in the study included 578 men who developed prostate cancer over a 13-year period and a set of 1,294 matched controls (age, marital status, and smoking). A significantly lower mean lycopene level was found in the prostate cancer patients than in the controls, with a p value for the trend of 0.04. The odds ratio for all prostate cancers declined slightly with increasing quintile of plasma lycopene with a trend p value of 0.12. Prostate cancer was reduced in each lycopene quintile relative to men with low lycopene and placebo. Lycopene plasma levels were strongly related to lowered prostate cancer risk in aggressive cancers, with a p=0.006 (Gann et al, 1999).

An epidemiological study of members of a health professional's follow-up study showed that lycopene ingestion was associated with a decreased risk of cancer. A statistically significant (p=0.04) trend toward reduced prostate cancer risk was associated with self-reported intake of various fruits and vegetables containing lycopene. The differences were between the first and fifth quintiles of the study group. This same group was studied to determine if there was a significant difference in the risk of getting cancer depending on the food eaten. There was a statistically significant difference for Tomato sauce, Tomatoes, and pizza but not Tomato juice (p=0.01, 0.3, 0.05, and 0.67, respectively. The categories included in the trend were: no servings, 1 to 3 servings a month, 1 serving a week, 2 to 4 servings per week, and greater than 5 servings per week. Other carotenoids were also examined; no statistically significant differences were found for these agents (Giovannucci & Clinton, 1998).

INDICATIONS AND USAGE

With studies showing a relationship between high tomato consumption and lower levels of cancer, complementary and alternative medicine practitioners have suggested increasing consumption of tomato and other fruits and vegetables high in lycopene to their patients. Lycopene may help support prostate function and is often used as an adjunctive therapy in treating prostate cancer. Many combination products for support of the prostate include lycopene and other nutrients such as zinc and saw palmetto.

Unproven Uses: In folk medicine, Tomato is used externally for sore eyes (extract) and inflammations of the mouth and throat (decoction).

Indian Medicine: Tomato is used for ''flu'' infections (tea), and for flatulence, atonic dyspepsia, and anorexia.

Homeopathic Uses: Lycopersicon esculentum is used to treat rheumatic conditions, colds, chills and digestive disorders.

PRECAUTIONS AND ADVERSE REACTIONS

Drug-Food Interactions

Dietary interactions with lycopene are possible. For example, daily olestra consumption of 18 g/d may significantly reduce serum lycopene levels. As much as a 30% reduction has been noted after 16 weeks of olestra (Clinton, 1998). Lycopene requires fat for absorption and transport in the body. It will dissolve in olestra and will not be absorbed. Patients should eat foods that contain olestra at a different time of day than when they take lycopene supplements or eat lycopene-rich foods (Tomatoes and Tomato sauce as well as apricots, cranberries, eggplant, grapes, papaya, peaches, guava, and watermelon).

Lycopene levels are inconsistently affected by ingestion of alcohol or by smoking. Often patients with increased lipid levels will have lowered lycopene levels; Gerster, 1997).

OVERDOSAGE

Signs of poisoning are not to be expected with less than 100 g of the fresh leaves (or green Tomatoes) and for that reason is unlikely. Symptoms would be severe mucous membrane irritation (vomiting, diarrhea, and colic). Following absorption, dizziness, stupor, headache, bradycardia, respiratory disturbances, mild spasms and, in very severe cases, death through respiratory failure could occur.

DOSAGE

Mode of Administration: The drug is commonly used in homeopathic dilutions.

Preparation: The mother tincture is produced by maceration or percolation of the fresh or dried drug, with an ethanol content of 45%. Lycopene from Tomato is available as a dietary supplement.

Daily Dose: When lycopene is supplemented on its own, dosing recommendations range from 5 to 10 mg daily

Hypercholesterolemia: 60 mg daily (Fuhrman et al, 1997).

Homeopathic Dosage: 5 drops, 1 tablet or 10 globules every 30 to 60 minutes (acute) or 1 to 3 times daily (chronic); parenterally: 1 to 2 mL SC (acute), 3 times daily; chronic: once a day (HAB1).

LITERATURE

Agarwal S, Rao AV. Tomato lycopene and low density lipoprotein oxidation: a dietary human intervention study. *Lipids* 33(10):981-984. 1998.

Agudo A, Esteve MG, Pallares C, et al: Vegetable and fruit intake and the risk of lung cancer in women in Barcelona, Spain. *Eur J Cancer* 33(8):1256-1261. 1997.

Amir H, Karas M, Giat J, et al: Lycopene and 1,25-dihydroxyvitamin D3 cooperate in the inhibition of cell cycle progression and induction of differentiation in HL-60 leukemic cells. *Nutr Cancer* 33(1):105-112. 1999.

Anon. Tomaten als Krebsschutz. *DAZ* 134(6):485. 1994

Batieha AM, Armenian HK, Norkus EP, et al: Serum micronutrients and the subsequent risk of cervical cancer in a population-based nested case-control study. *Cancer Epidemiol Biomarkers, Prev* 2(4):335-339. 1993.

Boeing H, Jedrychowski W, Wahrendorf J, et al: Dietary risk factors in intestinal and diffuse types of stomach cancer: a multicenter case-control study in Poland. *Cancer Causes Control* 2(4):227-233. 1991.

Bohm V, Bitsch R. Intestinal absorption of lycopene from different matrices and interactions to other carotenoids, the lipid status, and the antioxidant capacity of human plasma. *Eur J Nutr* 38(3):118-125. 1999.

Boosalis MG, Snowdon DA, Tully CL, et al: Acute phase response and plasma carotenoid concentrations in older women: findings from the nun study. *Nutrition* 12(7-8):475-478. 1996.

Brady WE, Mares-Perlman JA, et al: Human plasma carotenoid response to the ingestion of controlled diets high in fruits and vegetables. *J Nutr* 126:129-137. 1996.

Brown ED, Micozzi MS, Craft NE, et al: Plasma carotenoids in normal men after a single ingestion of vegetables or purified beta-carotene. *Am J Clin Nutr* 49:1258-1265. 1989.

Brown LM, Blot WJ, Schuman SH, et al: Environmental factors and high risk of esophageal cancer among men in coastal South Carolina. *J Natl Cancer Inst* 80:1620-1625. 1988.

Bueno de Mesquita HB, Maisonneuve P, et al: Intake of foods and nutrients and cancer of the exocrine pancreas: a population-based case-control study in The Netherlands. *Int J Cancer* 48(4):540-549. 1991.

Buiatti E, Palli D, Decarli A, et al: A case-control study of gastric cancer and diet in Italy. *Int J Cancer* 44(4):611-616. 1989.

Burney PG, Comstock GW, Morris JS. Serologic precursors of cancer: serum micronutrients and the subsequent risk of pancreatic cancer. *Am J Clin Nutr* 49(5):895-900. 1989.

Campbell DR, Gross MD, Martini MC, et al: Plasma carotenoids as biomarkers of vegetable and fruit intake. *Cancer Epidemiol Biomarkers Prev* 3(6):493-500. 1994.

Candelora EC, Stockwell HG, Armstrong AW, et al: Dietary intake and risk of lung cancer in women who never smoked. *Nutr Cancer* 17(3):263-270. 1992.

Clinton SK. Lycopene: chemistry, biology, and implications for human health and disease. *Nutr Rev* 56(2):35-51. 1998.

Colditz GA, Branch LG, Lipnick RJ, et al: Increased green and yellow vegetables intake and lowered cancer deaths in an elderly population. *Am J Clin Nutr* 41(1):32-36. 1985.

Comstock GW, Alberg AJ, Huang HY, et al: The risk of developing lung cancer associated with antioxidants in the blood: ascorbic acid, carotenoids, alpha-tocopherol, selenium, and total peroxyl radical absorbing capacity. *Cancer Epidemiol Biomarkers Prev* 6(11):907-916. 1997.

Dorgan JF, Sowell A, Swanson CA, et al: Relationships of serum carotenoids, retinol, alpha-tocopherol, and selenium with breast cancer risk: results from a prospective study in Columbia, Missouri. *Cancer Causes Control* 9(1):89-97. 1998.

Dugas TR, Morel DW, Harrison EH. Dietary supplementation with beta-carotene, but not with lycopene, inhibits endothelial cell-mediated oxidation of low-density lipoprotein. *Free Radical Biol Med* 26(9/10):1238-1244. 1999.

Forman MR, Johnson EJ, Lanza E, et al: Effect of menstrual cycle phase on the concentration of individual carotenoids in lipoproteins of premenopausal women: a controlled dietary study. *Am J Clin Nutr* 67(1):81-87. 1998.

Forman MR, Yao SX, Graubard BI, et al: The effect of dietary intake of fruits and vegetables on the odds ratio of lung cancer among Yunnan tin miners. *Int J Epidemiol* 21(3):437-441. 1992.

Franceschi S, Bidoli E, Baron AE, et al: Nutrition and cancer of the oral cavity and pharynx in north-east Italy. *Int J Cancer* 47(1):20-25. 1991.

Franceschi S, Bidoli E, La Vecchia C et al: Tomatoes and risk of digestive-tract cancers. *Int J Cancer* 59(2):181-184. 1994.

Franceschi S, Favero A, La Vecchia C, et al: Food groups and risk of colorectal cancer in Italy. *Int J Cancer* 72(1):56-61. 1997.

Fraser GE, Beeson WL, Phillips RL. Diet and lung cancer in California Seventh-day Adventists. *Am J Epidemiol* 133(7):683-693. 1991.

Fuhrman B, Elis A, Aviram M. Hypocholesterolemic effect of lycopene and beta-carotene is related to suppression of cholesterol synthesis and augmentation of LDL receptor activity in macrophages. *Biochem Biophys Res Commun* 233(3):658-662. 1997.

Gann PH, Ma J, Giovannucci E et al: Lower prostate cancer risk in men with elevated plasma lycopene levels: results of a prospective analysis. *Cancer Res* 59(6):1225-1230. 1999.

Gartner C, Stahl W, Sies H. Lycopene is more bioavailable from Tomato paste than from fresh Tomatoes. *Am J Clin Nutr* 66(1):116-122. 1997.

Gaziano JM, Hohnson EJ, Russell RM, et al: Discrimination in absorption or transport of beta-carotene isomers after oral supplementation with either all-trans or 9-cis beta-carotene. *Am J Clin Nutr* 61(6):1248-1252. 1995.

Gerster H. The potential role of lycopenes for human health. *J Am Coll Nutr* 16(2):109-126. 1977.

Giovannucci E, Clinton SK. Tomatoes, lycopene, and prostate cancer. *Proc Soc Exp Biol Med* 218(2):129-139. 1998.

Giovannucci E. Tomatoes, Tomato-based products, lycopene, and cancer: review of the epidemiologic literature. *J Nat Cancer Instit* 91(4):317-331. 1999.

Giuliano AR, Neilson EM, Ypa HH, et al: Quantitation of an inter/intra-individual variability of major carotenoids of mature human milk. *J Nutr Biochem* 5:551-556. 1994.

Gonzales CA, Sanz JM, Marcos G, et al: Dietary factors and stomach cancer in Spain: a multi-centre case-control study. *Int J Cancer* 49:513-519. 1991.

Harris RW, Key TJ, Silcocks PB, et al: A case-control study of dietary carotene in men with lung cancer and in men with other epithelial cancers. *Nutr Cancer* 15:63-68. 1991.

Helzlsourer KJ, Alberg AJ, Norkus EP, et al: Prospective study of serum micronutrients and ovarian cancer. *J Natl Cancer Inst* 88(1):32-37. 1996.

Hoppe PP, Kramer K, van den Berg H, et al: Synthetic and Tomato-based lycopene have identical bioavailability in humans. *Eur J Nutr* 42:272-278. 2003.

Hsing AW, Comstock GW, Abbey H, et al: Serologic precursors of cancer. Retinol, carotenoids, and tocopherol and risk of prostate cancer. *J Natl Cancer Inst* 82(11):941-946. 1990.

Hughes DA, Wright AJA, Finglas PM, et al: Comparison of effects of beta-carotene and lycopene supplementation on the expression of functionally associated molecules on human monocytes. *Biochem Soc Trans* 16(2):25. 1997.

Jarvinen R, Knekt P, Seppanen R, et al: Diet and breast cancer risk in a cohort of Finnish women. *Cancer Lett* 114(1-2):251-253. 1997.

Johnson EJ. Human studies on bioavailability and plasma response of lycopene. *Proc Soc Exp Biol Med* 218(2):115-120. 1998.

Johnson EJ, Qin J, Krinsky NI, et al: Ingestion by men of a combined dose of beta carotene and lycopene does not affect the absorption of beta-carotene but improves the absorption of lycopene. *J Nutr* 127(9):1833-1837. 1997.

Johnson EJ, Suter PM, Sahyoun N, et al: The relationship between beta-carotene intake and plasma and adipose tissue concentrations of carotenoids and retinoids. *Am J Clin Nutr* 62:598-603. 1995.

Kanetsky PA, Gammon MD, Mandelblatt J, et al: Dietary intake and blood levels of lycopene: association with cervical dysplasia among non-Hispanic, black women. *Nutr Cancer* 31(1):31-40. 1998.

Khachik F, Beecher GR, Smith Jr JC. Lutein, lycopene, and their oxidative metabolites in chemoprevention of cancer. *J Cell Biochem* 22(suppl):236-246. 1995.

Khachik F, Pfander H, Traber B. Proposed mechanisms for the formation of synthetic and natural occurring metabolites of lycopene in Tomato products and human serum. *J Agric Fd Chem* 46:4885-4890. 1998.

Kim Y, English C, Reich P, et al: Vitamin A and carotenoids in human milk. *J Agric Fd Chem* 38(10):1930-1933. 1990.

Klebanov GI, Kapitanov AB, Teselkin YO, et al: The antioxidant properties of lycopene. *Membr Cell Biol* 12(2):287-300. 1998.

Kohlmeier L, Kark JD, Gomez-Gracia E, et al: Lycopene and myocardial infarction risk in the EURAMIC study. *Am J Epidemiol* 146(8):618-626. 1997.

Krutovskikh V, Asamoto M, Takasuka N, et al: Differential dose-dependent effects of alpha-, beta-carotenes and lycopene on gap-junctional intercellular communication in rat liver in vivo. *Jpn J Cancer Res* 88(12):1121-1124. 1997.

Kvale G, Bjelke E, Gart JJ: Dietary habits and lung cancer risk. *Int J Cancer* 31(4):397-405. 1983.

Le Marchand L, Hankin JH, Kolonel LN, et al: Intake of specific carotenoids and lung cancer risk. *Cancer Epidemiol Biomarkers Prev* 2(3):183-187. 1993.

Le Marchand L, Hankin JH, Kolonel LN, et al: Vegetable and fruit consumption in relation to prostate cancer risk in Hawaii: a re-evaluation of the effect of dietary beta-carotene. *Am J Epidemiol* 133(3):215-219. 1991.

Le Marchand L, Oshizawa CN, Kolonel LN et al: Vegetable consumption and lung cancer risk: a population-based case-control study in Hawaii. *J Nat Cancer Inst* 1989; 81(15):1158-1164.

Levy J, Bosin E, Feldman B et al: Lycopene is a more potent inhibitor of human cancer cell proliferation than either alpha-carotene or beta-carotene. *Nutr Cancer* 24(3):257-266. 1995.

Li Y, Elie M, Blaner WS, et al: Lycopene, smoking and lung cancer (abstr). *Proc Ann Meet Am Assoc Cancer Res* 38:A758. 1997.

Lyle BJ, Mares-Perlman JA, Klein BK, et al: Serum carotenoids and tocopherols and incidence of age-related nuclear cataract. *Am J Clin Nutr* 69(2):272-277. 1999.

Marangon K, Herbeth B, Lecomte E, et al: Diet, antioxidant status, and smoking habit in French men. *Am J Clin Nutr* 67(2):231-239. 1998.

Mayne ST, Cartmel B, Silva F, et al: Plasma lycopene concentrations in humans are determined by lycopene intake, plasma cholesterol concentrations, and selected demographic factors. *J Nutr* 129(4):849-854. 1999.

Mayne ST, Janerich DT, Greenwald P, et al: Dietary beta carotene and lung cancer risk in U.S. nonsmokers. *J Natl Cancer Inst* 86(1):33-38. 1994.

Modan B, Cuckle H, Lubin F. A note on the role of dietary retinol and carotene in human gastro-intestinal cancer. Int J Cancer 1981; 28(4):421-424. 1981.

Muscat JE, Huncharek M. Dietary intake and the risk of malignant mesothelioma. *Br J Cancer* 73:1122-1125. 1996.

Nguyen ML, Schwartz SJ. Lycopene: chemical and biological properties. *Food Technol* 53(2):38-45. 1999.

Okajima E, Ozono S, Endo T, et al: Chemopreventive efficacy of piroxicam administered alone or in combination with lycopene with beta-carotene on the development of rat urinary bladder carcinoma after n-butyl-N-(4-hydroxybutyl)nitrosamine treatment. *Jpn J Cancer Res* 88(6):543-552. 1997.

O'Neill ME, Thurnham DI. Intestinal absorption of beta-carotene, lycopene and lutein in men and women following a standard mal: response curves in the triacylclycerol-rich lipoprotein fraction. *Br J Nutr* 79(2):149-159. 1998.

Paetau I, Khachik F, Brown ED, et al: Chronic ingestion of lycopene-rich Tomato juice or lycopene supplements significantly increases plasma concentrations of lycopene and related Tomato carotenoids in humans. *Am J Clin Nutr* 68(6):1187-1195. 1998.

Paetau I, Rao D, Wiley ER, et al: Carotenoids in human buccal mucosa cells after 4 wk of supplementation with Tomato juice or lycopene supplements. *Am J Clin Nutr* 70(4):490-494. 1999.

Palan PR, Chang CJ, Mikhail MS, et al: Plasma concentrations of micronutrients during a nine-month clinical trial of beta-carotene in women with precursor cervical cancer lesions. *Nutr Cancer* 30(1):46-52. 1998.

Palan PR, Mikhail MS, Goldberg GL, et al: Plasma levels of beta-carotene, lycopene, canthaxanthin, retinol, and alpha- and gamma-tocopherol in cervical intraepithelial neoplasia and cancer. *Clin Cancer Res* 2(1):181-185. 1996.

Pastori M, Pfander H, Boscoboinik D, et al: Lycopene in association with alpha-tocopherol inhibits at physiological concentrations proliferation of prostate carcinoma cells. *Biochem Biophys Res Comm* 250(3):582-585. 1998.

Peng YM, Peng YS, Lin Y, et al: Concentrations and plasma-tissue diet relationships of carotenoids, retinoids, and tocopherols in humans. *Nutr Cancer* 23(3):233-246. 1995.

Pierce JP, Faerber S, Wright FA, et al: Feasibility of a randomized trial of a high-vegetable diet to prevent breast cancer recurrence. *Nutr Cancer* 28(3):282-288. 1997.

Porrini M, Riso P, Testolin G: Absorption of lycopene from single or daily portions of raw and processed Tomato. *Br J Nutr* 80(4):353-361. 1998.

Potischman N, Herrero R, Brinton LA, et al: A case-control study of nutrient status and invasive cervical cancer II. Serological indicators. *Am J Epidemiol* 134(11):1347-1355. 1991.

Potischman N, Hoover RN, Brinton LA et al: The relations between cervical cancer and serological markers of nutritional status. *Nutr Can* 21(3):193-201. 1994.

Ramon JM, Serra L, Cerdo C, et al: Dietary factors and gastric cancer risk. A case-control study in Spain. *Cancer* 1993; 71(5):1731-1735. 1993.

Rao AV, Agarwal S. Bioavailability and in vivo antioxidant properties of lycopene from Tomato products and their possible role in the prevention of cancer. *Nutr Cancer* 31(3):199-203. 1998a.

Rao AV, Agarwal S. Effect of diet and smoking on serum lycopene and lipid peroxidation. *Nutr Res* 18(4):713-721. 1998.

Ribaya-Mercado JD, Garmyn M, Gilchrest BA, et al: Skin lycopene is destroyed preferentially over beta-carotene during ultraviolet irradiation in humans. *J Nutr* 125(7):1854-1859. 1995.

Riso P, Pinder A, Santangelo A, et al: Does Tomato consumption effectively increase the resistance of lymphocyte DNA oxidative damage? *Am J Clin Nutr* 69(4):712-718. 1999.

Sengupta A, Das S. The anti-carcinogenic role of lycopene, abundantly present in Tomato. *Eur J Cancer Prevention* 8(4):325-330. 1999.

Sharma SK, LeMaguer M. Lycopene in Tomatoes and Tomato pulp fractions. *Ital J Food Sci* 8(2):107-113. 1996.

Stahl W, Junghans A, de Boer B, et al: Carotenoid mixtures protect multilamellar liposomes against oxidative damage: synergistic effects of lycopene and lutein. *FEBS Lett* 427(2):305-308. 1998.

Stahl W, Sies H. Uptake of lycopene and its geometrical isomers is greater from heat-processed than from unprocessed Tomato juice in humans. *J Nutr* 122(11):2161-2166. 1992.

Steinmetz KA, Potter JD, Folsom AR: Vegetables, fruit, and lung cancer in the Iowa Women's Health Study. *Cancer Res* 53(3):536-543. 1993.

Suganuma H, Inakuma T. Protective effect of dietary Tomato against endothelial dysfunction in hypercholesterolemic mice. *Biosci Biotechnol Biochem* 63(1):78-82. 1999.

Sutherland WF, Walker RJ, DeJong SA, et al: Supplementation with Tomato juice increases plasma lycopene but does not alter susceptibility to oxidation of low-density lipoproteins from renal transplant recipients. *Clin Nephrol* 52(1):30-36. 1999.

Tuyns AJ, Kaaks R, Haelterman M. Colorectal cancer and the consumption of foods: a case-control study in Belgium. *Nutr Cancer* 11(3):189-204. 1988.

van den Berg H & van Vliet T. Effect of simultaneous, single oral doses of beta-carotene with lutein or lycopene on the beta-carotene and retinyl ester responses in triacylglcerol-rich lipoprotein fraction of men. *Am J Clin Nutr* 68(1):82-89. 1998.

Vogel S, Contois JH, Tucker KL, et al: Plasma retinol and plasma and lipoprotein tocopherol and carotenoid concentrations in healthy elderly participants of the Framingham Heart Study. *Am J Clin Nutr* 66(4):950-8. 1997.

Weisburger JH, Dolan L, Pittman B. Inhibition of PhIP mutagenicity by caffeine, lycopene, daidzein, and genistein. *Mutat Res* 416(1-2):125-128. 1998.

Yeum KJ, Booth SL, Sadowski JA, et al: Human plasma carotenoid response to the ingestion of controlled diets high in fruits and vegetables. *Am J Clin Nutr* 64(4):594-602. 1996.

Zarling EJ, Mobarhan S, Bowen P, et al: Pulmonary pentane excretion increases with age in healthy subjects. *Mech Aging Dev* 67(1-2):141-147. 1993.

Zhang S, Tang G, Russell RM, et al: Measurement of retinoids and carotenoids in breast adipose tissue and a comparison of concentrations in breast cancer cases and control subjects. *Am J Clin Nutr* 66(3):626-632. 1997,

Zheng T, Boyle P, Willett WC, et al: A case-control study of oral cancer in Beijing, People's Republic of China. Associations with nutrient intakes, foods and food groups. *Eur J Cancer B Oral Oncol* 29B(1):44-45. 1993.

Tonka Beans

Dipteryx odorata

DESCRIPTION

Medicinal Parts: The medicinal part is the seeds.

Flower and Fruit: The beans are usually 2 to 5 cm long and 1 cm in diameter. They have a grayish or black color.

Characteristics: The bean has a characteristic odor, like new-mown hay.

Habitat: South America

Production: Tonka Beans are the seeds of *Dipteryx odorata.*

Other Names: Tonquin Bean

ACTIONS AND PHARMACOLOGY

COMPOUNDS

Coumarin (1-3% to 10%)

Fatty oil

EFFECTS

Tonka Beans have a tonic and aromatic effect.

INDICATIONS AND USAGE

Unproven Uses: Whooping cough (no longer used).

PRECAUTIONS AND ADVERSE REACTIONS

Health risks or side effects following the proper administration of designated therapeutic dosages are not recorded. The therapeutic administration of drugs containing coumarin can lead to slight liver damage (elevated liver enzyme values in the blood) in a very small number of patients; the damage is reversible following discontinuation of the drug.

OVERDOSAGE

The intake of very high dosages (4 g coumarin, equivalent to 150 g of the drug) could bring about stupor, headache, nausea, and vomiting.

DOSAGE

Mode of Administration: Tonka Beans are obsolete as a drug.

LITERATURE

Kalume DE, Sousa MV, Morhy L, Purification characterization sequence determination and mass spectrometric analysis of a trypsin inhibitor from seeds of the Brazilian tree Dipteryx alata (Leguminosae). *J Protein Chem*, 14:685-93, Nov. 1995.

Lewin L, Gifte und Vergiftungen, 6. Aufl., Nachdruck, Haug Verlag, Heidelberg 1992.

Roth L, Daunderer M, Kormann K, Giftpflanzen, Pflanzengifte, 4. Aufl., Ecomed Fachverlag Landsberg Lech 1993.

Steinegger E, Hänsel R, Pharmakognosie, 5. Aufl., Springer Verlag Heidelberg 1992.

Sullivan G, *J Agric Food Chem* 30(3):609. 1968

Teuscher E, Lindequist U, Biogene Gifte - Biologie, Chemie, Pharmakologie, 2. Aufl., Fischer Verlag Stuttgart 1994.

Tragacanth

Astragalus gummifer

DESCRIPTION

Medicinal Parts: The medicinal product of the plant is the gumlike exudation from the trunk and branches.

Flower and Fruit: The axillary flowers are solitary or in groups of 2 or 3 and are sessile. The calyx is 6 to 7 mm long and densely pubescent. The corolla is yellowish to white and sometimes has bluish or reddish veins. The standard, wings, and carina are each 9 to 10 mm long. The fruit is ovoid, 4 mm long with dense, silky hairs. The seed is oval, smooth, and about 3 mm long.

Leaves, Stem and Root: Astralagus gummifer is a low shrub that grows up to 30 cm high and has gray branches that become glabrous. The older branches have scalelike remains of the stipules from the previous year, which disappear later, and a 1- to 4-cm long perennial, thorny leaf column. The 8 to 14 leaflets are folded, oblong-ovate, 2.5 to 6 mm long, and 0.7 to 2.5 mm wide. They are blue-gray and glabrous or sparsely pubescent beneath.

Habitat: The plant grows in Turkey, Syria, Lebanon, northwest Iraq, and the border area between Iran and Iraq.

Production: Tragacanth is the latex that exudes primarily from immediately under the bark of *Astralagus gummifer* and other varieties. It is extracted by making an incision in the trunk and branches of shrubs growing in the wild. When dried, it forms flakes that swell in water to form a gelatinous mass.

Other Names: Gum Dragon

ACTIONS AND PHARMACOLOGY

COMPOUNDS

Polysaccharides (water-soluble part, approximately 40%): tragacanthine, which can decompose into tragacanthic acid (galacturonane with side chains consisting of D-xylose, L-fucose, D-galactose)

Arabino-galactane-protein complex (non-water soluable part, approximately 60%): containing bassorin, a composition similar to that of tragacanthine

EFFECTS
Tragacanth has a laxative effect, primarily due to stimulating stretching of the intestinal wall, which results in increased peristalis.

INDICATIONS AND USAGE
Unproven Uses: Tragacanth is used as a laxative. Folk medicine uses in Europe and the Arab world have included treatment for tumors of the eyes, liver, and throat. Efficacy has not been proved.

PRECAUTIONS AND ADVERSE REACTIONS
No health hazards or side effects are known in conjunction with the proper administration of designated therapeutic dosages. Allergic reactions have been observed in rare cases. Insufficient fluid supply following intake of large quantities of tragacanth can lead to obstruction ileus, as well as to esophageal closure.

DOSAGE
Mode of Administration: Tragacanth is used in various combinations and preparations.

Daily Dosage: Recommended daily dosage is not specified. A typical single dose is 1 tsp. granulated drug (approximately 3 g) added to 250 to 300 mL liquid for oral administration.

Storage: Tragacanth cannot be stored for any significant length of time because of its instability.

LITERATURE
Anderson DMW, Bridgeman MME, *PH* 24:2301-2304. 1985.

Srimal RC, Dhawan CN, *J Pharm Pharmacol* 25: 447. 1973

Whistler RL et al., *Adv Carbohydr Chem Biochem* 32: 235. 1976

Trailing Arbutus

Epigae repens

DESCRIPTION
Medicinal Parts: The medicinal parts are the fresh or dried leaves.

Flower and Fruit: The flowers are in apical dense racemes. They are white with a reddish tinge and are very fragrant. They are divided at the tip into 5 segments, which open in a star shape.

Leaves, Stem, and Root: The plant is a fragrant evergreen branching shrub with rust-colored, pubescent, round stems. Roots develop at the stem nodes, which spread quickly. The leaves are petioled, broadly ovate, 2.5 to 4 cm long, and about 2 cm wide. They are coriaceous, entire-margined, reticulate, with a cordate base, a short pointed apex, and short hairs on the undersurface. The branches, petioles, and leaf nerves are very pubescent.

Characteristics: The plant has a similar action to Buchu on the urinary system.

Habitat: Indigenous to North America, established as an ornamental plant in Europe.

Production: Trailing Arbutus is the aerial part of *Epigae repens.*

Other Names: Gravel Plant, Ground Laurel, Mountain Pink, Water Pink, Winter Pink

ACTIONS AND PHARMACOLOGY
COMPOUNDS
Arbutin (hydroquinone glucoside)

Tannins

EFFECTS
Eleuthero has astringent and diuretic properties.

INDICATIONS AND USAGE
Unproven Uses: Trailing Arbutus is used for urinary tract conditions.

PRECAUTIONS AND ADVERSE REACTIONS
Health risks or side effects following the proper administration of designated therapeutic dosages are not recorded. Nausea and vomiting can also occur with stomach sensitivity in children. Liver damage, cachexia, hemolytic anemia, and depigmentation of the hair is possible with long-term use of the drug.

OVERDOSAGE
Overdosages could lead to inflammatory reactions of the mucous membranes of the bladder and urinary passages, accompanied by strangury and possible blood in the urine.

DOSAGE
Mode of Administration: Trailing Arbutus is available as an infusion or extract for internal use.

LITERATURE
Kern W, List PH, Hörhammer L (Hrsg.), Hagers Handbuch der Pharmazeutischen Praxis, 4. Aufl., Bde. 1-8, Springer Verlag Berlin, Heidelberg, New York, 1969.

Traveller's Joy

Clematis vitalba

DESCRIPTION
Medicinal Parts: The medicinal parts of the plant are the fresh leaves.

Flower and Fruit: The flowers are arranged in leafy cymes. The blossoms are small and white with 4 downy, revolute or splayed bracts. The stamens and ovaries are numerous. The fruit is a red-brown, long-tailed nut.

Leaves, Stem, and Root: The plant grows to about 1.5 to 5 m high. The leaves are petiolate and 5-pinnate. The leaflets are ovate or slightly cordate, acute, and lobed. The petioles are clinging and the stems climbing and grooved, at first leafy then woody.

Characteristics: The flowers have a slight scent resembling white thorn. The plant is poisonous if ingested in large amounts.

Habitat: The plant is indigenous to Europe.

ACTIONS AND PHARMACOLOGY

COMPOUNDS

Protoanemonine-forming agents: In the freshly harvested plant, it is presumably the glycoside ranunculin that changes enzymatically when the plant is cut into small pieces, and probably also when it is dried. It then changes into the pungent, volatile protoanemonine, which is severely irritating to skin and mucous membranes but quickly dimerizes to anemonine; when dried, the plant is not capable of protoanemonine formation.

Saponins

EFFECTS

No information is available.

INDICATIONS AND USAGE

Unproven Uses: The drug causes blistering and was formerly used to treat diseases of the male genitals, as well as for poorly healing wounds. Today, it is used in small doses, both internally and externally, for migraine.

PRECAUTIONS AND ADVERSE REACTIONS

No health hazards or side effects are known in conjunction with the proper administration of designated therapeutic dosages of the dehydrated drug.

Extended skin contact with the freshly harvested, bruised plant can lead to treatment-resistant blisters and cauterizations due to the release of protoanemonine, which is severely irritating to skin and mucous membranes. If taken internally, severe irritation to the gastrointestinal tract, combined with colic, diarrhea, and irritation of the urinary drainage passages, are possible. Symptomatic treatment for external contact should consist of irrigation with diluted potassium permanganate solution followed by mucilage.

OVERDOSAGE

Ingestion of the drug should be treated with gastric lavage followed by activated charcoal. Death by asphyxiation following the intake of large quantities of protoanemonine-forming plants has been observed in animal experiments. The toxicity of this plant is less than that of many other Ranunculaceae (Anemones nemorosae) due to the relatively low levels of protoanemonine-forming agents.

DOSAGE

Mode of Administration: The drug is used topically and is also available in alcoholic extracts.

LITERATURE

Bonora A et al., *PH* 26:2277. 1987.

Frohne D, Pfänder HJ: Giftpflanzen - Ein Handbuch für Apotheker, Toxikologen und Biologen, 4. Aufl., Wiss. Verlagsges. mbH Stuttgart 1997.

Kern W, List PH, Hörhammer L (Hrsg.), Hagers Handbuch der Pharmazeutischen Praxis, 4. Aufl., Bde 1-8, Springer Verlag Berlin, Heidelberg, New York, 1969.

Lewin L, Gifte und Vergiftungen, 6. Aufl., Nachdruck, Haug Verlag, Heidelberg 1992.

Roth L, Daunderer M, Kormann K: Giftpflanzen, Pflanzengifte, 4. Aufl., Ecomed Fachverlag Landsberg Lech 1993.

Southwell IA et al., Protoanemonin in australian Clematis. In: *PH* 33:1099. 1993.

Teuscher E, Lindequist U, Biogene Gifte - Biologie, Chemie, Pharmakologie, 2. Aufl., Fischer Verlag Stuttgart 1994.

Tree of Heaven

Ailanthus altissima

DESCRIPTION

Medicinal Parts: The medicinal parts are the dried trunk and root bark.

Flower and Fruit: The small, greenish-yellow flower is in branched axillary or terminal panicles. Some of the flowers are male, some female, and some androgynous. The calyx is short and has 5 glandular, fused sepals. The sepals are much longer than the corolla and have 5 hollow, splayed petals. There are 10 stamens, often only 5 in the androgynous and rudimentary remains in the female flowers. There are 5 obovate, compressed ovaries with 5 splayed stigmas. There is a narrow, oblong-lanceolate schizocarp, 4 to 5 cm by 1 cm. It is winged above and below, first green then brown-red and finally brown. The seed is orbicular and found in the middle of the fruit section. It is thin-skinned, without any recognizable endosperm, and has an ovate, flat cotyledon.

Leaves, Stem, and Root: Ailanthus altissima is a beautiful, fast-growing tree, up to 30 m high. The bark is smooth, pale and vertically striated. The branches are initially fine haired, yellow or red-brown. The leaves are up to 1 m long and odd-pinnate. The upper surface of the leaves is dark green and the under-surface is light gray-green. The leaflets are ovate to oblong-lanceolate. The shallow, cordate base of the leaflets has 1 to 3 small lobes at either side, each with 1 gland. The wood surface is satiny and white.

Characteristics: The flowers have a strong elderflower scent. The fresh bark and leaves give off an unpleasant, nauseating smell.

Habitat: The tree was originally indigenous to China. Today it grows in the wild and is cultivated in tropical and subtropical eastern Asia, northern Europe, and North America.

Production: Tree of Heaven bark is the trunk and branch bark of *Ailanthus altissima*. The bark is gathered year-round. The outer bark is removed and dried in the sun. After drying, there is a process of sorting and removing foreign bodies, washing, macerating and a second drying.

Other Names: Ailanto, Chinese Sumach, Vernis de Japon

ACTIONS AND PHARMACOLOGY

COMPOUNDS

Quassinoids: including ailanthone, quassin

Indole alkaloids of the beta-carbolic type

Tannins

EFFECTS

An antimalarial action is being tested in an in-vitro trial. The active agents also have astringent, antipyretic, and antispasmodic properties.

INDICATIONS AND USAGE

Unproven Uses: In Africa, Tree of Heaven is used for cramps, asthma, tachycardia, gonorrhea, epilepsy, and tapeworm infestation. It is increasingly used in the treatment of malaria.

Chinese Medicine: The drug is used for pathological leukorrhea, diarrhea, chronic dysentery, and dysmenorrhea.

PRECAUTIONS AND ADVERSE REACTIONS

Large doses of the drug are said to lead to queasiness, dizziness, headache, tingling in the limbs, and diarrhea.

OVERDOSAGE

Fatal poisonings have been observed in animal experiments. Treatment of poisonings should be conducted symptomatically, following stomach and intestinal emptying.

DOSAGE

Mode of Administration: Tree of Heaven is still being researched as a drug; up until now it has only been used in folk medicine.

Daily Dosage: 6 to 9 g of drug

Storage: Keep in a dry, well-ventilated area away from moths.

LITERATURE

Bourke CA. Lack of toxicity of *Ailanthus altissima* (tree-of-heaven) for goats. Aust Vet J, 74:465, Dec 1996

Bray DH, et al., *Phytother Res* 1(1):22. 1987

Bucar F, Roberts MF. β-Carboline Alkaloids from *Ailanthus altissima* (Mill.) SWINGLE Tissue Cultures. *Sci Pharm.* 62; 107. 1994

Crespi Perellino N, Guicciardi A, Minghetti A, Speroni E. Comparison of biological activity induced by *Ailanthus altissima* plant or cell cultures extracts. *Pharmacol Res Commun*, 20 Suppl 5:45-8, Dec 1988

Ishibashi M, et al., *Bull Chem Soc Jpn* 58:2723-2724. 1985

Ishibashi M, et al., *Chem Pharm Bull* 31:2179-2182. 1983

Ishibashi M, et al., *Tetrahedron Lett*:1205-1206. 1985

Kubota K, Fukamiya N, Hamada T, Okano M, Tagahara K, Lee KH. Two new quassinoids ailantinols A and B and related compounds from *Ailanthus altissima. J Nat Prod,* 59:683-6, Jul 1996

Niimi Y, et al., *Chem Pharm Bull* 35:4302-4306. 1987

Polonski J, *Prog Chem Org Nat Prod* 47:221. 1985

Yeoman CL, Homeyer BC, Roberts MF, Phillipson JD. The Effect of Yeast Glucan Elicitation on Alkaloid Production during the Growth cycle of *Ailanthis altissima* cell Suspensions. *J Pharm Pharmacol.* 42; Suppl.; 98P. 1990

Trifolium pratense

See Red Clover

Trigonella foenum-graecum

See Fenugreek

Trillium erectum

See Beth Root Stock

Triticum

Agropyron repens

DESCRIPTION

Medicinal Parts: The medicinal part is the rhizome collected in spring or autumn.

Flower and Fruit: Five to 7 flowered spikelets in groups of 20 form a 10 cm-long ear. The ears are usually short, upright, and usually dense green and inconspicuous grass with a 5-veined, lanceolate, sharply keeled glume. The spike stem is glabrous. The glume is 8 to 11 mm long, acuminate, or awned. The anthers are 5 to 6 mm. The fruit is 6 to 7 mm long, flat to the front with 1 groove.

Leaves, Stem and Root: Triticum is a 0.2- to 1.5-m perennial plant with a hardy creeping rhizome. The rhizome has long white runners, is segmented, and hollow. The leaves are thin, flat, grass-green, or gray-green. The upper surface is rough and often covered in solitary, long hairs.

Characteristics: The spikelets have their broad side turned toward the wavelike curved main axis. The plant is odorless; the taste sweetish.

Habitat: Indigenous to the temperate regions of the Northern Hemisphere. Introduced to Greenland, South America, Australia, and New Zealand.

Production: Triticum rhizome consists of the rhizome, roots and short stems of *Agropyron repens,* harvested in spring before the blade develops, as well as its preparations. The rhizomes are collected after the fields are harrowed. They are cleaned, washed and dried at approximately 35° C.

Not to be Confused With: The rhizomes of Cynodon dactylon, Poaceae and Carex species (a frequent occurrence).

Other Names: Couch Grass, Cutch, Dog-Grass, Durfa Grass, Quack Grass, Quickgrass, Quitch Grass, Scotch Quelch, Twitch-Grass, Witch Grass

ACTIONS AND PHARMACOLOGY

COMPOUNDS

Mucilages

Triticin (polyfructosan)

Sugar alcohols

Soluble silicic acid

Volatile oil: including carvacrol and carvone-containing P-hydroxyalkyl cinnamic acid alkyl ester

EFFECTS

The essential oil has an antimicrobial effect.

INDICATIONS AND USAGE

Approved by Commission E:

- Infections of the urinary tract
- Kidney and bladder stones

Triticum is used as an irrigation therapy, for inflammatory diseases of the urinary tract and the prevention of kidney gravel.

Unproven Uses: The drug is also used for cystitis, kidney stones, gout, rheumatic pain, and chronic skin disorders. Due to the high mucilage content, the drug is used as a soothing cough remedy. The infusion is used for constipation. It is also used as fructose-containing additive for diabetics.

Homeopathic Uses: Agropyron repens is used to treat urinary tract infections.

CONTRAINDICATIONS

No irrigation therapy if edema is present due to cardiac or renal insufficiency.

PRECAUTIONS AND ADVERSE REACTIONS

No health hazards or side effects are known in conjunction with the proper administration of designated therapeutic dosages. For irrigation therapy, ensure copious fluid intake.

DOSAGE

Mode of Administration: Comminuted herb decoctions and other galenic preparations for internal use.

Preparation: Liquid extract: 1:1; Tincture: 1:5; Tea: Pour boiling water over the drug and strain after 10 minutes.

Daily Dosage: The average single dose is 3 to 10 g of drug in 1 cup of boiling water; average daily dose is 6 to 9 g of drug.

Tea: 12 to 24 g fresh several times a day; Liquid extract: 4 to 8 mL 3 times daily; Tincture: 5 to 15 mL 3 times daily.

Homeopathic Dosage: 5 drops, 1 tablet, 10 globules every 30 to 60 minutes (acute) or 1 to 3 times a day (chronic); Parenterally: 1 to 2 mL sc acute, 3 times daily; Chronic: once a day (HAB1).

Storage: The drug must be kept in sealed containers, protected from light and moisture.

LITERATURE

Bell EA, Jansen DH, *Nature* 229:136. 1971

Koetter U, et al., Isolierung und Strukturaufklärung von p-Hydroxyzimtsäurealkylesterverbindungen aus dem Rhizom von *Agropyron repens*, 2. Mitt. In: *PM* 60(5):488. 1994.

Koetter U, Kaloga M, Schilcher H, Isolierung und Strukturaufklärung von p-Hydroxyzimtsäurealkylester-Verbindungen aus dem Rhizom von *Agropyron repens*; 1. Mitt. In: PM 59(3):279. 1993.

Schilcher H, Boesel R, Effenberger ST, Segebrecht S, Neuere Untersuchungsergebnisse mit aquaretisch, antibakteriell und prostatotrop wirksamen Arzneipflanzen. In: ZPT 10(3):77. 1989.

Triticum aestivum

See Wheat

Trollius europaeus

See Globe Flower

Tropaeolum majus

See Nasturtium

Tropical Almond

Terminalia chebula

DESCRIPTION

Medicinal Parts: The medicinal part of the tree is the fruit.

Flower and Fruit: The flowers are arranged in 5- to 7-cm axillary spikes. The flowers are small and fused, and arranged in fives. The sepals are almost glabrous and yellowish-white; the calyx tube has 5 tips. There are no petals, but there are 10 stamens and a single-chambered, inferior ovary. The style is long and projects out of the bud. The fruit is a glabrous, ovoid drupe, yellow to orange-brown when ripe and 2 to 4 cm long.

Leaves, Stem, and Root: Tropical Almond is a tree that grows up to 25 m high. The leaves are alternate or opposite, 7 to 18 cm long, 4 to 6 cm wide, and coriaceous. The petiole is approximately 2.5 cm long, with 2 glands at the upper end. The lamina is ovate or elliptical, blunt and orbicular at the base. It is finely crenate and woolly pubescent beneath. The branches are rust colored, woolly or glabrous, and the trunk has a brown, longitudinally fissured bark.

Habitat: India

Production: Tropical Almond fruit is the dried ripe fruit of *Terminalia chebula.*

Not to be Confused With: Can be confused with emblica and *Terminalia bellirica.*

Other Names: Black Myrobalan, Chebulic Myrobalan, Myrobalan

ACTIONS AND PHARMACOLOGY

COMPOUNDS

Tannins (20 to 45%): gallotannins, including terchebulin, terflavin A, punicalagin, corilagin, chebulic acid, and chebulinic acid

Monosaccharides/oligosaccharides (9%): including D-glucose, D-fructose, saccharose

Fruit acids: including quinic acid (1.5%), shikimic acid (2%)

Fatty oil (in the seeds, to 40%)

EFFECTS

Its high tannin content explains the use of the drug as an astringent. A variety of experiments have demonstrated antibacterial, cardiotonic, and antiarteriosclerotic effects for the drug.

INDICATIONS AND USAGE

Chinese Medicine: Tropical Almond is used for chronic diarrhea, chronic dysentery, rectal prolapse, loss of voice because of chronic coughs, blood in the stool, leukorrhea, night sweats, and undesired discharges.

Indian Medicine: The drug is used in the treatment of wounds, ulcers, gingivitis, excitation, gastric complaints, anorexia, worm infestation, flatulence, hemorrhoids, jaundice, for liver and spleen disease, pharyngodynia, hiccups, coughs, epilepsy, eye disease, skin changes, leprosy, intermittent fever, cardiac dysfunction, gastritis, and neuropathy.

PRECAUTIONS AND ADVERSE REACTIONS

No health hazards are known in conjunction with the proper administration of designated therapeutic dosages, although even therapeutic dosages could lead to constipation, due to the high tannin content (administration as an antidiarrheal).

OVERDOSAGE

The administration of extremely high doses (25% of the fodder) over a period of 4 weeks to rats led to kidney and liver damage; mice developed liver tumors in a related experiment (750 mg/kg body weight of the tannin fraction over a period of 12 weeks).

DOSAGE

Mode of Administration: Whole herb preparations for internal and external use.

Daily Dosage: 3 to 9 g

Storage: Should be stored in a dry and cool place.

LITERATURE

el-Mekkawy S, Meselhy MR, Kusumoto IT, Kadota S, Hattori M, Namba T, Inhibitory effects of Egyptian folk medicines on human immunodeficiency virus (HIV) reverse transcriptase. *Chem Pharm Bull* (Tokyo), 20:641-8, Apr. 1995

Grover IS, Bala S, Antimutagenic activity of *Terminalia chebula* (myroblan) *in Salmonella typhimurium. Indian J Exp Biol*, 30:339-41, Apr. 1992

Hamada S, Kataoka T, Woo JT, Yamada A, Yoshida T, Nishimura T, Otake N, Nagai K, Immunosuppressive effects of gallic acid and chebulagic acid on CTL-mediated cytotoxicity. *Biol Pharm Bull*, 20:1017-9, Sep. 1997

Jiang JY, Influence of processing methods on the quality of *Terminalia chebula. Chung Yao Tung Pao*, 20:24-6, Sep. 1986

Kurokawa M, Nagasaka K, Hirabayashi T, Uyama S, Sato H, Kageyama T, Kadota S, Ohyama H, Hozumi T, Namba T, et al Efficacy of traditional herbal medicines in combination with acyclovir against herpes simplex virus type 1 infection in vitro and in vivo. *Antiviral Res*, 45:19-37, May. 1995

Miglani BD, Sen P, Sanyal RK, Purgative action of an oil obtained from *Terminalia chebula. Indian J Med Res*, 20:281-3, Feb. 1971

Phadke SA, Kulkarni SD, Screening of in vitro antibacterial activity of *Terminalia chebula, Eclapta alba* and *Ocimum sanctum. Indian J Med Sci,* 43:113-7, May. 1989

Sato Y, Oketani H, Singyouchi K, Ohtsubo T, Kihara M, Shibata H, Higuti T, Extraction and purification of effective antimicrobial constituents of *Terminalia chebula* Retz. against methicillin-resistant *Staphylococcus aureus. Biol Pharm Bull,* 20:401-4, Apr. 1997

Shin TY, Jeong HJ, Kim DJ, Kim SH, Lee JK, Kim DK, Chae BS. Inhibitory action of water soluble fraction of *Terminalia chebula* on systemic and local anaphylaxis. *J Ethnopharmacol* 74(2); 133-140. 2001

Shiraki K, Yukawa T, Kurokawa M, Kageyama S, Cytomegalovirus infection and its possible treatment with herbal medicines. *Nippon Rinsho*, 56:156-60, Jan. 1998

Shiraki K, Yukawa T, Kurokawa M, Kageyama S, Influence of processing methods on the quality of *Terminalia chebula. Chung Yao Tung Pao*, 56:24-6, Sep. 1986

Sohni YR, Bhatt RM, Activity of a crude extract formulation in experimental hepatic amoebiasis and in immunomodulation studies. *J Ethnopharmacol*, 45:119-24, Nov. 1996

Sohni YR, Kaimal P, Bhatt RM, The antiamoebic effect of a crude drug formulation of herbal extracts against *Entamoeba histolytica* in vitro and in vivo. *J Ethnopharmacol*, 45:43-52, Jan. 1995

Thakur CP, Thakur B, Singh S, Sinha PK, Sinha SK, The Ayurvedic medicines Haritaki, Amala and Bahira reduce cholesterol-induced atherosclerosis in rabbits. *Int J Cardiol*, 21:167-75, Nov. 1988

Yukawa TA, Kurokawa M, Sato H, Yoshida Y, Kageyama S, Hasegawa T, Namba T, Imakita M, Hozumi T, Shiraki K, Effect of tannins from *Terminalia chebula* Retz. on the infectivity of potato virus X. *Acta Microbiol Pol B*, 32:127-32, 1970.

Yukawa TA, Kurokawa M, Sato H, Yoshida Y, Kageyama S, Hasegawa T, Namba T, Imakita M, Hozumi T, Shiraki K, Prophylactic treatment of cytomegalovirus infection with traditional herbs. *Antiviral Res*, 32:63-70, Oct. 1996

Tsuga canadensis

See Pinus Bark

Tulip Tree

Liriodendron tulipifera

DESCRIPTION

Medicinal Parts: The bark is said to have medicinal properties.

Flower and Fruit: The flowers are apical, single with 3 revolute, greenish-white sepals. There are 6 petals, 4 to 5 cm long, greenish-yellow with orange bands near the base on the inside, similar to the tepals of the tulip. The flower has numerous stamens and numerous apocarpic ovaries on a spindle-shaped column. The small, single-seeded nut with pointed wings is in a 6 to 8 cm long, conelike, aggregate fruit that is light green when ripe.

Leaves, Stem, and Root: Liriodendron tulipifera is a tree that grows up to 60 m high. The leaves are alternate with saddle-shaped middle lobes and 2 large lateral lobes, almost square in outline, 8 to 15 cm long and wide, and usually rounded at the base. The upper leaf surface is fresh green, the lower surface a weak blue. The petioles are 5 to 10 cm long. The young branches are yellow-green in summer and reddish-brown in winter and spotted with lenticles. The young trunks are dark green to gray and spotted white with lenticles. The trunks (up to 3 m thick) of older trees have a brown, deeply grooved bark.

Characteristics: The leaves are bright golden-yellow in autumn.

Habitat: Indigenous to North America, Europe, and China.

Production: The Tulip Tree bark is the peeled and dried branch bark of *Liriodendron tulipifera*.

Other Names: Yellow Poplar

ACTIONS AND PHARMACOLOGY

COMPOUNDS

Isoquinoline alkaloids (0.1%), particularly of the aporphine type: including remerine, lysicamine, liriodenine, lanugosine

Lignans (0.1%): including liriodendrin

Volatile oil (0.1%): chief components cis-beta-ocimene, beta-pinene, bornyl acetate

Hydroxycumarins: esculetin methyl and dimethyl esters

EFFECTS

The alkaloids contained in the drug are antimicrobial in effect, and a positively inotropic effect has been described. Its usefulness as a tonic and a stimulant appears to be plausible, based upon its qualities as a bitter substance.

INDICATIONS AND USAGE

Unproven Uses: Folk medicine indications have included fever, menstrual complaints, insomnia, and malaria.

PRECAUTIONS AND ADVERSE REACTIONS

The drug is considered toxic, due to its alkaloid content. Administration in animal experiments led to coma (exact details unavailable). No case of poisoning among humans has been recorded.

DOSAGE

Preparation: There is no information in the literature.

Daily dosage: Powder: 4 to 8 g daily; decoction (30:500) 60 g daily.

LITERATURE

Doskotch RW, el-Feraly FS, Antitumor agents. II. Tulipinolide, a new germacranolide sesquiterpene, and constunolide. Two cytotoxic substances from *Liriodendron tulipifera L. J Pharm Sci,* 28:877-80, Jul. 1969

Hufford CD, Funderburk MJ, Morgan JM, Robertson LW, Two antimicrobial alkaloids from heartwood of *Liriodendron tulipifera L. J Pharm Sci,* 64:789-92, May. 1975

Rzedowski M, Furmanowa M, Molak W, Liriodenine in tissue culture of *Liriodendron tulipifera L.* II. Quantitative analysis and antifungal effect. *Acta Pol Pharm,* 42:300-4, 1985.

Schulz HK, Hausen BM, White wood allergy (author's transl) *Derm Beruf Umwelt,* 28:158-60, 1980.

Turkey Corn

Dicentra cucullaria

DESCRIPTION

Medicinal Parts: The medicinal part is the dried tuber.

Flower and Fruit: The inflorescence is racemous. The 4 to 10 flowers are odorless, white, and often tinged pink. The flowers are hanging, with yellow to yellow-orange tips and widely splayed spurs. The fruit is oval and 9 to 13 mm long. The seeds are reniform, 2 mm long, black, and glossy.

Leaves, Stem, and Root: Turkey Corn is a delicate, glabrous, 15- to 40-cm high plant on a tawny yellow, tuberous rhizome. The rhizome has subglobular, pink, smaller tubers about 0.5 cm in diameter, with a scar on both depressed sides. All the leaves are basal and almost triangular in outline. They are tripinnate and bluish-green on the underside.

Characteristics: The taste of the tuber is bitter.

Habitat: Canada and U.S.

Production: Turkey Corn root is the root of *Dicentra cucullaria.*

Other Names: Bleeding Heart, Corydalis, Dutchman's Breeches, Squirrel Corn, Staggerweed

ACTIONS AND PHARMACOLOGY

COMPOUNDS

Isoquinoline alkaloids: including bicuculline, corlumine, protopine, cryptopine, cularine

EFFECTS

Diuretic and tonic

INDICATIONS AND USAGE

Unproven Uses: Turkey corn is used for digestive disorders, urinary tract diseases, menstrual disorders, and skin rashes. It was formerly used for syphilis.

PRECAUTIONS AND ADVERSE REACTIONS

Health risks or side effects following the proper administration of designated therapeutic dosages are not recorded. Bicuculline is a centrally acting, spasmogenic antagonist of gamma-aminobutyric acid (GABA). Due to the bicuculline component, poisonings are possible if higher dosages are consumed, but none has been reported to date.

DOSAGE

Mode of Administration: The drug is available as a liquid extract.

LITERATURE

Kanamori H, Sakamoto I, Mizuta M, *Chem Pharm Bull* 34:1826. 1986.

Tusboi NS, J Labelled compd *Radiopharm* 13:353. 1977.

Turmeric

Curcuma domestica

DESCRIPTION

Medicinal Parts: The medicinal parts are the stewed and dried rhizome.

Flower and Fruit: The inflorescence is conelike, 10 to 15 cm long, and is attached to a stem enclosed in a sheathing petiole. The flower has 2 pale green bracts, which are 5 to 6 cm long. The covering bracts are whitish, often red-tinged. The individual flowers are yellowish-white or yellow. The flowers have a tubular, 3-lobed calyx, and funnel-shaped, 3-tipped corolla. The fruit is a gobular capsule.

Leaves, Stem, and Root: Curcuma domestica is a perennial, erect, leafy plant with very large, lilylike leaves up to 1.2 m long. The leaf blade is ovate-lanceolate, thin, entire-margined, and narrows to a long sheathlike petiole. The main rhizome is thickened to a tuber and has numerous roots. The roots in turn terminate in partially elliptical tubers. The secondary rhizomes are digit-shaped with no roots. All rhizomes are yellowish-brown with stipules and appear transversely ringed when they die.

Habitat: Turmeric is probably indigenous to India; it is cultivated today in India and other tropical regions of Southeast Asia.

Production: Turmeric root consists of the fingerlike scalded and dried rhizomes of *Curcuma longa*. It is harvested from February to April. The rhizomes are boiled in water for 5 to 10 minutes and then dried in the sun.

Adulterations: The synthetic color pigments azo and anilin are sometimes added to the herb.

Not to be Confused With: Curcuma xanthorrhiza, Curcuma aromatica, and *Curcuma zedoaria*

ACTIONS AND PHARMACOLOGY

COMPOUNDS

Volatile oil (3-5%): alpha- and beta-tumerone (aroma source), artumerone, alpha- and gamma-atlantone, curlone, zingiberene, curcumol

Curcuminoids (3-5%): including curcumin, demethoxy curcumin, bidemethoxy curcumin

1,5-diaryl-penta-1,4-dien-3-one derivatives

Starch (30-40%)

EFFECTS

Turmeric has antihepatotoxic, antihyperlipidemic, antithrombotic, and anti-inflammatory effects. It is also antioxidative, antitumoral and antimicrobial (in particular, the sesquiterpene derivatives). It has insect repellent and antifertile effects. It also inhibits prostaglandin formation, *in vitro*.

Anti-Inflammatory Effects: The anti-inflammatory effects of turmeric are thought to be due to inhibition of leukotriene biosynthesis, and through this inhibition, a change in prostaglandin production. Alpha tumerone blocks the proliferation of human lymphocytes and decreases the activity of natural killer cells. Ukonan A (a polysaccharide) has phagocytic effects when tested in mice (Bisset, 1994).

Turmeric binds to estradiol and progesterone receptors and may have weak estrogenic activity in vivo. Turmeric had an estradiol binding capacity in vitro of 0.5 mcg of estradiol binding equivalent per 2 g of dried herb and 4 mcg of progesterone binding activity per 2 g of dried herb. After ingestion, saliva was used to obtain these phytoestrogens and phytoprogesterones. The substances isolated were used to detect bioavailability and bioactivity of phytoestrogens and phytoprogesterones in turmeric. Breast cancer cell lines were used to evaluate growth rate changes induced by this herb, but the differences were not significant (Zava et al, 1998).

Curcumin has antineoplastic effects through an antiproliferative mechanism. Part of this effect may be due to curcumin's effect on various kinases. Curcumin was found to be an inhibitor of highly purified protein kinase A (Ka), protein kinase C (Kc), protamine kinase (PK), phosphorylase kinase (PHK), autophosphorylation-activated protein kinase (AAPK), and pp60-tyrosine kinase (TK). The amount of inhibition varied, with phosphorylase kinase being the most effected at lower doses of curcumin. A dose of 0.1 mmol of curcumin produced the following reductions: PHK (98%), TK (40%), Kc (15%), Ka (10%), AAPK (1%), and PK (0.5%). PHK is a key regulatory enzyme in glycogen metabolism, which may result in antiproliferation effects if it is inhibited (Reddy & Aggarwal, 1994). Curcumin also inhibits the expression of several proto-oncogenes (c-jun, c-fos, c-myc) in mouse skin cells and transcription factor AP-1 (Sikora et al, 1997). The antiproliferative effect of curcumin on transformed and nontransformed cancer cells was measured in vitro. In all experiments, curcumin caused slight-to-moderate inhibition of the proliferation of leukemia hematopoietic cell types but not fibroblasts (Gautam et al, 1998).

Curcumin I and curcumin III are two antineoplastic chemicals found in curcumin. Curcumin I inhibited benzopyrene-induced forestomach and benzopyrene-initiated, tetradeconyl-phorbol-acetate-promoted skin tumors in Swiss mice. Curcumin II inhibited dimethylbenzathracene-induced skin tumors in Swiss bald mice. Both compounds demonstrated in vitro cytotoxicity against human chronic myeloid leukemia in a dose dependent manner. Using in vivo carcinogen metabolism enzyme studies and 3H-benzopyrene-DNA studies, curcumins were shown to inhibit cancer at the initiation, promotion, and progression stages of development. Altering of the activation and/or detoxification process of carcinogen metabolism was reported (Nagabhushan & Bhide, 1992).

Antioxidant Effects: Curcumin provides an antioxidant and anti-inflammatory effect by inhibiting the binding of transcription factor AP-1 to DNA and activation of NF-kappaB. These two substances control many endothelial genes such as plasminogen activator factor-1, tissue factor, endothelin-1, and interleukin 6 & 8. Via its AP-1 inhibitory activity, curcumin inhibits both cell growth and cell death (Bierhaus et al, 1997; Sikora et al, 1997; Singh & Aggarwal, 1995). Curcumin inhibits epidermal arachidonic acid metabolism by means of lipoxygenase and cyclooxygenase pathways and reduces the inflammatory effects of arachidonic acid and tetradeconylphorbol-acetate (TPA) (Stoner & Mukhtar, 1995).

Tumerone has anti-snake venom properties, blocking the hemorrhagic effects of Bothrops venom and reducing the lethality of Crotalus venoms (Bisset, 1994). Specific studies could not be found, but maybe due to an antithrombotic effect (Bierhaus et al, 1997; Sikora et al, 1997).

CLINICAL TRIALS

Turmeric is frequently cited as a mild and effective anti-inflammatory for such conditions as postoperative inflammation, osteoarthritis, and rheumatoid arthritis (Yarnell, 2006).

Ulcerative Colitis

A double-blind, multi-center placebo-controlled trial in 89 Japanese adults with ulcerative colitis in a period of relative quiet found that Curcumin was promising and relatively free of side-effects in maintaining remission. The Curcumin dosage of 2 grams daily in combination with the standard medicines sulfasalazine (SZ) or mesalamine was effective, with only 2 of 43 patients randomized to the Curcumin regimen relapsing during the 6 months of therapy, while eight of 39 patients receiving placebo with SZ or mesalamine did so. The regimen proved to be significantly superior in preventing relapse as compared with SZ and mesalamine alone, or placebo alone. Also, the Curcumin regimen resulted in significantly improved index designed to measure clinical activity (clinical activity index; P=.038) and endoscopic index (EI; P=.0001). The Curcumin was well tolerated, with none of the participants reporting serious side effects—a notable finding given the many unpleasant side effects such as rash, headache, fever, and increased risk of kidney inflammation typically associated with conventional medicines used to treat ulcerative colitis (Hanai, 2006).

Ulcers

One study demonstrated that turmeric was not better than controls in healing duodenal ulcers. The study was a double-blind, prospective, placebo-controlled, multicenter trial of 118 patients who received 6 g/d of turmeric. No H2-receptor antagonists, anticholinergics, or other antiulcer drugs were used during the study or for a week before the study began. The follow-up endoscopy and x-rays were done after 28 and 56 days. The ulcer healing rate of placebo was 29% and that of turmeric was 27% (Van Dau et al, 1998).

Chronic Anterior Uveitis

Marked improvement was seen in 32 patients with chronic anterior uveitis (CAU) who received 375 mg curcumin daily for 12 weeks. Patients were divided into 2 groups. Group A (n=18) received topical mydriatic agents, local hot fomentation and curcumin. Patients in group B (n=14) were treated with antitubercular drugs (rifampicin 10 mg/kg plus INH 5 mg/kg plus pyrazinamide 30 mg/kg daily), local mydriatics, hot fomentation, and curcumin. In Group B, curcumin was administered for 12 weeks but antitubercular medications were continued for one year. Symptomatic improvement was observed in both groups. Patients in group A experienced improved vision, pain relief, decreased redness and lacrimation, regression in circumciliary congestion, keratic precipitates, aqueous flare, and vitreous turbidity. Complete remission of CAU was observed in 12 of 14 patients in group B within 12 weeks of beginning therapy (Lal et al, 1999).

INDICATIONS AND USAGE

Approved by Commission E:

- Dyspeptic complaints
- Loss of appetite

Turmeric is used for dyspeptic disorders, particularly feelings of fullness after meals and regular abdominal distention due to gas.

Unproven Uses: The drug is also used for diarrhea, intermittent fever, edema, bronchitis, colds, worms, leprosy, kidney inflammation, and cystitis. Other uses include headaches, flatulence, upper abdominal pain, chest infections, colic, amenorrhea, and flushing. It is used externally for bruising, leech bites, festering eye infections, inflammation of the oral mucosa, inflammatory skin conditions, and infected wounds.

Chinese Medicine: Turmeric is used for pains in the chest, ribs, abdomen, liver and stomach; nosebleeds, vomiting with bleeding, and heat stroke.

Indian Medicine: Turmeric is used for inflammation, wounds and skin ulcers, itching, stomach complaints, flatulence, conjunctivitis, constipation, ringworm infestation, and colic.

CONTRAINDICATIONS

Turmeric should not be used by people with gallstones or bile duct obstruction. It should also not be used by patients with hyperacidity or gastrointestinal ulcers.

Pregnancy: Not to be used during pregnancy. Turmeric has emmenagogic and abortifacient effects from its uterine stimulant activity.

PRECAUTIONS AND ADVERSE REACTIONS

Stomach complaints can occur following extended use or in the case of overdose. One case of acute contact dermatitis was reported following a 6-month occupational exposure to turmeric (Kiec-Swierczynska & Krecisz, 1998).

DRUG INTERACTIONS

MODERATE RISK

Anticoagulants, Antiplatelet Agents, Low Molecular Weight Heparins, and Thrombolytic Agents: Theoretically, curcumin may add to the effect of these medications and increase the risk of bleeding. Curcumin inhibited platelet aggregation in animals and in vitro (Srivastava et al, 1995; Srivastava et al, 1985), which may result in prolonged bleeding times if taken with drugs known to affect platelet function. *Clinical Management:* Caution is advised if curcumin and any of these agents are used concomitantly. Monitor bleeding time and signs and symptoms of excessive bleeding.

DOSAGE

Mode of Administration: Whole, cut and powdered drug available as capsules, solution, coated tablets, and compound preparations.

Preparation: To prepare a tea, scald 0.5 to 1 g drug in boiling water, cover, draw for 5 minutes and then strain. The tincture strength is 1:10.

Daily Dosage: The average dose is 1.5 to 3 g of drug. The powder should be taken 2 to 3 times daily after meals; the tea (2 to 3 cups) should be taken between meals. The tincture dose is 10 to 15 drops 2 to 3 times daily.

Storage: Turmeric should be protected from light.

LITERATURE

Ammon HP, Wahl MA. Pharmacology of *Curcuma longa*. In: *Planta Med,* 57:1-7, 1991.

Ammon HPT, Anazodo MI, Safayhi H et al. In: *Planta Med* 58:226, 1992.

Ammon HPT, Wahl MA. Pharmacology of *Curcuma longa*. In: *Planta Med* 57:1-7, 1991.

Anto RJ, George J, Babu KV, RaJasekharan KN, Kuttan R. Antimutagenic and anticarcinogenic activity of natural and synthetic curcuminoids. In: *Mutat Res*, 42:127-31, 1996.

Apisariyakul A, Vanittanakom N, Buddhasukh D. Antifungal activity of Turmeric oil extracted from Curcuma longa (Zingiberaceae). In: *J Ethnopharmacol*, 30:163-9, 1995.

Babu PS, Srinivasan K. Hypolipidemic action of curcumin the active principle of Turmeric (Curcuma longa) in streptozotocin induced diabetic rats. In: *Mol Cell Biochem*, 30:169-75, 1997.

Banz (Federal German Gazette) No. 223; published 30 Nov 1985; revised 1 Sept 1990.

Basu AB. *Ind J Pharm* 33:131, 1971.

Bierhaus A, Zhang Y, Quehenberger et al. The dietary pigment curcumin reduces endothelial tissue factor gene expression by inhibitingbinding of AP-1 to the DNA and activaton of NF-kappaB. In: *Thromb Haemost* 77(4):772-782, 1997.

Bonte F, Noel-Hudson MS, Wepierre J, Meybeck A. Protective effect of curcuminoids on epidermal skin cells under free oxygen radical stress. In: *Planta Med,* 8:265-6, 1997.

Chan MM. Inhibition of tumor necrosis factor by curcumin a phytochemical. In: *Biochem Pharmacol*, 42:1551-6, 1995.

Chen HW & Huang HC. Effect of curcumin on cell cycle progression and apoptosis in vascular smooth muscle cells. In: *Br J Pharm* 124(6):1029-1040, 1998.

Charles V, Charles SX. The use and efficacy of Azadirachta indica ADR (''Neem'') and Curcuma longa (''Turmeric'') in scabies. A pilot study. In: *Trop Geogr Med*, 30:178-81, 1992.

Dhar ML. et al *Indian J Exp Biol* 6:232, 1968.

Donatus IA, SardJoko, Vermeulen NP. Cytotoxic and cytoprotective activities of curcumin. Effects on paracetamol-induced cytotoxicity lipid peroxidation and glutathione depletion in rat hepatocytes. In: *Biochem Pharmacol*, 39:1869-75, 1990.

Ferreira LA, Henriques OB, Andreoni AA, Vital GR, Campos MM, Habermehl GG, de Moraes VL. Antivenom and biological effects of ar-turmerone isolated from *Curcuma longa* (Zingiberaceae). In: *Toxicon*, 30:1211-8, 1992.

Ferreira LA, Henriques OB, Andreoni AA, Vital GR, Campos MM, Habermehl GG, de Moraes VL. Toxicity studies on *Alpinia galanga* and *Curcuma longa*. In: *Planta Med*, 30:124-7, 1992.

Garg SK. *Planta Med* 26:225, 1974.

Gautam SC, Xu YX, Pindolia KR et al. Nonselective inhibition of proliferation of transformed and nontransformed cells by the anticancer agent curcumin (diferuloylmethane). In: *Biochem Pharm* 55(8):1333-1337, 1998.

Hanai H, Iida T, Takeuchi K, et al. Curcumin maintenance therapy for ulcerative colitis: randomized, multicenter, double-blind, placebo-controlled study. *Clin Gastroent Hepatol*; 4 (12): 1502-1506. 2006.

Hanif R, Qiao L, Shiff SJ, Rigas B. Curcumin a natural plant phenolic food additive inhibits cell proliferation and induces cell cycle changes in colon adenocarcinoma cell lines by a prostaglandin-independent pathway. In: *J Lab Clin Med*, 42:576-84, 1997.

Hasmeda M, Polya GM. Inhibition of cyclic AMP-dependent protein kinase by curcumin. In: *Phytochemistry*, 42:599-605, 1996.

Huang HC, Jan TR, Yeh SF. Inhibitory effect of curcumin an anti-inflammatory agent on vascular smooth muscle cell proliferation. In: *Eur J Pharmacol*, 54:381-4, 1992.

Inagawa H et al. Homeostasis as regulated by activated macrophage. II. LPS of plant origin other than wheat flour and their concomitant bacteria. In: *Chem Pharm Bull* (Tokyo), 54:994-7, 1992.

Kiec-Swierczynska M & Krecisz B: Occupational allergic contact dermatitis due to curcumin food colour in a pasta factory worker. In: *Contact Dermatitis*, 39(1):30-31, 1998.

Lal B, Kapoor AK, Asthana OP et al. Efficacy of curcumin in the management of chronic anterior uveitis. In: *Phytother Res* 13:318-322, 1999.

Limtrakul P, Lipigorngoson S, Namwong O, Apisariyakul A, Dunn FW. Inhibitory effect of dietary curcumin on skin carcinogenesis in mice. In: *Cancer Lett,* 8:197-203, 1997.

Masuda T et al. Anti-oxidative and anti-inflammatory curcumin-related phenolics from rhizomes of Curcuma domestica. In: *Phytochemistry* 32:1557, 1986.

Mehta K, Pantazis P, McQueen T, Aggarwal BB. Antiproliferative effect of curcumin (diferuloylmethane) against human breast tumor cell lines. In: *Anticancer Drugs*, 8:470-81, 1997.

Mukhopadhyay A, Basu N, Ghatak N et al. Anti-inflammatory and irritant activities of curcumin analogs in rats. In: *Agents Actions* 12(4):508-515, 1982.

Nagabhushan M & Bhide SV. Curcumin as an inhibitor of cancer. In: *J Am Coll Nutr* 11(2):192-198, 1992.

Nagarajan K, Arya VP. *J Sci Ind Res* 41:232, 1982.

Nakayama R et al. Two curcuminoid pigments from *Curcuma domestica*. In: *Phytochemistry* 33:501, 1993.

Polasa K, Sesikaran B, Krishna TP, Krishnaswamy K. Turmeric (*Curcuma longa*)-induced reduction in urinary mutagens. In: *Food Chem Toxicol*, 47:699-706, 1991.

Priyadarsini KI. Free radical reactions of curcumin in membrane models. In: *Free Radic Biol Med,* 54:838-43, 1997.

Rafatullah S, Tariq M, Al-Yahya MA, Mossa JS, Ageel AM. Evaluation of Turmeric (*Curcuma longa*) for gastric and duodenal antiulcer activity in rats. In: *J Ethnopharmacol,* 47:25-34, 1990.

Ravindranath V, Satyanarayana MN. *Phytochemistry* 19:2031, 1980.

Reddy S & Aggarwal BB. Curcumin is a non-competitive and selective inhibitor of phosphorylase kinase. In: *FEBS Lett* 341(1):19-22, 1994.

Ruby AJ, Kuttan G, Babu KD, RaJasekharan KN, Kuttan R. Anti-tumour and antioxidant activity of natural curcuminoids. In: *Cancer Lett*, 42:79-83, 1995.

Selvam R, Subramanian L, Gayathri R, Angayarkanni N. The anti-oxidant activity of Turmeric (*Curcuma longa*). *J Ethnopharmacol,* 47:59-67, 1995.

Sikora E, Bielak-ZmiJewska A, Piwocka K, Skierski J, Radziszewska E. Inhibition of proliferation and apoptosis of human and rat T lymphocytes by curcumin a curry pigment. In: *Biochem Pharmacol,* 54:899-907, 1997.

Singh S & Aggarwal BB. Activation of transcription factor NF-kappaB is suppressed by curcumin. In: *J Biol Chem* 270(42):24995-25000, 1995.

Soni KB, RaJan A, Kuttan R. Reversal of aflatoxin induced liver damage by Turmeric and curcumin. In: *Cancer Lett*, 66:115-21, 1992.

Srimal RC, Dhawan CN. *J Pharm Pharmacol* 25:447, 1973.

Srinivas L, Shalini VK, ShylaJa M. Turmerin: a water soluble antioxidant peptide from Turmeric Curcuma longa. In: *Arch Biochem Biophys*, 30:617-23, 1992.

Srivastava KC, Bordia A, Verma SK. Curcumin a major component of food spice Turmeric (Curcuma longa) inhibits aggregation and alters eicosanoid metabolism in human blood platelets. In: *Prostaglandins Leukot Essent Fatty Acids*, 52:223-7, 1995.

Srivastava R, Dikshit M, Srimal RC et al. Anti-thrombotic effects of curcumin. In: *Thromb Res* 40(3):413-417, 1985.

Srivastava R, Puri V, Srimal RC et al. Effect of curcumin on platelet aggregation and vascular prostacyclin synthesis. In: *Arnzmittelforschung* 36(4):715-717, 1986.

Steinegger E, Hänsel R. *Pharmakognosie,* 5. Aufl.; Springer Verlag Heidelberg 1992.

Stoner GD & Muktar H. Polyphenols as cancer chemopreventive agents. In: *J Cell Biochem Suppl* 22:169-180, 1995.

Tang W, Eisenbrand G. *Chinese Drugs of Plant Origin*. Springer Verlag Heidelberg, 1992.

Van Dau N, Ham NN, Khac DH et al. The effects of a traditional drug, turmeric (*Curcuma longa*), and placebo on the healing of duodenal ulcers. In: *Phytomedicine* 5:29-34, 1998.

Veit M. Beeinflussung der Leukotrien-Biosynthese durch Curcumin. In: *Z Phytother* 14:46, 1993.

Verma SP, Salamone E, Goldin B. Curcumin and genistein plant natural products show synergistic inhibitory effects on the growth of human breast cancer MCF-7 cells induced by estrogenic pesticides. In: *Biochem Biophys Res Commun*, 233:692-6, 1997.

Wagner H et al. 6th Int Conf. Prostaglandins and Related Compounds. Florence, Italy. Pub. Fondzione Giovanni Lorenzini. June 3-6, 1986.

Yarnell E, Abascal K. Herbs for curbing inflammation. *Alt Comp Med*; 22-28. 2006.

Zava DT, Dollbaum CM & Blen M. Estrogen and progestin bioactivity of foods, herbs, and spices. In: *Proc Soc Exp Biol Med* 217(3):369-378, 1998.

Turnera diffusa

See Damiana

Tussilago farfara

See Colt's Foot

Ulmus minor

See Elm Bark

Ulmus rubra

See Slippery Elm

Uncaria species

See Gambir

Uncaria tomentosa

See Cat's Claw

Urginea indica

See Indian Squill

Urginea maritima

See Squill

Urtica dioica

See Stinging Nettle

Usnea

Usnea species

DESCRIPTION

Medicinal Parts: Research into this species is not yet complete, making it difficult to establish which lichens are used for the extraction of which drug, and which lichens have been described by earlier botanists.

Flower and Fruit: Mycelia flourishes on a variety of trees (on the trunk and branches) as a whitish, reddish, or black lichen.

Habitat: Usnea is found worldwide in cool, damp places.

Production: Usnea consists of the dried thallus of *Usnea* species, primarily of *Usnea barbata, Usnea florida, Usnea hirta* and *Usnea plicata.*

Other Names: Beard Moss, Tree Moss, Old Man's Beard

ACTIONS AND PHARMACOLOGY

COMPOUNDS

Lichen acids (polyketides): including among others (+)-usnic acid, thamnolic acid (hirtellic acid), usnaric acid (salazinic acid), lobaric acid, stictinic acid, protocetraric acid, everninic acid, barbatinic acid (rhizonic acid), diffractaic acid (dirhizonic acid), barbatolic acid. The lichen acid spectrums of the different species vary from one another, with usnic acid the chief constituent.

Mucilage

EFFECTS

The drug is antimicrobial, and has shown both antifungal and antiviral effects in vitro.

INDICATIONS AND USAGE

Approved by Commission E:

- Inflammation of the mouth and pharynx

PRECAUTIONS AND ADVERSE REACTIONS

No health hazards or side effects are known in conjunction with the proper administration of designated therapeutic dosages. Following overdosage, signs of poisoning could appear. These signs have yet to be described.

DOSAGE

Mode of Administration: The drug is available as lozenges and equivalent solid forms of medication.

Daily Dose: The daily dose is 600 mg. For lozenge preparations, use the equivalent of 100 mg of herb; take 1 lozenge 3 to 6 times daily.

LITERATURE

Fournet A, Ferreira ME, Rojas de Arias A et al. Activity of compounds isolated from Chilean lichens against experimental cutaneous Leishmaniasis. *Comp Biochem Physiol.*; 116C: 51-54. 1997

Ghione M, Parrello D, Grasso L. Usin acid revisited, its activity on oral flora. *Chemoterapia.*; 7: 302-325 1988

Hahn M, Lischka G, Pfeifle J, Wirth V. A case of contact dermatitis from lichens in South Germany. *Contact Dermatitis.*; 32: 55-56. 1995

Okuyama E et al., Usnic acid and diffractic acid as analgesic and antipyretic components of *Usnea diffracta*. In: *PM* 61(2):113-115. 1995.

Usnea species

See Usnea

Utricularia vulgaris

See Bladderwort

Uva-Ursi

Arctostaphylos uva-ursi

DESCRIPTION

Medicinal Parts: The medicinal parts of the plant are the dried leaves and preparations of the fresh leaves.

Flower and Fruit: The flowers are on 3 to 12 short, hanging stalks, where they are in clusters at equal length and distance on the terminal end of the stalks. The pedicle has 2 small, ciliate, oval-shaped leaves at the base with the subtending flower clusters. The calyx is 1 mm long, palmate, and has 5 membranous tips. The corolla (fused petals of the inner whorl) is ovoid to jug-shaped, white or reddish with a red border, 5 to 6 mm long with 5 short tips rolled backward. The 10 stamens are half the length of the corolla tube. The filaments are heavily thickened at the base. The crimson anthers have porous openings and a long, whiplike, curling appendage. The ovaries are 5- to 7-valved, and the style is longer than the stamens. The fruit is a globular, pea-sized, scarlet, floury drupe. The fruit has 5 to 7 stone seeds, 4 mm in length, which are kidney-shaped and also compressed at the sides.

Leaves, Stem, and Root: The plant is a decumbent, creeping espalier that grows up to 1.5 m long with elastic, red-brown branches. The leaves are alternate, coriaceous, short-petioled, spatulate-obovate, or wedge-shaped, entire-margined, and slightly revolute. They are 12 to 30 mm long by 4 to 15 mm wide, glabrous, glossy, and evergreen. The underside is distinctly reticulate, and the midrib and the margins are often downy.

Characteristics: The leaves have a bitter, astringent taste. They are distinguished from the cranberry by the reticulate vein structure and nonglandular spots beneath.

Habitat: The plant has spread from the Iberian Peninsula across Central Europe north to Scandinavia and east to Siberia. The plant is also found in the Altai mountains, the Himalayas, and in North America.

Production: Uva-Ursi (Bearberry) leaves consist of the fresh or dried leaves of *Arctostaphylos uva-ursi,* which are gathered in the wild. The arbutin content is highest in December and January and also when the leaves are dried rapidly. The main sources are Spain, Italy, Austria, Switzerland, Scandinavia, Poland, Russia, and Bulgaria.

Not to be Confused With: The leaves are sometimes confused with the leaves of other Ericaceae, such as Buxus sempervirens.

Other Names: Arberry, Bearberry, Arbutus Uva-Ursi, Bear's Grape, Common Bearberry, Kinnikinnick, Mealberry, Mountain Box, Mountain Cranberry, Red Bearberry, Red-Beery, Red-Berried Trailing Arbutus, Redberry Leaves, Rockberry, Sagackhomi, Sandberry, Upland Cranberry

ACTIONS AND PHARMACOLOGY

COMPOUNDS

Hydroquinone glycosides: arbutin (arbutoside, hydroquinone-O-beta-D-glucoside, 5-16%), methyl arbutin (O-methyl hydroquinone-O-beta-D-glycoside, up to 4%), galloyl derivatives of arbutin (0.05%): O-galloyl hydroquinone-O-beta-D-glucoside (p-galloyl oxyphenyl-O-beta-D-glucoside), 2''O- galloyl arbutin, 6''O-galloyl arbutin, free hydroquinone (usually under 0.3%) as decomposition product of arbutin, emerging as the leaves age or during dehydration

Piceoside: (4-hydroxyacetophenone-O-beta-D-glucopyranoside)

Phenol carboxylic acids: including gallic acid (free 180 mg/100 g), p-coumaric acid (18.0 mg/100 g), syringic acid (16.8 mg/100 g), salicylic acid (12.0 mg/100 g), p-hydroxybenzoic acid (9.6 mg/100 g), ferulic acid (6.0 mg/100 g), caffeic acid (6.0 mg/100 g), lithospermic acid (dimeric caffeic acid)

Tannins (15-20%): gallo tannins including penta-O-galloyl-beta-D-Glucose and hexa-O-galloyl-beta-D-glucose; ellagitannins, including corilagin (1-0-galloyl-3, 6-di-O-hexahydroxydophenol-beta-D-gulcoside); condensed tannins, chiefly proanthocyanidins and their monomerics, including cyanidin, delphinidin

Iridoide: monotropein (0.025%)

Flavonoids: flavonol glycosides, including hyperoside (0.8-1.5%) which is the chief flavonol glycoside, quercitrin-3-beta-D-O-6''galloyl galactoside, quercitrin, isoquercitrin, myricitrin, myricetin-3-O-beta-D-galactoside, 2 isomeric quercetin arabinosides, aglycones of these compounds

Enzymes: including a beta-glucosidase (arbutase), that is rendered inactive with dehydration and processing of the drug, due to the high tannin content

Triterpenes: including among others ursolic acid (0.4-0.8%), alcohol uvaol, beta-amyrin

EFFECTS

The tannins in Uva-ursi act as an astringent, and the phenol glucosides and their aglyca have an antibacterial effect. The antimicrobial effect is associated with the aglycon hydroquinone released from arbutin (transport form) or arbutin waste products in the alkaline urine. The drug has urine-sterilizing properties that are attributed to bacteriostatic hydroquinones, conjugates of glucuronic acid and sulfuric acid.

Based on pharmacological studies, some practitioners recommend that Uva-ursi be used internally and externally as adjuvant treatment of inflammatory conditions, such as contact dermatitis, edema, arthritis, and in hyperpigmentation disorders (Mills & Bone, 2000).

Antimicrobial Effects: The effect of aqueous extracts of Uva-ursi leaves to decrease surface hydrophobicity of 155 *Escherichia coli* strains was determined in cattle. The adhesion of microbes on host cells is important for development of gram-negative microbe-induced infections and is influenced by the surface hydrophobicity of the microbial cell. Bactericidal action of Uva-ursi was low, but the decrease in cell surface hydrophobicity may influence the bacteria's virulent properties (Turi, 1997).

The aqueous extract of Uva-Ursi leaves was also studied in *Helicobacter pylori* strains to determine possible changes in cell surface hydrophobicity. The tannic acid in the Uva-Ursi was determined to have the highest activity of decreasing cell surface hydrophobicity as well as antibacterial activity against H. Pylori (Annuck, 1999)

A decoction of Uva-ursi leaves enhanced cell aggregation of various *Helicobacter pylori* strains, and possessed a remarkable bacteriostatic activity in vitro (Annuk et al, 1999).

Hyperpigmentation Effects: The leaves of Uva-ursi, particularly species *Arctostaphylos patula and A viscida,* can be applied as a whitening agent for the skin. In a study, an ethanol extract of dried leaves of 5 species of Uva-ursi were freeze-dried and lyophilized for the study. All extracts showed strong superoxide dismutase-like activity. No correlation was found between the arbutin content of the extracts and their anti-tyrosinase activity. The authors conclude that Uva-ursi is a promising cosmetic whitening agent because of its potent anti-tyrosinase activity, inhibition of melanin production, superoxide dismutase-like activity, and ability to absorb ultraviolet light (Matsuda et al, 1996).

CLINICAL TRIALS

Cystitis

Uva-ursi (as UVA-E) had a prophylactic effect on recurrent cystitis in a double-blind, prospective, randomized study of 57 women. The patients had suffered at least 3 episodes of cystitis in the year preceding the study and at least 1 episode in the previous 6 months that had been successfully treated with antibiotics. Patients received either 3 tablets of uva-E (containing a hydroalcoholic extract of Uva-ursi leaves with a standardized content of arbutin and methylarbutin, and Dandelion root and leaves) or placebo 3 times daily for 1 month. After 7 and 12 months the patients were examined and during the year any occurrences of cystitis were treated with antibiotics. At the end of the year none of the patients in the Uva-ursi group had had a recurrence of cystitis compared to 23 percent of the placebo group ($p<0.05$). The authors noted that Uva-ursi is not the treatment of choice for acute cystitis but consider it to have a possible prophylactic role in the treatment of recurrent urinary tract infections. This study used a combination product and although the results are likely attributable to the effect of Uva-ursi, this conclusion cannot be stated with certainty (Larsson et al, 1993).

Diuresis

Uva-ursi has a diuretic effect in rats. A single intraperitoneal dose of Uva-ursi (50 mg/kg) was administered to rats with hydrochlorothiazide (10 mg/kg) used as a reference and hypotonic saline used as a control. Immediately after injection, urine was collected and the volume measured hourly for 8 hours and at 24 hours. Urine electrolyte determinations were made at 8 and 24 hours. Uva-ursi caused significant diuresis compared to control from hours 2 through 24 ($p<0.001$ to 0.05). Uva-ursi eliminated 100% of the hypotonic saline solution overload at 5.75 hours compared to 5.33 hours for hydrochlorothiazide. Uva-ursi did not increase sodium or potassium excretion while hydrochlorothiazide had a natriuretic effect ($p<0.001$). The authors conclude that the use of Uva-ursi as a diuretic agent is justified by the study results (Beaux et al, 1999).

INDICATIONS AND USAGE

Approved by Commission E:

- Infections of the urinary tract

Uva-Ursi is used for inflammatory disorders of the efferent urinary tract.

Unproven Uses: In folk medicine, the herb is used for all forms of urogenital and biliary tract disease.

Homeopathic Uses: The herb is used for inflammations of the efferent urinary tract.

CONTRAINDICATIONS

Uva-ursi is not for unsupervised, prolonged use.

Individuals with kidney disorders, irritated digestive disorders, and acidic urine should not take Uva-ursi. It should not be administered with any substances that cause acidic urine since this reduces its antibacterial effect (Blumenthal et al, 2000).

Pregnancy: Not to be used during pregnancy.

Breastfeeding: Not to be used while breastfeeding.

Pediatrics: Not to be used in children under 12.

PRECAUTIONS AND ADVERSE REACTIONS

Individuals with gastric sensitivity may experience nausea, vomiting, and/or stomachache following intake of preparations made from the drug due to its high tannin content.

Hepatic Effects: Liver damage is conceivable in connection with administration of the drug over extended periods, particularly with children, due to the possible hepatotoxicity of the hydroquinones released

DRUG INTERACTIONS

POTENTIAL INTERACTIONS

Iron: The tannin content of Uva-ursi may complex with concomitantly administered iron, resulting in nonabsorbable insoluble complexes and may result in adverse sequelae on blood components. *Clinical Management:* Until more is known, patients who need iron supplementation should be advised to separate administration times of these compounds by 1 to 2 hours.

Thiazide and Loop Diuretics: The sodium sparing effect of Uva-Ursi may offset the diuretic effect of thiazide and loop diuretics. *Clinical Management:* Avoid concomitant use. Uva-Ursi preparations should not be administered with any substance that causes acidic urine since this reduces the antibacterial effect. Because the urine-disinfecting effect of the hydroquinones released in the urinary tract only occurs in an alkali environment, the simultaneous administration of medication or food that increase uric acid levels in the bladder is to be avoided.

OVERDOSAGE

Overdosage can lead to inflammation and irritation of the bladder and urinary tract mucous membranes. Liver damage is conceivable in connection with administration of the drug over extended periods, particularly with children, due to the possible hepatotoxicity of the hydroquinones released.

DOSAGE

Mode of Administration: Uva-Ursi is available as comminuted drug, drug powder, or dried extract for infusions or cold macerations, and also as extracts and solid forms for oral administration. It is also a component of urologic combination and single-component preparations.

How Supplied:

Capsules - 150 mg, 455 mg, 505 mg

Teas

Solutions

Preparation: To make a tea, pour boiling water over 2.5 g finely cut or coarse powdered drug (1 teaspoonful is equivalent to 2.5 g drug.), or place the drug in cold water that is rapidly brought to a boil. The tea should steep (to extract the essence) for 15 minutes and then be strained. Teas may contain up to 30% Uva-Ursi in combination with other drugs. For higher Uva-Ursi content, prepare cold macerate (over 6 to 12 hours) to lower the tannin content.

Daily Dosage: The daily dosage of finely cut or powdered drug is 10 g (corresponding to arbutin content of 400 to 840 mg) or 0.4 g dry extract in a single dose. A single dose of liquid extract is 2 g. Daily dosages of an infusion or cold maceration are 3 g drug to 150 mL water as an infusion or cold maceration up to 4 times a day or 400 to 840 mg hydroquinone derivatives calculated as water-free arbutin. The urine should be alkaline.

Homeopathic Dosage: 5 to 10 drops, 1 tablet, or 5 to 10 globules 1 to 3 times daily or 1 mL injection solution twice weekly sc (HAB1).

Storage: Store in well-sealed containers protected from light.

LITERATURE

Annuk H, Hirmo S, Turi E et al., Effect on cell surface hydrophobicity and susceptibility *of Helicobacter pylori* to medicinal plant extracts. In: *FEMS Microbiol Lett*;172(1):41-5, Mar 1, 1999.

Beaux D, Fleurentin J, Mortier F, Effect of extracts of *Orthosiphon stamineus Benth, Hieracium pilosella L., Sambucus nigra L.* and *Arctostaphylos uva-ursi* (L.) Spreng. in rats. In: *Phytother Res*;13(3):222-5, May 1999.

Britton G, Haslam E, *J Chem Soc* (London): 7312. 1965.

Constantine GH, Cataglomo P, Sheth K et al, Phytochemical investigation of *Arctostaphylos columbiana Piper* and *Arctostaphylos patula Greene* (Ericaceae). In: *J Pharm Sci*; 55:1378-1382, 1966.

Denford KE, *Experientia* 29:939, 1973.

Frohne D, *Planta Med* 18:1, 1970.

Frohne D, Arctostaphylos uva-ursi: Die Bärentraube. In: *Z Phytother* 7:45-47, 1986.

Grases F, Melero G, Costa-Bauza A et al., Urolithiasis and phytotherapy. In: *Int Urol* Nephrol;26(5):507-11, 1994.

Hiller K, Pharmazeutische Bewertung ausgewählter Teedrogen. In: *DAZ* 135(16):1425-1440. 1995.

Ihring M, Blume H, Zur pharmazeutischen Qualität von Phytopharmaka 2. Mitt.: Vergleichende Bewertung von Arbutin enthaltenden Urologika. In: *PZW* 135(6)267. 1990.

Jahodar L et al., *Pharmazie* 33(8):536, 1978.

Jahodar L et al., *Pharmazie* 36(2):294, 1981.

Jahodar L et al., *Cesk Farm.* 34(5):174, 1985.

Kraus L, *DAZ* 111:1225. 1974.

Kubo M et al., Pharmacological studies on leaf of *Arctostaphylos uva-ursi*: Combined effect of 50% methanolic extract from *Arctostaphylos uva-ursi* and prednisolone on immuno-inflammation. In: *Pharmazie*; 33(8):536-7, Aug 1978.

Larsson B, Jonasson A & Pianu S, Prophylactic effect of UVA E in women with recurrent cystitis: A preliminary report. In: *Curr Ther Res Clin Exp*; 53(4):441-443, 1993.

Matsuda H et al., Pharmacological studies on leaf of *Arctostaphylos uva-ursi*: Effect of 50% methanolic extract from Arctostaphylos uva-ursi on melanin synthesis. In: *Yakugaku Zasshi*, 112:276-82, Apr 1992.

Matsuda H et al., Pharmacological studies on leaf of *Arctostaphylos uva-ursi*: Effect of water extract from Arctostaphylos uva-ursi on the antiallergic and anti-inflammatory activities of dexamethasone ointment. In: *Yakugaku Zasshi*, 112:673-7, Sep 1992.

Matsuda H, Higashino M, Nakai Y et al: Studies of cuticle drugs from natural sources IV. Inhibitory effects of some Arctostaphylos plants on melanin biosynthesis. In: *Biol Pharm Bull;* 19(1):153-156, 1996.

Matsuda H, Nakata H, Tanaka T, Kubo M, Phenolic acids in leaves *of Arctostaphylos Uva-ursi L. Vaccinium vitis'idaea L.* and *Vaccinium myrtillus L.* In: *Pharmazie*, 110:680-1, Sep 1991.

Matsuda H, Tanaka T, Kubo M, Pharmacological studies on leaf of *Arctostaphylos uva-ursi* (L.) Spreng. III. Combined effect of arbutin and indomethacin on immuno-inflammation. *Yakugaku Zasshi*, 111:253-8, Apr-May 1991.

Matsuda H, Nakata H, Tanaka T, Kubo M, Pharmacological study on *Arctostaphylos uva-ursi* (L.) Spreng. II. Combined effects of arbutin and prednisolone or dexamethazone on immuno-inflammation. In: *Yakugaku Zasshi,* 110:68-76, Jan 1990.

Matsuo K, Kobayashi M, Takuno Y, Kuwajima H, Ito H, Yoshida T, Anti-tyrosinase activity constituents of *Arctostaphylos uva-ursi. Yakugaku Zasshi,* 117:1028-32, Dec 1997.

Ng TB et al., Examination of coumarins, flavonoids and polysaccharopeptides for antibacterial activity. In: *General Pharmacology* 27(7):1237-1240, 1996.

Paper DH, Koehler J, Franz G, Bioavailalibilty of drug preparations containing a leaf extract of *Arctostaphylos uva-ursi* (Uvae Ursi Folium). In: *PM* 59(7):A589,1993.

Thesen R, Phytotherapeutika-nicht immer harmlos. In: *ZPT* 9(49):105, 1988.

Turi M, Turi E, Koljalg S et al., Influence of aqueous extracts of medicinal plants on surface hydrophobicity of *Escherichia coli* strains of different origin. *APMIS*; 105(12):956-62, Dec 1997.

Uzara

Xysmalobium undulatum

DESCRIPTION

Medicinal Parts: Different varieties are used for drug extraction depending on the area. The drug is therefore easier to categorize according to its definitive active substances (bitters) than to its particular varieties.

Flower and Fruit: The root has a weak and unusual odor. The taste is bitter, followed by a burning sensation after it has been chewed for a long time.

Habitat: South Africa

Production: Uzara root consists of the dried, underground parts of 2- to 3-year-old plants of *Xysmalobium undulatum*.

ACTIONS AND PHARMACOLOGY

COMPOUNDS

Cardioactive steroid glycosides (cardenolides, mixture referred to as uzarone or xysmalobin): including uzarin (5.5%), xysmalorin (1.5%), allo-uzarine, allo-xysmalobin, urezin, uzaroside, ascleposide, glucoascleposide

Pregnane derivatives: delta5-pregnene-3beta-ol-20-one glucoside, 5alpha-pregnane-3beta-ol-20-one glucoside

EFFECTS

Uzara inhibits intestinal motility. In high dosages, it has digitalislike effects on the heart.

INDICATIONS AND USAGE

Approved by Commission E:

- Diarrhea

CONTRAINDICATIONS

Uzara should not be administered concomitantly with other cardioactive glycosides.

PRECAUTIONS AND ADVERSE REACTIONS

General: No health hazards or side effects are known in conjunction with the proper administration of designated therapeutic dosages.

DRUG INTERACTIONS

POTENTIAL INTERACTIONS

Cardioactive Glycosides (Digitoxin, Digoxin): Concurrent use may result in false high serum concentrations of digitoxin and digoxin.

OVERDOSAGE

Because the glycosides are absorbed only with difficulty and because their cardiac effect is minimal, poisonings following oral intake are unlikely, although conceivable. There have been cases of fatalities following parenteral application of Uzara drugs.

DOSAGE

Mode of Administration: The drug is available as ethanol-water extracts in liquid form or as dry extracts for internal use. Pharmaceutical forms include coated tablets, drops, and compound preparations.

Daily Dose: The daily dose should be equivalent to 45 to 90 mg of total glycosides, calculated as uzarin. Follow the manufacturer's dosing instructions.

LITERATURE

Ghorbani M, Kaloga M, Frey HH, Mayer G, Eich E. Phytochemical Reinvestigation of *Xysmalobium undulatum* (Uzara). *Planta Med.* 63 (4); 343-346. 1997

Kannacher M. Uzara - *Xysmalobium undulatum*; Pachycarpus (=Gomphocarpus) schinizianus. *Volksheilkunde* 45; H.12; 22. 1993

Kormann K, Giftpflanzen, Pflanzengifte, 4. Aufl., Ecomed Fachverlag Landsberg Lech 1993.

Pauli G, Schiller H, Asymmetric key position in Uzara steroids. In: PM 62, Abstracts of the 44th Ann Congress of GA, 113. 1996.

Vaccinium macrocarpon

See Cranberry

Vaccinium myrtillus

See Bilberry

Vaccinium uliginosum

See Bog Bilberry

Vaccinium vitis-ideae

See Alpine Cranberry

Valerian

Valeriana officinalis

DESCRIPTION

Medicinal Parts: The medicinal parts are the carefully dried underground parts and the dried roots.

Flower and Fruit: The androgynous, bright, pink-to-white flowers are in panicled cymes. The calyx consists of 10 revolute tips. The corolla is funnel-shaped with a 5-sectioned margin. The tube has a bump at the base. There are 3 stamens. The ovary is inferior and has 3 chambers. The fruit is ovate-oblong, yellow, indehiscent, and has a 10-rayed tuft of white hair.

Leaves, Stem, and Root: The plant is 50 to 100 cm high and has a short, cylindrical rhizome with finger-length, bushy round roots. The stem is erect and unbranched. The leaves are odd-pinnate with 11 to 23 lanceolate, indented-dentate leaflets. The lower ones are petiolate and the upper ones sessile and clasping with a white sheath.

Characteristics: The flowers are fragrant and the rhizome smells strongly when dried. The odor is not present in the fresh plant. Hydrolysis of components in the root form isovaleric acid, which is responsible for the offensive smell.

Habitat: The plant is found in Europe and in the temperate regions of Asia. It is cultivated mainly in central Europe, England, France, Eastern Europe, Japan and the U.S.

Production: Valerian root, consisting of fresh underground plant parts, or parts carefully dried below 40° C of the species *Valeriana officinalis.* Cultivation is possible in low-lying, sandy, humus soil that is well supplied with lime and situated in a damp area. The root is harvested in September. The fresh roots are washed, chopped, and carefully dried in circulating air under 40° C.

Not to be Confused With: Confusion with other species seldom occurs since the plant is primarily supplied via cultivation. The most dangerous adulteration of the plant occurs with the addition of the roots of *Veratrum album.*

Other Names: All-Heal, Amantilla, Capon's Tail, Heliotrope, Setewale, Setwall, Vandal Root

ACTIONS AND PHARMACOLOGY

COMPOUNDS

Iridoids: valepotriates (Valeriana-epoxy-triacylates, iridoide monoterpenes, 0.5-2.0%) chief components (50-80%), isovaltrate (up to 46%), isovaleroxyhydroxy didrovaltrate (IVDH-valtrate, 10-20%), including among others, didrovaltrate, acevaltrate

Volatile oil (0.2-1.0%): chief components (-)-bornyl isovalerenate and isovalerenic acid (both aroma-carriers), including, among others, (-)-bornyl acetate, isoeugenyl valerenate, isoeugenyl isovalerenate, also with some strains valerenal, valeranone, cryptofaurinol

Sesquiterpenes: valerenic acid (0.1-0.9%), 2-hydroxyvalerenic acid, 2-acetoxy-valerenic acid

Pyridine alkaloids (traces, cat pheromone): actinidine, Valerianine, alpha-methylpyrrylketone

Caffeic acid derivatives: chlorogenic acid.

The subspecies within the collective species differ in their constituent substances spectra.

EFFECTS

In animal experiments, the interaction of the various constituents is centrally depressive, sedative, anxiolytic, spasmolytic, muscle relaxing, and anti-ulcerogenic. The pharmacological efficacy is heavily dependent on the quality of the extract used. The main effect in humans is to reduce sleep induction time. In vitro the valerenic acid components have been shown to decrease the degradation of gamma-aminobutyric acid (GABA.) Animal experiments have demonstrated an increase of GABA at the synaptic cleft via inhibition of re-uptake and an increase in secretion of the neurotransmitter. The increase of available GABA is one factor that may be responsible for the sedative properties of Valerian root (Houghton, 1998; Santos et al, 1994) One other mechanism that may contribute to the sedative properties of Valerian could be the high levels of glutamine present in the extract Unlike GABA, glutamine more effectively crosses the blood-brain barrier where it can be taken up by the nerve terminals and converted to GABA (Santos, Fero, 1994)

Sedative Effects: While numerous studies have shown that Valerian extract possesses mild sedative and tranquilizing characteristics, the mechanism of action for this effect has not been clarified. Some constituents may influence the brain GABA metabolism and the properties of the cortical membrane receptors (Andreatini & Leite, 1994).

Spasmolytic Effects: The traditional use of Valerian preparations in gastroenteropathy is probably attributable to its content of valerenic acid, which exerts a spasmolytic effect (Hoelzl, 1996).

CLINICAL TRIALS

Most human clinical trials have been of short duration with a small defined population. This along with the widely varying differences in Valerian preparations has made the evaluation process difficult and not well defined.

Anxiety Disorders

A Cochrane Collaboration review of the effectiveness of Valerian for treating anxiety disorders identified one quality randomized clinical trial for inclusion—a four-week pilot study of Valerian, diazepam, and placebo (n=12 for each group). Based on this limited research, the reviewers write that there is insufficient evidence to draw any conclusions regarding the safety or efficacy of Valerian compared with placebo or diazepam for anxiety disorders (Miyasaka, 2007).

Sleep Quality

A systematic review and meta-analysis of randomized, placebo-controlled trials of extracts of Valerian root for improving the quality of sleep identified 16 eligible studies for inclusion (total of 1,093 patients). While the findings overall indicate that Valerian might improve sleep quality without simultaneously causing side effects, the broad range in dosages used and lack of standardization for Valerian preparations and sleep quality measurement limited the authors' ability to make conclusions (Bent, 2006).

In an earlier study, improvements in sleep quality ratings were demonstrated in a well-constructed, randomized, placebo-controlled, multicenter study involving 121 patients. Subjects were given either 600 mg of a 70% ethanol extract (5:1, n = 61) of Valerian root that was standardized to 0.4 - 0.6% valerenic acid or placebo (n=60) 1 hour before bedtime for 28 consecutive nights. Patients were given 2 standardized sleep questionnaires; one that measured the depression/mood scale and another global clinical impression scale. Sixty-six percent of the Valerian treatment arm rated the therapeutic effect as either good or very good at the end of the 28-day trial. This compared to only a 29% equally positive rating by the placebo participants. (Vorbach, 1996).

Another small preliminary trial reported that Valerian treatment reduced sleep difficulties in children (ages 5 to 14 years) with intellectual and neurologic deficits. In an 8-week, randomized, double-blind, placebo controlled, crossover study (n=5), children with intellectual deficits (IQ<70) and severe sleep difficulties underwent a 2-week baseline measurement period and then were assigned to receive placebo or Valerian (20 mg/kg once daily at least 1 hour prior to assigned bedtime) for 2 weeks. Valerian was from dried and crushed whole root from *Valeriana edulis* plants (1.1.% valtrate/isovaltrate). Following a 7-day washout period, patients crossed over to the other treatment arm for 2 weeks and then underwent another 7-day washout period. Patient sleep patterns and behavior were assessed via a daily diary of 21 questions completed by parents over the 8-week period. As compared to baseline or placebo, Valerian treatment had a significantly better effect on time spent awake during the night (p=0.008), total sleep time (p=0.030), and parent-rated sleep quality (p=0.002). Initial analysis of the data did not find a significant treatment effect for sleep latency; however, post-hoc Least Significant Difference comparisons did show a significant reduction in sleep latency in patients given Valerian as compared to baseline (p=0.05). Additional studies are needed to substantiate these findings (Francis et al, 2002).

INDICATIONS AND USAGE

Approved by Commission E:

- Restless states and difficulties falling asleep caused by nervousness

Unproven Uses: Valerian is used for mental strain, lack of concentration, excitability, stress, headache, neurasthenia, epilepsy, hysteria, nervous cardiopathy, menstrual states of agitation, pregnancy, menopause, neuralgia, fainting, nervous stomach cramps, colic, uterine spasticity, and states of anxiety.

CONTRAINDICATIONS

Hepatotoxic reactions have been reported with Valerian, but causality is uncertain. Monitor patients for signs and symptoms of hepatotoxicity. Avoid use in patients with preexisting liver disease.

PRECAUTIONS AND ADVERSE REACTIONS

In rare cases, gastrointestinal complaints have been reported. Very rarely, contact allergies have occurred.

With long-term administration, the following can occasionally appear: headache, restless states, sleeplessness, mydriasis, disorders of cardiac function.

When large skin injuries or acute skin illnesses, severe feverish or infectious diseases, cardiac insufficiency or hypertonia are present, entire-body baths with the addition of the volatile oil or of extracts from the drug should be avoided.

Pregnancy: Long-term observations in humans have demonstrated no teratogenic or embryotoxic properties (Fachinfo Valdispert 125(R), 1996), but more research is needed.

During pregnancy, Valerian should not be used without medical advice (ABDA-Datenbank, 1996).

Breastfeeding: During lactation, Valerian should not be used without medical advice (ABDA-Datenbank, 1996).

Children: Valerian should not be used in children 14 years of age and younger without medical supervision.

DRUG INTERACTIONS

MAJOR RISK

Hepatotoxic Agents: Concurrent use of Valerian and hepatotoxic drugs or other herbs with the potential to cause hepatotoxicity (including but not limited to chaparral, Russian comfrey, coltsfoot, germander, jin bu huan, kava, pennyroyal, petasites and skullcap) may result in increased risk of hepatotoxicity. *Clinical Management:* Caution is advised if patients take Valerian with other drugs or herbs with potential for hepatotoxicity. Monitor for signs and symptoms of hepatotoxicity.

MODERATE RISK

Alcohol: Concurrent use of Valerian and alcohol may result in increased sedation. *Clinical Management:* Because of the sedative effects associated with Valerian, caution patients against driving or operating machinery following Valerian intake, and to avoid alcohol use.

Barbiturates: Increased central nervous system depressant effects, specifically sedation, may be encountered if Valerian and barbiturates are taken together. *Clinical Management:* Avoid concomitant use of Valerian with barbiturates. If therapy with Valerian and a barbiturate is initiated, monitor patients for signs of excessive central nervous system (CNS) depression.

Benzodiazapines: Valerian intake may result in increased CNS depression or reduced effectiveness of the benzodiazepine. *Clinical Management:* Caution is advised if Valerian and a benzodiazepine are taken concomitantly. Patients should be advised to avoid operating heavy machinery until the magnitude of the interaction is known. Monitor for altered effectiveness of the benzodiazepine.

Iron: The tannin content of Valerian may complex with concomitantly administered iron, possibly resulting in nonabsorable insoluble complexes and decreased iron absorption. *Clinical Management:* Until more is known, patients who need iron supplementation should be advised to separate administration times of these two compounds by one to two hours.

Loperamide: Valerian taken concomitantly with loperamide may result in delirium with symptoms of confusion, agitation, and disorientation. *Clinical Management:* Caution is advised if Valerian and loperamide are taken together. Monitor the patient closely for signs of altered mental status.

Opioid Analgesics: Concurrent use of Valerian and opioid analgesics may result in additive CNS depression. *Clinical Management:* Avoid concomitant use of valerian opioid analgesics. For patients who chose to use the combination despite this advice, monitor closely for sedation, drowsiness, slowed reflexes, and other indicators of CNS depression. Advise against activities that require mental and psychomotor acuity (e.g., handling of heavy machinery).

DOSAGE

Mode of Administration: Valerian is used internally as expressed juice from fresh plants, tincture, extracts, and other galenic preparations. Externally, it is used as a bath additive, though efficacy has not been proved for this indication.

How Supplied:

Capsules - 100 mg, 250 mg, 380 mg, 400 mg, 445 mg, 450 g, 475 mg, 493 mg, 495 mg, 500 mg, 530 mg, 550 mg, 1000 mg

Liquid - 1:1

Tablets - 160 mg, 550 mg

Tea Bags

Preparation: To prepare an infusion, use 2 to 3 g of drug per cup. A tea is prepared by adding 1 teaspoonful (3 to 5 g) of drug to 150 mL of hot water and strain after 10 to 15 minutes. An extract is prepared by mixing 2 parts root powder to 6 parts spirit of wine and 9 parts water. For external use, 100 g of comminuted drug is mixed with 2 liters hot water; this is then added to the bath.

Daily Dosage: The daily dose of Valerian extract ranges from 100 mg to 1800 mg, depending on the manufacturer. Total internal daily dose is 15 g of root powder. For restlessness: 220 mg of extract three times daily. As a sleep aid: 400 mg to 900 mg of extract 30 minutes before bedtime.

External use - As a bath according to preparation instructions above.

Extract - see Daily Dosage listed above.

Infusion - 2 to 3 g (1 teaspoonful) of drug per cup (150 mL), 2 to 3 times daily and before bedtime.

Plant juice - Adults take 1 tablespoonful 3 times daily. Children take 1 teaspoonful 3 times daily.

Tea - 2 to 3 g (1 teaspoonful) of drug per cup (150 mL) 2 to 3 times daily and before bedtime.

Tincture - 1/2 to 1 teaspoonful (1 to 3 mL) one to several times per day.

Tincture (1:5) - 15 to 20 drops in water several times daily.

Storage: Must be kept from sources of light; tinctures and extracts should be stored at room temperature in tightly closed, non-plastic containers.

LITERATURE

ABDA-Datenbank: Valerianae radix monograph. WuV, Eschborn and Micromedex, Inc, 1996.

Abebe W: Herbal medication: potential for adverse effects with analgesic drugs. In: *J Clin Pharm Ther*; 27:391-401, 2002.

Andreatini R & Leite JR: Effect of valepotriates on the behavior of rats in the elevated plus-maze during diazepam withdrawal. In: *Eur J Pharmacol*; 260(2-3):233-235,1994.

Anonym, Phytotherapeutika: Nachgewiesene Wirkung, aber wirksame Stoffe meist nicht bekannt. In: *DAZ* 137(15):1221-1222. 1997.

Banz (Federal German Gazette) No. 90; published May 15, 1985; revised Mar 13, 1990.

Becker H et al., *Planta Med* 49(1):64, 1983.

Bent S, Padula A, Moore D, et al. Valerian for sleep: a systematic review and meta-analysis. *Am J Med.* 119(12)1005-1012. 2006.

Bodesheim U, Hölzl J, Isolation and receptor binding properties of alkaloids and lignans *from Valeriana officinalis L.* in: *PA* 52(5):386-391. 1997.

Bos R et al., *Phytochemistry* 22 (6):1505, 1983.

Bos R et al., Seasonal variation of the essential oil, valerenic acid derivatives, and valepotriates in *Valeriana officinalis* roots. In: *PM* 59(7):A698. 1993.

Bounthanh C et al., *Planta Med* 41:21, 1981.

Bounthanh C et al., *Planta Med* 49:138, 1983.

Bounthanh C, Bergmann C, Beck JP, Haag-Berrurier M, Anton R, Valepotriates, a new class of cytotoxic, antitumor agents. *Planta Med* 41:21-28, 1981.

Braun R et al., *Dtsch Apoth Ztg* 122:1109, 1982.

Braun R et al., *Planta Med* 1, 1984.

Braun R, Dittmar W, Machut M, Weickmann S, Valepotriate mit Epoxidstruktur - beachtliche Alkylantien. *Dtsch Apoth Z* 122:1109-1113, 1982.

Braun R, Dittmar W, von der Hude W, Scheutwinkel-Reich M, Bacterial mutagenicity of the tranquilizing constituents of Valerianaceae roots. Naunyn- Schmiedeberg's Arch Pharmacol Suppl 329:R28, 1985.

Donath F, Roots I, Untersuchung zur Erfassung der Wirkung von Baldrianextrakt (LI 156) auf das Pharmako-EEG bei 16 Probanden. Z Phytother Abstractband, S. 10, 1995.

Eickstedt KW von, *Arzneim Forsch* 19:995, 1969.

Eickstedt KW von, Rahmann R, Psychopharmakologische Wirkungen von Valepotriaten. *Arzneim-Forsch* 19:316-319, 1969.

Fachinformation: Valdispert 125(R), Valerian extract. Duphar Arzneimittel GmbH, Hannover, Germany, 1996.

Francis AJP & Dempster RJW, Effect of Valerian, Valeriana edulis, on sleep difficulties in children with intellectual deficits: randomised trial. *Phytomedicine*; 9:273-279, 2002.

Funk ED, Friedrich H, *Planta Med* 28:215, 1975.

Gross D et al., *Arch Pharm* 304:19, 1971.

Grusla D, Nachweis der Wirkung eines Baldrianextraktes im Rattenhirn mit der 14C-2-Desoxyglucose-Technik. Dissertation, Phillipps-Universität, Marburg, 1987.

Hänsel R, Bewertung von Baldrian-Präparaten: Differenzierung wesentlich: *Dtsch Apoth Z* 124:2085, 1984.

Hänsel R, Pflanzliche Beruhigungsmittel Möglichkeiten und Grenzen der Selbstmedikation. In: *DAZ* 135(32):2935-2943. 1995.

Hänsel R, Pflanzliche Sedativa. In: *ZPT* 11(1):14. 1990.

Hänsel R, Schultz J, *Dtsch Apoth Ztg* 122(5):215, 1982.

Hänsel R, Schulz J, Valerensäuren und Valerenal als Leitstoffe des offizinellen Baldrians. *Dtsch Apoth Z* 122:215-219, 1982.

Hänsel R, Schulz J, Beitrag zur Qulaitätssicherung von Baldrianextrakten. *Pharm Industrie* 47:531-533, 1985.

Hardy M, Kirk-Smith MD, Stretch DD, Replacement of drug treatment for insomnia by ambient odour. *Lancet* 346:701, 1995.

Hazelhoff B, Phytochemical, Pharmacological Aspects of Valeriana compounds. Dissertation, Universität Groningen, 1984.

Hazelhoff B et al., *Pharm Weekbl Sci Ed.* 1:71, 1979.

Hendricks H, Bruins AB, *J Chromatogr* 190:321, 1980.

Hendricks R et al., *Phytochemistry* 16:1853, 1977.

Hendriks H et al., *Planta Med* 42(1):62, 1981.

Hendriks H et al., Central nervous depressant activity of valerenic acid in the mouse. In: *Planta Med* (3):28, 1985.

Hendriks H, Bos R, Woerdenbag HJ, Koster AS, Central Nervous Depressant Activity of Valerenic Acid in the Mouse. *Planta Med* 51:28-31, 1985.

Hiller K-O & Zetler G, Neuropharmacological studies on ethanol extracts of *Valeriana officinalis L*: behavioral and anticonvulsant properties. In: *Phytother Res;* 10:145-151,1996.

Hiller KO, Kato G, Anxiolytic activity of psychotropic plant extracts. I. Test of ethanolic Valeriana extract STEI Val. In: PM 62, Abstracts of the 44th Ann Congress of GA, 65. 1996.

Holzl J, Baldrian - Ein Mittel gegen Schlafstoerungen und Nervositaet. In: *Dtsch Apoth Ztg*; 136(10):17-25,1996.

Holzl J & Godau P, Receptor bindings studies with *Valeriana officinalis* on the benzodiazepine receptor. In: *Planta Med*; 55:642, 1989.

Jansen W, Doppelblindstudie mit Baldrisedon. *Therapiewoche* 27:2779-2786, 1977.

Khawaja IS, Marotta RF & Lippmann S, Herbal medicines as a factor in delirium (letter). In: *Psych Serv;* 50(7):969-970, 1999.

Leuschner J, Mueller J & Rudmann M, Characterization of the central nervous depressant activity of a commercially available Valerian root extract. *Arzneimittelforschung*; 43:638-641, 1993.

Kamm-Kohl AV, Jansen W Brockmann P, Moderne Baldriantherapie gegen nervöse Störungen im Senium. *Med Welt* 35:1450-1454, 1984.

Krieglstein J, Grusla D, Zentraldämpfende Inhaltsstoffe im Baldrian. *Dtsch Apoth Z* 128:2041-2046, 1988.

Kubitschek J, Baldrian beeinflu bt die Melatoninwirkung. In: *PZ* 142(6):433 1997.

Leathwood PD et al., *Pharmacol Biochem Behav* 17:65, 1982.

Leathwood PD, Chauffard F, *J Psychiatr Res* 17(2):115, 1983.

Leathwood PD, Chauffard F, Quantifying the effects of mild sedatives. *J Psychiat Res* 17:115-122, 1983.

Leathwood PD, Chauffard F, Aqueous extract of Valerian reduces latency to fall asleep in man. *Planta Med* 50:144-148, 1984.

MacGregor FB, Abernethy VE, Dahabra S et al., Hepatotoxicity of herbal remedies. In: *BMJ*; 299:1156-1157, 1989.

Meier B, Linnenbrink N, Status und Vergleichbarkeit pflanzlicher Arzneimittel. In: *DAZ* 136(47):4205-4220. 1996.

Miyasaka LS, Atallah AN, Soares BGO. Valerian for anxiety disorders. *Cochrane Database Syst Rev* 4:CD004515, Oct 18, 2006.

Müller-Bohn T, Pflanzliche Sedativa und Antidepressiva. In: *DAZ* 136(24):2032-2033. 1996.

Orth-Wagner S, Ressin WJ, Friedrich I, Phytosedativum gegen Schlafstörungen. In: *ZPT* 16(3):147-156. 1995.

Petkov V: Plants with hypotensive, anti-atheromatous and coronary dilatating action. *In: Am J Chin Med;* 7(3):197-236, 1979.

Popov S et al., *Phytochemistry* 13:2815, 1974.

Reidel E et al., Planta Med 46:219, 1982.

Riedel E, Hänsel R, Ehrke G, Hemmung des Gamma-Aminobuttersäureabbaus durch Valerensäurederivate. *Planta Med* 46:219-220, 1982.

Santos MS, Ferreira F, Cunha AP et al., An Aqueous Extract of Valerian Influences the Transport of GABA in Synaptosomes. *Planta Med* 60:278-279, 1994.

Schilcher H, Pflanzliche Psychopharmaka. Eine neue Klassifizierung nach Indikationsgruppen. In: DAZ 135(20):1811-1822. 1995.

Schimmer O, Röder A, Valerensäuren in Fertigarzneimitteln und selbst bereiteten Auszügen aus der Wurzel von Valeriana officinalis L.s.l. In: *PZW* 137(1):31-36. 1992.

Schulz H, Jobert M, Die Darstellung sedierender/ Tranquilisierender Wirkungen von Phytopharmaka im quantifizierten EEG Z Phytother Abstractband, S. 10, 1995.

Schulz H, Stolz C, Müller J, The effect of a Valerian extract on sleep polygraphy in poor sleepers. A pilot study. *Pharmacopsychiat* 27:147-151, 1994.

Schulz V, Hübner WD, Ploch M, Klinische Studien mit Psycho-Phytopharmaka. In: *ZPT* 18(3):141-154. 1997.

Sprecher E, Pflanzliche Geriatrika. In: *ZPT* 9(2):40. 1988.

Sprecher E, Über die Qualität von Phytopharmaka. In: *ZPT* 12(4):105. 1991.

Thies PW, Funke S, *Tetrahedron Letters* 11:1155, 1966.

Torii S, Fukuda H, Kanemoto H, Miyanchi R, Hamauzu Y, Kawasaki M, Contingent negative variation (CNV), the psychological effects of odour. In: Van Toller St, Dodd GH (eds) Perfumery, The psychology, biology of fragrance. Chapman, Hall, London New York, S 107-146, 1988.

Trossell K, Wahlberg K, *Tetrahedron Letters* 4:445, 1966.

Tyler VE, *The New Honest Herbal. A Sensible Guide to Herbs and Related Remedies*, 2nd ed. Stickley Co., Philadelphia, 125-126, 1987.

Van Meer JH, Labadine RP, *J Chromatogr.* 205(1):206, 1981.

Veith J et al., *Planta Med* (3):179, 1986.

Vorbach EU, Arnold KH, Wirksamkeit und Verträglichkeit von Baldrianextrakt (LI 156) versus Placebo bei behandlungsbedürftigen Insomnien. *Z Phytother Abstractband*, S 11, 1995.

Vorbach EU, Gortelmeyer R & Bruning J, Therapie von Insomnien. Wirksamkeit und Vertraeglichkeit eine Baldrianpraeparats. *Psychopharmakotherapie*; 3:109-115, 1996.

Werner, Arzneipflanzen in der Volksmedizin. In: *DAZ* 130(45):2510. 1990.

Wichtl M, Volksmedizinisch verwendete pflanzliche Arzneimittel. In: *ZPT* 11(3):71. 1990.

Valeriana officinalis

See Valerian

Venus Flytrap

Dionaea muscipula

DESCRIPTION

Medicinal Parts: The entire fresh plant is used medicinally.

Flower and Fruit: The peduncles are leafless, up to 45 cm long with 3 to 10 radial flowers arranged in an umbelliferous raceme. The sepals are fused, and the 5 petals are free and white. There are 15 to 20 stamens and 5 superior carpels. The styles are fused to a column with 5 stigmas on the tip. The fruit is an ovoid capsule, which splits when ripe. The numerous seeds are ovoid, black, and smooth.

Leaves, Stem, and Root: This herbaceous perennial grows up to 45 cm high with leaves that are arranged in a basal rosette. The leaves are 6.5 to 13 cm long, have a cuneiform, broad petiole and an orbicular lamina with 2 sides forming a trap. The leaf sides have 15 to 20 stiff bristles on the edge and 3 sensitive bristles on the surface. The nectar glands are on the periphery and the digestive glands toward the center. When the sensitive bristles are stimulated, the lamina halves snap shut and the bristles on the edge lock together. Digestion of the trapped insect takes approximately 6 days after which the trap slowly opens again. The fully grown plant has only adventitious roots.

Characteristics: The plant is carnivorous.

Habitat: Dionaea muscipula is native to North America.

Production: Venus flytrap herb is the whole fresh, aerial plant of *Dionaea muscipula*, which is harvested shortly before the flowering season and processed immediately.

ACTIONS AND PHARMACOLOGY

COMPOUNDS

Naphthalene derivatives: napthoquinones, including hydroplumbagin-4-O-beta-glucoside, (0.6%), plumbagin (0.2%)

Flavonoids: including quercetin-3-O-galactoside, quercetin-3-O-glucoside, kaempferol-3-O-galactoside, kaempferol-3-O-glucoside

Phenol carboxylic acids: glucosides of gallic acid, ellagic acid, 3-O-methyl-ellagic acid and 3,3-dimethyl ellagic acid

Enzymes (in the secretions of the digestive glands): proteases, phosphatases, nucleases

EFFECTS

The pressed fresh plant (chief active ingredient plumbagin) is immunostimulating, antineoplastic, and spasmogenic due to the lysophosphatidinic acid component.

INDICATIONS AND USAGE

Unproven Uses: The drug extracted from the plant is used chiefly in the treatment of malignant conditions such as tumors in advanced stages (mammary carcinoma, bladder carcinoma, prostate carcinoma, and osteosarcoma) and also for hematological systemic conditions (such as Hodgkin and non-Hodgkin lymphoma) as well as solid tumors.

PRECAUTIONS AND ADVERSE REACTIONS

Parenteral administration of medicinal preparations made from the fresh plant led to elevated body temperature, chills, and circulatory damage. Circulatory collapse, possibly as a result of contamination with endotoxins, is possible. Skin contact with the fresh plant may cause irritation.

DOSAGE

Mode of Administration: Preparations of the pressed juice have been administered orally, by inhalation and parenterally.

How Supplied: Availability of the pressed juice of the fresh plant in two commercial preparations was halted in 1986.

Daily Dosage: Juice from the fresh plant used orally and as an inhalant: 50 to 60 drops 5 times daily p.o.; 25 drops with 1 ml physiological NaCl in a cold atomizer. Injection solution: initial dose is 2 mL ampule daily for 14 days. Maintenance dose: 1 ampule every second to third day I.M.

LITERATURE

Blaschek W, Hänsel R, Keller K, Reichling J, Rimpler G, Schneider G (Eds), Hagers Handbuch der Pharmazeutischen Praxis. Folgebände 1 und 2. Drogen A-Z. Springer. Berlin, Heidelberg 1998.

Veratrum album

See White Hellebore

Veratrum luteum

See False Unicorn Root

Veratrum viride

See American Hellebore

Verbascum densiflorum

See Mullein

Verbena officinalis

See Vervain

Veronica beccabunga

See Brooklime

Veronica officinalis

See Speedwell

Vervain

Verbena officinalis

DESCRIPTION

Medicinal Parts: The medicinal parts are the dried aerial parts collected during the flowering season, the fresh, flowering herb, the flowers and the whole fresh plant.

Flower and Fruit: The small flowers are pale lilac and arranged in thin, paniculate spikes. The calyx is fused to a short, 5-tipped tube. The corolla has a 5-tipped, bent tube, and a bilabiate margin. The mouth of the tube is closed by crosshairs. There are 4 stamens and 1 ovary, which breaks up into four single-seeded mericarps. These are oblong-cylindrical, 1.5 to 2 mm long, warty on the inside, reticulately grooved and light brown on the outside. The seeds are grooved on the inside and have very little endosperm.

Leaves, Stem, and Root: The true variety is an annual or biennial to perennial with a fusiform, branched, whitish root. The stem is erect, rigid, quadrangular, and branched above. The leaves are opposite, dull green, ovate-oblong, and have a short broad petiole. They are deeply divided in 3 with notched, crenate tips. They are wrinkled and roughly bristled.

Habitat: The plant is probably indigenous to the Mediterranean region. It is cultivated worldwide, but mainly in eastern Europe.

Production: Verbena herb consists of the above-ground parts of *Verbena officinalis*. The herb is predominantly cultivated in eastern Europe. It is collected in the wild and harvested in southeastern Europe. After being cut, the drug is hung in bunches to dry.

Note: Improper drying leads to hydrolytic decomposition of verbenalin.

Not to be Confused With: Lippiae triphyllae folium

Other Names: Enchanter's Plant, Herb of Grace, Herb of the Cross, Juno's Tears, Pigeon's Grass, Pigeonweed, Simpler's Joy

ACTIONS AND PHARMACOLOGY

COMPOUNDS

Iridoide monoterpenes (0.2-0.5%): including among others verbenalin (cornin, 0.15%), hastatoside (0.08%), dihydroverbenalin (0.01%)

Flavonoids: including among others luteolin, scutellarin and 6-hydroxy-luteolin glycosides, artemitin, sorbifolin, pedalitin, nepetin (eupafolin)

Caffeic acid derivatives: verbascoside 0.8%), eucovoside, artynoside

EFFECTS

The amaroidlike affect of the iridoid glycosides explains its use as an astringent. The drug is weakly antiedemic, analgesic, cytotoxic, and antitumoral. The verbenalin has antitussive, secretolytic, and lactation-promoting properties.

INDICATIONS AND USAGE

Unproven Uses: Preparations of Vervain are used for diseases and ailments of the oral and pharyngeal mucosa, such as sore throat, and for diseases of the respiratory tract, such as coughs, asthma, and whooping cough. In addition, the drug is used internally for pain, cramps, fatigue, nervous disorders, and digestive disorders. The drug is used externally as a gargle for cold symptoms and for diseases of the oral and pharyngeal cavity.

Vervain is also used for antipruritic treatment of skin diseases and minor topical burns (in France) and for arthritis, rheumatism, dislocations, and contusions.

Chinese Medicine: The herb is used for edema, chronic malaria, dysmenorrhea, and carbuncles.

Homeopathic Uses: The herb is used for bruising and cerebral convulsions.

CONTRAINDICATIONS

Vervain should not be used during pregnancy.

PRECAUTIONS AND ADVERSE REACTIONS

No health hazards or side effects are known in conjunction with the proper administration of designated therapeutic dosages.

DOSAGE

Mode of Administration: Vervain is available as whole, cut and powdered drug for internal and external use.

Preparation: The ratio for the liquid extract is 1:1 in 25% ethanol; the tincture should be mixed with 40% ethanol. An infusion is prepared by adding 5 to 20 g drug to 1 liter water.

Daily Dosage: For the liquid extract, take 2 to 4 mL daily. For the tincture, take 5 to 10 mL up to 3 times per day. For the infusion, take 2 to 4 g up to 3 times per day.

Chinese Medicine Dosage: The daily dose is 4.5 to 9 g of the drug.

Homeopathic Dosage: 5 to 10 drops, 1 tablet, or 5 to 10 globules 1 to 3 times daily; parenterally: 1 mL injection solution sc twice weekly (HAB34).

Storage: Vervain must be stored in a dry environment to avoid hydrolytic decomposition of verbenalin.

LITERATURE

Carnat A, Carnat AP, Chavignon O, Heitz A, Wylde R, Lamaison JL. Luteolin-7-Diglucuronide, the Major Flavonoid from *Aloysia triphylla* and *Verbena officinalis*. *Planta Med.* 61 (5); 490. 1995.

Ernst E, März R, Sieder C. A controlled multi-centre study of herbal versus synthetic secretolytic drugs for acute bronchitis. *Phytomedicine* 4 (4); 287-293. 1997

McIlroy RJ, In: The Plant Glycosides, Arnold, London 1951.

Pozo MD et al. Allergic contact dermatitis from *Verbena officinalis L.* Contact Dermatitis 31; 200-201. 1994.

Reynaud J et al., Pharm Acta Helv 67:216. 1992.

Weber R, Dissertation Marburg. 1995.

Yip L, Pei S, Hudson JB, Towers GHN, Screening of medicinal plants from Yunnan Province in southwest China for antiviral activity. In: *ETH* 34:1-6. 1991.

Viburnum prunifolium

See Black Haw

Vicia faba

See Broad Bean

Vinca minor

See Periwinkle

Viola odorata

See Sweet Violet

Viola tricolor

See Heartsease

Virola

Virola theiodora

DESCRIPTION

Medicinal Parts: The medicinal part of the plant is the bark.

Flower and Fruit: The flowers are in panicles. The male inflorescence has numerous flowers and is brown, gold-yellow, and pubescent. The female flowers are either single or in clusters of 2 to 10 flowers. They are fused and have 3 to 5 stamens. The ovary develops from only 1 carpel with 1 ovule. The fruit is orbicular-oval, 10 to 20 mm long, and 8 to 15 mm wide.

Leaves, Stem, and Root: Virola theiodora is a diclinous tree that grows up to 23 m high. The leaves are alternate, 9 to 35 cm long, and 4 to 12 cm wide; the lamina is simple, elongate to wide-oval, acute, entire, and paperlike. The trunk is approximately 0.5 m thick and cylindrical with a smooth, brown-speckled bark with gray spots.

Characteristics: The flowers have sharply astringent fragrance.

Habitat: Amazon region

Production: Virola bark is the dried bark of *Virola theiodora.*

There are various methods of production. Either the bark is scraped off, dried over a fire, and powdered, or the outer bark is peeled off before sunrise and the inner bark with the resin is scraped off and cooked to a syrup. The syrup is pulverized after drying in the sun.

ACTIONS AND PHARMACOLOGY

COMPOUNDS

Tryptamine derivatives: particularly N,N-dimethyl tryptamine, 5-methoxy-NN-dimethyl tryptamine (5-MeO-DMT)

EFFECTS

Due to its psychotropic and narcotic-hallucinogenic characteristics (tryptamine alkaloids), the drug is chiefly used in the form of a snuff powder in connection with ritual and religious ceremonies. The resin is also administered topically to yeast infections of the skin and for the promotion of the healing of wounds.

INDICATIONS AND USAGE

Unproven Uses: Virola is used for skin disease and fungal skin diseases, to speed the healing of wounds, and to clean infected wounds (South America).

PRECAUTIONS AND ADVERSE REACTIONS

The drug is not used as a medication. The drug has a psychomimetic effect when administered through the nasal mucous membrane.

OVERDOSAGE

Signs of poisoning include nausea, increased irritability, numbness in the limbs, coordination disorders, and hallucinations. The tryptamine derivatives are resorbed only to a very limited extent following oral administration.

DOSAGE

Preparation: There is no information in the literature.

LITERATURE

de Smet PA, A multidisciplinary overview of intoxicating snuff rituals in the Western Hemisphere. *J Ethnopharmacol*, 13:3-49, Mar. 1985

Hänsel R, Keller K, Rimpler H, Schneider G (Ed), Hagers Handbuch der Pharmazeutischen Praxis, 5. Aufl., Bde 4 - 6 (Drogen), Springer Verlag Berlin, Heidelberg, New York, 1992-1994.

MacRae WD, Towers GH, *Justicia pectoralis*: a study of the basis for its use as a hallucinogenic snuff ingredient. *J Ethnopharmacol*, 12:93-111, Oct. 1984

MacRae WD, Towers GH, Phytochemical investigation of *Virola peruviana*, a new hallucinogenic plant. *J Pharm Sci,* 12:1561-3, Sep. 1973

McKenna DJ, Towers GH, Abbott FS, Alkaloids in certain species of Virola and other South American plants of ethnopharmacologic interest. *Acta Chem Scand*, 12:903-16, 1969.

McKenna DJ, Towers GH, Abbott FS, Monoamine oxidase inhibitors in South American hallucinogenic plants. Part 2: Constituents of orally active Myristicaceous hallucinogens. *J Ethnopharmacol*, 12:179-211, Nov. 1984

Plotkin MJ, Schultes RE, Virola: a promising genus for ethnopharmacological investigation. *J Psychoactive Drugs,* 22:357-61, Jul-Sep. 1990

Virola theiodora

See Virola

Viscum album

See European Mistletoe

Vitex agnus-castus

See Chaste Tree

Vitis vinifera

See Grape

Wafer Ash

Ptelea trifoliata

DESCRIPTION

Medicinal Parts: The medicinal parts are the leaves, the young bark, and the root bark. The plant is also used in homeopathic medicine.

Flower and Fruit: The small, greenish-white flowers are in loose, terminal cymes and are dioecious. The 4- to 5-sepaled calyx and the 4 to 5 petals are downy on the outside. There are 4 to 5 stamens whose filaments are hairy at the base. The compressed ovary has a short style and stigma, which is divided in two. The fruit is circular and winged with a broad, greenish-white, later ochre-colored margin.

Leaves, Stem, and Root: The plant is a bush or small tree up to 4 m high with glabrous, smooth, dark or red-brown branches. The younger branches, leaves and petioles are downy. The large leaves have 3 lobes, are lanceolate, entire, dark green above, lighter beneath, and covered with numerous fine glandular spots.

Characteristics: The flowers are pleasantly perfumed and the fruit is bitter-tangy.

Habitat: The plant is indigenous to Eastern North America and is cultivated in Europe as an ornamental bush.

Production: Wafer Ash is the root-bark of *Ptelea trifoliata.*

Other Names: Pickaway Anise, Prairie Grub, Scubby Trefoil, Stinking Prairie Bush, Swamp Dogwood, Three-Leafed Hop Tree, Wingseed

ACTIONS AND PHARMACOLOGY

COMPOUNDS

Furoquinoline alkaloids: including kokusaginine, skimmianine (beta-fagarine), ptelein, dictamnine, and maculosidine

Furanocoumarins: including isopimpinellin, marmesin, and phellopterin

EFFECTS

Wafer Ash is antimicrobial. The alkaloid content acts against microbes; pteleatinium chloride acts against *mycobacterium tuberculosis* and yeast fungus.

INDICATIONS AND USAGE

Unproven Uses: Wafer Ash is used for stomach complaints, gallstones, and rheumatism. Its root bark is used as a tonic.

PRECAUTIONS AND ADVERSE REACTIONS

No health hazards or side effects are known in conjunction with the proper administration of designated therapeutic dosages. The plant could trigger phototoxicosis through skin contact, possibly also through internal ingestion of larger quantities.

DOSAGE

Mode of Administration: Wafer Ash is available as an extract.

LITERATURE

Kern W, List PH, Hörhammer L (Hrsg.), Hagers Handbuch der Pharmazeutischen Praxis, 4. Aufl., Bde. 1-8, Springer Verlag Berlin, Heidelberg, New York, 1969.

Neville CF, Reisch J. Biosynthesis of Quinoline Alkaloids of *Ptelea trifoliata. Arch Pharm* (Weinheim) 320; 977. 1987

Petit-Paly G, Montagu M, Merienne C, Ambrose JD, Rideau M, Viel C, Chenieux JC. New Alkaloids from *Ptelea trifoliata. Planta Med.* 55; 209-210. 1989

Roth L, Daunderer M, Kormann K, Giftpflanzen, Pflanzengifte, 4. Aufl., Ecomed Fachverlag Landsberg Lech 1993.

Wahoo

Euonymus species

DESCRIPTION

Medicinal Parts: The medicinal parts are the trunk, root bark, and the fruit.

Flower and Fruit: The flowers are yellowish-green, small, and flat in double cymes with few blossoms. There are 4 sepals, 4 petals, 4 stamens, and 4 styles on a glandular disc, which surrounds the ovary. The fruit is a 4-lobed, obtuse, pink capsule, which bursts open at the tip showing the seeds covered in an orange-yellow skin.

Leaves, Stem, and Root: The plant is an unwieldy shrub up to 3 m high with green rectangular young branches. The older branches are light gray. The leaves are opposite, oblong-lanceolate or elliptical, acuminate, finely serrate, and glabrous.

Characteristics: The seeds are poisonous.

Habitat: The plant grows in the Eastern and Central U.S. and Canada.

Production: Wahoo root bark is the bark of the root and young branches of *Euonymus atropurpureus*. Wahoo fruit is the fruit of *Euonymus europaeus*.

Other Names: Burning Bush, Fusanum, Fusoria, Gadrose, Gatten, Gatter, Indian Arrowroot, Pigwood, Prickwood, Skewerwood, Spindle Tree

ACTIONS AND PHARMACOLOGY

COMPOUNDS: WAHOO ROOT BARK (EUONYMUS ATROPURPUREUS)

Cardioactive steroids (cardenolides) in the root: including euatroside, euatromonoside

COMPOUNDS: WAHOOO FRUIT (EUONYMUS EUROPAEUS)

Cardioactive steroids (cardenolides) in the seeds: including evonoside, evobioside, evomonoside, evolonoside, glucoevonoloside, glucoevonogenin

Alkaloids: polyester from a sesquiterpene polyol with pyrridine carbon acids (for example, evonine)

Peptide alkaloids: including frangula amine, franganin, frangufolin

1-benzyl-tetrahydro-isoquinoline alkaloids

Purine alkaloids: caffeine, theobromine

EFFECTS: WAHOO ROOT BARK AND FRUIT

The drug is reported to be a laxative and a choleretic. Larger doses have an effect on the heart.

INDICATIONS AND USAGE

Unproven Uses: In the past, the drug was used as a cholagogue, laxative, diuretic, and tonic, and for dyspepsia. Today, it is used in homeopathy.

PRECAUTIONS AND ADVERSE REACTIONS

Poisonings caused by the berries have been recorded. A fatal dose of *Euonymus europaeus* is said to be 36 berries. After a latency period of several hours, intestinal colic, severe, sometimes bloody diarrhea, elevation of body temperature, shortness of breath, and circulatory disorders with signs of collapse occur. Often there is elevation of cerebrospinal pressure with increasing stupor that may progress unconsciousness. The first measures to be taken with poisonings are gastric lavage, intestinal emptying, the instillation of activated charcoal, and shock prophylaxis (which includes quiet, heat and the possible administration of a plasma volume expander). All other measures depend on the symptoms. For loss of potassium, careful replenishment of potassium should be undertaken. Lidocaine can be administered for ventricular extrasystole; atropine for partial atrioventricular block. For elimination of the glycosides hemoperfusion is possible, as is the administration of cholestyramine to interrupt enterohepatic circulation. Intubation and oxygen respiration may also be necessary in cases of asphyxiation.

DOSAGE

Mode of Administration: Wahoo root bark and fruit are not recommended for use, as the drug is considered too dangerous.

LITERATURE

Gazzinelli RT, Romanha AJ, Fontes G, Chiari E, Gazzinelli G, Brenner Z, Distribution of carbohydrates recognized by the lectins

Euonymus europaeus and concanavalin A in monoxenic and heteroxenic trypanosomatids. *J Protozool*, 38:320-5, Jul-Aug, 1991.

Nickrent DL, Franchina CR, Phylogenetic relationships of the Santalales and relatives. J Mol Evol, 26:294-301. Oct, 1990.

Roussel F, Dalion J, Wissocq JC, Cytotoxic cardenolides from woods of *Euonymus alata*. Chem Pharm Bull (Tokyo), 26:615-7. Mar, 1996.

Roussel F, Dalion J, Wissocq JC, *Euonymus europaeus* lectin as an endothelial and epithelial marker in canine tissues. Lab Anim, 26:114-21. Apr, 1992.

Roussel F, Dalion J, Wissocq JC, Lectin binding defines and differentiates M-cells in mouse small intestine and caecum. *Histochem Cell Biol*, 26:161-8. Aug, 1995

Roussel F, Dalion J, Wissocq JC, Occupational wood-dust sensitivity from *Euonymus europaeus* (spindle tree) and investigation of cross reactivity between *E.e.* wood and *Artemisia vulgaris* pollen (mugwort). *Allergy*, 26:186-90. Apr, 1991.

Wallflower

Cheiranthus cheiri

DESCRIPTION

Medicinal Parts: The medicinal parts are the dried flowers, the dried ripe seeds, and the fresh aerial parts of the erect plant before flowering.

Flower and Fruit: The flowers are golden yellow to orange-yellow in dense racemes on 10 to 14 cm long, pubescent, erect stems. The sepals are 9 to 11 mm long, linear-lanceolate, with a membranous border. The stigma is curled back. The fruit is a pod, which has no beak but has distinct ribs. The seeds are arranged in 1 row, are 3 mm long, oblong, narrowly winged, and light brown.

Leaves, Stem, and Root: The plant grows from about 30 to 70 cm. The stems are woody below and shrublike, with gray-appressed hairs and thick foliage above. The leaves are lanceolate with revolute tip, short-petioled, entire-margined, and hairy.

Characteristics: The plant has a pleasant fragrance.

Habitat: The plant is probably only indigenous to the eastern Mediterranean region, but is cultivated today in Europe, northern Africa, western Asia, Japan, and New Zealand.

Production: Wallflower can be obtained from commercial growers (cultivated regions).

Other Names: Beeflower, Gillyflower, Giroflier, Handflower, Keiri, Wallstock-Gillofer,

ACTIONS AND PHARMACOLOGY

COMPOUNDS

Cardioactive steroid glycosides (cardenolids): in particularly high concentration in the seeds (0.5%), including cheirotoxin, erysimoside, glucoerysimoside, and cheiroside A

Glucosinolates: glucocheiroline, glucoiberin, which yield the isothiocyanates cheiroline and iberin

Fatty oil (in the seeds)

EFFECTS

The drug has cardiac effects similar to digitaloid drugs, due to the cardenolide glycosides. Its application for constipation is plausible because of the inhibition of Na^+ and H_2O absorption and the stimulating effect on the smooth muscles of the gastrointestinal tract.

INDICATIONS AND USAGE

Unproven Uses: Wallflower is used for cardiac insufficiency, as a laxative, and to encourage menstruation.

Homeopathic Uses: The herb is used for wisdom tooth pain.

PRECAUTIONS AND ADVERSE REACTIONS

No health hazards or side effects are known in conjunction with the proper administration of designated therapeutic dosages.

OVERDOSAGE

For possible symptoms of overdose and treatment of poisonings see *Digitalis folium*. Despite the strong efficacy of the drug's cardioactive steroid glycosides in parenteral application, serious poisoning is not expected due to the presumably low resorption rate following oral administration.

DOSAGE

Mode of Administration: Wallflower is used internally in drops and an infusion as well as in some combination preparations.

Preparation: To make an infusion from the flowers, mix 2 to 3 g of drug per 100 mL of water.

Daily Dosage: Drink 3 to 4 cups of the infusion daily.

LITERATURE

Hänsel R, Keller K, Rimpler H, Schneider G (Hrsg.), Hagers Handbuch der Pharmazeutischen Praxis, 5. Aufl., Bde 4-6 (Drogen): Springer Verlag Berlin, Heidelberg, New York, 1992-1994.

Kumar P, Dixit VP, Khanna P. Antifertility Studies of Kaempferol: Isolation and Identification from Tissue Culture of Some Medicinally Important Plant Species. *Plant med et phyt.* 23; 193-201. 1989

Madaus G, Lehrbuch der Biologischen Arzneimittel, Bde 1-3, Nachdruck, Georg Olms Verlag Hildesheim 1979.

Roth L, Daunderer M, Kormann K, Giftpflanzen, Pflanzengifte, 4. Aufl., Ecomed Fachverlag Landsberg Lech 1993.

Teuscher E, Lindequist U, Biogene Gifte - Biologie, Chemie, Pharmakologie, 2. Aufl., Fischer Verlag Stuttgart 1994.

Walnut

Juglans regia

DESCRIPTION

Medicinal Parts: The medicinal parts are the feathery leaflets without the rachis and the green fruit shells.

Flower and Fruit: The flowers are green and appear before the leaves. They are monoecious. The male flowers are 10 cm long, sessile, globular-cylindrical, limp, hanging catkins. The female flowers are in groups of 1 to 3 at the tip of annual growth. They are greenish with a glandular pubescent calyx and 2 large, curved, warty, reddish stigmas. The fruit is globular or oblong-globular with a smooth, green, white-spotted outer shell and a wooden, wrinkled inner shell.

Leaves, Stem, and Root: The plant grows to 25 m and has a broad, loose-branched crown. The bark is smooth and ash gray at first; later dark and fissured. The leaves are large, long petioled, odd-pinnate with 7 to 9 oblong or ovate, entire-margined leaflets. The leaflets are spotted with glands when young. The terminal leaflet is the largest and is petiolate.

Characteristics: The leaves are aromatic when rubbed. The taste is bitter.

Habitat: The walnut is indigenous to the Middle East and Iran. Today, it is cultivated in many regions.

Production: Walnut leaf consists of the dried leaf of *Juglans regia.*

Other Names: Caucasian Walnut, Circassian Walnut, English Walnut, Persian Walnut

ACTIONS AND PHARMACOLOGY

COMPOUNDS

Tannins (galloylglucose, ellagitannins)

Naphthalene derivatives: The fresh leaves and the fruit peels contain 1,4,5- trihydroxynaphthalene-4-beta-D-glucoside, which is transformed into juglone through bruising or drying. Juglone polymerizes readily into yellow or brown products (that stain the skin), so there can be hardly any juglone present in the drug itself.

Flavonoids: including, among others, hyperoside, quercitrin

EFFECTS

Walnut is astringent and fungistatic. The juglone content in the walnut hulls has been linked to mutagenic action. The topical use of walnut hulls has been linked to cancer of the tongue and leukoplakia of the lips. The main active principles are the tannins and juglone. There is an astringent effect because of the tannins. The antifungal effect comes from the juglone content and the essential oil.

INDICATIONS AND USAGE

Approved by Commission E:

- Inflammation of the skin
- Excessive perspiration

Externally, Walnut is used for mild, superficial inflammation of the skin and excessive perspiration.

Unproven Uses: Internally, the drug is used for gastrointestinal catarrh and as a blood purifier.

Chinese Medicine: In China, Walnut is used to treat asthma, lumbago, beriberi, impotence, and constipation.

Indian Medicine: In India, Walnut is used for alternating rheumatic complaints, and the oil of the seeds is used for tapeworms. The seeds are said to have an aphrodisiac effect and are also used for dysentery and colic.

PRECAUTIONS AND ADVERSE REACTIONS

No health hazards or side effects are known in conjunction with the proper administration of designated therapeutic dosages.

DOSAGE

Mode of Administration: Comminuted drug for decoctions and other galenic preparations for external use.

Preparation: To prepare a decoction, soak 2 teaspoonfuls of drug in 1 cup of water, boil and strain. An infusion is prepared by using 1.5 g of finely cut drug, soaked in cold water, brought to simmer and strained after 3 to 5 minutes.

Daily Dosage: The average daily dose for external use is 3 to 6 g of drug.

LITERATURE

Carnat A, Petitjean-Freytet C, Muller D, Lamaison JL. Teneurs en principaux constituants de la Feuille de Noyer *Juglans regia L. Plant med et phyt.* 26; 332-339. 1993

Hasler A, Meier B, Sticher O. Quantitative HPLC Analysis of Flavonoid Aglycones in Different Medicinal Plants. *Planta Med.* 56; 575-576. 1990

Özürk Y, Aydin S, Arslan R, Baser KHC, Kurtar-Öztürk N. Thyroid Hormone enhancing Activity of the Fruits of *Juglans regia L.* in Mice. *Phytother Res.* 8 (5); 308-310. 1994

Willuhn G, Pflanzliche Dermatika. Eine kritische Übersicht. In: *DAZ* 132(37):1873. 1992.

Water Avens

Geum rivale

DESCRIPTION

Medicinal Parts: The medicinal parts are the dried, underground parts of the plant, the fresh, flowering plant, and the roots.

Flower and Fruit: The flowering peduncle usually sprouts singly from the axils of the rosette leaves. It is often tinged red-brown and is downy. The flowers and subinflorescences are on long, dense, and glandular-haired pedicles. The 5 sepals are red-brown. The 5 petals are pale yellow and tinged dirty pink. The flower remains attached long after flowering. The carpel axis is stemmed and villous, and stretches when mature. The fruit is hooked at the tip.

Leaves, Stem, and Root: The plant is a 30 to 100 cm high semirosette shrub with adventitious roots. The rhizome is simple, thick, cylindrical, and crooked with a terminal rosette. The rosette leaves are long-petioled, irregularly lyre-shaped, and pinnate. The upper surface is glandular and hairy. The underside is heavily ciliated along the veins.

Habitat: The plant is found in Europe, temperate Asia and North America.

Production: Water Avens root is the root of *Geum rivale*.

Other Names: Chocolate Root, Cure All, Drooping Avens, Indian Chocolate, Nodding Avens, Purple Avens, Throat Root, Water Chisch, Water Flower

ACTIONS AND PHARMACOLOGY

COMPOUNDS: IN THE FRESHLY HARVESTED RHIZOME

Gein (eugenol vicianoside): transformed into eugenol through drying or cutting into small pieces

Tannins

COMPOUNDS: IN THE DRIED RHIZOME AND ROOT

Volatile oil (traces): chief component eugenol

Tannins (15-20%)

EFFECTS

See Geum urbanum; overall, Water Avens has very weak action.

INDICATIONS AND USAGE

Unproven Uses: Uses are the same as for Geum urbanum.

PRECAUTIONS AND ADVERSE REACTIONS

Health risks or side effects following the proper administration of designated therapeutic dosages are not recorded.

DOSAGE

No information is available.

LITERATURE

Hänsel R, Keller K, Rimpler H, Schneider G (Hrsg.), Hagers Handbuch der Pharmazeutischen Praxis, 5. Aufl., Bde 4-6 (Drogen). Springer Verlag Berlin, Heidelberg, New York, 1992-1994.

Madaus G, Lehrbuch der Biologischen Arzneimittel, Bde 1-3, Nachdruck, Georg Olms Verlag Hildesheim 1979.

Water Dock

Rumex aquaticus

DESCRIPTION

Medicinal Parts: The medicinal parts are the dried roots.

Flower and Fruit: The inflorescence is a large, dense panicle. The pedicles are filiform and up to 2.5 times as long as the capsules. The capsules are 6 to 8 mm long, ovate-triangular, fairly acute, elongated, and entire-margined.

Leaves, Stem, and Root: The herb is perennial and has an erect 100 to 200 cm high stem. The leaves are 7.5 to 10 cm wide with curly margins. The basal leaves are triangular, acute, deeply cordate at the base, and 1.5 to 2.5 times as long as they are wide. The petiole is at least as long as the leaf blade. The rhizome is dark brown to blackish on the outside and porous.

Habitat: The plant is common in Europe.

Production: The root material is sliced and then dried in the shade.

ACTIONS AND PHARMACOLOGY

COMPOUNDS

Oxalates: oxalic acid, calcium oxalate

Tannins

Anthracene derivatives: including anthranoids

EFFECTS

The active agents are quercitrin, protein, fat, starch, essential oil and tannin. The herb acts as an aid to digestion.

INDICATIONS AND USAGE

Unproven Uses: Water Dock is used for blood purification and constipation.

PRECAUTIONS AND ADVERSE REACTIONS

No health hazards or side effects are known in conjunction with the proper administration of designated therapeutic dosages.

OVERDOSAGE

Oxalate poisonings are conceivable, but only with the consumption of very large quantities of the leaves.

DOSAGE

Mode of Administration: The drug is used internally and externally as a liquid extract or as a powder. Use of the herb went out of favor during the 18th century.

LITERATURE

Kern W, List PH, Hörhammer L (Hrsg.), Hagers Handbuch der Pharmazeutischen Praxis, 4. Aufl., Bde. 1-8: Springer Verlag Berlin, Heidelberg, New York, 1969.

Sharma M et al., *Indian J Chem Sect B* 15B:544. 1977.

Water Dropwort

Oenanthe crocata

DESCRIPTION

Medicinal Parts: The medicinal part is the rhizome.

Flower and Fruit: The flowers are in terminal umbels. The flowering shoots are longer than the 10 to 40 pedicled rays, which do not thicken in the fruiting phase. The cylindrical fruit is 4 to 6 mm long.

Leaves, Stem, and Root: The plant is a branched, stout perennial up to 150 cm high. The roots are fleshy and pale yellow. They have obovoid or ellipsoid tubers close to where they attach to the stem. The stems are hollow, striate, and grooved. The basal leaves are 3- to 4-pinnate. The lobes of the basal leaves are ovate to suborbicular, cuneate at base. The lobed, crenate, cauline leaves are 2- to 3-pinnate and almost sessile. The lobes of the cauline leaves are ovate to linear, and the segments are closer and sharper than the basal leaves.

Characteristics: The plant is extremely poisonous.

Habitat: The plant grows around ditches and ponds in the U.S., and parts of Europe, excluding Scandinavia, Holland, Germany, Russia, Turkey, and Greece.

Production: Water Dropwort is the root of *Oenanthe crocata*, which is collected in the wild.

Other Names: Dead Men's Fingers, Dead Tongue, Five-Fingered Root, Hemlock Water Dropwort, Horsebane, Water Lovage

ACTIONS AND PHARMACOLOGY

COMPOUNDS

Polyynes: including among others the highly toxic oenanthotoxin as well as oenanthetol, oenanthetone, dihydrooenanthotoxin

EFFECTS

The pharmacologically active substances of the root drug are the toxic oenanthotoxin and the less toxic polyacetylenes oenanthetol and oenantheton. Oenanthotoxin caused an irreversible inhibition of loading transfer and sodium inflow at the nerve fibers of frogs.

INDICATIONS AND USAGE

Homeopathic Uses: Homeopathic uses include epilepsy and cerebral convulsions.

PRECAUTIONS AND ADVERSE REACTIONS

Use of the drug can no longer be recommended because of its severe toxicity, due to the oenanthotoxin content.

OVERDOSAGE

Symptoms of poisoning include a burning sensation in the mouth and nose, dizziness, weakness, chills, mild twitching, and speech disorders. Higher dosages may produce tonic-colonic spasms, temporarily slowed cardiac activity, unconsciousness, bloody foam at the mouth, and death through respiratory failure.

Following gastrointestinal emptying (inducement of vomiting, gastric lavage with burgundy-colored potassium permanganate solution and sodium sulfate), and the administration of activated charcoal, the therapy for poisonings consists of treating spasms with thiobarbiturates (diazepam is said to be less effective); hemodialysis or hemperfusion have been applied successfully.

DOSAGE

Mode of Administration: The drug is obsolete except in homeopathy.

Homeopathic Dosage: Adult dosages are 5 drops, 1 tablet, or 10 globules every 30 to 60 minutes (acute) or 1 to 3 times daily (chronic); from D4 parenterally: 1 to 2 mL sc IV, IM. acute, 3 times daily; chronic: once a day. Children up to 6 years old are given a maximum of half the adult dose; children up to 12 are given a maximum of two-thirds the adult dose (HAB34).

LITERATURE

Anet E, Lythgoe B, Silk MH, Tripett S, The chemistry of oenanthotoxin and cicutoxin. In: *Chem Ind* 31:757. 1952.

Bohlmann F, Rode KM, Polyacetylenic compounds: CXVII. Polyynes of *Oenanthe crocata*. In: *Chem Ber* 101(4):1163-1175. 1968.

Grindy HF, Howarth F, Pharmacological studies on hemlock water dropwort. In: *Brit J Pharmacol* 11:225-30. 1956.

Mitchell MJ, Routledge PA, Hemlock water dropwort poisoning - a review. In: *Clin Toxicol* 12(4):417-426. 1978.

Water Fennel

Oenanthe aquatica

DESCRIPTION

Medicinal Parts: The medicinal parts of the plant are the ripe seeds.

Flower and Fruit: The flowers are white and grow in many-rayed compound umbels opposite the leaves. There is no involucre but there is a small epicalyx. The calyx is distinct with an irregular corolla and petals that have a distinct border. The calyx narrows at the base and has an involute tip. The style is long. The fruit is 5 mm long, 1.5 mm wide, with 5 broad obtuse ribs.

Leaves, Stem, and Root: The plant grows from 30 to 120 cm high. The stem is angularly branched, hollow, and soft. The lower end of the 3-cm thick stem, which grows underwater, has long roots at the nodes. Above water, the stem grows to only 6 mm thick. The leaves are double pinnate, pinnatifid to pinnatisect, with splayed leaflets, which are often turned backward and have lanceolate, deeply indented-serrate tips. The underwater leaves have a threadlike tip.

Habitat: Found near ponds and ditches in both the U.S. and Europe.

Production: Water Fennel fruit are the ripe seeds of *Oenanthe aquatica*, which are collected in the wild.

Not to be Confused With: Mistaken identity can occur with *Cicuta virosa, Sium latifolium*, or *Perculanum palustre*.

Other Names: Horsebane, Water Dropwort

ACTIONS AND PHARMACOLOGY

COMPOUNDS

Volatile oil (1-2.5%): including among others (+)-beta-phellandrene, dillapiol, myristicin, 1-nonen-3-ol (androle), volatile polyynes, undecen-4-ole, camphene, isopropyl cyclohexene-2-ole

Polyynes: including among others all-trans-pentadeca-2,8,10-trien-4,6-diin-12-on

Fatty oil (20%)

Lignans: including arctigenin, matairesinol, dimethyl matairesinol, secoisolariciresinol

EFFECTS

The drug's expectorant and antitussive effects are probably due to the essential oil. The active agents are the essential and fatty oil, resin, wax, galacton, and mannan and rubber substances. There is no further information available.

INDICATIONS AND USAGE

Unproven Uses: Water Fennel is used in folk medicine as an expectorant and for the relief of coughs due to inflammation of the bronchial mucous membranes or asthma. It is also used for gastrointestinal disorders.

Homeopathic Uses: Inflammation of the respiratory tract and breast pain in nursing mothers are indications for use in homeopathy.

PRECAUTIONS AND ADVERSE REACTIONS

No health hazards or side effects are known in conjunction with the proper administration of designated therapeutic dosages.

DOSAGE

Mode of Administration: Ground, as an extract and as a tea.

Preparation: A tincture is prepared using the drug in a 1:5 ratio with 70% ethanol (m/m)

Daily Dosage: The recommended daily dose is 4 to 5 g drug.

Homeopathic Dosage: Adult dosage is 5 drops, 1 tablet, or 10 globules every 30 to 60 minutes (acute) or 1 to 3 times daily (chronic); from D4 parenterally: 1 to 2 ml sc IV, IM acute, 3 times daily; chronic: once a day. Children up to 6 years are given half the dose, children up to 12 are given a maximum of two-thirds the adult dosage (HAB1).

LITERATURE

Ram AS, Devi HM, *Indian J Bo*t 6(1):21. 1983

Vincieri FF, Mazzi G, Mulinazzi N, Coran SA, Bambagiotti-Alberti M. Permeation of *Oenanthe aquatica* fruit tincture - β-Cyclodextrin Complex through artificial Membranes. *Il Farmaco* 49; 63-67. 1994

Vincieri FF, Coran SA, Mulinacci N, Bambagiotti-Alberti M. An Insight into *Oenanthe aquatica L.* Fruit Tincture through the MS Identification of its Gaschromatigraphable Compounds. *Pharm Acta Helv.* 64; 30-32. 1989

Wagner H, Wiesenauer M, Phytotherapie. Phytopharmaka und pflanzliche Homöopathika, Fischer-Verlag, Stuttgart, Jena, New York 1995.

Water Germander

Teucrium scordium

DESCRIPTION

Medicinal Parts: The medicinal parts are the herb harvested during or shortly before the flowering season and the fresh flowering herb.

Flower and Fruit: The flowers are light red, 8 to 10 mm long, with short pedicles. They are in inconspicuous clusters in 1- to 4-blossomed cymes between bracts, which are longer than the flowers. The calyx has 5 tips and is campanulate-tubular with a touch violet. It appears to have 5 lobes. After flowering, the head drops. There are 4 stamens. The nutlets are 1 mm long and punctate-reticulate.

Leaves, Stem, and Root: The plant is a perennial, downy herb that smells of garlic. The rhizome creeps in mud and produces above-round runners, which immediately turn into leaves and flower shoots. The stems are unbranched or branched, erect, round, and villous with soft-hairs. The leaves are sessile, oblong-oval, and crossed opposite.

Characteristics: The plant has an odor similar to garlic and a bitter taste.

Habitat: The plant is indigenous to most of Europe as far as northern Africa and central Asia.

Production: Water Germander is the aerial part of *Teucrium scordium*. It is picked during or shortly before flowering.

ACTIONS AND PHARMACOLOGY

COMPOUNDS

Diterpenes: including among others, 6,20-bisdeacetylteupy-reinidin, 6-deacetylteupyreinidin, 2beta, 6beta-dihydroxy-teuscordin, 2beta,6beta-dihydroxyteuscordin, dihydroteugin, teuflidin, teucrin E, teugin, 2-keto-19-hydroxyteuscordin

EFFECTS

See other *Teucrium* species.

INDICATIONS AND USAGE

Unproven Uses: The herb is used for the treatment of festering and inflamed wounds, bronchial ailments, diarrhea, fever, hemorrhoids, and intestinal parasites.

PRECAUTIONS AND ADVERSE REACTIONS

No health hazards or side effects are known in conjunction with the proper administration of designated therapeutic dosages.

DOSAGE

Mode of Administration: Water Germander is used internally and externally.

Daily Dosage: Four teaspoonfuls of the herb (7.2 g) is taken daily as an infusion. The same preparation can be used internally or externally.

LITERATURE

Fikenscher LH, Hegnauer R, *Plant Med Phytother* 3(3):183.

Hänsel R, Keller K, Rimpler H, Schneider G (Hrsg.), Hagers Handbuch der Pharmazeutischen Praxis, 5. Aufl., Bde 4-6 (Drogen): Springer Verlag Berlin, Heidelberg, New York, 1992-1994.

Madaus G, Lehrbuch der Biologischen Arzneimittel, Bde 1-3, Nachdruck, Georg Olms Verlag Hildesheim 1979.

Papanov GY et al., *PH* 24:297-299. 1985.

Singh S et al., *Fitoteràpia* 63:555. 1992.

Watercress

Nasturtium officinale

DESCRIPTION

Medicinal Parts: The medicinal parts are the aerial parts collected during the flowering season and the entire flowering plant.

Flower and Fruit: On the leading and side shoots there are terminal, racemelike inflorescences, which are slightly um-belliferous and consist of small, white, solitary flowers. The 4

white sepals are 2 to 3 mm long and glabrous. The 4 white petals are 2.5 to 5 mm long and turn lilac. There are 2 to 4 stamens with yellow anthers and filaments, which also turn lilac. The fruit is 13 to 18 mm long, with a glabrous pod on an 8 to 12 cm stem. The seeds are flat, ovate, 1 mm long, 0.8 to 0.9 mm wide, and roughly reticulate. There are about 25 sections on each seed surface.

Leaves, Stem, and Root: The plant is a perennial that grows from 25 to 90 cm and has creeping runners. The stem is angular, hollow, decumbent, rooting, and branched. The somewhat fleshy leaves are alternate, usually odd-pinnate, lyrate, and petiolate. They remain grass-green in winter. They have broad-elliptical, entire-margined, or sweeping-crenate leaflets and roundish, broadly cordate terminal leaflets.

Characteristics: The plant has a radish-like taste and smells tangy when rubbed.

Habitat: The plant is found almost all over the world and is cultivated in many regions.

Production: Watercress consists of the fresh or dried above-ground parts of *Nasturtium officinale*. The fresh herb is collected in the wild and dried in shady, well-aired conditions.

Not to be Confused With: Berula erecta or *Cardamine amara*

Other Names: Indian Cress

ACTIONS AND PHARMACOLOGY

COMPOUNDS

Glucosinolates in the fresh, unbruised plant (0.9% of fresh weight): chief components gluconasturtiin (80%), which releases during the course of cell destruction the mustard oil phenyl ethyl isothiocyanate, from which 3-phenyl propionitrile, among other substances, spontaneously arises; additionally glucotropaeolin (yielding benzyl isothiocyanate), as well as 7-methyl thioheptyl glucosinolate, 8-methyl thiooctyl glucosinolate

Flavonoids

Vitamin C (80 mg/100 g)

EFFECTS

Watercress has antibiotic, antitumoral, and diuretic actions. The diuretic effect is probably due to the mustard oil content. As an amaroid drug, it stimulates appetite and digestion.

INDICATIONS AND USAGE

Approved by Commission E:

■ Cough/bronchitis

Unproven Uses: Internally, the plant is used for catarrh of the respiratory tract, as an appetite stimulant and for digestion complaints. Externally, a decoction of the leaves in poultices and compresses is used for arthritis.

Homeopathic Uses: Watercress is used to treat irritation of the efferent urinary tract.

CONTRAINDICATIONS

Contraindications include stomach or intestinal ulcers and inflammatory renal diseases.

PRECAUTIONS AND ADVERSE REACTIONS

General: No health hazards or side effects are known in conjunction with the proper administration of designated therapeutic dosages. The intake of large quantities of the freshly harvested plant (e.g., in salad) could lead to gastrointestinal complaints due to the mucous membrane-irritating effect of the mustard oil.

Pediatric Use: The drug should not be administered to children under 4 years old.

Pregnancy: The drug should not be used during pregnancy.

DOSAGE

Mode of Administration: The comminuted herb, freshly pressed juice, as well as other galenic preparations of the plant, are for internal use.

How Supplied:

Capsules — 500 mg

Preparation: To make a tea, pour 150 mL boiling water over 2 g drug (1 to 2 teaspoonfuls), cover for 10 to 15 minutes and strain.

Daily Dosage: The daily dosage is 2 to 3 cups of the tea before meals, 4 to 6 g of the dried herb, 20 to 30 g of the fresh herb, or 60 to 150 g of freshly pressed juice. Externally, the drug is applied as a poultice or a compress.

Homeopathic Dosage: 5 drops, 1 tablet, or 10 globules every 30 to 60 minutes (acute) or 1 to 3 times daily (chronic); parenterally: 1 to 2 mL sc, acute, 3 times daily; chronic: once a day (HAB1).

LITERATURE

Cruz A. Marked antimitotic activity of watercress (*Nasturtium officinale*) in various experimental tumors. Hospital (Rio de Janeiro).; 77: 943-52. 1970

Diamond SP, Wiener SG, Marks JG. Allergic contact dermatitis to nasturtium. *Dermatol Clin.*; 8:77-80. 1990

Goda Y, Hoshino K, Akiyama H et al. Constituents in watercress: inhibitors of histamine release from RBL-2H3 cells induced by antigen stimulation. *Biol Pharm Bull.*; 22:1319-26. 1999

Hecht SS, Chung FL, Richie JP et al. Effects of watercress consumption on metabolism of a tobacco-specific lung carcinogen in smokers. *Cancer Epidemiol Biomarkers Prevent.*; 4:877-84. 1995

Wheat

Triticum aestivum

DESCRIPTION

Medicinal Parts: The medicinal parts are the fruit wall, seed shell, and outer layers of the endosperm.

Flower and Fruit: The inflorescence is a 4 to 18 cm long, 4-sided, double-rowed awnless spike (occasionally with an awn up to 16 cm long). The spikelet has 2 to 6 flowers, 2 to 4 of which are sterile. Each spikelet has 2 glumes at the base, is approximately 10 mm long, blunt, keeled at the tip with a blunt or acute tooth. The flowers are surrounded by 2 bracts; the first is bulbous and coriaceous, the second is smaller and membranous. There are 3 stamens and an ovary with 2 featherlike styles. The fruit is a yellow, red, or brown orbicular to elongate oval caryopse.

Leaves, Stem, and Root: The herb grows up to 1.5 m high. The leaves are arranged in two rows, are parallel-veined, and 5 to 15 mm wide. The leaf base clasps the stem, the ligule is short with a ciliate eyelet. The stem is thin-walled, hollow, and glabrous at the nodes.

Habitat: Asia, North America, and Europe

Production: Wheat bran is the fruit wall, seed shell, and outer layers of the endosperm of *Triticum aestivum*. Wheat germ oil is the fatty oil derived from cold-pressing the embryo of *Triticum aestivum* in a filter press.

Not to be Confused With: Wheat bran is sometimes confused with rye bran; wheat germ oil with other oils such as sesame oil.

Other Names: Wheat Bran, Wheat Germ Oil

ACTIONS AND PHARMACOLOGY

COMPOUNDS: WHEAT BRAN

Polysaccharides

Glucans: starch (15 to 20%), cellulose (30 %)

Heteroglycans (10%): complex arabinoxylans, to some extent water-soluble

Fatty oil (2%)

Phospolipids (1%)

Glycolipids (0.5%): particularly acyldigalactosyl glycerols

Steroids (0.3%): sterol esters

Proteins (20%)

Lignin

Alkyl resorcinols (0.1 to 0.2%): chiefly with C21- or C17-side chains

EFFECTS: WHEAT BRAN

Wheat bran is laxative in effect through expanding polysaccharides, which, through an increased level of fullness pressure, stimulate intestinal peristalsis and markedly shorten the transition time. At the same time, a measurable bonding of bile acids and their elimination from the enterohepatic circulation takes place. In addition, a significant reduction of postprandial lipid levels is exhibited. The topical application of the drug as a bath additive for injured or irritated skin (due to the carbohydrates and proteins it contains) leads to milieu changes in the epidermis and thus to a reconstitution of the callous layer.

COMPOUNDS: WHEAT GERM OIL

Fatty oil: triacylglycerols (60 to 75%), diacylglycerols (to 4%): chief fatty acids linoleic acid (50 to 65%), oleic acid (15 to 22%), palmitic acid (7 to 18%), linolenic acid (5 to 8%)

Phospholipids (9 to 14%)

Glycolipids (0 to 2%): particularly acyldigalaktosyl glycerols

Free fatty acids (1 to 2%)

Steroids: sterol esters (2.5 to 3%), particularly those of beta-sitosterol and campesterol

Tocopherols (vitamin E, 0.2 to 0.3%): particularly alpha-tocopherol (share 60 to 70%), as well as beta-tocopherol, gamma-tocopherol, alpha-tocotrienol, beta-tocotrienol

Carotinoids (0.15 to 0.25%)

EFFECTS: WHEAT GERM OIL

Wheat germ oil protects and nurtures the skin, is a laxative and reduces lipids. It is a valuable dietetic because of the high level of polyunsaturated fatty acids and vitamin E.

INDICATIONS AND USAGE

WHEAT BRAN

Unproven Uses: Folk medicine internal uses include constipation. Externally, bran has been used for itching and inflammatory dermatoses (as a bran bath).

Chinese Medicine: Used to treat night sweats.

Indian Medicine: Flatulence, constipation, itching, and menorrhagia are indications for use in Indian medicine. Efficacy for constipation and dermatoses seems plausible, but efficacy for the other indications has not been sufficiently proved.

WHEAT GERM OIL

Unproven Uses: Used as a dietary agent because of the high level of polyunsaturated fatty acids and vitamin E.

PRECAUTIONS AND ADVERSE REACTIONS

WHEAT BRAN AND WHEAT GERM OIL

No health hazards are known in conjunction with the proper administration of designated therapeutic dosages.

DOSAGE

WHEAT BRAN

Mode of Administration: Whole drug preparations are for internal and external use.

How Supplied:

Capsules: 500 mg, 770 mg

Daily Dosage: As a laxative, the dose is 15 to 40 g 1 to 2 times daily, taken with meals and plenty of liquid. For a full/partial bath: minimum 0.34 g aqueous extract to 1 L water

Chinese Medicine Daily Dosage: 9 to 15 g drug

WHEAT GERM OIL

Mode of Administration: Soft gelcaps or oil for internal and external use.

Storage: Store tightly sealed in a cool place.

LITERATURE

Andre F, Andre C, Colin L, Cacaraci F, Cavagna S. Role of new allergens and of allergens consumption in the increased incidence of food sensitizations in France. *Toxicology* 93; 77-83. 1994

Blaschek W, Hänsel R, Keller K, Reichling J, Rimpler G, Schneider G, (Eds) Hagers Handbuch der Pharmazeutischen Praxis. Folgebände 1 und 2. Drogen A-Z. Springer. Berlin, Heidelberg 1998.

Goff DJ, Kull FJ, The inhibition of human salivary alpha-amylase by type II alpha-amylase inhibitor from *Triticum aestivum* is competitive, slow and tight-binding. *J Enzyme Inhib*, 252:163-70, 1995.

Kluge M, Grambow HJ, Sicker D. (2R)-2-β-D-Glucopyranosyloxy-4,7-Dimethoxy-2H-1,4-Benzoxacin- 3(4H)-one from *Triticum aestivum. Phytochemistry* 44 (4); 639-641. 1997

Kuninori T, Nishiyama J. Separation and Quantitation of Ferulic Acid and Tyrosine in Wheat Seeds (*Triticum aestivum*) by reversed-phase High-performance liquid Chromatography. *J Chromatogr*. 362, 255-262. 1986

White Bryony

Bryonia alba

DESCRIPTION

Medicinal Parts: The medicinal part is the root.

Flower and Fruit: The plant is monoecious, occasionally dioecious. The male flowers are in long-peduncled racemes, which are 10 to 12 mm wide and shed easily. The female flowers are in short-stemmed umbel-like clusters. The sepals are almost as long as the corolla. The 5-petaled corolla is yellowish-white and has green veins. The 3 styles are almost completely free. The stigmas are glabrous. The 2 fused, inferior ovaries are triple-valved. The fruit is a 1- to 2-seeded, thin-skinned, 7 to 8 mm thick, globose black berry.

Leaves, Stem, and Root: White Bryony is an extremely fast-growing perennial. It has a thick, tuberous root. The root is fleshy, wrinkled horizontally, yellowish-gray on the outside, and white and slimy on the inside. The grooved, angular stems are climbing, branched, and have long internodes and simple screwlike climbers. They grow up to 4 m long. The leaves are short-petioled, broadly cordate, pentagonal to 5-lobed, and covered with short bristles on both sides.

Characteristics: The root is bitter and spicy. The plant is categorized as extremely poisonous.

Habitat: Indigenous from northeastern and southeastern Europe and also Iran.

Production: Bryonia root consists of the dried taproot of *Bryonia alba*, which is cultivated.

Other Names: Devil's Turnip, English Mandrake, Ladies' Seal, Tamus, Tetterberry, Wild Hops, Wild Nep, Wild Vine, Wood Vine

ACTIONS AND PHARMACOLOGY

COMPOUNDS

Cucurbitacins: including cucurbitacins B, D, E, I, J, K, L, 23,24-dihydro-cucurbitacins, 1,2,23,24-tetrahydrocucurbitacins, 22-deoxycucurbitacins and bryodulcigenin; cucurbitacin glycosides, including bryonin, elaterinide, bryonosid, bryodulcigenin, cucurbitacin glycosides

Triterpenes with unusual structure: for example, bryonolic acid

Steroids: including sterols like C-4- and/or C-24-methylated or ethylated cholest-7-en-3-beta-oles

Polyhydroxy fatty acids: including 9,12,13-trihydroxy-octadeca-10 (E)-15(Z)-dienic acid.

Lectins

EFFECTS

The mainly glycosidically bonded cucurbitanes contained in the drug have a strong toxic and cytotoxic effect; in topical application they are irritating to the skin and mucous membranes. Various aqueous extracts of the drug display an antitumoral effect in animal tests. The resin is a drastic purgative. The methanol extracts have a strong hypoglycemic affect. Use of the drug as an emetic and purgative has become obsolete because of the toxicity.

INDICATIONS AND USAGE

Unproven Uses: Because of its strong purgative and emetic effect, use of the drug cannot be recommended. Bryonia root has been used as a laxative, emetic and diuretic in the treatment of various disorders of the gastrointestinal tract and respiratory tract and for rheumatic disorders. It has also been used prophylactically and therapeutically for metabolic disorders, liver disease, and acute and chronic infectious disease.

PRECAUTIONS AND ADVERSE REACTIONS

The drug is highly toxic when freshly harvested. The toxicity of the drug declines rapidly with dehydration and storage because of the instability of the cucurbitacins. Due to the cucurbitacin content, the drug has a severely irritating effect on skin and mucous membranes. Contact between skin and the juice of the plant can lead to rash, infection, blister formation, and necroses.

OVERDOSAGE

The intake of toxic dosages can lead to vomiting, bloody diarrhea, colic, kidney irritation, anuria, collapse, spasms, paralysis and, under certain conditions, to death. Following gastric lavage, the treatment for poisonings should proceed symptomatically. Consumption of 40 berries is presumed fatal for an adult; 15 for a child.

DOSAGE

Mode of Administration: Since the efficacy of Bryonia preparations for the claimed applications is not documented, and since the use of it as a drastic laxative and emetic is obsolete, a therapeutic administration cannot be justified because of the risks involved.

Bryonia is found occasionally in some pharmaceutical preparations.

Preparation: A decoction is prepared by adding 0.5 to 1 g drug to 1 cup water.

Daily Dosage: Dosage of the powder is 0.3 to 0.5 g as an emetic and purgative.

LITERATURE

Konopa J et al., Cucurbitacins, Cytotoxic and Antitumor Substances from *Bryonia alba L.* Part I: Isolation and Identification. *Arzneim Forsch.* 24; 1554-1557. 1974

Krauze-Baranowska M, Cisowski W. Flavone C-Glycosides from *Bryonia alba* and *B. dioica. Phytochemistry* 39 (3); 727-729. 1995

Miro M. Cucurbitacins and their Pharmacological Effects. *Phytother Res.* 9 (3); 159-168. 1995

Oobayashi K, Yoshikawa K, Arihara S, Structural revision of Bryonoside and structure elucidation of minor saponins from *Bryonia dioica*. In: *PH* 31:943-946. 1992.

Orekhov AN, Panossian AG. Trihydroxyoctadecadienoic acids exhibit antiatherosclerotic and antiatherogenic activity. *Phytomedicine* 1; 123-126. 1994

Pohlmann J, The cucurbitacins in *Bryonia alba* and *Bryonia dioica*. In: *PH* 14(7):1587-1589. 1980.

Withmarsh TE, Coleston-Shields DM, Steiner TJ. Double-blind randomized placebo-controlled study of homoeopathic prophylaxis of migraine. *Cephalgia* 17; 600-604. 1997

White Fir

Abies alba

DESCRIPTION

Medicinal Parts: The medicinal part of the trees is needles and branch tips, from which essential oil is extracted.

Flower and Fruit: The ovules are in pairs on the upper surface of the seed scales, in axils of the spirally arranged covering scales, which are in turn fused into cones. The cones are 10 to 16 cm long and 3 to 5 cm thick, with protruding surface scales that are green and tinged brown-red before ripening. The stamens are arranged like catkins. The fruit is diclinous, monoecious. The seeds are long-winged on one side.

Leaves, Stem, and Root: The tree grows up to 50 m and occasionally up to 75 m tall. The needles are 1 to 3 cm long, 1.8 to 2.3 mm wide. The needles are dark green on the upper surface with two white stripes on the lower surface. They are divided with a blunt apex indented at the tip. The trunk is initially grayish, later scaly.

Habitat: White Fir is found in the Balkan countries. It originated from former Yugoslavia, Bulgaria, Poland, Romania, and Albania.

Production: The essential oil of White Fir is extracted from the needles and branch tips by aqueous steam distillation for 5 to 6 hours.

Not to be Confused With: May occur with turpentine oils, cone oils, fir needle oils, camphors, bornyl acetate, and various *Pinaceae* oils.

Other Names: Common Silver Fir, Swiss Pine

ACTIONS AND PHARMACOLOGY

COMPOUNDS

Limonene (25 to 55%)

Alpha-pinene (6 to 35%)

Camphene (9 to 20%)

Bornyl acetate (2 to 10%)

Santene (2 to 3%)

Tricyclene (1.0 to 2.5%): including among others beta-pinene, beta-phellandrene and delta3-carene

EFFECTS

The essential oil has secretolytic and mildly antiseptic effects on the bronchial mucous membranes and hyperemic effects on the skin. The constituents' camphene, limonene, and alpha-pinene are responsible for the strong expectorate effect connected with its inhalation.

INDICATIONS AND USAGE

Approved by Commision E:

- Neuralgia
- Rheumatism

Unproven Uses: Internally, the drug is used for catarrh of the respiratory tract. Externally, it can be used for nervous unrest and neuralgic pain. It can also be used for sprains, strains, bruises, and as a prophylactic treatment for bedsores.

CONTRAINDICATIONS

The plant is contraindicated for conditions like bronchial asthma, other obstructive bronchial diseases and whooping cough. Whole-body baths involving the essential oil should only be undertaken in consultation with a physician in the presence of larger skin injuries, severe feverish or infectious diseases, cardiac insufficiency, or hypertonia. Inhalation is to be avoided when the patient suffers from acute infections of the respiratory passages.

PRECAUTIONS AND ADVERSE REACTIONS

No health hazards are known in conjunction with the proper administration of designated therapeutic dosages. Bronchial spasms could become worse following administration of the drug.

OVERDOSAGE

Poisonings are possible in connection with overdose and large-area external administration, including injuries to the kidneys and the CNS. The use of outdated essential oils with unsaturated terpene carbohydrates could lead to severe irritation of the skin and mucous membranes.

Severe poisonings are possible following the ingestion of very large doses, leading to nausea, vomiting, reddening of the face, salivation, throat soreness, thirst, diarrhea, intestinal colic, dyspnea, dizziness, staggering walk, twitching, stranguria, dysuria, hematuria, albuminuria, and skin efflorescence. Ingestion should be followed with gastric lavage with sodium sulfate solutions, intestinal emptying through administration of sodium sulfate, instillation of paraffin oil and medicinal charcoal, and shock prophylaxis (suitable body position, quiet, warmth).

The treatment for poisonings consists of the treatment of spasms with diazepam (IV), electrolyte substitution and the countering of any acidosis imbalance that may appear through sodium bicarbonate infusions. In the event of shock, plasma volume expanders should be infused. Monitoring of kidney function is necessary. Intubation and oxygen respiration may also be required.

DOSAGE

Mode of Administration: Liquid preparations for internal and external use.

Daily Dosage:

Drops — 4 drops, 3 times daily in water or with sugar

Inhalation — add a few drops to hot water; and inhale several times daily

Lotion — rub into the affected parts

Storage: Keep sealed tightly and protected from light.

LITERATURE

Aronow WS, Starling L, Etienne F, D'Alba P, Edwards M, Lee NH, Parungao RF, Sales FF. Risk factors for atherothrombotic brain infarction in persons over 62 years of age in a long-term healthcare facility. *J Am Geriatr Soc*, 35:1-3, Jan. 1987

Faure-Raynaud M, Determination of the chitinolytic activity of "*Abies alba Mill*". litter microorganisms: bacteria and yeasts (author's transl) *Ann Microbiol* (Paris), 132B:267-79, Sep-Oct. 1981.

Faure-Raynaud M, Study of volatile oil from *Abies alba Miller*. I. Study of raw material. *Acta Pol Pharm*, 132B:71-7, 1970.

Faure-Raynaud M, Study of volatile oil from sprigs of *Abies alba Miller*. II. Study of monoterpene fractions of oil. *Acta Pol Pharm*, 132B:155-62, 1970.

Faure-Raynaud M, Study of volatile oil of fir branches *Abies alba Miller*. III. Study of non-monoterpene fraction and gas chromatography of oil. *Acta Pol Pharm*, 132B:301-5, 1970.

Hänsel R, Keller K, Rimpler H, Schneider G (Ed) Hagers Handbuch der Pharmazeutischen Praxis. 5. Aufl., Bde 4 - 6 (Drogen), Springer Verlag Berlin, Heidelberg, New York, 1992-1994.

White Hellebore

Veratrum album

DESCRIPTION

Medicinal Parts: The medicinal parts are the rhizome and root.

Flower and Fruit: The flowers are in racemes that form a 30- to 60-cm panicle. The pedicles are much shorter than the flowers. The yellowish-white flowers consist of 6 similar tepals, which are oblong-lanceolate, acute, denticulate, and broadly splayed. There are 6 stamens, which are shorter than the perigone, and 3 styles. The fruit is capsulelike.

Leaves, Stem, and Root: The plant is roughly 60 to 120 cm high. The rhizome is short, cylindrical, and stunted. It has numerous, long, thick and fleshy root fibers. The round, canelike, glabrous stem is almost completely surrounded by the tight sheaths of the basal leaves. The basal leaves are whorled, broad, elliptical to linear-lanceolate, and heavily ribbed.

Habitat: The plant is found from Lapland to Italy but not on the British Isles.

Production: White Hellebore rootstock is the rhizome of *Veratrum album.*

ACTIONS AND PHARMACOLOGY

COMPOUNDS

Steroid alkaloids (mixture is referred to as veratrine, 0.8-2.5%): C-nor-D-homo-sterane type-including protoverine, protoveratrines A and B, germerine, jervine, protoverine, veratroyl zygadenine

Solidane type-including isorubijervine, rubijervine

EFFECTS

Internally, the drug reduces blood pressure and heart rate, inhibits respiration in higher doses, and has an aconitine-like effect on the conductor system. Externally, the drug causes severe irritation to the skin, including numbing and poisoning through absorption.

INDICATIONS AND USAGE

Unproven Uses: Internally, White Hellebore is used for the treatment of vomiting, cramps, diarrhea, cholera, and bradycardia, and Graves' disease. Externally, the drug is used for neuralgia, rheumatism, joint pain and gout pain.

Homeopathic Uses: White Hellebore is used for neuralgia, infections, diarrhea, hypotension, and as a stimulant.

PRECAUTIONS AND ADVERSE REACTIONS

The drug is severely toxic and has numerous severe side effects, even at therapeutic dosages. It is no longer administered in allopathic medicine for that reason. The veratrum alkaloids severely irritate mucous membranes. By inhibiting inactivation of sodium ion channels, the resorption of alkaloids has a paralyzing effect on numerous excitable cells, particularly those governing cardiac activity.

OVERDOSAGE

The first symptoms of poisoning are sneezing, lacrimation, salivation, vomiting, diarrhea, a burning sensation in the mouth and pharyngeal cavity, and inability to swallow. Then, following resorption, paresthesia, vertigo, possible blindness, paralysis of the limbs, mild convulsions, lowering of cardiac frequency, cardiac arrhythmias, and hypotension occur. Death occurs either through systolic cardiac arrest or through asphyxiation. The lethal dosage is between 10 and 20 mg of the alkaloid mixture, corresponding to 1 to 2 g of the drug. The alkaloids can be absorbed through uninjured skin.

Treatment of poisoning consists of gastrointestinal emptying (inducement of vomiting, gastric lavage with burgundy-colored potassium permanganate solution, sodium sulphate), administration of activated charcoal and shock prophylaxis (appropriate body position, quiet, warmth). Thereafter, spasms should be treated with diazepam or barbiturates (IV), bradycardia should be treated with atropine, hypotension should be treated with peripherally active circulatory medications, electrolyte substitution should be employed, and possible cases of acidosis should be treated with sodium bicarbonate infusions. Intubation and oxygen respiration may also be necessary.

DOSAGE

Mode of Administration: The drug is used in powders, tinctures and homeopathic dilutions for internal use; preparations made with fatty oils are used externally.

Preparation: Mix 5 g drug with 10 g lanolin and 20 g fat for topical application.

Daily Dosage: Internally, the drug is administered as 0.02 to 0.1 g of powder or 20 to 60 drops of tincture. Externally, the drug is applied as a poultice or compress.

Homeopathic Dosage: 5 drops, 1 tablet, or 10 globules every 30 to 60 minutes (acute) and 1 to 3 times daily (chronic); parenterally: 1 to 2 mL s.c., acute: 3 times daily; chronic: once a day (HAB34). The globules are from D2; all others are from D4.

LITERATURE

Atta-Ur-Rahman, Ali RA, Choudhary MI, New steroidal alkaloids from rhizomes of *Veratrum album*. In: *JNP* 55:565-570. 1992.

Atta-Ur-Rahmann, Ali RA, Gilani A, Choudhary MI, ASftab K, Sener B, Turkz S, Isolation of antihypertensive alkaloids from rhizomes of *Veratrum album*. In: *PM* 59(6):569. 1993.

Atta-Ur-Rahman et al., Alkaloids from *Veratrum album*. In: *PH* 30(1):368. 1991.

Brossi, Buch. In: Brossi A, Cordell GA (Eds), The Alkaloids. Vol. 41. Academic Press, 1250 Sixth Avenue, San Diego, CA 92101. 1992.

Festa M, Andreetto B, Ballaris MA, Panio A, Piervittori R, A case of *Veratrum poisoning. Minerva Anestesiol*, 62:195-6, May. 1996

Fogh A, Kulling P, Wickstrom E, Veratrum alkaloids in sneezing-powder a potential danger. *J Toxicol Clin Toxicol*, 20:175-9, Apr. 1983

Garnier R, Carlier P, Hoffelt J, Savidan A, Acute dietary poisoning by white hellebore (*Veratrum album L.*). Clinical and analytical data. A propos of 5 cases. *Ann Med Interne* (Paris), 136:125-8, 1985.

Hruby K, Lenz K, Krausler J, *Veratrum album* poisoning (author's transl). *Wien Klin Wochenschr*, 93:517-9, 1981 Sep 4.

Jaspersen-Schib R, Theus L, Guirguis-Oeschger M, Gossweiler B, Meier-Abt PJ, Serious plant poisonings in Switzerland 1966-1994. Case analysis from the Swiss Toxicology Information Center. *Schweiz Med Wochenschr*, 60:1085-98, Jun 22. 1996

Marinov A, Koev P, Mirchev N, Electrocardiographic studies of patients with acute hellebore (*Veratrum album*) poisoning. Vutr Boles, 26:36-9, 1987.

White Lily

Lilium candidum

DESCRIPTION

Medicinal Parts: The medicinal part is the fresh and dried bulb.

Flower and Fruit: The inflorescence has 5 to 20 blossoms. The flowers are white, occasionally striped or spotten crimson, and very fragrant. They are on erect pedicles, the lower ones nodding. The tepals are obtuse, the anthers yellow. The style is as long as the sepals. The fruit is obovate and is seldom developed.

Leaves, Stem, and Root: The plant is perennial and grows to 60 to 150 cm high. It has a broad, ovate, scaled, yellow bulb. The stem is rigid, erect, and leafy. The leaves are oblong to linear-lanceolate and glabrous. The entire plant survives winter. The bulb consists of imbricate, fleshy, lanceolate, and bent scales, which are 3.25 cm long and 2.5 cm wide at the broadest point.

Characteristics: The bulbs are odorless and have a mildly bitter and unpleasant flavor.

Habitat: The plant is indigenous to Mediterranean regions and is cultivated in many other regions.

Production: Baurenlilien (Farmer's Lily) root is the subterranean part (onion) of *Lilium candidum*.

Other Names: Madonna Lily, Meadow Lily

ACTIONS AND PHARMACOLOGY

COMPOUNDS

Flavonoids: including isorhamnetin glycosides

Gamma-methylene glutamic acid

Soluble polysaccharides: glucomannans

Starch

Tuliposide

The constituents of the drug have not been investigated extensively.

EFFECTS

The plant has astringent, anti-inflammatory, pain reliever, diuretic, and expectorant properties.

INDICATIONS AND USAGE

Unproven Uses: Internally for gynecological disorders and externally for ulcers, inflammation, furuncles, finger ulcers, reddened skin, burns, and injuries.

PRECAUTIONS AND ADVERSE REACTIONS

No health hazards or side effects are known in conjunction with the proper administration of designated therapeutic dosages.

DOSAGE

Mode of Administration: An infusion made from the ground drug is used internally. The drug is also used externally as a wet compress (paste).

Daily Dosage: Apply a thick paste, made from fresh or cooked bulbs in the form of a compress or poultice, to the affected area. This should be done several times during the day.

LITERATURE

Kern W, List PH, Hörhammer L (Hrsg.), Hagers Handbuch der Pharmazeutischen Praxis, 4. Aufl., Bde. 1-8, Springer Verlag Berlin, Heidelberg, New York, 1969.

Masterova I et al., *Phytochemistry* 26(6):1844. 1987

Nagy E et al., *Z Naturforsch* 39B(12):1813. 1984

White Mustard

Sinapis alba

DESCRIPTION

Medicinal Parts: The medicinal parts are the dried seeds.

Flower and Fruit: The flowers form an umbelliferous-racemous inflorescence. The flowers are on 3 to 7 mm long, stiff-haired pedicles. When in bloom the 4 narrow, obtuse sepals lie horizontally. There are 3 green, ovate nectaries at the base of the stamens. The fruit is a 2-to 4-cm long bristly pod, divided into two chambers. Each chamber contains two to three 2.5 mm thick seeds. The chamber ends as a large curled lip. The seeds vary from brown to white and are arranged in opposite rows.

Leaves, Stem, and Root: Sinapis alba is an annual plant. The lower part of the plant is covered in stiff, single hairs. The thin root is yellow to white and branched. The root produces a 30 to 60 cm high, erect, grooved, and branched stem. The leaves are 4 to 10 cm long, petiolate, lyrate, pinnatifid to pinnatesect, and always have 2 to 3 indented-dentate lobed pinna.

Habitat: The plant has been introduced and naturalized in all of Europe and in Siberia, east Asia and America. The areas of cultivation are western and northern Europe and the northern U.S.

Production: White Mustard seed consists of the ripe, dried seed of *Sinapis alba*.

Not to be Confused With: Other Sinapis or Brassica species. Artificial colorings such as butter yellow or turmeric may be added.

Other Names: Mustard

ACTIONS AND PHARMACOLOGY

COMPOUNDS

Glucosinolates: chiefly sinalbin (p-hydroxybenzylglucosinolates, 2.5%), grinding the seeds into powder and then rubbing with warm water (not with hot water – enzymes would be destroyed), as well as chewing, releases the non-volatile mustard oil p-hydroxybenzyl isothiocyanate

Fatty oil (20-35%)

Proteins (40%)

Phenyl propane derivatives: including among others sinapine (choline ester of sinapic acid, 1.5%)

EFFECTS

The p-hydroxybenzyl mustard oil that results from fermentation of sinalbin is bacteriostatic, irritating to the skin and hyperemic (as an additive in 35° to 40° C baths).

INDICATIONS AND USAGE

Approved by Commission E:

- Common cold
- Cough/bronchitis
- Rheumatism

Externally, White Mustard is used in poultices for congestion of the respiratory tract, for topical hyperemization of the skin as well as for segment therapy of chronic degenerative diseases affecting the joints and soft tissue.

Unproven Uses: In folk medicine, Mustard is used to clear the voice. It is also used in Mustard plasters and poultices as a counter-irritant. Mustard is used in footbaths, and for the treatment of paralytic symptoms in the form of Mustard baths.

Chinese Medicine: In China, White Mustard is used to treat painfully swollen ribs and chest, coughs, vomiting, regurgitation, ulcerous swelling, and rheumatic pains.

Homeopathic Uses: Sinapis alba is used to treat inflammation of the gastrointestinal tract and the respiratory tract.

CONTRAINDICATIONS

White Mustard is contraindicated in gastrointestinal ulcers and inflammatory kidney diseases. The drug should not be given to children under 6 years of age.

PRECAUTIONS AND ADVERSE REACTIONS

General: No health hazards or side effects are known in conjunction with the proper administration of designated therapeutic dosages. The danger of nerve damage exists with long-term intake. Long-term external application carries the danger of skin injury. The drug possesses minimal potential for sensitization (possible cause of food allergies).

Pediatric Use: White Mustard preparations should not be used in children under 6 years of age.

OVERDOSAGE

Gastrointestinal complaints could appear following the intake of large quantities, due to the mucous membrane-irritating effect of the Mustard oil.

DOSAGE

Mode of Administration: The drug is used internally as well as externally. Ground or powdered seeds are used for poultices.

Preparation: To prepare an external footbath, 20 to 30 g of the Mustard flour in 1 liter of water is used. To prepare a Mustard bath, 150 g of the Mustard flour in a pouch is used in the bathwater.

Daily Dosage: The average daily dose of the drug is 60 to 240 g. To brighten and clear the voice, Mustard flour is stirred with honey and formed into balls. One to 2 of these are taken orally on an empty stomach.

For external use, just prior to application, mix 50 to 70 g of the powdered seeds with warm water to prepare a poultice. The poultice is applied for 10 to 15 minutes for adults and for 5 to 10 minutes for children, except for those with sensitive skin where the usage should be shortened. Treatment should not exceed 2 weeks.

Homeopathic Dosage: 5 drops, 1 tablet, or 10 globules every 30 to 60 minutes (acute) or 1 to 3 times daily (chronic); parenterally: 1 to 2 mL sc, acute: 3 times daily; chronic: once a day (HAB34)

Storage: The drug must be protected from light and moisture.

LITERATURE

Josefsson E, *J Sci Food Agric* 21:94. 1970.

Meding B. Immediate hypersensitivity to mustard and rape. *Contact Dermatitis* 13; 121-122. 1985

White Nettle

Lamium album

DESCRIPTION

Medicinal Parts: The medicinal parts are the flowers and leaves.

Flower and Fruit: The white, fairly large bilabiate flowers are in axillary false whorls of 6 to 16 flowers. The campanulate calyx is green and has 5 tips. The tube of the corolla is bent like a knee and the curved upper lip has a ciliate margin. The lower lip is gordate. The tube has 1 large and 1 small tip; there are 2 long and 2 short stamens under the upper lip. The calyx remains after flowering and protects the small nut. When the nut is ripe, slight pressure is sufficient to fling out the seeds.

Leaves, Stem, and Root: The plant is 30 to 50 cm high with an underground creeping stem from which the aerial stems grow. These are erect, quadrangular, grooved, hollow, and noded. The leaves are crossed opposite, petiolate, ovate to cordate, acuminate, and serrate. The plant has no nettle hairs. The plant is similar to the stinging nettle but has a different stem.

Characteristics: The flowers have a weak honeylike fragrance and a slimy-sweet taste.

Habitat: The plant is common in Europe and central and northern Asia.

Production: White Nettle flower consists of the dried petal with attached stamens of *Lamium album* as well as its preparations.

Other Names: Archangel, Bee Nettle, Blind Nettle, Dead Nettle, Deaf Nettle, Dumb Nettle, Stingless Nettle, White Archangel

ACTIONS AND PHARMACOLOGY

COMPOUNDS

Iridoide monoterpenes: including among others lamalbide, caryoptoside, alboside A and B

Triterpene saponins

Caffeic acid derivatives: including among others rosmaric acid, chlorogenic acid

Flavonoids: including among others kaempferol glycosides

Mucilages

EFFECTS

Because of the mucins and saponins the drug is expectorant. It is astringent because of the tannins.

INDICATIONS AND USAGE

Approved by Commission E:

- Inflammation of the skin
- Cough/bronchitis
- Inflammation of the mouth and pharynx

Unproven Uses: Internally, the herb is used for catarrh of the upper respiratory passages and gastrointestinal disorders such as gastritis, bloating, and flatulence. Externally, it is used for leukorrhea. In folk medicine used for climacteric complaints and complaints of the urogenital tract.

Chinese Medicine: In Chinese medicine, White Nettle is used for fractures, carbuncles, lumbago, and inflammation of wounds.

PRECAUTIONS AND ADVERSE REACTIONS

No health hazards or side effects are known in conjunction with the proper administration of designated therapeutic dosages.

DOSAGE

Mode of Administration: Comminuted drug for infusions and other galenic preparations for internal applications, rinses, baths and moist compresses; occasionally used as a constituent of sedative teas and bronchial teas.

Preparation:

Infusion — Pour one cup of water over 1 g drug, leave to draw for 5 minutes and strain.

Extract for poultices — Scald 50 g of flowers with 500 mL of water, draw for 5 minutes and strain.

Daily Dosage: For internal use, the average daily dose is 3 g drug. For external use, 5 g drug is added to a bath.

LITERATURE

Damtoft S, Iridoid glucosides from *Lamium album*. In: *PH* 31(1):175. 1992.

Gora J et al., Chemical comparative studies of the herb and flowers of *Lamium album L.* In: *Acta Pol Pharm* 40(3):389-393. 1983.

Kern W, List PH, Hörhammer L (Hrsg.), Hagers Handbuch der Pharmazeutischen Praxis, 4. Aufl., Bde. 1-8, Springer Verlag Berlin, Heidelberg, New York, 1969.

Madaus G, Lehrbuch der Biologischen Arzneimittel, Bde 1-3, Nachdruck, Georg Olms Verlag Hildesheim 1979. Skrypczak L et al., Phenylpropanoid esters and flavonoids in taxonomy of *Lamium* species. In: *PM* 61(Abstracts of 43rd Ann Congr):70. 1995.

Wichtl M (Hrsg.), Teedrogen, 4. Aufl., Wiss. Verlagsges. Stuttgart 1997.

White Willow

Salix species

DESCRIPTION

Medicinal Parts: The medicinal part is the bark. Salix nigra is American Willow.

Flower and Fruit: The male flowers are yellow and the female green. They are dioecious and appear at the same time as the leaves on leafy stems in erect catkins. The male catkins are densely blossomed and cylindrical, up to 6.5 cm by 1 cm and have 2 stamens. The female catkins are cylindrical, 4.5 cm by 7 mm. The seeds have a tuft of hair.

Leaves, Stem, and Root: Silver Willow is a 6- to 18-m high tree or bush with fissured gray bark. The leaves are short-petioled, lanceolate, acuminate, and become cuneate at the base. They are finely serrate, silky-haired, and tomentose underneath, and blue-green matte in color.

Characteristics: The annual twigs are not easy to break off at the base.

Habitat: The plant is indigenous to central and southern Europe.

Production: White Willow bark consists of the bark of the young, 2- to 3-year-old branches harvested during early spring of *Salix alba, Salix purpurea, Salix fragilis,* and other comparable *Salix* species.

Other Names: Black Willow, Cartkins Willow, European Willow, Pussywillow, Salicin Willow, Withe Withy,Withy

ACTIONS AND PHARMACOLOGY

COMPOUNDS

Glycosides and esters yielding salicylic acid (1.5-12%): salicin (0.1-2%), salicortin (0.01-11%) and salicin derivatives acylated to the glucose residue (up to 6%, including fragilin, populin)

Tannins (8-20%)

Flavonoids

EFFECTS

The efficacy of the drug is due mainly to the proportion of salicin present. After splitting of the acyl residue, the salicin glycosides convert to salicin, the precursor of salicylic acid. Salicylic acid is antipyretic, antiphlogistic and analgesic. White Willow bark is the phytotherapeutic precursor to acetylsalicylic acid (aspirin).

The salicin component is responsible for the anti-inflammatory and antipyretic effects. The tannin content has astringent properties on mucous membranes.

INDICATIONS AND USAGE

Approved by Commission E:

- Rheumatism
- Pain

Salicin is useful in diseases accompanied by fever, rheumatic ailments, headaches and pain caused by inflammation.

Unproven Uses: Folk medicine uses include toothache, gout, gastrointestinal disorders, diarrhea, and wound healing.

CONTRAINDICATIONS

Willow Bark is contraindicated in patients that have a hypersensitivity to salicylates. Salicylates should not be used in children with flulike symptoms due to the association of salicylates with Reye's Syndrome.

Patients with an active gastric or duodenal ulcer, hemophilia, asthma, or diabetes should avoid Willow Bark preparations.

Pregnancy: Salicylates should be avoided during pregnancy.

Nursing Mothers: Salicylates have been associated with rashes in breastfed infants; use is not recommended.

PRECAUTIONS AND ADVERSE REACTIONS

General: No health hazards are known in conjunction with the proper administration of designated therapeutic dosages. Stomach complaints could occur as a side effect due to the tannin content.

There have been reports of metabolic acidosis in children with normal renal and hepatic function who were treated with salicylates and carbonic anhydrase inhibitors for joint pain and glaucoma. This combination should be avoided (Cowan, 1984).

DRUG INTERACTIONS

POTENTIAL INTERACTIONS

Due to the salicin component of White Willow, caution should be exercised when used in combination with salicylates and other nonsteroidal anti-inflammatory drugs. There are reports that salicylate decreased serum naproxen concentrations markedly and increased serum naproxen clearance by as much as 56% (Furst, 1987).

Though there are no reports of interactions with drugs that affect blood-clotting times, and some studies suggest that thrombocyte inhibition is unlikely. Antiplatelet medications and any medication that prolongs the PT time should not be used with Willow Bark (Wichtl & Bisset, 1994).

Alcohol and barbiturates may mask the symptoms of salicylate overdosage and may enhance the toxicity of salicylates.

DOSAGE

Mode of Administration: Liquid and solid preparations for internal use. Combinations with diaphoretic drugs could be considered. Drug extracts are contained in some standardized preparations of analgesics/antirheumatics, hypnotics/sedatives, and gastrointestinal remedies.

Preparation: To prepare an infusion, use 2 to 3 g of finely cut or coarsely powdered drug in cold water, boil, allow to steep for 5 minutes, then strain.

Daily Dosage: 6 to 12 g (average daily dose corresponding to 60-120 mg total salicin).

Infusion–1 cup 3 to 4 times daily. (1 teaspoonful = 1.5 g drug)

Liquid Extract–(1:1 in 25% alcohol) 1 to 3 mL 3 times daily.

Powder–1 to 2 g, several times a day.

LITERATURE

Amling R, Phytotherapeutika in der Neurologie. In: ZPT 12(1):9. 1991.

Anonym, Phytotherapie:Pflanzliche Antirheumatika - was bringen sie? In: DAZ 136(45):4012-4015. 1996.

Cowan, RA, Hartnell G, Lowdell C, Baird I, Leak A, Metabolic acidosis induced by carbonic anhydrase inhibitors and salicylates in patients with normal renal function. In: *BMJ* (*Clin Res Ed*) 289(6441):347-8, Aug 11, 1984.

Furst DE, Sarkissian E, Blocka K et al., Serum concentrations of salicylate and naproxen during concurrent therapy in patients with rheumatoid arthritis. In: *Arthritis Rheum* 30(10):1157-61, Oct, 1987.

Kreymeier J, Rheumatherapie mit Phytopharmaka. In: DAZ 137(8):611-613. 1997.

Meier R et al., A chemotaxonomic survey of phenolic compounds in swiss willow species. In: *PM* 58(7):A698. 1992.

Schmid B, Heide L, The use of Salicis cortex in rheumatic disease: phytotherapie with known mode of action? In: *PM* 61(Abstracts of 43rd Ann Congr):94. 1995.

Schmid B, Heide L, Wirksamkeit und Verträglichkeit von Weidenrinde bei Arthrose: Design und Durchführung einer klinischen Studie. In: *PUZ* 26(1):33, Jahrestagung der DPhG, Berlin, 1996. 1997.

Wild Carrot

Daucus carota

DESCRIPTION

Medicinal Parts: The medicinal part is the root.

Flower and Fruit: The flowers are in compact, terminal umbels or flattened, compound capitula. The peduncle divides in raylike fashion from one particular point. Each ray divides and forms further umbels with white flowers. The outer flowers are irregular and larger than the others. The florets are small. When in bloom, the flower head is flattened or slightly convex. When they are ripe, the flowers draw together to form a cuplike structure. The double achenes are formed in the fruit umbel. They are slightly flattened and have numerous bristles arranged in 5 rows.

Leaves, Stem, and Root: The Wild Carrot is a biennial, 30-cm to 1-m high cultivated plant with a fusiform, usually red root and numerous pinnate, segmented, hairy leaves. In the second year, the plant produces a branched, angular stem with alternate jointed leaves, which terminates in the flowering umbels.

Habitat: Now found in its cultivated form all over the world.

Production: Wild Carrots are the roots of *Daucus carota*. The ripe roots are harvested.

Other Names: Bees' Nest, Bird's Neat, Birds' Nest, Carrot, Philtron, Queen Anne's Lace

ACTIONS AND PHARMACOLOGY

COMPOUNDS

Carotinoids: including alpha-, beta-, gamma-, zeta-carotene, lycopene

Volatile oil (very little): including among others p-cymene, limonene, dipenten, geraniol, alpha- and beta- caryophyllene

Polyynes: including falcarinol (carotatoxin)

Mono and oligosaccharides: glucose, saccharose

EFFECTS

Wild Carrot has anthelmintic and antimicrobial activity. It is also a mild vermifuge. The essential oil has an initially stimulating, paralyzing effect on worms. In controlled animal tests, a temporary reduction of arterial blood pressure was observed. The pectin content is probably responsible for the severe constipating effect of the Carrot. The essential oil has a mild bactericidal effect, especially on gram-positive bacteria. The drug has a positive effect on visual acuity and scotopic (twilight) vision, as well as being a mild diuretic.

INDICATIONS AND USAGE

Unproven Uses: The Wild Carrot is an unreliable adjuvant in the treatment of oxyuriasis. It is a useful drug in pediatrics for tonsillitis, nutritional disorders, and as a dietary agent for digestive disorders. It is also used in medicinal preparations for dermatological conditions such as photodermatosis and pigment anomalies. It is used in teas for intestinal parasites.

PRECAUTIONS AND ADVERSE REACTIONS

Health risks or side effects following the proper administration of designated therapeutic dosages are not recorded. The drug has a low potential for sensitization through skin contact.

DOSAGE

Mode of Administration: The drug is taken in a ground form or consumed as a juice or vegetable. It is found in ready-made medicinal preparations.

Preparation: The Carrot is finely grated and made into a juice or syrup.

LITERATURE

Cao G, Sofic E, Prior RL. Antioxidant Capacity of Tea and Common Vegetables. *J Agric Food Chem.* 44 (11); 3426-3431. 1996

Chandra A, Nair MG. Supercritical Fluid Carbon Dioxide Extraction of à- and β-Carotene from Carrot (*Daucus carota L.). Phytochem Anal.* 8; 244-246. 1997

Cu JQ, Perineuae F, Delmas M, Gaset A. Comparison of the Chemical Composition of Carrot Seed Essential Oil by Different Solvents. *Flav Fragr J.* 4; 225-231. 1989

Foulds I, Sadhra S. Allergic contact dermatitis from carrots. *Contact Dermatitis* 23; 261. 1990

Kilibarda V, Nanusevic N, Dogovic N, Ivanic R, Savin K. Content of the essential oil of the carrot and its antibacterial activity. *Pharmazie* 51 (10); 777-778. 1996

Hausen B, Allergiepflanzen, Pflanzenallergene, ecomed Verlagsgesellsch. mbH, Landsberg 1988.

Harborne JB, In: The Biology and Chemistry of the Umbelliferae, Ed. VN Heywood, Academic Press, London, 1971.

Kern W, List PH, Hörhammer L (Hrsg.), Hagers Handbuch der Pharmazeutischen Praxis, 4. Aufl., Bde 1-8, Springer Verlag Berlin, Heidelberg, New York, 1969.

Leung AY, Encyclopedia of Common Natural Ingredients Used in Food Drugs and Cosmetics, John Wiley & Sons Inc., New York 1980.

Saad HE, El-Sharkawy SH, Halim AF. Essential oils of *Daucus carota ssp. maximus. Pharm Acta Helv.* 70; 79-84. 1995

Wild Cherry

Prunus serotina

DESCRIPTION

Medicinal Parts: The medicinal part is the inner tree bark, which has an odor similar to almonds, which dissipates on drying.

Flower and Fruit: The racemes are 6 to 15 cm long with about 30 flowers. The perianth remains when the fruit ripens. The 3 to 4 tepals are denticulate and creamy white. The fruit is 8 mm across, depressed-globose, and purple-black. The endocarp is smooth.

Leaves, Stem, and Root: Wild Cherry is a deciduous tree up to 20 m high with aromatic bark. The leaves are obovate to elliptical-oblong, acute, and finely serrate with flattened, forwardly directed teeth. The leaves are dark, glossy green above, paler and slightly pubescent beneath.

Habitat: Prunus serotina originates from North America but is cultivated in Europe.

Production: Wild Cherry bark is the bark of *Prunus serotina.*

Other Names: Black Choke, Choke Cherry, Rum Cherry, Virginian Prune, Wild Black Cherry

ACTIONS AND PHARMACOLOGY

COMPOUNDS

Cyanogenic glycosides: prunasin yielding 0.05 to 0.15%, 5 to 15 mg HCN/100 g

Tannins

EFFECTS

Wild Cherry bark is an astringent, antitussive, and sedative.

INDICATIONS AND USAGE

Unproven Uses: Wild Cherry bark is used for coughs, bronchitis, and whooping cough. It is also used in the treatment of nervous digestive disorders and diarrhea.

PRECAUTIONS AND ADVERSE REACTIONS

No health hazards or side effects are known in conjunction with the proper administration of designated therapeutic dosages. Cyanide poisonings from the drug are unlikely, due to both its low cyanogenic glycoside content and the lack of inclination to ingest it.

DOSAGE

Mode of Administration: Wild Cherry bark is available as syrup or tincture for internal use and also available in commercial compounded preparations.

LITERATURE

Frohne D, Pfänder HJ, Giftpflanzen - Ein Handbuch für Apotheker, Toxikologen und Biologen, 4. Aufl., Wiss. Verlags-Ges. Stuttgart 1997.

Kern W, List PH, Hörhammer L (Hrsg.), Hagers Handbuch der Pharmazeutischen Praxis, 4. Aufl., Bde. 1-8, Springer Verlag Berlin, Heidelberg, New York, 1969.

Leung AY, Encyclopedia of Common Natural Ingredients Used in Food, Drugs and Cosmetics, John Wiley & Sons Inc., New York 1980.

Roth L, Daunderer M, Kormann K, Giftpflanzen, Pflanzengifte, 4. Aufl., Ecomed Fachverlag Landsberg Lech 1993.

Santamour jr, FS. Amygdalin in *Prunus* Leaves. *Phytochemistry* 47 (8); 1537-1538. 1998

Wild Daisy

Bellis perennis

DESCRIPTION

Medicinal Parts: The medicinal part is the whole flowering plant.

Flower and Fruit: The flower heads are usually found singly at the end of the sharply angular stem. The flower is small- to medium-sized and heterogamous. The epicalyx is semispherical to bell-shaped. The sepals of the epicalyx are more or less double-rowed. The receptacle is conical and glabrous when bearing fruit. The 1- to 2-rowed female ray flowers are linguiform, white, pink, purple, or bluish and distinctly longer than the epicalyx. The disc flowers are androgynous, tubular, and have 5 tips. The achenes are obovate, very flattened, ribless, and have side veins. The flower has no pappus but may have short, brittle bristles.

Leaves, Stem, and Root: Wild Daisy is a 10- to 15-cm high perennial plant that has basal leaves in rosettes or alternate leaves at the lower part of the stem; its roots are short and cylindrical. The rosette leaves are circular to spatulate or heart-shaped, dentate, and occasionally entire-margined with a single rib; they have vertical hairs on both sides.

Habitat: The plant is distributed from Portugal to the Moscow region and Asia Minor. It is also found from Great Britain to Ireland and southern Scandinavia, and as far south as the Mediterranean, with the exception of the Balearic Islands and the islands of Sardinia, Sicily, Crete, and Cyprus.

Production: The capitula and short stems of the plant are picked and dried in either the sun or shade.

Other Names: Bruisewort, Daisy, Garden Daisy

ACTIONS AND PHARMACOLOGY

COMPOUNDS

Triterpene saponins (2.7%): bisdemosides of the bayogeninic and polygalic acid (the latter acylated)

Polyynes: including trans-lachnophyllum ester

Flavonoids: including cosmosiin

EFFECTS

The drug acts as an astringent, reduces mucous production, and also has anti-inflammatory and fever-reducing effects, possibly due to the triterpene saponin content.

INDICATIONS AND USAGE

Unproven Uses: Wild Daisy is used as an expectorant and for easing diarrhea and gastrointestinal catarrh. It is also used for treating wounds, skin diseases, coughs and bronchitis, disorders of the liver and kidneys, and inflammation.

Homeopathic Uses: Wild Daisy is used for bruises, bleeding, muscular pain (after injuries), purulent skin diseases, and rheumatism.

PRECAUTIONS AND ADVERSE REACTIONS

No health hazards or side effects are known in conjunction with the proper administration of designated therapeutic dosages.

DOSAGE

Mode of Administration: The drug is used topically, as an extract, in teas, and in poultices of pressed leaves for the treatment of skin diseases. A decoction can be used for wound poultices.

Preparation: An infusion or cold extract is prepared by adding 2 teaspoonfuls of drug to 2 cups of water, then allowing it to draw for 20 minutes. A decoction is made from the green leaves.

Daily Dosage: The daily dose of the infusion is 2 to 4 cups per day.

Homeopathic Dosage: 5 to 10 drops, 1 tablet, or 5 to 10 globules 1 to 3 times daily; parenterally: 1 mL sc injection solution twice weekly; ointments: 1 to 2 times daily (HAB1).

LITERATURE

Avato P, Vitali C, Mongelli P, Tava A. Antimicrobial Activity of Polyacetylenes from *Bellis perennis* and their Synthetic Derivatives. *Planta Med.* 63 (6); 503-507. 1997

Avato P, Tava A. Acetylenes and Terpenoids from *Bellis perennis. Phytochemistry* 40 (1); 141-147. 1995

Avato P, Vitali C, Tava A, New acetylenic compounds from *Bellis perennis L.* and their antimicrobial activity. In: *PM* 61(Abstracts of 43rd Ann Congr):49. 1995.

Desevedavy C, Amoros M, Girre L, Lavaud C, Massiot G. Antifungal Agents: In Vitro and in vivo Antifungal Extract from the Common Daisy, *Bellis perennis. Planta Med.* 52 (1); 184-185. 1989

Schöpke T, Wray V, Hiller K, Triterpenoid saponins of plants of the Asteraeae tribe (Asteraceae). In: *PM* 59(7):A591. 1992.

Schöpke Th et al., Saponin composition of the *Bellis* genus and related species. In: *PM* 61(Abstracts of 43rd Ann Congr):68. 1995.

Willigmann I et al., Antimycotic compounds from different *Bellis perennis* varieties. In: *PM* 58(Suppl.7):A636. 1993.

Wild Indigo

Baptisia tinctoria

DESCRIPTION

Medicinal Parts: The medicinal part of the plant is the root.

Flower and Fruit: The flowers are terminal and axillary in 7- to 10-cm long, lightly flowered racemes. The pedicles are 3 to 5 cm long. The calyx is 4 to 5 mm long and glabrous with a slight fringe. The corolla is yellow. The standard is circular with convoluted sides and is slightly shorter than the oblong wings. The 10 stamens are freestanding. The ovary is stemmed, elliptoid, drawn together at the style and stigma, and is glabrous. The fruit is a blue-black, ovoid, slightly swollen pod, 7 to 15 mm long, with a sharp tip. The seeds are yellowish-brown, kidney-shaped, and 2 mm long.

Leaves, Stem, and Root: The shrug is many-branched and grows to 1 m high with woody rootstock and knotty branches. The stem is 1 to 3 mm thick, round, slightly grooved, and glabrous. The alternating leaves are trifoliate and have a 1 to 3 mm long petiole. The stipules are small and arrow-shaped, and drop early. The leaflets are 1 to 4 cm long, and 0.6 to 1 cm wide, ovate, almost sessile, and entire-margined. They are wedge-shaped at the base and rounded at the tip. The distinct midrib on the lower surface is pubescent. The leaves are brittle. The roots vary in diameter from 0.2 to 1.5 cm. The outer surface is brownish, vertically wrinkled and grooved. It is also warty due to root fibers sticking to the surface. The tissue is solid and fibrous. The transverse fracture shows a thick bark and whitish wood with concentric rings.

Characteristics: The taste is bitter and acrid; the odor is faint. The leaves yield an indigo dye; the wood a red dye.

Habitat: Wild Indigo is indigenous to southern Canada and the eastern and northeastern U.S.

Production: Wild indigo root is the underground part of *Baptisia tinctoria*, which is collected and dried in autumn from plants growing in the wild.

Not to be Confused With: Wild Indigo can be confused or adulterated with the root of *Baptisia australis* (false blue indigo) and *Baptisia alba.*

Other Names: Baptisia, Horse-Fly Weed, Indigo Broom, Rattlebush, Yellow Indigo

ACTIONS AND PHARMACOLOGY

COMPOUNDS

Water-soluble polysaccharide: in particular arabinogalactans

Glycoproteins

Quinolizidine alkaloids: including cytisine, N-methyl cytisine, anagyrine, sparteine

Isoflavonoids: formononetin baptigenin, pseudobaptigenin, maackiain, formononetin and their glycosides baptisin, pseudobaptisin, trifolirhizin

Hydroxycumarins: including scopoletine

EFFECTS

The ethanol extract has had a significantly positive effect on the phagocytosis of human erythrocytes. It has also been found to raise the leukocyte count and to improve the endogenous defense reaction. Wild Indigo has a mild estrogenic effect. In animal experimentation, the polysaccharide and glycoprotein fraction contained in the drug demonstrated an immune-stimulating effect. Changes in mice included an increase of phagocytosis activity of Kupffer's cells; a significant, dose-dependent stimulation of lymphocytes; and release of interleukin-1 macrophages. Antiviral effects have been shown when Wild Indigo is used in combination with Echinacea and Thuja.

INDICATIONS AND USAGE

Unproven Uses: Wild Indigo root is used for septic and typhoid cases with prostration and fever, such as diphtheria, influenza, malaria, and typhus. It is used internally for infections of the upper respiratory tract, the common cold, tonsillitis, stomatitis, fever, lymphadenitis, and furunculosis. It is used externally as an ointment for painless ulcers, inflamed nipples, and as a douche for leukorrhea. The efficacy of the drug has not been proved. Native America Indians traditionally have used the root to make a tea to treat fever, scarlet fever, typhoid, and pharyngitis and externally as an ointment for sores. Water in which the root has been soaked is used to clean open and inflamed wounds. Canadian Indians used the plant for treating gonorrhea and disease of the kidneys and as an expectorant.

Homeopathic Uses: Uses in homeopathy include severe febrile infections, states of confusion and blood poisoning.

CONTRAINDICATIONS

Use of the drug is contraindicated during pregnancy.

PRECAUTIONS AND ADVERSE REACTIONS

No health hazards or side effects are known in conjunction with the proper administration of designated therapeutic dosages.

OVERDOSAGE

Only very high dosages (for example, 30 g of the drug) lead to signs of poisoning (vomiting, diarrhea, gastrointestinal complaints, spasms), due to the quinolizidine alkaloid content.

DOSAGE

Mode of Administration: Wild Indigo is not common as a drug, but is found in combination preparations; taken internally as a tea and tincture; and used externally as an ointment.

How Supplied:

Drops

Injection solutions

Liquid — 1:1 and 1:2, with and without alcohol.

Suppositories

Tablets

Preparation: To prepare an ointment, use 1 part liquid extract to 8 parts ointment base. A tincture may be prepared using the liquid extract in 60% alcohol 1:1.

Daily Dosage: Dosage for a single dose is 0.5 g to 1 g of the dried drug as decoction, to be taken 3 times daily.

Homeopathic Dosage: 5 to 10 drops, 1 tablet, or 5 to 10 globules 1 to 3 times daily or 1 mL injection solution twice weekly sc (HAB34).

LITERATURE

Beuscher H, Kopanski L, Modulation of the immune response by polymeric substances from *Baptisia tinctoria* and *Echinacea angustifolia*. In: *Pharm Weekblad Sci Ed.* 9:229. 1987.

Beuscher N, Beuscher HU, Bodinet C, Enhanced Release of Interleukin-1 from Mouse Macrophages by Glykoproteins and Polysaccharides from *Baptisia tinctoria* and *Echinacea* Species. In: PM, Abstracts of the 37th Annual Congress on Medicinal Plant Research Braunschwe.

Beuscher N, Bodinet C, Willigmann I, Harnischfeger G, Biologiocal activity of *Baptisia tinctoria* extracts. In: Inst. für Angew. Botanik der Univ. Hamburg, Angewandte Botanik, Berichte 6, 46-61. 1997.

Beuscher N, Scheit KH, Bodinet C, Egert D, Modulation der körpereigenen Immunabwehr durch polymere Substanzen aus *Baptisia tinctoria* und *Echinacea purpurea.* In: Immunotherapeutic prospects of infectious diseases, Hrsg. Masihi KN, Lange W. Springer, Heidel.

Beuscher N, Scheit KH, Bodinet C, Kopanski L, Immunologisch aktive Glykoproteine aus Baptisia tinctoria. In: PM 55:358-363. 1989.

Bodinet C, Beuscher N, Kopanski L, Purification of Immunologically Active Glycoproteins from *Baptisia tinctoria* Roots by Affinity Chromatography and Isoelectric Focussing. In: PM, Abstracts of the 37th Annual Congress on Medicinal Plant Research Braunschwe.

Egert D, Beuscher N. Studies on Antigen Specifity of Immunoreactive Arabinogalactan Proteins extracted from *Baptisia tinctoria* and *Echinacea purpurea. Planta Med.* 58; 163-165. 1992

Henneicke-von Zepelin HH et al. Efficacy and safety of a fixed combination phytomedicine in the treatment of the common cold (acute viral respiratory tract infection): results of a randomised, double blind, placebo controlled, multicentre study. *Cur Med Res* 15-3..1999

Hentschel C et al. Akute virale Atemwegsinfekte. Wirksamkeit und Sicherheit eines phytotherapeutischen Kombinationspräparats in der Erkältungsbehandlung. Fortschritte der Medizin. Originalien 118, 1. 2000

Wild Mint

Mentha aquatica

DESCRIPTION

Medicinal Parts: The medicinal part is the dried leaf.

Flower and Fruit: The flowers are in 2 to 3 dense false axillary whorls with inconspicuous bracts. The upper ones are fused into a terminal, globular, or ovate capitulum. The calyx is tubular, with 13 ribs, and glabrous interior. The tips are awl-shaped to triangular. The pedicles are pubescent. The corolla is violet with a ring of hair in the tube. The fruit is hard with an ovoid, light brown nutlet.

Leaves, Stem, and Root: Wild Mint is a perennial, 20 to 80 cm high plant with a branched underground rhizome and an erect stem with alternate sessile curly leaves. The stem is branched in the upper half and terminates in spikes of blue flowers. The leaves are ovate and serrated.

Characteristics: The whole plant smells of caraway. The plant is a result of many crossbreedings in gardens and fields.

Habitat: The plant grows in Europe, northern Africa and western Asia. In has been introduced to America, Australia, and Madiera.

Production: Wild Mint is the aerial part of *Mentha aquatica*. The drug is derived from the dried leaves.

Other Names: Hairy Mint, Marsh Mint, Water Mint

ACTIONS AND PHARMACOLOGY

COMPOUNDS

Volatile oil: chief components - menthofurane, beta-caryophyllene, 1,8-cineole, germacren D, limonene, viridiflorol, a chemotype contains isopinocamphone as chief constituent (according to older references, also linalool, linalyl acetate, cineole, menthone)

Tannins

EFFECTS

The drug is an astringent and a stimulant.

INDICATIONS AND USAGE

Unproven Uses: Water Mint is used for diarrhea and dysmenorrhea.

PRECAUTIONS AND ADVERSE REACTIONS

No health hazards or side effects are known in conjunction with the proper administration of designated therapeutic dosages.

DOSAGE

Mode of Administration: Ground drug is used as an infusion.

Preparation: Add approximately 30 g of the drug to 500 mL of water.

Daily Dosage: As a daily dose, drink a wineglassful during the course of the day.

LITERATURE

Avato P, Sgarra G, Casadoro G. Chemical composition of the essential oils of *Mentha* species cultivated in Italy. *Sci Pharm.* 63; 223-230. 1995

Hänsel R, Keller K, Rimpler H, Schneider G (Hrsg.), Hagers Handbuch der Pharmazeutischen Praxis, 5. Aufl., Bde 4-6 (Drogen), Springer Verlag Berlin, Heidelberg, New York, 1992-1994.

Wild Radish

Raphanus raphanistrum

DESCRIPTION

Medicinal Parts: The medicinal part is the fresh plant before flowering.

Flower and Fruit: The flowers are bright yellow, sometimes white with violet veins. The form of the flower corresponds to that of the Cruciferae. The calyx is erect. The pods are cylindrical with vertical grooves between which the seeds are tied (like a string of pearls). The pods fall apart at these points.

Leaves, Stem, and Root: The leaves are petiolate and lyrate; the upper ones are lanceolate. The leaves and lower part of the stem are covered in stiff hair.

Habitat: The plant has been cultivated for a very long time and is grown in all parts of the world, especially in temperate regions.

Production: Wild Radish is the fresh plant of *Raphanus raphanistrum* before flowering.

Other Names: Jointed-Podded Charlock

ACTIONS AND PHARMACOLOGY

COMPOUNDS

Glucosinolates in the freshly harvested, unbruised plant: chief component glucoputranjivine, which yields isopropyl mustard oil as the cells are destroyed.

EFFECTS

No information is available.

INDICATIONS AND USAGE

Unproven Uses: Wild Radish is used for skin conditions and stomach disorders.

PRECAUTIONS AND ADVERSE REACTIONS

No health hazards or side effects are known in conjunction with the proper administration of designated therapeutic dosages. Administration of high dosages of the freshly harvested plant can lead to mucous membrane irritation of the gastrointestinal tract.

DOSAGE

Mode of Administration: Wild Radish is administered ground and as an alcoholic extract.

LITERATURE

Daria V et al. New Contribution to the Ethnopharmacological Study of the Canary Islands. *J Ethnopharmacol.* 25; 77-92. 1989

Kern W, List PH, Hörhammer L (Hrsg.), Hagers Handbuch der Pharmazeutischen Praxis, 4. Aufl., Bde. 1-8: Springer Verlag Berlin, Heidelberg, New York, 1969.

Wild Service Tree

Sorbus torminalis

DESCRIPTION

Medicinal Parts: The medicinal parts are the ripe fruit.

Flower and Fruit: The flowers are in erect, loose umbelliferous panicles on loosely tomentose pedicles, which later become glaborous. The petals are white and the anthers light yellow. The false fruit is orbicular-oblong and 1.5 cm long. The fruit is initially reddish-yellow, later brown, and speckled. The 4 seeds are oblong, deltoid, 7 mm long, and dark red-brown.

Leaves, Stem, and Root: The tree may sometimes grow up to 22 m with a widely domed crown. The bark is dark brown or gray. It is cracked into scaly plates. The older branches are glabrous, gray-brown, glossy, and angular with lighter lenticles. The younger branches are loosely tomentose, greenish, later turning reddish-brown. The buds are broad ovoid and glabrous with shiny green scales. The buds are brown at the edge and loosely pubescent or glabrous. The leaves have 5 cm long, thin, downy, loosely tomentose petioles, which are fresh green. The petioles turn blood-red in autumn.

Habitat: The plant is common in northern temperate zones. It is cultivated in many regions.

Production: Wild Service Tree berries are the fruits of *Sorbus torminalis*.

Other Names: Ash, Wild Sorvice

ACTIONS AND PHARMACOLOGY

COMPOUNDS

Sugar alcohols: sorbitol

The fruits do not contain parasorboside, in contrast to those of *Sorbus aucuparia*.

The drug has not been fully researched.

EFFECTS

No information is available.

INDICATIONS AND USAGE

See Mountain Ash Berry (*Sorbus aucuparia*).

PRECAUTIONS AND ADVERSE REACTIONS

No health hazards or side effects are known in conjunction with the proper administration of designated therapeutic dosages.

DOSAGE

Mode of Administration: See Mountain Ash Berry (*Sorbus aucuparia*).

LITERATURE

Kokubun T, Harborne JB, Waterman PG. Antifungal Biphenyl Compounds are the Phytoalexins of the Sapwood of *Sorbus aucuparia. Phytochemistry* 40 (1); 57-59. 1995

Wild Thyme

Thymus serpyllum

DESCRIPTION

Medicinal Parts: The medicinal parts are the dried aerial parts, the aerial shoots collecting during the flowering season and dried, the fresh aerial parts of the flowering plant, and the whole plant.

Flower and Fruit: The inflorescence is globular to very elongated, often interrupted in false whorls, which are separate from each other. The calyx is tubular-campanualte with 10 distinct ribs. The 3 tips of the upper lip are short and ciliate. The 2 lower tips are awl-shaped, longer than the upper tips, and ciliate. The corolla is 3 to 6 cm long with a short tube. It is light to dark purple, occasionally white.

Leaves, Stem, and Root: The plant is a slightly woody subshrub that grows from 10 to 30 cm high. The flowering stems are erect. The nonflowering stems are decumbent, round, or mildly quadrangular, pubescent all around and rooting at all points. The leaves are small, linear or elliptical, and obtuse. The leaves are also flat, narrowing to the petiole, ciliate at the base, glabrous or rough-haired, with protruding nerves.

Characteristics: The odor is aromatic.

Habitat: The plant is found in all temperate regions of Eurasia.

Production: Wild thyme consists of the steamed distillation the dried, flowering, above-ground parts of *Thymus serpyllum.*

Not to be Confused With: Herba Thymi (thymian)

Other Names: Creeping Thyme, Mother of Thyme, Serpyllum, Shepherd's Thyme, White Thyme

ACTIONS AND PHARMACOLOGY

COMPOUNDS

Volatile oil (0.2-0.6%): as a collective species, Thymus serpyllum (over 20 subspecies) encompasses a large number of chemical strains with different volatile oil make-up; chief component is usually carvacrol, further containing, among others, borneol, isobutyl acetate, caryophyllene, 1,8-cineole, citral, citronellal, citronellol, p-cymene, geraniol, geranyl acetate, linalool, linalyl acetate, alpha-pinene, gamma-terpinene, alpha-terpineol, terpinyl acetate and thymol

Flavonoids: including among others scutellarenine-7-O-glucoside-4-O-rhamnoside

Caffeic acid derivatives: in particular rosmarinic acid (2.3%)

EFFECTS

In animal experiments, an antihormonal and thyroid hormone-like effect on the pituitary has been demonstrated. The herbs efficacy for treating conditions of the upper respiratory tract is due to the presence of the aromatic and spicy smelling essential oil.

INDICATIONS AND USAGE

Approved by Commission E:

- Cough
- Bronchitis

The herb is used internally for catarrhs of the upper respiratory tract.

Unproven Uses: Kidney and bladder disorders, and as a stomachic, carminative, and expectorant. It is also used internally for dysmenorrhea, coliclike pain, and whooping cough. The herb is used externally in herbal cures, baths (especially for respiratory tract conditions), and alcoholic extracts, as well as in embrocations for rheumatic disorders and sprains.

Chinese Medicine: The herb is used for vomiting, diarrhea, flatulence, coughs, toothache, itching, and general pain syndrome.

PRECAUTIONS AND ADVERSE REACTIONS

No health hazards or side effects are known in conjunction with the proper administration of designated therapeutic dosages.

DOSAGE

Mode of Administration: Wild Thyme is administered as a comminuted drug for infusions, teas, and other preparations internally. The drug is a component of various standardized preparations of antitussives. Alcoholic extracts of the herb are contained in cough drops.

Preparation: To make an infusion, pour boiling water over 1.5 to 2 g finely cut drug, steep for 10 minutes, then strain (1 teaspoonful = 1.4 g drug). For a liquid extract, use a ratio of 1:1 with either 45% ethanol or 20% ethanol. For a tincture, use a ratio of 1:10 with 70% ethanol. To make a bath, add 1 g drug (or equivalent of 0.004 g Wild Thyme oil) to 1 liter water, filter, then add to bath water.

Daily Dosage: The average daily dosage is 4 to 6 g of herb. As a stomachic, drink one cup of tea before meals. Other daily dosages are as follows: powder: take 2 g drug mixed with honey; infusion: single dose, 0.6 to 4 g, 2 to 3 cups per day; liquid extract: single dose, 0.4 to 4 mL 3 times daily; liquid extract: daily dose, 5 to 15 g (1 g or 30 drops).

Storage: Protect from light.

LITERATURE

Adzet T et al., Chromatographic Analysis of Polyphenols of some Iberian Thymus species. *Pharm Weekbl Sci Ed.* 9; 218. 1987.

Bellomaria B, Valentin G, Arnold HJ. Composition and variation of essential oil of *Thymus integer* Griseb. of Cyprus. *Pharmazie* 49; 684-688. 1994

Broucke CO van den, Lemli JA. Pharmacological and Chemical Investigations of Thyme Liquid Extracts. *Planta Med.* 41; 129-135. 1981

Wild Turnip

Brassica rapa

DESCRIPTION

Medicinal Parts: The medicinal part of the plant is the root.

Flower and Fruit: The flowers are in racemes. There are 4 almost horizontally splayed sepals. The 4 petals are yellow, 11 to 14 mm long, approximately 1.5 times as long as the calyx, with an orbicular-elliptical plate. There are 2 short and 4 long stamens. The 4-carpeled ovary is superior and fused. The fruit is 4.5 to 6.5 cm long, a dehiscent pod opening on 2 sides with a septum and 15 to 25 seeds. The seeds are globose and reticulate with a diameter of approximately 1.5 to 3 mm.

Leaves, Stem, and Root: Turnip is an annual or biennial herb, and grows up to 0.8 m high. The leaves are alternate, grass-green, with a slight bluish bloom and always bristly pubescent. The lower ones are petiolate, pinnatisect with a terminal lobe; the middle and upper leaves are sessile, simple, dentate, or entire. The stem of the larger plants is branched. The root is thin and spindle-shaped.

Habitat: Europe, North Africa, and the U.S.

Production: The seeds are cold-pressed and then refined. Rapeseed oil is the cold-pressed and refined oil from the ripe seeds of *Brassica napus* and *Brassica rapa.*

Not to be Confused With: Rapeseed oil may be adulterated with resins and mineral oil. *Sinapis arvensis* is a permitted substitute

Other Names: Chinese Cabbage, Field Mustard, Oilseed Turnip, Turnip Rape, Turnip Greens,

ACTIONS AND PHARMACOLOGY

COMPOUNDS

Fatty oil: chief fatty acids: oleic acid (45 to 65%), linoleic acid (18 to 32%), linolenic acid (10%), including as well palmitic acid, stearic acid, eicosanoic acid, behenic acid; varieties with high erucic acid content (40 to 50%) are no longer cultivated (reduction of the erucic acid content in the Common Market countries to below 5%)

Sterols: beta-sitosterol, campesterol, brassicasterol, estered to some extent

EFFECTS

Rapeseed oil, when ingested in high dosages over an extended period of time, is cardiotoxic. The drug is chiefly used as a substitute for olive oil and in the manufacture of salves and liniments.

INDICATIONS AND USAGE

No medicinal indications

PRECAUTIONS AND ADVERSE REACTIONS

No health hazards are known in conjunction with the proper administration of designated therapeutic dosages of the oil, which is low on erucic acid.

DOSAGE

Storage: Store in the dark, in well-filled containers.

LITERATURE

Butcher RD, Goodman BA, Deighton N, Smith WH. Evaluation of the allergic/irritant potential of air pollutants: detection of proteins modified by volatile organic compounds from oilseed rape (*Brassica napus ssp. oleifera*) using electrospray ionization-mass spectrometry. *Clin Exp Allergy*, 25. 1995

Gatti GL, Michalek H. Investigations on Rapseed Oil Toxicology. *Arzneim Forsch.* 25 (1); 1639-1642. 1975

Hänsel R, Keller K, Rimpler H, Schneider G (Ed), Hagers Handbuch der Pharmazeutischen Praxis, 5. Aufl., Bde 4 - 6 (Drogen), Springer Verlag Berlin, Heidelberg, New York, 1992-1994.

Kull D, Pfander H. Isolation and Identification of Carotenoids from Petals of Rape (*Brassica napus*). *J Agric Food Chem.* 43 (11); 2854-2857. 1995

Inamori Y, Muro C, Sajima E, Katagiri M, Okamoto Y, Tanaka H, Sakagami Y, Tsujibo H, Biological activity of purpurogallin. *Biosci Biotechnol Biochem*, 61:890-2, May 1997

Wild Yam

Dioscorea villosa

DESCRIPTION

Medicinal Parts: The medicinal part is the dried rhizome with the roots.

Flower and Fruit: The plant has small greenish-yellow flowers. The male flowers are in drooping panicles; the female ones in drooping spicate racemes.

Leaves, Stem, and Root: Dioscorea villosa is a perennial vine. It has a pale brown, cylindrical, twisted, tuberous rhizome and a thin, woolly, reddish-brown stem that measures up to 12 m long. The leaves are broadly ovate, usually alternating, cordate and 6 to 14 cm long. The upper surface of the leaves is glabrous and they are pubescent beneath. The fracture is short and hard.

Characteristics: The taste is insipid at first, then acrid. The leaves are odorless.

Habitat: The plant is indigenous to the Southern U.S. and Canada. It is now widely cultivated in many parts of the world in tropical, subtropical, and temperate regions.

Production: Wild Yam root is the root and rhizome of *Dioscorea villosa*.

Other Names: China Root, Colic Root, Devil's Bones, Rheumatism Root, Yuma

ACTIONS AND PHARMACOLOGY

COMPOUNDS

Saponins: including dioscin (aglycone diosgenin)

Isoquinuclidine alkaloids: including dioscorin

Pyrridinal alkaloids: including dioscorine

EFFECTS

Wild Yam has an antispasmodic, and a mild diaphoretic effect. The root of the plant is used as a precursor for manufacturing progesterone and estrogen. Though the diosgenin component has been promoted as a ''natural progesterone,'' diosgenin does not have any progesterone-like effects. The body does not convert diosgenin into estrogen or any other steroid.

Anti-Inflammatory Effect: In the rat model, diosgenin has been found to decrease the intestinal inflammation that accompanies indomethacin use.

Biliary Cholesterol Elimination Effect: Diosgenin has been shown to markedly increase the biliary output of cholesterol and lipid lamellar structures in the rat model. Diosgenin also has a cytoprotective effect on the rat liver that is subjected to obstructive cholestasis.

Estrogenic Effect: Diosgenin has been found to have an estrogenic effect on mouse mammary epithelium. Ovariectomized mice that received diosgenin (sc) at dosage levels between 20 and 40 mg/kg for 15 days had significant increases in mammary development scores. When administered estrogen and diosgenin, an augmentation of the estrogenic effect was recorded.

INDICATIONS AND USAGE

Unproven Uses: Wild Yam is used for rheumatic conditions, gallbladder colic, dysmenorrhea, and cramps.

Wild Yam is used industrially as an active agent in the half-synthesis of steroid hormones and for the manufacture of homeopathic preparations.

PRECAUTIONS AND ADVERSE REACTIONS

General: Health risks or side effects following the proper administration of designated therapeutic dosages are not recorded.

DRUG INTERACTIONS

POTENTIAL INTERACTIONS

There is evidence that the diosgenin component of Wild Yam may decrease the anti-inflammatory effect of indomethacin by increasing the elimination constant and reducing plasma levels of indomethacin. Wild Yam may have an additive estrogenic effect when administered with estrogen containing drugs.

OVERDOSAGE

Poisoning is conceivable with overdosages because of the picrotoxin-like effect of dioscorin (see Cocculi fructus).

DOSAGE

Mode of Administration: Liquid extract.

How Supplied:

Capsules—200 mg, 400 mg, 505 mg, 535 mg

Liquid—1:1; 1:2; 250 mg/mL

LITERATURE

Hegnauer R, Chemotaxonomie der Pflanzen, Bde 1-11, Birkhäuser Verlag Basel, Boston, Berlin 1962-1997.

Kern W, List PH, Hörhammer L (Hrsg.), Hagers Handbuch der Pharmazeutischen Praxis, 4. Aufl., Bde 1-8, Springer Verlag Berlin, Heidelberg, New York, 1969.

Madaus G, Lehrbuch der Biologischen Arzneimittel, Bde 1-3, Nachdruck, Georg Olms Verlag Hildesheim 1979.

Willow Herb

Epilobium species

DESCRIPTION

Medicinal Parts: The medicinal parts are the herb and the roots of the drug containing Epilobium varieties.

Flower and Fruit: The flowers are arranged in terminal clusters in the axils of foliage supporting the leaves. The receptacle extends over the ovary. There are 4 sepals that are often colored and 8 stamens. The petals are purple to pink seldom white or yellow. The style is erect or curved downwards. The stigma is capitual or club-like and has 4 grooves or is divided into 4. The fruit is long, linear capsule-like, quadrangular, 4-valved and opens with 4 bending valves. The seeds are numerous and smooth or they may be covered in tiny warts with a white, often short-stemmed, tuft of hair.

Leaves, Stem and Root: The species includes perennial herbs and occasionally up to 2 m high sub-shrubs with underground creeping rhizomes. The stems are erect, glabrous or covered with simple hairs or glandular hairs. The leaves are entire-margined or dentate. They are alternate or opposite and in whorls of 3, which are flat or occasionally with a turned-back border.

Habitat: The plant is found all over Europe, Asia, Africa and America, Australia, Tasmania, and New Zealand.

Production: Willow Herb is the aerial part of *Epilobium parviflorum* and other small-blossomed Willow Herbs. The herb is dried in the open air in the shade.

Other Names: Blood Vine, Blooming Sally, Rose Bay Willow Herb, Willow-Herb

ACTIONS AND PHARMACOLOGY

COMPOUNDS: ANGUSTIFOLIUM VARIETY

Flavonoids: in particular myricitrin, isoquercitrin, quercitrin, guaiaverin, quercetin-3-O-beta-D-glucuronide

Palmitate

Steroids: in particular beta-sitosterol and its ester, including among others beta-sitosterol caproate

Tannins

COMPOUNDS: HIRSUTUM VARIETY

Flavonoids: in particular guaiaverin, hyperoside, myricitrin, quercetin-3-O-beta-D-glucuronide, quercetin-3-O-alpha-L-arabinofuranoside

Steroids: in particular beta-sitosterol

Tannins

COMPOUNDS: PARVIFLORUM VARIETY

Flavonoids: in particular guaiaverin, quercetin-3-O-beta-D-glucuronide, quercitrin

Palmitate

Steroids: in particular beta-sitosterol and its ester, including among others beta-sitosterol caproate

Tannins

EFFECTS

Willow Herb is reported to have antiphlogistic, antiexudative, antimicrobial, and tumor-inhibiting effects. A watery infusion revealed a significant inhibitory effect on edema in rat paws. The methanol infusion had a distinctly weaker effect. Antimicrobial effects have also been demonstrated. A suspension of the fresh drug in ethanol stunts the growth of the bacteria of *Pseudomonas pyocyanea.* Tincture and the liquid extract showed anti-microbial effect against *Candida albicans*, *Staphylococcus albus* and *Staphylococcus aureus*. The dried residue of a maceration, which is fixed on filter paper, shows a weak effect against *Bacillus subtilis*, *Escherichia coli*, *Mycobacterium smegmatis*, *Shigella flexneri*, *Shigella sonnei* and *Staphylococcus aureus*. An extra fraction of the drug (insufficiently chemically defined) showed a tumor-inhibiting effect on transplanted tumors in mice and rats. The drug was helpful in treating benign prostate hyperplasia and certain micturition disorders.

INDICATIONS AND USAGE

Unproven Uses: Willow Herb fever, rheumatic complaints, headache, and general pain relief.

PRECAUTIONS AND ADVERSE REACTIONS

Health risks or side effects following the proper administration of designated therapeutic dosages are not recorded.

DOSAGE

Mode of Administration: The drug is not available as a ready made medicinal preparation; only as a tea, watery extract or as a vegetable.

LITERATURE

Ducrey B et al., Inhibition of 5alpha-Reduktase and aromatase by ellagitannins oenothein A and eonothein B from Epilobium species. In: *PM* 63(2):111-114. 1997.

Hänsel R, Keller K, Rimpler H, Schneider G (Hrsg.), Hagers Handbuch der Pharmazeutischen Praxis, 5. Aufl., Bde 4-6

(Drogen), Springer Verlag Berlin, Heidelberg, New York, 1992-1994.

Hiemann A, Mayr K, *Sci Pharm* 53:39. 1985.

Hiermann A, *Sci Pharm* 63:135. 1995.

Lesuisse D et al., Determination of Oenothein B as the active 5-alpha-reductase-inhibiting principles of the folk medicine *Epilobium parvifloruam*. In: *JNP* 59(5):490-492. 1996.

Slacanin I et al., *J Chromatogr* 557:391. 1991.

Wichtl M (Hrsg.), Teedrogen, 4. Aufl., Wiss. Verlagsges. Stuttgart 1997.

Winter Cherry

Physalis alkekengi

DESCRIPTION

Medicinal Parts: The medicinal parts are the ripe fruit and the leaves.

Flower and Fruit: The whitish, long-pedicled flowers are solitary and nodding. The calyx is fused and 5-tipped. The corolla is fused with a slightly 5-tipped margin. There are 5 stamens and 1 superior ovary. The fruit is a cherry-sized, globular, scarlet berry, enclosed in the swollen, orange-red calyx. It contains numerous flat, reniform seeds.

Leaves, Stem, and Root: The plant is a perennial and grows from 30 to 60 cm. The stems are erect or ascending and angular with opposite, long-petioled, entire-margined leaves.

Characteristics: Winter Cherry has a lantern-like, enlarged calyx when the fruit is ripe.

Habitat: The plant is indigenous to central and southern Europe, China, and Indochina and is naturalized in the U.S.

Production: Winter Cherry fruits are the ripe fruits of *Physalis alkekengi.*

Other Names: Cape Gooseberry, Coqueret, Strawberry Tomato

ACTIONS AND PHARMACOLOGY

COMPOUNDS

Whitasteroids: among others physalines A-C, F, L-O

Carotinoids: including zeaxanthine dipalmitic acid ester (red)

EFFECTS

No information is available.

INDICATIONS AND USAGE

Unproven Uses: Winter Cherry is used as a diuretic in kidney and bladder conditions and in the treatment of gout and rheumatism.

PRECAUTIONS AND ADVERSE REACTIONS

The ripe fruit is edible, but unripe fruit can cause poisoning in animals.

DOSAGE

Mode of Administration: The drug is administered in a ground form and as an extract.

LITERATURE

Dornberger K, Untersuchungen über potentiell antineoplastisch wirksame Inhaltsstoffe von *Physalis alkekengi* L. var. franchettii MAST. In: PA 41:265. 1986.

Vessal M, Mehrani HA, Omrani GH, Effects of an aqueous extract of Physalis alkekengi fruit on estrus cycle, reproduction and uterine craetive kinase BB-isoenzyme in rats. In: ETH 34(1):69-78. 1991.

Völksen W, Zur Kenntnis der Inhaltsstoffe und arzneilichen Verwendung einiger Physalisarten - Ph. alkekengi, Ph. franchettii, Ph. peruviana. In: DAZ 117(30):1199-1203. 1977.

Winter's Bark

Drimys winteri

DESCRIPTION

Medicinal Parts: The medicinal part is the dried bark of the trunk and larger branches.

Flower and Fruit: The flowers are solitary or in umbels and often in clusters at the tips of the branches. They are fragrant and white. The sepals are membranous, broadly ovate to reniform. The 4 to 14 petals are also membranous, oblong to narrow-ovate. The 15 to 40 stamens are in 2 to 4 rows. The 2 to 10 carpels are free, ovate, or elliptical. There are 9 to 18 ovules on a short seed stalk. The fruit is berrylike, black to violet, fleshy, and usually contains 2 or 3 seeds.

Leaves, Stem, and Root: The plant is an evergreen tree or shrub, with brownish or gray wrinkled branches. The bark is aromatic and smooth. The leaf blade is coriaceous, oblong-ovate to elliptical, with a somewhat revolute margin. The undersurface is usually punctate.

Characteristics: Winter's Bark has an astringent taste and mild smell.

Habitat: The plant is found from central Chile to Cape Horn and in neighboring Argentina.

Production: Genuine Winter's Bark is the bark of *Drimys winteri*. The bark is collected from the dried trunk or produced from the stronger branches. It is collected in uncultivated regions.

Not to be Confused With: The drug is often confused with *Cortex Canellae albae* and with the bark of *Cinnamodendron corticosum.*

Other Names: Pepper Bark, Wintera Aromatica, Wintera, Winter's Cinnamon

ACTIONS AND PHARMACOLOGY

COMPOUNDS

Sesquiterpenes: including drimenol, drimenin, confertifoline, polygodial, isodrimenine, winterin, valdiviolide, fuegin, futranolide, cryptomeridiol, 1beta-p-cumaroyloxypolygodial, a trimeric sesquiterpene lactone

Volatile oil: chief components eugenol, caryophyllene, 1,8-cineol, pinenes

EFFECTS
The drug has carminative, stomachic, and tonic effects due to the sesquiterpenes (bitter effect) and tannins.

INDICATIONS AND USAGE
Unproven Uses: In South America, the drug is used for toothache and for dermatitis.

PRECAUTIONS AND ADVERSE REACTIONS
Health risks or side effects following the proper administration of designated therapeutic dosages are not recorded.

DOSAGE
Mode of Administration: As an infusion and domestic herb.

LITERATURE
Hänsel R, Keller K, Rimpler H, Schneider G (Hrsg.), Hagers Handbuch der Pharmazeutischen Praxis, 5. Aufl., Bde 4-6 (Drogen): Springer Verlag Berlin, Heidelberg, New York, 1992-1994.

Hegnauer R, Chemotaxonomie der Pflanzen, Bde 1-11, Birkhäuser Verlag Basel, Boston, Berlin 1962-1997.

Morton JF, An Atlas of Medicinal Plants of Middle America, Charles C. Thomas USA 1981.

Wintergreen

Gaultheria procumbens

DESCRIPTION
Medicinal Parts: The medicinal parts of the plant are the leaves and the oil extracted from them, as well as the fruit.

Flower and Fruit: The 7.5 mm long, solitary, hanging flowers grow from the base of the leaves. They are white or pale pink and campanulate. The fruit is the enlarged calyx. The scarlet berries are dull red and about 0.5 cm in diameter when dried. They are fleshy, globular, bilocular, and contain numerous whitish, ovoid, flattened seeds.

Leaves, Stem, and Root: Gaultheria procumbens is a bushy evergreen plant with procumbent stems and upright rigid branches up to 15 cm high. It grows best under trees and shrubs. The branches bear clusters of leaves at their tips. The leaves are coriaceous, oval, 3 to 5 cm long, glabrous and glossy above, paler beneath, long and solitary.

Characteristics: Wintergreen has an aromatic odor; the taste of the whole plant is astringent.

Habitat: Gaultheria procumbens is indigenous to the northern United States and Canada.

Production: Wintergreen leaves are the leaves of *Gaultheria procumbens.*

Other Names: Canada Tea, Checkerberry, Deerberry, Ground Berry, Hillberry, Mountain Tea, Partridge Berry, Spiceberry, Wax Cluster, Boxberry, Teaberry

ACTIONS AND PHARMACOLOGY
COMPOUNDS: FRESHLY HARVESTED PLANT
Monotropitoside (Gaultherin): changing into methyl salicylate when the plant is dried

COMPOUNDS: DRIED PLANT
Volatile oil: chief component methyl salicylate (96-98%), in addition to oenanthic alcohol (n-heptan-1-ol) and its ester (which contributes to the odor of the volatile oil)

EFFECTS
The essential oil has a rubefacient effect.

INDICATIONS AND USAGE
Unproven Uses: Wintergreen was previously used as a carminative, tonic, antiseptic and aromatic. The drug was also used for neuralgia (particularly sciatica), gastralgias, pleurisy, pleurodynia (especially for medium stage pain), ovarialgia, orchitis, epidydimitis, diaphragmitis, uratic arthritis, and dysmenorrhea. Folk medicine indications also include asthma and use of wintergreen as an antiseptic. The drug is administered externally in the treatment of rheumatoid arthritis and related conditions.

PRECAUTIONS AND ADVERSE REACTIONS
Health risks or side effects following the proper administration of designated therapeutic dosages are not recorded. The drug and its volatile oil can, however, trigger contact allergies.

OVERDOSAGE
Signs of poisoning such as severe stomach and kidney irritation appear with overdosages of the drug. Fatal poisonings can occur through oral and percutaneous administration of the pure volatile oil, often following are signs of central nervous system distress, lung edema, and collapse. Poisonings with fatal results have been observed following the oral intake of as little as 4 to 6 g of the volatile oil.

DOSAGE
The drug is seldom used today. The active ingredient, methyl salicylate, is produced synthetically at a lower cost. Methyl salicylate is a constituent of liniments and bath additives.

LITERATURE
Frohne D, Pfänder HJ, Giftpflanzen - Ein Handbuch für Apotheker, Toxikologen und Biologen, 4. Aufl., Wiss. Verlagsges. mbH Stuttgart 1997.

Kern W, List PH, Hörhammer L (Hrsg.), Hagers Handbuch der Pharmazeutischen Praxis, 4. Aufl., Bde. 1-8, Springer Verlag Berlin, Heidelberg, New York, 1969.

Leung AY, Encyclopedia of Common Natural Ingredients Used in Food Drugs and Cosmetics, John Wiley & Sons Inc., New York 1980.

Lewin L, Gifte und Vergiftungen, 6. Aufl., Nachdruck, Haug Verlag, Heidelberg 1992.

Madaus G, Lehrbuch der Biologischen Arzneimittel, Bde 1-3, Nachdruck, Georg Olms Verlag Hildesheim 1979.

Roth L, Daunderer M, Kormann K, Giftpflanzen, Pflanzengifte, 4. Aufl., Ecomed Fachverlag Landsberg Lech 1993.

Steinegger E, Hänsel R, Pharmakognosie, 5. Aufl., Springer Verlag Heidelberg 1992.

Witch Hazel

Hamamelis virginiana

DESCRIPTION

Medicinal Parts: The medicinal parts are the plant's hamamelis water, which is distilled from various plant parts; the bark; the fresh and dried leaves; the fresh bark of the roots and branches; and the dried bark of the trunk and branches.

Flower and Fruit: The androgynous and unisexual flowers grow in light to golden yellow, short-stemmed clusters on the trees before the leaves come out. The inflorescence is a small, head-like spike in the axils of the dropping leaves, with 5 to 8 flowers. The 4 sepals are ovate or triangular, curved outward, yellow-brown to brown on the inside. The petals are bright yellow, long, narrow-linear, rolled to a spiral in the bud and crushed like tissue paper when open. The ovary is villous, bivalvular with 2 anatropic ovules. Fertilization takes place during the spring that follows 5 to 7 months after pollination. The fruit capsule is woody, ovate, sectioned and divided, hazelnut-like, 12 to 15 mm long and thickly pubescent. It bursts so dramatically in autumn that the 2 dark seeds are projected up to 4 m away from the plant.

Leaves, Stem and Root: The plant is a tree-like deciduous bush that typically grows 2 to 3 m high (but sometimes reaches heights up to 10 m) with a trunk diameter of 40 cm. The bark is thin, brown on the outside, reddish on the inside. The older branches are bushy, divided and silver-gray to gray-brown. The younger branches are yellowish-brown with hairs. The alternate leaves have stipules. The leaf margin is roughly crenate, bluntly indented to irregularly sweeping.

Habitat: Witch Hazel originated in the deciduous forests of Atlantic North America. The tree is common in European gardens and parks, and is also cultivated in subtropical countries.

Production: Witch Hazel leaf is obtained from the leaves of Hamamelis virginiana, which are collected in autumn and dried rapidly. Witch Hazel bark is the dried bark of the trunk and branches of Hamamelis virginiana.

Not to be Confused With: Witch Hazel is sometimes confused with Hazelnut bark, to which it bears a resemblance. Confusion can arise between Witch Hazel leaves and the leaves of Corylus avellana (hazelnut leaves), which are sometimes substituted as an adulteration.

Other Names: Hamamelis, Hazel Nut, Snapping Hazel, Spotted Alder, Striped Alder, Tobacco Wood, Winterbloom

ACTIONS AND PHARMACOLOGY

COMPOUNDS: WITCH HAZEL BARK

Tannins (up to 12%): including hamamelitannin, monogalloyl hamameloses

Catechins: including (+)-catechin, (+)-gallocatechin, (-)-epicatechin gallate(III), (-)-epigallocatechin gallate(III)

Oligomeric procyanidins

EFFECTS: WITCH HAZEL BARK

Witch Hazel bark is astringent, anti-inflammatory and locally hemostatic.

COMPOUNDS: WITCH HAZEL LEAF

Tannins (5%): including hamamelitannin

Catechins: including (+)-catechin, (+)-gallocatechin, (-)-epicatechin gallate(III), (-)-epigallocatechin gallate(III)

Oligomeric procyanidins

Volatile oil (0.01 to 0.5%): steam distillate, consisting chiefly of aliphatic carbonyl compounds, for example hex-2-en-1-ale, 6-methyl-hepta-3,5-dien-2-one aliphatic alcohols, aliphatic esters

Flavonoids: including quercitrin, isoquercitrin

EFFECTS: WITCH HAZEL LEAF

The tannins and tannin elements have an astringent, anti-inflammatory and locally hemostatic effect.

INDICATIONS AND USAGE

Approved by Commission E:

- Hemorrhoids
- Inflammation of the mouth and pharynx (leaf only)
- Inflammation of the skin
- Venous conditions
- Wounds and burns

Unproven Uses: Witch Hazel leaf and bark are used internally in folk medicine for non-specific diarrheic ailments (such as inflammation of the mucous membrane of the large intestine and colon), hematemesis, hemoptysis and also for menstrual complaints. Efficacy in the treatment of diarrhea seems plausible because of the tannin content. Witch Hazel is used externally for minor injuries of the skin, localized inflamed swelling of the skin and mucous membranes, hemorrhoids and varicose veins. It is also used in folk medicine for inflammation of the mucosa of the colon, hematemesis and hemoptysis.

Homeopathic Use: Applications for use of Witch Hazel bark in homeopathy include hemorrhoids, varicose veins, skin inflammation and bleeding of the mucous membranes.

PRECAUTIONS AND ADVERSE REACTIONS

Health risks following the proper administration of designated therapeutic dosages are not recorded. If taken internally, the tannin content of the drug can lead to digestive complaints. Liver damage is conceivable following long-term administration, but rare.

DOSAGE

WITCH HAZEL BARK

Mode of Administration: Witch Hazel Bark is available as comminuted drug or extract for internal and external use as galenic preparations. A steam distillate of the fresh leaves and bark is used for internal and external application.

How Supplied: Forms of commercial pharmaceutical preparations include: cream; gel; ointment; suppositories.

Preparation: Various formulations of Witch Hazel are prepared as follows:

External–aqueous steam distillate (Witch Hazel water) undiluted, or diluted 1:3 with water.

For poultices–20 to 30% in semi-solid preparations.

Extract preparations–semi-solid and liquid preparations, corresponding to 5 to 10% drug.

Compresses and rinses–decoctions of 5 to 10 g of herb per cup (250 ml) of water.

Ointment/gel–5 g Witch Hazel extract in 100 g ointment base.

Suppositories–Use 0.1 to 1 g drug.

Daily Dosage: Suppositories can be used 1 to 3 times a day.

Homeopathic Dosage: 5 drops, 1 tablet or 10 globules every 30 to 60 minutes (acute) or 1 to 3 times daily (chronic); parenterally: 1 to 2 ml sc acute, 3 times daily; chronic: once a day, suppositories 2 to 3 times per day and ointment 1 to 2 times daily (acute and chronic); for the external application, 1 dessertspoonful to be mixed with 250 ml water and then used as a wash or poultice (HAB1).

Storage: Store Witch Hazel bark protected from exposure to light.

WITCH HAZEL LEAF

Mode of Administration: Witch hazel leaf is available as comminuted drug or extract for internal and external use as galenic preparations. A steam distillate of the fresh leaves and bark is used for internal and external applications.

How Supplied:

Liquid –1:1 liquid

Preparation:

Liquid extract–1:1 with 45% ethanol (PF X).

Stabilized liquid extract–100 g of leaf powder are moistened with 45 g 1:2 90% ethanol:water and subsequently percolated with 540 g 1:2 90% ethanol:water. Separation into 85 g forerun and the residue, which is evaporated until dry. The dried substance is dissolved with 15 g ethanol:water and is then mixed with the forerun. This solution is kept for 8 days at 2 to 8° C and then filtered at the same temperature. Tea: pour 150 ml boiling water over 2 to 3 g drug and strain after 10 minutes.

Daily Dosage:

Decoction–250 ml water with 5 to 10 g drug for washes or poultices; 2 to 3 g to 150 ml water as a gargle solution.

Suppositories–0.1 to 1 g drug/supp. 3 times daily.

Tea–1 cup 2 to 3 times daily between meals.

Liquid extract–2 to 4 ml 3 times daily.

Storage: Protect Witch Hazel leaf from light and moisture when stored.

LITERATURE

WITCH HAZEL BARK AND LEAF

Dorsch W., Neues über antientzündliche Drogen. *Z Phytother* 14: 26. 1993.

Erdelmeier CAJ et al, Antiviral and antiphlogistic activities of *Hamamelis virginiana* bark. *Planta Med* 62: 241-245. 1996.

Friedrich H, Krüger N, *Planta Med* 25: 138. 1974.

Haberland C, Kolodziej H, Novel galloylhamamelose from *Hamamelis virginiana. Planta Med* 59:A608. 1993.

Hartisch C et al., Dual inhibitory activities of tannins from *Hamamelis virginiana* and related polyphenols on 5-lipoxygenase and Lyso-PAF: Acetyl-CoA-Acetyltransferase. *Planta Med* 63: 106-110.

Hartisch C et al., Proanthocyanidin pattern in Hamamelis virginiana. Planta Med 62 (Abstracts of the 44th Ann Congress of GA) 119. 1996.

Hartisch C et al., Study on the localisation and composition of the volatile fraction *of Hamamelis virginiana. Planta Med* 62 (Abstracts of the 44th Ann Congress of GA) 133. 1996.

Hughes-Formella BJ, Filbry A, Gassmueller J, Rippke F. Anti-inflammatory efficacy of topical preparations with 10 % *hamamelis destillate* in a UV erythema test. *Skin Pharmacol Appl Skin Physiol.* 15:125-132. 2002.

Knoch HG, Hämorrhoiden I. Grades, Wirksamkeit einer Salbe auf pflanzlicher Basis 31/32: 481-484. 1991

Korting HC, Schäfer-Korting M, Hart H et al., Anti-inflammatory activity of hamamelis distillate applied topically to the skin. Influence of vehicle and dose. *Eur J Clin Pharmacol* 44 315-318: 1993.

Laux P, Oschmann R, Die Zaubernuβ - Hamamelis virginiana L. Z Phytother 14: 155-166. 1993.

Mennet-von Eiff M, Meier B, Phytotherapie in der Dermatologie. *Z Phytother* 16: 201-210. 1995.

Schulz R, Hänsel R, Rationale Phytotherapie. Springer Verlag Heidelberg 1996.

Sorkin B, Hametum-Salbe, eine kortikoidfreie antiinflammatorische Salbe. *Phys Med Rehab* 21: 53-57. 1980.

Wood Anemone

Anemone nemorosa

DESCRIPTION

Medicinal Parts: The medicinal parts are the fresh plant gathered shortly before the flowers open as well as the dried aerial parts of the plant.

Flower and Fruit: The white flowers are solitary and located at the end of a long stem. The stem is erect when in flower, white to reddish-violet, and has a diameter of 1.5 to 4 cm. The bracts (usually 6 but possibly 5 to 9) are oblong-ovate, entire-margined, and glabrous. The flowers have numerous yellow stamens. The 10 to 20 carpels are oblong with a short curved beak. They are downy and 4 to 5 mm long. The fruit is a drooping compound with a roughly haired fruitlet.

Leaves, Stem, and Root: Anemone nemorosa is a perennial plant, 6 to 30 cm high with a horizontally creeping roundish rhizome that is yellow to dark brown. The stems are usually solitary, erect, glabrous, or sparsely pubescent. There is usually a long-stemmed basal leaf. The leaf is tripinnate and pinnatifid-serrate. The first row of pinna are stemmed and have horizontal pinna sections, each with 1 pinna of the second level. There are cauline rosettes of 3 leaflike bracts, which have a 2-cm long petiole. The bracts do not generally have axillary buds, and are palmate and pinnatifid-serrate.

Habitat: The plant is spread almost all over Europe as far as the Volga region except in the Mediterranean and northern Lapland.

Production: Wood Anemone is the aerial part of *Anemone nemorosa*, collected shortly before the flowers open.

Other Names: Crowfoot, Pasque Flower, Smell Fox, Wind Flower

ACTIONS AND PHARMACOLOGY

COMPOUNDS

Protoanemonine-forming agents (yielding approximately 300 mcg protoanemonine per gram of fresh weight): presumably, the glycoside ranunculin, which changes enzymatically when the plant is cut into small pieces (and probably also when it is dried) into the pungent, volatile protoanemonine that quickly dimerizes to anemonine; when dried, the plant is not capable of protoanemonine formation

EFFECTS

No information is available.

INDICATIONS AND USAGE

Unproven Uses: The drug is used for stomach pains, delayed menstruation, gout, whooping cough, and asthma.

PRECAUTIONS AND ADVERSE REACTIONS

No health hazards or side effects are known in conjunction with the proper administration of designated therapeutic dosages.

Prolonged skin contact with the freshly harvested plant can lead to slow-healing blisters and cauterizations due to the formation of protoanemonine, which is severely irritating to skin and mucous membranes. If taken internally, severe irritation to the gastrointestinal tract and urinary drainage passages, as well as colic and diarrhea, are possible. Symptomatic treatment for external contact should consist of irrigation with diluted potassium permanganate solution followed by mucilage.

OVERDOSAGE

In case of internal contact, administer gastric lavage followed by activated charcoal. Death by asphyxiation following the intake of large quantities of protoanemonine-forming plants has been observed in animal experiments. The ingestion of 30 freshly harvested plants is considered the fatal level for humans.

DOSAGE

Mode of Administration: The drug can be found in dilute homeopathic preparations of the mother tincture.

LITERATURE

Bulatovic V, Gorunovic M. Flavonoids of wood anemone (*Anemone nemorosa L.,* Ranunculaceae). Pharm Acta Helv. 70; 219-221. 1995

Frohne D, Pfänder HJ, Giftpflanzen - Ein Handbuch für Apotheker, Toxikologen und Biologen, 4. Aufl., Wiss. Verlags-Ges Stuttgart 1997.

Hänsel R, Keller K, Rimpler H, Schneider G (Hrsg.), Hagers Handbuch der Pharmazeutischen Praxis, 5. Aufl., Bde 4-6 (Drogen): Springer Verlag Berlin, Heidelberg, New York, 1992-1994.

Lewin L, Gifte und Vergiftungen, 6. Aufl., Nachdruck, Haug Verlag, Heidelberg 1992.

Madaus G, Lehrbuch der Biologischen Arzneimittel, Bde 1-3, Nachdruck, Georg Olms Verlag Hildesheim 1979.

Roth L, Daunderer M, Kormann K, Giftpflanzen, Pflanzengifte, 4. Aufl., Ecomed Fachverlag Landsberg Lech 1993.

Ruijgrok HWL, PM 11:338-347. 1963.

Teuscher E, Lindequist U, Biogene Gifte - Biologie, Chemie, Pharmakologie, 2. Aufl., Fischer Verlag Stuttgart 1994.

Wood Betony

Betonica officinalis

DESCRIPTION

Medicinal Parts: The medicinal part is the herb, including the basal leaves.

Flower and Fruit: The flowers are crimson and labiate in a terminal, spikelike, irregular formation. The calyx, with 5 even, triangular tips, has long ciliate hairs and is shorter than the corolla tube. The corolla is curled downward, and the white tube has no ring of hair. The upper lip is erect, and the lower lip has 3 lobes, with the middle one being broad. There are 4 stamens.

Leaves, Stem, and Root: The plant grows to a height of about 30 to 100 cm. The stem is erect, unbranched, quadrangular, bristly-haired, and usually only has 2 distal pairs of leaves. The basal leaves are rosettelike. The leaves are elongate-ovate with a cordate base and crenate. The lower ones are larger and long-petioled, and the upper ones are smaller and shorter.

Habitat: The plant grows in Europe.

Production: Wood Betony is the flowering plant of *Betonica officinalis* collected from June to August at flowering time. The herb, including the basal leaves, is collected and dried in the shade at a maximum temperature of 40° C.

Not to be Confused With: Stachys alpina

Other Names: Betony, Bishopswort

ACTIONS AND PHARMACOLOGY

COMPOUNDS

Betaine: including betonicine [(-)-oxystachydrine), (-)- stachydrine), ((+)oxystachydrine]

Caffeic acid derivatives: including chlorogenic acid, isochlorogenic acid, rosemary acid iridoid glycosides *Diterpene lactone*

Iridoids: iridoid glycosides, including harpagide

Flavonoids

EFFECTS

The drug is said to act as a tranquilizer, a disinfectant and an astringent. It contains glycosides with hypotensive characteristics.

INDICATIONS AND USAGE

Unproven Uses: Wood Betony is an astringent. As an expectorant, it is used for coughs, bronchitis, and asthma. It is contained in combination preparations as a sedative and for the treatment of neuralgia and anxiety. In folk medicine, it is used as an antidiarrheal agent, a carmative, and a sedative, and for catarrh, lung catarrh, heartburn, gout, nervousness, bladder and kidney stones, and inflammation of the bladder.

Homeopathic Uses: Betonica officinalis is used in homeopathy for asthma and general states of debility.

PRECAUTIONS AND ADVERSE REACTIONS

No health hazards or side effects are known in conjunction with the proper administration of designated therapeutic dosages.

DOSAGE

Mode of Administration: The herb is used topically, as an extract and an infusion. The fresh leaves are also used.

Daily Dosage: The infusion can be taken daily. The total daily dosage of the powder is 1 to 2 g, to be taken in 3 separate doses. The fresh leaves may be boiled and used for wounds and swelling.

LITERATURE

Hoppe HA, Drogenkunde, 8. Aufl., Bde 1-3, W. de Gruyter Verlag, Berlin, New York. 1975-1987

Kern W, List PH, Hörhammer L (Hrsg.), Hagers Handbuch der Pharmazeutischen Praxis, 4. Aufl., Bde. 1-8, Springer Verlag Berlin, Heidelberg, New York, 1969.

Madaus G, Lehrbuch der Biologischen Arzneimittel, Bde 1-3, Nachdruck, Georg Olms Verlag Hildesheim 1979.

Sattar AA, Bankova V, Kujumgiev A, Galabov A, Ignatova A, Todorova C, Popov S. Chemical composition and biological activity of leaf exudates from some Lamiaceae plants. Pharmazie 50; 62-65. 1995

Wood Sage

Teucrium scorodonia

DESCRIPTION

Medicinal Parts: The medicinal parts are the herb, the fresh aerial parts of the flowering plant, and the whole flowering plant.

Flower and Fruit: The flowers are approximately 1 cm long, pale yellow or greenish-yellow. They are solitary or in pairs on short pedicles in one-side-inclined, terminal racemes. The calyx of the labiate flower is tubular-campanulate and bilabiate with an undivided upper and a 4-tipped lower lip. The stamens are pubescent and the anthers are violet. The nutlet is round, about 2 mm long, and almost smooth.

Leaves, Stem, and Root: The plant is erect, 30 to 60 cm high and has far-reaching runners. The stem is erect, paniculate-branched above, quadrangular and soft-pubescent. The leaves are petiolate, opposite, wrinkled, ovate or oblong, unevenly crenate, and have a shallowly cordate base.

Characteristics: The plant smells faintly of leeks when being dried.

Habitat: The plant is common to large parts of western and central Europe including the Mediterranean region. It is rarely found in eastern Europe and Scandinavia but it has naturalized there.

Production: Wood Sage is the aerial part of *Teucrium scorodonia.*

Other Names: Ambroise, Garlic Sage, Hind Heal, Large-Leaved Germander, Wood Germander

ACTIONS AND PHARMACOLOGY

COMPOUNDS

Volatile oil (0.3%): containing among others, alloaromadendrene, aristolene, beta-caryophyllene, alpha-caryophyllene (humulene), spathulenone, caryophyllene epoxide

Iridoide monoterpenes: including among others, acetyl harpagide, reptoside

Diterpenes: the spectrum varies greatly according to strain, including among others teuscorodal, teuscorodin, teuscorodol, teuscorodonin, teuflin, teuscorolide, teupolin I

Flavonoids: including among others, cirsiliol, cirsimaritin, luteolin

EFFECTS

The expectorant effect attributed to the drug may be due to the amaroids and the essential oil. See other *Teucrium* species for the toxic effect.

INDICATIONS AND USAGE

Unproven Uses: Wood Sage is used for the treatment of tuberculosis, chronic bronchial catarrh, inflammation of mucous membranes of the nose and throat, spasms, hypertension, wounds, and liver disorders.

Homeopathic Uses: The herb is used for chronic inflammation of the respiratory tract.

PRECAUTIONS AND ADVERSE REACTIONS

No health hazards or side effects are known in conjunction with the proper administration of designated therapeutic dosages.

DOSAGE

Mode of Administration: Wood Sage is obsolete as a drug in most countries, but it can be found as cut drug in capsules and drops.

Preparation: To treat bronchitis, a tea is made using 2 teaspoons of herb per cup.

LITERATURE

Bruno M et al., *Phytochemistry* 24(11):2597. 1985.

Hänsel R, Keller K, Rimpler H, Schneider G (Hrsg.), Hagers Handbuch der Pharmazeutischen Praxis, 5. Aufl., Bde 4-6 (Drogen): Springer Verlag Berlin, Heidelberg, New York, 1992-1994.

Madaus G, Lehrbuch der Biologischen Arzneimittel, Bde 1-3, Nachdruck, Georg Olms Verlag Hildesheim 1979.

Marco JL et al., PH 21:2567. 1982.

Marco JL et al., PH 22:727-731. 1983.

Velasco-Negueruela A et al., PH 29:1165-1169. 1990.

Wagner H, Wiesenauer M, Phytotherapie. Phytopharmaka und pflanzliche Homöopathika, Fischer-Verlag, Stuttgart, Jena, New York 1995.

Wood Sorrel

Oxalis acetosella

DESCRIPTION

Medicinal Parts: The medicinal part is the fresh flowering plant with the root.

Flower and Fruit: The solitary flower is white or reddish-white and red-veined with yellow spots. The pedicle is longer than the leaves. There are 5 sepals and 5 petals, 10 stamens, and 1 ovary with 5 styles. The fruit is an ovate capsule. It is pentangular, tearing open in long slits when ripe, thus freeing the seeds.

Leaves, Stem, and Root: The plant grows to a height of between 5 and 12 cm tall. The leaves are basal, tender, long-petioled, and trifoliate. The leaflets are broad, obovate-cordate, downy, and often tinged red underneath. The stem is leafless apart from bracts above the middle, which are fused at the base.

Characteristics: The plant has a pleasant, rather sour odor.

Habitat: The plant is commonly found in woods and forests throughout Europe.

Production: Wood Sorrel is the aerial part of *Oxalis acetosella*, which is harvested while the plant is in blossom.

Other Names: Cuckoo Bread, Cuckowes Meat, Fairy Bells, Green Sauce, Hallelujah, Shamrock, Sour Trefoil, Stickwort, Stubwort, Surelle, Three-Leaved Grass, Wood Sour

ACTIONS AND PHARMACOLOGY

COMPOUNDS

Oxalic acid (0.3-1.25%): especially present as potassium salt

EFFECTS

The drug, including the green parts of the plant, contains clover acid that, in small amounts, affects gallbladder activity by acting as a diuretic. The fresh plant provides a substantial source of vitamin C.

INDICATIONS AND USAGE

Unproven Uses: Wood Sorrel is no longer used as a remedy, but previously was used for liver and digestive disorders. Also, in the past, the fresh leaves were used to treat scurvy and inflammation of the gums.

PRECAUTIONS AND ADVERSE REACTIONS

No health hazards or side effects are known in conjunction with the proper administration of designated therapeutic dosages.

OVERDOSAGE

Oxalic acid poisonings could occur only through the ingestion of very large quantities of the leaves, for example as in salad. The poisonings mentioned in older scientific literature seem dubious.

DOSAGE

Mode of Administration: Ground and as an extract. Wood Sorrel is no longer used as a remedy.

LITERATURE

Kern W, List PH, Hörhammer L (Hrsg.), Hagers Handbuch der Pharmazeutischen Praxis, 4. Aufl., Bde. 1-8, Springer Verlag Berlin, Heidelberg, New York, 1969.

Madaus G, Lehrbuch der Biologischen Arzneimittel, Bde 1-3, Nachdruck, Georg Olms Verlag Hildesheim 1979.

Roth L, Daunderer M, Kormann K, Giftpflanzen, Pflanzengifte, 4. Aufl., Ecomed Fachverlag Landsberg Lech 1993.

Teuscher E, Lindequist U, Biogene Gifte - Biologie, Chemie, Pharmakologie, 2. Aufl., Fischer Verlag Stuttgart 1994.

Tosto DS, Hopp HE, Sequence analysis of the 5.8S ribosomal DNA and internal transcribed spacers (ITS1 and ITS2) from five species of the *Oxalis tuberosa* alliance. *DNA Seq,* 6:361-4. 1996.

Tschesche R, Struckmeyer K, (1976) Chem Ber. 109:2901.

Wormseed

Artemisia cina

DESCRIPTION

Medicinal Parts: The medicinal parts are closed flower-buds, that have not yet blossomed.

Flower and Fruit: The numerous flower heads are about 2 mm long with a diameter of 1.5 mm. They are ovoid and greenish-yellow when fresh, later brownish-green. They contain three to five minute, tubular, androgynous florets with a slim, cylindrical, and glabrous receptacle. The epicalyces have numerous oblong-obtuse, imbricate scales.

Leaves, Stem, and Root: Artemisia cina is an evergreen, perennial semi-shrub, 30 to 60 cm high with many slim sprouting stems. The gnarled rhizome produces numerous leaf and flower branches. The stems are smooth and woody and the leaves pinnatifid on the nonflowering branches. The leaves on the flowering branches are small and entire-margined.

Characteristics: The odor is aromatic and the taste bitter.

Habitat: The plant is indigenous to Iran, Turkestan, and the Kirghizin Steppes around Buchara.

Production: Wormwood flowers are the inflorescent buds of *Artemisia cina* (occasionally incorrectly called Wormseed), which are cultivated and gathered in the wild.

Not to be Confused With: Refined mustard flour

Other Names: Levant, Santonica, Sea Wormwood

ACTIONS AND PHARMACOLOGY

COMPOUNDS

Sesquiterpene lactones: especially alpha-santonin, in addition to artemisin and beta-santonin

EFFECTS

The anthelmintic and antipyretic effect of the drug can be attributed to its alpha-santonin content. The drug acts as a vermifuge action for ascarids, including intestinal parasitic worms, whose muscles are paralyzed by the santonin. The worms are then forced into the large intestine where they are removed by means of a laxative. In rats, the rectal temperature was lowered during fevers that had been induced by brewer's yeast injections. This leads to the speculation that santonin effects body temperature in a similar manner to dopamine.

INDICATIONS AND USAGE

Unproven Uses: The drug is used for ascarid and oxyuris infestations.

Homeopathic Uses: Uses in homeopathy include fevers, tendency to convulsions and worms.

PRECAUTIONS AND ADVERSE REACTIONS

Even with the therapeutic dose there is a danger of poisoning. Side effects may resemble those of the alpha-santonins: kidney irritation, gastroenteritis, stupor, visual disorders (xanthopsia), muscle twitching and epileptiform spasms. Administration in allopathic dosages is to be avoided.

OVERDOSAGE

Deadly poisonings following the intake of less than 10 g of the drug are known.

DOSAGE

Preparation: Wormwood is considered completely obsolete as a drug, occasionally available as a powder for use when more modern antithelmintic agents fail. Symptoms of poisoning are possible even in therapeutic dosages.

Daily Dosage: The drug is always used in combination with a laxative. The average single dose is 0.025 g for adults. For children, take the child's age in years, and double this amount in milligrams of the drug. According to the Austrian pharmacopoeia, the single dose is 1 to 2 g. The powder is administered in the morning and followed later by castor oil or sodium sulfate. The remedy is repeated on the following day.

Homeopathic Dosage: 5 to 10 drops, 1 tablet, 5 to 10 globules, 1 to 3 times a day or 1 mL injection solution twice weekly sc (HAB34).

LITERATURE

Frohne D, Pfänder HJ: Giftpflanzen - Ein Handbuch für Apotheker, Toxikologen und Biologen, 4. Aufl., Wiss. Verlagsges. mbH Stuttgart 1997.

Hänsel R, Keller K, Rimpler H, Schneider G (Hrsg.), Hagers Handbuch der Pharmazeutischen Praxis, 5. Aufl., Bde 4-6 (Drogen): Springer Verlag Berlin, Heidelberg, New York, 1992-1994.

Lewin L, Gifte und Vergiftungen, 6. Aufl., Nachdruck, Haug Verlag, Heidelberg 1992.

Madaus G, Lehrbuch der Biologischen Arzneimittel, Bde 1-3, Nachdruck, Georg Olms Verlag Hildesheim 1979.

Roth L, Daunderer M, Kormann K, Giftpflanzen, Pflanzengifte, 4. Aufl., Ecomed Fachverlag Landsberg Lech 1993.

Teuscher E, Lindequist U, Biogene Gifte - Biologie, Chemie, Pharmakologie, 2. Aufl., Fischer Verlag Stuttgart 1994.

Teuscher E, Biogene Arzneimittel, 5. Aufl., Wiss. Verlagsges. mbH Stuttgart 1997.

Wormseed Oil

Chenopodium ambrosioides

DESCRIPTION

Medicinal Parts: The plant's medicinal parts are the seeds and the herb, including the flowers.

Flower and Fruit: The numerous small flowers are yellowish-green and form small racemes or roundish spikes in the axils of the apical leaves. The calyx is divided into 5; the lobes are ovate and pointed. There are 5 stamens. The ovary has small, oblong, stemmed glands at the tip. The angular fruit is enclosed in the calyx. The small seeds are achaenes, smooth, and black.

Leaves, Stem and Root: The plant is an annual that grows to about 1 m in height with a branched, reddish stem. The stem is covered in alternate-linear to lanceolate leaves.

Characteristics: The whole plant gives off a pleasant fragrance. The oil is dangerously explosive.

Habitat: Wormseed originated in Mexico and South America but has spread to the eastern U.S.

Production: Wormseed Oil is the seed oil of *Chenopodium ambrosioides*.

Other Names: American Wormseed, Jesuit's Tea, Mexican Tea

ACTIONS AND PHARMACOLOGY

COMPOUNDS

Ascaridiole (chief constituent - up to 80%): including, according to variety and breed, p-cymene, L-pinocarvone, alpha-pinenes and/or alpha-terpenes, limonene. The combination creates a volatile, explosive oil.

EFFECTS

Wormseed Oil acts as an anthelmintic that causes flight and defensive reactions in worms. This is due to the main constituent of the terpene fraction, which is ascaridole, a monoterpene. This constituent is highly toxic.

INDICATIONS AND USAGE

Unproven Uses: Although considered obsolete as a drug, Wormseed Oil is used against roundworms and hookworms, if other, more modern anthelmintic drugs fail. The leaves and seeds have long been used in South American medicine as a vermifuge, stimulant, antiasthmatic and abortifacient for cramps, paralysis and asthmatic complaints.

Chinese Medicine: The Chinese have used Wormseed Oil for rheumatism of the joints, metrorrhagia, eczema, and bites.

PRECAUTIONS AND ADVERSE REACTIONS

Even the administration of therapeutic dosages can lead to disorders of the central nervous system, including spasms, signs of paralysis, and Pachymeningitis haemorrhagica. Damage to the Nervus cochlearis is frequent, leading to buzzing in the ears and hearing impairment (sometimes lasting for years). In addition, the oil is dangerously explosive.

OVERDOSAGE

Cases of death have been observed following intake of 10 mg of the oil by adults, and much less for children. For that reason, an administration in allopathic dosages is to be avoided.

DOSAGE

Mode of Administration: Wormseed Oil is obsolete as a drug. In clinically described cases, which are exceptional, it can be used in combination with a fast-acting and powerful purgative.

Daily Dosage: Typical adult daily dosage is 20 drops taken in the morning on an empty stomach. Two hours later, a purgative is taken. Pediatric dosage is two single doses of drops taken one hour apart. Each dose has one drop per year of the child's age.

LITERATURE

Bombardelli E et al., *Fitoterapia* 47:3. 1976

Chan, EH et al., (Eds), Advances in Chinese Medicinal Materials Research, World Scientific Pub. Co. Singapore 1985.

Chantraine JM, Laurent D, Ballivian C, Saavedra G, Ibanez R, Vilaseca LA. Insecticidal Activity of Essential Oils on Aedes aegypti Larvae. *Phytother Res.* 12 (5); 350-354. 1998

Franca F, Lago EL, Marsden PD. Plants used in the treatment of leishmanial ulcers due to Leishmania (Viannia) braziliensis in an endemic area of Bahia Brazil. *Rev Soc Bras Med Trop,* 29:229-32, May-Jun 1996

Leung AY, Encyclopedia of Common Natural Ingredients Used in Food Drugs and Cosmetics, John Wiley & Sons Inc., New York 1980.

Lewin L, Gifte und Vergiftungen, 6. Aufl., Nachdruck, Haug Verlag, Heidelberg 1992.

Madaus G, Lehrbuch der Biologischen Arzneimittel, Bde 1-3, Nachdruck, Georg Olms Verlag Hildesheim 1979.

Roth L, Daunderer M, Kormann K, Giftpflanzen, Pflanzengifte, 4. Aufl., Ecomed Fachverlag Landsberg Lech 1993.

Wormwood

Artemisia absinthium

DESCRIPTION

Medicinal Parts: The medicinal parts are the aerial shoots and leaves of the plant.

Flower and Fruit: The numerous flower heads are short-stemmed and hang in a many-flowered panicle. The capitula are small, globular, inclined and nearly as long as their 3 to 4 mm width. The bracts are gray and silky-pubescent with a rounded tip. The outer bracts are linear-oblong and pubescent, while the inner ones are ovate, obtuse, broad and have a transparent, membranous margin. The receptacle is rough-haired. The flowers are yellow and fertile. The disc florets are androgynous; the ray florets are female with an extending style stem. The fruit is about 1.5 mm long.

Leaves, Stem, and Root: This semishrub grows from 60 to 120 cm in height with a woody, hardy rosette and a high-branch bearing stem. The stem is usually erect and leafy. The alternate, long-petioled leaves are silky pubescent on both sides. The lower leaves are abrupt pinnate and the upper ones simple. The leaf tips are lanceolate to linear-lanceolate, obtuse to acuminate, and 2 to 3 mm wide.

Characteristics: The plant has an aromatic odor and a very bitter taste.

Habitat: Wormwood grows in Europe, northern Africa, parts of Asia, and North and South America.

Production: Wormwood consists of the fresh or dried upper shoots and leaves, the fresh or dried basal leaves, or a mixture of the aerial plant parts from *Artemisia absinthium,* harvested during flowering season from cultivated or wild plants.

Other Names: Absinthe, Green Ginger

ACTIONS AND PHARMACOLOGY

COMPOUNDS

Volatile oil: with a high level (varies a great deal among different strains) of (+)-thujone, cis-epoxy ocimene, trans-sabinyl acetate or chrysanthenyl acetate

Sesquiterpene bitter principles: including absinthine, anabsinthine, artabsine, and matricine

EFFECTS

The cholagogic, digestive, appetite-stimulating, and wound-healing effects ascribed to the drug are attributed to the essential oils and amaroids. A significant increase of alpha-amylase, lipase, bilirubin, and cholesterol has been observed during the 70 to 100 minutes during which patients with liver disorders were given a suspension of 20 mg extract in 10 mL water via a duodenal probe. In rabbits, fever induced through yeast injection was reduced by using an esophageal probe to administer diverse fractions of the drug. In vitro, a watery extract of the whole drug is supposed to retard the growth of *Plasmodium falciparum*. The essential oil of the drug may possess an antimicrobial effect. The drug also stimulates the bitter receptors in the taste buds of the tongue. When bitter agents are introduced into the mouth, they trigger a reflexive increase of stomach secretion with higher acid concentration.

Anticancer Effects: A combination of dihydroartemisinin (200 mcmol) and halotransferrin (12 mcmol) selectively killed tumor cells over control cells. Addition of dihydroartemisinin to tumor cell (molt-4 lymphocytes) culture resulted in 50% decreased growth in 8 hours. Dihydroartemisinin alone had a similar effect on normal cells (lymphocytes) but cell death was not enhanced by the addition of halotransferrin. This technique may be effective for the treatment for cancers that express a large number of transferrin receptors because it allows the concentration of iron in the tumor cells. This allows a more directed approach in that free radicals are formed preferentially in the tumor cells where cell killing is wanted. This formation of free radicals is dependent on the endoperoxide bridge of artemisinin (Lai & Singh, 1995).

Antiparasitic Effects: Artemisia compounds become concentrated in parasite-infected erythrocytes where they are thought to cause free-radical damage to parasite membranes. The parasite is then phagocytosed and cleared by leukocytes. Drug activity is potentiated by oxidant drugs and oxygen. Derivatives of artemisinin (arteether, artesunate, and artemether) are 20x to 100x more active in vitro than artemisinin (Hien & White, 1993).

CLINICAL TRIALS

Crohn's Disease

Results of a five-center, randomized, placebo-controlled, and double-blind trial in 40 individuals with Crohn's disease (CD) strongly suggest that wormwood has a steroid-sparing effect. All participants began with 3 x 500 mg/daily capsules of an herbal blend containing Wormwood or placebo in addition to continuing basic CD treatment. Tapering of a daily and stable equivalent of 40 mg or less of corticosteroids (prednisone) started after week 2 and was completed at week 10 in 90 percent (18) of the participants assigned to wormwood treatment. At week 10, 65% (13) of patients in the Wormwood-treatment group had almost complete remission of symptoms as compared to zero in the placebo group. In a subgroup of these patients, a possible "curative" effect was observed given that there was no need to restart corticosteroids in the follow-up weeks, and no remission of disease over the ensuring 10 weeks of wormwood treatment. Results also suggest improvement in mood and quality of life with wormwood treatment (Omer, 2007).

Malaria

A randomized, double-blind study adults found artemether more rapid than quinine in treating apparent drug-resistant malaria in 560 adults. Quinine provided a more rapid recovery for patients with cerebral malaria. Patients received 4 mg/kg artemether intramuscularly, followed by 2 mg/kg every 8 hours, or 20 mg/kg intramuscular quinine, followed by 10 mg/kg every 8 hours for a minimum of 72 hours. There was no significant difference in mortality between groups, with an overall rate of 15%, but multiple logistic-regression model associated artemether with a lower mortality (p=0.028). Parasite clearance times were 72 hours for artemether and 90 hours for quinine. Fever resolution times were 127 hours for artemether and 90 hours for quinine. Recovery from coma was 66 hours for artemether and 48 hours for quinine. Side effects for quinine included hypoglycemia. Culture negative pyuria was a side effect in the artemether group (Hien et al, 1996).

A randomized study involving 160 children found intramuscular artemether to be effective in treating cerebral malaria. This study compared artemether (3.2 mg/kg on day 1, followed by 1.6 mg/kg daily) with intravenous quinine (20 mg/kg on day 1, followed by 10 mg/kg every 8 hours) and found both to be equally effective. One hundred percent parasite clearance time was 39.5 hours for artemether and 48 hours for quinine. Fever clearance was 32 hours in both groups. Coma resolution was 12 hours with artemether and 13 hours with quinine. Mortality was 20% in the artemether group and 11.3% in the quinine group (not significant). Most deaths in the artemether group were in patients with respiratory distress. Both treatments were given until parasitemia had cleared (at least 3 doses), after which pyrimethamin-sulfadoxine was given. This study was done in Africa where quinine resistance is not a significant problem. The authors recommend that quinine be the drug of choice for treating severe malaria in African children (Murphy et al, 1996).

INDICATIONS AND USAGE

Approved by Commission E:

- Loss of appetite
- Dyspeptic complaints
- Dyskinesia of the bile ducts

Unproven Uses: In folk medicine, wormwood preparations are used internally for gastric insufficiency, intestinal atonia, gastritis, stomachache, liver disorders, bloating, anemia, irregular menstruation, intermittent fever, loss of appetite, and worm infestation. Externally, the drug is applied for poorly healing wounds, ulcers, skin blotches and insect bites.

Efficacy in the above-mentioned popular uses is insufficiently documented.

CONTRAINDICATIONS

Wormwood is contraindicated in people with a history of seizures, and stomach or intestinal ulcers.

Pregnancy: Wormwood should not be used during pregnancy.

Breastfeeding: Wormwood should not be used while breastfeeding.

PRECAUTIONS AND ADVERSE REACTIONS

Continuous use of wormwood is not advisable. Due to the drug's thujone content, the internal administration of large doses can lead to vomiting, stomach and intestinal cramps, headache, dizziness and disturbances of the central nervous system.

DRUG INTERACTIONS

MODERATE RISK

Phenobarbital: Wormwood contains thujones, which may lower the seizure threshold, thereby reducing the clinical efficacy of phenobarbital (Tyagi & Delanty, 2003; Miller, 1998). *Clinical Management:* Avoid coadministration of Wormwood and phenobarbital.

POTENTIAL INTERACTIONS

Iron: The tannin content of wormwood may complex with concomitantly administered iron, resulting in nonabsorbable insoluble complexes and may result in adverse sequelae on blood components. *Clinical Management:* Until more is known, patients who need iron supplementation should be advised to separate administration times of these compounds by 1 to 2 hours.

DOSAGE

Mode of Administration: Comminuted herb is used for infusions and decoctions. Powdered herb, extracts and tinctures in liquid or solid forms are used for oral administration. Combination with other bitters or aromatics is common.

Preparation: To prepare an infusion, pour 150 mL boiling water over 1/2 teaspoonful of the drug, strain after 10 minutes. A decoction is prepared by adding 1 handful of drug to 1 liter of boiling water for 5 minutes. To prepare a tea, use 1 g drug in 1 cup water.

Daily Dose: The total daily dose is 3 to 5 g of the herb as an aqueous extract. Internal dose of the infusion is 1 cup freshly prepared tea taken 30 minutes before each meal. The tincture dosage is 10 to 30 drops in sufficient water taken 3 times daily. The liquid extract dosage is 1 to 2 ml taken 3 times daily. Externally, a decoction is used for healing of wounds and insect bites.

Storage: Wormwood must be kept in sealed containers and protected from light.

LITERATURE

Akhmedov IS et al., *Khim Prir Soedin* 6:691, 1970.

Akhmedov IS et al., (Artabin, a new lactone from *Artemisia absinthium*). In: *Khim Prid Soed* 5:622. 1970.

Baumann IC et al., *Z Allg Med* 51 (17):784, 1975.

Beauhaire J et al., *Tetrahedron Letters* 22 (24):2269, 1981.

Beauhaire J, Fourrey JL, *J Chem Soc Perk Trans*: 861, 1982.

Del Castillo J et al., *Nature* 253:365, 1975.

Dermanovic S et al., *zit CA* 87:98796h, 1976.

Greger H, Hofer O, New unsymmetrically substituted tetrahydrofuran lignans from Artemisia absinthium. In: *Tetrahedron* 36(24):3551. 1980.

Greger H, *Phytochemistry* 17:806, 1978.

Hien TT & White NJ, Drug Profiles: Qinghaosu. In: *Lancet*; 341:603-608, 1993.

Hoffman B, Herrmann K. *Z Lebensm* Unters Forsch 174 (3):211, 1982.

Kasimov Ah Z et al., Anabsin-a new diguaianolide from Artemisia absinthium. In: *Khim Prid Soed* 4:495. 1979.

Kasymov SZ et al., *Khim Prir Soed* 5:658, 1979.

Kennedy AI et al., Volatile oils from normal and transformed roots of Artemisia absinthium. In: *PH* 32:1449. 1993.

Kinloch JD, Practitioner 206:44, 1971.

Lai H & Singh NP, Selective cancer cell cytotoxicity from exposure to dihydroartemisinin and holotransferrin. In: *Cancer Lett*; 91(1):41-46, 1995.

Lemberkovics E et al., Some phytochemical characteristics of essential oil of *Artemisia absinthium L.* In: *Herba hung* 21(3):197-215. 1982.

Marles RJ, Kaminski J, Arnason JT, Pazos-Sanou L, Heptinstall S, Fischer NH, Crompton CW, Kindack DG, A bioassay for inhibition of serotonin release from bovine platelets. In: *JNP* 55:1044-1056. 1992.

Miller L, Herbal medicinals: selected clinical considerations focusing on known or potential drug-herb interactions. In: *Arch Intern Med*; 158:2200-2211, 1998.

Murphy S, English M, Waruiru C et al: An open randomized trial of artemether versus quinine in the treatment of cerebral malaria in African children. *Trans R Soc Trop Med Hyg* 1996; 90:298-301.

Omer B, et al. Steroid-sparing effect of wormwood (Artemisia absinthium) in Crohn's disease: A double-blind placebo-controlled study. *Phytomedicine* 14 (2-3): 87, 95, 2007

Rucker G, Manns D, Wilbert S, Peroxides as constituents of plants. 10. Homoditerpene peroxides from *Artemisia absinthium*. In: *PH*:31(1):340. 1992.

Schneider Von G, Mielke B, *Deutsch Apoth Ztg* 119 (25):977, 1979.

Stahl E, Gerard D, *Z Lebensm Unters Forsch* 176 (1):1, 1983.

Swiatek L, Dombrowicz E, *Farm Pol* 40 (2):729, 1984.

Taylor TE, Wills BA, Kazembe P et al. Rapid coma resolution with artemether in Malawian children with cerebral malaria. *Lancet* 1993; 341(8846):661-662.

Tyagi A & Delanty N, Herbal remedies, dietary supplements, and seizures. In: *Epilepsia*; 44(2):228-235, 2003.

Vostrowski O et al., *Z NaturForsch* (C) 36 (5/6):369, 1981.

Vostrowski O et al., Über die Komponenten des ätherischen Öls aus Artemisia absinthium L. In: Z Naturforsch 36(5/6):369. 1981.

White NJ, Waller D, Crawley J et al: Comparison of artemether and chloroquine for severe malaria in Gambian children. *Lancet* 1992; 339:317-321.

Zafar MM, Hamdard ME, Hameed A, Screening of *Artemisia absinthium* for antimalarial effects on Plasmodium berghei in mice: Preliminary report. In: *ETH* 30(2):223. 1990.

Zakirov SK et al., *Khim Prir Soedin* 4:548, 1976.

Wormwood Grass

Spigelia anthelmia

DESCRIPTION

Medicinal Parts: The whole fresh plant, the juice prepared from the fresh plant and the dried leaves are used medicinally.

Flower and Fruit: The inflorescences are terminal or axillary, 5 to 12 cm long spikes turned to one side. They are often involute. The flowers in the axils of the bracts are sessile. The flowers are radial and their structures are in fives. The sepals are free, linear-lanceolate, and 2 to 5 mm long. The 5 petals are fused with a 6.5 to 15 mm long, lilac, pink or white, funnel-shaped corolla. There are 5 stamens and a 2-chambered ovary. The fruit is a capsule approximately 5 mm long and 5 mm wide. The seeds are 2 to 3 mm long, elliptical or ovoid, dark brown, and warty.

Leaves, Stem, and Root: The herb grows upright to a height of up to 60 cm. The leaves are opposite and, because of short internodes, appear to be in whorls. They are 4 to 18 cm long, 2 to 6 cm wide, very short petiolate, simple, entire, ovate-lanceolate to elongate-ovate, and long acuminate. The stipules are fused, membranous, broad, and triangular. The stem and lateral branches are almost leafless, usually terminating in a 4-leafed whorl.

Habitat: Spigelia anthelmia is indigenous to North, Central, and South America.

Production: Wormwood Grass herb is the dried aerial part of *Spigelia anthelmia*, which is collected in the wild and cultivated in tropical and subtropical regions of America.

Other Names: Annual Wormwood Grass, American Wormwood Grass, Demerara Pinkroot, Pink Root,

ACTIONS AND PHARMACOLOGY

COMPOUNDS

Flavonoids: including hyperoside, quercetin-di-O-glucoside, quercetin-O-rhamnoglucoside

Phenol carboxylic acids: vanillic acid, dihydroxy benzoic acid, caffeic acid

Caffeic acid derivatives: chlorogenic acid

Amines: isoquinoline

Monoterpene alkaloids: actinidine

EFFECTS

The choline esters contained in the drug are possibly hypertensive in effect. Depending upon the dosage level, isoquinoline is positively inotropic in effect on isolated gerbil hearts. The experimental results in this area require further testing. The vermifugal action mechanism credited to the drug has not yet been proved. The isoquinoline found in the drug is not present at levels required for protoplasma-destroying effect.

INDICATIONS AND USAGE

Unproven Uses: Traditional folk medicine has included use for worm infestation.

Homeopathic Uses: Homeopathic uses include angina pectoris, neuralgia and headache, acute carditis, and worm infestation.

PRECAUTIONS AND ADVERSE REACTIONS

General: The drug is considered to be severely poisonous. Animal poisonings were described in older literature sources, as was deliberate use to poison humans. The toxin is said to be a nonvolatile alkaloid. Human consumption of large quantities of the drug is said to lead to vomiting, myositis, dyspnea, and spasms.

Homeopathic Precautions: No health hazards are known in conjunction with the proper administration of designated homeopathic dosages.

DOSAGE

How Supplied: Whole and cut drug.

Daily Dosage: The literature has no information.

LITERATURE

Achenbach H, H bner H, Vierling W, Brandt W, Reiter M, Spiganthine, the cardioactive principle of *Spigelia anthelmia. J Nat Prod*, 58:1092-6, Jul. 1995

Hänsel R, Keller K, Rimpler H, Schneider G (Ed), Hagers Handbuch der Pharmazeutischen Praxis, 5. Aufl., Bde 4 - 6 (Drogen), Springer Verlag Berlin, Heidelberg, New York, 1992-1994.

Wagner H, Seegert K, Gupta MP, Avella ME, Solis P, Cardiotonic active principles from *Spigelia anthelmia. Planta Med,* 378-81, Oct. 1986

Woundwort

Stachys palustris

DESCRIPTION

Medicinal Parts: The medicinal part is the fresh and dried herb.

Flower and Fruit: The closely sessile flowers have very small bracteoles. They are arranged in false whorls of 6 florets joined in groups of 10 to 20 into a spike. The calyx is tubular-campanulate, violet-tinged with awned tips. The corolla is dull violet and the style pink. The nutlet is globular, 2 mm long, lightly striped, and glossy dark brown.

Leaves, Stem, and Root: The plant is a perennial, with long runners and barrel-like white swellings between the nodes. The shoots are usually loose and have partly appressed, partly patent silky hairs. They are pubescent or almost glabrous and almost odorless. The stems are erect or ascendent from the ground, 30 to 60 cm high, simple or branched, tough, usually with pubescent edges. The internodes are 2 to 10 cm long. The leaves are sessile or very short-petioled, usually clasping, ribbed, matte green, and loosely appressed pubescent on both surfaces.

Habitat: The plant is common in Europe.

Production: Woundwort is the aerial part of *Stachys palustris* or *Stachys sylvatica.*

Not to be Confused With: S. palustris is Marsh Woundwort and *S. sylvatica* is Hedge Woundwort. Several other plants have the name Woundwort, among them, *Prunella vulgaris* and *Achillea millefolium.*

Other Names: Clown's Woundwort, Hedge Woudwort, Marsh Stachys, Marsh Woundwort

ACTIONS AND PHARMACOLOGY

COMPOUNDS

Iridoide monoterpenes

Betaines: (-)- and (+)stachydrine

Flavonoids: including among others palustrin

EFFECTS

Woundwort is said to be a disinfectant, an antispasmodic, and a cure for wounds.

INDICATIONS AND USAGE

Unproven Uses: The herb is used externally for the treatment of wounds and internally for abdominal pain, cramps, dizziness, fever, gout, and menstrual disorders.

PRECAUTIONS AND ADVERSE REACTIONS

No health hazards or side effects are known in conjunction with the proper administration of designated therapeutic dosages.

DOSAGE

Mode of Administration: As an extract or poultice for external application.

LITERATURE

Barberan FAT, *Fitoterapia* 57(2):67. 1986

Hegnauer R, Chemotaxonomie der Pflanzen, Bde 1-11: Birkhäuser Verlag Basel, Boston, Berlin 1962-1997.

Kern W, List PH, Hörhammer L (Hrsg.), Hagers Handbuch der Pharmazeutischen Praxis, 4. Aufl., Bde 1-8: Springer Verlag Berlin, Heidelberg, New York, 1969.

Xysmalobium undulatum

See Uzara

Yagé

Banisteriopsis caapi

DESCRIPTION

Medicinal Parts: The medicinal part of the plant is the bark.

Flower and Fruit: The inflorescence is multi-flowered. The flowers are 10 to 15 mm wide with pale pink petals. Their structures are arranged in fives. The fruit, which resembles that of the maple, is up to 4 mm long and 0.4 mm wide. Each of the 3 schizocarps has an 18 to 42 mm long and 8 to 22 mm wide wing.

Leaves and Stem: Banisteriopsis caapi is a hardy tree. The leaves are opposite, 8 to 18 cm long, 3.5 to 8 cm wide, ovate, and entire. The stem is woody with a brown, smooth bark.

Habitat: The plant is native to jungle areas of the Amazon basin.

Production: Yagé bark is the dried or fresh trunk bark of *Banisteriopsis caapi.*

Other Names: Ayahuasca, Vine of the Souls

ACTIONS AND PHARMACOLOGY

COMPOUNDS

Indole alkaloids (beta-carboline type): particularly harmine (0.5 to 5.9%), harmaline (0.5 to 3.8%), tetrahydroharmine (0.3 to 3.3%), harmol (0.05 to 1.2%), harmalol (up to 0.4%)

Pyridine alkaloids: shinunine, dihydroshinunine

EFFECTS

The alkaloid-containing drug is psychotropic and hallucinogenic in effect, due to the harmine and harmaline it contains (pronounced MAO-inhibition in vitro and in animal experiments). Lower dosages bring on euphoric states in humans, while higher dosages have hallucinogenic effects.

INDICATIONS AND USAGE

Unproven Uses: The plant contains psychoactive substances, which intensify dreams and experiences.

PRECAUTIONS AND ADVERSE REACTIONS

The drug is not in medicinal use. Extracts of the drug (ayahuasca, 5 mg alkaloids/mL), ingested orally in low doses, have hallucinogenic and euphoric effects. These effects are primarily due to monoamine oxidase inhibition; later the effect becomes sedative.

OVERDOSAGE

The intake of higher dosages (corresponding to levels starting at approximately 0.3 g alkaloids) leads to vomiting, nausea, ringing of the ears and tendency to collapse.

DOSAGE

Mode of Administration: Fresh or dried herb powder and liquid preparations for internal use.

Preparation: The fresh or dried cut bark is macerated for several hours resulting in a bitter syrup, which is then consumed in small amounts. In addition, some of the bark is pulverized, mixed with water and then consumed in larger amounts. The juice can be kept for up to 6 months in tightly sealed containers.

LITERATURE

McKenna DJ, Towers GH, Abbott F, Monoamine oxidase inhibitors in South American hallucinogenic plants: tryptamine and beta-carboline constituents of ayahuasca. *J Ethnopharmacol,* 10:195-223, Apr. 1984

McKenna DJ, Towers GH, Abbott F, Ritual and medicinal plants of the Ese'ejas of the Amazonian rainforest (Madre de Dios, Peru). *J Ethnopharmacol,* 10:45-51, May 1996

Yarrow

Achillea millefolium

DESCRIPTION

Medicinal Parts: The dried flower clusters and above-ground parts of the herb are used medicinally.

Flower and Fruit: The plant has white, pink or purple composite flowers in dense cymes with small capitula. The bracts are imbricate, long, thorn-tipped, and taper to a point. There are 5 white female florets. The disc florets are tubular, yellowish-white, and androgynous. The fruit is 1.5 to 2 mm long.

Leaves, Stem, and Root: Achillea millefolium are 0.1 to 1.5 m high plants with hardy, horizontal rhizomes, which grow from underground runners. The stem is simple, erect, and hairy. The leaves are lanceolate and multipinnate with short acute tips.

Habitat: The numerous subspecies of the *Achillea millefolium* group are found in various regions. They mainly grow in regions of eastern, southeastern, and central Europe, as well as on the southern edge of the Alps from Switzerland to the Balkans.

Production: Yarrow herb consists of the fresh or dried, above-ground parts of *Achillea millefolium,* harvested at flowering season. Yarrow flower consists of the dried inflorescence of *Achillea millefolium.*

Other Names: Band Man's Plaything, Bloodwort, Carpenter's Weed, Devil's Nettle, Devil's Plaything, Knight's Milfoil, Milfoil, Nose Bleed, Old Man's Pepper, Sanguinary, Soldier's Woundwort, Staunchweed, Thousand Weed, Thousand Seal, Noble Yarrow, Yarroway

ACTIONS AND PHARMACOLOGY

COMPOUNDS

Volatile oil (0.2-1.0%): chief components (rendered through steam distillation) are chamazulene (blue, 6-19%, maximum 40%), camphor (up to 20%), beta-pinene (up to 23%), 1,8-cineole (up to 10%), caryophyllene (up to 10%), alpha-pinene (up to 5%), isoartemisiaketon (up to 8%). The composition depends greatly on the variety, and the volatile oil of some strains is free of chamazulene.

Sesquiterpene lactones: Mainly guaianolides including, achillicin, 8-alpha-angeloyloxy-10-epi-artabsin, 2,3-dihydro-desacetoxy-matricin, alpha-peroxyachifolide. There are also germacranolides such as millefoild and 3-oxaguaianolides. Some sesquiterpenes are transformed through steam distillation into chamazulene (proazulenes).

Polyynes: including pontica epoxide

Alkamids: including tetradeca-4,6-diin-10,12-dien acetyl isobutylamides

Flavonoids: including apigenine-7-O-glucoside, luteolin-7-O-glucoside, rutin

Betaine: including L-stachydrine, L-hydrostachydrine (betonicine)

EFFECTS

The herb has a cholagogue (stimulates the flow of bile) effect due to the guaianolide and germacranolide content. The flavonoid content exerts a spasmolytic effect, while the proazulene fraction has an anti-edema and anti-inflammatory effect. The effect probably results from the interaction of various structured bonds with the chamazulene and flavonoids. The plant has similar effects to those observed in Chamomile flowers, since some of their components are identical.

Anti-inflammatory Effects: Yarrow contains salicylate-like derivatives that may contribute to its anti-inflammatory effects (Kelley et al, 1988; Chandler et al, 1982). Stigmasterol and beta-sitosterol contribute to the anti- inflammatory effects.

Antimicrobial Effects: Extracts from several Yarrow species, *including Achillea millefolium, Achillea atrata,* and *Achillea fragrantissima,* exhibit bacteriostatic or bacteriocidal activity against a broad range of gram-positive and gram-negative organisms, as well as *Candida albicans* (Alijancic et al, 1999; Barel et al, 1991; Moskalenko, 1986). Yarrow species *Achillea millefolium* and *Achillea fragrantissima* contain terpinen-4-ol, which has bacteriostatic activity against *Escherichia coli, Salmonella typhosa, Shigella sonnei, Staphylococcus aureus,* and *C albicans* (Barel et al, 1991).

Cardiovascular Effects: An extract from Yarrow species, *Achillea wilhemsii,* lowered blood pressure in hypertensive subjects and decreased LDL cholesterol and triglycerides while raising HDL in hyperlipidemic subjects (Asgary et al, 2000).

CLINICAL TRIALS

Hyperlipidemia

A 70% (1:8) ethanolic extract of Yarrow species *Achillea wilhelmsii* had favorable lipid-lowering effects in subjects with hyperlipidemia. Sixty subjects with a total cholesterol between 200 and 300 mg/dL and a triglyceride reading between 200 and 400 mg/dL were randomized to receive 15 to 20 drops twice daily of either the extract or an alcoholic placebo for 6 months. Compared with placebo, the extract significantly decreased LDL by a mean 31.7 mg/dL at 4 months and 38.8 mg/dL at 6 months (p=0.001 and p<0.0001, respectively). Significant decreases in triglycerides occurred as early as 2 months after beginning treatment (p=0.05), to a significant 75.3 mg/dL at 6 months (p<0.0001). HDL increased but did not become significant until 6 months (20.4 mg/dL versus -4.3 for placebo, p<0.001) (Asgary et al, 2000).

Hypertension

A 70% (1:8) ethanolic extract of Yarrow species *Achillea wilhemsii* had blood pressure-lowering effects in subjects with Stage I hypertension. Sixty subjects with a systolic blood pressure (SBP) between 140 and 160 mm Hg and a diastolic blood pressure (DBP) between 90 and 95 mm Hg were randomized to receive 15 to 20 drops twice daily of either the extract or an alcoholic placebo for 6 months. Compared with placebo, the extract significantly decreased DBP as early as 2 months after starting treatment (8.3 mm Hg, p=0.003) by a mean 14.7 mm Hg at 6 months of treatment (versus 2.6 mm Hg for placebo; p<0.0001). SBP did not decrease significantly until 6 months post-treatment (by a mean 14.1 mm Hg versus 3.8 mm Hg for placebo, p=0.005) (Asgary et al, 2000).

Liver Cirrhosis

Liv-52 is an herbal blend commonly used in Indian traditional medicine. It contains five herbal extracts including Yarrow (*Achillea millefolium*), as well as *Mandur basma* and *Tamarix gallica*. The efficacy of Liv-52 for liver cirrhosis was investigated in 36 patients in a double-blind, placebo-controlled study. At month 6, the placebo group showed no significant improvements in measures of liver status. But the group treated with Liv-52 had a significant decrease in serum alanine aminotransferase and aspartate aminotransferase levels as compared to baseline. They also had significantly better Child-Pugh scores and decreased ascites. The researchers conclude that the hepatoprotective actions of Liv-52 may be due to its anti-inflammatory, anti-oxidative, diuretic, and immunomodulating and restorative effects. (Huseini et al, 2005).

Wound Care

The chloroform extract of Yarrow species *Achillea ageratum* has topical anti-inflammatory effects. The dried aerial parts of *Achillea ageratum* were extracted chloroform and dried. The terpenic compounds stigmasterol and beta-sitosterol were isolated from this extract and additionally tested. Effect on inflammation was determined using the 12-O-tetradecanoylphorbol acetate-induced mouse ear edema model. The chloroform extract was applied topically to the affected ear at doses of 1,3, and 5 mg per ear and stigmasterol and beta-sitosterol were each applied at 0.5 mg per ear. Compared with the control, the chloroform extract inhibited both acute inflammation in a dose-dependent fashion (from 50.6% with 1 mg to 82.5% with 5 mg, p<0.01 to 0.001). The 5-mg dose also inhibited chronic inflammation by 26.3% (p<0.001). Stigmasterol and beta-sitosterol inhibited both acute inflammation (by 59% and 64.9%, respectively; p<0.001) and chronic inflammation (by 36.4% and 40.6%, respectively; p<0.001) (Gomez et al, 1999).

INDICATIONS AND USAGE

Approved by Commission E:

- Loss of appetite
- Dyspeptic complaints (mild, spastic gastrointestinal discomfort)
- Externally, in a hip bath for female functional lower abdominal complaints

Unproven Uses: Yarrow is also used externally as a palliative treatment for liver disorders and for the healing of wounds. In folk medicine, it is used for bleeding hemorrhoids, menstrual complaints, and as a bath for the removal of perspiration. It is contained in other cholagogic preparations and biliary tract therapeutic agents. It is also used as an adjuvant in preparations for many other indications such as laxatives, cough treatments, gynecological agents, cardiac agents, and preparations for varicose veins.

Homeopathic Uses: Achillea millefolium is used in varicose veins, arterial bleeding, convulsions.

CONTRAINDICATIONS

Pregnancy: Not to be used during pregnancy.

Breastfeeding: Not to be used while breastfeeding; Yarrow contains trace amounts of the neurotoxin thujone (Newall et al, 1996).

PRECAUTIONS AND ADVERSE REACTIONS

The drug possesses a weak to medium-severe potential for sensitization resulting in contact dermatitis. The main compound responsible for the sensitization is a sespuiterpene lactone, alpha-peroxyachfolid (Hausen, 1991; Rucker, 1991).

Fertility: Yarrow is believed to have abortifacient activity.

DRUG INTERACTIONS

POTENTIAL INTERACTIONS

Iron: The tannin content of Yarrow may complex with concomitantly administered iron, resulting in nonabsorbable insoluble complexes and may result in adverse sequelae on blood components. *Clinical Management:* Until more is known, patients who need iron supplementation should be advised to separate administration times of these two compounds by one to two hours.

DOSAGE

How Supplied:

Capsules - 340 mg, 350 mg

Liquid - 1:1, 250 mg/mL

Mode of Administration: As a comminuted drug for teas and other galenic preparations for internal use and for sitz baths. The pressed juice of fresh plants is used internally. The drug is contained in standardized preparations of cholagogic and gallbladder therapeutics and as an adjunct in many other preparations, such as laxatives, antitussives, gynecological products, cardiac remedies, and preparations for varicose veins.

Preparation: To make a tea, place 2 g of finely cut drug in boiling water, cover, leave to steep for 10 to 15 minutes, and then strain. For sitz baths, use 100 g Yarrow per 20 liters of water.

Daily Dosage:

Infusion - 4.5 gm Yarrow herb or 3 g Yarrow flowers.

Tea - A cup of freshly made tea to be drunk 3 to 4 times daily between meals.

External application - 100 g Yarrow to be drawn in 1 to 2 liter of water for 20 minutes and added to the bath water.

Homeopathic Dosage: 5 to 10 drops 1 to 3 times daily; 1 tablet or 5 to 10 globules; injection solution 1 mL 1/week sc (HAB1).

Storage: The herb must be protected from light and moisture. The essential oil should not be stored in synthetic containers.

LITERATURE

Ageel AM, Mossa JS, Al-Yahya MA et al., Experimental studies on antirheumatic crude drugs used in Saudi traditional medicine. In: *Drugs Exptl Clin Res;* XV(8):368-372, 1989.

Al-Hindawi MK, Al-Deen HIS, Nabi MHA et al., Anti-inflammatory activity of some Iraqi plants using intact rats. In: *J Ethnopharmacol*; 26(2):163-168, 1989.

Aljancic I, Vajs V, Menkovic N et al., Flavones and sesquiterpene lactones from *Achillea atrata* subspecies multifida: antimicrobial activity. In: *J Nat Prod;* 62(6):909-911, 1999.

Asgary S, Naderi GH, Sarrafzadegan N et al., Antihypertensive and antihyperlipidemic effects of *Achillea wilhemlsii. Drugs Exptl Clin Res*; XXVI(3):89-93, 2000.

BAnz (Federal German Gazette) No. 22a; published Feb 1, 1990.

Barel S, Segal R & Yashphe J, The antimicrobial activity of the essential oil from *Achillea fragrantissima.* In: *J Ethnopharmacol*; 33:187-191, 1991.

Chandler RF, Hooper SN & Harvey MJ, Ethnobotany and phytochemistry of yarrow, *Achillea millefolium,* Compositae. In: *Econ Bot*; 36(2):203-222, 1982.

Cuong BN et al., *Phytochemistry* 18: 331, 1979.

Goldberg AS, Mueller EC, Eigen E et al., Isolation of the anti-inflammatory principles *from Achillea millefolium* (Compositae). In: *J Pharm Sci*; 58(8):938-941,1969.

Gomez MA, Saenz MT, Garcia MD et al., Study of the topical anti-inflammatory activity of Achillea ageratum on chronic and acute inflammation models. In: *Z Naturforsch*; 54c(11):937-941, 1999.

Hausen BM, Breuer J, Weglewski J et al., Alpha-peroxyachifolid and other new sensitizing sequiterpene lactones from yarrow (*Achillea millefolium L,* Compositae). In: *Contact Dermatitis*; 24(4):274- 280, 1991.

Huseini HF, Alavian SM, Heshmat R, et al. The efficacy of Liv-52 on liver cirrhotic patients: a randomized, double-blind, placebo-controlled first approach. *Phytomed.* 12 (9): 619, 624. 2005.

Kastner U et al., Anti-edematous activity of sesquiterepene lactones from different taxa of the *Achillea millefolium* group. In: *PM* 59(7):A669. 1993.

Kastner U, Glasl S, Jurenitsch J, Achillea millefolium - ein Gallentherapeuticum. In: *ZPT* 16(1):34-36. 1995.

Kastner U, Glasl S, Jurentisch J, Kubelka W, Isolation and structure elucidation of the main proazulenes of the cultivar *Achillea collina* "Proa". In: *PM* 58(7):A718. 1992.

Kastner U, Jurenitsch J, Lehner S, Baumann A, Robien W, Kubelka W, The major proazulenes from *Achillea collina* BECKER: a revision of structure. In: *Pharm Pharmacol Letters* 1(1):27. 1991.

Kelley BD, Appelt GD & Appelt JM, Pharmacological aspects of selected herbs employed in hispanic folk medicine in the San Luis Valley of Colorado, USA: II. *Ascepias asperula* (immortelle) and *Achillea lanulosa* (plumajillo). In: *J Ethnopharmacol*; 22(1):1-9, 1988.

Miller FM & Chow LM, Alkaloids of *Achillea millefolium L.* I. Isolation and characterization of achilleine. In: *J Am Chem Soc*; 76(5):1353-1354, 1954.

Moskalenko SA, Preliminary screening of Far-Eastern ethnomedicinal plants for antibacterial activity. In: *J Ethnopharmacol*; 15:231-259, 1986.

Müller-Jakic B et al., In vitro inhibition of cyclooxygenase and 5-lipoxygenase by alkamides from Echinacea and Achillea species. In: *PM* 60:37. 1994.

Ochir G, Budesinsky M, Motl O, 3-Oxa-guaianolides from Achillea-millefolium. In: *PH* 30(12):4163. 1991.

Orth M, van den Berg T, Czygan FC, Die Schafgarbe - Achillea millefolium L. In: *ZPT* 15(3):176-182. 1994.

Rucker G, Manns D, Breuer J, Peroxides as plant constituents. 8. Guaianolide-peroxides from yarrow, *Achillea millefolium L.*, a soluble component causing yarrow dermatitis. In: Arch Pharm (Weinheim) 324(12):979-81, Dec 1991.

Schmidt M, Phytotherapie: Pflanzliche Gallenwegstherapeutika. In: *DAZ* 135(8):680-682. 1995.

Smolenski SJ et al., *Lloydia* 30: 144, 1967.

Tewari JP, Srivastava MC & Bajpai JL, Phytopharmacologic studies of *Achillea millefolium Linn.* In: *Indian J Med Sci*; 28(8):331-336, 1974.

Verzăr-Petri G et al., Herba Hung. 18 (2): 83, 1979.

Yellow Dock

Rumex crispus

DESCRIPTION

Medicinal Parts: The medicinal parts are the fresh and dried roots.

Flower and Fruit: The green androgynous flowers are in panicles. The inner tips of the perigone are entire-margined, orbicular, or ovate. Otherwise the flower is the same as *R. acetosa* in that there is a 6-tepalled perigone. The inner tepals are longer than the outer ones and grow closer together. The ripe fruit is usually red-tinged, membranous, entire-margined, and has a downward curved, scalelike welt at the base. The outer 3 tips are revolute. There are 6 stamens and 3 styles with stigmas that resemble paintbrushes. The fruit is a triangular, brown-black nut, which is enclosed by the winglike enlarged inner tepal.

Leaves, Stem, and Root: The plant is about 100 cm high and has a carrotlike rhizome. The roots are 20 to 30 cm long, about 1.25 cm thick, fleshy, and unbranched. The roots are rusty brown on the outside, whitish on the inside, and have a relatively thick bark. The stems are angular, grooved, and usually branched from the base up. The lower leaves are large and have flat petioles. They are supported at the base or almost cordate, lanceolate acute, undate-curly at the margins, and alternate. The upper leaves are smaller and narrow-lanceolate.

Habitat: The plant is indigenous to Europe and Africa, but grows wild in many regions of the world.

Production: Yellow Dock root is the fresh root harvested in spring from *Rumex acetosa*.

Other Names: Curled Dock

ACTIONS AND PHARMACOLOGY

COMPOUNDS

Oxalates: oxalic acid, calcium oxalate

Tannins (3-6%)

Flavonoids: including among others, quercitrin

Anthracene derivatives (0.9-2.5%): anthranoids, aglycones physcion, chryosphanol, emodin, aloe-emodin, rhein, their glucosides

Naphthalene derivatives: neopodin 8-glucoside, lapodin

EFFECTS

No documentation is available, but laxative and mildly tonic characteristics have been attributed to *Rumex crispus*.

INDICATIONS AND USAGE

Unproven Uses: Yellow Dock is used for acute and chronic inflammation of the nasal passages and respiratory tract. It is also used as an adjuvant in antibacterial therapy. The plant has traditionally been used like the Red Dock (*R. aquatica*) for its similar properties, in decoctions for scurvy and other skin eruptions, and as a ''blood cleanser.''

PRECAUTIONS AND ADVERSE REACTIONS

No health hazards or side effects are known in conjunction with the proper administration of designated therapeutic dosages. However, mucous membrane irritation accompanied by vomiting is possible following intake of the fresh rhizome, due to its anthrone content. The anthrones are oxidized to anthraquinones after dehydration and storage.

OVERDOSAGE

Oxalate poisonings are conceivable primarily with the consumption of numerous leaves eaten as salad. One case of death following consumption of a soup made from the leaves of the curled Yellow Dock has been described (see Frohne).

DOSAGE

Mode of Administration: Preparations are available in ground form or as an extract.

How Supplied:

Capsules – 500 mg, 505 mg

Liquid – 1:1

LITERATURE

Dabi-Lengyel E, Jamber E, Danos B, Tetenyi P. Chemical Composition and Biological Activity of the *Rumex crispus L. Crop. Herba Hung.* 30 (1-2); 91-95. 1991

Demirezer LÖ. Anthraquinone derivatives in *Rumex gracilescens* (Rech.) and *Rumex crispus L. Pharmazie* 49; 378-379. 1994

Demirezer LÖ. Comparison of Two Rumex Species with a Spectrophotometric Method and Chromatographic Identification with Regard to Anthraquinone Derivatives. *Planta Med.* 59; A630. 1993

Frohne D, Pfänder HJ, Giftpflanzen - Ein Handbuch für Apotheker, Toxikologen und Biologen, 4. Aufl., Wiss. Verlags-Ges. Stuttgart 1997.

Kern W, List PH, Hörhammer L (Hrsg.), Hagers Handbuch der Pharmazeutischen Praxis, 4. Aufl., Bde. 1-8: Springer Verlag Berlin, Heidelberg, New York, 1969.

Madaus G, Lehrbuch der Biologischen Arzneimittel, Bde 1-3, Nachdruck, Georg Olms Verlag Hildesheim 1979.

Morton JF, An Atlas of Medicinal Plants of Middle America, Charles C Thomas Pub. USA 1981.

Teuscher E, Lindequist U, Biogene Gifte - Biologie, Chemie, Pharmakologie, 2. Aufl., Fischer Verlag Stuttgart 1994.

Koukol J, Dugger WM Jr, Anthocyanin formation as a response to ozone and smog treatment in *Rumex crispus, L. Plant Physiol*, 42:1023-4, Jul 1967.

Yellow Gentian

Gentiana lutea

DESCRIPTION

Medicinal Parts: The medicinal parts of the plant are the dried or fresh underground plant organs.

Flower and Fruit: The flowers are yellow, terminal, pedicled, and axillary in cymelike false whorls. The calyx is deeply divided in 2. The corolla is rotate and divided almost to the base into 5 or 6 lanceolate tips. There are 5 stamens with 8 mm long anthers and 1 superior ovary. The fruit is 6 cm long and capsule shaped. The numerous seeds are flat, oblong or round, with a membranous edge.

Leaves, Stem, and Root: Yellow Gentian is a completely glabrous perennial plant that grows to 140 cm high. The rhizome has a number of heads, and the top of the rhizome can attain the thickness of an arm. The main root is a taproot, which grows up to 1 m long. The stem is round, unbranched, hollow, and grooved in the upper region to finger thickness. The leaves are elliptical, bluish-green, have strongly curved ribs and grow up to 30 cm long and 15 cm wide.

Characteristics: The drug has a weak, sweetish odor. It tastes metallic/sweet at first, then bitter.

Habitat: The plant is indigenous to the mountainous regions of central and southern European, and cultivated in many other regions.

Production: The roots are collected from spring through October, cleaned, and swiftly dried. Extended, slower drying causes the roots to ferment. The roots become brittle through drying, swollen and spongy through contact with moisture.

Not to be Confused With: The roots of *Rumex alpinus* or *Gentiana asclepiadea*

Other Names: Bitter Root, Bitterwort, English Gentian, Field Gentian, Gentian Root, Pale Gentian

ACTIONS AND PHARMACOLOGY

COMPOUNDS

Iridoide monoterpenes (bitter principles): amarogentin (determines the value), gentiopricroside, swertiamarine, sweroside

Monosaccharides/Oligosaccharides: saccharose, gentianose (somewhat bitter), gentiobiose (bitter)

Pyrridine alkaloids

Xanthone derivatives (colored yellow): including gentisin, gentisein, isogentisin, 1,3,7-trimethoxyxanthone

Volatile oil (traces)

EFFECTS

The essential active principles are the bitter substances contained in the herb. These bring about a reflex stimulation of the taste receptors, leading to increased secretion of saliva and the digestive juices. Gentian root is therefore considered to be not simply a pure bitter, but also a restorative and tonic. There is also a possible cholagogic effect, although it is not clear if the mode of action is sensory-reflexive. In addition, a fungistatic effect has been proved for the gentian extract.

INDICATIONS AND USAGE

Approved by Commission E:

- Dyspeptic complaints
- Loss of appetite
- Flatulence

The drug is used as a tonic and in teas to stimulate bile secretion and alleviate loss of appetite, fullness, and flatulence.

Homeopathic Uses: Yellow Gentian is used in homeopathy for digestive disorders.

CONTRAINDICATIONS

The drug's stimulation of gastric juice secretion rules out its administration in the presence of stomach or duodenal ulcers.

PRECAUTIONS AND ADVERSE REACTIONS

Health risks or side effects following the proper administration of designated therapeutic dosages are not recorded.

DOSAGE

Mode of Administration: Comminuted drug and dried extracts for infusions and teas. Forms of commercial pharmaceutical preparations include digestives, drops, and coated tablets.

Preparation: Tea is prepared by pouring boiling water over 1/2 teaspoon of the drug (1 to 2 g) and allowing it to steep for 5 to 10 minutes. The tea may be sweetened with honey to alleviate the bitter taste. Decoctions are made using 1 g of the drug to 1 cup boiled water.

Daily Dosage: The average single dose is 1 g of the drug; daily dose is 2 to 4 g. The average daily dose of tincture is 1 to 4 mL 3 times daily. Liquid extract: 2 to 4 g; root: 2 to 4 g. A one-cup dose of cold or lukewarm tea is taken several times a day, including 1/2 hour before meals.

Homeopathic Dosage: 5 drops, 1 tablet, or 10 globules every 30 to 60 minutes (acute) or 1 to 3 times daily (chronic); parenterally: 1 to 2 mL sc acute, 3 times daily: chronic: once a day (HAB1)

Storage: The drug must be stored away from light sources.

LITERATURE

Ernst E, März R, Sieder C. A controlled multi-centre study of herbal versus synthetic secretolytic drugs for acute bronchitis. *Phytomedicine* 4 (4); 287-293. 1997

Heymons S, Hölzl J, Weber HC. Va-Mycorrhiza in *Gentiana lutea*, the Importance of Cultivation and Influence on Constituents. *Planta Med.* 52; 510. 1986

Öztürk N, Herekman-Demir T, Öztürk Y, Bozan B, Baser KHC. Choleretic Activity of *Gentiana lutea ssp.* symphyandra in rats. *Phytomedicine* 5 (4); 283-288. 1998

Yellow Jessamine

Gelsemium sempervirens

DESCRIPTION

Medicinal Parts: The medicinal part of the plant is the dried rhizome with the roots.

Flower and Fruit: Yellow, strongly perfumed, 2.5 to 4 cm, funnel-shaped, long flowers grow in axillary or terminal cymes of 2 to 5 blooms. The fruit consists of 2 separable, connected pods containing numerous flat-winged seeds.

Leaves, Stem, and Root: The plant is a perennial evergreen vine on a tortuous, smooth root with a thin bark and woody center, showing broad medullary rays. The stem is slender, woody, and up to 6 m high. The leaves are opposite, lanceolate to ovate-lanceolate, short-stemmed, entire-margined, 2.5 to 10 cm long, dark green above, and paler green beneath.

Habitat: The plant is indigenous to southern North America, along the coast from Virginia to Florida, and Mexico.

Production: Gelsemium root consists of the rhizome and roots of *Gelsemium sempervirens*.

Not to be Confused With: The plant should not be confused with yellow flowering Jasmine (*Jasminum odoratissimum*), which is also called True Yellow Jasmine or Gelsemium.

Other Names: False Jasmine, Gelsemin, Yellow Jasmine, Woodbine

ACTIONS AND PHARMACOLOGY

COMPOUNDS

Indole alkaloids: main alkaloid gelsemin, including among others 21-oxygelsemine, gelsemicin, gelsidin, gelsevirin, sempervirin

Hydroxycoumarins: including scopoletine (gelseminic acid), fabiatrin

Anthracene derivatives: emodin monomethyl ether

Volatile oil

EFFECTS

In animal tests, the following effects on the autonomic nervous system have been documented: inhibition of cholinesterase; cardiac-circulatory effects (vasodilatory, hypotensive); a bronchodilatory effect on respiration; an effect on the smooth muscle; and an analgesic effect, as well as mydriasis on rabbits' eyes.

INDICATIONS AND USAGE

Unproven Uses: The drug is used for neuralgia, headache, gastric disorders, nervous stomach, feelings of fullness, and heartburn.

CONTRAINDICATIONS

Particular dangers are associated with administration of the drug in the presence of cardiac weakness.

PRECAUTIONS AND ADVERSE REACTIONS

Health risks following the proper administration of designated therapeutic dosages are not recorded. The following side effects could appear: heaviness of the eyelids, inhibition of movement of the eyeball, double vision, hypocyclosis, dryness of the mouth, and vomiting. Particular dangers lie with administration in the presence of cardiac weakness.

OVERDOSAGE

Poisonings through overdosages, sometimes with fatal outcome, are possible. Extracts corresponding to approximately 0.5 g of the drug can kill a child, 2 to 3 g can be fatal for an adult. Initial side effects can include heaviness of the eyelids, inhibition of movement of the eyeball, double vision, hypocyclosis, dryness of the mouth, swallowing difficulties, or vomiting. They may progress to symptoms of poisoning that can include headache, dizziness, loss of speech ability, vision weakness or double vision, pupil enlargement, trembling of the limbs, paralysis or stiffening of the muscles, cyanosis, shortness of breath, and coma.

The therapy for poisonings, following stomach emptying (gastric lavage with burgundy-colored potassium permanganate solution), consists of prophylaxis for shock, diazepam for spasms, electrolyte replenishment and sodium bicarbonate infusions for any acidosis that may arise. Intubation and oxygen respiration may also be necessary.

DOSAGE

Medicinal preparations are obsolete. Yellow Jessamine is currently used in homeopathic dilutions only.

LITERATURE

Frohne D, Pfänder HJ, Giftpflanzen - Ein Handbuch für Apotheker, Toxikologen und Biologen, 4. Aufl., Wiss. Verlagsges. mbH Stuttgart 1997.

Jensen SR et al., () Phytochemistry 26(6):1725. 1987

Kern W, List PH, Hörhammer L (Hrsg.), Hagers Handbuch der Pharmazeutischen Praxis, 4. Aufl., Bde 1-8, Springer Verlag Berlin, Heidelberg, New York, 1969.

Leung AY, Encyclopedia of Common Natural Ingredients Used in Food Drugs and Cosmetics, John Wiley & Sons Inc., New York 1980.

Lewin L, Gifte und Vergiftungen, 6. Aufl., Nachdruck, Haug Verlag, Heidelberg 1992.

Madaus G, Lehrbuch der Biologischen Arzneimittel, Bde 1-3, Nachdruck, Georg Olms Verlag Hildesheim 1979.

Roth L, Daunderer M, Kormann K, Giftpflanzen, Pflanzengifte, 4. Aufl., Ecomed Fachverlag Landsberg Lech 1993.

Wagner H, Wiesenauer M, Phytotherapie. Phytopharmaka und pflanzliche Homöopathika, Fischer-Verlag, Stuttgart, Jena, New York 1995.

Yellow Lupin

Lupinus luteus

DESCRIPTION

Medicinal Parts: The medicinal parts are the seeds and the aerial parts of the plant.

Flower and Fruit: The terminal flowers are almost sessile. They are arranged in numerous, distinct whorls. They have dropping, silky-haired bracts. The corolla is bright yellow with a blunted boat-shaped tip. The fruit is an oblong-lanceolate, 5 to 7 cm by 1 cm, densely pubescent pod with nodes. It contains 4 to 7 yellowish, reddish-white, black or dark violet marbled seeds 5.5 to 6.5 mm long.

Leaves, Stem, and Root: The plant is an annual with up to a 1 m long taproot, which contains numerous lateral roots. The stem is light green and pubescent with numerous side shoots. The 5 to 10 leaves are oblong-obovate to lanceolate, 4 to 8 cm long, acuminate, and pubescent on both sides.

Habitat: The plant is indigenous to Europe, Asia, and North and South America.

Production: Lupin herb and seeds are the aerial part and seeds of *Lupinus luteus* and other *Lupinus species*.

ACTIONS AND PHARMACOLOGY

COMPOUNDS: IN THE FOLIAGE

Quinolizidine alkaloids (0.6-1.6%): sparteine (55-70%), lupinine (20-30%), p-cumaroyllupinine (10%); in cultivated strains (sweet lupins), alkaloid content is 0.01-0.8%

COMPOUNDS: IN THE SEEDS

Quinolizidine alkaloid (0.4-3.3%): lupinine (60%), sparteine (30%); in some cultivated strains, gramine; in cultivated strains (sweet lupins), alkaloid content is less than 0.1%

Fatty oil (4-6%)

Carbohydrates: including stachyose (6%)

Proteins (36-48%)

EFFECTS

There has been no research on the effects of the drug; however, an anthelmintic effect has been established for the constituents lupinin and benzolylupinin.

INDICATIONS AND USAGE

Unproven Uses: Yellow Lupin is used externally for ulcers. It is used internally for urinary tract disorders and worm infestation.

PRECAUTIONS AND ADVERSE REACTIONS

See Overdosage section.

OVERDOSAGE

Symptoms of poisoning include salivation, swallowing difficulties, vomiting, diarrhea, headaches, hypocyclosis, double vision, cardiac rhythm disorders, and prickling sensation in the extremities. In cases of severe poisoning, symptoms include ascending paralysis and possible death through respiratory failure within a few hours. The intake of a single seed of a bitter lupin is said to be toxic for a child. In one case, a small child died following intake of several seeds. The intake of more than one pod of the plant or 10 seeds by an adult is said to trigger vomiting and should be treated with administration of activated charcoal. Following gastrointestinal emptying (inducement of vomiting, gastric lavage with burgundy-colored potassium permanganate solution, sodium sulfate) and installation of activated charcoal, the therapy for severe poisonings consists of electrolyte substitution, treating possible cases of acidosis with sodium bicarbonate infusions, and administering orciprenaline or lidocaine for cardiac rhythm disorders. In case of shock, plasma volume expanders should be administered. Intubation and oxygen respiration may also be necessary.

The lupinosis seen in animals is caused by mycotoxins that are formed from the fungus *Phomopsis leptostromiformis*, which can live as an endophyte in lupins.

DOSAGE

Mode of Administration: The drug is used internally as an infusion, and externally in poultices.

LITERATURE

Plakhota VA, Berezyuk NK, Oleinik GV, Boiko VP. Poisoning of animals with lupins. In: *Veterinariya,* Moscow, USSR, No. 8, 79-81. 1966

Frohne D, Pfänder HJ, Giftpflanzen - Ein Handbuch für Apotheker, Toxikologen und Biologen, 4. Aufl., Wiss. Verlags-Ges Stuttgart 1997.

Schmeller Th et al., Binding of quinolizidine alkaloids to nicotinic and muscarinic acetylcholine receptors. In: *JNP* 57(9):1316-1319. 1994.

Seeger R, Lupanin und Anagyrin. In: *DAZ* 133(17):35. 1993.

Yellow Toadflax

Linaria vulgaris

DESCRIPTION

Medicinal Parts: The medicinal part is the fresh or dried herb.

Flower and Fruit: The flowers are in terminal dense racemes. They are sulfur yellow and remain closed until a bee gains entry. The calyx is only fused at the base and is 5-tipped. The corolla has a long sharp spur and is bilabiate with orange edges. There are 2 large and 2 small stamens and 1 superior ovary. The fruit is an orbicular, dry capsule with some chambers, which open when ripe, flinging out the seeds. The seeds are flattened and are in the middle of a circular wing.

Leaves, Stem, and Root: A number of slim, glabrous, erect, simple stems 30 to 60 cm high grow from a perennial creeping root. The numerous leaves are alternate, sessile, very long, and narrow. The leaves and stems are pale blue and completely glabrous.

Habitat: The plant is indigenous to the northern hemisphere and the southwest U.S.

Production: True Toadflax is the flowering herb of *Linaria vulgaris*.

Other Names: Brideweed, Butter and Eggs, Buttered Haycocks, Calves' Snout, Churnstaff, Devil's Head, Devil's Ribbon, Doggies, Dragon-Bushes, Eggs and Bacon, Eggs and Collops, Flaxweed, Fluellin, Gallwort, Larkspur Lion's Mouth, Monkey Flower, Pattens and Clogs, Pedlar's Basket, Pennywort, Rabbits, Ramsted, Snapdragon, Toadpipe, Yellow Rod

ACTIONS AND PHARMACOLOGY

COMPOUNDS

Iridoide monoterpenes: chief component - antirrhinoside

Flavonoids: including among others linarin, pectolinarin, linariin (pectolinarigenin-7-rhamnoglucoside- acetate)

Aurones: including among others aureusin, bracteatin-6-O-glucoside

Quinazoline alkaloids: peganine (vasicin)

EFFECTS

The main active agents are the flavon glycosides linarin and pectolinarin, pectin, phytosterol, tannic acid, and vitamin C.

The drug is anti-inflammatory. Diaphoretic and diuretic effects have been documented.

INDICATIONS AND USAGE

Unproven Uses: Yellow Toadflax is used internally to aid digestion problems and urinary tract disorders. Externally, the herb is used for hemorrhoids, ablution of festering wounds, skin rashes, and ulcus cruris.

PRECAUTIONS AND ADVERSE REACTIONS

No health hazards or side effects are known in conjunction with the proper administration of designated therapeutic dosages.

DOSAGE

Mode of Administration: The powdered form and the extract are used as a diuretic and a mild laxative (tea). Externally the herb is used in poultices.

Preparation: Tea infusion is prepared from 1 to 2 teaspoonfuls of the drug and 2 to 4 cups of boiling water left to steep for 18 minutes.

Daily Dosage: Drink the tea during the course of the day.

LITERATURE

Hegnauer R, Chemotaxonomie der Pflanzen, Bde 1-11, Birkhäuser Verlag Basel, Boston, Berlin 1962-1997.

Ilieva E et al., 5-O-Allosylantirrinoside from *Linaria* species. In: PH 32:1068. 1993.

Kern W, List PH, Hörhammer L (Hrsg.), Hagers Handbuch der Pharmazeutischen Praxis, 4. Aufl., Bde. 1-8, Springer Verlag Berlin, Heidelberg, New York, 1969.

Madaus G, Lehrbuch der Biologischen Arzneimittel, Bde 1-3, Nachdruck, Georg Olms Verlag Hildesheim 1979.

Pauli F, Ofterdinger-Dasegel S, Teborg D. Digitalis, Scophularia & Co.= Dtsch Apoth Ztg. 135; 111-124. 1995

Yerba Santa

Eriodictyon californicum

DESCRIPTION

Medicinal Parts: The medicinal parts are the dried leaves.

Flower and Fruit: The flowers are tubular to funnel-shaped, lavender or white, and clustered at the top of the plant. The calyx is ciliate. The fruit is a small, oval, grayish-brown seed capsule containing shriveled, almost black seeds.

Leaves, Stem, and Root: The plant is a 2.5 m high, sticky, evergreen shrub, with woody rhizomes. The trunk is smooth and usually branched near the ground. It is completely covered in sticky resin. The leaves are up to 15 cm long and about 2 cm broad. They are thick, coriaceous, glabrous, greenish white, lanceolate, and irregularly dentate at the margins. The upper surface appears to be varnished with resin, the lower surface is reticulate and tomentose.

Characteristics: The taste is balsamic and the odor, pleasant and aromatic.

Habitat: The plant grows in California, Oregon, and parts of Mexico.

Production: Yerba Santa is the aerial part of *Eriodictyon californicum.*

Other Names: Bear's Weed, Consumptive's Weed, Eriodictyon, Gum Bush, Holy Herb, Mountain Balm, Sacred Herb, Tarweed

ACTIONS AND PHARMACOLOGY

COMPOUNDS

Flavonoids: including eriodictyonin, eriodictyol, chrysoeriodictyol, xanthoeriodictyol

Resinous substances: made up of flavonone and flavone aglycones

Volatile oil (very little)

Tannins

EFFECTS

Yerba Santa is mildly diuretic and masks bitter tastes.

INDICATIONS AND USAGE

Unproven Uses: The drug is used as a constituent of antiasthmatic treatments and painted on medicines to counteract bitter tastes.

PRECAUTIONS AND ADVERSE REACTIONS

Health risks or side effects following the proper administration of designated therapeutic dosages are not recorded.

DOSAGE

Mode of Administration: As an additive to mask bitter flavors and for painting on as *Tinctura Eriodictyonis.*

How Supplied:

Liquid – 1:5

LITERATURE

Johnson ND, *Biochem Syst Ecol* 11:211. 1983.

Kern W, List PH, Hörhammer L (Hrsg.), Hagers Handbuch der Pharmazeutischen Praxis, 4. Aufl., Bde 1-8, Springer Verlag Berlin, Heidelberg, New York, 1969.

Liu YL, Ho DK, Cassady JM, Isolation of potential cancer chemopreventive agents from *Eriodictyon californicum.* In: *JNP* 55(3):357-363. 1992.

Yew

Taxus baccata

DESCRIPTION

Medicinal Parts: The medicinal parts are the fresh leaves, the branch twig tips, and the branches.

Flower and Fruit: The flowers are inconspicuous and dioecious. The male florets appear in autumn in yellowish catkins in the axils of the annual needle. The female florets, with only 1 pistil, are on short pedicles, which have scalelike high leaves. The hard, pea-sized, dark-brown seed is surrounded by a crimson, pulpy, beaker-shaped, sweet, and edible aril.

Leaves, Stem, and Root: The Yew may be a bush or small tree approximately 17 m high with a trunk diameter of over 1 m. The trunk has red-brown bark. The numerous branches are crowded and evergreen. The needles are 2 to 3 cm long, arranged in double rows, soft, and acute. They are glossy dark green above, have a distinct midrib, and are lighter green beneath, matte, with no resin.

Characteristics: Yew is poisonous.

Habitat: The plant is common in large areas of Europe as far as Anatolia and Sicily.

Production: Yew leaves are the needles of *Taxus baccata.*

Other Names: Chinwood, Common Yew, English Yew, European Yew

ACTIONS AND PHARMACOLOGY

COMPOUNDS

Diterpene esters of the taxane-type (mixture is known as taxine, 0.6-2.0%): including among others, taxine A, taxine B, taxol

Flavonoids: including among others, sciadopytisin, ginkgetin, sequoia flavone (biflavonoids)

EFFECTS

In animal experiments, the taxin, a mixture of different ester alkaloids, leads to an improvement in cardiac metabolism. The motility-inhibiting effect may be attributable to the biflavonoid fraction. In higher doses the drug is cardiotoxic and can cause tachycardiac arrhythmia leading to diastolic cardiac arrest.

INDICATIONS AND USAGE

Unproven Uses: The cooked Yew leaves are used to promote menstruation; to treat diphtheria, epilepsy, worm infestation, and tonsillitis; and as an abortifacient. The plants are highly toxic and their use is not recommended.

Homeopathic Uses: The drug is used for poor digestion and skin pustules.

CONTRAINDICATIONS

The drug is considered an abortifacient and therefore should not be used during pregnancy.

PRECAUTIONS AND ADVERSE REACTIONS

General: The drug is severely toxic: 50-100 g Yew needles (fresh weight) are fatal for an adult. The red seed coat of the berries, although not the green seed, is free of toxic taxane derivatives.

Use in Pregnancy: The drug is used as an abortifacient.

OVERDOSAGE

Symptoms of poisoning include queasiness, vomiting, severe abdominal pain, and feelings of vertigo, followed later by unconsciousness, mydriasis, reddening of the lips, tachycardia, and superficial breathing. Death results from asphyxiation and diastolic cardiac arrest.

Following gastrointestinal emptying (inducement of vomiting, gastric lavage with burgundy-colored potassium permanganate solution, sodium sulphate) and use of activated charcoal, treatment for poisonings consists of treating spasms with diazepam or barbital (IV). In case of shock, plasma volume expanders should be infused. The administration of lidocaine has proven effective in cardiac rhythm disorders. Monitoring of kidney function, blood coagulation and liver values is necessary. Intubation and oxygen respiration may also be necessary.

DOSAGE

Mode of Administration: Yew is used in homeopathic dilutions of the mother tincture.

Homeopathic Dosage: 5 drops, 1 tablet, or 10 globules, every 30 to 60 minutes (acute) or 1 to 3 times daily (chronic); parenterally: 1 to 2 ml sc, acute: 3 times daily; chronic: once a day (HAB1).

Storage: The mother tincture should be protected from light.

LITERATURE

Aljancic I, Popovic K, Stefanovic M. Biflavone from *Taxus baccata L. J Serb Chem Soc.* 60; 265-267. 1995

Aljancic I, Popvic K, Gasic MJ, Stefanovic M. Investigation of the extract of the needles of the domestic *Taxus baccata L. J Serb Chem Soc.* 61 (11); 947-950 1996

Breeden SW, Jordan AM, Lawrence NJ, McGown AT. 2'-Deacetoxyaustrospicatine from the Stem Bark of *Taxus baccata. Planta Med.* 62 (1); 94-95. 1996

Chattopadhyay SK, Saha GC, Sharma RP, Kumar S, Roy R. A Rearranged Taxane from the Himalayan Yew *Taxus wallichiana. Phytochemistry* 42 (3); 787-788. 1996

Das B, Padma Rao S, Srinivas KV, Yadav JS, Das R. A Taxoid from Needles of Himalayan *Taxus baccata. Phytochemistry* 38; 671-674. 1995

Das B, Padma Rao S, Srinivas KV, Yadav JS. Lignans, Bioflavones and Taxoids from Himalayan *Taxus baccata. Phytochemistry* 38; 715-717. 1995

Denis JN, Greene AE. Preparation of a Novel Paclitaxel / Docetaxel Derivative from Taxagifine. *Nat Prod Lett.* 8; 27-32. 1996

Gabetta B, Orsini P, Peterlongo F, Appendino G. Paclitaxel Analogues from Taxus baccata. Phytochemistry 47 (7); 1325-1329 (1998)

Guo Y, Vanhaelen-Fastre R, Diallo B, Vanhaelen M. Immunoenzymatic Methods Applied to the Search for Bioactive Taxoids from *Taxus baccata. J Nat Prod.* 58 (7); 1015-1023. 1995

Guo Y, Daillo B, Jaziri M, Vanhaelen-Fastre R, Vanhaelen M. Two New Taxoids from the Stem Bark of *Taxus baccata. J Nat Prod.* 58 (12); 1906-1912. 1995

Guo Y, Diallo B, Jazir M, Vanhaelen-Fastre R, Vanhaelen M. Immunological Detection and Isolation of a New Taxoid from the Stem Bark of *Taxus baccata. J Nat Prod.* 59 (2); 169-172. 1996

Jenniskens LHD, Identification of six taxine alkaloids from *Taxus baccata* needles. In: *JNP* 59(2):117-123. 1996.

Kelsey RG, Vance NC, Taxol and cephalomannine concentrations in the foliage and bark of shade-grown and sun-exposed *Taxus baccata* trees. In: *JNP* 55:912-917. 1992.

Kingston DGI, Sorties and surprises: unexpected reactions of taxol. In: PM 62, Abstracts of the 44th Ann Congress of GA, 5. 1996.

Kongreβbericht, Taxol in der onkologischen Therapie. In: ZPT 15(2):114. 1994.

Kubitschek J, Eibenwirkstoff gegen Malaria. In: PZ 140(8):684. 1995.

Ma W et al., New bioactive taxoids from cell cultures of *Taxus baccata*. In: *JNP* 57(1):116. 1994.

Poupat Ch et al., Noveau taxoide basique isolé des feuilles D'if, *Taxus baccata*: La 2-désacétyltaxine A. In: *JNP* 57(10):1468-1469. 1994.

Schneider B, Taxol, ein Arzneistoff der Eibe. In: *DAZ* 134(36):3389. 1994.

Vanek T et al., Study of the influence of year season on taxanes content in *Taxus baccata* bark. In: *PM* 59(7):A699. 1993.

Vidensek N, Lim P, Campbell A, Carlson C, Taxol content in bark, wood, root, leaf, twig and seedling from several *Taxus* species. In: *JNP* 53:1609-1610. 1994.

Yohimbe Bark

Pausinystalia yohimbe

DESCRIPTION

Medicinal Parts: The medicinal part is the bark.

Flower and Fruit: The inflorescence consists of racemes of yellow blooms.

Leaves, Stem, and Root: The evergreen tree grows up to 30 m in height. The bark is gray-brown, fissured and split, and is often spotted. The inner fracture is reddish brown and grooved. The leaves are oblong or elliptical.

Characteristics: The taste is bitter, and the plant is odorless.

Habitat: The plant grows in the jungles of West Africa, Cameroon, Congo, and Gabon.

Production: Yohimbe bark consists of the dried bark of the trunk and/or branches of *Pausinystalia yohimbe*.

ACTIONS AND PHARMACOLOGY

COMPOUNDS

Indole alkaloids (2.7-5.9%): including among others Yohimbine (quebrachine) and its stereoisomers alpha-yohimbine (rauwolscine), beta-yohimbine, and allo-yohimbine. Including also, ajamalicine, dihydroyohimbine, corynantheine, dihydrocorynantheine, corynanthine (rauhimbin)

Tannins

EFFECTS

A potent alpha-2-adrenoncepter blocker and a weak alpha-1-adrenergic antagonist with some antidopaminergic properties (Langer, 1980), yohimbine interacts with adrenoreceptors that are selectively stimulated by clonidine, alpha-methylnorepinephrine, tramazoline, guanabenz, guanfacine, B-HT 920, B-HT 933, M7, and also with compounds that are nonselectively stimulated by norepinephrine and epinephrine. These receptors are selectively blocked by rauwolscine, nonselectively blocked by phentolamine and tolazoline, and are resistant to blockade by prazosin and corynanthine. Based on radioligand and pharmacological studies, yohimbine can interact with alpha-1 adrenoreceptors. At high concentrations yohimbine may interact with serotonin and dopamine receptors and at very high concentrations it may have a nonspecific local anesthetic action (Goldberg & Robertson, 1983).

Yohimbine is a relatively safe medication that has a modest beneficial effect in the management of erectile dysfunction. No effect on sexual drive in humans has been adequately demonstrated. The therapeutic gain achieved with yohimbine in clinical trials is more effective in patients with psychogenic erectile disorder than with organic disorder. Most trials have shown some degree of benefit of yohimbine relative to placebo, particularly in psychogenic erectile disorder but results have not always been statistically significant. All the trials reported on yohimbine in erectile dysfunction can be criticized on methodological grounds. It is not known if yohimbine has a role in the prevention of myocardial infarction, stroke, or orthostatic hypotension due to autonomic failure.

Alpha-2 adrenergic Antagonist/Norepinephrine Release Effects: Rauwolscine is a selective alpha-2 adrenergic receptor antagonist. Yohimbine increases plasma norepinephrine (NE) levels by stimulating the rate of norepinephrine release from sympathetic nerves (alpha-2 adrenergic antagonist) (Murburg, 1991). Plasma concentrations of 3-methoxy-4-hydroxyphenylglycol (MHPG), the major central nervous system metabolite of NE, also increase with yohimbine (Piletz, 1998). Central noradrenergic stimulation of yohimbine results in the enhancement of recall and recognition of emotional material (O'Carroll, 1999).

Analgesic Effects: Yohimbine significantly enhanced the overall analgesic effect of morphine with postoperative dental pain (Gear, 1995).

Cardiovascular/Hemodynamic Effects: In a dose-ranging study in normal men yohimbine hydrochloride caused dose-related rises in mean, systolic, and diastolic pressures. Associated with the rise in blood pressure were enhanced pressor and heart rate responses to the cold pressor, isometric handgrip, and Valsalva maneuvers (Goldberg et al, 1983). Yohimbine given in moderate doses increases systolic blood pressure in patients with orthostatic hypotension due to primary autonomic failure (Jordan, 1998). Yohimbine-induced enhancement of sympathetic tone in patients with neurally mediated syncope improves orthostatic tolerance (Mosqueda-Garcia, 1998).

Effects on Sexual Function: Because of the alpha-2 adrenergic blockade, the drug may be an effective treatment for sexual side effects, such as decrease libido and decreased sexual response, caused by selective serotonin reuptake inhibitors (Jacobsen, 1992; Hollander, 1992). There was no therapeutic response to yohimbine in women with hypoactive sexual desire (Piletz, 1998).

Hormonal Effects: In a double-blind, crossover study of normal men, yohimbine raised plasma norepinephrine and altered mood. When prolactin, cortisol, ACTH, beta-endorphin, TSH, and growth hormone were measured after 45 minutes of yohimbine infusion, there were no changes from baseline. The results suggested that alpha-2 adrenoreceptors in the hypothalamus, adenohypophysis, or other brain areas do not tonically modulate release of these hormones into the blood (Goldberg et al, 1986).

Salivary Effects: Yohimbine (18 mg daily) increases salivary flow in patients treated with psychotropic drugs (tricyclic antidepressants or neuroleptics) suffering from xerostomia (Bagheri, 1997).

CLINICAL TRIALS

Body composition/exercise performance

Twenty athletes (top-level male soccer players) were allocated to two randomly assigned trials to investigate the effects of yohimbine supplementation on body composition and exercise performance. Subjects ingested tablets that contained either yohimbine at a dose of 20 mg/day in two equal doses or cellulose (placebo) for 21 days. No statistically different changes in body mass, muscle mass, and performance indicators were found within or between trials (P>0.05). In contrast, fat mass was significantly lower in the yohimbine group in comparison to placebo (P<0.05) (Ostojic, 2006).

Depression

A six-week, randomized, double-blind, placebo-controlled clinical trial examined the effects of combining Yohimbine, an alpha2-antagonist, with fluoxetine, a selective serotonin reuptake agent (SSRI). Fifty subjects with a DSM-IV diagnosis of major depressive disorder confirmed by SCID interview were randomly assigned to receive either 20 mg fluoxetine plus placebo or 20 mg fluoxetine plus a titrated dose of Yohimbine. The results showed that addition of Yohimbine to fluoxetine results in a more rapid onset of antidepressant action as compared to SSRI alone (Sanacora et al, 2004).

Erectile Dysfunction

Yohimbine hydrochloride improved organic erectile dysfunction in 50% of subjects (n=9) ages 34 to 69 years. Eighteen subjects received Yohimbine hydrochloride 5.4 mg orally 3 times daily for 4 weeks and 10.8 mg orally 3 times daily for 4 more weeks. Nonsmoking subjects without major psychiatric problems who had normal initial serum testosterone and prolactin levels and an organic cause of erectile dysfunction were enrolled in the study. A sexual questionnaire was administered and nocturnal penile tumescence and rigidity testing was performed before treatment and after 4 weeks and 8 weeks of treatment. Four parameters of base and tip tumescence and rigidity were measured at baseline and after taking 5.4 mg and 10.8 mg Yohimbine hydrochloride. Responders demonstrated an increase in these parameters that either achieved significance or demonstrated a trend toward significance compared to non-responders. Responders were defined as those achieving successful intercourse for at least 75% of endeavors. It was less difficult obtaining an erection for intercourse taking Yohimbine hydrochloride 10.8 mg compared with baseline (p=0.011) (Guay et al, 2002).

Yohimbine was found superior to placebo (odds ratio 3.85, 95% CI 6.67-2.22) in a meta-analysis of 7 randomized, double-blind, placebo-controlled clinical trials involving male erectile dysfunction. Computerized literature searches were performed on all randomized controlled trials of Yohimbine for erectile dysfunction. Articles that scored less than 3 points out of 5 on the Jadad scale assessing methodological quality were excluded. Inclusion criteria included only randomized, placebo-controlled, double-blind trials that used adequate statistical evaluation. All studies examined found a positive response of Yohimbine versus placebo. Few adverse events were reported, with only 8 withdrawals due to adverse effects overall (Ernst & Pittler, 1998).

Hypotension

In 35 patients with severe orthostatic hypotension due to multiple system atrophy or pure autonomic failure, the effect was determined on seated systolic blood pressure (SBP) of placebo, phenylpropanolamine (12.5 mg and 25 mg), Yohimbine (5.4 mg), indomethacin (50 mg), ibuprofen (600 mg), caffeine (250 mg), and methylphenidate (5 mg). The pressor response was significant for phenylpropanolamine, Yohimbine, and indomethacin compared with placebo. In a subgroup of patients, the pressor effect was confirmed of phenylpropanolamine, Yohimbine, and indomethacin corresponding to a significant increase in standing SBP. The pressor responses to ibuprofen, caffeine, and methylphenidate were not significantly different from placebo, and phenylpropanolamine and midodrine exerted similar pressor responses (Jordan, 1998).

Syncope

Yohimbine significantly improved hemodynamic and sympathetic tilt response in neurally mediated syncope subjects (NMS) (n=8). All subjects experienced an upright tilt at 15-degree intervals every 3 minutes until reaching a 75 degree tilt. Subjects were placed in a supine position when presyncope or syncope developed. Blood samples of plasma catecholamines were obtained during tilting and after presyncope or syncope. Tilting was repeated after subjects had been supine for 3 hours. Patients developed a significant decrease in blood pressure that slowly worsened, resulting in syncope between 45 degrees and 75 degrees. Yohimbine significantly increased norepinephrine (p less than 0.05), epinephrine (p value not provided), muscle sympathetic nerve activity (p<0.01), systolic blood pressure (p<0.02), diastolic blood pressure (p<0.01), and heart rate (p<0.02) in NMS subjects compared to baseline (Mosqueda-Garcia et al, 1998).

INDICATIONS AND USAGE

Unproven Uses: Yohimbe bark is used as an aphrodisiac, and for debility and exhaustion.

CONTRAINDICATIONS

The drug should not be used by patients with liver and kidney diseases or chronic inflammation of the sexual organs or prostate gland, or with a history of gastric or duodenal ulcers. Yohimbine is not for use in psychiatric patients. Not recommended for long-term use.

Pregnancy: Not to be used during pregnancy.

Breastfeeding: Not to be used while breastfeeding.

Pediatrics: Not to be used by children under 12.

Tyramine-Containing Foods (such as wine and aged cheese): Due to its monoamine oxidase inhibitory effect, Yohimbine is contraindicated with tyramine-containing foods (Langer, 1980).

PRECAUTIONS AND ADVERSE REACTIONS

Side effects that can appear include anxiety states, elevated blood pressure, exanthema, nausea, insomnia, tachycardia, tremor, and vomiting.

Anxiety: Yohimbine was reported to exacerbate anxiety/panic and PTSD-specific symptoms after oral ingestion of the drug (Southwick, 1997, 1999). Patients with agoraphobia with panic attacks had greater autonomic anxiety symptoms, increase in SBP and cortisol responses to Yohimbine than healthy patients. Yohimbine also induced panic episodes in these patients (Gurguis, 1997). Patients with Parkinson's disease have demonstrated a vulnerability to Yohimbine-induced somatic symptoms such as panic attacks (Richard, 1999).

Hypertension: Yohimbine increased blood pressure in hypertensive and normotensive patients in several studies (Musso et al, 1995; Grossman et al, 1993; Damase-Michel et al, 1993; Goldstein et al, 1991; Murburg et al, 1991).

Mania: Yohimbine precipitated a manic episode in a depressed patient taking desipramine. The authors concluded that patients with a bipolar diathesis may be predisposed to the psychogenic effect of Yohimbine (Price et al, 1984).

DRUG INTERACTIONS

MODERATE RISK

Alcohol: Concurrent use of Yohimbine and alcohol significantly increased intoxication and also increased symptoms of anxiety and blood pressure in humans (McDougle et al, 1995). *Clinical Management:* Avoid concomitant use. Patients taking Yohimbine should avoid alcohol ingestion. If patients elect to use alcohol despite this advice, activities which require alertness (i.e. driving, operating heavy machinery) should be avoided.

Antihypertensive Agents (including Alpha-1 adrenergic blockers, Angiotensin Converting Enzyme (ACE) inhibitors, Angiotensin II receptor antagonists, Beta-adrenergic blockers, Calcium channel blockers, Diuretics, Hydralazine, Methyldopa): Theoretically, Yohimbine may counteract the hypotensive effect of these medications, resulting in inadequate blood pressure control. *Clinical Management:* Avoid concomitant use of Yohimbine and these agents.

Carbamazepine: Yohimbine may exacerbate bipolar disorder by precipitating manic episodes. This effect has been noted in 3 case reports, generally within 1 to 2 hours of Yohimbine administration (Price et al, 1984). *Clinical Management:* Avoid Yohimbine use in patients taking carbamazepine for treatment of bipolar disorder.

Clomipramine: Concurrent use of Yohimbine and clomipramine may result in increased risk of hypertension. *Clinical Management:* Monitor orthostatic and sitting blood pressure in patients taking clomipramine who initiate therapy with Yohimbine, as Yohimbine may increase blood pressure.

Clonidine: Concurrent use of Yohimbine and clonidine may result in a reduced antihypertensive effect of clonidine. *Clinical Management:* Avoid concomitant use.

Desipramine: Concurrent use may result in an increased risk of manic episodes. *Clinical Management:* Avoid concomitant use.

Guanabenz, Guanadrel, Guanethidine, and Guanfacine: Theoretically, Yohimbine may counteract the antihypertensive effect of these substances. *Clinical Management:* Avoid concomitant use.

Lithium: Yohimbine may exacerbate bipolar disorder by precipitating manic episodes. This effect has been noted in 3 case reports, generally within 1 to 2 hours of Yohimbine administration (Price et al, 1984). *Clinical Management:* Avoid concomitant use of Yohimbine and lithium.

Minoxidil: Theoretically, Yohimbine may counteract the antihypertensive effect of minoxidil. Opposing mechanisms of action resulted in opposite effects on blood pressure by Yohimbine and clonidine (Charney et al, 1983). *Clinical Management:* Avoid concomitant use.

Morphine: Yohimbine may enhance and/or prolong the analgesic effect of morphine. Pretreatment with Yohimbine prior to dental surgery enhanced the analgesic effect of morphine in patients (Gear et al, 1995). *Clinical Management:* Patients taking Yohimbine and morphine concomitantly should be monitored closely for analgesic effect and adverse effects. Patients taking morphine chronically should be advised not to self-initiate Yohimbine without close medical monitoring.

Naloxone: Yohimbine may increase symptoms of nervousness, anxiety, tremors, palpitations, nausea, hot and cold flashes, and increased plasma cortisol levels when taken concomitantly with naloxone. *Clinical Management:* Use caution if initiating treatment with naloxone in patients taking Yohimbine. Concomitant treatment with Yohimbine and naloxone has been proposed as a treatment for male erectile dysfunction. However, at the doses studied, the combination of Yohimbine and naloxone resulted in greater nervousness, anxiety, tremors, palpitations, nausea, hot and cold flashes, and increased plasma cortisol levels over that with either agent alone.

Naltrexone: Yohimbine and naltrexone administered concomitantly may symptoms of anxiety or nervousness, which may decrease compliance with treatment. *Clinical Management:* Use with caution.

Reserpine: Concurrent use of Yohimbine and reserpine may result in reduced reserpine effectiveness. *Clinical Management:* Avoid concomitant use.

Sibutramine: Concomitant use may result in adverse cardiovascular effects (Jordan & Sharma, 2003). *Clinical Management:* Avoid concomitant use.

Valproic Acid: Yohimbine may exacerbate bipolar disorder by precipitating manic episodes. *Clinical Management:* Avoid Yohimbine use in patients taking valproic acid for treatment of bipolar disorder.

POTENTIAL INTERACTIONS

OTC Stimulants: These may have alpha-1 adrenergic receptor activity to potentiate hypertension when Yohimbine is given concomitantly. *Clinical Management:* Avoid concomitant use.

OVERDOSAGE

Overdosage leads to salivation, mydriasis, evacuation, hypotension and disorders of the cardiac impulse-conducting system with negative-inotropic effect. Death occurs through cardiac failure.

Treatment of overdosage includes gastrointestinal emptying (inducement of vomiting, gastric lavage with burgundy-colored potassium permanganate solution, sodium sulfate) and administration of activated charcoal. For cardiac rhythm disorders, treat with lidocaine; possibly using physostigmine for its anticholinergic effect and electrolyte substitution. For cases of acidosis, treat with sodium bicarbonate infusions. In case of shock, plasma volume expanders should be infused.

DOSAGE

How Supplied:

Capsule - 500 mg

Liquid - 1000 mg/mL

Tablet - 5.4 mg, 800 mg

Daily Dosage:

Erectile Dysfunction - Yohimbine hydrochloride was effective for nonorganic erectile dysfunction administered as 30 mg daily (10 mg 3 times daily). Given up to 30 mg daily and 36 mg daily, Yohimbine, showed no effect for mixed-type impotence and erectile problems (Kunelius, 1997; Rowland, 1997). For erectile impotence, Yohimbine 5.4 mg (1 tablet) three times daily is recommended, and if side effects of nausea, dizziness or nervousness are reported, reduce to one-half tablet three times daily. Gradually increase to 1 tablet three times daily and therapy should not exceed 10 weeks (Prod Info Yocon®, 1985).

Xerostomia Treatment (for increasing salivary flow in patients treated with psychotropic drugs): 6 mg 3 times daily (Bagheri, 1997).

LITERATURE

Adler LE, Hoffer L, Nagamoto HT et al., Yohimbine impairs P50 auditory sensory gating in normal subjects. *Neuropsychopharmacology*;10(4):249-57, Jul 1994.

Bagheri H, Schmitt L, Berlan M, Montastruc J, A comparative study of the effects of Yohimbine and anetholtrithione on salivary secretion in depressed patients treated with psychotropic drugs. *Eur J Clin Pharmaco l*; 52(5):339-42, 1997.

Berlin I, Crespo-Laumonnier B, Cournot A et al., The alpha-2 adrenergic receptor antagonist Yohimbine inhibits epinephrine-induced platelet aggregation in healthy subjects. *Clin Pharmacol Ther;* 49(4):362-369, 1991.

Bharucha AE, Novak V, Camilleri M et al., Alpha-2 adrenergic modulation of colonic tone during hyperventilation. *Am J Physiol*; 273(5 Pt 1):G1135-40, Nov 1997.

Buffum J, *J Psychoactive Drugs* 17:131, 1982.

Charney DS, Heninger GR & Redmond DE, Yohimbine-induced anxiety and increased noradrenergic function in humans: effects of diazepam and clonidine. *Life Sci*; 33(1):19-29, 1983.

Charney DS, Heninger GR & Sternberg DE, Assessment of alpha-2 adrenergic autoreceptor function in humans: effect of oral Yohimbine. *Life Sci*; 30(23):2033-2041, 1982.

Clark JT et al., *Science* 225:847.

Damase-Michel C, Tran MA, Llau ME et al., The effect of Yohimbine on sympathetic responsiveness in essential hypertension. *Eur J Clin Pharmacol.* 1993;44(2):199-201.

Ernst E & Pittler MH, Yohimbine for erectile dysfunction: A systematic review and meta-analysis of randomized clinical trials. *J Urol.* 1998;159:433-436.

Gear RW, Gordon NC, Heller PH, Levine JD, Enhancement of morphine analgesia by the alpha 2-adrenergic antagonist Yohimbine. *Neuroscience*; 66(1):5-8, May 1995.

Goldberg MR & Robertson D, Yohimbine: a pharmacological probe for study of the alpha-2-adrenoreceptor. *Pharmacol Rev;* 35(3):143-180, 1983.

Goldstein DS, Grossman E, Listwak S et al., Sympathetic reactivity during a Yohimbine challenge test in essential hypertension. *Hypertension*; 18(Suppl 5): III40-48, 1991.

Grossman E, Rosenthal T, Peleg E et al., Oral Yohimbine increased blood pressure and sympathetic nervous outflow in hypertensive patients. *J Cardiovasc Pharmacol*; 22(1):22-26, 1993.

Guay AT, Spark RF, Jacobson J et al., Yohimbine treatment of organic erectile dysfunction in a dose-escalation trial. *Int J Impot Res*; 14(1):25-31, 2002.

Gurguis GN, Vitton BJ, Uhde TW, Behavioral, sympathetic and adrenocortical responses to Yohimbine in panic disorder patients and normal controls. *Psychiatry Res*; 71(1):27-39, Jun 16, 1997.

Hollander E, McCarley A, Yohimbine treatment of sexual side effects induced by serotonin reuptake blockers. *J Clin Psychiatry*; 53(6):207-9, Jun 1992.

Jordan J, Shannon JR, Biaggioni I et al., Contrasting actions of pressor agents in severe autonomic failure. *Am J Med*; 105(2):116-24, Aug 1998.

Jordan J & Sharma AM, Potential for sibutramine-Yohimbine interaction. *Lancet*; 2003;361(9371):1826.

Kunelius P, Hakkinen J, Lukkarinen O, Is high-dose Yohimbine hydrochloride effective in the treatment of mixed-type impotence? A prospective, randomized, controlled double-blind crossover study. *Urology*; 49(3):441-4, Mar 1997.

Langer SZ, Presynaptic regulation of the release of catecholamines. *Pharmacol Rev*; 32(4):337-362, 1980.

Liu N, Bonnet F, Delaunay L et al., Partial reversal of the effects of extradural clonidine by oral Yohimbine in postoperative patients. *Br J Anaesth*; 70(5):515-8, 1993 May.

McDougle CJ, Krystal JH, Price LH et al., Noradrenergic response to acute ethanol administration in healthy subjects: comparison with intravenous Yohimbine. *Psychopharmacology* (Berl); 118(2):127-35, Mar 1995.

Mosqueda-Garcia R, Fernandez-Violante R, Tank J et al., Yohimbine in neurally mediated syncope. Pathophysiological implications. *J Clin Invest*; 102(10):1824-30, Nov 15, 1998.

Murburg MM, Villacres EC, Ko GN, Veith RC, Effects of Yohimbine on human sympathetic nervous system function. *J Clin Endocrinol Metab*; 73(4):861-5, Oct 1991.

Mosqueda-Garcia R, Fernandez-Violante R, Tank J et al: Yohimbine in neurally mediated syncope. *J Clin Invest.* 1998; 102(10):1824-1830.

Musso NR, Vergassola C, Pende A, Lotti G, Yohimbine effects on blood pressure and plasma catecholamines in human hypertension. *Am J Hypertens*; 8(6):565-71, Jun 1995.

Ostojic SM. Yohimbine: the effects on body composition and exercise in soccer players. *Res Sports Med*: 14(4): 289-299. 2006.

Piletz JE, Segraves KB, Feng YZ et al., Plasma MHPG response to Yohimbine treatment in women with hypoactive sexual desire. *J Sex Marital Ther*;24(1):43-54, Jan-Mar 1998.

Price LH, Charney DS & Heninger GR., Three cases of manic symptoms following Yohimbine administration. *Am J Psychiatry*; 141(10):1267-1268, 1984.

Product Information Yocon® (Yohimbine hydrochloride tablets). Glenwood, Tenafly, NJ, USA, 1985.

Richard IH, Szegethy E, Lichter D et al., Parkinson's disease: a preliminary study of Yohimbine challenge in patients with anxiety. *Clin Neuropharmacol*;22(3):172-5, May-Jun 1999.

Rosen MI, Kosten TR, Kreek MJ. The effects of naltrexone maintenance on the response to Yohimbine in healthy volunteers. *Biol Psychiatry*; 45(12):1636-45, Jun 15, 1999.

Rowland DL, Kallan K, Slob AK, Yohimbine, erectile capacity, and sexual response in men. *Arch Sex Behav*; 26(1):49-62, Feb 1997.

Sanacora G, Berman RM, Cappielo A, et al. Addition of the alpha2-antagonist Yohimbine to fluoxetine: effects on rate of antidepressant response. *Neuropsychopharmacology*; 29(6): 1166-1171. 2004.

Southwick SM, Morgan CA III, Charney DS, High JR, Yohimbine use in a natural setting: effects on posttraumatic stress disorder. *Biol Psychiatry*; 46(3):442-4, Aug 1, 1999.

Southwick SM, Krystal JH, Bremner JD et al., Noradrenergic and serotonergic function in posttraumatic stress disorder. *Arch Gen Psychiatry*; 1997;54(8):749-58.

Vogt HJ, Brandl P, Kockott G et al. Double-blind, placebo-controlled safety and efficacy trial with Yohimbine hydrochloride in the treatment of nonorganic erectile dysfunction. *Int J Impot Res*. 1997;9(3):155-61.

Yucca filamentosa

See Adam's Needle

Zanthoxylum americanum

See Northern Prickly Ash

Zea mays

See Corn Silk

Zedoary

Curcuma zedoaria

DESCRIPTION

Medicinal Parts: The medicinal part is the dried tuberous part of the rhizome, cut in transverse slices or in longitudinal quarters.

Flower and Fruit: The inflorescences are on 5 to 15 cm long, obtuse and silky involucre bracts. The spikelike inflorescences are 7.5 to 12.5 cm long and 5 to 7.5 cm wide. The bracts bearing the flowers are ovate with revolute tips, pale green with a reddish border, densely punctuated with glands. There are stiff hairs on the surface, in particular at the tip. The bracts at the tip of the inflorescence are 5 cm long, initially white, turning pink to crimson. The flowers are pale yellow. The calyx is 8 mm long, obtuse, and 3-tipped. The tips of the corolla are broadly triangular and pale pink at the extreme tips. The labellum is light yellow, fluorescent yellow in the center with very slightly reddish tinged borders at the lower part. The ovary is 4 to 5 mm long and very weakly pubescent. The fruit is an ovate, thin, smooth, and irregularly opening capsule. The elliptical seeds have a white aril.

Leaves, Stem, and Root: Curcuma zedoaria is a perennial, erect, leafy plant. The rhizome has a grayish outer surface and is ovate to pear-shaped, thick, and branched downwards. It is whitish-yellow, with numerous thin roots, and it has a strong smell of camphor. The roots are partially thickened to ovate, white tubers. The leaves, in groups of 4 and 6 on the rhizome, are up to 1 m long. The 20 to 60 cm long and 8 to 10 cm wide leaf blade is oblong-ovate, glabrous, and has a purple mark in the middle of the leaf.

Characteristics: The taste is bitter. The smell is like camphor and is reminiscent of cardamom and ginger.

Habitat: The plant is indigenous to northeast India and is also found in the Moluccas, the Philippines, and New Guinea.

Production: Zedoary rhizome consists of the dried rhizome of *Curcuma zedoaria* and its preparations. After the root tubers have been harvested they are washed, cut, and dried.

Other Names: Turmeric

ACTIONS AND PHARMACOLOGY

COMPOUNDS

Volatile oil (1.0-1.5%): chief components zingiberene, 1,8-cineole, D-camphor, D-camphene, D-borneol, alpha-pinene, also including among others curcumol, zederone, curcumeneol, curculone, furanodienone, isofuranodienone

Curcuminoids: curcumin, desmethoxycurcumin, bisdesmethoxycurcumin

Starch (50%)

EFFECTS

Main active principles: essential oil, tannins, mucilage, small-grained starch. In animal tests, the drug has a choleretic, mildly antacid, and spasmolytic effect, as well as increasing intestinal transit time. The ethanol extract (main active principle p-methoxy cinnamic acid ethyl ester) is a strong fungicide. An antitumoral effect has also been proved.

INDICATIONS AND USAGE

Unproven Uses: Zedoary is used as a stomachic for digestive debility, colic, and spasms (stomachic, carminative). In folk medicine, it is also used as a remedy for nervous diseases.

Indian Medicine: In India, the drug is used for loss of appetite, tuberculosis, wounds, fever, bronchitis, and asthma.

PRECAUTIONS AND ADVERSE REACTIONS

General: No health hazards or side effects are known in conjunction with the proper administration of designated therapeutic dosages.

Pregnancy: Not to be used during pregnancy.

DOSAGE

Mode of Administration: Zeodary is available as solid and liquid dosage forms for oral intake.

How Supplied: Capsules: 300 mg, 450 mg; liquid: 1:4.

Preparation: Extracts of the drug are contained in numerous combination preparations for gastrointestinal indications and as cholagogues. To prepare an infusion, pour boiling water over 1 to 1.5 g of comminuted or powdered drug, or put in cold water and strain after 3 to 5 minutes (1 teaspoonful = 3 g of drug).

Daily Dosage: Drink 1 cup as an aromatic bitter at meals.

LITERATURE

Gupta SK et al., Isolation of Ethyl-p-Methoxycinnamat, the Major Antifungal Principle of *Curcuma zedoaria. J Nat Prod.* 39; 218-222. 1976.

Hänsel R, Keller K, Rimpler H, Schneider G (Hrsg.), Hagers Handbuch der Pharmazeutischen Praxis, 5. Aufl., Bde 4-6 (Drogen): Springer Verlag Berlin, Heidelberg, New York, 1992-1994.

Latif MA et al., *Br J Nutr* 41:57. 1979.

Matthes HWD et al., *Phytochemistry* 19:2643. 1980

Shiobara Y et al., *Phytochemistry* 24(11):2629. 1985

Takano I, Yasuda I, Takeya K, Itokawa H. Guaiane Sesquiterpene Lactones from *Curcuma aeruginosa. Phytochemistry* 40 (4); 1197-1200. 1995

Zingiber officinale

See Ginger

Zyzyphus jujube

See Jujube (Da-Zao)

Nutritional Supplement Monographs

Alpha Lipoic Acid

DESCRIPTION

Alpha lipoic acid (ALA) is a vitamin-like substance used as a primary clinical nutrient in several areas of complementary care. ALA supports blood sugar metabolism and increases insulin sensitivity. In diabetic neuropathy, ALA improves blood flow to peripheral nerves with the goal of stimulating nerve fiber regeneration. In heavy metal toxicity, ALA is used for its free-radical scavenging qualities and its mechanism for improving glutathione levels in the body. The same mechanisms support the use of ALA in the treatment of acquired immunodeficiency syndrome to prevent potential viral replication. The daily use of alpha lipoic acid as an antioxidant is uncommon due to the cost.

Other Names: 2-dithiolane-3 penatanoic acid, 1,2-dithiolane-3 valeric acid, 6,8-thioctic acid, Acidum thiocticum, Alpha liponacid, Alpha-Liponsaeure, Lipoaminsaeure, Lipoate, Pyruvate oxidation factor, Thioctic acid, Thioctsaeure

ACTIONS AND PHARMACOLOGY

EFFECTS

ALA is an important coenzyme and has antioxidant and antidiabetic properties. It is a biologically occurring substance that acts as a cofactor in the pyruvate-dehydrogenase complex, the alpha-ketoglutarate-dehydrogenase complex, and the amino acid hydrogenase complex. Reduced levels of ALA have been found in patients with liver cirrhosis, diabetes mellitus, atherosclerosis, and polyneuritis. During metabolism, ALA may be transformed from its oxidized form (with the disulfide bridge in the molecule) to its reduced dihydro form with two free sulfide groups. Both forms have strong antioxidant effects. They protect the cell from free radicals that result from intermediate metabolites, from the degradation of exogenous molecules, and from heavy metals.

Antioxidant Effects: Dihydrolipoic acid scavenges superoxide radicals and hydroxyl radicals and prevents lipid peroxidation (Fachinfo: Thioctacid 1996; Kagan et al 1992; Suzuki et al 1992). Oxygen-derived free radicals produced during biological activation of drugs damage red blood cells, causing aging and hemolysis. In vitro reduced and oxidized enantiomeric forms of lipoic acid protected against 2,2 azobis (2-amidionpropane) dihydrochloride-induced hemolysis of human erythrocytes in a concentration-dependent manner (Constantinescu et al 1994). Dihydrolipoate is a potent radical scavenger and the uptake of exogenous lipoate and reduction to dihydrolipoate by normal human erythrocytes may contribute to oxidant protection in the human bloodstream (Constantinescu et al 1995).

Hypoglycemic Effects: ALA is synergistic with insulin, resulting in more efficient glucose utilization. In animals, it reduces blood sugar and increases liver glycogenesis; in humans, it decreases serum concentrations of pyruvic acid (Fachinfo: Thioctacid 1996). It also improves insulin action of skeletal muscle glucose transport and metabolism in human and animal models of insulin resistance (Henriksen et al 1997). ALA facilitates glucose uptake into cells by an unknown mechanism (Bashan et al 1993).

CLINICAL TRIALS

Cognitive Impairment

Although ALA has been used for the treatment of human immunodeficiency virus (HIV)-associated cognitive impairment, clinical studies have not shown a beneficial effect. In a 10-week multicenter, double-blind trial, 36 patients with HIV dementia were randomized to one of the following treatment groups: placebo, selegiline alone, ALA alone, or selegiline plus ALA. The dose of selegiline was 2.5 mg orally three times a week; the dose of ALA was 600 mg twice daily before meals. The selegiline group performed significantly better on tests of verbal memory, specifically on the Rey Auditory Verbal Learning Test total score ($p=0.002$) and trial 5 ($p=0.007$). Mood, neurologic examination, and functional status were not affected. ALA did not improve HIV-associated cognitive impairment (Anon 1998).

Diabetic Neuropathy

Oral Treatment

Results of a recently published study demonstrated the efficacy of once-daily oral administration of ALA for the treatment of neuropathic symptoms and deficits in patients with distal symmetric polyneuropathy (DSP). The second Symptomatic Diabetic Neuropathy (SYDNEY 2) trial was a multicenter, randomized, double-blind, placebo-controlled study that enrolled 181 diabetic patients with DSP in Russia and Israel. Subjects received once-daily oral doses of ALA 600 mg (n=45), ALA 1200 mg (n=47), ALA 1800 mg (n=46), or placebo (n=43). After an initial 1-week placebo run-in period, treatment continued for 5 weeks. During the study, 15 subjects discontinued treatment, mainly due to adverse effects; the most frequent of these was a dose-dependent increase in the incidence of nausea (Ziegler et al, 2006).

The primary outcome measure was the change from baseline in the Total Symptom Score (TSS), a scoring system that comprises the presence, severity, and duration of the four main positive neuropathic sensory symptoms of stabbing pain, burning pain, paresthesia, and asleep numbness. By study end, of the 166 evaluable subjects, the response rates (defined as a ≥50% reduction in TSS after 5 weeks) were 62% in the ALA 600 mg group, 50% in the ALA 1200 mg group, and 56% in the ALA 1800 mg group, compared with 26% in the placebo group ($p<0.05$).

Of note, a significant improvement in TSS was noted as early as the end of the first week of therapy with ALA 1800 mg, and after 2 weeks with ALA 600 mg and 1200 mg. This finding suggests that oral treatment with ALA in doses ranging from 600 mg to 1800 mg may be as effective as intravenous (IV) therapy using 600 mg/day over 3 weeks. However, since the higher doses administered in this study were more frequently associated with the reported adverse effects, the investigators concluded that once-daily oral treatment with 600 mg ALA appears to be the most appropriate dose.

Intravenous Use/Combination with Oral Therapy

A meta-analysis reviewed four randomized, double-masked, placebo-controlled, parallel-group trials: the first SYDNEY trial, ALADIN I, ALADIN III, and NATHAN II. Comprising 1258 diabetic patients with symptomatic DSP, it reviewed data on those who had received IV treatment with either ALA 600 mg (n=716) or placebo (n=542). The objectives of the analysis were to compare the differences in TSS from baseline to end of treatment between the two groups and to measure the daily changes in TSS response rates and other values. Overall, the analysis suggested that treatment with 600 mg ALA administered daily via IV infusion for 3 weeks reduced pain, paresthesia, and numbness to a clinically meaningful extent. Specifically, the relative difference in favor of ALA vs. placebo was 24.1% (13.5, 33.4 [geometric mean with 95% confidence interval]) for TSS. Response rates (≥ 50% improvement in TSS) were 52.7% in the ALA group and 36.9% in the placebo group. In addition, there was an accompanying improvement of neuropathic deficits, suggesting that ALA may influence the underlying neuropathy in a favorable way (Ziegler et al 2004).

Earlier studies on the efficacy of ALA in diabetic neuropathy yielded conflicting results. When ALA was administered intravenously (IV) for 3 weeks followed by ALA orally for 6 months, it demonstrated no effect compared to placebo on symptoms of neuropathy in type 2 diabetics with polyneuropathy. A total of 509 subjects were enrolled in a 7-month multicenter, double-blind, placebo-controlled study (Alpha Lipoic Acid in Diabetic Neuropathy [ALADIN] III Study). Subjects were randomized into 3 groups to sequentially receive: ALA 600 mg/day IV for 3 weeks, followed by ALA 600 mg 3 times a day orally for 6 months (n=167); ALA 600 mg/day IV for 3 weeks, followed by placebo orally 3 times a day for 6 months (n=174); and placebo IV daily for 3 weeks, followed by placebo orally 3 times a day for 6 months (n=168). An intercenter variability in symptom scoring may be responsible for the nondistinguishable effect on neuropathic symptoms between ALA and placebo. This regimen, however, demonstrated a beneficial effect on a secondary outcome: neuropathic assessment of muscle weakness and stretch reflex and perceptions to touch-pressure, vibration, joint position, and pinprick (Ziegler et al, 1999).

In a study including 260 adult patients with non-insulin–dependent diabetes mellitus, ALA 600 mg per day, administered intravenously for 3 weeks, decreased peripheral neuropathy symptoms (numbness, paresthesia, pain, and burning) vs placebo (p=0.002). In this multicenter, double-blind, placebo-controlled trial (Alpha Lipoic Acid in Diabetic Neuropathy; ALADIN), subjects were randomized to ALA 1200 mg (n=86), 600 mg (n=77), 100 mg (n=81), or placebo (n=82) in 0.9% isotonic saline solution 250 mL. Treatment was administered over 30 minutes, 5 days a week, for 3 weeks. After 19 days, the response rates (defined as TSS improvement of at least 30%) were ALA 200 mg (70.8%), 600 mg (82.5%), 100 mg (65.2%), and placebo (57.6%) (Ziegler et al, 1995).

Finally, an earlier study found ALA to be more effective than thiamine for the treatment of diabetic neuropathy. In patients with diabetic neuropathy, greater symptomatic improvement occurred during treatment with ALA compared with thiamine therapy. Twenty-three patients received ALA 300 mg twice daily intravenously for 3 weeks followed by identical dosages orally for another 12 weeks; or thiamine 200 mg twice daily intramuscularly for 3 weeks, followed by 12 weeks of the same dose orally. After 3 and 15 weeks, there were significant improvements in overall pain and paresthesia in the ALA group as compared to those in the thiamine group. There were no significant differences between the two groups in motor and sensory nerve conduction and autonomic nerve function (Ziegler et al, 1993).

INDICATIONS AND USAGE

Findings on the efficacy of ALA for treating complications of diabetes mellitus continue to emerge. ALA may be beneficial for alleviating pain and paresthesia caused by diabetic neuropathy. It is probably ineffective for the treatment of alcohol-related liver disease, Amanita (''death cap'' mushroom) poisoning, and HIV-associated cognitive impairment. More placebo-controlled trials are needed.

CONTRAINDICATIONS

The injection contains benzyl alcohol and should not be used in neonates or premature babies.

PRECAUTIONS AND ADVERSE REACTIONS

Because ALA can cause hypoglycemia, patients with diabetes may need their blood sugar monitored. Symptoms of paresthesia may temporarily worsen at the beginning of therapy; some research shows that antidepressants or neuroleptics may be used concurrently to treat the pain (Fachinfo Thioctacid 1996). Nausea has been reported with the oral formulation. Adverse events associated with the intravenous injection include platelet disorders, purpurea, headache, diplopia, shortness of breath, injection site reactions, and muscle cramps.

The bioavailability of ALA is decreased with food.

Pregnancy: No US FDA rating is available for thioctic acid.

Nursing: Infant risk cannot be ruled out. Available evidence and/or expert consensus is inconclusive or is inadequate for determining infant risk when thioctic acid is used during breast-feeding. The potential benefits of treatment should be weighed against the potential risks before prescribing thioctic acid during breast-feeding.

DRUG INTERACTIONS

MODERATE RISKS

Cisplatin: ALA antagonizes the action of cisplatin and may result in decreased cisplatin effectiveness. *Clinical Management:* Avoid concomitant use.

MINOR RISKS

Antidiabetic agents: Additive hypoglycemic effects may occur with concurrent use of antidiabetic agents and ALA. Close monitoring of blood sugar control is recommended when starting therapy with ALA. *Clinical Management:* If ALA and an antidiabetic are used together, monitor blood glucose levels and signs and symptoms of hypoglycemia regularly.

POTENTIAL INTERACTIONS

ALA intravenous solutions are incompatible with Ringer solutions; solutions that react with disulfide bridges; and solutions with metallic ion complexes, e.g., cisplatin (Fachinfo Pleomix-Alpha 1996).

OVERDOSAGE

ALA is generally safe in prescribed dosages. Allergic skin conditions are among the few reported side effects of ALA administration in humans. The LD50 was 400 to 500 mg/kg after an oral dosage in dogs.

DOSAGE

Mode of Administration: Oral, intramuscular, intravenous

How Supplied: Tablet, IV solution

Daily Dosage: Diabetic neuropathy

Oral – Daily starting dose: 600 mg daily in two or three divided doses. Maintenance therapy: 200 to 600 mg daily in single or divided doses. In severe neuropathy, it is recommended that treatment be initiated with IV infusions (Fachinfo Pleomix-Alpha 1996; Fachinfo Thioctacid 1996). ALA tablets should be taken on an empty stomach.

IM Injection – Usual dose: 300 to 600 mg (12 to 24 mL) daily for 2 to 4 weeks. Maximum dose: 50 mg (2 mL) per injection site. Several injections should be given when larger doses are used (Fachinfo Pleomix-Alpha 1996; Fachinfo Thioctacid 1996). Maintenance therapy is administered orally.

IV Injection – Usual starting dose: 300 to 600 mg (12 to 24 mL) daily for 2 to 4 weeks. Maintenance therapy: 200 to 400 mg per day orally. IV injection should be given slowly at a maximum rate of 2 mL per minute (Fachinfo Pleomix-Alpha 1996; Fachinfo Thioctacid 1996).

IV Infusion – This is the preferred method of administration. Mix the dose in 100 to 250 mL of normal saline and infuse over 30 minutes. Parenteral therapy has the advantage of ensuring absorption and maintaining constant blood levels in patients with autonomic gastrointestinal neuropathy. If parenteral therapy must be interrupted for an extended period (for example, on weekends), 600 mg per day orally may be given (Fachinfo Pleomix-Alpha 1996; Fachinfo Thioctacid 1996). If there is no improvement after 2 weeks of parenteral therapy, thiamine 100 to 300 mg/day orally for 2 weeks should be added to the regimen (Fachinfo Pleomix-Alpha 1996; Fachinfo Thioctacid 1996).

Storage: ALA is photo-labile. Intravenous infusions should be covered with aluminum foil. When protected from light, the infusion solution is stable for approximately 6 hours (Fachinfo Pleomix-Alpha 1996; Fachinfo Thioctacid 1996).

LITERATURE

Anon: Monograph: Alpha Lipoic Acid. *Alt Med Rev*; 3(4):308-311. 1998

Bashan N, Burdett E, Klip A: Effect of thioctic acid on glucose transport, in Gries/Wiesel (eds): *Stellenwert von Antioxidantien beim Diabetes mellitus*. pmi Verlag GmbH, Frankfurt, Germany, 1993.

Constantinescu A, Pick U, Handelman GJ et al: Reduction and transport of lipoic acid by human erythrocytes. *Biochem Pharmacol*; 50(2):253-261. 1995

Constantinescu A, Tritschler H, Packer L: Alpha-lipoic acid protects against hemolysis of human erythrocytes induced by peroxyl radicals. *Biochem Mol Biol Int*; 33(4):669-679. 1994

Fachinformation: Pleomix-Alpha®, alpha-Liponsaeure. Illa Health Care GmbH, Geretsried, 1996.

Fachinformation: Thioctacid®, alpha-Liponsaeure. Asta Medica AG, Frankfurt, Germany, 1996.

Henriksen EJ, Jacob S, Streeper RS et al: Stimulation by alpha-lipoic acid of glucose transport activity in skeletal muscle of lean and obese Zucker rats. *Life Sci*; 61(8):805-812. 1997

Kagan V, Shvedova A, Serbinova E et al: Dihydrolipoic acid–a universal antioxidant both in the membrane and in the aqueous phase: reduction of peroxyl ascorbyl and chromanoxyl radicals. *Biochem Pharmacol*; 44(8):1637-1649. 1992

Suzuki YJ, Aggarwal BB & Packer L: alpha-Lipoic acid is a potent inhibitor of NF-kappaB activation in human T cells. *Biochem Biophys Res Commun*; 189(3):1709-1715. 1992

Ziegler D, Mayer P, Muehlen H et al: Effekte einer Therapie mit alpha-Liponsaeure gegenueber Vitamin B1 bei der diabetischen Neuropathie. *Diabetes Stoffwechsel*; 2:443-448. 1993

Ziegler D, Hanefeld M, Ruhnau K et al: Treatment of symptomatic diabetic peripheral neuropathy with the anti-oxidant alpha-lipoic acid. *Diabetologia*; 38(12):1425-1433. 1995

Ziegler D, Hanefeld M, Ruhnau K et al: Treatment of symptomatic diabetic polyneuropathy with the antioxidant alpha-lipoic acid. A 7-month multicenter randomized controlled trial (ALADIN III Study). *Diabetes Care*; 22(8):1296-1301. 1999

Ziegler D, Nowak H, Kempler P, et al: Treatment of symptomatic diabetic polyneuropathy with the antioxidant a-lipoic acid: a meta-analysis. *Diabet Med*; 21:114-121. 2004

Ziegler D, Ametov A, Barinov A, et al: Oral treatment with α-lipoic acid improves symptomatic diabetic polyneuropathy: the SYDNEY 2 trial. *Diabetes Care*; 29(11):2365-2370. 2006

Androstenedione

DESCRIPTION

Androstenedione and its derivatives (androstenediol, norandrostenedione, and norandrostenediol) are prohormones for both androgens (testosterone) and estrogens. Androstenedione is thought to increase testosterone levels by about 15% and is marketed as a natural alternative to anabolic steroids. Innately produced by the adrenal glands and gonads, androstenedione is also produced by some plants. The supplement has gained popularity among athletes and body builders who are interested in augmenting testosterone levels, improving performance, and increasing muscle mass and strength. Research on androstenedione does not support the product claims for increasing muscle size and strength or improving overall performance.

Androstenedione is banned by the National Football League, the International Olympic Committee, the National Collegiate Athletic Association, high school athletic associations, and professional tennis (NCAA 2004; WADA 2004).

Other Names: andro; androstene; androst-4-ene-3,17-dione

ACTIONS AND PHARMACOLOGY

EFFECTS

Androstenedione and related molecules, if given in sufficient quantities and for sufficient duration, are likely to cause androgenic or estrogenic effects in humans. The biochemical evidence supporting the effect of androstenedione to raise circulating levels of testosterone and estrogen is strong (FDA 2004). Whether androstenedione supplementation can increase muscle mass and enhance performance is unknown.

CLINICAL TRIALS

Anabolic Effect

There is no reliable evidence that androstenedione aids athletic performance. It appears that androstenedione increases testosterone to some extent in certain people, but only for a few hours at a time. It is unclear if this increase significantly alters muscle development.

Androstenedione did not increase serum testosterone or enhance skeletal muscle adaptation in two separate controlled trials. The first trial consisted of 10 men randomly assigned one 100 mg oral dose of androstenedione or placebo. In the second trial, 20 men were randomized to receive androstenedione 300 mg daily or placebo in addition to performing 8 weeks of whole-body resistance training. Main outcome measures included changes in serum testosterone, muscle strength, muscle fiber cross-sectional measurement, body composition, blood lipids, and liver transaminase activity. Androstenedione supplementation did not increase serum testosterone concentrations or enhance skeletal muscle adaptations to resistance training. It did, however, increase serum estradiol levels by about 50% in the group taking 300 mg daily. No adverse effects were reported (King et al 1999).

Increased Hormonal Levels

Mild increases in testosterone were found 120 minutes after oral administration of 200 mg of either androstenedione or androstenediol in eight healthy males (Earnest et al 1999). More dramatic increases were seen in a two-period crossover study of 10 healthy young women given 100 mg of androstenedione or placebo. Over a period of 24 hours, the women receiving androstenedione had a 16-fold increase in testosterone versus the placebo-treated group (Kicman et al 2003).

Another study treated healthy men aged 20 to 40 years with androstenedione 100 mg daily (n=15), 300 mg daily (n=14), or nothing (n=13) for 7 days. Although there was no increase in testosterone at the 100-mg dose, there was a mean testosterone increase of about 35% at the 300-mg dose. Additionally, serum estradiol levels were elevated 42% and 128%, respectively, at the low and high doses of androstenedione (Leder et al 2000).

Other studies have found androstenedione to have no significant effect on testosterone levels. Plasma testosterone concentrations did not increase in 10 males who received oral androstenedione 200 mg daily for 2 days in combination with heavy resistance exercise (Ballantyne et al 2000). Likewise, no effect on testosterone was noted in six healthy males given 100-mg oral doses of androstenedione for 5 days (Bizeau et al 1999).

INDICATIONS AND USAGE

Proponents claim that taking androstenedione increases testosterone levels and muscle mass and enhances athletic performance. There is some evidence that it may increase testosterone levels for short periods of time, but there are no definitive studies that show increases in muscle mass or improved performance. Anecdotal reports have cited both positive and negative results. The potential hormonal effects of androstenedione taken long-term could result in serious adverse events in children and adults of both sexes (FDA 2004).

CONTRAINDICATIONS

Pregnant or lactating women should not take androstenedione.

PRECAUTIONS AND ADVERSE REACTIONS

The use of androstenedione for increasing muscle mass or strength should be discouraged. Although serum testosterone levels may rise temporarily, the potential health risks outweigh any possible benefits. Adverse reactions can occur at normal doses, and long-term use may impair liver function and glucose metabolism, reduce HDL cholesterol, and increase the risk of heart disease and certain cancers (breast, prostate, and pancreatic).

The side effects of androstenedione have not been well-documented but are thought to be similar to those of testosterone, namely liver cancers, hair loss in men, hirsutism, aggressive behavior, gynecomastia, testicular atrophy, altered blood lipids, cystic acne, and premature termination of growth in adolescents (Zurer 1998; FDA 2004). Priapism has been reported with androstenedione. (Kachhi 2000). Side effects reported with nasal spray formulations include nasal irritation, decreased sense of smell, and headache. Taking androstenedione could increase serum testosterone levels and result in a positive testosterone assay (Cummings et al 1998).

DOSAGE

Mode of Administration: oral, sublingual, intranasal

How Supplied: Capsules, tablets, sublingual tablets, and nasal spray

Daily Dosage: For muscle gain, most manufacturers recommend a maximum of 100 mg per day, taken with water on an empty stomach, 30 minutes prior to physical activity; a few advocate using higher doses. For maintenance of normal testosterone levels in women, the usual dose is 25 mg of nasal spray (1 spray) per day, no more than 5 days per week.

Storage: Store at room temperature, away from heat, moisture, and direct light.

LITERATURE

Ballantyne CS, Phillips SM, MacDonald JR et al: The acute effects of androstenedione supplements in healthy young males. *Can J Appl Physiol*; 25(1):68-78. Feb 2000

Bizeau, Hazel (abstract): Experimental biology 99. Washington, DC USA. April 17-21, 1999. Abstracts, Part I. *FASEB J*; Mar 12;13(4):A1-646. 1999

Cummings EA, Salisbury SR, Givner ML et al: Testosterone - associated high androgen levels: a pharmacologic effect or a laboratory artifact? *J Clin Endocrinol Metab*; 83(3):784-787. 1998

Earnest CP, Olson MA, Broeder CE et al: In vivo 4-androstene-3,17-dione and 4-androstene-3 beta, 17 beta-diol supplementation in young men. *Eur J Appl Physiol;* 81:229-232. Feb 2000

FDA White Paper. Health effects of androstenedione. March 11, 2004. Available at: http /www.fda.gov/oc/whitepapers/andro.html. Accessed 7/30/04

Josefson D: Concern raised about performance enhancing drugs in the US. *BMJ*; 317(7160):702. 1998

Kachhi PN, Henderson SO: Priapism after androstenedione intake for athletic performance enhancement. *Ann Emerg Med*; 35(4):391-393. 2000

Kicman AT, Bassindale T, Cowan DA et al: Effect of androstenedione ingestion on plasma testosterone in young women. *Clinical Chemistry*; 49:167-169. 2003

King DS, Sharp RL, Vukovich MD et al: Effect of oral androstenedione on serum testosterone and adaptations to resistance training in young men. *JAMA*; 281(21):2020-2028. 1999

Leder BZ, Longcope C, Catlin DH et al: Oral androstenedione administration and serum testosterone concentrations in young men. *JAMA*; Feb 9;283(6):779-782. 2000

NCAA Drug-Testing Program. Banned Drug List. Available at: www1.ncaa.org/membership/ed__outreach/health-safety/drug__testing/index.html. Accessed 7/30/04.

World Anti-Doping Agency. The 2004 Prohibited List. Available at: www.wada-ama.org/en/t1.asp?p=29626&x=1&a=75704. Accessed 7/30/04.

Zurer P: Androstenedione: out of the park or out in left field? *Science Insights*; 76:102-104. 1998

Bee Pollen

DESCRIPTION

This nutritive substance is a mixture of bee saliva, nectar, and flower pollen that sticks to the bees' legs and other body parts as they collect the nectar from flowers. The yellow-orange pollen granules contain a wide variety of nutrients and are a food source for male drones (Leung et al 1996; Pedersen 1994). Bee pollen products have been known to provoke allergic reactions, since there's no way of knowing whether they contain a common allergen such as ragweed.

Bee pollen granules have a protective coating that can be dissolved by bee saliva or human digestive enzymes (Pedersen 1994). It can contain a wide variety of chemical ingredients depending on the species from which the pollen was collected, the season, and the method of collection (by bees or by man) (Linskens et al 1997). Ingredients include heterosidic flavonols (0.5%), water (3% to 16%), protein (5.9% to 28.3%), all 22 amino acids (14.6 % to 21.9%), more than 25 minerals (especially calcium, magnesium, and zinc), rutin, enzymes, lipids or fatty acids (1% to 20%), carbohydrates (1% to 50%), simple sugars (4% to 10%), and vitamins (Leung et al 1996; Pedersen 1994; Kamen 1991; Murray 1991; de Graca Ribeiro Campos et al 1990; Guan et al 1984).

Bee pollen has more amino acids and vitamins than other amino-acid-containing products like beef, eggs, or cheese. Bee pollen is one of the few vegetable sources of vitamin B12 (Scheer 1992). A tablespoonful of bee pollen contains about 45 calories and is 15% lecithin (which is required for normal fat metabolism) by weight (Kamen 1991).

Names: bee bread, buckwheat pollen, maize pollen, pollen, rape pollen, songhuuafen

ACTIONS AND PHARMACOLOGY

EFFECTS

Bee pollen is claimed to have anti-inflammatory, antineoplastic, desensitizing, immune-stimulating, rejuvenating, and adaptogenic properties. Studies on the biological effects of bee pollen are difficult to evaluate since most pollen mixes vary from study to study (Leung et al 1996). Medicinal claims for bee pollen, outside of its nutritive value, have yet to be proven.

CLINICAL TRIALS

Altitude Sickness

Bee pollen is thought to aid in adapting to high altitudes. Two studies determined that people who ingested pollen 3 to 7 days before moving to an altitude above 5,000 meters (about 16,250 feet) were asymptomatic or had fewer symptoms than those who did not receive the pollen (Linskens et al 1997).

Athletic Performance

The use of bee pollen does not significantly enhance athletic performance but it may improve recovery time and prevent illness. The number of missed training days due to colds and upper respiratory infections was reduced in a study of adolescent swimmers who took bee pollen (Pollitabs®, strength unknown) versus placebo. Athletes trained daily during the 6-week, double-blind trial. There was no significant difference in maximal oxygen uptake or forced expiratory volume in 1 second (FEV1) between the two groups. However, vital capacity increased in the athletes taking bee pollen ($p=0.05$) but not placebo. The number of training days missed in the bee pollen group was 4 compared to 27 in the placebo group (Maughan et al 1982).

Desensitizing Therapy

Although supplemental bee pollen has been used to decrease allergic responses to a number of pollens, controlled studies have not found it to be an effective desensitizer (Leung et al 1996; Taudorf 1983). Some anecdotal reports describe a desensitizing action with oral bee pollen (Cooper et al 1984).

Gastric Ulcers

One small study showed improvement in gastric ulcers after bee pollen supplementation. Forty patients with bleeding gastric ulcers improved after twice-daily administration of 250 milligrams of bee pollen (Linskens et al 1997).

Side Effects of Cancer Treatment

Bee pollen was effective in reducing adverse effects of cancer treatment in a double-blind, placebo-controlled study of 25 women with inoperable uterine cancer. The stresses and adverse effects of radiation, such as anorexia, nausea, alopecia, inflammation, and sleeplessness, were decreased in patients taking bee pollen. Leukocyte concentrations were also higher (Murray 1991).

INDICATIONS AND USAGE

Unproven Uses: Bee pollen is taken to enhance athletic stamina, aid in recovery from illness, and provide rejuvenating and tonifying effects. It is often used as a pollen and spore antidote during allergy season. It may aid in respiratory complaints such as bronchitis, sinus congestion, and common rhinitis. Limited evidence suggests it may help prevent altitude sickness and the side effects of cancer radiation treatment.

Bee pollen is thought to balance the endocrine system and provide specific benefits for menstrual and prostate disorders. Proponents also claim that bee pollen can improve sexual performance, prevent infection and cancer, prolong life, produce weight loss or weight gain, and aid the treatment of renal disease, colitis, and skin blemishes (Mirkin 1989; Mansfield et al 1981).

Chinese Medicine: Bee pollen is used for building blood, reducing cravings for sweets and alcohol, as a radiation protectant, cancer inhibitor, a nutritive, a diuretic, and hemostatic agent. It has been recommended for treatment of abdominal pain, amenorrhea, bloody diarrhea, dysmenorrhea, dysuria, hematemesis, oral sores, and trauma (Leung et al 1996).

PRECAUTIONS AND ADVERSE REACTIONS

Allergic reactions have been reported, including abdominal pain, asthma, decreased memory, diarrhea, dyspnea, facial itch, facial swelling, gastrointestinal upset, grand mal seizures, headache, hypereosinophilia, hypotension, nausea, pruritus, sore throat, and stridor.

As its name suggests, bee pollen contains large amounts of pollen—a known allergen—from varying sources. Individuals allergic to airborne pollens should exercise caution when ingesting large amounts of bee pollen since it can retain its allergenic potential, as demonstrated in a recent study using skin prick testing (SPT). The study enrolled 202 subjects: 145 (71.8%) atopic individuals and 57 (28.2%) nonatopic individuals assigned to the control group. Five homemade extracts of bee pollen in a concentration of 0.02 g/mL (dilution in glycerine 1:2) were used to perform SPT. Although there were no reactions in the control group, 73% of atopic individuals reacted to one or more of the bee pollen extracts. Further studies evaluating the safety of supplemental bee pollen in pollen-sensitive individuals are warranted. (Pitsios et al 2006).

DRUG INTERACTIONS

No human interactions information is available.

DOSAGE

Mode of Administration: Oral

How Supplied: Capsule, granule, tablet

Daily Dosage: Athletic stamina enhancement: 400 mg daily. Gastric ulcers: 500 mg daily.

LITERATURE

Cooper PJ, Derbyshire J, Nunn AJ et al: A controlled trial of oral hyposensitization in pollen asthma and rhinitis in children. *Clin Allergy*; 14(6):541-550. 1984

de Graca Ribeiro Campos M, Sabatier S, Amiot M-J et al: Characterization of flavonoids in three hive products: bee pollen, propolis, and honey. *Planta Med*; 56(6):580-581. 1990

Guan F, Hong B, Shi X et al: Composition analysis and application of natural bee pollen. *Shipin Kexue (Beijing)*; 57:18-21. 1984

Kamen B: Bee pollen: from principles to practice. *Health Foods Business* (April):66-67. 1991

Leung AY, Foster S (eds): *Encyclopedia of Common Natural Ingredients Used in Food, Drugs, and Cosmetics.* John Wiley & Sons Inc., New York, NY, 1996.

Linskens HF, Jorde W: Pollen as food and medicine - a review. *Econ Bot*; 51(1):78-87. 1997

Mansfield LE, Goldstein GB: Anaphylactic reaction after ingestion of local bee pollen. *Ann Allergy*; 47:154-156. 1981

Maughan JR, Evans SP: Effects of pollen extracts upon adolescent swimmers. *Br J Sports Med*; 16(3):142-145. 1982

Mirkin G: Can bee pollen benefit health? *JAMA*; 262(13):1854. 1989

Murray F: Get the buzz on bee pollen. *Better Nutr*; May:20-21,31. 1991

Pedersen M: *Nutritional Herbology: A Reference Guide to Herbs.* Wendell W. Whitman Co., Warsaw, IN, 1994.

Pitsios C, Chliva C, Mikos N: Bee pollen sensitivity in airborne pollen allergic individuals. *Ann Allergy Asthma Immunol*; 97:703-706. 2006

Taudorf E, Weeke B: Orally administered grass pollen. *Allergy*; 38(8):561-564. 1983

Beta-Carotene

DESCRIPTION

Beta-carotene is the most active precursor of vitamin A (Wang et al 1998). It is a naturally occurring carotenoid pigment found in fresh fruits and green and yellow vegetables. Beta-carotene is converted to vitamin A in vivo. The best dietary sources of beta-carotene include carrots, dark green leafy vegetables such as spinach, green leafy lettuce, sweet potatoes, broccoli, cantaloupe, and winter squash. Ordinary cooking does not destroy beta-carotene (USP DI 2004).

Beta-carotene is often used in complementary clinical settings. It is useful in diminishing the photosensitivity reactions that occur in patients with erythropoietic protoporphyria. Much controversy surrounds the clinical utility of beta-carotene in the prevention and treatment of cancer. Still, it remains a frequently used supplement in many individuals.

Other Name: provitamin A

ACTIONS AND PHARMACOLOGY

EFFECTS

Beta-carotene is a natural precursor of vitamin A that has antioxidant and pro-oxidant properties, and may also have photoprotective effects in erythropoietic protoporphyria.

Antioxidants Effects: Beta-carotene can function as both an antioxidant and a pro-oxidant. Beta-carotene shows radical-scavenging activity under physiologic oxygen partial pressures (less than 100 mm Hg). When exposed to hyperoxic partial pressures (greater than 150 mm Hg) beta-carotene shows pro-oxidant properties with a loss of its antioxidant capacity (Powers et al 1999).

Another study concluded there was no antioxidant effect. An in vitro experiment conducted in cells loaded with beta-carotene and then exposed to peroxyl radicals concluded that beta-carotene did not provide any antioxidant protection to live cells under normobaric oxygen tension (Day et al 1998). Experimental data show beta-carotene acts as an antioxidant in vitro, but in vivo data are less convincing. Pro-oxidant data are based on high oxygen tension levels, giving little support that beta-carotene acts as a pro-oxidant in the body (Krinsky 1998).

CLINICAL TRIALS

Asthma

Beta-carotene exerted a protective effect against exercise-induced asthma (EIA) in a randomized, double-blind, placebo-controlled trial of 38 subjects aged 8 to 33 with proven EIA. Beta-carotene 64 mg daily or placebo was given for 1 week and pulmonary function was tested. This protocol was completed twice with a 4-week washout period. Postexercise forced expiratory volume in 1 second (FEV-1) was reduced by more than 15% in all participants taking placebo. In the beta-carotene treated group, 53% showed a postexercise FEV-1 reduction of less than 15%. Strenuous exercise may promote increased free-radical production resulting in lipid peroxidation and tissue damage. It is believed the antioxidant properties associated with beta-carotene may protect against some of this damage (Neuman et al 1999).

Cancer Prevention

Prostate Cancer

Heavy use of multivitamins, including beta-carotene, may increase the risk of advanced and fatal prostate cancer, according to an article in the *Journal of the National Cancer Institute*. Investigators involved in the National Institutes of Health—AARP Diet and Health Study screened men (n=295,344) at entry for self-reported multivitamin use and followed them for 5 years; 47% of subjects reported taking beta-carotene supplements more than 7 times per week, compared with 20% who reported never taking beta-carotene. By study end, an association was found between the frequent use of beta-carotene supplements in combination with either selenium or zinc and an increased risk of advanced and fatal prostate cancers. However, a similar pattern for localized prostate cancer was not observed (Lawson et al 2007).

Conversely, supplementation with beta-carotene in individuals having low plasma levels of the antioxidant may confer protection against less advanced forms of the disease. In one study, the effects of intakes of vitamin E, beta-carotene, and vitamin C on risk of prostate cancer were examined in 29,361 men followed for 8 years (average follow-up was 4.2 years); of these, 42% reported taking beta-carotene supplements. Those men with low dietary intakes of beta-carotene who took the supplement form of the antioxidant (calculated at about 2000 mg/day) had a decreased risk of prostate cancer. By study end, just 1,338 men had been diagnosed with prostate cancer (38.9% with the advanced form of the disease). However, no association was found between supplementation with beta-carotene and risk of prostate cancer in men with normal baseline plasma levels of the antioxidant (Kirsh et al 2006). This finding parallels that of the Physician's Health Study, which showed that although beta-carotene supplementation did significantly reduce the risk of prostate cancer in men with low baseline plasma levels of the antioxidant, it had no effect on men with higher baseline plasma levels (Cook et al 1999). No association was found between supplementation with beta-carotene and prostate cancer risk in the β-Carotene and Retinol Efficacy Trial (CARET; Omenn et al 1996).

Skin Cancer

Within the Physician's Health Study—a large, randomized, placebo-controlled trial with 12 years of follow-up—a nested case-control study was conducted to examine the effects of supplemental beta-carotene on the risk of developing nonmelanoma skin cancer (NMSC) in subjects with low baseline plasma levels of the antioxidant. Beta-carotene 50-mg was administered on alternate days to 1,338 men, most of whom subsequently developed NMSC over the 12-year follow-up, specifically, basal cell carcinoma (BCC, n=1156) and squamous cell carcinoma (SCC, n=166). An age- and smoking-matched control group (n=1338) remained free of NMSC at the time of diagnosis of the case, and both groups had similar mean baseline levels of beta-carotene. Following conclusion of the 12-year study, no positive effects of supplementation with beta-carotene on the risk of NMSC, BCC and SCC were observed among subjects. No association between plasma levels of beta-carotene and risk of NMSC was found (Schaumberg et al 2004).

Earlier trials yielded similar results, including 2 that showed no statistically significant benefit of supplemental beta-carotene for basal or squamous cell skin cancers (Frieling et al 2000, Green et al 1999). The Skin Cancer Prevention Study followed men who had received treatment for an earlier skin cancer, and interceded with beta-carotene supplementation (50 mg/day) to observe the effect of supplementation on the development of subsequent NMSC. After 5 years, a 10-fold increase of plasma levels of beta-carotene were noted in the men; however, there was no effect on skin cancer (Greenberg et al 1990).

Various Cancers

No statistically significant benefit associated with beta-carotene supplementation has been found for the following cancers: colorectal (Bjelakovic et al 2006, Albanes et al 2000, Cook et al 2000); gastric (Plummer et al 2007); lung (Cook et al 2000, Omenn et al 1996); pancreatic (Rautalahti et al 1999); renal cell (Virtamo et al 2000); or urothelial cell (Virtamo et al 2000). Several large studies of beta-carotene supplementation show no beneficial effect on the prevention of malignant neoplasms (Hennekens et al 1996).

Beta-carotene supplementation appeared to increase the risk of lung cancer among smokers in one study (Albanes et al 1996). The CARET trial reported that male smokers receiving a combination of supplemental beta-carotene and retinyl palmitate (vitamin A) had a 39% greater incidence of lung cancer (CARET; Omenn et al 1996). In the Alpha-Tocopherol, Beta-Carotene Cancer Prevention Study, male smokers aged 50-69 years (n=29,133) were randomly assigned to treatment with 1 of 4 regimens. Those receiving supplementation with beta-carotene (20 mg) had a 16% greater incidence of lung cancer (Heinonen et al 1994). Taking beta-carotene supplements did not appear to have a direct effect on precancerous conditions such as cervical dysplasia and HPV infection (Romney et al 1997).

Diabetes

Evidence suggests that serum beta-carotene levels may be reduced in diabetic patients. A case-controlled study assessed the effects of diabetes on vitamin A, beta-carotene, alpha-tocopherol, and retinol binding protein (RPB). Patients with type 2 diabetes (n=107) and a control group (n=143) received a dietary assessment, fasting blood levels, and a 10-hour urinalysis. Serum beta-carotene was significantly higher in the control group (p=0.002). The diabetic group had a significantly higher serum and urine RPB concentration (p=0.0001). Diabetic patients with renal impairment had a significantly higher urinary excretion of RPB (p=0.0001). Serum retinol concentrations in patients with diabetes were normal. There was a negative correlation between fasting blood glucose and serum beta-carotene (p=0.008) (Abahusain et al 1999).

In another study, beta-carotene supplementation was ineffective in reducing the risk of developing type 2 diabetes in a 12-year, randomized, double-blind, placebo-controlled study. The incidence of type 2 diabetes was not significantly different: 396 men in the beta-carotene group and 402 men in the placebo group developed type 2 diabetes. The two groups were comparable in terms of age, body mass index, smoking status, alcohol intake, physical activity, and other variables (Liu et al 1999).

Immune Function

Studies of beta-carotene's effects on immune function have yielded conflicting results. In one placebo-controlled crossover study (n=25), supplementation with beta-carotene 15 mg daily for 26 days resulted in an elevated expression of peripheral blood monocyte surface molecules involved in initiating immune responses and an increased secretion of tumor necrosis factor alpha. All participants were nonsmokers (Hughes et al 1997).

However, other short- and long-term trials show that beta-carotene supplementation has no effect on T-cell mediated immunity. Twenty-five healthy elderly women were given placebo or beta-carotene 90 mg daily for 23 days. Beta-carotene supplementation had no effect on delayed-type hypersensitivity, in vitro lymphocyte proliferation, production of interleukin 2, or production of prostaglandin E2. In a long-term (12-year) randomized, placebo-controlled trial from a subset (n=54) of the Physician's Health Study, men receiving beta-carotene 50 mg every other day showed no differences from the placebo group in the profile of lymphocyte subsets or in percentages of natural killer cells and activated lymphocytes (Santos et al 1997).

Ocular Disorders

Night Vision

A study conducted to assess the effects of carotenes on night vision showed no effects. Subjects in the Blue Mountain Eye Study (n=3,654) were interviewed for nutrient and food intake by questionnaire. Self-reported poor night vision in women was associated with higher intakes of beta-carotene (p=0.03) and total vitamin A (p=0.048). There was no association between night vision and beta-carotene or vitamin A intake in men. The study concluded that perceived poor night vision caused an increase in carrot consumption in women (Smith et al 1999).

Photosensitivity

Oral carotenoids (25 mg daily) or carotenoids plus vitamin E (500 IU daily) reduced ultraviolet light (UV)-induced erythema in 17 healthy volunteers with skin type I or II. After 12 weeks of supplementation, approximate sun protection factors

(SPF) of 2.4 and 3.0 were estimated for carotenoids alone and for carotenoids plus vitamin E, respectively (Stahl et al 2000).

Beta-carotene alone or in combination with canthaxanthin was administered to 36 patients with erythropoietic protoporphyria. Daily doses of 50 mg to 200 mg were given during the summer months. Eighteen patients reported being symptom-free, 16 patients improved, and two patients improved only slightly. Carotenemia was the only side effect reported (Thomsen et al 1979).

Overall Mortality

One recent meta-analysis suggests that supplementation with beta-carotene may increase overall mortality (Bjelakovic et al 2007). Data was extracted from 385 publications involving 68 randomized trials with a total of 232,606 subjects. Using statistical analysis and other methodology to review the medical literature, the authors concluded that supplementation with beta-carotene, either alone or in combination with other antioxidants, was significantly associated with increased all-cause mortality (dose range=1.2 mg to 50 mg in studies examined). Further studies are warranted to examine whether a correlation exists between supplementation with beta-carotene and increased risk of death. Distinctions should be made between the clinical utility of supplementation in persons with a deficiency of beta-carotene, and its possible deleterious effects in persons with adequate plasma levels of the antioxidant.

Pregnancy-Related Mortality

Vitamin A or beta-carotene supplementation of Nepalese women of childbearing age significantly reduced mortality during pregnancy and through 12 weeks postpartum. Of more than 44,000 women who were given weekly vitamin A supplements of 23,300 IU (7,000 mcg retinol equivalents, as retinyl palmitate), or trans-beta-carotene (7,000 mcg retinol equivalents, assuming a conversion ratio to retinol of 6 to 1 after uptake), or placebo, more than 7,000 women per treatment group became pregnant. Mortality per 100,000 pregnancies was 426 in the vitamin A group, 361 in the beta-carotene group, and 704 in the placebo, yielding relative risks of 0.60 (p=0.04) and 0.51 (p=0.01) for vitamin A and beta-carotene. Mortality among women in the vitamin A group was not different from that among women in the beta-carotene group. This suggests that the risk of maternal death among women who are deficient in vitamin A can be substantially reduced by modest increases in vitamin A or beta-carotene intake (West et al 1999).

INDICATIONS AND USAGE

Accepted Uses: Beta-carotene supplementation can be used for prophylaxis of vitamin A deficiency, although dietary improvement is preferable. For treatment of documented vitamin A deficiency, vitamin A supplements are preferred. Beta-carotene is also used for photosensitivity reactions in erythropoietic protoporphyria (prophylaxis and treatment) and severe polymorphous light eruption (prophylaxis and treatment) (USP DI 2004).

Unproven Uses: Although research is ongoing, supplemental beta-carotene has also been used for the following: angina, asthma, cancer prevention, cardiovascular disease, cataract prevention, diabetes, free-radical reduction during bone marrow transplantation, immunostimulation, night vision, and oral leukoplakia.

PRECAUTIONS AND ADVERSE REACTIONS

Beta-carotene supplements are not recommended for patients with lung cancer or asbestosis (Albanes et al 1996; Chuwers et al 1997). Caution is also advised in patients with impaired renal function, impaired liver function, hypervitaminosis A, and anorexia (USP DI 2004).

Beta-carotene may cause yellow skin discoloration due to carotenodermia (USP DI 2004; Product Info: Solatene 1996). This condition may be differentiated from jaundice by the lack of pigmentation in the sclera and represents a therapeutic response to the drug. The protective response from the drug will not be seen until the carotenemic effect becomes apparent. It is usually first seen as yellowness of the palms and soles (Product Info: Solatene 1996). Hypervitaminosis A does not result from the carotenemic condition (Gilman et al 1980; Mathews-Roth et al 1974).

Slight diarrhea or loose stools could occur during beta-carotene therapy but may not require drug withdrawal (Product Info: Solatene 1996; Mathews-Roth et al 1974). Although rare, the manufacturer has reported the occurrence of ecchymoses and arthralgia during beta-carotene administration (USP DI 2004; Product Info: Solatene 1996).

Pregnancy: FDA-rated as Pregnancy Category C. Beta-carotene crosses the placenta. No problems with pregnancy have been documented in women taking up to 30 mg (5,000 retinol equivalents) of beta-carotene daily (USP DI 2004).

Breastfeeding: Beta-carotene is safe in normal dietary amounts.

DRUG INTERACTIONS

MINOR RISKS

Orlistat: Concurrent use of orlistat and beta carotene may result in decreased beta carotene efficacy. *Clinical Management:* Patients should be instructed to space the administration of orlistat and beta carotene by at least two hours.

POTENTIAL INTERACTIONS

Cholestyramine, Colestipol, Mineral Oil, and Neomycin: Concurrent use may interfere with the absorption of beta-carotene or vitamin A (USP DI 2004). *Clinical Management:* Vitamin A requirements may be increased; monitor for deficiency.

OVERDOSAGE

Vitamin A toxicity has been reported in a 20-year-old Japanese woman whose diet included an excessive amount of beta-carotene-rich foods. Her symptoms included low-grade fever, cheilitis, dry skin, limb edema, and headache. It is unclear whether the toxicity symptoms were due to beta-carotene or vitamin A consumption (Nagai et al 1999).

DOSAGE

Mode of Administration: Oral

How Supplied: Tablets, capsules, liquid

Daily Dosage: The preferred way of designating vitamin A activity is in retinol equivalents (RE); 6 mcg of beta-carotene is equivalent to 1 RE and 10 units of vitamin A activity (USP DI 2004).

Erythropoietic Protoporphyria – Adults: 30 to 300 mg daily in single or divided doses. Children under 14 years old: 30 to 150 mg daily.

Extended therapy (2 to 6 weeks) is needed to accumulate enough beta-carotene in the skin to exert a protective effect. If an adult dose of 180 mg daily for 3 months (serum level at 800 mcg/100 mL) does not provide a clinical response, then it may be concluded that beta-carotene supplementation will be of no benefit. Patients who develop carotenodermia should be instructed to increase exposure to sunlight gradually until individual exposure limits are established (Product Info: Solatene 1996).

Vitamin A Deficiency (prophylaxis) – Adults and adolescents: 1,000 to 2,500 RE (the equivalent of 10,000 to 25,000 units of vitamin A activity) or 6 to 15 mg of beta-carotene daily.

Children: 500 to 1,000 RE (the equivalent of 5,000 to 10,000 units of vitamin A activity) or 3 to 6 mg of beta-carotene per day (USP DI 2004).

LITERATURE

Abahusain MA, Wright J, Dickerson JWT et al: Retinol, alpha-tocopherol and carotenoids in diabetes. *Eur J Clin Nutr*; 53(8):630-635. 1999

Albanes E, Heinonen OP, Taylor PR et al: Alpha-tocopherol and beta-carotene supplements and lung cancer incidence in the alpha-tocopherol, beta-carotene cancer prevention study: effects of base-line characteristics and study compliance. *J Natl Cancer Inst*; 88(21):1560-1570. 1996

American Society of Health-System Pharmacists (ASHP): *American Hospital Formulary Service Drug Information.* ASHP, Bethesda, MD; 1997.

Bjelakovic G, Nagorni A, Nikolova D, et al. Meta-analysis: antioxidant supplements for primary and secondary prevention of colorectal adenoma. *Aliment Pharmacol Ther*; 24:281-291, 2006

Bjelakovic G, Nikolova D, Gluud LL, et al: Mortality in randomized trials of antioxidant supplements for primary and secondary prevention. Systemic review and meta-analysis. *JAMA*; 297:842-857. 2007

Briggs GG, Freeman RK, Yaffe SJ: *Drugs in pregnancy and lactation: A Reference Guide to Fetal and Neonatal Risk*, 3rd ed. Williams & Wilkins, Baltimore, MD; 1998.

Chuwers P, Barnhart S, Blanc P et al: The protective effect of beta-carotene and retinol on ventilatory function in an asbestos-exposed cohort. *Am J Respir Crit Care Med*; 155:1066-1071. 1997

Cook NR, Lee I-M, Manson JE et al: Effects of beta-carotene supplementation on cancer incidence by baseline characteristics in the Physicians' Health Study (United States). *Cancer Causes Control*; 11:617-626. 2000

Cook NR, Stampfer MJ, Ma J et al: Beta-carotene supplementation for patients with low baseline levels and decreased risks of total and prostate carcinoma. *Cancer*; 86(9):1783-1792. 1999

Day B, Bergamini S, Tyurina U et al: β-Carotene: An antioxidant or a target of oxidative stress in cells? *Subcell Biochem*; 30:209-217. 1998

Green A, Williams G, Neale R et al: Daily sunscreen application and beta-carotene supplementation in prevention of basal-cell and squamous-cell carcinomas of the skin. *Lancet*; 354(9180):723-729. 1999

Greenberg ER, Baron JA, Stukel TA, et al, and The Skin Cancer Prevention Study Group. A clinical trial of β-carotene to prevent basal-cell and squamous-cell cancers of the skin. *N Engl J Med*; 323:789-795. 1990

Greenwald P, Anderson D, Nelson SA, et al. Clinical trials of vitamin and mineral supplements for cancer prevention. *Am J Clin Nutr*; 85(suppl):314S-317S. 2007

Heinonen OP, Huttunen JK, Albanes D -for the a-Tocopherol b-Carotene Cancer Prevention Study Group. The effect of vitamin E and b-carotene on the incidence of lung cancer and other cancers in male smokers. *N Engl J Med*; 330:1029-1035. 1994

Hennekens CH, Buring JE, Manson JE et al: Lack of effect of long-term supplementation with beta carotene on the incidence of malignant neoplasms and cardiovascular disease. *N Engl J Med*; 334:1145-1149. 1996

Hughes DA, Wright AJA, Finglas PM et al: The effect of beta-carotene supplementation on the immune function of blood monocytes from healthy male nonsmokers. *J Lab Clin Med*; 129:309-317. 1997

Kirsh VA, Hayes RB, Mayne ST, et al. Supplemental and dietary vitamin E, β-carotene, and vitamin C intakes and prostate cancer risk. *J Natl Cancer Inst*; 98:245-254. 2006

Lawson KA, Wright ME, Subar A, et al: Multivitamin use and risk of prostate cancer in the National Institutes of Health—AARP Diet and Health Study. *J Natl Cancer Inst*. 99:754-764. 2007

Liu S, Ajani U, Chae C et al: Long-term beta-carotene supplementation and risk of type 2 diabetes mellitus. *JAMA*; 282(11):1073-1075. 1999

Mathews-Roth MM, Pathak UA, Fitzpatrick TB et al: Beta-carotene as an oral photoprotective agent in erythropoietic protoporphyria. *JAMA*; 228:1004-1008. 1974

Nagai K, Hosaka H, Kubo S et al: Vitamin A toxicity secondary to excessive intake of yellow-green vegetables, liver and laver. *J Hepatol*; 31:142-148. 1999

Neuman I, Nahum H, Ben-Amotz A: Prevention of exercise-induced asthma by a natural isomer mixture of β-carotene. *Ann Allergy Asthma Immunol*; 82:549-553. 1999

Omenn GS, Goodman GE, Thornquist MD et al: Risk factors for lung cancer and for intervention effects in CARET, the β-Carotene and Retinol Efficacy Trial. *J Natl Cancer Inst*; 88:1550-1559. 1996

Omenn GS, Goodman GE, Thornquist MD et al: Effects of a combination of beta carotene and vitamin A on lung cancer and cardiovascular disease. *N Engl J Med*; 334:1150-1155. 1996

Plummer M, Vivas J, Lopez G, et al. Chemoprevention of precancerous gastric lesions with antioxidant vitamin supplementation: a randomized trial in a high-risk population. *J Natl Cancer Inst*; 99:137-146; 2007

Powers S, Hamilton K: Antioxidants and exercise. *Clin Sports Med*; 18(3):525-536. 1999

Product Information: Lumitene® (beta-carotene). (Tishcon Corp., Westbury, NY, 1996.

Product Information: Solatene® (beta-carotene). Roche Laboratories, Nutley, NJ, 1996.

Product Information: Xenical® (orlistat). Roche Laboratories Inc, Nutley, NJ, 1999.

Rautalahti MT, Virtamo JRK, Taylor PR et al: The effects of supplementation with alpha-tocopherol and beta-carotene on the incidence and mortality of carcinoma of the pancreas in a randomized, controlled trial. *Cancer*; 86:37-42. 1999

Romney SL, Ho GYF, Palan PR et al: Effects of betacarotene and other factors on outcome of cervical dysplasia and human papillomavirus infection. *Gynecol Oncol*; 65:483-492. 1997

Santos MS, Leka LS, Ribaya-Mercado D et al: Short- and long-term beta-carotene supplementation do not influence T cell-mediated immunity in healthy elderly persons. *Am J Clin Nutr*; 66:917-924. 1997

Schaumberg DA, Frieling UM, Rifai N, et al: No effect of β-carotene supplementation on risk of nonmelanoma skin cancer among men with low baseline plasma β-carotene. *Cancer Epidemiol Biomarkers Prev*; 13:1079-1080. 2004

Smith W, Mitchell P, Lazarus R: Carrots, carotene and seeing in the dark. *Aust N Z J Ophthalmol*; 27:200-203. 1999

Stahl W, Heinrich U, Jungmann H et al: Carotenoids and carotenoids plus vitamin E protect against ultraviolet light-induced erythema in humans. *Am J Clin Nutr*; 72:795-798. 2000

Swanbeck G, Wennersten G: Effect of beta-carotene on photohomolysis. *Acta Derm Venereol Suppl (Stockh)*; 653:283. 1973

Thomsen K, Schmidt H, Fischer A: Beta-carotene in erythropoietic protoporphyria: 5 years' experience. *Dermatologica*; 159:82-86. 1979

United States Pharmacopoeial Convention, Inc. *USP DI. Volume I: Drug Information for the Health Care Professional,* 24th ed. Thomson Micromedex, Greenwood Village, CO; 2004.

Virtamo J: Vitamins and lung cancer. *Proc Nutr Soc*; 58:329-333. 1999

Wang XD, Krinsky N: The bioconversion of beta-carotene into retinoids. *Subcell Biochem*; 30:159-180. 1998

West KP, Katz J, Khatry S et al: Double blind, cluster randomized trial of low dose supplementation with vitamin A or beta carotene on mortality related to pregnancy in Nepal. *BMJ*; 318:570-575. 1999

Bromelain

DESCRIPTION

Bromelain is a concentrated mixture of proteolytic enzymes derived from the pineapple plant *Ananas comosus*. Commercial bromelain is not a chemically homogeneous substance because if the enzyme is highly purified it loses its stability and most of its physiological activity. The main ingredient is a proteolytic enzyme (a glycoprotein), but it also contains small amounts of an acid phosphatase, a peroxidase, several protease inhibitors, and organically bound calcium (Hatano et al 1996; Taussig 1980).

Stem: Pineapple stem cysteine proteinases include bromelain, comosain, and ananain. Bromelain has a structural similarity to comosain but not ananain (Napper et al 1994).

Crude Extract: The crude extract of bromelain is a combination product containing enzymes, proteins, carbohydrates, and seven protease inhibitors that are active against bromelain, papain, and ficin (Cooreman et al 1976).

Other Names: Ananas comosus, bromelins

ACTIONS AND PHARMACOLOGY

EFFECTS

Bromelain is a proteolytic enzyme that has anti-inflammatory, antitumor, and digestive properties.

Anti-Inflammatory Effects: Bromelain selectivity inhibits the biosynthesis of pro-inflammatory prostaglandins (Taussig 1980). Bromelain lowers kininogen and bradykinin in serum and tissues and may alter prostaglandin synthesis (Lotz-Winter 1990). The action of bromelain can be compared to endogenous protease plasmin because it acts on fibrinogen to stimulate the biosynthesis of anti-inflammatory prostaglandins. Bromelain inhibits prostaglandin E(2), which does not block the synthesis of all pro-inflammatory and anti-inflammatory prostaglandins as in the case of aspirin, but instead results in a partial inhibition of thromboxane synthetase. This partial and dose-dependent inhibition decreases the total amount of pro-inflammatory prostaglandins and improves the ratio of anti-inflammatory prostaglandins (Taussig 1980).

Antitumor Effects: In vitro studies with bromelain indicate specific retardation of Lewis lung carcinoma, YC-8 lymphoma, and MCA-1 ascitic tumor cells, as well as a human gastric carcinoma cell line (KATO III). Fractionation of bromelain by ultra-filtration produces a high molecular weight fraction (greater than 30,000) and a low molecular weight fraction (5,000). Only the high molecular weight fraction contains proteases that retard Lewis lung tumor growth (Batkin et al 1988). Bromelain also induces cytokine production in peripheral blood mononuclear cells in vitro. A polyenzymatic preparation that included bromelain had a synergistically increased immunomodulatory effect when used in combination with interferon-gamma, with respect to tumor necrosis factor production (Desser et al 1993).

Debridement Effects: Bromelain effectively degrades third-degree burn eschar fragments at 37° to 38° Celsius when oxygen is excluded to avoid enzyme inactivation. Investigators propose that bromelain activates collagenase in the living tissue to hydrolyze the denatured collagen at the interface of the eschar and the live tissue (Felton 1980). The debridement activity of bromelain appears to be enhanced by mercaptans such as N-acetylcysteine, penicillamine, and cysteine (Levenson et al 1981).

Digestive Effects: When administered orally to piglets in vivo, bromelain inhibited the attachment of enterotoxigenic *Escherichia coli* to the small intestine. Therefore, bromelain therapy may be useful for the prevention of enterotoxigenic *E. coli*-induced diarrhea (Mynott et al 1996). When bromelain was compared to gastric and intestinal proteases in digestive functions, it had equivalent casein-splitting activity at pH 3.3 as gastric proteases and at pH 6.0 as the intestinal proteases with almost the same rate, suggesting that bromelain can take over full digestive functions in the stomach as well as in the intestine (Hennrich et al 1965).

Fibrinolytic Activity/Platelet Aggregation: Numerous clinical studies have shown that bromelain possesses fibrinolytic activity, apparently via an indirect mechanism (substituting for the inhibited plasmin), which increases both anti-inflammatory and serum fibrinolytic activity. The physiological activity of bromelain resides in its protease fraction, as measured by inhibition of adenosine diphosphate-stimulated human platelet aggregation (Taussig 1980).

In contrast, bromelain does not inhibit aggregation of washed platelets, indicating that it might act on fibrinogen to yield peptides that affect the arachidonate cascade. It has been proposed that the plasmin cleaves Hageman factor, leading to a strong release of kallikrein but a weak release of thrombin, which seems to be sufficient enough to stimulate the release of the prostaglandins that increase cyclic-adenosine monophosphate. The mechanism of action in this regard needs further investigation for a better assessment (Taussig 1980).

CLINICAL TRIALS

Analgesic/Anti-Inflammatory Effects

Clinical studies in humans have demonstrated analgesic and anti-inflammatory effects such as reduced swelling, pain, and tenderness (Kelly 1996). The reduction of edema and bruising was more rapid in bromelain-treated patients than those taking placebo. In rats, the anti-inflammatory effects of bromelain are comparable to those of prednisolone (Kelly 1996). Bromelain-treated patients showed a clear reduction in all parameters at all time points as compared with baseline in an open, uncontrolled study of 59 patients with blunt injuries to the musculoskeletal system who were treated with orally administered enteric-coated bromelain. High-dose Bromelain-POS® (exact dose not specified) was administered according to the nature and severity of the lesion between 1 and 3 weeks. On the day of injury and on 5 subsequent days, the patients were evaluated for swelling, pain at rest, pain during movement, and tenderness. The preparation was well-tolerated and patient compliance was high (Masson 1995). It should be noted that some studies were poorly designed and yielded inconclusive results. More controlled studies are necessary.

Enhanced Antibiotic Absorption

Antibiotic absorption differs widely among individuals but may be improved by the addition of bromelain. Bromelain (as part of a multiple-enzyme treatment product) was a significant adjuvant to antibiotic therapy in a randomized, double-blind, placebo-controlled study. Fifty-six patients with adnexitis were treated for 28 days with antibiotic therapy (doxycycline) plus placebo, or the same antibiotic therapy plus a multiple enzyme preparation (Wobenzyme®) containing bromelain 45 mg, pancreatin 100 mg, papain 60 mg, lipase 10 mg, amylase 10 mg, trypsin 24 mg, chymotrypsin 1 mg, and rutin 50 mg. Significant improvement in individual scores and the adnexitis score was seen in both groups but there was a significant difference between the two groups. By the end of the study, the advantage of enzymes combined with antibiotic therapy compared to placebo was highly significant (p=7.45x10-10). The effect due to just bromelain was not established. Measures used to evaluate the effect were body temperature, white blood cell count, ESR, tenderness scores, and vaginal discharge (Dittmar et al 1992).

Fibrocystic Mastopathy

Enzyme treatment improved symptoms of fibrocystic mastopathy in a double-blind, placebo-controlled, randomized study using the enzyme preparation Wobenzyme®. The regimen was 10 tablets a day for 6 weeks. Each tablet contained pancreatin 100 mg, papain 60 mg, bromelain 45 mg, lipase 10 mg, amylase 10 mg, trypsin 24 mg, chymotrypsin 1 mg, and rutin 50 mg. Enzyme treatment of 96 women with fibrocystic mastopathy resulted in reduced size of cysts (p=0.003), lower score of complaints (p=0.001), and less subjective disturbance by symptoms (p=0.001). The number of cysts was not altered (p=0.695). The profiles of the active-treatment and control groups were similar (Dittmar et al 1993). The effect of bromelain by itself was not evaluated.

Osteoarthritis

The role of bromelain in the treatment of osteoarthritis remains inconclusive. A recently published randomized, double-blind, placebo-controlled trial studied the effectiveness of bromelain in treating osteoarthritis (OA) of the knee. Forty-seven subjects with a confirmed diagnosis of knee OA (moderate to severe in nature) were enlisted; 31 completed the trial. Of these, 14 received bromelain 800 mg/day, and the remaining 17 received placebo. After 12 weeks of treatment, no statistically significant differences between groups were noted for the primary outcome measure (the change in total WOMAC score from baseline to end of treatment) (Brien et al 2006).

An earlier review by the same primary author concluded that bromelain may have potential for the treatment of OA of the knee, but noted that further studies were warranted. Out of the 10 studies identified in the review that assessed the efficacy of bromelain in OA of the knee, several were suspected to have been underpowered, and the findings inconclusive. Additionally, in many of the studies, the treatment period did not parallel that used in clinical practice, being of much shorter duration. In one study, there was no control group; in another, no formal medical diagnosis of knee pain for those enrolled. However, two comparative studies cited in the review showed reduced symptoms of pain (Brien et al 2004).

INDICATIONS AND USAGE

Approved by Commission E

■ Wounds and burns

Bromelain may be of therapeutic value in modulating inflammation, edema, tumor growth, blood coagulation, and debridement of third-degree burns. It could possibly enhance absorption of some drugs, including antibiotics.

CONTRAINDICATIONS

Bromelain is contraindicated in patients who have severe liver or kidney impairment or who need dialysis. The supplement should also be avoided by patients who have a coagulation disorder such as hemophilia or who have demonstrated hypersensitivity to bromelain, pineapple, or the inactive ingredients of enzyme preparations.

PRECAUTIONS AND ADVERSE REACTIONS

Bromelain is capable of inducing IgE-mediated respiratory and gastrointestinal allergic reactions. Human subjects can exhibit a cross-reaction between the two plant proteases bromelain and papain (Baur et al 1979). Hypersensitivity reactions have been reported, including skin rashes and asthma. There is some evidence for sensitization due to bromelain inhalation that resulted in occupationally acquired asthma. This has not been reported after ingestion (Gailhofer et al 1988).

Bromelain may increase heart rate at higher doses. It should be used cautiously (doses less than 500 mg per day) in patients with heart palpitations or tachycardia (Kelly 1996).

DRUG INTERACTIONS

MODERATE RISK

Anticoagulants, Low-Molecular-Weight Heparins, and Thrombolytic Agents: Concurrent use of bromelain and these agents may result in an increased risk of bleeding. *Clinical Management:* Caution is advised if bromelain is taken with these medications. Monitor the patients for signs and symptoms of bleeding.

OVERDOSAGE

The LD50 intravenously was 30 to 35 mg/kg (mice) and 20 mg/kg (rats). The LD50 after intraperitoneal administration to mice was 36.7 mg/kg and in rats was 85.2 mg/kg (Cooreman et alb 1976).

DOSAGE

Mode of Administration: Oral, topical

How Supplied: Capsules, cream, suspension, tablets

Daily Dosage: Available preparations of bromelain tablets vary widely in their concentrations, and caution must be exercised in determining dosage regimens. For best results, the total daily dosage should be divided into 4 doses and taken an hour before or after food (Kelly 1996).

General use – 500 to 2,000 mg daily.

Carpal tunnel syndrome – 1,000 mg (with a potency of at least 3,000 microunits/gram) given 3 times a day, between meals (Miller et al 1997).

Inflammation – 500 to 2,000 mg per day (Kelly 1996). A European manufacturer recommends 450 to 1,500 Federation Internationale Pharmaceutique (FIP) units divided into 3 daily doses and administered over 8 to 10 days (Fachinfo: Traumanase/forte 1997).

Pediatric dosage – 150 to 300 FIP units daily, divided into 3 doses.

Storage: Store at room temperature, away from heat, moisture, and direct light. The shelf-life of bromelain is 5 years (Fachinfo: Traumanase/forte 1997).

LITERATURE

Batkin S, Taussig S, Szekerczes J: Modulation of pulmonary metastasis (Lewis Lung Carcinoma) by bromelain, an extract of the pineapple stem (*Ananas comosus*). *Cancer Invest*; 6:241-242. 1988

Baur X: Studies on the specificity of human IgE-antibodies to the plant proteases papain and bromelain. *Clin Allergy*; 9:451-457. 1979

Blumenthal M, Busse WR, Goldberg A et al: Bromelain, in *The Complete German Commission E Monographs.* American Botanical Council, Austin, TX; 1998.

Brien S, Lewith G, Walker AF, et al: Bromelain as an adjunctive treatment for moderate-to-severe osteoarthritis of the knee: a randomized placed-controlled pilot study. *Q J Med*; 99:841-850. 2006

Brien S, Lewith G, Walker AF, et al: Bromelain as a treatment for osteoarthritis: a review of clinical studies.*eCAM*; 1:251-257. 2004

Cooreman WM, Scharpe S, Demester J et al: Bromelain, biochemical and pharmacological properties. *Pharm Acta Helv*; 51:73-97. 1976

Desser L, Rehberger A, Kokron E et al: Cytokine synthesis in human peripheral blood mononuclear cells after oral administration of polyenzyme preparations. *Oncology*; 50:403-407. 1993

Dittmar FW, Luh W: Treatment of fibrocystic mastopathy with hydrolytic enzymes. *Int J Exper Clin Chemother*; 6:9-20. 1993

Dittmar FW, Weissenbacher ER: Therapy of adnexitis - enhancement of the basic antibiotic therapy with hydrolytic enzymes. *Int J Exper Clin Chemother*; 5:73-81. 1992

Fachinformation: Traumanase®/forte (bromelain). Rhone-Poulenc Rorer, A Nattermann & Cie. GmbH, Koeln, 1997.

Gailhofer G, Wilders-Trusching M, Smolle J et al: Asthma caused by bromelain: an occupational allergy. *Clin Allergy*; 18:445-450. 1988

Galleguillos F, Rodriguez C: Asthma caused by bromelain inhalation. *Clin Allergy*; 8:21-24. 1978

Hatano K, Kojima M, Tanokura M et al: Solution structure of bromelain inhibitor VI from pineapple stem: structure similarity with Bowman-Birk trypsin/chymotrypsin inhibitor from soybean. *Biochemistry*; 35:5379-5384. 1996

Hennrich N, Huffman A, Lange H: Eignung der Pflanzenprotease Bromelin fuer die Substitutionstherapie von Verdauungsstoerungen. *Arzneimittelforschung*; 15:434-437. 1965

Kalimanovska V, Whitaker KB, Moss DW: Effect of bromelain on alkaline phosphatases of intestinal and non-intestinal tissues and serum. *Clin Chim Acta*; 170:219-226. 1987

Kane S, Goldberg MJ. Use of bromelain for mild ulcerative colitis. *Ann Intern Med*; 132: 680. 2000

Kelly GS: Bromelain: a literature review and discussion of its therapeutic applications. *Altern Med Rev*; 1:243-257. 1996

Kottel RH, Hanford WC: Differential release of membrane-bound alkaline phosphatase isoenzymes from tumor cells by bromelain. *J Biochem Biophys Methods*; 2:325-330. 1980

Levenson SM, Gruber DK, Gruber C et al: Chemical debridement of burns: mercaptans. *J Trauma*; 21:632-644. 1981

Lotz-Winter H: On the pharmacology of bromelain: an update with special regard to animal studies on dose-dependent effects. *Planta Med*; 56:249-253. 1990

Maurer HR. Bromelain: biochemistry, pharmacology and medical use. *Cell Mol Life Sci*; 58: 1234-45. 2001

Masson M. Bromelain in blunt injuries of the locomotor system. A study of observed applications in general practice. [English translation of German title] *Fortschr Med*; Jul 10;113(19):303-6. 1995

Mattei O, Fabri G, Farina G: Industrial medicine experience in relation to four cases of occupational asthma due to bromelain. [English translation of Italian title]. *Med Lav*; 5:404-409. 1979

Miller AL, Birdsall TC: Etiology and conservative treatment of carpal tunnel syndrome. *Altern Med Rev*; 2:26-35. 1997

Mynott TL, Luke RKJ, Chandler DS: Oral administration of protease inhibits enterotoxigenic *Escherichia coli* receptor activity in piglet small intestine. *Gut*; 38:38-32. 1996

Taussig S: The mechanism of the physiological action of bromelain. *Med Hypotheses*; 6:99-104. 1980

Taussig SJ, Batkin S: Bromelain, the enzyme complex of pineapple (*Ananas comosus*) and its clinical application: an update. *J Ethonopharmacol*; 191-203. 1988

Calcium

DESCRIPTION

Calcium is an essential mineral. Average adult weight is made up of about 2% calcium, most of which is stored in the skeleton and teeth. A small amount of calcium circulates in the blood, muscles, and fluid between cells to help transmit nerve impulses. Along with keeping teeth and bones strong, calcium also promotes blood coagulation and plays an essential role in enabling muscles, including the heart, to relax and contract. Food sources of calcium include dairy products (milk, yogurt, cheese), sea vegetables, sardines, almonds, hazelnuts, legumes, collards, kale, parsley, and tofu (Pitchford 1993).

The scope of this discussion will be limited to the oral salt formulations, including carbonate, citrate, glubionate, gluconate, lactate, phosphate, and other calcium salts. (Calcium acetate, calcium chloride, calcium gluceptate, and calcium gluconate may be administered intravenously.) Because calcium salts are bound with other molecules such as oxygen and carbon, supplements often list the percentage of elemental calcium in each tablet along with the total salt weight, usually in milligrams. The table below lists common examples.

Type of oral calcium salt	**Elemental calcium per 1,000 mg (percentage and weight)**
Carbonate	40% (400 mg)
Citrate	21% (210 mg)
Lactate	13% (130 mg)
Gluconate	9% (90 mg)

Other Names: Ca, calcium carbonate, calcium chloride, calcium citrate, calcium gluceptate, calcium gluconate, calcium malate

ACTIONS AND PHARMACOLOGY

EFFECTS

Calcium has anti-osteoporotic, antihypertensive, antihyperlipidemic, and possible anticarcinogenic properties. It is an electrolyte, a nutrient, and a mineral. Calcium functions as a regulator in the release and storage of neurotransmitters and hormones, in the uptake and binding of amino acids, and in vitamin B12 absorption and gastrin secretion. Calcium is required to maintain the function of the nervous, muscular, and skeletal systems and cell membrane and capillary permeability. It is an activator in many enzyme reactions and is essential in the transmission of nerve impulses; contraction of cardiac, smooth, and skeletal muscles; respiration; blood coagulation; and renal function (Product Info: Calcium gluconate 1992; AHFS 1979).

Antiproliferative Effects: Calcium precipitates soluble colonic luminal surfactants (bile acids and free fatty acids) resulting in reduced cytolytic activity of these substances and, consequently, reduced epithelial damage and colonic proliferation. This antiproliferative effect was found for calcium provided as milk, calcium carbonate, and calcium phosphate and may explain the inverse association between calcium intake and colorectal neoplasia reported in some studies (Govers et al 1994).

CLINICAL TRIALS

Colorectal Polyps/Cancer

Large clinical trials found that calcium supplementation decreased the risk of recurrent colorectal adenomas. In the Calcium Polyp Prevention Study, 930 patients with a recent history of colorectal adenomas were randomized to treatment with calcium carbonate (1200 mg/day) or placebo. Following 4 years of treatment, those who received calcium had a 17% lower risk of one or more colorectal adenomas compared with those in the placebo group (Baron et al 1999). A subsequent study enrolled the same patients to examine the effects of calcium supplementation on colorectal lesions. Using data obtained from the Calcium Polyp Prevention Study, the analysis revealed an even larger reduction in the risk of advanced adenomas. This effect was most pronounced in those with high intakes of dietary calcium and fiber and low intakes of fat, although these interactions were not statistically significant (Wallace et al 2004).

However, in the Women's Health Initiative study involving 36,282 postmenopausal women, a combined regimen of calcium and vitamin D supplementation for 7 years had no effect on the incidence of colorectal cancer. This large-scale placebo-controlled trial, primarily designed to study this regimen for the prevention of osteoporosis, investigated its impact on rates of colorectal cancer as well. Participants were randomized to active treatment received 1000 mg calcium and 400 IU vitamin D daily (n=18,176) or placebo (n=18,106). Although no positive association was found with supplementation, the authors point out that the long latency of colorectal cancer development, coupled with the lengthy duration of the trial, may have contributed to these null findings (Wactawski-Wende et al 2005).

Finally, the Calcium Follow-up Study recently reported its findings regarding the effects of long-term calcium supplementation on the recurrence of colorectal adenomas. Designed as an observational phase of the Calcium Polyp Prevention Study, the goal was to explore the effect of supplementation post-treatment for an average of 7 years. It found that the protective effect of calcium supplementation observed in the initial trial extended up to 5 years after treatment stopped (Grau et al 2007).

Complications and Outcomes of Pregnancy

The World Health Organization (WHO) conducted a randomized, placebo-controlled, double-blind trial in an attempt to clarify whether calcium supplementation in expectant mothers with a deficiency of the mineral reduced rates of pre-eclampsia and preterm delivery. Women who enrolled prior to gestational week 20 were randomized to treatment with 1.5 mg/day calcium (n=4151) or placebo (n=4161) throughout the remainder of pregnancy. Although supplementation did not prevent pre-eclampsia, it did reduce its severity and reduced its incidence by about 10%; however, this did not approach statistical significance. Maternal morbidity and neonatal mortality were improved in the group receiving calcium supplementation, with reductions observed in the severe maternal morbidity and mortality index (risk ratio [RR], 0.80; 95% CI, 0.70-0.91) and the neonatal mortality rate (RR, 0.70; 95% CI, 0.56-0.88). A Cochrane review cited in this article, involving more than 15,000 pregnant women, found an overall protective effect of calcium supplementation on pre-eclampsia (RR, 0.78; 95% CI, 0.68-0.89) (Villar et al 2006).

An earlier meta-analysis of studies evaluating the effect of calcium supplementation on pregnancy-related hypertension and pre-eclampsia raised controversy. The meta-analysis (n=2,260 subjects) reported a significant and substantial 62% reduction in risk of pre-eclampsia as well as decreases in both systolic (-5.4 mm Hg) and diastolic (-3.4 mm Hg) blood pressure with calcium supplementation (typically, 1 to 2 g per day). Many of the studies reviewed were conducted in countries where there is low dietary calcium intake. The authors acknowledged insufficient data hindered their ability to determine whether calcium supplementation affects the meaningful outcomes of maternal and fetal morbidity and mortality. Nevertheless, they suggested a policy of offering calcium supplementation to all pregnant women in whom there is a concern about the development of pre-eclampsia (Bucher et al 1996). Numerous criticisms of the authors' methods of analysis, of their conclusions, and of their advice have been offered (Cher 1997; Cappuccio 1996; Roberts et al 1996; Levine et al 1996).

A review article explored the effect of maternal calcium supplementation on the blood pressure of offspring. Data were examined from 2 randomized trials and 3 observational studies; follow-up among children ranged from birth to 9 years across studies. Although higher intakes of calcium during pregnancy were associated with lowered systolic blood pressure among offspring in all studies, these effects were statistically significant in just 3 studies. The largest randomized trial observed a clinically and statistically significant reduction in the incidence of hypertension in offspring 7 years of age (RR, 0.59; 95% CI, 0.39-0.90). The reviewers concluded that evidence exists to support an association between maternal calcium intake during pregnancy and offspring blood pressure, although additional research is warranted (Bergel and Barros 2007).

Fluorosis

A combination of calcium, ascorbic acid, and vitamin D3 reversed dental, clinical, and early skeletal fluorosis in children in a double-blind, placebo-controlled study. Twenty-five children (aged 6 to 12 years), living in an area where the drinking water contained fluorides at a concentration of 4.5 mg/liter (mg/L), were administered either placebo (n=10) or ascorbic acid 250 mg and calcium compound (125 mg elemental calcium) twice a day and vitamin D3 60,000 IU once a week (n=15) for 180 days. Intake of fluoride-rich water continued as usual. At the end of the treatment period, there was significant improvement in dental, clinical, and skeletal grades of fluorosis in the treated children (p=0.05) but not in the placebo group. There were significantly reduced fluoride levels in the blood and serum and increased urinary fluoride levels in the treated group (p=0.05 for all three parameters) but not in the placebo group, indicating increased removal of fluoride from the body. The results of this small study indicate that calcium, ascorbic acid, and vitamin D3 supplementation can reverse fluorosis in children (Gupta et al 1996).

Osteoporosis/Fractures

A meta-analysis examined the effects of calcium supplementation on risk of fracture in children of both genders. Studies meeting inclusion criteria were randomized, placebo-controlled trials of at least 3 months duration with bone measurements taken at baseline and again after at least 6 months follow-up. Of the 19 studies identified involving 2,859 children, no effect of calcium supplementation on bone mineral density (BMD) was found at the hip or lumbar spine—common sites of fractures. A slight effect was observed on total bone mineral content and upper limb BMD. Although the effect to the upper limb persisted after supplementation ceased, it is of little clinical importance, since it is unlikely to result in an overall decrease in fracture risk among children (Wizenberg et al 2007).

One study found that 1200 mg/day calcium reduced the risk of osteoporotic fractures in elderly women compliant with the 5-year regimen. The double-blind, placebo controlled trial corresponded in length to the 5-year risk of fracture, projected to be 15% among this group of women (older than 70 years). Those taking calcium (n=730) noted improvements in quantitative ultrasonography findings of the heel, femoral neck, and whole-body dual x-ray absorptiometry data compared with those randomized to placebo (n=730). Calcium supplementation was also associated with greater bone strength (Prince et al 2006). Another 5-year study in a similar number of postmenopausal women found that 1 g/day of calcium citrate taken for 5 years led to significant positive effects on bone density, including a sustained reduction in bone loss and turnover and cumulative benefits to the proximal femur. The effect on fracture risk was less certain, since fractures still occurred in both groups. This may have been the result of decreasing compliance over the 5-year regimen, possibly due in part to a higher incidence of diarrhea reported among supplement users vs those receiving placebo (18% vs 11%, p=.0002). Given the positive cumulative and sustained effects observed among supplement users in this study, the authors suggest that continuous, long-term calcium supplementation can lead to even greater effects on bone density (Reid et al 2006).

An earlier review of studies in which postmenopausal women were treated with antiresorptive drugs (estrogen or calcitonin) or with antiresorptive drugs plus calcium showed greater increases in bone mass when treatment included supplemental calcium. Calcitonin alone stopped bone loss in the spine, but calcitonin plus calcium increased bone mass of the spine (Nieves et al 1998).

Intermittent fluoride treatment plus calcium increased BMD and was associated with a lower fracture rate than calcium supplementation alone in men with idiopathic osteoporosis. Fifty men with osteoporosis but no history of vertebral fractures were given either calcium 1,000 mg/day, or intermittent monofluorophosphate (MFP, 114 mg=15 mg fluoride ions daily, 3 months on, 1 month off) plus calcium 950 to 1,000 mg/day for 36 months. There was a progressive decrease in back pain in the MFP group over the three years, whereas there was no significant change in the calcium-only group. The fracture rate (new fractures per 100 patient-years) at the end of 3 years was 4.9 for the MFP group and 20.5 for the calcium-only group (Ringe et al 1998).

Although some earlier studies have shown a reduction in fractures associated with concurrent use of vitamin D and calcium, a more recent study examining older community-dwelling women (n=3,314) differed in its findings. Subjects included women aged 70 and above with one or more risk factors for fracture of the hip; all received an informational leaflet on calcium intake and how to reduce falls. Those in the treatment group (n=1,321) were instructed to take the combined daily regimen of 1000 mg calcium and 800 IU vitamin D_3 (cholecaliferol), while the control group (n=1,993) received the leaflet only. After 2 years, although clinical fracture rates were lower than anticipated in both groups, the researchers found no evidence of reduced risk with supplementation. However, the lack of a placebo arm and the fact that the study was underpowered may have limited the study's findings (Porthouse et al 2005).

In a smaller 3-year study involving 318 women and men over the age of 65 who lived at home, calcium 500 mg/day (as calcium citrate malate) plus 700 IU of cholecalciferol/day, in comparison to placebo, reduced the rate of bone loss in both men and women and significantly reduced the incidence of nonvertebral fractures. Rates of loss of bone mass were lower for femoral neck, spine, and total body in treatment groups after 1 year. However, significant differences between treatment groups in years 2 and 3 were maintained only for total-body BMD (Dawson-Hughes et al 1997).

In a larger study, concurrent administration of oral vitamin D3 and calcium reduced the incidence of nonvertebral fractures and hip fractures and increased bone density of the total proximal femoral region in elderly women (mean age 84 years). Compared with the placebo group (n=888), the treated women (n=877) had 32% fewer nonvertebral fractures and 43% fewer hip fractures. Eighteen months of treatment resulted in an increase of 2.7% in bone density of the total proximal femoral region compared with a decrease of 4.6% in the placebo group ($p<0.001$). The dosage of vitamin D3 was 20 mcg (800 IU)/day and elemental calcium was 1.2 g/day (Chapuy et al 1992).

Premenstrual Pain

Calcium supplementation was effective in reducing premenstrual pain, but not menstrual pain, in a prospective, randomized, double-blind, placebo-controlled, parallel-group, multicenter clinical trial of premenstrual syndrome. Subjects (n=497) were given calcium 1,200 mg daily or placebo for three menstrual cycles. Outcome measures included a daily subjective rating scale with 17 core symptoms, of which three were pain-related, and four symptom factors, of which one was pain-related. Significantly lower scores occurred for all pain measures in the treatment group during the luteal phase of the third menstrual cycle (p=0.001) while scores did not change significantly in controls. Pain scores did not decrease significantly during the menstrual phase of the third menstrual cycle for both calcium and placebo groups (Thys-Jacobs et al 1998).

INDICATIONS AND USAGE

Approved by the FDA:

- Prophylaxis of calcium deficiency and treatment of osteoporosis
- Calcium acetate: Treatment of hyperphosphatemia related to renal failure and hemodialysis
- Calcium carbonate: Used alone or in combination products as an antacid to relieve symptoms of heartburn, acid indigestion, and stomach upset

Unproven Uses: Calcium supplementation may reduce premenstrual pain, total and LDL cholesterol, hypertension, and the occurrence of colorectal polyps. Studies show it may also reverse fluorosis in children (when combined with vitamins C and D), control age-related increases in parathyroid hormone, and reduce plasma bilirubin in patients with Crigler-Najjar syndrome (calcium phosphate only).

Weaker evidence shows calcium supplementation may be helpful for leg cramps, pre-eclampsia, and prophylaxis of urinary crystallization of calcium oxalate in patients with nephrolithiasis (calcium citrate only).

CONTRAINDICATIONS

Calcium supplements are contraindicated in patients with hypercalcemia (Gilman et al 2001).

PRECAUTIONS AND ADVERSE REACTIONS

Calcium enhances the effect of cardiac glycosides on the heart and may precipitate arrhythmias (Dukes 1980).

Oral calcium supplementation can cause constipation. Additionally, oral calcium—including antacids containing calcium carbonate or other absorbable calcium salts—can cause hypercalcemia (especially in patients with hypothyroidism) and milk-alkali syndrome with doses higher than 4 g daily. Hypercalcemia may result in nephrolithiasis, anorexia, nausea, vomiting, and ocular toxicity. Symptoms of milk-alkali syndrome include hypercalcemia, uremia, calcinosis, nausea, vomiting, headache, weakness, azotemia, and alterations in taste.

High intake of calcium, whether from food alone or including supplements, was associated in an epidemiological study with an increased incidence of prostate cancer, possibly due to calcium's inhibitory effect on vitamin D conversion (Giovannucci et al 1998).

Pregnancy: FDA-rated as Pregnancy Category C. Calcium is safe in normal dietary amounts.

Breastfeeding: Calcium is safe in normal dietary amounts.

Dairy foods: Phosphorus, found in dairy products, may inhibit calcium absorption by forming insoluble compounds with calcium ions. This binds the mineral into a form that is poorly absorbed through the intestinal wall. *Clinical Management:* Calcium products should not be taken within 2 hours of a dairy product or other foods high in phosphorous.

Foods containing oxalic acid or phytic acid: Oxalic acid (found in foods such as spinach, parsley, rhubarb, and beans) and phytic acid (found in bran and whole cereals) may inhibit calcium absorption by forming insoluble compounds with calcium ions. This binds the mineral into a form that is poorly absorbed through the intestinal wall. *Clinical Management:* Calcium products should not be taken within 2 hours of eating foods high in oxalic acid or phytic acid.

Iron: Concurrent use may result in reduced absorption of iron, although the effect is usually not clinically significant.

Zinc: Concurrent use may result in reduced absorption of zinc, although the effect is usually not clinically significant.

DRUG INTERACTIONS

CONTRAINDICATED

Digitoxin: Coadministration of digitoxin and parenteral calcium is contraindicated (Product Info: Crystodigin 1995). Early case reports describe cardiovascular collapse after administration of intravenous calcium in patients receiving digitalis. *Clinical Management:* Administration of parenteral calcium to digitoxin-treated patients is contraindicated.

Digoxin: Most textbooks and reviews state that a contraindication exists in giving calcium intravenously in the presence of digitalis glycosides, though this is based on relatively few reports. The similar actions of digitalis glycosides and calcium are documented, and deaths have occurred during simultaneous administration. *Clinical Management:* If calcium is needed in a digitalized patient, it should be infused over several hours or given orally.

MAJOR RISKS

Gentamicin: A retrospective study conducted on 267 patients who had undergone elective coronary artery bypass graft (CABG) surgery showed an increased incidence of renal failure in patients who had received gentamicin and bypass prime solutions containing high amounts of calcium (Schneider et al 1996). *Clinical Management:* Avoid concurrent use of gentamicin and solutions containing a high amount of calcium during CABG surgery.

MODERATE RISKS

Aspirin: Concurrent use may result in decreased effectiveness of aspirin due to increased urinary pH and subsequent increased renal elimination of salicylates. *Clinical Management:* Monitor for reduced aspirin effectiveness upon initiation of calcium-containing products or for possible aspirin toxicity upon withdrawal of calcium-containing products. Adjust the dose accordingly. Using buffered aspirin may limit the degree to which the urine is alkalinized.

Cefpodoxime: Concomitant use may result in decreased effectiveness of cefpodoxime. *Clinical Management:* Concurrent administration of cefpodoxime and calcium-containing products is not recommended. If concurrent use cannot be avoided, cefpodoxime should be taken at least 2 to 3 hours before the administration of calcium. Because staggered administration may not be completely reliable, aggressively monitor patients for continued antibiotic efficacy. Alternative antibiotic therapy (eg, another third-generation cephalosporin or a second-generation cephalosporin with similar activity) may need to be considered.

Diuretics: Thiazide and thiazide-like diuretics may cause hypercalcemia by decreasing renal calcium excretion. Concomitant ingestion of calcium salts and thiazide diuretics may predispose patients to developing the milk-alkali syndrome. *Clinical Management:* Instruct patients to avoid excessive ingestion of calcium in any form (eg, antacids, dairy products) during thiazide diuretic therapy. Consider monitoring the patient's serum calcium level and/or parathyroid function if calcium replacement therapy is clinically necessary.

Fluoroquinolones: Concomitant use may result in decreased effectiveness of fluoroquinolones such as ciprofloxacin and enoxacin. *Clinical Management:* Concurrent administration of fluoroquinolones with calcium—including calcium-fortified foods and drinks such as orange juice—should be avoided. Fluoroquinolones may be taken 2 hours before or 6 hours after taking calcium-containing products.

Itraconazole: Concomitant use may result in decreased effectiveness of itraconazole. *Clinical Management:* Calcium-containing products should be taken at least 1 hour before or 2 hours after itraconzaole.

Ketoconazole: Concomitant use may result in decreased effectiveness of ketoconazole. *Clinical Management:* Concurrent administration of ketoconazole and calcium-containing products is not recommended. If concurrent use cannot be avoided, ketoconazole should be taken at least 2 hours before calcium-containing products. Because staggered administration may not be completely reliable, aggressively monitor patients for continued antifungal efficacy.

Levothyroxine: Concurrent use with calcium carbonate may result in decreased absorption of levothyroxine. *Clinical Management:* Separate the administration of levothyroxine and calcium carbonate by at least 4 hours.

Polystyrene Sulfonate: Concomitant administration of calcium-containing antacids and sodium polystyrene sulfonate resin therapy has resulted in the elevation of serum carbon dioxide content levels, associated with varying degrees of metabolic alkalosis. *Clinical Management:* Separate the oral administration of sodium polystyrene sulfonate and calcium-containing products by as much time as possible. Another alternative is to administer the sodium polystyrene sulfonate rectally. If concurrent oral administration cannot be avoided, monitor the patient for evidence of alkalosis.

Tetracyclines: Concurrent use may result in decreased effectiveness of tetracyclines. *Clinical Management:* Concurrent administration of any of the tetracyclines and calcium-containing products is not recommended. If concurrent use cannot be avoided, tetracyclines should be taken at least 1 to 3 hours before calcium-containing products. Because staggered administration may not be completely reliable, aggressively monitor patients for continued antibiotic efficacy.

Ticlopidine: Concurrent use may result in decreased effectiveness of ticlopidine. *Clinical Management:* Concurrent administration of ticlopidine and calcium-containing products is not recommended. If concurrent use cannot be avoided, ticlopidine should be taken at least 1 to 2 hours before the administration of calcium.

Verapamil: Concomitant use may result in decreased effectiveness of verapamil, a calcium channel blocker, and result in reversal of hypotensive effects. *Clinical Management:* Calcium generally is given to reverse hypotension and improve cardiac conduction defects. Monitor the patient for expected cardiovascular response.

Zalcitabine: Concurrent use may result in decreased effectiveness of zalcitabine. *Clinical Management:* Separate the administration of zalcitabine and calcium-containing products as far apart as possible.

MINOR RISKS

Atenolol: Concomitant use may decreased bioavailability of atenelol. *Clinical Management:* Instruct patients to avoid taking atenolol and calcium-containing products at the same time. Atenolol should be administered 2 hours before or 6 hours after calcium-containing products.

Bismuth Subcitrate: Concomitant use may result in decreased effectiveness of bismuth subcitrate. *Clinical Management:* Bismuth subcitrate and calcium-containing products should be administered at least 30 minutes apart.

Bisphosphonates: Concurrent use may interfere with the absorption of bisphosphonates such as alendronate, etidronate, and risedronate. *Clinical Management:* Administer bisphosphonates 2 hours before and 3 to 4 hours after a dose of calcium.

Hyoscyamine: Concomitant use may result in decreased absorption of hyoscyamine. *Clinical Management:* Hyoscyamine should be taken prior to meals and calcium-containing products should be taken after meals.

Methscopolamine: Concomitant use may result in decreased absorption of methscopolamine, although the effect is minor. *Clinical Management:* Monitor the patient for drug effectiveness.

Ranitidine bismuth citrate: Concurrent use may result in decreased plasma concentrations of ranitidine; however, the effect is clinically insignificant.

Sucralfate: Concurrent use may result in decreased effectiveness of sucralfate. *Clinical Management:* Calcium-containing products should not be taken 30 minutes before or after sucralfate administration.

POTENTIAL INTERACTIONS

Sulfasalazine: Concomitant sulfasalazine and calcium gluconate therapy has been reported to result in delayed absorption of sulfasalazine.

OVERDOSAGE

Active treatment is required when serum calcium levels reach 12 mg/dL, and intensive treatment is necessary for levels greater than 15 mg/dL (AMA 1980).

DOSAGE

Mode of Administration: Oral

How Supplied: Capsule, liquid, tablet

Daily Dosage: The National Institute of Medicine recommends the following Adequate Intakes (AIs) for males and females: *0 to 6 months* — 210 mg/day; *7 to 12 months* — 270 mg/day; *1 to 3 years* — 500 mg/day; *4 to 8 years* — 800 mg/day; *9 to 18 years* — 1,300 mg/day; *19 to 50 years* — 1,000 mg/day; *51+ years* — 1,200 mg/day. The same AIs apply to pregnant or lactating women.

ADULTS

Colorectal cancer prevention: 1,200 to 2,000 mg/d (Hofstad et al 1998; Duris et al 1996; Lipkin & Newmark 1993; Zimmerman 1993).

Crigler-Najjar Syndrome: 4,000 mg/d (Van der Veere et al 1997).

Dysmenorrhea: 1,000 to 1,300 mg/d (Penland et al 1993; Thys-Jacobs et al 1989).

Hypercholesterolemia: 250 to 400 mg/d with meals (Denke et al 1993; Bell et al 1992; Karanja et al 1994).

Hyperphosphatemia: 1,334 mg of calcium acetate with each meal initially. Most patients will require 2,001 to 2,668 mg with each meal. The dosage may be increased as necessary to obtain serum phosphate levels below 6 mg/dL as long as hypercalcemia does not occur (Product Info: PhosLo 1996); or alternatively, 1 to 17 grams of calcium carbonate daily in divided doses (Malberti et al 1988; Slatopolsky et al 1986).

Hyperphosphatemia of renal failure and hemodialysis: 4,000 to 8,000 mg/d of calcium acetate (Product Info: PhosLo 1996) or 2,500 to 8,500 mg/d of calcium carbonate (Malberti et al 1988; Slatopolsky et al 1986).

Hypertension, idiopathic: 1,000 to 2,000 mg/d (Bucher et al 1996; Takagi et al 1991; Lyle et al 1987; Tabuchi et al 1986).

Hypertension, pregnancy-related: 1,000 to 2,000 mg/d (Bucher et al 1996).

Hypocalcemia: calcium carbonate, 1 to 2 grams 3 times a day with meals (AMA 1986); calcium citrate, 950 mg to 1.9 g given 3 or 4 times a day after meals (AMA 1986); calcium gluconate, 15 g daily in divided doses (AMA 1986); calcium lactate, 7.7 grams daily in divided doses with meals (USPDI 2004; AMA 1980); calcium glubionate, 15 grams/d in divided doses (AMA 1986); dibasic calcium phosphate, 4.4 g daily in divided doses with or after meals (USPDI 2004; AMA 1980); tribasic calcium phosphate, 1.6 grams twice daily with or after meals (USPDI 2004).

Nephrolithiasis, prevention: 200 to 300 mg with meals or as the citrate salt between meals (Liebman et al 1997; Levine et al 1994; Barilla et al 1978).

Osteoporosis, glucocorticoid-induced, prevention of bone loss:1,000 mg/d (Buckley et al 1996).

Osteoporosis, idiopathic, prevention of bone loss and fractures: 500 to 2,400 mg/d including a bedtime dose (Nieves et al 1998; Dawson-Hughes et al 1997; Fujita et al 1997; McKane et al 1996; Blumsohn et al 1994; Reid et al 1993; Chapuy et al 1992).

Pre-eclampsia, prevention: 1,000 to 2,000 mg/d (Bucher et al 1996).

Premenstrual syndrome: 1,000 to 1,200 mg/d (Thys-Jacobs et al 1998; Penland et al 1993; Thys-Jacobs et al 1989).

PEDIATRICS

Bone mass accretion (adolescents): 500 mg/d (Lloyd et al 1993).

Fluorosis: 250 mg/d (Gupta et al 1996).

Hypertension, prevention: 600 mg/d (Gillman et al 1995).

Hypocalcemia: calcium chloride, 200 mg/kg/d in divided doses every 4 to 6 hours (Benitz et al 1988); calcium glubionate: infants up to 1 year old should receive 1.8 grams of calcium glubionate 5 times a day before meals, and children 1 to 4 years old should receive 3.6 grams 3 times a day before meals. Children over age 4 should receive adult and adolescent doses (USPDI 2004); calcium gluconate, 200 to 800 mg/kg/d in divided doses (USPDI 2004; Benitz et al 1988); calcium lactate, 500 mg/kg/24 hours given orally in divided doses (USPDI 2004; Benitz et al 1981; Shirkey 1980; AMA 1980; Pagliaro et al 1979); calcium levulinate: 500 mg/kg/24 hours (12 g/square meter/24 hours) given orally in divided doses (Shirkey 1980); dibasic calcium phosphate: 200 to 280 mg/kg of body weight a day, in divided doses with or after meals (USPDI 2004).

LITERATURE

American Society of Health-System Pharmacists (AHFS): *American Hospital Formulary Service Drug Information.* ASHP, Bethesda, MD; 1997.

AMA Department of Drugs: *AMA Drug Evaluations,* 4th ed. American Medical Association, Chicago, IL, USA; 1980.

Baron J, Beach M, Mandel J et al: Calcium supplements for the prevention of colorectal adenomas. *N Engl J Med*; 340:101-107, 1999

Bell L, Halstenson CE, Halstenson CJ et al: Cholesterol-lowering effects of calcium carbonate in patients with mild to moderate hypercholesterolemia. *Arch Intern Med*; 152(12):2441-2444. 1992

Benitz WE, Tatro DS: *The Pediatric Drug Handbook,* 2nd ed. Year Book Medical Publishers, Chicago, IL, USA; 1988.

Bergel E, Barros AJD: Effect of maternal calcium intake during pregnancy on children's blood pressure: a systematic review of the literature. *BMC Pediatrics*; 7:15. 2007

Blumsohn A, Herrington K, Hannon RA et al: The effect of calcium supplementation on the circadian rhythm of bone resorption. *J Clin Endocrinol Metab*; 79(3):730-735. 1994

Bucher HC, Cook RJ, Guyatt GH et al: Effects of dietary calcium supplementation on blood pressure - a meta-analysis of randomized controlled trials. *JAMA*; 275(13):1016-1022. 1996

Bucher HC, Guyatt GH, Cook RJ et al: Effect of calcium supplementation on pregnancy-induced hypertension and preeclampsia. *JAMA*; 275(14):1113-1117. 1996

Buckley LM, Leib ES, Cartularo KS et al: Calcium and vitamin D3 supplementation prevents bone loss in the spine secondary to low dose corticosteroids in patients with rheumatoid arthritis: a randomized, double-blind placebo-controlled trial. *Ann Intern Med*; 125(12):961-968. 1996

Cappuccio FP, Markandu ND, Singer DRJ et al: Does oral calcium supplementation lower high blood pressure? A double blind study. *J Hypertens*; 5(1):67-71. 1987

Chapuy MC, Arlot ME, Duboeuf F et al: Vitamin D3 and calcium to prevent hip fractures in elderly women. *N Engl J Med*; 327(23):1637-1642. 1992

Cher DJ: Dietary calcium and blood pressure (letter). *JAMA*; 126(6):492. 1997

Dawson-Hughes B, Harris SS, Krall EA et al: Effect of calcium and vitamin D supplementation on bone density in men and women 65 years of age or older. *N Engl J Med*; 337(10):670-676. 1997

Denke MA, Fox MM, Schulte MC: Short-term dietary calcium fortification increases fecal saturated fat content and reduces serum lipids in men. *J Nutr*; 123(6):1047-1053. 1993

Deroisy R, Zartarian M, Meurmans L et al: Acute changes in serum calcium and parathyroid hormone circulating levels induced by the oral intake of five currently available calcium salts in healthy male volunteers. *Clin Rheumatol*; 16(3):249-253. 1997

Dukes MNG: *Meyler's Side Effects of Drugs,* vol 9. Excerpta Medica, New York, NY; 1980.

Duris I, Hruby D, Pekarkova B et al: Calcium chemoprevention in colorectal cancer. *Hepatogastroenterology*; 43(7):152-154. 1996

Fujita T, Ohgitani S, Fujii Y: Overnight suppression of parathyroid hormone and bone resorption markers by active absorbable algae calcium: a double-blind crossover study. *Calcif Tissue Int*; 60(6):506-512. 1997

Gilman AG, Hardman JG, Limbird LE (eds): *Goodman & Gilman's The Pharmacological Basis of Therapeutics,* 10th ed. McGraw-Hill, New York, NY; 2001.

Giovannucci E, Rimm EB, Wolk A et al: Calcium and fructose intake in relation to risk of prostate cancer. *Cancer Res*; 58(3):442-447. 1998

Govers MJAP, Termont DSML, Van der Meer R: Mechanism of the antiproliferative effect of milk mineral and other calcium supplements on colonic epithelium. *Cancer Res*; 54(1):95-100. 1994

Grau MV, Baron JA, Sandler RS et al: Prolonged effect of calcium supplementation on risk of colorectal adenomas in a randomized trial. *J Natl Cancer Inst*; 99:129-136. 2007

Gupta SK, Gupta RC, Seth AK et al: Reversal of fluorosis in children. *Acta Paediatr Jpn*; 38(5):513-519. 1996

Harvey JA, Kenny P, Poindexter J et al: Superior calcium absorption from calcium citrate than calcium carbonate using external forearm counting. *J Am Coll Nutr*; 9(6):583-587. 1990

Heaney RP, Smith KT, Recker RR et al: Meal effects on calcium absorption. *Am J Clin Nutr*; 49(2):372-376. 1989

Hofstad B, Almendingen K, Vatn M et al: Growth and recurrence of colorectal polyps: a double-blind 3-year intervention with calcium and antioxidants. *Digestion*; 59(2):148-156. 1998

Ivanovich P, Fellows H, Rich C: The absorption of calcium carbonate. *Ann Intern Med*; 66(5):917-923. 1967

Karanja N, Morris CD, Rufolo P et al: Impact of increasing calcium in the diet on nutrient consumption, plasma lipids, and lipoproteins in humans. *Am J Clin Nutr*; *59(4):900-907.* 1994

Levine BS, Rodman JS, Wienerman S et al: Effect of calcium citrate supplementation on urinary calcium oxalate saturation in female stone formers: implications for prevention of osteoporosis. *Am J Clin Nutr*; 60(4):592-596. 1994

Levine R, DerSimonian R: Effects of calcium supplementation on pregnancy-induced hypertension (letter). *JAMA*; 276(17):1387. 1996

Liebman M, Chai W: Effect of dietary calcium on urinary oxalate excretion after oxalate loads. *Am J Clin Nutr*; 65(5):1453-1459. 1997

Lipkin M, Newmark H: Calcium and colon cancer (letter). *Nutr Rev*; 51(7):213-214. 1993

Lloyd T, Andon MB, Rollings N et al: Calcium supplementation and bone mineral density in adolescent girls. *JAMA*; 270(7):841-844. 1993

Lopez-Jaramillo P, Delgado F, Jacome P et al: Calcium supplementation and the risk of preeclampsia in Ecuadorian pregnant teenagers. *Obstet Gynecol*; 90(2):162-167. 1997

Lyle RM, Melby CL, Hyner GC et al: Blood pressure and metabolic effects of calcium supplementation on normotensive white and black men. *JAMA*; 257(13):1772-1776. 1987

Malberti F, Surian M, Poggio F et al: Efficacy and safety of long-term treatment with calcium carbonate as a phosphate binder. *Am J Kidney Dis*; 12(6):487-491. 1988

McKane WR, Khosla S, Egan KS et al: Role of calcium intake in modulating age-related increases in parathyroid function and bone resorption. *J Clin Endocrinol Metab*; 81(5):1699-1703. 1996

Newmark K, Nugent P: Milk-alkali syndrome: a consequence of chronic antacid abuse. *Postgrad Med*; 93(6):149-150, 156. 1993

Nieves JW, Komar L, Cosman F et al: Calcium potentiates the effect of estrogen and calcitonin on bone mass: review and analysis. *Am J Clin Nutr*; 67(1):18-24. 1998

Penland JG, Johnson PE: Dietary calcium and manganese effects on menstrual cycle symptoms. *Am J Obstet Gynecol*; 168(5):1417-1423. 1993

Parfitt K (ed): *Martindale: The Complete Drug Reference.* London: Pharmaceutical Press (electronic version). Thomson Micromedex, Greenwood Village, CO, 2000.

Pitchford P: *Healing with Whole Foods.* North Atlantic Books, Berkeley, CA; 1993.

Porthouse J, Cockayne S, King C et al: Randomised controlled trial of calcium and supplementation with cholecalciferol (vitamin D_3) for prevention of fractures in primary care. *BMJ*; 330:1003. 2005

Prince RL, Devine A, Dhaliwal SS, Dick IM: Effects of calcium supplementation on clinical fracture and bone structure. Results of a 5-year, double-blind, placebo-controlled trial in elderly women. *Arch Intern Med*; 166:869-875. 2006

Product Information: Calcium gluconate. LyphoMed, Deerfield, IL; 1992.

Product Information: Crystodigin (digitoxin). Eli Lilly and Company, Indianapolis, IN; 1995.

Product Information: PhosLo (calcium acetate). Braintree Laboratories, Braintree, MA; 1996.

Recker RR: Calcium absorption and achlorhydria. *N Engl J Med*; 313(2):70-73. 1985

Reid IR, Mason B, Horne A, et al. Randomized controlled trial of calcium in healthy older women. *Am J Med*; 119:777-785. 2006

Reid IR, Ames RW, Evans MC et al: Effect of calcium supplementation on bone loss in postmenopausal women. *N Engl J Med*; 328(7):460-464. 1993

Riley BB: Incompatibilities in intravenous solutions. *J Hosp Pharm*; 28:228-240. 1970

Ringe JD, Dorst A, Kipshoven C et al: Avoidance of vertebral fractures in men with idiopathic osteoporosis by a three year therapy with calcium and low-dose intermittent monofluorophosphate. *Osteoporos Int*; 8(1):47-52. 1998

Roberts JM, D'Abarno J: Effects of calcium supplementation on pregnancy-induced hypertension (letter). *JAMA*; 276(17):1386-1387. 1996

Schneider M, Valentine S, Clarke G et al: Acute renal failure in cardiac surgical patients, potentiated by gentamicin and calcium. *Anaesth Intensive Care*; 24:647-650. 1996

Shirkey HC: *Pediatric Dosage Handbook.* American Pharmaceutical Association, Washington, DC, USA; 1980.

Slatopolsky E, Weerts C, Lopez-Hilker S et al: Calcium carbonate as a phosphate binder in patients with chronic renal failure undergoing dialysis. *N Engl J Med*; 315(3):157-161. 1986

Tabuchi Y, Ogihara T, Hashizume K et al: Hypotensive effect of long-term oral calcium supplementation in elderly patients with essential hypertension. *J Clin Hypertens*; 2:254-262. 1986

Takagi Y, Fukase M, Takata S et al: Calcium treatment of essential hypertension in elderly patients evaluated by 24 h monitoring. *Am J Hypertens*; 4(10 pt 1):836-839. 1991

Thys-Jacobs S, Ceccarelli S, Bierman A et al: Calcium supplementation in premenstrual syndrome: a randomized crossover trial. *J Gen Intern Med*; 4(3):183-189. 1989

Thys-Jacobs S, Starkey P, Bernstein D et al: Calcium carbonate and the premenstrual syndrome: effects on premenstrual and menstrual symptoms (Premenstrual Syndrome Study Group). Am J Obstet Gynecol; 179(2):444-452. 1998

United States Pharmacopeial Convention, Inc.: *USP DI: Drug Information for the Health Care Professional,* 24th ed. Thomson Micromedex, Greenwood Village CO; 2004.

Van der Veere CN, Jansen PL, Sinaasappel M et al: Oral calcium phosphate: a new therapy for Crigler-Najjar disease? *Gastroenterology*; 112(2):455-462. 1997

Villar J, Abdel-Aleem H, Merialdi M et al: World Health Organization randomized trial of calcium supplementation among low calcium intake pregnant women. *Am J Obstet Gynecol*; 194:639-649. 2006

Wabner CL, Pak CYC: Modification by food of the calcium absorbability and physicochemical effects of calcium citrate. *J Am Coll Nutr*; 11(5):548-552. 1992

Wactawski-Wende J, Kotchen JM, Anderson GL et al. Calcium plus vitamin D supplementation and the risk of colorectal cancer. *N Engl J Med*; 354:684-696. 2006

Wallace K, Baron JA, Cole BF et al: Effect of calcium supplementation on the risk of large bowel polyps. *J Natl Cancer Inst*; 96:921-925. 2004

Wizenberg T, Shaw K, Fryer J, Jones G: Effects of calcium supplementation on bone density in healthy children: meta-analysis of randomized controlled trials. *BMJ*; 2006

Young LY, Koda-Kimble MA: *Applied Therapeutics: The Clinical Use of Drugs,* 6th ed. Applied Therapeutics, Inc, Vancouver, WA, USA; 1995.

Zimmerman J: Does dietary calcium supplementation reduce the risk of colon cancer (letter)? *Nutr Rev*; 51(4):109-112. 1993

Chondroitin Sulfate

DESCRIPTION

Chondroitin sulfate is a mucopolysaccharide found in most mammalian cartilaginous tissues. It has a molecular configuration similar to sodium hyaluronate, although chondroitin has a considerably shorter chain length (Liesegang 1990). In clinical settings, chondroitin is commonly used as a viscoelastic agent during ophthalmic procedures. Its major use as a supplement is for relieving symptoms of osteoarthritis and rheumatic diseases. It has also been used to treat heart disease, nephrolithiasis, and hypercholesterolemia. The chondroprotective properties of chondroitin have led to speculative use in the prevention and/or treatment of disorders of other connective tissue structures such as the aorta, vascular tissues, and soft tissues involved in musculoskeletal trauma. Chondroitin has demonstrated some efficacy in small clinical trials for treating dry eyes, interstitial cystitis, and temporomandibular joint (TMJ) disorder.

Other Names: CDS, chondroitin sulfate A, chondroitin sulfate C, chondroitin-4-sulfate, chondroitin-6-sulfate, CSA, CSC, and galactosaminoglucuronoglycan sulfate

ACTIONS AND PHARMACOLOGY

EFFECTS

Chondroitin sulfate has protective effects on cartilage as well as viscoelastic effects. Preliminary evidence suggests it may also have antilipidemic, anticoagulant, and antithrombogenic properties.

Cardiovascular Effects: Chondroitin sulfate administered orally or parentally has been reported to produce beneficial effects on serum lipids and "lipid clearing." (Morrison 1971; Morrison 1969). In a 22-week evaluation, phospholipid levels were significantly reduced after 14 weeks of treatment with chondroitin sulfate. However, this benefit was not sustained through trial completion (Izuka et al 1968).

Chondroprotective Effects: Chondroitin sulfate is a galactosaminoglucuronoglycan sulfate (GAG) that has demonstrated some efficacy in the treatment of osteoarthritis. Exogenously administered GAGs concentrate in cartilage where they can be used in the synthesis of new cartilaginous matrix. The chondroprotective action of chondroitin sulfate has been demonstrated in vitro. Chondroitin sulfate inhibits the effect of leukocyte elastase, which can alter fundamental components of the cartilaginous matrix (proteoglycans and collagen fibers). Leukocyte elastase is found in high concentrations in the blood and synovial fluid of patients with rheumatic diseases (Shankland 1998; Morreale et al 1996; Pipitone 1991).

Viscoelastic Effects: Similar to sodium hyaluronate, chondroitin sulfate is used primarily as a viscoelastic agent for ophthalmic surgical procedures. Viscoelastic agents possess rheologic properties (e.g., viscosity, pseudoplasticity, and coatability) that make them amenable to ocular surgical procedures. Specifically, these agents are used to protect cells and tissues from mechanical trauma (coating actions), to allow space for surgical manipulation, to separate tissues and break adhesions, and to provide lubrication to manipulate tissue (Liesegang 1990; Barron et al 1985). Viscoelastic agents are also postoperatively employed to maintain space, diminish localized bleeding, and lubricate and separate tissues to prevent adhesions; they are also used as tissue substitutes (e.g., vitreous) (Liesegang 1990).

CLINICAL TRIALS

Interstitial Cystitis

According to a recent report, two nonrandomized, uncontrolled pilot studies noted an improvement in symptoms of interstitial cystitis (IC) associated with use of chondroitin sulfate. Both trials administered a bladder-instilled solution of chondroitin to subjects for over 1 year. The first trial enrolled 18 newly-diagnosed, untreated IC subjects who underwent weekly instillations (0.2% solution) for 4 consecutive weeks, followed by monthly treatments. Patients completing the trial used a scoring index to rate improvements: 46.2% gave a rating of "good," 15.4% rated them as "fair," 30.8% gave a "partial" rating, and 7.7% rated improvements as "none." In the other trial, 24 patients with IC of 1 to 20 years' duration were treated with a bladder-instilled solution of chondroitin after failing to respond to other therapies. Therapy began with instillations of 2.0% solution twice weekly for 2 weeks, followed by 0.2% solution for 4 weeks, and monthly thereafter. Of the 20 patients completing the trial, symptom improvement was noted in 73.1% (range, 50% to 95%). Most patients reported improvement of symptoms after 3 to 4 weeks (Palylyk-Colwell 2006).

In an earlier study, some benefit was noted for patients with interstitial cystitis after treatment with chondroitin sulfate. Eighteen patients with the disorder who tested positive to the potassium stimulation test received 40 mL chondroitin sulfate 0.2% intravesically once weekly for 4 weeks and then once monthly for 1 year in an open-label study. Of the 13 patients followed for the entire 13-month study, 6 showed good response, 4 had partial response, 2 had fair response, and 1 patient had no response. Patients with epithelial permeability as demonstrated by the positive potassium challenge test may be more likely to respond to treatment with glucosaminoglycans (Steinhoff et al 2002).

Osteoarthritis

A recent meta-analysis, which included 20 trials involving 3,846 subjects, reported that the symptomatic benefit of chondroitin for osteoarthritis of the knee or hip is minimal to nonexistent. Daily oral doses ranged from 800 mg to 2000 mg across studies. The systematic review included several large-scale, high-quality trials that showed minimal or no effect on joint pain with chondroitin (Reichenbach et al 2007). One well-designed study cited in the analysis enrolled 1,583 patients with symptomatic knee pain and randomly distributed them across 5 treatment groups: glucosamine 1500 mg/day (n=317), chondroitin sulfate 1200 mg/day (n=318), glucosamine plus chondroitin (n=317), celocoxib 200 mg/day (n=318) and placebo (n=313). Investigators were looking for a 20% decrease in Western Ontario and MacMaster Universities Osteoarthritis Index (WOMAC) pain score from baseline to week 24. Compared with the high rate of response to placebo (60.1%), rates of response were just 3.9 percentage points higher for glucosamine (p=0.30), 5.3 percentage points higher for chondroitin (p=0.17), and 6.5 points higher for the combination of the two (p=0.09). These results show that chondroitin sulfate, either alone or in combination with glucosamine, did not effectively reduce pain in the overall group of subjects studied (Clegg et al 2006).

An earlier meta-analysis of 15 randomized, placebo-controlled trials evaluated the structural and symptomatic efficacy of oral glucosamine or chondroitin in knee osteoarthritis. Glucosamine improved scores on all outcomes measures, including joint space narrowing. Chondroitin demonstrated improvement on two outcome measures: the Lequesne Index (e.g., distance walked, duration of morning stiffness, and discomfort) and a visual analog scale for pain and mobility. Safety was excellent for both compounds (Richy et al 2003).

Another meta-analysis of 16 studies on the use of chondroitin in osteoarthritis recognized a general positive trend, with supplementation demonstrating improvement in functional capacity, reduction of pain, reduction of nonsteroidal anti-inflammatory drugs (NSAIDs) or analgesic consumption, and tolerability. In each study, an analgesic or NSAID was concurrently used with chondroitin. However, nine of the trials in this analysis suffered from a variety of methodological problems and did not meet evaluation criteria. The authors concluded that larger long-term, randomized clinical trials are needed to define chondroitin's specific place in therapy (Leeb et al 2000).

Treatment with naproxen and chondroitin helped to decrease the number of joints affected by erosive osteoarthritis over a 2-year radiological investigation (n=24). However, chondroitin sulfate did not modify disease progression, and the authors concluded there was no overall clinical significance in this trial. Patient assessment of pain and adverse effects were not evaluated (Rovetta et al 2002).

Combination therapy with glucosamine, chondroitin, and manganese ascorbate improved symptoms of knee arthritis but had equivocal effects on low-back arthritis in a 16-week, randomized, double-blind, placebo-controlled, cross-over pilot study involving 34 men from the United States Navy. Subjects were randomized to receive either oral Cosamin (consisting of glucosamine hydrochloride 500 mg, chondroitin sulfate 400 mg, and manganese ascorbate 76 mg) or placebo three times daily for 8 weeks. Improvement under treatment was statistically significant by patient assessment of results (p=0.02) and the visual analog scale for pain, both recorded in examinations (p=0.02) or patient diaries (p=0.02). Running times and knee range of motion were unaffected by treatment, and trends in acetaminophen use, Lequesne scores, and patient and examiner assessment of severity did not reach significance (Leffler et al 1999).

TMJ

Decreased temporomandibular joint (TMJ) tenderness, fewer TMJ sounds, and fewer over-the-counter analgesics resulted with supplementation of glucosamine and chondroitin. In a 12-week, double-blind, placebo-controlled study, patients received 750 mg of glucosamine HCl and 600 mg of chondroitin sulfate twice daily (n=23) or placebo (n=22). Statistically significant improvements were demonstrated in one scale of the McGill Pain Questionnaire in the treatment group (evaluative pain rating index) and four scales in the placebo group (sensory, evaluative, number of words, and miscellaneous pain rating indices). There was also a significant decrease in the visual analog scale in the placebo group. TMJ noises significantly decreased in the treatment group with no change in patients in the control group. The mean number of over-the-counter medications (mainly acetaminophen) was significantly fewer in the treatment group (Nguyen et al 2001).

Administration of 1,600 mg of glucosamine HCl, 1,000 mg of calcium ascorbate, and a 1,200-mg mixture of chondroitin sulfate-4 and -6, all taken twice daily, produced beneficial effects in TMJ arthritis. Of the 50 participants in the uncontrolled, preliminary study, 80% reported a decrease in joint noises; 2% reported a worsening in symptoms of pain and/or swelling; 10% failed to comply with conditions of the study, and 8% reported no change. Responses were noted an average of 14 to 21 days after starting treatment; however, patients were allowed to take aspirin and ibuprofen when TMJ pain interfered with daily activities (Shankland 1998).

INDICATIONS AND USAGE

Approved by the FDA:

- For protection during cataract extraction with intraocular lens implantation
- For use as a corneal preservation medium

Unproven Uses: People with osteoarthritis and rheumatic diseases take chondroitin sulfate to reduce pain, improve functional capacity, and reduce the use of painkillers. Chondroitin therapy is sometimes used to treat the following: TMJ disorder, coronary heart disease, hypercholesterolemia, nephrolithiasis, interstitial cystitis (intravesical), dry eye syndrome (ophthalmic), snoring (intranasal), and to prevent or treat disorders of connective tissue structures such as the aorta, vascular tissues, and soft tissues involved in musculoskeletal trauma.

PRECAUTIONS AND ADVERSE REACTIONS

Intraocular pressure changes may occur when chondroitin is used in the eye. Patients with asthma may be at risk for symptom exacerbation when taking a combination of glucosamine and chondroitin (Tallia et al 2002).

Pregnancy and lactation: Scientific evidence for the safe use of chondroitin sulfate during pregnancy and lactation is not available.

DRUG INTERACTIONS

POTENTIAL INTERACTIONS

Antiplatelet and Anticoagulant Agents: Theoretically, concurrent use with chondroitin may increase the risk of bleeding.

DOSAGE

Mode of Administration: Intramuscular, intravenous, oral

How Supplied: Capsule, tablet, sterile solution derived from bovine tracheal cartilage or shark cartilage

Daily Dosage:

Cataract extraction/lens implantation (ophthalmic solution): 0.2 to 0.5 mL using standard sterile technique into the anterior chamber with the provided needle/cannula prior to capsulotomy.

Osteoarthritis: 800 to 1200 mg orally in single or divided doses

LITERATURE

Alpar JJ, Alpar AJ, Baca J et al: Comparison of Healon® and Viscoat® in cataract extraction and intraocular lens implantation. *Ophthalmic Surg*; 19(9):636-642. 1988

Bourne WM: Endothelial cell survival on transplanted human corneas preserved at 4 degrees C in 2.5% chondroitin sulfate for one to 13 days. *Am J Ophthalmol*; 102(3):382-386. 1986

Clegg DO, Reda DJ, Harris CL et al. Glucosamine, chondroitin sulfate, and the two in combination for painful knee osteoarthritis. *N Engl J Med*; 354(8):795-808. 2006

Cohen M, Wolfe R, Mai T et al: A randomized, double blind, placebo controlled trial of a topical cream containing glucosamine sulfate, chondroitin sulfate, and camphor for osteoarthritis of the knee. *J Rheumatol*; 30(3):523-528. 2003

Conte A, de Bernardi M, Palmieri L et al: Metabolic fate of exogenous chondroitin sulfate in man. *Arzneimittelforschung*; 41(7):768-772. 1991

Leeb BF, Schweitzer H, Montag K et al: A meta-analysis of chondroitin sulfate in the treatment of osteoarthritis. *J Rheumatol*; 27(1):205-211. 2000

Leffler CT, Philippi AF, Leffler SG et al: Glucosamine, chondroitin, and manganese ascorbate for degenerative joint disease of the knee or low back: a randomized, double-blind, placebo-controlled pilot study. *Mil Med*; 164(2):85-91. 1999

Liesegang TJ: Viscoelastic substances in ophthalmology. *Surv Ophthalmol*; 34(4):268-293. 1990

Mazieres B, Combe B, Phan Van A et al: Chondroitin sulfate in osteoarthritis of the knee: a prospective, double blind, placebo controlled multicenter clinical study. *J Rheumatol*; 28(1):173-178. 2001

Morreale P, Manopulo R, Galati M et al: Comparison of the antiinflammatory efficacy of chondroitin sulfate and diclofenac sodium in patients with knee osteoarthritis. *J Rheumatol*; 23(8):1385-1391. 1996

Nguyen P, Mohamed SE, Gardiner D et al: A randomized, double-blind clinical trial of the effect of chondroitin sulfate and glucosamine hydrochloride on temporomandibular joint disorder: a pilot study. *J Craniomandibular Pract*; 19(2):130-139. 2001

Palylyk-Colwell E: Chondroitin sulfate for treatment of interstitial cystitis (Issues in emerging health technologies issue 84), Ottawa-Canadian Agency for Drugs and Technologies in Health. 2006

Product Information: DuoVisc® Ophthalmic Viscosurgical Device; Alcon Labs, Fort Worth, TX, 2001.

Reichenbach S, Sterchi R, Scherer M et al: Meta-analysis: chondroitin for osteoarthritis of the knee or hip. *Ann Intern Med*; 146:580-590. 2007

Richy F, Bruyere O, Ethgen O et al: Structural and symptomatic efficacy of glucosamine and chondroitin in knee osteoarthritis. *Arch Intern Med*; 163(13):1514-1522. 2003

Rovetta G: Galactosaminoglycuronoglycan sulfate (matrix) in therapy of tibiofibular osteoarthritis of the knee. *Drugs Exp Clin Res*; 17(1):53-57. 1991

Rovetta G, Monteforte P, Molfetta G et al: Chondroitin sulfate in erosive osteoarthritis of the hands. *Int J Tissue React*; 24(1):29-32. 2002

Shankland WE: The effects of glucosamine and chondroitin sulfate on osteoarthritis of the TMJ: a preliminary report of 50 patients. *J Craniomandibular Pract*; 16(4):230-235. 1998

Steinhoff G, Ittah B, and Rowan S: The efficacy of chondroitin sulfate 0.2% in treating interstitial cystitis. *Can J Urol*; 9(1): 1454-1458. 2002

Tallia A, Cardone D: Asthma exacerbation associated with glucosamine- chondroitin supplement. *J Am Board Fam Pract*; 15(6):841-848. 2002

Verbruggen G, Goemaere S, Veys E: Chondroitin sulfate: S/MOAD (structure/disease modifying anti-osteoarthritis drug) in the treatment of finger joint OA. *Osteoarthritis Cartilage*; 6(suppl A): 37-38. 1998

Coenzyme Q10

DESCRIPTION

Coenzyme Q10 is a fat-soluble quinone that is synthesized intracellularly and participates in a variety of important cellular processes. It has vitamin-like characteristics and is structurally similar to vitamin K. Coenzyme Q10 is a vital component of the inner mitochondrial membrane, with the highest concentrations found in the heart, liver, kidneys, and pancreas. The total body content ranges from 0.5 to 1.5 grams (Lampertico et al 1993; Mortensen 1993; Beyer 1992; Greenberg et al 1990; Langsjoen et al 1988; Farah et al 1984). Its most common clinical use is for treating heart disease, hypertension, and immunodepression. Although coenzyme Q10 is necessary for energy production and function, further studies are needed to warrant its use for performance enhancement.

An endogenous deficiency of coenzyme Q10 has been suggested in a variety of disorders, including cancer, congestive heart failure, hypertension, chronic hemodialysis, mitochondrial disease, and periodontal disease (Lockwood et al 1994; Triolo et al 1994; Matthews et al 1993; Greenberg et al, 1990; Ogasahara et al 1986).

Other Names: Coenzyme Q, CoQ, CoQ10, ubidecarenone, ubiquinone, ubiquinone-Q10

ACTIONS AND PHARMACOLOGY

EFFECTS

Coenzyme Q10 is an antioxidant and cardiotonic. Some evidence suggests it may also have cytoprotective and neuroprotective qualities.

Cardiovascular Effects: The most extensive studies of coenzyme Q10 have been in cardiovascular disease, most specifically for its purported benefit in preventing cellular damage during myocardial ischemia and reperfusion (Mortensen 1993; Rengo et al 1993; Greenberg et al 1990). Numerous potential therapeutic mechanisms have been considered. The most notable of these are: (1) correction of coenzyme Q10 deficiency, (2) direct free-radical scavenging activity via semiquinone species, (3) direct membrane-stabilizing properties due to phospholipid protein interactions, (4) and correction of a mitochondrial "leak" of electrons during oxidative respiration (Ma et al 1996; Mortensen 1993; Rengo et al 1993; Greenberg et al 1990; Greenberg et al 1988). Other potential mechanisms include effects on prostaglandin metabolism, inhibition of intracellular phospholipases, and stabilization of the integrity of calcium-dependent slow channels (Greenberg et al 1990).

Migraine Prophylaxis: Because some migraine sufferers show dysfunction in mitochondrial energy metabolism, researchers speculate that coenzyme Q10 reduces migraine frequency by improving mitochondrial oxidative phosphorylation (Rozen et al 2002).

Mitochondrial Electron Transfer Effects: Coenzyme Q10 has a significant role in mitochondrial electron transfer and the synthesis of adenosine triphosphate (ATP). The oxidation-reduction cycling of coenzyme Q10 during electron transport has been directly observed. Coenzyme Q10 may also have direct membrane-stabilizing properties as well as free-radical scavenging abilities, especially against lipid peroxidation (Lampertico et al 1993; Matthews et al 1993; Beyer 1992; Permanetter et al 1992; Greenberg et al 1990).

CLINICAL TRIALS

Cardiac Surgery/Heart Failure

Raising plasma coenzyme Q10 levels may lead to improvements in left ventricular (LV) function. Evidence exists that these levels are decreased in patients with advanced chronic heart failure (CHF). One recent, double-blind, placebo-controlled study enrolled 23 patients in a crossover design to determine if supplementation with oral coenzyme Q10 could lead to improvements in cardiocirculatory efficiency and endothelial function. Patients with stable CHF (NYHA class II and III) were assigned to each of the four treatments: oral coenzyme Q10 (100 mg tid); coenzyme Q10 plus supervised exercise training (ET), 5 times a week; placebo; and placebo plus ET. Each phase lasted for 4 weeks. Among the 21 subjects completing the study, supplementation with coenzyme Q10 led to a four-fold increase in plasma levels of the antioxidant; ET amplified this effect. Other favorable improvements were noted as well: coenzyme Q10 treatment increased HDL cholesterol (+3%, p=0.0588) and decreased levels of uric acid in plasma (-3%, p<0.0001). The investigators concluded that oral coenzyme Q10 improves functional capacity, endothelial function, and LV contractility in patients with CHF, and when paired with ET, results are even more pronounced (Belardinelli et al 2006).

Orally administered coenzyme Q10 leads to a corresponding increase in the levels of this antioxidant in human myocardium and mitochondria, which may offer protection to the myocardium during cardiac surgery. One study examined the effect of preoperative oral administration of coenzyme Q10 in patients undergoing elective cardiac surgery. Patients were randomized to treatment with either coenzyme Q10 300 mg/d (n=62) or placebo (n=59) for 2 weeks prior to surgery. Following treatment, levels of coenzyme Q10 were increased in the serum (p=.001), myocardium (p=.0001) and mitochondria (p=.0002) of those receiving oral coenzyme Q10 compared with those receiving placebo. Mitochondrial efficiency was improved with coenzyme Q10, and myocardial tolerance to in vitro hypoxia-reoxygenation stress was increased (Rosenfeldt et al 2005).

In a 3-month, randomized, placebo-controlled study of 27 end-stage heart failure patients awaiting heart transplantation, coenzyme Q10 supplementation led to significant improvements in functional status, clinical symptoms, and quality of life. However, no significant changes in echocardiography parameters or plasma levels of atrial natriuretic factor (ANF) and tumor necrosis factor (TNF) were noted, leaving cardiac status unchanged following treatment. Still, the authors suggest that coenzyme Q10 may be considered an optional addition to the medical regimen in this patient population (Berman et al 2004).

Earlier controlled studies had reported an improvement in quality of life and a significant reduction in hospitalizations for patients with worsening heart failure who took coenzyme Q10 (Morisco et al 1993; Mortensen 1993). Beneficial effects were attributed to enhanced myocardial contractility, with the most benefit appearing in patients with severe heart failure (NYHA class III or IV) and in those with dilated cardiomyopathy and the lowest plasma or tissue levels of coenzyme Q10. A meta-analysis of eight of these clinical trials concluded that addition of coenzyme Q10 to standard CHF regimens was associated with significant improvements in ejection fraction, stroke volume, and cardiac output (Soja et al 1997).

Numerous open studies of patients with congestive heart failure, some involving more than 1,000 participants, have reported clinical benefits with oral coenzyme Q10 added to conventional therapy such as digitalis, diuretics, and ACE inhibitors. Trials were both short-term (1 to 4 weeks) and long-term (3 months to 6 years), with typical doses ranging from 50 to 100 mg (Baggio et al 1993; Lampertico et al 1993; Mortensen 1993; Greenberg et al 1990; Langsjoen et al 1990; Langsjoen et al 1988; Mortensen et al 1985; Ishiyama et al 1976). Most placebo-controlled studies support these findings, demonstrating a significant improvement in left-ventricular ejection fraction, stroke volume, clinical symptoms, and functional status during coenzyme Q10 add-on therapy (100 to 150 mg daily for up to 1 year) in chronic heart failure patients (Morisco et al 1993; Mortensen 1993; Rengo et al 1993; Greenberg et al 1990).

Migraine prophylaxis

A randomized, double-blind, placebo-controlled trial examined the effect of supplemental coenzyme Q10 on migraine prophylaxis. Patients with migraine were randomized to treatment with either coenzyme Q10 100 mg tid (n=21) or placebo (n=21). By month 3 of treatment, the response rates (decrease in headache frequency $\geq$ 50%) were 47.6% in the coenzyme Q10 group and 14.4% in the placebo group. Other measures improved as well; supplemental coenzyme Q10 was superior to placebo in reducing attack frequency, headache-days and days-with-nausea. (Sandor et al 2005). This study confirmed the results of an earlier open-label study by Rozen and colleagues. In that trial, coenzyme Q10 reduced migraine frequency in 29 of 31 patients with episodic migraine (with or without aura). Subjects took 150 mg of coenzyme Q10 daily with breakfast for 3 months after a 1-month baseline period. Average headache frequency was reduced from 7.34 days during the 30-day baseline to 2.95 days during the last 60 days of treatment ($p<0.002$). However, headache intensity was not affected. No side effects were observed (Rozen et al 2002).

Parkinson's Disease

In one study, coenzyme Q10 appeared to slow the progression of Parkinson's disease (PD) in patients with early-stage disease. The randomized, double-blind, placebo-controlled trial enrolled 80 patients, who were randomly assigned to daily treatment with 300, 600 or 1200 mg coenzyme Q10 or placebo for 16 months. Follow-up continued for 16 months post-treatment. All 3 groups receiving coenzyme Q10 showed a slowing of the functional decline associated with PD; this effect was most pronounced in the group receiving the highest dosage of 1200 mg. When the 3 groups receiving coenzyme Q10 were compared to placebo, a significant difference between the group receiving 1200 mg and those receiving placebo was noted ($p=.04$) (Shults et al 2002).

Another study examined the effect of orally administered coenzyme Q10 (360 mg/day for 4 weeks) on symptomatic response in patients with PD. In this parallel-group, placebo-controlled, double-blind trial, 28 patients were scored on PD symptoms and visual function, using the Farnsworth-Munsell 100 Hue test (FMT). Compared with placebo, supplementation with coenzyme Q10 resulted in a significant ($p=0.01$) mild symptomatic improvement in PD symptoms and a significantly better improvement of FMT performance ($p=0.008$) (Muller et al 2003).

INDICATIONS AND USAGE

Approved by the FDA:

- For use as an orphan product in the treatment of Huntington's disease and mitochondrial cytopathies

Unproven Uses: Coenzyme Q10 is used mainly for the treatment of congestive heart failure and cardiomyopathy. Studies have shown it may benefit patients having cardiovascular surgery such as cardiac valve replacement, coronary artery bypass grafting, and repair of abdominal aortic aneurysms. Coenzyme Q10 has also been used for asthenozoospermia, central nervous system problems, and muscle disorders. Athletes sometimes take it to improve performance, but current evidence does not justify this use.

PRECAUTIONS AND ADVERSE REACTIONS

Hepatic failure is a precaution for use, since the primary site of metabolism is the liver. However, coenzyme Q10 has a very low toxicity profile, and higher plasma levels seem to be well-tolerated. There have been no reports of overt hepatotoxicity with coenzyme Q10.

Gastrointestinal problems are the most common adverse effects (less than 1% in large studies), including nausea, epigastric discomfort, diarrhea, heartburn, and appetite suppression. Rare side effects may include skin rash, pruritus, photophobia, irritability, agitation, headache, and dizziness.

Transient minor abnormalities of urinary sediment (protein, granular, and hyaline casts) were reported in patients with Parkinson's disease given doses of 400 to 800 mg of coenzyme Q10 daily for 1 month. Problems resolved following discontinuation of therapy (Shults et al 1998).

Fatigue and increased involuntary movements were reported in patients with Huntington's chorea taking high doses (Feigin et al 1996).

DRUG INTERACTIONS

MODERATE RISK

Anticoagulants: Concurrent use of anticoagulants and Coenzyme Q10 may result in reduced anticoagulant effectiveness. *Clinical Management:* Caution is advised if Coenzyme Q10 and warfarin are taken together. Monitor the INR to determine continued therapeutic effect.

POTENTIAL INTERACTIONS

HMG-CoA Reductase Inhibitors (e.g., lovastatin, simvastatin): Use of these drugs may inhibit the natural synthesis of coenzyme Q10. Reduced levels of coenzyme Q10 may place patients at risk for side effects of HMG-CoA reductase inhibitors, particularly myopathy (Mortensen et al 1997; Bargossi et al 1994; Watts et al 1993; Folkers et al 1990).

Oral Hypoglycemic Agents and Insulin: Dosage adjustment may be necessary, since coenzyme Q10 could reduce insulin requirements.

DOSAGE

Mode of Administration: Intravenous, oral, topical

How Supplied: Capsule, gelcap, solution

Daily Dosage:

Note: For best absorption, coenzyme Q10 should be taken with food.

ADULTS

Angina (stable): 150 to 600 mg orally in divided doses; 1.5 mg/kg IV once daily for 7 days.

Cardiac Surgery: 100 mg daily for 14 days before surgery, followed by 100 mg daily for 30 days postoperatively.

Congestive Heart Failure: 50 to 150 mg daily in two or three divided doses; 50 to 100 mg IV daily for 3 to 35 days.

Migraine Prevention: 150 mg daily.

Neurological Disease: (associated with mitochondrial ATP-producing deficiency): 150 mg or more daily.

Parkinson's Disease/Huntington's Disease: 800 to 1200 mg daily.

Periodontal Disease: 25 mg twice daily; or topical solution consisting of 85 mg/mL in soybean oil applied twice daily.

PEDIATRIC

General Use: 2.4 to 3.8 mg/kg daily.

Pediatric Mitochondrial Encephalomyopathy: 30 mg daily.

Storage: Store at room temperature away from heat, moisture, and direct light.

LITERATURE

Baggio E, Gandini R, Plancher AC et al: Italian multicenter study on the safety and efficacy of coenzyme Q10 as adjunctive therapy in heart failure (interim analysis). *Clin Invest*; 71:145-149. 1993

Baggio E, Gandini R, Plancher AC et al: Italian multicenter study on the safety and efficacy of coenzyme Q10 as adjunctive therapy in heart failure. *Mol Aspects Med*; 15(suppl):S287-S294. 1994

Belardinelli R, Mucaj A, Lacalaprice F, et al: Coenzyme Q10 and exercise training in chronic heart failure. *Eur H J*; 27:2675-2681. 2006

Berman M, Erman A, Ben-Gal T, e al: Coenzyme Q10 in patients with end-stage heart failure awaiting cardiac transplantation: a randomized, placebo-controlled study. *Clin Cardiol*; 27:295-299. 2004

Beyer RE: An analysis of the role of coenzyme Q in free radical generation and as an antioxidant. *Biochem Cell Biol*; 70:390-403. 1992

Farah AE, Alousi AA, Schwarz RP: Positive inotropic agents. *Ann Rev Pharmacol Toxicol*; 24:275-328. 1984

Feigin A, Kieburtz K, Como P et al: Assessment of coenzyme Q10 tolerability in Huntington's disease. *Movement Disord*; 11:321-323. 1996

Folkers K, Langsjoen P, Willis P et al: Lovastatin decreases coenzyme Q levels in humans. *Proc Natl Acad Sci USA*; 87:8931-8934. 1990

Greenberg S, Frishman WH: Co-enzyme Q10: a new drug for cardiovascular disease. *J Clin Pharmacol*; 30:596-608. 1990

Ishiyama T, Morita Y, Toyama S et al: A clinical study of the effect of coenzyme Q on congestive heart failure. *Jpn Heart J*; 17:32-42. 1976

Kamikawa T, Kobayashi A, Tamashita T et al: Effects of coenzyme Q10 on exercise tolerance in chronic stable angina pectoris. *Am J Cardiol*; 56:247-251. 1985

Lampertico M, Comis S: Italian multicenter study on the efficacy and safety of coenzyme Q10 as adjuvant therapy in heart failure. *Clin Invest*; 71:129-133. 1993

Langsjoen H, Langsjoen P, Langsjoen P et al: Usefulness of coenzyme Q10 in clinical cardiology: a long-term study. *Mol Aspects Med* 1994; 15(suppl):S165-S175.

Langsjoen PH, Folkers K, Lyson K et al: Effective and safe therapy with coenzyme Q10 for cardiomyopathy. *Klin Wochenschr*; 66:583-590. 1988

Langsjoen PH, Langsjoen A, Willis R et al: Treatment of hypertrophic cardiomyopathy with coenzyme Q10. *Mol Aspects Med*; 18(suppl):S145-S151. 1997

Langsjoen PH, Langsjoen PH; Folkers K: Isolated diastolic dysfunction of the myocardium and its response to CoQ10 treatment. *Clin Invest*; 71(suppl):S140-S144. 1993

Langsjoen PH, Langsjoen PH, Folkers K: Long-term efficacy and safety of coenzyme Q10 therapy for idiopathic dilated cardiomyopathy. *Am J Cardiol*; 65:521-523. 1990

Lockwood K, Moesgaard S, Folkers K: Partial and complete regression of breast cancer in patients in relation to dosage of coenzyme Q10. *Biochem Biophys Res Commun*; 199:1504-1508. 1994

Lockwood K, Moesgaard S, Hanioka T et al: Apparent partial remission of breast cancer in high risk patients supplemented with nutritional antioxidants, essential fatty acids and coenzyme Q10. *Mol Aspects Med*; 10(suppl):S231-S240. 1994

Ma A, Zhang W, Liu Z: Effect of protection and repair of mitochondrial membrane-phospholipid on prognosis in patients with dilated cardiomyopathy. *Blood Press*; 5:53-55. 1996

Matthews PM, Ford B, Dandurand RJ et al: Coenzyme Q10 with multiple vitamins is generally ineffective in treatment of mitochondrial disease. *Neurology*; 43:884-890. 1993

Morisco C, Trimarco B, Condorelli M et al. Effect of coenzyme Q10 therapy in patients with congestive heart failure: a long-term, multicenter, randomized study. *Clin Investig*; 71(suppl 8):S134-136. 1993.

Mortensen SA, Leth A, Agner E et al: Dose-related decrease of serum coenzyme Q10 during treatment with HMG-CoA reductase inhibitors. *Mol Aspects Med*; 18(Suppl):137-144. 1997

Mortensen SA: Perspectives on therapy of cardiovascular diseases with coenzyme Q10 (Ubiquinone). *Clin Invest*; 71:116-123. 1993

Muller T, Buttner T, Gholipour AF et al: Coenzyme Q10 supplementation provides mild symptomatic benefit in patients with Parkinson's disease. *Neurosci Lett*. 341:201-204. 2003

Ogasahara S, Nishikawa Y, Yorifuji S et al: Treatment of Kearns-Sayre syndrome with coenzyme Q10. *Neurology*; 36:45-53. 1986

Permanetter B, Rossy W, Klein G et al: Ubiquinone (coenzyme Q10) in the long-term treatment of idiopathic dilated cardiomyopathy. *Eur Heart J*; 13:1528-1533. 1992

Rengo F, Abete P, Landino P et al: Role of metabolic therapy in cardiovascular disease. *Clin Invest*; 71:124-128. 1993

Rosenfeldt F, Marasco S, Lyon W: Coenzyme Q10 therapy before cardiac surgery improves mitochondrial function and in vitro contractility of myocardial tissue. *J Thor Cardiovasc Surg*; 129:25-32. 2005

Rozen TD, Oshinsky ML, Gebeline CA et al: Open label trial of coenzyme Q10 as a migraine preventive. *Cephalalgia*; 22:137-141. 2002

Sandor PS, Di Clemente L, Coppola G et al: Efficacy of coenzyme Q10 in migraine prophylaxis: a randomized controlled trial. *Neurology*; 64:713-715. 2005

Schults CW, Oakes D, Kieburtz K et al: Effects of coenzyme Q10 in early Parkinson's disease: evidence of slowing the functional decline. *Arch Neurol*; 59:1541-1550. 2002

Shults CW, Beal MF, Fontaine D et al: Absorption, tolerability, and effects on mitochondrial activity of oral coenzyme Q10 in parkinsonian patients. *Neurology*; 50:793-795. 1998

Soja AM, Mortensen SA: Treatment of congestive heart failure with coenzyme Q10 illuminated by meta-analyses of clinical trials. *Mol Aspects Med*; 18(suppl):S159-S168. 1997

Triolo L, Lippa S, Oradei A et al: Serum coenzyme Q10 in uremic patients on chronic hemodialysis. *Nephron*; 66:153-156. 1994

Watts GF, Castelluccio C, Rice-Evans C et al: Plasma coenzyme Q (Ubiquinone) concentrations in patients treated with simvastatin. *J Clin Pathol*; 46:1055-1057. 1993

Zimmerman JJ: Therapeutic application of oxygen radical scavengers. *Chest*; 100:189-192. 1991

Folic Acid

DESCRIPTION

Folic acid is a water-soluble B vitamin found in a variety of foods, especially green leafy vegetables. Folium, the Latin word for leaf, is the source of the term folic acid. This vitamin is required for DNA synthesis and a variety of other key reactions in normal metabolism.

Folic acid has emerged as an important preventive nutrient, most notably for neural tube defects in pregnancy and atherosclerotic disease due to elevated homocysteine. Sexually active women of child-bearing potential should be encouraged to use folic acid supplements if dietary intake is not sufficient. Individuals with vascular disease risks should be tested for hyperhomocysteinemia or given prophylactic supplementation. Cancer prevention is inadequately supported, yet intriguing relationships exist at several sites, including the cervix, colon, and lung.

As a therapeutic intervention, the treatment of megaloblastic anemia has been the primary application of folic acid supplementation for some time in both traditional and alternative medicine, though a concerted attempt to rule out vitamin B_{12} deficiency is required before initiating monotherapy with folic acid. Deficiencies secondary to pharmaceutical therapy with anticonvulsants and oral contraceptives increase the need for folic acid supplementation. Topical folic acid solutions for use in periodontal disease are available but remain underutilized.

Other Names: folate, folinic acid, pteroylglutamic acid, vitamin B9

ACTIONS AND PHARMACOLOGY

EFFECTS

Folic acid has the following effects: antidepressant, antiproliferative, antiteratogenic, antihomocysteinemic, and anti-inflammatory (gingival). The coenzymes formed from folic acid are instrumental in the following intracellular metabolisms: conversion of homocysteine to methionine, conversion of serine to glycine, synthesis of thymidylate, histidine metabolism, synthesis of purines, and utilization or generation of formate (Gilman et al 2001).

CLINICAL TRIALS

Cardiovascular Disease

Low folic acid status has been associated with cardiovascular disease (CVD) (Omenn et al 1998), and earlier epidemiological studies suggested that folic acid supplementation was associated with reduced risk of coronary heart disease (Rimm et al 1998). Prior to its institution, the plan to fortify cereal-grain products with 140 mcg of folate per 100 grams was projected to reduce the U.S. population risk of coronary artery disease by 5% (Tucker et al 1996), presumably by lowering blood homocysteine levels (Boers 1998).

Since hyperhomocysteinemia is an independent risk factor for CVD, it was believed that reducing plasma homocysteine levels with folic acid could reduce atherosclerosis progression and the risk of cardiovascular events. Unfortunately, current findings from clinical studies do not support this idea. A 2006 meta-analysis showed that folic acid supplementation conferred no benefits to those with preexisting vascular disease; the risk of CVDs or all-cause mortality remained unchanged during supplementation (Bazzano et al 2006). The analysis reviewed data from 12 randomized, controlled trials involving 16,958 subjects with a history of cardiovascular or renal disease who received supplemental folic acid for a period ranging from 6 months to 5 years. Dosages of folic acid used in the studies ranged from 0.5 mg/day to 15 mg/day. Folic acid supplementation reduced homocysteine levels in all trials (range: -1.5 to -26.0 μmol/L), but did not prevent cardiovascular events or reduce all-cause mortality. One multicenter trial mentioned in the analysis, the Atherosclerosis and Folic Acid Supplementation Trial (ASFAST), examined 315 patients with chronic renal failure (CRF). Patients in the folic acid group (n=156) received 15 mg/day; at median follow-up 3.6 years later, plasma homocysteine levels were reduced by 19% in those receiving active treatment as compared to the group randomized to placebo (n=159). However, folic acid supplementation did not slow the progression of atherosclerosis, nor did it reduce cardiovascular events (Zoungas et al 2006). Even a large trial such as the Heart Outcomes Prevention Evaluation 2 study (HOPE-2)—which followed 5,522 subjects—yielded similar results. That study examined the effect of combined folic acid and vitamins B_{12} and B_6 on cardiovascular events in patients with preexisting vascular disease. Although mean levels of plasma homocysteine were reduced, the risk of major cardiovascular events was not (Lonn et al 2006). Given the discrepancies between results from earlier observational studies and those from clinical trials, the role of folic acid supplementation in primary prevention of vascular disease needs to be explored. Studies to date have only examined its effects in secondary prevention.

Other studies show that folic acid supplementation safely reduces elevated plasma homocysteine levels (Villa et al 2007; Huemer et al 2005). One review examined the effect of folic acid supplementation on plasma homocysteine levels in postmenopausal women and observed the relationship between supplementation with folic acid and various metabolic parameters. In one randomized, placebo-controlled study cited in the review, postmenopausal women were assigned to one of two groups: Group A (n=10) received folic acid 7.5 mg/day, and Group B (n=10) received placebo. By study end, Group A had lower plasma homocysteine levels compared with Group B. In addition, although some lipid profiles remained unchanged, significant improvements vs baseline were noted in levels of high-density lipoprotein (HDL, $p<0.01$), as well as in the ratios of total cholesterol/HDL cholesterol (HDL-C) and low-density lipoprotein cholesterol (LDL-C)/HDL-C ($p<0.02$ and $p<0.03$, respectively), insulin sensitivity ($p<0.02$), and hepatic clearance of insulin ($p<0.01$). It was also noted that folic acid supplementation modifies impaired endothelial function due to hyperhomocysteinemia (Villa et al 2007). Interestingly, another study observed this effect independent of homocysteine-lowering. The randomized, placebo-controlled, crossover study enrolled 19 patients with type 2 diabetes; active treatment was 10 mg/day of folic acid for 2 weeks. Two weeks of folic acid supplementation was shown to improve endothelial dysfunction in these subjects, but no relationship was observed between changes in homocysteine levels and the significant improvements noted in flow-mediated dilatation (Title et al 2006). Another double-blind, randomized study examining children with epilepsy (n=123) found that of those receiving antiepileptic drugs (AEDs), 15.5% had elevated plasma homocysteine levels (ie, hyperhomocysteinemia). Supplementation with 1 mg/day of folic acid for 3 months significantly reduced plasma homocysteine levels, while significantly increasing blood concentrations of folate. Levels of both remained unchanged in the group receiving placebo (Huemer et al 2005).

A 2005 meta-analysis studied the effect of folic acid supplementation, with and without vitamins B_{12} and B_6, on levels of plasma homocysteine. Various doses were examined among the 25 randomized controlled trials involving 2,596 subjects. The authors concluded that, in general, daily doses of >0.8 mg folic acid are needed to achieve the maximal reduction in plasma homocysteine levels produced with supplementation. Doses of 0.2 and 0.4 mg/day correlate with 60% and 90% of the maximal effect, respectively. When vitamin B_{12} was combined with folic acid, an additional 7% reduction in plasma homocysteine levels was noted (Homocysteine Lowering Trialists' Collaboration, 2005). In earlier studies, folic acid was combined with vitamin B_6 and vitamin B_{12} for greater effect on homocysteine levels. A meta-analysis of 12 trials examining the effects of supplemental folic acid on plasma homocysteine levels showed that supplements of 0.5 to 5 mg of folic acid could be expected to reduce plasma levels of homocysteine by a quarter to a third. Addition of vitamin B_{12} reduced plasma homocysteine concentrations by another 7%. Vitamin B_6 did not lower these levels any further when added to the mix (Anon 1998).

Contraceptive-Induced Folic Acid Deficiency

Using oral contraceptives may result in folic acid deficiency that may occasionally manifest as megaloblastic anemia and thrombocytopenia. Administration of folic acid can correct the folic acid deficiency and thereby promptly reverse any abnormalities associated with the deficiency (Lewis 1974; Luhby et al 1971). The FDA-approved minimum optimal dose of oral folic acid is 2 milligrams/day for oral contraceptive-induced folate deficiency.

Depression

Folic acid deficiency may cause psychiatric disturbances such as depression. Low folate status is more common in depressed patients and has been linked with poor response to antidepressant therapy. Two controlled studies have suggested that supplementation of folate or its derivatives may improve clinical outcomes in the treatment of depression (Alpert et al 1997; Bottiglieri 1996).

Lung Cancer

Low folate status may increase lung cancer risk, and large doses may reduce precancerous changes in bronchial tissues. Epidemiological studies have suggested a relationship between low folate status and cancer of the lung (Glynn et al 1994). One study found that folic acid (10 mg) with vitamin B_{12} (500 mcg) reduced evidence of atypical bronchial squamous metaplasia in smokers. However, the authors cautioned that the spontaneous variation in sputum cytology results along with other limitations of this study temper the significance of these findings (Heimberger et al 1988).

Methotrexate Toxicity

A randomized study compared the effects of 5 mg/day of either folic acid or folinic acid added to current methotrexate (MTX) therapy on purine metabolism in patients with rheumatoid arthritis (RA). Specifically, researchers wanted to observe the effects of supplementation on urinary 5-amino-imidazole-4-carboxamide (AICA) and urinary adenosine excretion, two markers for MTX interference with purine metabolism. Blockages along this pathway may in turn affect immune cell function. Supplementation began concurrent with the sixth dose of MTX. Of the 40 subjects, 21 were randomized to treatment with folic acid and 19 were randomized to folinic acid. During MTX therapy, folinic acid, but not folic acid, normalized urinary AICA levels (Morgan et al, 2004). An earlier meta-analysis of published double-blind, randomized, controlled trials (n=7) testing the influence of folate supplementation in RA patients treated with MTX showed an 80% reduction of side effects (mainly gastrointestinal) with folic acid supplementation and no compromise of MTX efficacy. However, high-dose folinic acid was associated with an increase in tender and swollen joints (Ortiz et al 1998).

A more recently published study found that psoriasis patients treated with MTX had a marked deterioration in the disease following folic acid supplementation. This 12-week, double-blind clinical trial was originally designed to determine the effects of folic acid on the efficacy of MTX and its bearing on the frequency of side effects associated with MTX. Patients receiving long-term MTX therapy for their psoriasis were randomized to active treatment with 5 mg folic acid or placebo daily (n=11 in both groups). The addition of folic acid was associated with a decline in the efficacy of MTX for the treatment of psoriasis as measured by specific indices and visual analog scales. Given the small sample size and short duration of the trial, no conclusions could be made regarding the effect of folic acid on side effects associated with MTX therapy (Salim et al, 2006).

Prevention of Neural Tube Defects/Congenital Anomalies

The use of folic acid supplements by pregnant women to prevent neural tube defects is well established and supported by extensive clinical literature. Less known is the potential for reducing other congenital anomalies with folic acid supplementation. A 2006 meta-analysis reported that the use of folic acid—fortified multivitamins, beginning prior to conception and continuing throughout the first trimester of pregnancy, consistently provided protection against several serious congenital anomalies. In addition to neural tube defects, these included cardiovascular defects, limb defects, urinary tract anomalies, congenital hydrocephalus, and oral clefts. The meta-analysis identified 41 studies for inclusion, including 27 case-control studies, 10 cohort studies, and 4 randomized, controlled trials. All trials supplied a folic acid—fortified multivitamin to a group of pregnant subjects (Goh et al 2006). Oral clefts such as cleft palate alone (CP) or as cleft lip with or without cleft palate (CLP) are embryologically related to neural tube defects. A 2007 meta-analysis suggests that folic acid supplements taken during pregnancy protect against the development of oral clefts. From the 5 prospective studies that were analyzed, combined relative risks among those receiving supplementation were reported as 0.51 (95% CI: 0.32, 0.95) for CLP; 1.19 (95% CI: 0.43, 3.28) for CP; and 0.55 (95% CI: 0. 32, 0.95) for all clefts. From the 12 case-control studies, these combined risks were 0.77 (95% CI: 0.65, 0.90) for CLP; 0.80 (95% CI: 0.69, 0.93) for CP; and 0.78 (95% CI: 0. 71, 0.85) for all clefts. Although a negative association between supplementation and risk of CP was observed in 3 of the prospective studies, the reviewers note these studies, being the fewest in number, were underpowered. For those women receiving supplementation in the case-control studies, the likelihood of having a child with an oral cleft was 33% less for any oral cleft, 29% less for CLP, and 20% less for CP. For their counterparts in the prospective studies, the likelihood of having a child with an oral cleft was 45% less for any oral cleft and 49% less for CLP. However, women in this group were 19% more likely to have a child with CP. This may be due to study limitations or the variation among studies regarding the distinction between syndromic vs nonsyndromic clefts (Badovinac et al 2007). The 2006 meta-analysis by Goh and colleagues, having been published just a few months earlier, was not included in this report (Goh et al 2006). It found that taking folic acid—fortified multivitamins beginning prior to conception and continued through the first trimester of pregnancy provided consistent protection against the development of cleft palate across studies. Case-control studies included in the analysis showed OR 0.76 (95% CI: 0.62-0.93) for CP; cohort and randomized, controlled trials showed OR 0.42 (95% CI: 0.06-2.84). For CLP, case-control studies showed OR 0.63 (95% CI: 0.54-0.73) while cohort and randomized, controlled trials showed OR 0.58 (95% CI: 0.28-1.19).

The 2006 meta-analysis by Goh and colleagues also showed that supplementation with folic acid–fortified multivitamins protects against neural tube defects (Goh et al 2006). For each study included in the analysis, odds ratios (ORs) and 95% confidence intervals (CIs) were calculated. Among the eight case-control studies and 11 cohort and randomized, controlled trials included, women beginning supplementation prior to conception and taking it through the first trimester were consistently protected against neural tube defects (OR 0.67, 95% CI 0.58-0.77 in case-control studies; OR 0.52, 95% CI 0.39-0.69 in cohort and randomized, controlled trials). In six case-control studies, protection was even conferred to women who began supplementation in the first trimester, after learning they were pregnant (OR 0.80; 95% CI 0.72-0.89).

Ideally, folic acid should be administered at least 1 month before and during the first 3 months of pregnancy. The Centers for Disease Control and Prevention and various other committees recommend that all women of childbearing age who are capable of becoming pregnant receive 400 mcg/day. The reduction in neural tube defects in patients receiving folic acid therapy has been 60% to 70% (NHMRC 1994). Patients with previous history of neural tube defects during pregnancy should receive 4 milligrams/day starting 1 month before pregnancy and throughout the first 3 months of pregnancy (NHMRC 1991 and 1994; AAP 1993; Mulinare 1993).

In an earlier study, neural tube defects were decreased by approximately 60% in 3,051 pregnant mothers treated with 0.4 milligram of folic acid during the periconceptional period (28 days before the last menstrual period through 28 days after the last menstrual period) (Werler et al 1993).

A significant reduction in risk for first-time occurrence of neural tube defects was observed in 18,508 pregnant women consuming folic acid-containing multivitamins compared to no folic acid consumption (Milunsky et al 1989). Similar results were reported in another study (Czeizel et al 1992).

Ulcerative Colitis and Colonic Adenomas

Folate supplementation can reduce cell abnormalities in the rectal mucosa of patients with ulcerative colitis. Folic acid 15 mg/day (as calcium folate) or a placebo was taken (double-blind) for 3 months by 24 patients with UC of more than 7 years' duration. Patients had been in remission (no acute inflammation) for more than 1 month. In the placebo group, there was no difference in proliferative index between baseline and 3-month measures. In the folate group, proliferation was significantly reduced at 3 months compared to baseline (Biasco et al 1997).

Epidemiological studies have suggested a relationship between low folate status and colorectal cancer (Glynn et al, 1994). Folic acid supplementation had a nonsignificant but dose-response effect on protecting ulcerative colitis patients against colonic neoplasia. Use of higher doses (1,000 mcg daily) of folic acid was associated with greater risk reduction (46%, nonsignificant) (Lashner et al 1997).

INDICATIONS AND USAGE

Approved by the FDA

- Prevention of neural tube defects in pregnancy
- Treatment of megaloblastic anemias caused by folic acid deficiency
- Treatment of folic acid deficiency caused by oral contraceptive or anticonvulsant therapy

Unproven Uses: Strong evidence shows that folic acid therapy can reduce high levels of homocysteine, which has been linked to coronary heart disease. Other studies have suggested that folic acid supplementation may be helpful for atherosclerosis, colon cancer prevention, coronary heart disease, depression, gingival hyperplasia, hyperhomocysteinemia, iron-deficiency or sickle-cell anemia, lung cancer prevention, methotrexate toxicity, prevention of restenosis following coronary angiography, ulcerative colitis, and vitiligo. Weaker evidence suggests that folic acid may be of some benefit for cervical cancer prevention (some studies were inconclusive), aphthous ulcers, geriatric memory deficit, and prevention of fragile X syndrome in children.

CONTRAINDICATIONS

Pernicious anemia and megaloblastic anemia caused by vitamin B_{12} deficiency (Prod Info: Folic acid tablets 1995).

PRECAUTIONS AND ADVERSE REACTIONS

Folic acid doses above 0.1 mg/day may obscure pernicious anemia. Side effects of folic acid therapy include erythema, pruritus, urticaria, irritability, excitability, nausea, bloating, and flatulence.

A variety of central nervous system effects have been reported following 5 mg of folic acid three times a day, including altered sleep patterns, vivid dreaming, irritability, excitability, and overactivity (Hunter et al 1970). Discontinuation of the drug usually results in rapid improvement but in some cases may require 3 weeks before complete restoration.

Gastrointestinal disturbances following oral doses of 5 mg three times daily have been reported and include nausea, abdominal distention, discomfort, flatulence, and a constant bad or bitter taste in the mouth (Prod Info: Folic acid tablets 1995).

High-dose folic acid has been associated with zinc depletion. (Kakar et al 1985). Evidence suggests that up to 5 to 15 milligrams daily of folic acid does not have significant adverse effects on zinc status in healthy, nonpregnant individuals (Butterworth et al 1989).

Pregnancy: FDA-rated as Pregnancy Category A (relatively safe) at doses below 0.8 mg/day; doses higher than this are rated as Pregnancy Category C (effects unknown).

DRUG INTERACTIONS

MODERATE RISK

Phenytoin and fosphenytoin: Concurrent use may decrease phenytoin or fosphenytoin levels, respectively, and increase seizure frequency. *Clinical Management:* If folic acid is added to phenytoin therapy, monitor patients for decreased seizure control.

Pyrimethamine: Concurrent use may reduce the effectiveness of pyrimethamine. *Clinical Management:* Folic acid should not be used as a folate supplement during pyrimethamine therapy as it is ineffective in preventing megaloblastic anemia. Leucovorin (folinic acid) may be added to pyrimethamine therapy to prevent hematologic toxicity without affecting pyrimethamine efficacy. However, the use of leucovorin may worsen leukemia.

MINOR RISKS

Sulfasalazine: Concurrent use may decrease the absorption of folic acid. *Clinical Management:* Monitor patient for signs of deficiency.

POTENTIAL INTERACTIONS

Colestipol: In vitro data has shown that colestipol may bind to cyanocobalamin/intrinsic factor complex, Folic Acid and iron citrate.Concurrent administration may decrease the bioavailability of vitamin and mineral preparations (Leonard et al, 1979).

Pancreatic enzymes: Concurrent use may interfere with the absorption of folic acid. *Clinical Management:* Patients taking pancreatin may require folic acid supplementation.

Triamterine: Concurrent use may cause decreased utilization of dietary folate. *Clinical Management:* Monitor patient for signs of deficiency.

DOSAGE

Mode of Administration: Intramuscular, intravenous, oral, subcutaneous

How Supplied: Capsule, tablet, sterile solution for injection

Daily Dosage: All doses are for oral administration unless otherwise noted.

ADULTS

Recommended dietary allowance (RDA): *adults and adolescents ≥ 14 years* — 400 mcg/day; *pregnancy* — 600 mcg/day; *lactation* — 500 mcg/day.

Anticonvulsant-induced folate deficiency: 15 mg daily.

Aphthous ulcers (canker sores): treat folic acid deficiency.

Hyperhomocysteinemia: 500 to 5,000 mcg daily.

Methotrexate toxicity: 5 mg orally per week.

Oral contraceptive-induced folate deficiency: 2 mg daily.

Periodontal disease: 2 mg twice daily, or 5 mL of 0.1% topical mouth rinse twice daily.

Prevention of birth defects: 400 to 4,000 mcg orally daily beginning 1 month before conception.

Prevention of cerebrovascular disease: treat folic acid deficiency or hyperhomocysteinemia.

Prevention of cervical cancer: 800 to 10,000 mcg daily.

Prevention of colorectal cancer: 1 to 5 mg daily.

Prevention of lung cancer: 10 mg daily.

Prevention of neural tube defects (first occurrence prevention): 0.4 mg of folic acid daily. Doses from 0.5 to 1 mg daily are often administered during pregnancy.

Prevention of neural tube defects (prevention of recurrence): Patients with a previous history of neural tube defects during pregnancy should receive 4 mg daily starting 1 month before pregnancy and throughout the first 3 months of pregnancy.

Prevention of restenosis following coronary angiography: 1 mg in combination with 400 mcg vitamin B_{12} and 10 mg vitamin B_6 daily.

Sickle cell anemia: 1 mg daily.

Treatment of folic acid deficiency (intramuscular, intravenous, or oral): Up to 1 mg daily until clinical symptoms of deficiency have resolved and blood levels have returned to normal.

Ulcerative colitis: 15 mg daily.

Vitiligo: 2,000 to 10,000 mcg daily.

PEDIATRICS

Recommended dietary allowance (RDA): *Infants and children: 0 to 6 months* — 65 mcg/day; *7 to 12 months* — 80 mcg/day; *1 to 3 years* — 150 mcg/day; *4 to 8 years* — 200 mcg/day; *9 to 13 years* — 300 mcg/day.

Anticonvulsant-induced folate deficiency: 5 mg daily.

Folic acid deficiency (intramuscular, intravenous, subcutaneous, or oral): Up to 1 mg daily until clinical symptoms of deficiency have resolved and blood levels have returned to normal.

Folic acid deficiency in preterm neonates (intramuscular): 100 mcg daily from day 7 until discharge from hospital.

Gingival hyperplasia: 5 mg daily (Backman et al 1989).

Hyperhomocysteinemia: 500 to 5,000 mcg daily.

Storage: Store oral and parenteral folic acid at room temperature.

LITERATURE

Alpert JE, Fava M: Nutrition and depression: the role of folate. *Nutr Rev*; 55(5):145-149. 1997

American Academy of Pediatrics (AAP): AAP Committee on Genetics: folic acid for the prevention of neural tube defects. *Pediatrics*; 92(3):493-494. 1993

Anon: Lowering blood homocysteine with folic acid based supplements: meta-analysis of randomized trials. Homocysteine Lowering Trialists' Collaboration. *BMJ*; 316(7135):894-898. 1998

Anon: Use of folic acid for prevention of spina bifida and other neural tube defects: 1983-1991. *MMWR*; 40(30):513-516. 1991

Anon: Vitamin supplements. *Med Lett Drugs Ther*; 27(693):66-68. 1985

Backman N, Holm A-K, Hanstrom L et al: Folate treatment of diphenylhydantoin-induced gingival hyperplasia. *Scand J Dent Res*; 97(3):222-232. 1989

Bailey LB: Evaluation of a new recommended dietary allowance for folate. *J Am Diet Assoc*; 92(4):463-468, 471. 1992

Bazzano LA, Reynolds K, Holder KN, He J. Effect of folic acid supplementation on risk of cardiovascular diseases: a meta-analysis of randomized controlled trials. *JAMA*; 296:2720-2726. 2006

Berg MJ, Rivey MP, Vern BA et al: Phenytoin and folic acid: individualized drug-drug interaction. *Ther Drug Monit*; 5(4):395-399. 1983

Biasco G, Zannoni U, Paganelli GM et al: Folic acid supplementation and cell kinetics of rectal mucosa in patients with ulcerative colitis. *Cancer Epidemiol Biomarkers Prev*; 6(6):469-471. 1997

Boers G: Moderate hyperhomocysteinemia and vascular disease: evidence, relevance and the effect of treatment (review). *Eur J Pediatr*; 157(suppl 2):S127-S130. 1998

Bottiglieri T: Folate, vitamin B_{12}, and neuropsychiatric disorders. *Nutr Rev*; 54(12):382-390. 1996

Butterworth CE Jr: Folate status, women's health, pregnancy outcome, and cancer. *J Am Coll Nutr*; 12(4):438-441. 1993

Butterworth CE Jr, Hatch KD, Gore H et al: Improvement in cervical dysplasia associated with folic acid therapy in users of oral contraceptives. *Am J Clin Nutr*; 35(1):73-82. 1982

Czeizel AE, Dudas I: Prevention of the first occurrence of neural-tube defects by periconceptional vitamin supplementation. *N Engl J Med*; 327(26):1832-1835. 1992

Dickinson CJ: Does folic acid harm people with vitamin B_{12} deficiency (review)? *QJM*; 88(5):357-364. 1995

Gilman AG, Hardman JG, Limbird LE (eds): *Goodman & Gilman's The Pharmacological Basis of Therapeutics,* 10th ed. McGraw-Hill, New York, NY; 2001.

Glynn SA, Albanes D: Folate and cancer: a review of the literature. *Nutr Cancer*; 22:101-119. 1994

Goh YI, Bollano E, Einarson TR, Koren G. Prenatal multivitamin supplementation and rates of congenital anomalies: a meta-analysis. *J Obstet Gynaecol Can*; 28(8):680-689. 2006

Guidolin L, Vignoli A, Canger R: Worsening in seizure frequency and severity in relation to folic acid administration. *Eur J Neurol*; 5(3):301-303. 1998

Heimburger DC, Alexander CB, Birch R et al: Improvement in bronchial squamous metaplasia in smokers treated with folate and vitamin B_{12}: report of a preliminary randomized double-blind intervention trial. *JAMA*; 259(10):1525-1530. 1988

Homocysteine Lowering Trialists' Collaboration. Dose-dependent effects of folic acid on blood concentrations of homocysteine: a meta-analysis of the randomized trials. *Am J Clin Nutr*; 82:806-812. 2005

Huemer M, Ausserer B, Graninger G et al. Hyperhomocysteinemia in children treated with antiepileptic drugs is normalized by folic acid supplementation. *Epilpepsia*; 46(10):1677-1683. 2005

Hunter R, Barnes J, Oakeley HF et al: Toxicity of folic acid given in pharmacological doses to healthy volunteers. *Lancet*; 1(7637):61-63. 1970

Kakar F, Henderson MM: Potential toxic side effects of folic acid (letter). *J Natl Cancer Inst*; 74(1):263. 1985

Lashner BA, Heidenreich PA, Su GL et al: The effect of folate supplementation on the incidence of dysplasia and cancer in chronic ulcerative colitis: a case-control study. *Gastroenterology*; 97(2):255-59. 1989

Lashner BA, Provencher KS, Seidner DL et al: The effect of folic acid supplementation on the risk for cancer or dysplasia in ulcerative colitis. *Gastroenterology*; 112(1):29-32. 1997

Leung CF, Lao TT, Chang AMZ: Effect of folate supplement on pregnant women with beta-thalassaemia minor. *Eur J Obstet Gynecol Reprod Biol*; 33(3):209-213. 1989

Lonn E, Yusuf S, Arnold MJ et al. Homocysteine lowering with folic acid and B vitamins in vascular disease. *N Engl J Med*; 354:1567-1577. 2006

Melikian V, Paton A, Leeming RJ et al: Site of reduction and methylation of folic acid in man. *Lancet*; 2(7731):955-957. 1971

Milunsky A, Jick H, Jick SS et al: Multivitamin/folic acid supplementation in early pregnancy reduces the prevalence of neural tube defects. *JAMA*; 262(20):2847-2852. 1989

Morita H, Tagushi J, Kurihara H et al: Genetic polymorphism of 5, 10-methylenetetrahydrofolate reductase (MTHFR) as a risk factor for coronary artery disease. *Circulation*; 95(8):2032-2036. 1997

Morgan SL, Oster RA, Lee JY et al. The effect of folic acid and folinic acid supplements on purine metabolism in methotrexate-treated rheumatoid arthritis. *Arthritis & Rheumatism*; 50(10):3104-3111. 2004

Mulinaire J: Epidemiologic associations of multivitamin supplementation and occurrence of neural tube defects. *Ann N Y Acad Sci*; 678:130-136. Mar 15, 1993

National Health and Medical Research Council (NHMRC): Prevention of neural tube defects: results of the Medical Research Council Vitamin Study, MRC Vitamin Study Research Group. *Lancet*; 338(8760):131-137. 1991

National Health and Medical Research Council (NHMRC): Revised statement on the relationship between dietary folic acid and neural tube defects such as spina bifida. *J Paediatr Child Health*; 30:476-477. 1994

Nguyen TT, Dyer DL Dunning DD et al: Human intestinal folate transport: cloning, expression, and distribution of complementary RNA. *Gastroenterology*; 112(3):783-791. 1997

Omenn GS, Beresford SAA, Motulsky AG: Preventing coronary heart disease: B vitamins and homocysteine. *Circulation*; 97(5):421-424. 1998

Pack ARC: Folate mouthwash: effects on established gingivitis in periodontal patients. *J Clin Periodontol*; 11(9):619-628. 1984

Pack AR, Thomson ME: Effects of topical and systemic folic acid supplementation on gingivitis in pregnancy. *J Clin Periodontol*; 7(5):402-414. 1980

Prakash R, Petrie WM: Psychiatric changes associated with an excess of folic acid. *Am J Psychiatry*; 139(9):1192-1193. 1982

Product Information: Folic acid tablets, USP. Halsey Drug Co, Inc, Brooklyn, NY; 1995.

Product Information: Folvite® (folic acid). Lederle Labs, Pearl River, NY; 1990.

Rieder MJ: Prevention of neural tube defects with periconceptual folic acid. *Clin Perinatol*; 21(3):483-503. 1994

Rimm EB, Willett WC, Hu FB: Folate and vitamin B_6 from diet and supplements in relation to risk of coronary heart disease among women. *JAMA*; 279(5):359-364. 1998

Russell RM, Dutta SK, Oaks EV et al: Impairment of folic acid absorption by oral pancreatic extracts. *Dig Dis Sci*; 25(5):369-373. 1980

Salim A, Tan A, Ilchyshyn, Berth-Jones J. Folic acid supplementation during treatment of psoriasis with methotrexate: a randomized, double-blind, placebo-controlled trial. *Br J Dermatol*; 154:1169-1174. 2006

Skoutakis VA, Acchiardo SR, Meyer MC et al: Folic acid dosage for chronic hemodialysis patients. *Clin Pharmacol Ther*; 18(2):200-204. 1975

Thomson ME, Pack ARC: Effects of extended systemic and topical folate supplementation on gingivitis of pregnancy. *J Clin Periodontol*; 9(3):275-280. 1982

Title LM, Ur E, Giddens K et al. Folic acid improves endothelial dysfunction in type 2 diabetes—an effect independent of homocysteine-lowering. *Vasc Med*; 11:101-109. 2006

Tucker KL, Mahnken B, Wilson PWF et al: Folic acid fortification of the food supply: potential benefits and risks for the elderly population. *JAMA*; 276(23):1879-1885. 1996

Villa P, Suriano R, Constantini B et al. Hyperhomocysteinemia and cardiovascular risk in postmenopausal women: the role of folate supplementation. *Clin Chem Lab Med*; 45(2):130-135. 2007

Werler MM, Shapiro S, Mitchell AA: Periconceptional folic acid exposure and risk of occurrent neural tube defects. *JAMA*; 269(10):1257-1261. 1993

Zoungas S, McGrath BP, Branley P et al. Cardiovascular morbidity and mortality in the Atherosclerosis and Folic Acid Supplementation Trial (ASFAST) in chronic renal failure: a multicenter, randomized, controlled trial. *J Am Coll Cardiol*; 47:1108-1116. 2006

Glucosamine

DESCRIPTION

Glucosamine is an endogenous aminomonosaccharide synthesized from glucose and utilized for biosynthesis of two larger compounds, glycoproteins and glycosaminoglycans. These compounds are necessary for the construction and maintenance of virtually all connective tissues and lubricating fluids in the body (Reichelt et al 1994; Reuser 1994; Setnikar et al 1993). The sulfate salt of glucosamine forms half of the disaccharide subunit of keratan sulfate, which is decreased in osteoarthritis, and of hyaluronic acid, which is found in both articular cartilage and synovial fluid (Leffler et al 1999).

Supplemental glucosamine is generally used to reduce pain and immobility associated with osteoarthritis, especially in the knee joint. The supplements are usually derived from crab shells, although a corn source is also available. Most studies of osteoarthritis have used the sulfate form of glucosamine (D'Ambrosio et al 1981; Pujalte et al 1980). Other forms include glucosamine hydrochloride and N-acetyl glucosamine.

Other Names: 2-amino-2-deoxy-beta-D-glucopyranose, chitosamine, glucosamine hydrochloride, glucosamine sulfate, N-acetyl glucosamine (NAG)

ACTIONS AND PHARMACOLOGY

EFFECTS

Anti-arthritic Effects: Preclinical studies with glucosamine have suggested tropism for cartilage and bone. Glucosamine seems to enhance cartilage proteoglycan synthesis, thereby inhibiting deterioration of cartilage brought about by osteoarthritis and helping to maintain equilibrium between cartilage catabolic and anabolic processes (Setnikar et al 1993; D'Ambrosio et al 1981; Vidal y Plana et al 1980, 1978). Exogenous administration of glucosamine in animals has been reported to retard cartilage degradation and rebuild experimentally damaged cartilage tissue (D'Ambrosio et al 1981; Pujalte et al 1980; Crolle et al 1980). Protection against metabolic impairment of cartilage induced by nonsteroidal anti-inflammatory drugs and corticosteroids has been described. An anti-inflammatory action of glucosamine has also been proposed, unrelated to cyclo-oxygenase inhibition (Reichelt et al 1994).

Glucose Metabolism Effects: It has been hypothesized that glucosamine may impair insulin secretion through competitive inhibition of glucokinase in pancreatic beta cells and/or alteration of peripheral glucose uptake (Monauni et al 2000; Balkan et al 1994).

Wound Healing Effects: Hyaluronic acid (HA), which is synthesized by fibroblasts, promotes proliferation of epithelial cells. Oral glucosamine may enhance HA synthesis, thus accelerating healing and minimizing scarring in fresh wounds (McCarty 1996).

CLINICAL TRIALS

Knee Pain/Osteoarthritis

Results continue to vary among studies investigating the efficacy of glucosamine for the treatment of knee osteoarthritis. While the findings of one study suggest that oral glucosamine is more effective than placebo (Beaumont et al 2007), an earlier study found no difference between the two (McAlindon et al 2004). In the more recent study, subjects were randomized to receive 1500 mg/day glucosamine (n=106), 3 gm/day acetaminophen (used as a side comparator, [n=108]), or placebo (n=104). Nearly one-half of the glucosamine group reported decreased pain above the threshold for a minimally clinically-important improvement, while just slightly more than 30% of the placebo group did (p=0.023). In the other study, patients were randomized to treatment with 1.5 g/day glucosamine (n=101) or placebo (n=104). No difference was observed between the two groups in any of the outcome measures during the study. Another article reporting on the evidence from two 3-year studies suggests that long-term administration of glucosamine can delay the structural progression of knee osteoarthritis in postmenopausal women and may lead to improvement of symptoms (Bruyere et al 2004).

One study enrolled 1,583 patients with symptomatic knee pain and randomly distributed them across 5 treatment groups: glucosamine 1500 mg/day (n=317), chondroitin sulfate 1200 mg/day (n=318), glucosamine plus chondroitin (n=317), celocoxib 200 mg/day (n=318) and placebo (n=313). Investigators were looking for a 20% decrease in Western Ontario and MacMaster Universities Osteoarthritis Index (WOMAC) pain score from baseline to week 24. Compared with the high rate of response to placebo (60.1%), rates of response were just 3.9 percentage points higher for glucosamine (p=0.30), 5.3 percentage points higher for chondroitin (p=0.17), and 6.5 points higher for the combination of the two (p=0.09). These results showed that glucosamine, either alone or in combination with chondroitin sulfate, did not effectively reduce pain in the overall group of subjects in this study (Clegg et al 2006).

Another group of investigators used a unique approach to study glucosamine's effects. Their randomized, double-blind trial enrolled 137 subjects with knee osteoarthritis who had been taking glucosamine for relief of painful symptoms and had experienced moderately beneficial results. Subjects were continued on an equivalent dose of glucosamine (n=71) or assigned to placebo (n=66). Disease flare was noted in 42% of those receiving placebo and 45% of those receiving glucosamine (p=0.76). In summary, no evidence of symptomatic benefit from continued use of glucosamine was found compared to placebo (Cibere et al 2004).

In another randomized, placebo-controlled study, a benefit was observed with glucosamine: patients reported improvement in unspecified knee pain and function after supplementation. Glucosamine hydrochloride 2,000 mg (n=24) or placebo (n=22) was given once daily in the morning for 3 months. Between the groups, there was no difference in joint line palpation, duck walk, or stair-climb results. There were significant improvements in the glucosamine group on the knee pain scale at week 8 of evaluation (p=0.004) and on the knee injury and osteoarthritis outcome score (KOOS) on weeks 8 and 12 (p=0.038). Self-reported improvements in perceived pain began to occur between weeks 4 and 8 and at week 12. Eighty-eight percent of patients who were receiving glucosamine reported some level of pain relief, compared to 17% in the placebo group. Side effects were reported as mild and short-lived, with gastrointestinal effects and headache cited most frequently and occurring equally in both groups (Braham et al 2003).

A meta-analysis of 15 randomized, placebo-controlled trials evaluating the structural and symptomatic efficacy of oral glucosamine and chondroitin in knee osteoarthritis demonstrated efficacy for glucosamine on joint space narrowing (JSN) and WOMAC. Similar efficacies were demonstrated for chondroitin and glucosamine on the Lequesne Index (LI) and visual analog scale (VAS) for pain and mobility. Joint cartilage degeneration was slowed by the long-term daily administration of oral glucosamine at the minimal dose of 1,500 mg during a minimal period of 3 years (Richy et al

2003). An earlier meta-analysis of 16 randomized, controlled trials found glucosamine to be safe and effective for the treatment of osteoarthritis. In 12 of 13 studies comparing it to placebo, glucosamine demonstrated superior pain relief. In four studies comparing glucosamine to NSAIDs, results of efficacy with each agent were evenly divided (Towheed et al 2001).

A topical preparation of glucosamine, chondroitin, and shark cartilage reduced pain associated with osteoarthritis of the knee. Sixty-three patients were randomized to receive a water-soluble cream (30 mg/g of glucosamine sulfate; 50 mg/g of chondroitin sulfate, 140 mg/g of shark cartilage, 32 mg/g of camphor, and 9 mg/g of peppermint oil) or placebo for 8 weeks. Both groups reported improvement on the visual analog scale pain scores, with the treatment group improving a further 1.2 points (p=0.03) at 4 weeks and 1.8 points (p=0.002) at 8 weeks compared to the placebo group. Patients were instructed to apply cream generously to painful joints, gently massage until cream disappears, and repeat as necessary (Cohen et al 2003).

Two randomized, double-blind, parallel trials of glucosamine reported no improvement in osteoarthritis of the knee. In the first, patients were randomized to receive 500 mg of glucosamine three times daily (n=49) or a placebo (n=49) for 2 months. No statistical difference was noted between the groups in mean scores for resting and walking after 30 and 60 days (Rindone et al 2000). In the second study, glucosamine was no better than placebo as an analgesic for knee pain due to osteoarthritis. In the 6-month evaluation, patients with varying degrees of pain were randomized to receive 500 mg of glucosamine sulfate three times daily (n=38) or placebo (n=37). There were no differences between the groups in any assessment marker at any time during the trial. The authors suggested that their results differ from previous glucosamine studies because the patients in this trial were more symptomatic and had more structural damage than patients in trials with positive glucosamine results. In addition, this trial had a high placebo response of 33%, perhaps an indication of selection bias to those who have an affinity for complementary therapies (Hughes et al 2002).

Osteoarthritis

Oral glucosamine was effective for osteoarthritis of the spine in a multicenter, randomized, double-blind, placebo-controlled trial. Subjects (n=160) with symptomatic cervical and/or lumbar spine osteoarthritis of at least 6 months' duration received 1,500 mg of glucosamine sulfate daily or placebo for 6 weeks. Outcome measures included visual analog scales and/or clinical measurements for pain, morning stiffness, tenderness, and mobility. Analysis of variance found significant improvement compared to placebo at both locations for pain at rest and at night, tenderness and lateral flexion, and at the lumbar level for pain on active movement, flexion, rotation, and morning stiffness. Improvement persisted 4 weeks after discontinuation of treatment (Giacovelli et al 1993).

Temporomandibular Joint (TMJ) Disorder

A randomized, double-blind study involving 45 subjects with TMJ disorder compared glucosamine and ibuprofen for the treatment of pain. Researchers were looking for a 20% or greater reduction in TMJ pain during common activities (eg, chewing, speaking). After 90 days of treatment, no significant difference in outcomes between groups was observed. (Thie et al 2001). Another study published in the same year showed a benefit for the combined regimen of glucosamine and chondroitin. In that 12-week, double-blind, placebo-controlled study, patients received 750 mg of glucosamine hydrochloride and 600 mg of chondroitin sulfate twice daily (n=23) or placebo (n=22). Statistically significant improvements were seen in measures of joint tenderness and jawbone noises (eg, cracking). In addition, the mean number of over-the-counter analgesics (mainly acetaminophen) used was significantly lower in the treatment group (p=0.03). Adverse effects were mainly gastrointestinal, which were reported as transient and resolved spontaneously (Nguyen et al 2001).

INDICATIONS AND USAGE

Unproven Uses: Glucosamine, especially the sulfate form, is a popular treatment for pain and immobility associated with osteoarthritis. Glucosamine is classified by the European League Against Rheumatism (EULAR) as a Symptomatic Slow-Acting Drug in Osteoarthritis. This drug group is characterized by slow-onset improvement in osteoarthritis with persistent benefits after discontinuation (Jordan et al 2003). Whether long-term use of glucosamine can reverse the course of osteoarthritis still remains to be proven. Supplemental glucosamine has also been used for articular injury repair, TMJ, and cutaneous aging (wrinkles).

PRECAUTIONS AND ADVERSE REACTIONS

Glucosamine should be used with caution in patients with an allergy to shellfish and shellfish products. Asthma patients may be at risk for symptom exacerbation when taking the combination of glucosamine and chondroitin. Patients with diabetes should also be cautious, since glucosamine may affect insulin sensitivity or glucose tolerance.

The most commonly reported adverse effects are gastrointestinal disturbances, including nausea, dyspepsia, heartburn, vomiting, constipation, diarrhea, anorexia, and epigastric pain. Less than 1% of patients have reported edema, tachycardia, drowsiness, insomnia, headache, erythema, and pruritus.

Pregnancy and Lactation: Scientific evidence for the safe use of glucosamine sulfate during pregnancy and lactation is not available

DRUG INTERACTIONS

MODERATE RISKS

Doxorubicin, Etoposide, and Teniposide: Concurrent use may result in reduced effectiveness of these drugs. *Clinical Management:* Avoid concomitant use.

Warfarin: Concurrent use may result in elevations of International Normalized Ratio (INR) serum values and potentiation of anticoagulant effects. *Clinical Management:* Warfarin dosage adjustments may be required when glucosamine therapy is initiated or modified during concomitant treatment. During concurrent treatment, closely monitor the prothrombin time or INR.

MINOR RISKS

Antidiabetic Agents: Concurrent use may result in reduced antidiabetic agent effectiveness. *Clinical Management:* Glucosamine is likely safe for patients with diabetes that is well-controlled with diet only or with one or two oral antidiabetic agents (HbA1c less than 6.5%). In patients with higher HbA1c concentrations or for those requiring insulin, closely monitor blood glucose concentrations.

OVERDOSAGE

In mice, the LD50 for glucosamine hydrochloride is 15 g/kg oral, 1,100 mg/kg intravenous, and 6,200 mg/kg subcutaneous (RTECS 2001). No mortality in mice or rats resulted from glucosamine sulfate at doses of 5,000 mg/kg oral, 3,000 mg/kg intramuscular, and 1,500 mg/kg intravenous (Kelly 1998).

DOSAGE

Mode of Administration: Intra-articular, intramuscular, intravenous, oral, topical

How Supplied: Cream, liquid, tablet, solution

Daily Dosage: Osteoarthritis

Oral: 1,500 mg in single or three divided doses daily. Results were seen after a minimum of 4 weeks and up to 3 years later (Pavelka et al 2002; Reginster et al 2001; Noack et al 1994).

Intramuscular: 400 mg of glucosamine sulfate once daily (Reichelt et al 1994; D'Ambrosio et al 1981; Crolle et al 1980). A regimen of 400 mg twice weekly for 6 weeks has also been given (Reichelt et al 1994).

LITERATURE

Balkan B, Dunning BE: Glucosamine inhibits glucokinase in vitro and produces a glucose-specific impairment of in vivo insulin secretion in rats. *Diabetes*; 43(10):1173-1179. 1994

Braham R, Dawson B, Goodman C et al: The effect of glucosamine supplementation on people experiencing knee pain. *Br J Sports Med*; 37(1):45-49. 2003

Bruyere O, Pavelka K, Rovati LC et al: Glucosamine sulfate reduces osteoarthritis progression in postmenopausal women with knee osteoarthritis: evidence from two 3-year studies. Menopause; 11(2):138-143. 2004

Cibere J, Kopec JA, Thorne A et al: Randomized, double-blind, placebo-controlled glucosamine discontinuation trial in knee osteoarthritis. *Arthritis & Rheumatism*; 51(5):738-745. 2004

Clegg DO, Reda DJ, Harris CL et al. Glucosamine, chondroitin sulfate, and the two in combination for painful knee osteoarthritis. *N Engl J Med*; 354(8):795-808. 2006

Cohen M, Wolfe R, Mal T et al: A randomized, double blind, placebo controlled trial of a topical cream containing glucosamine sulfate, chondroitin sulfate, and camphor for osteoarthritis of the knee. *J Rheumatol*; 30(3):523-528. 2003

Crolle G, D'Este E: Glucosamine sulphate for the management of arthrosis: a controlled clinical investigation. *Curr Med Res Opin*; 7(2):104-109. 1980

D'Ambrosio E, Casa B, Bompani R et al: Glucosamine sulphate: a controlled clinical investigation in arthrosis. *Pharmatherapeutica* 1981; 2(8):504-508.

Giacovelli G, Rovati LC: Clinical efficacy of glucosamine sulfate in osteoarthritis of the spine (abstract). *Rev Esp Rheumatol*; 20(suppl 1):325. 1993

Herrero-Beumont G, Ivorra JAR, Trabado M et al: Glucosamine sulfate in the treatment of knee osteoarthritis symptoms. *Arthritis & Rheumatism*; 56(2):555-567. 2007

Higgins G: Optimistic look for disease modifiers in osteoarthritis. *Inpharma*; 896:3-4. 1993

Hughes R, Carr A. A randomized, double-blind, placebo-controlled trial of glucosamine sulphate as an analgesic in osteoarthritis of the knee. *Rheumatology (Oxford).* Mar;41(3):279-84. 2002

Jordan KM, Arden NK, Doherty M et al: EULAR Recommendations 2003: an evidence based approach to the management of knee osteoarthritis: Report of a Task Force of the Standing Committee for International Clinical Studies Including Therapeutic Trials (ESCISIT). *Ann Rheumatic Dis*; 62:1145-1155. 2003

Kelly G: The role of glucosamine sulfate and chondroitin sulfates in the treatment of degenerative joint disease. *Alt Med Review*; 3(1):27-39. 1998

Leffler CT, Philippi AF, Leffler SG et al: Glucosamine, chondroitin, and manganese ascorbate for degenerative joint disease of the knee or low back: a randomized, double-blind, placebo-controlled pilot study. *Mil Med*; 164(2):85-91. 1999

McCarty MF: Glucosamine for wound healing. *Med Hypotheses*; 47:273-275. 1996

McAlindon T, Formica M, LaValley M et al: Effectiveness of glucosamine for symptoms of knee osteoarthritis: results from an internet-based randomized double-blind controlled trial. *Am J Med*; 117:643-639. 2004

Monauni T, Zenti MG, Cretti A et al: Effects of glucosamine infusion on insulin secretion and insulin action in humans. *Diabetes*; 49(6): 926-935. 2000

Nguyen P, Mohamed SE, Gardiner D et al: A randomized, double-blind clinical trial of the effect of chondroitin sulfate and glucosamine hydrochloride on temporomandibular joint disorder: a pilot study. *J Craniomandibular Pract*; 19(2):130-139. 2001

Noack W, Fischer M, Foerster KK et al: Glucosamine sulfate in osteoarthritis of the knee. *Osteoarthritis Cartilage*; 2:51-59. 1994

Pavelka K, Gatterova J, Olejarova M et al: Glucosamine sulfate use and delay of progression of knee osteoarthritis: a 3-year, randomized, placebo-controlled, double-blind study. *Arch Intern Med*;162(18):2113-2123. 2002

Pujalte JM, Llavore EP, Ylescupidez FR: Double-blind clinical evaluation of oral glucosamine sulphate in the basic treatment of osteoarthrosis. *Curr Med Res Opin*; 7(2):110-114. 1980

Reginster JY, Deroisy R, Rovati LC et al: Long-term effects of glucosamine sulfate on osteoarthritis progression: a randomized, placebo-controlled clinical trial. *Lancet*; 357(9252):251-256. 2001

Reichelt A, Forster KK, Fischer M et al: Efficacy and safety of intramuscular glucosamine sulfate in osteoarthritis of the knee: a randomised, placebo-controlled, double-blind study. *Arzneimittelforschung*; 44(1):75-80. 1994

Reuser AJJ, Wisselaar HA: An evaluation of the potential side-effects of alpha-glucosidase inhibitors used for the management of diabetes mellitus. *Eur J Clin Invest*; 24(suppl 3):19-24. 1994

Richy F, Bruyere O, Ethgen O et al: Structural and symptomatic efficacy of glucosamine and chondroitin in knee osteoarthritis. *Arch Intern Med*; 163(13):1514-1522. 2003

Rindone JP, Hiller D, Collacott E, et al. Randomized, controlled trial of glucosamine for treating osteoarthritis of the knee. *West J Med.* Feb;172(2):91-4. 2000.

RTECS: Registry of Toxic Effects of Chemical Substances. National Institute for Occupational Safety and Health, Cincinnati, OH (internet version), Thomson Micromedex, Greenwood Village, CO; 2001.

Setnikar I, Palumbo R, Canali S et al: Pharmacokinetics of glucosamine in man. *Arzneimittelforschung*; 43(10):1109-1113. 1993

Thie NMR, Prasad NG, Major PW. *J Rheumatol*; 28:1347-1355. 2001

Towheed TE, Anastassiades TP, Shea B et al: Glucosamine therapy for treating osteoarthritis. *Cochrane Databasa Syst Rev*; 1:CD002946. 2001

Vidal y Plana RR, Karzel K: Glukosamin. Seine Bedeutung fuer den Knorpelstoffwechsel der Gelenke. 2. Gelenkknorpel-Untersuchungen. *Fortschr Med*; 21:801-806. 1980

Glutamine

DESCRIPTION

Glutamine has traditionally been considered a nonessential amino acid. It is the most abundant amino acid in the body. It is produced in skeletal muscle from glutamate and ammonia catalyzed by glutamine synthetase. Skeletal muscle contains up to 60% of total-body glutamine stores. Glutamine is manufactured in the liver from glutamate, cysteine, and glycine. It is an important substrate in supporting liver detoxification processes and acts as a powerful antioxidant that protects hepatocytes. Glutamine supplementation has been shown to preserve glutathione liver stores and protect the liver from free radical damage after acute toxicity from acetaminophen poisoning and high-dose cytotoxic therapy during bone marrow transplants (Hong et al, 1992; Brown et al, 1998).

Glutamine serves as metabolic fuel for rapidly proliferating cell lines such as enterocytes, colonocytes, fibroblasts, lymphocytes, and macrophages (Fraga Fuentes et al 1996). It is essential for maintaining intestinal function, the immune response, and amino acid homeostasis. Glutamine is released into circulation during metabolic stress, trauma, and surgery. The concentration of glutamine in the muscle is affected by injury, sepsis, prolonged stress, and starvation (Miller 1999). Plasma glutamine levels decrease after severe organic injuries, partly because the small intestine uses it faster than it can be produced by skeletal muscle (Cukier et al 1999).

Clinical studies suggest that glutamine may be helpful for treating impaired intestinal permeability, short-bowel syndrome, cancer, critical illness and trauma, infection, and as an adjunct and protective agent during chemotherapy and radiation therapy. Further research is required to validate its effectiveness for these indications, as most human studies have used a small number of patients.

Other Names: levoglutamide, levoglutamine, L-glutamic acid, 5-amide, L-glutamine, L-(+)-2-aminoglutaramic acid

ACTIONS AND PHARMACOLOGY

EFFECTS

Human and animal studies have shown that glutamine has antioxidant, antitumor, chemoprotective, and immunostimulant effects.

Antioxidant Effects: Glutamine supplementation has been shown to preserve stores of glutathione (an important hepatic antioxidant) and protect the liver from free radical damage after acute toxicity from acetaminophen poisoning and high-dose cytotoxic therapy during bone marrow transplants (Brown et al 1998; Hong et al 1992).

Antitumor/Chemoprotective Effects: Serum levels of glutamine in gastric carcinoma patients were reduced when compared to controls in a Russian study (Anderson et al 1998). Glutamine supplementation also increased the cytotoxicity of methotrexate. A preclinical animal study showed a 300% increase in the therapeutic delivery of methotrexate to targeted tumor cells. Based on these findings, a subsequent trial in nine breast cancer patients showed that supplemental glutamine decreased methotrexate toxicity and increased methotrexate concentration in tumor cells (Rubio et al 1998).

Immunostimulant Effects: Lymphocyte reactivity was higher after mice received a diet enriched in glutamine (13.3 g/kg) for 2 weeks. Increasing the amount of dietary glutamine increased the ability of T-lymphocytes to respond to mitogenic stimulation. Increasing the oral availability of glutamine may promote the T-cell immune response (Kew et al 1999). An in vitro study found that glutamine increased the production of interleukin-2 and gamma interferon, which is important for optimal lymphocyte proliferation (Rohde et al 1996). Additionally, glutamine-supplemented parenteral nutrition prevented the reduction of both B- and T-cell lines when compared to glutamine deficient parenteral nutrition in an animal study (Alverdy et al 1992). A human study also showed that glutamine supplementation caused an increase in T-cell synthesis in postoperative surgical patients receiving total parenteral nutrition (O'Riordain et al 1994).

CLINICAL TRIALS

Cancer

Glutamine appears to exert a protective effect when administered with chemotherapy. Five cancer patients developed moderate to severe joint and muscle pain 24 to 36 hours after receiving their initial course of paclitaxel. During the next course of paclitaxel treatment, patients received 10 g of glutamine three times daily 24 hours after receiving paclitaxel. None of these patients developed myalgia or arthralgia with glutamine supplementation (Savarese et al 1998).

Glutamine had a positive effect on decreasing methotrexate toxicity and increasing the concentration of methotrexate in tumor cells. Nine patients with breast cancer received 0.5 g/kg/day of oral glutamine during methotrexate treatment. Glutamine supplementation was given 4 days prior to starting chemotherapy and for 1 week after the treatment course. Patients in this study did not develop any symptoms of chemotherapy-related toxicity, including neutropenia or liver and kidney toxicity. Chemotherapy did not have to be withheld or delayed. No toxicity related to glutamine administration was found in this study (Rubio et al 1998).

Duration and severity of oral stomatitis and mouth pain were reduced with glutamine treatment in a randomized, double-blind, crossover study of patients undergoing chemotherapy. Eight adults and 16 children received either a placebo or an oral suspension of 2 g/m2 of glutamine twice daily to swish and swallow on chemotherapy administration days and for the following 14 days. Glycine was used as the placebo treatment. Glutamine reduced the duration of mouth pain by 4.5 days ($p=0.0005$) compared to placebo. The severity of oral pain was also significantly reduced ($p=0.002$), allowing patients to resume oral intake 4 days earlier than the placebo group. These results are based on paired data analysis using patients as their own control (n=13). Others were unable to complete the experiment for various reasons. No significant adverse reactions were reported (Anderson et al 1998).

Glutamine protected lymphocytes and intestinal integrity in patients with advanced esophageal cancer in a randomized, placebo-controlled study. Patients receiving active treatment (n=7) were given 30 g of oral glutamine daily for 28 days at the start of radiochemotherapy. Placebo-treated patients (n=6) received a standard amino acid solution. All patient received 5-fluorouracil and cisplatin plus mediastinal irradiation. Blood chemistries, lymphocyte counts, and gut barrier functions were completed before treatment and on days 7, 14, and 28. Glutamine prevented a reduction in lymphocyte count on day 7 ($p<0.05$) but there were no differences between groups on days 14 and 28. Blast formation of lymphocytes was maintained by glutamine on days 7 and 14 ($p<0.05$). Urinary excretion of phenolsulfonphthalein was greater in the control group on day 7 only ($p<0.05$). The study concluded that glutamine supplementation may protect gut integrity and T-cell functioning during radiochemotherapy (Yoshida et al 1998).

Glutamine supplementation improved some outcome parameters in patients receiving allogenic bone marrow transplants. In this prospective, double-blind, controlled trial, 45 adult patients with hematologic malignancies received either total parenteral nutrition (TPN; control) or TPN plus glutamine (TPN-GLN) 0.57 g/kg/day starting the day after bone marrow transplantation. During the first week of TPN, plasma GLN levels rose by 40% in the TPN-GLN group, but a significant treatment effect could only be recorded in the bilirubin concentration (14 micromoles/L in the control versus 18 micromoles/L in the TPN-GLN group; $p=0.044$). The number of days until leukocyte recovery did not differ significantly between groups. The incidence of positive microbial cultures was significantly reduced in the supplemented group (42%) versus the control group (5%) ($p<0.005$). Clinical infections occurred in 10 control patients (43%) but only 3 TPN-GLN patients (3%; $p=0.041$). Nitrogen retention was markedly better in the TPN-GLN group. This group also had a significantly reduced hospital stay of 29 days versus 36 days for the control group ($p=0.017$). However, overall 100-day survival rates were similar. No significant side effects were attributed to GLN administration (Ziegler et al 1992).

HIV Infection

In a double-blind, placebo-controlled trial, glutamine supplementation in addition to antioxidants increased body mass in 26 HIV-positive patients suffering from weight loss. Patients received 40 g of glutamine plus antioxidants daily in divided doses or placebo (40 g of glycine) for 12 weeks. Over this time period, the glutamine-antioxidant group gained an average of 2.2 kg of body weight compared with 0.3 kg in the control group ($p=0.04$). Body cell mass and intracellular water also increased in the glutamine-antioxidant group with little or no change in the control group (Shabert et al 1999).

Infection

Glutamine had beneficial results in the treatment of trauma patients in a randomized, placebo-controlled study evaluating infection rates in acute multiple trauma. Patients with multiple trauma were randomly assigned to receive an enriched enteral feeding with 30.5 g of glutamine per 100 g of protein (n=29) or a control feeding (n=31) along with usual care. An assessment for infection was conducted every 8 hours for at least 5 days. Five glutamine-treated patients (17%) developed pneumonia compared to 14 patients (45%) in the control group ($p<0.02$). Two patients in the glutamine group (7%) developed bacteremia compared to 13 (42%) in the control group ($p<0.005$). One patient developed sepsis in the glutamine group compared to 8 (26%) in the control group ($p<0.02$). Glutamine-treated patients had increased plasma glutamine concentrations as well as increased concentrations of both citrulline and arginine, suggesting that glutamine caused stimulation of renal production of arginine. Arginine has been shown to stimulate lymphocyte immune responses and wound healing. Soluble tumor necrosis factors p55 and p75 were also lower compared to controls, suggesting a lower systemic inflammatory response. All of these were found parallel with a decreased number of infectious complications (Houdijk et al 1998).

INDICATIONS AND USAGE

Unproven Uses: Research suggests that supplemental glutamine may have beneficial effects in the treatment of cancer due to its protective action during chemotherapy. Supplementation with glutamine may also enhance T-cell functioning, which could be beneficial for critically ill and trauma patients. In ''wasting'' diseases such as AIDS, glutamine is used to support T-cell function, augment lean muscle mass, and decrease cachexia. Glutamine may also be helpful for acute toxicity from acetaminophen poisoning and high-dose cytotoxic therapy during bone marrow transplants.

Glutamine has also been used for the following: environmental and multiple-chemical sensitivity; as a biomarker in determining and treating diseases of aging; as support for phase II liver detoxification pathways; as a muscle enhancer and athletic recovery aid; and to promote the release of growth hormone.

CONTRAINDICATIONS

Patients with liver disease should not use glutamine. This supplement is also contraindicated for patients with any condition that puts them at risk for accumulation of nitrogenous wastes in the blood&emdash;such as Reye's syndrome or cirrhosis&emdash;since it can lead to ammonia-induced encephalopathy and coma.

PRECAUTIONS AND ADVERSE REACTIONS

Patients who are taking glutamine and have chronic renal failure should have their kidney function monitored. Extreme caution is also advised when adding glutamine to the total parenteral nutrition of cancer patients, since glutamine serves as the main substrate for many tumors (Fischer et al 1990). The most common side effects of supplemental glutamine are constipation, gastrointestinal upset, and bloating.

DOSAGE

Mode of Administration: Oral, enteral, parenteral

How Supplied: Crystalline powder, solution, tablet

Daily Dosage: Dosages are for oral administration unless otherwise noted.

ADULTS

Cancer: 30 g daily, usually taken in 3 divided doses; for intravenous administration, 50 g of glycl-L-glutamine daily or glutamine 0.57 g/kg/day.

Chemoprotective: 10 g daily taken in 3 divided doses, or 0.5 g/kg/day.

Critical Illness (enteral): 5 g per each 500 mL of enteral feeding solution.

Infection (enteral): 12 to 30.5 g in an enteral feeding solution.

Immune-System Enhancement (intravenous): 0.18 g/kg/day in a total parenteral nutrition solution.

Intestinal Permeability: 7 to 21 g daily in single or divided doses.

Short-Bowel Syndrome: 0.4 to 0.63 g/kg/day.

Stomatitis (oral solution): 2 g twice daily used as a mouthwash and then swallowed.

CHILDREN

Stomatitis (oral solution): 2 g twice daily used as a mouthwash and then swallowed.

LITERATURE

Alverdy JA, Aoys E, Weiss-Carrington P et al: The effect of glutamine-enriched TPN on gut immune cellularity. *J Surg Res*; 52(1):34-38. 1992

Anderson P, Schroeder G, Skubitz K: Oral glutamine reduced the duration and severity of stomatitis after cytotoxic cancer chemotherapy. *Cancer*; 83:1433-1439. 1998

Brown SA, Goringe A, Fegan C et al: Parenteral glutamine protects hepatic function during bone marrow transplantation. *Bone Marrow Transplant*; 22:281-284. 1998

Cukier C, Waitzberg DL, Borges VC et al: Clinical use of growth hormone and glutamine in short bowel syndrome. *Rev Hosp Clin Fac Med Sao Paulo*; 54(1):29-34. 1999

Fischer J, Chance W: Total parenteral nutrition, glutamine, and tumor growth. *J Parenter Enteral Nutr*; 14(4):86S-89s. 1990

Fraga Fuentes MD, de Juana Velasco P, Pintor Recuenco YR: Papel metabolico de la glutamina y su importancia en la terapia nutricional. *Nutr Hosp*; 11(4):215-225. 1996

Fraser CL, Arieff AI: Hepatic encephalopathy. *N Engl J Med*; 313(14):865-873. 1985

Hong RW, Rounds JD, Helton WS et al: Glutamine preserves liver glutathione after lethal hepatic injury. *Ann Surg*; 215:114-119. 1992

Houdijk A, Rijnsburger E, Jansen J: Randomized trial of glutamine-enriched enteral nutrition on infectious morbidity in patients with multiple trauma. *Lancet*; 352:772-776. 1998

Jones C, Palmer A, Griffiths F et al: Randomized clinical outcome study of critically ill patients given glutamine-supplemented enteral nutrition. *Nutrition*; 15:108-115. 1999

Kew S, Wells S, Yaqoob P et al: Dietary glutamine enhances murine t-lymphocyte responsiveness. *J Nutr*; 129:1524-1531. 1999

Klimberg VS, Kornbluth J, Cao Y et al: Glutamine suppresses PGE2 synthesis and breast cancer growth. *J Surg Res*; 63(1):293-297. 1996

Lacey J, Wilmore D: Is glutamine a conditionally essential amino acid? *Nutr Rev*; 48(8):297-307. 1990

MacLennan P, Smith K, Weryk B et al: Inhibition of protein breakdown by glutamine in perfused rat skeletal muscle. *FEBS Lett*; 237 (1,2):133-136. 1988

Miller A: Therapeutic considerations of L-glutamine: a review of the literature. *Altern Med Rev*; 4:239-248. 1999

Noyer C, Simon D, Borcxuk A et al: A double-blind placebo-controlled pilot study of glutamine therapy for abnormal intestinal permeability in patients with AIDS. *Am J Gastoenterol*; 93:972-975. 1998

O'Riordain M, Fearon K, Ross J et al: Glutamine-supplemented total parenteral nutrition enhanced T-lymphocyte response in surgical patients undergoing colorectal resection. *Ann Surg*; 220(2):212-221. 1994

Rhoads JM, Keku EO, Quinn J et al: L-glutamine stimulates jejunal sodium and chloride absorption in pig rotavirus enteritis. *Gastroenterology*; 100(3):683-691. 1991

Rohde T, Maclean D, Pedersen B: Glutamine, lymphocyte proliferation and cytokine production. *Scand J Immunol*; 44:648-650. 1996

Rubio I, Cao Y, Hutchins L et al: Effect of glutamine on methotrexate efficacy and toxicity. *Ann Surg*; 227 (5):772-780. 1998

Savarese D, Boucher J, Corey B: Glutamine treatment of paclitaxel-induced myalgias and arthralgias. *J Clin Oncol*; 16(12):3918-3919. 1998

Shabert JK, Winslow C, Lacey JM et al: Glutamine-antioxidant supplementation increases body cell mass in AIDS patients with weight loss: a randomized, double-blind controlled trial. *Nutrition*; 15(11-112):860-864. 1999

Ward E, Picton S, Reid U et al: Oral glutamine in paediatric oncology patients: a dose finding study. *Eur J Clin Nutr*; 57(1):31-36. 2003

Yoshida S, Matsui M, Shirouzu Y et al: Effects of glutamine supplements and radiochemotherapy on systemic immune and gut barrier function in patients with advanced esophageal cancer. *Ann Surg*; 227(4):485-491. 1998

Ziegler T, Young L, Benfell K et al: Clinical and metabolic efficacy of glutamine-supplemented parenteral nutrition after bone marrow transplantation. A randomized, double-blind, controlled study. *Ann Intern Med*; 116:821-828. 1992

Iron

DESCRIPTION

Iron is an essential trace mineral involved in the entire process of respiration, including oxygen and electron transport. The function and synthesis of hemoglobin, which carries most of the oxygen in the blood, is dependent on iron. Iron is also involved in the production of cytochrome oxidase, myoglobin, L-carnitine, and aconitase, all of which are involved in energy production in the body. In addition to its fundamental roles in energy production, iron is involved in DNA synthesis and may also play roles in normal brain development and immune function. Iron is also involved in the synthesis of collagen and the neurotransmitters serotonin, dopamine, and norepinephrine.

Iron-deficiency anemia is the most common nutritional disorder in the world. Although about 25% of the world's population is iron deficient, it should be noted that anemia is not always associated with iron deficiency. Low iron levels can occur from insufficient dietary intake, impairment of iron absorption, or loss of iron through bleeding. It is important to determine the cause before treating. Whether to treat iron deficiency (ferritin <20 mcg/L) in the absence of anemia (hemoglobin 11 g/dL or greater) is controversial. Preliminary data from NHANES III demonstrate that the prevalence of iron-deficiency anemia in the United States is very low. There is no known benefit of high iron storage status, and some evidence exists that a moderate increase in iron stores is a possible risk factor for ischemic heart disease and cancer. The safe upper range of iron intake is difficult to specify due to the complexity of the Western diet and iron physiology (Lynch et al 1996).

The best dietary sources of iron are green vegetables, legumes, and meat. Much of the iron ingested in the American diet in the form of enriched breads and cereals is not well absorbed. The average dietary intake of iron in the United States ranges from 10 to 20 mg daily. Some individuals, including adolescents and pregnant and lactating women, may be at risk for iron deficiency.

ACTIONS AND PHARMACOLOGY

EFFECTS

Iron has putative immune-enhancing, anticarcinogenic, and cognition-enhancing activities.

Antibacterial Effects: The role of iron in resistance to infection is complex. Iron deficiency is known to impair response of T lymphocytes to mitogens and to decrease the bactericidal activity of neutrophils. On the other hand, bacteria require iron for growth, and bacterial virulence is enhanced by increased iron availability. Also, the presence of infection or inflammation changes the cytokine-mediated metabolism of iron, which complicates attempts to define the relative benefits and hazards of iron therapy for prophylaxis of infectious disease (Walter et al 1997). Some studies have shown that iron supplementation given to infants reduces the incidence of respiratory infections. Other studies have found no difference in groups of infants given either iron or a placebo. Adult studies cited in this review found no benefit of iron use for reducing infection rates, and suggested that more illness may occur with supplementation (Oppenheimer 2001).

Cardiac Effects: Breath-holding spells in children have been overcome by iron supplementation. Along with improved iron status in these children, autonomic cardiovascular control during sleep was improved (i.e., increased heart rate variability, reduced ratio of low-frequency/high-frequency powers) (Orii et al 2002).

Oxidative Effects: Researchers have theorized that excess iron could play a role in the etiology of cancer and coronary heart disease. Iron is able to catalyze reactions that produce free radical metabolites, which may damage cell membranes, cause chromosomal mutations, or oxidize low-density lipoproteins (LDL) into more atherogenic particles (Sempos et al 1996; Minotti 1993; Imlay et al 1988). Animal studies have confirmed that atherosclerotic plaques contain a high concentration of iron, and rats given large amounts of iron have increased LDL lipid peroxidation. In human studies, atherosclerosis has been associated with increased iron levels (Meyers 2000).

CLINICAL TRIALS

Cognitive Function/Children & Adolescents

One review assessed the various benefits of iron supplementation in early childhood based on reports from 26 studies of iron supplementation in children aged 0 to 4 years. Among the eight randomized, controlled trials addressing developmental issues, some positive effects on a variety of developmental outcomes, including cognitive function, were noted in five. A meta-analysis of randomized, clinical trials cited in the review found significant beneficial effects on mental development with supplementation—especially among those identified as anemic or iron deficient at baseline. In addition, the meta-analysis revealed that all children >7 years old significantly benefited from iron supplementation, obtained from either oral doses, fortified food and milk, or through parenteral administration. Lower, longer-term, doses (2-12 months) seemed to provide greater benefit than very short courses of therapy (Iannotti et al 2006).

One trial in the review cited above bears mention. A randomized, double-blind, placebo-controlled trial of iron administration among preschoolers aged 3-4 years old (n=49) showed that 15 mg of iron supplementation in iron-deficient anemic subjects resulted in cognitive improvements including discrimination and information processing. Supplemented children exhibited 8% higher accuracy ($p<0.05$) and were significantly more efficient (mean difference = 1.09, $p<0.05$) than their untreated anemic counterparts, and made significantly fewer errors of commission (14% higher specificity, $p<0.05$). These effects did not extend to those preschoolers with adequate iron status (Metallinos-Katsaras et al 2004).

Iron supplementation improved hematological status and some measures of cognitive functioning in a double-blind, placebo-controlled study of 81 iron-deficient, nonanemic adolescent girls. Participants were randomly assigned to receive oral ferrous sulfate 650 mg twice daily or placebo for 8 weeks. Four tests of attention and memory were administered before and after the intervention. The supplemented group had significantly higher serum ferritin levels and performed significantly better than controls on a test of verbal learning and memory. Other measures of attention and learning were unchanged (Bruner et al 1996).

Positive results were also found in a randomized, double-blind, placebo-controlled study of 59 primarily nonanemic girls aged 16 or 17 years who took 105 mg daily of elemental iron as a liquid syrup or placebo. After 2 months, iron supplementation significantly improved subjective reports of lassitude, ability to concentrate in school, and mood. The majority of subjects reporting improvement had been hypoferremic prior to treatment. Physical fitness scores and subjective measures of appetite and sleep quality were unaffected by iron therapy (Ballin et al 1992).

Cognitive Function/Adults

One 3-year study demonstrated a relationship between iron status and cognitive abilities in young women of reproductive age—a group vulnerable to iron-deficiency. In this randomized, controlled trial, 152 women were assigned to one of three iron-status groups: iron sufficient (control group, CN); nonanemic, but with iron deficiency (ID group); or iron deficiency with anemia (IDA group). The groups were blinded to treatment with iron supplements or placebo. Significant improvements in serum ferritin following treatment were associated with a 5- to 7-fold improvement in cognitive performance, while faster completion of cognitive tasks was associated with significant improvements in hemoglobin levels (Murray-Kolb and Beard 2007).

Fatigue

Iron supplementation may reduce unexplained fatigue in nonanemic women. In a randomized, double-blind, placebo-controlled trial, 144 nonanemic women (aged 18 to 55 years, hemoglobin above 11.7 g/dL) with fatigue as a primary complaint were given placebo or long-acting ferrous sulfate providing 80 mg of elemental iron per day for 4 weeks. On a 10-point visual analog scale, fatigue scores at 1 month, relative to baseline, were reduced significantly more in the iron group than in the placebo group ($p=0.004$). After adjustments for age, depression and anxiety, and serum ferritin concentration, iron supplementation was the variable most associated with decrease in fatigue. Younger age was associated with a greater decrease in intensity of fatigue (Verdon et al 2003).

Iron-Deficiency Anemia

In adult and pediatric trials, both oral and intravenous iron supplementation were shown to overcome documented iron-deficiency anemia (Komolafe et al 2003; Shobha et al 2003; Kianfar et al 2000; Fridge et al 1998; Singh et al 1998). Athough an earlier study found that intravenous iron sucrose therapy was safer, more effective, and more convenient than oral ferrous sulfate in the treatment of severe anemia in pregnant women (Al-Momen et al 1996), a more recent trial reported equivalent short-term efficacy and overall tolerability with either route of administration. However, in this randomized, controlled study of anemic patients with inflammatory bowel disease (n=46), a better gastrointestinal tolerability for iron sucrose was observed (Schroder et al 2005). One large review found that levels of hemoglobin were consistently increased in iron-supplemented children who were anemic or had iron-deficient anemia at baseline (Iannotti et al 2006).

Prenatal Studies

A Cochrane review of the effects of oral iron supplementation with or without folic acid during pregnancy identified 40 trials for inclusion involving 12,706 women. An overall lack of data on clinical maternal and infant outcomes precluded the reviewers from making definitive conclusions regarding the effects of supplementation on these parameters. The types of treatments studied were four main regimens of daily or intermittent iron, with or without folic acid, compared to placebo or each other. Weekly (intermittent) supplementation appeared to be as effective at preventing low hemoglobin levels as daily dosing (Pena-Rosas and Viteri 2006). A randomized, controlled study published around the same time as the review enrolled pregnant women of less than 20 weeks' gestation and randomized 429 of those with adequate hemoglobin and ferritin levels to treatment with a multivitamin containing 30 mg of ferrous sulfate (n=218) or placebo (n=211). Mean birth weights increased by 108 g (p=.03) among the offspring of mothers receiving iron compared to the offspring of placebo-treated subjects. Additionally, the incidence of premature delivery was lower in the supplemented group compared to the control group (8% vs 14%; p=.05). These observations suggest a prophylactic role for iron supplementation started in early pregnancy beyond the commonly reported reduction of iron-deficiency anemia (Siega-Riz et al 2006).

Pediatric Studies

The frequency of breath-holding spells (BHS) diminished significantly in children with this disorder (n=33) given iron 5 mg/kg/day for 16 weeks compared with controls (n=34). Some 88% of those given iron had complete or partial responses compared with 6% in the placebo group (Daoud et al 1997). In another study, children receiving iron supplements showed improved autonomic cardiovascular control during sleep (eg, increased heart rate variability and reduced ratio of low-frequency/high-frequency powers) (Orii et al 2002).

INDICATIONS AND USAGE

Approved by the FDA:

- Iron-deficiency anemia (prophylaxis and treatment)

Unproven Uses: Limited research suggests that supplemental iron could be helpful for reducing the frequency of breath-holding spells in children. It may also enhance cognition in children and adolescents who have a documented iron deficiency. Likewise, iron may have some favorable effects on immunity and exercise performance—but again, these benefits are most likely limited to those with acute or borderline iron deficiency. Iron supplementation has also been used for the following: Plummer-Vinson syndrome, malaria, herpes simplex outbreaks, pediatric diarrhea, intestinal helminth infection, microcephaly prophylaxis, and decreased thyroid function during very-low-calorie diets.

CONTRAINDICATIONS

Iron supplements are contraindicated in patients with hemochromatosis and hemosiderosis. They are also contraindicated for treating anemias not caused by iron deficiency, such as hemolytic anemia or thalassemia, due to the risk of excess iron storage.

Parenteral preparations are not for subcutaneous administration. Sustained-release dosage forms should be avoided in patients who have conditions associated with intestinal strictures.

PRECAUTIONS

Treatment of iron-deficiency anemia must only be done under medical supervision. Iron supplements should be used with extreme caution in those with chronic liver failure, alcoholic cirrhosis, chronic alcoholism, and pancreatic insufficiency. Iron should also be used cautiously in those with a history of gastritis, peptic ulcer disease, and gastrointestinal bleeding. Patients with elevated serum ferritin levels should generally avoid iron supplements, as should those with an active or suspected infection.

In addition, patients should be aware that a moderate increase in iron stores has been associated with an increased risk of ischemic heart disease and cancer (Lynch et al 1996).

The most common side effects of iron supplements are gastrointestinal problems, including nausea, vomiting, bloating, abdominal discomfort, black stools, diarrhea, constipation, and anorexia. Enteric-coated iron preparations may prevent some of the gastrointestinal complaints associated with iron therapy. Temporary staining of teeth may occur from iron-containing liquids. Adverse effects from intramuscular iron injections include cutaneous pigmentation with iron deposits, sarcoma, nausea, vomiting, fever, chills, backache, headache, myalgia, malaise, and dizziness.

Pregnancy: FDA-rated as Pregnancy Category C. Pregnant women should not use supplemental doses of iron higher than RDA amounts (27 mg daily) unless their physician recommends it.

Breastfeeding: Nursing mothers should not use supplemental doses of iron higher than RDA amounts (9 or 10 mg daily, depending on age) unless their physician recommends it.

Pediatrics: Iron supplements can be highly toxic or lethal to small children. Those who take iron supplements should use childproof bottles and store them away from children.

Potential Supplement Interactions

Beta-carotene, l-cysteine, n-acetyl-l-cysteine: Using iron with these supplements may result in enhanced absorption of iron

Inositol hexphosphate, vanadium: Using iron with these supplements may result in decreased absorption of iron:

Copper: Using iron with copper may result in decreased copper status.

Tocotrienols, tocopherols (alpha-tocopherol, gamma-tocopherol, mixed tocopherols)): Concomitant use of iron and nonesterified tocopherols and tocotrienols, which are typically used in their nonesterified forms, may cause oxidation of tocotrienols and tocopherols.

Potential Food Interactions

Caffeine: Concomitant use may decrease the absorption of iron.

Dairy Foods: Concomitant use may decrease the absorption of iron.

Oxalic Acid (contained in spinach, sweet potatoes, rhubarb, beans): Concomitant use may decrease the absorption of iron.

Phytic Acid (contained in unleavened bread, raw beans, seeds, nuts and grains, soy isolates): Concomitant use may decrease the absorption of iron.

Teas and Other Tannin-Containing Herbs: Concomitant use may cause decrease the absorption of iron.

DRUG INTERACTIONS

MODERATE RISKS

Captopril: Concurrent use may result in decreased unconjugated captopril levels resulting in possible blood pressure elevations. *Clinical Management:* An alternative angiotensin converting enzyme (ACE) inhibitor may need to be prescribed to avoid interaction with iron preparations.

Cefdinir: Concurrent use may result in decreased cefdinir efficacy. *Clinical Management:* The administration of cefdinir and iron supplements or vitamins containing iron should be separated by at least 2 hours.

Enoxacin: Concurrent use may result in decreased enoxacin effectiveness. *Clinical Management:* Avoid concurrent use. However, if used concurrently, the dose of the iron salt should be given at least 6 hours before or 4 hours after the enoxacin dose.

Etidronate: Concurrent use may result in decreased etidronate absorption. *Clinical Management:* The administration of etidronate and iron or any supplement containing iron should be separated by at least 2 hours.

Levodopa: Concurrent use may result in decreased levodopa effectiveness. *Clinical Management:* If products containing iron, such as vitamins or iron supplements, are used in a patient receiving levodopa, monitor for an increase in Parkinson's disease symptoms. If symptoms worsen, consider adjusting the levodopa dose or avoiding iron-containing products, if possible.

Levothyroxine: Concurrent use may result in worsened hypothyroidism. *Clinical Management:* Separate the administration of iron salts and levothyroxine as much as possible. Monitor thyroid function tests.

Methyldopa: Concurrent use may result in decreased methyldopa effectiveness. *Clinical Management:* Monitor for decreased methyldopa efficacy if both drugs are administered concurrently.

Mycophenolate mofetil: Concurrent use may result in decreased mycophenolate mofetil efficacy. *Clinical Management:* The administration of mycophenolate mofetil and iron supplements or vitamins containing iron should be separated by at least 2 hours.

Penicillamine: Concurrent use may result in decreased penicillamine effectiveness. *Clinical Management:* If penicillamine and iron are used concurrently, separate administration of each by at least 2 hours.

Quinolones (ciprofloxacin, gatifloxacin, grepafloxacin, levofloxacin, lomefloxacin, moxifloxacin, norfloxacin, ofloxacin, sparfloxacin, temafloxacin, trovafloxacin): Concomitant use may decrease the absorption of both the quinolone and iron supplement. *Clinical Management*: If possible, avoid concurrent use. If both agents are administered together, separate doses by 2 to 6 hours before and 2 to 8 hours after, depending on dosing schedule.

Tetracyclines (demeclocycline, doxycycline, methacycline, minocycline, oxytetracycline, rolitetracycline, tetracycline): Concomitant use may decrease the absorption of both the tetracycline and iron supplement. *Clinical Management:* If both medicines must be used concurrently, iron salts should be given not less than three hours before or two hours after the tetracycline dose.

Trientine: Concurrent use may result in decreased gastrointestinal absorption of both drugs. *Clinical Management:* If it is necessary to administer iron supplements during trientine therapy, allow a minimum of 2 hours between administrations of each drug.

MINOR RISKS

Aluminum, calcium or magnesium containing products: Concomitant use may result in decreased iron effectiveness. *Clinical Management:* Concurrent administration of iron salts and aluminum, calcium, or magnesium containing products is not recommended. If concurrent use cannot be avoided, iron salts should be taken at least one hour before or two hours after aluminum, calcium or magnesium containing products.

Chloramphenicol: Concurrent use may result in decreased iron effectiveness.*Clinical Management:* Avoid chloramphenicol in patients receiving iron therapy for iron deficiency anemia.

Cholestyramine: Concurrent use may result in decreased iron effectiveness. *Clinical Management:* To prevent cholestyramine from binding dietary iron, separate administration of each drug by at least 4 hours.

Gossypol: Concurrent use may result in reduced iron absorption. *Clinical Management:* Increased iron dosage may be required by patients who take gossypol with iron supplements.

Proton Pump Inhibitors (PPIs) (esomeprazole, lansoprazole, omeprazole, pantoprazole, rabeprazole): Concurrent use may result in reduced iron bioavailability. *Clinical Management:* Monitor the patient for iron efficacy if a PPI is used concomitantly.

Zinc: Concurrent use may result in decreased gastrointestinal absorption of zinc and/or iron. *Clinical Management:* Separate administration of zinc and iron by at least 2 hours.

POTENTIAL INTERACTIONS

Acetohydroxamic Acid: Concurrent use may result in reduced absorption of both iron and acetohydroxamic acid.

Allopurinol: Concurrent use may result in increased liver iron stores.

Ascorbic Acid: Concurrent use may result in enhanced absorption of iron.

Bismuth Subcitrate: Concurrent use may result in decreased absorption of iron.

Calcium: Concurrent use may result in reduced iron absorption.

Cimetidine: Concurrent use may result in decreased iron effectiveness.

Colestipol: Concurrent use may result in decreased bioavailability of iron.

Pancreatin: Concurrent use may result in inhibition or iron absorption.

Sodium bicarbonate: Concurrent use may result in poor iron absorption.

Sulfasalazine: Concurrent use may result in a decrease in sulfasalazine concentration.

OVERDOSAGE

Acute iron overdose can be divided into four stages. In the first, which occurs up to 6 hours after ingestion, the principal symptoms are vomiting and diarrhea. Other symptoms include hypotension, tachycardia, and CNS depression ranging from lethargy to coma. The second phase may occur at 6 to 24 hours after ingestion and is characterized by a temporary remission. In the third phase, gastrointestinal symptoms recur accompanied by shock, metabolic acidosis, coma, hepatic necrosis and jaundice, hypoglycemia, renal failure, and pulmonary edema. The fourth phase may occur several weeks after ingestion and is characterized by gastrointestinal obstruction and liver damage.

In a young child, 75 mg/kg is considered extremely dangerous. A dose of 30 mg/kg can lead to symptoms of toxicity. The lethal dosage range is estimated at ≥ 180 mg/kg. A peak serum iron concentration of 5 mcg/mL or more is associated with moderate to severe poisoning.

DOSAGE

Mode of Administration: Intramuscular, oral

How Supplied: Capsule, elixir, suspension, tablet

Ferrous fumarate is available in the following forms and strengths:

Chewable tablets — 100 mg
Suspension — 100 mg/5 mL
Tablets — 200 mg, 300 mg, 325 mg, 350 mg

Ferrous gluconate is available in the following forms and strengths:

Enteric-coated tablets — 325 mg
Tablets — 300 mg, 320 mg, 324 mg, 325 mg

Ferrous sulfate is available in the following forms and strengths:

Capsules, extended-release — 250 mg
Enteric-coated tablets — 324 mg, 325 mg
Elixir — 220 mg/5 mL
Liquid — 75 mg/0.6 mL
Tablets — 195 mg, 300 mg, 324 mg, 325 mg

Exsiccated ferrous sulfate is available in the following forms and strengths:

Capsules — 150 mg, 159 mg
Enteric-coated tablets — 200 mg
Tablets — 200 mg
Tablet, extended-release — 160 mg

The following lists the elemental iron content of various forms:

Iron Salt % Iron
Ferrous fumarate 33
Ferrous gluconate 11.6
Ferrous sulfate 20
Ferrous sulfate, anhydrous 30

Daily Dosage: All doses are for oral administration unless otherwise note. Iron supplementation should be done only under a physician's supervision.

The following lists the Recommended Dietary Allowance (RDA) for iron:

Males and females — Infants to 6 months: 0.27 mg/d; *7 to 12 months:* 11 mg/d; *1 to 3 years:* 7 mg/d; *4 to 8 years:* 10 mg/d; *9 to 13 years:* 8 mg/d.

Males — 14 to 18 years: 11 mg/d; ≥ *19 years*: 8 mg/d

Females — 14 to 18 years: 15 mg/d; *19 to 50 years:* 18 mg/d; ≥ 51 years: 8 mg/d

Pregnancy — all ages: 27 mg/d

Lactation — 14 to 18 years: 10 mg/d; *19 to 50 years:* 9 mg/d

ADULTS

Decreased Thyroid Function During Very-Low-Calorie Diets: 9 mg/d or more to bring total iron intake to 1.5 times the RDA.

Impaired Athletic Performance: Treat only confirmed iron deficiency.

Inflammatory Bowel Disease: Treat only confirmed iron deficiency.

Iron-Deficiency Anemia (intramuscular injection): The total parenteral dose required for restoration of hemoglobin and body stores of iron can be approximated using the following formula: Adults and children over 15 kg: dose (mL) = 0.0442 (desired hemoglobin - observed hemoglobin) x lean body weight in kg + (0.26 x lean body weight in kg).

Iron Deficiency In Pregnancy: 60 to 100 mg/d.

Iron Insufficiency Therapy: immediate-release dosage forms: 2 to 3 mg/kg daily in 3 divided doses; sustained-release dosage forms: 50 to 100 mg daily.

Plummer-Vinson Syndrome: 2 to 3 mg/kg/d.

Prevention of Iron Deficiency in Pregnancy: 400 to 1,000 mg daily.

PEDIATRICS

Adolescent Girls With Low Ferritin: 105 to 260 mg daily.

Breath-Holding Syndrome (ferrous sulfate solution): 5 mg/kg daily.

Cognitive Function: 105 to 260 mg daily.

Iron Deficiency: 6 mg/kg/d for 2 to 3 months; absorption of iron is increased if given with a source of vitamin C.

Iron-Deficiency Anemia: *premature infants*, 2 to 4 mg/kg/d in 2 to 4 divided doses, up to a maximum of 15 mg/d; *children*, 3 to 6 mg/kg/d in 1 to 3 divided doses. *Intramuscular injection:* The total parenteral dose required for restoration of hemoglobin and body stores of iron can be approximated using the following formula: Children 5 to 15 kg: dose (mL) = 0.0442 (desired hemoglobin - observed hemoglobin) x weight in kg + (0.26 x weight in kg).

LITERATURE

Abdel-Salam G, Czeizel AE: A case-control etiologic study of microcephaly. *Epidemiology*; 11(5):571-575. 2000

Al-Momen A, Al-Meshari A, Al-Nuaim L et al: Intravenous iron sucrose complex in the treatment of iron deficiency anemia during pregnancy. *Eur J Obstet Gynecol*; 69:121-124. 1996

Anderson BD, Turchen SG, Manoguerra AS et al: Retrospective analysis of ingestions of iron containing products in the United States: are there differences between chewable vitamins and adult preparations? *J Emerg Med*; 19(3):255-258. 2000

Anon: NKF-DOQI clinical practice guidelines for the treatment of anemia of chronic renal failure. *Am J Kidney Dis*; 30:S137-S192. 1997

Anon: Routine iron supplementation during pregnancy: policy statement: US Preventive Task Force. *JAMA*; 270(23):2846-2848. 1993

Baker WF: Iron deficiency in pregnancy, obstetrics, and gynecology. *Hematol Oncol Clin North Am*; 14(5):1061-1077. 2000

Ballin A, Berar M, Rubinstein U et al: Iron state in female adolescents. *Am J Dis Child*; 146(7):803-805. 1992

Beard J, Borel M & Peterson FJ: Changes in iron status during weight loss with very-low-energy diets. *Am J Clin Nutr*; 66(1):104-110. 1997

Beard JL: Iron deficiency anemia: reexamining the nature and magnitude of the public health problem. *J Nutr*; 131:568S-580S. 2001

Brolin RE, Gorman JH, Gorman RC et al: Prophylactic iron supplementation after Roux-en-Y gastric bypass: a prospective, double-blind, randomized study. *Arch Surg*; 133:740-744. 1998

Bruner AB, Joffe A, Duffan AK: Randomized study of cognitive effects of iron supplementation in non-anemic iron-deficient adolescent girls. *Lancet*; 348(9033):992-996. 1996

Campbell NRC, Hasinoff BB: Iron supplements: a common cause of drug interactions. *Br J Clin Pharmacol*; 31(3):251-255. 1991

Cogswell ME, Parvanta I, Ickes L et al: Iron supplementation during pregnancy, anemia, and birth weight: a randomized controlled trial. *Am J Clin Nutr*; 78:773-781. 2003

Dantas RO & Villanova MG: Esophageal motility impairment in Plummer-Vinson syndrome: correction by iron treatment. *Dig Dis Sci*; 38(5):968-971. 1993

Daoud AS, Batieha A, Al-Sheyyab M et al: Effectiveness of iron therapy on breath-holding spells. *J Pediatr*; 130(4):547-550. 1997

Herrinton LJ, Friedman GD, Baer D, et al: Transferrin saturation and risk of cancer. *Am J Epidemiol*; 142(7):692-698. 1995

Hoffman RM, Jaffe PE: Plummer-Vinson syndrome: a case report and literature review. *Arch Intern Med*; 155(18):2008-2011. 1995

Horl WH, Cavill I, Macdougall IC et al: How to diagnose and correct iron deficiency during r-huEPO therapy — a consensus report. *Nephrol Dial Transplant*; 11(2):246-250. 1996

Hurrell RF: Bioavailability of iron. *Eur J Clin Nutr*; 51(suppl 1):S4-S8. 1997

Iannotti LL, Tielsch JM, Black MM, Black RE: Iron supplementation in early childhood: health benefits and risks. *Am J Clin Nutr*; 84:1261-1276. 2006

Kianfar H, Kimiagar M & Ghaffarpour M: Effect of daily and intermittent iron supplementation on iron status of high school girls. *Int J Vitam Nutr Res*; 70(4):172-177. 2000

Knekt P, Reunanen A, Takkunen H et al: Body iron stores and risk of cancer. *Int J Cancer*; 56(3):379-382. 1994

LaManca JJ & Haymes EM: Effects of iron repletion on VO2max, endurance, and blood lactate in women. *Med Sci Sports Exerc*; 25(12):1386-1392. 1993

Looker AC, Dallman PR, Carroll MD et al: Prevalence of iron deficiency in the United States. *JAMA*; 277(12):973-976. 1997

Lynch SR & Baynes RD: Deliberations and evaluations of the approaches, endpoints and paradigms for iron dietary recommendations. *J Nutr*; 126(9 suppl):2404S-2409S. 1996

Lynch SR: Interactions of iron with other nutrients. *Nutr Rev*; 55(4):102-110. 1997

Lynch SR: The effect of calcium on iron absorption. *Nutr Res Rev*; 13(2):141-158. 2000

Makrides M, Crowther CA, Gibson RA et al: Efficacy and tolerability of low-dose iron supplements during pregnancy: a randomized controlled trial. *Am J Clin Nutr*; 78:145-153. 2003

Makrides M, Leeson R, Gibson RA et al: A randomized controlled clinical trial of increased dietary iron in breast-fed infants. *J Pediatr*; 133:559-562. 1998

Meyers DG: The iron hypothesis: does iron play a role in atherosclerosis? *Transfusion*; 40(8):1023-1029. 2000

Metallinos-Katsaras, Valassi-Adam E, Dewey KG, et al: Effect of iron supplementation on cognition in Greek preschoolers. *Eur J Clin Nutr*; 58:1532-1542. 2004

Milman N, Bergholt T, Byg KE et al: Iron status and iron balance during pregnancy. A critical reappraisal of iron supplementation. *Acta Obstet Gynecol Scand*; 78(9):749-757. 1999

Murray-Kolb LE, Beard JL: Iron treatment normalizes cognitive functioning in young women. *Am J Clin Nutr* ; 85:778-787. 2007

Nelson RL: Iron and colorectal cancer risk: human studies. *Nutr Rev*; 59(5):140-148. 2001

Nishiyama S, Inomoto T, Nakamura T et al: Zinc status relates to hematological deficits in women endurance runners. *J Am Coll Nutr*; 15(4):359-363. 1996

Oppenheimer SJ: Iron and its relation to immunity and infectious disease. *J Nutr*; 131(2s-2):616S-635S. 2001

Orii KE, Kato Z, Osamu F et al: Changes of autonomic nervous system function in patients with breath-holding spells treated with iron. *J Child Neurol*; 17:337-340. 2002

Pena-Rosas JP, Viteri FE. Effects of routine oral iron supplementation with or without folic acid for women during pregnancy. *Cochrane Database of Systemic Reviews*; Issue 3. Art. No.: CD004736. 2006

Salonen JT, Nyyssonen K, Korpela H et al: High stored iron levels are associated with excess risk of myocardial infarction in eastern Finnish men. *Circulation*; 86(3):803-811. 1992

Schroder O, Mickisch O, Seidler U et al: Intravenous iron sucrose versus oral iron supplementation for the treatment of iron deficiency anemia in patients with inflammatory bowel disease—a randomized, controlled, open-label, multicenter study. *Am J Gastroenterol*; 100:2503-2509. 2005

Sempos CT, Looker AC, Gillum RF: Iron and heart disease: the epidemiologic data. *Nutr Rev*; 54(3):73-84. 1996

Shobha S & Sharada D: Efficacy of twice weekly iron supplementation in anemic adolescent girls. *Indian Pediatr*; 40:1186-1190. 2003

Siega-Riz AM, Hartzema AG, Turnbull C, et al: The effects of prophylactic iron given in prenatal supplements on iron status and birth outcomes: a randomized controlled trial. *Am J Obstet Gynecol*; 194:512-519. 2006

Stellon AJ & Kenwright SE: Iron deficiency anaemia in general practice: presentations and investigations. *Br J Clin Pract*; 51(2):78-80. 1997

Stevens RG, Graubard BI, Micozzi MS et al: Moderate elevation of body iron level and increased risk of cancer occurrence and death. *Int J Cancer*; 56(3):364-369. 1994

Tam DA, Rash FC: Breath-holding spells in a patient with transient erythroblastopenia of childhood. *J Pediatr*; 130(4):651-653. 1997

Tseng M, Sandler RS, Greenberg ER et al: Dietary iron and recurrence of colorectal adenomas. *Cancer Epidemiol Biomarkers Prev*; 6(12):1029-1032. 1997

Tzonou A, Lagiou P, Trichopoulou A et al: Dietary iron and coronary heart disease risk: a study from Greece. *Am J Epidemiol*; 147(2):161-166. 1998

Ullen H, Augustsson K, Gustavsson C et al: Supplementary iron intake and risk of cancer: reversed causality? *Cancer Lett*; 114(1-2):215-216. 1997

van Asperen IA, Feskens EJ, Bowles CH et al: Body iron stores and mortality due to cancer and ischaemic heart disease: a 17-year follow-up study of elderly men and women. *Int J Epidemiol*; 24(4):665-670. 1995

Verdon F, Burnand B, Fallab Stubi CL et al: Iron supplementation for unexplained fatigue in non-anaemic women: double blind randomised placebo controlled trial. *BMJ*; 326:1124-1126. 2003

Walter T, Olivares M, Pizarro F et al: Iron, anemia, infection. *Nutr Rev*; 55(4):111-124. 1997

Young YE, Koda-Kimble M: *Applied Therapeutics: The Clinical Use of Drugs*, 6th ed. Applied Therapeutics, Inc, Vancouver, WA; 1995.

Zhu YI, Haas JD: Iron depletion without anemia and physical performance in young women.

Lutein

DESCRIPTION

Lutein is a naturally occurring carotenoid used to improve eye health, especially in people with age-related macular degeneration (ARMD) and cataracts. Studies show that the retina selectively accumulates two carotenoids, lutein and its chemical cousin zeaxanthin. Within the central macula, zeaxanthin is the dominant component (up to 75%), whereas in the peripheral retina, lutein predominates (greater than 67%). The macular concentration of lutein and zeaxanthin is so high that they are visible as a dark yellow spot called the macular pigment. Because these carotenoids are powerful antioxidants and absorb blue light, researchers have hypothesized that they protect the retina. While both are abundant in green and yellow fruits and vegetables, lutein is the carotenoid most often used as a supplement. Dietary intake of lutein and zeaxanthin is estimated at 1 to 3 mg daily (Landrum et al 2001). Sources include spinach, collard greens, corn, kiwis, zucchini, pumpkins, squash, peas, cucumbers, green peppers, and egg yolks.

ACTIONS AND PHARMACOLOGY

EFFECTS

Lutein is an antioxidant that has immunostimulant and photoprotectant properties.

Immunomodulatory Effects: Animal studies show that lutein appears to modulate cellular and humoral-mediated immune responses. Cats supplemented with 10 mg of lutein daily for 12 weeks had significantly increased peripheral blood CD4+T and CD21+B lymphocytes compared to controls, suggesting that lutein affects cell surface marker expression (Kim et al 2000). Similar effects were found in a study of dogs treated for 12 weeks (Kim et al 2000). Lutein also stimulated phytohemagglutinin-induced lymphocyte proliferation in a small study of mice fed a semipurified diet with 0.1% and 0.4% lutein for 2 or 4 weeks (Chew et al 1996).

Photoprotective Effects: Lutein may protect against photooxidation because of its ability to absorb light, especially blue light. It may also provide photoprotection through its antioxidant effects, including the ability to scavenge free radicals/ reactive oxygen species and reduce peroxidation of membrane phospholipids (Beatty et al 2001; Landrum et al 2001; Mares-Perlman et al 2001).

CLINICAL TRIALS

Cancer Prevention

Daily dietary intake of lutein (5,921 mcg to more than 7,300 mcg) appears to be protective against various types of cancer. As revealed by logistic regression analysis, lutein/zeaxanthin intake of more than 7,300 mcg daily was associated with a 70% reduction in the risk for developing endometrial cancer compared with consumption of less than 3,501 mcg daily in a case-controlled study (McCann et al 2000). A multivariate risk analysis showed that the highest quintile intake of lutein (>5,921 mcg of lutein daily for women and 6,701 mcg daily for men) was associated with a nonsignificant 19% reduction in lung cancer risk compared with the lowest quintile intake, based on pooled results from two prospective United States cohort studies (Michaud et al 2000). In addition, lutein/zeaxanthin intake of >7,162 mcg daily was associated with a 53% reduction (p=0.001) in the risk of developing breast cancer compared with consumption of <3,652 mcg daily in a population-based case-controlled study of premenopausal women over age 40 (Freudenheim et al 1996).

Cataracts

Consumption of more than 2.4 mg of lutein/zeaxanthin daily from foods and supplements was significantly correlated with reduced incidence of nuclear lens opacities, as revealed from data collected during a 13- to 15-year period in the Nutrition and Vision Project (NVP). However, these results were insignificant after adjustment for other nutrients. The authors state that due to study limitations, an inverse relationship between lutein/zeaxanthin intake and nuclear lens opacities cannot be ruled out with certainty (Jacques et al 2001).

In a prospective cohort study of male healthcare professionals aged 45 to 75 years (n=36,664), men consuming the highest amounts of lutein and zeaxanthin had a 19% reduction in cataract development risk requiring extraction compared with men who had the lowest consumption. Subjects were followed from 1986 to 1994 or until cataract extraction, cancer, or death occurred. Eating vegetables high in lutein (broccoli and spinach) was also associated with reduced cataract development risk, but increased consumption of fruits and vegetables was not associated with a risk reduction, suggesting that the effect is specific to lutein (Brown et al 1999).

Macular Degeneration, Age-Related

The Lutein Antioxidant Supplementation Trial (LAST) examined the effect of lutein alone or in combination with antioxidants, vitamins and minerals on atrophic age-related macular degeneration (ARMD). This 12-month, randomized, double-masked, placebo-controlled trial enrolled 90 veterans from two veterans' medical facilities. Patients were randomized to three groups: Group 1 (n=29) received lutein 10 mg; Group 2 (n=30) received the combination of lutein 10 mg plus antioxidants/vitamins/minerals in a broad-spectrum formulation; Group 3 (n=31) received placebo. The objective was to note any improvements in visual function and symptoms related to supplementation with lutein.

Ophthalmic testing occurred at baseline and at 4, 8, and 12 months in all subjects. Measures included macular pigment optical density (MPOD), monocular visual acuity at distance, and contrast sensitivity function (CSF). By treatment end, improvements were noted in MPOD for both Groups 1 and 2: mean eye MPOD increased approximately 0.09 log units from baseline measures. Specifically, mean eye MPOD improved 36% in Group 1 and 43% in Group 2. MPOD was mildly decreased in the placebo group. Snellen equivalent visual acuity improved 5.4 letters for Group 1 and 3.5 for group 2; contrast sensitivity was improved in both groups. Subjects receiving placebo (Group 3) had no significant changes in any of the measured findings.

The investigators concluded that, in this study, lutein supplementation improved visual function. The authors point out that the sample included in the study was comprised mostly of male subjects (n=86), although the prevalence of ARMD is generally higher among older women. Therefore, larger studies with more female subjects are required to assess the long-term beneficial effects of lutein supplementation for the treatment of atrophic ARMD (Richer et al 2004).

On average, lutein and zeaxanthin concentrations in donor eyes from individuals with AMD were lower in the inner, medial, and outer areas of the retina than levels found in control eyes (n=112). Using the outer portion of the retina (considered a more reliable predictor of AMD), the risk of developing AMD after logistic regression analysis was 82% less in those with the highest concentrations of lutein/zeaxanthin compared to donors with the lowest concentrations (Bone et al 2001).

Intake of food high in carotenoids decreased neovascular AMD in a multicenter study of individuals with advanced AMD (n=356; aged 55 to 80 years) compared with matched controls (n=520). The researchers also controlled for smoking and other risk factors using multiple logistic regression analysis. Individuals with the highest intake of carotenoids had a 43% lower risk of developing AMD compared to individuals who consumed the lowest amount (p = 0.02). The strongest association was found between increased intake of lutein/zeaxanthin and reduced risk for AMD (p=0.001) (Seddon et al 1994).

However, in the third National Health and Nutrition Examination Survey of individuals over 40 years of age (n=8,222), dietary intake and serum levels of lutein/zeaxanthin were not inversely correlated with early or late AMD diagnosed by photographic evidence. Inverse relationships were noted in certain subgroups of the overall study group. Intake of lutein/zeaxanthin were inversely correlated with pigment abnormalities in at-risk individuals aged 40 to 59 and late AMD in at-risk individuals aged 60 to 79. A direct correlation was reported between intake of lutein/zeaxanthin and soft drusen (the most common type of early AMD). This finding was inconsistent with other evidence and may be due to increases in intake of fruits and vegetables as a result of diagnosed retinal abnormalities (Mares-Perlman et al 2001).

Retinitis Pigmentosa

A double-masked, randomized, placebo-controlled phase I/II clinical trial examined the effect of lutein supplementation in patients with retinitis pigmentosa (RP). The primary objective was to observe the effect of lutein in preserving visual function. The study employed a crossover design: 34 adult subjects with RP were randomized to two groups. One group (n=16) was randomized to treatment with lutein for the first 24 weeks (10 mg/day for 12 weeks followed by 30 mg/day for 12 weeks) before switching to placebo for another 24 weeks. The other group (n=18) was randomized to placebo for the initial 24 weeks prior to receiving the lutein regimen for the remaining 24 weeks. By treatment end, the investigators observed a statistically significant effect of lutein on visual field ($p = 0.038$); this effect increased in a model assuming a 6-week delay in the effect of lutein supplementation. These results suggest that lutein supplementation in patients with RP improves visual field and may lead to slight improvements in visual acuity (Bahrami et al 2006).

INDICATIONS AND USAGE

Unproven Uses: Increased consumption of lutein may prevent, delay, or modify the course of age-related macular degeneration, although conclusive evidence is not available. Lutein has also been used to help prevent or treat various cancers, including breast, ovarian, endometrial, lung, and prostate. Some advocates have promoted lutein as a general antiaging supplement.

PRECAUTIONS AND ADVERSE REACTIONS

No data on side effects is available.

Scientific evidence for the safe use of Lutein during pregnancy and breast-feeding is not available.

DRUG INTERACTIONS

No human drug interaction information is available.

DOSAGE

Mode of Administration: Oral

How Supplied: Capsule

Daily Dosage: For prevention of macular degeneration, the standard supplemental dose is 10 mg daily (Berendschot et al 2000). For cancer prevention, a daily dietary intake of 5,921 mcg to more than 7,300 mcg appears to be protective against various types of cancer (McCann et al 2000, Michaud et al 2000; Freudenheim et al 1996).

LITERATURE

Bahrami H, Melia M, Dagnelie G: Lutein supplementation in retinits pigmentosa: PC-based vision assessment in a randomized double-masked placebo-controlled clinical trial [NCT000299289]. *BMC Ophthalmol*; 6:23. 2006

Beatty S, Murray IJ, Henson DB et al: Macular pigment and risk for age-related macular degeneration in subjects from a northern European population. *Invest Ophthalmol Vis Sci*; 42(2):439-446. 2001

Berendschot TTJM, Goldbohm RA, Klopping WAA et al: Influence of lutein supplementation on macular pigment, assessed with two objective techniques. *Invest Ophthalmol Vis Sci*; 41(11):439-446. 2000

Bone RA, Landrum JT, Dixon Z et al: Lutein and zeaxanthin in the eyes, serum and diet of human subjects. *Exp Eye Res*; 71(3):239-245. 2000

Bone RA, Landrum JT, Mayne ST et al: Macular pigment in donor eyes with and without AMD: a case-control study. *Invest Ophthalmol Vis Sci*; 42(1):235-240. 2001

Brown L, Rimm EB, Seddon JM et al: A prospective study of carotenoid intake and risk of cataract extraction in US men. *Am J Clin Nutr*; 70(4):517-524. 1999

Chew BP, Wong MW, Wong TS: Effects of lutein from marigold extract on immunity and growth of mammary tumors in mice. *Anticancer Res*; 16(6B):3689-3694. 1996

Freudenheim JL, Marshall JR, Vena JE et al: Premenopausal breast cancer risk and intake of vegetables, fruits, and related nutrients. *J Natl Cancer Inst*; 88(6):340-348. 1996

Hammond BR, Johnson EJ, Russell RM et al: Dietary modification of human macular pigment density. *Invest Ophthalmol Vis Sci*; 38(9):1795-1801. 1997

Hankinson SE, Stampfer MJ, Seddon JM et al: Nutrient intake and cataract extraction in women: a prospective study. *BMJ*; 305(6849):335-339. 1992

Jacques PF, Chylack LT, Hankinson SE et al: Long-term nutrient intake and early age-related nuclear lens opacities. *Arch Ophthalmol*; 119(7):1009-1019. 2001

Johnson EJ, Hammond BR, Yeum KJ et al: Relation among serum and tissue concentrations of lutein and zeaxanthin and macular pigment density. *Am J Clin Nutr*; 71(6):1555-1562. 2000

Kim HW, Chew BP, Wong TS et al: Dietary lutein stimulates immune response in the canine. *Vet Immunol Immunopathol*; 74(3-4):315-327. 2000

Kim HW, Chew BP, Wong TS et al: Modulation of humoral and cell-mediated immune responses by dietary lutein in cats. *Vet Immunol Immunopathol*; 73(3-4):331-341. 2000

Landrum JT, Bone RA: Lutein, zeaxanthin, and the macular pigment. *Arch Biochem Biophysc*; 385(1):28-40. 2001

Mares-Perlman JA, Brady WE, Klein R et al: Serum antioxidants and age-related macular degeneration in a population-based case-control study. *Arch Ophthalmol*; 113(12):1518-1523. 1995

Mares-Perlman JA, Fisher AI, Klein R et al: Lutein and zeaxanthin in the diet and serum and their relation to age-related maculopathy in the third national health and nutrition examination survey. *Am J Epidemiol*; 153(5):424-432. 2001

McCann SE, Freudenheim JL, Marshall JR et al: Diet in the epidemiology of endometrial cancer in western New York (United States). *Cancer Causes Control*; 11(10):965-974. 2000

Michaud DS, Feskanich D, Rimm EB et al: Intake of specific carotenoids and risk of lung cancer in 2 prospective US cohorts. *Am J Clin Nutr*; 72(4):990-997. 2000

Olmedilla B, Granado F, Gil-Martinez E et al: Supplementation with lutein (4 months) and alpha-tocopherol (2 months), in separate or combined oral doses, in control men. *Cancer Lett*; 114(1-2):179-181. 1998

Richer S, Stiles W, Statkute L, et al: Double-masked, placebo-controlled, randomized trial of lutein and antioxidant supplementation in the intervention of atrophic age-related macular degeneration: the Veterans LAST study (Lutein Antioxidant Supplementation Trial). *Optometry*; 75:216-230. 2004

Seddon JM, Ajani UA, Sperduto RD et al: Dietary carotenoids, vitamins A, C, and E, and advanced age-related macular degeneration. Eye Disease Case-Control Study Group. *JAMA*; 272(18):1413-1420. 1994

Sommerburg O, Keunen JEE, Bird AC et al: Fruits and vegetables that are sources for lutein and zeaxanthin: the macular pigment in human eyes. *Br J Ophthalmol*; 82(8):907-910. 1998

van het Hof KH, West CE, Weststrate JA et al: Dietary factors that affect the bioavailability of carotenoids. *J Nutr*; 130(3):503-506. 2000

Lysine

DESCRIPTION

Lysine is an essential amino acid involved in many biological processes, including receptor affinity, protease-cleavage points, retention of endoplasmic reticulum, nuclear structure and function, muscle elasticity, and chelation of heavy metals. Like other amino acids, the metabolism of free lysine follows two principal paths, protein synthesis and oxidative catabolism. It is required for biosynthesis of such substances as carnitine, collagen, and elastin. Because the body cannot manufacturer lysine, it must be provided in the diet. Lysine is found mostly in protein-rich food such as beef, pork, fish, poultry, eggs, and dairy products. Grain and cereal products are usually poor sources of lysine, with the exception of wheat germ and brewer's yeast. The terms L-lysine and lysine are used interchangeably. The D-stereoisomer (D-lysine) is not biologically active.

Supplemental lysine has been used with varying success to treat and prevent outbreaks of herpes simplex virus (Flodin 1997). Lysine also appears to increase the absorption of calcium in women with osteoporosis (Civitelli et al 1992). Intravenous lysine acetylsalicylate has been useful in treating pain due to rheumatoid arthritis, surgery, migraine headache, dental ailments, and renal colic (Limmroth et al 1999). Because of its role in muscle repair, lysine supplements are sometimes used by athletes and bodybuilders.

Other Names: 2,6-diaminohexanoic acid, alpha-epsilon-diaminocaproic acid, L-lysine, lysine hydrochloride, lysine monohydrochloride

ACTIONS AND PHARMACOLOGY

EFFECTS

Lysine appears to have antiviral, anti-osteoporotic, cardiovascular, and lipid-lowering effects, although more controlled human studies are needed.

Anti-Osteoporotic Effects: Improving the biological value of protein with supplemental lysine may improve utilization of dietary calcium, perhaps by enhancing production of one of the calcium-binding proteins by enterocytes (Flodin 1997).

Antiviral Effects: Lysine demonstrated antiviral action when introduced in vitro to green monkey kidney cells inoculated with approximately 500 plaque-forming units (PFU) of herpes simplex virus (Griffith et al 1981). Human research suggests that adequate serum levels of lysine inhibit the virus, although results are contradictory (Griffith et al 1987; Simon et al 1985; DiGiovanna et al 1985; Thein et al 1984; DiGiovanna et al 1984).

Blood Lipid Effects: Decreased cholesterol and triglyceride levels have been documented in humans and rats given oral L-lysine monochloride. The increased biological value of dietary protein resulting from lysine supplementation may leave fewer amino acids in the digestive tract for conversion to cholesterol and triglycerides (Flodin 1997).

Cardiovascular Effects: Limited human and animal studies suggest that a high-lysine diet or L-lysine monochloride supplements may have a moderating effect on blood pressure and the incidence of stroke (Flodin 1997).

CLINICAL TRIALS

Acute Migraine Attack

A randomized, double-blind, parallel-group phase II study comparing the efficacy and tolerability of intravenous (IV) valproate (iVPA) with IV lysine-acetylsalicylic acid (iLAS) in acute migraine attacks concluded that although both were effective, there was a trend in favor of iLAS. Forty patients with acute migraine attacks alternately received iVPA 800 mg and iLAS 1000 mg. The primary outcome measures were the percentage of patients who reported pain relief after 1 hour and those who remained pain-free for 24 hours after treatment. Percentage of pain relief after 1 hour was 25% in the iVPA group and 30% in the iLAS group. Pain relief was sustained for 24 hours in 20% of the iVPA group and in 30% of the iVLAS group. Associated migrainous symptoms were improved with both treatments, without significant differences over the course of 24 hours; however, a trend favoring iLAS was observed (Leniger et al 2005).

An earlier randomized, double-blind, crossover trial in 56 patients with acute migraine (112 attacks total) compared pain relief with intravenous L-lysine-monoacetylsalicylate (LAS) 1,000 mg and subcutaneous ergotamine 0.5 mg. Both agents achieved similar headache relief after 120 minutes; however, LAS showed significantly faster pain relief (p=0.017), probably due to IV administration. By 120 minutes after drug administration, 68% of patients treated with LAS and 59% treated with ergotamine reported improvement in nausea and vomiting. Photophobia and phonophobia improved in 68% of LAS-treated patients and 54% of ergotamine-treated patients (Limmroth et al 1999).

Anxiety

The results of a recently published, randomized double-blind, placebo-controlled trial suggest that oral treatment with a combined regimen of L-lysine and L-arginine reduces anxiety and basal cortisol levels in healthy human subjects. The investigators studied the effect of the oral dosage (2.64 g/day for each, administered over 1 week) in 108 Japanese adults. The combined regimen was found to reduce both trait anxiety and state anxiety induced by cognitive stress in both genders. Men in the study were also observed to have reduced basal levels of salivary cortisol and chromogranin-A, a salivary marker of the sympatho-adrenal system (Smriga et al 2007).

These findings are in line with an earlier randomized, double-blind, placebo-controlled study in which 29 healthy subjects were administered a mixture of L-lysine and L-arginine (3 g/day each) for 10 days. Subjects were all at the upper limit of the normal range on a scale measuring trait anxiety, and were challenged with a psychological stress procedure based on public speaking following administration of the amino acid mixture. Post-treatment, enhanced levels of adrenocorticotropic hormone, cortisol, adrenaline and nonadrenaline, and galvanic skin responses were noted, as compared to the placebo group. These findings suggest that the combined regimen modifies hormonal responses to psychological stress in humans (Jezova et al 2005).

Herpes Simplex Virus (HSV)

Lysine was superior to placebo in treating HSV in a randomized, double-blind, placebo-controlled study involving 114 patients (42% had genital herpes, 44% facial-oral herpes, and 14% had both). Subjects were randomly assigned to receive 500 milligrams of L-lysine or placebo; subjects were instructed to take 2 tablets three times daily with meals and to record any occurrences of herpes outbreaks. After 6 months of treatment with lysine, the frequency of HSV attacks was nearly half the amount experienced in the previous year. In the lysine group, 63% reported improved symptoms, 8% reported worse symptoms, and 29% experienced no change. In the placebo group, 36% reported improved symptoms, 16% reported worse symptoms, and 48% reported no change. In the group taking lysine, 74% rated their treatment as effective or very effective compared to 28% of the placebo group (Griffith et al 1987).

Osteoporosis

Two studies by Civitelli and colleagues suggested a potential benefit of supplemental lysine for increasing calcium absorption in women with and without osteoporosis. The first trial enrolled 15 women with diagnosed osteoporosis and 15 women without the condition. All subjects were given 3 g of calcium with or without 400 mg of lysine. Serum calcium levels significantly increased in both groups regardless of the addition of L-lysine. However, in the non-osteoporotic control group taking lysine, urinary excretion of calcium was decreased, suggesting an interruption of calcium excretion. In the second study, 45 postmenopausal women with diagnosed osteoporosis were given a blind compound containing 800 mg of lysine, valine, or tryptophan to be taken daily for 3 consecutive days. After 3 days of treatment, intestinal calcium absorption was significantly increased in the lysine group ($p<0.01$), while calcium absorption did not change in the groups taking valine or tryptophan (Civitelli et al 1992).

Post-Surgical Pain

A double-blind study compared the effectiveness of a continuous intravenous infusion of lysine acetyl salicylate (LAS) with an infusion of morphine for the treatment of pain following pulmonary surgery. Mean pain scores in the two groups were not significantly different at any stage during the 24-hour period after anesthesia wore off. LAS was not associated with any significantly greater blood loss in the period after surgery. The incidence of drowsiness, nausea and vomiting, and the need for antiemetic medication were similar in both groups (Jones et al 1985).

INDICATIONS AND USAGE

Unproven Uses: The most popular use of supplemental lysine is for preventing and treating episodes of herpes simplex virus. Lysine has been used in conjunction with calcium to prevent and treat osteoporosis. It has also been used for treating pain, migraine attacks, rheumatoid arthritis, and opiate withdrawal.

CONTRAINDICATIONS

Patients who have kidney or liver disease should not use lysine.

PRECAUTIONS AND ADVERSE REACTIONS

Patients with hypercholesterolemia should be aware that supplemental lysine has been linked to increased cholesterol levels in animal studies (Kritchevsky et al 1984; Leszczynski et al 1982). However, other studies have shown lysine can also decrease cholesterol levels (Flodin 1997).

DRUG INTERACTIONS

MAJOR RISKS

Aminoglycoside Antibiotics: Concurrent use of Lysine and aminoglycosides may result in an increased risk of nephrotoxocity. *Clinical Management:* Avoid use of lysine with aminoglycoside antibiotics if possible. If both agents are used, monitor renal function closely.

OVERDOSAGE

Research indicates that individuals who eat a balanced American diet can safely ingest up to 3 g/day of lysine, divided and taken with meals, as a long-term supplement. Until more data are available, dosages exceeding 3 g/day should be monitored by a physician (Flodin 1997).

DOSAGE

Mode of Administration: Intramuscular, intravenous, oral

How Supplied: Capsule, powder, solution, tablet

Daily Dosage:

ADULTS

Herpes Simplex Virus: 1 to 3 g daily, divided and taken with meals (Flodin 1997).

Migraine Headache: Oral sachet of lysine acetylsalicylate 1,620 mg plus metoclopramide 10 mg (Pradalier et al 1999); intravenous solution of D,L-lysine-monoacetylsalicylate 1,000 mg (Limmroth et al 1999).

Opiate Detoxification (intravenous solution): Lysine acetylsalicylate 80 mg/kg/day for 2 days; then 50 mg/kg/day for 2 days; and then orally for 5 more days at 1,800 mg/day (Vescovi et al 1984).

Osteoporosis Prophylaxis (tablet or capsule): Lysine 400 to 800 mg daily taken with calcium (Civitelli et al 1992).

Post-Surgical Pain (intravenous solution): Lysine acetylsalicylate 1.8 g over 5 minutes followed by a 24-hour infusion, for a total administered dose of 7.2 g (Jones et al 1985).

CHILDREN

Hyperargininemia (oral): Lysine 250 mg/kg/day with ornithine 100 mg/kg/day (Kang et al 1983).

Storage: Store at room temperature, away from heat, moisture, and direct light.

LITERATURE

Civitelli R, Villareal DT, Agnusdei D et al: Dietary l-lysine and calcium metabolism in humans. *Nutrition*; 8(6):400-405. 1992

DiGiovanna JJ, Blank H: Failure of lysine in frequently recurrent herpes simplex infection. *Arch Dermatol*; 120:48-51. 1984

DiGiovanna JJ, Wesley MN, Blank H: Reply (letter). *Arch Dermatol*; 121:167-168. 1985

Fico ME, Hassan AS, Milner JA: The influence of excess lysine on urea cycle operation and pyrimidine biosynthesis. *J Nutr*; 112:1854-1861. 1982

Flodin NW: The metabolic roles, pharmacology and toxicology of lysine. *J Am Coll Nutr*; 16(1):7-21. 1997

Griffith RS, Walsh DE, Myrmel KH et al: Success of l-lysine in frequently recurrent herpes simplex infection. *Dermatologica*; 175(4):183-190. 1987

Jezova D, Makatsori A, Smriga M, et al: Subchronic treatment with amino acid mixture of L-lysine and L-arginine modifies neuroendocrine activation during psychosocial stress in subjects with high trait anxiety. *Nutr Neurosci*. 8(3):155-160. 2005

Jones RM, Cashman JN, Foster JMG et al: Comparison of infusions of morphine and lysine acetyl salicylate for the relief of pain following thoracic surgery. *Br J Anaesth*; 57:259-263. 1985

Kagan C: Failure of lysine? *Arch Dermatol*; 121:21. 1985

Kang S-S, Wong PWK, Melyn MA: Effect of ornithine and lysine supplementation. *J Pediatr*; 103(5):763-765. 1983

Kritchevsky D, Weber MM, Klurfeld DM: Gallstone formation in hamsters: influence of specific amino acids. *Nutr Rep Int*; 29(1):117-121. 1984

Leniger T, Pageler L, Stude P et al: Comparison of intravenous valproate with intravenous lysine-acetylsalicylic acid in acute migraine attacks. *Headache*; 45(1):42-46. 2005

Leszczynski DE, Kummerow FA: Excess dietary lysine induces hypercholesterolemia in chickens. *Experientia*; 38(38):266-267. 1982

Limmroth V, May A, Diener H-C: Lysine-acetylsalicylic acid in acute migraine attacks. *Eur Neurol*; 41:88-93. 1999

Pradalier A, Chabriat H, Danchot J et al: Safety and efficacy of combined lysine acetylsalicylate and metoclopramide: Repeated intakes in migraine attacks. *Headache*; 39:125-131. 1999

Racusen LC, Whelton A, Solez K: Effects of lysine and other amino acids on kidney structure and function in the rat. *Am J Pathol*; 120(3):436-442. 1985

Roby KA, Segal S: Cystine and lysine reabsorption in the isolated perfused rat kidney. *Am J Physiol*; 256(suppl F):F901-F908. 1989

Simon CA, Van Melle GD, Ramelet AA et al: Failure of lysine in frequently recurrent herpes simplex infection. *Arch Dermatol*; 121:167. 1985

Smriga M, Ando T, Akutsu M et al: Oral treatment with L-lysine and L-arginine reduces anxiety and basal cortisol levels in healthy humans. *Biomed Res*. 28(2):85-90. 2007

Thein DJ, Hurt WC: Lysine as a prophylactic agent in the treatment of recurrent herpes simplex labialis. *Oral Surg Oral Med Oral Pathol*; 58(6):659-666. 1984

Vescovi PP, Donati C, Gerra G et al: Heroin detoxification by lysine acetylsalicylate. *Curr Ther Res*; 35(5):826-831. 1984

Magnesium

DESCRIPTION

Magnesium is an essential mineral. Average daily intakes of dietary magnesium have declined in recent years due to processing of food. The average daily intake has been estimated to be approximately 300 to 360 mg. Some experts suggest an increased daily intake of 440 to 490 mg, especially if the patient is pregnant, taking potent loop diuretics, or rarely eating a well-balanced meal containing green leafy vegetables, legumes, nuts, or animal protein (Whang et al, 1994).

Magnesium sulfate is used for replacement therapy for hypomagnesemia; in total parenteral nutrition to correct or prevent deficiencies; to control or prevent seizures in preeclampsia; and in the oral form as a cathartic. Magnesium may also be effective in treating certain cardiac arrhythmias, in asthma when unresponsive to other treatments, during alcohol withdrawal, and for ischemic heart disease.

Patients with congestive heart failure often take medications that may deplete magnesium to the extent that arrhythmias occur or are worsened. Magnesium therapy has inconsistent effects on hypertension, but should be considered in those at risk of deficiency, including women and patients taking magnesium-depleting medications.

The scope of this discussion will be limited to the oral formulations.

ACTIONS AND PHARMACOLOGY

EFFECTS

Magnesium is said to exhibit anti-osteoporotic activity; anti-arrhythmic, antihypertensive, glucose regulatory, bronchodilator. It is an electrolyte, a nutrient, and a mineral.

Magnesium is important as a cofactor in many enzymatic reactions in the body (Gilman et al, 1990; Havel et al,1989). There are at least 300 enzymes that are dependent upon magnesium for normal functioning. Actions on lipoprotein lipase have been found to be important in reducing serum cholesterol (Davis et al, 1984). Magnesium is necessary for maintaining serum potassium and calcium levels due to its effect on the renal tubule (Rasmussen et al, 1988).

In the heart magnesium acts as a calcium channel blocker. It also activates sodium-potassium ATPase in the cell membrane to promote resting polarization and reduce arrhythmias (Shattock et al, 1987).

CLINICAL TRIALS

Diabetes

According to a recent meta-analysis, supplementation with oral magnesium (Mg) may be effective in reducing plasma glucose levels, although it was not shown to produce significant reductions in levels of glycated hemoglobin (HbA_{1C}). Nine randomized, double-blind, controlled studies including 370 patients with type 2 diabetes were identified for inclusion in the review. The median dose of supplemental Mg was 360 mg/day in the groups receiving active treatment. Although no significant differences were observed between groups in post-intervention HbA1c after a median term of 12 weeks, the weighted mean post-intervention fasting glucose was significantly lower in the treatment groups vs the control groups (—0.56 mmol/l; p for heterogeneity = 0.02). The reviewers conceded that since most of the studies cited in the meta-analysis were short-term trials, the results provided may underestimate the actual effect of magnesium supplementation on long-term glycemic control. Additional large-scale trials of longer duration are therefore warranted. (Song et al, 2006)

High doses of magnesium significantly reduced plasma fructosamine in type 2 diabetics, but did not affect fasting glucose or HbA1c; half of that dose was without effect on any of those parameters. In a randomized, double-blind trial, 128 type 2 diabetics with poor glycemic control while being treated by diet or diet plus hypoglycemic drugs were given placebo, magnesium (as MgO) 20.7 mmol/day, or Mg 41.4 mmol/day for 30 days. Before supplementation, 31% of subjects had low intramononuclear Mg levels, compared to a control group of blood donors. In the 29 patients with peripheral neuropathy, intracellular Mg was significantly lower ($p<0.05$) than in those without it. After 30 days, no change in plasma or intracellular Mg or improvement in glycemic control was evident in the placebo group or the lower dose Mg group. In the higher dose Mg group, fructosamine fell from 4.1 to 3.8 mmol ($p<0.05$) and urinary Mg increased. There were no significant changes in plasma or intracellular Mg, HbA1, or fasting glucose (Lima et al, 1998).

Three months of magnesium supplementation 15 mmol/day did not improve glycemic control in insulin-requiring type 2 diabetics. Fifty patients who were not necessarily hypomagnesemic but had used insulin for at least 6 months were randomized to receive magnesium as Mg-asparate-HCl or placebo. Plasma Mg concentration and urinary Mg excretion were significantly higher in the Mg group than in the placebo group after 3 months' treatment ($p<0.05$ and $p=0.004$, respectively), but there were no differences between the groups in plasma glucose, HbA1c, plasma cholesterol, or plasma triglycerides (de Valk et al, 1998).

A randomized, double-blind, cross-over study was conducted to assess effects of magnesium in noninsulin-dependent diabetes. Patients with type 2 diabetes (n=9) treated by diet only received either 15.8 mmol Mg daily or a placebo for 4 weeks. Serum levels were measured after each treatment period. Increased plasma Mg levels, total body glucose disposal ($p<0.005$) and glucose oxidation ($p<0.01$) were observed with Mg supplementation (Paolisso et al, 1994).

A randomized, double-blind, placebo-controlled study was done to assess effects of magnesium treatment in type 2 diabetes. Patients with type 2 diabetes (n=40) were given 30 mmol Mg daily or a placebo for 3 months. Serum and urine measurements were done at the beginning, and at 2 and 3 months. Plasma Mg levels increased after the 3-month treatment but declined to pretreatment levels after 6 months (Eibl et al, 1995).

Hypertension

Uncertainty remains as to the clinical utility of supplemental magnesium for controlling blood pressure (BP). A recent Cochrane review of the effectiveness of magnesium supplementation for the management of primary hypertension in adults identified 12 randomized, controlled trials (total n=545) for inclusion. Combined trial results from hypertensive subjects receiving magnesium showed no significant reductions in systolic BP as compared to controls. Although small, significant reductions in diastolic BP were noted in those receiving magnesium, the reduction was small (2.2 mm Hg) and may not last beyond 26 weeks. Lacking a clear, sustained effect on BP, the reviewers concluded that evidence from the trials was not strong enough to establish an association between magnesium supplementation and BP reduction. Additionally, they state that the reduction in diastolic BP may be the result of bias. Larger, randomized, double-blind, placebo-controlled studies with longer follow-up are needed (Dickinson et al, 2007).

An earlier meta-analysis of randomized studies investigating the effects of magnesium supplementation on BP showed a dose-dependent effect. Twenty trials (total n=1,220), including 14 trials with hypertensive subjects, met inclusion criteria, including randomization, use of a control group, magnesium as the sole treatment, and sufficient data to calculate the difference in BP change between the active and control treatments. The dose of magnesium varied from 10 to 40 mmol/day. For every 10-mmol increase in daily Mg intake, there was a reduction in systolic BP of 4.3 mm Hg ($p<0.001$) and in diastolic BP 2.3 mm Hg ($p=0.09$). This result still remains to be confirmed by adequately powered trials (Jee et al, 2002).

However, in the Cochrane review by Dickinson noted above, several limitations to the meta-analysis by Jee are noted, including the fact that it was not restricted to trials involving hypertensive populations, nor did it exclude trials in which subjects received various antihypertensive medications during the trials. Some studies included in the meta-analysis by Jee had less than 8 weeks of follow-up, hindering observations on sustained effects. Nevertheless, both the meta-analysis by Jee and the Cochrane review by Dickinson are consistent in one regard: the finding that overall, magnesium supplementation had little effect on the BP of subjects with hypertension.

Migraine

A recent review of natural or alternative treatments for prevention of migraine cited one randomized, double-blind, placebo-controlled trial that showed no significant superiority of magnesium over placebo. In this study of children aged 3 to 17 years, active treatment consisted of daily magnesium oxide 9 mg/kg in three divided doses. Among the subjects completing the study (about 75%), a significant downward trend in headache days was observed in the active treatment (magnesium) group vs placebo; however, the lack of any difference in the slope of treatment trends precluded the authors from making any claims of significant superiority for magnesium(Evans and Taylor, 2006).

Oral magnesium was effective in reducing the frequency of migraine headaches in an earlier 12-week, multicenter, placebo-controlled, double-blind study. Of 81 patients, 43 were administered magnesium 600 mg (24 mmol) (trimagnesium dicitrate) every day for 12 weeks and 38 were given placebo. After 9 weeks of therapy, the average frequency of attacks was reduced in the Mg-treated group compared with the placebo-treated group (41.6% vs 15.8%, $p=0.03$) and compared with baseline ($p=0.04$). The number of days with migraine was also reduced in the Mg group (52.3%) compared with placebo (19.5%) ($p=0.03$). The average duration of attack, pain intensity, and amount of acute medication required per person were also reduced in the treatment group compared with placebo; these differences were not statistically significant. The major adverse events reported consisted of diarrhea and gastric irritation (Peikert et al, 1996).

A similarly designed study showed no difference between magnesium and placebo treatment in prevention of migraine. Sixty-nine patients with confirmed history of migraine without aura were randomly assigned to a 12-week treatment of either 20 mmol Mg-L-aspartate-hydrochloride twice daily (n=35) or an identical-appearing placebo (n=34). Responders were identified as those with a 50% reduction in the duration of migraine in hours or in the intensity of migraine at the end of the third month of treatment in comparison to baseline values. There were 10 responders in each group; specifically, the responder rate was 28.6% in the group receiving magnesium and 29.4% in subjects receiving placebo. There was no difference between groups in the absolute number of migraine days or the number of migraine attacks during the study. Although physicians' assessments of efficacy were nearly the same for the two treatments, 33% of the magnesium group and only 11% of the placebo group regarded the study medication to be superior to previously used migraine prophylactics. The authors mentioned that some patients started using sumatriptan to treat migraine attacks; this may have biased outcomes. They recommended that future studies provide a standardized scheme for treatment of attacks during the study (Pfaffenrath et al, 1996).

Osteoporosis

Magnesium supplementation was associated with accrual of bone mass in one study. A small cohort of healthy 8- to 14-year-old girls with suboptimal intakes of dietary magnesium was enrolled in this randomized, placebo-controlled study. Girls were assigned to 12 months of treatment with either 300 mg/day supplemental magnesium (n=23) or placebo (n=27). By treatment end, significantly increased accrual in integrated hip bone mineral content (BMC) was observed in the magnesium-supplemented group compared with placebo ($p=0.05$), an approximate 3% increase compared with baseline measurements. A slightly greater, though not statistically significant, mean incremental gain in spinal BMC was noted in the magnesium-supplemented group as well (Carpenter et al, 2006).

A cross-sectional analysis was conducted to assess dietary components in bone mineral density (BMD). Cohorts in a heart study were analyzed for changes in BMD and dietary intake. Baseline BMDs were obtained in individuals (n=628) and dietary intake was assessed by questionnaires. Changes in a 4-year period were analyzed in BMD. Greater magnesium intake was associated with a lesser decline in BMD (Tucker et al, 1999).

Patients with gluten-sensitive enteropathy (sprue) and associated osteoporosis showed increases in BMD after 2 years of magnesium therapy. Five patients took magnesium 504 to 576 mg daily, as either Mg chloride or Mg lactate, for 2 years. Erythrocyte magnesium concentrations rose from 137 microM at baseline to 193 microM at 2 years ($p<0.02$) (normal 202 ± 6 microM). Serum parathyroid hormone rose from 37 to 63 pg/mL at the 3-month point ($p<0.04$) (normal 10 to 55 pg/mL). BMD increased at all sites measured–significantly, so at both the femoral neck and proximal femur ($p<0.04$). Increases in BMD correlated well ($r=0.95$) with the rise in erythrocyte magnesium, which had been significantly below normal at the start of study (Rude & Olerich, 1996).

INDICATIONS AND USAGE

Approved by the FDA:

- Magnesium sulfate (Epsom salt) is approved as a laxative for the temporary relief of constipation.

Unproven Uses: Magnesium is used for migraine, bone resorption, diabetes, hypertension, arrhythmias, PMS, nephrolithiasis, spasms, and leg cramps during pregnancy.

CONTRAINDICATIONS

Magnesium is not to be used in the presence of heart block, severe renal disease, or toxemia in the 2 hours preceding delivery.

PRECAUTIONS AND ADVERSE REACTIONS

Side effects include blurred vision, photophobia, diarrhea, hypermagnesemia, hypotension, increased bleeding times, neuromuscular blockade (in higher doses), and vasodilation.

Administration of magnesium, especially in renally impaired patients, may lead to loss of deep tendon reflexes, hypotension, confusion, respiratory paralysis, cardiac arrhythmias, or cardiac arrest. Increased bleeding time has been reported. Monitor to avoid magnesium toxicity.

Concurrent use of magnesium-containing products and dairy foods may result in altered serum calcium concentrations.

Pregnancy: Rickets in the newborn may result from prolonged magnesium sulfate administration in the second trimester of pregnancy.

DRUG INTERACTIONS

MAJOR RISKS

Levomethadyl: Concomitant use with magnesium may precipitate QT prolongation. *Clinical Management:* Caution should be used when prescribing concomitant drugs known to induce hypokalemia or hypomagnesemia, such as laxatives, as they may precipitate QT prolongation and interact with levomethadyl.

MODERATE RISKS

Aminoglycosides: Concomitant use with magnesium may precipitate neuromuscular weakness and possibly paralysis. *Clinical Management:* Monitor patients for respiratory dysfunction and apnea. If neuromuscular blockade occurs, discontinue the aminoglycoside and change antibiotic therapy. Patients receiving large cumulative doses of aminoglycosides should have serum calcium, magnesium, potassium, and creatinine monitored.

Calcium channel blockers: Concomitant use with magnesium may enhance hypotensive effects. *Clinical Management:* Monitor blood pressure closely when adding or deleting calcium channel blockers in patients receiving magnesium

Doxercalciferol: Concurrent use of doxercalciferol and magnesium may result in hypermagnesemia. *Clinical Management:* Avoid concomitant use.

Fluoroquinolones: Concomitant use with magnesium may decrease absorption and effectiveness. *Clinical Management:* Fluoroquinolones should be administered at least 4 hours before magnesium or any product containing magnesium.

POTENTIAL INTERACTIONS

Labetalol: Concomitant use with magnesium may cause bradycardia and reduced cardiac output. *Clinical Management:* Myocardial function should be monitored when using concomitant magnesium sulfate and labetalol.

Neuromuscular blockers: Concomitant use with magnesium may enhance neuromuscular blocking effects. *Clinical Management:* The dose of neuromuscular blocker may need to be adjusted downward in patients receiving large doses of magnesium salts administered for toxemia of pregnancy.

OVERDOSAGE

Hypermagnesemia from magnesium administration is most commonly seen in patients with renal insufficiency. Hypermagnesemia presents as muscle weakness, electrocardiogram changes, sedation, hypotension, and confusion. These symptoms will progress to absent deep-tendon reflexes, respiratory paralysis, and heart block (Gilman et al, 1990).

Respiratory paralysis occurs at 12 to 15 mEq/L, while concentrations greater than 15 mEq/L result in cardiac conduction abnormalities and cardiac arrest (Gilman et al, 1990).

DOSAGE

Mode of Administration: Intramuscular, intravenous, oral, topical

How Supplied: Capsule, cream, solution, tablet

Daily Dosage: The following chart lists the Recommended Dietary Allowance (RDA) for magnesium:

Age	Males	Females	Pregnancy	Lactation
0 to 6 months	30 mg/day	30 mg/day		
7 to 12 months	75 mg/day	75 mg/day		
1 to 3 years	80 mg/day	80 mg/day		
4 to 8 years	130 mg/day	130 mg/day		
9 to 13 years	240 mg/day	240 mg/day	400 mg/day	400 mg/day
14 to 18 years	410 mg/day	360 mg/day	400 mg/day	360 mg/day
19 to 30 years	400 mg/day	310 mg/day	350 mg/day	310 mg/day
31+ years	420 mg/day	320 mg/day	360 mg/day	320 mg/day

ADULTS

Abdominal and Perineal Incision Wound Healing (magnesium hydroxide ointment, topical): apply twice daily along with zinc chloride spray for 7 days.

Congestive Heart Failure (enteric-coated magnesium chloride): 3,204 mg/d in divided doses (equal to 15.8 mmol elemental Mg).

Dentine Hypersensitivity: 4% Magnesium sulfate solution applied by iontophoresis.

Detrusor Instability (magnesium hydroxide): 350 mg for 4 weeks; double after 2 weeks if there is an unsatisfactory response.

Diabetes Mellitus Type 2: 15.8 to 41.4 mmol/d.

Dietary Supplement: 54 to 483 mg daily in divided doses.

Dyslipidemia (enteric-coated magnesium chloride): a mean dose of 17.92 mmol for a mean duration of 118 days; OR magnesium oxide, 15 mmol/d for 3 months.

Hypertension: 360 to 600 mg/d.

Migraine Prophylaxis: 360 to 600 mg/d.

Mitral Valve Prolapse (magnesium carbonate capsules): During the first week of treatment, 21 mmol/d is used; then 14 mmol/d is used during the second to fifth weeks.

Nephrolithiasis Prophylaxis (magnesium hydroxide): 400 to 500 mg/d.

Osteoporosis: 250 mg taken at bedtime on an empty stomach, increased to 250 mg three times daily for 6 months, followed by 250 mg daily for 18 months.

Premenstrual Syndrome: 200 to 360 mg/d.

PEDIATRICS

Deficiency: The oral dose of magnesium sulfate to treat hypomagnesemia in children is 100 to 200 mg/kg four times daily.

Dietary Supplement: 3 to 6 mg/kg body weight per day in divided doses 3 to 4 times daily, up to a maximum of 400 mg daily.

Laxative: The recommended dose of magnesium citrate for children 2 to 5 years of age is 2.7 to 6.25 g daily as a single or divided dose. For children 6 to 11 years of age, the dose is 5.5 to 12.5 g daily in single or divided doses.

LITERATURE

Abraham GE. Nutritional factors in the etiology of the premenstrual tension syndromes. *J Reprod Med;* 28(7):446-464. 1983

de Valk HW, Verkaaik R, van Rijn HJM et al. Oral magnesium supplementation in insulin-requiring type 2 diabetic patients. *Diabet Med;* 15:503-507. 1998

Carpenter TO, DeLucia MC, Zhang JH, et al. A randomized controlled study of effects of dietary magnesium oxide supplementation on bone mineral content in healthy girls. *J Clin Endocrinol Metab*; 91:4866-4872. 2006

Dickinson HO, Nicolson DJ, Campbell F, et al. Magnesium supplementation for the management of primary hypertension in adults (review). *Cochrane Database of Systematic Reviews;* 3:CD004640. 2006

Davis WH, Leary WP, Reyes AJ et al. Monotherapy with magnesium increases abnormally low high density lipoprotein cholesterol: a clinical assay. *Curr Ther Res*; 36:341-346. 1984

Eibl NL, Kopp HP, Nowak HR et al. Hypomagnesemia in type II diabetes: Effect of a 3-month replacement therapy. *Diabetes Care*; 18(2):188-192. 1995

Evans RW, Taylor FR. ''Natural'' or alternative medications for migraine prevention. *Headache*; 46:1012-1018. 2006

Gilman AG, Rall TW, Nies AS et al (eds). Goodman and Gilman's The Pharmacological Basis of Therapeutics, 8th ed. Pergamon Press, New York, NY, 1990.

Havel RJ, Calloway DH, Gussow JD et al. Recommended Dietary Allowances, 10th ed. National Academy Press, Washington, DC, 1989.

Lima M, Cruz T, Pousada JC et al. The effect of magnesium supplementation in increasing doses on the control of type 2 diabetes. *Diabetes Care*; 21:682-686. 1998

Jee SH, Miller ER III, Guallar E et al. The effect of magnesium supplementation on blood pressure: a meta-analysis of randomized clinical trials. *Am J Hypertens*; 15(8):691-696. 2002

Paolisso G, Scheen A, Cozzolino D et al. Changes in glucose turnover parameters and improvement of glucose oxidation after 4-week magnesium administration in elderly noninsulin-dependent (type II) diabetic patients. *J Clin Endocrinol Metab*; 78:1510-514. 1994

Peikert A, Wilimzig C & Kohne-Volland R. Prophylaxis of migraine with oral magnesium: results from a prospective, multi-center, placebo-controlled and double-blind randomized study. *Cephalagia*; 16:257-263. 1996

Pfaffenrath V, Wessely P, Meyer C et al. Magnesium in the prophylaxis of migraine–a double-blind, placebo-controlled study. *Cephalagia*; 16:436-440. 1996

Rasmussen HS, Aurup P, Goldstein K et al. Influence of magnesium substitution therapy on blood lipid composition in patients with ischemic heart disease. *Arch Intern Med*; 149:1050-1053. 1989

Rasmussen HS, Cintin C, Aurup P et al. The effect of intravenous magnesium therapy on serum and urine levels of potassium, calcium, and sodium in patients with ischemic heart disease, with and without acute myocardial infarction. *Arch Intern Med*;148:1801-1805. 1988

Rude RK & Olerich M. Magnesium deficiency: possible role in osteoporosis associated with gluten-sensitive enteropathy. *Osteoporos Int*; 6(6):453-461. 1996

Rude RK. Physiology of magnesium metabolism and the important role of magnesium in potassium deficiency. *Am J Cardiol*; 63(14):31G-34G. 1989

Shattock MJ, Hearse DJ & Fry CH. The ionic basis of the anti-ischemic and anti-arrhythmic properties of magnesium in the heart. *J Am Coll Nutr*; 6:27-33. 1987

Song Y, He K, Levitan EB, et al. Effects of oral magnesium supplementation on glycaemic control in Type 2 diabetes: a meta-analysis of randomized double-blind controlled trials. *Diabet Med*; 23:1050-1056. 2006

Stendig-Lindberg G, Tepper R & Leichter. Trabecular bone density in a two-year controlled trial of peroral magnesium in osteoporosis. *Mag Res*; 6(2):155-163. 1993

Stuart A, Smellie A, O'Reilly J et al. Magnesium replacement and glucose tolerance in elderly subjects. *Am J Clin Nutr*; 57(4):594-595. 1993

Tucker AK, Hannan MT, Chen H et al. Potassium, magnesium, and fruit and vegetable intakes are associated with greater bone mineral density in elderly men and women. *Am J Clin Nutr*; 69:727-736. 1999

Whang R, Hampton EM & Whang DD. Magnesium homeostasis and clinical disorders of magnesium deficiency. *Ann Pharmacother*; 28:220-226. 1994

Melatonin

DESCRIPTION

Melatonin (N-acetyl-5-methoxytryptamine) is a neurohormone produced by pinealocytes in the pineal gland during the dark hours of the day-night cycle. Serum levels of melatonin are very low during most of the day, and it has been labeled the "hormone of darkness." Melatonin is involved in the induction of sleep, may play a role in the internal synchronization of the mammalian circadian system, and may serve as a marker of the "biologic clock" (Haimov & Lavie, 1995; Garfinkel et al, 1995; Dollins et al, 1994; Tzischinsky & Lavie, 1994; Jan et al, 1994; Cavallo, 1993; Short, 1993).

Other Names: N-acetyl-5-methoxytryptamine

ACTIONS AND PHARMACOLOGY

EFFECTS

Melatonin is thought to have antioxidant, immunomodulator, and hypnotic effects.

In general, the pineal gland (projecting from diencephalon into third ventricle) is a neuroendocrine transducer, related to its secretion of melatonin. The hormone serves as a messenger to the neuroendocrine system regarding environmental conditions (especially the photoperiod). Putative functions of endogenous melatonin in this regard include regulation of sleep cycles, hormonal rhythms, and body temperature (Deacon et al, 1994; Dollins et al, 1993; Cavallo, 1993). Melatonin may also have a role in influencing the maturation and function of the hypothalamic-pituitary-gonadal axis and in determining the onset of puberty (Cavallo, 1993).

Production of melatonin is regulated by postsynaptic receptors originating in the superior cervical ganglion, which innervate the pineal gland. The suprachiasmatic nucleus of the hypothalamus (entrained by the light-dark cycle and considered the anatomic site for the biologic clock) receives stimuli from the retina (retinohypothalamic tract), and during dark hours the suprachiasmatic nuclei forward a stimulus to the superior cervical ganglion and pineal gland, resulting in melatonin secretion (Haimov & Lavie, 1995; Cavallo, 1993). This stimulatory activity is suppressed by light, especially bright light (Thalen et al, 1995; Cavallo, 1993; Strassman et al, 1987). Melatonin synthesis in the pinealocyte is dependent upon noradrenergic stimulation (Cavallo, 1993). The normal endogenous production rate is 28 to 30 mcg/d (Short, 1993; Lane & Moss, 1985). Production of the hormone is reduced in cirrhotic patients (12 mcg/day) (Lane & Moss, 1985) and in the elderly (Garfinkel et al, 1995).

Antioxidant Effects: Melatonin possesses free-radical scavenging properties, protecting cells against many oxidative agents. The mechanism of free-radical scavenging action is not well elucidated. Melatonin reacts with nitric oxide in the presence of doublet oxygen, producing N-nitrosomelatonin. Since nitric oxide can cause some cellular destruction, melatonin may protect the cell against such oxidative damage (Turjanski et al, 2000). Melatonin also inhibits the production of nitric oxide by inhibiting nitric oxide synthase. Nitric oxide's damaging effects are mediated through its reaction with superoxide to form peroxynitrite. Peroxynitrite stimulates lipid peroxidation, inactivates various enzymes, and depletes glutathione (Cuzzocrea et al, 2000).

Antitumor Effects: In vitro and animal studies have reported that melatonin is capable of inducing direct cytostatic actions on some human cancer cell lines, stimulating host immune responses, and inhibiting release of somatomedin-C (Lissoni et al, 1995; Lissoni et al, 1991). Melatonin has been used alone and in combination with interleukin-2 as an immunotherapeutic regimen in the treatment of cancer (Lissoni et al, 1995; Lissoni et al, 1994).

Sleep-Regulating Effects: Prolonged administration of oral melatonin has reportedly induced phase-setting effects on circadian rhythms, such as the sleep-wake cycle and rest-activity. The hormone has been reported to produce re-entrainment of circadian rhythms after time-zone shifts, and entrainment of previously free-running rhythms in the blind (Dollins et al, 1993; Cavallo, 1993; Dahlitz et al, 1991; Arendt et al, 1988; Arendt et al, 1986).

CLINICAL TRIALS

Cancer

Findings from several studies have established a link between low serum levels of melatonin and high cancer risk, through the disruption of circadian rhythms. One update to the literature examined several studies of melatonin in the treatment of advanced cancer. In one randomized, controlled trial mentioned involving 30 patients with colorectal cancer, subjects received treatment with irinotecan alone (n=16) or with concomitant oral melatonin (20 mg/day, administered in the evening). A 4% disease control rate was observed in those receiving melatonin in addition to chemotherapy (12/14 vs 7/16, $p<0.05$). Overall, most studies of exogenous melatonin, given alone or in combination, showed increased survival rates and at least a partial response to therapy (Mahmoud et al 2005).

A systematic review examined 10 randomized trials published between 1992-2003 involving 643 subjects with solid tumors. Researchers investigated the effects of melatonin, given at bedtime, on treatment of cancer or supportive care and 1-year survival rates. Dosages ranged from 10-40 mg/day across all studies. In addition to being well tolerated, melatonin diminished the risk of mortality at 1 year, without severe adverse events (Mills et al 2005).

Tumor regression rate and 5-year survival results were significantly increased in metastatic non-small cell lung cancer subjects who were concomitantly treated with chemotherapy and melatonin. One hundred subjects were randomized to receive chemotherapy only or chemotherapy and melatonin. Chemotherapy subjects received cisplatin 20 mg/m^2 per day intravenously and etoposide 100 mg/m^2 per day intravenously for 3 consecutive days. Four chemotherapy cycles were planned at 21-day intervals. Melatonin 20 mg orally was given 7 days every evening before chemotherapy and was continued after chemotherapy. Toxicity and clinical response were evaluated according to criteria of the World Health Organization. A complete response (CR) was achieved in 2 of 49 (4%) subjects treated with chemotherapy and melatonin. No patient achieved a CR with only chemotherapy. Fifteen of 49 (31%) subjects treated with chemotherapy and melatonin achieved a partial response (PR) compared to 9 of 51 (18%) chemotherapy-only subjects. Disease progression occurred in 20 of 51 chemotherapy-only subjects while 6 of 49 chemotherapy-melatonin subjects had progression ($p<0.01$). At 5 years, chemotherapy plus melatonin compared to chemotherapy alone improved survival (3 vs 0, $p<0.001$). Chemotherapy treatment was also better tolerated in subjects treated concomitantly with melatonin (Lissoni et al, 2003).

Sixteen patients with glioblastoma who were treated with melatonin 20 mg/d and radiotherapy (RT) experienced prolonged overall survival time compared to 14 patients given RT alone. Both groups were given steroids and anticonvulsants. The melatonin-treated group had a higher rate of survival at 1 year than did the RT-only group ($p<0.02$). Patients with RT alone experienced a significantly higher number of infections compared to melatonin plus RT group ($p<0.025$) (Lissoni et al, 1996a).

Tamoxifen and melatonin administered to 25 patients with metastatic solid tumors showed beneficial effects in terms of controlling cancer-cell proliferation or improving performance status. Patients included those diagnosed with melanoma, uterine cervix carcinoma, pancreatic cancer, heptocarcinoma, ovarian cancer, small cell cancer, or unknown primary tumor. Tamoxifen 20 mg and melatonin 20 mg were given daily. In 3 patients (12%) a partial response was seen. Stable disease was observed in 13 patients (52%) with the remaining 9 patients demonstrating progressive disease. No toxicity was seen (Lissoni et al, 1996b).

Other studies have reported significantly prolonged survival and greater improvement in performance status with oral melatonin plus supportive care compared to supportive care alone in patients with non-small cell lung cancer (n=63) (Lissoni et al, 1992a) and brain metastases of solid tumors (n=50) (Lissoni et al, 1994a). In the non-small cell lung cancer patients, a dose of 10 mg daily for 21 of 28 days was administered. No complete or partial responses were observed, although stable disease was achieved in significantly more patients treated with melatonin (32% versus 9%). A dose of 20 mg daily until progression was given to patients with brain metastases; the free-from-progression period was greater and the frequency of steroid-induced metabolic and infective complications was significantly lower with melatonin therapy relative to supportive care alone in this study. In both studies, patients had failed or progressed on prior chemotherapy, although details of previous therapy or criteria for failure were not provided. Methods of randomization and pretreatment clinical status of patients (such as underlying conditions) in each group, which could affect outcome, were also not specified, and the numbers of patients may have been too small for adequate statistical analysis. The same group of investigators conducted all studies.

The combination of subcutaneous recombinant interleukin-2 (aldesleukin) given 5 or 6 days/week for 4 weeks, plus oral melatonin 10 to 50 mg daily produced complete or partial tumor responses in 23% of pretreated patients with various digestive tract tumors (ie, colorectal, gastric, hepatic, or pancreatic carcinoma) (Lissoni et al, 1993a), 21% with solely metastatic gastric carcinoma and low performance status (Lissoni et al, 1993), and 20% of patients with non-small cell lung cancer (first-line therapy) (Lissoni et al, 1992) in small uncontrolled studies. A partial response rate was also observed with this combination in 3 of 12 previously treated or untreated patients (25%) with locally unresectable or metastatic endocrine tumors; responses occurred in carcinoid tumor, neuroendocrine lung tumor, and pancreatic islet cell tumor (Lissoni et al, 1995).

Chemotherapy-Induced Toxicity

Evening administration of melatonin throughout chemotherapy treatment and every day thereafter resulted in significant reductions in manifestations of chemotherapy-induced toxicity. Eighty patients were given melatonin 20 mg/d concomitantly with chemotherapy or chemotherapy only. Supportive care was the same in both groups of patients. Thrombocytopenia was significantly less ($p<0.006$) in the group receiving melatonin. Leukopenia and anemia were also less frequent. Asthenia and malaise were significantly less frequent ($p<0.006$) in the melatonin group. Stomatitis, neuropathy, and cardiac complications also occurred less frequently in the group receiving concomitant melatonin than in the group receiving chemotherapy alone. There was no difference between groups in the frequency of alopecia, nausea and vomiting, or diarrhea. The antitumor activity of cytotoxic drugs was not negatively influenced by concomitant administration of melatonin (Lissoni et al, 1997b).

Headache

Melatonin reduced the number of daily attacks of cluster headache and the consumption of analgesics in acute sufferers. In a double-blind study of 20 sufferers of cluster headaches, subjects were given either melatonin 10 mg in a single evening dose or placebo for 2 weeks, during a cluster period. Fifty percent of melatonin-treated patients responded. Improvement began 3 days after the onset of treatment, and responders were free of headaches after 5 days. There was no improvement in the placebo group. Discontinuation of treatment by responders was followed by gradual recurrence of cluster attacks, obliging re-institution of treatment (Leone & Bussone, 1998; Leone et al, 1996).

Melatonin eliminated the occurrence of headaches of various kinds (migraine, cluster, tension headache) in 5 patients with delayed sleep phase syndrome. Each patient received either melatonin 5 mg or a placebo nightly for 14 days, followed by the other treatment for 14 days. Thereafter, each patient took melatonin nightly for at least 3 months. Melatonin was given 5 hours before the time when endogenous melatonin reached 10 picograms/mL. The endogenous nocturnal melatonin level of all subjects was normal and did not differ from those of patients who had delayed sleep phase syndrome without headache, suggesting that the headaches were not caused by melatonin deficiency. Rather, relief from headaches may have been a result of increased sleep and synchronicity of the biological clock to lifestyle (Nagtegaal et al, 1998).

Jet Lag/Sleep Restriction

A meta-analysis examining the effect of exogenous melatonin on sleep onset latency in those with sleep disorders accompanying sleep restriction found no evidence of efficacy with supplementation. Nine randomized trials involving 427 participants were studied. However, two systematic reviews cited in the analysis, including a large Cochrane review, concluded that melatonin was effective in alleviating jet lag. This disparity may have been the result of an aspect overlooked in the meta-analysis—namely, measures of daytime fatigue—which was examined in the studies reporting a benefit with melatonin (Buscemi et al 2006). Another study used exogenous melatonin administration combined with exposure to light and physical exercise to hasten resynchronization after transmeridian flights (comprising 12-13 time zones). Improvements were noted after about 2 days of treatment, compared with an average resolution occurring over 8 to 10 days following such a flight (Cardinali et al 2006).

In some earlier jet lag studies, melatonin was not statistically superior to placebo (Claustrat et al, 1992; Petrie et al, 1989). In particular, mood, sleep quality, and morning sleepiness were not altered significantly in one study (Claustrat et al, 1992). Effective doses of melatonin have been either 5 mg daily (at various times) for 3 days prior to the flight, then the same dose for 4 additional days, or an 8 mg dose on the day of the flight and for 3 further days. The former regimen appears more effective.

Nocturnal Hypertension

A controlled-release formulation of melatonin (2 mg) administered nightly reduced nocturnal systolic and diastolic blood pressure in patients with confirmed nocturnal hypertension. The double-blind study randomized patients to treatment with melatonin 2 hours before bedtime (n=19) or placebo (n=19) for 4 weeks. Melatonin treatment significantly reduced nocturnal systolic BP from 136±9 to 130±10 mm Hg (p=.011) and diastolic BP from 72±11 to 69±9 mm Hg (p=.002). No effect on nocturnal blood pressure was observed with placebo (Grossman et al 2006).

Daily nighttime melatonin decreased sleep systolic and diastolic blood pressure in subjects with untreated mild to moderate essential hypertension in a randomized, double-blind, placebo-controlled, crossover trial. Sixteen men (aged 36 to 68 years) were orally supplemented with melatonin 2.5 mg or placebo 1 hour before bedtime one time only (acute); this dosage was then repeated daily for 3 weeks. Twenty-four hour ambulatory blood pressure and sleep quality were evaluated for both the acute and repeated treatment period. A significant decrease in sleep systolic (6 mm Hg) and diastolic (4 mm Hg) blood pressure was demonstrated during the 3 weeks of melatonin compared to placebo (p=0.046 and p=0.020). The 1-day only treatment had no effect on systolic and diastolic blood pressures while asleep (p=0.89 and p=0.86, respectively). No significant improvement in awake systolic and diastolic blood pressure was demonstrated during the 3 weeks of melatonin compared to placebo. Repeatedly used melatonin significantly increased sleep efficiency (p=0.017) and sleep time (p=0.013) (Scheer et al, 2004).

Sedation and Anxiolysis

Contrary to earlier findings in younger subjects, a prospective, double-blind, randomized trial involving elderly subjects (>65 years old) concluded that melatonin was no more effective than placebo in reducing anxiety prior to elective surgery. Subjects were randomized to receive 10 mg melatonin (n=67) or placebo (n=71). Preoperative anxiety at 90 minutes decreased by 33% in the melatonin group and 21% in the placebo group, a nonsignificant finding. The authors point out that the differences they observed compared to earlier studies may be attributable to the higher mean age of subjects and the inclusion of males in this study, and their failure to measure plasma melatonin levels (Capuzzu et al 2006).

In a randomized, double-blind, dose-ranging study, melatonin (MLN) was as efficacious as midazolam (MZ) and more efficacious than placebo in provoking sedation and anxiolysis in preoperative surgical patients. Adult women scheduled for laparoscopic surgery were assigned to receive 1 of the following 7 sublingual premedication regimens (n=12 each group): MZ 0.05, 0.1, or 0.2 mg/kg; MLN 0.05, 0.1, or 0.2 mg/kg; or placebo. All patients were premedicated 2 hours prior to surgery; in each case, the patient was instructed to avoid swallowing the sublingual preparation of their respective study drug for 3 minutes after dosing, after which they were allowed to swallow. Sedation and anxiety were measured by a 4-point sedation scale and a visual analog scale, respectively. Both MZ and MLN induced significantly greater reductions in preoperative anxiety when compared with placebo ($p<0.05$), and sedation was attained at 60 and 90 minutes after dosing by significantly more patients receiving

MZ and MLN than placebo ($p<0.02$). With the exception of patients receiving MZ 0.2 mg/kg, there were no differences between groups with regard to the level of postoperative sedation; patients receiving MZ 0.2 mg/kg experienced an increased depth of sedation compared with patients receiving MLN 0.05 and 0.1 mg/kg. Postoperative pain scores were not different between groups at any time during postanesthesia recovery (Naguib & Samarkandi, 2000).

Sleep Disorders/Delayed Sleep

A retrospective study examined the effect of long-term administration of melatonin (3 to 5 mg/day) in adolescents with delayed sleep phase syndrome. Subjects were treated for an average of 6 months as investigators evaluated changes in sleep parameters following treatment and assessed its impact on school performance and behavior. Doses of melatonin were taken 2 hours prior to bedtime in 33 subjects, and subsequently, difficulty falling asleep resolved in all of them. In this sample of patients, treatment with melatonin improved sleep-wake patterns, was accompanied by a reduction in sleep-related symptoms, and appeared to decrease the proportion of subjects who misbehaved at school (Szeinberg et al 2006). These findings are consistent with an earlier study, which found that melatonin advanced sleep onset in subjects with delayed sleep phase syndrome. When administered 5 hours before endogenous melatonin secretion, a dose of 5 mg melatonin advanced sleep onset and improved quality of life for 16 patients (Smits & Nagtegaal, 2000). One study found melatonin to be statistically and clinically superior to placebo in reducing initial insomnia, which is common among those with ADHD. In this trial, 27 children with ADHD and initial insomnia who were taking prescription stimulants were treated with sleep hygiene methods; those not responding to this treatment were randomized to treatment with melatonin (5 mg). Full remission of sleep disorders was obtained with sleep hygiene or both treatments in 71% of subjects. The response rate was significant—81% of the total sample noted clinically meaningful improvements with sleep hygiene, melatonin, or both (Weiss et al 2006). The authors of another study recommended melatonin as first-line treatment to resolve sleep disturbances in children with Sanfilippo syndrome, based on their observations of this sample population (Fraser et al 2005).

Nine patients with periodic limb movement disorder showed improvements when given melatonin for 6 weeks in an open trial. Patients were given melatonin 3 mg taken 30 minutes before bedtime, between 10 and 11 p.m. for 6 weeks. Polysomnography was performed at baseline and during the last week of treatment. A wrist actigraph was worn during 2 weeks prior to treatment and during the last 14 days of supplementation in order to measure motor activity during sleep. Seven patients subjectively reported feelings of improved daytime symptoms of fatigue and excessive sleepiness within 7 days of treatment. Polysomnographic recordings reported significant decreases in parameters of periodic limb movements ($p<0.05$), which were confirmed through actigraphy. The investigators hypothesized that a resynchronization of circadian rhythms enhanced REM sleep and produced the observed effects (Kunz & Bes, 2001).

Improved sleep parameters were seen when melatonin was given to schizophrenic patients with insomnia in a randomized, double-blind, placebo-controlled, crossover study. Nineteen subjects were given either controlled-release melatonin 2 mg or placebo 2 hours before bedtime for 3 weeks, with a 1 week washout between the treatments. Wrist actigraphs were used to assess sleep quality for 3 nights during the last week of each treatment period. Sleep efficiency was significantly improved in the melatonin group compared to placebo ($p=0.038$). There was an insignificant decrease in sleep latency and increased total sleep time with melatonin versus placebo. Twenty-seven patients entered the study, but only 19 were assessed due to lack of compliance (n=4) and technical problems with the actigraphs (n=4) (Shamir et al, 2000).

Melatonin was effective in improving the sleep of patients with major depressive disorder. This double-blind, placebo-controlled study treated 24 outpatients with fluoxetine 20 mg and either slow-release melatonin 2.5 to 10 mg or placebo nightly for 4 weeks. No other medications were used. Patients treated with melatonin showed significant improvement in sleep variables compared with controls ($p=0.01$). No effect of melatonin on depression symptoms was found (Dolberg et al, 1998).

Limited data suggest benefits of oral melatonin in blind adults with free-running sleep-wake rhythms (Haimov & Lavie, 1995; Cavallo, 1993; Arendt et al, 1988). Sleep problems in these patients were considered related to an inability to remain synchronized to the normal 24-hour day, due at least in part to lack of light-dark perception. Therapy with melatonin resulted in normal sleep (without early awakening and day sleeps), attributed to resynchronization of the sleep-wake activity cycle. Effective doses have been 5 mg nightly at normal bedtime.

Ten children with neurologic and developmental disorders were given 3 mg melatonin 1 to 2 hours before bedtime and monitored for a mean of 7.5 months. In eight (80%) of the children, the average number of hours of sleep, average number of nighttime awakenings, average number of nights with early morning arousal, and average number of nights with delayed sleep onset greatly improved after treatment. Use of melatonin also improved daytime activities and behaviors (Jan, 2000). Another study examining 5 severely psychomotor retarded children showed improved sleep patterns after 4 weeks of treatment with 3 mg melatonin given every day at 6:30 p.m. (Pillar et al, 2000).

In a study of 100 pediatric patients (ages 3 months to 21 years) with chronic sleep disorders, 54% were visually impaired and 85% had multiple neurodevelopmental disabilities (including visual loss, deafness, blindness, mental retardation, cerebral palsy, epilepsy, chromosomal abnormalities, head injuries, degenerative central nervous system disorders, autism, and brain tumors). Of the 15 patients not having the above conditions, diagnoses were attention deficit hyperactive disorder, anxiety, bowel disorders, and nocturnal seizures. Treatment with oral melatonin doses of 2.5 to 10 mg resulted in improved sleep in 82% of these patients. Factors involved in non-response were recurrent pain, malfunction or absence of the suprachiasmatic nucleus, noisy sleep environments, psychological reasons for delayed sleep onset, multiple medications, and organically driven behavior. In 2 children with pineal glands destroyed by brain tumor or trauma, oral melatonin doses of 25 mg were required to produce a beneficial improvement in sleep quality. A secondary benefit was that improved patient sleep allowed caretakers to also have improved sleep (Jan & O'Donnell, 1996).

Tinnitus

Patients reported more subjective improvement in tinnitus with melatonin than with placebo in a randomized, crossover study. Twenty-three subjects were given melatonin 3 mg or placebo, to be taken 1 to 2 hours before retiring, for 30 days. After a 7-day washout, patients took the alternate treatment for 30 days. Average improvements in Tinnitus Handicap Inventory (THI) scores were significant and were the same with melatonin and placebo. However, on a follow-up questionnaire, 39% of patients reported an overall improvement with melatonin, whereas only 17% reported improvement with placebo. Among those reporting difficulty sleeping due to their tinnitus, 46.7% had overall improvement with melatonin and 20% with placebo ($p=0.04$). Eight of 16 patients with bilateral tinnitus reported improvement with melatonin and only 3 of the 16 had improvement with placebo. Overall, 35% of subjects had a decrease in loudness of their tinnitus with melatonin, compared with 13% with placebo. The only side effect reported in the study was bad dreams, which was equally distributed between the melatonin and placebo trials (Rosenberg et al, 1998).

INDICATIONS AND USAGE

Melatonin is used as a sleep aid, in the treatment of a variety of solid tumors (in combination with interleukin-2), and can be used to improve thrombocytopenia and other toxicities induced by cancer chemotherapy and from other conditions. Melatonin is also used for cluster headaches and tinnitus.

PRECAUTIONS AND ADVERSE REACTIONS

Adverse effects of exogenous melatonin have generally been minimal. Drowsiness, fatigue, headache, confusion, gastrointestinal complaints, and reduced body temperature have been reported. Melatonin has exacerbated dysphoria in depressed patients and has caused mood swings. It has caused depressive symptoms and fever when used with interleukin-2 in cancer therapy. Rarely, tachycardia, seizures, acute psychotic reactions, autoimmune hepatitis, and pruritus have been reported.

DRUG INTERACTIONS

MODERATE RISKS

Warfarin: Concomitant use may result in an increased risk of bleeding. *Clinical Management:* Avoid concomitant use of melatonin and warfarin. If both agents are taken together, monitor prothrombin time, INR, and signs and symptoms of excessive bleeding frequently. Only adjust the warfarin dose if the patient takes a consistent dosage of melatonin with a consistent and standardized brand.

MINOR RISKS

Fluvoxamine: Concomitant use may result in increased central nervous system depression. *Clinical Management:* Monitor patients taking fluvoxamine with melatonin supplementation for changes in sleep patterns and signs of excessive central nervous system depression. Downward titration of melatonin dosages may be required during concomitant administration with fluvoxamine.

Nifedipine: Concomitant use may result in increased blood pressure. *Clinical Management:* Close monitoring of blood pressure is advised with appropriate dose adjustment of nifedipine or withdrawal of melatonin.

DOSAGE

Mode of Administration: intramuscular, intravenous, oral, oral transmucosal, transdermal

How Supplied: tablet, tincture

Daily Dosage:

Cancer as combination therapy: 40 or 50 mg oral tablets given once daily at night, initiated 7 days prior to interleukin-2 and continued throughout the cycle

Cancer as single agent therapy: Melatonin 20 mg intramuscularly daily for 2 months (induction phase), followed by oral doses of 10 mg daily until progression, has been given for the treatment of solid tumors

Chronic insomnia: 1 to 10 mg orally daily

Delayed sleep phase syndrome: 5 mg orally daily

Jet lag: 5 mg orally daily for 3 days prior to departure, then 5 mg for 4 additional days

Normalization of nocturnal levels: constant intravenous daytime infusion of melatonin 4 mcg/hour for 5 hours (0.1 and 0.3 mg oral tablets have also been used)

Sleep disorders: 5 mg at the usual bedtime

Pediatric Dosage:

Congenital sleep disorder: 2.5 mg oral tablet

Neurological disability: 0.5 to 10 mg oral tablet at bedtime

Sleep-wake cycle disorder (controlled release tablets, oral: An average of 5.7 mg was used in children ages 4 to 21 years

LITERATURE

Arendt J, Aldhous J & Marks V. Alleviation of jet lag by melatonin: preliminary results of controlled double blind trial. *BMJ*; 292(6529):1170. 1986

Arendt J, Aldhous M & Wright J. Synchronisation of a disturbed sleep-wake cycle in a blind man by melatonin treatment (letter). *Lancet*; 1(8588):772-773. 1988

Buscemi N, Vandermeer B, Hooton N, et al. Efficacy and safety of exogenous melatonin for secondary sleep disorders and sleep disorders accompanying sleep restriction: meta-analysis. *BMJ*; 332:385-393.

Capuzzo M, Zanardi B, Schiffino E et al. Melatonin does not reduce anxiety more than placebo in elderly undergoing surgery. *Anesth Analg;* 103:121-123. 2006

Cardinali DP, Furio AM, Reyes MP, Brusco LI. The use of chronobiotics in the resynchronization of the sleep—wake cycle. *Cancer Causes Control*; 17:601-609. 2006

Cavallo A. The pineal gland in human beings: relevance to pediatrics. *J Pediatr*; 123(6):843-851. 1993

Claustrat B, Brun J, David M et al. Melatonin and jet lag: confirmatory result using a simplified protocol. *Biol Psychiatry*; 32(8):705-711. 1992

Cuzzocrea S, Constantino G, Gitto E et al. Protective effects of melatonin in ischemic brain injury. *J Pineal Res*; 29(4):217-227. 2000

Dahlitz M, Alvarez B, Vignau J et al. Delayed sleep phase syndrome response to melatonin. *Lancet*; 337(8750):1121-1124. 1991

Deacon S, English J & Arendt J. Acute phase-shifting effects of melatonin associated with suppression of core body temperature in humans. *Neuroscience*; 178(1):32-34. 1994

Dolberg OT, Hirschmann S & Grunhaus L. Melatonin for the treatment of sleep disturbances in major depressive disorder. *Am J Psychiatry*; 155(8): 1119-1121. 1998

Dollins AB, Lynch HJ, Wurtman RJ et al. Effect of pharmacological daytime doses of melatonin on human mood and performance. *Psychopharmacology* (Berl); 112(4):490-496. 1993

Dollins AB, Zhdanova IV, Wurtman RJ et al. Effect of inducing nocturnal serum melatonin concentrations in daytime on sleep, mood, body temperature, and performance. *Proc Natl Acad Sci USA*; 91(5):1824-1828. 1994

Dollins AB, Zhdanova IV, Wurtman RJ et al. Effect of inducing nocturnal serum melatonin concentrations in daytime on sleep, mood, body temperature, and performance. *Proc Natl Acad Sci USA*; 91(5):1824-1828. 1994

Fraser J, Gason AA, Wraith JE, Delatycki MB. Sleep disturbance in Sanfilippo syndrome: a parental questionnaire study. *Arch Dis Child*; 90:1239-1242. 2005

Garfinkel D, Laudon M, Nof D et al. Improvement of sleep quality in elderly people by controlled-release melatonin. *Lancet*; 346(8974):541-544. 1995

Grossman E, Laudon M, Yalcin R, et al. Melatonin reduceds night blood pressure in patients with nocturnal hypertension. *Am J Med*; 119:898-902. 2006

Haimov I & Lavie P. Potential of melatonin replacement therapy in older patients with sleep disorders. *Drugs Aging*; 7(2):75-78. 1995

James SP, Mendelson WB, Sack DA et al: The effect of melatonin on normal sleep. *Neuropsychopharmacology*; 1(1):41-44. 1988

Jan JE & O'Donnell ME. Use of melatonin in the treatment of paediatric sleep disorders. *J Pineal Res*; 21(4):193-199. 1996

Jan JE, Espezel H & Appleton RE. The treatment of sleep disorders with melatonin. *Dev Med Child Neurol*; 36(2):97-107. 1994

Kunz D & Bes F. Exogenous melatonin in periodic limb movement disorder: an open clinical trial and a hypothesis. *Sleep*; 24(2):183-187. 2001

Lane EA & Moss HB. Pharmacokinetics of melatonin in man: first pass hepatic metabolism. *J Clin Endocrinol Metab*; 61(6):1214-1216. 1985

Lissoni P, Barni S, Ardizzoia A et al. A randomized study with the pineal hormone melatonin versus supportive care alone in patients with brain metastases due to solid neoplasms. *Cancer* 1994a; 73(3):699-701.

Lissoni P, Barni S, Ardizzoia A et al. Randomized study with the pineal hormone melatonin versus supportive care alone in advanced nonsmall cell lung cancer resistant to a first-line chemotherapy containing cisplatin. *Oncology*; 49(5):336-339. 1992a

Lissoni P, Barni S, Cattaneo G et al. Clinical results with the pineal hormone melatonin in advanced cancer resistant to standard antitumor therapies. *Oncology*; 48(6):448-450. 1991

Lissoni P, Chilelli M, Villa S et al. Five years survival in metastatic non-small cell lung cancer patients treated with chemotherapy alone or chemotherapy and melatonin: a randomized trial. *J Pineal Res*; 35(1):12-15. 2003

Lissoni P, Meregalli S, Nosetto L et al. Increased survival time in brain glioblastomas by a radioneuroendocrine strategy with radiotherapy plus melatonin compared to radiotherapy alone. *Oncology*; 53(1):43-46. 1996a

Lissoni P, Paolorossi F, Tancini G et al. A phase II study of tamoxifen plus melatonin in metastatic solid tumor patients. *Br J Cancer*; 74(9):1466-1468. 1996b

Lissoni P, Tancini G, Barni S et al. Treatment of cancer chemotherapy-induced toxicity with the pineal hormone melatonin. *Support Care Cancer*; 5(2):126-129. 1997b

Lissoni P, Barni S, Tancini G et al. A randomised study with subcutaneous low-dose interleukin 2 alone vs interleukin 2 plus the pineal neurohormone melatonin in advanced solid neoplasms other than renal cancer and melanoma. *Br J Cancer*; 69(1):196-199. 1994

Mahmoud F, Sarhill N, Mazurczak MA. The therapeutic application of melatonin in supportive care and palliative medicine. *Am J Hosp Pallative Med*; 22(4):295-309. 2005

Mallo C, Zaidan R, Galy G et al. Pharmacokinetics of melatonin in man after intravenous infusion and bolus injection. *Eur J Clin Pharmacol*; 38(3):297-301. 1990

MacFarlane JG, Cleghorn JM, Brown GM et al. The effects of exogenous melatonin on the total sleep time and daytime alertness of chronic insomniacs: a preliminary study. *Biol Psychiatry*; 30(4):371-376. 1991

Mills E, Wu P, Seely D, Guyatt G. Melatonin in the treatment of cancer: a systematic review of randomized controlled trials and meta-analysis. *J Pineal Res*; 329:360-366. 2005

Naguib M & Samarkandi AH. The comparative dose-response effects of melatonin and midazolam for premedication of adult patients: a double-blinded, placebo-controlled study. *Anesth Analg*; 91:473-479. 2000

Nagtegaal JE, Smits MG, Swart ACW et al. Melatonin-responsive headache in delayed sleep phase syndrome: preliminary observations. *Headache*; 38(4):303-307. 1998

Rosenberg SE, Silverstein H, Rowan PT et al. Effect of melatonin on tinnitus. *Laryngoscope*; 108(3):305-310. 1998

Petrie K, Conaglen JV, Thompson L et al: Effect of melatonin on jet lag after long haul flights. *BMJ*; 298(6675):705-707. 1989

Pillar G, Shahar E, Peled N et al. Melatonin improves sleep-wake patterns in psychomotor retarded children. *Pediatr Neurol*; 23(3):225-228. 2000

Scheer F, Van Montfrans G, van Someren E et al. Daily nighttime melatonin reduces blood pressure in male patients with essential hypertension. *Hypertension*; 43(2):192-197. 2004

Shamir E, Barak Y, Shalman I et al. Melatonin treatment for tardive dyskinesia. *Arch Gen Psychiatry*; 58(11):1049-1052. 2001

Strassman RJ, Peake GT, Qualls CR et al. A model for the study of the acute effects of melatonin in man. *J Clin Endocrinol Metab*; 65(5):847-852. 1987

Szeinberg A, Borodkin K, Dagan Y. Melatonin treatment in adolescents with delayed sleep phase syndrome. *Clin Pediatr;* 45:809-818. 2006

Thalen BE, Kjellman BF, Morkrid L et al. Melatonin in light treatment of patients with seasonal and nonseasonal depression. *Acta Psychiatr Scand*; 92(4):274-284. 1995

Tzischinsky O & Lavie P. Melatonin possesses time-dependent hypnotic effects. *Sleep*; 17(7):638-645. 1994

Waldhauser F, Waldhauser M, Lieberman HR et al. Bioavailability of oral melatonin in humans. *Neuroendocrinology*; 39(4):307-313. 1984

Weiss MD, Wasdell MB, Bomben MM, et al. Sleep hygiene and melatonin treatment for children and adolescents with ADHD and initial insomnia. *J Am Acad Child Adolesc Psychiatry*; 45(5):512-519. 2006

Probiotics (Lactobacilli)

DESCRIPTION

Lactobacillus products are often called probiotics, translated as ''for life,'' a popular term used to refer to bacteria in the intestine considered beneficial to health. At least 400 different species of microflora colonize the human gastrointestinal tract. The most important commercially available lactobacillus species are *L acidophilus* and *L casei GG.* Other lactobaccilli inhabiting the human gastrointestinal tract include *L brevis, L cellobiosus, L fermentum, L leichmannii, L plantarum,* and *L salivaroes.*

As the intestinal flora is intimately involved in the host's nutritional status and affects immune system function, cholesterol metabolism, carcinogenesis, toxin load, and aging, lactobacillus supplementation is often used to promote overall good health. The primary areas of use by alternative medicine providers are in the promotion of proper intestinal environment, recovery from any diarrheal disease, prevention and treatment of ''yeast overgrowth syndrome'' (a controversial diagnosis), antibiotic-induced diarrhea, vaginal bacteria and yeast infections, urinary tract infections, and cancer prevention.

Other Names: Lactobacillus acidophilus, Lactobacillus casei strain GG, *Lactobacillus bulgaricus*

ACTIONS AND PHARMACOLOGY

EFFECTS

Possible mechanisms for the effective action of lactobacilli in the treatment of various gastrointestinal (GI) tract pathologies include replacement of pathogenic organisms in the GI tract by lactobacilli, elicitation of an immune response, lowering of fecal pH, and interfering with the ability of pathogenic bacteria to adhere to intestinal mucosal cells (Bezkorovainy, 2001).

Commercially available *lactobacillus* products are designed to be taken orally with the intent to colonize the intestine and establish a balanced ecosystem. The mechanism of action may involve acid production and competition. Some metabolic byproducts of lactobacilli, such as lactic acid and hydrogen peroxide, may contribute to the ability to help maintain a healthy urogenital tract. It has been proposed that lactobacilli must possess properties including adhesion, competitive exclusion, and inhibitor production to colonize a mucosal surface (Reid et al, 1990).

Antidiarrheal Effects: Lactobacillus acidophilus LA-1 inhibited cell association and cell entry of bacterial enteropathogens associated with diarrhea. Such inhibition could have resulted from steric hindrance of apical enterocytic receptors of the pathogens by *lactobacillus* or an antimicrobial substance secreted by the *lactobacillus* or by intestinal cells after *lactobacillus* binding (Bernet et al, 1994).

Antimicrobial Effects: Several studies have reported isolation of antimicrobial substances from lactobacilli. An inhibitory substance was isolated from *Lactobacillus* strain GG that was active against a broad spectrum of gram-negative and gram-positive bacteria. The substance was not lactic or acetic acid. Based on molecular weight it could not be considered a bacteriocin but more closely resembled a microcin (Silva et al, 1987). The growth of enterococci was inhibited by 4 of 13 strains of lactobacilli. The activity was not due to pH, acid production or hydrogen peroxide production but was considered bacteriocin-like in nature (McGroarty & Reid, 1988). Lactobacilli produced a substance that inhibited *Escherichia coli,* which was not lactic acid or hydrogen peroxide (McGroarty & Reid, 1988a) and demonstrated the ability to coaggregate with uropathogens (Reid et al, 1988). *Lactobacillus acidophilus* strain LB produced antibacterial activity against gram-negative and gram-positive pathogens. Once again, lactic acid and hydrogen peroxide were not responsible for the antimicrobial activity. The antimicrobial component appeared different from bacteriocins and microcins. The substance was more effective in vitro against the invasive process of *Salmonella typhimurium* than against the adhesive process and appeared to have in vivo activity against this organism in mice when administered orally (Coconnier et al, 1997). Bacteriocin production by lactobacilli has also been demonstrated. *Lactobacillus acidophilus* LF221 isolated from feces produced 2 new bacteriocins. Activity was demonstrated against some pathogenic and food spoilage bacteria (Bogovic-Matijasic et al, 1998).

Lactobacilli may protect vaginal epithelium through barrier and interference mechanisms. Vaginal lactobacilli strongly adhered to vaginal epithelial cells and interfered with adherence of genito-urinary pathogens. Lactobacilli recovered from other sources, such as dairy products, adhered in lower numbers. *Lactobacillus acidophilus* and *Gardnerella vaginalis* may bind to the same receptors on the surface of vaginal epithelial cells, with *lactobacillus* having a higher affinity (Boris et al, 1998). Adhesion of lactobacilli to the Caco-2 cell line, an in vitro model for intestinal epithelium, has been shown to be concentration dependent (Tuomola & Salminen, 1998).

Anticarcinogenic Effects: Oral administration of lactobacilli has been shown to significantly reduce activity of beta-glucuronidase, nitroreductase, and azoreductase, enzymes that are known to transform fecal procarcinogens to the active form. Continuous consumption is necessary to maintain the effect (Kasper et al, 1998). Oral administration of a milk base inoculated with *Lactobacillus acidophilus* LA-2 had a beneficial impact on fecal mutagenicity (Hosoda et al, 1998).

Effects Against Colitis: The protective effects of probiotics against experimental colitis in the mouse are mediated by bacterial DNA, rather than by bacterial metabolites or ability of the bacteria to colonize the colon. Both viable and irradiated (nonviable) probiotic bacteria attenuated the severity of experimental colitis (induced by dextran sodium sulfate or trinitrobenzene sulfonic acid) in mice. The probiotic product used in this study contained 4 strains of lactobacilli (*L casei, L plantarum, L acidophilus,* and *L delbrueckii*), 3 strains of bifidobacteria (*B longum, B breve, and B infantis*), and 1 strain of *Streptococcus salivarius subsp. Thermophilus* (Rachmilewitz et al, 2004). Although human TLR9 has 76% identity to mouse TLR9, the CpG motifs to which the two respond are not identical (Takeshita et al, 2001), and it remains to be seen whether human TLR9 is responsive to probiotic DNA.

CLINICAL TRIALS

Bacterial Vaginosis

A vaginal *lactobacillus* preparation was significantly more effective than placebo in the treatment of bacterial vaginosis in a multicenter, randomized, placebo-controlled trial involving 34 nonmenopausal women. The test preparation (Gynoflor®) contained 50 mg of a lyophilisate of one selected strain of hydrogen peroxide producing *Lactobacillus acidophilus* (corresponding to at least 10 million viable bacteria per tablet) and 0.03 mg estriol. Patients administered 1 or 2 vaginal tablets daily before bed for 6 days. Intra-group analysis found no difference in effectiveness between groups using a 1-tablet or 2-tablet dose. Patients receiving the *Lactobacillus* preparation had a significantly better cure rate (77% at day 15 and 88% at day 28) compared with the placebo group (25% at day 15 and 22% at day 28) ($p<0.05$) (Parent et al, 1996).

Vaginal application of yogurt containing *Lactobacillus acidophilus* was found to be significantly more effective than acetic acid tampons or no treatment in a randomized comparison in the treatment of bacterial vaginosis in pregnancy. Patients randomized to the yogurt group received 10 to 15 mL of commercially available yogurt (based on *Lactobacillus acidophilus* more than 100 million per mL) twice daily for 7 days, with the regimen repeated 1 week later. Clinical improvement was significantly better in the yogurt group compared with the acetic acid group ($p=0.04$) and controls receiving no therapy ($p<0.0005$). An evaluation of patients for the absence of bacterial vaginosis 2 months after treatment also found that yogurt treated patients had significant improvement compared with the acetic acid group ($p=0.04$) and controls ($p<0.0005$) (Neri et al, 1993).

Bladder Cancer, Prevention of

Regular consumption of fermented milk products (possibly containing *Lactobacillus casei*) may reduce the risk of bladder cancer. One hundred eighty (180) subjects (mean age=67 years) diagnosed with primary bladder cancer (transitional cell carcinoma) and 445 controls (matched by age and gender) were enrolled in a case-control study. Subjects were asked 81 questions including past and present smoking, food consumption frequency 10 to 15 years ago (dairy products and milk, fermented milk products [yogurt or fermented milk drinks, such as Yakult]), and a generalized health description. There was no difference in most dietary habits between subjects and controls 10 to 15 earlier except with dairy product consumption Yakult was consumed more often by controls than subjects ($p=0.07$). The difference between groups was greater ($p=0.027$) when all fermented milk products were considered. Subjects smoked more than controls ($p=0.01$). The odds ratio demonstrated that smoking, low levels of consumption of all fermented milk products, and low levels of consumption of Yakult were associated with subjects rather than controls. There was little change in these results after smoking status adjustments (Ohashi et al, 2002).

Candidal Vaginitis

No efficacy was found for *lactobacillus* in the prevention of post-antibiotic vulvovaginitis in one randomized, placebo-controlled, double-blind study. Following enrollment, *lactobacillus* preparations were taken orally, vaginally, or both until 4 days following antibiotic therapy. Overall, 23% of women developed vulvovaginal candidiasis during the trial, which was terminated early due to a lack of treatment effect. (Pirotta et al 2004). In an earlier study, 28 women with recurrent vaginitis used glycerol suppositories impregnated with 10 billion *lactobacillus* GG organisms twice a day for 7 days. Specimens were taken from the posterior fornix at the start and after the treatment period. All women reported subjective improvement; on physical exam, a decrease in erythema and discharge were noted. Five of the women had significant colony counts on *Candida albicans,* which may have been secondary to prior treatment with antifungal agents (Hilton, 1995).

Constipation

Daily consumption of a beverage containing *Lactobacillus caseii Shirota* (LcS) improved stool frequency and consistency and sense of well-being in patients with chronic constipation. In a randomized, double-blind, placebo-controlled trial 70 men and women with chronic idiopathic constipation received LcS 65 mL or 65 mL of a sensorially equivalent placebo daily for 4 weeks. Both beverages contained protein 1.3 g, fat 0.004 g, carbohydrates 18 g per 100 mL, and lactic acid 580 mg. The daily dose of LcS beverage contained at least 6.5 x 10^9 colony forming units of LcS. In the LcS group, the occurrence of moderate or severe constipation decreased during treatment from 96% at baseline to 34%; occurrence in the placebo group was unchanged ($p<0.001$). The occurrence of hard stools decreased in the LcS group but not in the placebo group ($p<0.001$). Differences between the groups were significant starting in the second week of treatment. Flatulence occurred in 47% of patients at baseline; at the end of the study, 6% of the LcS group and 17% of the placebo group reported flatulence (treatment effect not statistically significant). Self-reported general well-being was distinctly improved in the treatment group and not in the placebo group ($p=0.008$). The treatment tolerability was rated as "very good" or "good" by 91% of the patients (Koebnick et al, 2003).

Diarrhea, Antibiotic-Associated

According to one recent review, the probiotic organism *Saccharomyces boulardii* can prevent antibiotic-associated diarrhea (AAD), as demonstrated by several controlled trials. In an earlier study of 180 hospitalized patients, AAD occurred in 22% of those receiving placebo and in 9% of those who received *S boulardii*. More recently, *S boulardii* reduced AAD in patients being treated for *Helicobacter pylori*. Another randomized controlled trial showed similar benefits in a pediatric population (Huebner and Surawicz 2006).

A meta-analysis of randomized, double-blind, placebo-controlled trials (n=9), published between 1966 and 2000 and studying the effects of concurrent administration of probiotics on the occurrence of antibiotic-induced diarrhea, showed an overall odds ratio of 0.37 (95% confidence interval 0.26 to 0.53) in favor of active treatment over placebo. In the 5 studies that employed*lactobacillus* organisms (n=4) or enterococci (n=1), the odds ratio was 0.34 (95% confidence interval 0.19 to 0.61) in favor of active treatment for prevention of antibiotic-induced diarrhea (D'Souza et al, 2002).

On the contrary, a 14-day course of *Lactobacillus* GG (20 x 10^9 CFU) did not reduce the occurrence of antibiotic-associated diarrhea in hospitalized adult patients receiving a variety of antibiotics, based on a double-blind, randomized, controlled trial (n=267). Enrollees were patients admitted to a general internal medicine inpatient ward who received intravenous or oral antibiotics. Within 24 hours of initiation of antibiotic therapy, patients began placebo tablets or *lactobacillus* GG 1 capsule twice daily for 14 days (each capsule contained 10 x 10^9 CFU live *Lactobacillus*); patients continued the study medication even if discharged within the 14-day treatment period. Diarrhea occurred in 39 of 133 patients (29.3%) in the *Lactobacillus* group and in 40 of 134 patients (29.9%) in the control group ($p=0.93$). *Lactobacillus* did not affect either the consistency of stools or the frequency of stools. Similar frequencies of diarrhea occurred in *lactobacillus* and placebo-treated patients among those treated with beta-lactam antibiotics and those treated with non-beta-lactam antibiotics (Thomas et al, 2001).

Lactobacillus GG effectively ameliorated the frequency of diarrhea in a randomized, double-blind trial of 202 children (aged 6 months to 10 years) being treated with a 10-day course of oral antibiotics for minor infections. *Lactobacillus* was dosed once daily with food as 10 billion CFU for body weight under 12 k and 20 billion CFU for weight above 12 kg. Active and placebo groups did not differ significantly with respect to type of infection or antibiotic used. Eight percent of *Lactobacillus* and 26% of placebo recipients developed diarrhea (at least 2 liquid stools/day on at least 2 observation periods). Mean diarrhea duration was of borderline significance (4.7 vs 5.9 days for active and placebo groups, $p=0.05$). Stool consistency scores and number of stools/day favored *Lactobacillus* therapy ($p<0.02$ by day 10) (Vanderhoof et al, 1999).

Diarrhea, Infants and Children

According to one recent review, several placebo-controlled studies showed efficacy for *Lactobacillus* GG in reducing the severity and duration of acute diarrhea in infants and children. A meta-analysis of 18 studies concluded that the duration of acute diarrheal illness is reduced by about 1 day with probiotic therapy. Other controlled studies suggested a benefit for *Lactobacillus* GG in the prevention of community-acquired acute diarrhea, and for combination probiotic therapy in the prevention of nosocomial diarrhea. (Huebner and Surawicz 2006).

Bouts of acute diarrhea were lessened with *S boulardii* in one study of hospitalized children. This randomized, placebo-controlled trial assigned subjects to treatment with a daily dose of 250 mg *S boulardii* (n=100) or placebo (n=100) for 5 days. Following treatment, the duration of diarrhea was significantly reduced in the group receiving active treatment compared to the placebo group (4.7 vs 5.5 days; $p=0.03$). In addition, the duration of hospital stay was shorter in *S boulardii*—treated subjects compared with placebo subjects (2.9 vs 3.9 days; $p<0.001$) (Kurugol and Koturoglu 2005).

One controlled study examined the effect of 2 different species of probiotics in preventing infections in 201 infants among 14 child-care centers in Israel. Infants fed a formula supplemented with *Lactobacillus reuteri* or *Bifidobacterium lactis* for 12 weeks had fewer and shorter episodes of diarrhea compared to control subjects, although no effect was noted on the primary outcome of respiratory illness. There was a greater association of these findings with *Lactobacillus reuteri,* which also improved additional morbidity parameters. This was the first study of its kind to compare two commonly used probiotic organisms side by side (Weizman et al 2005).

Randomized, blinded, placebo-controlled trials have shown that treatment with *Lactobacillus casei* strain GG (LGG) can reduce the duration of watery diarrhea, including rotavirus-caused diarrhea in infants (Shornikova et al, 1997b; Isolauri et al, 1994; Isolauri et al, 1991). Typical dosages of LGG were 10 billion to 200 billion CFU/day for 5 days after rehydration therapy. Improvement was evident after 1 day of LGG treatment, and duration of diarrhea was reduced by about a day. LGG was not effective in the treatment of bacteria-caused diarrhea or bloody diarrhea. Not all trials with LGG have shown a beneficial effect (Costa-Ribeiro, 2003; Pearce & Hamilton, 1974). *Lactobacillus reuteri* in protocols similar to those with LGG has also produced reduction in duration of watery diarrhea (Shornikova et al, 1997a,c).

Diarrhea, Infectious

A Cochrane review reporting on the effects of probiotics in infectious diarrhea suggests that they are a useful addition to rehydration therapy. Adults and children were included in the total number of subjects studied (n=1,917) in the 23 randomized, controlled trials included for review. Random effects modeling of 15 studies showed the risk of diarrhea was reduced with probiotics at 3 days (relative risk [RR] 0.66, 95% confidence interval [CI] 0.55 to 0.77). In addition, the mean duration of diarrhea was reduced by 30.58 hours (95% CI 18.51 to 42.46 hours, random effect model, 12 studies) (Allen et al 2006).

Cow's milk containing added lactobacilli of specific strains or added *Saccharomyces* was effective in reducing persistent diarrhea in young children in comparison to cow's milk without additives. In a randomized, double-blind, placebo-controlled trial, 89 children (ages 6 to 24 months) with diarrhea for the previous 14 or more days were given pasteurized cow's milk 175 g twice daily for 5 days or the same dosage of pasteurized cow's milk containing lyophilized *Saccharomyces boulardii* 0.1 g/mL (with 1 g of powder containing 10^{10} colony-forming units [CFU]) or lyophilized *Lactobacillus casei* CERELA strain and *Lactobacillus acidophilus* CERELA strain (10^{10} to 10^{12} CFU/g). Prior to receiving the study medication, children with mild or moderate dehydration were rehydrated. By day 5, the average number of stools was 2 in the *S boulardii* group and 1.5 in the lactobacilli group, compared to 5.2 in the placebo group ($p<0.001$). Diarrhea did not stop by day 5 for 17% of the patients in the *S boulardii* group, 10% in the lactobacilli group, and 90% in the placebo group. Most children in the placebo group continued to have diarrhea up to 12 days. Both active treatments were effective in rotavirus-positive and rotavirus-negative subjects (Gaon et al, 2003).

Diarrhea Prevention

One randomized, double-blind, placebo-controlled study reported no impact on the prevention of diarrhea with a fermented infant formula containing *Bifidobacterium breve C50* and *Streptococcus thermophilus 065*. Infants ranging in age from 4 to 6 months were randomized to feeding with the fermented formula (FF group, n=464) or standard formula (control group, n=449) for 5 months. Although the incidence, duration of diarrhea episodes, and number of hospitalizations did not differ significantly between groups, episodes were of lesser severity in the FF group (Thibault et al 2004).

In an earlier study, milk fermented with yogurt cultures plus *Lactobacillus casei* strain DN-114 001 (3.2 x 10^8 CFU/mL) (Actimel®) decreased the incidence but not duration of diarrhea in healthy children (ages 6 to 24 months) attending daycare centers in France. In a randomized, double-blind trial (n=928 enrolled, 779 evaluable), Actimel or traditional yogurt were given twice daily, 5 days/week for 12 weeks followed by a 6-week observation period. Diarrhea occurred in 16% and 22% of the Actimel and yogurt groups, respectively, during the initial supplementation phase ($p=0.03$). Corresponding rates during the observation phase were statistically insignificant (1.9% vs 3.8%, respectively). The average durations of diarrhea were similar (3.95 vs 3.53 days for active and control groups, respectively) (Pedone et al, 2000).

Helicobacter pylori Infection

A meta-analysis investigated whether the addition of probiotics to therapy aimed at *H pylori* eradication could improve eradication rates and reduce side effects associated with therapy, thereby enhancing its effectiveness. The analysis identified 14 randomized trials involving 1,671 patients for inclusion. In intent-to-treat analysis, pooled *H pylori* eradication rates were 83.6% and 74.8% for patients with or without probiotics, respectively (odds ratio, 1.84). The occurrence of total side effects observed were 24.7% and 38.5% for groups with or without probiotics, especially for diarrhea. These findings provide evidence that the use of probiotics can inhibit *H pylori* colonization and may improve side effects (Tong et al 2007).

Fermented milk containing *Lactobacillus johnsonii* reduced the severity and activity of antrum inflammation and increased mucus thickness but did not eradicate *Helicobacter pylori* in asymptomatic, *H pylori*-infected patients. In a randomized, double-blind, placebo-controlled trial, 50 asymptomatic patients shown by serology, a C-urea breath test, histology, and culture to be infected with *H pylori* were given a fermented milk preparation either with or without *L johnsonii.* Patients were to ingest 125 g of the preparation twice daily for the first 3 weeks and then once daily through the 16th week of treatment. The product containing *L johnsonii* provided 10^6 to 10^7 CFU/g. *H pylori* was not eradicated in any patient over the 16 weeks of treatment. By 16 weeks, the inflammatory cell score in the antrum decreased modestly but significantly in the treatment group compared to baseline values (5.3 vs 6.0, p=0.04) and compared to the placebo-treated group (5.3 vs 6.4, p=0.002). Inflammatory cell score in the corpus was unchanged in both groups over the treatment period. Mucus thickness was increased in both the antrum and the corpus with 16 weeks of active treatment but not with placebo treatment (p=0.03). *H pylori* density decreased a small but statistically significant amount in the antrum (p=0.02) but not in the corpus of *L johnsonii*-treated subjects. *H pylori* density was unchanged in the placebo group (Pantoflickova et al, 2003).

INDICATIONS AND USAGE

Lactobacilli are used primarily for diarrhea. Other uses include treatment of irritable bowel syndrome, urinary tract infection, and vaginal candidiasis, and bacterial vaginosis.

CONTRAINDICATIONS

Lactobacillus is contraindicated in patients who have a hypersensitivity to lactose or milk. Over-the-counter commercial preparations are not to be used in children less than 3 years old unless under the direction of a physician.

PRECAUTIONS AND ADVERSE REACTIONS

Vomiting, diarrhea, burping, flatulence, hiccups, increased phlegm production, and rash were reported infrequently with oral administration. Disagreeable sensation and burning is possible with vaginal tablet. Stupor with EEG-slowing with high oral doses in patients with hepatic encephalopathy.

DRUG INTERACTIONS

No human drug interaction information is available.

DOSAGE

Mode of Administration: oral, vaginal

How Supplied: tablet, capsule, powder, dairy products, vaginal tablets

Daily Dosage:

ADULTS

Radiation-induced diarrhea (oral capsule): *Lactobacillus rhamnosus* (Antibiophilus®) 1.5 x 10^9 colony forming units 3 times daily for up to 1 week.

Uncomplicated diarrhea (oral): 1 to 2 billion viable cells of *L acidophilus* or other *Lactobacillus* species daily.

PEDIATRIC:

Note: Over-the-counter commercial preparations are not to be used in children under the age of 3 unless directed by a physician.

Diarrhea in undernourished children (oral, powder): *Lactobacillus rhamnosus* GG 37 billion organisms daily 6 days per week up to 15 months.

Infantile diarrhea (oral solution): *Lactobacillus reuteri* 10^{10} CFU daily for up to 5 days. *Lactobacillus* strain GG 5 x 10^9 CFU daily for up to 5 days.

LITERATURE

Allen SJ, Okoko B, Martinez E, et al. Probiotics for treating infectious diarrhea. *Cochrane Database Syst Rev*; 2:CD003048. 2004

Bernet MF, Brassart D, Neeser JR et al. Lactobacillus acidophilus LA-1 binds to cultured human intestinal cell lines and inhibits cell attachment and cell invasion by enterovirulent bacteria. *Gut*; 35(4):483-489. 1994

Bezkorovainy A. Probiotics: determinant of survival and growth in the gut. *Am J Clin Nutr*; 73(suppl):339S-405S. 2001

Bogovic-Matijasic B, Rogelj I, Nes IF et al. Isolation and characterization of two bacteriocins of Lactobacillus acidophilus LF221. *Appl Microbiol Biotechnol*; 49(5):606-612. 1998

Boris S, Suarez JE, Vazquez F et al. Adherence of human vaginal Lactobacilli to vaginal epithelial cells and interaction with uropathogens. *Infect Immun*; 66(5):1985-1989. 1998

Charteris WP, Kelly PM, Morelli L et al. Development and application of an in vitro methodology to determine the transit tolerance of potentially probiotic Lactobacillus and Bifidobacterium species in the upper human gastrointestinal tract. *J Appl Microbiol*; 84(5):759-768. 1998

Clements ML, Levine MM, Ristaino PA et al. Exogenous lactobacilli fed to man - their fate and ability to prevent diarrheal disease. *Prog Food Nutr Sci*; 7(3-4):29-37. 1983

Coconnier M-H, Lievin V, Bernet-Camard M-F et al. Antibacterial effect of the adhering human Lactobacillus acidophilus strain LB. *Antimicrob Agents Chemother*; 41(5):1046-1052. 1997

Costa-Ribeiro H, Ribeiro TCM, Mattos AP et al. Limitations of probiotic therapy in acute, severe dehydrating diarrhea. *J Pediatr Gastroenterol Nutr*; 36:112-115. 2003

D'Souza A, Rajkumar C, Cooke J et al. Probiotics in prevention of antibiotic associated diarrhoea: meta-analysis. *BMJ*; 324:1361. 2002

Elmer GW, Surawicz CM & McFarland LV. Biotherapeutic agents: a neglected modality for the treatment and prevention of selected intestinal and vaginal infections. *JAMA*; 275(11):870-876. 1996

Gaon D, Garcia H, Winter L et al. Effect of Lactobacillus strains and Saccharomyces boulardii on persistent diarrhea in children. *Medicina* (B Aires); 63:293-298. 2003

Hawrelak J. Probiotics: Choosing the right one for your needs. *J Austral Tradition Med Soc*; 9(2):67-75. 2003

Hilton E, Isenberg HD, Alperstein P et al. Ingestion of yogurt containing lactobacillus-acidophilus as prophylaxis for candidal vaginitis. *Ann Intern Med*; 116(5):353-357. 1992

Hilton E, Rindos P & Isenberg H. Lactobacillus GG Vaginal suppositories and vaginitis. *J Clin Microbiol*; 33(5):1433. 1995

Hosoda M, Hashimoto H, He F et al. Inhibitory effects of fecal lactobacilli and bifidobacteria on the mutagenicities of Trp-P-2 and IQ. *Milchwissenschaft*; 53(6):309-313. 1998

Huebner ES, Surawicz CM. Probiotics in the prevention and treatment of gastrointestinal infections. *Gastroenterol Clin N Am*; 35:355-365. 2006

Kasper H. Protection against gastrointestinal diseases–present facts and future developments. *Int J Food Microbiol*; 41(2):127-131. 1998

Koebnick C, Wagner I, Leitzmann P et al. Probiotic beverage containing *Lactobacillus casei Shirota* improves gastrointestinal symptoms in patients with chronic constipation. *Can J Gastroenterol*; 17(11):655-659. 2003

Kurugol Z, Koturoglu G. Effect of *S boulardii* in children with acute diarrhea. *Acta Paediatrica*; 94:44-47, 2005

McGroarty JA & Reid G. Detection of a Lactobacillus substance that inhibits *Escherichia coli. Can J Microbiol*; 34(8):974-978. 1988a

McGroarty JA & Reid G. Inhibition of Enterococci by Lactobacillus species in vitro. *Microb Ecol Health Dis*; 1:215-219. 1988

Neri A, Sabah G & Samra Z. Bacterial vaginosis in pregnancy treated with yoghurt. *Acta Obstet Gynecol Scand*; 72(1):17-19. 1993

Nielsen OH, Jorgensen S, Pedersen K et al. Microbiological evaluation of jejunal aspirates and faecal samples after oral administration of bifidobacteria and lactic acid bacteria. *J Appl Bacteriol*; 76(5):469-474. 1994

Ohashi Y, Nakai S, Tsukamoto T et al. Habitual intake of lactic acid bacteria and risk reduction of bladder cancer. *Urol Int*; 68(7):273-22002

Pantoflickova D, Corthesy-Theulaz I, Dorta G et al. Favourable effect of regular intake of fermented milk containing *Lactobacillus johnsonii* on *Helicobacter pylori*-associated gastritis. *Aliment Pharmacol Ther*; 18:805-813. 2003

Parent D, Bossens M, Bayot D et al. Therapy of bacterial vaginosis using exogenously-applied *Lactobacilli acidophili* and a low dose of estriol. *Arzneimittelforschung*; 46(1):68-73. 1996

Pearce JL & Hamilton JR. Controlled trial of orally administered lactobacilli in acute infantile diarrhea. *J Pediatr*; 84(2):261-262. 1974

Pedone CA, Arnaud CC, Postaire ER et al. Multicentric study of the effect of milk fermented by *Lactobacillus casei* on the incidence of diarrhea. *Int J Clin Pract*; 54(9):568-571. 2000

Pirotta M, Gunn J, Chondros P, et al. Effect of lactobacillus in preventing post-antibiotic vulvovaginal candidiasis: a randomized controlled trial. *BMJ*; August 27 2004

Read AE, McCarthy CF, Heaton KW et al. Lactobacillus acidophilus (Enpac) in treatment of hepatic encephalopathy. *BMJ*; 1(5498):1267-1269. 1966

Reid G, Bruce AW, McGroarty JA et al. Is there a role for Lactobacilli in prevention of urogenital and intestinal infections? *Clin Microbiol Rev*; 3(4):335-344. 1990

Reid G, McGroarty JA, Angotti R et al. Lactobacillus inhibitor production against Escherichia coli and coaggregation ability with uropathogens. *Can J Microbiol*; 34(3):344-351. 1988

Shornikova AV, Casas IA, Mykkanen H et al. Bacteriotherapy with *Lactobacillus reuteri* in rotavirus gastroenteritis. *Pediatr Infect Dis J*; 16(12):1103-1107. 1997a

Silva M, Jacobus NV, Deneke C et al. Antimicrobial substance from a human Lactobacillus strain. *Antimicrob Agents Chemother*; 31(8):1231-1233. 1987

Takeshita F, Leifer CA, Gursel I et al. Cutting edge: role of toll-like receptor 9 in CpG DNA-induced activation of human cells. *J Immunology*; 167:3555-3558. 2001

Thibault H, Aubert-Jacquin C, Goulet O. Effects of long-term consumption of a fermented infant formula (with *Bifidobacterium breve C50* and *Streptococcus thermophilus* 065) on acute diarrhea in healthy infants. *J Pediatr Gastroenterol Nutr*; 39:147-152. 2004

Thomas MR, Litin SC, Osmon DR et al. Lack of effect of Lactobacillus GG on antibiotic-associated diarrhea: a randomized, placebo-controlled trial. *Mayo Clin Proc*; 76:883-889. 2001

Tong JL, Ran ZH, Shen J et al. Meta-analysis: the effect of supplementation with probiotics on eradication rates and adverse events during *Helicobacter pylori* eradication therapy. *Aliment Pharmacol Ther*; 25:155-168. 2007

Tuomola EM & Salminen SJ. Adhesion of some probiotic and dairy Lactobacillus strains to Caco-2 cell cultures. *Int J Food Microbiol*; 41(1):45-51. 1998

Vanderhoof JA, Whitney DB, Antonson DL et al. Lactobacillus GG in the prevention of antibiotic-associated diarrhea in children. *J Pediatr* 1999; 135:564-568.

Weizman Z, Ghaleb A, Alsheikh A. Effect of a probiotic infant formula on infections in child care centers: comparison of two probiotic agents. *Pediatrics*;115:5-9. 2005

Quercetin

DESCRIPTION

Quercetin is a bioflavonoid with antioxidant capacities. The highest quercetin concentrations are found in beer, wine, tea, coffee, onions, kale, French beans, broccoli, lettuce, apples, and tomatoes (Formica & Regelson, 1995).

Other Names: 2-(3,4-dihydroxyphenyl)-3,5,7,trihydroxy-4H-1-benzopyran-4-one; 3,3′,4′,5,7-pentahydroxyflavone; Flavan-3,4-diols; Vitamin P

ACTIONS AND PHARMACOLOGY

EFFECTS

Quercetin may have antioxidant, antineoplastic, anti-inflammatory, and antiviral activity. As an anticancer agent, quercetin interrupts cell cycles, ATPase activity, signal transduction, and phosphorylation. Some activity had been found against viral reverse transcriptases.

Anti-Enzymatic Effects: Inhibition of liver glutathione-S-transferase activity has been demonstrated. This enzyme plays an important part in the development of resistance to various cancer chemotherapy agents (Pickett & Lu, 1989; Das et al, 1986). Quercetin is also a potent inhibitor of p-form phenol-sulfotransferase, an enzyme used to sulfonate various drugs and environmental chemicals. (Walle et al, 1995).

Antioxidant Effects: Low-density lipoproteins are oxidatively modified by macrophages in the formation of foam cells and atherosclerotic plaque. Quercetin inhibited oxidative modification with an effective dose concentration 50% of about 2 mmol/liter. Based on the results of several studies, it appears that quercetin donates an electron to enzyme-bound alpha tocopherol, preventing LDL oxidation (Frankel et al, 1993a, Frankel et al, 1993b, De Walley et al, 1990).

Anti-Inflammatory Effects: Quercetin, like most flavonoids, modified acute inflammatory responses by suppressing macrophage phagocytosis. Quercetin also decreased the release of oxidants by phagocytosizing neutrophils and by macrophages phagocytosizing latex particles, and activation of mast cells (Daniel et al, 1988; Busse et al, 1984). A specific anti-inflammatory response may be more complicated since many of quercetin's functions are biphasic with lymphocyte proliferation and function stimulated at low doses but inhibited at larger doses (Formica & Regelson, 1995). Quercetin inhibits both lung and intestinal mast cell reactivity to histamine release (Middleton & Ferriola, 1988; Pearce et al, 1984).

Antiviral Effects: Antiviral activity has been demonstrated. Quercetin's antiviral activity may be related to its ability to bind viral protein coat and to interfere with viral nucleic acid synthesis (DNA) (Formica & Regelson, 1995).

Effects with Iron: Quercetin acts as an iron-chelating agent (Sestili et al, 1998). This was demonstrated in an iron-loaded preparation of rat hepatocytes. Quercetin prevented lipid peroxidation and enzyme leakage in this preparation (Morel et al, 1993). Quercetin has a pro-oxidant effect and will increase the iron-dependent DNA damage induced by bleomycin. Quercetin may reduce iron to the ferrous state, which allows bleomycin to complex more readily with oxygen and produce more efficient DNA damage (Laughton et al, 1991). A biphasic pro-oxidant effect with bleomycin has been demonstrated. At low concentrations increased DNA damage was noted, and at higher doses less DNA damage was noted.

CLINICAL TRIALS

Cancer Treatment

Lymphocyte protein kinase phosphorylation was inhibited by quercetin in 9 of 11 cancer patients in a phase I clinical trial. Fifty-one patients with microscopically confirmed cancer not amenable to standard therapies and with a life expectancy of at least 12 weeks participated in this trial. The patients had not received any other form of chemotherapy, immunotherapy, or radiotherapy for 3 to 6 weeks (depending on the agent). The patients were treated at 3-week intervals at the beginning of the study. Quercetin was administered intravenously as quercetin dihydrate and administered at a concentration of 50 mg/mL for doses up to 945 mg/m2, and at 100 mg/mL for doses above this. The maximum allowed dose was reached when 2 of 3 patients on each dose schedule reached grade 3 or 4 general toxicity, or grade 2 renal toxicity, cardiac toxicity, or neurotoxicity. Phosphorylation was inhibited at 1 hour and persisted for 16 hours. In one patient with ovarian cancer refractory to cisplatin, CA 125 fell from 295 to 55 units/mL after treatment with two courses of quercetin (totaling 420 mg/m2). Also in this group of study patients, a hepatoma patient had serum alpha-fetoprotein fall (Ferry et al, 1996).

Cardiovascular Disease

Epidemiological studies suggest that quercetin protects against cardiovascular disease. Long-term flavone and flavonol dietary intake was strongly inversely proportional to thrombotic stroke. One study involved a cohort of 552 middle-aged men without history of stroke. The men were divided into quartiles of flavonol and flavone intake and followed for 15 years. During these years, 42 men had a first stroke. The association was not affected by other risk factors. In the top quartile, those that were taking over 30 mg daily had about one-third the risk of stroke (Hertog & Hollman, 1996).

Prostatitis

Quercetin improved symptoms of benign prostatic hyperplasia in a small double-blind, placebo-controlled study. Thirty men with category IIIa and IIIb chronic pelvic pain were randomized to receive placebo or 500 mg quercetin twice daily for a month. All of the patients in the quercetin group finished the study while 2 of the 15 placebo subjects withdrew due to increased symptoms. Improvement was measured on the NIH symptom score. Twenty percent of patients taking placebo and 67% of those taking the quercetin had symptom improvement of at least 25% (p=0.003) (Shoskes et al, 1999).

INDICATIONS AND USAGE

Unproven Uses: Quercetin may protect against the development of cardiovascular disease and alleviate the symptoms of prostatitis.

PRECAUTIONS AND ADVERSE REACTIONS

Side effects include pain, flushing, dyspnea, and emesis after intravenous injection.

Nephrotoxicity has been a dose-limiting side effect of quercetin administration in humans.

Drug Interactions:

Cyclosporine: Concomitant use may reduce cyclosporine effectiveness. *Clinical Management:* Monitor serum concentrations of cyclosporine and signs and symptoms of loss of efficacy in patients taking quercetin and cyclosporine.

Floroquinolones: Concomitant use may reduce effectiveness of fluoroquinolones. *Clinical Management:* Patients taking fluoroquinolones and quercetin concomitantly should be monitored for signs of decreased activity of fluoroquinolones.

DOSAGE

Mode of Administration: Oral, intravenous

How Supplied: Intravenous solution in ethanol or DMSO, capsule, tablet, food and drink.

Daily Dosage: 400 to 500 mg orally 3 times daily is recommended by practitioners of natural medicine. If the water soluble quercetin chalcone is used the dose is reduced to about 250 mg 3 times daily.

Prostatitis: 500 mg orally of quercetin twice daily.

Cancer (quercetin dihydrate in ethanol or DMSO): An intravenous bolus dose of 1400 mg/m^2 given at 3-week intervals (from a phase 1 study) (Ferry et al, 1996).

Storage: Quercetin tablets and capsules should be stored at room temperature, away from heat, moisture, and direct light.

LITERATURE

Beretz A, Stierle A, Anton R et al. Role of cyclic AMP in the inhibition of human platelet aggregation by quercetin, a flavonoid that potentiates the effect of prostacyclin. *Biochem Pharmacol*; 31(22):3597-3600. 1982

Busse WW, Kopp DE & Middleton E Jr. Flavonoid modulation of human neutrophil function. *J Allergy Clin Immunol*; 73(6):801-809. 1984

Christensen RL, Shade DL & Graves CB. Evidence that protein kinase C is involved in regulating glucose transport in the adipocyte. *Int J Biochem*; 19(3):259-265. 1987

Daniel PT, Holzschuh J & Berg PA. Interference of the flavonoid compound cianidanol with macrophage function and lymphocyte activating mechanisms. In: Cody V, Middleton Jr E, Harborne JB (eds): Progress in Clinical and Biological Research; vol. 280, pp. 205-209, Alan R. Liss, New York, NY, 1988.

De Walley CV, Rankin SM, Hoult JRS et al. Flavonoids inhibit the oxidative modification of low density lipoproteins by macrophages. *Biochem Pharmacol*; 39(11):1743-1750. 1990

Fawzy AA, Vishwanath BS & Franson RC. Inhibition of human non-pancreatic phospholipases A2 by retinoids and flavonoids. Mechanism of action. *Agents Actions*; 25(3-4):394-400. 1988

Ferry DR, Smith A, Malkhandi J et al. Phase I clinical trial of the flavonoid quercetin. Pharmacokinetics and evidence for in vivo tyrosine kinase inhibition. *Clin Cancer Res*; 2(4):659-668. 1996

Formica JV & Regelson W. Review of the biology of quercetin and related bioflavonoids. *Fd Chem Tox*; 33(12):1061-1080. 1995

Frankel EN, Kanner J, German JB et al. Inhibition of oxidation of human low-density lipoprotein by phenolic substances in red wine. *Lancet*; 341(8843):454-457. 1993a

Frankel EN, Waterhouse AL & Kinsella JE. Inhibition of human LDL oxidation by resveratrol. *Lancet*; 341(8852):1103-1104. 1993b

Gorman RR, Bunting S & Miller OV. Modulation of human platelet adenylate cyclase by prostacyclin. *Prostaglandins*; 13(3):377-388. 1977

Havsteen B. Flavonoids, a class of natural products of high pharmacological potency. *Biochem Pharmcol*; 32(7):1141-1448. 1983

Hertog MGL & Hollman PCH. Potential health effects of the dietary flavonol quercetin. *Eur J Clin Nutr*; 50(2):63-71. 1996

Lanza F, Beretz A, Stierle A et al. Cyclic nucleotide phosphodiesterase inhibitors prevent aggregation of human platelets by raising cyclic AMP and reducing cytoplasmic free calcium mobilization. *Thrombosis Res*; 45(5):477-484. 1987

Laughton MJ, Evans PA, Moroney MA et al. Inhibition of mammalian 5-lipoxygenase and cyclo-oxygenase by flavonoids and phenolic dietary additives. *Biochem Pharmacol*; 42(9):1673-1681. 1991

Lee T-P, Matteliano ML & Middleton E Jr. Effect of quercetin on human polymorphonuclear leukocyte lysosomal enzyme release and phospholipid metabolism. *Life Sci*; 31(24):2765-2774. 1982

Middleton E Jr & Ferriola P. Effect of flavonoids on protein kinase C, relationship to inhibition of human basophil histamine release. In: Cody V, Middleton Jr E, Harborne JB (eds): Progress in Clinical and Biological Research; vol. 280, pp. 251-266, Alan R. Liss, New York, NY, 1988.

Morel I, Lescoat G, Cogrel P et al. Antioxidant and iron-chelating activities of the flavonoids catechin, quercetin and diosmetin on iron-loaded rat hepatocyte cultures. *Biochem Pharmcol*; 45(1):13-19. 1993

Pearce FL, Befus AD & Bienenstock J. Mucosal mast cells. III. Effect of quercetin and other flavonoids on antigen-induced histamine secretion from rat intestinal mast cells. *J Allergy Clin Immunol*; 73(6):819-823. 1984

Pickett CB & Lu AY. Glutathione S-transferase: gene structure, regulation and biological function. *Ann Rev Biochem*; 58:743-764. 1989

Robinson DR, Curran DP & Hamer PJ. Prostaglandins and related compounds in inflammatory rheumatic diseases. In: Ziff M, Vilo GP & Gorini S (eds): Advances in Inflammatory Research. vol. 3, Raven Press, NY, NY; 1982: 17-27.

Sestili P, Guidarelli A, Dacha M et al. Quercetin prevents DNA single strand breakage and cytotoxicity caused by tert-butylhydroperoxide: free radical scavenging versus iron chelating mechanism. *Free Rad Bio Med*; 25(2):196-200. 1998

Shoskes DA, Zeitlin SI, Shahed A et al. Quercetin in men with category III chronic prostatitis: a preliminary prospective, double-blind, placebo-controlled trial. *Urology*; 54(6):960-963. 1999

Walle T, Eaton A & Walle UK. Quercetin, a potent and specific inhibitor of the human p-form phenolsulfotransferase. *Biochem Pharmacol*; 50(5):731-734. 1995

S-adenosylmethionine (SAMe)

DESCRIPTION

SAMe is a naturally occurring substance present in virtually all body tissues and fluids. It is derived from adenosine triphosphate and the amino acid l-methionine (Osman et al, 1993). SAMe was discovered in 1952 but it was not until the mid-1970s that a stable salt of the molecule was made available for clinical investigation. The first indication of an antidepressive action was reported in 1976. Injectable forms of SAMe have been available on the pharmaceutical market since the late 1970s (Di Padova, 1987).

Other Names: Ademethionine, Adomet, S-adenosyl-L-methionine

ACTIONS AND PHARMACOLOGY

EFFECTS

SAMe is primarily used for the treatment of depression. In addition to its antidepressant action SAMe has been used to relieve symptoms of osteoarthritis and fibromyalgia and to combat the clinical and biochemical abnormalities of chronic alcoholic and nonalcoholic liver disease. SAMe promotes bile flow and may relieve cholestasis. It is claimed that SAMe may increase the detoxification and elimination of pharmaceuticals from the body.

There is also evidence that SAMe may lessen the severity of chronic liver disease and, in animal studies, prevent liver cancer. SAMe is produced in the body from the amino acid methionine and adenosine triphosphate. It serves as a source of methyl groups in numerous biochemical reactions involving the synthesis, activation, and metabolism of hormones, proteins, catecholamines, nucleic acids, and phospholipids. Release of methyl groups also promotes the formation of glutathione, the chief cellular antioxidant, thereby favoring detoxification processes. SAMe is closely linked with the metabolism of folate and vitamin B_{12}, which accounts for its ability to lower excessive homocyteine serum concentrations resulting from a deficiency of one or both of these nutrients (Osman et al, 1993; Bottiglieri et al, 1990). SAMe is postulated to increase the turnover of the neurotransmitters dopamine and serotonin in the central nervous system. It has been shown to increase the levels of the serotonin metabolite 5-hydroxyindoleacetic acid in the cerebrospinal fluid (Pies, 2000).

Antidepressant Effects: A low level of SAMe in the cerebrospinal fluid (CSF) of some depressed patients suggests a possible disorder of methylation in the central nervous system and provides a rational basis for using SAMe therapeutically (Bottiglieri et al, 1994, 1990). Parenterally administered SAMe crosses the blood-brain barrier and, when present in high levels in the CSF, increases the CSF concentrations of 5-hydroxyindoleacetic acid and homovanillic acid while reducing serum prolactin levels, reflecting increased turnover of serotonin and dopamine.

There is evidence that SAMe increases the turnover of serotonin, inhibits reuptake of the catecholamine norepinephrine, and enhances dopaminergic activity. SAMe also increases levels of folate, which may have a role in depression (Rosenbaum et al, 1990). SAMe increases the fluidity of cell membranes by increasing the conversion of phosphatidylethanolamine (PtdEth) to phosphatidylcholine (PtdCho) and thereby could alter the functioning of receptors and ion channels. The stimulation of phospholipid methylation by beta-adrenergic agonists is regulated by SAMe, suggesting a possible common path whereby amines and SAMe interact in depression (Bressa, 1994; Kagan et al, 1990). Studies following the time course of changes in SAMe and melatonin in the rat pineal gland suggest an association between the concentration of SAMe and melatonin synthesis. Because disordered circadian rhythm is common in depression, the antidepressant action of SAMe may result from its ability to alter these rhythms through regulating melatonin synthesis in the pineal gland (Sitaram et al, 1995).

Anti-Inflammatory Effects: The action of SAMe in relieving symptoms of primary fibromyalgia may result from its effectiveness in lessening the depressive state that can accompany fibromyalgia (Tavoni et al, 1987). SAMe also has antidepressive and mood-elevating effects in patients with rheumatoid arthritis and osteoarthritis (Koenig, 1987). SAMe exerts both anti-inflammatory and analgesic effects, which may possibly explain its efficacy in relieving symptoms of osteoarthritis. Its anti-inflammatory activity is not reliant on conversion to methionine. SAMe does not appear to act in the same way as nonsteroidal anti-inflammatory drugs. It increases the formation of native proteoglycans in human chondrocytes, which may have positive effects on the metabolism of joint tissue (Di Padova, 1987). SAMe counters the effects of tumor necrosis factor-alpha by decreasing the proliferation of synovial cells and fibronectin synthesis, suggesting a protective effect of joint cells against the activity of pro-inflammatory mediators (Gutierrez et al, 1997).

Hepatoprotective Effects: Several mechanisms for the hepatoprotective effect of SAMe have been proposed. The release of methyl groups from SAMe activates the transsulfuration pathway and leads to formation of glutathione, a key cellular antioxidant that promotes detoxifying processes. In cirrhosis, both transmethylation and transsulfuration are impaired and there are abnormally low amounts of SAMe synthetase, an enzyme needed to form SAMe. Glutathione levels also are reduced in cirrhosis, reflecting decreased synthesis of SAMe (Osman et al, 1993). In chronic liver disease, cholesterol is deposited in liver-cell membranes as well as those of red blood cells and kidney cells. An elevated cholesterol content in cell-surface membranes reduces membrane fluidity and this effect might be reduced when SAMe is available to reverse cholesterol accumulation (Rafique et al, 1992).

Estrogen reduces the membrane fluidity of liver cells, possibly contributing to the accumulation of bile in the liver of pregnant women with intrahepatic cholestasis. SAMe may improve those affected by lessening cholesterol saturation of the bile. SAMe also promotes the formation of thiols by enhancing transsulfuration, which aids in detoxification (Frezza et al, 1988). Feeding rats a methyl-deficient diet is carcinogenic and also reduces the amount of SAMe present. Providing SAMe exogenously prevents precancerous and cancerous lesions in the rat liver. It is possible that inadequate methylation of growth-related genes leads to their overexpression and the overgrowth of precancerous liver tissue (Pascale et al, 1993). Rats given a chemical that induces malignant changes in liver cells over-expressed several proto-oncogenes. Providing adequate SAMe inhibited the expression of these genes and prevented malignant lesions (Simile et al, 1994). The preventive effect of SAMe against induced cancer in the rat liver may be related to the production of 5′-methylthioadenosine, a product of SAMe metabolism that inhibits cell growth (Pascale et al, 1992).

CLINICAL TRIALS

Depressive disorders

Evidence exists demonstrating the efficacy and tolerability of SAMe as an antidepressant. Parenteral and oral formulations of SAMe exhibited comparable efficacy to imipramine in two multicenter studies, with fewer side effects. One study involved orally administered SAMe at a dose of 1600 mg/day (n=143) for 6 weeks compared to 150 mg/day of oral imipramine (n=138). In a second study, SAMe was given via the intramuscular route at a dose of 400 mg/day (n=147) for 4 weeks, while another group received 150 mg/day of oral imipramine (n=148). The results of treatment with SAMe demonstrated comparable efficacy with oral imipramine; measures of efficacy did not differ significantly between groups. However, significantly less adverse events were noted in the patients treated with SAMe (Delle Chiaie et al, 2002).

One review reports that of seven studies examined, depression ratings were improved after administration of SAMe on at least one measure in six of the trials (Sarac and Gur, 2006)

Three separate meta-analyses of the studies on SAMe assessing the efficacy of this compound in the treatment of depression compared with placebo and standard tricyclic antidepressants showed a greater response rate with SAMe when compared with placebo, with a global effect size ranging from 17% to 38%, depending on the definition of response, and an antidepressant effect comparable with that of standard tricyclic antidepressants. The efficacy of SAMe in treating depressive syndromes and disorders is superior with that of placebo and comparable to that of standard tricyclic antidepressants (Bressa GM, 1994). The following describes each meta-analysis in this study:

A meta-analysis of the effects of SAMe in patients with depressive syndromes included 6 prospective studies which used oral and parenteral SAMe and compared it with placebo. One of the criteria for inclusion in the study was that the SAMe dosage was greater than or equal to 200 mg daily parenterally or greater than or equal to 1600 mg daily orally.

Another meta-analysis of 6 trials in the partial to full response outcome group, which was a part of a controlled study comparing SAMe with placebo, found a global response of 70% for SAMe and 30% for placebo with a highly significant global p value ($p<0.00001$). Five of the 6 studies found a greater full or partial response rate with SAMe than with placebo. The full response outcome comparing SAMe to placebo showed a global response of 38% for SAMe and 22% for placebo and a significant global p value ($p<0.05$) and 17% global effect size.

A third meta-analysis of 6 trials in the partial to full response outcome group, which was a part of the controlled study comparing SAMe with antidepressants, showed SAMe to have a global response of 92% and 85% for tricyclic antidepressants and a nonsignificant global p value and a global effect size of 7%. The full response outcome in the meta- analysis comparing SAMe to antidepressants showed a global response of 61% for SAMe and 59% for antidepressants. There was a non-significant global p value and a global effect size of 1%.

SAMe appears to have a rapid onset of effect in the treatment of depression. In an open, multicenter study, 195 patients were given 400 mg of SAMe, administered parenterally, for 15 days, depressive symptoms remitted after both 7 and 15 days of treatment with SAMe, and no serious adverse events were reported (Fava et al, 1995).

In a double-blind, placebo-controlled study of 80 postmenopausal women, between the ages of 45 and 59, who were diagnosed as having DSM-III-R major depressive disorder or dysthymia between 6 and 36 months following either natural menopause or hysterectomy, underwent 1 week of single-blind placebo washout, followed by 30 days of double-blind treatment with either SAMe 1,600 mg/day or placebo. There was a significantly greater improvement in depressive symptoms in the group treated with SAMe compared to the placebo group from day 10 of the study. Side effects were mild and transient (Salmaggi P et al, 1993).

Liver Disease

A recent review of the potential efficacy and safety of 7 nutritional supplements reported the effects of SAMe on liver function (Hanje et al, 2006). One study of alcoholic patients treated with parenteral SAMe (2 d/day for 15 days IV) noted improved erythrocyte glutathione (GSH) concentrations. Patients with alcoholic and primary biliary cirrhosis demonstrated similar improvements in another study cited. Improvements in serum transaminase and bilirubin have been observed in patients with intrahepatic cholestasis when treated with SAMe. One pivotal study reported that supplementation with SAMe (1200 mg/day) in patients with less severe alcoholic cirrhosis led to improved mortality and decreased the need for liver transplantation. The 2-year, multicenter, randomized, placebo-controlled trial enrolled a total of 123 patients.

SAMe reduced pruritus associated with gestational cholestasis but did not improve serum bile acid concentrations in a randomized, open-label trial of 46 women with gestational cholestasis who were diagnosed before 36 weeks of gestation. They were given either SAMe 500 mg twice daily or oral ursodeoxycholic acid 300 mg twice daily until delivery. Treatment lasted for 4 to 54 days (mean 18 days) for the SAMe group and 3 to 63 days (mean 27 days) for the ursodeoxycholic acid group ($p=0.04$). Pruritus improved equally for the 2 treatments. Laboratory values (bile acids, serum bilirubin, serum liver enzymes) improved with ursodeoxycholic acid but not with SAMe (Roncaglia et al, 2004).

Nine patients with alcoholic liver disease and 7 patients with nonalcoholic liver disease received 1.2 g of SAMe orally for 6 months, after which time hepatic glutathione levels were significantly increased compared to those in matched control subjects. The results suggested that SAMe may reverse hepatic glutathione depletion in patients with liver disease (Vendemiale et al, 1989).

Mood Disorders

SAMe significantly improved quality of life and behavior in subjects (aged 55 to 80 years) with mild mood disorders. One hundred ninety-two subjects, who did not meet DSM-IV criteria for major depression or qualify for psychotropic medication, received SAMe 100 mg 2 times a day orally for 2 months in an open-label, multicenter trial. Subjects were administered two self-assessment questionnaires at prestudy and at 1 and 2 months post treatment in order to evaluate physical, mental, and social behaviors and to rate drug efficacy and tolerability. Subjects reported improvement in all measurable parameters of the questionnaires compared to baseline ($p<0.001$) (Pancheri, 2002). Open label depression studies are often subject to a large placebo effect, suggesting that the results of this study should be cautiously interpreted.

Fibromyalgia

A recent review of treatments for fibromyalgia found that SAMe decreased the number of tender points or intensity of tender point scores in 5 of 7 clinical trials, 4 of which were randomized, control trials (Sarac and Gur, 2006).

In an earlier study, SAMe significantly decreased tender points and improved pain and fatigue in patients with primary fibromyalgia as compared to transcutaneous electrical nerve stimulation (TENS). Thirty patients were randomly assigned to receive SAMe or TENS in a 6-week controlled study. Patients daily received 200 mg intramuscularly and 400 mg orally of SAMe. TENS patients received 5 morning sessions each week. Four tender points, selected by the investigator after discussion with the patient, were chosen at each session. Both groups had a manual assessment of the pain of each tender point, which was graded on a scale of 0 (no tenderness) to 4 (maximum tenderness). The SAMe group showed a significant decrease in the total number of tender points ($p<0.01$). At the end of treatment the two groups differed significantly ($p=0.05$) in the total number of tender points ($p<0.05$). Both treatments were well tolerated without side effects (Di Benedetto et al, 1993).

In yet an earlier study involving 44 patients with primary fibromyalgia who took 800 mg of oral SAMe daily, benefits were observed in the active-treatment group compared with the placebo group. In this double-blind, placebo-controlled study, fatigue, morning stiffness, and clinical disease activity decreased in the actively treated patients, as did the amount of pain experienced in the past week. Mood, as assessed using the Face Scale, improved in patients given SAMe compared to placebo recipients. There were no group differences in tender points or muscle strength. Beck depression ratings did not differ between the SAMe-treated and placebo patients. Eight actively treated patients experienced side effects. Of this group, 7 patients had gastrointestinal symptoms and 1 patient experienced dizziness. The placebo group reported similar side effects (Jacobsen et al, 1991).

Osteoarthritis

A randomized, double-blind crossover study comparing SAMe (1200 mg/day) with celecoxib (200 mg/day) found both were effective at relieving symptoms associated with osteoarthritis of the knee. Sixty-one adults were enrolled; of these, 56 completed the study. Treatment was administered for 16 weeks, with a 1-week washout between the two 8-week phases. On the first month, there was significantly more pain reduction with celocoxib vs SAMe ($p=0.024$); however, by the second month of Phase I, no significant differences were observed between groups ($p<0.01$). Functional measures were improved from baseline in both groups following treatment; but again, no significant differences were observed between groups. Testing of isometric joint function appeared to show continual improvement over the course of treatment with either agent. The findings from this study show that although it had a slower onset of action, SAMe was as effective as celecoxib in managing symptoms of knee osteoarthritis. (Najm et al, 2004)

INDICATIONS AND USAGE

The clinical application of SAMe centers on the treatment of depression, pain disorders, and liver toxicity.

PRECAUTIONS AND ADVERSE REACTIONS

For patients with bipolar disorder, only under strict medical supervision should SAMe be considered (Kagan et al, 1990).

Reported side effects are rare and include anxiety, headache, urinary frequency, pruritus, nausea, and diarrhea.

DRUG INTERACTIONS

MODERATE RISKS

Tricyclic Antidepressants: Concurrent use of SAMe and tricyclic antidepressants may result in an increased risk of serotonin syndrome (hypertension, hyperthermia, myoclonus, mental status changes). *Clinical Management:* If SAMe and a tricyclic antidepressant are used together, use low doses of each and titrate upward slowly, while monitoring closely for early signs of serotonin syndrome such as increasing anxiety, confusion, and disorientation.

DOSAGE

Mode of Administration: oral, intravenous, intramuscular

How Supplied: enteric-coated tablet, solution for parenteral administration

Daily Dosage: Tablets containing 768 mg of sulfo-adenosyl-L-methionine (SAMe) sulfate-p- toluenesulfonate are equivalent to 400 mg of SAMe.

Arthritis: 600 to 800 mg daily, sometimes reduced to 400 mg daily when patients began responding (Jacobsen et al, 1991; Konig, 1987).

Depression: 200 to 1600 mg orally daily in the form of enteric-coated tablets; dosage often is graduated in increments of 200 mg (Bell et al, 1994; Bressa, 1994; Bottiglieri et al, 1990). Intramuscular or intravenous injection of 45 mg to 400 mg. The most frequent dose by either route is 200 mg daily (Bressa, 1994).

Fibromyalgia: 600 or 800 mg daily, sometimes reduced to 400 mg daily when patients began responding (Jacobsen et al, 1991; Konig, 1987). 200 mg daily by intramuscular injection (Tavoni et al, 1987).

Liver toxicity, estrogen-related: Women treated for estrogen-related liver toxicity received 800 mg of SAMe daily by the oral route (Frezza et al, 1988). In general, the minimum recommended daily dose by mouth is 1600 mg but no dose-finding studies have been done in patients with liver disease. Possibly patients with less well-compensated disease will require larger doses (Osman et al, 1993).

Mood disorders, mild: Standard dosing regimens are not available. However, an open-label study (n=192) demonstrated improved mild mood disorders in subjects (55 to 80 years) treated with ademetionine (SAMe) 100 mg orally 2 times a day for 2 months (Pancheri, 2002).

LITERATURE

Bell KM, Potkin SG, Carreon D et al. S-adenosylmethionine blood levels in major depression: changes with drug treatment. *Acta Neurol Scand Suppl*; 154:15-18. 1994

Bressa GM. S-adenosyl-l-methionine (SAMe) as antidepressant: meta-analysis of clinical studies. *Acta Neurol Scand Suppl*; 154:7-14. 1994

Bottiglieri T, Hyland K & Reynolds EH. The clinical potential of ademetionine (S-adenosylmethionine) in neurological disorders. *Drugs*; 48(2):137-152. 1994

Bottiglieri T, Godfrey P, Flynn T et al. Cerebrospinal fluid S-adenosylmethionine in depression and dementia: effects of treatment with parenteral and oral S-adenosylmethionine. *J Neurol Neurosurg Psychiatry*; 53(12):1096-1098. 1990

Delle Chiaie R, Pancheri P, Scapicchio P. Efficacy and tolerability of oral and intramuscular *S*-adenosylmethionine 1,4-butanedisulfonate (SAMe) in the treatment of major depression: comparison with imipramine in 2 multicenter studies. *Am J Clin Nutr*; 76(suppl):1172S-1176S. 2002

Di Benedetto R, Iona LG & Zidarich V. Clinical evaluation of S-adenosyl-L-methionine versus transcutaneous electrical nerve stimulation in primary fibromyalgia. *Curr Ther Res*; 53(2):222-229. 1993

Di Padova C. S-adenosylmethionine in the treatment of osteoarthritis: review of the clinical studies. *Am J Med*; 83(suppl 5A):60-65. 1987

Fava M, Giannelli A, Rapisarda V, Patralia A, Guaraldi GP. Rapidity of onset of the antidepressant effect of parenteral S-adenosyl-L-methionine. *Psychiatry Res* Apr 28;56(3):295-7. 1995

Frezza M, Tritapepe R, Pozzato G et al. Prevention by S-adenosylmethionine of estrogen-induced hepatobiliary toxicity in susceptible women. *Am J Gastroenterol*; 83(10):1098-1102. 1988

Gutierrez S, Palacios I, Sanchez-Pernaute O et al. SAMe restores the changes in the proliferation and in the synthesis of fibronectin and proteoglycans induced by tumour necrosis factor alpha on cultured rabbit synovial cells. *Br J Rheumatol*; 36(1):27-31. 1997

Hanje AJ, Fortune B, Song M, et al. The use of selected nutrition supplements and complementary and alternative medicine in liver disease. *Nutr Clin Pract*.; 21:255-272. 2006

Jacobsen S, Danneskiold-Samsoe B & Andersen RB. Oral S-adenosylmethionine in primary fibromyalgia: double-blind clinical evaluation. *Scand J Rheumatol*; 20(4):294-302. 1991

Kagan BL, Sultzer DL, Rosenlicht N et al. Oral S-adenosylmethionine in depression: a randomized, double-blind, placebo-controlled trial. *Am J Psychiatry*; 147(5):591-595. 1990

Konig B. A long-term (two years) clinical trial with S-adenosylmethionine for the treatment of osteoarthritis. *Am J Med*; 83(5A):89-94. 1987

Najm WI, Reinsch S, Hoehler F, et al. S-Adenosyl methionine (SAMe) versus celecoxib for the treatment of osteoarthritis symptoms: a double-blind cross-over trial. [ISRCTN36233495]. *BMC Musculoskeletal Disorders*; 5:6. 2004

Osman E, Owen JS & Burroughs AK. Review article: S-adenosyl-L-methionine - a new therapeutic agent in liver disease? *Aliment Pharmacol Ther*; 7(1):21-28. 1993

Pancheri P. Effects of a low dose of oral ademetionine (SAMe) on behaviour and quality of life in elderly patients with mild mood disorders. *Clin Drug Invest*; 22(5):321-327. 2002

Pancheri P, Scapicchio P & Delle Chiaie R. A double-blind, randomized parallel-group, efficacy and safety study of intramuscular S-adenosyl-L-methionine 1,4-butanedisulphonate (SAMe) versus imipramine in patients with major depressive disorder. *Int J Neuropsychopharmacol*; 5:287-294. 2002

Pascale RM, Marras V, Simile MM et al. Chemoprevention of rat-liver carcinogens by S-adenosyl-L-methionine: a long-term study. *Cancer Res*; 52(18):4979-4986. 1992

Pascale RM, Simile MM & Feo F. Genomic abnormalities in hepatocarcinogenesis: implications for a chemopreventive strategy. *Anticancer Res*; 13(5A):1341-1356. 1993

Pies R. Adverse neuropsychiatric reactions to herbal and over-the-counter antidepressants. *J Clin Psychiatry*; 61(11):815-820. 2000

Rafique S, Guardascione M, Osman E et al. Reversal of extrahepatic membrane cholesterol deposition in patients with chronic liver diseases by S-adenosyl-L-methionine. *Clin Sci (Colch)*; 83(3):353-356. 1992

Roncaglia N, Locatelli A, Arreghini A et al. A randomised controlled trial of ursodeoxycholic acid and S-adenosyl-L-methionine in the treatment of gestational cholestasis. *BJOG*; 111:17-21. 2004

Salmaggi P, Bressa GM, Nicchia G, Coniglio M, La Greca P, Le Grazie C. Double-blind, placebo-controlled study of S-adenosyl-L-methionine in depressed postmenopausal women. *Psychother Psychosom;* 59(1):34-40. 1993

Simile MM, Pascale R, De Miglio MR et al. Correlation between S-adenosyl-L-methionine content and production of c-myc, c-Ha-ras, and c-Ki-ras mRNA transcripts in the early stages of rat liver carcinogenesis. *Cancer Lett*; 79(1):9-16. 1994

Sitaram BR, Sitaram M, Traut M et al. Nyctohemeral rhythm in the levels of S-adenosylmethionine in the rat pineal gland and its relationship to melatonin biosynthesis. *J Neurochem*; 65(4):1887-1894. 1995

Surac AJ, Gur A. Complementary and alternative medical therapies in fibromyalgia. *Curr Pharma Design*; 12:47-57. 2006

Tavoni A, Vitali C, Bombardieri S et al. Evaluation of S-adenosylmethionine in primary fibromyalgia: a double-blind crossover study. *Am J Med*; 83(5A):107-110. 1987

Vendemiale G, Altomare E, Trizio T et al. Effects of oral S-adenosyl-L-methionine on hepatic glutathione in patients with liver disease. *Scand J Gastroenterol*; 24(4):407-415. 1989

Vitamin C

DESCRIPTION

Vitamin C is an important biological antioxidant and has been a popular nutritional supplement for decades. Vitamin C is often used to prevent or ameliorate a wide variety of infections and to enhance the effectiveness of the immune system. It is popular as a promoter of connective-tissue health in conditions such as minor trauma and capillary fragility.

Other Names: ascorbic acid, calcium ascorbate

ACTIONS AND PHARMACOLOGY

EFFECTS

Vitamin C has antioxidant, atherogenic, anticarcinogenic, antihypertensive, antiviral, antihistamine, immunomodulatory, ophthalmoprotective, airway-protective, and heavy-metal detoxifying properties.

Antioxidant effects have been demonstrated as increased resistance of red blood cells to free radical attack in elderly persons and reduced activated oxygen species in patients receiving chemotherapy and radiation. Antioxidant mechanisms have been shown in the reduction of LDL oxidation as well, though studies on the prevention of heart disease and stroke are conflicting.

CLINICAL TRIALS

Alzheimer's Disease

Vitamin C and vitamin E supplements in combination were associated with reduced prevalence and incidence of Alzheimer's disease (AD) in a cross-sectional, prospective study. A population of 4,740 adults 65 years of age and older were assessed for cognitive status, and their use of vitamin supplements was determined. Vitamin C users were those who took at least 500 mg of ascorbic acid, either as a single supplement or as part of a multivitamin preparation. Vitamin E users were defined as those who took a multivitamin preparation or an individual vitamin E supplement providing more than 400 IU per day. Multiple vitamin users were those whose preparation provided lower amounts of vitamin E and vitamin C. There were 200 prevalent cases of AD in the starting population. At the end of follow-up (up to 5 years), there were 104 incident cases of AD and 3,123 subjects who were free of dementia. The group of 1,429 people lost to follow-up comprised individuals who were older, less educated, and had performed less well on their cognitive screen than those who completed the protocol. Hence, AD incidence during the follow-up period may have been underestimated. After adjustment for age, sex, education, and apolipoprotein E genotype, prevalence analysis showed a significant inverse relation between prevalence of AD and vitamin E and multivitamin use. Vitamin E alone, vitamin C alone, or vitamin C in combination with multivitamins were not associated with AD prevalence. The strongest association was with the combination of vitamin E and vitamin C, with or without multivitamins (multivariate adjusted odds ratio, 0.22; 95% confidence interval (CI), 0.05 to 0.6). The combination of vitamin E and vitamin C also apparently reduced incidence (adjusted hazard ratio, 0.36; 95% CI, 0.09 to 0.99). For incidence, associations were not significant for vitamin E alone, vitamin C alone, multivitamin use alone or in combination (Zandi et al, 2004).

Antioxidant Defense Status

Supplementation with antioxidant vitamins, including vitamin C, improved antioxidant defense status in elderly subjects. Eighty-one subjects were stratified by sex and age and randomized to receive daily either placebo, a mineral combination (20 mg zinc, 100 mcg selenium), a vitamin combination (120 mg vitamin C, 6 mg beta-carotene, 15 mg vitamin E) or both combinations for a period of 2 years. Antioxidant defense, measured by in vitro challenge of red blood cells with free radicals, was improved in the vitamin group only (Girodon et al, 1997).

Supplementation with antioxidant vitamins, including vitamin C, prior to conditioning therapy (chemotherapy and radiation) for bone-marrow transplantation resulted in less of a rise in plasma lipid hydroperoxides than did conditioning therapy without presupplementation. Sixteen patients with leukemia were supplemented with alpha-tocopherol 825 mg, beta-carotene 45 mg, and ascorbic acid 450 mg for 3 weeks before beginning conditioning therapy. Ten other patients received conditioning therapy without supplementation with antioxidant vitamins. The rise in plasma lipid hydroperoxide level between the start of conditioning therapy and the completion of transplantation was from 20.1 to 36.2 mmol/liter in the supplemented group and from 23.3 to 83.5 mmol/liter in the unsupplemented group. The increase was significant ($p<0.05$) only in the unsupplemented group. Conditioning therapy causes delayed toxic effects in several tissues, which is thought to be caused by free-radical damage. The authors speculated that reducing lipid peroxide formation may reduce the toxicity of conditioning therapy (Clemens et al, 1997).

Vitamin C Deficiency

Serum concentrations of vitamin C rose sharply in one group of subjects receiving high-dose vitamin C (500 mg/day; n=161). Those who completed 5 years' supplementation with the high-dose form had significant increases in serum levels of vitamin C; mean levels differed significantly from those observed at baseline ($p<0.05$) (Kim et al, 2004).

Ascorbic acid deficiency in the institutionalized elderly may be corrected by daily vitamin C supplements. In a double-blind, placebo-controlled trial of 94 elderly inpatients with low levels of plasma and leukocyte vitamin C, patients received placebo or vitamin C 1 g for 60 days. Plasma and leukocyte vitamin C levels rose significantly during therapy. Treated patients showed significant increases in the mean values of body weight (0.41 kg), plasma albumin (0.46 g/liter), and prealbumin (25.4 mg/liter), and untreated patients showed decreases of these values, 0.6 kg, 0.53 g/liter, and 7 mg/liter, respectively. Reductions in purpura and petechial hemorrhages were also noted in the vitamin C group; however, no change in mood or mobility was observed (Schorah et al, 1981).

Cardiovascular Disease Protection

A 2006 review noted that levels of vitamin C are reduced in heart failure. In patients with chronic cardiac failure (CCF), IV or oral administration of vitamin C has been associated with sharp improvements in vasomotor function as reported in 2 studies cited. Administration of vitamin C in patients with CCF may reduce endothelial and cardiomyocyte apoptosis. Another study mentioned in the review found that oral administration of vitamin C reversed endothelial vasomotor dysfunction in patients with coronary artery disease (CAD), with benefits observed after 30 days (Witte and Clark, 2006).

Discrepancies exist between studies of subjects with adequate plasma levels of vitamin C and those obtaining vitamin C from diet or supplementation. For example, in a 2005 review, several studies with conflicting results are mentioned. One study examining older adults (aged 74-84 years) found a marked inverse trend for plasma levels of vitamin C and all-cause and cardiovascular disease (CVD) mortality. Following adjustments for CVD risk factors and variations in diet, subjects with higher plasma levels of vitamin C (>66 mm) were observed to have about half the mortality risk as subjects with lower plasma levels of vitamin C (<17 mm). However, in this study, no association was found between dietary intakes of vitamin C and all-cause or CVD mortality. The Nurses' Health Study examined the association between levels of vitamin C (obtained from either diet or supplementation) and risk of coronary heart disease (CHD). A group of women representing 1,240,566 person-years was followed; by study end, the investigators observed that although supplementation with vitamin C was associated with a significantly reduced risk of CHD, no association could be found between dietary vitamin C and risk of CHD. Another study of postmenopausal women with type 2 diabetes found just the opposite. In that study, subjects were from the Iowa Women's Health Study Cohort, and had high intakes of vitamin C. After adjusting for CVD risk factors and variations in diet, the authors found that total vitamin C and supplemental vitamin C were positively associated with risk of CVD mortality, whereas dietary vitamin C was not. Finally, a pooled analysis of 9 older cohort studies cited in the review inferred that supplemental vitamin C was associated with a reduced relative risk of CHD (Baldwin et al, 2005).

In a Finnish prospective population study (n=1605), subjects with low plasma vitamin C (less than 11.4 mmol/liter, or 2 mg/liter) had a relative risk of acute myocardial infarction of 2.5 compared with those who were not deficient, after adjustments of the model for the strongest risk factors of myocardial infarction. The authors suggest that supplementation of vitamin C may be beneficial in individuals with low plasma levels but not in those whose plasma levels are above 2 mg/liter (Nyyssonen et al, 1997).

Cold Symptoms

Unlike some other studies, one double-blind, randomized trial found an inverse relationship between supplementation with vitamin C and common cold incidence, but reported no effect of supplementation on cold duration or severity. Among subjects who completed the 5-year study, the low-dose group received 50 mg/day vitamin C (n=120) and the high-dose group received 500 mg/day (n=124). By study end, the total number of common colds (per 1000 person-months) was 21.3 in the low-dose group and 17.1 in the high-dose group. These findings differ from other studies, and should be interpreted cautiously. The authors point out several disadvantages of the study, including the lack of a placebo arm, the limitations of self-reporting, a relatively small sample size, and a large dropout rate (Sasazuki et al 2006).

Different findings were reported in an update to a recent Cochrane review. Three meta-analyses of placebo-controlled studies using doses of 200 mg or more of vitamin C were presented. Distinctions were made between using vitamin C as continuous prophylaxis or after the onset of cold symptoms. For the incidence of colds during prophylaxis, 29 studies involving 11,077 subjects were identified for inclusion in the review. Although doses as high as 2 g/day did not affect incidence in a subgroup of 23 community studies (n=10,435), a subgroup of 6 studies (n=642) showed a 50% reduction in common cold incidence among runners, skiers, and soldiers exposed to significant cold and/or stress. Duration of colds occurring during prophylaxis was examined in 30 studies involving 9,676 subjects; of these, 12 involved children (n=2,434) and 18 involved adults (n=7,242). Supplementation with vitamin C was associated with significant reductions in duration in both groups. The average reduction in symptom days was 14% in children and 8% in adults. Finally, of the 7 studies that evaluated the duration of colds treated at onset of symptoms, no benefits were observed for duration of episodes in the 3,294 adult participants (Douglas and Hemila, 2005).

These findings are more in line with other controlled trials, which found no significant effect of ascorbic acid on the incidence of colds, except for individuals under heavy acute physical stress. According to these earlier studies, the effect of ascorbic acid supplementation on severity and duration of cold symptoms has been repeatedly, though not consistently, shown to be measurable and statistically significant, with a median decrease of 22% compared to placebo (Hemila, 1997a). Some authorities have called these effects minor at best (AMA, 1986).

Three earlier studies reported significant reductions in incidence of pneumonia with ascorbic acid supplementation, including a randomized, double-blind, placebo-controlled trial (Hemila, 1997b). These studies were again cited in a recent Cochrane review, which searched the literature from 1945 to 2006 for trials examining the use of vitamin C to prevent and/or treat pneumonia. In the 3 prophylactic trials included in the review, 37 cases of pneumonia were identified in a total of 2,335 subjects. Subjects who received vitamin C had an 80% or greater reduction in the incidence of pneumonia. Only 2 therapeutic trials were identified, involving 197 patients with pneumonia. Of these, just one was a double-blind, randomized trial. One trial examined elderly subjects and found that administration of vitamin C was associated with lower mortality and reduced respiratory symptom scores among those most ill; the other study found a dose-dependent reduction in recovery time with 2 doses of vitamin C (Hemila and Louhiala, 2007).

Fluorosis

A combination of calcium, ascorbic acid, and vitamin D_3 reversed dental, clinical, and early skeletal fluorosis in children in a double-blind, placebo-controlled study. Twenty-five children (aged 6 to 12 years) living in an area where the drinking water contained 4.5 mg fluoride/liter were administered either placebo (n=10) or ascorbic acid 250 mg and calcium compound (125 mg elemental calcium) twice a day and vitamin D_3 60,000 IU once a week (n=15) for 180 days. Intake of fluoride-rich water continued as usual. At the end of the treatment period, there was significant improvement in dental, clinical, and skeletal grades of fluorosis in the treated children (p<0.05) but not in the placebo group. There were significantly reduced fluoride levels in the blood and serum and increased urinary fluoride levels in the treated group (p<0.05 for all 3 parameters) but not in the placebo group, indicating increased removal of fluoride from the body. The results of this small study indicate that calcium, ascorbic acid, and vitamin D_3 supplementation can reverse fluorosis in children (Gupta et al, 1996).

Hypertension

Oral ascorbic acid reduced blood pressure and arterial stiffness in patients with type 2 diabetes. In a randomized, double-blind, placebo-controlled trial, 30 patients (aged 45 to 70 years) with type 2 diabetes that was controlled with diet or hypoglycemic agents received either placebo or oral ascorbic acid 500 mg daily. After 4 weeks of treatment, mean brachial systolic pressure was reduced from 142 to 132 mm Hg in the ascorbic acid group (p=0.001 in comparison to baseline), and brachial diastolic pressure was reduced from 83.9 to 79.5 (p=0.003 in comparison to baseline). In the placebo group, blood pressure was not changed. The difference between treatments was statistically significant (p<0.001). The aortic augmentation index and the time to wave reflection, both indicators of aortic stiffness, showed improvement in the ascorbic acid group but not in the placebo group. Differences between treatments were significant (p=0.026 and p<0.01, respectively) (Mullan et al, 2002).

Vitamin C reduced daytime ambulatory but not nighttime blood pressure in older persons with hypertension; blood pressure of normotensive older persons was unaffected. In a double-blind, randomized, placebo-controlled crossover study (1 week washout between treatments), 40 nonsmokers between the ages of 60 and 80 years took ascorbic acid 250 mg twice daily or placebo, each for 3 months. Within the group of 17 participants who were hypertensive (systolic blood pressure 140 mm Hg or greater), SBP decreased significantly, by 3.7 mm Hg (95% confidence interval 1.5 to 5.9 mm Hg), with ascorbic acid treatment. Ascorbic acid treatment also increased HDL cholesterol in women but not in men (Fotherby et al, 2000).

Ascorbic acid 500 mg per day reduced systolic, diastolic, and mean blood pressure in healthy hypertensive individuals. In a randomized, double-blind trial, 39 hypertensive patients were given ascorbic acid 500 mg or placebo for 1 month. At the end of treatment, systolic blood pressure had been reduced from 155 to 142 mm Hg in the ascorbic acid group (p<0.001) and mean blood pressure from 110 to 100 mm Hg (p<0.001). The changes were significantly greater than those in the placebo group (p=0.03 and p=0.02, respectively). Heart rate was not affected by ascorbic acid treatment (Duffy et al, 1999).

Trauma Support

Early administration of vitamin C and vitamin E to critically ill patients who had experienced trauma or were to undergo surgery reduced the incidence of multiple organ failure and the length of time required in the intensive care unit (ICU). Eligible patients (n=595) were randomized within 24 hours of injury or emergency operation to receive antioxidant supplementation or standard care. d,l-alpha-tocopheryl acetate 1000 IU was given by naso- or orogastric tube every 8 hours, and ascorbic acid 1000 mg was given intravenously in 100 mL D5W (5% dextrose in water) every 8 hours for the shorter of either 28 days or the time in the ICU. The relative risk of pulmonary morbidity (acute respiratory distress syndrome or pneumonia) in patients receiving antioxidants was 0.81 (95% confidence interval (CI) 0.6-1.1). The relative risk of multiple organ failure was 0.43 (95% CI, 0.19-0.96). Patients in the antioxidant group required 1.2 fewer days in the ICU (95% CI, 0.81-1.5) and 0.4 fewer days in the hospital (95% CI: -0.2-1.0). There were no difference between groups in occurrence of renal failure, and there were no other adverse effects attributable to the antioxidants (Nathens et al, 2002).

INDICATIONS AND USAGE

FDA-approved:

- Prophylaxis of Vitamin C deficiency
- Iron absorption

Unproven Uses: Vitamin C has been used in the prevention of heart disease, pneumonia, sunburn, and hyperlipidemia, and for cancer prevention, muscle soreness, asthma, common cold, erythema (after CO2 laser skin resurfacing), fluorosis, wound healing after severe trauma, and as an antioxidant.

PRECAUTIONS AND ADVERSE REACTIONS

Avoid rapid intravenous injections. Adverse effects of parenteral vitamin C include faintness or dizziness, hemolysis, renal failure, and injection site pain. Adverse effects of oral vitamin C include diarrhea, esophagitis (rare), and intestinal obstruction (rare).

Use cautiously in patients with preexisting kidney stone disease, erythrocyte G6PD deficiency, hemochromatosis, thalassemia, or sideroblastic anemia.

Avoid supplemental vitamin C before conducting laboratory examinations for acetaminophen, AST (SGOT), bilirubin, carbamazepine, creatinine, glucose, LDH, stool guiac, theophylline, and uric acid.

DRUG INTERACTIONS

MAJOR RISKS

Amygdalin: Concurrent use of amygdalin and ascorbic acid may result in increased metabolism of amygdalin, leading to increased cyanide levels. *Clinical Management:* Use amygdalin and ascorbic acid concomitantly with caution or use a therapeutic alternative. High doses of ascorbic acid may increase the hydrolysis of amygdalin, leading to increased levels of the metabolite hydrogen cyanide, and also reduce body stores of cysteine, which is used to detoxify cyanide. Monitor the patient for signs of cyanide toxicity, including headache, tachycardia, confusion, convulsions, and cardiac arrhythmias.

MODERATE RISKS

Indinavir: Concurrent use of ascorbic acid and indinavir may result in decreased indinavir plasma concentrations. *Clinical Management:* Advise patients to use caution with ascorbic acid (Vitamin C) doses above the recommended daily allowance. Decreased indinavir plasma concentrations may occur, potentially making indinavir less effective.

MINOR RISKS

Antacids: Concurrent use of ascorbic acid and antacids may result in aluminum toxicity (personality changes, seizures, coma). *Clinical Management:* Concurrent administration of antacids and high-dose ascorbic acid is not recommended, especially in patients with renal insufficiency. If concurrent use cannot be avoided, monitor patients for possible acute aluminum toxicity (e.g., encephalopathy, seizures, or coma) and adjust the doses accordingly.

Cyanocobalamin: Concurrent use of ascorbic acid and cyanocobalamin may result in reduced amounts of cyanocobalamin available for serum and body stores. *Clinical Management:* Ascorbic acid (Vitamin C) should be administered 2 or more hours after a meal or vitamin B12 supplements.

POTENTIAL INTERACTIONS

Aspirin: Increased ascorbic requirements with concomitant use. *Clinical Management:* Increased dietary or supplemental vitamin C intake (100 to 200 mg daily) should be considered for patients on chronic high-dose aspirin.

DOSAGE

Mode of Administration: oral, intramuscular, intravenous

How Supplied: capsule, injectable, lozenge, solution, tablet

Daily Dosage: The following chart lists the Recommended Dietary Allowance (RDA) for vitamin C. Individuals who smoke require an additional 35 mg/day of vitamin C over the established RDA.

Age	Males	Females	Pregnancy	Lactation
0 to 6 months	40 mg/day	40 mg/day		
7 to 12 months	50 mg/day	50 mg/day		
1 to 3 years	15 mg/day	15 mg/day		
4 to 8 years	25 mg/day	25 mg/day		
9 to 13 years	45 mg/day	45 mg/day	80 mg/day	115 mg/day
14 to 18 years	75 mg/day	65 mg/day	80 mg/day	115 mg/day
19 years and older	90 mg/day	75 mg/day	85 mg/day	120 mg/day

ADULTS

Oral

Antioxidant effects: 120 to 450 mg/day (Girodon et al, 1997; Clemens et al, 1997).

Asthma: 500 to 2000 mg/day or prior to exercise (Cohen et al, 1997; Bielory & Gandhi, 1994).

Atherosclerosis prevention: 45 to 1000 mg/day (Jialal & Fuller, 1995; Gale et al, 1995; Kritchevsky et al, 1995).

Delayed-onset muscle soreness: 3000 mg/day (Kaminski & Boal, 1992).

Gastric cancer: 50 mg/day (Anon, 1993).

Histamine detoxification: 2000 mg/day (Johnston et al, 1992).

Hypercholesterolemia: 300 to 3000 mg/day (Simon, 1992).

Respiratory Infection: 1000 to 2000 mg/day (Hemila, 1997a; Hemila, 1997b).

Scurvy: The recommended dose for the treatment of scurvy is 1 to 2 g administered intravenously or orally for the first 2 days, then 500 mg intravenously or orally daily for a week (Oeffinger, 1993). However, the AMA recommends 100 mg 3 times a day for 1 week then 100 mg daily for several weeks until tissue saturation is normal (AMA, 1990).

Sunburn prevention: 2000 mg/day (Eberlein-Konig et al, 1998).

Urine acidification: 3 to 12 g/day titrated to desired effect (Krupp & Chatton, 1980) and given as divided doses every 4 hours (AMA, 1980).

Wound healing: 1000 to 1500 mg/day (Mazzotta, 1994).

Intramuscular

Scurvy: The recommended dose for the treatment of scurvy in adults and children is 100 mg 3 times a day for 1 week, then 100 mg daily for several weeks until tissue saturation is normal. This dosage can be administered intramuscularly, intravenously, or orally (AMA, 1990).

Vitamin deficiency: 100 to 500 milligrams/day (Krupp & Chatton, 1980).

Intravenous

Cancer: A dosing protocol for adjunctive therapy for cancer, based on more than 20 years of experience and isolated case reports (Riordan et al, 2003) is as follows: By intravenous (IV) drip (not push) week 1: 15 g/d IV 2 to 3 times/week ; week 2: 30 g/day IV 2 to 3 times/week; week 3: 65 g/day IV 2 to 3 times/week; week 4: 100 g/day IV 2 to 3 times/week; The dose should then be adjusted to achieve transient plasma concentrations of 400 mg/dL, or 200 mg/dL if lipoic acid (300 mg twice daily) is also being given. This protocol should be continued for at least a year. Patients are advised to supplement orally with at least 5 g daily when no infusion is given to maintain basal tissue levels and to prevent a rare but possible rebound scurvy.

Scurvy: The recommended dose for the treatment of scurvy is 1 to 2 g administered intravenously or orally for the first 2 days then 500 mg orally or intravenously daily for a week (Oeffinger, 1993). However, the American Medical Association recommends 100 mg 3 times a day for 1 week then 100 mg daily for several weeks until tissue saturation is normal (AMA, 1990).

Topical

Topical wound healing, skin erythema, aqueous solution: 10% solution applied once daily (Alster & West, 1998).

PEDIATRICS

Oral

The recommended prophylactic dose for infants on formula feedings is 35 mg/day orally or intramuscularly for the first few weeks of life. If the formula contains 2 to 3 times the amount of protein in human milk, the dose should be 50 mg/day orally or intramuscularly (AMA, 1980).

Infants and children require 30 to 60 mg of crystalline ascorbic acid daily. This may be taken as oral tablets or as part of the normal diet (i.e., 2 to 4 oz. of orange juice) (AMA, 1980).

Flourosis: 500 mg/day (Gupta et al, 1996).

Scurvy: The recommended dose for the treatment of scurvy in adults and children is 100 mg 3 times a day for 1 week, then 100 mg daily for several weeks until tissue saturation is normal. The regimen may be administered intramuscularly, intravenously, or orally (AMA, 1990).

Intramuscular

Scurvy: See Adult Dosage. The recommended prophylactic dose for infants on formula feedings is 35 mg/day orally or intramuscularly for the first few weeks of life. If the formula contains 2 to 3 times the amount of protein in human milk, the dose should be 50 mg/day orally or intramuscularly (AMA, 1980).

Intravenous

Scurvy: See Adult Dosage. In patients 17 years and younger, ascorbic acid should be diluted in at least an equal volume of fluid and infused over a minimum of 10 minutes. Direct intravenous push is not recommended. The final solution should be protected from light (Anon, 1984). The maximum recommended intravenous dose for ascorbic acid in pediatric patients (17 years and younger) is 100 mg/kg/day up to 6 g/day (Anon, 1984).

LITERATURE

Alster TS, West TB. Effect of topical vitamin C on postoperative carbon dioxide laser resurfacing erythema. *Dermatol Surg*; 24(3):331-334. 1998

AMA Council on Drugs. AMA Drug Evaluations, 4th ed. American Medical Association, Chicago, IL, USA, 1980.

AMA. AMA Drug Evaluations Subscription, vol 2. American Medical Association, Chicago, IL, USA, 1990.

AMA Department of Drugs. AMA Drug Evaluations, 6th ed. American Medical Association, Chicago, IL, USA, 1986.

Angel J, Alfred B, Leichfter J et al. Effect of oral administration of large quantities of ascorbic acid on blood levels and urinary excretion of ascorbic acid in healthy men. *J Vitam Nutr Res*; 45(2):237-243. 1975

Anon. ''Little doubt'' over gastric cancer link with diet low in vitamin C. *Pharm J*; 830. 1993

Anon. Guidelines for Administration of Intravenous Medications to Pediatric Patients, 2nd ed. American Society of Hospital Pharmacists, Bethesda, MD, USA, 1984a.

Baldwin CM, Bootzin RR, Schwenke DC et al. Antioxidant nutrient intake and supplements as potential moderators of cognitive decline and cardiovascular disease in obstructive sleep apnea. *Sleep Med Rev*; 9:459-476. 2005

Clemens MR, Waladkhani AR, Bublitz K et al. Supplementation with antioxidants prior to bone marrow transplantation. *Wien Klin Wochenschr*; 109(19):771-776. 1997

Cohen HA, Neuman I, Nahum H. Blocking effect of vitamin C in exercise-induced asthma. Arch Pediatr Adolesc Med; 151(4):367-370. 1997

Dawson EB, Harris WA, Rankin WE et al. Effect of ascorbic acid on male infertility. *Ann NY Acad Sci*; 498:312-323. 1987

Douglas RM, Hemila H. Vitamin C for preventing and treating the common cold. *PLoS Med*; 2(6):e168. 2005

Duffy SJ, Gokce N, Holbrook M et al. Treatment of hypertension with ascorbic acid (letter). *Lancet*; 354(9195):2048-2049. 1999

Fotherby MD, Williams JC, Forster LA et al. Effect of vitamin C on ambulatory blood pressure and plasma lipids in older persons. *J Hypertens*; 18(4):411-415. 2000

Gale CR, Martyn CN, Winter PD et al. Vitamin C and risk of death from stroke and coronary heart disease in cohorts of elderly people. *BMJ*; 310(6994):1563-1566. 1995

Girodon F, Blache D, Monget AL et al. Effect of a two-year supplementation with low doses of antioxidant vitamins and/or minerals in elderly subjects on levels of nutrients and antioxidant defense parameters. *J Am Coll Nutr*; 16(4):357-365. 1997

Gupta SK, Gupta RC, Seth AK et al. Reversal of fluorosis in children. *Acta Paediatr Jpn*; 38(5):513-519. 1996Hemila H. Vitamin C intake and susceptibility. *Pediatr Infect Dis J*; 16(9):836-837. 1997b

Hemila H. Vitamin C supplementation and the common cold—was Linus Pauling right or wrong? *Int J Vitam Nutr Res*; 67(5):329-335. 1997a

Hemila H, Louhiala P. Vitamin C for preventing and treating pneumonia. *Cochrane Database Syst Rev*; Jan 24;(1):CD005532. 2007

Jialal I, Fuller CJ. Effect of vitamin E, vitamin C and beta-carotene on LDL oxidation and atherosclerosis. *Can J Cardiol*; 11(suppl G):97G-103G. 1995

Johnston CS, Retrum KR, Srilakshmi JC. Antihistamine effects and complications of supplemental vitamin C. *J Am Diet Assoc*; 92(8):988-989. 1992

Kaminski M, Boal R. An effect of ascorbic acid on delayed-onset muscle soreness. *Pain*; 50(3):317-321. 1992

Kim MK, Sasaki S, Sasazuki S et al. Long-term vitamin C supplementation has no markedly favourable effect on serum lipids in middle-aged Japanese subjects. *Br J Nutr*; 91:81-90. 2004

Kodama H, Yamaguchi R, Fukuda J et al. Increased oxidative deoxyribonucleic acid damage in the spermatozoa of infertile male patients. *Fertil Steril*; 68(3):519-524. 1997

Kritchevsky SB, Shimikawa T, Tell GS et al. Dietary antioxidants and carotid artery wall thickness: the ARIC Study. *Circulation*; 92(8):2142-2150. 1995

Krupp MA, Chatton MJ. Current Medical Diagnosis and Treatment. Lange Medical Publications, Los Altos, CA, USA, 1980.

Mazzotta MY. Nutrition and wound healing. *J Am Podiatr Med Assoc*; 84(9):456-462. 1994

Mullan BA, Young IS, Fee H et al. Ascorbic acid reduces blood pressure and arterial stiffness in type 2 diabetes. *Hypertension*; 40:804-809. 2002

Nathens AB, Neff MJ, Jurkovich GJ et al. Randomized, prospective trial of antioxidant supplementation in critically ill surgical patients. *Ann Surg*;236(6):814-822. 2002

Nyyssonen K, Parviainen MT, Salonen R et al. Vitamin C deficiency and risk of myocardial infarction: prospective population study of men from eastern Finland. *BMJ*; 314(7081):634-638. 1997

Oeffinger KC. Scurvy: more than historical relevance. *Am Fam Physician*; 48(4):609-613. 1993

Riordan HD, Hunninghake RB, Riordan NH et al. Intravenous ascorbic acid: protocol for its application and use. *Puerto Rico Health Sci J*; 22(3):2003. 2003

Sasazuki S, Sasaki S, Tsubono Y et al. Effect of vitamin C on common cold: a randomized controlled trial. *Eur J Clin Nutr*; 60:9-17. 2006

Schorah CJ, Tormey WP, Brooks GH et al. The effect of vitamin C supplement on body weight, serum proteins, and general health of an elderly populatin. *Am J Clin Nutr*; 34(5):871-876. 1981

Simon JA. Vitamin C and cardiovascular disease: a review. *J Am Coll Nutr*; 11(2):107-125. 1992

Vilter RW. Nutritional aspects of ascorbic acid: uses and abuses. *West J Med*; 133(6):485-492. 1980

White JD: No ill effects from high-dose vitamin C (letter). *N Engl J Med*; 304(24):1491-1492. 1981

Will JC & Byers T. Does diabetes mellitus increase the requirement for vitamin C*? Nutr Rev*; 54(7):193-202. 11. 1996

Witte KK, Clark AL. Micronutrients and their supplementation in chronic cardiac failure. An update beyond theoretical perspectives. *Heart Fail Rev*; 11:65-74. 2006

Zandi PP, Anthony JC, Khachaturian AS et al. Reduced risk of Alzheimer disease in users of antioxidant vitamin supplements. *Arch Neurol*; 61:82-88. 2004

Vitamin E

DESCRIPTION

Vitamin E is a fat-soluble vitamin chemically known as tocopherol. Vitamin E is extremely versatile in both preventive and therapeutic applications, though it is rarely used alone. Vitamin E appears to be safe, except when normal coagulation mechanisms are impaired. While the synthetic vitamin has been effective when used in clinical trials, the natural stereoisomer may be superior in bioavailability.

Several forms of vitamin E exist: Alpha-tocopherol (Farrell & Roberts, 1994); d-alpha tocopherol (also termed RRR-alpha tocopherol) is an unesterified natural product derived from soybean oil; d-alpha tocopheryl (acetate or succinate) is an esterified form of the natural product; dl-alpha tocopheryl (acetate or succinate) is an esterified form of synthetic vitamin E (also termed all-rac-alpha tocopherol). Mixed tocopherols is a mixture of unesterified natural isomers including alpha, beta, delta, and gamma tocopherol.

Tocophero Equivalents (Farrell & Roberts, 1994):
1 mg dl-alpha tocopheryl acetate = 1 IU
1 mg dl-alpha tocopherol = 1.1 IU
1 mg d-alpha tocopheryl acetate = 1.36 IU
1 mg d-alpha tocopherol = 1.49 IU
1 mg d-alpha tocopheryl acid succinate = 1.21 IU
1 mg dl-alpha tocopheryl acid succinate = 0.89 IU

Other Names: Alpha-tocopherol, D-alpha tocopherol, D-alpha tocopheryl acid succinate, Dl-alpha tocopheryl acetate, D-alpha tocopherol,Dl-alpha tocopheryl acid succinate, D-alpha tocopheryl acetate

ACTIONS AND PHARMACOLOGY

EFFECTS

Vitamin E has antioxidant, immunomodulation, and antiplatelet effects.

Antioxidant Effects: Vitamin E appears to act as an antioxidant within membranes by preventing propagated oxidation of unsaturated fatty acids (Spielberg et al, 1979). Vitamin E is hypothesized to reduce atherosclerosis and subsequent coronary heart disease by preventing oxidative changes to low-density lipoproteins (LDL). Oxidized LDL particles are more readily converted by macrophages than native LDL to the cholesterol-loaded foam cells found in the fatty streak of early atherosclerosis. Atherogenesis may also be promoted by oxidized LDL's chemotactic action on monocytes, its cytotoxicity to endothelial cells, its stimulation of the release of growth factors and cytokines, its immunogenicity, and its possible arterial vasoconstrictor actions (Rimm et al, 1993; Stampfer et al, 1993).

Immunomodulating Effects: Vitamin E appears to enhance lymphocyte proliferation, decrease production of immunosuppressive prostaglandin E2, and decrease levels of immunosuppressive serum lipid peroxides (Meydani, 1995b).

Antiplatelet Effects: Vitamin E inhibits platelet adhesion measured in a laminar flow chamber using blood from patients who have taken vitamin E supplements. This effect appears to be related to a reduction in the development of pseudopodia, which normally occurs upon platelet activation. This effect of vitamin E may be related to changes in fatty acylation of structural platelet proteins. Although vitamin E inhibits platelet aggregation in vitro, its effect in vivo has not been consistently shown. Thromboembolic disease may be prevented with vitamin E supplementation (Calzada et al, 1997; Steiner, 1993).

Platelet Adhesion Effects: Vitamin E administration at 200 IU daily for 2 weeks has resulted in reduction of platelet adhesion by 44% to 75%. After an additional 2 weeks at a dose of 400 IU, platelet adhesion reduction was 77% to 82% (Steiner, 1993; Jandak et al, 1989). A related study found no dose-dependent downward trend in platelet adhesion at vitamin E doses between 400 IU and 1600 IU (Jandak et al, 1988). The effects of vitamin E on platelet adhesion appear to be independent of the effects of aspirin on platelet aggregation (Steiner et al, 1995).

CLINICAL TRIALS

Alzheimer's Disease/Cognitive Function

Although earlier studies showed that vitamin C and vitamin E supplements in combination offered some benefit to patients with Alzheimer's disease (AD), more recent studies showed no benefits on cognitive function with supplemental vitamin E given alone. The Women's Health Study (WHS), a randomized, double-blind, placebo-controlled trial, examined the effects of supplementation with 600 IU vitamin E on alternating days on cardiovascular disease and cancer in 39,876 healthy older women. A substudy of that larger trial examined its effects on cognitive function in a subset of women (n=6,377). Of these, one group received vitamin E, and the other, placebo. Patients received 10 years of treatment with 4 years of follow-up. No overall benefit on cognitive function was found at study end, and there were no differences in global score between the vitamin E and placebo groups. (Kang et al, 2006)

The Alzheimer's Disease Cooperative Study Group enrolled 769 subjects in double-blind fashion to examine the effects of 3 years' treatment with 2000 IU vitamin E daily, 10 mg donepezil daily, or placebo. Once again, no benefits on cognitive function were observed among those receiving vitamin E (Petersen et al, 2005).

Vitamin C and vitamin E supplements in combination were associated with reduced prevalence and incidence of AD in an earlier cross-sectional, prospective study. A population of 4,740 adults 65 years of age and older were assessed for cognitive status, and their use of vitamin supplements was determined. Vitamin C users were those who took at least 500 mg of ascorbic acid, either as a single supplement or as part of a multivitamin preparation. Vitamin E users were defined as those who took a multivitamin preparation or an individual vitamin E supplement providing more than 400 IU per day. Multiple vitamin users were those whose preparation provided lower amounts of vitamin E and vitamin C. There were 200 prevalent cases of AD in the starting population. At the end of follow-up (up to 5 years), there were 104 incident cases of AD and 3,123 subjects who were free of dementia. The group of 1,429 people lost to follow-up comprised individuals who were older, less educated, and had performed less well on their cognitive screen than those who completed the protocol. Hence, AD incidence during the follow-up period may have been underestimated. After adjustment for age, sex, education, and apolipoprotein E genotype, prevalence analysis showed a significant inverse relation between prevalence of AD and vitamin E and multivitamin use. Vitamin E alone, vitamin C alone, and vitamin C in combination with multivitamins were not associated with AD prevalence. The strongest association was with the combination of vitamin E and vitamin C, with or without multivitamins (multivariate adjusted odds ratio, 0.22; 95% confidence interval (CI), 0.05 to 0.6). The combination of vitamin E and vitamin C also apparently reduced incidence (adjusted hazard ratio, 0.36; 95% CI, 0.09 to 0.99). For incidence, associations were not significant for vitamin E alone, vitamin C alone, multivitamin use alone, or in combination (Zandi et al, 2004).

In an epidemiological study of elderly Japanese-American men, long-term use of vitamin E and/or vitamin C was associated with reduced incidence of vascular and mixed dementia and with higher cognitive function among those without dementia; however, there was no effect of vitamin usage on frequency of development of Alzheimer's dementia. Supplemental vitamin use was determined from an examination given between 1980 and 1982 and again in a questionnaire administered in 1988. Cognitive function and dementia were assessed between 1991 and 1993. Combined vitamin E and C supplement use was associated with an 88% reduction in the frequency of subsequent vascular dementia. Use of either vitamin resulted in better cognitive performance among non-demented subjects (OR, 1.25, 95% confidence interval, 0.995 to 1.5) (Masaki et al, 2000).

Antioxidation

Supplementation of vitamin E intake of smokers decreased susceptibility of their erythrocytes to hydrogen peroxide-induced lipid peroxidation. Fifty male smokers were given daily supplements of 70, 140, 560, or 1050 mg of d-alpha-tocopheryl acetate for 20 weeks. Erythrocyte vitamin E levels rose in a dose-dependent manner, and peroxidizability of erythrocytes decreased significantly with each dose ($p<0.001$). Nonsmokers also showed decreased erythrocyte peroxidizability with increasing vitamin E, except at the 1050-mg dose, at which they displayed significantly increased peroxidizability ($p<0.001$). Increases in red-cell vitamin E were associated with decreases in plasma ascorbate. The percentage increase in red cell peroxidizability was positively correlated with the percentage decrease in plasma ascorbate ($r=0.767$, $p<0.001$) in nonsmokers consuming 1050 mg d-alpha-tocopheryl acetate daily for 20 weeks (Brown et al, 1997).

Supplementation with antioxidant vitamins, including vitamin E, prior to conditioning therapy (chemotherapy and radiation) for bone marrow transplantation resulted in less of a rise in plasma lipid hydroperoxides than did conditioning therapy without presupplementation. Sixteen patients with leukemia were supplemented with alpha-tocopherol 825 mg, beta-carotene 45 mg, and ascorbic acid 450 mg for 3 weeks before beginning conditioning therapy. Ten other patients received conditioning therapy without supplementation with antioxidant vitamins. The rise in plasma lipid hydroperoxide level between the start of conditioning therapy and the completion of transplantation was from 20.1 to 36.2 mmol/liter in the supplemented group and from 23.3 to 83.5 mmol/liter in the unsupplemented group. The increase was significant ($p<0.05$) only in the unsupplemented group. Conditioning therapy causes delayed toxic effects in several tissues, which are thought to be caused by free-radical damage. The authors speculated that reducing lipid peroxide formation may reduce the toxicity of conditioning therapy (Clemens et al, 1997).

The addition of vitamin E to aspirin therapy reduced the incidence of ischemic cerebrovascular events among patients with a history of transient ischemic attacks (TIAs). One hundred TIA patients randomly received either aspirin 325 mg per day plus placebo or aspirin plus vitamin E 400 IU daily in a double-blind fashion. After 2 years, the aspirin-only group had experienced 6 ischemic attacks and 2 recurrent TIAs while the combination treatment group experienced 1 ischemic attack and 1 recurrent TIA (p less than 0.05). There was no difference in incidence of hemorrhagic events (Steiner et al, 1995).

Atherosclerosis

The combination of vitamin E and vitamin C slowed the progression of atherosclerosis in hypercholesterolemic subjects. In the Antioxidant Supplementation in Atherosclerosis Prevention (ASAP) study, 520 smoking and nonsmoking men and postmenopausal women aged 45 to 69 years with serum cholesterol above 193 mg/dL were stratified by sex and smoking habits and then randomly assigned to receive twice daily, with a meal, alpha-tocopherol 91 mg (136 IU of vitamin E), slow-release ascorbic acid (vitamin C) 250 mg, the combination of both vitamin doses, or placebo. Administration was double-blinded for 3 years. At the end of 3 years, all supplemented subjects were eligible to continue open supplementation with the combination for 3 more years. The placebo subjects continued without supplementation. Four hundred forty subjects were included in the intent-to-treat analysis at 6 years. Over 6 years, the mean annual increase in the common carotid artery intima-media thickness (CCA-IMT) (difference of first and last measures) was 0.0162 mm/yr in nonsupplemented males and 0.0103 mm/yr in supplemented males, a 37% treatment effect ($p=0.028$). In women, CCA-IMT increased 0.0111 mm/yr in the nonsupplemented group and 0.0102 in the supplemented group ($p=0.625$), a 14% treatment effect (not significant). When the first and second 3-year periods were compared, the treatment effect in men was significant only in the second period ($p=0.029$). The treatment effect was greater in subjects who already had plaques at baseline than in those without. The treatment effect was principally confined to subjects who had baseline plasma vitamin C levels below the median (less than 71 mmol/liter) (Salonen et al, 2003).

Higher dietary intake of vitamin E and high plasma levels of vitamin E were weakly associated with lowered risk of atherosclerosis in men but not in women. No benefit was seen from supplemental antioxidant vitamin use. In a study of more than 1,000 asymptomatic subjects, with equal numbers in age deciles of 27 to 77 years, the relationships of carotid intima-media wall thickness (IMT) and focal plaque to dietary intake of antioxidant vitamins and plasma vitamin concentrations were examined. In men, there was a progressive decrease in mean IMT with increasing quartiles of dietary vitamin E intake ($p=0.02$) and a nonsignificant trend for women ($p=0.10$). There were no significant relationships between dietary vitamin A, beta-carotene, or vitamin C and IMT. Plasma levels of lycopene were inversely correlated with mean carotid artery IMT in women ($p=0.047$). The prevalence of carotid artery plaque decreased with increasing quartiles of dietary vitamin E in women ($p=0.03$), but there was no significant association between plaque and dietary intake of any antioxidant vitamin in men. The prevalence of carotid artery plaque decreased with increasing plasma levels of alpha-carotene ($p=0.03$) and lycopene ($p=0.001$) in women and with vitamin A ($p=0.02$) and lycopene ($p=0.001$) in men. However, when adjusted for other risk factors (eg, age, smoking, hypertension, total energy intake), there were no residual associations between any dietary or plasma antioxidant vitamins or supplemental vitamin use and the risk of focal plaque in men and women (McQuillan et al, 2001).

Platelet Aggregation

Vitamin E at daily dosages of 400 IU to 1200 IU for 6 weeks produced no significant effects on platelet aggregation induced by collagen, ADP, or epinephrine in a controlled study of 47 healthy volunteers (Steiner, 1983). However, another controlled study of 40 healthy subjects found that vitamin E 300 mg daily for 8 weeks significantly decreased platelet aggregation in response to ADP and arachidonic acid, increased platelet sensitivity to inhibition by PGE1, decreased plasma beta-thromboglobulin concentration, and decreased ATP secretion (Calzada et al, 1997).

Cancer

Although the clinical utility of vitamin E for the prevention and treatment of cancer remains in dispute, findings from several studies bear mention.

Heavy use of vitamin E may increase the risk of localized prostate cancer, according to an article in the *Journal of the National Cancer Institute.* Investigators involved in the National Institutes of Health—AARP Diet and Health Study screened men (n=295,344) at entry for self-reported multivitamin use and followed them for 5 years; 78.2% of subjects reported taking vitamin E supplements more than 7 times per week, compared with 18.8% who reported never taking vitamin E. By study end, those who reported frequent use of vitamin E were observed to have an increased risk of localized prostate cancer (Lawson et al 2007).

Three studies (see *Cardiovascular Disease,* below) examined the effects of vitamin E on cancer and cardiovascular disease; none reported overall benefits on cancer prevention (Buring JE, 2006; Lee et al 2005, Lonn et al, 2005). A review of the literature, including 38 studies, failed to justify the use of vitamin E supplements for the prevention or treatment of cancer, as no statistically significant effects associated with supplementation were observed. One notable exception mentioned in the review is a study published in 1998, which showed a benefit of vitamin E supplementation on the prevention of new tumors in patients with prostate cancer (Coulter ID et al, 2006).

One study examining the effects of intakes of vitamin E, beta-carotene, and vitamin C on risk of prostate cancer enrolled 29,361 men who were followed for 8 years (average follow-up was 4.2 years). Of these, 52% reported taking vitamin E supplements. Within this group, male smokers who took high-dose vitamin E supplements (>400 mg/day) for at least 10 years had a reduced risk of advanced prostate cancer, although they may be at increased risk for nonadvanced forms of the disease. By study end, 1338 men had been diagnosed with prostate cancer, of these, 38.9% had the advanced form of the disease. According to the author, these findings parallel results from two earlier studies. In one including only smokers, the protective effect of vitamin E was limited to more aggressive forms of prostate cancer (stages II-IV). In the other, while a decreased risk of metastatic or fatal prostate cancers was observed among smokers taking vitamin E, an increased risk was noted for supplement users who never smoked (Kirsh et al, 2006).

A meta-analysis examining the effect of multivitamin supplementation on the prevention of colorectal adenoma found no significant beneficial effects associated with vitamin E, given alone or in combination with other vitamins. However, one study of male smokers cited in the analysis showed that vitamin E had a significantly harmful impact on the development of colorectal adenoma. The meta-analysis included 8 randomized trials comprising 17,620 subjects (Bjelakovic et al, 2006).

In yet an earlier, multicenter, double-blind, placebo-controlled trial of 540 patients with stage I or II head and neck cancer treated by radiation therapy, those who received vitamin E supplements (400 IU daily) had a higher rate of second primary cancers compared with those receiving placebo. However, upon cessation of treatment with vitamin E, these rates were lower in the group that had received supplementation vs those who had received placebo. Subjects were followed for a median of 52 months. Similarly, recurrence rates were observed to be higher during supplementation with vitamin E, but lowered once supplementation stopped. The study concluded that supplementation with vitamin E in this group of subjects produced adverse effects on the occurrence of second primary cancers and on cancer-free survival—results that surprised the investigators (Bairati et al, 2005).

Finally, data supporting a role for vitamin supplementation in the prevention and treatment of gastric cancers is lacking. No effect was found in one randomized, double-blind chemoprevention study (Plummer et al 2007). Here, 990 subjects were randomized to treatment with a combination of vitamin C (750 mg/day), vitamin E (600 mg/day) and beta-carotene (18 mg/day) for 3 years; an equal number of participants received placebo. Given the slow transitional changes that occur in the gastric mucosa between healthy tissue and the development of cancerous tissue, the investigators examined whether vitamin supplementation could offer a protective effect. Instead, they concluded that no statistically significant association could be found between vitamin supplementation for 3 years and progression or regression of precancerous gastric lesions.

Cardiovascular Disease

Two recently published articles do not support a role for vitamin E in the primary prevention of cardiovascular (CV) disease. Buring and Lee each reviewed data from the Women's Health Study (WHS), a 10-year-long, randomized, double-blind, placebo-controlled trial that examined the effects of vitamin E (600 IU on alternating days) on CV disease in 39,876 healthy women aged 45 years and older. Participants received treatment with either vitamin E (n=19,937) or placebo (n=19,939); vitamin E was found to have very little effect in preventing CV events. Of the total number of events that occurred during the study (n=999), 48% (n=482) occurred in the group receiving vitamin E compared with 51.8% (n=517) in the group receiving placebo; a nonsignificant 7% difference in risk between groups (relative risk [RR], 0.93; 95% confidence interval [CI] 0.82-1.05; p=.26). However, both articles point out a decrease in CV events and death rates in the WH Study among a small subset of women older than 65 years of age who were receiving vitamin E (Buring JE, 2006; Lee et al 2005).

Another study reports similar findings. The HOPE-TOO trial, a trial extension of the earlier Heart Outcomes Prevention Evaluation (HOPE) study, examined the effects of long-term supplementation with vitamin E on CV events. The initial HOPE study was a randomized, double-blind, placebo-controlled trial involving patients aged 55 and older with vascular disease or diabetes mellitus (n=9,541); it found no significant effect of vitamin E on CV events. In HOPE-TOO, of the 7,030 patients enrolled at participating centers, 3,994 continued taking the study intervention and 738 agreed to follow-up (median duration 7 years). At study conclusion, no differences in major CV events were observed in those who had received supplementation with vitamin E. However, higher rates of heart failure and hospitalizations were observed in the vitamin E group (Lonn et al, 2005).

A meta-analysis of large studies investigating the use of vitamin E for the prevention of CV disease showed no benefit relative to placebo for mortality. Seven trials involving vitamin E alone or in combination with other antioxidants were analyzed. Daily doses of vitamin E ranged from 50 IU to 800 IU. Duration of studies ranged from 1.4 to 12 years. All studies were randomized, placebo-controlled trials with intention-to-treat analyses and included 1,000 or more subjects each (total number of subjects = 81,788). Vitamin E did not lower all-cause mortality (11.3% vs 11.1%; odds ratio (OR) 1.02, 95% CI 0.98-1.06) or cardiovascular mortality (6.0% vs 6.0%; OR 1, 95% CI 0.96-1.06) relative to placebo. The incidence of cerebrovascular accidents did not differ between vitamin E-treated and placebo-treated patients (3.6% vs 3.5%; OR 1.02, 95% CI 0.92-1.12). When primary and secondary prevention studies were analyzed separately, no improvement in all-cause mortality was observed with vitamin E treatment for either category (Vivekananthan et al, 2003).

High-dose vitamin E from natural sources (400 IU daily) for an average of 4.5 years did not reduce the incidence of CV events in subjects at high risk. In a double-blind, randomized, 2-by-2 factorial design study, the Heart Outcomes Prevention Evaluation (HOPE) Study, 9,541 subjects were given vitamin E (from natural sources) or placebo and ramipril or placebo. Primary CV events (myocardial infarction, stroke, and death from cardiovascular causes) occurred in 16.2% of patients who received vitamin E and 15.5% of those who received placebo (relative risk 1.05; 95 percent confidence interval, 0.95 to 1.16). There were no significant differences due to vitamin E treatment for any of the specific CV events. Likewise, there were no differences due to vitamin E with respect to secondary outcomes (death from any cause, unstable angina, congestive heart failure, revascularization or limb amputation, nephropathy or the need for dialysis) (HOPE Study Investigators, 2000).

Mortality

One recent meta-analysis suggests that supplementation with vitamin E may increase overall mortality (Bjelakovic et al 2007). Data was extracted from 385 publications involving 68 randomized trials with a total of 232,606 subjects. Using statistical analysis and other methodology to review the medical literature, the authors concluded that supplementation with vitamin E, either alone or in combination with other antioxidants, significantly increases all-cause mortality (dose range=10 IU to 5,000 IU in studies examined). This finding follows a prior meta-analysis, which found that doses of vitamin E higher than 400 IU per day might increase all-cause mortality (Miller et al, 2005). Further studies are warranted to examine whether a correlation exists between supplementation with vitamin E and increased risk of death. Distinctions should be made between the clinical utility of supplementation in persons with a deficiency of the vitamin, and its possible deleterious effects in persons with adequate plasma levels of vitamin E. Dietary intake of sources rich in vitamin E remains the most ideal method of supplementation.

INDICATIONS AND USAGE

Accepted Uses: Supplementation is indicated for prevention and treatment of vitamin E deficiency. However, dietary improvement is preferred for prophylaxis, while vitamin E supplements are preferred for treating a deficiency (USP DI 2004).

Unproven Uses: Vitamin E is used to prevent coronary heart disease, ischemic cerebrovascular events (in conjunction with aspirin), and cancer of the oropharynx, prostate, and upper gastrointestinal tract. Vitamin E is also used to prevent exercise-induced tissue damage, nitrate tolerance, sunburn, some types of senile cataracts, other cancers, as well as to enhance immune function in the elderly, intermittent claudication, osteoarthritis, and some types of male infertility. Along with other therapies, vitamin E may be an important adjunctive treatment in Alzheimer's disease, diabetes, hemodialysis, premenstrual syndrome, tardive dyskinesia, and some cases of variant angina. Conditions such as dysmenorrhea, epilepsy, fibromyalgia, rheumatoid arthritis, and vasomotor menopausal symptoms may respond to vitamin E, but further investigation is needed into these applications.

CONTRAINDICATIONS

Oral use is contraindicated in coagulation disorders or anticoagulant therapy. Topical use is contraindicated after recent chemical peel or dermabrasion.

PRECAUTIONS AND ADVERSE REACTIONS

Thrombophlebitis has been reported in patients at risk of small-vessel disease who were taking 400 IU or more. In patients with blood clotting disorders or those taking anticoagulant medication, bleeding time should be monitored (Kappus & Diplock, 1992)

Pregnancy: Nutritional supplement doses of vitamins and minerals are generally considered safe during pregnancy. Daily dietary Vitamin E requirements are the same during pregnancy (dietary reference intake of 15 milligrams alpha-tocopherol equivalents) as those recommended in nonreproducing adult women (Picciano, 2003). Doses of Vitamin E above the recommended daily allowance should not be used in women during pregnancy.

Nursing: Infant risk cannot be ruled out. Available evidence and/or expert consensus is inconclusive or is inadequate for determining infant risk when Vitamin E is used during breastfeeding. Weigh the potential benefits of treatment against potential risks before prescribing Vitamin E during breastfeeding.

DRUG INTERACTIONS

MAJOR RISKS

Dicumarol: Concurrent use of dicumarol and Vitamin E may result in an increased risk of bleeding. *Clinical Management:* Monitor PT (prothrombin time ratio) more closely in patients taking Vitamin E at doses greater than 300 mg to 400 mg daily.

MODERATE RISKS

Warfarin: Concurrent use of warfarin and Vitamin E may result in an increased risk of bleeding. *Clinical Management:* In patients receiving oral anticoagulant therapy with warfarin, the prothrombin time ratio or international normalized ratio (INR) should be closely monitored with the addition and withdrawal of treatment with greater than 300 International Units daily of Vitamin E, and should be reassessed periodically during concurrent therapy. Adjustments of the warfarin dose may be necessary in order to maintain the desired level of anticoagulation.

Anisindione: Vitamin E has been shown to enhance the response to oral anticoagulants, perhaps due to an interference with the effect of vitamin K in clotting factor synthesis. *Clinical Management:* Concomitant use of oral anticoagulants and Vitamin E should be avoided if possible. If these drugs are used together, careful monitoring is called for (Hansen & Horn, 1989; Hansten, 1981).

MINOR RISKS

Cholestyramine: Concomitant administration of cholestyramine resin and fat-soluble vitamins may cause malabsorption of these vitamins. *Clinical Management:* Concomitant administration of cholestyramine and fat-soluble vitamins should be avoided if possible. If these drugs are used together, careful monitoring is called for (Hansen & Horn, 1989; Hansten, 1981).

Colestipol: Concomitant use may result in decreased Vitamin E effectiveness. *Clinical Management:* Since colestipol may interfere with absorption of vitamin E, try to separate administration of doses as much as possible.

Orlistat: Concomitant use may result in decreased Vitamin E efficacy. *Clinical Management:* Patients should be instructed to space the administration of orlistat and vitamin E by at least two hours.

Phenprocoumon: Vitamin E has been shown to enhance the response to oral anticoagulants, perhaps due to an interference with the effect of vitamin K in clotting factor synthesis (Anon, 1982; Corrigan & Marcus, 1974). *Clinical Management:* Concomitant use of oral anticoagulants and vitamin E should be avoided if possible. If these drugs are used together, careful monitoring is called for.

OVERDOSAGE

Vitamin E plasma concentrations greater than 3.5 mg/dL may result in toxicity (Lemons & Maisels, 1985). Prolonged vitamin E plasma levels of approximately 4.5 mg/dL were associated with an increased incidence of bacterial sepsis and necrotizing enterocolitis (Meyers et al, 1986).

DOSAGE

Mode of Administration: Oral, topical, intramuscular

How Supplied: Tablet, capsule, ointment, suspension

Daily Dosage: 1 mg of alpha-tocopherol is approximately equal to 1.5 International Units (IU). Recommended Dietary Allowance (RDA): *adults and adolescents 14 years and older* – 15 mg (22 IU) daily. *During pregnancy* – 15 mg/day; *during lactation* – 19 mg/day. *Infants and children: 0 to 6 months* – 4 mg/day; *7 to 12 months* – 5 mg/day; *1 to 3 years* – 6 mg/day; *4 to 8 years* – 7 mg/day; *9 to 13 years* – 11 mg/day.

ADULTS

Deficiency: 32 to 50 mg daily. The usual oral dose for vitamin E deficiency is 4 to 5 times the RDA. Doses as high as 300 mg may be necessary (Gilman et al, 1985; Alpers et al, 1983).

Alzheimer's disease: 2000 IU daily (Sano et al, 1997).

Anemia in hemodialysis patients: 500 mg/day (Cristol et al, 1997).

Angina pectoris: 50 to 300 mg/day (Rapola et al, 1996; Miwa et al, 1996).

Antioxidant effects: 100 to 800 mg/day (Brown et al, 1997; Clemens et al, 1997; Girodon, et al, 1997; Prieme et al, 1997).

Antiplatelet effects: 200 to 400 IU/day (Calzada et al, 1997; Steiner, 1993).

Cerebrovascular disease: 400 IU/day with aspirin 325 mg/day (Steiner et al, 1995).

Colorectal cancer prevention: 50 mg/day (Anon, 1994).

Coronary heart disease prevention: 100 to 800 IU/day (Kushi et al, 1996; Azen et al, 1996; Stephens et al, 1996; Takamatsu et al, 1995; Rimm et al, 1993; Stampfer et al, 1993).

Cystic fibrosis: 50 mg/day for correction of anemia (Anon, 1988; Nasr et al, 1993).

Diabetes: 100 to 900 IU/day for improving glucose tolerance and reducing protein glycation in insulin-dependent (and some non-insulin dependent) diabetics (Jain et al, 1996; Duntas et al, 1996; Paolisso et al, 1993; Paolisso et al, 1993a).

Dysmenorrhea: 150 mg/day (Butler & McKnight, 1955).

Exercise-induced tissue damage, prevention: 500 to 1200 IU/ day (McBride et al, 1998; Rokitzki et al, 1994; Meydani et al, 1993).

Exercise performance at high altitude: 400 mg/day (Simon-Schnass & Pabst, 1988).

Fibromyalgia: 300 IU/day (Steinberg, 1949).

Immune system support in geriatric patients: 200 mg daily (Meydani et al, 1997).

Infertility, male: 200 to 300 mg/day (Kodama et al, 1997; Suleiman et al, 1996; Geva et al, 1996).

Intermittent claudication: 600 to 1600 mg/day (Piesse, 1984; Williams et al, 1971; Williams et al, 1962; Livingstone & Jones, 1958).

Menopause: 75 to 100 mg/day (Finkler, 1949; Rubenstein, 1948).

Nitrate tolerance: 600 mg/day (Watanabe et al, 1997).

Oral leukoplakia and oropharyngeal cancer (prevention): 800 IU/day (Benner et al, 1993; Gridley et al, 1992). Osteoarthritis: 400 to 1200 IU/day (Scherak et al, 1990; Blankenhorn, 1986; Machtey & Ouaknine, 1978).

Premenstrual symptoms: 150 to 600 IU/day (London et al, 1987; London et al, 1983a; London et al, 1983b).

Rheumatoid arthritis: 800 to 1200 IU/day (Edmonds et al, 1997; Kolarz et al, 1990).

Stomach and esophageal cancer, prevention: 30 mg/day with 15 mg beta-carotene and 50 micrograms selenium (Taylor et al, 1994; Blot et al, 1993).

Sunburn, prevention: 1000 IU/day with 2000 mg vitamin C (Eberlein-Konig et al, 1998).

Tardive dyskinesia: 1200 to 1600 IU/day (Lohr & Caligiuri, 1996; Egan et al, 1992; Elkashef et al, 1990; Lohr et al, 1987).

PEDIATRICS

Premature or low-birth-weight neonates: vitamin E 25 to 50 units/day results in normal plasma tocopherol levels in 1 week (Taketomo et al, 2003). (1 unit = 1 mg alpha tocopheryl acetate).

Children with malabsorption syndrome: water-miscible vitamin E 1 unit/kg/day (to raise plasma tocopherol to within the normal range within 2 months and to maintain normal plasma concentrations) (Taketomo et al, 2003).

LITERATURE

Anon. Vitamin E therapy in cystic fibrosis. Nutr Rev 1988; 46(8):289-290. 89. Jain SK, McVie R, Jaramillo JJ et al. Effect of modest vitamin E supplementation on blood glycated hemoglobin and triglyceride levels and red cell indices in type 1 diabetic patients. *J Am Coll Nutr*; 15(5):458-461. 1996

Bairati I, Meyer F, Gelinas M, et al. A randomized trial of antioxidant vitamins to prevent second primary cancers in head and neck cancer patients. *J Natl Cancer Inst*; 97(7):481-488. 2005

Benner SE, Winn RJ, Lippman SM et al. Regression of oral leukoplakia with alpha-tocopherol: a Community Clinical Oncology Program Chemoprevention study. *J Natl Cancer Inst*; 85(1):44-47. 1993

Bjelakovic G, Nagorni A, Nikolova D, et al. Meta-analysis: antioxidant supplements for primary and secondary prevention of colorectal adenoma. *Aliment Pharmacol Ther*; 24:281-291, 2006

Bjelakovic G, Nikolova D, Gluud LL, et al: Mortality in randomized trials of antioxidant supplements for primary and secondary prevention. Systemic review and meta-analysis. *JAMA*; 297:842-857. 2007

Blankenhorn G. Clinical effectiveness of Spondyvit (Vitamin E) in activated arthroses: a multicenter placebo-controlled double-blind study (German). *Z Orthop*; 124(3):340-343. 1986

Blot WJ, Li JY, Taylor PR, et al. Nutrition intervention trials in Linxian, China: supplementation with specific vitamin/mineral combinations, cancer incidence, and disease-specific mortality in the general population. *J Natl Cancer Inst*; 85(18):1483-1492. 1993

Brown KM, Morrice PC & Duthie GG. Erythrocyte vitamin E and plasma ascorbate concentrations in relation to erythrocyte peroxidation in smokers and nonsmokers: dose response to vitamin E supplementation. *Am J Clin Nutr*; 65(2):496-502. 1997

Buring JE, Aspirin prevents stroke but not MI in women; vitamin E has no effect on CV disease or cancer. *Cleve Clin J Med*; 73:863-870. 2006

Butler EB & McKnight E. Vitamin E in the treatment of primary dysmenorrhea. *Lancet*; 1(Apr Jun 2):844-847. 1955

Calzada C, Bruckdorfer KR, Rice-Evans CA. The influence of antioxidant nutrients on platelet function in healthy volunteers. *Atherosclerosis*; 128(1):97-105. 1997

Clemens MR, Waladkhani AR, Bublitz K et al. Supplementation with antioxidants prior to bone marrow transplantation. *Wien Klin Wochenschr*; 101(19):771-776. 1997

Coulter ID, Hardy ML, Morton SC, et al. Antioxidants vitamin C and vitamin E for the prevention and treatment of cancer. *J Gen Intern Med*; 21:735-744. 2006

Cristol JP, Bosc JY, Badiou S et al. Erythropoietin and oxidative stress in haemodialysis: beneficial effects of vitamin E supplementation. *Nephrol Dial Transplant*; 12(11):2312-2317. 1997

Duntas L, Kemmer TP, Vorberg B et al. Administration of d-alpha-tocopherol in patients with insulin-dependent diabetes mellitus. *Curr Ther Res Clin Exp*; 57(9):682-690. 1996

Eberlein-Konig B, Placzek M & Przybilla B. Protective effect against sunburn of combined systemic ascorbic acid (vitamin C) and d-alpha-tocopherol (vitamin E). *J Am Acad Dermatol*; 38(1):45-48. 1998

Edmonds SE, Winyard PG, Guo R et al. Putative analgesic activity of repeated oral doses of vitamin E in the treatment of rheumatoid arthritis: results of a prospective placebo controlled double blind trial. *Ann Rheum Dis*; 56(11):649-655. 1997

Egan MF, Hyde TM, Albers GW et al. Treatment of tardive dyskinesia with vitamin E. *Am J Psychiatry*; 149(6):773-777. 1992

Elkashef AM, Ruskin PE, Bacher N et al. Vitamin E in the treatment of tardive dyskinesia. *Am J Psychiatry*; 147(4):505-506. 1990

Farrell PM & Roberts RJ. Vitamin E, in Shils ME, Olsen JA & Shike M (eds): Modern Nutrition in Health and Disease, 8th ed. Lea & Febiger, Philadelphia, PA, USA, 1994:326-341.

Finkler RS. The effect of vitamin E in the menopause. *J Clin Endocrinol Metab*; 9(1):89-94. 1949

Geva E, Bartoov B Zabludovsky N et al. The effect of antioxidant treatment on human spermatazoa and fertilization rate in an in vitro fertilization program. *Fertil Steril*; 66(3):430-434. 1996

Gilman AG, Goodman LS, Rall TW et al (eds). Goodman and Gilman's The Pharmacological Basis of Therapeutics, 7th ed. Macmillan Publishing Co, New York, NY, USA, 1985.

Girodon F, Blache D, Monget AL et al. Effect of a two-year supplementation with low doses of antioxidant vitamins and/or minerals in elderly subjects on levels of nutrients and antioxidant defense parameters. *J Am Coll Nutr*; 16(4):357-365. 1997

Gridley G, McLaughlin JK, Block G et al. Vitamin supplementation use and reduced risk of oral and pharyngeal cancer. *Am J Epidemiol*; 135(10):1083-1092. 1992

Heinonen OP, Albanes D, Virtamo J et al. Prostate cancer and supplementation with alpha-tocopherol and beta-carotene: incidence and mortality in a controlled trial. *J Natl Cancer Inst*; 90(6):440-446. 1998

The Heart Outcomes Prevention Evaluation Study Investigators: Vitamin E supplementation and cardiovascular events in high-risk patients. *N Engl J Med*; 342(3):154-160. 2000

Kang JH, Cook N, Manson J, et al. A randomized trial of vitamin E supplementation and cognitive function in women. *Arch Intern Med*; 166:2462-2468. 2006

Kappus H & Diplock AT: Tolerance and safety of vitamin E: a toxicological position report. Free Radic Biol Med 1992; 13(1):55-74.

Kirsh VA, Hayes RB, Mayne ST, et al. Supplemental and dietary vitamin E, β-carotene, and vitamin C intakes and prostate cancer risk. *J Natl Cancer Inst*; 98:245-254. 2006

Kodama H, Yamaguchi R & Fukuda J et al. Increased oxidative deoxyribonucleic acid damage in the spermatozoa of infertile male patients. *Fertil Steril*; 68(3):519-524. 1997

Kolarz G, Scherak O, El-Shohoumi M et al. High dose vitamin E in rheumatoid arthritis (German). *Aktuel Rheumatol*; 15(6):233-237. 1990

Kushi LH, Folsom AR, Prineas RJ et al. Dietary antioxidant vitamins and death from coronary heart disease in postmenopausal women. *N Engl J Med*; 334(18):1156-1162. 1996

Lawson KA, Wright ME, Subar A, et al: Multivitamin use and risk of prostate cancer in the National Institutes of Health—AARP Diet and Health Study. *J Natl Cancer Inst*. 99:754-764. 2007

Lee I-M, Cook NR, Gaziano JM, et al. Vitamin E in the primary prevention of cardiovascular disease and cancer. The Women's Health Study: A randomized controlled trial. *JAMA*; 294:56-65. 2005

Lemons JA & Maisels MJ. Vitamin E-how much is too much? *Pediatrics*; 76(4):625-627. 1985

Livingstone PD & Jones C. Treatment of intermittent claudication with vitamin E. *Lancet*; 2(1 Sept):602-604. 1958

Lohr JB & Caligiuri MP. A double-blind placebo controlled study of vitamin E treatment of tardive dyskinesia. *J Clin Psychiatry*; 57(4):167-173. 1996

Lohr JB, Cadet JL, Lohr MA et al. Alpha-tocopherol in tardive dyskinesia (letter). *Lancet*; 1(8538):213-214. 1987

Lonn E, Bosch J, Yusuf S for the HOPE and HOPE-TOO Trial Investigators: Effects of long-term vitamin E supplementation on cardiovascular events and cancer. A randomized controlled trial. *JAMA;* 293:1338-1347. 2005

London RS, Murphy L, Kitlowski KE et al. Efficacy of alpha-tocopherol in the treatment of the premenstrual syndrome. *J Reprod Med*; 32(6):400-404. 1987

London RS, Sundaram GS, Murphy L et al. Evaluation and treatment of breast symptoms in patients with the premenstrual syndrome. *J Reprod Med*; 28(8):503-508. 1983a

London RS, Sundaram GS, Murphy L et al. The effect of alpha-tocopherol on premenstrual symptomatology: a double-blind study. *J Am Coll Nutr*; 2(2):115-122. 1983b

London RS, Sundaram GS, Murphy L et al. The effect of vitamin E on mammary dysplasia: a double-blind study. *Obstet Gynecol*; 65(1):104-106. 1985

Machtey I & Ouaknine L. Tocopherol in osteoarthritis: a controlled pilot study. J Am Geriatr Soc; 26(7):328-330. 1978

McBride JM, Kraemer WJ, Triplett-McBride T et al. Effect of resistance exercise on free radical production. *Med Sci Sports Exerc*; 30(1):67-72. 1998

McQuillan BM, Hung J, Beilby JP et al. Antioxidant vitamins and the risk of carotid atherosclerosis: The Perth Carotid Ultrasound Disease Assessment Study (CUDAS). *J Am Coll Cardiol*; 38(7):1788-1794. 2001

Meydani M, Evans WJ, Handelman et al. Protective effect of vitamin E on exercise-induced oxidative damage in young and older adults. *Am J Physiol*; 264(5 pt 2):R992-R998. 1993

Meydani SN, Meydani M, Blumberg JB et al. Vitamin E supplementation and in vivo immune response in healthy elderly subjects: a randomized controlled trial. *JAMA*; 277(17):1380-1386. 1997

Meydani SN. Vitamin E enhancement of T-cell mediated function in healthy elderly: mechanisms of action. *Nutr Rev*; 53(4 pt 2):S52-S58. 1995b

Miller ER, Pastor-Barriuso R, Dalal D, et al. Meta-analysis: high-dosage vitamin E supplementation may increase all-cause mortality. *Ann Intern Med*; 142:37-46. 2005

Miwa K, Miyagi Y, Igawa A et al. Vitamin E deficiency in variant angina. *Circulation*; 94(1):14-18. 1996

Ogunmekan AO. Plasma vitamin E (alpha-tocopherol) levels in normal children and in epileptic children with and without anticonvulsant drug therapy. *Trop Geogr Med*; 37:175-177. 1985

Paolisso G, D'Amore A, Galzerano D et al. Daily vitamin E supplements improve metabolic control but not insulin secretion in elderly type II diabetic patients. *Diabetes Care*; 16(11):1433-1437. 1993a

Paolisso G, D'Amore A, Giugliano D et al. Pharmacologic doses of vitamin E improve insulin action in healthy subjects and non-insulin-dependent diabetic patients. *Am J Clin Nutr*; 57(5):650-656. 1993

Petersen RC, Thomas RG, Grundman M, et al for the Alzheimer's Disease Cooperative Study Group. Vitamin E and donepezil for the treatment of mild cognitive impairment. *N Engl J Med*; 352:2379-2388. 2005

Piesse JW. Vitamin E and peripheral vascular disease. *Int Clin Nutr Rev*; 4(4):178-182. 1984

Plummer M, Vivas J, Lopez G, et al. Chemoprevention of precancerous gastric lesions with antioxidant vitamin supplementation: a randomized trial in a high-risk population. *J Natl Cancer Inst*; 99:137-146; 2007

Prieme H, Loft S, Nyssonen K et al. No effect of supplementation with vitamin E, ascorbic acid, or coenzyme Q10 on oxidative DNA damage estimated by 8-oxo-7,8-dihydro-2′-deoxyguanosine excretion in smokers. *Am J Clin Nutr*; 65(2):503-507. 1997

Rapola JM, Virtamo J, Haukka JK et al. Effect of vitamin E and beta carotene on the incidence of angina pectoris: a randomized, double-blind, controlled trial. *JAMA*; 275(9):693-698. 1996

Rimm EB, Stamper MJ, Ascherio A et al: Vitamin E consumption and the risk of coronary heart disease in men. *N Engl J Med*; 328(20):1450-1456. 1993

Rokitzki L, Logemann E, Huber G et al. Alpha-tocopherol supplementation in racing cyclists during extreme endurance *training. Int J Sport Nutr*; 4(3):253-264. 1994

Rubenstein BB. Vitamin E diminishes the vasomotor symptoms of menopause (abstract). *Fed Proc*; 7:106. 1948

Salonen RM, Nyyssonen K, Kaikkonen J et al. Six-year effect of combined vitamin C and E supplementation on atherosclerotic progression. *Circulation*; 107:947-953. 2003

Sano M, Ernesto C, Thomas RG et al. A controlled trial of selegiline, alpha-tocopherol, or both as treatment for Alzheimer's disease: the Alzhmeier's Disease Cooperative Study. *N Engl J Med*; 336(17):1216-1222. 1997

Scherak O & Kolarz G. Vitamin E and rheumatoid arthritis (letter). *Arthritis Rheum*; 34(9):1205-1206. 1991

Simon-Schnass I & Pabst H. Influence of vitamin E on physical performance. *Int J Vitam Nutr Res*; 58(1):49-54. 1988

Spielberg SP, Boxer LA, Corash LM et al. Improved erythrocyte survival with high-dose vitamin E in chronic hemolyzing G6PD and glutathione synthetase deficiencies. *Ann Intern Med*; 90(1):53-54. 1979

Stampfer MJ, Hennekens CH, Manson JE et al. Vitamin E consumption and the risk of coronary disease in women. *N Engl J Med*; 328(20):1444-1449. 1993

Steinberg CL. Vitamin E and collagen in the rheumatic diseases. *Ann NY Acad Sci*; 52(3):380-389. 1949

Steiner M, Glantz M & Lekos A. Vitamin E plus aspirin compared with aspirin alone in patients with transient ischemic attacks. *Am J Clin Nutr*; 62(6 suppl):1381S-1384S. 1995

Steiner M. Vitamin E: more than an antioxidant. *Clin Cardiol*; 16(4 suppl 1):I16-I18. 1993

Stephens NG, Parsons A, Schofield PM et al. Randomized controlled trial of vitamin E in patients with coronary disease: Cambridge Heart Antioxidant Study (CHAOS). *Lancet*; 347(9004):781-786. 1996

Suleiman SA, Ali ME, Zaki ZM et al. Lipid peroxidation and human sperm motility: protective role of vitamin E. *J Androl*; 17(5):530-537. 1996

Takamatsu S, Takamatsu M, Satoh K et al. Effects on health of dietary supplementation with 100 mg d-alpha tocopheryl acetate daily for 6 years. *J Intern Med Res*; 23(5):342-357. 1995

Taketomo CK, Hodding JH & Kraus DM (eds). Pediatric Dosage Handbook, 9th edition, 2002-2003. Lexi-Comp, Inc.

Taylor PR, Li B, Dawsey SM et al. Prevention of esophageal cancer: the nutrition intervention trials in Linxian, China, Linxian Nutrition Intervention Trials Study Group. *Cancer Res*; 54(7 suppl):2029S-2031S. 1994

Vivekananthan DP, Penn MS, Sapp SK et al. Use of antioxidant vitamins for the prevention of cardiovascular disease: meta-analysis of randomised trials. *Lancet*; 361:2017-2023. 2003

Watanabe H, Kakihana M, Ohtsuka S et al. Randomized, double, blind, placebo-controlled study of supplemental vitamin E on attenuation of the development of nitrate tolerance. *Circulation*; 96(8):2545-2550 1997

Williams HT, Clein LJ & Macbeth RA. Alpha tocopherol in the treatment of intermittent claudication. *Can Med Assoc J*; 87(10):538-540. 1962

Williams HT, Fenna D & Macbeth RA. Alpha tocopherol in the treatment of intermittent claudication. *Surg Gynecol Obstet*; 132(4):662-666. 1971

Zandi PP, Anthony JC, Khachaturian AS et al. Reduced risk of Alzheimer disease in users of antioxidant vitamin supplements. *Arch Neurol*; 61:82-88. 2004

Zinc

DESCRIPTION

Zinc is an essential trace element. Zinc salts are used for supplementation to correct zinc-deficiency conditions such as acrodermatitis enteropathica, as an astringent to relieve minor eye irritations, and for therapy with penicillamine (e.g., such as that used for Wilson's disease). Other disease entities associated with zinc-depletion are anorexia nervosa, arthritis, diarrhea, eczema, recurrent infections, and recalcitrant skin problems. Other illnesses where efficacy, safety, and standardized dose of zinc have yet to be established include sickle cell disease, thalassemia, senile dementia, the common cold, diabetes mellitus, virile potency disturbances, acne vulgaris, neoplasia, and infertility. However, the mechanisms of action of zinc have to be further clarified and more studies are needed to determine its specific place in therapy.

Other Names: Zinc can be administered as zinc sulfate, zinc acetate, zinc chloride, zinc-D-gluconate, zinc carbonate, zinc oxide, zinc aspartate, bis(L-histidinato)zinc or zinc orotate. A

220-mg dose of zinc sulfate is equivalent to 50 mg of elemental Zinc (Alpers et al, 1995).

ACTIONS AND PHARMACOLOGY

EFFECTS

Zinc is thought to have antimicrobial, anti-sickling, cell-protective, copper-absorbing, enzyme-regulating, and growth-stimulating effects.

Antimicrobial Effects: Zinc may reduce the growth rate of plaque bacteria and thus decrease oral plaque growth (Cohen et al, 1986; Harrap et al, 1984).

Anti-sickling Effects: Zinc increases the filterability of partially deoxygenated cells in vitro. It decreases calcium-induced hemoglobin binding to red cell membranes and antagonizes the echinocyte-promoting effect of calcium. Thus, it can be used as an anti-sickling agent (Gupta & Choubey, 1987).

Cell-Protective Effects: Zinc exerts a protective effect in maintaining the integrity of both cellular and organelle membranes. Zinc deficiency can cause increased membrane peroxidation and subsequent membrane damage and abnormalities of cellular transport with decreased enzyme activity (Gupta & Choubey, 1987).

Copper-Absorbing Effects: Zinc inhibits copper absorption and induces a negative copper balance, which is the primary goal in the treatment of Wilson's disease (Hoogenraad & Van Hattum, 1988). It is thought that zinc causes copper malabsorption by preventing serosal transfer of copper secondary to induction of the intestinal copper-binding protein metallothionein and the copper is thus excreted in the feces (Friedman, 1993; Brewer et al, 1987).

Enzyme-Regulating Effects: Zinc is an integral part of several enzymes necessary for protein and carbohydrate metabolism. It is required for synthesis and mobilization of retinol-binding protein.

Growth-Stimulating Effects: Zinc supplementation may increase hepatic synthesis of somatomedin-C; it may accelerate growth response to growth hormone, or it can be involved directly in promoting growth. Studies are needed to establish the relationship of growth hormone, somatomedin, and zinc in beta thalasemia major (Arcasoy et al, 1987).

CLINICAL TRIALS

Common Cold

Results of a prospective study in children suggest a prophylactic role for zinc sulphate in decreasing the occurrence and severity of common cold and in shortening its mean duration. This randomized, double-blind, placebo-controlled study enrolled 200 healthy children, who were evenly assigned to treatment with either oral zinc sulphate syrup (providing 15 mg of zinc) or placebo syrup. Treatment was administered once daily for 7 months; this dosage was increased to twice daily at the onset of cold, until a reduction in symptoms was observed. Results showed that the mean number of colds was significantly reduced in the zinc group compared to the placebo group (mean 1.2 vs 1.7 cold per child; p=0.003), as was the mean duration of cold symptoms (4.7 days in the zinc group, compared to 5.3 days in the placebo group; p<0.0001). Total severity scores for cold symptoms were also decreased with supplementation vs placebo (p<0.0001) (Kurugol et al 2006).

Zinc lozenges have been reported to be effective in some studies and ineffective in others. Efficacy may depend on whether the zinc is provided in a molecular form, as demonstrated by a re-analysis of findings from 10 double-blind, placebo-controlled trials published between 1984 and 2004. Taking a fresh look at the data, the investigator found a statistically significant correlation between total daily dosages of positively charged zinc species and reductions in median (p=0.005) and mean (p<0.02) duration of common colds in the trials studied (Eby 2004). Similar outcomes were noted in a 2004 review on the medicinal value of zinc for the treatment of the common cold. That review found that zinc effectively reduced the duration and severity of common cold when administered within 24 hours following onset of symptoms (Husliz 2004).

A prospective phase IV study examined the prophylactic and therapeutic effects of a specific brand of zinc lozenges (Cold-Eeze®) on common cold in 134 children aged 12 to 18 years. Therapeutic use (4 lozenges per day) resulted in a significant reduction in average cold duration vs placebo (mean, 6.9 days vs 9.0 days; p<0.001). Prophylactic use during the cold season (once daily) resulted in a 25% reduction in cold incidence and overall, two-thirds of treated subjects had only one cold or none at all (McElroy and Miller 2003). A randomized, controlled study conducted in geriatric subjects (aged 60 to 91 years) found similar benefits, and concluded that use of zinc gluconate glycine lozenges is safe and well tolerated in this population (Silk and LeFante 2005).

An earlier meta-analysis of 6 clinical trials evaluated the effectiveness of zinc salts lozenges in the common cold; all studies included had consistent moderate quality scores. The summary odds ratio for the incidence of any cold symptom was reported to be 0.50, but this did not reach statistical significance (Jackson et al, 1997).

Positive results were reported in a double-blind, placebo-controlled study of 100 patients. Zinc gluconate therapy was initiated within 24 hours of symptom onset. One zinc gluconate lozenge containing 13.3 mg of zinc was administered every 2 hours while awake for the duration of cold symptoms in 50 patients. The zinc-treated group had a significantly shorter time to symptom resolution than the placebo group (4.4 versus 7.6 days, p<0.001). Coughing, headache, hoarseness, nasal congestion and drainage, and sore throat were the symptoms that responded to zinc treatment. Nausea (10 vs 2 patients) and bad-taste reactions (39 vs 15 patients) were significantly more common in the zinc-treated group than the placebo group; one zinc-treated patient withdrew because of intolerance to the lozenge (Mossad et al, 1996).

Herpes Simplex Virus/Oral Herpes (Cold Sores)

Treatment with systemic zinc sulphate led to a reduction in the number of episodes and time to recovery associated with herpes labialis in one pilot study. Twenty patients with a history of the disease (>6 episodes per year) were treated with 22.5 mg zinc sulphate twice daily for 2 consecutive months, followed by a 5-month break, and then treated again for 2 consecutive months. After 1 year, investigators noted a reduction in flare-ups among subjects, with episodes declining to <4 episodes (average, 3). In addition, each episode lasted less than 7 days (Femiano et al 2005).

A randomized, double-blind, placebo-controlled trial involving 46 subjects examined the effect of a topical formulation of zinc oxide/glycine cream on facial and circumoral herpes infection (cold sores). Subjects were instructed to apply the cream within 24 hours after symptoms manifested, and to continue treatment every 2 hours until the lesion resolved, for up to 3 weeks; the control group was treated with a placebo cream. Cold sores occurring in the zinc treatment arm were of a significantly shorter duration following treatment (mean, 5 days) compared with the placebo arm (mean, 6.5 days). Application of the cream was also associated with a reduction in the severity of signs and symptoms of oral herpes, including blistering, soreness, itching, and tingling (Godfrey et al 2001).

A solution of 0.25% zinc sulfate can cause clearing of herpes simplex lesions, but solutions of 0.025% to 0.05% were ineffective as treatment for acute attacks or as prophylaxis for recurrent infections. Zinc sulfate gel 103 mg/g applied topically every 2 hours was more effective than placebo in clearing herpes simplex labialis infections in a controlled double-blind trial with 80 patients. Symptoms were milder and lesions healed more rapidly with zinc sulfate gel than with placebo gel. (Kneist et al, 1995)

In another study, 200 patients with herpes simplex showed clearing of lesions within 3 to 6 days of treatment with 0.25% zinc sulfate in camphor water USP applied 8 to 10 times per day beginning within 24 hours after the appearance of the lesions (Finnerty, 1986).

Immune Function

Zinc supplementation in a population of elderly subjects significantly decreased the incidence of infection in one randomized, double-blind, placebo-controlled trial. Study participants (age range, 55-87 years) were assigned to daily treatment with either 45 mg oral zinc gluconate (n=24) or placebo (n=25). Following 1 year of treatment, the group receiving zinc supplementation had significantly fewer infections than their unsupplemented counterparts (0.29±0.46 vs 1.4±0.95, respectively; p<0.01). The generation of tumor necrosis factor alpha and oxidative stress markers was significantly lowered by zinc supplementation in this study compared to placebo, and plasma levels of zinc were significantly increased from baseline with supplementation (Prasad et al 2007).

Zinc supplementation may improve cell-mediated immunity and leukocyte chemotaxis independently of zinc depletion. The cell-mediated immune response determined by CD4, DR, T-cells and cytotoxic T-lymphocytes was improved after zinc supplementation in a randomized, double-blind, placebo-controlled study of 118 patients older than 65 years. Patients received 25 mg of zinc sulfate per day; 800 mcg of retinol palmitate; 25 mg of zinc per day plus 800 mcg of retinol palmitate; or placebo. Significant increases in the zinc group were observed for CD4 + DR + T-cells (P=0.016) and cytotoxic t-lymphocytes (P=0.005). For vitamin A, reductions in the counts of CD3 + T-cells (P=0.012) and CD4 + T-cells (P=0.0129) were reported (Fortes et al, 1998).

The rate of infection was significantly reduced by zinc and selenium supplementation in a 2-year randomized, placebo-controlled study of 81 institutionalized elderly patients. Daily doses of 20 mg of zinc plus 100 mcg of selenium or the same doses of trace elements plus daily doses of 120 mg of vitamin C, 6 mg of beta-carotene, and 15 mg of alpha-tocopherol were equally effective in correcting deficiencies after 6 months and in preventing infectious events (Girodon et al, 1997).

Macular Degeneration

Zinc supplementation has yet to be proven useful in age-related macular degeneration (ARMD). Prospective, randomized, controlled trials have been conducted investigating the role of zinc in ARMD using doses 5.3 times the RDA of zinc for men and 6.7 times the RDA of zinc for women. Beneficial results from one small trial could not be confirmed in the much larger AREDS trial (see below), which failed to find a significant reduction in visual acuity loss after zinc therapy.

The Age-Related Eye Disease Study report 8 (AREDS) was an 11-center, double-blind, prospective trial designed to evaluate the effect of high-dose vitamins C and E, beta-carotene, and zinc supplementation on ARMD progression and visual acuity. Three thousand six hundred forty (3,640) participants aged 55 to 80 years were enrolled. All subjects had extensive small drusen, intermediate drusen, large drusen, noncentral geographic atrophy, or pigment abnormalities in one or both eyes, or advanced ARMD or vision loss due to ARMD in one eye. At least one eye had best corrected visual acuity of 20/32 or better. Participants were randomized to 1 of 4 treatment groups: antioxidants (500 mg vitamin C, 400 IU vitamin E, and 15 mg beta-carotene daily); zinc oxide and cupric oxide (80 mg elemental zinc and 2 mg elemental copper daily); antioxidants plus zinc; or placebo. The total daily dosage of each supplement was taken orally by each participant in 2 divided doses with food to avoid potential gastrointestinal irritation by zinc. The main outcome measures included photographic assessment of progression to or treatment for advanced ARMD and at least moderate visual acuity loss from baseline (15 or more letters from the Snellen eye chart). Comparison with placebo demonstrated a statistically significant odds ratio (OR) reduction for the development of advanced AMD with antioxidants plus zinc (0.72, 99% confidence interval (CI) 0.52-0.98, p<0.007). The ORs for zinc alone (0.75, 99% CI 0.55-1.03, p<0.02) and antioxidants alone (0.80, 99% CI 0.59-1.09, p less than 0.07) were not found to be statistically significant (Anon, 2001b).

INDICATIONS AND USAGE

Approved by the FDA for:

■ Zinc deficiency

Unproven Uses: Zinc supplements are used for numerous conditions, including the following: acne vulgaris, acrodermatitis enteropathica, Alzheimer's disease, common cold, dental hygiene, diabetes mellitus, diarrhea, eczema, eye irritation, growth, Hansen's disease, herpes simplex infection, hypertension, hypogeusia (decreased sense of taste), immunodeficiency, impotence, infertility, leg ulcers, lipid peroxidation, macular degeneration, necrolytic migratory erythema, parasites, peptic ulcer disease, psoriasis, scalp dermatoses, schistosomiasis, sepsis, sickle cell anemia, stomatitis, thalassemia major, trichomoniasis, Wilson's disease, and wound healing.

PRECAUTIONS AND ADVERSE REACTIONS

Zinc ophthalmic solution should be used cautiously in patients with glaucoma.

Side effects include gastrointestinal discomfort, nausea, vomiting, headaches, drowsiness, and metallic taste. Do not use zinc ophthalmic solutions that have changed color.

Breastfeeding: Zinc should not be used in doses greater than the RDA during lactation.

Caffeine: Concurrent administration with zinc reduces zinc absorption. Coffee reduces zinc absorption by up to 50%. Wait 1 to 2 hours before drinking coffee after zinc administration (Pecoud et al, 1975).

Foods containing high amounts of phosphorous, calcium (dairy), or phytates (e.g., bran, brown bread) may reduce absorption.

DRUG INTERACTIONS

MAJOR RISKS

Gatifloxacin: Concurrent use may result in decreased gatifloxacin effectiveness. *Clinical Management:* Gatifloxacin should be administered 4 hours before or 4 hours after zinc or any product containing zinc.

Levofloxacin: Concurrent use may result in decreased levofloxacin effectiveness. *Clinical Management:* Administer levofloxacin at least 2 hours before or 2 hours after zinc or a multiple ingredient product which contains zinc.

MODERATE RISKS

Grepafloxacin: Concurrent use may result in decreased efficacy of grepafloxacin. *Clinical Management:* Zinc supplements or zinc-containing products should be administered 4 hours before or 4 hours after grepafloxacin.

Moxifloxacin: Concurrent use may result in decreased efficacy of moxifloxacin. *Clinical Management:* Moxifloxacin should be administered at least 4 hours before or 8 hours after zinc.

Norfloxacin: Concurrent use may result in decreased efficacy of norfloxacin. *Clinical Management:* Avoid concurrent use. However, if used concurrently, the dose of the zinc salt should be given at least 6 hours before or 4 hours after the norfloxacin dose.

Ofloxacin: Concurrent use may result in decreased efficacy of ofloxacin. *Clinical Management:* Zinc supplements or zinc-containing products should be administered 2 hours before or 2 hours after ofloxacin.

Sparfloxacin: Concurrent use may result in decreased efficacy of sparfloxacin. *Clinical Management:* If sparfloxacin and a product containing zinc must be taken concurrently, administer the zinc-containing preparation 4 hours after the sparfloxacin is given.

Tetracyline: Concurrent use may result in decreased tetracycline effectiveness. *Clinical Management:* Administer tetracycline at least 2 hours before or 3 hours after zinc.

MINOR RISKS

Ciprofloxacin: Concurrent use may result in decreased ciprofloxacin effectiveness. *Clinical Management:* Zinc salts or vitamins containing zinc should be given 2 hours after or 6 hours before oral ciprofloxacin.

Copper: Concurrent administration with zinc may inhibit the absorption of copper or zinc. *Clinical Management:* Optimal dosage separation time has not been determined. Space administration of zinc and copper as far apart as possible.

Penicillamine: Concurrent administration with zinc reduces zinc absorption. *Clinical Management:* Optimal dosage separation time has not been determined. Space administration of zinc and penicillamine as far apart as possible.

POTENTIAL INTERACTIONS

Doxycycline: Concurrent use may result in impaired tetracycline absorption.

Iron: Concurrent use may result in decreased gastrointestinal resorption.

Methacycline: Concurrent use may result in decreased absorption.

Temafloxacin: Concurrent use may result in decreased absorption of temafloxacin.

OVERDOSAGE

Intravenous overdose has been associated with thrombocytopenia, hypotension, cardiac arrhythmias, oliguria, hyperamylasemia, diarrhea, jaundice, and pulmonary edema, sideroblastic anemia, microcytic anemia secondary to zinc-induced copper deficiency anemia, copper deficiency, hemorrhagic gastric erosions, and lymphocytoma cutis.

DOSAGE

Mode of Administration: oral, topical, intramuscular

How Supplied: tablet, cream, gel

Daily Dosage: Recommended Dietary Allowance (RDA): *Men and adolescent boys 14 and older* – 11 mg/day; *adolescent girls 14 to 18 years* – 9 mg/day; *women 19 years and older* – 8 mg/day; *pregnancy (19 years and older)* – 11 mg/day; *lactation (19 years and older)* – 12 mg/day. *Infants and children: 7 months to 3 years* – 3 mg/day; *4 to 8 years* – 5 mg/day; *9 to 13 years* – 8 mg/day.

ADULTS

Dietary supplement: daily oral doses range from 9 to 25 mg

Acne and dermatitis: a topical preparation (cream or gel) of 10 mg zinc sulfate per gram or 27 to 30 mg zinc oxide per gram used several times daily.

Acne: 90 to 135 mg orally daily

Zinc deficiency/acrodermatitis: maximum doses up to 40 mg orally daily

Wilson's Disease, tablet: 300 mg to 1200 mg orally daily in divided doses

PEDIATRICS

Acne: 135 mg orally daily.

Zinc deficiency: daily doses ranging from 1.5 to 12 mg, depending on age.

Supplementation (intramuscular injection): 100 mcg per kg body weight per day for children up to 5 years old.

Wilson's disease (intramuscular injection): 25 mg 3 times daily for children 10 years and older.

LITERATURE

Alpers DH, Stenson WF & Bier DM. Manual of Nutritional Therapeutics, 3rd ed. Little, Brown & Co, Boston, MA, 1995

Anon. A randomized, placebo-controlled, clinical trial of high-dose supplementation with vitamins C and E, beta-carotene, and zinc for age-related macular degeneration and vision loss: AREDS report no. 8. *Arch Ophthalmol*; 119(10):1417-1436. 2001

Arcasoy A, Cavdar A, Cin S et al. Effects of zinc supplementation on linear growth in beta-thalasemia (a new approach). *Am J Hematol*; 24(2):127-136. 1987

Brewer GJ, Yuzbasiyan-Gurkan V, Johnson V et al. Treatment of Wilson's disease with zinc, XII: dose regimen requirements. *Am J Med Sci*; 305(4):199-202. 1993

Cohen DW, Hangorsky U, Emling RC et al. Clinical evaluations of a zinc sulfate/ascorbic acid mouthrinse. *Clin Prev Dent*; 8(6):5-12. 1986

Eby GA. Zinc lozenges: cold cure or candy? Solution chemistry determinations.*Biosci Rep*; 24(1):23-39. 2004

Femiano F, Gombos F, Scully C. Recurrent herpes labialis: a pilot study of the efficacy of zinc therapy. *J Oral Pathol Med*; 34(7):423-425. 2005

Finnerty EF. Topical zinc in the treatment of herpes simplex. Cutis 1986; 37(2):130-131.

Fortes C, Forastiere F, Agabiti N et al. The effect of zinc and vitamin A supplementation on immune response in an older population. *J Am Geriatr Soc*; 46(1):19-26. 1998

Friedman LS. Zinc in the treatment of Wilson's disease: how it works. *Gastroenterology*; 10495):1566-1575. 1993

Fung EB, Ritchie LD, Woodhouse LR et al. Zinc absorption in women during pregnancy and lactation: a longitudinal study. *Am J Clin Nutr*; 66(1):80-88. 1997

Girodon F, Lombard M, Galan P et al. Effect of micronutrient supplementation on infection in institutionalized elderly subjects: a controlled trial. *Ann Nutr Metab*; 41(2):98-107. 1997

Godfrey HR, Godfrey NJ, Godfrey JC, Riley D. A randomized clinical trial on the treatment of oral herpes with topical zinc oxide/glycine. *Altern Ther Health Med*; 7(3):49-56. 2001

Gupta VL & Choubey BS. RBC survival, zinc deficiency, and efficacy of zinc therapy in sickle cell disease. *Birth Defects*; 23(5A):477-483. 1987

Haeger K, Lanner E & Magnusson PO. Oral zinc sulfate in the treatement of venous leg ulcers, in Pories WJ, Strain WH, Hwu JM et al (eds): Clinical applications of zinc metabolism. CC Thomas, Springfield, IL:158-167. 1974

Harrap GJ, Best JS & Saxton CA. Human oral retention of zinc from mouthwashes containing zinc salts and its relevance to dental plaque control. *Arch Oral Biol*; 29(2):87-91. 1984

Henderson LM, Brewer GJ, Dressman JB et al. Effect of intragastric pH on the absorption of oral zinc acetate and zinc oxide in young healthy volunteers. *J Parenter Enteral Nutr*; 19(5):393-397. 1995

Hulisz D. Efficacy of zinc against common cold viruses: an overview. *J Am Pharm Assoc*; 44(5):594-603. 2004

Jackson JL, Peterson C & Lesho E. A meta-analysis of zinc salts lozenges and the common cold. *Arch Intern Med*; 157(20):2373-2376. 1997

Kneist W, Hempel B & Borelli S. Klinische Doppelblindpruefung mit Zinksulfat topisch bei Herpes labialis recidivans (German). *Arzneimittelforschung*; 45(5):624-626. 1995

Krieger I. Picolinic acid in the treatment of disorders requiring zinc supplementation. *Nutr Rev*; 38(4):148-149. 1980

Kurugol Z, Akilli M, Bayram N, Koturoglu G. The prophylactic and therapeutic effectiveness of zinc sulphate on common cold in children. *Acta Paediatrica*; 95:1175-1181, 2006.

Silk R, LeFante C. Safety of zinc gluconate glycine (Cold-Eeze) in a geriatric population: a randomized, placebo-controlled, double-blind trial. *Am J Ther*; 12(6):612-617, 2005

McElroy BH, Miller SP. An open-label, single-center, phase IV clinical study of the effectiveness of zinc gluconate lozenges (Cold-Eeze®) in reducing the duration and symptoms of the common cold in school-aged subjects. *Am J Ther*; 10(5):324-329. 2003

Mossad SB, Macknin ML, Medendorp SV et al. Zinc gluconate lozenges for treating the common cold: a randomized, double-blind, placebo-controlled study. *Ann Intern Med*; 125(2):81-88. 1996

Naveh Y, Schapira D, Ravel Y et al. Zinc metabolism in rheumatoid arthritis: plasma and urinary zinc and relationship to disease activity. *J Rheumatol*; 24(4):643-646. 1997

Prasad AS, Beck WJ, Bao B et al. Zinc supplementation decreases incidence of infections in the elderly: effect of zinc on generation of cytokines and oxidative stress. *Am J Clin Nutr*; 85:837-844. 2007

Product Information: Galzin™, zinc acetate. Gate Pharmaceuticals, Sellersville, PA, USA, 1997

Product Information. Visine AC®, zinc sulfate and tetrahydrozoline hydrochloride. Pfizer Consumer Health Care, Parsippany, NJ, USA, 1994

Wood RJ & Zheng JJ. High dietary calcium intakes reduce zinc absorption and balance in humans. *Am J Clin Nutr*; 65(6):1803-1809. 1997